Werner and Ingbar's
The Thyroid

Werner and Ingbar's The Thyroid

A Fundamental and Clinical Text

SEVENTH EDITION

EDITED BY

LEWIS E. BRAVERMAN, MD
Professor of Medicine, Nuclear Medicine, and Physiology
Director, Division of Endocrinology and Metabolism
Chairman, Department of Nuclear Medicine
University of Massachusetts Medical School, Worcester, Massachusetts

ROBERT D. UTIGER, MD
Clinical Professor of Medicine, Harvard Medical School
Deputy Editor, New England Journal of Medicine, Boston, Massachusetts

With 130 Contributors

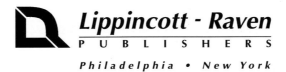

Lippincott - Raven
PUBLISHERS
Philadelphia • New York

Acquisitions Editor: Lisa McAllister
Sponsoring Editor: Anne Sydor
Project Editor: Sandra Cherrey Scheinin
Production Manager: Helen Ewan
Production Coordinator: Kathryn Rule
Design Coordinator: Doug Smock
Indexer: Sandra King

Werner and Ingbar's the thyroid: a fundamental and clinical text. — 7th ed. / edited by Lewis E. Braverman, Robert D. Utiger; with 130 contributors.

    p. cm
    Includes biographical references and index.
    ISBN 0-397-51406-9 (alk. paper)
    1. Thyroid gland—Diseases. 2. Thyroid gland—Physiology. I. Werner, Sidney C. II. Ingbar, Sidney H. III. Braverman, Lewis E.,. IV. Utiger, Robert D.
    [DNLM: 1. Thyroid Diseases. 2. Thyroid Gland—physiology. WK 200 W492 1996]
RC665.W39 1996
616.4'4—dc20
DNLC/DLC
for Library of Congress   95-39527
                     CIP

The material contained in this volume was submitted as previously unpublished material, except in the instances in which credit has been given to the source from which some of the illustrative material was derived.

Great care has been taken to maintain the accuracy of the information contained in the volume. However, neither Lippincott–Raven Publishers nor the editors can be held responsible for errors or for any consequences arising from the use of the information herein.

The authors and publisher have exerted every effort to ensure that drug selection and dosage set forth in this text are in accord with current recommendations and practice at the time of publication. However, in view of ongoing research, changes in government regulations, and the constant flow of information relating to drug therapy and drug reactions, the reader is urged to check the package insert for each drug for any change in indications and dosage and for added warnings and precautions. This is particularly important when the recommended agent is a new or infrequently employed drug.

Materials appearing in this book prepared by individuals as part of their official duties as U.S. Government employees are not covered by the above-mentioned copyright.

9 8 7 6 5 4 3 2 1

∞ This paper meets the requirements of ANSI/NISO Z39.48-1992 (Permanence of Paper).

CONTRIBUTORS

Jack E. Ansell, M.D.
Professor of Medicine
Vice Chairman for Clinical Affairs
Department of Medicine
Boston University School of
Medicine
Boston, Massachusetts

Rebecca S. Bahn, M.D.
Professor of Medicine
Mayo Medical School
Consultant, Division of
Endocrinology
Mayo Medical Center
Rochester, Minnesota

Douglas W. Ball, M.D.
Assistant Professor of Medicine and
Oncology
The Johns Hopkins University School
of Medicine
Baltimore, Maryland

Daniel T. Baran, M.D.
Professor of Medicine,
Orthopedics, and Cell Biology
University of Massachusetts Medical
Center
Worcester, Massachusetts

Charles P. Barsano, M.D., Ph.D.
Professor of Medicine, Pharmacology
and Molecular Biology
Vice Chairman, Department of
Medicine
Finch University of Health
Sciences/The Chicago Medical
School
Associate Chief of Staff for Academic
Affairs
North Chicago Veterans Affairs
Medical Center
North Chicago, Illinois

Luigi Bartalena, M.D.
Assistant Professor of Endocrinology
Institute of Endocrinology
University of Pisa
Pisa, Italy

Nesli Basgoz, M.D.
Instructor in Medicine
Harvard Medical School
Assistant in Medicine
Massachusetts General Hospital
Boston, Massachusetts

Stephen B. Baylin, M.D.
Professor of Oncology and Medicine
The Johns Hopkins University School
of Medicine
Associate Director for Research
Chief, Cancer Biology
Johns Hopkins Comprehensive
Cancer Center
Baltimore, Maryland

Jeffrey D. Bernhard, M.D.
Professor of Medicine
Director, Division of Dermatology
University of Massachusetts Medical
School
Worcester, Massachusetts

Lewis E. Braverman, M.D.
Professor of Medicine, Nuclear
Medicine, and Physiology
Director, Division of Endocrinology
and Metabolism
University of Massachusetts Medical
School
Worcester, Massachusetts

Gregory A. Brent, M.D.
Associate Professor of Medicine
University of California, Los Angeles
Assistant Chief of Endocrinology and
Metabolism
West Los Angeles Veterans Affairs
Medical Center
Los Angeles, California

Henry B. Burch, M.D.
Assistant Professor, Department of
Medicine
Uniformed Services University of the
Health Sciences
Assistant Chief, Endocrine-Metabolic
Service
Walter Reed Army Medical Center
Washington, D.C.

Albert G. Burger, M.D.
Professor of Endocrinology
Thyroid Research Unit
Division of Endocrinology
Department of Medicine
Geneva University Hospital
Geneva, Switzerland

Ulrich Bürgi, M.D.
Professor of Medicine
University of Bern Medical School
Head, Endocrine and Diabetes
Division
University Hospital (Inselspital)
Bern, Switzerland

Andree de Bustros, M.D.
Clinical Associate Professor of
Medicine
University of Illinois School of
Medicine
Section Head, Endocrinology
Christ Hospital
Chicago, Illinois

Bernard Caillou, M.D.
Chief, Histopathology
Institut Gustave Roussy
Villejuif, Cedex, France

Charles C. Capen, D.V.M., Ph.D.
Professor and Chairman
Department of Veterinary Biosciences
The Ohio State University College of
Veterinary Medicine
Columbus, Ohio

Ralph R. Cavalieri, M.D.
Professor of Medicine and Radiology
University of California, San Francisco
Consultant, Nuclear Medicine
Veterans Affairs Medical Center
San Francisco, California

Inder J. Chopra, M.D.
Professor of Medicine
University of California, Los Angeles
  School of Medicine
Staff Physician
University of California, Los Angeles
  Center for the Health Sciences
Los Angeles, California

Orlo H. Clark, M.D.
Professor of Surgery
University of California, San
  Francisco School of Medicine
Chief of Surgery
UCSF/Mount Zion Medical Center
San Francisco, California

Vivian Cody, Ph.D.
Senior Research Scientist
Hauptman-Woodward Medical
  Research Institute, Inc.
Buffalo, New York

David S. Cooper, M.D.
Associate Professor of Medicine
Director, Thyroid Clinic
The Johns Hopkins University
  School of Medicine
Director, Division of Endocrinology
Sinai Hospital of Baltimore
Baltimore, Maryland

Gilbert H. Daniels, M.D.
Associate Professor of Medicine
Harvard Medical School
Co-Director, Thyroid Associates
Physician, Massachusetts General
  Hospital
Boston, Massachusetts

Terry F. Davies, M.D., F.R.C.P.
Baumritter Professor of Medicine
Director, Division of Endocrinology
  and Metabolism
Mount Sinai School of Medicine
Attending Physician
Mount Sinai Hospital
New York, New York

François M. Delange, M.D.
Executive Director
International Council for Control of
  Iodine Deficiency Disorders
Brussels, Belgium

G. Robert DeLong, M.D.
Associate Professor of Pediatrics
Attending Physician
Duke University Medical Center
Durham, North Carolina

Robert G. Dluhy, M.D.
Associate Professor of Medicine
Harvard Medical School
Brigham and Women's Hospital
Boston, Massachusetts

Ann D. Dunn, Ph.D.
Research Associate Professor of Medicine
University of Virginia School of
  Medicine
Charlottesville, Virginia

John T. Dunn, M.D.
Professor of Medicine
University of Virgina School of
  Medicine
Attending Physician
University of Virginia Hospital
Charlottesville, Virginia

Charles H. Emerson, M.D.
Professor of Medicine and Physiology
University of Massachusetts Medical
  School
Worcester, Massachusettes

André-Marie Ermans, M.D.
Universite Libre de Bruxelles
Former Head, Department of Nuclear
  Medicine
University Hospital Saint-Pierre
Brussels, Belgium

James A. Fagin, M.D.
Heady Professor of Medicine
Volunteer Professor of Cell Biology,
  Neurobiology, and Anatomy
Director, Division of Endocrinology
  and Metabolism
University of Cincinnati College of
  Medicine
Cincinnati, Ohio

Giovanni Faglia, M.D.
Professor of Endocrinology
Head, Institute of Endocrine Sciences
University of Milan
Milan, Italy

Vahab Fatourechi, M.D.
Associate Professor of Medicine
Mayo Medical School
Consultant
Division of Endocrinology/
  Metabolism, and Internal Medicine
Mayo Clinic
Rochester, Minnesota

Delbert A. Fisher, M.D.
Professor Emeritus
Pediatrics and Medicine
University of California, Los Angeles
  School of Medicine
Los Angeles, California
Chief Science Officer
Corning-Nichols Institute
San Juan Capistrano, California

Thomas P. Foley, Jr., M.D.
Professor of Pediatrics
University of Pittsburgh School of
  Medicine
Director, Division of Endocrinology,
  Metabolism, and Diabetes Mellitus
Department of Pediatrics
Childrens Hospital of Pittsburgh
Pittsburgh, Pennsylvania

Irwin M. Freedberg, M.D.
George Miller MacKee Professor and
  Chairman
The Ronald O. Perelman Department
  of Dermatology
New York University School of
  Medicine
New York, New York

Steven R. Gambert, M.D.
Professor and Acting Chairman
Department of Medicine
New York Medical College
Valhalla, New York

James A. Garrity, M.D.
Associate Professor of
  Ophthalmology
Mayo Medical School
Consultant, Division of
  Ophthalmology
Mayo Clinic
Rochester, Minnesota

Hans Gerber, M.D.
Professor
University of Bern Medical School
Head, Division of Protein
  Chemistry
Department of Clinical Chemistry
University Hospital (Inselspital)
Bern, Switzerland

Neil Gesundheit, M.D., M.P.H.
Attending Physician
Santa Clara Valley Medical Center
San Jose, California
Vice President for Clinical and
  Regulatory Affairs
Vivus, Inc.
Menlo Park, California

Colum A. Gorman, M.D., B.Ch.
Professor of Medicine
Mayo Medical School
Consultant, Division of
  Endocrinology
Mayo Clinic
Rochester, Minnesota

William L. Green, M.D.
Professor of Medicine
State University of New York
Health Science Center, Brooklyn
Associate Chief of Staff, Research
Veterans Affairs Medical Center
Brooklyn, New York

Monte A. Greer, M.D.
Professor of Medicine and Physiology
Oregon Health Sciences University
Portland, Oregon

Torsten Grunditz, M.D., Ph.D.
Lund University
Department of Otorhinolaryngology
University Hospital, MAS
Malmo, Sweden

Joel I. Hamburger, M.D.
West Bloomfield, Michigan

Ian D. Hay, M.D., Ph.D.
Professor of Medicine
Mayo Medical School
Consultant
Division of Endocrinology and
Internal Medicine
Mayo Clinic
Rochester, Minnesota

Jerome M. Hershman, M.D.
Professor of Medicine
University of California, Los Angeles
School of Medicine
Chief, Endocrinology and
Metabolism Division
West Los Angeles Veterans Affairs
Medical Center
Los Angeles, California

Eva Horvath, Ph.D.
Associate Professor of Pathology
University of Toronto
Research Associate
St. Michael's Hospital
Toronto, Ontario, Canada

David H. Ingbar, M.D.
Associate Professor of Medicine
University of Minnesota School of
Medicine
Director, Medical Intensive Care
Unit
University of Minnesota Hospital
and Clinic
Minneapolis, Minnesota

Anthony S. Jennings, M.D.
Clinical Assistant Professor of
Medicine
University of Pennsylvania School of
Medicine
Presbyterian Medical Center of
Philadelphia
Philadelphia, Pennsylvania

Michael M. Kaplan, M.D.
Associate Endocrinologists
West Bloomfield, Michigan
Division of Endocrinology,
Department of Medicine
William Beaumont Hospital
Royal Oak, Michigan

Irwin Klein, M.D.
Professor of Medicine and Cell
Biology
New York University School of
Medicine
Chief, Division of Endocrinology
North Shore University Hospital
Manhasset, New York

Robert Z. Klein, M.D.
Professor of Pediatrics
Dartmouth Medical School
Lebanon, New Hampshire

Josef Koehrle, Dr. rer. nat. Dipl.
Biochem.
Professor
Med Poliklinik Wurzburg
Wurzburg, Germany

Kalman Kovacs, M.D., Ph.D.
Professor of Pathology
University of Toronto
St. Michael's Hospital
Toronto, Ontario, Canada

Paul W. Ladenson, M.D.
John Eager Howard Professor
of Endocrinology and
Metabolism
The Johns Hopkins University School
of Medicine
Director, Division of Endocrinology
and Metabolism
The Johns Hopkins Hospital
Baltimore, Maryland

Stephen LaFranchi, M.D.
Professor of Pediatrics
Head, Pediatric Endocrinology
Oregon Health Sciences
University
Doernbecher Children's Hospital
Portland, Oregon

P. Reed Larsen, M.D.
Professor of Medicine
Harvard Medical School
Chief, Thyroid Division
Brigham and Women's Hospital
Boston, Massachusetts

John H. Lazarus, M.D., F.R.C.P.
Senior Lecturer in Medicine
Department of Medicine
University of Wales College of
Medicine
Heath Park
Cardiff, Wales

Jack L. Leonard, Ph.D.
Professor of Nuclear Medicine and
Physiology
University of Massachusetts Medical
School
Worcester, Massachusetts

Gerald S. Levey, M.D.
Provost, Medical Sciences
Dean
University of California, Los Angeles
School of Medicine
Center for the Health Sciences
Los Angeles, California

Jonathan M. Links, Ph.D.
Associate Professor
Environmental Health Sciences and
Radiology
The Johns Hopkins University School
of Medicine
Baltimore, Maryland

Virginia A. LiVolsi, M.D.
Professor of Pathology and
Laboratory Medicine
University of Pennsylvania
Vice Chair, Anatomic Services
University of Pennsylvania Medical
Center
Philadelphia, Pennsylvania

John N. Loeb, M.D.
Professor of Medicine
College of Physicians and
Surgeons
Columbia University
Attending Physician
The Presbyterian Hospital in the City
of New York
New York, New York

Christopher Longcope, M.D.
Professor of Obstetrics and
Gynecology and Medicine
University of Massachusetts Medical
School
Worcester, Massachusetts

Jonathan S. LoPresti, M.D., Ph.D.
Associate Professor of Clinical
Medicine
University of Southern California
School of Medicine
Los Angeles, California

James A. Magner, M.D.
Professor of Medicine
East Carolina University School of
Medicine
Greenville, North Carolina

Scott H. Mandel, M.D.
Associate Professor of Pediatrics
Division of Endocrinology
Oregon Health Sciences University
Doernbecher Children's Hospital
Portland, Oregon

Enio Martino, M.D.
Professor of Endocrinology
University of Pisa
Pisa, Italy

Harry R. Maxon, III, M.D.
Professor of Radiology
Director, Division of Nuclear Medicine
Department of Radiology
University of Cincinnati College of
  Medicine
Cincinnati, Ohio

Ernest L. Mazzaferri, M.D.
Professor of Medicine and
  Physiology
Chairman of Internal Medicine
The Ohio State University Medical
  Center
Columbus, Ohio

I. Ross McDougall, M.D., Ch.B., Ph.D.
Professor of Radiology and Medicine
Stanford University School of Medicine
Stanford, California

J. Maxwell McKenzie, M.D.
Kathleen and Stanley Glaser
  Professor of Medicine
Dpartment of Medicine
University of Miami School of
  Medicine
Staff Physician
University of Miami Hospital and
  Clinics
Jackson Memorial Hospital
Miami, Florida

Sandra M. McLachlan, Ph.D.
Professor of Medicine (Adjunct)
University of California, San Francisco
San Francisco, California

Christoph A. Meier, M.D.
Clinique de Medecine II
Thyroid Research Unit
Division of Endocrinology
Department of Medicine
Geneva University Hospital
Geneva, Switzerland

Marvin L. Mitchell, M.D.
Associate Professor of Medicine
Tufts University School of Medicine
Boston, Massachusetts

John C. Morris, M.D.
Associate Professor of Medicine
Mayo Medical School
Consultant
Division of Endocrinology and
  Internal Medicine
Mayo Clinic
Rochester, Minnesota

Arnold M. Moses, M.D.
Professor of Medicine
State University of New York
Health Sciences Center, Syracuse
Attending Physician
University Hospital
Syracuse, New York

Shigenobu Nagataki, M.D., Ph.D
Chairman and Professor
The First Department of Internal
  Medicine
Nagasaki Univeristy School of
  Medicine
Nagasaki, Japan

John T. Nicoloff, M.D.
Professor of Medicine
University of Southern California
  School of Medicine
Los Angeles, California

Kaie Ojamaa, Ph.D.
Assistant Professor of Medicine
  and Pediatrics
New York University School of
  Medicine
Director, Laboratory of Molecular
  Endocrinology
North Shore University Hospital
Manhasset, New York

Jack H. Oppenheimer, M.D.
Cecil J. Watson Professor of Medicine,
  Cell Biology and Neuroanatomy
University of Minnesota School of
  Medicine
Director, Thyroid Research Unit
University of Minnesota Hospitals
  and Clinics
Minneapolis, Minnesota

Hans Jakob Peter, M.D.
Head, Division of Internal Medicine
University Hospital (Inselspital)
Bern, Switzerland

Aldo Pinchera, M.D.
Professor of Endocrinology
Chairman, Institute of Endocrinology
University of Pisa
Pisa, Italy

John E. Pintar, M.D.
Department of Neuroscience and
  Cell Biology
UMDNJ-Robert Wood Johnson
  Medical School
Piscataway, New Jersey

Basil Rapoport, M.B., Ch.B.
Professor of Medicine
University of California, San Francisco
Staff Physician
Veterans Affairs Medical Center
San Francisco, California

H. Lester Reed, M.D., COL., MC USA
Associate Professor of Medicine
Uniformed Services University of the
  Health Sciences
Bethesda, Maryland
Chief, Department of Medicine
Madigan Army Medical Center
Tacoma, Washington

Samuel Refetoff, M.D.
Professor of Medicine and
  Pediatrics
The University of Chicago School of
  Medicine
Chicago, Illinois

E. Chester Ridgway, III, M.D.
Professor of Medicine
Head, Division of
  Endocrinology, Metabolism and
  Diabetes
Senior Associate Dean of Academic
  Affairs
University of Colorado Health
  Sciences Center
Denver, Colorado

Richard S. Rivlin, M.D.
Professor of Medicine and Chief,
  Nutrition Division
The New York Hospital-Cornell
  Medical Center
Program Director, Clinical Nutrition
  Research Unit
GI-Nutrition Service
Memorial Sloan-Kettering Cancer
  Center
New York, New York

Jacob Robbins, M.D.
Scientist Emeritus, Genetics and
  Biochemistry Branch
National Institute of Diabetes
  and Digestive and Kidney
  Diseases
National Institutes of Health
Bethesda, Maryland

Elaine Ron, Ph.D.
Radiation Epidemiology Branch
National Cancer Institute
National Institutes of Health
Bethesda, Maryland

Douglas S. Ross, M.D.
Assistant Professor of Medicine
Harvard Medical School
Co-Director, Thyroid Associates
Massachusetts General Hospital
Boston, Massachusetts

Elio Roti, M.D.
Investigator
Centro per lo Studio Prevenzione
Diagnosi e Cura delle Tireopatie
Universita degli Studi di Parma
Parma, Italy

Eugene L. Saenger, M.D.
Professor Emeritus of
  Radiology
Director Emeritus, Division of
  Nuclear Medicine
University of Cincinnati College of
  Medicine
Cincinnati, Ohio

Clark T. Sawin, M.D.
Professor of Medicine
Boston University School of Medicine
Chief, Endocrine-Diabetes Section
Boston Veterans Affairs
  Medical Center
Boston, Massachusetts

Maurice F. Scanlon, M.D., F.R.C.P.
Professor of Endocrinology
Department of Endocrinology,
  Metabolism and Diabetes
University of Wales College
  of Medicine
Cardiff, Wales

Steven J. Scheinman, M.D.
Professor of Medicine
Chief, Nephrology Division
State University of New York
Health Science Center, Syracuse
Attending Physician
University Hospital
Syracuse, New York

Martin Schlumberger, M.D.
Chief, Nuclear Medicine Department
Institut Gustave Roussy
Villejuif, Cedex, France

Arthur B. Schneider, M.D., Ph.D.
Professor of Medicine
Chief, Section of Endocrinology and
  Metabolism
University of Illinois College of
  Medicine
Michael Reese Hospital
Chicago, Illinois

Harold L. Schwartz, Ph.D.
Associate Professor of Medicine,
  Cell Biology and Neuroanatomy
University of Minnesota School of
  Medicine
Minneapolis, Minnesota

Joseph H. Sellin, M.D.
Professor of Medicine
Chief, Division of Gastroenterology
University of Texas Medical
  School
Houston, Texas

J. Enrique Silva, M.D.
Professor of Medicine
McGill University
Director, Division of Endocrinology
Sir Mortimer B. Davis Jewish General
  Hospital
Montreal, Quebec, Canada

Allan E. Siperstein, M.D.
Assistant Professor of Surgery
University of California, San Francisco
  School of Medicine
Mt. Zion Medical Center
San Francisco, California

Robert C. Smallridge, M.D.
Colonel, Medical Corps
Professor of Medicine
Director, Endocrinology Division
Uniformed Services University of
  Health Sciences
Bethesda, Maryland
Director, Division of Medicine
Walter Reed Army Institute of
  Research
Washington, D.C.

Terry J. Smith, M.D.
Professor of Medicine, Biochemistry
  and Molecular Biology, and
  Opthalmology
Head, Division of Molecular and
  Cellular Medicine
Albany Medical Center
Staff Physician
Veterans Affairs Medical Center
Albany, New York

Peter J. Snyder, M.D.
Professor of Medicine
University of Pennsylvania School of
  Medicine
Philadelphia, Pennsylvania

Stephen W. Spaulding, M.D.
Professor of Medicine
State University of New York,
  Buffalo
Associate Chief of Staff for Research
  and Development
Buffalo Veterans Affairs Medical
  Center
Buffalo, New York

Carole A. Spencer, Ph.D., M.T.
Professor of Medicine
University of Southern California
  School of Medicine
Los Angeles, California

Lucia Stefaneanu, Ph.D.
Assistant Professor of Pathology
University of Toronto
Research Associate
St. Michael's Hospital
Toronto, Ontario, Canada

Jan R. Stockigt, M.D., F.R.A.C.P.
Director, Ewen Downie Metabolic
  Unit
Alfred Hospital
Professor of Medicine
Monash University
Melbourne, Australia

Kevin A. Strait, Ph.D.
Assistant Professor of Medicine
  and Cell Biology and
  Neuroanatomy
University of Minnesota School of
  Medicine
Minneapolis, Minnesota

Frank Sundler, M.D., Ph.D.
Department of Physiology and
  Neuroscience
Lund University
Lund, Sweden

Morton N. Swartz, M.D.
Professor of Medicine
Harvard Medical School
Chief, Emeritus, Infectious Disease Unit
Massachusetts General Hospital
Boston, Massachusettes

Alvin Taurog, Ph.D.
Professor Emeritus of Pharmacology
University of Texas Southwestern
  Medical Center
Dallas, Texas

Anthony D. Toft, C.B.E., M.D.
Consultant Physician
Royal Infirmary
Edinburgh, Scotland

W. Michael G. Tunbridge, M.D., F.R.C.P.
Director of Postgraduate Medical
  Education and Training
University of Oxford
Honorary Consultant Physician
Radcliffe Infirmary
Oxford, United Kingdom

Robert D. Utiger, M.D.
Deputy Editor, New England Journal
  of Medicine
Clinical Professor of Medicine
Harvard Medical School
Boston, Massachusetts

Apostolos G. Vagenakis, M.D.
Professor and Chairman
Department of Medicine
University of Patras Medical School
Patras, Greece

Mark P.J. Vanderpump, M.D., M.R.C.P.
Senior Medical Registrar
Department of Endocrinology and
  Diabetes
City General Hospital
Stoke-on-Trent, United Kingdom

Rena Vassilopoulou-Sellin, M.D.
Associate Professor of Medicine
Section of Endocrinology
The University of Texas
M.D. Anderson Cancer Center
Houston, Texas

Jan J.M. de Vijlder, Ph.D.
Academic Medical Center
University of Amsterdam
Department of Pediatric
  Endocrinology
EMMA Children's Hospital
Amsterdam, The Netherlands

Louis N. Vogel, M.D.
Clinical Assistant Professor of
 Dermatology
New York University School of
 Medicine
Tisch Hospital
New York, New York

Thomas Vulsma, M.D., Ph.D.
Academic Medical Center
University of Amsterdam
Department of Pediatric
 Endocrinology
EMMA Children's Hospital
Amsterdam, The Netherlands

Leonard Wartofsky, M.D.
Professor of Medicine and Physiology
Uniformed Services University of the
 Health Sciences
Clinical Professor of Medicine
Georgetown University School of
 Medicine
Chairman, Department of Medicine
Washington Hospital Center
Washington, D.C.

Anthony P. Weetman, M.D., DSc
Professor of Medicine
University of Sheffield
Honorary Consultant
 Physician
Northern General Hospital
Sheffield, United Kingdom

Bruce D. Weintraub, M.D.
Professor of Medicine
University of Maryland School of
 Medicine
Chief, Laboratory of Glycoprotein
 Hormones
Institute of Human Virology
Baltimore, Maryland

Peter C. Whybrow, M.D.
Ruth Meltzer Professor and Chairman
Department of Psychiatry
University of Pennsylvania School of
 Medicine
Psychiatrist-in-Chief
Hospital of the University of
 Pennsylvania
Philadelphia, Pennsylvania

Fredric E. Wondisford, M.D.
Assistant Professor of Medicine
Harvard Medical School
Chief, Thyroid Unit
Beth Israel Hospital
Boston, Massachusetts

Naokata Yokoyama, M.D.
Assistant Professor
The First Department of Internal
 Medicine
Nagasaki University School of
 Medicine
Nagasaki, Japan

Margita Zakarija, M.D.
Professor of Medicine and
 Microbiology and Immunology
University of Miami School of
 Medicine
Staff Physician
University of Miami Hospital and
 Clinics
Jackson Memorial Hospital
Miami, Florida

PREFACE

More than 40 years ago, the late Sidney Werner perceived the need for a comprehensive textbook of thyroidology that would contain contributions from multiple authors, each an authority in the subject he or she would be addressing. The success of the first edition of *The Thyroid*, published in 1955, indicated the wisdom of his perception. As knowledge about the thyroid and its diseases has grown, the book's scope and magnitude have increased substantially. Through the next 40 years and its succeeding editions, *The Thyroid* has become what many throughout the world consider to be the standard textbook of thyroid physiology and disease.

It is with sadness that we note the death of Dr. Werner at the age of 84 in 1994, and we wish to dedicate this edition of *The Thyroid* to him. Dr. Werner not only conceived the book but also guided it through its first two editions. He was joined by Dr. Sidney H. Ingbar as co-editor for the third and fourth editions, and then chose to relinquish his editorial role in the book. Dr. Ingbar's role continued through the fifth edition, which was completed two years before his untimely death in 1988.

Sidney Werner's vision and skill in creating the book and developing its basic organization undoubtedly contributed much to its rapid acceptance and continued value. Indeed, the basic organization has changed little from what he created, although individual chapters about particular topics have been added and subtracted in later editions. Even after stepping down as editor, he continued to contribute to the book as both an advisor to the editors and an author.

The creation of this book was but one of Dr. Werner's many contributions to thyroidology. As a faculty member of the Columbia University College of Physicians and Surgeons and director of its thyroid clinic for over 40 years, he educated scores of young physicians and cared for thousands of patients. During this same interval he made many contributions to many different areas of thyroidology. He was among the first to demonstrate that repeated injections of thyrotropin led to antibody formation, and he was one of the first to study the biology of thyrotropic tumors in animals. Long interested in Graves' disease, Dr. Werner carried out many of the early studies of the therapeutic efficacy and side effects of radioiodine therapy for Graves' hyperthyroidism, and he was one of the first to question whether Graves' hyperthyroidism was a pituitary disease. He devised one of the earliest tests—the triiodothyronine suppression test—to detect thyroid autonomy, and used this test to obtain results supporting his view that Graves' disease was not a pituitary disease. Dr. Werner also devised one of the first methods for measuring serum triiodothyronine. He was responsible for the first system for classifying and quantitating the ocular manifestations of Graves' disease, and he carried out many studies of the pathogenesis and therapy of Graves' ophthalmopathy. Dr. Werner was a long-time member of the American Thyroid Association, a member of its board of directors from 1968 to 1974, and its president from 1972 to 1973. In short, he was a leader in the field of thyroidology for many, many years.

In his preface to the first edition, which is reprinted on the following pages, Dr. Werner commented that the book "is intended for those who must deal with the problems of thyroid function and thyroid disease in man." We can put it no better than that. But to be more specific, we would like *The Thyroid* to be useful to basic scientists and clinicians interested in all aspects of the thyroid gland and of its secretions and their actions; to research and clinical fellows just entering the field, and, we hope, caught up in its excitement; and maybe even to younger students at the time of their first exposure to thyroidology. Although this new edition of *The Thyroid* owes much to its predecessors, it has been changed in a number of ways that we hope enhances its value to all readers. The authorship has become increasingly international. There are new chapters on environmental effects on thyroid physiology, the role of oncogenes in thyroid carcinoma, and infectious thyroiditis. As in the past, we have tried to minimize overlap among different chapters, but some is certainly inevitable and probably essential. For example, iodine has so many and such diverse actions in normal subjects and in patients with different thyroid diseases, that its effects must be considered in many chapters.

Thyroid research has remained vibrant and productive in recent years. Much has been learned about the structure and actions of the nuclear receptors for thyroid hormone, and, therefore, about the mechanisms of action of the hormone; the chapter on thyroid hormone actions has become The Molecular Basis of Thyroid Hormone Actions, and one of the longest in the book as well. The genes for the thyrotropin receptor, thyroid peroxidase, thryoxine 5′-deiodinase and the major thyroid hormone binding proteins have been cloned. Many mutations of these genes have been identified, resulting in a great increase in our understanding of structure–function relationships in these areas, providing explanations for many different clinical findings, and leading to the identification of new disorders of thyroid hormone secretion and action. With respect to the common thyroid diseases, iodine deficiency un-

doubtedly remains the most common, not because of lack of understanding but, instead, because of lack of will to provide adequate prophylaxis against it. While understanding of the pathogenesis of the autoimmune thyroid diseases has increased as increasingly sophisticated immunological methods are used to study them, we still know little about how they are initiated or why they subside, and our methods of treatment remain somewhat archaic.

But enough; it is our colleagues who have done the work, and we hope the reader will learn from and, more important, be stimulated by them. We want to thank them all, old and new. They worked hard to be sure that what they wrote was up to date, and they met their deadlines exceedingly well. We tried to guide them, but not with too heavy a hand; they have tolerated our reviews and requests with good humor and with alacrity, and we have learned a great deal. We are pleased with the results, and hope that readers will be as well.

Last, but by no means least, we wish to acknowledge the help and encouragement provided by Ms. Melissa James and Ms. Sandra Cherrey Scheinin at Lippincott-Raven Publishers. They have contributed much to the production of the book, and we thank them.

Lewis E. Braverman, MD
Robert D. Utiger, MD

PREFACE
TO THE FIRST EDITION

This book is intended for those who must deal with the problems of thyroid function and thyroid disease in man. It is designed for use in the clinic and in the basic science laboratory connected with the clinic. The information made available has been brought together from widely diverse sources, and in some instances is reported here for the first time. Many subjects have been presented both in broad outline and in more comprehensive detail to meet differing requirements. It has been planned to provide sufficient documentation to satisfy most needs and, for more exhaustive requirements, to provide a bibliography adequate enough to initiate a search of the literature.

The introduction of a book into a field of clinical medicine today requires considerable justification. In the thyroid field particularly, there already is a profusion of books including the almost classic works of Means in this country and of Joll in England, recently and capably revised by Rundle. Nevertheless, the recent growth of medical knowledge in general, and about the thyroid in particular, appears to have created need for a new volume constructed on a somewhat different basis from those of previous works.

Barry Wood has compared the growth of medical information to that of bacteria. Bacteria show a lag at the beginning of growth and then multiply at a logarithmic rate. Wood considers the growth of current-day medicine to have reached the logarithmic phase. The accumulation of data about the thyroid provides a good example of this acceleration. One author of a recent review claims to have unearthed 3000 new references pertaining to the gland and published during the single year before he wrote his article. *The Quarterly Cumulative Index Medicus* offers about 7800 references to the thyroid in the past decade. More than this, the thyroid field is perme-ated by contributions from the cardiologist, neurologist, muscle physiologist, and many others, bringing the highly unique technics of their particular specialties to bear on the subject.

It is evident that the ability of any one individual to follow progress in all directions at once has all but vanished. As a consequence, marked subspecialization of interest has developed and advances have come to depend upon the interchange of information among many specialists, each providing his own orientation.

This trend has suggested that the information in a book about the healthy and diseased thyroid should also be subjected to the process of sifting and appraising through many eyes. The various specialists present material with which they have had direct experience, and the editor functions as the overseer to provide orientation and preserve the inherent orderliness of the entire subject. The total clinical and research experience made available in this way exceeds that of one person alone. Each topic can be subjected to the critique of a man who has worked intensively with the problem. Finally, a book of this sort can be readily kept current, because of the authors' continued contact with investigation and the fact that there are no large sections to be rewritten by any one individual.

Every effort has been made to make available sufficient basic and clinical knowledge to satisfy curiosity about either of these aspects. For example, sections on the fundamental properties of radioiodine that permit the use of the isotope and on the instrumentation that facilitates such use are presented as well as a discussion of the clinical application. Most basic sections are separated from the clinical material, but are incorporated with it where this has seemed reasonable.

The fundamental aspects of thyroid function in man and the mechanisms which control the activity of the gland; the biochemistry of the hormone; and histology and comparative anatomy make up Part I. The mechanisms of action of the anti-thyroid drugs are included because of the intimate relationship of their effects to the problems of basic physiology.

Part II presents the laboratory methods which supplement the clinical appraisal of thyroid secretory activity. The presentations of the basic principles involved in radioiodine usage and the instrumentation which is employed are included within the laboratory section and are available here for later reference when the therapeutic as well as diagnostic use of the isotope are considered.

The diseases of the thyroid are considered in Part III. The disorders first described are those in which the level of thyroid hormone in the circulation and tissues is within normal limits—euthyroidism. After this come the derangements in which hormone levels are increased—toxic goiter or hyperthyroidism—or decreased—hypothyroidism or myxedema. The effects of hyperthyroidism and of hypothyroidism upon the individual body systems have been subjected to fairly detailed analysis.

The plan to arrange disease by functional categories breaks down in relation to inflammations of the thyroid including the peculiar composite entity, chronic thyroiditis. Inflammations of the thyroid tend to inactivate the gland but chronic thyroiditis is almost as often associated with evidence of hyperthyroidism as with hypothyroidism. The inflammations have been placed under a separate heading on this account.

Before the disease states are presented, several important preliminary subjects are considered in Part III. The normal and abnormal developments of the gland are described, together with the surgical anatomy and a method of physical examination that is an essential procedure because of the accessibility of the thyroid to this approach. The pathology is presented in its entirety in the introductory sections and is not dispersed among the various diseases. A concept of change in thyroid disease emerges in this way which could not otherwise become evident.

A major goal throughout the volume has been to assess the validity of the facts on which current information or procedure is based. Corroborative information is often documented beyond reasonable doubt, but too often is based only on speculation or custom or is wanting altogether. The fact that a critical appraisal has been accomplished is a tribute to the contributors. The world today, as in the past, is threatened by prejudice, of which racial, social and economic prejudices are but a few. Equally influential, but less well recognized, is the prejudice of "experience," derived from uncritical or uncontrolled observation, from the word of an "authority," or from emotional bias.* Fortunately there are those who are willing to give time and effort to seek out and correct such distortions of the truth.

Considerable aid has come to the editor from several sources. Dr. John Stanbury has been particularly helpful. The members of the Thyroid Clinic at the Presbyterian Hospital need recognition for their influence upon the formulation of many of the views presented herein. Credit must be given to the patience and forbearance of the many contributors who tolerated changes in style and length of manuscript in the interest of creating an integrated volume out of a series of individual essays. The editor's wife has acted as guardian of clarity, upon the thesis that even the layman should be able to read and understand a well-written article. Miss Anne Powell, of the librarian staff at P. & S., was extremely generous with her time. Finally, Mrs. R. Levine and Mrs. K. Sorensen were more than patient with the secretarial details.

Sidney C. Werner
New York City

---

*"*Conviction is by no means devoid of emotion but it is a disciplined and differentiated emotion, pointed to the removal of a realistic obstacle. By contrast, the emotion behind prejudice is diffused and overgeneralized, saturating unrelated objects.*"—Gordon W. Allport: The Nature of Prejudice.*

CONTENTS

PART FIVE   THYROID DISEASES: HYPOTHYROIDISM   735

PART SIX   THYROID DISEASES: NONTOXIC DIFFUSE AND MULTINODULAR GOITER   **889**

Werner and Ingbar's
The Thyroid

ONE

The Normal Thyroid

Werner and Ingbar's The Thyroid, Seventh Edition,
edited by Lewis E. Braverman and Robert D. Utiger.
Lippincott–Raven Publishers, Philadelphia, © 1996

Section A
History, Ontogeny, and Anatomy

1

The Heritage of the Thyroid

Clark T. Sawin

Goiter was no surprise to Europeans living 2000 years ago, especially to those living in the Alps. They did not know, however, that goiter was related to the thyroid gland, nor did they know that the thyroid gland existed.[1] All they knew was that there was a swelling in the neck that was called "bronchocele" (ancient Greek for tracheal outpouching), a name that was still applied in 19th century England despite the anatomic discovery of the thyroid gland 200 years earlier (Fig 1-1).

Not until the Renaissance and the expansion of inquiry into the human body was the gland identified, probably by Leonardo da Vinci about the year 1500 and definitely by Vesalius in 1543 (although he called them "laryngeal glands"). By the early 1600s, anatomists finally identified the gland in humans and saw that its enlargement caused clinically evident goiter, as documented by Fabricius in 1619. Only later was the gland called "thyroid" (from the Greek word meaning "shield-shaped") by Thomas Wharton in 1656, not by virtue of its own shape, but because the thyroid cartilage was nearby (Wharton, 1643). Alpine travelers' observations of cretinism, a thyroid-linked disorder, can be traced to the 13th century, but clinically relevant descriptions appeared only in the 16th century, when Paracelsus (ca. 1527) and Platter (in 1562) made the connection between goiter and cretinism.[2]

Until the 19th century, such was the extent of our knowledge of thyroid physiology and disease. Medical theories of disease causation were humorally based; an imbalance of the four humors (blood, phlegm, bile, and black bile) caused illness. Some thought that goiter was due to an excess of phlegm. Treatment was empiric, however. Remedies for goiter were numerous; some were complex mixtures of seaweed and marine sponge. These aquatic substances were well known in medieval Europe and were used a thousand years earlier in China (some historians believe that the Europeans may have learned of these substances from the Chinese indirectly via traders).

After Courtois discovered iodine in the residue of burnt seaweed (ca. 1812), Coindet, an Edinburgh-trained physician working among the goitrous population of Geneva, Switzerland, considered iodine to be the active ingredient of the empiric therapies. In 1820, he gave it to goitrous patients, mostly as the potassium salt, and their goiters shrunk remarkably.[3] To his chagrin, he also saw major toxic effects in some patients (not his own) who probably used too much of the astonishing remedy, which consequently fell into disfavor. Iodine continued to be used for other disorders,[4] such as scrofula, syphilis, and tuberculosis (which explains the use of iodine compounds for bronchial disorders up through the 1980s). In fact, Coindet's toxicity was the earliest description of any form of thyrotoxicosis—in this case, iodine-induced—although neither he nor anyone else recognized the toxicity as thyrotoxicosis until some decades later. Despite the controversy over the use of iodine in Geneva, the therapy represented a shift from an empiric, "folk" medicine to a rational treatment of a defined illness with a specific substance.

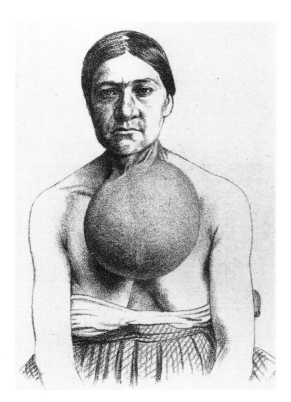

FIGURE 1-1. Large goiter in a woman from an area with a high rate of endemic goiter (Bern, Switzerland). The woman was a patient of the Bern surgeon, E. Theodor Kocher, a Nobel laureate. (Kocher T. Zur Pathologie and Therapie des Kropfes. Deutsche Zeitschrift f. Chirurgie 1874;4:417)

The use of iodine as a drug, even if effective, did not ensure that practitioners knew the treatment was replacing a deficiency: for most of the 19th century, few accepted the idea that disease could be due to the lack of something. Although the use of iodine as a goiter preventive was proposed in 1831, based on observations in Colombia, South America,[5] and later in 1850 by Chatin, a Parisian pharmacist, botanist, and physician,[6] these suggestions were discarded. Most believed that goiter must be due to something in the water—a toxin, a bacterium, or a parasite. The issue was not resolved until the early 20th century when small amounts of iodine were found to prevent goiter in schoolgirls in Akron, Ohio.[7] Even then, the girls were not shown to be iodine-deficient (proof of such deficiency was not established for another decade or so).

What has happened since the 1920s is curiously reminiscent of the 19th century, when iodine replacement never became widespread and was eventually abandoned because it was seen as toxic or irrational. This attitude resulted in continued goiter and the associated, but less common, cretinism. In the 1900s, after the Akron experiment, the notion of deficiency was accepted, but iodine replacement still did not become widespread for decades. Proof that iodine in small amounts prevents goiter and cretinism has still not been translated into worldwide prevention. The lesson of the 19th century —that iodine is useful prophylaxis against and therapy for goiter—has not been thoroughly learned. Today, an international consortium (the International Council for the Control of Iodine Deficiency Disorders) attempts to move social, cultural, and scientific levers to provide sufficient iodine to literally hundreds of millions of people.

The thyroid dysfunctions we know as hypothyroidism and thyrotoxicosis were not thought to be thyroid diseases when described in the 19th century. There was instead a slow amalgamation of clinical and physiologic evidence that gradually defined these conditions as we know them today.

Coindet was not the only one to describe thyrotoxicosis without realizing it. Parry, who saw spontaneous thyrotoxicosis before Coindet but whose observations went unpublished until after his death[8] (and then in an obscure book, rather than a journal), saw a few patients with rapid heartbeat, goiter, and sometimes exophthalmos. (Exophthalmos was not described by Coindet). He thought that the constellation of signs represented a heart disease. A few years later, Graves described, in his Meath Hospital lectures, three women who seemed alike (they had goiter and palpitations). His published lectures[9] included a fourth patient who also had exophthalmos. This patient had been mentioned to him by his student, friend, and colleague Stokes. Both Graves and Stokes believed that the illness was cardiac. Graves' description was not widely known on the European continent, so when Basedow reported his patients in 1840,[10] he was thought to be the first to describe the illness. As a result, most Europeans still use the term "Basedow's disease." Even after Basedow's report, however, the goiter itself was not considered of much importance. The belief that the syndrome was due to a heart disease faded after about 1860, in part because of Charcot's emphasis on the nervousness of most patients;[11] a neurologic hypothesis was dominant for the rest of the 19th century. The disorder was not yet thought to be a thyroid disease.

By the 1880s, surgeons were able to remove the goiters, at least partially, in these nervous, overactive patients without killing too many of them. Interestingly, the nervousness often disappeared in the survivors. This fact, plus the observation in the 1890s that too much thyroid extract led to similar nervousness and weight loss, brought a shift in thinking toward the thyroid origin of the syndrome. Only in reference to the 1890s and early 1900s can we speak of thyrotoxicosis, because only then did the concept of an excessive amount of thyroid hormone come into existence. The concept was applied to both the spontaneous disease and the disease induced by desiccated thyroid. Note that the term *thyrotoxicosis* is based on another idea of the 1890s, namely, that the thyroid in this syndrome either secretes or fails to inactivate a toxin (i.e., a deleterious substance not found in a normal person). The word is still in common use, but it does not reflect the actual pathophysiology. The success of partial thyroidectomy over 100 years ago helped focus attention on the thyroid gland, eventually leading to the now more commonly used treatments, radioiodine[12,13] and antithyroid drugs.[14]

Hypothyroidism as a clinical syndrome was recognized even later, and its cause was equally obscure. First defined in London in the 1870s,[15] it was named "myxoedema" because of the swollen skin ("oedema") and its excess content of mucin ("myx-").[16] It was considered either a neurologic or a skin disease; there was no cure. At about the same time, it became evident that the same surgical skill that allowed thyrotoxic patients to survive the operation allowed even better survival after thyroidectomy in goitrous patients who were not nervous and overactive. Almost no patients died in the hands of good surgeons. The ability to remove the entire thyroid gland, however, led to a peculiar and disastrous outcome: the patient lived but became puffy-faced, slow of mind, and socially nonfunctional.[17,18] Again, no one knew why, and again there was no cure.

The Swiss, writing in German or French, and the English, writing in English, did not read each other's reports; thus, neither was aware of the other's work. That situation changed when Felix Semon, an immigrant Prussian practicing laryngology in London, mentioned at a meeting of the Clinical Society of London that the Swiss patients who had undergone total thyroidectomy seemed quite similar to the English ones with myxedema. Scoffed at, Semon persisted, and a committee was named to investigate his observation. The report was finished 5 years later, in 1888, and is now considered a classic.[19] Cretinism, myxedema, and the postthyroidectomy changes were all seen to result from "the annihilation of the function of the thyroid body."[19]

Despite this major step in understanding, the report did not offer an effective therapy. In 1889, however, Brown-Séquard's work in Paris on the rejuvenating effects of testicular extracts[20] led to the use of extracts of other tissues as treatments for a wide variety of diseases. Most were eventually found to be ineffective, but the idea indirectly led to the successful and remarkable cure of myxedema by the use of injected thyroid extract by Murray in 1891.[21] A year later, the treatment was made even easier by simply eating ground or fried sheep thyroid, or tablets of dried thyroid tissue. This affirmation that Brown-Séquard's organotherapy was effective in at least one serious illness was the origin of modern endocrinology.

Nevertheless, no one knew just why this peculiar treatment worked, even though it was extended in 1894 to the successful treatment of goiter.[22] (The 15th century Chinese may have used the same therapy for goiter on the basis of "like treating like."[23]) A vigorous search for the "active principle" took place, but nothing was discovered until 1895, when Baumann, to his great surprise, found iodine in the thyroid gland.[24] Twenty years later, Kendall at the Mayo Clinic used iodine as a marker for the isolation of the active substance and succeeded in isolating bioactive crystalline material on Christmas Day, 1914.[25] He and his associate, Osterberg, named it "thyroxin," while waiting for a train in Chicago; the name was a contraction of "thyroxyindole," a term that resulted from Kendall's erroneous belief that the compound had an indole nucleus with three iodine atoms per molecule. Kendall never changed his ideas, despite repeated failures to synthesize an active molecule. He was much disappointed when, in 1926 and 1927, Harington found the correct structure, showed that it had four (not three) iodine atoms per molecule, and synthesized it.[26,27] Harington also added an "e," calling it "thyroxine" to fit the convention at the time for naming amino acid derivatives; Kendall agreed with this change. The correct spelling is thus "thyroxine."

Kendall's extracted thyroxine was patented and commercially licensed, but was far more expensive and not as effective as desiccated thyroid. (In the 1920s, no one knew that thyroxine as the free acid is not well absorbed). Even Harington's synthetic product was too costly. Therefore, until the 1960s, therapy for thyroid deficiency and goiter consisted only of the administration of desiccated thyroid; for some older patients, this is still the therapy. The successful synthesis of thyroxine in high yield in 1949[28] made therapy with it (in the form of sodium L-thyroxine) economically sensible; thyroxine is used now in almost all treatment with thyroid hormone.

Both Kendall and Harington suspected that there might be another thyroid hormone, other than thyroxine, but they were never able to find it. Kendall moved on to work with adrenal steroids, which won him a Nobel prize. Harington gave up the idea of a second thyroid hormone and became director of London's National Institute for Medical Research. He was much surprised when his associates, Rosalind Pitt-Rivers, and her postdoctoral fellow, Jack Gross, found and synthesized triiodothyronine (T_3) and showed it to be more active than thyroxine in a bioassay.[29,30] Harington was elated when, with Gross on a vacation in France, the bioassay was successfully repeated and confirmed the high biologic activity of T_3. T_3 was found almost simultaneously across the English Channel in Paris by Roche, Lissitsky, and Michel.[31,32] There was indeed a second thyroid hormone.

While we may not completely understand why spontaneous hypothyroidism occurs, thyroxine treatment has made the task of management easier, particularly after the development of reliable assays for the measurement of serum thyrotropin (TSH) and the demonstration that thyroxine suppresses to normal the raised concentrations of TSH characteristic of primary hypothyroidism.[33,34]

Gaps in our knowledge remain, for example, an identification of the cause of goiter in the absence of iodine deficiency, or an explanation of the initial causes of thyrotoxicosis. The record of the past does suggest a certain optimism; at least some of these gaps will be filled in.

Only Kocher, among all those mentioned earlier, won a Nobel prize for work in the area of thyroid studies, although several others were considered "worthy" by one or another Nobel Committee. No matter; our patients are still the better for it.

References

1. Sawin CT. Goiter. In: Kiple KF, ed. Cambridge world history of human disease. Cambridge: Cambridge University Press, 1993:750
2. Cranefield PF. The discovery of cretinism. Bull Hist Med 1962;36:489
3. Coindet J-F. Découverte d'un nouveau remède contre le goitre. Annales Chim Phys 1820;15:49 (originally published in the Swiss Bibliotèque Universelle, 1820, and reprinted in its entirety in J Pharmacie 1820;6:485)
4. Lugol JGA. Mémoire sur l'emploi de l'iode dans les maladies scrophuleuses. Paris. 1829
5. Boussingault J-B. Recherches sur la cause qui produit le Goître dans les Cordilières de la Nouvelle-Grenade. Annales Chim Phys 1831;48:41
6. Chatin A. Existence de l'iode dans les plantes d'eau douce: Consequences de ce fait pour le géognosie, la physiologie végétale, la thérapeutique et peut-être pour l'industrie. Compt Rend Acad Sci 1850;30:352
7. Marine D, Kimball OP. Prevention of simple goiter in man. Arch Intern Med 1920;25:661
8. Parry CH. Collections from the unpublished medical writings. London: Underwoods, 1825:111

9. Graves RJ. Clinical Lectures delivered by Robert J. Graves, M.D., at the Meath Hospital during the Session of 1834-5. London Med Surg J 1835;7:516

10. Basedow CA. Exophthalmos durch hypertrophie des Zellgewebes in der Augenhohle. Wschr f d ges Heilkunde 1840;6:197,220

11. Charcot JM. Mémoire sur une affection caractérisée par des palpitations du coeur et des artères, la tumefaction de la glande thyroïde et une double exophthalmie. Compt Rend Soc Biol 1857;3(2nd ser):43

12. Hertz S, Roberts A. Radioactive iodine in the study of thyroid physiology. vii. The use of radioactive iodine therapy in hyperthyroidism. JAMA 1946;131:81

13. Chapman E, Evans RD. The treatment of hyperthyroidism with radioactive iodine. JAMA 1946;131:86

14. Astwood EB. Treatment of hyperthyroidism with thiourea and thiouracil. JAMA 1943;122:78

15. Gull WW. On a cretinoid state supervening in adult life in women. Trans Clin Soc Lond 1874;7:180

16. Ord WM. On myxoedema, a term proposed to be applied to an essential condition in the "cretinoid" affection occasionally observed in middle-aged women. Med-chir Trans 1878;61:57

17. Reverdin JL. Accidents consécutifs à l'ablation totale du goitre. Rev Méd Suisse Romande 1882;2:539

18. Kocher T. Ueber Kropfexstirpation und ihre Folgen. Archiv f klin Chir 1883;29:254

19. Ord WM (chairman). Report of a committee of the Clinical Society of London nominated December 14, 1883, to investigate the subject of myxoedema. Trans Clin Soc Lond 1888;21(Supplement)

20. Brown-Séquard CE. Des effets produits chez l'homme par les injections sous-cutanées d'un liquide retiré des testicules frais de cobaye et de chien. Compt Rend Soc Biol 1889;41:415

21. Murray GR. Note on the treatment of myxoedema by hypodermic injections of an extract of the thyroid gland of a sheep. Br Med J 1891;2:796

22. Bruns P. Ueber die Kropfbehandlung mit Schildrusenfutterung. Deut Mediz Wschr 1894;41:785

23. Needham J. Proto-endocrinology in medieval China. In: Needham J, Ling W, Gwei-Djen L, Ping-Yu H. Clerks and craftsmen in China and the West. Cambridge: Cambridge University Press, 1970:294

24. Baumann E. Ueber das normale Vorkommen von Jod im Thierkorper. Hoppe-Seyler's Z fur Physiol Chem 1895;21:319

25. Kendall EC. The isolation in crystalline form of the compound which occurs in the thyroid: its chemical nature and physiologic activity. JAMA 1915;64:2042

26. Harington CR. Chemistry of thyroxine. II. Constitution and synthesis of desiodo-thyroxine. Biochem J 1926;20:300

27. Harington CR, Barger G. Chemistry of thyroxine. III. Constitution and synthesis of thyroxine. Biochem J 1927;21:169

28. Chalmers JR, Dickson GT, Elks J, Hems BA. The synthesis of thyroxine and related substances. Part V. A synthesis of L-thyroxine from L-tyrosine. J Chem Soc 1949;3424

29. Gross J, Pitt-Rivers R. The identification of 3:5:3′-L-triiodothyronine in human plasma. Lancet 1952;1:439

30. Gross J, Pitt-Rivers R. Physiological activity of 3:5:3′-L-triiodothyronine. Lancet 1952;1:593

31. Roche J, Lissitsky S, Michel R. Sur la triiodothyronine, produit intermédiaire de la transformation de la diiodothyronine en thyroxine. Compt Rend Acad Sci 1952;234:997

32. Roche J, Lissitzky S, Michel R. Sur la presence de triiodothyronine dans la thyroglobuline. Compt Rend Acad Sci 1952;234:1228

33. Utiger RD. Radioimmunoassay of human plasma thyrotropin. J Clin Invest 1965;44:1277

34. Odell WD, Wilber JF, Paul WE. Radioimmunoassay of human thyrotropin in serum. Metabolism 1965;14:465

Suggested Readings

In addition, readers will find more historical detail in the following:

Harington CR. The thyroid gland: its chemistry and physiology. London: Oxford University Press, 1933

Pitt-Rivers R, Vanderlaan WP. The therapy of thyroid disease. In: Parnham MJ, Bruinvels J, eds. Discoveries in pharmacology. Vol 2. Amsterdam: Elsevier, 1984:391

Rolleston HD. The endocrine organs in health and disease with an historical review. London: Oxford University Press, 1936

Sawin CT. Defining thyroid hormone: its nature and control. In: McCann SM, ed. Endocrinology: people and ideas. Bethesda, MD: American Physiological Society, 1988:149

Werner and Ingbar's The Thyroid, Seventh Edition,
edited by Lewis E. Braverman and Robert D. Utiger.
Lippincott–Raven Publishers, Philadelphia, © 1996

2

Normal Development of the Hypothalamic-Pituitary-Thyroid Axis

John E. Pintar

The function of the adult thyroid gland is primarily regulated by thyroid-stimulating hormone (TSH; thyrotropin) released from the pituitary gland, which itself is regulated by additional peptides and amines secreted from the hypothalamus. Thus, appropriate regulation of adult thyroid function depends on the normal maturation during development of three separate components: (1) morphologic and biochemical differentiation of the thyroid follicle itself, which includes the production of thyroglobulin (Tg) and thyroperoxidase, the uptake systems for iodine, and finally, the formation and secretion of triiodothyronine (T_3) and thyroxine (T_4); (2) the normal development in the pituitary of cells that secrete TSH (thyrotrophs); and (3) the differentiation of cells that secrete thyrotropin-releasing hormone (TRH) in the hypothalamus. The initial differentiation of these three components occurs independently, and the maturation of the entire integrated system occurs over a prolonged period that extends well into neonatal life. This chapter reviews knowledge about the morphogenesis and differentiation of these cell populations; it focuses on humans as much as possible but also includes relevant experimental data from other vertebrate species.

MORPHOLOGIC AND BIOCHEMICAL DIFFERENTIATION

Formation of the Neural Tube, Neural Crest, and Hypothalamus

The neural plate progenitor of the central and peripheral nervous systems begins to form in humans on embryonic day 17 and can be identified as a thickening of the midline ectoderm that overlies the notochord. The interaction of the notocord and overlying ectoderm has been classically viewed as essential for neural cell induction, although the possibility that neural differentiation represents a default pathway in the ectoderm, rather than an induced state, is currently receiving experimental support.[1] (Fig 2-1*a*). During the next 10 days, this region of thickened ectoderm gradually forms neural folds that fuse to form the neural tube (see Fig 2-1*b–e*). Some cells in the dorsal region of this tube, the neural crest, leave this region (see Fig 2-1*c–e*) to form numerous derivatives, including neurons and glia of the peripheral nervous system, melanocytes, connective tissue of the head, and numerous endocrine derivatives, such as the calcitonin-producing parafollicular cells of the thyroid. The colonization of the thyroid by these cells is described later in this chapter.

The remainder of the neural tube gives rise to the central nervous system. More anterior regions of this tube give rise to the early subdivisions of the brain, including (from anterior to posterior) the prosencephalon, mesencephalon, and rhombencephalon. Quail-chick chimera studies indicate that the presumptive hypothalamic area initially occupies the most rostral region of the neural tube[2] (Fig 2-2) and subsequently assumes a more caudal and ventral position. The hypothalamus proper begins to develop from the ventral caudal prosencephalon (diencephalon) during the 6th week of gestation in humans (Fig 2-3). An evagination from the ventral hypothalamus, the infundibulum, gives rise to multiple structures, including the posterior pituitary, the median eminence, and the pituitary stalk, which connects the hypothalamus and pituitary (Fig 2-4). The median eminence has an important physiologic role because it serves as the termination site for nerve fibers whose

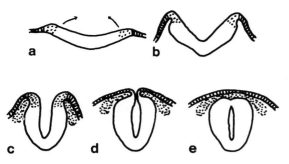

FIGURE 2-1. Diagram of cross sections of the dorsal ectoderm of the human embryo between 18 and 24 days' gestation, illustrating the derivation of the neural tube and neural crest as follows: (*a*) neural plate stage: *white area*—neural plate, *dotted areas*—future neural crest, *hatched areas*—somatic ectoderm; (*b–d*) neural groove stages; (*e*) neural tube stage. Fusion of the neural folds begins in the region of the first occipital somite and proceeds both rostrally and caudally thereafter. Future neural crest cells at the margins of the neural folds are not included in the wall of the neural tube or in the overlying somatic ectoderm.

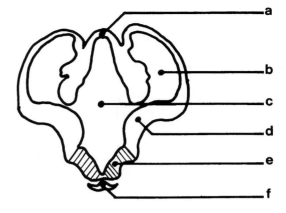

FIGURE 2-3. Diagram of a human embryo of about 50 days. Coronal section at the level of the pituitary: (a) roof of diencephalon; (b) lateral ventricle; (c) third ventricle; (d) corpus striatum; (e) hypothalamus; (f) pituitary. (Modified from Tuchmann-Duplessis H, Auroux M, Haegel P. Illustrated human embryology. Vol 3. Nervous system and endocrine glands. New York: Springer-Verlag, 1974)

cell bodies originate in the hypothalamus proper and release neurosecretory material into the veins of the primary portal plexus that develops in this area.

The hypothalamus in humans can be recognized as a discrete brain region at about 3 weeks of gestation. The nuclear groups synthesizing peptides that control pituitary function first appear about 2 or 3 weeks after the hypothalamus can be recognized.[3] In humans, the first hypothalamic nuclei appear

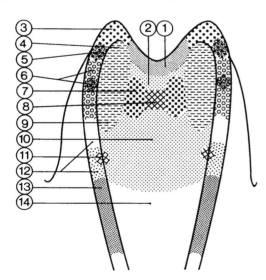

FIGURE 2-2. Mapping of the anterior neural primordium at the three-four somite stage in the avian embryo. (1) Adenohypophysis; (2) hypothalamus; (3) ectoderm of the naval cavity; (4) floor of the telencephalon; (5) olfactory placode; (6) ectoderm of the upper beak and egg tooth; (7) optic vesicles; (8) neurophysis; (9) roof of the telencephalon; (10) diencephalon; (11) hemiepiphysis; (12) ectoderm of the calvaria and caudal prosencephalon (*lightly spotted area*); (13) rostral mesencephalic neural crest (*densely stippled area*); (14) mesencephalon. (Couly G, LeDouarin NM. Mapping of the neural primordium in quail-chick chimeras. II. The prosencephalic neural plate and neural folds: implications for the genesis of cephalic congenital abnormalities. Dev Bio 1987;120:213)

at 55 days; the remaining nuclei appear over a protracted developmental period, but all can be recognized by the 16th week. Thus, a small but morphologically mature hypothalamus is present by the 4th month and serves as a template for further neuronal and glial differentiation and for formation of appropriate synapses and fiber tracts.

The tripeptide TRH is the major positive regulator of pituitary TSH synthesis and release.[4] In human adults, the highest concentrations of TRH immunoreactivity are found in hypothalamic areas, including the upper pituitary stalk, the posterior nucleus, and the anterior hypothalamus.[5] Immunoreactive TRH, however, is widespread throughout the brain, and greater than 70% of total immunoreactive TRH is found outside the hypothalamus in both brain and spinal cord (intermediolateral) sites.[4,6] Initial immunohistochemical studies demonstrated that the highest density and number of TRH neurons are present in the dorsal part of the dorsomedial hypothalamic nucleus.[7] Subsequently, more effective fixation procedures that prevent TRH diffusion and effectively crosslink the small TRH peptide demonstrated another major concentration of TRH cell bodies in the parvocellular parts or the paraventricular nucleus.[8] These neurons project primarily to the medial region of the external layer of the median eminence and are thus the likely major regulators of TSH release. Immunoreactive TRH fibers in the median eminence of rats disappear when the anterior periventricular hypothalamic region is lesioned, and this loss likely results from an interruption of at least some fiber tracts that originate in more rostral areas.[8]

Immunoreactive TRH has been detected at as early as 30 days of gestation in whole brain extracts and in the isolated hypothalamus and cerebellum by 9 weeks[9]; after this time, TRH concentration remains constant throughout gestation. The ontogeny of immunoreactive TRH neurons within any area has unfortunately not yet been reported, probably because appropriate fixation conditions have not yet been used. TRH can cross the placenta, but maternal TRH levels do not appear sufficient to stimulate pituitary TSH release.[10,11] Although significant amounts of TRH are produced in islet cells

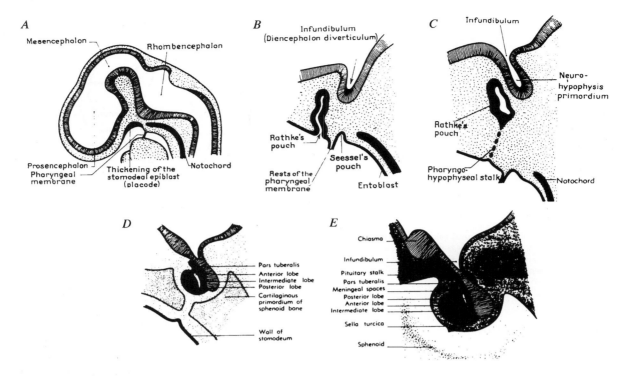

FIGURE 2-4. Diagrammatic representation of pituitary development in sagittal sections of human embryos of 22 days (*A*), 42 days (*B*), 60 days (*C*), 2 months (*D*), and 3 months (*E*). The diencephalon arises from subdivision of the prosencephalon, Rathke's pouch from the stomadeum epiblast. (Tuchmann-Duplessis H, Auroux M, Haegal P. Illustrated human embryology. Vol 3. Nervous system and endocrine glands. New York: Springer-Verlag, 1974)

of the human fetal pancreas as early as the 6th week of gestation,[12,13] it is thought that rapid degradation (within seconds) of TRH in serum would prohibit peripheral or maternal TRH from affecting pituitary function.[14] Although the primary negative regulator of TSH secretion is direct feedback inhibition of thyroid hormone on the pituitary, dopamine and somatostatin also inhibit TSH secretion, and neurons containing these transmitters differentiate and have nerve terminals that enter the median eminence within the first trimester.

For TRH to regulate pituitary function, it not only must be synthesized, but also must reach the pituitary. The conduit for this pathway consists of the TRH fibers that enter the median eminence and release TRH into the portal system. Although the time at which TRH fibers reach the median eminence has not been examined in the human fetus, fluorescent fibers from catecholamine-containing neurons reach the median eminence by the 13th week.[15] The development of the portal system is discussed in more detail later in this chapter.

Hypophyseal Portal Circulation

The hypophyseal portal circulation links the median eminence (into which hypothalamic peptides that modulate pituitary hormone synthesis and secretion are released) with the pituitary (Fig 2-5). Two distinct capillary plexuses form, one in the median eminence (primary plexus) and a second in the pituitary (secondary plexus); the pituitary plexus develops from a network of vessels derived from the internal carotids and the floor of the diencephalon.[16] The two components of the portal system develop gradually in all species, including humans, and the exact time at which a functional connection between the two is established remains unknown. Initial morphologic studies[17] found that the secondary plexus in the anterior pituitary developed by the 4th month, and that the primary plexus, which links the median eminence with the secondary plexus, was the last component of this portal system to develop and was observed at about 6 months. It now appears, however, that a rudimentary portal circulatory system is established much earlier. Human fetuses as young as 11.5 weeks have been perfused with siliconized rubber, and blood vessels containing silicone have been visualized histologically. In all specimens examined, ranging in age from as early as 11.5 weeks of gestation to 16 weeks of gestation, impregnated vessels were observed throughout the median eminence, infundibulum, and in all regions of the pituitary.[18] Thus, it appears likely, but is not yet proved, that by the time TRH fibers in the hypothalamus reach the median eminence, any released TRH has direct access to the pituitary through this route.

Alternative routes by which TRH could reach the pituitary also exist. For example, if TRH fibers have not yet reached the medial eminence, TRH released in the hypothalamus could diffuse to the pituitary. Alternatively, TRH released from the intermediolateral cell column of the spinal cord[6] could reach the pituitary through the cerebrospinal fluid (CSF). The fact that TRH and other releasing factors are found in adult CSF supports this possibility.[19] Finally, the pia-arachnoid membrane surrounds the pituitary, and blood vessels entering the anterior pituitary lobe are accompanied by the subarachnoid

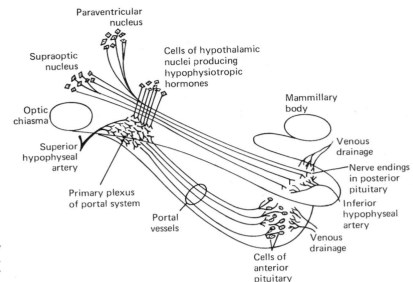

FIGURE 2-5. Diagram of hypothalamus and pituitary gland showing the portal system of the vasculature. (Villee DB. Human endocrinology: a developmental approach: Philadelphia: WB Saunders, 1975)

space of Virchow-Robin.[20] Material injected into this subarachnoid space enters the anterior lobe along with the blood vessels, and it presumably could reach the entire pituitary.

The Anterior Pituitary

Both the anterior and intermediate pituitary lobes are derived from Rathke's pouch, which is an invagination of the ectodermal lining of the buccopharyngeal cavity (see Fig 2-4). This ectodermal region, at least in lower vertebrates, has been shown to originate from the anterior neural ridge in a region that is adjacent to the presumptive hypothalamic region[2] (see Fig 2-2). During subsequent development, this region is separated from the hypothalamic primordium and becomes located in the roof of the mouth. Rathke's pouch itself first appears in humans at gestational day 21 at the junction between the ectodermal and endodermal linings of the buccal cavity just anterior to the notochord.[21,22] From the initial stages of its formation, this structure is in contact with the presumptive posterior lobe or infundibulum; thus, contact between the presumptive hypothalamus and pituitary, which was disrupted, is reestablished. This interaction is maintained in species that have an intermediate lobe, but in humans the intermediate lobe is transitory and disappears soon after birth. The anterior wall of the pouch proliferates extensively and gives rise to the anterior lobe, which contains multiple hormone cell types, including the cells that produce TSH. Initial morphologic studies showed that cells of the basophilic family, which include the TSH cells, can be detected at as early as 10 weeks of gestation in humans.[23] Other characteristics of TSH cells, including staining by the aldehyde-thionine procedure[23] and Alcian blue[21] and their distinctive polyhedral shape, appear by 13 and 28 weeks, respectively. Immunoreactive TSH cells have been observed in the human pituitary at least as early as 13 weeks,[24] confirming that presumptive thyrotrophs identified histologically are indeed TSH cells.

The appearance of TSH pituitary cells during the 13th week of gestation coincides with the time at which TSH has been detected by bioassay and radioimmunoassay, not only in the pituitary but also in the serum.[25–28] Because at least some nerve fibers have reached the median eminence by this age, it is possible that the initial stages of thyroid regulation by hypothalamic TRH are beginning. Even so, most evidence suggests that in the absence of TRH, thyroid development can proceed normally for at least a few weeks (see later in chapter).

Although fetal pituitary TSH synthesis can be detected by immunoprecipitation by 13 weeks, levels remain low until the 18th week of gestation. At that point, and continuing throughout the month that follows, levels of pituitary and serum TSH increase dramatically,[25,26] and this increase is followed by increases in both serum total T_4 and serum free T_4. It appears that the increase in circulating TSH represents a continuing maturation of the hypothalamic-pituitary axis. Either this increase could represent the development of a mature secretory response to TRH by the pituitary TSH population, or, alternatively, it could result from the more mature state of the portal system that delivers TRH to the pituitary (discussed later). Other pituitary cell types apparently increase their secretion during the midgestational period (weeks 18–24)[29] while the thyroid itself increases iodine concentration by about threefold during this period.[30]

The Thyroid

MORPHOGENESIS

The thyroid gland is the earliest endocrine glandular structure to appear in mammalian development.[31] Early studies of thyroid development described both its early morphogenesis from the embryonic endoderm and the subsequent appearance of morphologic features that indicate function, such as the accumulation of colloid. In higher vertebrates, the mature thyroid gland has a dual embryonic origin from two distinct regions of the endodermal pharynx. The median anlage arises from a thickening in the midline of the anterior pharyngeal floor[32,33] (Figs 2-6 through 2-8A); this thickening is located in the region between branchial arches 1 and 2 (see Fig 2-7) and is adjacent

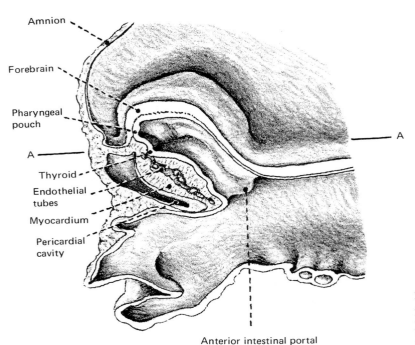

Amnion

Forebrain

Pharyngeal
pouch

A

Thyroid

Endothelial
tubes

Myocardium

Pericardial
cavity

A

Anterior intestinal portal

FIGURE 2-6. Drawing of a midsagittal model of a two-somite embryo (17 days), showing the early thyroid anlage. (Modified from Boyd JD. Development of the human thyroid gland. In: Pitt-Rivers R, Trotter WR, eds. The thyroid. Vol 1. Washington, DC: Butterworths, 1964:9)

to the newly differentiating myocardium (see Fig 2-8*A*). The two lateral anlagen (ultimobranchial bodies) have had a more controversial history and are now thought to develop as caudal projections from the fourth or fifth pharyngeal pouch[32–34] (Fig 2-9). In lower vertebrates, these cell populations are not incorporated into the thyroid and exist as independent structures. In higher vertebrates, however, they contain the precursors of the parafollicular cells (see later in chapter).

Formation of the Medial Anlage. The medial anlage appears first and becomes a visible outpocketing in humans during gestational days 16 and 17 (see Figs 2-6 and 2-7). The inductive factors responsible for formation and growth of this anlage remain unknown, but they may involve a stimulus from the adjacent mesenchyme, because transplants of the presumptive thyroid region form typical thyroid tissue only when the mesenchyme is present;[35] further experimental studies are needed. The thyroid diverticulum continues to expand ventrally, with the most rapid proliferation at its distal tip, but it remains attached to the pharyngeal floor by the stalk, now called the thyroglossal duct (see Fig 2-8*B*). Continued proliferation by the thyroid progenitors soon obliterates the lumen of the outpocketing, which becomes filled with cords of cells. The thyroid rudiment then begins to expand laterally, which leads to formation of the characteristic bilobed structure. Because this medial component of the thyroid is closely associated with the developing heart (see Fig 2-8*B*), the thyroid is essentially pulled to its position near the base of the neck as a consequence of the continuing descent of the heart during these early stages of thyroid formation. This caudal displacement is accompanied by the rapid elongation of the thyroglossal duct, which eventually fragments and, in general, incompletely degenerates.[32,33]

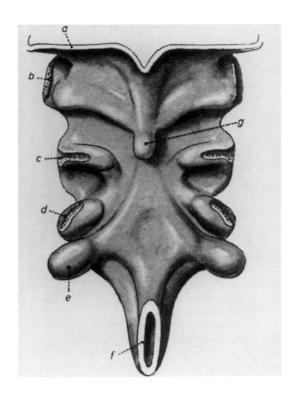

FIGURE 2-7. Ventral aspect of pharyngeal endoderm in a late-somite human embryo, based on a model by Weller: (a) buccal epithelium; (b–d) lateral extremities of first, second, and third pharyngeal pouches; (e) fourth pharyngeal pouch; (f) esophagus; (g) median thyroid diverticulum. Stippled areas indicate areas of contact with the corresponding ectodermal grooves.

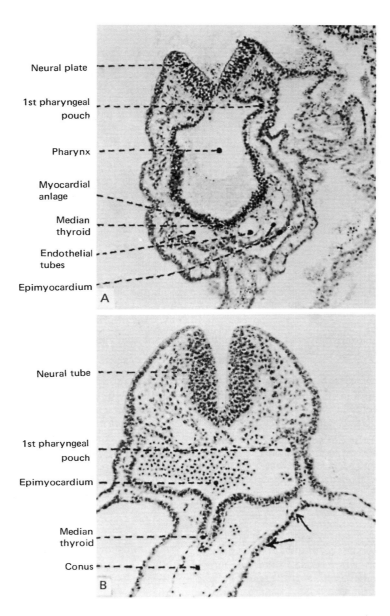

Neural plate

1st pharyngeal
pouch

Pharynx

Myocardial
anlage

Median
thyroid

Endothelial
tubes

Epimyocardium

A

Neural tube

1st pharyngeal
pouch

Epimyocardium

Median
thyroid

Conus

B

FIGURE 2-8. (*A*) Plane of section through embryo shown in Figure 2-6 (lines A and A) (×150). (*B*) Transverse section through a 10-somite embryo; plane of section passes through the median thyroid (×150).

Because these critical events in thyroid morphogenesis occur during the first 2 months of gestation, most developmental thyroid abnormalities result from morphogenetic errors during this period that lead to displacement of cells derived from this medial anlage. Ectopic thyroid tissue can result from abnormal medial thyroid migration that is secondary to abnormal heart morphogenesis, or from abnormal interactions between the thyroid primordium and the heart. As a result, ectopic thyroid cells have been found throughout the regions through which their displacement occurs and thus have been observed in sublingual, high cervical, mediastinal, and even intracardiac locations. In the first three cases, interaction between the heart and medial anlage is abrogated earlier in development than normal, while in the last case, thyroid tissue differentiates within the cardiac endothelium. Finally, in some cases, the thyroglossal duct does not degenerate and instead persists as a fistulous tract.[36]

Formation of the Ultimobranchial Bodies. The formation of the presumptive lateral thyroids as diverticula from the fourth or fifth pharyngeal pouch begins as the medial thyroid anlage begins its descent.[32,34] These ultimobranchial bodies ultimately separate from the pharyngeal pouches and fuse with the lateral parts of the medial thyroid (see Fig 2-9). The connections of the lateral lobes with the rest of the pharynx degenerate, and the tissue derived from the lateral anlage is surrounded by cells derived from the differentiating medial anlage. In humans the contribution of this population to the thyroid mass is minimal (about 10%). The association between the medial and lateral thyroid anlage is complete by 8 to 9 weeks of gestation, at which time the thyroid has assumed its definitive form.

An additional common abnormality results from abnormal lateral lobe development and is characterized by the failure of the lateral thyroid anlage (ultimobranchial body) to fuse with the median thyroid. As a result, there are larger than normal

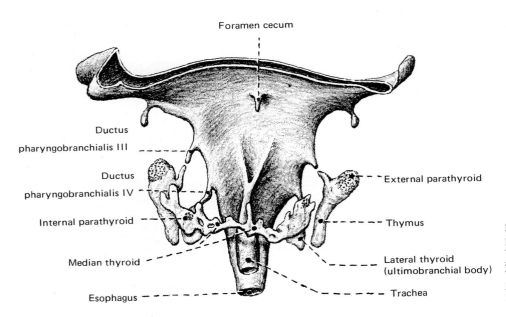

Foramen cecum

Ductus
pharyngobranchialis III

Ductus
pharyngobranchialis IV

Internal parathyroid

Median thyroid

Esophagus

External parathyroid

Thymus

Lateral thyroid
(ultimobranchial body)

Trachea

FIGURE 2-9. Ventral view of model of pharynx of 14.5-mm embryo (early in 7th week). (Rogers WM. Normal and anomalous development of the thyroid. In: Werner SC, Ingbar SH, eds. The thyroid. 3rd ed. Hagerstown, MD: Harper & Row, 1971)

amounts of presumptive parafollicular tissue that can become neoplastic.[36]

Origin of Parafollicular Cells. The lateral thyroid anlage in the human fetus corresponds to the ultimobranchial body of lower species, but the fate of its component cells has had a controversial history. The parafollicular calcitonin-producing cells (C cells) of the thyroid have been conclusively shown to be the only mature thyroid cells to originate from this presumptive thyroid primordium. Historically, parafollicular cells had alternatively been thought to arise from follicular cells, cells of the thyroglossal duct, connective tissue cells, or Feyter system endocrine cells.[33]

The parafollicular cells in the thyroid derive from cells associated with the fourth or fifth pharyngeal pouch, which contributes to the ultimobranchial body. This derivation was first shown by demonstrating that 5-HTP and L-dopa injected into pregnant rodents traversed the placenta and could be converted into histochemically demonstrable serotonin and dopamine in numerous cell groups, including those in the fourth endodermal pouch. Cells that retained these characteristics were identified in the outgrowths of the pharyngeal pouches as ultimobranchial bodies formed and were ultimately traced into the thyroid.[37]

Cells of the ultimobranchial bodies have been shown to originate not only from pharyngeal endoderm but also from the neural crest, at least in birds and probably in rodents. A series of quail-chick chimera experiments have shown that grafted quail neural crest cells, which can readily be identified histologically, contribute to the ultimobranchial body.[38] In addition, mouse neural crest cells that exhibit dopa-induced fluorescence have been followed from their site of origin to the foregut and into the developing ultimobranchial body.[39] In the human embryo, suitable markers have not been used to investigate this problem, and controversy about the origin of the ultimobranchial body continues. For example, morphologic observations suggest that as the fifth endodermal pouch approaches the ectodermal surface, cells of ectodermal origin become incorporated into the evagination and ultimately give rise to parafollicular cells[34]; however, the fate of this ectodermal cell population has not yet been followed histochemically.

A molecular basis for the initiation of thyroid morphogenesis and differentiation is beginning to emerge. For example, both the homeodomain-containing thyroid transcription factor 1 (TTF-1) and a member of the paired box family of DNA-binding proteins, Pax-8, are expressed in the medial anlage of the fetal mouse when evagination begins.[40,41] Expression of both genes continues through development, and PAX-8 expression has also been documented in the adult human thyroid.[42] Two prospective target genes (Tg and thyroperoxidase) that are expressed in derivatives of the medial thyroid contain overlapping TTF-1 and Pax-8 binding domains in their promotors, and activation of these genes by Pax-8 has been documented in cotransfection experiments.[43] Taken together, these data indicate that TTF-1 and Pax-8 may have central roles in establishing or maintaining cell-type–specific thyroid functions, or in both, although there is a significant delay between the times at which TTF-1 and Pax-8 are first expressed and the onset of Tg gene expression in the fetal mouse thyroid.

Histogenesis of the Thyroid Follicle

The basic unit of cellular organization in the mature thyroid is the thyroid follicle, which consists of a lumen filled with viscous colloid that is surrounded by a single layer of epithelial cells enclosed by a basement membrane. Parafollicular cells are found within this basement membrane and are in contact with follicular cells, but themselves do not abut the lumen.[32] During development, the histologic differentiation of the follicular cells can be considered to pass through three stages,[44,45] depending on the general level of colloid development: (1) the precolloid stage (7–13 weeks), (2) the beginning colloid stage (13–14 weeks), and (3) the follicular stage (>14 weeks). Because new cells are constantly being added, however, all older fetal ages also include follicles at less advanced histogenetic stages.

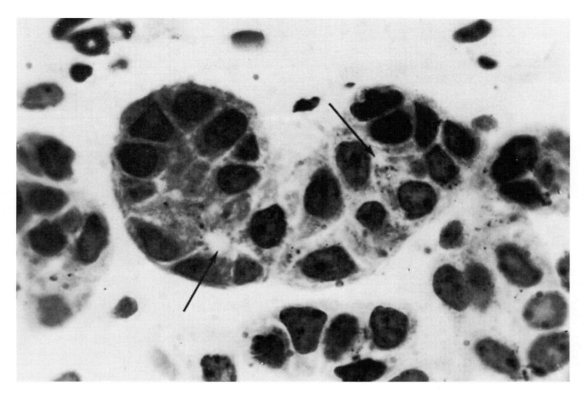

FIGURE 2-10. Photomicrograph of thyroid tissue from a human fetus of 50-mm crown-to-rump length. Arrows indicate two intracellular canaliculi ($\times$ 2400). (Shepard TH. Onset of function in the human fetal thyroid: biochemical and radioautographic studies from organ culture. J Clin Endocrinol Metab 1967;27:945)

These histologic stages are characterized by the changes in an initially intracellular compartment, the canaliculus, which is thought to be an extension of the smooth endoplasmic reticulum. As the presumptive follicle cells begin to mature in the beginning colloid stage, the canaliculi become dilated by accumulation of increasingly electron-dense material[44] (Figs 2-10 and 2-11). The contents of these primitive secretory granules are subsequently discharged to the extracellular space. This secreted material is retained in this location because desmosomes hold the edges of adjacent cells together and limit the spread of extruded material from this progenitor of the central colloid space (Fig 2-12). During the follicular phase, there is a progressive increase in diameter of the follicle and an increase in colloid storage. Intracellularly, the most marked and likely significant change is an increase in the number of lysosomes within the follicle cells. This increase may mediate the liberation of already formed T_4 and T_3 from Tg that is endocytosed from the colloid in preparation for its release to the circulation.[33]

Biochemical Differentiation of Follicular Cells

The importance of fetal thyroid function on development has been most dramatically shown in sheep, in which removal of the fetal thyroid results in prolonged pregnancy and a 33% drop in birth weight.[46] The synthesis of the precursor of iodothyronine, Tg, has been detected in the thyroid as early as the 5th gestational week, when morphogenesis is still occur-

ring.[47] Iodine trapping and the first indication of T_4 production do not occur until 5 to 7 weeks later. This period corresponds to the final stages of follicular lumen formation, when colloid is detectable extracellularly in the cloverleaf pattern[25,44] (see Fig 2-12). Precocious follicle formation and iodine fixation result from TSH, cAMP, or administration of forskolin to fetal rat thyroids in vitro,[48] which suggests that TSH may be a limiting step during early stages of follicle development. There appear to be numerous developmental changes in posttranslational modifications of Tg during gestation. For example, it appears that the level of Tg iodination is relatively low in the fetus, as it is in the neonate.[49] In addition, evidence suggests that the Tg dimer characteristic of adult thyroid colloid is not present, even by 28 weeks, even though colloid was abundant.[50]

The most recent studies of Tg expression in rodents have refined understanding of the posttranslational changes in Tg that occur during ontogeny. For example, although the appearance of 12S Tg appears concurrently with Tg RNA, formation of 19S Tg, which requires iodination, does not occur until near birth.[51]

Thyroxine is first detected in human fetal serum at about 11 to 13 weeks, slightly later than it is first detected in the thyroid. Total serum T_4 increases throughout gestation and maintains a general correlation to rump-to-crown length. There is some controversy over the levels of free T_4, because T_4 radioimmunoassays can be influenced by differences in thyroxine-binding globulin (TBG) between the fetal and adult stages.[52] Although previous studies showed that TSH was correlated with free T_4, but not total T_4, more recent studies suggest instead that the levels of total T_4, TSH, and TBG are

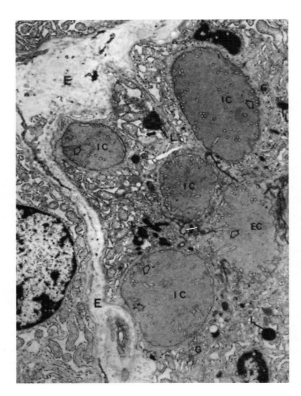

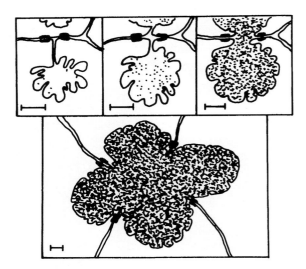

FIGURE 2-12. Diagrammatic drawing of the histogenesis of the human thyroid's central colloid cavity. In the bottom panel, the intracellular canaliculi are shown in the final phase of union. Desmosomes, indicated by short parallel marks, play an important part in the final organization of these cells by containing the disgorged contents of the canaliculi. The marker is a diagrammatic representation of 1 μm. The final stage resembles a clover leaf in cross section. (Shepard TH. Onset of function in the human thyroid: biochemical and radioautographic studies from organ culture. J Clin Endocrinol Metab 1967;27:945)

FIGURE 2-11. Electron micrograph of a group of follicular cells from the thyroid gland of a fetus several weeks before the expected date of birth. Prominent, dilated intracellular cavities (IC), lines by microvilli (*arrowheads*), fill a major part of the cell profiles. At this stage, colloid production is beginning. An expanding extracellular luminal cavity (EC), bordered by four follicular cells, is also shown. Also seen in this field are lysosomal bodies (L), Golgi complex (G), and extracellular space (E) (× 15,000). (Nunez EA, Gershon MD. Development of follicular and parafollicular cells of the mammalian thyroid gland. In: Greenfield LD, ed. Thyroid cancer. West Palm Beach, FL: CRC Press, 1978)

correlated. TSH values are higher than adult levels throughout gestation.

Onset of Calcitonin Secretion

The number of parafollicular cells in the human fetus is higher than in the adult,[33] and secretory granules in these cells, which are likely to contain calcitonin, are present by midgestation.[53] Calcitonin, however, if present in the fetal circulation during human fetal development, must be present at low levels. No estimates of calcitonin levels have been reported until birth, when higher levels are found in the umbilical serum than in the maternal serum.[54] Morphologic evidence suggests that there is an increase of secretory activity of parafollicular cells in dogs at birth.[55] In humans, there are higher levels of calcitonin in the neonate than in the adult.[56] Taken together, these observations have led to the suggestion that calcitonin has an important, but still poorly defined, role at the time of parturition.[33]

Appearance of Iodothyronine-Binding Proteins

Numerous circulating proteins bind T_4 and T_3. All iodothyronine-binding proteins have been detected by midgestation, al-

though the levels of each appear to change in relation to each other during the prenatal period. Thus, the levels of TBG parallel the rise in serum T_4[28,52]; T_4-binding prealbumin, or transthyretin, and T_4-binding albumin reach term levels by 14 to 24 weeks of gestation[28]; serum protein-bound iodine has been detected by the 13th week.[57] The time at which T_3 is first synthesized is not known, but the relative ratios of serum T_4 to T_3 are always high during prenatal life, primarily because of lower levels of outer ring 5′-deiodinase activity in peripheral tissues, which results in decreased peripheral conversion of T_4 to T_3[26,58] (Fig 2-13). In addition, there are increased circulating levels of the metabolically inactive iodothyronine reverse T_3 (rT_3) during fetal stages, again because of decreased 5′-deiodinase activity and, therefore, decreased clearance of rT_3.[25]

FUNCTIONAL DIFFERENTIATION OF THE HYPOTHALAMIC-THYROID-PITUITARY AXIS

Influence of the Maternal Environment on Fetal Thyroid Function

The maturation of the human fetal hypothalamic-pituitary-thyroid unit is complex, and the role of the maternal environment is still somewhat uncertain. It is generally agreed that human TSH does not cross the placenta,[13,25] nor does endogenous TRH cross the placenta in sufficient amounts to increase thyroid function, although high doses of exogenous TRH administered to the mother can increase fetal TSH levels.[13] The general consensus from numerous early studies was that endogenous or exogenous maternal T_3 and T_4 have limited, if any, access to

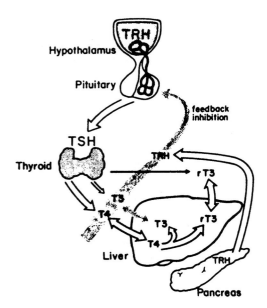

FIGURE 2-13. The hypothalamic-pituitary-thyroid axis in the late-gestation fetus. The complexity of the system is illustrated by the several levels of control and modulation. Function of the system is controlled by hypothalamic TRH production and transport through the pituitary portal vascular system to the anterior pituitary gland. TRH production from the fetal pancreas and other tissues probably plays a role at midgestation. Maturation of thyroid hormone feedback control of pituitary TSH and maturation of thyroid responsiveness to TSH stimulation occur during the later phase of gestation. T_4 is deiodinated in peripheral tissues (here shown as liver) to active T_3 and inactive rT_3. The enzyme deiodinase systems mature during the last third to half of gestation and in the early neonatal period. (Fisher DA, Polk DH. Development of the thyroid. Ballieres Clin Endocrinol Metab 1989;3:628)

the fetus during most of development.[11] In human fetuses, before the appearance of T_4 in the thyroid at 11 weeks, T_4 and T_3 present at normal maternal levels have not been detected in fetal serum. The placenta contains relatively high levels of an iodothyronine inner-ring monodeiodinase that can convert T_4 to inactive rT_3 and also deiodinate T_3 into inactive diiodothyronine.[11] This activity may protect the fetus from high T_4 levels and may be responsible for the high rT_3 levels in amniotic fluid.[10,11,25] More recent evidence suggests that some T_4, T_3, and rT_3 may be transported across the placenta, at least during late gestation, because detectable levels of these hormones can be found in the serum of athyrotic human neonates.[59] Even at late stages, however, most estimates suggest that most fetal T_4 is of fetal origin. In contrast to the absence of proven maternal T_4 in early human fetuses, studies have shown that T_3 and T_4 are found in rat embryos at embryonic day 9 (well before the onset of fetal thyroid function at embryonic day 18), and that maternal thyroidectomy delays fetal development.[60] Thus, in rats at least, maternal iodothyronines may functionally affect the fetus at early stages, and the possibility that a similar situation exists in humans cannot be excluded.

The most significant aspect of fetal thyroid development that depends on the placenta is the provision of sufficient iodine for T_4 production in Tg; maternal hypothyroidism resulting from iodine deficiency leads to fetal cretinism. Fetal iodine

is actively transported through the placenta and has a fetal serum concentration at midgestation four to five times that of maternal blood.[10]

FUNCTIONAL MATURATION OF THE FETAL HYPOTHALAMIC-PITUITARY-THYROID AXIS

The ontogenesis of the hypothalamic-pituitary-thyroid axis is summarized in Figure 2-14, and the major features of the axis present at late fetal stages are summarized in Figure 2-13. These data suggest that the interaction between these different components is present at late gestational ages. For example, numerous genetic deficits in T_4 biosynthesis exist, and all are accompanied by goiter formation and hypothyroidism, which indicates that the rest of the hypothalamic-pituitary-thyroid axis is intact.[57]

In contrast, little evidence suggests that this interdependence exists from the earliest stages of development. In the most dramatic case, decapitation of chick embryos does not impair thyroid function until late prehatching stages, days after the initiation of thyroid function.[61] In humans, numerous cases of abnormal nervous system and pituitary development suggest that thyroid function can also differentiate independently of TSH. In cases in which the pituitary is absent, such as in cyclocephaly, and in cases in which there is partial agenesis of the anterior pituitary,[62–64] the thyroid undergoes normal development initially. In these cases, however, as in others in which pituitary development is experimentally delayed or abolished, the thyroid does exhibit reduced size and functional activity at later developmental stages.[65,66] Whether these deficits specifically result from loss of TSH is unclear.

A similar finding emerges from the study of human anencephalic infants exhibiting abnormal development of the hypothalamus. In these cases, both the anterior pituitary and the thyroid are relatively normal. In fact, thyroid hormone synthesis may be enhanced, because the cells appear hyperactive and contain less of some thyroid hormones than normal, which suggests that they may be secreted.[67,68]

More experimental analysis, however, shows that there is a gradual maturation of cellular interactions during development that depends both on the levels of hormone found in individual cells and on the maturation of functional receptor systems that transduce secretagogue binding into TSH or T_4 release. Some evidence suggests that maximal ability to release functional TSH in response to TRH develops independently of the ability to release TSH basally. Thus, when fetal rat pituitaries and thyroids from embryos of different ages are cocultured, for a short time (embryonic days 15–16), exogenous TRH cannot increase the amount of functional TSH secretion above basal levels, as assessed by the lack of additional increase in the size of the adjacent thyroids.[69] Because maturation of thyroid hormone levels in humans coincides with the abrupt increase in pituitary TSH levels at about 18 weeks,[25] these data suggest that increases in pituitary TRH receptor function may contribute to the increase in fetal TSH synthesis and release that occurs during midgestation. Furthermore, because the TSH/T_4 ratio is higher in the fetus than in the adult, maturation of posttranslational modifica-

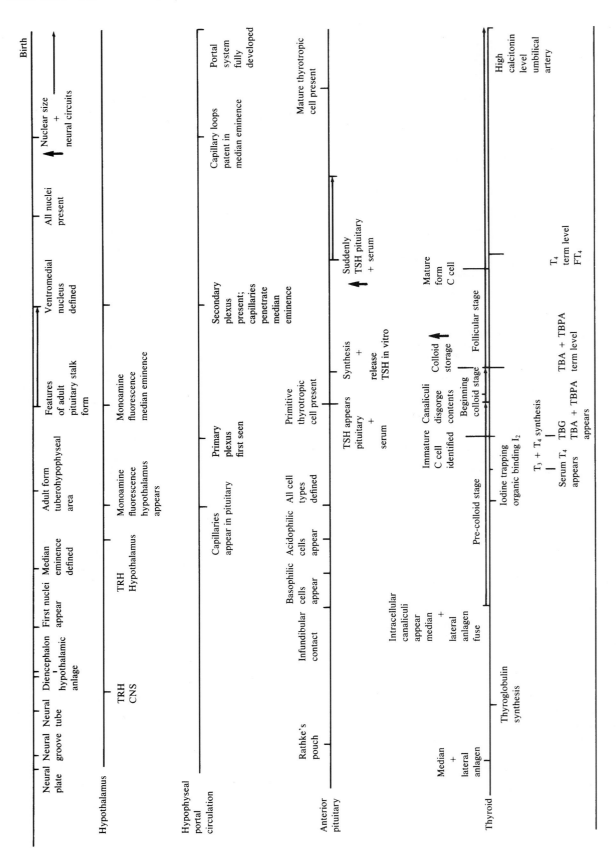

FIGURE 2-14. Summary of the ontogenesis of the hypothalamic-pituitary-thyroid axis.

tion of Tg (discussed earlier) may also represent a mechanism by which relatively constant TSH levels can mediate the continuing increase in fetal T_4 that occurs until birth.

Finally, comprehensive measurement of serum TSH, of serum total and free T_3 and T_4, and of serum TBG over the period from 12 to 37 weeks of gestation has been carried out, using direct measurement of umbilical cord blood through cordocentesis. Significantly, the levels of TSH rose coordinately with T_4, suggesting that negative feedback is either limited or counterbalanced by increasing TRH secretion from the pituitary.[70]

References

1. Hemmati-Brivanlou A, Melton DA. Inhibition of activin receptor signaling promotes neuralization in Xenopus. Cell 1994;77:273
2. Couly G, Le Douarin NM. Mapping of the neural primordium in quail-chick chimeras. II. The prosencephalic neural plate and neural folds: implications for the genesis of cephalic congenital abnormalities. Dev Biol 1987;120:198
3. Papez JW. The embryological development of the hypothalamic area in mammals. In: The hypothalamus and central levels of autonomic function. Res Publ Assoc Res Nerv Ment Dis 1940;20:31
4. Jackson IMD. Thyrotropin releasing hormone. N Engl J Med 1982;306:145
5. Brownstein MJ, Palkovits M, Saavedra JM, et al. Thyrotropin-releasing hormone in specific nuclei of rat brain. Science 1974;185:267
6. Lechan RM, Snapper SB, Jacobson S, Jackson IMD. The distribution of thyrotropin releasing hormone (TRH) in the rhesus monkey spinal cord. Peptides 1984;5:185
7. Johansson O, Hokfelt T. Thyrotropin releasing hormone, somatostatin, and enkephalin: distribution studies using immunohistochemical techniques. J Histochem Cytochem 1980;28:364
8. Lechan RM, Jackson IMD. Immunohistochemical localization of thyrotropin releasing hormone in the rat hypothalamus and pituitary. Endocrinology 1982;111:55
9. Winters AJ, Eskay RL. Porter JC. Concentration and distribution of TRH and LRH in the human fetal brain. J Clin Endocrinol Metab 1974;39:960
10. Roti E. Regulation of thyroid-stimulating hormone (TSH) secretion in the fetus and neonate. J Endocrinol Invest 1988;11:145
11. Roti E, Gnudi A, Braverman LE. The placental transport, synthesis, and metabolism of hormones and drugs which affect thyroid function. Endocr Rev 1981;4:131
12. Leduque P. Aratan-Spire S, Czernichow P, Dubois PM. Ontogenesis of thyrotropin releasing hormone in human fetal pancreas. J Clin Invest 1986;78:1028
13. Martino E, Grasso S, Bambini G, et al. Ontogenetic development of pancreatic thyrotropin-releasing hormone in human foetuses and in infants. Acta Endocrinol 1986;112:372
14. Mulchahey JJ, Di Blasio AM, Martin MC, Blumenfeld Z, Jaffe RB. Hormone production and peptide regulation of the human fetal pituitary gland. Endocr Rev 1987;8:406
15. Hyppa M. Hypothalamic monoamines in human fetuses. Neuroendocrinology 1972;9:257
16. Hamilton WJ, Mossman HW. Human embryology. 4th ed. Baltimore: Williams & Wilkins, 1972
17. Niemineva K. Observations on the development of the hypophysial-portal system. Acta Paediatr Scand 1950;39:366
18. Thliveris JA. Currie RW. Observations on the hypothalamic-hypophyseal portal vasculature in the developing human fetus. Am J Anat 1980;157:441
19. Oliver C, Charvet JP, Codaccioni JL, et al. TRH in CSF. Lancet 1974;1:873
20. Hughson W. Meningeal relations of the hypophysis cerebri. Johns Hopkins Hosp Bull 1924;35:232
21. Conklin JL. The development of the human fetal adenohypophysis. Anat Rec 1968;160:79
22. Falin LI. The development of human hypophysis and differentiation of cells of its anterior lobe during embryonic life. Acta Anat (Basel) 1961;44:188
23. Rosen F, Ezrin C. Embryology of the thyrotroph. J Clin Endocrinol Metab 1966;26:1343
24. Baker BL, Jaffe RB. The genesis of cell types in the adenohypophysis of the human fetus as observed with immunocytochemistry. Am J Anat 1974;143:137
25. Fisher DA, Duseault JH. Development of the mammalian thyroid gland. In: Greer MA, Solomon DH, eds. Handbook of physiology, Sec 7, Endocrinology. Vol III. The thyroid. Washington DC: American Physiological Society, 1974
26. Fisher DA, Polk DH. Development of the thyroid. Ballieres Clin Endocrinol Metab 1989;3:67
27. Fukuchi M, Inque T, Abe H, Kumahara Y. Thyrotropin in human fetal pituitaries. J Clin Endocrinol Metab 1970;31:565
28. Greenberg AH, Czernichow P, Reba RC, et al. Observations on the maturation of thyroid function in early fetal life. J Clin Invest 1970;49:1990
29. Levina SE. Endocrine features in development of human hypothalamus, hypophysis, and placenta. Gen Comp Endocrinol 1968;11:151
30. Evans TC, Kretzchmar M, Hodges RD, Song CW. Radioiodine uptake studies in the human fetal thyroid. J Nucl Med 1967;8:157
31. Staglitzer KE. Contribution to the study of the thyroid gland. J Anat 1941;75:389
32. Boyd JD. Development of the human thyroid gland. In: Pitt-Rivers R, Trotter WR, eds. The thyroid. Vol 1. Washington, DC: Butterworths, 1964:9
33. Nunez EA, Gershon MD. Development of follicular and parafollicular cells of the mammalian thyroid gland. In: Greenfield LD, ed. Thyroid cancer. West Palm Beach, FL: CRC Press, 1978:1
34. Merida-Velasco JA, Garcia-Garcia JD, Espin-Ferra J, Linares J: Origin of the ultimobranchial body and its colonizing cells in human embryos. Acta Anat 1989;136:325
35. Dossal WE. Effects of depletion and substitution of perivascular mesenchyme upon the development of the thyroid primordium. J Elisha Mitchell Sci Soc 1957;73:244
36. Rogers WM. Normal and anomalous development of the thyroid. In: Werner SC, Ingbar SH, eds. The thyroid. 3rd ed. Hagerstown, MD:: Harper & Row, 1971
37. Pearse AGE, Carvalheira AF. Cytochemical evidence for an ultimobranchial origin of rodent thyroid C cells. Nature 1967;214:929
38. Le Douarin NM, Fontaine J, Le Lievre C. New studies on the neural crest origin of the avian ultimobranchial glandular cells: interspecific combinations and cytochemical characterization of C cells based on the uptake of biogenic amine precursors. Histochemie 1974;38:297
39. Pearse AGE. Pollack JM. Cytochemical evidence for the neural crest origin of mammalian ultimobranchial body C-cells. Histochemie 1971;27:96
40. Lazzaro D, Price M, De Felice M, Di Lauro R. The transcription factor TTF-1 is expressed at the onset of thyroid and lung morphogenesis and in restricted regions of the foetal brain. Development 1991;113:1093
41. Plachov D, Chowdhury K, Walther C, Simon D, Guenet J-L, Gruss. PAX-8, a murine paired box gene expressed in the devel-

oping excretory system and thyroid gland. Development 1990; 110:643

42. Poleev A, Fickenscher H, Mundlos S, Winterpacht A, Zabel B, Fidler A, Gruss P, Plachov D. PAX-8, a human paired box gene: isolation and expression in developing thyroid, kidney and Wilms' tumor. Development 1992;116:611

43. Zannini M, Prancis-Lang H, Plachov D, Di Lauro R. Pax-8, a paired domain-containing protein, binds to a sequence overlapping the recognition site of a homeodomain and activates transcription from two thyroid-specific promoters. Mol Cell Biol 1992;12:4230

44. Shepard TH. Onset of function in the human fetal thyroid: biochemical and radioautographic studies from organ culture. J Clin Endocrinol Metab 1967;27:945

45. Shepard TH. The thyroid. In: DeHaan AC, Ursprung H, eds. Organogenesis. New York: Holt, Rinehart & Winston, 1965

46. Chard T. Hormonal control of growth in the human fetus. J Endocrinol 1989;123:3

47. Gitlin D, Biasucci A. Ontogenesis of immunoreactive thyroglobulin in the human conceptus. J Clin Endocrinol Metab 1969;29:849

48. Pic P, Michel-Bechet M, El Atiq F, Athouel-Haon AM. Forskolin stimulates cAMP production and the onset of the functional differentiation in the fetal rat thyroid in vitro. Biol Cell 1986; 57:231

49. Etling N. Concentration of thyroglobulin, iodine contents of thyroglobulin and of iodoaminoacids in human neonate thyroid glands. Acta Paediatr Scand 1977;66:97

50. Sinadinovic J, Savin S, Micic JV. Some characteristics of soluble thyroid proteins in human fetus during morphogenesis of follicular structure. Exp Clin Endocrinol 1986;88:346

51. Rodrigues M, Santisteban P, Acebron A, Hernandez LC, del Valle M, Jolin T. Expression of thyroglobulin gene in maternal and fetal thyroid in rats. Endocrinology 1992;131:415

52. Ballabio M, Nicolini U, Jowett T, Ruiz de Elvira MC, Ekins RP, Rodeck CH. Maturation of thyroid function in normal human foetuses. Clin Endocrinol 1989;31:565

53. Chan AS, Conen PE. Ultrastructural observations on cytodifferentiation of parafollicular cells in the human fetal thyroid. Lab Invest 1971;25:249

54. Samaan NA, Anderson GD, Adam-Mayne ME. Immunoreactive calcitonia in the mother, neonate, child and adult. Am J Obstet Gynecol 1975;121:622

55. Nunez EA, Gershon MD. Secretion by parafollicular cells beginning at birth: ultrastructural evidence from the developing canine thyroid. Am J Anat 1976;14:375

56. Wolfe HJ, De Lellis RA, Voelkel EF, Tashjian AH Jr. Distribution of calcitonin-containing cells in the normal neonatal human thyroid gland: a correlation of morphology with peptide content. J Clin Endocrinol Metab 1975;41:1076

57. Andraoli M, Robbins J: Serum proteins and thyroxine-protein interaction in early human fetuses. J Clin Invest 1962;41:1070

58. Villes DB. Human endocrinology: a developmental approach. Philadelphia: WB Saunders, 1975

59. Vulsma T, Gons MH, De Vijlder JJM. Maternal fetal transfer of thyroxine in congenital hypothyroidism due to a total organification defect or thyroid agenesis. N Engl J Med 1989;321:13

60. Morreale de Escobar G, Obregon MJ, Escobar del Rey F. Fetal and maternal thyroid hormones. Horm Res 1987;26:12

61. Hilfer SR, Searis RL. Differentiation of the thyroid in the hypophysectomized chick embryo. Dev Biol 1980;79:107

62. Brewer DB. Congenital absence of the pituitary gland and its consequences. J Pathol 1957;73:59

63. Browne EJ. The anencephalic syndrome in its relation to apituitarism. Edinburgh Med J 1920;25:296

64. Reid JR. Congenital absence of the pituitary gland. J Pediatr 1960;56:658

65. Fisher DA, Klein AH. Thyroid development and disorders of thyroid function in the newborn. N Engl J Med 1981;304:702.

66. Jost A. Anterior pituitary function in fetal life. In: Harris GW, Donovan BT, eds. The pituitary gland. Vol II. Berkeley: University of California Press, 1966

67. Allen JP, Greer MA, McGilvra R, et al. Endocrine function in an anencephalic infant. J Clin Endocrinol Metab 1974;38:94

68. Herlant M. Etude endocrinologique d'un cas'anencephalic. Ann Endocrinol (Paris) 1953;14:899

69. Takizawa T, Yamamoto M, Arishima K, Eguchi Y. Effect of thyrotropin-releasing hormone on development of the pituitary-thyroid system in fetal rats in organ culture. Anat Rec 1987; 218:441

70. Thorpe-Beeston JG, Nicolaides KH, Felton CV, Butler J, McGregor AM. Maturation of the secretion of thyroid hormone and thyroid-stimulating hormone in the fetus. N Engl J Med 1991; 324:532

Werner and Ingbar's The Thyroid, Seventh Edition,
edited by Lewis E. Braverman and Robert D. Utiger.
Lippincott–Raven Publishers, Philadelphia, © 1996

3

Anatomy

COMPARATIVE ANATOMY AND PHYSIOLOGY

Charles C. Capen

GROSS ANATOMY

The thyroid is the largest endocrine gland in humans, weighing about 20 g in an adult. The normal weight of the thyroid often is given as being considerably greater because thyroid enlargement ("goiter") is quite common. It is frequently stated that the thyroid is so named because of its shield-shaped configuration. However, this bilobed structure bears no resemblance to a shield but is named because of its topographic relationship to the laryngeal thyroid cartilage, which does look like a Greek shield.[1]

The thyroid parenchyma is mostly derived from the endoderm at the base of the tongue. It may remain attached to this region even in adult life if the embryonic thyroglossal duct persists. More often, only portions of this duct survive as the pyramidal lobe extending upward from the narrow isthmus connecting the two lobes of the thyroid. The differential growth of the neck structures occasionally results in displacement of the thyroid to a level below the larynx. The isthmus of the thyroid normally overlies the second or third cartilaginous rings of the trachea in humans. Some or all thyroid tissue occasionally remains embedded in the base of the tongue as a lingual thyroid. The thyroid also includes epithelial structures derived from the ultimobranchial bodies that are described later.

ORGANOGENESIS

The thyroid gland originates as a thickened plate of epithelium in the floor of the pharynx (Fig 3-1). It is intimately related to the aortic sac in its development and this association leads to the frequent occurrence of accessory thyroid parenchyma in the mediastinum. A portion of the thyroglossal

duct may persist postnatally and form a cyst owing to the accumulation of proteinic material secreted by the lining epithelium. Thyroglossal duct cysts develop in the anterior cervical region. Their lining epithelium may undergo neoplastic transformation and give rise to follicular cell carcinomas.

Accessory thyroid tissue is common (nearly 100%), particularly in certain animal species such as the dog, and may be located anywhere from the larynx to the diaphragm. About 50% of adult dogs have accessory thyroids embedded in the fat on the intrapericardial aorta. They are completely lacking in C- (parafollicular) cells, but their follicular structure and function are the same as those of the main thyroid lobes. Such dogs under experimental conditions cannot be made hypothyroid by surgical ablation of the two lateral thyroid lobes alone.

The postnatal human thyroid gland contains solid cell nests in the middle to upper third of the lateral lobes that are derived from the ultimobranchial body.[2] The solid cell nests are approximately 1 mm in diameter and composed of nonkeratinizing epidermoid cells that lack intercellular bridges.[3] Histochemical analysis revealed the presence of mucoid material in 73%, calcitonin (CT)-immunoreactive cells in 36%, and both carcinoembryonic antigen and high–molecular-weight cytokeratin proteins in 85.7% of epidermoid cells. A central lumen in the solid cell nests usually is surrounded by mucinous cells and may contain desquamated cells, cell debris, periodic acid–Schiff (PAS)-positive granular material, and colloid. Follicles containing Alcian blue-positive acid mucins also are present in the solid cell nests of the human thyroid.[4] These follicles were composed of or related to CT-positive cells (by immunohistochemistry) and intermixed with alcianophilic mucinous cells. These findings support the hypothesis that mucoepidermoid carcinomas of the thyroid are of ultimobranchial tissue origin.[2]

Cysts derived from remnants of the ultimobranchial body are observed frequently in the postnatal thyroid of rats lined by squamous epithelium and containing keratin debris.[5] Occasional follicles derived from ultimobranchial primordia contain a heterogeneous material in the lumen and scattered ciliated epithelial cells in the follicular wall. In Wistar rats, CT-immunoreactive cells have been demonstrated in the wall of the

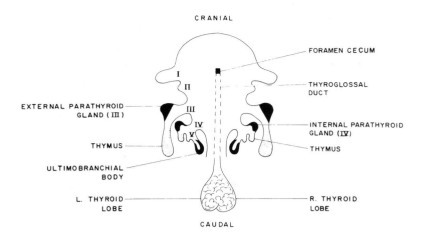

FIGURE 3-1. Embryology of thyroid and parathyroid glands and the relationship to primordia for the ultimobranchial body.

ultimobranchial tubule as well as thyroglobulin-positive staining in adjacent follicles and solid clusters.[6] These findings plus the presence of numerous mitosis and PAS-positive microfollicles support the hypothesis that the ultimobranchial body contributes to the formation of follicles in certain areas of the thyroid lobes.

To investigate cell function and proliferation of human thyroid follicles, an experimental system has been established to culture thyrocytes in collagen gel suspended in serum-free medium.[7] The human thyrocytes were functional as determined by their time- and dose-dependent response to thyroid-stimulating hormone (TSH), which consisted of a 15-fold increase in iodide uptake and organification, triiodothyronine (T_3) secretion, and cyclic adenosine monophosphate (cAMP) production. The same in vitro system also permits measurement of cell proliferation as indicated by ^3H incorporation and DNA content. Normal cell polarity, which is essential for thyroid follicle function, was maintained by the use of collagen gel and serum-free medium. The development of an in vitro system using thyroid cells of human origin should be of considerable use in future studies on thyroid pathophysiology in humans. Isolated thyroid follicular cells of human and porcine origin cultured in three-dimensional collagen gel have characteristic structural polarity, respond to TSH, and produce thyroid hormones.[8,9] Thyroid follicular cells formed follicles in collagen gel culture by (1) cell division of cavity-associated single cells, and (2) through aggregation and linkage to adjacent cells.[9]

HISTOLOGY AND ULTRASTRUCTURE

The thyroid gland is the largest of the organs that function exclusively as an endocrine gland. The basic structure of the thyroid is unique for endocrine glands, consisting of follicles of varying size that contain colloid produced by the follicular cells (Fig 3-2). During folliculogenesis an intracytoplasmic cavity develops initially in individual cells. Follicles appear to grow during development by proliferation of component cells and coalescence of adjacent colloid-containing microfollicles in individual cells.[10,11] Folliculogenesis stimulated by TSH in vitro appears to require integrity of both microfilaments and microtubules because chemicals (vinblastine and colchicine) that disorganize these organelles block follicle formation.[12] Studies have shown that protein tyrosine phosphorylation and microfilament integrity are essential for thyroid cells to

spread on a substrate.[13] These are potential intracellular loci where TSH and intercellular contact may regulate adhesion of follicular cells to extracellular matrix and influence thyroid cell behavior.

Studies in Wistar rats have shown that the volumetric fractions of the different histologic components (follicular cells, C cells, colloid, and interstitial tissue) change considerably during development (birth to 120 days of age).[14] The fraction of follicular cells decreased from 61% at birth to 37.2% at 4 months. C cells increased from 2.9% in newborns to 4% at 15 days, with no further change at 4 months. Colloid and stroma together represented 36% at birth and increased to 59% at 120 days. During the first 4 months of life in rats, the absolute volumes occupied by follicular cells, C cells, colloid, and stroma increased 13.3, 30.8, 39, and 34 times, respectively.[14] Delverdier and colleagues[15] have shown that the limits of thyroid follicles were more clearly defined in both silver-impregnated, paraffin-embedded and resin-embedded semithin sections than in routinely stained paraffin-embedded sections, permitting the more accurate measurements of thyroid structures essential during morphometric evaluation.

Thyroid follicular cells are cuboidal to columnar and their secretory polarity is directed toward the lumen of the follicles. Polarity of follicular cells is important for iodine uptake, but the follicle structure is required for the synthesis of thyroid hormones.[16] The luminal surfaces of follicular cells protrude into the follicular lumen and have numerous microvillar projections that greatly increase the surface area in contact with colloid (see Fig 3-2). An extensive network of interfollicular and intrafollicular capillaries provides the follicular cells with an abundant blood supply.

Follicular cells have long profiles of rough endoplasmic reticulum and a large Golgi apparatus in their cytoplasm for synthesis and packaging of substantial amounts of protein that are then transported into the follicular lumen (Fig 3-3). Numerous electron-dense lysosomal bodies are present in the cytoplasm, which are important in the secretion of thyroid hormones. The interface between the luminal side of follicular cells and the colloid is modified by numerous microvilli (see Fig 3-3).

The biosynthesis of thyroid hormones is also unique among endocrine glands because the final assembly of the hormones occurs extracellularly within the follicular lumen. Essential raw materials, such as iodide, are trapped efficiently

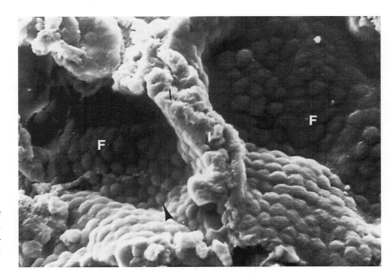

FIGURE 3-2. Scanning electron micrograph of thyroid gland of a dog with two opened follicles (F). The luminal aspect of individual follicular cells protrudes into the follicular lumen (*arrowhead*). Interfollicular space (I) with connective tissue and capillaries is present.

at the basilar aspect of follicular cells from interfollicular capillaries, transported rapidly against a concentration gradient to the lumen, and oxidized by a thyroid peroxidase in microvillar membranes to reactive iodine (I_2) (Fig 3-4). The assembly of thyroid hormones within the follicular lumen is made possible by a unique protein (thyroglobulin) synthesized on the rough endoplasmic reticulum and packaged in the Golgi apparatus of follicular cells.

Thyroglobulin is a high–molecular-weight glycoprotein synthesized in successive subunits on the ribosomes in follicular cells. The constituent amino acids (tyrosine and others) and carbohydrates come from the circulation. Recently synthesized thyroglobulin (17S) leaving the Golgi apparatus is packaged in apical vesicles and extruded into the follicular lumen. Human thyroglobulin contains complex carbohydrate units with up to four sulfate groups and units with both sulfate and sialic acid.[17] The amino acid tyrosine is incorporated within the molecular structure of thyroglobulin. Iodine is bound to tyrosyl residues in thyroglobulin at the apical surface of follicular cells to form, successively, monoiodotyrosine (MIT) and diiodotyrosine (DIT). The resulting MIT and DIT combine to form the two biologically active iodothyronines (thyroxine [T_4] and T_3) secreted by the thyroid gland.

The extracellular storage of thyroglobulin in the follicle lumen is essential for maintaining constant blood levels of thyroid hormones in vertebrates under conditions of varied intake of and varying requirements for T_4 and T_3. Storage of large amounts of thyroglobulin is made possible by compaction or the tight packing of thyroglobulin molecules in the follicular lumen.[18] Protein concentrations as high as 100 to 400 mg/mL have been reported in colloid collected by micropuncture techniques from the lumens of single thyroid follicles. The luminal content of follicles consists of discrete globules (20–120 μm in diameter) that, by scanning electron microscopy, show a unique cobblestone-like surface pattern from impressions of microvilli of the apical plasma membranes of thyrocytes. Thyroglobulin in isolated globules was highly iodinated (~ 55 iodine atoms per 12S subunit), suggesting that covalent nondisulfide cross-linking occurs during iodination of thyroglobulin and that this process involves the formation of intermolecular dityrosine bridges.[18]

Most of the epithelial cells and the functionally most important cells of the thyroid are the follicular cells (Fig 3-5). They vary in height, depending on the intensity of stimulation by pituitary TSH, between low cuboidal and tall columnar. Follicular size and shape are quite variable in the human thyroid and there is no discernible pattern in the distribution of small and large follicles within the gland. Peripherally situated follicles in rats tend to be large and central ones small. Uchiyama and coworkers[19,20] reported that distinct variations occur morphometrically in volume and numerical densities of follicles during a 24-hour period in rats and reflect changes in subcellular organelles of follicular cells. Follicular cells in the human thyroid are relatively flat compared with those of the rat, reflecting the different plasma half-life of thyroid hormones in rat (short) compared to humans (long).

The histologic appearance of the thyroid is dramatically influenced by the level of circulating TSH from the adenohy-

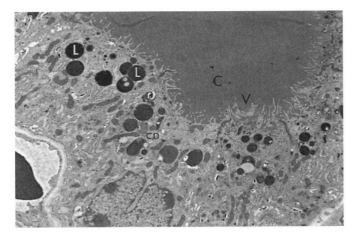

FIGURE 3-3. Electron micrograph of normal thyroid follicular cells with long microvilli (V) that extend into the luminal colloid (C). Pseudopods from the apical plasma membrane surround a portion of the colloid to form an intracellular colloid droplet (CD). Numerous lysosomes (L) are present in the apical cytoplasm in proximity to the colloid droplets. An intrafollicular capillary is visible in the lower left.

FOLLICULAR   LUMEN

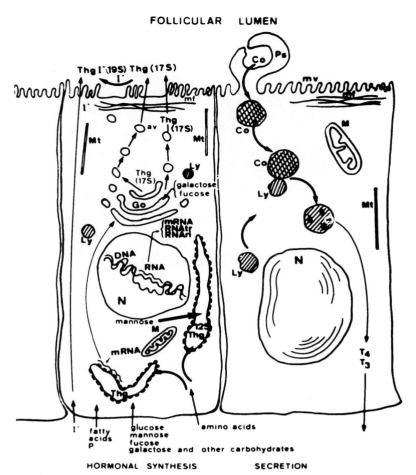

FIGURE 3-4. Thyroid follicular cells illustrating two-way traffic of materials from capillaries into the follicular lumen. Raw materials, such as iodide ion (I⁻), are concentrated by follicular cells and rapidly transported into the lumen (*left side of the drawing*). Amino acids (tyrosine and others) and sugars are assembled by follicular cells into thyroglobulin (Thg), packaged into apical vesicles (av), and released into the lumen. The iodination of tyrosyl residues occurs within the thyroglobulin molecule to form thyroid hormones in the follicular lumen. Elongation of microvilli and endocytosis of colloid by follicular cells occurs in response to TSH stimulation (*right side of drawing*). The intracellular colloid droplets (Co) fuse with lysosomal bodies (Ly); active thyroid hormone is enzymatically cleaved from thyroglobulin; and free T$_4$ and T$_3$ are released into the cytosol and eventually into the circulation. Mt, microtubules; M, mitochondria; mf, microfilaments. (Bastenie PA, Ermans AM, Bonnyns M, Neve P, Delespese G: Molecular pathology. Springfield, IL: Charles C Thomas, 1975:243)

pophysis.[10] Thyrotropin binds to the basilar aspect of thyroid follicular cells, activates adenylate cyclase with accumulation of cAMP, and increases the rate of biochemical reactions concerned with biosynthesis and secretion of thyroid hormones.[21] One of the initial structural responses by follicular cells to TSH

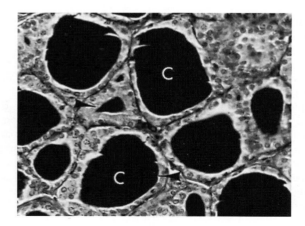

FIGURE 3-5. Normal rat thyroid gland illustrating basic histologic structure of colloid-filled (C) follicles of varying size lined by cuboidal follicular cells. An extensive network of capillaries is present between the thyroid follicles. Periodic acid-Schiff reaction.

is the formation of numerous cytoplasmic pseudopods, resulting in increased endocytosis of colloid and release of preformed thyroid hormone stored within the follicular lumen (Fig 3-6). Nilsson and colleagues[22] reported that follicular cells do not respond in an all-or-none mode to acute TSH stimulation; rather, the response (i.e., numbers of pseudopods formed after 20 minutes) was graded depending on the level of TSH.

If the secretion of TSH is sustained (hours or days), thyroid follicular cells become more columnar and follicular lumens become smaller and appear as slit-like spaces because of increased endocytosis of colloid[10,23,24] (Fig 3-7). Numerous PAS-positive colloid droplets are present in the luminal aspect of the hypertrophied follicular cells. TSH stimulation not only elicits a highly individual macropinocytotic response among different follicular cells but, in addition, the fraction of TSH-responsive cells is also a function of dose.[25]

Iodine deficiency in the diet resulting in diffuse thyroid hyperplasia was common in animals and humans in many goitrogenic areas throughout the world before the widespread addition of iodized salt to the diet (Fig 3-8). Marginal iodine-deficient diets containing certain goitrogenic compounds may result in thyroid follicular cell hypertrophy and hyperplasia with clinical evidence of goiter with hypothyroidism. These goitrogenic substances include thiouracil, sulfonamides, anions of the Hofmeister series, and a number of plants from the genus *Brassica*, among others.

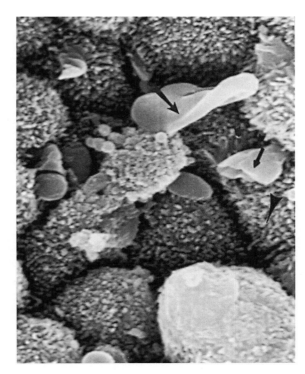

FIGURE 3-6. Scanning electron micrograph of apical surface of hypertrophied thyroid follicular cell 4 hours after TSH stimulation. Numerous elongated microvilli and cytoplasmic projections (*arrows*) extend into the follicular lumen to engulf colloid as part of the initial stages of thyroid hormone secretion in response to TSH. (Collins WT, Capen CC. Ultrastructure and functional alterations of the rat thyroid gland produced by polychlorinated biphenyls compared with iodide excess and deficiency, and thyrotropin and thyroxine administration. Virchows Arch [B] 1980;33:213)

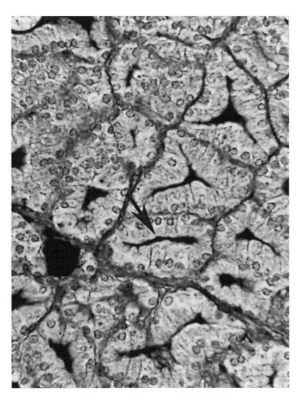

FIGURE 3-7. Response of thyroid follicular cells 8 hours after TSH stimulation. The follicular cells are hypertrophic and columnar. Many follicles are nearly depleted of colloid and are partially collapsed (*arrow*).

In response to long-term stimulation of follicular cells by TSH, as occurs with chronic iodine deficiency, both lateral lobes of the thyroid are uniformly enlarged (see Fig 3-8). The enlargements may be extensive and result in prominent swelling in the cranial cervical area. The affected lobes are firm and dark red because an extensive interfollicular capillary network develops under the influence of long-term TSH stimulation. The thyroid enlargements are the result of intense hypertrophy and hyperplasia of follicular cells, often with the formation of papillary projections into the lumens of follicles or multiple layers of cells lining follicles (Fig 3-9). Endocytosis of colloid usually proceeds at a rate greater than synthesis, resulting in progressive depletion of colloid. Thyroid follicles become smaller than normal and there may be a partial collapse of follicles owing to the lack of colloid (see Fig 3-9). The hypertrophic lining follicular cells are columnar with a deeply eosinophilic cytoplasm and small hyperchromatic nuclei that often are situated in the basilar part of the cell. The follicles are lined by either single or multiple layers of hyperplastic follicular cells that in some follicles form papillary projections into the lumen (see Fig 3-9).

The converse of what has just been described occurs in follicular cells as a response to an increase in circulating thyroid hormones and a corresponding decrease in circulating pituitary TSH (e.g., after exogenous thyroxine therapy), or in patients with a large space-occupying pituitary lesion that markedly decreases the ability to secrete TSH.[10,26] Thyroid follicles become greatly enlarged and distended with densely staining colloid as a result of decreased TSH-mediated endocytosis of colloid. Follicular cells lining the involuted follicles are low cuboidal and there are few endocytotic vacuoles at the interface between the colloid and follicular cells (Fig 3-10). The luminal surface of follicular cells is flattened. Microvilli extending into the colloid are widely separated and short in response to a long-standing decreased secretion of TSH (Fig 3-11).

The thyroid stroma is exceptionally rich in blood vessels that form extensive interfollicular capillary plexuses lying close to the follicular basement membranes. There is also a network of lymphatics in the gland. The stroma encloses a number of nerve fibers, some of which are parasympathetic, but most are sympathetic. These nerves terminate on blood vessels or in apposition to follicular cells.

Much less numerous, especially in the human thyroid, are cells concerned with the secretion of the peptide hormone of the mammalian thyroid. CT has been shown to be secreted by a second endocrine cell population in the mammalian thyroid gland. C cells (parafollicular or light cells) are distinct from follicular cells in the thyroid that secrete T_4 and T_3.[27] They are situated either within the follicular wall immediately beneath the basement membrane or between follicular cells (Fig 3-12) and as small groups of cells between thyroid follicles. C cells do not border the follicular

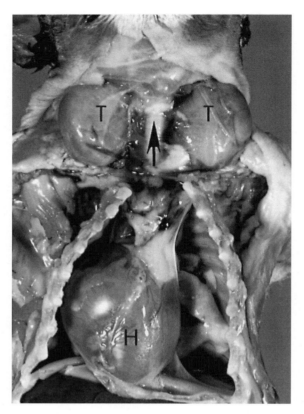

FIGURE 3-8. Diffuse hyperplastic goiter in a pup, resulting in prominent symmetric enlargements of both thyroid lobes (T). The hyperplastic thyroids were freely movable from the trachea (*arrow*) in the cervical region. H, heart.

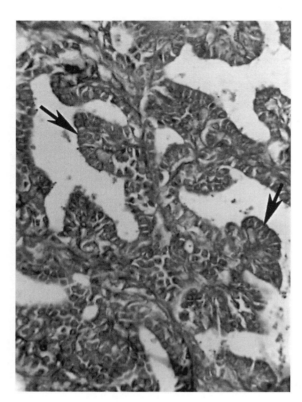

FIGURE 3-9. Diffuse hyperplastic goiter (see Fig 3-8) illustrating papillary projections of thyroid follicular cells (*arrows*) into follicular lumens in response to long-term TSH stimulation. Partial collapse of follicles is due to increased endocytosis of colloid.

colloid directly and their secretory polarity is oriented toward the interfollicular capillaries (see Fig 3-12). The distinctive feature of C cells, compared to thyroid follicular cells, is the presence of numerous, small membrane-limited secretory granules in the cytoplasm. Immunocytochemical techniques have localized the CT activity of C cells to these secretory granules.[28]

Calcitonin-secreting thyroid C cells have been shown to be derived embryologically from cells of the neural crest. Primordial cells from the neural crest migrate ventrally and become incorporated within the last (ultimobranchial) pharyngeal pouch (Fig 3-13). They move caudally with the ultimobranchial body to the point of fusion with the midline primordia that gives rise to the thyroid gland (see Fig 3-13). The ultimobranchial body fuses with and is incorporated into the thyroid near the hilus in mammals, and C cells subsequently are distributed throughout the gland. Although C cells are present throughout the thyroid gland of humans and most other mammals in postnatal life, they often remain more numerous near the hilus and point of fusion with the ultimobranchial body. Under certain conditions, colloid-containing follicles lined by follicular cells also can differentiate from cells of ultimobranchial origin.[29]

In submammalian species C cells and CT activity remain segregated in the ultimobranchial gland, which is anatomically distinct from both the thyroid and the parathyroid glands (Fig 3-14). In the avian ultimobranchial gland a network of stellate cells with long cytoplasmic processes supports the C-cells.[30]

In contrast to the iodothyronines (T_4 and T_3) produced by follicular cells, CT is a polypeptide hormone composed of 32 amino acid residues arranged in a straight chain.[31] The concentration of calcium ion in plasma and extracellular fluids is the principal physiologic stimulus for the secretion of CT by C cells. CT is secreted continuously under conditions of normocalcemia, but the rate of secretion of CT is increased greatly in response to elevations in blood calcium.

C cells store substantial amounts of CT in their cytoplasm in the form of membrane-limited secretory granules (see Fig 3-12). In response to hypercalcemia there is a rapid discharge of stored hormone from C cells into interfollicular capillaries. The hypercalcemic stimulus, if sustained, is followed by hypertrophy of C cells and an increased development of cytoplasmic organelles concerned with the synthesis and secretion of CT. C-cell hyperplasia occurs in response to long-term hypercalcemia. When the blood calcium is lowered, the stimulus for CT secretion is diminished and numerous secretory granules accumulate in the cytoplasm of C cells. The storage of large amounts of preformed hormone in C cells and its rapid release in response to moderate elevations in blood calcium probably reflect the physiologic role of CT as an "emergency" hormone to protect against the development of hypercalcemia.

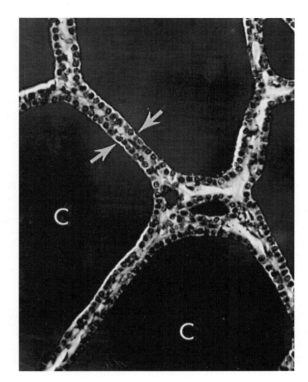

FIGURE 3-10. Response of thyroid follicular cells to long-term decreased levels of TSH. The follicular cells (*arrows*) are low-cuboidal, and thyroid follicles are distended with dense colloid (C) in response to decreased TSH secretion.

HISTOCHEMISTRY AND HISTOPHYSIOLOGY

Follicular cells show striking polarity orientated toward the follicular lumen (Fig 3-15). Varying numbers of lysosomes, histochemically stainable for enzymes such as acid phosphatase, are found in the apical portion of the cell.[32,33] Soon after stimulation by TSH in follicular cells, intracellular droplets (phagosomes), corresponding to those demonstrated light microscopically by the PAS reaction and representing ingested colloid, are more numerous than in the resting state.[33] Some of these form phagolysosomes in follicular cells by fusion with lysosomes.

The apical portion of the follicular cell develops prominent elongations of microvilli shortly after stimulation by TSH that form cytoplasmic processes (pseudopods) that surround portions of the follicular colloid (see Fig 3-15). Pseudopods appear to collect thyroglobulin located at some distance from the apical surface and may provide a mechanism of selective macropinocytosis by which newly synthesized thyroglobulin recently delivered to the follicle lumen is prevented from undergoing immediate reuptake[34] (Fig 3-16). This process, termed "endocytosis," results in the formation of colloid droplets in the cytoplasm of follicular cells.[33,35,36] In addition, small, clathrin-containing coated vesicles appear to be involved in the uptake and transport of iodinated thyroglobulin from the follicular lumen to the lysosomal compartment of thyroid follicular cells.[37] This process of receptor-mediated endocytosis of colloid ("micropinocytosis") may be a major pathway of thyroglobulin uptake in the normal thyroid gland

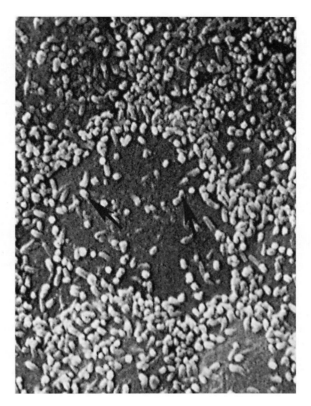

FIGURE 3-11. Scanning electron micrograph of luminal surface of thyroid follicular cells from a rat that was given 100 μg of T_4 daily for 4 weeks. In response to decreased TSH levels, microvilli (*arrows*) are widely separated and short. There is no evidence of formation of cytoplasmic pseudopodia into the luminal colloid, as occurs in actively secreting thyroid follicles (contrast with Fig 3-6). (Collins WT, Capen CC. Ultrastructural and functional alterations of the rat thyroid gland produced by polychlorinated biphenyls compared with iodide excess and deficiency, and thyrotropin and thyroxine administration. Virchows Arch [B] 1980;33:213)

under conditions in which the demands for thyroid hormone secretion are low. During the vesicular transport of thyroglobulin through the cytoplasm of follicular cells ("transcytosis"), the molecule does not undergo cleavage and its electrophoretic mobility remains unchanged.[38] Thyroglobulin may be released as an intact molecule into the circulation in small quantities by this TSH-regulated transepithelial vesicular transport. Clearance of thyroglobulin from the circulation with release of thyroid hormones occurs in the liver by macrophages (Kupffer cells).[39]

Microtubules and microfilaments in the cytoplasm of follicular cells beneath the apical plasma membrane are important in moving colloid droplets into close proximity to lysosomal bodies.[40] The membranes of these two organelles fuse, resulting in the local release of enzymes that break down the colloid and release T_4 and T_3 into the cytosol.

The active thyroid hormones subsequently diffuse out of the cell and enter the abundant interfollicular capillaries, which have a fenestrated endothelial lining. The iodinated tyrosines (MIT and DIT) released from the colloid droplets are deiodinated enzymatically and the iodide generated either is recycled to the lumen to iodinate new tyrosyl residues or released into the circulation. These unique structural and functional charac-

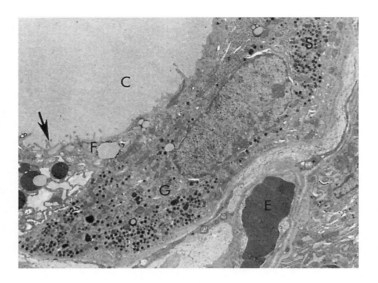

FIGURE 3-12. Electron micrograph of thyroid, illustrating a C cell in the wall of a follicle, wedged between several follicular cells (F). Follicular cells line the follicle directly and extend microvilli (*arrow*) into the colloid (C). The cytoplasm of C cells has many calcitonin-containing secretion granules (S) and a prominent Golgi apparatus (G). The secretory polarity of C cells is directed toward interfollicular capillaries (E), rather than toward the follicle lumen, as with follicular cells.

teristics of the phylogenetically oldest endocrine gland suggest that the thyroid may have evolved toward a more "ideal" structure to perform its vital metabolic functions.[41]

The functionally most important enzyme in the thyroid hormone synthetic pathway is present in the apical plasma membrane and microvilli as well as in other structures of the follicular cells[42,43] (Fig 3-17). Thyroperoxidase in the human thyroid is a membrane-bound, heme-containing glycoprotein composed of 933 amino acids with a transmembrane domain.[44] This important enzyme oxidizes iodide ion (I^-) taken up by follicular cells into reactive iodine, which binds to the tyrosine residues in the thyroglobulin. Iodine is incorporated not

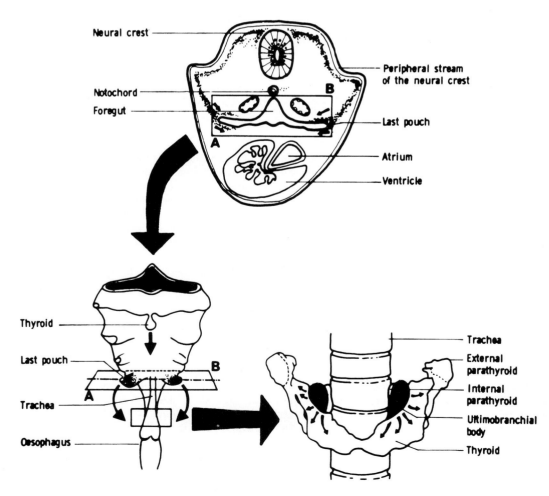

FIGURE 3-13. Schematic representation of neural crest origin of calcitonin-secreting C cells. Primordial cells arising from neural crest migrate ventrally during embryonic life to become incorporated in the last (ultimobranchial) pharyngeal pouch. The ultimobranchial body fuses with primordia of the thyroid and distributes C cells throughout the mammalian thyroid gland. (Foster GV, Byfield PGH, Gudmundsson TV. Calciton. Clin Endocrinol Metab 1972;1:93)

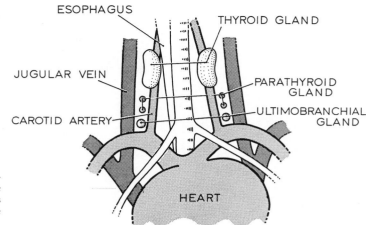

FIGURE 3-14. Calcitonin-secreting C cells in submammalian vertebrates remain in an anatomically distinct endocrine organ separate from the thyroid gland. The ultimobranchial gland in chickens is caudal to the two pairs of parathyroids and thyroid gland along the carotid artery.

only into newly synthesized thyroglobulin recently delivered to the follicular lumen but into molecules already stored in the lumen.[45] Thyroperoxidase also functions as a "coupling" enzyme to combine MIT and DIT to form T_3 or two DITs to form T_4.

The follicular cell of the thyroid is involved concurrently in luminally directed processes of thyroglobulin synthesis and exocytosis as well as basally directed processes of colloid endocytosis with breakdown and eventual release of thyroid hormones into the interfollicular capillaries. Radioautographs prepared at increasing time intervals after pulse labeling of thyroids with a radioactive amino acid such as ^{3}H-leucine (Fig 3-18) have shown that its incorporation into peptides occurs in the rough endoplasmic reticulum. Labeled material subsequently appears in the Golgi region, then over vesicles between the Golgi apparatus and the lumen, and finally in the lumen.[46] With the use of tritiated monosaccharides, it can be shown that the synthesis of the carbohydrate chains of thyroglobulin starts in the endoplasmic reticulum and is completed in the Golgi apparatus.[47]

The thyroid takes up iodine in the form of iodide ion. Although the active transport of iodide occurs at the base of the follicular cells near the interfollicular capillaries, iodide that has entered the thyroid cell is transported rapidly to the follicular lumen[48] (Fig 3-19). Iodide in the thyroid is oxidized to a higher valence state by the thyroperoxidase in microvilli. This oxidized form of iodine becomes rapidly attached to the tyrosyl residues in thyroglobulin in proximity to the apical microvilli.[49,50]

COMPARATIVE ASPECTS OF THYROID

Comparative studies of thyroid structure and function have contributed, to an important and often not fully appreciated degree, to mammalian and clinical thyroidology. The first iodoproteins and their incorporated iodotyrosines were discovered in invertebrate organisms long before their association was known with the thyroid gland. The relationship between iodine lack and thyroid hypertrophy was first worked out in hatchery trout and was quickly applied to clinical situations in human patients.[51]

Morphology

The thyroid in all adult vertebrates has a basic follicular pattern and it would be difficult, with few exceptions, to differentiate among species solely on the basis of thyroid histology. Similarity in thyroid structure has been found between lower vertebrates and mammals at the ultrastructural level as well[52] (Fig 3-20).

The macroscopic shape of the thyroid is formed by amalgamation of the numerous histologic units (i.e., follicles) and can vary quite considerably among the different vertebrate species (Fig 3-21). However, the function of the thyroid gland as a whole is not influenced by its macroscopic shape, which suggests this anatomic variation among species is not of fundamental evolutionary significance.[51]

There is not an organized thyroid in the adult cyclostomes (lampreys, hagfish) and teleost fish. However, follicles occur scattered in the subpharyngeal connective tissue in a pattern roughly approximating the ventral aorta and its principal branches into the gills. In a few species of teleosts (parrotfish, swordfish), most thyroid follicles may be gathered into an organized gland. An interesting finding in fish is the occurrence of thyroid follicles in nonpharyngeal areas. The most frequent location of heterotopic follicles in teleosts is in the kidney; other, less common sites include the eye, brain, heart, esophagus, and spleen.

The thyroid in elasmobranch fishes usually is aggregated into a single encapsulated organ near the tip of the lower jaw (see Fig 3-21). In amphibians there are two rounded thyroid lobes, often quite widely separated and associated with branches of the hyoid cartilage. Thyroid shape in reptiles is variable, with turtles having a large disc of thyroid tissue immediately in front of the heart at the branching of the two systemic aortae. Lizards have a bilobed gland connected by an isthmus that crosses the trachea. Birds have two widely separated, rounded thyroid lobes, one on each side of the trachea at the level of the clavicles (see Figs. 3-14 and 3-21). Mammals are fairly consistent in the well known pattern that consists of two lobes connected by an isthmus.

Physiology

Marine algae are efficient concentrators of iodine, indicative of some kind of iodide or halide pump.[53] Most groups of invertebrates are able to form iodoproteins, usually in skeletal or fibrous scleral layers. As a rule, iodination of such rigid proteins does not go beyond formation of diiodotyrosine,[54,55] presumably because the iodotyrosines are not free to couple. There

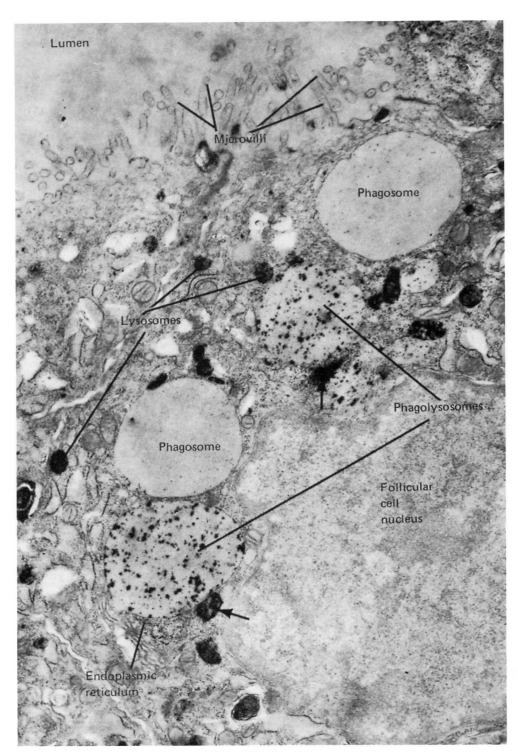

FIGURE 3-15. Electron micrograph of the apical portion of a follicular cell stained for acid phosphatase. The enzyme is present in the darkly stained lysosomes, some of which are attached to colloid droplets (phagosomes, *arrows*). The large droplets with irregular black material are phagolysosomes, whose colloid has become intermingled with lysosomal contents. (Wetzel BK, Spicer CC, Wollman SH. Changes in fine structure and acid phosphatase localization in rat thyroid cells following thyrotropin administration. J Cell Biol 1965;25:593)

are reports of formation of significant proportions of T_4 in certain invertebrate genera, such as in *Musculium* (small freshwater clams). This cannot be taken as a significant finding because in vitro iodination of pure proteins under oxidative conditions yields a certain amount of T_4.

Although there has been no conclusive evidence of a function for thyroid hormones in invertebrates despite the general occurrence of iodotyrosines and T_4, there is evidence from coelenterates of the metabolism of iodine to T_4.[56] Data from one of the most primitive invertebrate groups support the conclusion that T_4 formation is an ancient biochemical phenomenon in animals and that T_4 may have a function in some invertebrates. However, T_4 in many of the primitive forms may be merely an accidental product of the oxidative iodination of proteins exposed to high levels of environmental iodine.

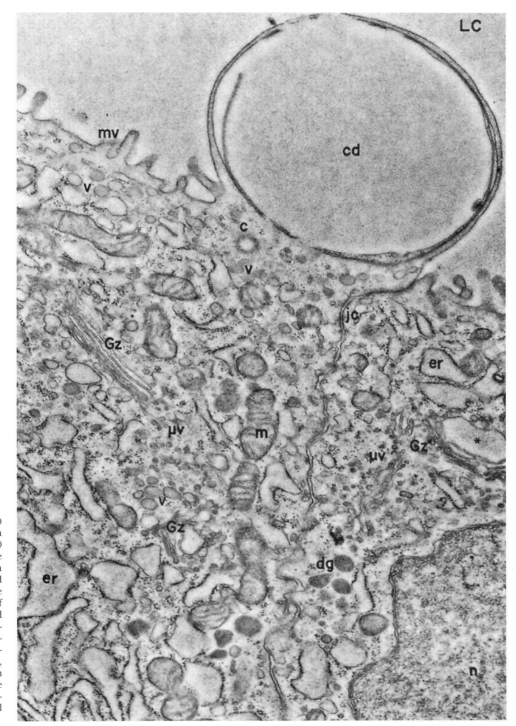

FIGURE 3-16. Colloid droplet (cd) enclosed within a thin pseudopod on apical surface of a follicular cell 30 minutes after TSH injections. Note dense granules (dg), mitochondria (m), endoplasmic reticulum (er), and centriole (c). Vesicles (v) of moderate size with contents similar to those of the luminal colloid (LC) are clustered about the Golgi zones (Gz) and beneath the apical membrane. (MV, microvilli; JC, junctional complex; n, nucleus; uv, microvesicles). (Wetzel; BK, Spicer SS, Wollman SH. Changes in fine structure and acid phosphatase localization in rat thyroid cells following thyrotropin administration. J Cell Biol 1965;25:593)

THYROID IODOPROTEINS IN LOWER VERTEBRATES

Molecular variations have not been reported in the structure of T_4 and T_3 among animals. All vertebrates that metabolize iodine into an organic form, whether in a thyroid or in any other pharyngeal epithelial structure, form T_4 and variable proportions of a triiodinated form of the thyronine molecule.

Iodination of tyrosine molecules appears to take place in a characteristic protein, which in the mammalian thyroid is thyroglobulin. However, mammals and a few species of birds, reptiles, amphibians, elasmobranchs, and teleosts that have been studied also synthesize lesser amounts of 12S and 27S iodoproteins.[57,58] Smaller thyroproteins also have been identified with iodination to various degrees in different species and referred to as "5S" or "3-8S" fractions.

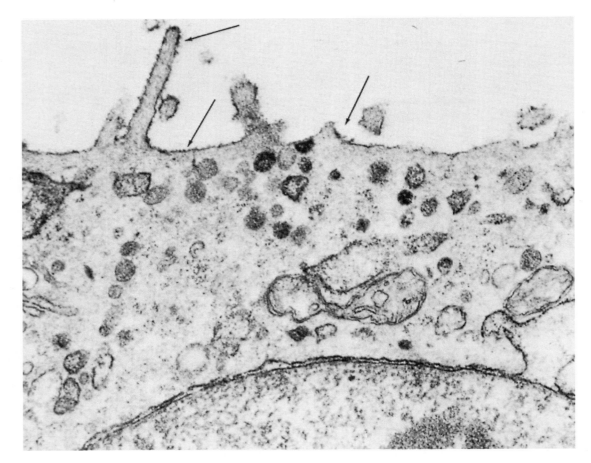

FIGURE 3-17. Rat thyroid cytochemically stained to demonstrate the distribution of peroxidase. Precipitate corresponding to the location of the enzyme is most evident in the apical membrane, including the portion lining a microvillus (*arrows*). There is also some precipitate in apical vesicles. (Tice LW, Wollman SH. Ultrastructural localization of peroxidase activity on some membranes of the typical thyroid epithelial cell. Lab Invest 1972;26:23. Courtesy of US–Canadian Division of the International Academy of Pathology)

The thyroid iodoproteins of the Agnatha are of special interest because they come from the most primitive existing vertebrates. Conflicting reports that the principal thyroid iodoprotein was 12S in one species of lamprey and 19S in another most likely are the result of procedural differences. This is suggested by the finding of 19S thyroglobulin in thyroid tissue of the Pacific lamprey (*Entosphenus tridentatus*) on sucrose density gradient centrifugation, but 12S on fractional precipitation and then purification with ammonium sulfate.[59,60]

The findings of mean T_4 levels of 1.5 μg/dL in leopard frogs, 3.4 μg/dL in Pacific hagfish, 0.5 μg/dL in migrating adult lampreys,[61] and 3.7 μg/dL in a Japanese hagfish offer little opportunity for generalizations except that marine fish have higher circulating levels of T_4 than freshwater fish. Functions for T_4 have been demonstrated in teleosts, and a negative feedback for T_4 has been observed on TSH secretion. In agnathans there is no demonstrated action of T_4 and no evidence for TSH production with feedback control.[52]

Regard and colleagues[62] and others[63] have reported a surge in both T_3 and T_4 at the time of metamorphosis in several species of amphibians. They speculated that because their assay failed to detect measurable plasma T_3 and T_4 in post-metamorphic or adult amphibians, there may be no function for thyroid hormones in adults.[62] However, it is known that the adult amphibian thyroid gland actively metabolizes iodine and responds to goitrogenic treatment.[63,64] In addition, there are reported actions of thyroidectomy and thyroid hormones on skin, nervous function, and intermediary metabolism in amphibians.

In anuran amphibia, metamorphosis is accompanied by alterations in thyroid hormone receptor concentration and marked changes in the activities of the iodothyronine deiodinase systems.[65] All of these changes contribute to enhancing the peripheral sensitivity to circulating T_4. The Mexican axolotl, *Ambystoma mexicanum*, is a neotenous salamander that rarely undergoes anatomic metamorphosis but can be induced to undergo metamorphosis by the administration of T_4.[65] The neoteny results primarily from low levels of plasma T_4 secondary to a low secretory rate of TSH from the pituitary. Tissues of the Mexican axolotl do not undergo specific changes that enhance the physiologic response to T_4 (summarized previously), as in anuran amphibia.[65]

Metamorphosis in amphibians is a complex metabolic process controlled by thyroid hormones. The limbs of *Xenopus laevis* grow and differentiate concomitant with the formation of

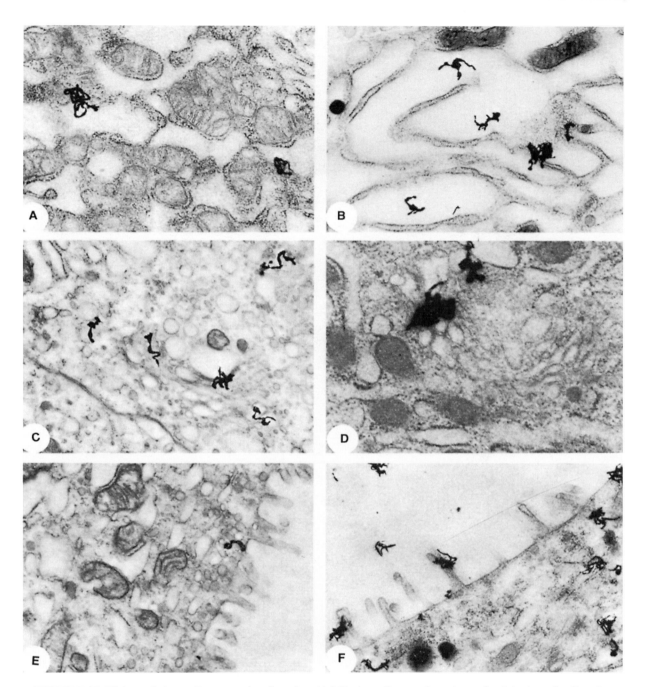

FIGURE 3-18. High-resolution radioautographs of rat thyroid follicular cells at various times after injection of radioactive precursors of thyroglobulin. (*A*) Thyroid 10 minutes after ³H-leucine injection. Silver gains over ribosomes studding the membranes of the rough endoplasmic reticulum indicate that the synthesis of thryoglobulin starts in association with the ribosomes. (*B*) Thyroid 30 minutes after ³H-leucine injection. Silver grains over the cisternae of the endoplasmic reticulum indicate that the newly synthesized protein portion of thyroglobulin migrates from the ribosomes to the cisternae. (*C*) Thyroid 1 hour after ³H-leucine injection. Silver grains in association with Golgi zone indicate that the newly synthesized protein molecule is transported from the endoplasmic reticulum to the Golgi apparatus. (*D*) Thyroid 15 minutes after ³H-galactose injection. Note silver grains in association with the Golgi zone. (*E*) Thyroid 2 hours after ³H-leucine injection. Silver grains over the region of apical vesicles indicate that the glycoprotein molecules emerge from the Golgi apparatus contained in vesicles that move to the apical surface of follicular cells. (*F*) Thyroid 4 hours after ³H-leucine injection. Silver grains over the colloid in the lumen indicate that thyroglobulin is secreted by the follicular cells into the colloid of the lumen (*A* through *C*, courtesy of Dr. B.A. Young; *D*, courtesy of Dr. E.J.H. Nathaniel)

the thyroid gland and increasing levels of thyroid hormones. More than 120 genes are up-regulated within 24 hours after induction of metamorphosis by thyroid hormone.[66] Some of the genes respond directly, but most appear to be secondary response genes judging from their delayed kinetics and cyclohexamide sensitivity. Up-regulation of nuclear thyroid hormone

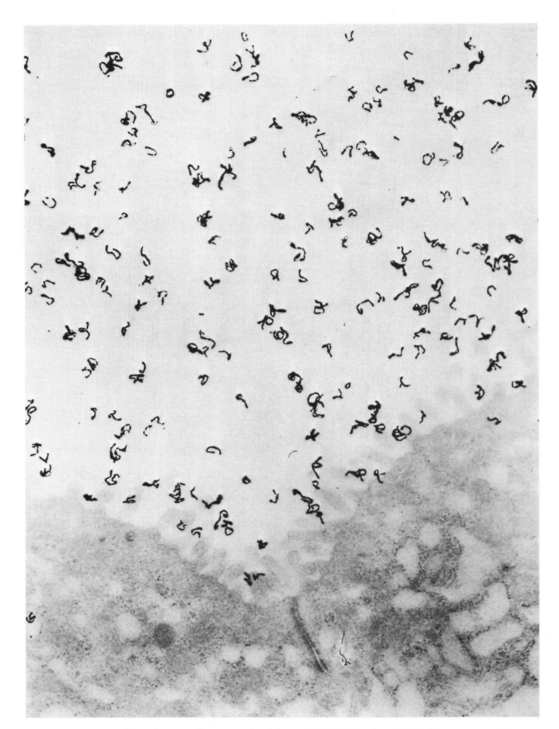

FIGURE 3-19. High resolution radioautograph of thyroid follicle. The thyroid gland was removed from a rat 1 minute after injection of a tracer dose of [125]I. With few exceptions, the silver grains are located over the colloid in the follicular lumen, indicating that iodination of thyroglobulin takes place in the lumen near the apical surface. (Courtesy of Dr. Huberta van Heyningen)

receptor mRNA is one of the earliest changes in gene expression in *Xenopus* tadpoles in response to thyroid hormones, which correlates closely with the progress of metamorphosis.[67]

A 56-kd protein composed of four identical subunits has been reported in the plasma of the bullfrog (*Rana catesbeiana*), the amino acid composition of which was highly ho-

mologous with the mammalian transthyretins (e.g., T_4-binding prealbumin).[68] In contrast to mammalian transthyretins, the affinity of bullfrog transthyretin for T_3 was 360 times greater than for T_4. These findings suggest that bullfrog transthyretin plays an important role in transporting T_3 in the blood during metamorphosis.[68] In turtles (*Trachemys scripta*), plasma T_4 is

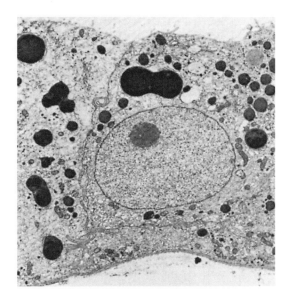

FIGURE 3-20. Electron micrograph of thyroid epithelial cells of a hag-fish (*Eptatretus stouti*). The follicular lumen contains no colloid, but colloid-like secretion droplets are numerous in the cytoplasm. Other structures, including the microvilli of the apical surface, are similar to the equivalent ones in thyroid cells of higher vertebrates. (Courtesy of N.E. Henderson, University of Calgary).

bound principally to a relatively high-affinity, low-capacity T_4-binding protein.[69] Because of the low concentrations of albumin in turtle blood (~ 10 mg/mL), T_4-binding protein appears to account for a greater proportion of T_4 binding than T_4-binding globulin (TBG) in humans.

A surge in plasma T_4 or T_3, or both, occurs in developing salmon at the stage when the "parr" becomes a "smolt."[70] The exact timing of the smoltification T_4 surge appears to be keyed to the phase of the moon.[71] There are sev-

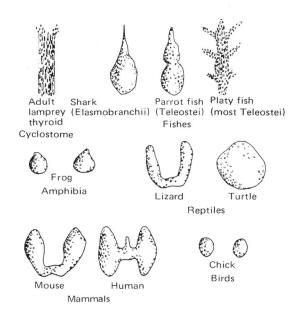

FIGURE 3-21. Distribution of thyroid follicles and their organization into thyroid glands of different characteristic shapes in vertebrates.

eral reports that peripheral deiodination of T_4 to T_3 appears at the time of amphibian metamorphosis,[72] and a similar phenomenon occurs in developing salmonids.[73] Deiodination of T_3 during parr–smolt transformation in Atlantic salmon proceeds exclusively through an inner ring deiodinase pathway, which permits regulation of T_3 degradation independently of the outer ring deiodinase pathway responsible for T_3 formation.[74] By comparison, deiodination of reverse T_3 in salmon occurs primarily through an outer ring deiodinase pathway, but reverse T_3 inner ring deiodinase activity does occur in some tissues.

The actions of thyroid hormones in different animal groups and species reflect adaptiveness in the evolutionary sense.[51] Particular target tissues for T_3 and T_4 appear to vary in their sensitivity to these hormones at different stages of development. For example, brain and gut are sensitive to T_4 in tadpoles but are much less so in adult frogs.[75,76] The characteristic action of thyroid hormone in stimulating oxygen consumption and heat production in mammals is absent or different in the cold-blooded vertebrates. Most of the actions of thyroid hormones eventually are explicable on the basis of translation of specific ribonucleic acid messages for synthesis of particular structural or enzyme proteins. It appears from the multiplicity of actions of thyroid hormones that cellular receptors are widespread and that receptor protein synthesis is relatively easily evoked (or suppressed) during evolution or ontogenetic development.[51]

CONTROL OF THYROID ACTIVITY

Different elements in the thyroid control system have been subjected to evaluation in nonmammalian vertebrates, with some interesting differences detected. Hypophyseal thyrotropic activity has been demonstrated in most vertebrate groups.[77] In the cartilaginous elasmobranch fishes, evidence indicates that TSH is synthesized primarily in the "ventral lobe" of the pars distalis.[78] Definitive chemical identification of thyrotropin-releasing hormone (TRH) in the hypothalamus has been achieved for several mammalian species and in the salamander.[79] However, TRH was found distributed through all parts of the brain and in the pituitary of rats, chickens, snake (*Thamnophis*), leopard frogs and their tadpoles, and Atlantic salmon, as well as in the "head region" of Amphioxus.[80] Frog hypothalamic extract had TRH biologic activity in rats in proportion to its immunoreactive TRH content. Recent studies have reported that TRH, corticotropin-releasing hormone (ovine), and gonadotropin-releasing hormone (mammalian) all stimulated the secretion of bioactive TSH by frog (*Rana esculenta*) pituitary glands in vitro.[81] Preincubation with T_4 for 6 hours suppressed the TRH- and corticotropin-releasing hormone–induced secretion of TSH but did not affect the response to gonadotropin-releasing hormone, whereas preincubation with T_3 reduced both the TRH- and gonadotropin-releasing hormone–stimulated release of TSH. The results suggest that thyroid hormones exert a negative feedback control on the secretion of TSH in adult frogs by a direct action on the pituitary.

The action of T_4 on TSH secretion in amphibians indicates negative but no positive feedback.[82,83] Thus, the surging high plasma levels of T_4 in metamorphosing tadpoles may reflect extreme changes in the set point for negative feedback during development, analogous to the changes in sex steroid feedback on gonadotropins during puberty in mammals.[51]

In the turtle, *Pseudemys scripta*, hypothyroidism induced by surgical thyroidectomy or a goitrogen (methimazole) resulted in marked depression of plasma binding of T_4, and T_4 treatment restored binding after 4 to 6 weeks.[84] The T_4-binding protein in turtles has a high degree of structural homology (68% of NH_2 terminal region) to the mammalian vitamin D-binding protein (rat, mouse, and human) rather than mammalian TBG.[85] Binding studies confirmed that the turtle T_4-binding protein likely also represents the major vitamin D-binding protein and is electrophoretically distinct from the sex hormone-binding proteins.[86] T_4 tends to enhance the affinity and the capacity for transporting vitamin D_3 in this species. Therefore, turtles have a single binding protein, resembling vitamin D-binding protein, that performs two major functions that are normally served by proteins representing different multigene families in mammals.[85]

Pathology

Although the basic hypothalamic–pituitary–thyroid axis functions in a similar manner in animals and humans, there are important differences between species that are significant when extrapolating data from chronic toxicity and carcinogenicity studies of drugs and chemicals in animals for human risk assessment.[41,87] Long-term perturbations of the pituitary–thyroid axis by various xenobiotics or physiologic alterations (e.g., iodine deficiency, partial thyroidectomy) are more likely to predispose laboratory rodents (e.g., rat and mouse) to a higher incidence of proliferative lesions (e.g., hyperplasia and tumors) of follicular cells than in the human thyroid.[88] This appears to be particularly true in the male rat, in which there usually are higher circulating levels of TSH than in females. The greater sensitivity of the rodent thyroid to derangement by drugs, chemicals, and physiologic perturbations also is related to the shorter plasma half-life of T_4 than in humans, which results, in part, from the considerable differences between species in the transport proteins for T_4.

The plasma half-life of T_4 in rats is considerably shorter (12–24 hours) than in humans (5–9 days). This is related in part to differences between species in the transport proteins for T_4 and T_3.[89] In human beings and the monkey, circulating T_4 is bound primarily to TBG; however, this high-affinity binding protein for T_4 is not present in rodents, birds, amphibians, or fish. The binding affinity of TBG for T_4 is approximately 1000 times higher than for transthyretin. The percentage of unbound active T_4 is lower in species with high levels of TBG than in animals in which T_4 binding is limited to albumin and transthyretin.

Although T_4 is the principal secretory product of the thyroid, it functions primarily as a prohormone and undergoes a single deiodination of the phenolic ring in extrathyroidal tissues to form the metabolically more active T_3.[90] T_3 is transported bound to TBG and albumin in human beings, monkey, and dog but only to albumin in mouse, rat, and chicken. These differences in plasma half-life of thyroid hormones and binding to transport proteins between rats and humans may be one factor in the greater propensity of the rat thyroid to development of hyperplastic or neoplastic lesions in response to chronic TSH stimulation.

Many chemicals and drugs disrupt one or more steps in the synthesis and secretion of thyroid hormones or enhance the metabolism of thyroid hormones, especially those that increase hepatic cytochrome P450 T_4-metabolizing enzymes. This results in subnormal levels of T_4 and T_3 associated with a compensatory increased secretion of pituitary TSH in long-term rodent studies for safety assessment of a particular chemical for humans.[91–96] When tested in highly sensitive species, such as rats and mice, these compounds result in early follicular cell hypertrophy/hyperplasia and increased thyroid weights, and long-term studies show an increased incidence of thyroid tumors by a secondary (indirect) mechanism associated with hormonal imbalances.

In the secondary mechanism of thyroid oncogenesis in rodents, the specific xenobiotic chemical or physiologic perturbation evokes another stimulus (e.g., chronic hypersecretion of TSH) that promotes the development of nodular proliferative lesions (initially hypertrophy, followed by hyperplasia, subsequently adenomas, infrequently carcinomas) derived from follicular cells. Thresholds for a no-effect on the thyroid gland can be established by determining the dose of xenobiotic that fails to elicit an elevation in the circulating level of TSH. Compounds acting by this indirect (secondary) mechanism with hormonal imbalances usually show little or no evidence for mutagenicity or for producing DNA damage.

In humans who have markedly altered changes in thyroid function and elevated TSH levels, as in areas with a high incidence of endemic goiter due to iodine deficiency, there is little if any increase in the incidence of thyroid cancer.[97,98] The relative resistance to the development of thyroid cancer in humans with elevated plasma TSH levels is in marked contrast to the response of the thyroid gland to chronic TSH stimulation in rats and mice. The human thyroid is much less sensitive to this pathogenetic phenomenon than rodents.[99]

Although numerous in vitro thyroid follicular cell culture systems have been described,[100–105] secretion of the thyroid hormones T_3 and T_4 is seldom measured in vitro because of the reduced ability of follicular cells growing in monolayer culture (i.e., lacking follicular organization) to concentrate and efficiently iodinate thyroglobulin. Thyroid function in vitro of-

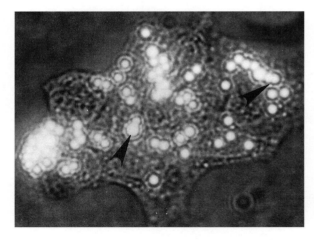

FIGURE 3-22. Fluorescence photomicrograph of a small cluster of FRTL-5 cells with numerous latex beads (*arrowheads*) located within the cytoplasm. The beads are approximately 2 μm in diameter. (Ozaki A, Sagartz JE, Capen CC. Phagocytic activity of FRTL-5 rat thyroid cells as measured by ingestion of fluorescent latex beads. Exp Cell Res 1995;219:547)

ten is assessed by evaluating specific phases of thyroid hormone synthesis, including iodide trapping[106]; thyroglobulin expression,[107–112] secretion,[113,114] and iodination[115,116]; thyroid peroxidase synthesis[117,118] and activity[119]; and TSH receptor expression. These functions are TSH-dependent and can be altered in response to various growth factors, hormones, second messengers, and xenobiotics.

The normal Fischer rat thyroid line (FRTL-5) cell line has most of the known in vivo functional responses to TSH and has thus been a useful model for the study of thyroid pathophysiology in vitro. Numerous TSH-induced functional responses have been described, including iodide influx, trapping, and efflux; thyroglobulin synthesis, secretion, and iodination; thyroid peroxidase synthesis and activity; thyroid hormone production; and morphologic differentiation. In addition to these functional responses, FRTL-5 cells have been used to measure the effects of TSH on cell growth.

Thyroid follicular cell phagocytic activity can be quantified by a sensitive nonradioactive assay using a normal rat thyroid follicular cell line (FRTL-5) with fluoresceinated latex beads and flow cytometry[120] (Fig 3-22). This in vitro assay permits discrimination of both the number of functionally active cells as well as the ability to estimate the level of activity of these cells. Electron microscopic studies demonstrated that latex beads were engulfed and located within cytoplasmic vacuoles of thyrocytes (Fig 3-23). Phagocytosis can be stimulated by forskolin, cholera toxin, 8-Br-cAMP, calcitriol, and transforming growth factor β. In contrast, phagocytosis was inhibited by insulin, NaI, $CaCl_2$, and aminotriazole.[121] The phagocytosis of latex beads was regulated in a manner similar to iodide trapping and could be altered by the addition of numerous compounds. Phagocytic activity was stimulated by both cAMP-dependent and cAMP-independent pathways. Flow cytometric evaluation of phagocytosis of fluorescent latex beads provides a simple, rapid, nonradioactive index of thyroid function in vitro after exposure to a variety of xenobiotic chemicals.

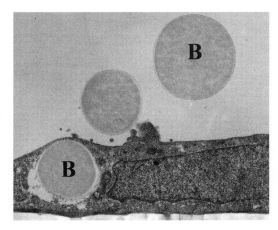

FIGURE 3-23. Phagocytosis of fluorescent latex beads by FRTL-5 rat thyroid follicular cell grown on polycarbonate membrane. Note the apical microvilli and the presence of a latex bead (B) within a cytoplasmic vacuole and on the cell surface. (Sagartz JE, Ozaki A, Capen CC. Phagocytosis of fluorescent T beads by rat thyroid follicular cells [FRTL-5]: comparison with iodide trapping as an index of functional activity of thyrocytes in vitro. Toxicol Pathol 1995;23. In press)

References

1. Halmi NS. Anatomy and histochemistry. In: Ingbar SH, Braverman LE, eds. Werner's the thyroid: a fundamental and clinical text. 5th ed. Philadelphia: JB Lippincott, 1986:24

2. Harach HR, Vujanic, Jasani B. Ultimobranchial body nests in human fetal thyroid: an autopsy, histological, and immunohistochemical study in relation to solid cell nests and mucoepidermoid carcinoma of the thyroid. J Pathol 1993;169:465

3. Harach HR. Solid cell nests of the thyroid. J Pathol 1988; 155:191

4. Harach HR. Thyroid follicles with acid mucins in man: a second kind of follicles? Cell Tissue Res 1985;242:211

5. Martin-Lacave I, Conde E, Moreno A, Utrilla JC, Galera-Davidson H. Evidence of the occurrence of calcitonin cells in the ultimobranchial follicle of the rat postnatal thyroid. Acta Anat (Basel) 1992;144:93

6. Conde E, Moreno AM, Martin-Lacave I, Fernandez A, Galera H. Immunocytochemical study of the ultimobranchial tubule in Wistar rats. Anat Histol Embryol 1992;21:94

7. Kraiem Z, Sadeh O, Yosef M. Iodide uptake and organification, tri-iodothyronine secretion, cyclic AMP accumulation and cell proliferation in an optimized system of human thyroid follicles cultured in collagen gel suspended in serum-free medium. J Endocrinol 1991;131:499

8. Toda S, Yonemitsu N, Hikichi Y, Sugihara H. Differentiation of human thyroid follicle cells from normal subjects and Basedow's disease in three-dimensional collagen gel culture. Pathol Res Pract 1992;188:874

9. Toda S, Yonemitsu N, Minami Y, Sugihara H. Plural cells organize thyroid follicles through aggregation and linkage in collagen gel culture of porcine follicle cells. Endocrinology 1993;133:914

10. Collins WT, Capen CC. Ultrastructural and functional alterations of the rat thyroid gland produced by polychlorinated biphenyls compared with iodide excess and deficiency, and thyrotropin and thyroxine administration. Virchows Arch [B] 1980;33:213

11. Toda S, Sugihara H. Reconstruction of thyroid follicles from isolated porcine follicle cells in three-dimensional collagen gel culture. Endocrinology 1990;126:2027

12. Pic P, Remy L, Athouel-Haon A-M, Mazzella E. Evidence for a role of the cytoskeleton in the in vitro folliculogenesis of the thyroid gland of the fetal rat. Cell Tissue Res 1984;237:499

13. Yap AS, Keast JR, Manley SW. Thyroid cell spreading and focal adhesion formation depend upon protein tyrosine phosphorylation and actin microfilaments. Exp Cell Res 1994;210:306

14. Conde E, Martin-Lacave I, Gonzalez-Campora R, Galera-Davidson H. Histometry of normal thyroid glands in neonatal and adult rats. Am J Anat 1991;191:384

15. Delverdier M, Cabanie P, Roome N, Enjalbert F, van Haverbeke G. Quantitative histology of the rat thyroid. Anal Quant Cytol Histol 1991;13:110

16. Takasu S, Ohno S, Komiya I, Yamada T. Requirements of follicle structure for thyroid hormone synthesis: cytoskeletons and iodine metabolism in polarized monolayer cells on collagen gel and in double layered, follicle-forming cells. Endocrinology 1992;131:1143

17. Sakurai S, Fogelfeld L, Ries A, Schneider AB. Anionic complex-carbohydrate units of human thyroglobulin. Endocrinology 1990;127:2056

18. Herzog V, Berndorfer U, Saber Y. Isolation of insoluble secretory product from bovine thyroid: extracellular storage of thyroglobulin in covalently cross-linked form. J Cell Biol 1992;118:1071

19. Uchiyama Y, Oomiya A, Murakami G. Fluctuations in follicular structures of rat thyroid glands during 24 hours: fine structural and morphometric studies. Am J Anat 1986;175:23

20. Uchiyama Y, Murakami G, Igarashi M. Changes in colloid droplets and dense bodies in rat thyroid follicular cells during 24 hours: fine structural and morphometric studies. Am J Anat 1986;175:15

21. Wynford-Thomas D, Smith P, Williams ED. Proliferative response to cyclic AMP elevation of thyroid epithelium in suspension culture. Mol Cell Endocrinol 1987;51:163

22. Nilsson M, Engström G, Ericson LE. Graded response in the individual thyroid follicle cell to increasing doses of TSH. Mol Cell Endocrinol 1986;44:165

23. Many M-C, Denef J-F, Haumont S, van den Hove-Vandenbroucke, Cornette C, Beckers C. Morphological and functional changes during thyroid hyperplasia and involution in C3H mice: effects of iodine and 3,5,3'-triiodothyronine during involution. Endocrinology 1985;116:798

24. Ericson LE, Engström G. Quantitative electron microscopic studies on exocytosis and endocytosis in the thyroid follicle cell. Endocrinology 1978;103:883

25. Gerber H, Peter HJ, Bachmeier C, Kaempf J, Studer H. Progressive recruitment of follicular cells with graded secretory responsiveness during stimulation of the thyroid gland by thyrotropin. Endocrinology 1987;120:91

26. Gerber H, Studer H, von Grünigen C. Paradoxical effects of thyrotropin on diffusion of thyroglobulin in the colloid of rat thyroid follicles after long term thyroxine treatment. Endocrinology 1985;116:303

27. Kalina M, Pearse AGE. Ultrastructural localization of calcitonin in C-cells of dog thyroid: an immunocytochemical study. Histochemie 1971;26:1

28. DeGrandi PB, Kraehenbuhl JP, Campiche MA. Ultrastructural localization of calcitonin in the parafollicular cells of the pig thyroid gland with cytochrome c-labeled antibody fragments. J Cell Biol 1971;50:446

29. Kameda Y, Ikeda A. Immunohistochemical study of the C-cell complex of dog thyroid glands with reference to the reactions of calcitonin, C-thyroglobulin and 19S thyroglobulin. Cell Tissue Res 1980;208:405

30. Youshak MS, Capen CC. Ultrastructural evaluation of ultimobranchial glands from normal and osteopetrotic chickens. Gen Comp Endocrinol 1971;16:430

31. Copp DH. Endocrine regulation of calcium metabolism. Annu Rev Physiol 1970;32:61

32. Wollman SH, Spicer SS, Burstone MS. Localization of esterase and acid phosphatase in granules and colloid droplets in rat thyroid epithelium. J Cell Biol 1964;21:191

33. Wetzel BK, Spicer SS, Wollman SH. Changes in fine structure and acid phosphatase localization in rat thyroid cells following thyrotropin administration. J Cell Biol 1965;25:593

34. Ericson LE, Ring KM, Öfverholm T. Selective macropinocytosis of thyroglobulin in rat thyroid follicles. Endocrinology 1983;113:1746

35. Björkman U, Ekholm R, Ericson LE. Effects of thyrotropin on thyroglobulin exocytosis and iodination in the rat thyroid gland. Endocrinology 1978;102:460

36. Ericson LE, Engstrom G, Ekholm R. Effect of cycloheximide on thyrotropin-stimulated endocytosis in the rat thyroid. Endocrinology 1980;106:1119

37. Bernier-Valentin F, Kostrouch Z, Rabilloud R, Munari-Silem Y, Rousset B. Coated vesicles from thyroid cells carry iodinated thyroglobulin molecules: first indication for an internalization of the thyroid prohormone via a mechanism of receptor-mediated endocytosis. J Biol Chem 1990;265:17373

38. Romagnoli P, Herzog V. Transcytosis in thyroid follicle cells: regulation and implications for thyroglobulin transport. Exp Cell Res 1991;194:202

39. Brix K, Herzog V. Extrathyroidal release of thyroid hormones from thyroglobulin by J774 mouse macrophages. J Clin Invest 1994;93:1388

40. Wolff J, Williams JA. The role of microtubules and microfilaments in thyroid secretion. Recent Prog Horm Res 1973; 29:229

41. Capen CC. Mechnistic considerations for thyroid gland neoplasia with FD and red 3. In: The toxicology forum: Proceedings of the 1989 annual winter meeting. The Toxicology Forum, Washington, DC, 1989:113

42. Tice LW, Wollman SH. Ultrastructural localization of peroxidase on pseudopods and other structures of the typical thyroid epithelial cell. Endocrinology 1974;94:1555

43. Mizukami Y, Matsubara F, Matsukawa S. Cytochemical localization of peroxidase and hydrogen-peroxide-producing NAD(P)H-oxidase in thyroid follicular cells of propylthiouracil-treated rats. Histochem 1985;82:263

44. Foti D, Rapoport B. Carbohydrate moieties in recombinant human thyroid peroxidase: role in recognition by antithyroid peroxidase antibodies in Hashimoto's thyroiditis. Endocrinology 1990;126:2983

45. Öfverholm T, Ericson LE. Intraluminal iodination of thyroglobulin. Endocrinology 1984;114:827

46. Nadler NJ, Young BA, Leblond CP, Mitmaker B. Elaboration of thyroglobulin in the thyroid follicle. Endocrinology 1964; 74:333

47. Whur P, Herscovics A, Leblond CP. Radioautographic visualization of the incorporation of galactose-^{3}H and mannose-^{3}H by rat thyroids in vitro in relation to the stages of thyroglobulin synthesis. J Cell Biol 1969;43:289

48. Loewenstein JE, Wollman SH. Distribution of ^{125}I and ^{127}I in the rat thyroid during equilibrium labeling as determined by autoradiography. Endocrinology 1967;81:1074

49. Öfverholm T, Björkman U, Ericson LE. Effects of TSH on iodination in rat thyroid follicles studied by autoradiography. Mol Cell Endocrinol 1985;40:1

50. Wollman SH, Ekholm R. Site of iodination in hyperplastic thyroid glands deduced from autoradiographs. Endocrinology 1981; 108:2082

51. Gorbman A. Comparative anatomy and physiology. In: Ingbar SH, Braverman LE, eds. Werner's the thyroid: a fundamental and clinical text. 5th ed. Philadelphia: JB Lippincott, 1986:43

52. Gorbman A. Thyroid function and its control in fishes. In: Hoar WS, Randall DJ, eds. Fish physiology. New York: Academic Press, 1969:241

53. Roche J, Fontaine M, Leloup J. Halides. In: Florkin M, Mason HS, eds. Comparative biochemistry. New York: Academic Press, 1963:493

54. Gorbman A, Clements, M, O'Brien R. Utilization of radioiodine by invertebrates with special study of several annelida and mollusca. J Exp Zool 1954;127:75

55. Roche J. Biochimie comparée des scléroprotéines des Anthozoaires et des Spongiaires. Experientia 1952;8:45

56. Spangenberg DB. Thyroxine induced metamorphosis in Aurelia. J Exp Zool 1972;178:183

57. Brisson A, Marchelidon J, Lachiver F. Comparative studies on the amino acid composition of thyroglobulins from various lower and higher vertebrates: phylogenetic aspect. Comp Biochem Physiol [B] 1974;49:51

58. Salvatore G. Thyroid hormone biosynthesis in Agnatha and Protochordata. Gen Comp Endocrinol [Suppl] 1969;2:535

59. Spangenberg DB. Thyroxine in early strobilation in *Aurelia aurita*. Am Zool 1974;14:825

60. Suzuki S, Gorbman A, Rolland M, Montort M, Lissitsky S. Thyroglobulins of cyclostomes and an elasmobranch. Gen Comp Endocrinol 1975;26:59

61. Packard GC, Packard MJ, Gorbman A. Serum thyroxine concentrations in the Pacific hagfish and lamprey and in the leopard frog. Gen Comp Endocrinol 1976;28:365

62. Regard E, Taurog A, Nakajima T. Plasma thyroxine and triiodothyronine levels in spontaneously metamorphosing *Rana*

catebeiana tadpoles and in adult anuran Amphibia. Endocrinology 1978;102:674

63. Leloup J, Buscaglia M. Thyroxine metabolism in *Xenopus laevis* tadpoles. In: Stockigt JR, Nagataki S, eds. Thyroid research. Canberra: Australian Academy of Science, 1980:233

64. Rosenkilde P. Regulation of thyrotropic function of the pituitary gland in Amphibia. In: Gaillard PJ, Boer HH, eds. Comparative endocrinology. Amsterdam: Elsevier, 1978

65. Galton VA. Thyroid hormone receptors and iodothyronine deiodinases in the developing Mexican axolotl, *Ambystoma mexicanum*. Gen Comp Endocrinol 1992;85:62

66. Buckbinder L, Brown DD. Thyroid hormone-induced gene expression changes in the developing frog limb. J Biol Chem 1992;267:25786

67. Kanamori A, Brown DD. The regulation of thyroid hormone receptor β genes by thyroid hormone in *Xenopus laevis*. J Biol Chem 1992;267:739

68. Yamauchi K, Kasahara T, Hayashi H, Horiuchi R. Purification and characterization of a 3,5,3′,-L-triiodothyronine-specific binding protein from bullfrog tadpole plasma: a homolog of mammalian transthyretin. Endocrinology 1993;132:2254

69. Glennemeier KA, Licht P. Binding affinities of thyroxine-binding proteins in turtle plasma. Gen Comp Endocrinol 1993; 90:78

70. Dickhoff WW, Folmar LC, Gorbman A. Changes in plasma thyroxine during smoltification of coho salmon, *Oncorhynchus kisutch*. Gen Comp Endocrinol 1978;36:229

71. Grau EG, Dickhoff WW, Nishioka RS, Folmar LC. Lunar phasing of the thyroxine surge preparatory to seaward migration of salmonid fish. Science 1981;211:607

72. Galton VA, Munck K. Metabolism of thyroxine in *Rana catesbeiana* tadpoles during metamorphic climax. Endocrinology 1981;109:1127

73. Eales JG. In vivo determination of thyroxine deiodination in rainbow trout, *Salmo gairdneri*. Gen Comp Endocrinol 1977; 32:89

74. Eales JG, Morin PP, Tsang P, Hara TJ. Thyroid hormone deiodination in brain, liver, gill, heart and muscle of Atlantic salmon (*Salmo salar*) during photoperiodically-induced parr-smolt transformation: II. outer- and inner-ring 3,5,3′-triiodo-l-thyronine and 3,3′,5′-triiodo-l-thyronine (reverse T$_3$) deiodination. Gen Comp Endocrinol 1993;90:157

75. Cohen PP. Biochemical differentiation during amphibian metamorphosis. Science 1970;168:533

76. Frieden E. Thyroid hormones and the biochemistry of amphibian metamorphosis. Recent Prog Horm Res 1967;23:139

77. Sage M. The evolution of thyroid function in fishes. Am Zool 1973;13:899

78. Jackson RG, Sage M. Regional distribution of thyroid stimulating hormone activity in the pituitary gland of the Atlantic stingray. Fishery Bulletin 1973;71:93

79. Grimm-Jorgensen Y, McElvy JF. Biosynthesis of thyrotropin-releasing factor by newt (*Triturus viridescens*) brain in vitro: isolation and characterization of thyrotropin-releasing factor. Neurochemistry 1974;23:471

80. Jackson IM, Reichlin S. Thyrotropin releasing hormone (TRH): distribution in hypothalamic and extrahypothalamic brain tissues of mammalian and submammalian chordates. Endocrinology 1974;95:854

81. Jacobs GFM, Kühn ER. Thyroid hormone feedback regulation of the secretion of bioactive thyrotropin in the frog. Gen Comp Endocrinol 1992;88:415

82. Kaye NW. Interrelationships of the thyroid and pituitary in embryonic and premetamorphic stages of the frog, *Rana pipiens*. Gen Comp Endocrinol 1961;1:1

83. Rosenkilde P. Role of feedback in amphibian thyroid regulation. Fortschr Zool 1974;22:99

84. Licht P, Denver RJ, Stamper DL. Relation of plasma thyroxine binding to thyroidal activity and determination of thyroxine binding proteins in a turtle, *Pseudemys scripta*. Gen Comp Endocrinol 1990;80:238

85. Licht P, Moore MF. Structure of a reptilian plasma thyroxine binding protein indicates homology to vitamin D-binding protein. Arch Biochem Biophys 1994;309:47

86. Licht P. Thyroxine-binding protein represents the major vitamin D-binding protein in the plasma of the turtle, *Trachemys scripta*. Gen Comp Endocrinol 1994;93:82

87. Zbinden G. Hyperplastic and neoplastic responses of the thyroid gland in toxicological studies. Arch Toxicol [Suppl] 1988; 12:98

88. Capen CC, Martin SL. The effects of xenobiotics on the structure and function of thyroid follicular and C-cells. Toxicol Pathol 1989;17:266

89. Döhler K-D, Wong CC, von zur Mühlen A. The rat as model for the study of drug effects on thyroid function: consideration of methodological problems. Pharmacol Ther 1979;5:305

90. Sharifi J, St. Germain DL. The cDNA for the type I iodothyronine 5′-deiodinase encodes an enzyme manifesting both high K$_m$ and low K$_m$ activity. J Biol Chem 1992;267:12539

91. Capen CC. Mechanisms of chemical injury of the thyroid gland. In: Spitzer HL, Slaga TJ, Greenlee WF, McClain M, eds. Receptor-mediated biological processes: implications for evaluating carcinogens. Proceedings of the Barton Creek conference on carcinogenesis and risk assessment. Progress in Clinical and Biological Research Series. Washington, DC: Wiley-Liss/ISLI Press, 1994:193

92. De Sandro V, Chevrier M, Boddaert A, Melcion C, Cordier A, Richert L. Comparison of the effects of propylthiouracil, amiodarone, diphenylhydantoin, phenobarbital, and 3-methylcholanthrene on hepatic and renal T$_4$ metabolism and thyroid gland function in rats. Toxicol Appl Pharmacol 1991;111:263

93. Saito K, Kaneko H, Sato K, Yoshitake A, Yamada H. Hepatic UDP-glucuronyltransferase(s) activity toward thyroid hormones in rats: induction and effects on serum thyroid hormone levels following treatment with various enzyme inducers. Toxicol Appl Pharmacol 1991;111:99

94. Smith PF, Grossman SJ, Gerson RJ, Gordon LR, DeLuca JG, Majka JA, Wang RW, Germershausen JI, MacDonald JS. Studies on the mechanism of simvastatin-induced thyroid hypertrophy and follicular cell adenoma in the rat. Toxicol Pathol 1991;19:197

95. Mori M, Naito M, Watanabe H, Takeichi N, Dohi K, Ito A. Effects of sex difference, gonadectomy, and estrogen on N-methyl-N-nitrosourea-induced rat thyroid tumors. Cancer Res 1990;50:7662

96. Sinha N, Lal B, Singh TP. Pesticides induced changes in circulating thyroid hormones in the freshwater catfish *Clarias batrachus*. Comp Biochem Physiol 1991;100C:107

97. Doniach I. Aetiological consideration of thyroid carcinoma. In: Smithers D, ed. Tumors of the thyroid gland. London: E & S Livingstone, 1970:55

98. Curran PG, DeGroot LJ. The effect of hepatic enzyme-inducing drugs on thyroid hormones and the thyroid gland. Endocr Rev 1991;12:135

99. McClain RM, Levin AA, Posch R, Downing JC. The effects of phenobarbital on the metabolism and excretion of thyroxine in rats. Toxicol Appl Pharmacol 1989;99:216

100. Ambesi-Impiombato FS. Living, fast-growing thyroid cell strain, FRTL-5. United States Patent #4,608,341

101. Brandi ML, Rotella CM, Mavilia C, Franceschelli F, Tanini A, Toccafondi R. Insulin stimulates all growth of a new strain of differentiated rat thyroid cells. Mol Cell Endocrinol 1987;54:91

102. Kowalski K, Babiarz D, Burke G. Phagocytosis of latex beads by isolated thyroid cells: effects of thyrotropin, prostaglandin E$_1$, and dibutyryl cyclic AMP. J Lab Clin Med 1972;79:258

103. Reader SCJ, Davison B, Ratcliffe JG, Robertson WR. Measurement of low concentration of bovine thyrotrophin by iodide uptake and organification in porcine thyrocytes. J Endocrinol 1985;106:13

104. Rodesch FR, Neve P, Dumont JE. Phagocytosis of latex beads by isolated thyroid cells. 1970;60:354

105. Smith P, Wynford-Thomas D, Stringer BMJ, Williams ED. Growth factor control of rat thyroid follicular cell proliferation. Endocrinology 1986;119:1439

106. Weiss SJ, Philp NJ, Grollman EF. Iodide transport in a continuous line of cultured cells from rat thyroid. Endocrinology 1984; 114:1090

107. Avvedimento VE, Monticelli A, Tramontano D, Polistina C, Nitsch L, DiLauro R. Differential expression of thyroglobulin gene in normal and transformed thyroid cells. Eur J Biochem 1985;149:467

108. Bone E, Kohn LD, Chomczynski P. Thyroblobulin gene activation by thyrotropin and cAMP in hormonally depleted FRTL-5 thyroid cells. Biochem Biophys Res Comm 1986;141:1261

109. Graves PN, Davies TF. A second thyroglobulin messenger RNA species (rTg-2) in rat thyrocytes. Mol Endocrinol 1990; 4:155

110. Isozaki O, Tsushima T, Emoto N, Saji M, Tsuchiya Y, Demura H. Sato Y, Shizume K, Kimura S, Kohn LD. Methimazole regulation of thyroblobulin biosynthesis and gene transcription in rat FRTL-5 thyroid cells. Endocrinology 1991;128:3113

111. Lee NT, Kamikubo K, Chai K-J, Kao L-R, Sinclair AJ, Nayfeh SN, Chae C-B. The deoxyribonucleic acid regions involved in the hormonal regulation of thyroglobulin gene expression. Endocrinology 1991;128:111

112. Santisteban P, Kohn LD, DiLauro R. Thyroblobulin gene expression is regulated by insulin and insulin-like growth factor I, as well as thyrotropin, in FRTL-5 thyroid cells. J Biol Chem 1987; 262:4048

113. Consiglio E, Acquaviva AM, Formisano S, Liguoro D, Gallo A, Vittorio T, Santisteban P, DeLuca M, Shifrin S, Yeh JC, Kohn LD. Characterization of phosphate residues on thyroglobulin. 1987; 262:10304

114. DiJeso B, Gentile F. TSH-induced galactose incorporation at the NH$_2$ terminus of thyroglobulin secreted by FRTL-5 cells. Biochem Biophys Res Comm 1992;189:1624

115. Leer LM, Ossendorp FA, de Vijlder JJM. TSH action on iodination in FRTL-5 cells. Horm Metab Res [Suppl] 1990;23:43

116. Ossendrop FA, Leer LM, Bruning PF, van den Brink JAM, Sterk A, de Vijlder JJM. Iodination of newly synthesized thyroglobulin by FRTL-5 cells is selective and thyrotropin dependent. Mol Cell Endocrinol 1989;66:199

117. Damante G, Chazenbalk G, Russo D, Rapoport B, Foti D, Filetti S. Thyrotropin regulation of thyroid peroxidase messenger ribonucleic acid levels in cultured rat thyroid cells: evidence for the involvement of a nontranscriptional mechanism. Endocrinology 1989;124:2889

118. Zarrilli R, Formisano S, DiJeso B. Hormonal regulation of thyroid peroxidase in normal and transformed rat thyroid cells. Mol Endocrinol 1990;4:39

119. Giraud A, Franc J-L, Long Y, Ruf J. Effects of deglycosylation of human thyroperoxidase on it enzymatic activity and immunoreactivity. J Endocrinol 1992;132:317

120. Ozaki A, Sagartz JE, Capen CC. Phagocytic activity of FRTL-5 rat thyroid follicular cells as measured by ingestion of fluorescent latex beads. Exp Cell Res 1995;219:547

121. Sagartz JE, Ozaki A, Capen CC. Phagocytosis of fluorescent beads by rat thyroid follicular cells (FRTL-5): comparison with iodide trapping as an index of functional activity of thyrocytes in vitro. Toxicol Path 1995;23 (in press)

ANATOMY AND PATHOLOGY OF THE THYROTROPHS

Kalman Kovacs
Eva Horvath
Lucia Stefaneanu

Although it had been known for a long time that the pituitary regulates the functional activity of the thyroid gland and produces a hormone called thyroid-stimulating hormone (thyrotropin; TSH), it was only about 50 years ago that the adenohypophysial cell type that produces TSH was morphologically identified. In studies of the pituitaries of rats that had altered function of the thyroid and other glands, using periodic acid—Schiff (PAS) and various trichrome, aldehyde fuchsin, and aldehyde thionin (AT) staining techniques, several investigators delineated the thyrotroph in the rat pituitary anterior lobe.[1,2] Subsequently, the fine structural features of rat thyrotrophs were revealed by transmission electron microscopy, and the ultrastructural alterations resulting from functional changes were disclosed.[3] Several attempts were also made, applying these and other staining procedures, to identify the thyrotrophs in the human pituitary, but real progress became possible only after the introduction of immunocytochemistry and electron microscopy.

DEVELOPMENT AND ANATOMY

The thyrotrophs can be detected by immunocytochemistry during the 12th week of gestation in the anteromedial zone of the fetal pituitary.[4] They become recognizable at about the same time as the gonadotrophs, after the appearance of the somatotrophs and corticotrophs and before that of the lactotrophs. Bioactive TSH is detected in the pituitary at 14 weeks of gestation. The thyrotrophs also develop in anencephalic fetuses, and tissue culture studies indicate that their differentiation and maturation are independent of the presence of hypothalamic hormones.[5,6] A recently discovered transcription factor, termed *pit-1*, plays a major role in the maturation of thyrotrophs as well as somatotrophs and lactotrophs.[7,8]

In the human pituitary, the thyrotrophs represent 1% to 5% of all adenohypophysial cell types. They are not randomly located throughout the gland but are concentrated in the anteromedial portion of the mucoid wedge of the anterior lobe; thus, they are not in proximity to the posterior lobe. In this well demarcated area, the thyrotrophs are the predominant cell type[9] (Fig 3-24). They contain PAS-, aldehyde fuchsin-, and AT-positive cytoplasmic granules, but they are less basophilic and less PAS-positive than the corticotrophs. They do not stain with acidophilic dyes, lead hematoxylin, erythrosin, or carmoisin. Immunocytochemistry is the most reliable method to reveal the presence of thyrotrophs by light microscopy (Fig 3-25). In situ hybridization reveals the presence of estrogen receptor mRNA in nontumorous and adenomatous thyrotrophs.[10]

CYTOLOGY

By electron microscopy, the thyrotrophs are medium-sized or large, elongated cells with conspicuous cytoplasmic processes and centrally located spherical or ovoid nuclei (see Fig 3-23). The cytoplasm is abundant and its rough-surfaced endoplasmic reticulum consists of randomly distributed, slightly dilated cisternae. The Golgi complex is located in the perinuclear area; its prominence varies depending on the hormonal activity of the cell. The mitochondria are rod shaped with regular transverse cristae and a moderately electron-dense matrix. Phagolysosomes are common. The secretory granules are small, most often measuring 100 to 200 nm. They are spherical, vary slightly in electron density, and are membrane bound with an electron-lucent halo between the electron-dense core

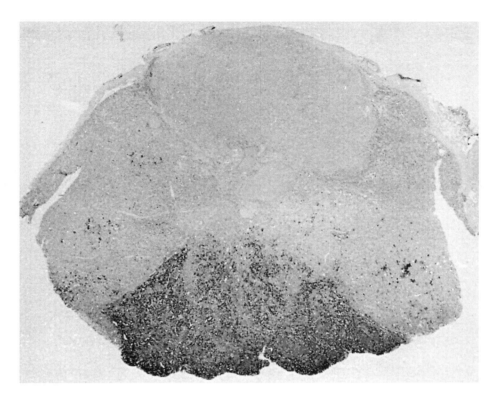

FIGURE 3-24. Photomicrograph of a human pituitary gland, showing thyrotrophs concentrated in the anteromedial portion of the gland. The section was immunostained for TSH using the avidin-biotin-perioxidase method (× 6).

and the limiting membrane. Secretory granule extrusions are not seen (Fig 3-26)

Immunocytochemistry shows strong immunoreactivity for the β-subunit of TSH and for the α-subunit, but not for other hormones.[9] Immunoelectron microscopy confirms that the thyrotrophs contain TSH localized in the secretory granules. In the rat pituitary, a few cells that contain both immunoreactive growth hormone and TSH can be identified,[11] suggesting a close link between somatotrophs and thyrotrophs and raising the possibility that somatotrophs can transform to thyrotrophs. Consistent with this suggestion, in the pituitaries of rats made hypothyroid by propylthiouracil administration, some somatotrophs degranulate and transform into thyroidectomy cells, exhibiting the ultrastructural signs of active secretion.[12] These

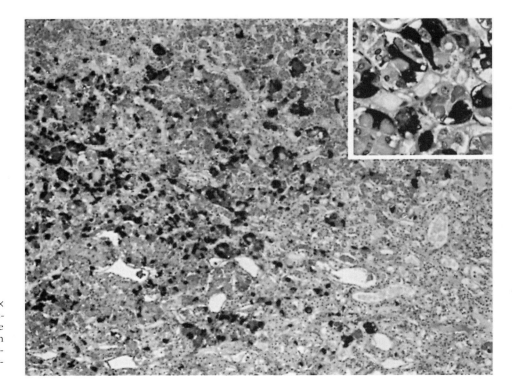

FIGURE 3-25. Low-magnification (× 250) and high-magnification (× 400, *inset*) photomicrographs of an area of the anterior lobe of a human pituitary rich in TSH-immunoreactive cells with long cytoplasmic processes (avidin-biotin-peroxidase method).

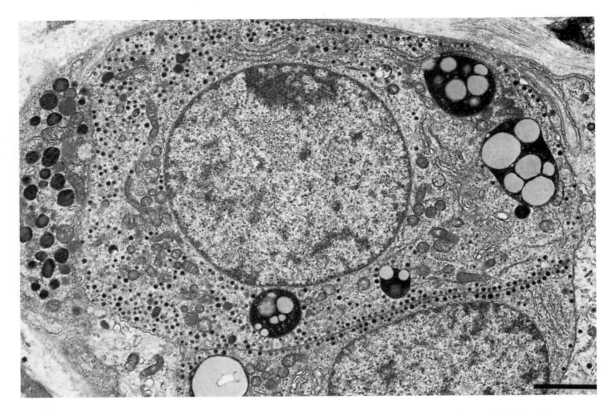

FIGURE 3-26. Electron photomicrograph of human thyrotrophs with euchromatic nuclei, well-developed cytoplasm, small secretory granules (100–200 nm), many of which are adjacent to the plasma membrane, and large phagolysosomes (× 11,000). Bar = 2 μm.

findings support the assumption that different adenohypophysial cell types cannot be conclusively separated and that under special conditions, one cell type may transform to another cell type and become able to produce the hormone characteristic of the latter cell type. Thus, the "one cell, one hormone" theory that dominated our thinking for several decades, which recognized five distinct cell types producing the six adenohypophysial hormones, is no longer accepted.[9,13,14]

The thyrotrophs can be demonstrated throughout life, and there are no major sex differences in their number, distribution, immunocytochemical profile, and histologic and ultrastructural features. They do not regress in old age and continue to produce and release TSH.[15] Indeed, the thyrotrophs are more prominent in older people in whom the incidence of subclinical and overt hypothyroidism is higher than in young or middle-aged people (see chap 26).

EFFECT OF THYROID DISORDERS ON PITUITARY MORPHOLOGY

Hypothyroidism

Changes in the secretion of TSH markedly affect the morphology of the thyrotrophs. In long-standing primary hypothyroidism, the thyrotrophs increase in number and size[16] (Figs 3-27 and 3-28). Reticulin stains show enlarged acinar structures without compression of surrounding tissue (Fig 3-29). The large thyrotrophs have an abundant vacuolated cytoplasm and long, prominent cytoplasmic processes, and they contain many large, strongly PAS-positive cytoplasmic globules, which are in fact large lysosomes. These latter structures, however, may occur in other conditions and in other cell types as well.[11,17]

Thyrotroph hyperplasia may be diffuse or nodular; the thyrotroph area within the anterior lobe enlarges, and the thyrotrophs extend to other parts of the anterior lobe. The extent of thyrotroph hypertrophy and hyperplasia may be sufficient to cause radiologically detectable enlargement of the pituitary and occasionally even optic nerve compression. Massive thyrotroph hyperplasia due to primary hypothyroidism thus may be difficult to distinguish clinically from a pituitary tumor causing secondary hypothyroidism. Also, several patients with marked thyrotroph hyperplasia have been misdiagnosed as having prolactin-producing pituitary adenomas because patients with long-standing primary hypothyroidism may have amenorrhea, galactorrhea, and hyperprolactinemia as well as pituitary enlargement.[18]

By electron microscopy, the hypertrophic and hyperplastic thyrotrophs of hypothyroid patients show different degrees of dilation and vesiculation of the endoplasmic reticulum, a prominent Golgi complex, and normal mitochondria. Also, compared with normal thyrotrophs, the secretory granules are less numerous and are similar in size or are slightly enlarged (Fig 3-30). No exocytosis is seen.[11]

In hypothyroid rats, the thyrotrophs also are large and have pale, vacuolated cytoplasm. Electron microscopy reveals prominent endoplasmic reticulum membranes and Golgi complexes. The endoplasmic reticulum is dilated and vesiculated.

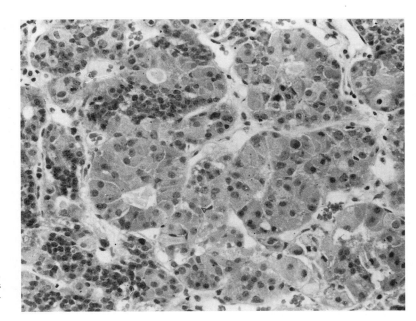

FIGURE 3-27. Photomicrograph of thyrotroph hyperplasia, showing large acinar structures formed by columnar cells possessing abundant, slightly vacuolated cytoplasm (hematoxylin and eosin; × 220).

The secretory granules in these thyrotrophs are small and sparse, measuring 50 to 150 nm.[11] These stimulated cells are called thyroidectomy or thyroid deficiency cells and are assumed to represent hyperactive cells due to protracted stimulation secondary to the lack of negative feedback action of thyroid hormones.[11] Occasionally, thyrotroph hyperplasia may progress to adenoma formation, suggesting that protracted stimulation may not only increase TSH synthesis and release and cell proliferation, but cause neoplastic transformation.

In humans and animals with primary hypothyroidism, thyroid hormone therapy results in regression of the morphologic changes in the pituitary, indicating that the hypertrophy and hyperplasia of thyrotrophs are reversible.

The morphology of thyrotrophs in thyrotropin-releasing hormone deficiency has not yet been described, nor have thyrotropin-releasing hormone–producing tumors been reported. In the former situation, TSH secretion is decreased, and one would expect this decrease to be accompanied by morphologic changes that reflect decreased functional activity. In a rare familial form of dwarfism accompanied by prolactin deficiency and hypothyroidism, the pituitary contains no somatotrophs, lactotrophs, and thyrotrophs.[19] This syndrome is

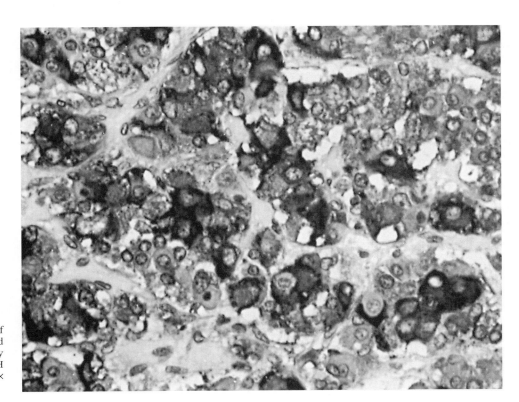

FIGURE 3-28. Photomicrograph of thyrotroph hyperplasia. The enlarged acini contain numerous cells intensely or moderately immunostained for TSH (avidin-biotin-peroxidase method; × 250).

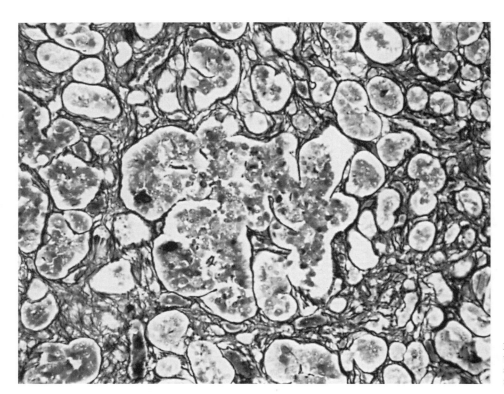

FIGURE 3-29. Reticulin-stained section of thyrotroph hyperplasia, showing enlarged acinar structures and loosened reticulin network (× 100).

assumed to be caused by mutation of the *pit-1* gene.[20,21] The simultaneous absence of somatotrophs, lactotrophs, and thyrotrophs in this uncommon type of hypopituitarism confirms the close relationship among these three adenohypophysial cell types.

Hyperthyroidism

Pituitary morphology has not been studied much in hyperthyroid patients. In 1966, Murray and Ezrin[22] described the light microscopic features of thyrotrophs in patients with hy-

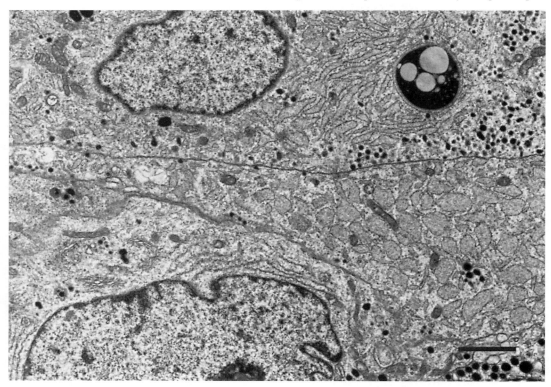

FIGURE 3-30. Electron photomicrograph of stimulated thyrotrophs in the pituitary of a patient with hypothyroidism. The rough endoplasmic reticulum is well-developed and dilated or vesiculated. A lactotroph is shown at the bottom of the micrograph (× 9000) Bar = 2 μm.

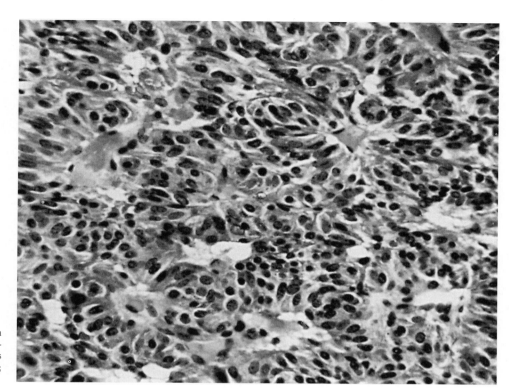

FIGURE 3-31. Photomicrograph of a thyrotroph adenoma. The chromophobic cells are disposed in pseudorosettes around vessels (hematoxylin and eosin; × 250).

perthyroidism due to Graves' disease. Using conventional histology as well as AT staining, they demonstrated regression of thyrotrophs in these patients. Well granulated thyrotrophs could not be identified, and the cells resembling thyrotrophs were decreased in size and had small nuclei, a thin rim of cytoplasm, and a few AT-positive vesicles. Studies using immunocytochemical techniques confirmed the re-

versible involution of thyrotrophs in patients with hyperthyroid Graves' disease.[23]

Other Conditions

In other endocrine or nonendocrine diseases, the thyrotrophs are not altered. For example, in patients with Addison's dis-

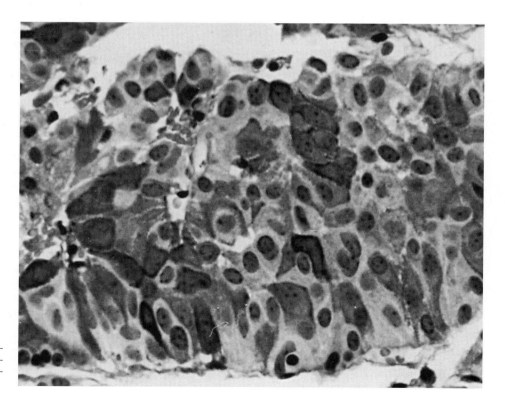

FIGURE 3-32. Photomicrograph of a thyrotroph adenoma. Most cells contain immunoreactive TSH (avidin-biotin-peroxidase method; × 250).

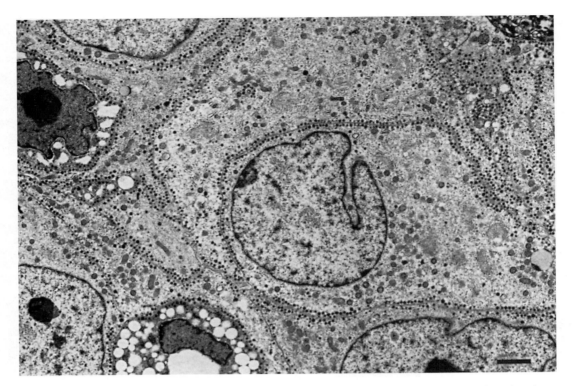

FIGURE 3-33. Electron photomicrograph of a thyrotroph adenoma, showing thyrotrophs with indented nuclei containing large nucleoli and long cytoplasmic processes. Small secretory granules are present at the periphery of the cytoplasm (× 5000). Bar = 2 μm.

ease or primary hypogonadism, the number, size, distribution, and morphologic appearance of the thyrotrophs are normal. Similarly the thyrotrophs are normal in patients with pituitary tumors not associated with TSH oversecretion.

Thyrotroph Adenomas

Thyrotroph adenomas occur but are the rarest type of anterior pituitary tumor.[17,24,25] One case of a thyrotroph carcinoma has been described.[26] It is not clear why adenomas arise less frequently in thyrotrophs than in other cell types. Thyrotroph adenomas may develop in association with hyperthyroidism (see chap 31) or hypothyroidism.[27–30] Morphologically, there is no consistent difference among the various forms.

At the time of discovery, thyrotroph adenomas in patients with hyperthyroidism range in size from microadenomas to large macroadenomas that occupy the entire sella turcica and may extend above it or invade neighboring structures. They are often well demarcated and surrounded by a pseudocapsule that consists of condensed reticulin fibers and a few rows of compressed nontumorous adenohypophysial cells. The adenoma cells are chromophobic (Fig 3-31) and contain a few small PAS-positive cytoplasmic granules or, occasionally, large PAS-positive lysosomal globules. Immunocytochemistry demonstrates the presence of TSH in the cytoplasm of the adenoma cells (Fig 3-32) of most tumors, but in some tumors the adenoma cells cannot be immunostained, suggesting either loss of TSH during fixation and embedding or production of an abnormal TSH that is not immunoreactive.[9] Nontumorous and adenomatous thyrotrophs express *pit-1*, the transcrip-

tion factor responsible for the development and maturation of thyrotrophs. *Pit-1*, however, plays no major role in the pathogenesis of thyrotroph adenomas.[31,32]

By electron microscopy, thyrotroph adenomas are composed of middle-sized or large, usually well differentiated, moderately polar, elongated cells that have spherical nuclei showing focal pleomorphism and prominent nucleoli as well as abundant cytoplasm with long cytoplasmic processes (Fig 3-33). The cytoplasm contains well developed rough endoplasmic reticulum membranes. The Golgi complexes, poorly represented in some tumors but well developed in others, are located in the perinuclear area and are composed of sacs, vesicles, and a few immature secretory granules. The mitochondria are ovoid or spherical, with transverse cristae and a moderately electron-dense matrix. The secretory granules are mostly spherical and usually small, measuring 100 to 200 nm in diameter (see Fig 3-33); occasionally, adenomas have larger secretory granules (up to 400 nm). The secretory granules accumulate in the cytoplasmic processes and are often located in a single row underneath the plasmalemma, but granule exocytosis is not seen.

Thyrotroph adenomas rarely contain thyroidectomy cells. In a few tumors, however, usually in hypothyroid or euthyroid patients, the adenoma cells have the appearance of typical thyroidectomy cells. The importance of thyroidectomy cells in thyrotroph adenomas is not known, but the finding could reflect the absence of thyroid hormone receptors in the tumors. The absence of thyroidectomy cells in most tumors may reflect immaturity or the absence of thyrotropin-releasing hormone receptors.[33]

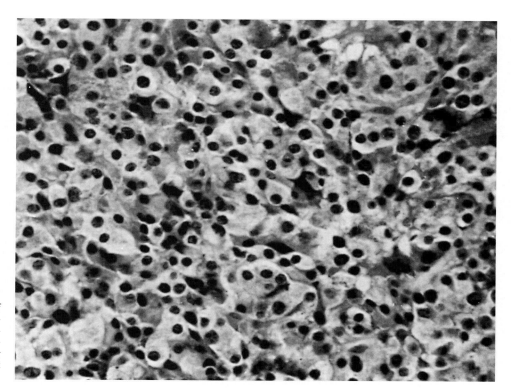

FIGURE 3-34. Photomicrograph of a glycoprotein-producing pituitary adenoma containing scattered TSH-immunoreactive cells (avidin-biotin-peroxidase method; × 250). This tumor also contained GH and α-subunit (not shown).

With the wider use of immunocytochemistry and electron microscopy, it has become evident that TSH-producing cells occur often in other hormone-secreting pituitary adenomas,[13,17,34,35] especially adenomas that contain growth hormone, TSH, and α-subunit. Most of these tumors are composed of densely granulated somatotrophs and are associated with acromegaly.[36] There also are adenomas that contain growth hormone or prolactin, or both, along with TSH and α-subunit, with the structural features of glycoprotein-producing adenomas[37] (Fig 3-34). Ultrastructurally, they are monomorphic adenomas that consist of cells with the characteristics of thyrotrophs.[17,37] Such tumors may be associated with

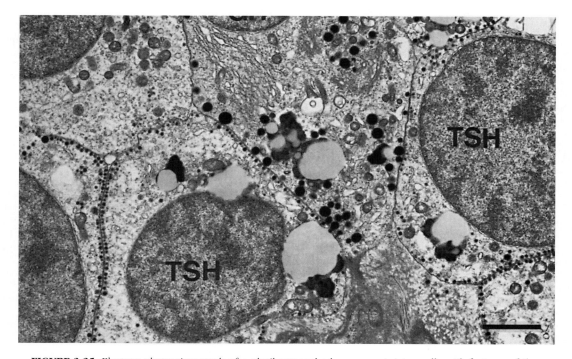

FIGURE 3-35. Electron photomicrograph of a plurihormonal adenoma containing cells with features of thyrotrophs (TSH) and somatotrophs (GH). The thyrotrophs contain small secretory granules lined up along the cell membranes. The cell with large secretory granules (up to 500 nm) and rough endoplasmic reticulum arranged in parallel stacks between the TSH cells is a somatotroph (× 9000). Bar = 2 μm.

acromegaly and hyperthyroidism.[17,36] Plurihormonal adenomas composed of different cell types indicating multidirectional differentiation have also been described[38] (Fig 3-35); usually, the expressed hormones are not secreted in clinically significant amounts. Null cell adenomas and oncocytomas often include a few scattered cells or groups of cells that contain immunoreactive TSH.[17] These clinically nonfunctioning tumors are thought to be derived from an uncommitted precursor cell, which may undergo multi- directional differentiation and produce various hormones, including TSH.

References

1. Halmi NS. Two types of basophils in anterior pituitary of rat and their respective cytophysiological significance. Endocrinology 1950;47:289

2. Purves HD. Cytology of the adenohypophysis. In: Harris GW, Donovan BT, eds. The pituitary gland. Vol 1. Anterior pituitary. London: Butterworths, 1966:147

3. Farquhar MG, Rinehart JF. Cytologic alterations in the pituitary gland following thyroidectomy: an electron microscopic study. Endocrinology 1954;55:857

4. Asa SL, Kovacs K, Singer W. Human fetal adenohypophysis: morphologic and functional analysis in vitro. Neuroendocrinology 1991;53:562

5. Dubois PM, Begeot M, Dubois MP, Herbert DC. Immunocytological localization of LH, FSH, TSH and their subunits in the pituitary of normal and anencephalic human fetuses. Cell Tissue Res 1978;191:249

6. Dubois PM, Hemming FJ. Fetal development and regulation of pituitary cell types. J Electron Microsc Tech 1991;19:2

7. Li S, Crenshaw EB III, Ranson EJ, Simmons DM, Swanson LW, Rosenfeld MG. Dwarf locus mutants lacking three pituitary cell types result from mutations in the POU-domain gene pit-1. Nature 1990;347:528

8. Pfäffle RW, DiMattia GE, Parks JS, et al. Mutation of the POU-specific domain of pit-1 and hypopituitarism without pituitary hypoplasia. Science 1992;257:1118

9. Kovacs K, Horvath E. Tumors of the pituitary gland. In Hartman WH, ed. Atlas of tumor pathology. 2nd series. Fascicle 21. Washington, DC: Armed Forces Institute of Pathology, 1986

10. Stefaneanu L, Kovacs K, Horvath E, et al. In situ hybridization study of estrogen receptor messenger ribonucleic acid in human adenohypophysial cells and pituitary adenomas. J Clin Endocrinol Metab 1994;78:83

11. Horvath E, Kovacs K. Fine structural cytology of the adenohypophysis in rat and man. J Electron Microsc Tech 1988;8:401

12. Horvath E, Lloyd RV, Kovacs K. Propylthiouracyl-induced hypothyroidism results in reversible transdifferentiation of somatotrophs into thyroidectomy cells: a morphologic study of the rat pituitary including immunoelectron microscopy. Lab Invest 1990;63:511

13. Kovacs K, Horvath E, Asa SL, Stefaneanu L, Sano T. Pituitary cells producing more than one hormone: human pituitary adenomas. Trends Endocrinol Metab 1989;1:95

14. Thapar K, Stefaneanu L, Kovacs K, Horvath E, Asa SL. Plurihormonal pituitary tumors: beyond the one cell—one hormone theory. Endocr Pathol 1993;4:1

15. Sano T, Kovacs K, Scheithauer BW, Young WF Jr. Aging and the human pituitary gland. Mayo Clin Proc 1993;68:971

16. Scheithauer BW, Kovacs K, Randall RV, Ryan N. Pituitary gland in hypothyroidism: histologic and immunocytologic study. Arch Pathol Lab Med 1985;109:499

17. Horvath E, Kovacs K. The adenohypophysis. In: Kovacs K, Asa SL, eds. Functional endocrine pathology. Boston: Blackwell, 1991:245

18. Khalil A, Kovacs K, Sima AAF, Burrow GN, Horvath E. Pituitary thyrotroph hyperplasia mimicking prolactin-secreting adenoma. J Endocrinol Invest 1984;7:399

19. Asa SL, Kovacs K, Halasz A, Toszegi AM, Szücs P. Absence of somatotrophs, lactotrophs, and thyrotrophs in the pituitary of two dwarfs with hypothyroidism: deficiency of pituitary transcription factor-1? Endocr Pathol 1992;3:93

20. Ingraham HA, Albert VR, Chen R, et al. A family of POU-domain and pit-1 tissue-specific transcription factors in pituitary and neuroendocrine development. Annu Rev Physiol 1990; 52:773

21. Simmons DM, Voss JW, Ingraham HA, et al. Pituitary cell phenotypes involve cell-specific pit-1 mRNA translation and synergistic interactions with other classes of transcription factors. Genes Dev 1990;4:695

22. Murray S, Ezrin C. Effects of Graves' disease on the "thyrotroph" of the adenohypophysis. J Clin Endocrinol Metab 1966; 26:287

23. Scheithauer BW, Kovacs KT, Young WF Jr, Randall RV. The pituitary gland in hyperthyroidism. Mayo Clin Proc 1992;67:22

24. Klibanski A, Zervas NT. Diagnosis and management of hormone-secreting pituitary adenomas. N Engl J Med 1991; 324:822

25. Thapar K, Kovacs K, Laws ER Jr, Muller PJ. Pituitary adenomas: current concepts in classification, histopathology, and molecular biology. Endocrinologist 1993;3:39

26. Mixson AJ, Friedman TC, Katz DA, et al. Thyrotropin-secreting pituitary carcinoma. J Clin Endocrinol Metab 1993;76:529

27. Beckers A, Abs R, Mahler C, et al. Thyrotropin-secreting pituitary adenomas: report of seven cases. J Clin Endocrinol Metab 1991; 72:477

28. Gesundheit N, Petrick PA, Nissim M, et al. Thyrotropin-secreting pituitary adenomas: clinical and biochemical heterogeneity. Case reports and follow-up of nine patients. Ann Intern Med 1989;111:827

29. Mindermann T, Wilson CB. Thyrotropin-producing pituitary adenomas. J Neurosurg 1993;79:521

30. Wynne AG, Charib H, Scheithauer BW, Davis DH, Horvath E. Hyperthyroidism due to inappropriate secretion of thyrotropin. Am J Med 1992;92:15

31. Lloyd RV, Jin L, Chandler WF, Horvath E, Stefaneanu L, Kovacs K. Pituitary specific transcription factor messenger ribonucleic expression in adenomatous and nontumorous human pituitary tissues. Lab Invest 1993;69:570

32. Pellegrini I, Barlier A, Gunz G, et al. Pit-1 gene expression in the human pituitary and pituitary adenomas. J Clin Endocrinol Metab 1994;79:189

33. Chanson P, Li JY, Le Dafniet M, et al. Absence of receptors for thyrotropin (TSH)-releasing hormone in human TSH-secreting pituitary adenoma associated with hyperthyroidism. J Clin Endocrinol Metab 1988;66:447

34. Felix I, Asa SL, Kovacs K, Horvath E, Smyth HS. Recurrent plurihormonal bimorphous pituitary adenoma producing growth hormone, thyrotropin, and prolactin. Arch Pathol Lab Med 1994; 118:66

35. Terzolo M, Orlandi F, Basetti M, et al. Hyperthyroidism due to a pituitary adenoma composed of two different cell types, one secreting alpha-subunit alone and another cosecreting alpha-subunit and thyrotropin. J Clin Endocrinol Metab 1991;72:415

36. Scheithauer BW, Horvath E, Kovacs K, Laws ER Jr, Randall RV, Ryan N. Plurihormonal pituitary adenomas. Semin Diagn Pathol 1986;3:69

37. Kovacs K, Horvath E, Ezrin C, Weiss MH. Adenoma of the human pituitary producing growth hormone and thyrotropin: a histologic, immunocytologic and fine-structural study. Virchows Arch [A] 1982;395:59

38. Horvath E, Kovacs K, Scheithauer BW, et al. Pituitary adenomas producing growth hormone, prolactin and one or more glycoprotein hormones: a histologic, immunohistochemical and ultrastructural study of four surgically-removed tumors. Ultrastruct Pathol 1983;5:171

Werner and Ingbar's The Thyroid, Seventh Edition,
edited by Lewis E. Braverman and Robert D. Utiger.
Lippincott–Raven Publishers, Philadelphia, © 1996

Section B
Hormone Synthesis and Secretion

4

Hormone Synthesis

HORMONE SYNTHESIS: THYROID IODINE METABOLISM

Alvin Taurog

Iodine enters the thyroid follicular cells as inorganic iodide and is transformed through a series of metabolic steps into the thyroid hormones thyroxine (T_4) and triiodothyronine (T_3). The individual steps in this metabolic sequence may be characterized as follows: (1) active transport of iodide; (2) iodination of tyrosyl residues of thyroglobulin (Tg); (3) coupling of iodotyrosine molecules within Tg to form T_4 and T_3; (4) proteolysis of Tg, with release of free iodotyrosines and iodothyronines, and secretion of iodothyronines into the blood; (5) deiodination of iodotyrosines within the thyroid and reuse of the liberated iodide; and (6) deiodination of T_4 to T_3 by an enzyme similar to the type I 5′-deiodinase that catalyzes T_4 to T_3 conversion in extrathyroidal tissue.

Each of these processes is discussed in this chapter. Because of my particular interests, special attention is given to thyroid peroxidase (TPO), and to its role in the mechanism of iodination, coupling, and antithyroid drug action. The subject of thyroid hormone biosynthesis has also been reviewed by Ekholm[1,2] and by Gentile and coworkers.[3]

The actions of thyroid-stimulating hormone (TSH; thyrotropin), which exerts a stimulatory effect on all steps of iodine metabolism, are discussed in chapter 11.

IODIDE TRANSPORT

Iodine may be classified as a trace element: Wolff[4] described the thyroid gland as "an efficient collector of a rare element." The first step in the synthesis and storage of thyroid hormone is a mechanism for concentrating iodide from the extracellular fluid, variably referred to as the iodide transport mechanism, the iodide-concentrating mechanism, the iodide pump, or the iodide trap.

Methods of Quantitating Thyroid Iodide Transport

Thyroid iodide transport may be measured either in vivo or in vitro. In both situations, the further metabolism of iodide in the tissue is usually blocked with propylthiouracil (PTU) or methimazole (MMI), agents that block organic iodine formation effectively. Studies with cultured rat thyroid cells (FRTL-5 cells), which are restricted in their ability to iodinate Tg, have shown that the I⁻ transport system is not affected by PTU.[5] The most commonly used measure of thyroid iodide transport is the thyroid-to-serum or medium iodide concentration ratio. For in vivo measurements, this is denoted as T/S. For in vitro measurements, the values are expressed as T/M for slice experiments and C/M for experiments with isolated cells. Values for T/S [I⁻], T/M [I⁻], and C/M [I⁻] are usually measured by use of radioactive iodine (RAI) and are defined as follows:

$$T/S[I^-] \text{ or}$$

$$T/M[I^-] = \frac{RAI/g \text{ thyroid tissue}}{RAI/mL \text{ serum or medium}}$$

$$C/M[I^-] = \frac{RAI/mL \text{ packed cells}}{RAI/mL \text{ medium}}$$

The thyroid is able to attain remarkably high concentration gradients for iodide, values for T/S [I$^-$] in excess of 400 having been recorded. Detailed instructions for measuring T/S [I$^-$], T/M [I$^-$], and C/M [I$^-$], together with an analysis of various factors that influence these measurements, are given by Wolff.[6]

T/S[I$^-$], T/M[I$^-$], and C/M[I$^-$] represent the balance between influx and efflux of iodide after equilibrium has been attained. Wollman and Reed[7] devised a simple two-compartment model for the study of iodide transport kinetics in vivo and demonstrated that

$$T/S[I^-] = \frac{C/m}{k_{TB}}$$

where C (μL/min) is the unidirectional clearance of radioiodide from serum by the thyroid, m (mg) is the mass of thyroid tissue, and k_{TB} (min^{-1}) is the fractional rate of efflux of radioiodide from thyroid to serum. C/m and k_{TB} can be separately measured by techniques described by Wollman and Reed.[7] They demonstrated that factors that influence T/S [I$^-$] may differently affect C/m and k_{TB}.

It is clear, however, that the two-compartment model represents an oversimplification. As indicated later, it is known from radioautographic studies that iodide concentrated by the intact thyroid is rapidly transferred into the follicular lumen. Wollman and Reed, therefore, proposed a three-compartment model,[7] in which the overall exit rate constant k_{TB} depends not only on transport of iodide from cell to serum but on transport of iodide from cell to lumen and from lumen to cell. In this model, $k_{TB} = k_{LC} \cdot k_{CB}/k_{CL}$, where k_{LC}, k_{CB}, and k_{CL} are the fractional rates of efflux of radioiodide from lumen to cell, cell to serum, and cell to lumen, respectively. It is not possible to measure these individual rate constants in the intact thyroid. However, it may be possible to make such measurements in systems now developed[8–10] in which polarized follicle cells are grown in monolayer on a semipermeable membrane in a bicameral chamber (see discussion later).

Iodide transport in the thyroid may also be measured in terms of K_m.[11] The K_m values derived in this manner are similar to the K_m values of classic enzyme kinetics and may be considered to represent the iodide concentration required for half-saturation of the assumed carrier system. Values of about 30 μmol/L have been reported for thyroid slices[11] and thyroid cells[5] and of about 20 μmol/L for iodide-accumulating reconstituted phospholipid vesicles.[12] A significantly lower value (about 5 μmol/L) was reported for thyroid plasma membrane vesicles.[13] The capacity of the normal thyroid to accumulate iodide actively is on the order of 1 to 5 mmol/L. (See Wolff[6] for a more detailed discussion.)

Extrathyroidal Iodide Transport

The thyroid gland is not unique in its ability to concentrate iodide. This process is shared by a number of other tissues, including gastric mucosa, salivary glands, mammary glands, choroid plexus, ovaries (lower species), placenta, and skin.[4]

Because saliva is readily collected in humans, and also because RAI is secreted in saliva only in the form of iodide, concentration of RAI by salivary tissue has useful clinical applications.[14] One is in the measurement of serum inorganic iodide. The inorganic iodide concentration in serum, a necessary measurement for estimating absolute iodide uptake by the thyroid,[15] is usually too low to measure accurately by direct chemical methods. It can, however, be calculated from the specific activity of salivary iodide after administration of RAI by using the following formula (assuming equal specific activities for labeled iodide in saliva and plasma):

$$\text{Serum inorganic iodide} = \frac{\text{Salivary }^{127}I \times \text{serum RAI}}{\text{Salivary RAI}}$$

Because the concentration of inorganic iodide in saliva is about 50 times greater than that in serum, the measurement of salivary ^{127}I is well within the range of usual laboratory methods. The mechanism of iodide concentration in extrathyroidal tissues resembles that in the thyroid in the following respects, as summarized by Wolff[4]: (1) inhibition by thiocyanate (SCN$^-$), perchlorate (ClO$_4^-$), tetrafluoroborate (BF$_4^-$), and nitrate (NO$_3^-$); (2) concentration of a number of anions other than I$^-$; (3) inhibition by dinitrophenol and by cardiac glycosides such as ouabain; (4) a requirement for K$^+$; (5) half-saturation with iodide near 3×10^{-5} mol/L I$^-$; and (6) a possible genetic relationship, as shown by the simultaneous loss of the ability to concentrate iodide by the thyroid and salivary glands and gastric mucosa in patients with a congenital defect in thyroid iodide transport (see discussion later). However, the anion transport system of extrathyroidal tissues appears to differ from that of the thyroid in that thiocyanate is not concentrated by thyroid tissue, whereas it is readily concentrated by salivary tissue and by gastric mucosa.[4]

Competing Anions

A number of anions act as competitive inhibitors of iodide transport by the thyroid. These have been discussed in detail by Wolff.[4] The most clinically useful of the competing anions are perchlorate, thiocyanate, and pertechnetate. The former two are used in the RAI discharge test for the diagnosis of organification defects in the thyroid.[16,17] Perchlorate is a potent inhibitor of I$^-$ transport (K$_i$ in sheep thyroid slices, 4×10^{-7} mol/L), and it has proved effective in the treatment of hyperthyroidism.[18] It acts by both decreasing unidirectional clearance and increasing efflux of I$^-$.[19,20] Pertechnetate, with a K$_m$ of about 4×10^{-7} mol/L for transport in sheep thyroid slices,[4] is widely used in the form of TcO$_4^-$ for thyroid scanning. Its short half-life (6 hours), absence of β emission, and 140-keV gamma ray make it ideal for this purpose. TcO$_4^-$ has also been recommended for uptake studies to measure thyroid function.[21,22] In humans, TcO$_4^-$ does not become bound in the thyroid to an appreciable extent.[23] Presumably, therefore, it measures only the anion transport function of the gland. The increased uptake in hyperthyroidism is attributable entirely to stimulation of unidirectional clearance.[23]

Anatomic Considerations

Follicular architecture is not essential for iodide transport, because it has been shown by several groups[5,24,25] that isolated thyroid cells are capable of concentrating iodide from the surrounding medium. It was previously thought that cellular integrity was required for the demonstration of iodide transport.[4] However, several groups of investigators have used model systems for studying iodide transport in membranes derived from disrupted thyroid cells.[12,13,26] Radioautographic studies, however, indicate that [131]I⁻ concentrated by the intact thyroid is rapidly transferred into the follicular lumen.[27,28] It seems likely from these studies and from the high concentration ratios attainable in vivo that follicular organization plays an important role in iodide transport in vivo.

The site of active iodide transport in thyroid epithelial cells is the basolateral membrane. This was first inferred from thyroid radioautographic studies in mice injected with ^{131}I after receiving an acute injection of PTU to block organic iodine formation.[29] More direct evidence was obtained in studies with polarized monolayers of porcine thyroid cells in culture.[8] In this system, a continuous epithelium consisting of polarized follicle cells, joined by tight junctions, is formed on a microporous filter, which separates the apical and basal compartments of the culture chamber. This system makes it possible to study separately the effects of various agents on the basolateral and apical membranes.

The interior of thyroid epithelial cells maintains a negative potential with respect to both the extracellular space and the follicular lumen.[30] There is little or no difference in potential between lumen and extracellular space; both are 40 to 50 mV-positive with respect to the cell interior. Accordingly, I⁻ that is concentrated against the electrical gradient at the basal membrane can flow downhill with the electrical gradient across the apical membrane into the lumen. In this way, follicular architecture facilitates iodide accumulation in the lumen.

Entry of I⁻ from cell to lumen is *acutely* (within minutes) stimulated by TSH. This was demonstrated by Nilsson and colleagues,[9,10] using the monolayer culture system already mentioned. They proposed the existence of a cyclic adenosine monophosphate (cAMP)-regulated iodide channel mediating TSH-stimulated efflux across the apical membrane. This is of particular interest because TPO and the H_2O_2-generating system are localized in the apical plasma membrane. An apically located iodide channel could function in synchronizing the availability of iodide with that of other components involved in thyroid hormone biosynthesis.

Mechanism of Active Transport

Wolff[4] summarized the evidence that thyroid I⁻ transport meets all the criteria for an active transport mechanism. Iodide transport in sheep thyroid slices is sensitive to ouabain.[11] A variety of cardiac glycosides that inhibited adenosine triphosphatase (ATPase) activity in thyroid and submaxillary tissue also inhibited iodide transport to about the same degree.[31] Thyroid ouabain-sensitive ATPase activity and iodide transport were correlated in several species.

Transport of I⁻ across the thyroid cell membrane is definitely linked to transport of sodium. This has been demonstrated in isolated cells[5,25,32] and in model systems[12,13,26] and has led to the concept of a Na⁺–I⁻ cotransport (symport) system, with the ion gradient generated by Na⁺–K⁺ ATPase as the driving force. Na⁺-dependent transport systems have also been described for amino acids and for glucose. Presumably, such systems depend on a transporter in the membrane, linked to both Na⁺ and to the substance being transported.

Saito and coworkers[12] prepared phospholipid vesicles from porcine thyroid membranes and soybean phospholipids, which are capable of accumulating I⁻ in the presence of external Na⁺. The degree of I⁻ concentration was much less than that in thyroid cells, but the system was Na⁺ dependent and was inhibited by ClO_4^- and SCN⁻. These workers[33] also obtained evidence that the iodide transporter is a protein rather than a phospholipid, as had been previously proposed.[34]

O'Neill and coworkers[13] pointed out some disadvantages of the use of the proteolysosome system of Saito and associates and described the use of thyroid plasma membrane vesicles for characterizing the iodide transport mechanism. They found that iodide transport is electrogenic and totally Na⁺ dependent, with a Na⁺:I⁻ flux ratio larger than 1. Nakamura and colleagues[35] analyzed the kinetic properties of I⁻ uptake in a similar system. Extending the findings of O'Neill and coworkers,[13] they proposed that binding of at least two Na⁺ to the carrier molecule was required for the transport of one I⁻, and that Na⁺ binding occurred before I⁻ binding. Kaminsky and associates[26] made the surprising observation that Na⁺–I⁻ symport activity was present in membrane vesicles from TSH-deprived FRTL-5 cells, which lack iodide transporting activity. They suggested that an inactive form of the Na⁺–I⁻ symporter constitutively resides in the thyroid basolateral membrane, and that it requires TSH for activation.

Vilijn and Carrasco[36] used fractions of poly(A⁺) ribonucleic acid (RNA) from FRTL-5 cells to express the transporter in *Xenopus laevis* oocytes. They obtained evidence suggesting that the mRNA encoding the message for the Na⁺–I⁻ symporter was 2.8 to 4 kb in length. More recent progress toward molecular characterization of the Na⁺–I⁻ symporter has been reviewed by Carrasco.[37]

A simplified model for I⁻ transport at the basolateral membrane is presented in Figure 4-1. The model (adapted from Wolff[38]) is based on evidence from many sources indicating

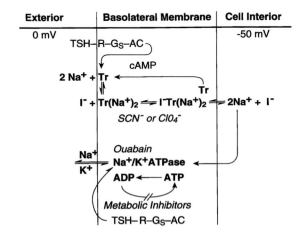

FIGURE 4-1. Proposed model for I transport at basolateral thyroid membrane. Transport components appear in bold type. Regulators appear in roman type, inhibitors in italics. Tr, transporter; R, receptor; Gs, GTP-binding protein; AC, adenylyl cyclase. (Adapted from Wolff J. Iodure. Le système de transport actif. In: Leclère J, Orgiazzi J, Rousset B, Schlienger J-L, Wémeau J-L, eds. La Thyroïde. Paris: Expansion Scientifique Française, 1992:17)

that the transport protein is a $Na^+–I^-$ symporter, which couples the inward movement of Na^+ down its electrochemical gradient to the simultaneous uphill translocation of I^- against its electrochemical gradient. The driving force for I^- uptake is the Na^+ gradient across the membrane generated by $Na^+–K^+$ ATPase.

Factors Influencing Iodide Transport

THYROID-STIMULATING HORMONE

Thyroid-stimulating hormone appears to be the most important factor affecting iodide transport in the thyroid. Values for T/S [I^-] are greatly decreased after hypophysectomy in rats and are restored or increased by injection of TSH[39,40] (Table 4-1). The response to injected TSH is biphasic—a transient depression reaching a minimal value in about 4 hours, followed by a slow increase. Halmi and coworkers[41] postulated that the initial depression in T/S [I^-] reflected an increase in k_{TB} and that the subsequent increase was the result of a slowly developed increase in C/M. The increase in k_{TB} was presumably caused by a rapid action of TSH on the cell membrane to accelerate iodide efflux. The slowly developed increase in C/M was thought to be related to the latent period required for the formation of a new enzyme or carrier involved in iodide transport. Evidence for this explanation of the biphasic response to TSH was obtained by Tong and coworkers using dispersed thyroid cells,[42] and by Weiss and coworkers using FRTL-5 cells.[43]

CYCLIC ADENOSINE MONOPHOSPHATE

The biphasic response of iodide transport to TSH in dispersed bovine thyroid cells is reproduced by dibutyryl cAMP,[42] suggesting that the effect of TSH on the iodide transport system is mediated entirely by cAMP. However, a dissociation between the acute effect of TSH on I^- efflux and on cAMP augmentation in FRTL-5 cells was reported by Weiss and coworkers.[44] Their results suggested that the TSH-induced iodide efflux is a Ca^{2+}-mediated response, independent of cAMP. In a later study from the same laboratory,[45] it was reported that in the presence of external Ca^{2+}, norepinephrine and arachidonic acid stimulated I^- efflux in FRTL-5 cells. The results with arachidonic acid suggested that TSH activated phospholipase A_2.

As mentioned earlier, Nilsson and colleagues,[9] using a monolayer of polarized porcine thyroid follicular cells in culture, observed that the stimulatory effect of TSH on iodide efflux at the apical membrane was cAMP dependent. Assuming that the I^- efflux observed by Weiss and coworkers in FRTL-5 cells (which are not polarized) is equivalent to the TSH-induced apical efflux demonstrated by Nilsson and colleagues with porcine thyrocytes, it appears that efflux in the two systems is regulated by different intracellular signals. However, it is not known whether this difference represents species variation or whether it reflects differences in regulation between thyrocytes in primary culture and a cell line obviously diverging from normal thyroid epithelium (e.g., by lack of cell polarity).

THYROID AUTOREGULATORY MECHANISM

Although TSH is the predominant factor affecting iodide transport, there is much evidence to indicate that the iodide transport system of the thyroid is subject to autoregulation by iodine, as are other facets of thyroid function.[46,47] This autoregulatory system, which is thought to be mediated by one or more forms of organic iodine, is responsible for the adaptation in iodide transport that occurs in response to chronic iodide administration.[48] The identity of the organic mediator has not been definitely established, but it was reported by Chazenbalk and colleagues[49] that iodide transport in calf thyroid slices can be inhibited by an iodinated form of arachidonic acid (see Effect of Iodine Excess). Both the intrinsic iodide transport activity and its responsiveness to TSH are sensitive to the total organic iodide concentration within the gland. (See Ingbar[46] and chap 13 for further discussions of thyroid autoregulation.)

Sherwin and Tong[50] developed a model for studying the autoregulatory phenomenon in dispersed thyroid cells. They studied the effects of I^- and of TSH on the thyroid iodide pump and concluded that iodide transport in the thyroid is

TABLE 4-1.
Kinetic Constants of Iodide Transport

Species	Diet and Treatment	T/S [I^-]	Unidirectional Clearance μL/mg/min	k_{TB}min^{-1}	Reference
Mouse	Iodine-sufficient	86	4.7	0.05	Wollman and Reed[7]
	Moderately iodine-deficient	192	9	0.041	Wollman and Reed[7]
	Hypophysectomized, moderately iodine-deficient	76	2.4	0.025	Wollman and Reed[7]
	Thiocyanate, moderately iodine-deficient	36	10	0.27	Wollman and Reed[7]
Rat	Iodine-sufficient	31	3.2	0.11	Wollman and Reed[7]
	Moderately iodine-deficient	115	15	0.12	Wollman and Reed[7]
	Hypophysectomized, moderately iodine-deficient	25	1.5	0.05	Wollman and Reed[7]
	Thiocyanate, moderately iodine-deficient	43	16	0.37	Wollman and Reed[7]
Guinea pig	Iodine-sufficient	~75			Wolff and Halmi[31]
	TSH-injected	400–500			Wolff and Halmi[31]
Human	Euthyroid	30–40	~0.8–2.5		Stanley and Astwood[39]

Adapted from Wolff J. Transport of iodide and other anions in the thyroid gland. Physiol Rev 1964;44:45

regulated by a complex dual-control system, with TSH increasing the maximum velocity (V_{max}) and iodide increasing the K_m.

Deficiency of Iodide Transport

Patients have been described who lack the ability to concentrate iodide in their thyroid glands.[34,51,52] Wolff[51] summarized information on 22 such patients and discussed the criteria for differentiating this condition from other defects in thyroid hormone biosynthesis (see chap 56). These patients usually lack the ability to concentrate iodide in saliva and gastric juice and respond favorably to treatment with large doses of iodide alone. Presumably, therefore, an active iodide transport mechanism is not absolutely essential for adequate thyroid hormone production. Under favorable conditions, enough I^- can be made to enter the gland by diffusion to allow production of normal amounts of thyroid hormone. However, long-term treatment of such patients is better accomplished with T_4.

CHEMICAL NATURE OF THYROID IODINE

19S Thyroglobulin

The greatest part of the iodine in normal thyroid glands exists in the form of Tg, a large dimeric protein molecule with a molecular weight of 660,000 and a sedimentation coefficient of 19S. Most of the Tg in the normal gland is present in the follicular lumen and has usually been assumed to be in soluble form. However, Herzog and coworkers[52a,52b] have provided evidence for an insoluble, covalently cross-linked form, which may comprise an appreciable fraction of luminal Tg in the thyroids of humans and other species. This insoluble form of Tg can be isolated as intact replicas of the luminal cavity of thyroid follicles. In humans, cross-linking occurs via disulfide bonds, and insoluble Tg constitutes, on average, about 34% of the total Tg in the lumen, varying between 3% and 85% in surgical material (Herzog V, personal communication). Tg does not have an unusual amino acid composition, but it is unique among body proteins in its content of iodinated amino acids. The structures of the iodoamino acids found in Tg are shown in Figure 4-2. The iodotyrosines, which form the most abundant iodinated amino acid components of Tg, have no biologic activity. They are considered to be the precursors of the biologically active hormones T_4 and T_3.

Purified Tg varies in total iodine content, depending on iodine intake. Normal human Tg varies widely in iodine content; values as low as 0.1%[53] and as high as 1.1% have been reported.[54] Reliable techniques for measuring the iodoamino acid distribution in Tg have been developed.[55] A careful analysis of normal human Tg containing 0.52% iodine yielded the following number of residues per molecule: monoiodotyrosine (MIT), 6.45; diiodotyrosine (DIT), 4.78; T_4, 2.28; T_3 0.29. These values correspond to a total of 27 atoms of iodine per molecule, of which 10 atoms, or 37%, are in the form of thyroid hormones, and 16 atoms, or 59%, are in the form of iodotyrosines. The slight discrepancy between total iodine and the sum of iodine in the form of iodinated amino acid is probably accounted for by deiodination during the proteolytic digestion of Tg. The iodoamino acid distribution in the thyroid varies with the degree of iodination of the Tg.[53,54,56,57] Further

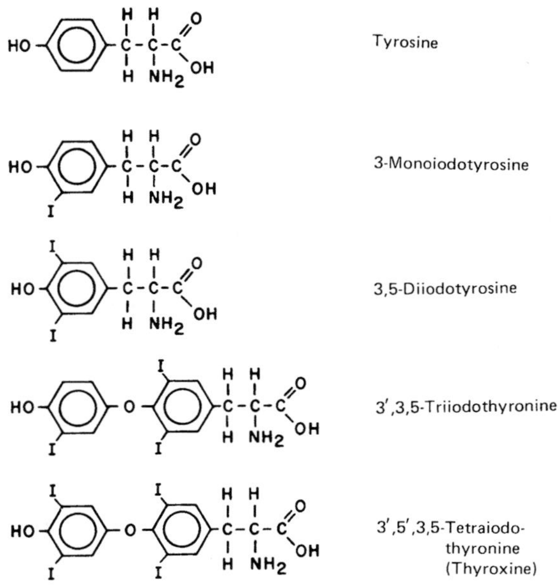

FIGURE 4-2. Structures of the major iodoamino acids found in thyroglobulin.

information about Tg is provided later in this chapter and in chapter 5.

Inorganic Iodide

The fraction of total glandular iodine present as inorganic iodide is usually low. In thyroids of iodine-sufficient rats, inorganic iodide comprises only about 0.25% of the total,[58] and even this low value may be an overestimate because of the difficulty of avoiding deiodination during the analytic procedure. Although inorganic iodide represents only a small fraction of the total iodine, its concentration in the thyroid is many-fold greater than that in the circulation.

Thyroid inorganic iodide is derived from two distinct sources: iodide transported from the serum (described previously), and iodide produced by deiodination of organic iodine compounds within the gland (internal iodide). The degree to which transported iodide and internal iodide are freely exchangeable has been a subject of controversy. Refinements in the measurement of radiolabeled internal iodide in rat thyroids have been reported by Hildebrandt and coworkers.[59,60] They concluded that iodide passes through a stage in which it is not available for organic binding,[59] but that it nevertheless does share a pool with external (transported) iodide.

Particulate-Bound Iodine

Particulate-bound iodine is usually measured as the iodine that sediments at 100,000 × g for 1 hour. The results obtained are influenced by homogenization techniques and other factors. A significant portion of total glandular iodine (about 10%) is frequently found in this fraction.[61] The physiologic significance of particulate-bound iodine is still under investigation. At least a portion of this iodine appears to be in the form of 19S Tg.[62,63] Whether this is Tg on its way into the follicular lumen or on its way out of the lumen has not been established, primarily because it has not been determined to what extent adventitious binding of Tg to cell membranes may occur during the homogenization procedure.

A 9S thyroid particulate iodoprotein, immunologically related to Tg, has been described in rats.[63] At isotopic equilibrium, it comprised 50% to 60% of the particulate ^{125}I in rats on a high-iodine intake but was almost absent in rats on a low-iodine intake. It appears to be a product of the partial degradation of Tg.

Free Iodinated Amino Acids and Iodinated Peptides

A small percentage of thyroid iodine is present in the form of free iodinated amino acids. In rat thyroids, values reported for MIT vary from about 0.01% to about 0.1%, and for DIT from about 0.03% to about 0.05% of total iodine.[58] For free T_4, a value of about 0.5% has been reported,[64] corresponding to a concentration about 100 times greater than that of circulating T_4. The presence in rat thyroids of numerous iodine-containing peptides, comprising about 5% of the total iodine, has also been described.[65] The suggestion that iodopeptides participate in a control mechanism for regulating thyroid hormone biosynthesis[66] requires confirmation.

27S Iodoprotein

A well defined iodoprotein with a sedimentation constant of 27S and a molecular weight of 1.2 million was first isolated from human and bovine thyroid glands by Salvatore and coworkers.[67] It constitutes 5% to 15% of the soluble thyroid protein in most animal species.[68] Although it was first reported that 27S iodoprotein has a much higher iodine and T_4 content than 19S Tg,[67,69] this was not found by other investigators.[62,70] This raises some doubt regarding the original suggestion[69] that 27S iodoprotein acts as a store for T_4 in the thyroid. Tg (19S) and 27S iodoprotein have similar, if not identical, solubilities, amino acid compositions, carbohydrate contents, and immunologic properties.[68] It has been suggested[68] that 27S iodoprotein is formed from 19S Tg by chemical alterations produced as a byproduct of iodination of tyrosyl residues, probably involving oxidative side reactions. The function of 27S iodoprotein remains unclear.

Nonthyroglobulin Iodinated Protein

The presence of soluble iodoprotein unrelated to Tg and containing 1% to 5% of the total iodine has been reported in normal rat thyroid glands. This component is largely iodinated serum albumin.[71] In congenital goiters and other abnormal thyroid conditions, an iodoprotein resembling iodinated serum albumin may become the dominant iodoprotein in the thyroid gland. Thyroid albumin originates from the circulation.[72,73]

THYROID PEROXIDASE

Iodide, the form in which iodine enters the thyroid gland, must first be oxidized to a higher oxidation state before it can act as an effective iodinating agent. Of the known biologic ox-

idizing agents, only H_2O_2 and O_2 are sufficiently potent to oxidize I^-.[74] It is not surprising, therefore, that iodination in the thyroid was previously thought to involve a peroxidase (see my earlier reviews).[58,75] The subject of TPO has been reviewed by Magnusson[76] and by McLachlan and Rapoport.[77]

Thyroid peroxidase is a membrane-bound, glycosylated, hemoprotein enzyme that plays a key role in thyroid hormone biosynthesis by catalyzing both the iodination of tyrosyl residues and the coupling of iodotyrosyl residues in Tg to form T_4 and T_3. Until 1985 this was considered to be its only role in the thyroid; it was then reported,[78–80] however, that TPO is closely related to, if not identical with, the thyroid microsomal antigen associated with the antithyroid microsomal autoantibodies found in the serum of many patients with autoimmune thyroid disease. The immunologic significance of TPO in relation to autoimmune thyroid disease is discussed elsewhere in this textbook (see chaps 21 and 55). This chapter deals with the structure and properties of TPO and with its role in thyroid hormone biosynthesis.

Purification and Properties

Purification of TPO was initially achieved after treatment of the thyroid membrane fraction with trypsin and detergent.[81–88] This procedure yields a large, solubilized tryptic fragment with high catalytic activity.[89] Such preparations, made from porcine thyroids, have been used in model systems to study the mechanisms of iodination and coupling (discussed later). More recently, detergent-solubilized native TPO has been prepared by monoclonal antibody-assisted affinity chromatography.[78,90,91] This procedure is much less time consuming and provides higher yields of purified enzyme. However, even though it has been reported that immunoaffinity-purified preparations of TPO display greater than 90% purity when analyzed by sodium dodecyl sulfate-gel electrophoresis,[91] the values for A_{412}/A_{280} (a standard measure of TPO purity) are only 0.25 to 0.26, compared to values of 0.5 to 0.6 for preparations purified after solubilization with trypsin and detergent. The specific activity of immunoaffinity-purified TPO, measured by different assays, is also considerably lower than that observed with trypsin-solubilized preparations.[91] These discrepancies have not been satisfactorily explained, although Ohtaki and coworkers[91] suggested that the protein content of immunoaffinity-purified TPO is overestimated by the Lowry method for protein determination. This implies that the tyrosine plus tryptophane content of intact human TPO (h-TPO) is proportionally greater than that of the trypsin fragment. However, this proposal is not in agreement with our characterization of the peptides cleaved during the trypsin treatment.[88]

Molecular cloning of h-TPO (see next section) has made it possible to prepare recombinant h-TPO. This has been accomplished in various systems, using CHO cells,[92,93] Hep G2 cells,[94] Sf9 cells,[95,96] and yeast cells.[97] Foti and coworkers[98] and Kaufman and associates[99] described the generation of a biologically active secreted form of h-TPO in CHO cells through use of a truncated cDNA. All of these recombinant h-TPO preparations show a high level of immunoreactivity with microsomal autoantibodies. Only those preparations expressed in CHO or Hep G2 cells displayed catalytic (guaiacol oxidation) activity. However, the level of catalytic activity was very low compared to TPO purified from thyroid glands and was not improved by the addition of hematin. Recombinant h-TPO has proved very useful for immunologic studies, but this technique has so far failed to generate a product with a useful level of catalytic activity.

Some of the properties of trypsin–deoxycholate-solubilized porcine TPO prepared in my laboratory[86,89] are as follows:

- Molecular weight about 90,000 (compared with estimated 110,000 for native porcine TPO)
- A_{412}/A_{280} = 0.50 to 0.54
- Carbohydrate content about 10%
- Isoelectric pH of 5.75
- $K_m[I^-]$, iodination of goiter Tg—0.1 mmol/L
- Turnover number, iodination of goiter Tg—1.8×10^4/min
- Turnover number, oxidation of guaiacol—7.1×10^4/min

The nature of the heme in TPO is controversial. Early studies in my laboratory[83,86] suggested that the heme in TPO is not identical to protoporphyrin IX, the heme found in horseradish peroxidase (HRP), hemoglobin, and many other hemoproteins. However, Ohtaki and coworkers[100] subsequently presented evidence favoring the view that the heme in TPO is protoporphyrin IX.

There is evidence to suggest that TPO in its native form exists as a dimer. Baker and colleagues,[101] confirming and extending previous observations, reported that Western blots obtained with detergent-treated human thyroid microsomes under nonreducing conditions, displayed a band at 220 to 230 kd, in addition to the expected bands at 105 to 110 kd. The 220- to 230-kd band was also observed after immunoprecipitation. The higher–molecular-weight band disappeared on Western blots under reducing conditions. These observations led to the suggestion that the membrane form of h-TPO is a disulfide-linked dimer, resembling the known structure of myeloperoxidase.[102] Additional evidence supporting this view was reported by Nishikawa and coworkers.[102a]

Structure and Molecular Biology

Thyroid peroxidase was the first animal peroxidase whose primary amino acid sequence was deduced from its nucleotide sequence. Shortly thereafter, the primary amino acid sequence of myeloperoxidase (MPO) was determined in the same manner,[103,104] and, more recently,[105] that of lactoperoxidase (LPO). Before the sequence of LPO was published, Kimura and Ikeda-Saito[106] compared the sequences of TPO and MPO and concluded that, even though the two enzymes have distinctly different physiologic functions, they are evolution-related members of the same gene family. It now appears that this family must be extended to include LPO, and also eosinophil peroxidase.[105]

The full-length primary amino acid sequences of porcine,[107] human,[108–110] rat,[111] and mouse[112] TPO, deduced from cDNA cloning experiments, are shown in Figure 4-3. A high degree of homology is apparent, particularly in the first two thirds of the molecule. The potential glycosylation sites are indicated. The location and nature of the N-linked oligosaccharide units have been determined only for porcine TPO. Porcine TPO contains about 10% carbohydrate. Four of the five potential glycosylation sites are actually glycosylated (Asn residues 129, 277, 307, and 342), and the oligosaccharide

units are of the high-mannose type.[113]

Figure 4-4 presents a simplified model of native porcine TPO showing its presumed orientation at the apical membrane. The model is drawn to depict the generally held view that iodination of Tg occurs on the luminal side of the apical membrane.[114] Immunocytochemical studies using IgG-coated colloidal gold particles[115] provide support for this orientation. Further evidence was obtained by Foti and coworkers,[98] who generated a mutated, secreted form of human TPO, lacking the transmembrane domain, which they expressed in Chinese hamster ovary cells. Also shown in Figure 4-4 are the location of N-linked oligosaccharides and the sites of cleavage in the trypsin-solubilized enzyme. The heme binding site is likely located within the disulfide loop, on the amino-terminal side of the trypsin cleavage site at residue 561.[88] Based on homology with myeloperoxidase, Kimura and Ikeda-Saito[106] suggested that the proximal histidine, linked to the iron center of the heme, is located at residue 407.

Two forms of h-TPO cDNAs were found by Kimura and coworkers[108] in a cDNA library prepared from mRNA isolated from the thyroid of a patient with Graves' disease. The longest cDNA encoded a protein of 933 amino acids, referred to as human TPO-1 (see Fig. 4-3). The shorter cDNA encoded a similar protein lacking 57 amino acids in the middle of the sequence, referred to as TPO-2. The two TPOs likely are generated through alternative splicing of the same gene. The TPO gene was mapped to the short arm of chromosome 2. More recently, Elisei and coworkers[116] provided evidence that TPO-2 also exists in normal thyroid tissue.

Kimura and associates[117] described the cloning and complete exon structure of the h-TPO gene. They showed that the gene consists of 17 exons and 16 introns and covers at least 150 kb pairs. Although TPO and MPO display a high degree of sequence similarity and are evolution related, the gene for h-MPO (10 kb pairs) is less than one tenth the length of the h-TPO gene.[117]

Libert and coworkers[117a] also studied the possible evolutionary homology between TPO and MPO. The primary structure of the first 735 amino acids of TPO is 42% homologous with human MPO. They suggested that TPO acquired a 197-residue C-terminal extension. This extension includes the membrane-spanning region (residues 848–871) and short regions of homology with the C4b-β_2-glycoprotein family and with the epidermal growth factor–low-density lipoprotein receptor family. In addition, the sequence from residues 510 to 567 in h-TPO is significantly homologous to a segment of cytochrome C oxidase, a polypeptide encoded in the mitochondrial genome. Based on these observations, Libert and coworkers[117a] proposed that TPO may be a paradigm for a new type of mosaic protein.

A number of patients have been described with severe congenital hypothyroidism attributed to an identified mutation in the TPO gene.[118–120] These mutations are described in detail in chapter 56.

Regulation of Gene Expression

It has long been known that TPO activity in the thyroid gland of rats is stimulated by administration of TSH.[121] Many studies have been performed to examine the regulation of TPO gene expression in thyroid cells. TSH increases the level of TPO

trations, I^- competes with tyrosine for the second site on TPO, and this gives rise to two I· radicals, which add to form I_2. The evidence favoring the radical mechanism has been summarized by Nunez and Pommier.[130] Although this mechanism is still cited,[3] the prevailing evidence[87,134,138–141] indi-

Dunford[138] in a kinetic study involving stopped flow techniques. L-Tyrosine was iodinated at a significantly higher rate than D-tyrosine, providing evidence for a binding site for tyrosine on the enzyme. Earlier studies in my laboratory[135] raised the possibility that enzyme-bound hypoiodite might also be

ese and French investigators relate to the nature of the NADPH oxidase, the pathway of electron transport from NADPH to O_2, and the site of action of Ca^{2+}. The Japanese group have suggested that the NADPH oxidase in the thyroid

only with labeled iodide. In short-term experiments, this would apply only to iodide recently transported into the cell. If there is a second pool of iodide in the gland that is not in rapid equilibrium with transported iodide,[181,182] then second-

```
HUM  MRALAVLSVTLVMACTEAFFPFISRGKELLWGKPEESRVSSVLEESKRLVDTAMYATMQR  60        VSNVFSTAAFRFGHATIHPLVRRLDASFQEHPDLPGLWLHQAFFSPWTLLRGGGLDPLIR 540
     :: :::: ::: :: : :::::: : : :: ::  :: : :::  :  ::: : ::  :        ::::::::::::::::::::::::: ::::: :  : ::: :: ::: :: ::  :
PIG  MGARAVLGVTLAVACAGAFFASILRRKDLLGGDTEASGVAGLVEASRLLVDEAIHTIMRR  60        VSNVFSTAAFRFGHATIHPLVRRLDARFQEHPGSHLP LRAAFFQPWRLLREGGVDPVLR 538
     :  : :   :: ::  :: : :: :: : :     ::::  :: ::::: :: : :::        ::::::::::::: :::::::: :: :    :  : ::::: ::: ::  :
RAT  MRTLGAMAVMLVVMGTAIFLPFLLRSRDILGGKTMTSHVISVVETSQLLVDNAVYNTMKR  60        VSNVFSTAAFRFGHATVHPLVRRLNTDFQDHTELPRLQLHDVFFRPWRLIQEGGLDPIVR 528
MUS  --------I-------V---S-I-------C----K-----A------M-----------  60        ---I---------------------E---------R------------------- 528

HUM  NLKKRGILSGAQLLSFSKLPEPTSGVIARAAEIMETSIQAMKRKVNLKTQQSQHPTDALS 120       GLLARPAKLQVQDQLMNEELTERLFVLSNSSTLDLASINLQRGRDHGLPGYNEWREFCGL 600
     :: :::: : :::::::::: ::::: :::::::: : ::  ::: :::  ::: ::        :::::::::::::::::::: :::::::::::::::::::::::::::::::::::::::
PIG  NLRKRGIFSPSOLLSFSKLPEPTSRTASRAAEIMETAVOEVKRRVCRRRDTDOLPTDVLS 120       GLLARPAKLOVODOLMNEELTERLFVLSNSGTLDLASINLQRGRDHGLPGYNEWREFCGL 598
```

the intermediate in TPO-catalyzed iodination of tyrosine and Tg at pH 7.0, although with LPO-catalyzed iodination the evidence favored free hypoiodous acid as the active iodinating intermediate. Results consistent with a diffusible iodinating

In later studies with rat FRTL-5 cells,[160] Björkman and Ekholm observed that H_2O_2 generation is regulated by the cAMP pathway as well as by the Ca^{2+}/phosphatidylinositol cascade. Regulation of H_2O_2 generation thus appears to be different in porcine and rat thyroids. In porcine thyrocytes only

pool iodide may not be labeled at early intervals after injection of radioactive iodide (except, perhaps, in highly activated thyroids with minimal stores of Tg). Iodination that involves second-pool iodide might not, therefore, be readily detected by autoradiography. Thus, although the results of autoradiography provide evidence against intracellular sites of iodination, they do not completely exclude this possibility. The most recent evidence,[59] however (discussed earlier), opposes the two-pool hypothesis. Moreover, iodination of Tg requires that four separate components be brought into close proximity (TPO, H_2O_2, iodide, Tg).[183] Evidence from various sources indicates that the apical membrane is the most likely site for this to occur.

Histochemical localization of TPO within the thyroid follicle has also been used to provide information on the site of the iodination. One would expect that TPO would be localized at or close to the site of iodination; however, its localization need not be restricted to such sites. Use of a procedure for localizing TPO, based on the incubation of fixed blocks of thyroid tissue with H_2O_2 and 3,3′-diaminobenzidine, has revealed stained material at numerous sites within the cell, including the rough-surfaced endoplasmic reticulum, nuclear envelope, Golgi apparatus, lateral vesicles, apical vesicles, and apical cell surface.[183–190] The presence of stained material at the apical cell surface supports the view that the apical membrane with its associated microvilli is the site for iodination of Tg, as suggested on the basis of the radioautographic findings already described. Localization of TPO in the apical membrane with a membrane-immunofluorescent technique using a monoclonal antibody has been described.[191]

Evidence for an intracellular site for iodination in the thyroid has also been reported by some investigators, based on autoradiography of rat thyroid glands,[192] or on studies with thyroid slices[193] or isolated thyroid cells.[194,195] Studies of localization of ^{125}I binding by electron microscopic radioautography in follicles and in isolated thyroid cells demonstrated that the site of iodination in follicles is the same in vitro as it is in vivo, namely, the apical surface.[178] Isolated cells with preserved polarity also showed labeling associated with remaining microvilli. In isolated cells with lost polarity, however, ^{125}I was localized over intracellular lumens, which were common in such cells.

The bulk of the evidence favors the view that iodination in vivo occurs at the cell–lumen interface.[196] It seems likely that this also applies to normally polarized cells in vitro.[178]

Iodination Defects

A number of patients have been described with congenital goitrous hypothyroidism attributable to defective iodination in the thyroid. The defect is characterized by a positive perchlorate discharge test, a diagnostic procedure that measures the proportion of accumulated radioiodine in the thyroid that is abruptly discharged by administration of perchlorate. This agent discharges only radioiodine that has remained in the form of iodide, normally a negligible fraction of the total thyroid radioiodine accumulated after a labeling period of several hours. In patients with an iodination defect, however, a good part or all of the accumulated radioiodine is discharged soon after administration of perchlorate.[17] Defective organification of iodine may involve TPO absence or deficiency, abnormal

TPO, impairment in H_2O_2 generation, or cytostructural defects. Many examples of familial iodination defects have been reported. These are discussed more fully in chapter 56 and in other reviews.[197,198]

MECHANISM OF IODOTHYRONINE FORMATION

The suggestion that diiodotyrosine is the biologic precursor of T_4 was first made by Harington and Barger in 1927.[199] A mechanism for the coupling of two molecules of DIT to form T_4 was first proposed by Johnson and Tewkesbury in 1942[200] and extended soon after by Harington.[201] It involved oxidation of DIT to a free radical and interaction of two DIT radicals through a quinol ether intermediate to form T_4. This formulation of the coupling reaction involved free DIT. Later studies indicated that peptide-linked DIT is the precursor of T_4 and that coupling of two molecules of DIT occurs within the Tg molecule. Harington[202] initially suggested that the conversion of DIT to T_4 need not require any special enzyme, only an oxidized form of iodine, but newer evidence indicates that TPO catalyzes intramolecular coupling.

In my laboratory, a model system involving purified porcine TPO and human goiter Tg has been used to provide information on intramolecular coupling. A similar system was used by Nunez and Pommier.[130] Results obtained with this model system form the basis for most of the material presented in this section.

Formation of T_4 and T_3 in the Model Incubation System

Figure 4-6 shows the time course of protein iodination and of DIT, MIT, T_4, and T_3 formation in the model iodination system. Formation of ^{131}I-MIT occurred more rapidly than ^{131}I-DIT formation, and iodotyrosine formation occurred more rapidly than iodothyronine formation, resembling the results obtained after administration of ^{131}I to intact animals. A lag was observed in the formation of T_4, as would be expected from the fact that DIT is the precursor of T_4. Sufficient DIT must first accumulate within the Tg before T_4 formation can occur. After this brief lag period, formation of MIT, DIT, and T_4 occurred simultaneously. Dème and coworkers[203] reported that the duration of the lag period is constant (3–5 minutes) and independent of the rate or degree of iodination of the Tg. These observations could not be confirmed in my laboratory.

Figure 4-6 also shows the relationship between the degree of iodination of Tg and the content of the various iodoamino acids. As in Tg isolated from normal thyroid glands, MIT and DIT represented the most abundant iodoamino acids, and the DIT/MIT ratio increased with the degree of iodination. The content of all the iodoamino acids except T_3 increased with increasing degree of iodination. In incubation systems containing a lower concentration of iodide (e.g., 10 μM), T_3 formation became more significant,[204] as it does in the thyroids of rats on an iodine-deficient diet.[57,205,206] However the ratio of T_3 to T_4 in the model iodination system, even under conditions of low iodide concentration, does not attain the high values seen in thyroids of severely iodine-deficient rats.[207,208] This suggests that, in vivo, factors other than

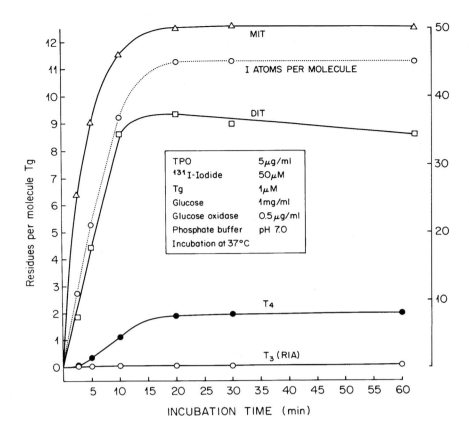

FIGURE 4-6. Time course of iodination and of formation of DIT, MIT, T_4 and T_3 in goiter thyroglobulin iodinated under the conditions indicated. The goiter thyroglobulin contained 0.038% I (2 atoms I per molecule). The value for A_{410}/A_{280} for TPO was 0.38. The reaction was started by addition of glucose oxidase (100 U/mg). Samples were taken from the incubation mixture at intervals and analyzed for PB[131]I and for ^{131}I-iodoamino acid distribution as previously described.[208]

iodide availability (e.g., high degree of TSH stimulation) are important in regulating T_3 formation relative to T_4 formation.

Coupling in the model iodination system is markedly stimulated by a low concentration of free DIT, as illustrated in Figure 4-7. A stimulatory effect of free DIT on the rate of T_4 formation was first reported by Dème and coworkers.[209] The results in Figure 4-7 indicate that a low concentration of free DIT stimulated not only the rate but the extent of T_4 and T_3 formation in the model iodination system. These effects occurred without any increase in the degree of iodination of Tg.

Catalytic Role of Thyroid Peroxidase in the Coupling Reaction

Evidence for a catalytic role for TPO in the coupling reaction was obtained in experiments in which the effect of TPO on coupling in prelabeled Tg was determined.[210] Results of one such experiment are shown in Figure 4-8. The content of labeled T_4 and T_3 increased markedly when the labeled Tg was incubated with TPO plus glucose–glucose oxidase. This increase could not be attributed to a change in the level of iodination of Tg because the coupling system, in contrast to the iodination system, contained no added iodide. Moreover, the increase in labeled T_4 and T_3 was accompanied by a corresponding decrease in labeled DIT, indicating conversion of DIT to T_4 and T_3. The increase in T_4 and T_3 was also readily demonstrable by radioimmunoassay. These results provide convincing evidence that TPO catalyzes the coupling reaction per se and does not serve merely to catalyze formation of the precursors of T_4 and T_3. Evidence for a catalytic role for TPO in the coupling reaction, derived primar-

ily from kinetic data, has also been reported by Pommier and coworkers.[129]

It may also be noted in Figure 4-8 that free DIT (1 µmol/L) was effective in stimulating both T_4 and T_3 formation in the coupling system. Experiments with ^{14}C-DIT showed that the added free DIT was not itself converted to iodothyronines. Its mode of action, therefore, must be through stimulation of intramolecular coupling, involving preformed iodotyrosyl residues within Tg. Dème and coworkers[209] suggested that the stimulatory effect of DIT on coupling might involve a regulatory action of DIT on TPO. We reported observations that were not consistent with this view.[211] Subsequently, Virion and coworkers reported[212] that free DIT is oxidized when it acts as a stimulator of coupling, and that the oxidized form acts to facilitate transfer of electrons from peptide-linked DIT to the heme in TPO. We have confirmed and extended this view (see Mechanism of the Coupling Reaction).

Specificity of Thyroid Peroxidase

As indicated in the section on Mechanism of Iodination, LPO and MPO are also efficient catalysts for iodination. They have been compared to TPO with respect to their ability to catalyze iodination and coupling.[126,127] These studies indicate that TPO possesses no marked specificity in its ability to catalyze iodination and coupling, although in a comparison with LPO,[126] TPO was slightly more effective in catalyzing iodination of Tg at concentrations of iodide in the physiologic range (10–40 µmol/L). It must be remembered, however, that results obtained with purified TPO may not reflect factors that could be important in vivo, for example, membrane binding of TPO. It

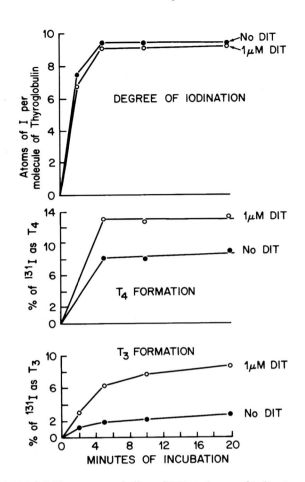

FIGURE 4-7. Time course of effect of DIT on degree of iodination and on T_3 and T_4 formation in goiter Tg iodinated with the TPO system. The incubation samples contained 5 μg/mL of TPO (A_{410}/A_{280} = 0.38), 1 μmol/L of goiter Tg (0.038% I), 10 μmol/L of ^{131}I-iodide, 1 mg/mL of glucose, and 39 mU/mL of glucose oxidase. (Taurog A, Nakashima T. Dissociation between degree of iodination and iodoamino acid distribution in thyroglobulin. Endocrinology 1978;103:632. Copyright by the Endocrine Society)

seems likely that, for in vivo function, TPO may possess advantages over LPO and MPO not disclosed by the model system.

Dème and coworkers[149] compared TPO and LPO in an iodination system, and found that at pH 7.4, TPO and LPO were equally effective in forming T_4 and T_3. When the pH was lowered to 6.6, however, TPO was more efficient than LPO in forming T_4 and T_3. They concluded that TPO plays an important role in the selection of the tyrosine residues of Tg that undergo iodination and that are then able to couple to form T_4 and T_3. However, in a study in my laboratory comparing chemical and enzymatic iodination of human goiter Tg,[213] it was concluded that selection of hormonogenic sites for iodination depends much more on the structure of Tg than on the enzymatic properties of TPO.

Role of Thyroglobulin Structure

Thyroglobulin is the polypeptide matrix necessary for the biosynthesis of thyroid hormones. It is a high–molecular-weight glycoprotein (660 kd, 10% carbohydrate), consisting of two identical subunits. The entire amino acid sequence has been deduced from cDNA cloning experiments for bovine,[214] human,[215] and rat[216] Tg (Di Lauro, personal communication, 1989) More extensive information on Tg can be found in chapter 5.

Studies performed in various laboratories have provided evidence that the native structure of Tg plays a major role in the coupling reaction.[217–222] Because T_4 formation occurs in a variety of proteins iodinated with the TPO system,[58,75,217] Tg is not unique in its ability to form T_4. Tg is, however, the most efficient of all the proteins tested, especially in terms of ability to form T_4 at relatively low levels of iodination.[210,217–221] Disruption of the native structure of Tg by exposure to 5 mol/L guanidine did not interfere with the extent of TPO-catalyzed iodination or formation of MIT and DIT, but it markedly reduced T_4 formation.[217] These results leave little doubt that the efficiency of the coupling reaction depends on the native structure of Tg.

A possible explanation for the higher efficiency of T_4 formation in Tg compared with other proteins was obtained in a double-labeling study in which it was shown that the tyrosine residues in Tg that are first iodinated are also those that are most readily converted to T_4.[223] In agreement with this in vitro observation, Palumbo and coworkers[224] demonstrated that the earliest site of iodination in Tg of iodine-deficient rats is tyr 5, known to be the most important hormonogenic acceptor site.

Human Tg contains 134 tyrosyl residues per 660-kd dimer.[215] Based on the iodoamino acid distribution presented earlier (see Chemical Nature of Thyroid Iodine), only about 18 of these residues are iodinated, on the average, in normal human Tg containing 0.5% iodine. This suggests that only tyrosines at particular sites in the molecule are available for iodination under physiologic conditions.

Coupling involves a reaction between two DIT residues, or between one MIT and one DIT residue, in Tg, to form T_4 and T_3, respectively (see following section). The iodotyrosyl residue contributing the phenolic outer ring is known as the "donor," whereas the DIT residue contributing the inner ring is known as the "acceptor." Both acceptor and donor sites are referred to as hormonogenic sites. The location of specific hormonogenic sites in Tg has been the subject of numerous investigations (see chap 5 for further discussion). One of the earliest investigations of this type, performed when only a partial cDNA sequence of bovine Tg was available, is shown in Figure 4-9. This figure shows the deduced primary structure of the amino-terminal portion of bovine Tg.[225] Independently, Rawitch and coworkers determined the sequence of a T_4-rich peptide of 19 amino acids from bovine Tg.[226] This peptide was obtained by trypsin digestion of a 10-kd peptide linked to Tg by disulfide bonds. The sequence of the 19–amino-acid peptide corresponded exactly to positions 1 through 19 of the sequence derived from the cDNA (see Fig. 4-9), except that it contained T_4 at position 5, where the DNA-derived sequence showed tyrosine.[227] These observations indicated that tyrosine at position 5 in Tg is one of the principal sites of T_4 formation. The same 19–amino-acid sequence containing T_4 at position 5 was also found in human, ovine, and porcine Tg,[228] indicating that it is completely conserved among four species.

Two other T_4-rich peptides were isolated from porcine Tg after cyanogen bromide (CNBr) treatment.[229,230] The amino acid sequences that surround T_4 in these peptides are different from each other and different from the sequence described by

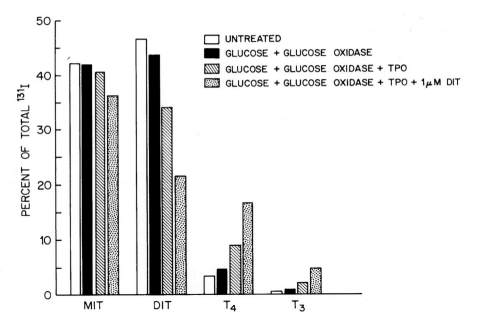

FIGURE 4-8. Effect of TPO on coupling reaction in prelabeled thyroglobulin with and without addition of 1 μM free DIT. The ^{131}I-prelabeled thyroglobulin was prepared by iodination of goiter Tg with ^{131}I- to a level of 23 atoms of iodine per molecule and was thoroughly dialyzed to remove inorganic I. The incubation mixture contained 5 μg/mL of TPO (A_{410}/A_{280} = 0.38), 1.5 μmol/L ^{131}I-Tg, 1 mg/mL glucose, and 50 mU/mL glucose oxidase. The ^{131}I-iodoamino acid distribution is shown for the ^{131}I-prelabeled Tg before and after incubation under various conditions. (Taurog A, Nakashima T. Dissociation between degree of iodination and iodoamino acid distribution in thyroglobulin. Endocrinology 1978;103:632. Copyright by the Endocrine Society)

Rawitch and coworkers.[228] From the amino acid sequence surrounding T_4, it was possible to assign the hormonogenic tyrosines to residues 2555 and 2569 in bovine Tg,[214] close to the carboxy-terminus (residue 2750). A T_3-containing peptide, the sequence of which corresponded to a unique T_3-forming tyrosine residue at position 2748[214] in bovine Tg, has also been described.[231] The tyrosine residues in Tg are distributed across the entire length of the polypeptide chain. It is of interest,

therefore, that the hormonogenic residues are located at or near the extreme ends of the molecule. This may facilitate proteolytic cleavage and release of T_4 and T_3.[232]

Dunn and coworkers[233] examined the sites of thyroid hormone formation in rabbit Tg, labeled in vivo with ^{125}I. The major hormonogenic site was tyrosine residue 5, which accounted for 44% of the ^{125}I-T_4 and 25% of the ^{125}I-T_3 in the Tg. The site corresponding to bovine residue 2555 contained

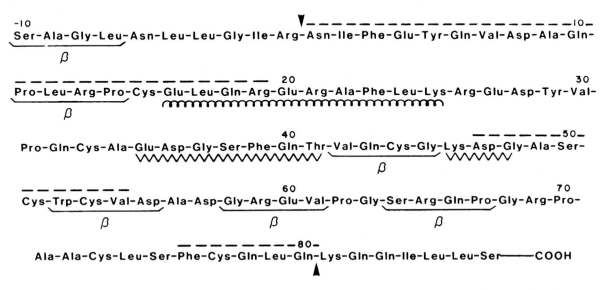

FIGURE 4-9. The N-terminal amino acid sequence proposed by Mercken and colleagues[225] from the cloned cDNA sequence of bovine thyroglobulin. The beginning and end of the 10K peptide previously described are indicated by the large arrowheads. The overscored residues (1–19) were independently established by amino acid sequencing of the intact 10K fragment or of tryptic peptides derived from it. (Rawitch AB, Mercken L, Hamilton JW, Vassart G. The structure of a naturally occurring 10K polypeptide derived from the amino terminus of bovine thyroglobulin. Biochem Biophys Res Commun 1984;119:335)

24% of the $^{125}I\text{-}T_4$ and 18% of the $^{125}I\text{-}T_3$. A major site for T_3 formation corresponded to bovine residue 2748, in agreement with the T_3 site reported by Marriq and coworkers[231] (mentioned earlier). A site not previously reported was tyrosine 1291, accounting for 17% of the $^{125}I\text{-}T_4$ in the Tg.

Less attention has been paid to the location of possible specific donor iodotyrosyl sites in Tg. Based on the well accepted view[234,235] that a dehydroalanine residue is formed at the position formerly occupied by the donor DIT residue, Palumbo[236] obtained evidence that donor sites in bovine Tg map at positions 2469 or 2522, or both. Ohmiya and coworkers,[237] however, using a different procedure to locate the dehydroalanine sites in bovine Tg, concluded that tyrosyl donor sites are located at positions 5,926, 1375, and either 986 or 1008. Marriq and coworkers[238] suggested that tyrosine 130 might act as the donor for the major hormone-forming acceptor tyrosine at position 5, based on studies involving the assumption that the cleavage site that gives rise to a hormone-rich, 26-kd peptide in iodinated human Tg is necessarily produced during the coupling reaction. Rawitch and coworkers[239] used a pulse/chase ^{125}I-labeling procedure involving TPO-catalyzed iodination of low-iodine human Tg and obtained evidence for a donor tyrosyl site at position 2553. It is apparent that there is much less agreement on the location of donor sites than acceptor sites in thyroid hormonogenesis in Tg. It may be that there is lower specificity among donor sites than acceptor sites, although it is not obvious why this should be the case. It seems more likely that the different results are related to the assumptions that underlie the different approaches used to determine the location of donor sites.

Thyroxine-rich peptides may be isolated from Tg after reduction and alkylation, procedures that would not be expected to cleave peptide bonds.[231,240,241] The source of these peptides has been a matter of controversy. Lejeune and coworkers[242] initially reported that these peptides are produced unavoidably by proteolysis during the process of Tg isolation because they are present in Tg domains that are especially susceptible to proteolysis. However, Chernoff and Rawitch[240] and Dunn and coworkers[241] disputed the view that the T_4-rich peptides are produced by postmortem hydrolysis. The latter group proposed that the peptides are produced during the process of iodination and raised the possibility that cleavage of peptide bonds associated with iodination may be a necessary condition for coupling.[243,244] Other groups[238,245] suggested that the origin of the T_4-rich peptides is associated with the coupling reaction itself.

Although it appears that Tg is a unique protein selected for maximum efficiency of T_4 formation at low levels of iodination, the biosynthesis of T_4 as currently visualized is energetically a rather inefficient process. It appears that the synthesis of a protein of molecular weight 660,000 is required for the synthesis and secretion into the circulation of only two to four molecules of T_4. This involves the expenditure of a considerable amount of energy, particularly because it is unlikely that peptide fragments of Tg proteolysis can be reused for Tg formation. Rather, it appears that Tg molecules must be formed de novo for iodination and T_4 formation. This same basic mechanism appears to be involved even at the lowest vertebrate levels, indicating that it has been conserved for hundreds of millions of years. It is not clear why nature has chosen this seemingly wasteful process for the synthesis of an

important hormone. Presumably, the large molecular size of Tg, as well as its structure, confers some special advantage in T_4 synthesis, storage, and release, thus permitting better-controlled regulation of thyroid hormone secretion under varying physiologic conditions.

Mechanism of the Coupling Reaction

A hypothetical coupling scheme compatible with the results obtained with TPO-catalyzed iodination is shown in Figure 4-10. This is an extension of the originally suggested free radical mechanism, which visualized the coupling reaction in terms of the conversion of free DIT to free T_4.[200,201] It is now clear, however, that iodination and coupling occur within the Tg molecule, and the scheme in Figure 4-10 depicts how the orig-

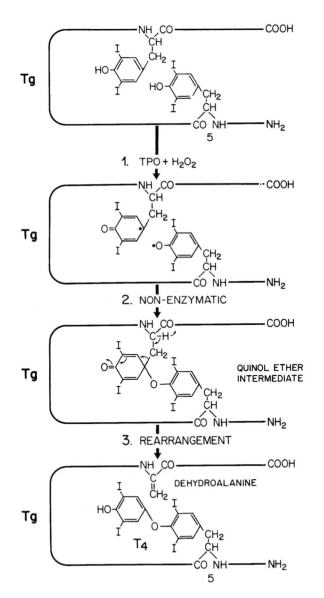

FIGURE 4-10. Proposed coupling scheme for intramolecular formation of T_4 within the thyroglobulin molecule. The major hormonogenic site at tyrosyl residue 5 is indicated.

inally postulated free radical mechanism might occur within the matrix of the protein. The mechanistic details were worked out by Dr. H. J. Cahnmann (personal communication).

Two basic ideas are involved in the mechanism. First, free DIT radicals are generated within the protein matrix through the action of TPO; second, two DIT radicals couple to form a quinol ether intermediate within the protein matrix. The splitting of the quinol ether to form a T_4 residue could occur in theory with the formation of either a dehydroalanine or a serine residue.[75] This can occur without the splitting of a peptide bond. Dehydroalanine residues are formed in Tg concomitantly with hormone residues in a molar ratio of 1,[234,235] thus indicating that dehydroalanine is the sole product of the alanine side chain that is eliminated during the coupling reaction.

Formation of T_3 may be visualized to occur by a scheme similar to that shown in Figure 4-10, except that in this case the coupling would occur between MIT (contributing the phenolic ring) and DIT. This would be consistent with the fact that the relative formation of T_3 is enhanced in iodine deficiency, a condition in which MIT is greatly increased relative to DIT[58] in Tg.

An alternative mechanism of coupling, based on an ionic rather than a radical mechanism, was proposed by Gavaret and coworkers.[246] Very recently, however, in collaboration with Dr. Dan Doerge, we presented evidence[247,248] favoring a radical mechanism for the coupling reaction. A major part of this evidence was based on the observation (discussed earlier) that the coupling reaction, catalyzed by TPO and other peroxidases, is markedly stimulated by a low concentration of free DIT. We proposed that free DIT, acting via the DIT radical, facilitates the transfer of oxidizing equivalents from compound I of the peroxidase to hormonogenic DIT residues in Tg, as shown in the following scheme:

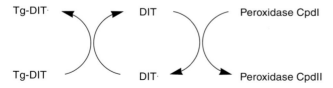

Tg-DIT represents a hormonogenic DIT residue in Tg, and Tg-DIT· a diiodotyrosyl residue radical, illustrated in Figure 4-10. Formation of Tg-DIT may also occur via reduction of compound II to the native enzyme. Under both sets of conditions, DIT molecules cycle between unoxidized and one-electron oxidized forms by successive peroxidase-mediated oxidation and hydrogen abstraction from hormonogenic DIT residues in Tg. This proposal is based, in part, on our observation that free DIT is an effective stimulator of coupling at substoichiometric concentrations, one molecule of DIT leading to the formation of as many as eight molecules of T_4+T_3.[247]

Further evidence for a radical mechanism in peroxidase-catalyzed coupling was obtained in single-turnover coupling experiments with HRP. The spectral properties of compounds I and II of HRP (unlike TPO and LPO), made it possible to correlate the kinetics and stoichiometry of T_4 and T_3 formation with spectral data. When preformed HRP compound I, in the presence of a low concentration of free DIT, was incubated with ^{125}I-Tg, containing almost all of its ^{125}I as MIT and DIT, nearly 100% of the oxidizing equivalents in HRP-compound I were used for T_4 and T_3 formation.[248] The yield of T_4+T_3 was

much lower in the absence of free DIT. The remarkable efficiency of the DIT-stimulated reaction supports the view that free DIT radicals act as a shuttle for transferring oxidizing equivalents from HRP-compound I to hormonogenic DIT residues in Tg. Evidence was obtained that HRP-compound II is an obligatory intermediate when coupling is initiated with HRP-compound I, a convincing argument that the reaction is radical mediated.

It has been suggested[249,250] that different forms of LPO (and of TPO) are used for iodination and coupling. The π-cation radical forms of LPO- and TPO-compound I, which are formed on addition of an equimolar amount of H_2O_2, are very unstable, and, as shown by Courtin and coworkers,[251,252] quickly isomerize to a protein radical form, in which an electron is transferred from a nearby aromatic amino acid to the porphyrin ring. The protein radical form, designated as TPO- or LPO-R·-Fe^{IV}=0, displays a visible spectrum very similar to that of HRP-compound II, but still retains two oxidation equivalents above the native enzyme. Dème and coworkers[249] proposed that coupling with LPO is mediated by the protein radical form of compound I, whereas iodination is initiated with the π-cation radical form. They showed that preformed LPO-R·-Fe^{IV}=0, in the presence of a low concentration of free DIT, reacted very efficiently with equimolar ^{125}I-Tg to form ^{125}I-T_4 and ^{125}I-T_3, but was ineffective in the iodination reaction. They obtained similar results with TPO.[250] However, in single turnover experiments with HRP-compound I, which exists only in the π-cation radical form, we observed[248] that the rate of coupling was much faster than that with LPO- or TPO-R·-Fe^{IV}=0. This raises the possibility that, under catalytic conditions, coupling with LPO (and also with TPO) may involve the π-cation radical form of compound I. The degree to which this occurs would depend on the relative rates of coupling by the π-cation radical form (which is formed before the protein radical form) and the rate of spontaneous conversion of the π-cation radical to the protein radical form. These relative rates are unknown. Based on our recent findings,[248] we believe that there is insufficient evidence to conclude that TPO- or LPO-catalyzed iodination and coupling are initiated by different forms of the enzyme. However, even if iodination and coupling are initiated by the same form of compound I, it is our view that iodination is a two-electron reaction, whereas coupling involves two successive one-electron reactions.

Coupling Defects

Among the types of familial goiter that have been described is one classified as a *coupling defect*. The name implies that there is a specific defect in coupling that is not secondary to some other factor important for normal T_4 formation in the thyroid. Diagnosis of a coupling defect was made in patients whose thyroids showed adequate formation of labeled DIT and MIT, but low formation of labeled T_4 and T_3 (see De-Groot[198] for references). The condition was associated with goiter, hypothyroidism, rapid uptake of radioiodine, and a negative perchlorate discharge test.[198] It was initially proposed[253] that the coupling defect involved impairment of "enzymatically controlled hormone synthesis." However, because most of these patients were described before the role of TPO in iodination and coupling had been elucidated, it was not possible to specify the nature of the enzymatic defect. Subsequently, Pommier and coworkers[254] reported a "coupling defect" in a patient with a partial organification defect, based on the observation that a partially purified TPO preparation from the patient's gland showed only a 30% reduction in iodination but a threefold to sixfold reduction in coupling (compared to purified porcine TPO). They suggested that the observed defects might involve a structural change in the patient's TPO. However, the finding that the Tg in the patient's gland contained only 0.02% to 0.04% total iodine and the observation of a positive perchlorate discharge test are inconsistent with a coupling defect as defined earlier. It seems unlikely that the coupling defect can be ascribed to a structural defect in TPO. Seven mutations in the human TPO gene have been described,[118–120] and all are associated with defects in iodide organification. Although it is conceivable that mutations can occur in TPO that affect coupling without affecting iodination, it seems more likely that coupling defects would involve Tg rather than TPO. As already mentioned,[220,221] disruption of the native structure of Tg does not interfere with TPO-catalyzed iodination, but markedly reduces T_4 formation. Many qualitative and quantitative defects in Tg have been described in humans,[255] including two mutations identified at the molecular level,[256,257] both resulting in congenital goitrous hypothyroidism. Several animal models of congenital defects in Tg synthesis have been described,[255] involving impairment of T_4 synthesis.

A coupling defect in rats secondary to iodine deficiency was described by Inoue and Taurog.[57] They used the molar ratio of DIT to T_4 as a measure of coupling efficiency. This ratio was depressed in extreme iodine deficiency and was restored to normal by a relatively small increase in iodine intake. The reduced coupling efficiency in severe iodine deficiency was attributed to the low degree of iodination of the Tg. Not only does poorly iodinated Tg contain relatively few iodotyrosine residues per molecule of protein, but the proportion present as DIT is markedly decreased. Because DIT is the precursor of T_4, this would be expected to reduce the probability of the T_4 coupling reaction (see Effect of Iodine Deficiency).

Similar findings have been reported for humans with nontoxic goiter.[53] The level of iodination in Tg obtained from a series of patients with nontoxic goiter averaged only 0.06%, compared with 0.23% for normal glands, and there was a significant fall in T_4 when the level of iodination of the Tg fell below 0.1%. The cause of the decreased level of iodination in these patients was unknown, although it was stated that the iodine intake in the Brussels, Belgium area (from which these patients came) is relatively low. The low T_4 formation likely was secondary to the decreased level of iodination of the Tg. It seems possible that relative iodine deficiency played a role in at least some of the patients previously diagnosed with a coupling defect. It is probably more accurate to describe this condition as a "coupling deficiency" rather than a "coupling defect." The term "coupling defect" may apply more specifically to patients with mutations in the Tg gene.

Effect of Iodine Deficiency

Adaptation to iodine deficiency in rats has been an area of active investigation for many years.[205] The effects of feeding iodine-deficient diets to rats include the following: (1) depletion of thyroidal iodine, (2) thyroid enlargement, (3) decrease in serum T_4, (4) increase in serum TSH, (5) decrease in the de-

gree of iodination of Tg, (6) increase in thyroidal MIT/DIT ratio, and (7) increase in thyroidal T_3/T_4 ratio. Although it may be decreased in severe iodine deficiency, serum T_3 is much less affected than serum T_4. The time course of these responses to a severely iodine-deficient Remington diet has been described in previous reports.[207,258–260]

Although studies in many laboratories[58] have established that iodine deficiency greatly alters the distribution pattern of administered ^{131}I among the various iodoamino acids of the thyroid, it is evident from the results of Table 4-2 that the nature and extent of this alteration are greatly affected by the degree of iodine deficiency. Both the severely and the moderately iodine-deficient diet produced enlargement of the thyroid, reduction of the iodine concentration in the thyroid, increase in MIT/DIT ratio, increase in T_3/T_4 ratio, and decrease in serum T_4. The effects produced by the severely iodine-deficient diet on all these parameters, however, were much greater. In one important respect, the percentage of ^{131}I-T_4 in the thyroid, severe and moderate iodine deficiencies had opposite effects. Severe iodine deficiency produced a marked lowering, whereas moderate iodine deficiency produced a slight elevation of ^{131}I-T_4.

Serum T_4 was reduced to undetectable levels in severely iodine-deficient rats but only to about half the normal level in moderately iodine-deficient rats. Serum T_3, on the other hand, remained in the normal range in the iodine-deficient group. Similar results were reported by Escobar del Rey and coworkers.[261] In other experiments with severely iodine-deficient rats,[207,259,260] we have seen a reduction in the serum T_3 level.

The response of rats to iodine-deficient diets can be markedly affected by nutritional factors other than the iodine content of the diet,[259] and also by the strain of rat.[260] These studies suggest that both hereditary and nutritional factors are involved in the variable responses of humans to iodine deficiency in endemic goiter areas (see subchapter on iodine deficiency in chap 14).

The major adaptation of rats to a severely iodine-deficient diet appears to be a shift from T_4 to T_3 formation in the thyroid and a dependence on circulating T_3 rather than circulating T_4. In rats on a normal iodine intake, most of the T_3 in the circulation is produced peripherally by T_4 to T_3 conversion. In rats on a severely limited iodine intake, on the other hand, most of the T_3 in the circulation arises directly from the thyroid,[206] most likely as a result of the great increase in thyroid type I 5′ deiodinase.[262] Severely iodine-deficient rats may show evidence of hypothyroidism, associated with decreased serum T_3 levels.[263] Tissue hypothyroidism may occur in iodine-deficient rats with markedly depressed serum T_4 levels even when circulating T_3 levels are normal.[261,264] These observations demonstrate the importance of local T_4-to-T_3 conversion in contributing to the action of T_3 at nuclear receptor sites.

Effect of Iodine Excess

ACUTE IODIDE EXCESS

Administration of small to moderate amounts of iodide to rats or to humans does not influence the uptake of simultaneously administered ^{131}I by the thyroid. As the iodide doses become progressively larger, however, inhibition of organic binding begins to occur. The decreasing yield of organic io-

TABLE 4-2.
Effect of Chronic Iodine Deficiency on Thyroid and Serum Iodine*

Experiment	Diet	Duration of Feeding	Thyroid Wt (mg/100 g)	Thyroid ^{127}I (μg/100 mg thyroid)
1	LID A†	5 mo	43 ± 9	0.63 ± 0.06
	LID A + KI‡	5 mo	4 ± 1	108 ± 30
2	LID A	3 mo	28 ± 8	0.29 ± 0.07
	LID B§	3 mo	10 ± 2	7.7 ± 7.1

Percentage of Total ^{131}I in Pronase Digest of Thyroid 24 h After ^{131}I Injection				Serum T$_4$ μg/100 mL (RIA)	Serum T$_3$ ng/100 mL (RIA)
MIT‖	DIT‖	T$_4$¶	T$_3$¶		
60 ± 2.8	12 ± 3.0	1.7 ± 0.01	9.2 ± 1.4	<0.25	51 ± 8
15 ± 2.2	49 ± 6.1	16 ± 4.0	2.8 ± 0.1	3.0 ± 0.4	52 ± 9
59 ± 2.5	14 ± 2.4	1.9 ± 0.5	9.7 ± 2.2	<0.25	
34 ± 3.5	23 ± 4.3	19 ± 4.3	11 ± 3.2	1.7 ± 0.8	

*Results expressed as mean ± SD.
†LID A contained about 15 μg I/kg.
‡KI added to drinking water at level of 1 μg/mL..
§LID B contained about 60 μg I/kg.
‖Measured by chromatography in collidine–NH$_4$OH.
‖Measured by chromatography in t-amyl alcohol–NH$_4$OH.

dine from increasing doses of inorganic iodide is termed the acute Wolff-Chaikoff effect, after the investigators who first described this phenomenon.[265] Detailed studies have revealed that small or moderate increments in available iodide result in augmented formation of thyroid hormone.[266] Only beyond a critical dose was hormone formation inhibited. The Wolff-Chaikoff effect depends on the attainment of a critical level of iodide in the thyroid rather than in the circulation.[267] The dose of iodide required to induce the Wolff-Chaikoff blockade in iodine-deficient rats (5–10 μg) is much lower than that required in iodine-sufficient rats (50–100 μg).[57,268]

It was early recognized that inhibition by a single large dose of iodide is only a transient phenomenon because hypothyroidism does not develop in rats exposed chronically to large doses of iodide. Despite the maintenance of high doses of circulating iodide, the thyroid escapes from inhibition after about 48 hours. This escape was shown by Braverman and Ingbar[48] to be related to adaptation of the iodide transport system, which results in lowering of the intracellular iodide concentration. Possible mechanisms for this adaptation have been proposed.[49,50] If, however, the mechanism for regulating intracellular iodide is impaired, as perhaps is the case in iodide-induced hypothyroidism,[269] then the resulting continued high level of intracellular iodide might be expected to cause persistent depression of hormone synthesis through inhibition of TPO-catalyzed iodination.

The mechanism by which iodination is acutely inhibited by excess iodide has been studied by several investigators.[129,270–273] Thyroid peroxide-catalyzed iodination of Tg or bovine serum albumin is inhibited by excess iodide.[270] A peak rate of iodination was reached between 0.3 and 1 mmol/L iodide. At iodide concentrations greater than 1 mmol/L, the iodination was inhibited, and at 10 mmol/L iodide, it was difficult to detect any iodination. The inhibitory effect of excess iodide on TPO-catalyzed iodination has been confirmed by Pommier and coworkers.[129]

An inhibitory effect of excess iodide on iodination was not found in an incubation system containing thyroid particles as the source of TPO instead of highly purified TPO,[271] suggesting that TPO acquires sensitivity to excess iodide as it becomes more highly purified. These results indicate that the Wolff-Chaikoff effect may involve an inhibitory effect of excess iodide on some process other than TPO-catalyzed iodination, for example, H$_2$O$_2$ generation. The Wolff-Chaikoff effect occurs in bovine thyroid slices,[272] and the inhibitory effect of excess iodide on iodination can be prevented by incubation in the presence of TSH or in the presence of an H$_2$O$_2$ generation system. These observations led to the suggestion that the Wolff-Chaikoff effect may be caused by diminished generation or a decreased availability of H$_2$O$_2$ in the thyroid.[272] This suggestion is supported by the demonstration that iodide inhibits H$_2$O$_2$ generation induced by a number of agents in dog thyroid slices.[273]

CHRONIC IODIDE EXCESS

When moderate or large doses of iodide are administered chronically to humans, adaptation occurs, as was discussed previously. This adaptation, however, is not complete, and the quantity of iodine accumulated and organified is well in excess of normal.[46] Nevertheless, the rate of secretion of T$_4$ is not enhanced. Both in animals and in humans,[268,274,275] during chronic iodide administration there is an increase in the release from the thyroid of noncalorigenic forms of iodine. This has been referred to as the "iodide leak" because it is believed that most of the iodine lost from the gland under these conditions is iodide. In normal subjects, the magnitude of this iodide leak varies directly with iodine intake.[275] In animals receiving excess iodine, the iodide generated by deiodination of iodotyrosines has been reported to be less efficiently organified than is iodide transported into the gland from the blood.[268] This could explain the observation that T_4 secretion does not increase despite increased absolute iodide uptake by the gland. This explanation assumes, however, at least transient compartmentalization between internally generated and transported iodide, a concept that gains some support from the studies of Hildebrandt and Halmi[59] (see Inorganic Iodide).

Excess iodide exerts an inhibitory effect on many aspects of iodine metabolism, including cAMP formation, thyroid growth, iodide transport, iodide organification, and H_2O_2 generation. Many investigators have reported that these effects are mediated by iodinated derivatives of arachidonic acid. Published studies provide further discussion.[47,276–283c]

MECHANISM OF ACTION OF ANTITHYROID DRUGS

The possibility that antithyroid compounds act as peroxidase inhibitors was suggested even before there was convincing evidence that peroxidase activity plays a role in thyroid hormone biosynthesis.[284] With the isolation and purification of TPO, it became clear that most compounds with antithyroid activity are inhibitors of TPO-catalyzed iodination. The data and the proposed mechanism of action of the drugs presented in this section are taken primarily from studies in my laboratory. Additional information on the pharmacology of these drugs may be found in several articles and reviews[285–290] (see also chap 14).

Effect of Various Compounds on Thyroid Peroxidase-Catalyzed Iodination

The drugs most commonly used for the treatment of hyperthyroidism are the thioureylene compounds, PTU, MMI, and carbimazole (CBZ). Figure 4-11 shows the inhibitory effect of these drugs on TPO-catalyzed iodination and guaiacol oxidation in a model system. Under these conditions, CBZ and MMI were about equally potent as inhibitors of iodination, whereas PTU had a somewhat lower potency. In humans, MMI and CBZ are more potent than PTU; in rats, PTU is more potent than MMI.[291] The results with CBZ in Figure 4-11 show that, in the in vitro system, this drug is an effective inhibitor of iodination without prior hydrolysis. CBZ is rapidly converted to MMI in vivo, however, and the antithyroid activity of CBZ under these conditions can be ascribed to the MMI that it forms.[292] Evidence for in vivo conversion of CBZ to MMI had previously been obtained by Marchant and coworkers.[293]

Table 4-3 shows the effect on the TPO model system of a variety of compounds, many of which have been reported to inhibit iodination in the thyroid. Thiourea, the prototype of the thioureylene drugs, is a potent inhibitor of TPO-catalyzed iodination, although its mechanism of action[294] is probably different from that of the thioureylene drugs. Thiocyanate, which is usually classified as an inhibitor of iodide transport, is also an effective inhibitor of iodination. Perchlorate, on the other hand, had little or no inhibitory effect, even at a concentration of 1000 μmol/L. The aromatic inhibitors of thyroid function probably owe their thyroid effects to inhibition of TPO-catalyzed iodination. The biologic reducing agents, glutathione, cysteine, ascorbic acid, NADPH, and NADH, were significantly inhibitory. Glutathione[295] and ascorbic acid[296]

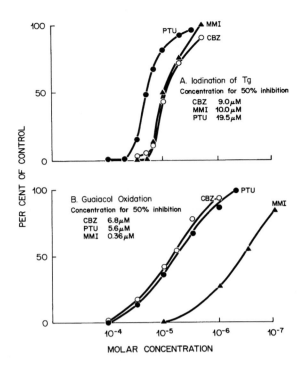

FIGURE 4-11. Dose-inhibition curves for inhibition by thioureylene drugs of TPO-catalyzed iodination of goiter thyroglobulin (*A*) and TPO-catalyzed oxidation of guaiacol (*B*). (Nakashima T, Taurog A. Rapid conversion of carbimazole to methimazole in serum: evidence for an enzymatic mechanism. Clin Endocrinol 1979;10:637)

have been suggested to play a physiologic role in the regulation of iodination reactions in the thyroid. The dose–inhibition relationships for the various compounds showed considerable lack of parallelism, most likely reflecting different mechanisms of inhibitory action.

Reversible and Irreversible Inhibition of Iodination By Thioureylene Drugs

The dose–inhibition curve shown in Figure 4-11 and data in Table 4-3 were based on 1-minute incubations and on initiation of the reaction by addition of H_2O_2. This procedure was useful for comparing the relative potency of various inhibitors of TPO-catalyzed iodination. For the study of the mechanism of action of the thioureylene drugs, however, it was preferable to use a model iodination system in which H_2O_2 was generated by glucose–glucose oxidase. Under these conditions, iodination could be sustained fairly linearly for 20 to 30 minutes, and the time course of inhibition by the drugs could be studied.

Figure 4-12 shows the time course of inhibition of TPO-catalyzed iodination by graded doses of MMI and PTU in the model iodination system. At the lower drug concentrations, the inhibition of iodination was transient. After a variable lag period, the duration of which was dependent on the drug concentration, there was escape of the iodination from inhibition. Under these conditions, inhibition was reversible. When the drug concentration was sufficiently high, however, there was no escape from inhibition with time, and iodination was irreversible. It is apparent from the curves in Figure 4-12 that conclusions regarding the inhibitory effects of the thioureylene drugs on iodination depend on the incubation time as well as

TABLE 4-3.
Effects of Various Agents on Thyroid Peroxidase–Catalyzed Iodination of BSA*

Compound Added (μmol/L)	Percentage of Control Iodination						
	1	2	10	30	100	300	1000
Thiourea	72	39	2	0.2			
Thiocyanate		82	57	25	6		
Perchlorate					94	94	83
Resorcinol	42	0.5					
p-Aminobenzoate	74	52	23	6.9			
Sulfathiazole		36	11	2	0.3		
Sulfadiazine		80	48	23	4.4		
3-Amino-1, 2, 4-triazole	33	8.4	0.5				
Cyanide		100	93	80	0.3		
Azide	29	2.7	0.1				
Iproniazid		98	85	47	9.5		
Glutathione		97	76	30	0.1		
Cysteine		100	85	68	0.2		
Ascorbic acid		97	79	21	0.15		
NADPH			84	3	0.4		
NADH			85	34	3.3		
Cobalt sulfate						98	102
Copper sulfate			89	65	49	47	

*The incubation system contained (in order of addition) 0.06 mol/L phosphate, pH 7, 0.5 mg/mL BSA, 100 μmol/L ^{131}-iodide, the test compound at the indicated concentration, and 1 μg/mL TPO (A_{410}/A_{380} 0.38). Exactly 5 minutes after addition of the TPO, the iodination was started at 24°C by addition of H_2O_2 (final concentration 0.1 mmol/L). The reaction was stopped after exactly 1 minute by rapid addition of methimazole (final concentration 5 mmol/L). Protein-bound ^{131}I was determined by paper chromatography.[210] The control rate of iodination was 31–35 nmol/mL/min iodine bound.

on the drug concentration. Consider, for example, the effect of 20 μmol/L MMI or 40 μmol/L PTU on the iodination of Tg. When the effect of the drug on iodination was studied for only 5 minutes, iodination was completely inhibited. On the other hand, when the reaction was studied at 60 minutes, there was little or no inhibition of iodination.

Another factor that plays an important role in determining whether inhibition of iodination is reversible or irreversible is the iodide concentration. This is illustrated in Table 4-4, which shows the effects of relative changes in inhibitor and iodide concentration on escape from inhibition by PTU and MMI in the model incubation system. At a low concentration of iodide (10 μmol/L), the inhibition produced by 10 μmol/L MMI or 20 μmol/L PTU was irreversible. Inhibition by these levels of MMI and PTU, however, was readily overcome, in time, by elevation of the I⁻ concentration to 100 μmol/L. Similarly, the irreversible inhibition produced by 20 μmol/L MMI or 50 μmol/L PTU in the presence of 100 μmol/L I⁻ was reversed, in time, when the iodide concentration was raised to 500 μmol/L. Inhibition by 100 μmol/L MMI or PTU, however, was not reversed by 1000 μmol/L I⁻. These and other results demonstrate that increases in iodide concentration can overcome competitively the inhibition of TPO-catalyzed iodination produced by lower concentrations of PTU and MMI. The type of inhibition, therefore, depends more on the drug-to-iodide concentration ratio than on the absolute concentration of drug or iodide.

The manner in which time and iodide concentration affect the type of inhibition produced by PTU and MMI is closely related to (1) the potential inactivation of TPO by MMI and PTU, and (2) iodide-dependent, TPO-catalyzed metabolism of these drugs.

Effect of Iodide Concentration on Inactivation of Thyroid Peroxidase by Methimazole and Propylthiouracil

The results in Figure 4-13 show that irreversible inhibition of iodination is related to inactivation of TPO by MMI and that this can be prevented by increasing the I⁻ concentration. Under the conditions of this experiment, iodination was irreversibly inhibited when the I⁻ concentration was 100 μmol/L. When the I⁻ concentration was raised to 500 μmol/L, however, there was escape from inhibition, similar to the results shown in Table 4-4. Also shown in Figure 4-13 is the residual guaiacol oxidation activity of TPO at intervals after initiation of the reaction with glucose oxidase. When the system contained 100 μmol/L I⁻ (irreversible inhibition), TPO was rapidly and completely inactivated. In the presence of 500 μmol/L I⁻ (reversible inhibition), however, TPO activity dropped to about 67% of the initial activity in 15 minutes and then began to level off. From these and similar results with both MMI and PTU, it became apparent that irreversible inhibition of iodination by thioureylene drugs was associated with rapid and complete inactivation of TPO, whereas reversible inhibition was associated with only partial inactivation of TPO. Under reversible conditions of inhibition, the drug was rapidly metabolized.

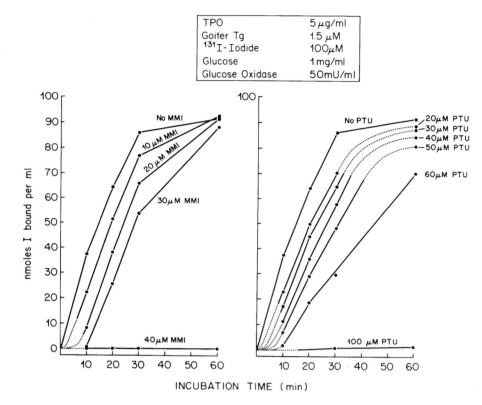

TPO	5 μg/ml
Goiter Tg	1.5 μM
^{131}I-Iodide	100μM
Glucose	1 mg/ml
Glucose Oxidase	50mU/ml

FIGURE 4-12. Time course of TPO-catalyzed iodination of goiter thyroglobulin in the model iodination system in the presence and absence of PTU and MMI. (Engler H, Taurog A, Dorris ML. Preferential inhibition of thyroxine and 3,5,3′-triodothyronin formation by propylthiouracil and methylmercaptoimidazole in thyroid peroxidase-catalyzed iodination of thyroglobulin. Endocrinology 1982; 110:190. Copyright by the Endocrine Society)

Metabolism of Methimazole and Propylthiouracil by the Thyroid Peroxidase Model System

Extensive studies have been performed in my laboratory[297–302] as well as by others[293,303–308] on the metabolism of radiolabeled MMI and PTU. Metabolism of the drugs by the TPO system is largely iodide dependent.

^{35}S-PROPYLTHIOURACIL METABOLISM

Figure 4-14 shows the time course of metabolism of ^{35}S-PTU by the TPO model system, determined by high-performance liquid chromatography (HPLC)[302] under conditions of reversible (see Fig. 4-14A) and irreversible (see Fig. 4-14B) inhibition of iodination. Under conditions of reversible inhibition of iodination, PTU itself disappeared rapidly, and PTU disulfide was the major early intermediate. An unidentified, less prominent early metabolite (31.2-minute peak) was also found. Its rate of formation and decrease roughly paralleled that of the disulfide. It could represent the sulfone or sulfoxide of PTU disulfide. Coincident with the decrease in the disulfide and the unidentified early metabolite was the appearance of three polar metabolites. These were identified as inorganic sulfate/sulfite, PTU sulfonate, and (tentatively) PTU sulfinate. It appears likely from the results in Figure 4-14A that PTU disulfide is an intermediate in the formation of the higher oxidation products.

The metabolic pattern under conditions of irreversible inhibition of iodination was different (see Fig. 4-14B). PTU decreased only to about 70% of its initial value during the first

10 minutes of incubation, and there was a corresponding increase in PTU disulfide. Thereafter, PTU was not further metabolized, but rather it was partially reformed as the disulfide decreased, probably by a nonenzymatic reaction.[302] The formation of sulfate/sulfite and PTU sulfonate was negligible under conditions of irreversible inhibition of iodination.

The metabolism of ^{35}S-MMI by the TPO model system[301] had essentially the same features as the metabolism of ^{35}S-PTU. Under conditions of reversible inhibition of iodination, MMI disappeared even more rapidly than PTU, and MMI disulfide was the first detectable intermediate. The disulfide was in turn converted to higher oxidation products, in this case, chiefly inorganic sulfate/sulfite. Under conditions of irreversible inhibition of iodination, MMI was enzymatically metabolized only to the stage of the disulfide. Nonenzymatic metabolism of the disulfide, with reformation of MMI, was more pronounced than in the case of PTU.

Effect of Other Factors on Inhibition by Thioureylene Drugs in the Model System[97]

THYROID PEROXIDASE CONCENTRATION

The concentration of TPO is a major factor in determining whether, at given drug and iodide concentrations, inhibition of iodination is reversible or irreversible. Increasing the TPO concentration favors reversible inhibition, whereas decreasing the TPO concentration favors irreversible inhibition.

TABLE 4-4.
Effects of Relative Changes in Inhibitor and Iodide Concentrations on Escape From Inhibition*

Inhibitor	Inhibitor Concentration (μmol/L)	I⁻Concentration (μmol/L)	Percentage of Control Iodination		
			10 MIN	30 MIN	60 MIN
Methimazole	10	10	0	0	0
	10	30	0	0	0
	10	100	49	67	86
	20	100		0.4	0.7
	20	500	10	58	78
	50	1000		10	45
	100	1000		0.2	1
Propylthiouracil	20	10	0.1	0.1	0.4
	20	30	0.2	78	93
	20	100	37	74	94
	50	100			0
	50	500			55
	100	1000			0

The incubation system contained 1 μg/mL thyroid peroxidase (A_{410}/A_{380} 0.38), 0.5 mg/mL BSA, 1 mg/mL glucose, and 39 mU/mL glucose oxidase. The reaction was carried out at 37°C and was initiated with glucose oxidase.

H_2O_2 CONCENTRATION

In contrast to the effect of iodide, an increase in H_2O_2 concentration had no significant effect on either drug oxidation or on escape of iodination from inhibition.[297]

ACCEPTOR CONCENTRATION

Tyrosine, rather than bovine serum albumin or Tg, was used in these experiments. Varying the concentration of tyrosine from 10 to 1000 μmol/L had no effect on the rate of MMI oxidation (10 μmol/L MMI); nor did it overcome the inhibitory effect of 20 μmol/L MMI, in contrast to the effect of increasing the iodide concentration.[297]

Proposed Hypothesis for the Mechanism of Inhibition of Thyroid Peroxidase-Catalyzed Iodination by Thioureylene Drugs

The scheme proposed in an earlier edition of this book, revised in accordance with new observations,[138,248,309] is shown in Figure 4-15. It is based on results obtained with ³⁵S-MMI,[301] but with only minor modifications it applies also to PTU. The reactions associated with reversible inhibition of iodination are shown in the left half of the diagram, and those with irreversible inhibition in the right half. An explanation of the various steps in the scheme follows:

1. Reaction 1 shows the two-electron oxidation of native TPO (ferric enzyme) by H_2O_2 to yield the π-cation radical form of compound I. As discussed earlier, this form of the enzyme converts rapidly and spontaneously to the protein radical form (TPO-compound I-R˙).
2. Reaction 2 shows that TPO can be inactivated by MMI.[298,310] The inactivation probably involves one or

both forms of compound I,[309] and is caused by covalent binding of an oxidized form of MMI to the heme group of TPO.[309–311]

3. Reaction 3 shows the oxidation of I⁻ by TPO-compound I-π˙ to form oxidized iodine. As indicated previously (see Mechanism of Iodination), this is generally considered to be a two-electron oxidation, yielding I⁺ or hypoiodous acid. The present scheme shows enzyme-bound hypoiodite ([EOI]⁻) as the active species.
4. Reactions 4 and 7 indicate that [EOI]⁻ acts both to oxidize the thioureylene drugs and to iodinate tyrosyl residues in Tg. Reversible inhibition depends on competition between MMI and tyrosyl for [EOI]⁻. Drug oxidation is the preferred reaction, and as long as sufficient drug is present, [EOI]⁻ is diverted from iodination to drug oxidation. The drug in this mechanism acts as an alternate substrate for [EOI]⁻. The enzyme itself is not inhibited, as is evident from the escape curves in Figure 4-12.
5. The earliest detectable ³⁵S-labeled metabolite, MMI disulfide, is found under conditions of both reversible and irreversible inhibition of iodination (reaction 4). Under reversible conditions, the disulfide is further oxidized by [EOI]⁻ to higher S oxidation products, especially sulfate/sulfite, and MMI completely disappears from the reaction mixture. Under irreversible conditions, however, TPO is rapidly inactivated (reaction 2), and only a small fraction of the disulfide is oxidized. Oxidation proceeds to the stage of the disulfide and possibly also as far as the sulfone or sulfoxide. The further transformation of the disulfide is nonenzymatic, and MMI is reformed (reaction 6).

According to the scheme in Figure 4-15, the relative rates of reactions 2 and 3 play a dominant role in determining

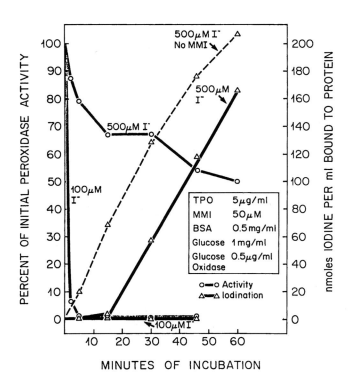

FIGURE 4-13. Effect of iodide concentration on inactivation of TPO by a fixed concentration of MMI (50 μmol/L). (Engler H, Taurog A, Luthy C, Dorris ML. Reversible and irreversible inhibition of thyroid peroxidase-catalyzed iodination by thioureylene drugs. Endocrinology 1983;112:86)

whether inhibition of iodination is reversible or irreversible. If reaction 2 is predominant, the TPO will be rapidly inactivated and inhibition of iodination will be irreversible. On the other hand, if reaction 3 is predominant, this will lead to extensive drug oxidation, permitting iodination to begin after a lag period during which the drug is metabolized. It is apparent from this scheme why the ratio of iodide to drug plays such an important role in determining the type of inhibition. A high ratio favors reaction 3 (and therefore reversible inhibition), whereas a low ratio favors reaction 2 (and therefore irreversible inhibition).

In Vivo Experiments With Propylthiouracil and Methimazole

The mechanism proposed in Figure 4-15 is based almost entirely on in vitro experiments with the model incubation system. Experiments have been performed with rats to test the physiologic relevance of this scheme. In an early study,[291] two features were tested: the effects of drug dosage and the effects of iodine deficiency. Marked inhibition of intrathyroidal drug metabolism occurred when drug dosage was increased. These results are similar to those obtained with the model system. Also, as expected from the in vitro findings, intrathyroidal metabolism of ^{35}S-PTU and ^{35}S-MMI was markedly reduced in iodine-deficient rats. The results of these rat studies, therefore, offer some support for the physiologic validity of the scheme proposed in Figure 4-15.

Figure 4-16 shows the HPLC profile of an ultrafiltrate prepared from the thyroid of a rat 19 hours after injection of ^{35}S-PTU (1 μmol/100 g). The intrathyroidal ^{35}S-labeled metabolites

are at least qualitatively the same as those formed in the model system (see Fig. 4-14), except that no peak for ^{35}S-PTU disulfide was found in the thyroid tissue. It seems most unlikely, however, that this early metabolite would be present in the thyroid after this long interval. Moreover, PTU disulfide does not survive the homogenization procedure that was used to prepare the tissue for HPLC analysis.[302] Comparison of the results in Figures 4-14 and 4-16 suggests that the pathways of PTU metabolism are similar in the thyroid and in the TPO model system. This implies that intrathyroidal metabolism of PTU is mediated primarily by TPO.

In an earlier study,[312] we observed that PTU had a surprisingly prolonged inhibitory effect on iodination in the rat thyroid. This led us to propose that TPO was inactivated by the drug, as in the in vitro model of irreversible inhibition (see Fig. 4-15). However, when this question was reexamined using improved methods for analysis of PTU metabolites in the rat thyroid, the results did not support the initial proposal, and it was withdrawn.[300] The new findings may be summarized as follows:

1. The peak for unchanged PTU in Figure 4-16 contained 6.4% of the total ^{35}S in the thyroid. The intracellular concentration of unchanged PTU was calculated to be about 20 μmol/L, a concentration that could explain the inhibition of iodination by the alternate substrate mechanism.
2. The intrathyroidal concentration of ^{35}S increased with time after injection up to at least 18 hours. The intrathyroidal concentrations of all the oxidation products of PTU, including sulfinate, sulfonate, and sulfate/sulfite increased markedly between 2 and 6 hours. Assuming that TPO is the major mediator of intrathyroidal PTU metabolism, these data indicate that active TPO must be present in the gland for many hours after administration of the drug. This observation is incompatible with the proposal that PTU inhibition of iodination occurs via inactivation of TPO.

Based on our most recent results,[300] we conclude that inhibition of iodination by PTU in the rat thyroid involves competition between PTU and tyrosyl residues of Tg for oxidized iodine, as initially proposed by Morris and Hager[144] and by Davidson and coworkers.[313] This corresponds to the reversible mechanism of iodination in the TPO model system (see Fig. 4-15). In a separate study,[301] we concluded that MMI also inhibits iodination in the rat thyroid through the reversible mechanism.

Both PTU and MMI are concentrated several fold by the rat thyroid.[285,291,293,303,304] Studies with analogues of PTU[314,315] and MMI[316] suggest that the concentration of these drugs by the thyroid is essential for their potent antithyroid activity. The mechanism of this concentration, however, is unknown. Studies in my laboratory[317] indicated that uptake of labeled PTU and MMI by thyroids of guinea pigs was increased sevenfold to eightfold by injection of TSH. Lang and colleagues[318,319] showed that variations in iodine intake, acutely and chronically, had considerable influence on thyroid accumulation and oxidation of ^{35}S-PTU and ^{35}S-MMI in rats. However, the mechanism by which iodine mediated these effects was not clarified.

Figure 4-17 shows the results of experiments[312] in which ^{35}S was measured in the thyroid and plasma of rats killed at in-

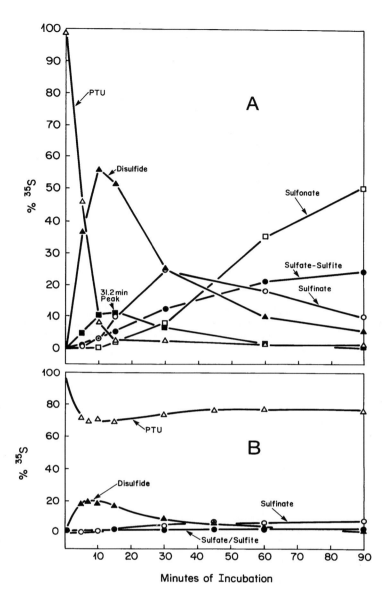

FIGURE 4-14. (*A*) ^{35}S-Labeled intermediates and end products formed during the metabolism of ^{35}S-PTU under contitions of *reversible* inhibition of iodination. The incubation mixture contained 100 μmol/L ^{35}S-PTU, 6.6 μg/mL TPO, 100 μmol/L KI, 1 mg/mL glucose and 0.5 μg/Ml glucose oxidase in 67 mol/L phospate buffer, pH 7. The reaction was started at 39°C with glucose oxidase, and aliquots were removed at intervals and rapidly frozen in liquid nitrogen for later analysis by high-performance liquid chromatography. (*B*) ^{35}S-Labeled intermediates and end products formed during the metabolism of ^{35}S-PTU under conditions of *irreversible* inhibition of iodination. The procedure and incubation conditions were the same as in *A*, except that the ^{35}S-PTU concentration was raised to 150 μmol/L. (Adapted from Taurog A, Dorris ML, Guiziec FS Jr, Uetrecht JP. Metabolism of [35]S- and ^{14}C-labeled propylthiouracil in a model *in vitro* system containing thyroid peroxidase. Endocrinology 1989;124:3030. Copyright by The Endocrine Society)

tervals ranging from 2 to 40 hours after injection of ^{35}S-PTU or ^{35}S-MMI (1 μmol/100 g). Thyroidal uptake of PTU was much greater than that of MMI. This most likely explains the greater antithyroid potency of PTU in the rat. Considering their rapid disappearance from plasma, both drugs showed a surprising ^{35}S accumulation in the thyroid. Similar results were reported by Marchant and coworkers.[285] The peak thyroidal ^{35}S concentration was at 18 hours, a time when plasma ^{35}S had decreased to 10% or less of the 2-hour value. Moreover, the thyroidal concentration of ^{35}S at 40 hours was not significantly different from that at 18 hours. The results in Figure 4-17 provide a striking example of dissociation between the half-life of a drug in the circulation and in its target tissue. Several groups of investigators[320–325] have reported that hyperthyroidism due to Graves' disease can be successfully controlled with single daily doses of PTU or MMI. The success of single–daily-dose treatment with MMI and PTU very likely reflects the concentration and retention of the drugs in the thyroid (see Figs. 4-16 and 4-17), despite their relatively short half-lives in the circulation (see chap 53).

Inhibition of Coupling by Propylthiouracil and Methimazole

Early investigations[326,327] with intact rats receiving graded doses of PTU showed that the formation of ^{131}I-T$_4$ in the thyroid is more sensitive than ^{131}I-DIT formation to the inhibitory action of the drug. Similar observations were made using the TPO model system.[75] Such findings[75,327] suggested that PTU had a specific inhibitory effect on the coupling reaction, independent of its inhibitory effect on iodination. This suggestion was questionable,[328] however, because T$_4$ formation involves a reaction between two molecules of DIT. The rate of this reaction, therefore, is second order with respect to DIT concentration. Inhibition of DIT formation by thioureylene drugs, therefore, would be expected to result in a disproportionately greater reduction in T$_4$ formation even if there were no specific inhibitory effect of the drugs on the coupling reaction.

Using graded doses of drugs in the model iodination system,[328] it was possible to show that, under certain conditions,

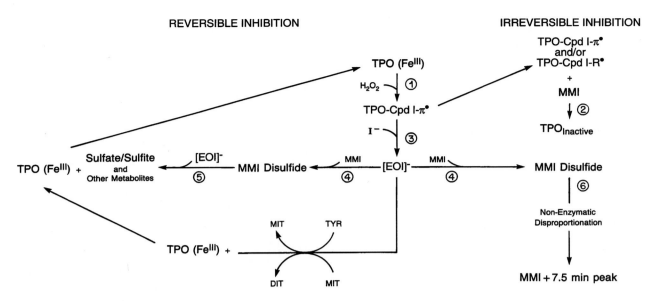

FIGURE 4-15. Scheme for mechanism of inhibition of TPO-catalyzed iodination by MMI. Cpd, compound. See text for further explanation. (Adapted from Taurog A, Dorris ML, Guziec FS Jr. Metabolism of [35]S- and ^{14}C-labeled 1-methyl-2-mercaptoimidazole *in vitro* and *in vivo*. Endocrinology 1989;124:30. Copyright by The Endocrine Society)

there was a clear inhibitory effect of PTU and MMI on coupling with no inhibitory effect on DIT formation. This observation, together with other data, led to the conclusion that, at least under some conditions in the in vitro system, the thioureylene drugs can selectively inhibit coupling independent of their inhibitory effect on iodination. This opens the

possibility that similar selective inhibition by these drugs may occur under some conditions in vivo.

Propylthiouracil or one of its metabolic products becomes bound to Tg in the thyroid gland of rats.[329] This binding could affect Tg structure in such a way as to inhibit the coupling reaction. Binding of both PTU and MMI (or their metabolic

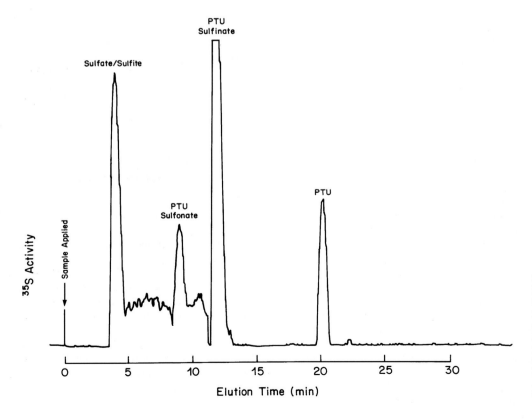

FIGURE 4-16. High-performance liquid chromatography analysis of thyroid ultrafiltrate 19 hours after injection of ^{35}S-PTU into normal rat (1 μmol/100 g). (Taurog A, Dorris ML. A reexamination of the proposed inactivation of thyroid peroxidase in the rat thyroid by propylthiouracil. Endocrinology 1989;124: 3038. Copyright by the Endocrine Society)

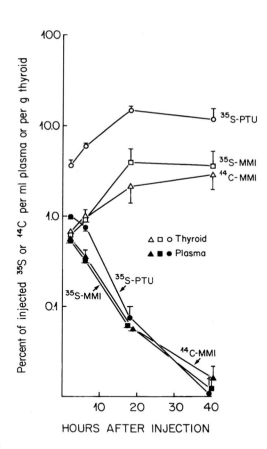

FIGURE 4-17. Plasma disappearance and thyroid accumulation of ^{35}S and ^{14}C after the injection of 1 μmol/100 g ^{35}S-PTU, ^{35}S-MMI or ^{14}C-MMI into normal rats. Each point represents the mean ± SD of three animals. (Shiroozu A, Taurog A, Engler H, Dorris ML. Mechanism of action of thioureylene antithyroid drugs in the rat: possible inactivation of thyroid peroxidase by propylthiouracil. Endocrinology 1983;113:362. Copyright by The Endocrine Society)

products) to Tg has also been observed both in vivo and in the TPO model system.[306,330] The significance of this binding, however, remains to be determined.

The entire emphasis in this discussion of the mechanism of action of thioureylene antithyroid drugs in the treatment of hyperthyroidism has been on their inhibitory effects on TPO-catalyzed reactions. However, from the point of view of attaining remission of Graves' disease, the immunosuppressive effects of the drugs have become a subject of great interest. Although there appears to be little doubt that immunomodulatory effects play an important role in the beneficial actions of PTU and MMI in Graves' disease, the mechanism of this immunosuppressive effect is a matter of controversy.[331–333] This topic is discussed more fully in chapter 53.

SUMMARY

Figure 4-18 presents a summary diagram of the major steps in thyroid hormone biosynthesis and release. The more important inhibitors of the various steps are also indicated.

The following comments are presented to help clarify some of the features of the diagram.

1. The role of TPO in the iodination of Tg is to generate an active iodinating species, indicated in the figure as [EOI]⁻, hypoiodous acid, or I⁺. [EOI]⁻ represents enzyme-bound hypoiodite. Although the question of whether iodination of Tg occurs on or off the enzyme is not resolved, a recent kinetic study on the mechanism of LPO-catalyzed iodination of tyrosine[138] favors the view that the iodinating species is [EOI]⁻, and that transfer of iodine occurs on the enzyme.

2. Colloid resorption occurs by both macropinocytosis and micropinocytosis. The relative importance of these alternate mechanisms appears to vary with the

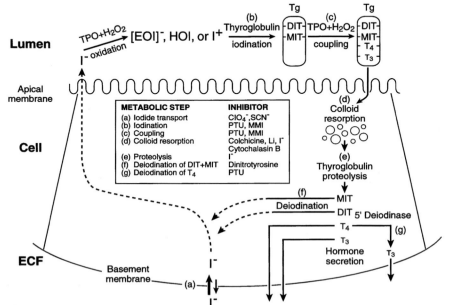

FIGURE 4-18. Summary diagram of the major steps in thyroid hormone biosynthesis and release. The more important inhibitors of the various steps are also indicated.

species and the physiologic state of the animal (see the second part of this chapter, Release and Secretion of Thyroid Hormone).

3. Iodide is shown to be an inhibitor of colloid resorption and of Tg proteolysis. It is generally believed, however, that I⁻ is not itself the active inhibitor but rather that the I⁻ must first become organically bound to form an inhibitory organic compound (see review by Wolff[277]).

4. A mechanism for H_2O_2 generation is not presented in Figure 4-18 because studies of this mechanism are not yet sufficiently advanced to provide a reliable model. There is good evidence that an NADPH oxidase is involved and that Ca^{2+} plays a regulatory role; however, further details of the biochemical pathway remain to be elucidated (see Fig. 4-5).

Acknowledgments

The author thanks Dr. Ronald P. Magnusson for the preparation of Figure 4-3, and Dr. Dan Doerge and Ms. Martha Dorris for helpful suggestions.

References

1. Ekholm R. Biosynthesis of thyroid hormones. Int Rev Cytol 1990;120:243

2. Björkman U, Ekholm R. Biochemistry of thyroid hormone formation and secretion. In: Greer MA, ed. The thyroid gland. New York: Raven Press, 1990:83

3. Gentile F, Di Lauro R, Salvatore G. Biosynthesis and secretion of thyroid hormones. In: DeGroot LJ, ed. Endocrinology. Vol I. 3rd ed. Philadelphia: WB Saunders, 1995:517

4. Wolff J. Transport of iodide and other anions in the thyroid gland. Physiol Rev 1964;44:45

5. Weiss SJ, Philp NJ, Grollman EF. Iodide transport in a continuous line of cultured cells from rat thyroid. Endocrinology 1984;114:1090

6. Wolff J. Iodide concentrating mechanism. In: Rall JE, Kopin IJ, eds. The thyroid and biogenic amines. Amsterdam: North-Holland, 1972:115

7. Wollman SH, Reed FE. Transport of radioiodide between thyroid and blood in mice and rats. Am J Physiol 1959;196:113

8. Chambard M, Verrier B, Gabrion J, Mauchamp J. Polarization of thyroid cells in culture: evidence for the basolateral localization of iodide "pumps" and of the thyroid-stimulating hormone receptor–adenyl cyclase complex. J Cell Biol 1972;96:1172

9. Nilsson M, Björkman U, Ekholm R, Ericson L. Iodide transport in primary cultured thyroid follicle cells: evidence of a TSH-regulated channel mediating iodide efflux selectively across the apical domain of the plasma membrane. Eur J Cell Biol 1990;52:270

10. Nilsson M, Björkman U, Ekholm R, Ericson L. Polarized efflux of iodide in porcine thyrocytes occurs via a c-AMP-regulated iodide channel in the apical plasma membrane. Acta Endocrinol (Copenh) 1992;126:67

11. Wolff J, Maurey J. Thyroidal iodide transport: II. comparison with non-thyroidal iodide concentrating tissues. Biochim Biophys Acta 1961;47:467

12. Saito K, Yamamoto K, Takai T, Yoshida S. The sodium-dependent iodide transport by phospholipid vesicles reconstituted with the thyroid plasma membrane. J Biochem (Tokyo) 1982;92:2001

13. O'Neill B, Magnolato D, Semenza G. The electrogenic, Na⁺-dependent I⁻ transport system in plasma membrane vesicles from thyroid glands. Biochim Biophys Acta 1987;896:263

14. Harden RMcG, Alexander WD. The salivary iodide trap in man: clinical applications. Proc R Soc Med 1968;61:647

15. Alexander WD, Koutras DA, Crooks J, et al. Quantitative studies of iodine metabolism in thyroid disease. Q J Med 1962;31:281

16. Ryan M, DeGroot LJ. Congenital defects in hormone formation and action. In: DeGroot LB, ed. Endocrinology. Vol 1. Philadelphia: WB Saunders, 1989:777

17. Stanbury JB. Familial goiter. In: Stanbury JB, Wyngaarden JB, Fredrickson DS, eds. Metabolic basis of inherited disease. 3rd ed. New York: McGraw-Hill, 1972:223

18. Morgans ME, Trotter WR. Potassium perchlorate in thyrotoxicosis. Br Med J 1960;2:1086

19. Scranton JR, Halmi NS. Thyroidal iodide accumulation and loss *in vitro*. Endocrinology 1965;76:441

20. Surks MI. Determination of iodide clearance and exit rate constants in incubated thyroid lobes. Endocrinology 1967;80:1020

21. Andros G, Harper PV, Lathrop KA, McArdle RJ. Pertechnetate-99m localization in man with applications to thyroid scanning and the study of thyroid physiology. J Clin Endocrinol Metab 1965;25:1067

22. Selby JB, Caldwell JG, Magoun SE, Beihn RM. The use of the ⁹⁹ᵐTc-pertechnetate neck/thigh ratio as a test of thyroid function. Radiology 1975;114:107

23. Shimmins J, Hilditch T, Harden RMcG, Alexander WD. Thyroidal uptake and turnover of the pertechnetate ion in normal and hyperthyroid subjects. J Clin Endocrinol Metab 1968;28:575

24. Tong W, Kerkof P, Chaikoff IL. Iodine metabolism of dispersed thyroid cells obtained by trypsinization of sheep thyroid glands. Biochim Biophys Acta 1962;60:1

25. Chow SY, Yen-Chow C, White HS, Woodbury DM. Effects of sodium on iodide transport in primary cultures of turtle thyroid cells. Am J Physiol (Endocrinol Metab) 1986;250:E464

26. Kaminsky S, Levy O, Salvador C, Dai G, Carrasco N. Na⁺–I⁻ symport activity is present in membrane vesicles from thyrotropin-deprived non-I⁻-transporting cultured thyroid cells. Proc Natl Acad Sci USA 1994;91:3789

27. Doniach I, Logothetopoulos JH. Radioautography of inorganic iodide in the thyroid. J Endocrinol 1955;13:65

28. Pitt-Rivers RV, Trotter WR. The site of accumulation of iodide in the thyroid of rats treated with thiouracil. Lancet 1953;2:918

29. Andros G, Wollman SH. Autoradiographic localization of radioiodide in the thyroid gland of the mouse. Am J Physiol 1967;213:198

30. Woodbury DM, Woodbury JW. Correlation of micro-electrode potential recordings with histology of rat and guinea pig thyroid glands. J Physiol (Lond) 1963;169:533

31. Wolff J, Halmi NS. Thyroidal iodide transport: V. the role of Na⁺-K⁺-activated ouabain-sensitive adenosine triphosphatase activity. J Biol Chem 1963;238:847

32. Bagchi N, Fawcett DM. Role of sodium ion in active transport of iodide by cultured thyroid cells. Biochim Biophys Acta 1973;318:235

33. Saito K, Yamamoto K, Takai T, Yoshida S. Characteristics of the thyroid iodide translocator and of iodide-accumulating phospholipid vesicles. Endocrinology 1984;114:868

34. Wolff J. Iodide transport. Anion selectivity and the iodide "trap." In: Reinwein D, Klein E, eds. Diminished thyroid hormone formation. Stuttgart: FK Schattauer Verlag, 1982:3

35. Nakamura Y, Ohtaki S, Yamazaki I. Molecular mechanism of iodide transport by thyroid plasmalemmal vesicles: cooperative sodium activation and asymmetrical affinities for the ions on the outside and inside of the vesicles. J Biochem 1988;104:544

36. Vilijn F, Carrasco N. Expression of the thyroid sodium/iodide symporter in *Xenopus laevis* oocytes. J Biol Chem 1989; 264: 11901

37. Carrasco N. Iodide transport in the thyroid gland. Biochim Biophys Acta 1993;1154:65

38. Wolff J. Iodure. Le système de transport actif. In: Leclère J, Orgiazzi J, Rousset B, Schlienger J-L, Wémeau J-L, eds. La thyroïde. Paris: Expansion Scientifique Française, 1992:17

39. Stanley MM, Astwood EB. The response of the thyroid gland in normal human subjects to the administration of thyrotropin as shown by studies with [131]I. Endocrinology 1949;44:49

40. Halmi NS. Factors influencing the thyroidal iodide pump. London: Ciba Foundation Colloquia on Endocrinology, JA Churchill, 1957:79

41. Halmi NS. Grammer DK, Doughman DJ, et al. Biphasic effect of TSH on thyroidal iodide collection in rats. Endocrinology 1960;67:70

42. Tong W. Actions of thyroid-stimulating hormone. In: Greep RO, Astwood EB, eds. Handbook of physiology. Vol III. Washington, DC: American Physiological Society, 1974:255

43. Weiss SJ, Philp NJ, Ambesi-Impiobato FS, Grollman EF. Thyrotropin-stimulated iodide transport mediated by adenosine $3',5'$-monophosphate and dependent on protein synthesis. Endocrinology 1984;114:1099

44. Weiss SJ, Philp NJ, Grollman EF. Effect of thyrotropin on iodide efflux in FRTL-5 cells mediated by Ca^{2+}. Endocrinology 1984; 114:1108

45. Marcocci C, Luini A, Santisteban P, Grollman EF. Norepinephrine and thyrotropin stimulation of iodide efflux in FRTL-5 thyroid cells involves metabolites of arachidonic acid and is associated with iodination of thyroglobulin. Endocrinology 1987; 120:1127

46. Ingbar SH. Autoregulation of the thyroid: response to iodide excess and depletion. Mayo Clin Proc 1972;47:814

47. Pisarev MA. Thyroid autoregulation. J Endocrinol Invest 1985; 8:475

48. Braverman LE, Ingbar SH. Changes in thyroidal function during adaptation to large doses of iodide. J Clin Invest 1963;42:1216

49. Chazenbalk GD, Valsecchi RM, Krawiec L, et al. Thyroid autoregulation: inhibitory effects of iodinated derivatives of arachidonic acid on iodine metabolism. Prostaglandins 1988;36:163

50. Sherwin JR, Tong W. The actions of iodide and TSH on thyroid cells showing a dual control system for the iodide pump. Endocrinology 1974;94:1465

51. Wolff J. Congenital goiter with defective iodide transport. Endocr Rev 1983;4:240

52. Saito K, Yamamoto K, Hoshida S, et al. Goitrous hypothyroidism due to iodide-trapping defect. J Clin Endocrinol Metab 1981; 53:1267

52a. Herzog V, Berndorfer U, Saber Y. Isolation of insoluble secretary product from bovine thyroid: extracellular storage of thyroglobulin in covalently cross-linked form. J Cell Biol 1992;118:1071

52b. Berndorfer U, Saber Y, Herzog V. Multimerization of thyroglobulin (Tg) by covalent cross-linking: a ubiquitous phenomenon and a prerequisite for the storage of Tg in osmotically inert form. Abstract No. 132. 11th International Thyroid Congress, Toronto, Canada, Sept. 10–14, 1995

53. Ermans AM, Kinthaert J, Camus M. Defective intrathyroidal iodine metabolism in nontoxic goiter: inadequate iodination of thyroglobulin. Endocrinology 1968;28:1307

54. DeCrombrugghe B, Edelhoch H, Beckers C, De-Visscher M. Effects of iodination on sedimentation and iodoamino acid synthesis. J Biol Chem 1967;242:5681

55. Sorimachi K, Ui N. Comparison of the iodoamino acid distribution in the thyroglobulin obtained from various animal species. Gen Comp Endocrinol 1974;24:38

56. Sorimachi K, Ui N. Comparison of the iodoamino acid distribution in various preparations of hog thyroglobulin with different iodine content and subunit structure. Biochim Biophys Acta 1974;342:30

57. Inoue K, Taurog A. Acute and chronic effects of iodide on thyroid radioiodine metabolism in iodine-deficient rats. Endocrinology 1968;83:279

58. Taurog A. Biosynthesis of iodoamino acids. In: Greep RO, Astwood EB, eds. Handbook of physiology. Vol III. Washington, DC: American Physiological Society, 1974:101

59. Hildebrandt JD, Halmi NS. Intrathyroidally generated iodide: the role of propylthiouracil-sensitive processes in its production. Endocrinology 1980;107:830

60. Hildebrandt JD, Scranton JR, Halmi NS. Intrathyroidally generated iodide: its measurement and origins. Endocrinology 1979; 105:618

61. Boat TF, Halmi NS. Studies of particulate iodoprotein in the rat thyroid. Endocrinology 1965;77:537

62. Gavaret J-M, Julien MF, Cadot M, et al. Relation entre teneur en iode et proprietes de thyroglobulines obtenues par la methode d'equilibrage isotopique. Biochim Biophys Acta 1971; 236:706

63. Gavaret J-M, Nunez J. 9S thyroid particulate iodoprotein. Biochim Biophys Acta 1975;405:353

64. Tong W, Taurog A, Chaikoff IL. Nonthyroglobulin iodine of the thyroid gland: II. free thyroxine and diiodotyrosine. J Biol Chem 1951;191:665

65. Simon C, Lissitzky S. Etude quantitative par la method d'equilibre isotopique avec le radioisotope [125]I. Biochim Biophys Acta 1964;93:494

66. Lissitzky S, Gregoire J, Gregoire J, Limozin M. The presence and *in vitro* activity of free iodinated peptides in the thyroid gland of mammals and man. Gen Comp Endocrinol 1961;1:519

67. Salvatore G, Vecchio G, Salvatore M. 27S thyroid iodoprotein. J Biol Chem 1965;240:2935

68. Frati L, Bilstad J, Edelhoch H, et al. Biosynthesis of the 27S thyroid iodoprotein. Arch Biochem Biophys 1974;162:126

69. Robbins J, Salvatore G, Vecchio G, Ui N. Thyroglobulin and 27S iodoprotein: iodination and ultracentrifugal heterogeneity. Biochim Biophys Acta 1966;127:101

70. Riesco G, Taurog A. Iodine and T_4 content of rat 27S thyroid iodoprotein. Abstract. 7th Annual Meeting of the European Thyroid Association, Helsinki, June 29–July 2, 1976

71. Torresani J, Roques M, Peyrot A, Lissitzky S. Mise in evidence, purification et proprietes d'une iodoalbumine, constitutant physiologique de la gland thyroide de rat. Acta Endocrinol (Copenh) 1968;57:153

72. Lissitzky S, Bismuth J, Codaccioni JI, Cartouzou G. Congenital goiter with iodoalbumin replacing thyroglobulin and defect of deiodination of iodotyrosines, serum origin of the thyroid iodoalbumin. J Clin Endocrinol Metab 1968;28:1797

73. de Vijlder JJM, Veenboer GJM, van Dijk JE. Thyroid albumin originates from blood. Endocrinology 1992;131:578

74. Taurog A. The biosynthesis of thyroxine. Mayo Clin Proc 1964; 39:569

75. Taurog A. Thyroid peroxidase and thyroxine biosynthesis. Recent Prog Horm Res 1970;26:189

76. Magnusson RP. Thyroid peroxidase. In: Everse J, Grisham MB, eds. Peroxidases in chemistry and biology. Vol I. Boca Raton, FL: CRC Press, 1990:199

77. McLachlan SM, Rapoport B. The molecular biology of thyroid peroxidase: cloning, expression and role as autoantigen in autoimmune thyroid disease. Endocr Rev 1992;13:192

78. Czarnocka B, Ruf J, Ferrand M, Carayon P, Lissitzky S. Purification of the human thyroid peroxidase and its identification as the microsomal antigen involved in autoimmune thyroid disease. FEBS Lett 1985;190:147

79. Portmann L, Hamada N, Heinrich G, DeGroot LJ. Antithyroid peroxidase antibody in patients with autoimmune disease: possible identity with anti-microsomal antibody. J Clin Endrocrinol Metab 1985;61:1001

80. Kotani T, Umeki K, Matsunaga S, Kato E, Ohtaki S. Detection of autoantibodies to thyroid peroxidase in autoimmune thyroid disease by micro-ELISA and immunoblotting. J Clin Endocrinol Metab 1986;62:928

81. Hosoya T, Morrison MM. The isolation and purification of thyroid peroxidase. J Biol Chem 1967;242:2828

82. Coval ML, Taurog A. Purification and iodinating activity of hog thyroid peroxidase. J Biol Chem 1967;242:5510

83. Taurog A, Lothrop ML, Estabrook RW. Improvements in the isolation procedure for thyroid peroxidase: nature of the heme prosthetic group. Arch Biochem Biophys 1970;139:221

84. Pommier J, DePrailaune S, Nunez J. Peroxydase particulaire thyroidienne. Biochimie 1972;54:483

85. Alexander NB. Purification of bovine thyroid peroxidase. Endocrinology 1977;100:1610

86. Rawitch AB, Taurog A, Chernoff SB, Dorris ML. Hog thyroid peroxidase: physical, chemical, and catalytic properties of the highly purified enzyme. Arch Biochem Biophys 1979; 194:244

87. Ohtaki S, Nakagawa H, Nakamura M, Yamazaki I. Reactions of purified hog thyroid peroxidase with H_2O_2, tyrosine, and methylmercaptoimidazole (goitrogen) in comparison with bovine lactoperoxidase. J Biol Chem 1982;257:761

88. Taurog A, Dorris ML, Yokoyama N, Slaughter C. Purification and characterization of a large, tryptic fragment of human thyroid peroxidase with high catalytic activity. Arch Biochem Biophys 1990;278:333

89. Yokoyama N, Taurog A. Porcine thyroid peroxidase: relationship between the native enzyme and an active, highly purified tryptic fragment. Mol Endocrinol 1988;2:838

90. Nakagawa H, Kotani T, Ohtaki S, Nakamura M, Yamazaki I. Purification of thyroid peroxidase by monoclonal antibody-assisted immunoaffinity chromatography. Biochem Biophys Res Commun 1985;127:8

91. Ohtaki S, Kotani T, Nakamura Y. Characterization of human thyroid peroxidase purified by monoclonal antibody-assisted chromatography. J Clin Endocrinol Metab 1986;63:570

92. Kaufman KD, Rapoport B, Seto P, Chazenbalk GD, Magnusson RP. Generation of recombinant, enzymatically-active, human thyroid peroxidase and its recognition by antibodies in the sera of patients with Hashimoto's thyroiditis. J Clin Invest 1989;84:394

93. Hata J-I, Yamashita S, Yagihashi S, et al. Stable high level expression of human thyroid peroxidase in cultured Chinese hamster ovary cells. Biochem Biophys Res Commun 1989;164:1268

94. Kimura S, Kotani T, Ohtaki S, Aoyama T. cDNA-directed expression of human thyroid peroxidase. FEBS Lett 1989;250:377

95. Kendler DL, Brennan V, Davies TF, Magnusson RP. Expression of human thyroid peroxidase in insect cells using recombinant baculovirus. Mol Cell Endocrinol 1993;93:199

96. Seto P, Nagayama Y, Foti D, McLachlan SM, Rapoport B. Autoantibodies in the sera of patients with autoimmune thyroid disease recognize a secreted form of human thyroid peroxidase generated in a baculovirus system. Mol Cell Endocrinol 1993;94:R-5

97. Wedlock N, Furmaniak J, Fowler S, et al. Expression of human thyroid peroxidase in the yeasts *Saccharomyces cerevisiae* and *Hansenula polymorpha*. J Mol Endocrinol 1993;10:325

98. Foti D, Kaufman KD, Chazenbalk GD, Rapoport B. Generation of a biologically active, secreted form of human thyroid peroxidase by site-directed mutagenesis. Mol Endocrinol 1990;4:786

99. Kaufman K, Foti D, Seto P, Rapoport B. Overexpression of an immunologically-intact, secreted form of human thyroid peroxidase in eukaryotic cells. Mol Cell Endocrinol 1991;78:107

100. Ohtaki S, Nakagawa H, Nakamura S, Nakamura M, Yamazaki I. Characterization of hog thyroid peroxidase. J Biol Chem 1985;260:441

101. Baker JR, Arscott P, Johnson J. An analysis of the structure and antigenicity of different forms of human thyroid peroxidase. Thyroid 1994;4:173

102. Zeng J, Fenna RE. X-ray crystal structure of canine myeloperoxidase at 3A° resolution. J Mol Biol 1992;226:185

102a. Nishikawa T, Rapoport B, McLachlan S. Exclusion of two major areas on thyroid peroxidase from the immunodominant region containing the conformational epitopes recognized by human auto-antibodies. J Clin Endocrinol Metab 1994;79:1648

103. Johnson KR, Nauseef WM, Care A, et al. Characterization of cDNA clones for human myeloperoxidase: predicted amino acid sequence and evidence for multiple mRNA species. Nucleic Acids Res 1987;15:2013

104. Morishita K, Kubota N, Asano S, Kaziro Y, Nagata S. Molecular cloning and characterization of cDNA for human myeloperoxidase. J Biol Chem 1987;262:3844

105. Dull TJ, Uyeda C, Strosberg AD, Nedwin G, Seilhamer JJ. Molecular cloning of cDNAs encoding bovine and human lactoperoxidase. DNA Cell Biol 1990;9:499

106. Kimura S, Ikeda-Saito M. Human myeloperoxidase and thyroid peroxidase, two enzymes with separate and distinct physiological functions, are evolutionarily related members of the same gene family. Proteins 1988;3:113

107. Magnusson RP, Gestautas J, Taurog A, Rapoport B. Molecular cloning of the structural gene for porcine thyroid peroxidase. J Biol Chem 1987;262:13885

108. Kimura S, Kotani T, McBride OW, et al. Human thyroid peroxidase: complete cDNA and protein sequence, chromosome mapping, and identification of two alternately spliced mRNA's. Proc Natl Acad Sci USA 1987;84:5555

109. Libert F, Ruel J, Ludgate M, et al. Complete nucleotide sequence of the human thyroperoxidase-microsomal antigen cDNA. Nucleic Acids Res 1987;15:6735

110. Magnusson RP, Chazenbalk GD, Gestautas J, et al. Molecular cloning of the complementary deoxyribonucleic acid for human thyroid peroxidase. Mol Endocrinol 1987;1:856

111. Derwahl M, Seto P, Rapoport B. Complete nucleotide sequence of the cDNA for thyroid peroxidase in FRTL-5 rat thyroid cells. Nucleic Acids Res 1989;17:8380

112. Kotani T, Umeki K, Yamamoto I, et al. Nucleotide sequence of the cDNA encoding mouse thyroid peroxidase. Gene 1993;123:289

113. Rawitch AB, Pollock G, Yang S-X, Taurog A. Thyroid peroxidase glycosylation: the location and nature of the N-linked oligosaccharide units in porcine thyroid peroxidase. Arch Biochem Biophys 1992;297:321

114. Ekholm R, Wollman SH. Site of iodination in the rat thyroid gland deduced from electron microscopic autoradiographs. Endocrinology 1975;97:1432

115. Nilsson M, Mölne J, Karlsson FA, Ericson LE. Immunoelectron microscopic studies on the cell surface location of the thyroid microsomal antigen. Mol Cell Endocrinol 1987;53:177

116. Elisei R, Vassart G, Ludgate M. Demonstration of the existence of the alternatively spliced form of thyroid peroxidase in normal thyroid. J Clin Endocrinol Metab 1991;72:700

117. Kimura S, Hong Y-S, Kotani T, Ohtaki S, Kikkawa F. Structure of the human thyroid peroxidase gene: comparison and relationship to the human myeloperoxidase gene. Biochemistry 1989;28:4481

117a. Libert F, Ruel J, Ludgate M, et al. Thyroperoxidase: an auto-antigen with a mosaic structure made of nuclear and mitochondrial gene modules. EMBO J 1987;6:4193

118. Abramowicz MJ, Targovnik HM, Varela V, et al. Identification of a mutation in the coding sequence of the human thyroid peroxidase gene causing congenital goiter. J Clin Invest 1992;90:1200

119. Bikker H, den Hartog MT, Baas F, et al. A 20-basepair duplication in the human thyroid peroxidase gene results in a total iodide organification defect and congenital hypothyroidism. J Clin Endocrinol Metab 1994;79:248

120. Bikker H, Vulsma T, Baas F, de Vijlder JJM. Identification of five novel inactivating mutations in the human thyroid peroxidase gene by denaturing gradient gel electrophoresis. Human Mutation 1995;6:9

121. Nagataki S, Uchimura H, Masuyama Y, Nakao K. Thyrotropin and thyroidal peroxidase activity. Endocrinology 1973;92:363

122. Gérard CM, Lefort A, Christophe D, et al. Distinct transcriptional effects of cAMP on 2 thyroid specific genes: thyroperoxidase and thyroglobulin. Horm Metab Res [Suppl] 1990;23:38

123. Abramowicz MJ, Vassart G, Christophe D. Functional study of the human thyroid peroxidase gene promoter. Eur J Biochem 1992;203:467

124. Aza-Blanc P, Di Lauro R, Santisteban P. Identification of a cis-regulatory element and a thyroid-specific nuclear factor mediating the hormonal regulation of rat thyroid peroxidase promoter activity. Mol Endocrinol 1993;7:1297

125. Damante G, Di Lauro R. Thyroid specific gene expression. Biochim Biophys Acta 1994;1218:255

126. Taurog A, Dorris ML, Lamas L. Comparison of lactoperoxidase- and thyroid peroxidase-catalyzed iodination and coupling. Endocrinology 1974;94:1286

127. Taurog A, Dorris ML. Myeloperoxidase-catalyzed iodination and coupling. Arch Biochem Biophys 1992;296:239

128. Roberts JE, Hoffman BM, Rutter R, Hager LP. Electron-nuclear double resonance of horseradish peroxidase compound I. J Biol Chem 1981;256:2118

129. Pommier J, Dème D, Nunez J. Effect of iodide concentration on thyroxine synthesis catalyzed by thyroid peroxidase. Eur J Biochem 1973;37:406

130. Nunez J, Pommier J. Formation of thyroid hormones. Vitam Horm 1982;39:175

131. DeGroot LJ, Niepomniszcze H. Biosynthesis of thyroid hormone: basic and clinical aspects. Metabolism 1977;26:665

132. Davidson B, Neary JT, Strout HV, Maloof F, Soodak M. Evidence for a thyroid peroxidase-associated "active iodine" species. Biochim Biophys Acta 1978;522:318

133. Morrison M, Schonbaum GR. Peroxidase-catalyzed halogenation. Annu Rev Biochem 1976;45:861

134. Ohtaki S, Nakagawa H, Kimura S, Yamazaki I. Analyses of catalytic intermediates of hog thyroid peroxidase during its iodinating reaction. J Biol Chem 1981;256:805

135. Magnusson RP, Taurog A, Dorris ML. Mechanisms of thyroid peroxidase- and lactoperoxidase-catalyzed reactions involving iodide. J Biol Chem 1984;259:13783

136. Dunford HB, Ralston IM. On the mechanism of iodination of tyrosine. Biochem Biophys Res Commun 1983;116:639

137. Huber RE, Edwards LA, Carne TJ. Studies on the mechanism of iodination of tyrosine by lactoperoxidase. J Biol Chem 1989;264:1381

138. Sun W, Dunford B. Kinetics and mechanism of the peroxidase-catalyzed iodination of tyrosine. Biochemistry 1993;32:1324

139. Roman R, Dunford B. pH dependence of the oxidation of iodide by compound I of horseradish peroxidase. Biochemistry 1972;11:2076

140. Björkstén F. The horseradish peroxidase-catalyzed oxidation of iodide: outline of the mechanism. Biochim Biophys Acta 1970;212:396

141. Kohler H, Taurog A, Dunford HB. Spectral studies with lactoperoxidase and thyroid peroxidase: interconversions between native enzyme, compound II, and compound III. Arch Biochem Biophys 1988;264:438

142. Nunez J. Iodination and thyroid hormone synthesis. In: DeVisscher M, ed. The thyroid gland. New York: Raven Press, 1980:39

143. Nunez J. Thyroid hormones: mechanism of phenoxyether formation. Methods Enzymol 1984;107:476

144. Morris DR, Hager LP. Mechanism of the inhibition of enzymatic halogenation by antithyroid agents. J Biol Chem 1966; 241:3852

145. Maloof F, Soodak M. The oxidation of thiourea, a new parameter of thyroid function. In: Cassano C, Andreoli M, eds. Current topics in thyroid research. New York: Academic Press, 1965:277

146. Nakamura M, Yamazaki I, Nakagawa H, Ohtaki S. Steady state kinetics and regulation of thyroid peroxidase-catalyzed iodination. J Biol Chem 1983;258:3837

147. Magnusson RP, Taurog A, Dorris ML. Mechanism of iodide-dependent catalytic activity of thyroid peroxidase and lactoperoxidase. J Biol Chem 1984;259:197

148. Morrison M, Bayse G. Specificity in peroxidase-catalyzed reactions. In: King TE, Mason HS, Morrison M, eds. Oxidases and related redox systems. Vol 1. Baltimore: University Park Press, 1971:375

149. Dème D, Pommier J, Nunez J. Specificity of thyroid hormone synthesis: the role of thyroid peroxidase. Biochim Biophys Acta 1978;540:73

150. Libby RD, Thomas JA, Kaiser LW, Hager LP. Chloroperoxidase halogenation reactions: chemical versus enzymic halogenating intermediates. J Biol Chem 1982;257:5030

151. Harrison JE, Schultz J. Studies on the chlorinating activity of myeloperoxidase. J Biol Chem 1976;251:1371

152. Neidleman SL, Geigert J. Biohalogenation: principles, basic roles and applications. Chichester: Ellis Horwood, 1986

153. Dziadik-Turner C, Rawitch AB. Iodination of tyrosyl residues and thyroid hormone production. In: Freedman RB, Hawkins HC, eds. The enzymology of post-translational modifications of proteins. Vol 2. London: Academic Press, 1985:95

154. Simon C, Roques M, Torresani J, Lissitzky S. Effect of propylthiouracil on the iodination and maturation of rat thyroglobulin. Acta Endocrinol (Copenh) 1966;53:271

155. Inoue K, Taurog A. Sedimentation pattern of soluble protein from thyroids of iodine deficient rats: acute effects of iodine. Endocrinology 1968;83:816

156. Corvilain B, Van Sande J, Laurent E, Dumont JE. The H_2O_2-generating system modulates protein iodination and the activity of the pentose phosphate pathway in dog thyroid. Endocrinology 1991;128:779

157. Björkman U, Ekholm R, Denef V-F. Cytochemical localization of hydrogen peroxide in isolated thyroid follicles. J Ultrastruct Res 1981;74:105

158. Björkman U, Ekholm R. Generation of H_2O_2 in isolated porcine thyroid follicles. Endocrinology 1984;115:392

159. Björkman U, Ekholm R. Accelerated exocytosis and H_2O_2 generation in isolated thyroid follicles enhance protein iodination. Endocrinology 1988;122:488

160. Björkman U, Ekholm R. Hydrogen peroxide generation and its regulation in FRTL-5 and porcine thyroid cells. Endocrinology 1992;130:393

161. Lippes HA, Spaulding SW. Peroxide formation and glucose oxidation in calf thyroid slices: regulation by protein kinase-C and cytosolic free calcium. Endocrinology 1986;116:1306

162. Björkman U, Ekholm R. Effect of P_1- purinergic agonist on thyrotropin stimulation of H_2O_2 generation in FRTL-5 and porcine thyroid cells. Eur J Endocrinol 1994;130:180

163. Raspé E, Laurent E, Corvilain B, et al. Control of the intracellular Ca^{2+}-concentration and the inositol phosphate accumulation in dog thyrocyte primary culture: evidence for different kinetics of Ca^{2+}-phosphatidylinositol cascade activation and for involvement in the regulation of H_2O_2 production. J Cell Physiol 1991; 146:242

163a. Raspé E, Dumont JE. Tonic modulation of dog thyrocyte H_2O_2 generation and I^- uptake by thyrotropin through the cyclic adenosine 3',5'-monophosphate cascade. Endocrinology 1995; 136:965

163b. Kimura T, Fumikazu O, Sho K, et al. Thyrotropin-induced hydrogen peroxide production in FRTL-5 cells is mediated not by adenosine 3',5'-monophosphate, but Aa^{2+} signaling followed by phospholipase-A_2 activation and potentiated by an adenosine derivative. Endocrinology 1995;136:116

164. Nakamura Y, Ogihara S, Ohtaki S. Activation by ATP of calcium-dependent NADPH-oxidase generating hydrogen peroxide in thyroid plasma membranes. J Biochem 1987;102:1121

165. Nakamura Y, Ohtaki S, Makino R, Tanaka T, Ishimura Y. Superoxide anion is the initial product in the hydrogen peroxide for-

mation catalyzed by NADPH oxidase in porcine thyroid plasma membrane. J Biol Chem 1989;264:4759

166. Nakamura Y, Makino R, Tanaka T, Ishimura Y, Ohtaki S. Mechanism of H_2O_2 production in porcine thyroid cells: evidence for intermediary formation of superoxide anion by NADPH-dependent H_2O_2-generating machinery. Biochemistry 1991;30:4880

167. Virion A, Michot JL, Dème D, Kaniewski J, Pommier J. NADPH-dependent H_2O_2 generation and peroxidase activity in thyroid particular fraction. Mol Cell Endocrinol 1984;36:95

168. Dème D, Virion A, Hammou NA, Pommier J. NADPH-dependent generation of H_2O_2 in a thyroid particulate fraction requires Ca^{2+}. FEBS Lett 1985;186:107

169. Dupuy C, Dème D, Kaniewski J, Pommier J, Virion A. Ca^{2+} regulation of thyroid NADPH-dependent H_2O_2 generation. FEBS Lett 1988;233:74

170. Dupuy C, Kaniewski J, Dème D, Pommier J, Virion A. NADPH-dependent H_2O_2 generation catalyzed by thyroid plasma membranes, studies with electron scavengers. Eur J Biochem 1989;185:597

171. Dupuy C, Virion A, Ohayon R, et al. Mechanism of hydrogen peroxide formation catalyzed by NADPH oxidase in thyroid plasma membrane. J Biol Chem 1991;266:3739

172. De Sandro V, Dupuy C, Kaniewski J, et al. Mechanism of NADPH oxidation catalyzed by horse-radish peroxidase and 2,4-diacetyl-[^{2}H] heme-substituted horse-radish peroxidase. Eur J Biochem 1991;201:507

173. Dupuy C, Virion A, de Sandro V, et al. Activation of the NADPH-dependent H_2O_2-generating system in pig thyroid particulate fraction by limited proteolysis and Zn^{2+} treatment. Biochem J 1992;283:591

174. Dème D, Doussiere J, de Sandro V, et al. The Ca^{2+}/NADPH-dependent H_2O_2 generator in thyroid plasma membrane: inhibition by diphenyleneiodonium. Biochem J 1994;301:75

175. Segal AW, Abo A. The biochemical basis of the NADPH oxidase of phagocytes. Trends in Biochemical Sciences 1993;18:43

176. Nadler N, Leblond CP. The site and rate of the formation of thyroid hormone. Brookhaven Symposia in Biology 1955; 7:40

177. Wollman SH, Wodinsky I. Localization of protein bound ^{131}I in the thyroid gland of the mouse. Endocrinology 1955;56:9

178. Ekholm R, Björkman U. Localization of iodine binding in the thyroid gland *in vitro*. Endocrinology 1984;115:1558

179. Nadler NJ. Anatomical features. In: Greep RO, Astwood EB, eds. Handbook of physiology. Vol III. Washington, DC: American Physiological Society, 1974:39

180. Stein O, Gross J. Metabolism of ^{125}I in the thyroid gland studied with electron microscopic autoradiography. Endocrinology 1964;75:787

181. Halmi NS, Pitt-Rivers R. The iodide pools of the rat thyroid. Endocrinology 1962;70:660

182. Nagataki S, Ingbar SH. Demonstration of a second thyroidal iodide pool in rat thyroid glands by double isotope labeling. Endocrinology 1963;73:479

183. Tice LW, Wollman SH. Ultrastructural localization of peroxidase on pseudopods and other structures of the typical thyroid epithelial cell. Endocrinology 1974;94:1555

184. Hosoya T, Matsukawa S, Kurata Y. Cytochemical localization of peroxidase in the follicular cells of pig thyroid gland. Endocrinol Jpn 1972;19:359

185. Hosoya T, Matsukawa G, Nagai Y. Further studies on the localization of peroxidase in pig thyroid cells. Endocrinol Jpn 1973; 20:555

186. Morrison M, Danner DJ, Bayse GS. Subcellular distribution and catalytic activity of thyroid peroxidase. In: Fellinger K, Hofer R, eds. Further advances in thyroid research. Vienna: Verlag der Wiener Medizinischen Akademie, 1971:741

187. Nakai Y, Fujita H. Fine structural localization of peroxidase in rat thyroid. Z Zellforsch 1970;107:104

188. Novikoff AB, Novikoff PM, Ma M, et al. Cytochemical studies of secretory and other granules associated with the endoplasmic reticulum in rat thyroid epithelial cells. Adv Cytopharmacol 1974;2:349

189. Strum JM, Karnovsky MJ. Cytochemical localization of endogenous peroxidase in thyroid follicular cells. J Cell Biol 1970; 44:655

190. Tice LW, Wollman SH. Ultrastructural localization of peroxidase activity on some membranes of the typical thyroid epithelial cells. Lab Invest 1972;26:63

191. Kotani T, Ohtaki S. Characterization of thyroid follicular cell apical plasma membrane peroxidase using monoclonal antibody. Endocrinol Jpn 1987;34:407

192. Croft CJ, Pitt-Rivers R. Radioautographic studies of the initial site of formation of protein-bound iodine in the rat thyroid gland. Biochem J 1970;118:311

193. Nunez J, Jacquemin D, Brun D, Roche J. Proteins iodees particulaire thyroidiennes: II. biosynthese proteique et iodination. Biochim Biophys Acta 1965;107:454

194. Rousset B, Poncet C, Dumont JE, Mornex R. Intracellular and extracellular sites of iodination in dispersed hog thyroid cells. Biochem J 1980;192:801

195. Kuliawat R, Arvan P. Intracellular iodination of thyroglobulin in filter-polarized thyrocytes leads to the synthesis and basolateral secretion of thyroid hormone. J Biol Chem 1994;269:4922

196. Ekholm R. Iodination of thyroglobulin, an intracellular or an extracellular process? Mol Cell Endocrinol 1981;24:141

197. Dumont JE, Vassart G, Refetoff S. Thyroid disorders. In: Scriver CR, Beaudet AL, Sly WS, Valle D, eds. The metabolic basis of inherited disease. 6th ed. New York: McGraw-Hill, 1989:1843

198. DeGroot LJ. Congenital defects in thyroid hormone formation and action. In: DeGroot LJ, ed. Endocrinology. Vol I. 3rd ed. Philadelphia: WB Saunders, 1995:871

199. Harington CR, Barger G. Chemistry of thyroxine: III. constitution and synthesis of thyroxine. Biochem J 1927;21:169

200. Johnson TB, Tewkesbury LB. The oxidation of 3,5-diiodotyrosine to thyroxine. Proc Natl Acad Sci USA 1942;28:73

201. Harington CR. Newer knowledge of the biochemistry of the thyroid gland. J Chem Soc (Part 1) 1944:193

202. Harington CR. Twenty-five years of research on the biochemistry of the thyroid gland. Endocrinology 1951;49:401

203. Dème D, Pommier J, Nunez J. Kinetics of thyroglobulin iodination and of hormone synthesis catalyzed by thyroid peroxidase: role of iodide in the coupling reaction. Eur J Biochem 1976; 70:435

204. Taurog A, Nakashima T. Dissociation between degree of iodination and iodoamino acid distribution in thyroglobulin. Endocrinology 1978;103:632

205. Studer H, Greer M. The regulation of thyroid function in iodine deficiency. Bern, Switzerland: Hans Huber, 1966

206. Abrams GM, Larsen PR. Triiodothyronine and thyroxine in the serum and thyroid glands of iodine-deficient rats. J Clin Invest 1973;52:2522

207. Riesco G, Taurog A, Larsen PR, Krulich L. Acute and chronic responses to iodine deficiency in rats. Endocrinology 1977; 100:303

208. Taurog A, Riesco G, Larsen PR. Formation of 3,3'-diiodothyronine and 3',5',3-triiodothyronine (reverse T_3) by thyroid glands of rats and in enzymatically iodinated thyroglobulin. Endocrinology 1976;99:281

209. Dème D, Fimiani E, Pommier J, Nunez J. Free diiodotyrosine effects on protein iodination and thyroid hormone synthesis catalyzed by thyroid peroxidase. Eur J Biochem 1975;51:329

210. Lamas L, Dorris ML, Taurog A. Evidence for a catalytic role for thyroid peroxidase in the conversion of diiodotyrosine to thyroxine. Endocrinology 1972;90:1417

211. Taurog A, Nakashima T. Mechanism of the stimulating effect of diiodotyrosine on thyroid peroxidase-catalyzed coupling. In: Stockigt JR, Nagataki S. eds. Thyroid research. Vol VIII. Canberra: Australian Academy of Science, 1980:121

212. Virion A, Dème D, Pommier J, Nunez J. The role of iodide and of free diiodotyrosine in enzymatic and non-enzymatic thyroid hormone synthesis. Eur J Biochem 1981;118:239

213. Taurog A, Rawitch AB, Dorris ML, Xiao S. Specificity in tyrosyl iodination sites in thyroglobulin: chemical versus enzymatic iodination. Thyroid 1992; (Suppl1):S88

214. Mercken L, Simons M-J, Swillens S, Massaer M, Vassart G. Primary structure of bovine thyroglobulin deduced from the sequence of its 8,431-base complementary DNA. Nature 1985; 316:647

215. Malthiery Y, Lissitzky S. Primary structure of human thyroglobulin deduced from the sequence of its 8448-base complementary DNA. Eur J Biochem 1987;165:491

216. Di Lauro R, Obici S, Condliffe D, et al. The sequence of 967 amino acids at the carboxyl-end of rat thyroglobulin: location and surroundings of two thyroxine-forming sites. Eur J Biochem 1985;148:7

217. Taurog A. Thyroid peroxidase-catalyzed iodination and thyroxine formation in various proteins. In: Fellinger K, Hofer F, eds. Further advances in thyroid research. Vienna: Verlag der Wiener Medizinischen Akademie, 1971:211

218. Rolland M, Montfort M-F, Lissitzky S. Efficiency of thyroglobulin as a thyroid hormone-forming protein. Biochim Biophys Acta 1973;303:338

219. Gavaret J-M, Dème D, Nunez J, Salvatore G. Sequential reactivity to tyrosyl residues of thyroglobulin upon iodination catalyzed by thyroid peroxidase. J Biol Chem 1977;252:3281

220. Lamas L, Taurog A. The importance of thyroglobulin structure in thyroid peroxidase-catalyzed conversion of diiodotyrosine to thyroxine. Endocrinology 1977;100:1129

221. Maurizis J-C, Marriq C, Rolland M, Lissitzky S. Thyroid hormone synthesis and reactivity of hormone-forming tyrosine residues of thyroglobulin. FEBS Lett 1981;132:29

222. Maurizis J-C, Marriq C, Michelot J, Rolland M, Lissitzky S. Thyroid peroxidase-induced thyroid hormone synthesis in relation to thyroglobulin structure. FEBS Lett 1979;102:82

223. Lamas L, Taurog A, Salvatore G, Edelhoch H. Preferential synthesis of thyroxine from early iodinated tyrosyl residues in thyroglobulin. J Biol Chem 1974;249:2732

224. Palumbo G, Gentile F, Condorelli GL, Salvatore G. The earliest site of iodination in thyroglobulin is residue number 5. J Biol Chem 1990;265:8887

225. Mercken L, Simons MJ, Vassart G. The 5'-end of bovine thyroglobulin mRNA encodes a hormonogenic peptide. FEBS Lett 1982;149:285

226. Rawitch AB, Chernoff SB, Litwer MR, Rouse JB, Hamilton JW. Thyroglobulin structure-function: the amino acid sequence surrounding thyroxine. J Biol Chem 1983;258:2079

227. Rawitch AB, Mercken L, Hamilton JW, Vassart G. The structure of a naturally occurring 10K polypeptide derived from the amino terminus of bovine thyroglobulin. Biochem Biophys Res Commun 1984;119:335

228. Rawitch AB, Litwer MR, Gregg J, Turner CD, Rouse JB, Hamilton JW. The isolation of identical thyroxine containing amino acid sequences from bovine, ovine and porcine thyroglobulin. Biochem Biophys Res Commun 1984;118:423

229. Lissitzky S. Thyroglobulin entering into molecular biology. J Endocrinol Invest 1984;7:65

230. Marriq C, Rolland M, Lissitzky S. Structure–function relationship in thyroglobulin: amino acid sequence of two different thyroxine-containing peptides from porcine thyroglobulin. EMBO J 1982;1:397

231. Marriq C, Rolland M, Lissitzky S. Amino acid sequence of the unique 3,5,3'-triiodothyronine-containing sequence from porcine thyroglobulin. Biochem Biophys Res Commun 1983;112:206

232. Vassart G, Brocas H, Cabrer B, et al. Structure and expression of the thyroglobulin gene. Progress in Endocrine Research and Therapy 1985;2:55

233. Dunn JT, Anderson PC, Fox JW, et al. The sites of thyroid hormone formation in rabbit thyroglobulin. J Biol Chem 1987; 262:16948

234. Gavaret J-M, Cahnmann HJ, Nunez J. The fate of the "lost side chain" during thyroid hormonogenesis. J Biol Chem 1979; 254:11218

235. Gavaret J-M, Nunez J, Cahnmann HJ. Formation of dehydroalanine residues during thyroid hormone synthesis in thyroglobulin. J Biol Chem 1980;255:2581

236. Palumbo G. Thyroid hormonogenesis: identification of a sequence containing iodophenyl donor site(s) in calf thyroglobulin. J Biol Chem 1987;262:17182

237. Ohmiya Y, Hayashi H, Kondo T, Kondo Y. Location of dehydroalanine residues in the amino acid sequence of bovine thyroglobulin, identification of "donor" tyrosine sites for hormonogenesis in thyroglobulin. J Biol Chem 1990;265:9066

238. Marriq C, Lejeune P-J, Venot, Vinet L. Hormone synthesis in human thyroglobulin: possible cleavage of the polypeptide chain at the tyrosine donor site. FEBS Lett 1989;242:414

239. Rawitch AB, Pollock G, Taurog A. Hormone forming sites in human thyroglobulin determined by pulse-chase experiments using ^{125}I and thyroid peroxidase. Abstract No 365. 10th International Thyroid Conference, The Hague, The Netherlands, Feb 3–8, 1991

240. Chernoff SB, Rawitch AB. Thyroglobulin structure–function: isolation and characterization of a thyroxine-containing peptide from bovine thyroglobulin. J Biol Chem 1981;256:9425

241. Dunn JT, Dunn AD, Heppner DG Jr, Kim PS. A discrete thyroxine-rich iodopeptide of 20,000 daltons from rabbit thyroglobulin. J Biol Chem 1981;256:942

242. Lejeune P-J, Marriq C, Rolland M, Lissitzky S. *In vitro* and *in vivo* iodination of human thyroglobulin in relation to hormone release. FEBS Lett 1983;156:77

243. Dunn JT, Dunn AD, Heppner DG Jr, Kim PS, Moore RC. The role of iodination in the formation of hormone-rich peptides from thyroglobulin. J Biol Chem 1983;258:9093

244. Dunn JT, Kim PS, Moore RC. Hormone-rich peptides of thyroglobulin: studies on their structure and origin. Progress in Endocrine Research and Therapy 1985;2:33

245. Turner CD, Chernoff SB, Taurog A, Rawitch AB. Differences in iodinated peptides and thyroid hormone formation after chemical and thyroid peroxidase-catalyzed iodination of human thyroglobulin. Arch Biochem Biophys 1983;222:245

246. Gavaret J-M, Cahnmann HJ, Nunez J. Thyroid hormone synthesis in thyroglobulin: the mechanism of the coupling reaction. J Biol Chem 1981;256:9167

247. Taurog A, Dorris M, Doerge DR. Evidence for a radical mechanism in peroxidase-catalyzed coupling: I. steady state experiments with various peroxidases. Arch Biochem Biophys 1994; 315:82

248. Doerge DR, Taurog A, Dorris ML. Evidence for a radical mechanism in peroxidase-catalyzed coupling: II. single turnover experiments with horseradish peroxidase. Arch Biochem Biophys 1994;315:90

249. Dème D, Virion A, Michot JL, Pommier J. Thyroid hormone synthesis and thyroglobulin iodination related to the peroxidase localization of oxidizing equivalents: studies with cytochrome c peroxidase and horseradish peroxidase. Arch Biochem Biophys 1985;236:559

250. Virion A, Courtin F, Dème D, Michot JL, Kaniewski J, Pommier J. Spectral characteristics and catalytic properties of thyroid peroxidase–H_2O_2 compounds in the iodination and coupling reactions. Arch Biochem Biophys 1985;242:41

251. Courtin F, Dème D, Virion A, et al. The role of lactoperoxidase–H_2O_2 compounds in the catalysis of thyroglobulin iodination and thyroid hormone synthesis. Eur J Biochem 1982;124:603

252. Courtin F, Michot JL, Virion A, Pommier J, Dème D. Reduction of lactoperoxidase–H_2O_2 compounds by ferrocyanide: indirect evidence of an apoprotein site for one of the two oxidizing equivalents. Biochem Biophys Res Commun 1984;121:463

253. Stanbury JB, Ohela K, Pitt-Rivers R. The metabolism of iodine in two goitrous cretins compared with that in two patients receiving methimazole. J Clin Endocrinol Metab 1955;15:54

254. Pommier J, Tourniaire J, Dème D, et al. A defective thyroid peroxidase solubilized from a familial goiter with iodine organification defect. J Clin Endocrinol Metab 1974;39:69

255. Medeiros-Neto G, Targovnik HM, Vassart G. Defective thyroglobulin synthesis and secretion causing goiter and hypothyroidism. Endocr Rev 1993;14:165

256. Ieiri T, Cochaux P, Targovnik H, et al. A 3′ splice site mutation in the thyroglobulin gene responsible for congenital goiter with hypothyroidism. J Clin Invest 1991;88:1901

257. Targovnik HM, Medeiros-Neto G, Varela V, et al. A nonsense mutation causes human hereditary congenital goiter with preferential production of a 171-nucleotide-deleted thyroglobulin ribonucleic acid messenger. J Clin Endocrinol Metab 1993;77:201

258. Fukuda H, Yasuda N, Greer MA, Kutas M, Greer SE. Changes in plasma thyroxine, triiodothyronine, and TSH during adaptation to iodine deficiency in rats. Endocrinology 1987;97:30

259. Okamura K, Taurog A, Krulich L. Elevation of serum 3,5,3′-triiodothyronine and thyroxine levels in rats fed Remington diets: opposing effects of nutritional deficiency and iodine deficiency. Endocrinology 1981;108:1247

260. Okamura K, Taurog A, Krulich L. Strain differences among rats in response to Remington iodine-deficient diets. Endocrinology 1981;109:458

261. Escobar del Rey F, Ruiz de Ona C, Bernal J, Obregon M, Morreale de Escobar G. Generalized deficiency of 3,5,3′-triiodo-L-thyronine (T₃) in tissues from rats on low iodine intake, despite normal circulating T₃ levels. Acta Endocrinol 1989;120:490

262. Pazos-Moura CC, Moura EG, Dorris ML, et al. Effect of iodine deficiency and cold exposure on 5′-deiodinase activity in various rat tissues. Am J Physiol 1991;260:E175

263. Okamura K, Taurog A, Krulich L. Hypothyroidism in severely iodine-deficient rats. Endocrinology 1981;109:464

264. Santisteban P, Obregon MJ, Rodriguez-Pena A, Lamas L, Escobar del Rey F, Morreale de Escobar G. Are iodine deficient rats euthyroid? Endocrinology 1982;110:1780

265. Wolff J, Chaikoff IL. Plasma inorganic iodide as a homeostatic regulator of thyroid function. J Biol Chem 1948;174:555

266. Nagataki S, Ingbar SH. Relation between qualitative and quantitative alterations in thyroid hormone synthesis induced by varying doses of iodide. Endocrinology 1964;74:731

267. Raben MS. The paradoxical effects of thiocyanate and of thyrotropin on the organic binding of iodine by the thyroid in the presence of large amounts of iodide. Endocrinology 1949;45:296

268. Nagataki S. Effect of excess of quantities of iodide. In: Greep RO, Astwood EB, eds. Handbook of physiology. Vol III. Washington, DC: American Physiological Society, 1974:329

269. Selenkow HS, Garcia AM, Bradley EB. An autoregulatory effect of iodide in diverse thyroid disorders. Ann Intern Med 1965;62:714

270. Taurog A. Thyroid peroxidase-catalyzed iodination of thyroglobulin: inhibition by excess iodide. Arch Biochem Biophys 1970; 139:212

271. Yamamoto K, DeGroot LJ. Function of peroxidase and NADPH-cyt c reductase during the Wolff-Chaikoff effect. Endocrinology 1973;93:822

272. Chiraseveenuprapund P, Rosenberg IN. Effects of hydrogen peroxide-generating systems on the Wolff-Chaikoff effect. Endocrinology 1981;109:2095

273. Corvilain B, Van Sande J, Dumont JE. Inhibition by iodide of iodide binding to proteins: the "Wolff-Chaikoff" effect is caused by inhibition of H₂O₂ generation. Biochem Biophys Res Commun 1988;154:1287

274. DeGroot LJ, Decostre P, Phair R. A mathematical model of human iodine metabolism. J Clin Endocrinol Metab 1971;32:757

275. Wartofsky L, Ingbar SH. Estimation of the rate of release of non-thyroxine iodine from the thyroid glands of normal subjects and patients with thyrotoxicosis. J Clin Endocrinol Metab 1971;33:488

276. Pisarev MA, Chazenbalk GD, Valsecchi RM, et al. Thyroid autoregulation: inhibition of goiter growth and of cyclic AMP formation in rat thyroid by iodinated derivatives of arachidonic acid. J Endocrinol Invest 1988;11:669

277. Wolff J. Excess iodide inhibits the thyroid by multiple mechanisms. In: Ekholm R, Kohn LD, Wollman SH, eds. Control of the thyroid gland. New York: Plenum Publishing, 1989:211

278. Dugrillon A, Bechtner G, Uedelhoven WM, Weber PC, Gärtner R. Evidence that an iodolactone mediates the inhibitory effect of iodide on thyroid cell proliferation but not on adenosine 3′,5′-monophosphate formation. Endocrinology 1990;127:337

279. Pereira A, Braekman J-C, Dumont JE, Boeynaems J-M. Identification of a major iodolipid from the horse thyroid gland as 2-iodohexadecanal. J Biol Chem 1990;265:17018

280. Krawiec L, Chester HA, Bocanera LV, et al. Thyroid auto-regulation: evidence for an action of iodoarachidonates and iodide at the cell membrane level. Horm Metab Res 1991;23:321

281. Pisarev MA, Bocanera LV, Chester HA, et al. Effect of iodoarachidonates on thyroid FRTL-5 cells growth. Horm Metab Res 1992;24:558

282. Pisarev MA, Krawiec L, Juvenal GJ, et al. Studies on the goiter inhibiting action of iodolactones. Eur J Pharmacol 1994;258:33

283. Panneels V, Van den Bergen H, Jacoby C, et al. Inhibition of H₂O₂ production by iodoaldehydes in cultured dog thyroid cells. Mol Cell Endocrinol 1994;102;167

283a. Dugrillon A, Uedelhoven WM, Pisarev MA, Bechtner G, Gärtner R. Identification of δ-iodolactone in iodide treated human goiter and its inhibitory effect on proliferation of human thyroid follicles. Horm Metab Res 1994;26:465

283b. Dugrillon A, Gärtner R. δ-Iodolactones decrease epidermal growth factor-induced proliferation and inositol-1,4,5-triphosphate generation in porcine thyroid follicles—a possible mechanism of growth inhibition by iodide. Eur J Endocrinol 1995; 132;735

283c. Boeynaems J-M, Van Sande J, Dumont JE. Which iodolipids are involved in thyroid autoregulation: iodolactones or iodaldehydes? Eur J Endocrinol 1995;132;733

284. Astwood EB. Mechanism of action of antithyroid compounds. Brookhaven Symp Biol 1955;7:61

285. Marchant B, Lees JFH, Alexander WD. Antithyroid drugs. Pharmacol Ther Part B 1978;3:305

286. Kampmann JP, Hansen JM. Clinical pharmacokinetics of antithyroid drugs. Clin Pharmacokinet 1981;6:401

287. Cooper DS. Antithyroid drugs. N Engl J Med 1984;311:1353

288. Cooper DS, Saxe VC, Meskell M, Maloof F, Ridgway EC. Acute effects of propylthiouracil (PTU) on thyroidal iodide organification and peripheral iodothyronine deiodination: correlation with serum PTU levels measured by radioimmunoassay. Endocrinology 1982;54:101

289. Halpern R, Cooper DS, Kieffer JD, et al. Propylthiouracil (PTU) pharmacology in the rat: I. serum and thyroid PTU measurements by radioimmunoassay. Endocrinology 1983; 113:915

290. Cooper DS, Kieffer JD, Halpern R, et al. Propylthiouracil (PTU) pharmacology function in the rat: II. effects of PTU on thyroid function. Endocrinology 1983;113:921

291. Nakashima T, Taurog A, Riesco G. Mechanism of action of thioureylene drugs: factors affecting intrathyroidal metabolism of propylthiouracil and methimazole in rats. Endocrinology 1978;103:2187

292. Nakashima T, Taurog A. Rapid conversion of carbimazole to methimazole in serum: evidence for an enzymatic mechanism. Clin Endocrinol 1979;10:637

293. Marchant B, Alexander WD, Lazarus JH, et al. The accumulation of ³⁵S-antithyroid drugs by the thyroid gland. J Clin Endocrinol Metab 1972;38:847

294. Davidson B, Soodak M, Strout HV, Neary JT, Nakamura C, Maloof F. Thiourea and cyanamide as inhibitors of peroxidase: the role of iodide. Endocrinology 1979;104:919

295. Schussler GC, Ingbar SH. The role of intermediary carbohydrate metabolism in regulating organic iodinations in the thyroid gland. J Clin Invest 1961;40:1394

296. Suzuki M, Nagashima M, Yamamoto K. Studies on the mechanism of iodination by the thyroid gland: iodide-activating enzyme and an intracellular inhibitor of iodination. Gen Comp Endocrinol 1961;1:103

297. Taurog A. The mechanism of action of the thioureylene antithyroid drugs. Endocrinology 1976;98:1031
298. Engler H, Taurog A, Luthy C, Dorris ML. Reversible and irreversible inhibition of thyroid peroxidase-catalyzed iodination by thioureylene drugs. Endocrinology 1983;112:86
299. Taurog A, Dorris ML. Propylthiouracil and methimazole display contrasting pathways of peripheral metabolism in both rat and human. Endocrinology 1988;122:592
300. Taurog A, Dorris ML. A reexamination of the proposed inactivation of thyroid peroxidase in the rat thyroid by propylthiouracil. Endocrinology 1989;124:3038
301. Taurog A, Dorris ML, Guziec FS Jr. Metabolism of ^{35}S- and ^{14}C-labeled 1-methy-2-mercaptoimidazole *in vitro* and *in vivo*. Endocrinology 1989;124:30
302. Taurog A, Dorris ML, Guziec FS Jr, Uetrecht JP. Metabolism of ^{35}S- and ^{14}C-labeled propylthiouracil in a model *in vitro* system containing thyroid peroxidase. Endocrinology 1989;124:3030
303. Marchant B, Alexander WD. The thyroid accumulation, oxidation and metabolic fate of ^{35}S-methimazole in the rat. Endocrinology 1972;91:747
304. Marchant B, Alexander WD, Robertson JWK, Lazarus JH. Concentration of ^{35}S-propylthiouracil by the thyroid gland and its relationship to anion trapping mechanism. Metabolism 1971;20:989
305. Patterson JR, Hood HT, Skellern GG. The role of porcine thyroid peroxidase and FAD-containing monooxygenase in the metabolism of 1-methyl-2-thioimidazole (methimazole). Biochem Biophys Res Commun 1983;116:449
306. Lindsey RH, Kelly K, Hill JB. Oxidative metabolites of [2-^{14}C] propylthiouracil in rat thyroid. Endocrinology 1979;104:1686
307. Skellern GG, Steer ST. The metabolism of [2-^{14}C] methimazole in the rat. Xenobiotica 1981;11:627
308. Edelhoch H, Irace G, Johnson ML, Michot JL, Nunez J. The effects of thioureylene compounds (goitrogens) on lactoperoxidase activity. J Biol Chem 1979;254:11822
309. Doerge DR. Mechanism-based inhibition of lactoperoxidase by thiocarbamide goitrogens, identification of turnover and inactivation pathways. Biochemistry 1988;27:3697
310. Engler H, Taurog A, Nakashima T. Mechanism of inactivation of thyroid peroxidase by thioureylene drugs. Biochem Pharmacol 1982;31:3801
311. Doerge DR. Mechanism-based inhibition of lactoperoxidase by thiocarbamide goitrogens. Biochemistry 1986;25:4724
312. Shiroozu A, Taurog A, Engler H, Dorris ML. Mechanism of action of thioureylene antithyroid drugs in the rat: possible inactivation of thyroid peroxidase by propylthiouracil. Endocrinology 1983;113:362
313. Davidson B, Soodak M, Neary JT, et al. The irreversible inactivation of thyroid peroxidase by methylmercaptoimidazole, thiouracil, and propylthiouracil *in vitro* and its relationship to *in vivo* findings. Endocrinology 1978;103:871
314. Nogimori T, Braverman LE, Taurog A, Fang S-L, Wright G, Emerson CH. A new class of propylthiouracil analogs: comparison of 5'-deiodinase inhibition and antithyroid activity. Endocrinology 1986;118:1598
315. Taurog A, Dorris ML, Hu W-X, Guziec FS Jr. The selenium analog of 6-propylthiouracil: measurement of its inhibitory effect on type I iodothyronine deiodinase and of its antithyroid activity. Biochem Pharmacol 1995;49:701
316. Taurog A, Dorris ML, Guziec LJ, Guziec FS Jr. The selenium analog of methimazole: measurement of its inhibitory effect on type I 5'-deiodinase and of its antithyroid activity. Biochem Pharmacol 1994;48:1447
317. Okamura K, Taurog A. Inhibitory action and intrathyroidal metabolism of propylthiouracil (PTU) and methimazole (MMI) in TSH-treated guinea pigs. Abstract No 104. Sixty-fourth Meeting of the Endocrine Society, San Francisco, June 16–18, 1982
318. Lang JCT, Lees JFH, Alexander WD, Ingbar SH. Effect of variations in acute and chronic iodine intake on the accumulation and metabolism of [^{35}S] propylthiouracil by the rat thyroid gland. Biochem Pharmacol 1983;32:233
319. Lang JCT, Lees JFH, Alexander WD, Ingbar SH. Effect of variations in acute and chronic iodine intake on the accumulation and metabolism of [^{35}S] methimazole by the rat thyroid gland: differences from [^{35}S] propylthiouracil. Biochem Pharmacol 1983;32:241
320. Greer MA, Meihoff WC, Studer H. Treatment of hyperthyroidism with a single daily dose of propylthiouracil. N Engl J Med 1965;272:888
321. Barnes HV, Bledsoe T. A simple test for selecting the thioamide schedule in thyrotoxicosis. J Clin Endocrinol Metab 1972;35:250
322. Bouma DJ, Kammer H. Single daily dose methimazole treatment of hyperthyroidism. West J Med 1980;132:13
323. Roti E, Gardini E, Minelli R, Salvi M, Robuschi G, Braverman LE. Methimazole and serum thyroid hormone concentrations in hyperthyroid patients: effects of single and multiple daily doses. Ann Intern Med 1989;111:81
324. Shiroozu A, Okamura K, Ikenoue H, et al. Treatment of hyperthyroidism with a small single daily dose of methimazole. J Clin Endocrinol Metab 1986;63:125
325. Wise PH, Marion M, Pain RW. Single dose, "block-replace" drug therapy in hyperthyroidism. Br Med J 1973;4:143
326. Iino S, Yamada T, Greer MA. Effect of graded doses of propylthiouracil on biosynthesis of thyroid hormones. Endocrinology 1961;68:582
327. Richards JB, Ingbar SH. The effects of propylthiouracil and perchlorate on the biogenesis of thyroid hormone. Endocrinology 1959;65:198
328. Engler H, Taurog A, Dorris ML. Preferential inhibition of thyroxine and 3,5,3'-triiodothyronine formation by propylthiouracil and methylmercaptoimidazole in thyroid peroxidase-catalyzed iodination of thyroglobulin. Endocrinology 1982; 110:190
329. Papapetrou PD, Mothons S, Alexander WD. Binding of ^{35}S-propylthiouracil by follicular thyroglobulin *in vivo* and *in vitro*. Acta Endocrinol (Copenh) 1975;79:248
330. Taurog A, Riesco G. Thyroid peroxidase-catalyzed oxidation of ^{35}S-propylthiouracil and binding of ^{35}S to thyroglobulin (abstract). Fed Proc 1974;33:249
331. Weetman AP. The immunomodulatory effects of antithyroid drugs. Thyroid 1994;4:145
332. Volpé R. Evidence that the immunosuppressive effects of antithyroid drugs are mediated through actions on the thyroid cell, modulating thyrocyte–immunocyte signaling: a review. Thyroid 1994;4:217
333. Volpe R. Immunomodulatory effects of antithyroid drugs. Thyroid 1994;4:507

RELEASE AND SECRETION OF THYROID HORMONE

Ann D. Dunn

THYROGLOBULIN RETRIEVAL AND THE ENDOCYTIC PATHWAY

Thyroid hormones (thyroxine [T$_4$] and triiodothyronine [T$_3$]) are stored as peptide-linked amino acids in thyroglobulin (Tg) and must be released before their secretion. The process begins with the retrieval of Tg from the follicular lumen. Two internalization mechanisms have been described: nonspecific bulk intake of Tg (macropinocytosis) and retrieval into small vesicles (micropinocytosis). Whereas macropinocytosis involves nonspecific resorption of luminal material, micropinocytosis can occur either by receptor-mediated uptake or by nonspecific fluid-phase endocytosis. The prevailing evidence suggests that each of these routes may occur to a variable extent, depending on the animal species involved and physiologic conditions.

Retrieval of Tg by macropinocytosis has been best documented in the hypophysectomized rat.[1] Within 10 minutes after thyroid-stimulating hormone (TSH) injection, pseudopods form at the apical surface of the thyroid cell, engulfing luminal material that soon appears intracellularly as large colloid droplets. These bodies then begin a basal migration and fuse with lysosomes to form so-called phagolysosomes, which continue the basal migration, gradually becoming smaller and more dense as colloid material disappears, indicating that Tg proteolysis has occurred. Several features of macropinocytosis suggest it may be of limited importance to the thyroid. The process has been documented only in the gland acutely stimulated with large doses of TSH, and pseudopods and colloid droplets are rare except in the rat. Also, bulk retrieval of material cannot explain the observation that more heavily iodinated Tg is preferentially internalized.[2]

Using microinjection techniques, Seljelid and coworkers[3] identified small endocytic vesicles in rat thyroids and suggested that these structures represented the normal transport system for Tg. The laboratory of Rousset and coworkers[4,5] recently reported Tg retrieval by micropinocytosis in both intact thyroid tissue and cultures of reconstituted pig thyroid follicles. Iodinated Tg was identified in apical coated vesicles, which are usually associated with the early stage of receptor-mediated and fluid-phase endocytosis. Using immunogold-labeled probes of Tg and intracellular enzyme markers, these investigators tracked the passage of Tg from these vesicles through an endosomal compartment and into lysosomes,[6] a common route in many cell types for internalized proteins destined for degradation. Tg immunogenicity diminished as it passed through the endosomal compartment, suggesting that some proteolytic processing occurred even before Tg entered the lysosomes. Endosomes contain lysosomal enzymes and may be important for proteolytic processing in other tissues.[7] In the same studies, TSH-stimulated endocytosis in reconstituted thyroid follicles at 37°C actually peaked before the appearance of pseudopods and took place in the absence of pseudopod formation at 20°C. Macropinocytosis was concluded to play only a minor role in the resting or moderately stimulated thyroid gland of the pig, and perhaps of most other mammals as well.

Because Tg exists in the thyroid lumen in highly concentrated form (100 mg/mL),[8] receptor-mediated endocytosis may not be necessary for efficient internalization of Tg, and, indeed, identification of a thyroglobulin receptor has proved difficult. Scheel and Herzog[9] described a cation-independent mannose-6-phosphate receptor on the apical surface of porcine thyroid cells and suggested that it participated in receptor-mediated endocytosis, but, more recently, the same group identified on the apical plasma membrane low-affinity binding sites that are distinct from the mannose-6-phosphate receptor.[10] Use of "inside-out follicles" with reversed polarity and monolayers of porcine thyrocytes in a bicameral system permitted access to the apical surface. Endocytosis of ^{125}I-Tg

was unaffected by mannose-6-phosphate but was strongly inhibited by excess Tg, indicating competition for receptor binding sites. The studies indicated cooperative and saturable binding of Tg to the apical cell membrane. The authors concluded that most of the Tg is internalized by receptor-mediated endocytosis but that a small component (up to 25%) cannot be inhibited by excess Tg and reflects fluid-phase endocytosis.

Kostrouch and coworkers,[11] however, found no evidence for the selective uptake of Tg by porcine thyroid cells. Reconstituted thyroid follicles were unable to distinguish between Tg and bovine serum albumin complexed to gold particles. Instead, sorting of Tg molecules occurred in early endosomes, with some protein being returned to the lumen. The authors suggested that Tg was internalized by fluid-phase endocytosis but that endosomal sorting could be selective by allowing normally iodinated Tg to proceed to lysosomal compartments and returning poorly iodinated protein back to the lumen for completion of hormone synthesis.

Not all internalized Tg reaches the lysosomes. Some is diverted to the bloodstream by transcytosis.[12] In inside-out porcine follicles using gold–Tg conjugates, ^{3}H-Tg, or cationized ferritin as probes, about 10% of endocytosed Tg is transported by small vesicles from the apical to basolateral cell surface, where it is released.[13] The process is stimulated by TSH and probably accounts for the appearance of Tg in the serum.

THYROGLOBULIN PROTEOLYSIS AND THE RELEASE OF THYROID HORMONES

Lysosomal enzymes play a major role in the intrathyroidal degradation of Tg. Purified lysosomes contain the full complement of proteases required for cleaving free iodoamino acids from Tg.[14,15] Their importance is underscored in the lysosomal storage disease caprine β-mannosidosis in which thyroid hormone release is significantly impaired.[16] Lysosomal proteases in the thyroid include the aspartic endopeptidase cathepsin D[17]; the cysteine endopeptidases cathepsins B, L, and H[18,19]; the exopeptidases dipeptidyl peptidases I and II[17,20]; a lysosomal dipeptidase I-like enzyme[21]; and a carboxyl exopeptidase designated N-acetyl-L-phenylalanyl-L-tyrosine hydrolase.[22] Cathepsins B, H, and L have been shown to coexist in colloid droplets and lysosome-like bodies in the rat thyroid by double immunostaining.[23] With the possible exception of N-acetyl-L-phenylalanyl-L-tyrosine hydrolase, all of these enzymes are widely distributed among mammalian cells and none is unique to the thyroid. Cathepsins D and L act primarily as endopeptidases, cleaving internal bonds to produce peptides of five or more residues, whereas cathepsins B and H act as both endopeptidases and exopeptidases, cleaving dipeptides or single amino acids, respectively, from larger peptides.

The relative importance of some of these enzymes for hormone release was assessed in lysosomal extracts from human thyroids incubated with rabbit ^{125}I-Tg as substrate together with enzyme-specific inhibitors.[15] Inhibitors of the cysteine endopeptidases cathepsin B and L (E64, N-Cbz-Phe-Ala-diazomethane) or of cathepsin L alone (N-Cbz-Phe-Phe-diazomethane) were much more effective in blocking Tg degradation and thyroid hormone release than was an inhibitor of cathepsin D (pepstatin). Blocking all endopeptidase activity by combining inhibitors completely prevented hormone release. The earliest products of digestion were peptide fragments of 50 kd or less that originated from both the C- and N-terminal regions of Tg and contained three of the major hormonogenic sites. It was concluded that the formation of discrete hormone-enriched peptides precedes the release of thyroid hormone from Tg and that the cysteine endopeptidases are more important than cathepsin D in this process. Dunn and colleagues[18] found that cathepsins B, D, and L isolated from human thyroid glands each process rabbit ^{125}I-Tg in a limited and distinctive manner, suggesting a synergistic action in vivo. Other studies suggest a synergy between cathepsin B and exopeptidases in releasing free T_4. Nakagawa and Ohtaki[24] isolated a cathepsin B-like enzyme (TP-2) that had little or no ability to release T_4 from intact Tg or its N-terminal peptide but facilitated the action of a second enzyme (TP-1) in releasing hormone from these substrates. Dunn and Crutchfield[25] identified a cathepsin B-generated T_4 dipeptide corresponding to residues 5 and 6 of intact human Tg that was further hydrolyzed by a lysosomal dipeptidase I-like enzyme to release free T_4.

Several additional lines of evidence suggest that Tg proteolysis selectively favors the early release of iodoamino acids. Tokuyama and coworkers[14] found that lysosomal extracts from hog thyroid glands released essentially all iodoamino acids from ^{131}I-Tg in 24 hours but left behind a substantial portion of noniodinated peptide fragments. Furthermore, Rousset and colleagues[26] found that nonreduced lysosomal Tg from hog thyroids had the same apparent molecular weight as intact Tg, but contained little iodide and had no detectable hormone. Under reducing conditions, lysosomal Tg fragmented into a number of smaller peptides. Tg proteolysis appeared to proceed in two steps, an initial rapid release of hormone followed by a delayed nonselective degradation of the remainder of the molecule. Additional evidence for a multistep process comes from studies of hormone release by a mouse macrophage cell line.[27] T_4 was released within 5 minutes of Tg's introduction to J774 cells, coincident with the arrival of the internalized protein to the endosomal compartment. T_3, on the other hand, was released more slowly (within 60 minutes), in parallel with the arrival of Tg in lysosomes. The generalized degradation of Tg occurred even more slowly. The authors suggested that macrophages, and specifically Kupffer cells that take up circulating Tg, represent an extrathyroidal source of thyroid hormones.

Once released from Tg, the thyroid hormones rapidly leave the cell and enter the circulation. It is not known whether the hormones are transported via a specific carrier system. Monoiodotyrosine and diiodotyrosine, in the meantime, are deiodinated by an iodotyrosine-specific deiodinase.[28] The iodide released by this action is partly reused for hormone synthesis; the remainder reenters the circulation. Some intrathyroidal conversion of T_4 to T_3 occurs. The thyroid gland contains an iodothyronine 5'deiodinase that resembles the type I enzyme found in peripheral tissue.[29] Its activity is enhanced in Graves' disease[29] and in experimentally induced iodine deficiency in rats,[30] and is stimulated by TSH[31] and by T_3 and T_4 in FRTL-5 rat thyroid cells.[32]

MODULATORS OF THYROID HORMONE SECRETION

The rapid effects of TSH in mobilizing structural components of the endocytic pathway have already been mentioned. TSH may also stimulate lysosomal enzymes independently. Its administration to rabbits increased cysteine endopeptidase activity in extracts of thyroid lysosomes, with peak activity 24 hours after injection.[33] Cathepsin D activity was stimulated to a lesser extent, and the activities of dipeptidyl peptidase II and acid phosphatase were unaffected. Cytochemical studies of cultured guinea pig thyroid fragments suggested that TSH promotes a rapid increase in the activities of the lysosomal enzymes N-acetyl-β-glucosaminidase, β-galactosidase, and leucyl-β-naphthylaminidase.[34] TSH induced a fivefold increase in cathepsin B mRNA in FRTL-5 cells cultured for up to 5 days.[35]

The release of thyroid hormone from the thyroid gland may be inhibited by a variety of agents, including iodide, which in high doses lessens thyroid hormone release in patients with hyperthyroidism and probably in euthyroid subjects (see chap 14). Several studies suggest a direct effect of iodide on proteolytic enzymes. Protease activity is markedly increased in preparations of thyroid lysosomes from patients with Graves' disease, but is normal in Graves' patients treated chronically with excess iodide.[36] Excess iodide administered in vivo for 3 days significantly reduced cathepsin D and β-glucuronidase activities in the thyroids but not the livers of rats.[37] Methimazole overcame the iodide-induced inhibition of hormone release in cultured rat thyroid lobes,[38] suggesting that an organic form of iodine is involved. Excess iodide can also inhibit TSH-stimulated colloid droplet formation in rat thyroids.[39] Because the same effect was observed with the administration of dibutyryl cyclic adenosine monophosphate (cAMP) in lieu of TSH, iodide probably exerted this effect at a step beyond the generation of cAMP. Lithium is also concentrated by the thyroid and can interfere with thyroid hormone release.[40] Perfusion studies in mouse thyroids suggest that lithium elicits its effect both by suppressing TSH-stimulated cAMP production and by inhibiting some step beyond cAMP generation.[41]

References

1. Wetzel BK, Spicer SS, Wollman SH. Changes in fine structure and acid phosphatase localization in rat thyroid cells following thyrotropin administration. J Cell Biol 1965;25:593

2. van den Hove M-F, Couvreur M, de Visscher M, Salvatore G. A new mechanism for the reabsorption of thyroid iodoproteins: selective fluid pinocytosis. Eur J Biochem 1982;122:415

3. Seljelid R, Reith A, Nakken KF. The early phase of endocytosis in rat thyroid follicle cells. Lab Invest 1970;23:595

4. Bernier-Valentin F, Kostrouch Z, Rabilloud R, Munari-Silem Y, Rousset B. Coated vesicles from thyroid cells carry iodinated thyroglobulin molecules. J Biol Chem 1990;265:17373

5. Bernier-Valentin F, Kostrouch Z, Rabilloud R, Rousset B. Analysis of the thyroglobulin internalization process using in vitro reconstituted thyroid follicles: evidence for a coated vesicle-dependent endocytic pathway. Endocrinology 1991;129:2194

6. Kostrouch Z, Munari-Silem Y, Rajas F, Bernier-Valentin F, Rousset B. Thyroglobulin internalized by thyrocytes passes through early and late endosomes. Endocrinology 1991;129:2202

7. Blum JS, Diaz R, Mayorga LS, Stahl PD. Reconstitution of endosomal transport and proteolysis. In: Bergeron JJM, Harris JR, eds.

Subcellular biochemistry. Vol 19. Endocytic components: identification and characterization. New York: Plenum Press, 1993:69

8. Smeds S. A microgel electrophoretic analysis of the colloid proteins in single rat thyroid follicles: II. the protein concentration of the colloid in single rat thyroid follicles. Endocrinology 1972;91:1288

9. Scheel G, Herzog V. Mannose 6-phosphate receptor in porcine thyroid follicle cells: localization and possible implications for the intracellular transport of thyroglobulin. Eur J Cell Biol 1989;49:140

10. Lemansky P, Herzog V. Endocytosis of thyroglobulin is not mediated by mannose-6-phosphate receptors in thyrocytes: evidence for low-affinity-binding sites operating in the uptake of thyroglobulin. Eur J Biochem 1992;209:111

11. Kostrouch Z, Bernier-Valentin F, Munari-Silem Y, Rajas F, Rabilloud R, Rousset B. Thyroglobulin molecules internalized by thyrocytes are sorted in early endosomes and partially recycled back to the follicular lumen. Endocrinology 1993;132:2645

12. Herzog V. Transcytosis in thyroid cells. J Cell Biol 1983; 97:607

13. Romagnoli P, Herzog V. Transcytosis in thyroid follicle cells: regulation and implications for thyroglobulin transport. Exp Cell Res 1991;194:202

14. Tokuyama T, Yoshinari M, Rawitch AB, Taurog A. Digestion of thyroglobulin with purified thyroid lysosomes: preferential release of iodoamino acids. Endocrinology 1987;121:714

15. Dunn AD, Crutchfield HE, Dunn JT. Proteolytic processing of thyroglobulin by extracts of thyroid lysosomes. Endocrinology 1991;128:3073

16. Boyer PJ, Jones MZ, Nachreiner RF, et al. Caprine β-mannosidosis: abnormal thyroid structure and function in a lysosomal storage disease. Lab Invest 1990;63:100

17. Dunn AD, Dunn JT. Thyroglobulin degradation by thyroidal proteases: action of purified cathepsin D. Endocrinology 1982; 111:280

18. Dunn AD, Crutchfield HE, Dunn JT. Thyroglobulin processing by thyroidal proteases: major sites of cleavage by cathepsins B, D, and L. J Biol Chem 1991;266:20198

19. Nakagawa H, Ohtaki S. Partial purification and characterization of two thiol proteases from hog thyroid lysosomes. Endocrinology 1984;115:33

20. Dunn AD, Dunn JT. Thyroglobulin degradation by thyroidal proteases: action of thiol endopeptidases in vitro. Endocrinology 1982;111:290

21. Loughlin RE, Trikojus VM. A metal-dependent peptidase from thyroid glands. Biochim Biophys Acta 1964;92:529

22. Dunn NW, McQuillan MT. Purification and properties of a peptidase from thyroid glands. Biochim Biophys Acta 1971; 235:149

23. Uchiyama Y, Watanabe T, Watanabe M, et al. Immunocytochemical localization of cathepsins B, H, L, and T_4 in follicular cells of rat thyroid gland. J Histochem Cytochem 1989; 37:691

24. Nakagawa H, Ohtaki S. Thyroxine (T_4) release from thyroglobulin and its T_4-containing peptide by thyroid thiol proteases. Endocrinology 1985;116:1433

25. Dunn AD, Crutchfield HE. Identification of two major thyroidal exopeptidases in the release of thyroglobulin's dominant T_4 (abstract). Presented at the Annual Meeting of the Endocrine Society, June 1991. Washington, DC. June 19–22, 1991

26. Rousset B, Selmi S, Bornet H, Bourgeat P, Rabilloud R, Munari-Silem Y. Thyroid hormone residues are released from thyroglobulin with only limited alteration of the thyroglobulin structure. J Biol Chem 1989;264:12620

27. Brix K, Herzog V. Extrathyroidal release of thyroid hormones from thyroglobulin by J774 mouse macrophages. J Clin Invest 1994;93:1388

28. Rosenberg IN, Goswami A. Purification and characterization of a flavoprotein from bovine thyroid with iodotyrosine deiodinase activity. J Biol Chem 1979;254:12318

29. Ishii H, Inadi M, Tanaka K, et al. Triiodothyronine generation from thyroxine in human thyroid: enhanced conversion in Graves' thyroid tissue. J Clin Endocrinol Metab 1981;52:1211

30. Pazos-Moura CC, Moura EG, Dorris ML, et al. Effect of iodine deficiency and cold exposure on thyroxine 5'-deiodinase activity in various rat tissues. Am J Physiol 1991;260:E175

31. Erickson VJ, Cavalieri RR, Rosenberg LL. Thyroxine-5'-deiodinase of rat thyroid, but not that of liver, is dependent on thyrotropin. Endocrinology 1982;111:434

32. Toyoda N, Nishikawa M, Horimoto M, et al. Synergistic effect of thyroid hormone and thyrotropin on iodothyronine 5'-deiodinase in FRTL-5 rat thyroid cells. Endocrinology 1990; 127:1199

33. Dunn AD. Stimulation of thyroidal thiol endopeptidases by thyrotropin. Endocrinology 1984;114:375

34. Perrild H, Hoyer PE, Loveridge N, Reader SCJ, Robertson WR. Acute in vitro thyrotropin regulation of lysosomal enzyme activity in the thyroid follicular cell. Mol Cell Endocrinol 1989;65:75

35. Phillips ID, Black EG, Sheppard MC, Docherty K. Thyrotrophin, forskolin and ionomycin increase cathepsin B mRNA concentrations in rat thyroid cells in culture. J Mol Endocrinol 1989;2:207

36. Yoshinari M, Inoue K, Nakashima T, et al. Acid protease activity in thyroid gland from patients with Graves' disease. Metabolism 1983;32:348

37. Starling JR, Hopps BA. Effect of excess iodine on thyroid and liver lysosomal enzymes. J Surg Res 1980;28:57

38. Bagchi N, Brown T, Shivers B, Mack RE. Effect of inorganic iodide on thyroglobulin hydrolysis in cultured thyroid glands. Endocrinology 1977;100:1002

39. Yamamoto K, Onaya T, Yamada T, Kotani M. Inhibitory effect of excess iodide on thyroid hormone release as measured by intracellular colloid droplets. Endocrinology 1972;90:986

40. Spaulding SW, Burrow GN, Bermudez F, Himmelhoch JM. The inhibitory effect of lithium on thyroid hormone release in both euthyroid and thyrotoxic patients. J Clin Endocrinol Metab 1972; 35:905

41. Mori M, Tajima K, Oda Y, Matsui I, Mashita K, Tarui S. Inhibitory effect of lithium on the release of thyroid hormones from thyrotropin-stimulated mouse thyroids in a perifusion system. Endocrinology 1989;124:1365

Werner and Ingbar's The Thyroid, Seventh Edition,
edited by Lewis E. Braverman and Robert D. Utiger.
Lippincott–Raven Publishers, Philadelphia, © 1996

5

Thyroglobulin: Chemistry and Biosynthesis

John T. Dunn

Thyroglobulin (Tg) is the most important protein of the thyroid gland. It provides a matrix for the synthesis of the thyroid hormones and a vehicle for their subsequent storage. It is also the most abundant of the thyroid's proteins, comprising the bulk of the follicular colloid as well as a substantial part of the thyroid's intracellular material. This chapter reviews Tg structure with particular emphasis on its role in hormone synthesis. Chapter 4 describes thyroid iodine metabolism and Tg proteolysis and chapter 20 its clinical relevance in serum. A large body of older work has been reviewed in previous editions of this book and elsewhere,[1] and is summarized only briefly here.

Table 5-1 lists some general features of Tg. It is a macromolecular glycoprotein of two apparently identical monomeric polypeptide chains that together make up the mature 660-kd 19S dimer. Its tyrosine content is not high, even though the iodination of tyrosine is Tg's only known biologic function. Also, most of its iodine is in the inactive hormone precursors monoiodotyrosine (MIT) and diiodotyrosine (DIT), rather than in triiodothyronine (T_3) and thyroxine (T_4). Tg's iodine content and the distribution of iodine among tyrosyls vary widely with iodine availability. Many observers have commented on the apparent inefficiency of synthesizing such a large molecule to achieve only a few residues of hormone. One explanation for this seeming excess is that iodine is not always readily available to land animals, and Tg can store it as MIT and DIT.

THE GENE AND ITS EXPRESSION

The human Tg (hTg) gene resides on the long arm of chromosome 8q24 distal to the c-*myc* oncogene,[2] and is linked with genes for carbonic anhydrase II and the *MOS* protooncogene. In the mouse the gene is located on chromosome 15,[3] in the rat on chromosome 7,[4] and in the cow on chromosome 14,

where synteny with the same three genes found in humans is preserved.[5]

Elucidation of the structure of the Tg gene has followed classical molecular biology techniques. Key work has come from several laboratories, principally those of Vassart (bovine),[6] Malthiery and Lissitzky (human),[7,8] Di Lauro (rat),[9] and DeVijlder (goats and humans).[2,10] In the human,[7] the successive steps included isolation of polysomal RNA from surgical thyroid samples of subjects with Graves' disease, purification of a mRNA sedimenting at 33S, synthesis and double stranding of complementary DNA, plasmid formation, cloning of fragments, nucleotide sequencing, and alignment of overlapping fragments. This procedure gave the 8.5-kb sequence for Tg's mRNA, from which the amino acid sequence of the translated Tg molecule was deduced.[11] A similar approach predicted the complete amino acid sequence of bovine Tg,[12] the first to be established, and a partial sequence in the rat.[13]

Only a small part of the chromosomal gene codes for Tg. The rest consists of large amounts of interspersed intronic material. For example, the rat gene has at least 170 kb, of which 9 are located in 42 exons of fairly homogeneous size.[14] The human gene has at least 260 kb, but the fraction in exons is less than 2% in the 3' region and about 10% in the 5' area.[2] Damante and Di Lauro[15] have reviewed recent information on the Tg promoter (Fig 5-1). It occupies a region of about 170 bases upstream from the transcription initiating site, and consists of three binding sites (A, B, and C) for thyroid transcription factor 1 (TTF-1). This phosphoprotein, whose mRNA codes for 371 amino acids, appears necessary for transcription activation, whereas another (TTF-2) is thought to affect hormonal regulation of the promoter. A third factor (Pax8) overlaps the response element of TTF-1 at binding site C. Other factors exist but are not well characterized and may compete with TTF-1. The promoter structure is highly conserved among human, rat,

TABLE 5-1.
General Features of Human Thyroglobulin

Usual Molecular Form	Dimer
Molecular weight	660 kd
Sedimentation coefficient	19S
Polypeptide chains	2
Carbohydrate content	10% of weight
Iodine content	0.1%–1.0% of weight
Residues per molecule of 660 kd Tg*	
Amino acids	5496
Tyrosine	134
MIT	5
DIT	4.5
T_4	2.5
T_3	0.7

*Values for iodoamino acids are typical for Tg of 0.5% iodine (26 atoms iodine per 660 kd molecule of Tg).

dog, and cow thyroids, but mutations at specific sites have differing effects on gene transcription among species.[16] The promoter for thyroperoxidase resembles the Tg promoter very closely and responds to the same transcription factors.

Thyroid-stimulating hormone (TSH; thyrotropin) influences transcription of the Tg gene. Hypophysectomy or T_3 treatment decreased transcription in rats, as measured by hybridization with Tg cDNA clones,[17] and injection of bovine TSH gave a prompt threefold rise.[18] Administration of cyclic adenosine monophosphate (cAMP) also stimulates transcription. Transcription in cell culture after TSH or cAMP is much slower than for other cAMP-dependent gene expressions, suggesting the synthesis of an intermediate protein.[19,20] Insulin also stimulates Tg gene transcription in FRTL-5 cells[21] and in dog thyroid cells.[19] The cytokine γ-interferon inhibits Tg gene expression in human[22] and FRTL-5[23] thyrocytes. DNA methylation of the promoter may be a mechanism to modify the rate of Tg gene expression.[24]

Most work so far has focused on the 8- to 9-kb mRNA that expresses the 300-kd Tg monomer. Graves and Davies[25] have described a 0.95-kb mRNA from FRTL-5 cells that codes for the N-terminal 193 amino acids of the Tg polypeptide chain, followed by a short string of nonhomologous coding and noncoding sequences. In the FRTL-5 cells this smaller mRNA was as abundant as the 9.0-kb material, but was much less abundant when isolated from normal Fisher and Buffalo rats. TSH stimulates expression of this gene.

Translation of cDNA from the cloned human Tg gene produces a polypeptide of 2767 amino acids[11] (2769 in the cow[12]), representing the Tg monomer of 300 kd. Its amino acid sequence is shown in Figure 5-2. (The amino acids in Figure 5-2 are numbered to include the 19-residue leader sequence, as published in data banks; the N-terminus of the mature Tg molecule is the asparagine at position 20; the designation of specific residues by various authors cited in this chapter has been altered to conform to this numbering.) The monomer contains 67 tyrosyls and 20 potential glycosylation sites. The N-terminal portion, through residue 1196, has a highly organized internal structure highlighted by a domain repeated 10 times, consisting of the sequence Cys-Trp/Tyr-Cys-Val-Asp and about 50 additional residues with Cys, Pro, and Gly in nonvarying positions. Another domain of 14 to 17 residues occurs three times between residues 1436 and 1483, and a third occurs five times between residues 1603 and 2186. The C-terminal part of the molecule has no homology with the N-terminal and only weakly repetitive domains. It is somewhat richer in tyrosine than the N-terminus.

The absence of homology between the N- and C-portions of Tg suggests that they arose from different ancestral genes. This conclusion is supported by the differences in intron size and restriction fragment length polymorphism.[2] A striking homology exists between the C-terminal 540 residues of Tg and about 90% of the sequence of acetylcholinesterases, both vertebrate and invertebrate.[26–28] The overall homology between these regions of Tg and acetylcholinesterase is about 28%, reaching 35% to 48% between residues 2292 and 2395. However, the homology does not extend to any of Tg's hormonogenic tyrosyls. Acetylcholinesterase binds to cell membranes, and a similar property has been postulated for the C-terminal region of Tg.[26,28] The homology between these two proteins provides exciting opportunities for studying the evolution and structure of Tg. For example, the homology includes six of eight cysteines, and the location of disulfides in cholinesterase[29] may well predict their location in the C-terminal portion of Tg. Mori and coworkers[26] use this homology to suggest a common evolutionary source for the endocrine and nervous systems, both having intracellular communication as their principal function. The homology extends to other esterases, all traced to an ancestral gene encoding a carboxyesterase.[30] Koch and colleagues[31] also noted homology between the repetitive domains in the N-terminal part of Tg and a domain of the Ia antigen in the major histocompatibility system.

CARBOHYDRATE, SULFATE, AND PHOSPHATE

The Tg gene codes for carbohydrate attachment sites by the sequence Asn-X-Ser/Thr, in common with the genes for most glycoproteins. Twenty such sites exist in the human Tg monomer,[11] as shown in Figure 5-2. Calculations from the total

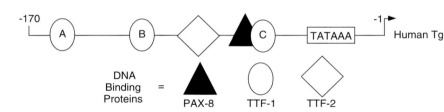

FIGURE 5-1. Proposed structure of the human thyroglobulin promoter, adapted by Damante and Di Lauro[15] from data of Donda and colleagues,[11] showing the binding sites of TTF-1 (◯), TTF-2 (◇), and PAX-8 (▲).

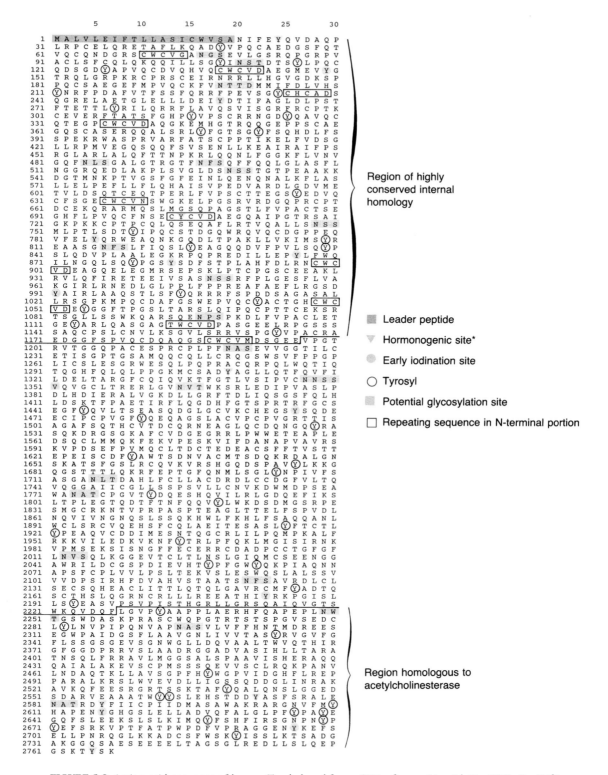

FIGURE 5-2. Amino acid sequence of human Tg, deduced from cDNA of gene. *A = 24; B = 2572; C = 2765; D = 1309; G = 2586; N = 704. (Adapted from Malthiery Y, Marriq C, BergeLefranc JL, et al. Thyroglobulin structure and function: recent advances. Biochimie 1989;71:195)

carbohydrate composition of the dimer indicate that about 15 of these sites are used.

Spiro and Spiro have contributed much of the available information on the structure and biosynthesis of Tg's carbohy-

drate units.[32] Two basic types of N-linked units exist, one variously designated as polymannose, simple, or type A, and the other complex, or type B (Table 5-2). Both are also found in many other glycoproteins. The polymannose unit contains

TABLE 5-2.
Carbohydrate Units of Human Thyroglobulin*

Feature	A (Polymannose)	B (Complex)	C	Chondroitin Sulfate
Molecular weight	1800	2100–3300	2000–3000	5750
Molecules unit/molecule 660 = kd Tg	7–8	22		1
Composition (residues/unit)			Incomplete	
N-acetylglucosamine	2	4–5		
Mannose	5–11	3		
Galactose		2–3		2
Fucose		1		
Sialic acid		1–2.5		
Galactosamine			13	11
Sulfate		0–4		14
Glucuronic acid				11
Xylose				1
Link to peptide	Asn-GlcNAc	Asn-GlcNAc	Ser-GaINAc	Ser-XYl-Gal

*All values are averages; widespread microheterogeneity exists in the carbohydrate units of Tg.
(Based on data from references 32 and 37.)

only mannose and N-acetyl glucosamine, through which it is linked to asparagine in the peptide chain. The complex unit has a similar asparagine-N-acetyl glucosamine link, and consists of a small core of three mannose residues, from which extend several chains of N-acetyl glucosamine-galactose-sialic acid or fucose. The complex units may contain up to four sulfate groups, and some have both sulfate and sialic acid.[33] Formation of the N-linked units occurs by transfer of a previously synthesized package of dolichol-linked oligosaccharides, including N-acetyl glucosamine, mannose, and glucose, to the asparagine link, subsequent removal of glucose and some mannose residues, and then completion of the terminal chains by addition of galactose, sialic acid, and fucose. The dolichol phosphate step appears central to the control of glycosylation both in vitro[34] and in vivo.[35]

Human Tg contains two additional carbohydrate units linked to the peptide chain through the hydroxyl group of serine or threonine[36,37] (see Table 5-2). One, unit C, contains galactosamine and has been incompletely characterized. The other, a chondroitin sulfate unit, has a molecular weight of almost 6000 and consists chiefly of galactosamine and glucuronic acid. These O-linked units have not been found in Tgs from other animals.

Of 20 potential glycosylation sites in the human Tg monomer (see Fig 5-2), actual utilization has been shown at asparagine 2581, linked to a polymannose unit,[38] and asparagines 76 and 110.[39] Each of the latter two can contain either the polymannose or the complex unit, indicating extensive microheterogeneity in use of these glycosylation sites. Rawitch and coworkers[40] carefully mapped bovine Tg and found that 13 of 14 potential sites were glycosylated, 9 with complex units and 4 with the simple unit. The latter were found only toward the C-terminus.

Human Tg contains sulfate in both the complex carbohydrate and the chondroitin sulfate units[37,41,42] (see Table 5-2). Sulfation of tyrosine was reported in one investigation[43] but not confirmed in another.[42] Addition of sulfate occurs as a late event in Tg maturation in the Golgi and involves complex carbohydrate units of at least three branches, perhaps in a terminal region of the Tg polypeptide chain.[42] Studies in vitro have shown wide variation over time in ^{35}S incorporation between the two units, with additional differences between normal and neoplastic thyroid tissue.[41] The biologic role of the sulfated carbohydrate unit is unknown. In general, such units may be involved with intracellular signalling, and perhaps they fill a similar role in Tg, but elucidation of their function requires much more investigation.

Thyroglobulin also contains phosphate.[44–46] Consiglio and coworkers[44] reported 10 to 12 moles of phosphate per mole 660-kd Tg, about 6 moles in the complex carbohydrate unit, 3 to 4 as phosphoserine, and 2 as phosphotyrosine. In studying Tg from human, bovine, porcine, or ovine Tg, Spiro and Gorski[45] found phosphate only in phosphoserine and none in tyrosine or carbohydrate. More recently, Sakurai and colleagues[47] concluded that some complex units can contain phosphodiesters as well as sulfate and sialic acid, and that the phosphodiesters occur in normal as well as neoplastic human thyroid tissue. Thus, from these reports, phosphate is clearly present in Tg, but its amount, distribution, and function remain to be established.

Thyroid-stimulating hormone and disease can affect glycosylation of Tg. Thyroids from rats treated with propylthiouracil had increased levels of mannosyl and galactosyl transferases,[48] suggesting that TSH stimulates these enzyme activities and promotes Tg glycosylation. In FRTL-5 cells, TSH appeared to increase the number of complex units (galactose-containing) while decreasing that of the simple units (mannose-rich).[49] In porcine thyroid cells, TSH administration in vitro appeared to shift capping from terminal α-galactose residues to sialic acid, with a resultant change in molecular charge.[50] Energy deprivation in vitro led to depletion of dolichyl phosphate,[34] the major limiting component in glycosylation,[51] and similar depletion or damage might plausibly occur in vivo. Ingenbleek[52] has postulated that vitamin A deficiency can impair thyroid hormonogenesis by reducing retinol-binding protein and consequent glycosylation of Tg and other proteins. This possibility has been used to explain the heightened severity of iodine-deficiency goitrogenesis in the presence of coexistent vitamin A deficiency.

The carbohydrates of Tg can vary in association with thyroid disease.[53] Yamamoto and colleagues[46] reported that Tg from papillary carcinoma contained less sialic acid than did normal Tg. This Tg had large, complex, highly branched carbohydrate units of 6 to 8 kd with repeating galactose-*N*-acetyl glucosamine moieties, and also contained a phosphodiester linkage in the complex (type B) unit. Adenoma or colloid nodules differed from normal tissue from the same glands by incorporating more sulfate into Tg and altering its distribution among the two types of sulfated carbohydrate units.[41]

IODINATION AND HORMONOGENESIS

Early work showed that only some of Tg's tyrosyls are available for iodination and hormonogenesis.[54,55] Further investigations[56-61] have established four major hormonogenic sites (designated A–D) in the Tg monomer, as well as three minor or limited ones (designated G, N, and R; Table 5-3 and Fig 5-2). Site A is the fifth residue from the N-terminus and the major T_4 site in most species. Site C, the third residue from the C-terminus, is favored for T_3 synthesis in some species, accounting for over 50% of Tg's newly formed T_3 in the rabbit and guinea pig.[56,57]

The use of the major and minor sites varies under differing physiologic conditions and among different species. For example, site B may contain more of Tg's newly formed T_4 than does site A on early iodination in several species.[58,61] Site D is a major hormonogenic tyrosyl in rabbit and guinea pig Tg iodinated in vivo, and TSH stimulated its use more heavily than at any other site[57]; however, site D was barely used in iodination of human Tg in vitro.[58] Site C appears more important for T_3 synthesis in guinea pigs, rabbits, and pigs than in humans and cows, perhaps related to a Ser-Tyr sequence in the first three species in contrast to a Thr-Tyr in the latter two.

Turtle Tg has tyrosine substituted for phenylalanine at position 632 in the human sequence, and this site (designated R) contained 12% of Tg's newly formed T_4.[61] In addition, turtle Tg showed significant differences from mammals in amino acid sequences and in hormonogenesis at sites A and C. Findings such as these show that many parts of the Tg molecule may be involved in hormone synthesis and processing, and their relative importance may vary with iodine availability, TSH stimulation, and species.

Thyroxine formation occurs by intramolecular coupling of two DIT residues, both in peptide linkage within Tg, leaving T_4 and dehydroalanine at the acceptor and donor positions respectively[62] (see chap 4). Mature Tg is a dimer of two monomeric chains, and it is not known whether iodotyrosyl coupling is intrachain, interchain, or both. Several tyrosyls have been proposed as possible donors of the iodothyronyl outer ring. Palumbo[63] reported treating bovine Tg with sodium [³H]borohydride, thus converting dehydroalanine to [³H]alanine, and localizing this presumed donor to tyrosyls corresponding to either Phe_{2486} or Tyr_{2539} in hTg. The same researcher also concluded that site A was the first tyrosyl iodinated in vivo in propylthiouracil-treated rats.[64] Ohmiya and coworkers[65] labeled dehydroalanine residues in bovine Tg with 4-aminothiophenol and identified tyrosyls at positions 5, 926, 1375, and 986 or 1008 in the bovine sequence as possible donors, corresponding respectively to positions 24, 945, 1393, 1004, and 1027 in hTg in Figure 5-2. Of these, only positions 5 and 986 have tyrosyls in the corresponding human sequence (see Fig 5-2). Lamas and coworkers[58] added iodine in vitro to hTg from a low-iodine goiter, and found initially more iodotyrosine formation at residues 2572 (site B), 704 (site N), 149, 866, and 1466 than at residue 24 (site A), but, with further iodine addition, noted more T_4 at site A than at any other tyrosyl. The tyrosyls at positions 149, 866, and 1466 were iodinated early but did not form inner iodothyronine rings on further iodination, making them attractive candidates for outer ring donors. Marriq and colleagues[66] iodinated in vitro an N-terminal fragment of hTg, consisting of residues 20 to 190 in Figure 5-2, and obtained a 26-kd iodopeptide, with T_4 at site A and Val_{148} at its C-terminus (the 26-kd peptide is described in more detail in the next section of this chapter). From this, they concluded that iodinated Tyr_{149} donated the outer ring for T_4

TABLE 5-3.
Hormonogenic Sites in Thyroglobulin, With Examples of Their Relative Utilization

Site	Location in hTg (residue #)*	Species	Fraction of Total T_4 of Tg (%)	
			HUMAN IN VITRO[58]	RABBIT IN VIVO[56]
A	24	h, rb, gp, t, b, o, p	36	44
B	2572	h, rb, gp, t	22	24
C	2765	h, rb, gp, p	15	7
D	1309	h, rb, gp	trace	17
G	2586	rb, p	trace	trace
N	704	h	12	—
R	(532)	t	—	—

Residues numbered to include 19 amino acid leader (see Fig. 5-2).
h, *human*; b, *bovine*; rb, *rabbit*; rt, *rat*; p, *pig*; gp, *guinea pig*; t, *turtle*; o, *sheep*.

formation at site A, leaving dehydroalanine and peptide bond cleavage at position 149. However, Rawitch and colleagues[67] repeated this work and found that Tyr_{149} was the acceptor rather than the donor. In another in vitro model, selective replacement of tyrosyl residues with phenylalanine by site-directed mutagenesis in the first N-terminal 198 residues of hTg did not decrease net hormone formation after iodination if tyrosyls 24, 128, and 149 remained intact; but replacement of only Tyr_{24} or of only Tyr_{149} also did not decrease T_4 formation.[68] Results such as these emphasize the need for caution in extrapolating from in vitro models to the intact thyroid.

The tyrosyls involved in early iodination and hormonogenesis of a low-iodine hTg fall into three consensus groups[58] as follows:

1. Asp/Glu-Tyr occurs at the three major T_4-forming sites, A, B, and D (tyrosyls 24, 2572, and 1309, respectively), as well as at two additional early iodination sites, tyrosyls 2586 and 991. One can speculate that the latter two might also form iodothyronine with further iodination and that the five other tyrosyls with this configuration are potential iodination sites. T_3 also forms at sites A, B, and D, particularly at low iodine levels.

2. Ser/Thr-Tyr-Ser occurs at site C (residue 2765), the major T_3 site in rabbits and guinea pigs, and this sequence was also associated with early iodination at residues 883 and 1466. These three sites are the only ones in the Tg monomer with this sequence. One of the proposed bovine donor sites also has this configuration.[65]

3. Glu-X-Tyr occurs seven times in the Tg monomer, each associated with early iodination. The three consensus sequences encompass most of Tg's known sites for early iodination and hormonogenesis.[58]

Results of these various studies are limited, of course, to their specific conditions of iodine addition and Tg substrate. Taken together, they suggest that Tg's structure permits hormonogenesis at several sites, and that their relative utilization can vary with physiologic conditions, such as TSH stimulation and iodine availability, and with structural differences, as among different species.

Further details of iodination of Tg and hormonogenesis are given in chapter 4.

THE MATURE THYROGLOBULIN MOLECULE

Thyroglobulin in its most stable form occurs as a 19S dimer of 660 kd. The two constituent monomeric polypeptide chains are believed to be identical when synthesized but heterogeneous after glycosylation and iodination. A number of studies have shown that iodine-poor dimer from animal thyroids dissociates easily (e.g., with cooling or low ionic strength). Increasing iodination in Tg produces more stable dimerization and less dissociation, reflecting the concomitant formation of interchain disulfide (and possibly other) bonds. TSH administration decreases dimer dissociation without change in the total iodine content of Tg.[69] Kim and Arvan[70,71] have carefully tracked the progress of newly synthesized Tg in thyrocyte cultures, beginning with a transient disulfide-linked aggregate and followed by an unstable monomer that dimerizes in the pre-Golgi complex. The molecular chaperones calnexin and BiP appear to act sequentially in folding of nascent Tg on the endoplasmic reticulum,[71] and other molecular chaperons (ERp72 and grp94) have also been found present.[72] Immature Tg is shuttled via an *N*-acetyl glucosamine-specific receptor from endosomes to apical membrane until glycosylation occurs, a process that protects it from the intracellular lysosomal digestion of the mature Tg.[73]

Edelhoch and coworkers[74] found that the iodine content of Tg varied reciprocally with sulfhydryl content, from six sulfhydryl residues per mole Tg of low iodine content (one atom iodine per mole), to two sulfhydryls in Tgs of 10 or more atoms iodine per mole (0.2% iodine by weight). Thus, several sulfhydryls are potentially available in Tg for producing interchain disulfide bonds. Both iodination and disulfide formation are oxidative processes and occur in parallel, so identification of the sulfhydryls involved in interchain bonds may help clarify the molecular mechanism of thyroid hormone formation.

Basic physicochemical features of the Tg molecule were presented in detail in previous editions of this book, and are summarized only briefly here. Tg has an isoelectric point of about 4.5 and is chemically stable over the pH range of 5 to 11. Electron microscopy of the dimer shows that normal Tg has an ovoid shape of approximately 150×300 angstroms, consisting of two symmetrical halves, each probably representing the monomer.[75] Low-iodine Tg has a cylindrical structure distinct from that found with normally iodinated Tg.

In addition to the 12S monomer and 19S dimer, about 10% of mature Tg is in the form of a 27S tetramer. The 27S is similar to the 19S dimer in amino acid composition and immunologic reaction, but it typically has much more iodine. Similar polymeric forms occur in other macroglobulins, such as α_2-macroglobulin and IgM. Shifrin and colleagues[76] reported the irreversible conversion of high-iodine 19S Tg to 27S by removal of its galactose and sialic acid. They concluded that the 27S and 19S forms had different attachment sites to thyroid membranes and were probably processed differently. Herzog and coworkers[77] have isolated globules of compacted Tg from bovine thyroid follicular lumina; these contained about 55 atoms of iodine per monomer, nearly twice the highest amount in soluble Tg as usually extracted from the gland. This high-iodine Tg was cross-linked by both disulfide and dityrosine bridges,[77] and dityrosine bridges have been described by others as well.[78]

Reduction of mature hTg's disulfide bonds produces iodopeptides of more than 300 kd, approximately 230 kd, approximately 45 kd, 26 kd, and 18 kd.[79] The 26- and 18-kd iodopeptides are of particular interest because, despite their small size, they together contain over one third of normal Tg's T_4. At lower contents of iodine, more than half of Tg's T_4 is in the 26-kd form. Incremental addition of iodine in vitro to low-iodine hTg from a goiter steadily increased the 26-kd iodopeptide's content of iodine, T_4, and peptide material, reaching a maximum after Tg's iodine content was about 30 atoms per 660-kd molecule (about 0.6% iodine content). Additional iodine produced no further increase in the 26-kd iodopeptide but markedly increased the 18-kd form. Because the amount of peptide material in the 26- and 18-kd forms increased *pari passu* with their iodine and T_4 contents, the process of iodination must be cleaving Tg's peptide bonds. Studies with 26-kd iodopeptide formation in vitro in hTg and in vivo in rat Tg support this conclusion.[80] Sequencing part of the 26-kd peptide and establishing the amino acid sequence of the Tg monomer from cDNA identified the peptide as Tg's N-terminus and its hormonogenic locus as site A.[81] The 18-kd iodopeptide has the same initial amino acid sequence as the 26-kd species, indicating it results from a further peptide cleavage in Tg's N-terminal region and that it also contains site A. If all the T_4 of the 26- and 18-kd forms is at site A, as seems likely, then the presence of nearly 2 moles iodothyronine per mole 660-kd Tg means that hormone formation at site A takes place on both chains of the Tg dimer, and that the tyrosyl at site A is unlikely to be a donor of the outer iodothyronine ring.

The same iodopeptide groups occur after disulfide reduction of Tgs from all vertebrates examined so far, including fish, reptiles, amphibia, birds, and a number of mammals.[82–84] Among these species, the 26-kd (range, 19–28 kd) and the 18-kd (range, 16–23 kd) iodopeptides contained from 25% to 63% of Tg's iodothyronines and about 1 mole each of Tg's peptide material per mole 660-kd Tg. Rawitch and coworkers[81] sequenced a 10-kd fragment from bovine reduced Tg and found it contained the protein's N-terminus, thus corresponding to a portion of the 18-kd and 26-kd forms in hTg. The C-terminus of the bovine 10-kd fragment was Gln-Leu-Gln, identical to residues 97 to 99 in hTg (see Fig 5-2), reflecting a cleavage between glutamine and lysine (residues 99 and 100). This area contained a high number of predicted β bends, suggesting a chain folding back on itself to produce a compact domain including site A.[81] An iodopeptide of 30 kd also occurs in bovine Tg and includes the N-terminus and site A.[85] Its cleavage from the remainder of the Tg monomer was localized to a Leu-Leu bond corresponding to residue 253 in hTg in Figure 5-2, a configuration with no obvious similarity to that producing the 10-kd peptide.

How peptide bonds break to produce the hormonogenic peptides remains unknown, and more than one mechanism may exist. The association of peptide bond cleavage with iodination was emphasized earlier. Use of enzyme inhibitors in Tg isolation makes postmortem proteolysis unlikely, and the known lysosomal proteases that normally process Tg apparently do not produce the 26-kd or 18-kd forms.[86] A possible parallel exists in the inactivation of bacteria by myeloperoxidase and halogens, a process thought to involve protein disruption. On the other hand, the cleavages in bovine Tg at Leu-Leu and Gln-Lys[85] suggest a mechanism different from that of the proposed iodination cleavage at donor tyrosyls in hTg. TSH in vivo also promotes the conversion of a 26-kd–like iodopeptide to an 18-kd–like iodopeptide in rabbits and guinea pigs, but does so without change in Tg's total iodine content.[57] Further study, particularly identification of donors for the outer iodothyronine rings, is needed to define how Tg's secondary and tertiary structure affects hormonogenesis, and how iodination and TSH participate in this process.

IMMUNOLOGY OF THYROGLOBULIN

Human Tg has many epitopes, as anticipated for a protein of its size. Numerous studies have described polyvalent and monoclonal antibodies to Tg. Interest in them stems from their use as tools in investigating Tg structure and from their role in thyroid diseases, particularly autoimmune thyroid disease and differentiated cancer (see chap 20).

Kurata and coworkers[87] prepared six monoclonal antibodies from "normal" hTg (0.5% iodine) and tested them against hTgs from healthy subjects and from patients with Graves' disease and papillary cancer. From binding studies, these investigators identified three types of Tg–antibody reaction, as follows: (1) reactivity with hTg only, independent of its iodine content; (2) reactivity with hTg or rat Tg, sensitivity increasing with Tg's iodine content, but activity not inhibited by any iodoamino acid; and (3) same as (2), but reactivity inhibited specifically by T_4 and not by other iodoamino acids. De Baets and colleagues[88] described 15 monoclonal antibodies raised against normal hTg (iodine content at least 0.5%). Of these, most cross-reacted with bovine, mouse, and rat Tgs, but with some differences in sensitivity. Four antibodies recognized iodothyronine sites, and disruption of Tg structure with cyanogen bromide abolished immunoreactivity with all but one antibody, emphasizing the importance of Tg's three-dimensional integrity. Other studies support the concept of several epitopes in hTg, variously related to animal species, iodination, hormone content, and tertiary structure. Dong and coworkers[89] attempted to localize epitopes in the Tg monomer by reacting rabbit antiserum with fragments from cDNA-derived hTg. They found 10 epitopes spread over the monomer chain, including site C but not site A. They noted that these fragments lack the iodine and carbohydrate that contribute to antibody recognition at some epitopes.

It has been known for a long time that subjects with autoimmune thyroid disease form autoantibodies to Tg. More recently, it has been recognized that healthy subjects also have Tg autoantibodies, but these are directed to different regions of the molecule.[90,91] Bouanani and coworkers[90] reported that the principal epitopes in healthy subjects involved Tg's tertiary structure, whereas subjects with autoimmune thyroid disease more commonly had autoantibodies against another immunologic domain. Using a panel of 20 monoclonal antibodies recognizing 12 determinant clusters, Bresler and colleagues[91] found that the antibodies of healthy subjects were directed chiefly at hormonogenic regions, whereas subjects with autoimmune thyroid disease had autoantibodies directed to the nonhormonogenic parts of Tg, which the researchers regarded as the most recently evolved and most species-specific parts. Another study with monoclonal antibodies to hTg fragments found an immunodominant region corresponding to residues 1130 to 1231 in the Tg monomer, and sera from subjects with autoimmune thyroid disease reacted more to this epitope than to others.[92] The importance of epitopes in the center of the Tg peptide chain was also reported by Henry and coworkers.[93] However, Dong and colleagues[89] did not find reactivity between the autoantibodies from autoimmune thyroid disease and the nonhormonogenic epitope fragments from cDNA-derived hTg described earlier. In still another study, autoantibodies from patients with Graves' disease reacted with Tgs from whales, pigs, chickens, and rats,[94] and they were not species specific.

It is surprising that the Tg source for antibody production has received little attention. Most experimental reports mention only that the Tg came from Graves' disease, surgery, autopsy, or some unnamed source, and provide no details of its composition or structure. In view of the complexity and apparent heterogeneity of Tg's antigenicity, more careful study of the Tg antigen would help explain its immunoreactivity and might resolve some of the apparent discrepancies among the studies just cited.

Thyroglobulin immunology has relevance for thyroid disease. For example, immunization of mice with human eye muscle membrane induced a monoclonal antibody that reacted with hTg and with Tgs of other species,[95] and mouse monoclonal antibodies against Tg also reacted against an antigen in human orbital connective tissue membranes.[96] Several authors have suggested that shared Tg antigens in orbit and thyroid could link these two targets of Graves' disease,[97,98] and, even more tenuously,[99] that the homologous regions of Tg and acetylcholinesterase may be the target epitope. Another example, discussed more fully in chapter 20, is the use of serum Tg as a marker for differentiated thyroid cancer. Several studies have found that Tg can have a low iodine content and altered protein structure in thyroid cancer and other diseases. Development of monoclonal antibodies directed at these altered features will help define the nature of these changes and will greatly improve the diagnostic value of the serum Tg test.

THYROGLOBULIN STRUCTURE IN DISEASE

Heterogeneity is a key feature of "normal" hTg, and involves its composition of carbohydrate, amino acids, iodine, and hormone as well as its three-dimensional structure and immunoreactivity. TSH stimulation can produce further changes in Tg (Table 5-4). New instances of heterogeneity are constantly being uncovered. Several studies have reported mRNAs distinct from the usual 8-kb form translating the usual Tg monomer.[25,100,101] Kim and coworkers[102] have reported some structural changes in Tg from glands in patients with Graves' disease (the source of the mRNA selected for cloning the hTg gene[11]), and the possibility of translating more than one mRNA for Tg clearly exists. Tg's large size, heterogeneity, and extensive posttranslational processing offer many opportunities for synthetic errors. The availability of several hormonogenic sites and the ability of TSH stimulation to cope with impaired hormonogenesis can mitigate the effects of many errors and allow the subject, although goitrous, to live and

---

TABLE 5-4.
Some Effects of Thyroid-Stimulating Hormone on Thyroglobulin

Enhances gene transcription

Enhances expression of 0.95 kb mRNA

Stimulates hexose transferases, promoting glycosylation

Shifts capping of carbohydrate units to sialic acid

Increases formation of T_3 relative to T_4

Shifts priority of iodination and hormonogenesis among tyrosyls

Promotes iodination cleavage of 26-kd N-terminal-peptide to 18 kd

Increases formation of interchain disulfide bonds

---

propagate genetic defects. Thus, a role for Tg in some thyroid diseases can be predicted with confidence.

The best examples of abnormal Tg leading to thyroid disease come from animal studies. Ricketts and colleagues[101] described an mRNA of 7.3 kb in thyroids from Afrikander cattle with hereditary goiter, in addition to the normal 8.4-kb messenger. They traced the defect to a mutation of cytosine to thymine, producing a stop codon that in turn led to excision of exon 9 and abnormal splicing. The same 7.3-kb mRNA was also found as a minor component in healthy thyroids. A recessive congenital goiter in mice (cog/cog) has been attributed to a defective gene, although its mRNA was of normal size.[3,103] The translated Tg differed immunologically from normal Tg and iodinated poorly. Investigation of hereditary goiter in Dutch goats found mRNA of normal size that translated a 35-kd fragment containing the N-terminal portion of the Tg monomeric chain.[2,10,104] These N-terminal fragments, which should contain site A, can form T_4, indicating that donors for the outer iodothyronine ring at site A can come from this part of the Tg chain, and that the entire monomer is not necessary for hormonogenesis. Oxidation of these fragments with peroxide, under conditions similar to those in the healthy thyroid, produced large disulfide-linked polymers in the colloidal spaces of the goiter. More recently, this group reported that the Tg defect that induces the Dutch goat goiter results from a C → G transition at position 945 in exon 8.[105]

Less is known about abnormal Tg in human thyroid disease. An early study found that Tg from human goiters differed from that of healthy subjects in composition of iodine, carbohydrate, and amino acids.[53] In general, the variability itself was more impressive than any consistent direction of change, although goiter Tg had more sialic acid and less iodine. Compositional changes have been described for Tgs from Pendred's syndrome[106] and metastatic thyroid cancer.[107] Many studies have reported diminished Tg synthesis associated with goiter[108] and neoplasia.[109] Other case reports have found goiters with various defects in Tg, including abnormal tertiary structure,[110] inability to couple iodotyrosines,[111] and defective glycosylation[112] or sialylation.[113]

More recently, the techniques of molecular genetics have been applied to the investigation of familial goiter.[108] Most studies have described decreased Tg production, but a few have reported abnormal mRNA. Ieiri and coworkers[114] found a guanine substituted for a cytosine in exon 4 of a subject with congenital goiter and hypothyroidism, resulting in a 200-bp deletion that translates a 68-residue peptide. The latter includes Tyr_{149}, which has been proposed as donor for T_4 formation at Tyr_{24}, and the investigators suggested that this genetic error caused the goiter. Mason and colleagues[115] reported that some clones from the Tg mRNA of two siblings with Pendred's syndrome had a 135-bp deletion that, if translated, would delete a segment between amino acid residues 2620 and 2666. They also found a two-base deletion at bp 7870 to 7871 in many clones from healthy and goitrous human thyroids; this deletion would result in a frame shift and degenerate amino acid sequence after residue 2610. These and other deviations were largely restricted to the 3' end of the message. Another patient with congenital goiter and hypothyroidism had a 171-bp deletion from positions 4567 to 4737 that would translate into a Tg lacking 57 residues from its midportion.[116] These and other studies clearly establish the existence of diversity in

Tg mRNA from both normal and diseased thyroids. How the presence of altered messages affects Tg synthesis and hormonogenesis will require further study of the translated protein. A more detailed discussion of inherited metabolic defects in thyroid hormone synthesis is given in chapter 56.

References

1. Eggo MC, Burrow GN. Thyroglobulin: the prothyroid hormone. Prog Endocr Res Therapy 1985;2:1.
2. De Vijlder JJM, Baas F, Kok K, et al. Molecular basis of thyroglobulin synthesis defects. Prog Endocr Res Therapy. 1985;2:69
3. Taylor BA, Rowe L. The congenital goiter mutation is linked to the thyroglobulin gene in the mouse. Proc Natl Acad Sci USA 1987;84:1986
4. Brocas H, Szpirer J, Lebo RV, et al. The thyroglobulin gene resides on chromosome 8 in man and on chromosome 7 in the rat. Cytogenet Cell Genet 1985;39:150
5. Threadgill DW, Fries R, Faber LK, et al. The thyroglobulin gene is syntenic with the MYC and MOS protooncogenes and carbonic anhydrase II and maps to chromosome 14 in cattle. Cytogenet Cell Genet 1990;53:32
6. Vassart G, Brocas H, Cabrer B, et al. Structure and expression of the thyroglobulin gene. Prog Endocr Res Therapy 1985;2:55.
7. Malthiery Y, Lissitzky S. On the structure of the messenger RNA of human thyroglobulin. In: Eggo MC, Burrow GN, eds. Thyroglobulin: the prothyroid hormone. Vol 2. Progress in Endoc Res and Therapy. 1985;2:77
8. Malthiery Y, Marriq C, Berge-Lefranc JL, et al. Thyroglobulin structure and function: recent advances. Biochimie 1989;71:195
9. Di Lauro R, Avvedimento EV, Cerillo R, et al. Structure and function of the rat thyroglobulin gene. Prog Endocr Res Therapy 1985;2:77
10. van Ommen G-JB, Sterk A, Mercken LOY, Arnberg AC, Baas F, De Vijlder JJM. Studies on the structures of the normal and abnormal goat thyroglobulin genes. Biochimie 1989;71:211
11. Malthiery Y, Lissitzky S. Primary structure of human thyroglobulin deduced from the sequence of its 8448-base complementary DNA. Eur J Biochem 1987;165:491
12. Mercken L, Simons M-J, Swillens S, Massaer M, Vassart G. Primary structure of bovine thyroglobulin deduced from the sequence of its 8,431-base complementary DNA. Nature 1985;316:647
13. Di Lauro R, Obici S, Condliffe D, et al. The sequence of 967 amino acids at the carboxyl-end of rat thyroglobulin: location and surroundings of two thyroxine-forming sites. Eur J Biochem 1985;148:7
14. Musti AM, Avvedimento EV, Polistina C, et al. The complete structure of the rat thyroglobulin gene. Proc Natl Acad Sci USA 1986;83:327
15. Damante G, Di Lauro R. Thyroid-specific gene expression. Biochim Biophys Acta 1994;1218:255
16. Donda J, Javaux F, Can Renterghem P, Gervy-Decoster C, Vassart G, Christophe D. Human, bovine, canine and rat thyroglobulin promoter sequences display species-specific differences in an in vitro study. Mol Cell Endocrinol 1993;90:R23
17. van Heuverswyn B, Streydio C, Brocas H, Refetoff S, Dumont J, Vassart G. Thyrotropin controls transcription of the thyroglobulin gene. Proc Natl Acad Sci USA 1984;81:5941
18. van Heuverswyn B, Lerich A, van Sande J, Dumont JE, Vassart G. Transcriptional control of thyroglobulin gene expression by cyclic AMP. FEBS Lett 1985;188:192
19. Gérard CM, Lefort A, Christophe D, et al. Control of thyroperoxidase and thyroglobulin transcription by cAMP: evidence for distinct regulatory mechanisms. Mol Endocrinol 1989;3:2110
20. Lee N-T, Nayfeh SN, Chae C-B. Induction of nuclear protein factors specific for hormone-responsive region during activation of thyroglobulin gene by thyrotropin in rat thyroid FRTL-5 cells. J Biol Chem 1989;264:7523
21. Santisteban P, Kohn LD, DiLauro R. Thyroglobulin gene expression is regulated by insulin and insulin-like growth factor I, as well a thyrotropin, in FRTL-5 thyroid cells. J Biol Chem 1987;262:4048
22. Nagayama Y, Izumi M, Ashizawa K, et al. Inhibitory effect of interferon-γ on the response of human thyrocytes to thyrotropin (TSH) stimulation: relationship between the response to TSH and the expression of DR antigen. J Clin Endocrinol Metab 1987;64:949
23. Graves P, Neufeld DS, Davies TF. Differential cytokine regulation of MHC class II and thyroglobulin mRNAs in rat thyroid cells. Mol Endocrinol 1989;3:758
24. Pichon B, Christophe-Hobertus C, Vassart G, Christophe D. Unmethylated thyroglobulin promoter may be repressed by methylation of flanking DNA sequences. Biochem J 1994;298:537
25. Graves PN, Davies TF. A second thyroglobulin messenger RNA species (rTg-2) in rat thyrocytes. Mol Endocrinol 1990;4:155
26. Mori N, Itoh N, Salvaterra M. Evolutionary origin of cholinergic macromolecules and thyroglobulin. Proc Natl Acad Sci USA 1987;84:2813
27. Schumacher M, Camp S, Maulet Y, et al. Primary structure of *Torpedo californica* acetylcholinesterase deduced from its cDNA sequence. Nature 1986;319:407
28. Swillens S, Ludgate M, Mercken L, Dumont JE, Vassart G. Analysis of sequence and structure homologies between thyroglobulin and acetylcholinesterase: possible functional and clinical significance. Biochem Biophys Res Commun 1986;137:142
29. Lockridge O, Adkins S, La Du BN. Location of disulfide bonds within the sequence of human serum cholinesterase. J Biol Chem 1987;262:12945
30. Takagi Y, Omura T, Go M. Evolutionary origin of thyroglobulin by duplication of esterase gene. FEBS Lett 1991;282:17
31. Koch N, Lauer W, Habicht J, Dobberstein B. Primary structure of the gene for the murine Ia antigen-associated invariant chains (Ii): an alternatively spliced exon encodes a cysteine-rich domain highly homologous to a repetitive sequence of thyroglobulin. EMBO J 1987;6:1677
32. Spiro MJ, Spiro RG. Synthesis and processing of thyroglobulin carbohydrate units. Prog Endocr Res Therapy. 1985;2:103
33. Sakurai S, Fogelfeld L, Ries A, Schneider A. Anionic complex-carbohydrate units of human thyroglobulin. Endocrinology 1990;127:2056
34. Spiro RG, Spiro MJ, Bhoyroo VD. Studies on the regulation of the biosynthesis of glucose-containing oligosaccharide–lipids. J Biol Chem 1983;258:9469
35. Eggo MC, Burrow GN. Glycosylation of thyroglobulin: its role in secretion, iodination, and stability. Endocrinology 1983;113:1655
36. Arima T, Spiro MJ, Spiro RG. Studies on the carbohydrate units of thyroglobulin. J Biol Chem 1972;247:1825
37. Spiro MJ. Presence of a glucuronic acid-containing carbohydrate unit in human thyroglobulin. J Biol Chem 1977;252:5424
38. Rawitch AB, Liao T-H, Pierce JG. The amino acid sequence of a tryptic glycopeptide from human thyroglobulin. Biochim Biophys Acta 1968;160:360
39. Franc J-L, Venot N, Marriq C. Characterization of the two oligosaccharides present in the preferential hormonogenic domain of human thyroglobulin. Biochem Biophys Res Commun 1990;166:937
40. Rawitch AB, Pollock HG, Yang S-X. Thyroglobulin glycosylation: location and nature of the N-linked oligosaccharide units in bovine thyroglobulin. Arch Biochem Biophys 1993;300:271
41. Schneider AB, Dudlak D. Differential incorporation of sulfate into the chondroitin chain and complex carbohydrate chains of

human thyroglobulin: studies in normal and neoplastic thyroid tissue. Endocrinology 1989;124:356

42. Spiro MJ, Spiro RG. Biosynthesis of sulfated asparagine-linked complex carbohydrate units of calf thyroglobulin. Endocrinology 1988;122:56, 1988

43. Herzog V. Secretion of sulfated thyroglobulin. Eur J Cell Biol 1985;39:399

44. Consiglio E, Acquaviva AM, Formisano S, et al. Characterization of phosphate residues on thyroglobulin. J Biol Chem 1987; 262:10304

45. Spiro MJ, Gorski KM. Studies on the posttranslational migration and processing of thyroglobulin: use of inhibitors and evaluation of the role of phosphorylation. Endocrinology 1986; 119:1146

46. Yamamoto K, Tsuji T, Tarutani O, Osawa T. Structural changes of carbohydrate chains of human thyroglobulin accompanying malignant transformations of thyroid glands. Eur J Biochem 1984; 143:133

47. Sakurai S, Fogelfeld L, Schneider AB. Anionic carbohydrate groups of human thyroglobulin containing both phosphate and sulfate. Endocrinology 1991;129:915

48. Spiro MJ. Preferential response of thyroid glycosyltransferases to changes in thyrotropin stimulation. Arch Biochem Biophys 1980; 202:35

49. Di Jeso B, Liguoro D, Ferranti P, et al. Modulation of the carbohydrate moiety of thyroglobulin by thyrotropin and calcium in Fisher rat thyroid line-5 cells. J Biol Chem 1992;267:1938

50. Ronin C, Fenouillet E, Hovsepian S, Fayet G, Fournet B. Regulation of thyroglobulin glycosylation. J Biol Chem 1986;261:7287

51. Spiro MJ, Spiro RG. Control of N-linked carbohydrate unit synthesis in thyroid endoplasmic reticulum by membrane organization and dolichyl phosphate availability. J Biol Chem 1986; 261:14725

52. Ingenbleek Y. Vitamin A deficiency impairs the normal mannosylation, conformation and iodination of thyroglobulin: a new etiological approach to endemic goitre. Experientia 1983; 39(Suppl 44):264

53. Dunn JT, Ray SC. Variations in the structure of thyroglobulins from normal and goitrous human thyroids. J Clin Endocrinol Metab 1978;47:861

54. Dunn JT. The amino acid neighbors of thyroxine in thyroglobulin. J Biol Chem 1970;245:5954

55. Lamas L, Taurog A, Salvatore G, Edelhoch H. Preferential synthesis of thyroxine from early iodinated tyrosyl residues in thyroglobulin. J Biol Chem 1974;249:2732

56. Dunn JT, Anderson PC, Fox JW, et al. The sites of thyroid hormone formation in rabbit thyroglobulin. J Biol Chem 1987; 262:16948

57. Fassler CA, Dunn JT, Anderson PC, et al. Thyrotropin alters the utilization of thyroglobulin's hormonogenic sites. J Biol Chem 1988;263:17366

58. Lamas L, Anderson PC, Fox JW, Dunn JT. Consensus sequences for early iodination and hormonogenesis in human thyroglobulin. J Biol Chem 1989;264:13541

59. Marriq C, Lejeune PJ, Rolland M, Lissitzky S. Structure of thyroid hormone-containing peptides in porcine and human thyroglobulins. Prog Endoc Res Therapy. 1985;2:21

60. Rawitch AB, Gregg J, Turner CD. Nature and location of hormonogenic sites within the structure of thyroglobulin. Prog Endoc Res Therapy. 1985;2:43

61. Roe MT, Anderson PC, Dunn AD, Dunn JT. The hormonogenic sites of turtle thyroglobulin and their homology with those of mammals. Endocrinology 1989;124:1327

62. Gavaret J-M, Nunez J, Cahnmann HJ. Formation of dehydroalanine residues during thyroid hormone synthesis in thyroglobulin. J Biol Chem 1980;255:5281

63. Palumbo G. Thyroid hormonogenesis: identification of a sequence containing iodophenyl donor sites(s) in calf thyroglobulin. J Biol Chem 1987;262:17182

64. Palumbo G, Gentile F, Condorelli GL, Salvatore G. The earliest site of iodination in thyroglobulin is residue number 5. J Biol Chem 1990;265:8887

65. Ohmiya Y, Hayashi H, Kondo T, Kondo Y. Location of dehydroalanine residues in the amino acid sequence of bovine thyroglobulin. J Biol Chem 1990;265:9066

66. Marriq C, Lejeune PJ, Venot N, Vinet L. Hormone formation in the isolated fragment 1-171 of human thyroglobulin involves the couple tyrosine 5 and tyrosine 130. Mol Cell Endocrinol 1991; 81:155

67. Rawitch AB, Taurog A, Xiao S, Dorris M. Formation of T_4 in an enzymatically iodinated N-terminal cNBR fragment derived from human goiter thyroglobulin (abstract). Thyroid 1993;3(Suppl):T-54

68. den Hartog MT, Sijmons CC, Bakker O, Ris-Stalpers C, de Vijlder JJM. The importance of the content and localization of tyrosine residues for thyroxine formation within the N-terminal part of human thyroglobulin. Eur J Endocrinol 1995;132:611

69. Dunn JT, Ray SC. Changes in thyroglobulin structure after TSH administration. J Biol Chem 1975;250:5801

70. Kim PS, Arvan P. Folding and assembly of newly synthesized thyroglobulin occurs in a pre-Golgi compartment. J Biol Chem 1991;266:12412

71. Kim PS, Arvan P. Calnexin and BiP act as sequential molecular chaperones during thyroglobulin folding in the endoplasmic reticulum. J Cell Biol 1995;128:29

72. Kuznetsov G, Chen LB, Nigam SK. Several endoplasmic reticulum stress proteins, including ERp72, interact with thyroglobulin during its maturation. J Biol Chem 1994;269:22990

73. Blanck O, Perrin C, Mziaut H, Darbon H, Mattei NG, Miquelis R. Molecular cloning, cDNA analysis, and localization of a monomer of the N-acetylglucosamine-specific receptor of the thyroid, NAGR1, to chromosome 19p13.3-13.2. Genomics 1994; 21:18 ·

74. Edelhoch H, Carlomagno MS, Salvatore G. Iodine and the structure of thyroglobulin. Arch Biochem Biophys 1969134:264

75. Berg G, Ekholm R. Electron microscopy of low iodinated thyroglobulin molecules. Biochim Biophys Acta 1975;386:422

76. Shifrin S, Consiglio E, Laccetti P, Salvatore G, Kohn LD. Bovine thyroglobulin: 27 S iodoprotein interactions with thyroid membranes and formation of a 27 S iodoprotein in vitro. J Biol Chem 1982;257:9539

77. Herzog V, Berndorfer U, Saber Y. Isolation of insoluble secretory product from bovine thyroid: extracellular storage of thyroglobulin in covalently cross-linked form. J Cell Biol 1992;118:1071

78. Leonardi A, Acquaviva R, Marinaccio M. Presence of dityrosine bridges in thyroglobulin and their relationship with iodination. Biochem Biophys Res Comm 1994;202:38

79. Dunn JT, Kim PS, Dunn AD. Favored sites for thyroid hormone formation on the peptide chains of human thyroglobulin. J Biol Chem 1982;257:88

80. Dunn JT, Kim PS, Dunn AD, Heppner DG Jr, Moore RC. The role of iodination in the formation of hormone-rich peptides from thyroglobulin. J Biol Chem 1983;258:9093

81. Rawitch AB, Mercken L, Hamilton JW, Vassart G. The structure of a naturally occurring 10K polypeptide derived from the amino terminus of bovine thyroglobulin. Biochem Biophys Res Commun 1984;119:335

82. Chernoff SB, Rawitch AB. Thyroglobulin structure-formation: isolation and characterization of a thyroxine-containing polypeptide from bovine thyroglobulin. J Biol Chem 1981; 256:9425

83. Dunn JT, Dunn AD, Heppner DG Jr, Kim PS. A discrete thyroxine-rich iodopeptide of 20,000 daltons from rabbit thyroglobulin. J Biol Chem 1981;256:942

84. Kim PS, Dunn JT, Kaiser DL. Similar hormone-rich peptides from thyroglobulins of five vertebrate classes. Endocrinology 1984; 114:369

85. Gregg JD, Dziadik-Turner C, Rouse J, Hamilton JW, Rawitch AB. A comparison of 30-kDa and 10-kDa hormone-containing fragments of bovine thyroglobulin. J Biol Chem 1988;263:5190

86. Dunn AD, Dunn JT. Thyroglobulin degradation by thyroidal proteases: action of thiol endopeptidases in vitro. Endocrinology 1982;111:290

87. Kurata A, Ohta K, Mine M, et al. Monoclonal antihuman thyroglobulin antibodies. J Clin Endocrinol Metab 1984;59:573

88. De Baets MH, Theunissen R, Kok K, De Vijlder JJM, van Breda Vriesman PJC. Monoclonal antibodies to human thyroglobulin as probes for thyroglobulin structure. Endocrinology 1987; 120:1104

89. Dong Q, Ludgate M, Vassart G. Towards an antigenic map of human thyroglobulin: identification of ten epitope-bearing sequences within the primary structure of thyroglobulin. J Endocrinol 1989;122:169

90. Bouanani M, Piechaczyk M, Pau B, Bastide M. Significance of the recognition of certain antigenic regions on the human thyroglobulin molecule by natural autoantibodies from healthy subjects. J Immunol 1989;143:1129

91. Bresler HS, Burek CL, Hoffman WH, Rose NR. Autoantigenic determinants on human thyroglobulin. Clin Immunol Immunopathol 1990;54:76

92. Henry M, Zanelli E, Piechaczyk M, Pau B, Malthiery Y. A major human thyroglobulin epitope defined with monoclonal antibodies is mainly recognized by human autoantibodies. Eur J Immunol 1992;22:315

93. Henry M, Malthiery Y, Zanelli E, Charvet B. Epitope mapping of human thyroglobulin. Heterogeneous recognition by thyroid pathologic sera. J Immunol 1990;145:3692

94. Kohno Y, Nakajima H, Tarutani O. Interspecies cross-reactive determinants of thyroglobulin recognized by autoantibodies. Clin Exp Immunol 1985;61:44

95. Tao T-W, Cheng P-J, Pham H, Leu S-L, Kriss JP. Monoclonal antithyroglobulin antibodies derived from immunizations of mice with human eye muscle and thyroid membranes. J Clin Endocrinol Metab 1986;63:577

96. Kuroki T, Ruf J, Whelan L, Miller A, Wall JR. Antithyroglobulin monoclonal and autoantibodies cross-react with an orbital connective tissue membrane antigen: a possible mechanism for the association of ophthalmopathy with autoimmune thyroid disorders. Clin Exp Immunol 1985;62:361

97. Ludgate ME, Dong Q, Soreq H, Mariotti S, Vassart G. The pathophysiological significance of a thyroglobulin–acetylcholinesterase shared epitope in patients with Graves' ophthalmopathy. Acta Endocrinol (Copenh) 1989;121(Suppl 2):38

98. Tao T-W, Leu S-L, Taylor P, Kriss JP. Reactivity to thyroglobulin and acetylcholinesterase: results with monoclonal antibodies raised against human thyroid, torpedo acetylcholinesterase, and human eye muscle and with affinity-purified, polyclonal, human anti-thyroglobulin. Acta Endocrinol (Copenh) 1989;121(Suppl 2):46

99. Hurel S, Wilkin TJ. Thyroglobulin antibodies cross-react with acetyl cholinesterase: a role in Graves' ophthalmopathy? (abstract 80) Ann Endocrinol 1988;49:210

100. Mercken L, Simons MJ, Brocas H, Vassart G. Alternative splicing may be responsible for heterogeneity of thyroglobulin structure. Biochimie 1989;71:223

101. Ricketts MH, Simons MJ, Parma J, Mercken L, Dong Q, Vassart G. A nonsense mutation causes hereditary goitre in the Afrikander cattle and unmasks alternative splicing of thyroglobulin transcripts. Proc Natl Acad Sci USA 1987;84:3181

102. Kim PS, Dunn AD, Dunn JT. Altered immunoreactivity of thyroglobulin in thyroid disease. J Clin Endocrinol Metab 1988; 67:161

103. Basche M, Beamer WG, Schneider AB. Abnormal properties of thyroglobulin in mice with inherited congenital goiter (cog/cog). Endocrinology 1989;124:1822

104. Sterk A, van Dijk JE, Veenboer GJM, Moorman AFM, De Vijlder JJM. Normal-sized thyroglobulin messenger ribonucleic acid in Dutch goats with a thyroglobulin synthesis defect is translated into a 35,000 molecular weight N-terminal fragment. Endocrinology 1989;124:477

105. Corral J, Martin C, Perez R, et al. Thyroglobulin gene point mutation associated with non-endemic simple goiter. Lancet 1993; 341:462

106. Cave WT Jr, Dunn JT. Studies on the thyroidal defect in an atypical form of Pendred's syndrome. J Clin Endocrinol Metab 1975; 41:590

107. Dunn JT, Ray SC. Changes in iodine metabolism and thyroglobulin structure in metastatic follicular carcinoma of the thyroid with hyperthyroidism. J Clin Endocrinol Metab 1973;36:1088

108. Medeiros-Neto G, Targovnik HM, Vassart G. Defective thyroglobulin synthesis and secretion causing goiter and hypothyroidism. Endocr Rev 1993;14:165

109. Ohta K, Endo T, Onaya T. The mRNA levels of thyrotropin receptor, thyroglobulin and thyroid peroxidase in neoplastic human thyroid tissues. Biochem Biophys Res Commun 1991; 174:1148

110. Kusakabe T. A goitrous subject with structural abnormality of thyroglobulin. J Clin Endocrinol Metab 1972;35:785

111. Silva JE, Santelices R, Kishihara M, Schneider A. Low molecular weight thyroglobulin leading to a goiter in a 12-year-old girl. J Clin Endocrinol Metab 1984;58:526

112. Lissitzky S, Torresani J, Burrow GN, Bouchilloux S, Chabaud O. Defective thyroglobulin export as a cause of congenital goitre. Clin Endocrinol 1975;4:363

113. Grollman EF, Doi SQ, Weiss P, Ashwell G, Wajchenberg BL, Medeiros-Neto G. Hyposialylated thyroglobulin in a patient with congenital goiter and hypothyroidism. J Clin Endocrinol Metab 1992;74:43

114. Ieiri T, Cochaux P, Targovnik HM, et al. A 3' splice site mutation in the thyroglobulin gene responsible for congenital goiter with hypothyroidism. J Clin Invest 1991;88:1901

115. Mason ME, Dunn AD, Wortsman J, et al. Thyroids from siblings with Pendred's syndrome contain thyroglobulin mRNA variants. J Clin Endocrinol Metab 1995;80:497

116. Targovnik HM, Medeiros-Neto G, Varela V, Cochaux P, Wajchenberg BL, Vassart G. A nonsense mutation causes human hereditary congenital goiter with preferential production of a 171-nucleotide-deleted thyroglobulin ribonucleic acid messenger. J Clin Endocrinol Metab 1993;77:210

Werner and Ingbar's The Thyroid, Seventh Edition,
edited by Lewis E. Braverman and Robert D. Utiger.
Lippincott–Raven Publishers, Philadelphia, © 1996

Section C
Peripheral Hormone Metabolism

6

Thyroid Hormone Transport Proteins and the Physiology of Hormone Binding

Jacob Robbins

The delivery system for the thyroid hormones in humans includes a set of circulating transport proteins that vary widely in concentration, affinity for thyroid hormone, and dissociation rate constants. The net result is that more than 99% of the circulating hormone is protein bound but can be liberated with great rapidity for entry into cells. Thyroxine-binding globulin (TBG), a minor component of the α-globulins, carries about 70% of the circulating thyroxine (T_4) and triiodothyronine (T_3) by virtue of its high affinity for the two hormones. It has no other known physiologic function. Transthyretin (TTR), or thyroxine-binding prealbumin, binds only about 10% to 15% of the hormones, but is responsible for much of the immediate delivery of T_4 and T_3 to cells because its affinity for the hormones is lower and therefore they dissociate from it more rapidly. TTR is the major thyroid hormone-binding protein in cerebrospinal fluid, where it may have a role in the distribution of T_4 and T_3 to the central nervous system. It also forms a complex with retinol-binding protein, and therefore is important for the transport of retinol (vitamin A) as well as T_4 and T_3. Albumin, a protein that carries a multitude of small molecules, binds 15% to 20% of the circulating T_4 and T_3. Its

affinity for the hormones is even lower than that of TTR, and the hormone–albumin complexes dissociate rapidly. The *lipoproteins* transport a minor fraction of circulating T_4 and T_3 through specific interactions with various apolipoproteins. Because these proteins are internalized by specific cell surface receptors, they may have a special role in thyroid hormone physiology. In autoimmune thyroid disease, there may be abnormal thyroid hormone binding to immunoglobulins.[1] These and other abnormalities in thyroid hormone transport are discussed in chapter 18 and in several reviews.[2–4]

All vertebrates have some form of thyroid hormone-binding protein in blood, but it is mainly higher mammals that have a high-affinity, low-capacity protein that resembles TBG. TTR is more widely distributed among species. The free T_4 concentration in serum of many animal species is similar to that in humans, despite wide variations in hormone binding.[5] This chapter is devoted to the proteins found in humans; the reader who is interested in the phylogenetic aspects of thyroid hormone transport will find a brief summary in a previous publication[6] and newer information in some more recent articles. For example, in turtles of the Emydidae family, the major transporter is a high-affinity

TABLE 6-1.
Physical Properties of the Major T_4 Transport Proteins in Human Serum*

	TBG[30,31,174]	TTR[23,24]	Albumin[16,177]
Size			
Monomer molecular mass	54 kd	13.5 kd	66 kd
Chains per molecule	1	4	1
Shape			
Relaxation ratio (ρ_h ρ_o)†	1.1	1.6	2.2
Tertiary structure			
α-Helix	55%	5%	50%
β-Structure	20%	55%	15%
S-S Bonds per molecule	2	0	17

*See also references 14, 175, and 176.
†ρ_h, relaxation time derived from polarization of fluorescence; ρ_o, relaxation time of a sphere of the same molecular weight. Rigid globular proteins have ratios between 1 and 2.
TBG, thyroxine-binding globulin; TTR, transthyretin.

protein with homology to vitamin D-binding protein and capable of carrying both T_4 and vitamin D.[7,8] In trout,[9] the major T_4 carriers are lipoproteins, especially high-density lipoproteins. T_4 transport by TTR in serum has been found in eutherians, diprotodont marsupials, and birds, but not in fish, toads, reptiles, or polyprotodont marsupials. TTR synthesis by choroid plexus apparently evolved before hepatic synthesis.[10]

The discovery that a major fraction of the circulating T_4 in humans is bound to an α-globulin was made in 1952,[11] and prealbumin was identified as a distinct thyroxine-binding protein in 1958.[12] T_4 binding to albumin also was recognized in these early studies, which have been reviewed in detail.[13] All three proteins have been isolated from serum and characterized.[14-18] The lipoproteins, also well characterized,[19,20] were more recently reinvestigated with respect to thyroid hormone binding.[21]

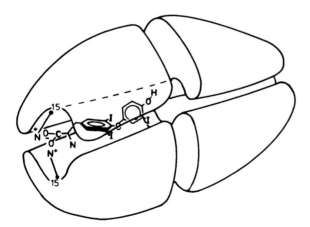

FIGURE 6-1. Schematic drawing of the transthyretin tetramer with T_3 occupying one of the two identical sites in the binding channel. The 3′-iodine is in the distal configuration. The side chain carboxylate is shown at the channel entrance interacting with the ε-amino group of lysine-15. (Jorgensen EC. Thyroid hormones and analogs. II. Structure–activity relationships. In: Li CH, ed. Hormonal proteins and peptides. Vol 6. New York: Academic Press, 1978:107. Drawn from the crystallographic data of Blake and colleagues)

MOLECULAR AND CHEMICAL PROPERTIES

Thyroxine-binding globulin, TTR, and albumin are compact, globular molecules of similar molecular weight (Table 6-1). Whereas TBG and albumin are composed of single polypeptide chains, TTR is a tetramer of identical subunits. These are arranged with twofold symmetry around a nearly cylindrical channel (Fig 6-1).[22-25] TTR has an unusually high content of β-structure, contributing to its extraordinary stability.[14,26,27] The tetramer is not dissociated by 0.1% sodium dodecyl sulfate,[14,26] and the subunits unfold slowly even in 6 mol/L guanidine.[27] Only one of the four sulfhydryl groups is easily detectable in the intact molecule.[28,29]

Thyroxine-binding globulin is a relatively unstable molecule with several unusual properties. It is irreversibly inactivated by dilute acid or guanidine, mild heating (>50°C), and mild mechanical agitation.[30,31] This transition destroys its ability to bind hormone, with only a minor loss in secondary or tertiary structure. When denatured by more concentrated guanidine, the unfolding can be reversed only to the first transition state. This suggests that TBG in serum may have acquired surface groups—perhaps carbohydrates—after folding to its native configuration in the liver cell.[18] Alternatively, intracellular conditions may assist the molecule to achieve the native state. The stability of TBG is significantly enhanced when its binding site for T_4 is occupied,[32] and slight conformational changes induced by hormone binding can be detected.

The complete amino acid sequence of these three proteins has been determined, permitting a search for homology with other proteins.[33-35] TBG was found to be a member of the serine protease inhibitor (serpin) superfamily,[35,36] which also includes corticosteroid-binding globulin (CBG).[37] Neither TBG nor CBG has antiprotease activity, but they share a structural feature in which the native protein exists in a stressed configuration (S).[36,38] In the case of $α_1$-antitrypsin, this results in an exposed peptide loop in which the two amino acid residues of the active center, Met-358 and Ser-359, are appropriately positioned (Fig 6-2). When this loop is cleaved by elastase, the antitrypsin molecule enters a relaxed configuration (R) and these two residues become widely separated. In the case of CBG, cleavage of the presumed loop by elastase results in a profound decrease in affinity for cortisol and an increase in thermal stability. In TBG, elastase increases the thermal stability but has no effect on T_4 binding. This molecular transition, therefore, differs from that induced in the TBG molecule by heat or acid. Although TBG crystals suitable for x-ray diffraction analysis have not yet been obtained, the homology between TBG and $α_1$-antitrypsin has permitted modeling of the TBG structure (Fig 6-3), with emphasis on the T_4-binding site (see below).[39,40]

The amino acid sequence of TTR has been known since 1974,[33] but only one report has suggested sequence homology with retinol-binding protein and the glucagon–secretin family of gastrointestinal hormones.[41] Albumin has substantial homology with α-fetoprotein and vitamin D-binding protein.[16,42] It has three major structural domains with repeating amino acid sequences, suggesting that they arose from gene duplication.[16] Each domain contains two helical subdomains. The crystallographic structure of albumin has been determined.[43]

Some features of the amino acid composition of TBG, TTR, and albumin are shown in Table 6-2. TTR has an unusu-

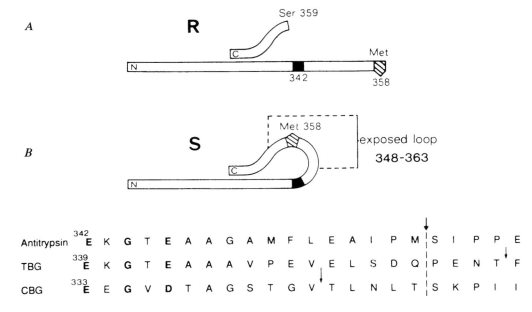

A

R

Ser 359

C

N ■ ▨ Met
342 358

B

S

Met 358

C

N ■

exposed loop
348-363

Antitrypsin ³⁴²E K G T E A A G A M F L E A I P M S I P P E

TBG ³³⁹E K G T E A A A V P E V E L S D Q P E N T F

CBG ³³³E E G V D T A G S T G V T L N L T S K P I I

FIGURE 6-2. The structure of the serpins based on the cleaved (R) form of α_1-antitrypsin shown diagrammatically (A). The native stressed (S) form has to be reconstructed by a deduced exposed loop that hinges near residue 342 (B). Alignment of the sequences of the exposed loop (based on hinge residues; *bold*) shows the sites of cleavage of TBG and corticosteroid-binding globulin (CBG) by neutrophil elastase (*arrows*). The dashed vertical line shows the putative reactive centers of TBG and CBG based on alignment with that of antitrypsin (*arrows*). (Pemberton PA, Stein, PE, Pepya MB, Potter JM, Carrell RW. Hormone binding globulins undergo serpin conformational change in inflammation. Nature 1988;336:257)

ally high content of aromatic amino acids, especially tryptophan, which may explain its sensitivity to altered nutrition. TBG has 2 disulfide bonds, TTR has none, and albumin has 17. The fluorescence properties of the single tryptophan (Trp214) in domain II of albumin have been used in binding studies.[44]

Of the three major T_4-binding proteins, only TBG is a glycoprotein (Table 6-3). It has on its surface four asparagine-linked complex oligosaccharides with branched chains and three slightly varying structures that contain an average of 10 terminal sialic acid groups (Fig 6-4).[45,46] These oligosaccha-

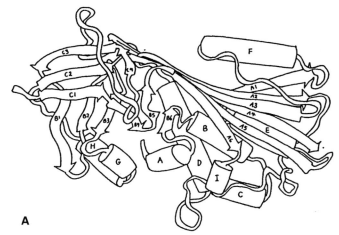

A

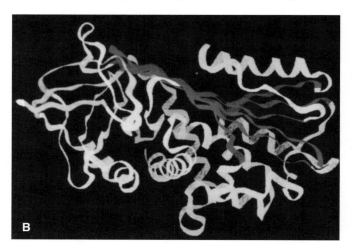

B

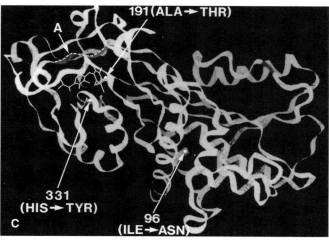

191(ALA→THR)

A

331
(HIS→TYR)

96
(ILE→ASN)

C

FIGURE 6-3. A structural model of TBG based on homology of α_1-antitrypsin. (A and B) The crystal coordinate structure of cleaved α_1-antitrypsin. The β-sheets are labeled A 1-6, B 1-3 and C 1-3. (C) The modeled structure of cleaved TBG with the T_4 molecule occupying the putative binding site. The T_4 binding site is in the β-barrel formed by β-sheets B and C and is not affected by cleavage. The peptide identified by affinity labeling[67] is indicated by A. Also identified are locations of mutations known to affect T_4 binding. These include Ala 191 → Thr, His 331 → Tyr, and Ile 96 → Asn. The latter is distant from the putative binding site but is associated with a major structural change in TBG. (Adapted from Jarvis JA, Munro SLA, Craik DJ. Homology model of thyroxine-binding globulin and elucidation of the thyroid hormone binding site. Protein Eng 1992;5:61)

TABLE 6-2.
Amino Acid Composition of the Major T_4 Transport Proteins in Human Serum*

	TBG[174]	TTR[33]	Albumin[16]
Residues per mol			
Basic			
Lys	28	32	58
Arg	6	16	23
His	11	16	16
Acidic			
Asp	36	32	54
Glu	25	48	30
Aromatic			
Tyr	9	20	18
Trp	4	8	1
Sulfuric			
Met	12	4	6
$\frac{1}{2}$-Cys	5	4	35
Free SH	1	4	1
N-terminal residue	Ala	Gly	Asp
C-terminal residue	Leu	Glu	Leu

See also references 144 and 175.

TABLE 6-3.
Carbohydrate Composition of TBG[45,46,54]

Number of chains	4
Total percentage by weight	15–21
Residues per mol	
Galactose	9–13
Mannose	10–11
Glucosamine (GlcNAc)	16–22
Sialic acid (NeuNAc)	10

rides are responsible for the acid isoelectric point and the microheterogeneity exhibited on isoelectric focusing.[47,48] Most studies reveal three to four major components and a variable number of minor bands with pI ranging from 4.2 to 5.0. Removal of sialic acid raises the pI to about 6 and gives a minimum of two residual components, which may represent charge heterogeneity of the polypeptide chain.[49–51] In males, who have only a single copy of the TBG gene on the X chromosome,[52] all TBG isoforms are present, arguing against a genetically determined polymorphism.[53] Removal of more than 80% of the carbohydrate does not prevent T_4 binding, although the affinity for T_4 is somewhat reduced[54] and the stability of the molecule is decreased.[55]

HORMONE BINDING

Thyroxine-Binding Globulin

About 70% of the T_4 in serum is carried by TBG, despite the fact that it is the least abundant of the three major transport proteins. This can be attributed to its extremely high affinity for T_4 (Table 6-4). Although the binding energy approaches that of a chemical bond, the interaction clearly is noncovalent. Indeed, the dissociation rate constant is rapid ($t\frac{1}{2}$ 39 seconds).[56,57] T_3 binds to TBG 10 to 20 times less avidly than T_4, and dissociates still more rapidly ($t\frac{1}{2}$ 4.2 seconds). The greater rate of dissociation is largely responsible for the lower affinity. In normal serum, about one fourth of the TBG molecules contain a T_4 molecule.

Representative data for the binding of thyroid hormone analogues to TBG are shown in Table 6-5.[13,58] Optimal binding requires an intact alanine side chain in the L-configuration, a phenolic hydroxyl that is ionized, a diphenyl ether oxygen (although a sulfur or methylene bridge is almost as good), and

four halogen atoms (either iodine or bromine). In other words, L-T_4 is the preferred ligand for the binding site of TBG, which therefore differs from the site on TTR or on the nuclear receptor.[58] Nevertheless, its specificity is broad enough to allow binding of many compounds that have only partial resemblance to T_4, such as phenytoin (5,5-diphenylhydantoin), fenclofenac, diazepam, and salicylates.[48,59] TBG also binds 1,8-anilinonaphthalene sulfonic acid (ANS), which is used for fluorescence analysis and to displace T_4 in immunoassays for the hormone.[60] 3,5-Diiodo-2′,3′-dimethylthyronine, which has the 3′-methyl in the "distal" configuration, is biologically more active than the 2′,5′-dimethyl analogue and also binds more strongly to TBG.[61]

Lacking a complete structural analysis for TBG, the information about the nature of its hormone-binding site is indirect. TBG appears to have only one binding site, which is shared by T_4, T_3, and other thyronine analogues.[62] The temperature dependence of binding suggests that hydrophobic forces between the hormone and the site are important,[62,63] which may be explained by the cluster of aromatic amino acids lining the proposed binding site.[40]

Affinity labeling of the site with N-bromoacetyl-T_4 indicates that a methionine is located near the side chain of T_4 because methionine constitutes 75% of the labeled residues[64]; it may, however, be outside the binding domain.[65] Other studies[30,66,67] indicate that a lysyl residue, possibly Lys 257, is on the surface of the β-barrel that constitutes the putative binding site (see Fig 6-3).[40] As shown by electron spin resonance analysis using "spin-labeled" analogues, T_4 is less rigidly bound in the TBG site than in the sites of TTR or albumin.[68] Furthermore, TBG can interact with small thyroxyl peptides.[69] Advances in defining the amino acid substitutions in genetically altered TBG should help to define the binding surface of this protein.[17,39,40]

Transthyretin

In contrast to the paucity of information concerning TBG, the T_4-binding site on TTR has been mapped in great detail. Each molecule contains two identical sites located in a central channel (see Fig 6-1).[23] The side-chain carboxyl and amino groups of T_4 are adjacent to Lys-15 and Glu-54, respectively, near the channel entrance, and the phenolic ring is in a hydrophilic patch near the center of the molecule, which consists of the hydroxyl groups of Ser-117 and Thr-119 and one or more water molecules. This is consistent with the normal pK of the hydroxyl group of T_4 when bound to TTR.[14,70] The iodine atoms

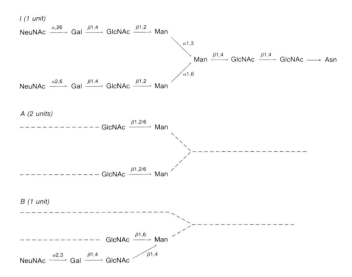

FIGURE 6-4. Structure of the oligosaccharide units of TBG. The dashed lines indicate structure identical to those in the top structure (1). Linkages designated β1,2/6 occur in A and B half in 1,2 linkages and half in 1.6 linkage. (Zinn AB, Marshall JS, Carlson DM. Carbohydrate structure on thyroxine-binding globulin and their effects of hepatocyte membrane binding. J Biol Chem 1978;253:6768)

appear to occupy four well defined hydrophobic pockets, accounting in part for the hydrophobic nature of the interaction.[70] The phenolic ring of T_3 can apparently bind in alternative positions, as shown by the variable location of the 3'-iodine in the TTR crystal.

Despite the now well established twofold symmetry of the TTR molecule, early evidence indicated that only one molecule of T_4 was bound.[29,71] This was later clarified when it was shown that there are in fact two sites, but that the second has an affinity two orders of magnitude lower than the first (see Table 6-4).[14,72] Together with evidence that some T_4 analogues

and ANS occupy the two sites with almost equal affinity, these findings are explained by strong negative cooperativity in the binding of T_4, T_3, and other analogues. The exact mechanism of this negative cooperativity is incompletely understood. The location of the ligands in the binding channel and a 0.4-nm constriction at the center of the molecule clearly exclude a steric effect.[23] The remaining possibilities are a charge–charge interaction between the ionized phenolic group of T_4[72] or a subtle allosteric effect of T_4 binding on the TTR molecule after the first site is occupied, which has been demonstrated by optical and enzymatic techniques.[73,74]

The affinity constant for the T_4–TTR interaction is intermediate between those for TBG and albumin (see Table 6-4), so that TTR transports about 10% to 15% of the T_4 in serum. Only the first site is occupied normally, and only 1 in 300 TTR molecules contains T_4. The affinity constant for T_3 is about 10-fold lower, but uncertainty exists as to exactly how much of the T_3 in serum is carried by TTR.[75] Because the dissociation rate constant for T_4–TTR is about fivefold greater than that of T_4–TBG, the contribution of T_4–TTR to the free hormone pool during capillary flow is about equal to that of T_4–TBG.[75,76]

Because about one third of the TTR molecules in normal serum carry a molecule of retinol-binding protein ([RBP], assuming that only one of the four sites for this protein is occupied), and because each molecule of RBP binds one molecule of vitamin A, the interplay between these carriers and ligands assumes importance.[15,77] Although the retinol—RBP—TTR interactions are mutually enhancing,[78–80] those of T_4—TTR—RBP do not seem to influence one another.[15] Crystallographic analysis has shown that two RBP molecules bind to one TTR dimer, which interferes with further RBP binding but not the T_4-binding channel.[80a] Thus, T_4 transport by TTR is independent of the concentration of RBP.

More recent work[81,82] has greatly amplified the earlier data[75] about the relative affinity of T_4 analogues for TTR, and offers the possibility of comparing the effects of these hormone modifications on their binding to TBG and to the nu-

TABLE 6-4.
Binding Characteristics, Concentration, and Hormone Distribution of T_4-Binding Proteins in Normal Serum at 37°C

	TBG	TTR		Albumin	
Association constant (M^{-1})*[75]					
K T_4	1.0×10^{10}	Site 1	7.0×10^7	Site 1	7.0×10^5
		Site 2	6.7×10^5	Sites 2–6	4.8×10^4
K T_3	4.6×10^8	Site 1	1.4×10^7	Site 1	1.0×10^5
		Site 2	5.5×10^5	Sites 2–6	6.9×10^3
Dissociation rate constant (sec^{-1})[76]					
k T_4	0.018	0.094			
k T_3	0.16	~0.69			
Concentration[75]					
mg/dL	1.5	25		4200	
μmol/L	0.27	4.6		640	
Hormone distribution (%)[75]					
T_4	68	11		20	
T_3	80	9		11	

*In PO$_4$-buffered 0.1 M NaCl at 37°C.

TABLE 6-5.
Relative Affinities of Selected T_4 Analogues for T_4-Binding Proteins

	TBG*	TTR (Site 1)†	ALB (Site 1)‡
T_4	100	100	100
Ring substitutions			
T_3	9	9.2 (8)	55
rT_3	38 (5)	33	100
$3,3'$-T_2	1.3	0.6	
$3',5'$-T_2	0.1	3.3	100
$3'$-isopropyl-T_3	3.5	0.8	
$3'$-methyl-T_3	0.3	0.4	
$3,5,3',5'$-methyl-T_4	0.3		
Side-chain substitutions			
D-T_4	54 (17)	3.7	
N-acetyl-T_4	25	(12)	
T_4-propionic acid	3.6	298 (160)	135
T_4-acetic acid	1.7	676 (160)	110
T_3-acetic acid	0.3	20	
Phenol substitutions			
$4'$-methyl-T_3	3.5		
$4'$-deoxy-T_3	1.9	0.4	
Ether bridge substitutions			
Sulfur bridge T_4	63		
Methylene bridge T_4	35		

*Data at pH 7.4 from reference 178. Data in parentheses from reference 65.
†Data at pH 8.0 from references 81 and 82. Data in parentheses, at pH 7.4, PO_4–Cl, 25°C, from 5.
‡Data at pH 7.4 from reference 179.

clear receptor. Representative data for the many compounds studied are shown in Table 6-5. All four iodine atoms, especially those in the phenolic ring, contribute favorably to binding to TTR; halogen substituents are more favorable than alkyl groups, despite their similar hydrophobic character; and the desamino analogues are bound with the highest affinity. These features differ in certain respects from those that govern binding to either TBG or the nuclear receptor.[58,83] The most striking differences are the decreased affinity of D-T_4 and L-T_3 for TBG but not for the receptor, and the decreased affinity of the desamino analogues for TBG but not for the receptor or TTR. Both the side-chain and the ring substituents are important in this respect.

Nonthyronine molecules also interact with the T_4-binding site of TTR. These include barbital, which explains the difficulties in demonstrating the presence of TTR in early electrophoretic experiments with this buffer[13]; ANS, which has been used in competitive binding studies[14]; 2,4-dinitrophenol; drugs such as salicylates and penicillin[48,59]; and naturally occurring plant pigments, the flavonoids, which also interact with iodothyronine deiodinase[84] (see chap 8).

Albumin

Human serum albumin has one relatively strong binding site for T_4 and T_3, in addition to at least five weaker sites (see Table 6-4). Few of the albumin molecules in serum carry the hormones, but the high albumin concentration results in the binding of about 15% to 20% of the circulating T_4 and possibly more of the T_3.[75] Both types of sites appear to be occupied at normal hormone concentrations. The dissociation rate constants have not yet been measured, but they clearly are more rapid than those of TBG and TTR. Hence, a large fraction of the hormone entering cells derives from the albumin-bound pool.[76,85]

Although the strong albumin site binds T_4 more avidly than T_3, other T_4 analogues are bound about equally (see Table 6-5). Fatty acids, other anions, and chloride decrease T_4 binding[86]; various substitution reactions on the protein also decrease binding.[75] The thyroid hormones and tryptophan are the only amino acids that bind noncovalently to albumin, and they share the same site, which appears to be near the surface of domain III of the albumin molecule.[16] T_4 also interacts with the warfarin site on domain II, so that it occupies the hydrophobic cavities on both subdomains IIA and IIIA that are the principal regions for multiple-ligand binding.[43] The latter appears to be the location of the high-affinity T_4-binding site.[87]

Lipoproteins

The lipoproteins are a heterogeneous group of complex particles consisting of various apolipoproteins, many of which have been well characterized,[19,20] and both polar and nonpolar lipids. In a study of all the lipoproteins in serum, differences in the distribution of T_4 and T_3 were found, but the high-density lipoproteins (HDL) were the major binders of both hormones.[21] HDL may carry about 3% of the T_4 and 6%

of the T_3 in serum, mainly in a very–high-density subfraction. Apolipoprotein binding of T_4 and T_3 is saturable.[88–90] The binding site for T_4 has been mapped by analyzing the ability of monoclonal antibodies to inhibit photoaffinity labeling with T_4. T_4 is bound to a single site in the N-terminal one third of apolipoprotein A-I, the major apoprotein of HDL.[91] Apolipoprotein B-100, the major protein of low-density lipoprotein (LDL), has a binding site for T_4 on each of its three domains.[92] In both apolipoproteins, the binding sites are in regions rich in β-structure, separate from regions that bind to lipoprotein receptors, and share amino acid homology with the T_4-binding domains of TBG, TTR, and albumin.[90] Apolipoprotein A-I binds T_4 with a K_a of 7.5×10^7 and has a similar affinity for D-T_4, T_3-acetic acid, and 3′,5′,3-triiodothyronine (rT_3), and a much lower affinity for T_3.[88]

GENE STRUCTURE AND INHERITED ABNORMALITIES

The gene for TBG occurs as a single, approximately 8-kb copy on the long arm of the X chromosome[52] and contains five exons, one of which is not translated.[35,93–95] The sequence of approximately 5 kb of the gene has been reported,[96] including 638 bases at the 5′ untranslated end and about 900 bases at the 3′ end. Both of these ends contain sequences that resemble thyroid hormone and estrogen response elements that might be sites for regulation of TBG synthesis by these hormones. There are two polyadenylation signals responsible for two mRNAs differing by 200 bases (1400 and 1600 bases in length).[97]

Inherited abnormalities that affect the transport of thyroid hormones in serum were first recognized for TBG.[98,99] Numerous mutations, some occurring in each of the four coding exons, of the TBG gene responsible for either quantitative or qualitative abnormalities in the proteins have been identified.[2,17,94] Most are single-base changes causing partial deficiency or polymorphism of TBG. In some cases, TBG deficiency is the result of reduced stability of the protein or reduced T_4 binding. In others, intracellular processing or secretion is impaired, perhaps because of altered glycosylation.[100] Complete TBG deficiency has been explained by deletions resulting in frameshift or premature termination of the transcript.[101,102] A catalogue of these abnormalities is provided in several reviews.[2,17,94] Newborn screening programs for hypothyroidism have identified TBG deficiency in about 1 of 5000 infants.[17] The defect is more commonly found in males (~1 in 2000) because hemizygosity leads to a more profound reduction in serum T_4.[103] TBG excess is much rarer (~1 in 25,000). Affected hemizygous males have serum TBG and T_4 concentrations two to three times normal. Gene duplication has been demonstrated in several patients with the syndrome.[103a,103b]

The TTR gene, also a single copy of ~approximately 7 kb, is on chromosome 18 and contains four exons.[104–106] Two unidentified open-reading frames exist within the gene on exons 1 and 4. The TTR genes in mice[107] and rats[108] are very similar to the human gene and contain highly conserved DNA regions in both the 5′ and 3′ ends. There are two categories of inherited variations in human TTR, those associated with amyloidosis, most of which are in families with familial amyloidotic polyneuropathy (FAP),[2,18] and those with hyperthyroxinemia, reported in only a few cases.[109,110] Although many of the FAP cases have decreased binding of T_4 to the abnormal

TTR,[111,112] hypothyroxinemia may not be evident because TTR carries less T_4 than TBG, and because the tetrameric TTR molecules in heterozygous subjects contain a mixture of normal and abnormal subunits, and the hybrid molecules have a higher affinity for T_4 than the homozygous tetramers.[111,113] Recombinant TTR molecules containing four abnormal subunits have been produced for study of T_4 binding.[113] The defects that have been described are single amino acid substitutions. In the Val 30 → Met variant associated with FAP and decreased T_4 binding, the defect is in the outer β sheet (Fig 6-5) and appears to deform the T_4 binding channel.[114] In the Ile 84 → Ser variant, associated with decreased binding of retinol-binding protein as well as decreased T_4 binding,[115] the defect is in the helix loop that connects strands E and F of the outer β sheet.

Three defects causing hyperthyroxinemia have been described. In one, Ala 109 → Thr, the increased affinity for T_4 has been explained by a change in the T_4 binding surface,[109,111,112,116] and the hybrid tetramers bind T_4 as strongly as homozygous tetramers.[113] In another, Thr 119 → Met, the increase in serum T_4 was attributed to an increase in the concentration of TTR in one study[110] but to increased affinity for T_4 in another.[117] The defect in this case is also located on the binding surface. In the third defect (Gly 6 → Ser), the mutation is on the N-terminal chain near the entrance to the binding channel,[118] but increased binding has not been confirmed with recombinant Ser 6 TTR.[113] Over 30 different point mutations have been found, and many are catalogued in several reviews.[2,18,111]

The single-copy human albumin gene consisting of 15 exons is on the long arm of chromosome 4, linked to the vitamin D-binding α_2-globulin gene. In mice, the albumin gene is on chromosome 5, close to the gene for α-fetoprotein. Many abnormal albumin genes have been characterized and are responsible for polymorphic forms of albumin in which there are differences in T_4 binding.[16,86] A rare abnormality, complete absence of albumin, or analbuminemia, also occurs. Of greater interest is the defect known as familial dysalbuminemic hyperthyroxinemia, which occurs with a prevalence varying from 0.01% to 1.8% in different populations.[2,119] Although earlier studies subdivided cases according to differences in T_4, T_3, and rT_3 binding,[2,18] more recent work has disclosed only a single albumin variant. A point mutation in exon 7, resulting in Arg 218 → His in subdomain IIA, has been identified in 24 subjects from 11 unrelated families.[119,120] The variant albumin comigrates with normal albumin in reverse-phase high-pressure liquid chromatography and sodium dodecyl sulfate-polyacrylamide gel electrophoresis, but fluorescence analysis suggests that the two forms are present in approximately equal amounts, the variant having an affinity for T_4 about 10 times normal.[2,18]

BIOSYNTHESIS AND METABOLISM

As for many of the serum proteins, hepatocytes are the source of TBG, TTR, and albumin.[14,16,18] TTR is also synthesized in pancreatic islet cells[121,122] and in the epithelium of the choroid plexus,[123,124] in which its production is regulated differently than in the liver.[18] Its high rate of synthesis in the choroid plexus[125] is responsible for the previously unexplained high relative concentration of TTR in cerebrospinal fluid.[18,126]

Precursor forms of TBG and TTR have not been identified,[123,127] but the relatively hydrophobic nature of their N-ter-

FIGURE 6-5. (*A*) Location of inherited amino acid substitutions in transthyretin. The figure shows the TTR tetramer with the T₄-binding channel running from left to right between the inner β-sheets (DAGH). (Hamilton JA, Steinrauf LK, Braden BC, et al. The x-ray crystal structure refinements of normal human transthyretin and the amyloidogenic Val 30 → Met variant to 1.7. A resolution. J Bio Chem 1993;268:2416) (*B*) Mutations on the outer β-sheet (Met 30) are associated with decreased T₄-binding and those on the helix-loop (Ser 84) are associated with both decreased T₄ and RBP binding. Two others (Tyr 77 and Ileu 122) also cause decreased binding of T₄. Mutations associated with increased T₄ binding are located on the inner β-sheet (Thr 109 and Met 119). (Adapted from Rosen HN, Moses AC, Murrell JR, et al. Thyroxine interactions with transthyretin: a comparison of 10 different naturally occurring human transthyretin variants. J Clin Endocrinol Metab 1993;77:370)

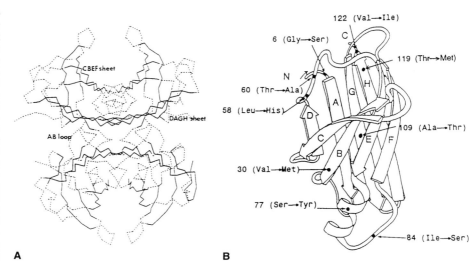

minal sequences may serve the role of signal peptides.[35,128,129] In the case of albumin, two exons at the 5′ end code for an 18-residue signal peptide.[16] In the embryo, as well as in some patients in whom albumin is genetically abnormal, proalbumin is secreted from the hepatocytes.[16]

Biosynthetic studies in the human hepatoma cell line, Hep G2, have shown a slower and more complex synthetic pathway for TBG compared with TTR and albumin, because only TBG is a glycoprotein.[18,130] Folding of the molecule into its native conformation occurs concomitantly with the addition of the carbohydrate chains and may depend on the glycosylation process.[18,131] Secretion of TBG also appears to require glycosylation,[131,132] although this may not be absolute.[130]

Both TTR and RBP are produced by hepatocytes. The release of the two proteins is not coupled, even though they are secreted in rather similar molar amounts.[133,134] RBP is secreted almost entirely as the holoprotein, and retinol is required for its release by a mechanism that remains unexplained.[134–136] TTR secretion does not depend on retinol.

The production rate of TTR in humans is 50 times greater than that of TBG (Table 6-6) but about 25 times less than that of albumin. TTR production is decreased in illness and malnutrition, possibly related to TTR's high tryptophan content. The situation with respect to RBP is similar.[14,137,138] When TTR secretion decreases, its serum concentration falls rapidly because the disappearance half-time (1–2 days) is not affected. Serum TTR measurements are therefore a sensitive indicator of protein-calorie malnutrition.

The rate of disappearance of TBG from plasma (t¹/₂ 5 days) is slower than that of TTR but considerably faster than that of albumin (t¹/₂ 13 days; see Table 6-6). Because TBG is a glycoprotein, the rate at which it leaves the circulation is related to the terminal sugar residues on the polysaccharide chains.[139] When sialic acid is removed and galactose becomes terminal, TBG is rapidly taken up by hepatocyte surface receptors.[45,47] This explains the earlier finding that a slowly migrating TBG (called sTBG) accumulates in the circulation of patients with liver failure.[4] Similarly, TBG components with a high isoelectric point accumulate in patients with liver disease.[49] sTBG is not the same as TBG-S, a slowly migrating TBG found in African Americans and other groups. TBG-S differs from normal (TBG-C) in a charged amino acid substitution rather than in carbohydrate composition.[17]

Pregnancy is associated with accumulation of a highly sialylated form of TBG.[140] Although TBG synthesis is increased by estrogen,[14] the reduced rate of metabolism of this highly sialylated TBG appears to be the major cause for increased serum TBG concentrations in pregnant women.

Thyroxine-binding globulin turnover in rhesus monkeys is affected by thyroid status,[141,142] the TBG production rate being decreased in both hypothyroidism and severe thyrotoxicosis. T₃ excess has a similar effect in Hep G2 cells.[143,143a] Thyroid status also affects the disappearance rate of TBG from plasma—it is slower in hypothyroidism and faster in thyrotoxicosis—and it also has small effects on the distribution space of TBG. These complicated effects of thyroid hormone may explain the variable changes in serum TBG concentrations in patients with thyroid disease.[144] Estrogen, dexamethasone, or T₃ do not affect activation of the TBG gene derived from human liver.[95] Although glucocorticoids decrease serum TBG and liver TBG mRNA in rats,[145] there are many differences between the regulation of TBG synthesis in rats and humans. In rats, T₃ has no effect on gene activation, even though it does cause down-regulation of TBG mRNA in vivo.[146,147]

Thyroxine-binding globulin synthesis in human Hep G2 cells is decreased by interleukin-6 at a pretranslational level,[148] whereas it decreases CBG synthesis at a posttranslational level.[149] Synthesis of other members of the serpin family of proteins is increased by this cytokine, as expected for acute-phase proteins, indicating very different regulation of the transport proteins.

PHYSIOLOGIC IMPLICATIONS

As discussed earlier, there are a number of clinically encountered genetic abnormalities associated with increased or, more often, with decreased concentrations of each of the thyroid hormone transport proteins in serum. None of them alters the thyroid state of the affected person, even when the protein is completely absent. TTR is the major thyroid hormone carrier protein in mice, and transgenic TTR-null mice are phenotypi-

TABLE 6-6.
Metabolism of T_4-Binding Proteins in Humans

	TBG*	TTR†	RBP[1] BOUND	RBP[1] FREE	Albumin[2]
Distribution					
volume	6.70	5.7			5.8–7.2
(L)‡	7.40	5–7.8			
Disappearance rate	0.14	0.36	2.7	19.1	0.054
(day⁻¹)	0.13	0.59			
Production rate (70-kg body weight)					
mg/d	17.5	679	336	294	14,000
	12.6	511			
μmol/d	0.32	13			
	0.23	9.5	16	14	212

Upper figures from reference 180; lower figures from reference 182.
†Upper figures from reference 181; lower figures from reference 183.
‡Recalculated from data in reference 144.

cally normal despite having low serum thyroid hormone and retinol concentrations.[150] Although there are no reported instances of a patient in whom all of the proteins capable of T_4 transport were absent, it is clear that no one of the transport proteins is required for good health. Despite large increases or decreases in serum total T_4 and T_3 concentrations in some of these patients, their serum free T_4 and T_3 concentrations are normal.[17] These results constitute strong evidence in support of the concept that homeostatic mechanisms are designed to maintain the normality of the free hormone concentration, and that this concentration determines a person's thyroid state.

Other inherited abnormalities create polymorphisms that do not affect either serum thyroid hormone concentrations or thyroid state, or that cause only changes in serum hormone concentrations. Included are the TBG polymorphism that affects African blacks,[53] a TTR polymorphism in rhesus monkeys,[151] and bisalbuminemia.[6]

Another kind of evidence supporting the concept that the transport proteins are not essential for thyroid hormone action is the correlation of thyroid hormone disposal rates with the serum concentrations of unbound thyroid hormone. As shown in Figure 6-6, T_4 and T_3 disposal rates are proportional to the serum free T_4 and free T_3 concentrations, respectively, rather than to the total concentrations.[152–154] Because the disposal rates are directly correlated with hormone action, it can be concluded that the free hormone concentration controls its action.

What, then, is the physiologic importance of the transport proteins? Three functions can be postulated: extrathyroidal storage of hormone; a buffering action, so that the stored hormone is released on demand while the tissues are protected from excessive hormone; and a hormone-releasing function that allows the minute free hormone pool to be continuously replenished and made available to the cells.

Thyroid homeostasis is characterized by the maintenance of a steady supply of hormone to tissues, resulting in steady hormone actions. Presumably, extrathyroidal storage contributes to this homeostasis. The ratio of the serum total T_4 concentration (100 nmol/L) to the free T_4 concentration (30 pmol/L) is an indi-

cator of the total storage function of the transport proteins with respect to the major secretory product of the thyroid gland. When serum is depleted of TBG, the ratio falls to one-third of normal (Fig 6-7), whereas depletion of TTR or albumin has only a small effect. It is thus evident that TBG is the major storage site for secreted hormone in the circulation. The ratio of total T_3 in serum (2 nmol/L) to free T_3 (8 pmol/L) is much less than that of T_4; although substantial, it is perhaps more related to the hormone delivery mechanism than to storage.

An important extension of our understanding of the storage function has been provided by liver perfusion experiments. Transport proteins are required for uniform distribution of hormone to all the cells of the hepatic lobules, because in the absence of transport proteins the first cells contacted take up the hormone during a single pass and fail to release it during a subsequent hour of perfusion.[153,155] Although albumin could also perform this storage and delivery function, the efficacy of TBG was less subject to physiologic variations in fatty acids.

To serve as an optimal buffer at the ambient free T_4 concentration in serum (3×10^{-11} mol/L), a binding protein should have a dissociation constant of the same magnitude. Thus, TBG (K_d 10^{-10} mol/L) is not the perfect buffer, but its K_d is much closer to the free T_4 concentration than that of either TTR or albumin (see Table 6-4). The buffering action of TBG in vivo has been supported by the demonstration that patients with genetically absent TBG have slightly elevated serum thyroglobulin concentrations.[156] This can be explained by postulating that the pituitary gland is exposed to fluctuating serum free T_4 concentrations, and so serum thyrotropin concentrations may fluctuate more than normal and net thyrotropin secretion is probably slightly increased. This increase would be responsible for the increase in serum thyroglobulin concentrations. The buffering action of TBG on T_4 also can be demonstrated by the theoretical calculations shown in Figure 6-8. When TBG is depleted from serum, there is a much greater increase in free T_4 concentration with increasing total T_4 concentration than when either TTR or albumin is depleted. In the presence of TBG, the plot of free T_4 concentration versus total T_4 concentration has an in-

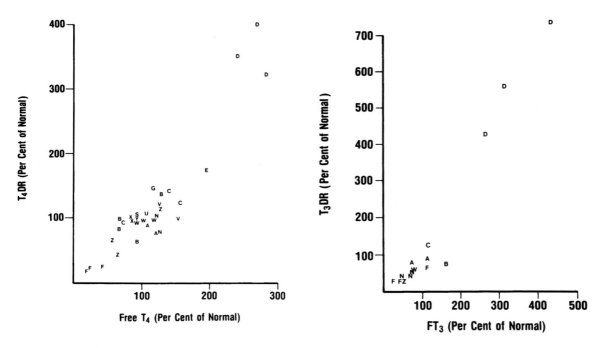

FIGURE 6-6. Correlation between serum free T_4 or T_3 concentrations and the disposal rate (DR) of T_4 or T_3 (both expressed as percentage of normal). Each data point is the mean for the group from an individual study; some groups were studied by multiple investigators. A, increased serum TBG; B, decreased serum TBG; C, familial dysalbuminemic hyperthroxinemia; D,E, thyrotoxicosis; F, hypothyroidism; G, treated thyrotoxicosis; X,Y,Z, nonthyroid illness (mild, moderate, severe); W, chronic renal failure; V, cirrhosis; U, hepatitis; S, ethanol abuse; N, caloric deprivation. (Mendel CM, Cavalieri R. Transport of thyroid hormones in health and disease: recent controversy surrounding the free hormone hypothesis. Thyroid Today 1988;11:3)

creasing slope over the normal range of total T_4 concentrations. This is a reflection of the fact that the molar concentration of TBG in serum is low relative to that of T_4, so that 25% of the T_4-binding sites are occupied. The physiologic implication of this amplification of free T_4 is uncertain.[157]

The buffering of T_3 is much less efficient that that of T_4, as expected from the fact that the free T_3 concentration (8×10^{-12} mol/L) is much lower than the dissociation constants, which range from 2.2×10^{-9} mol/L for TBG to 10^{-5} mol/L for albumin. Also, there is no curvilinear response of free T_3 with increasing total T_3.

The releasing function of the transport proteins has been the subject of considerable controversy.[158–160] Based on single-pass organ perfusion experiments in vivo, Pardridge and col-

leagues[85,158] concluded that T_4 bound to TBG is available for entry into some organs (e.g., liver) but not others (e.g., brain), that albumin-bound T_4 is the main source of hormone for all tissues, and that an alteration of binding that occurs within the capillaries enhances the liberation of hormone from the protein. Others have concluded from theoretical and other considerations that T_4 and T_3 dissociation from TBG is rapid enough and plentiful enough to meet the requirements of any tissue.[154,161] Owing to the more rapid dissociation rates from TTR (see Table 6-4) and probably from albumin, the latter proteins undoubtedly supply much of the hormone that enters the cells.[161]

An alternative mechanism that could account for selective cellular entry of T_4 and T_3 is the specific interaction of trans-

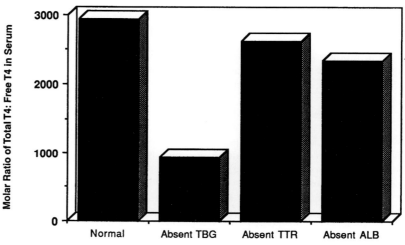

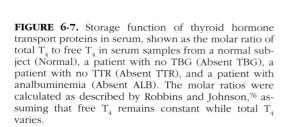

FIGURE 6-7. Storage function of thyroid hormone transport proteins in serum, shown as the molar ratio of total T_4 to free T_4 in serum samples from a normal subject (Normal), a patient with no TBG (Absent TBG), a patient with no TTR (Absent TTR), and a patient with analbuminemia (Absent ALB). The molar ratios were calculated as described by Robbins and Johnson,[76] assuming that free T_4 remains constant while total T_4 varies.

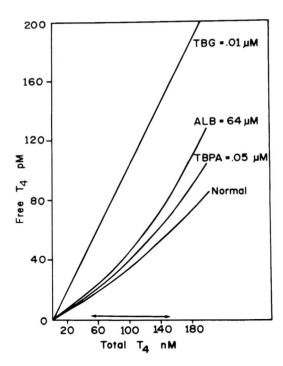

FIGURE 6-8. Theoretical curves showing the relation of free T_4 to total T_4 in normal serum and serum in which one thyroxine-binding protein is reduced to 10% of its normal concentration (the calculations are those of Robbins and Johnson.[76,161]) The horizontal arrow indicates the normal range of T_4. (Robbins J, Bartalena L. In: Hennemann G, ed. Plasma transport of thyroid hormones. New York: Marcel Dekker, 1986)

port proteins with cell surface receptors. A few reports have suggested that such receptors may exist in mononuclear cells for TBG,[162] in hepatocytes[163,164] and astrocytes[165] for TTR, and in fibroblasts for LDL.[166] Inasmuch as there also are cell surface receptors for free T_4 and T_3 that may be involved in cell entry,[167] the importance of receptors for the transport proteins is unclear. They could be involved in targeting the hormones to different subcellular sites, or they may be subject to specific regulation, as in the case of LDL, where the fibroblast receptors are upregulated by cholesterol deprivation, resulting in enhanced T_4 entry.[166]

With respect to the free hormone hypothesis, which states that the serum concentrations of T_4 and T_3 are directly related to the amount of hormone entering the cells and to their ultimate physiologic response,[13,75] it is important to realize that in an equilibrium mixture containing hormone and several binding proteins, the amount of hormone bound to a minor transport protein such as LDL will be proportional to the free hormone concentration. Thus

$$[T] = \frac{[TPi]}{ki\,[Pi]} = \frac{\Sigma[TPi]}{\Sigma ki\,[Pi]}$$

where the brackets indicate molar concentrations, T is free hormone, TPi is bound hormone or occupied binding sites of class i, P is unoccupied binding sites, and k is the intrinsic association constant.

Transthyretin may have a special role in facilitating the passage of T_4 across the choroid plexus and distributing it to the surface of the brain.[126,168,169] This might be an important

mechanism for entry of the hormone into the central nervous system,[170] and T_4 may indeed enter the cerebrospinal fluid by this pathway.[171,172] By comparing the distribution of T_4 and T_3 after intravenous or intrathecal injection, however, it is evident that most of the brain receives T_4 and T_3 via the general capillary circulation, whereas entry through the choroid plexus may provide more selective hormone distribution[173,174] and may also represent a more primitive pathway.[10,169]

Thyroid hormone transport proteins are an important aspect of thyroid physiology. Although they may not be essential for hormone action, they appear to be required for the smooth functioning of the thyroid gland and the actions of its hormones. As is evident in later chapters, an understanding of the basic properties of the transport system in serum is important for the appropriate evaluation and management of patients in whom the proteins are affected by physiologic alterations, pharmacologic agents, or disease (see chaps 7, 14, and 18).

References

1. Benvenga S, Trimarchi F, Robbins J. Circulating thyroid hormone autoantibodies. J Endocrinol Invest 1987;10:605
2. Bartalena L, Robbins J. Variations in thyroid hormone transport proteins and their clinical implications. Thyroid 1992;2:237
3. Bartalena L, Robbins J. Thyroid hormone transport proteins. Clin Lab Med 1993;13:583
4. Refetoff S, Larsen R. Transport, cellular uptake and metabolism of thyroid hormone. In: DeGroot LJ, ed. Endocrinology. 2nd ed, vol I. Philadelphia: WB Saunders, 1989:541
5. Refetoff S, Robin NI, Fang VS. Parameters of thyroid function in serum of 16 selected vertebrate species. Endocrinology 1970; 86:793
6. Robbins J, Bartalena L. Plasma transport of thyroid hormones. In: Hennemann G, ed. Thyroid hormone metabolism. New York: Marcel Dekker, 1986:3
7. Licht P. Thyroxine-binding protein represents the major vitamin D-binding protein in the plasma of the turtle, *Trachemys scripta*. Gen Comp Endocrinol 1994;93:82
8. Licht P, Moore MF. Structure of a reptilian plasma thyroxine binding protein indicates homology to vitamin D-binding protein. Arch Biochem Biophys 1994;309:47
9. Babin PJ. Binding of thyroxine and 3,5,3'-triiodothyronine to trout plasma lipoproteins. Am J Physiol 1992;262:E712
10. Richardson SJ, Bradley AJ, Duan W, et al. Evolution of marsupial and other vertebrate thyroxine-binding plasma proteins. Am J Physiol 1994;35:R1359
11. Gordon AH, Gross J, O'Connor D, Pitt-Rivers R. Nature of the circulating thyroid hormone–plasma protein complex. Nature 1952;169:19
12. Ingbar SH. Prealbumin: a thyroxine-binding protein of human plasma. Endocrinology 1958;63:256
13. Robbins J, Rall JE. Proteins associated with the thyroid hormones. Physiol Rev 1960;40:415
14. Robbins J, Cheng S-Y, Gershengorn MC, Glinoer D, Cahnmann HJ, Edelhoch H. Thyroxine transport proteins of plasma: molecular properties and biosynthesis. Recent Prog Horm Res 1978; 34:477
15. Goodman DS. Plasma retinol-binding protein. In: Sporn MB, Roberts AB, Goodman DS, eds. The retinoids. New York: Academic Press, 1984:41
16. Peters JT. Serum albumin. Adv Protein Chem 1985;37:161
17. Refetoff S. Inherited thyroxine-binding globulin abnormalities in man. Endocr Rev 1989;10:275
18. Bartalena L. Recent achievements in studies on thyroid-hormone binding proteins. Endocr Rev 1990;11:47
19. Albers JJ, Segrest JP. Plasma lipoproteins: Part B. characterization, cell biology and metabolism. Methods Enzymol 1986;129

20. Segrest JP, Albers JJ. Plasma lipoproteins: A. preparation, structure and molecular biology. Methods Enzymol 1986;128

21. Benvenga S, Gregg RE, Robbins J. Binding of thyroid hormones to human plasma lipoproteins. J Clin Endocrinol Metab 1988;67:6

22. Blake CCF, Geisow MJ, Swan IDA. Structure of human plasma prealbumin at 2.5A resolution: a preliminary report on the polypeptide chain conformation quaternary structure and thyroxine binding. J Mol Biol 1974;88:1

23. Blake CCF, Oatley SJ. Protein–DNA and protein–hormone interactions in prealbumin: a model of the thyroid hormone nuclear receptor? Nature 1977;268:115

24. Blake CCF, Geisow MJ, Oatley SJ, Rerat B, Rerat C. Structure of prealbumin: secondary, tertiary and quaternary interactions determined by Fourier refinement at 1.8A. J Mol Biol 1978; 121:339

25. Blake CCF, Burridge JM, Oatley SJ. Binding interactions with TBPA. In: Cumming TA, Funder JW, Mendelsohn FAO, eds. Endocrinology 1980. Canberra, Australia: Australian Academy of Science, 1980:417

26. Branch WT Jr, Robbins J, Edelhoch H. Thyroxine-binding prealbumin: conformation in aqueous solutions. J Biol Chem 1971; 246:6011

27. Branch WT, Robbins J, Edelhoch H. Thyroxine-binding prealbumin: conformation in urea and guanidine. Arch Biochem Biophys 1972;152:144

28. Rask L, Peterson PA, Nilsson SF. Subunit structure of human thyroxine-binding prealbumin. J Biol Chem 1971;251:6087

29. Raz A, Shiratori T, Goodman DS. Studies on the protein–protein and protein–ligand interactions involved in retinol transport in plasma. J Biol Chem 1970;245:1903

30. Gershengorn MC, Lippoldt RE, Edelhoch H, Robbins J. Structure and stability of human thyroxine-binding globulin. J Biol Chem 1977;252:8719

31. Johnson ML, Lippoldt RE, Gershengorn MC, Robbins J, Edelhoch H. Molecular transitions of human thyroxine-binding globulin. Arch Biochem Biophys 1980;200:288

32. Grimaldi S, Edelhoch H, Robbins J. Effects of thyroxine binding on the stability, conformation and fluorescence properties of thyroxine-binding globulin. Biochemistry 1982;21:145

33. Kanda Y, Goodman DH, Canfield RE, Morgan FJ. The amino acid sequence of human plasma prealbumin. J Biol Chem 1974; 249:6796

34. Brown JR, Shockley P, Behrens PQ. Albumin: sequence, evolution and structural models. In: Bing DH, ed. The chemistry and physiology of the human plasma proteins. New York: Pergamon Press, 1979:23

35. Flink IL, Bailey TJ, Gustefson A, Markham BE, Morkin E. Complete amino acid sequence of human thyroxine-binding globulin deduced from cloned DNA: close homology to the serine antiproteases. Proc Natl Acad Sci USA 1986;83:7708

36. Carrell RW, Pemberton PA, Boswell DR. The serpins: evolution and adaptation in a family of protease inhibitors. Cold Spring Harbor Symp Quant Biol 1987;52:527

37. Hammond GL, Smith CL, Goping IS, et al. Primary structure of human corticosteroid binding globulin deduced from hepatic and pulmonary cDNAs, exhibits homology with serine protease inhibitors. Proc Natl Acad Sci USA 1987;84:5153

38. Pemberton PA, Stein PE, Pepya MB, Potter JM, Carrell RW. Hormone binding globulins undergo serpin conformational change in inflammation. Nature 1988;336:257

39. Jarvis JA, Munro SLA, Craik DJ. Homology model of thyroxine-binding globulin and elucidation of the thyroid hormone binding site. Protein Eng 1992;5:61

40. Terry CJ, Blake CF. Comparison of the modelled thyroxine binding site in TBG with the experimentally determined site in transthyretin. Protein Eng 1992;5:505

41. Jornvall H, Carlstrom A, Pettersson T, Jacobson B, Persson M, Mutt V. Structural homologies between prealbumin, gastrointestinal prohormones and other proteins. Nature 1981;291:261

42. Cooke NE, Haddad JG. Vitamin D binding protein (Gc-globulin). Endocr Rev 1989;10:294

43. He XM, Carter DC. Atomic structure and chemistry of human serum albumin. Nature 1992;358:209

44. Dughi C, Bhagavan N, Jameson DM. Fluorescence investigations of albumin from patients with familial dysalbuminemic hyperthyroxinemia. Photochem Photobiol 1993;57:416

45. Zinn AB, Marshall JS, Carlson DM. Carbohydrate structure of thyroxine-binding globulin and their effects on hepatocyte membrane binding. J Biol Chem 1978;253:6768

46. Zinn AB, Marshall JS, Carlson DM. Preparation of glycopeptides and oligosaccharides from thyroxine-binding globulin. J Biol Chem 1978;253:6761

47. Marshall JS, Green AM, Pensky J, Williams J, Zinn A, Carlson DA. Measurement of circulating desialylated glycoprotein and correlation with hepatocellular damage. J Clin Invest 1974;54:555

48. Robbins J, Rall JE. The iodine containing hormones. In: Gray CH, James VHT, eds. Hormones in blood. 3rd ed, vol 4. London: Academic Press, 1983:219

49. Gartner R, Henze R, Horn K, Pickardt CR, Scriba PC. Thyroxine-binding globulin: investigation of microheterogeneity. J Clin Endocrinol Metab 1981;52:657

50. Grimaldi S, Bartalena L, Ramacciotti C, Robbins J. Polymorphism of human thyroxine-binding globulin. J Clin Endocrinol Metab 1983;57:1186

51. Lasne Y, Lasne F, Benzerara O. Microheterogeneity and polymorphism of human serum thyroxine-binding globulin: study by isoelectric focusing and radioprint immunofixation. Biochim Biophys Acta 1980;624:333

52. Trent JM, Flink IL, Morkin E, Van Tuinen P, Ledbetter DH. Localization of the human thyroxine binding globulin gene to the long arm of the X chromosome (Xq21–22). Am J Hum Genet 1987;41:428

53. Daiger SP, Wildin RS. Human thyroxine-binding globulin (TBG): heterogeneity within individuals and among individuals demonstrated by isoelectric focusing. Biochem Genet 1981;19:673

54. Cheng S-Y, Morrone S, Robbins J. Effect of deglycosylation on the binding and immunoreactivity of human thyroxine-binding globulin. J Biol Chem 1979;254:8830

55. Grimaldi S, Robbins J, Edelhoch H. The interaction of the carbohydrate and protein in thyroxine-binding globulin. Biochemistry 1985;24:3771

56. Hillier AP. Human thyroxine-binding globulin and thyroxine-binding prealbumin: dissociation rates. J Physiol 1971;217:625

57. Hillier AP. The rate of triiodothyronine dissociation from binding sites in human plasma. Acta Endocrinol 1975;80:49

58. Jorgensen EC. Thyroid hormones and analogs: II. Structure–activity relationships. In: Li W, ed. Hormonal proteins and peptides. Vol 6. New York: Academic Press, 1978:107

59. Cavalieri RR, Pitt-Rivers R. The effects of drugs on the distribution and metabolism of thyroid hormones. Pharmacol Rev 1981;33:55

60. Green AM, Marshall JS, Pensky J, Stanbury JB. Thyroxine-binding globulin: characterization of the binding site with a fluorescent dye as a probe. Science 1972;175:1378

61. Schussler GC. Thyroxine-binding globulin: specificity for the hormonally active conformation of triiodothyronine. Science 1972;178:172

62. Korcek L, Tabachnik M. Thyroxine–protein interactions: interaction of thyroxine and triiodothyronine with human thyroxine-binding globulin. J Biol Chem 1976;251:3558

63. Green AM, Marshall JS, Pensky J, Stanbury JB. Studies on thyroxine-binding globulin: IV. The interaction of thyroxine with thyroxine-binding globulin. Biochim Biophys Acta 1972;278:117

64. Erard F, Cheng S-Y, Robbins J. Affinity labeling of human serum thyroxine-binding globulin with N-bromoacetyl-L-thyroxine: identification of the labeled amino acid residues. Arch Biochem Biophys 1981;206:15

65. Siegel JS, Korcek L, Tabachnik M. Evaluation of N-bromoacetyl-L-thyroxine as an affinity label for the thyroxine (T_4)-binding site in human T_4-binding globulin. Endocrinology 1983;113:2173

66. Siegel JS, Korcek L, Tabachnik M. Modification of thyroxine-binding globulin with p-iodo-phenylsulfonyl (pipsyl) chloride and effect on thyroxine binding activity. FEBS Lett 1979; 102: 306

67. Tabachnik M, Perret V. Specific labeling of the thyroxine binding site in thyroxine-binding globulin. Biochem Int 1987;15:409

68. Cheng S-Y, Rakhit G, Erard F, Robbins J, Chignell CF. A spin label study of the thyroid hormone-binding sites in human plasma thyroxine transport proteins. J Biol Chem 1981;256:831

69. Tabachnik M, Hao YL, Korcek L. Effect of peptide derivatives of thyroxine on the binding of ^{125}I-thyroxine to purified human thyroxine-binding globulin. Endocrinology 1971;89:606

70. Nilsson SF, Peterson PA. Evidence for multiple thyroxine binding sites in human prealbumin. J Biol Chem 1971;246:6098

71. Pages RA, Robbins J, Edelhoch H. Binding of thyroxine and thyroxine analogues to human serum prealbumin. Biochemistry 1973;12:2773

72. Cheng S-Y, Pages RA, Saroff HA, Edelhoch H, Robbins J. Analysis of thyroid hormone binding to human serum prealbumin by 8-anilinonaphthalene-1-sulfonate fluorescence. Biochemistry 1977;16:3707

73. Irace G, Edelhoch H. Thyroxine-induced conformation changes in prealbumin. Biochemistry 1978;17:5729

74. Reid DG, MacLachlan LK, Voyle M, Leeson PD. A proton and fluorine-19 nuclear magnetic resonance and fluorescence study of the binding of some natural and synthetic thyromimetics to prealbumin (transthyretin). J Biol Chem 1989;264:2013

75. Robbins J, Rall JE. The iodine containing hormones. In: Gray CH, James VHT, eds. Hormones in blood. 3rd ed. Vol 1. London: Academic Press, 1979:576

76. Robbins J, Johnson ML. Theoretical considerations in the transport of the thyroid hormones in blood. In: Ekins R, Faglia G, Pennisi F, Pinchera A, eds. Free thyroid hormones. Amsterdam: Excerpta Medica, 1979:1

77. Soprano DR, Blaner WS. Plasma retinol binding protein. In: Sporn MB, Roberts AB, Goodman DS, eds. The retinoids. 2nd ed. New York: Raven Press, 1994:257

78. Noy N, Slosberg E, Scarlata S. Interactions of retinol with binding proteins: studies with retinol-binding protein and with transthyretin. Biochemistry 1992;31:11118

79. Zanotti G, Malpeli G, Berne R. The interaction of N-ethyl retinamide with plasma retinol-binding protein (RBP) and the crystal structure of the retinoid-RBP complex at 1.9-Å resolution. J Biol Chem 1993;268:24873

80. Sivaprasadarao A, Findlay JBC. Structure-function studies of human retinol-binding protein using site-directed mutagenesis. Biochem J 1994;300:437

80a. Monaco HL, Rizzi M, Coda A. Structure of a complex of two plasma proteins: transthyrotin and retinol binding protein. Science 1995;268:1039

81. Andrea TA, Cavalieri RR, Goldfine ID, Jorgensen EC. Binding of thyroid hormones and analogues to the human plasma protein prealbumin. Biochemistry 1980;19:55

82. Somack R, Andrea TA, Jorgensen EC. Thyroid hormone binding to human serum prealbumin and rat nuclear receptor: kinetics, contribution of the hormone phenolic hydroxyl group and accommodation of hormone side chain bulk. Biochemistry 1982;21:163

83. Cody V. Thyroid hormone interactions: molecular conformation, protein binding and hormone action. Endocr Rev 1980;1:140

84. Ciszak E, Cody V, Luft JR. Crystal structure determination at 2.3-Å resolution of human transthyretin-3′,5′-dibromo-2′,4,4′,6-tetrahydroxyaurone complex. Proc Natl Acad Sci USA 1992; 89:6644

85. Pardridge WM. Transport of protein-bound hormones into tissues in vivo. Endocr Rev 1981;2:103

86. Robbins J, Rall JE. The iodine containing hormones. In: Gray CH, Bacharach AL, eds. Hormones in blood. 2nd ed. London: Academic Press, 1967:383

87. Loun B, Hage DS. Characterization of thyroxine–albumin binding using high performance affinity chromatography. J Chromatogr 1992;579:225

88. Benvenga S, Cahnmann HJ, Gregg RE, Robbins J. Characterization of the binding of thyroxine to high density lipoproteins and apolipoprotein A-I. J Clin Endocrinol Metab 1989;68:1067

89. Benvenga S, Robbins J. Lipoprotein–thyroid hormone interactions. Trends Endocrinol Metab 1993;4:194

90. Benvenga S, Cahnmann HJ, Rader D, et al. Thyroid hormone binding to isolated human apolipoproteins A-II, C-I, C-II and C-III: homology in thyroxine binding sites. Thyroid 1994; 4:261

91. Benvenga S, Cahnmann HJ, Robbins J. The thyroxine-binding site of human apolipoprotein A-I: location in the N-terminal domain. Endocrinology 1991;128:547

92. Benvenga S, Cahnmann HJ, Robbins J. Localization of the thyroxine binding sites in apolipoprotein B-100 of human low-density lipoproteins. Endocrinology 1990;127:2241

93. Mori Y, Refetoff S, Flink I, et al. Detection of the thyroxine-binding globulin (TBG) gene in six unrelated families with complete TBG deficiency. J Clin Endocrinol Metab 1988;67:727

94. Janssen OE, Bertenshaw R, Takeda K, Weir R, Refetoff S. Molecular basis of inherited thyroxine-binding globulin defects. Trends Endocrinol Metab 1992;3:49

95. Hayashi Y, Mori Y, Janssen OE, et al. Human thyroxine-binding globulin gene: complete sequence and transcription regulation. Mol Endocrinol 1993;7:1049

96. Akbari MT, Kapadi A, Farmer MJ, et al. The structure of the human thyroxine binding globulin (TBG) gene. Biochim Biophys Acta 1993;1216:446

97. Kambi F, Seo H, Murata Y, Matsui N. Cloning of a complementary deoxyribonucleic acid coding for human thyroxine-binding globulin (TBG): existence of two TBG messenger ribonucleic acid species possessing different 3′-untranslated regions. Mol Endocrinol 1988;2:181

98. Refetoff S, Robin NI, Alper CA. Study of 4 new kindreds with inherited TBG abnormalities: possible mutations of a single gene locus. J Clin Invest 1972;51:848

99. Robbins J. Inherited variations in thyroxine transport. Mt Sinai J Med (NY) 1973;40:511

100. Kambi F, Seo H, Mori Y, et al. An additional carbohydrate chain in the variant thyroxine-binding globulin-Gary (TBG^{Asn-96}) impairs its secretion. Mol Endocrinol 1992;6:443

101. Janssen OE, Refetoff S. In vitro expression of thyroxine-binding globulin (TBG) variants. J Biol Chem 1992;267:13998

102. Miura Y, Kambe P, Yamamori I, et al. A truncated thyroxine-binding globulin due to a frameshift mutation is retained within the rough endoplasmic reticulum: a possible mechanism of complete thyroxine-binding globulin deficiency in Japanese. J Clin Endocrinol Metab 1994;78:283

103. Mandel S, Hanna S, Boston B, et al. Thyroxine-binding globulin deficiency detected by newborn screening. J Pediatr 1993; 122:227

103a. Mori Y, Miura Y, Takeuchi, H, et al. Gene amplification as a cause for inherited thyroxine-binding excess in two Japanese families. J Clin Endocrinol Metab 1995;80:3758

103b. Robbins J. Gene amplification as a cause for inherited thyroxine-binding globulin excess. J Clin Endocrinol Metab 1995;80:3425

104. Sasaki H, Yoshioka N, Takagi Y, Sakaki Y. Structure of the chromosomal gene for human serum prealbumin. Gene 1985; 37:191

105. Tsuzuki T, Mita S, Maeda S, et al. Structure of the human prealbumin gene. J Biol Chem 1985;260:12224

106. Wallace MR, Naylor SL, Kluve-Beckerman B, et al. Localization of the human prealbumin gene to chromosome 18. Biochem Biophys Res Commun 1985;129:753

107. Wakasugi S, Maeda S, Shimada K. Structure and expression of the mouse prealbumin gene. J Biochem 1986;100:49

108. Fung W-P, Thomas T, Dickson PW, et al. Structure and expression of the rat transthyretin (prealbumin) gene. J Biol Chem 1988;263:480

109. Moses AC, Rosen HN, Moller DE, et al. A point mutation in transthyretin increases affinity for thyroxine and produces euthyroid hyperthyroxinemia. J Clin Invest 1990;86:2025

110. Alves IL, Divino CM, Schussler GC, et al. Thyroxine-binding in a TTR Met 119 kindred. J Clin Endocrinol Metab 1993;76:484

111. Rosen HN, Moses AC, Murrell JR, et al. Thyroxine interactions with transthyretin: a comparison of 10 different naturally occurring human transthyretin variants. J Clin Endocrinol Metab 1993; 77:370

112. Steinrauf LK, Hamilton JA, Braden BC, et al. X-ray crystal structure of the Ala 109 → Thr variant of human transthyretin which produces euthyroid hyper-thyroxinemia. J Biol Chem 1993; 268:2425

113. Murrell JR, Schoner RG, Liepnieks JJ, et al. Production and functional analysis of normal and variant recombinant human transthyretin proteins. J Biol Chem 1992;267:16595

114. Hamilton JA, Steinrauf LK, Braden BC, et al. The x-ray crystal structure refinements of normal human transthyretin and the amiloidogenic Val-30 → Met variant to 1.7-Å resolution. J Biol Chem 1993;268:2416

115. Berni R, Malpeli G, Folli C, et al. The Ile 84 → Ser amino acid substitution in transthyretin interferes with the interaction with plasma retinol-binding protein. J Biol Chem 1994; 269:23395

116. Rosen HN, Murrell JR, Liepnieks JJ, et al. Threonine for alanine substitution at position 109 of transthyretin differentially alters human transthyretin's affinity for iodothyronines. Endocrinology 1994;134:27

117. Curtis AJ, Scrimshaw BJ, Topliss DJ, et al. Thyroxine-binding by human transthyretin variants: mutations at position 119, but not position 54, increase thyroxine binding affinity. J Clin Endocrinol Metab 1994;78:459

118. Fitch NJS, Akbari MT, Ramsden DB. An inherited non-amyloidogenic transthyretin variant, [Ser⁶]-TTR, with increased thyroxine-binding affinity characterized by DNA sequencing. J Endocrinol 1991;129:309

119. Sunthornthepvarakul T, Angkeow P, Weiss RE, et al. An identical missense mutation in the albumin gene results in familial dysalbuminemic hyperthyroxinemia in 8 unrelated families. Biochem Biophys Res Commun 1994;202:781

120. Petersen CE, Scottolini AG, Cody LR, et al. A point mutation in the human serum albumin gene results in familial dysalbuminemic hyperthyroxinemia. J Med Genet 1994;31:355

121. Jacobsson B, Collins VP, Grimelius L, et al. Transthyretin immunoreactivity in human and porcine liver, choroid plexus and pancreatic islets. J Histochem Cytochem 1989;37:31

122. Jacobsson B, Carlstrom A, Platz A, Collins VP. Transthyretin messenger ribonucleic acid expression in the pancreas and in endocrine tumors of the pancreas and gut. J Clin Endocrinol Metab 1990;71:875

123. Soprano DR, Herbert J, Soprano KJ, Schon EA, Goodman DS. Demonstration of transthyretin mRNA in the brain and other extrahepatic tissues in the rat. J Biol Chem 1985;260:11793

124. Dickson PW, Aldred AR, Marley PD, Bannister D, Schreiber G. Rat choroid plexus specializes in the synthesis and the secretion of transthyretin (prealbumin). J Biol Chem 1986;261:3475

125. Dickson PW, Schreiber G. High levels of messenger RNA for transthyretin (prealbumin) in human choroid plexus. Neurosci Lett 1986;66:311

126. Robbins J, Goncalves E, Lakshmanan M, Foti D. Thyroid hormone transport from blood to brain. In: DeLong GR, Robbins J, Condliffe P, eds. Iodine and the brain. New York: Plenum Press, 1989:39

127. Bartalena L, Tata JR, Robbins J. Characterization of nascent and secreted thyroxine-binding globulin in cultured human hepatoma (HepG2) cells. J Biol Chem 1984;259:13605

128. Mita S, Maeda S, Shimada K, Araki S. Cloning and sequence analysis of cDNA for human prealbumin. Biochem Biophys Res Commun 1984;124:558

129. Sasaki H, Sasaki Y, Matsuo H et al. Diagnosis of familial amyloidotic polyneuropathy by recombinant DNA techniques. Biochem Biophys Res Commun 1984;125:636

130. Bartalena L, Robbins J. Effect of tunicamycin and monensin on secretion of thyroxine binding globulin by cultured human hepatoma (HepG2) cells. J Biol Chem 1984;259:13610

131. Murata Y, Magner JA, Refetoff S. The role of glycosylation in the molecular conformation and secretion of thyroxine-binding globulin. Endocrinology 1986;118:1614

132. Murata Y, Sarne D, Horwitz AL, et al. Characterization of thyroxine-binding globulin (TBG) synthesis in a human hepatoma cell line. J Clin Endocrinol Metab 1985;60:472

133. Navab M, Smith JE, Goodman DS. Rat plasma prealbumin: metabolic studies on effects of vitamin A status and on tissue distribution. J Biol Chem 1977;252:5107

134. Smith JE, Borek C, Goodman DS. Regulation of retinol binding protein metabolism in cultured rat liver cell lines. Cell 1978; 15:865

135. Smith JE, Goodman DS. Retinol-binding protein and the regulation of vitamin A transport. Fed Proc 1979;38:2504

136. Soprano DR, Smith JE, Goodman DS. Effect of retinol status on retinol binding protein biosynthesis rate and translatable mRNA level in rat liver. J Biol Chem 1982;257:7693

137. Kanai M, Raz A, Goodman DS. Retinol binding protein: the transport protein for vitamin A in human plasma. J Clin Invest 1968;47:2025

138. Ingenbleek Y, Van Den Schrieck HG, De Nayer P, De Visscher M. Albumin, transferrin and the thyroxine-binding prealbumin/retinol-binding protein (TBPA-RBP) complex in assessment of malnutrition. Clin Chim Acta 1975;63:61

139. Refetoff S, Fang VS, Marshall JS. Studies on human thyroxine binding globulin (TBG): IX. Some physical, chemical and biological properties of radioiodinated TBG and partially desialylated TBG. J Clin Invest 1975;56:177

140. Ain KB, Mori Y, Refetoff S. Reduced clearance rate of thyroxine-binding globulin (TBG) with increased sialylation: a mechanism for estrogen-induced elevation of serum TBG concentration. J Clin Endocrinol Metab 1987;65:689

141. McGuire RA, Glinoer D, Albert MA, Robbins J. Comparative effects of thyroxine (T₄) and triiodothyronine on T₄-binding globulin metabolism in rhesus monkeys. Endocrinology 1982; 110:1340

142. Glinoer D, McGuire RA, Dubois A, Cogan JP, Robbins J, Berman M. Thyroxine binding globulin metabolism in rhesus monkeys: effects of hyper- and hypothyroidism. Endocrinology 1979; 104:175

143. Kobayashi M, Horiuchi R, Hachisu T, Takikawa H. Dualistic effects of thyroid hormone on a human hepatoma cell line: inhibition of thyroxine-binding globulin synthesis and stimulation of α₁-acid glycoprotein synthesis. Endocrinology 1988;123:631

143a. Crowe TC, Cowen NL, Loidl NM, Topliss DJ, Stockigt JR, Barlow JW. Down-regulation of thyroxine-binding globulin messenger ribonucleic acid by 3,5,3'-triiodothyronine in human hepatoblastoma cells. J Clin Endocrinol Metab 1995;80:2233

144. Gershengorn MC, Glinoer D, Robbins J. Transport and metabolism of thyroid hormones. In: De Visscher M, ed. The thyroid gland. New York: Raven Press, 1980:81

145. Emerson CH, Seiler CM, Alex S, et al. Gene expression and serum thyroxine-binding globulin are regulated by adrenal status and corticosterone in the rat. Endocrinology 1993;133:1192

146. Tani Y, Mori Y, Miura Y, et al. Molecular cloning of the rat thyroxine-binding globulin gene and analysis of its promoter activity. Endocrinology 1994;135:2731

147. Imamura S, Mori Y, Murata Y, et al. Molecular cloning and primary structure of rat thyroxine-binding globulin. Biochemistry 1991;30:5406

148. Bartalena L, Farsetti A, Flink IL, Robbins J. Effects of interleukin-6 on the expression of thyroid hormone-binding protein genes in cultured human hepatoblastoma-derived (HepG2) cells. Mol Endocrinol 1992;6:935

149. Bartalena L, Hammond GL, Farsetti A, et al. Interleukin-6 inhibits corticosteroid-binding globulin synthesis by human hepatoblastoma-derived (HepG2) cells. Endocrinology 1993;133:291

150. Episkopou V, Maeda S, Nishiguchi S, et al. Disruption of the transthyretin gene results in mice with depressed levels of plasma retinol and thyroid hormone. Proc Natl Acad Sci USA 1993;90:2375

151. Bernstein RS, Robbins J, Rall JE. Polymorphism of monkey thyroxine-binding prealbumin (TBPA): mode of inheritance and hybridization. Endocrinology 1970;86:383

152. Mendel CM, Cavalieri R. Transport of thyroid hormones in health and disease: recent controversy surrounding the free hormone hypothesis. Thyroid Today 1988;11:3

153. Mendel CM. The free hormone hypothesis: a physiologically based mathematical model. Endocr Rev 1989;10:232

154. Mendel CM, Cavalieri RR, Kohrle J. Thyroxine (T$_4$) transport and distribution in rats treated with EMD21388, a synthetic flavonoid that displaces T$_4$ from transthyretin. Endocrinology 1992; 130:1525

155. Mendel CM, Cavalieri RR, Weisiger RA. Uptake of thyroxine by the perfused rat liver: implications for the free hormone hypothesis. Endocrinology 1988;123:1817

156. Sarne D, Barokas K, Scherberg N, Refetoff S. Elevated serum thyroglobulin level in congenital thyroxine-binding deficiency. J Clin Endocrinol Metab 1983;57:665

157. DiStefano JJ, Fisher DA. Peripheral distribution and metabolism of thyroid hormones: a primarily quantitative assessment. In: Hershman JM, Bray GA, eds. The thyroid: physiology and treatment of disease. Oxford: Pergamon Press, 1979:47

158. Pardridge WM. Plasma protein-mediated transport of steroid and thyroid hormones. Am J Physiol 1987;252:E157

159. Ekins RP, Edwards PR. Plasma protein mediated transport of steroid and thyroid hormones: a critique. Am J Physiol 1988; 255:E403

160. Mendel CM, Cavalieri RA, Weisiger RA. On plasma-protein mediated transport of steroid and thyroid hormones. Am J Physiol 1988;255:E221

161. Robbins J, Johnson ML. Possible significance of multiple transport proteins for the thyroid hormones. In: Albertini A, Ekins RP, eds. Free hormones in blood. Venice: Elsevier Biomedical Press, 1982:53

162. Hashizume K, Sakurai A, Hiyamoto T, Yamauchi K, Nishii Y. Effect of thyroxine-binding globulin (TBG) on thyroxine (T$_4$) uptake by human peripheral mononuclear cells: evidence of TBG-dependent uptake of T$_4$. Endocrinol Jpn 1986;33:665

163. Azimova SS, Umarova OD, Petrova OS, Tukhtaev KR, Abdukarimov A. Nature of thyroid hormone receptors: translocation of thyroid hormones across plasma membrane. Biokhimya 1984; 49:1350

164. Divino CM, Schussler GC. Receptor-mediated uptake and internalization of transthyretin. J Biol Chem 1990;265:1425

165. Divino CM, Schussler GC. Transthyretin receptors on human astrocytoma cells. J Clin Endocrinol Metab 1990;71:1265

166. Benvenga S, Robbins J. Enhancement of thyroxine entry into low density lipoprotein (LDL) receptor-competent fibroblasts by LDL: an additional mode of entry of thyroxine into cells. Endocrinology 1990;126:933

167. Pontecorvi A, Robbins J. The plasma membrane and thyroid hormone entry into cells. Trends Endocrinol Metab 1989;1:90

168. Robbins J, Lakshmanan M. The movement of thyroid hormones in the central nervous system. Acta Med Austriaca 1992;19:21

169. Schreiber G, Aldred AR, Duan W. Choroid plexus, brain, protein-homeostasis and evolution. Today's Life Science 1992;September:22

170. Dickson PW, Aldred AR, Mentiny JGT, Marley PD, Sawyer WH, Schreiber G. Thyroxine transport in choroid plexus. J Biol Chem 1987;262:13907

171. Southwell BR, Duan W, Alcorn D, et al. Thyroxine transport to the brain: role of protein synthesis by the choroid plexus. Endocrinology 1993;133:2116

172. Chanoine JP, Alex S, Fang SL, et al. Role of transthyretin in the transport of thyroxine from the blood to the choroid plexus, the cerebrospinal fluid, and the brain. Endocrinology 1992; 130:933

173. Dratman MB, Crutchfield FL, Schoenhoff MB. Transport of iodothyronines from bloodstream to brain: contributions by blood: brain and choroid plexus: cerebrospinal fluid barriers. Brain Res 1991;554:229

174. Blay P, Nilsson C, Owman C, Aldred A, Schreiber G. Transthyretin expression in the rat brain: effect of thyroid functional state and role in thyroxine transport. Brain Res 1993; 632:114

175. Hocman G. Human thyroxine-binding globulin (TBG). Rev Physiol Biochem Pharmacol 1981;91:45

176. Robbins J. Thyroxine-binding proteins. In: Jamieson GA, Greenwalt TJ, eds. Trace components of plasma: isolation and clinical significance. New York: Alan R. Liss, 1976:331

177. Steiner RF, Edelhoch H. Fluorescent protein conjugates. Chem Rev 1962;62:457

178. Snyder SM, Cavalieri RR, Goldfine ID, Ingbar SH, Jorgensen EC. Binding of thyroid hormones and their analogues to thyroxine-binding globulin in human serum. J Biol Chem 1976; 251:6489

179. Tabachnik M, Giorgio NA. Thyroxine–protein interactions: II. The binding of thyroxine and its analogues to human serum albumin. Arch Biochem Biophys 1964;105:563

180. Cavalieri RR. Preparation of ^{125}I-labeled thyroxine-binding alpha-globulin and its turnover in normal and hypothyroid subjects. J Clin Invest 1975;56:79

181. Oppenheimer JH, Surks MI, Bernstein G, Smith JC. Metabolism of I131-labeled thyroxine-binding prealbumin in man. Science 1965;149:748

182. Refetoff S, Fang VS, Marshall JS, Robin NJ. Metabolism of thyroxine-binding globulin in man: abnormal rate of synthesis in inherited thyroxine-binding deficiency and excess. J Clin Invest 1976;57:485

183. Vahlquist AP, Peterson A, Wibell L. Metabolism of vitamin A transporting protein complex: I. Turnover studies in normal persons and in patients with chronic renal failure. Eur J Clin Invest 1973;3:352

Werner and Ingbar's The Thyroid, Seventh Edition,
edited by Lewis E. Braverman and Robert D. Utiger.
Lippincott–Raven Publishers, Philadelphia, © 1996

7

Nature, Source, and Relative Significance of Circulating Thyroid Hormones

Inder J. Chopra

In normal humans, the blood contains a variety of iodinated substances. They are present either as a result of their direct secretion from the thyroid, as products of the peripheral metabolism of the thyroid hormones, or both. The thyroid gland releases into the blood, in normal or abnormal circumstances, iodothyronines, iodotyrosines, iodoproteins such as thyroglobulin and iodoalbumin, and a small amount of inorganic iodide. Many of these substances also are formed in peripheral tissues, largely from thyroid precursors.

Of the various iodinated substances discussed in this chapter, only thyroxine (T_4) and 3,5,3'triiodothyronine (T_3) have traditionally been thought to have significant biologic activity. Whether T_4 has biologic activity has been questioned. Knowledge that a sizable fraction of T_4 is converted to T_3 in the peripheral tissues, together with the known greater biologic potency of T_3, has suggested that T_4 may be a prohormone that acts only after conversion to T_3. Data pertaining to this issue, as well as the significance of an alternate pathway of peripheral T_4 metabolism that leads to the formation of 3,3',5'-triiodothyronine (reverse T_3, rT_3), are discussed in the following section.

IODINATED SUBSTANCES WITH NO APPARENT BIOLOGIC ACTIVITY

Iodotyrosines

Monoiodotyrosine and diiodotyrosine (DIT) have long been known to be the major iodinated constituents of thyroglobulin (see chap 4). It was considered unlikely that they would be present in normal human serum, and early suggestions that they might be were disputed for several reasons. First, the thyroid

gland contains an iodotyrosine deiodinase that is believed to cause rapid and nearly complete deiodination of any free iodotyrosines within the gland before they can be released. Second, iodotyrosines are only weakly bound by serum proteins and should, therefore, be rapidly cleared by peripheral tissues. Finally, peripheral tissues contain a deiodinase similar to that present in the thyroid that is capable of rapidly deiodinating iodotyrosines.[1] In normal subjects, radioiodinated iodotyrosines disappear rapidly from the circulation after their intravenous administration, and all but a minute fraction of the radioactivity is soon excreted in the urine as iodide. The metabolic clearance rate of DIT in normal humans is about 79 to 153 L/d (mean, 122 L/d), and about 5% of the daily DIT production is excreted unchanged in urine.[2] In patients with one form of congenital goitrous cretinism, the iodotyrosine deiodinase activity in the thyroid or peripheral tissues is deficient or absent. When such patients are given either radioiodide or radioiodine-labeled iodotyrosines, the bulk of the radioactivity in serum or urine is in the form of iodotyrosines or their derivatives.[3–5] From 10% to 30% of the total organic iodine in normal serum is contained in iodotyrosines,[6–8] most covalently bound in albumin.[9,10] The concentration of noncovalently bound monoiodotyrosine when measured by radioimmunoassay in organic solvent extracts of serum approximated 250 ng/dL.[11] The normal serum DIT concentration is only about 7 to 9 ng/dL.[2,12] It is about 3-fold greater in hyperthyroidism, 1.5-fold greater in umbilical cord serum at birth, and lower in hypothyroidism and pregnancy. Low serum DIT levels are found in athyrotic patients receiving T_4 therapy, suggesting that little is formed from peripheral metabolism of T_4.[2] Furthermore, serum DIT levels are considerably higher in thyroid venous serum than in arterial serum. Some is detectable in serum from athyrotic patients, suggesting that there is some extrathyroidal production. The source may be de novo synthesis in extrathyroidal tissues, ether-link cleavage of iodothyronines in extrathyroidal tissues,[13] or catabolism of iodinated proteins in food. There is evidence that the ether-link cleavage of T_4 (or T_3) to DIT is markedly enhanced in bacterial sepsis.[14] The daily production rate of DIT in normal humans is about 10 μg/d (24 nmol/d).[2]

Iodoproteins

Serum contains iodine covalently bound to circulating proteins. The concentration of iodine in such iodoproteins usually has been measured by determining the difference between protein-bound iodine and butanol-extractable iodine or T_4 iodine concentrations.[15] The concentration of iodine in this form normally does not exceed 1.5 μg/dL. Higher values are found in the serum of patients with Hashimoto's thyroiditis, Graves' disease, thyroid cancer, and certain forms of congenital goiter.[5,15]

One iodoprotein of thyroid origin—thyroglobulin—can be measured in serum as such.[16–18] Thyroglobulin concentrations in normal serum were found to range from undetectable to 20 or 150 ng/mL in the initial studies,[17,19] but now the upper limit of the normal range is about 50 ng/mL in most laboratories. Serum thyroglobulin levels are somewhat higher in pregnant women and newborn infants,[19] and substantial elevations are characteristically found in patients with hyperthyroidism caused by Graves' disease, subacute thyroiditis, and metastatic thyroid carcinoma.[20] Serum thyroglobulin levels increase significantly in normal subjects after injection of thyroid-stimulating hormone (TSH; thyrotropin) or thyrotropin-releasing hormone,[18] and decrease when thyroid function is suppressed by administration of T_3.

The mechanism by which thyroglobulin reaches the circulation is unclear. High concentrations have been found in the lymph draining the thyroid, suggesting that thyroglobulin may leave the thyroid mainly by way of the lymphatics.[21,22] Alternatively, the high lymphatic fluid concentrations of thyroglobulin may reflect slower lymphatic fluid than venous blood flow. Chapters 4 and 5 provide a more extensive discussion of thyroglobulin physiology.

Besides thyroglobulin, iodinated albumin and iodinated polypeptides may be present in the serum. These substances are particularly likely to be found in the serum of patients with some types of goitrous cretinism, particularly those characterized by abnormal thyroglobulin synthesis, and patients with hyperthyroidism, chronic thyroiditis, or thyroid cancer.[5,23,24] That these substances originate in the thyroid is suggested by the finding of similar substances within the gland and by the demonstration that the thyroid is capable of synthesizing similar substances in vitro.[25,26] In both humans and rats, small amounts of iodoproteins also originate in peripheral tissues in the course of the metabolism of T_3 and T_4.[27–29] The electrophoretic characteristics and the kinetics of metabolism of the iodoprotein formed in this way in humans are similar to those of serum albumin.[27]

IODINATED SUBSTANCES WITH DEMONSTRABLE BIOLOGIC EFFECTS

Thyroxine

Thyroxine normally is the most abundant iodothyronine in thyroglobulin, being about 10 to 20 times more abundant than T_3, 20 to 100 times more abundant than rT_3,[30–34] 16 to 4500 times more abundant than thyronine (T_0),[35] and more than 1000 times more abundant than any other T_4 derivatives.[36–38] The serum concentrations and daily production rates of T_4 also are much greater than those of any other iodothyronine (Table 7-1). Iodine constitutes about 65% by weight of the T_4 molecule, and the iodine in T_4 normally constitutes about 30% to 40% of the iodine in thyroglobulin. The identification of T_4 in serum came from the studies of Taurog and coworkers,[39] who added radioactive T_4 to serum, extracted T_4 from serum, and recrystallized it to constant specific activity; subsequent studies indicated that T_4 accounts for up to 90% of the protein-bound iodine in serum.[40,41] The thyroid gland is the only known source of T_4 in the body.

In serum, T_4 is bound to three proteins, which are, in order of their affinity for T_4, thyroxine-binding globulin (TBG), thyroxine-binding prealbumin, and albumin.[42–47] The extent of overall binding is great, so that the serum free T_4 concentration is less than 0.1% of the total T_4 concentration. The physicochemical characteristics of these interactions and their profound effects on the physical state, concentration, and peripheral metabolism of T_4 in health and disease are discussed in chapters 6 and 8.

3,5,3′-Triiodothyronine

Triiodothyronine was first demonstrated in human serum in 1951,[48] after its discovery in the thyroid gland, and was soon found to be several times more potent than T_4 in producing the classic effects of thyroid hormone.[49–51] Like T_4, the key questions concerning T_3 have been as follows: what is the source of the T_3 present in serum, and to what extent does T_3 contribute to the overall action of thyroid hormone? Much of the remainder of this chapter is devoted to a discussion of these and related topics.

Like T_4, T_3 in the circulation is largely (> 99.5%) bound to TBG, thyroxine-binding prealbumin, and albumin, but its affinity for these proteins is less than that of T_4. The transport and peripheral metabolism of T_3 are discussed in chapters 6 and 8, and the clinical value of serum T_3 measurements in chapter 18. Techniques for measuring serum T_3 concentrations and the metabolic clearance rate of T_3 are briefly discussed here, because the results of these measurements can greatly influence the calculations that bear heavily on questions germane to this chapter: the rate of production of T_3, the fraction of T_3 production derived from the peripheral deiodination of T_4, and the relative contributions of T_3 and T_4 to the overall action of thyroid hormone.

The initial approaches to measurement of serum T_3 involved extraction of iodothyronines by various solvents, followed by separation of T_4 from T_3 by chromatography and subsequent quantitation of T_3 by either gas chromatography or competitive protein binding assay. The values for the mean serum T_3 concentration in normal subjects provided by these methods varied between 220 and 450 ng/dL.[52–54] Subsequent studies suggested that in these methods, there was inadequate separation of T_4 from T_3, with consequent contamination of T_3 by some T_4, and artifactual monodeiodination of T_4 to T_3 during the separation or analytic step.[55] Both phenomena would lead to falsely high T_3 estimates, which was confirmed when highly specific radioimmunoassays for T_3 in unmodified serum were developed. The mean serum total T_3 concentration in normal subjects as measured by most of these radioimmunoassays has varied between 110 and 180 ng/dL.[56–64]

TABLE 7-1.
Estimates of Mean Serum Concentration, Metabolic Clearance Rate (MCR), and Production Rates (PR) of Various Thyronine Derivatives in Normal Subjects*

Compound	Total Serum Concentration (ng/dL)	Total Serum Concentration (nmol/L)	MCR (L/d/70 kg)	PR† (nmol/d/70 kg)	References
T_4	8600	110	1.2	130	32
T_3	135	2.1	24	48	65, 98, 101, 104, 181–183
Reverse T_3	38	0.62	111	60	8, 32, 38, 97, 98, 100, 101
$3,3'$-T_2	3.1	0.058	857	50	8, 13, 38, 58, 114
$3,5$-T_2	2.9	0.055	117	6.4	8, 13
$3', 5'$-T_2	4.5	0.085	247	21	8, 13, 38, 58, 116
$3'$-T_1	2.3	0.059	510	30	8, 58
Tetrac	60	7.2‡	2.5	1.8	105, 112, 121, 184
Triac	2	2.8	222	5.8	117
T_3S	5.7	0.076	135	10	117, 119, 124
T_4S	1.9	0.019			118, 119
rT_3S	3.0	0.040			120

The results given represent the average of mean values of multiple studies.
†Conversion factors: T_4, 1 nmol = 0.78 µg; T_3 and rT_3, 1 nmol = 0.65 µg; T_2S, 1 nmol = 0.52 µg; T_1, 1 nmol = 0.40 µg; tetrac, 1 nmol = 0.84 µg; triac, 1 nmol = 0.71 µg; T_4S, 1 nmol = 0.87 µg; T_3S and rT_3S, 1 nmol = 0.75 µg.
‡Another study using a gas chromatographic method for measurement of tetrac levels reported a mean serum tetrac concentration in normal subjects of 0.12 nmol/L.[185]

Injected T_3 disappears from the circulation at a much faster rate than T_4; the difference is related in part at least to the lesser affinity of the binding proteins in serum for T_3. Analysis of the curve describing the disappearance of T_3 after intravenous injection of radiolabeled T_3 is complicated by the generation of radioactive iodoprotein, iodide, and other products.[27] This iodoprotein, a product of peripheral T_3 metabolism, is cleared much more slowly than T_3. The half-time of T_3 in serum varies between 1 and 1.5 days in most studies. Estimates of T_3 distribution space have varied between 38 and 46 L/d using single-compartment analysis.[65,66] The mean metabolic clearance rate of T_3 in normal subjects is about 24 L/d, whether determined by single injection or constant infusion techniques.[65–67]

Sources of Triiodothyronine

The possibility that conversion of T_4 to T_3 in peripheral tissues, in addition to direct thyroid secretion, might be a source of T_3 in the circulation was first suggested by Pitt-Rivers and colleagues in 1955.[68] Suggestive evidence of such conversion was obtained, but a subsequent, similar study did not confirm this finding.[69] The question lay fallow until 1970, when Braverman and associates[70] demonstrated the presence of substantial concentrations of both stable and labeled T_3 in the serum of athyrotic patients given stable and labeled T_4. This evidence for the peripheral conversion of T_4 to T_3 in humans was subsequently confirmed,[71,72] and the process was found to occur in several animal species, including frogs, birds, rats, and sheep.[37,73–78] It is, therefore, of more than theoretical interest to ascertain the extent to which thyroid secretion and peripheral generation from T_4 each contribute to the overall production of T_3.

Daily Production Rate of T_3. As with any other metabolite, the daily production rate of T_3 can be calculated as the product of its daily rate of clearance from the circulation (metabolic clearance rate) and its serum concentration. Production rates calculated in this way are referred to as blood production rates, because they are based solely on measurements made in the blood and do not take into account any hormone that is generated and then degraded in peripheral tissues without ever entering the circulation. Estimates of the daily T_3 production rate calculated in this way can readily be derived from available data. The metabolic clearance rate of T_3 in normal subjects varies from about 20 to 26 L/d, depending on the method of measurement, and the mean normal serum T_3 concentration varies from 110 to 180 ng/dL. Using the lower values for metabolic clearance rate and serum T_3 concentrations, the calculated production rate is 22 µg/d, whereas using the higher values, the calculated rate is 47 µg/d. This twofold variation indicates the uncertainties introduced by methodologic variations. For the present, it would appear that the best estimate of the mean T_3 production rate is 26 µg/d, based on a mean serum T_3 concentration of 110 ng/dL and a mean metabolic clearance rate of 24 L/d obtained by noncompartmental analysis.

Secretion Rate of T_3. No method as yet exists for directly measuring the rate of thyroid secretion of T_3, but it can be estimated indirectly. If T_4 and T_3 are assumed to be secreted in the same ratio as they are present in thyroglobulin within the gland, then the quantity of T_3 secreted daily can be calculated from the T_3∴T_4 ratio within the gland and the secretion rate for T_4. In steady-state conditions, the latter is reflected in the daily T_4 disposal rate, which, in contrast to the disposal rate for T_3, can be measured with considerable accuracy. The T_4 secretion rate in normal young and middle-aged adults is about 90 µg/d.[79,80] Immunoassay studies have yielded variable results for the intrathyroid $T_3::T_4$ ratio, the values ranging between 0.051 and 0.096.[32,33,81] When T_3 secretion rates are based on these data, the calculated thyroidal T_3 secretion rate varies from 4.6 to 8.4 µg/d. These estimates of the daily rate of direct T_3 secretion do not depend on measurement of the serum T_3 concentration or T_3 metabolic clearance rate. It is possible, then, to derive from these latter measurements limits for the fraction of total daily T_3 production contributed by direct thyroid secretion. Assuming the lowest T_3 production rate calculated above, 22 µg/d, and the higher limit for the thyroidal secretion rate, 8.4 µg/d, 38.2% of daily T_3 production could be ascribed to thyroid secretion. On the other hand, if the highest rate of T_3 production, 47 µg/d, is used together with the lower value for the thyroid rate, 4.6 µg/d, 9.8% of daily T_3 production could be ascribed to thyroid secretion. Although these estimates for the fraction of total T_3 production contributed by the thyroid vary widely and the true mean value is uncertain, they indicate that the generation of T_3 from T_4 peripherally accounts for most T_3 production in normal subjects.

These estimates of the rate of secretion of T_3 from the normal thyroid and the proportion of total T_3 production that this contributes are based on the presumption that T_4 and T_3 are secreted from the thyroid in the same proportion as exists in thyroglobulin. This assumption has not been verified in humans. In experimental animals (rats and dogs), the results are conflicting, some studies suggesting that the $T_3::T_4$ ratio in thyroid venous effluent is higher than in thyroglobulin, others that it is not.[82–85] There are several reasons to believe that the $T_3::T_4$ ratio of the total thyroid hormone secreted exceeds that found in thyroglobulin. First, thyroid contains type 1 5'-deiodinase (5'D-I), an enzyme that catalyzes the deiodination of T_4 to yield T_3.[73,86] Second, it is clear that the secretory product is derived from functionally heterogeneous intrathyroidal pools that differ with respect to the rate at which their iodinated compounds turn over. If the $T_3::T_4$ ratios in these several pools are not the same, as is likely, the $T_3::T_4$ ratio of the secretory product will not be the same as the overall $T_3::T_4$ ratio in the gland.

Several studies have produced new evidence that bears on the issue of the contribution of the thyroid versus nonthyroidal tissues to the daily production rate of T_3.[87–89] Thus, it has been demonstrated that the conversion of T_4 to T_3 is a function of at least two iodothyronine 5'-monodeiodinases (5'D-I and 5'D-II), and that among these two enzymes, 5'D-I contributes most of the T_3 produced in vivo. It turns out that 5'D-I is a selenoenzyme that is present in several tissues but is most abundant in the liver, the kidney, and the thyroid. Induction of selenium deficiency in the rat is associated with a marked decrease in the activity and the content of the 5'D-I in the liver and the kidney, but that in the thyroid remains relatively well maintained. Using selenium deficiency and thyroidectomy, it was determined that the thyroid is a major source of T_3 in the rat and that the intrathyroidal conversion of T_4 to T_3 may account for much of the T_3 released by the thyroid.[87,88] Similarly, the thyroid has been suggested to be the main source of the postnatal increase in serum T_3 in the rat.[89] Similar studies in other experimental animals would help establish the importance of intrathyroidal 5'D-I as a major contributor to the body pool of T_3 in most or all species.

3,3',5'-Triiodothyronine (Reverse Triiodothyronine)

Reverse T_3 (rT_3), which differs from T_3 in that iodine is missing from the inner or tyrosyl ring of T_4 rather than the outer or phenolic ring, was first found in both the blood and thyroglobulin of rats in 1956.[90] These findings stirred relatively little interest for two reasons: first, rT_3 has little or no calorigenic activity when administered to animals,[91,92] and second, its metabolism is so rapid that it seemed highly unlikely that significant or measurable quantities of rT_3 would be present in serum.[93] Renewal of interest in rT_3 stemmed from studies showing that rT_3 could be measured in human serum by radioimmunoassay and that its concentration varies in diverse pathologic states.[31,37,94–96]

The serum concentration of rT_3, as measured by various radioimmunoassays,[8,31,32,37,97–101] ranges from 15 to 40 ng/dL in normal adults, and is increased in hyperthyroidism and decreased in hypothyroidism. Reverse T_3 is readily detected in the serum of hypothyroid patients treated with T_4 and in euthyroid patients receiving suppressive doses of T_4 (Fig 7-1). Under these conditions, the serum rT_3 concentration approximates that in subjects with normally functioning thyroid tissue, suggesting that peripheral T_4 metabolism is the major source of rT_3.

Like T_4 and T_3, rT_3 in serum is almost completely bound to proteins, the free fraction being about 0.3%, a value similar to that for T_3.[37] Paper electrophoresis of serum containing radioiodine-labeled rT_3 indicates that like T_4, with which it shares two iodine atoms in the phenolic ring, rT_3 is bound by TBG, albumin, and thyroxine-binding prealbumin (Fig 7-2). As judged from the ability of T_4, T_3, and rT_3 to inhibit labeled rT_3 binding to TBG, rT_3 is bound to TBG much less firmly than T_4 (Fig 7-3).

After intravenous injection, rT_3 disappears from the circulation of normal subjects at a much faster rate than does T_3.[32] Because the overall serum binding of rT_3 and T_3 is similar, the difference probably reflects more rapid tissue metabolism of rT_3 than T_3. After intravenous injection of radioiodine-labeled rT_3 in normal subjects, most of the radioiodine is excreted in the urine as iodine within 24 hours. Rapid metabolism of rT_3 by tissues also is demonstrable in vitro. Both liver and kidney homogenates have monodeiodinating activity apparently due to 5'D-I, that rapidly metabolizes rT_3 to 3,3'-diiodothyronine (3,3'-T_2; see chap 8).[102] Estimates of the metabolic clearance rate of rT_3 in normal subjects have varied between 82 and 151 L/d in studies using noncompartmental analysis after a single injection of radioiodine-labeled rT_3.[8,32,97,98,100,101] The value was 131 L/d in another study using a constant infusion of radiolabeled rT_3.[38] The mean of these values was 111 L/d (see Table 7-1). The mean serum rT_3 concentration varied between 21 and 48 ng/dL (average, 38 ng/dL), whereas the mean daily production rate of rT_3 ranged between 21 and 52 µg/d (average, 39 µg [60 nmol]/d; see Table 7-1).

The concentration of rT_3 is much higher in umbilical cord serum than in serum obtained later in life (Figs 7-4 and 7-5). This finding is of particular interest because the concentration of T_3 in serum at birth is much lower than it is subsequently. Although serum T_3 concentrations in the newborn abruptly increase to normal adult levels or higher within a few hours after birth, serum rT_3 concentrations decline slowly and may reach normal adult levels by 30 days[94] (see Fig 7-4). The high concentrations of rT_3 in umbilical cord serum are not merely a phenomenon of

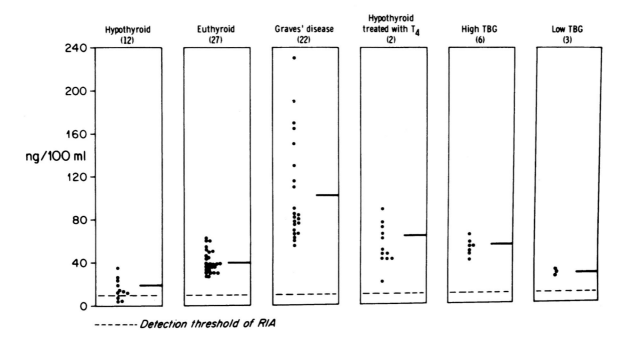

FIGURE 7-1. Serum concentrations of 3,3′,5′-triiodothyronine (reverse T$_3$, rT$_3$) in euthyroid subjects and patients with thyroid disease. The solid horizontal bars represent the mean values. (Chopra IJ. A radioimmunoassay for measurement of 3,3′,5′-triiodothyronine [reverse T$_3$]. J Clin Invest 1974;54:583)

the immediate prenatal period; rather, they are high throughout most of the last third of pregnancy.[37] In the human fetus, rT$_3$ concentrations in amniotic fluid are high as early as 15 weeks of gestation, and there is a decrease in amniotic fluid rT$_3$ concentrations as pregnancy advances. The values are higher in amniotic fluid than in maternal serum, even at term[103] (see chap 84).

As in the fetus and newborn, serum rT$_3$ concentrations are high and T$_3$ concentrations low in adults with a variety of nonthyroid disorders, including cirrhosis, neoplastic disease, congestive heart failure, burns, toxemia of pregnancy, febrile illnesses, and after major surgery (see Fig 7-5 and chaps 14 and 18),[104,105] but they usually are normal in chronic renal failure.[95,106,107] The serum free rT$_3$ concentrations are elevated in all the mentioned conditions, including chronic renal failure.[71,95] In

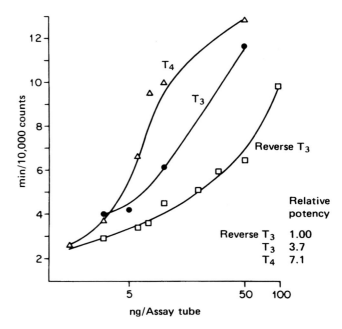

FIGURE 7-3. Dose-response curves of inhibition of the binding of ([125I] −rT$_3$ to thyroxine-binding globulin (TBG) by rT$_3$, T$_3$, and T$_4$. One to 32 (1/32) diluted normal human serum was the source of the TBG. The assay conditions were similar to those described previously for the competitive protein binding assay of T$_4$. (Murphy BEP. J Lab Clin Med 1965;66:161; Chopra IJ, unpublished data)

FIGURE 7-2. Radioautograph showing the electrophoretic patterns of binding of reverse T$_3$ (rT$_3$), T$_3$, and T$_4$ by the proteins in normal human serum. The serum was enriched with radioiodinated [125I] −rT$_3$, −T$_3$, and −T$_4$ and subjected to reverse-flow paper electrophoresis in 0.2 mol/L glycine acetate buffer, pH 9.0. (Chopra IJ, unpublished data)

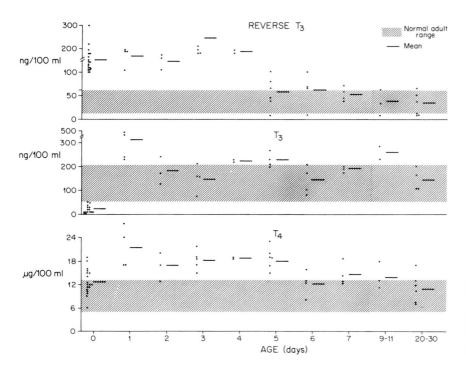

FIGURE 7-4. Serum rT_3, T_3, and T_4 concentrations from birth to 30 days of life. The horizontal bars indicate the mean values, and the shaded areas the normal adult ranges. (Chopra IJ, Sack J, Fisher DA. Circulating 3,3′,5′-triiodothyronine [reverse T_3] in the human newborn. J Clin Invest 1975; 55:1137)

normal-weight and obese people, serum T_3 concentrations decrease and rT_3 concentrations increase rapidly during caloric deprivation, and both changes are rapidly reversed by refeed-ing.[96,108,109] Similarly, serum rT_3 concentrations are increased in patients with protein-calorie malnutrition and return to normal during treatment.[95]

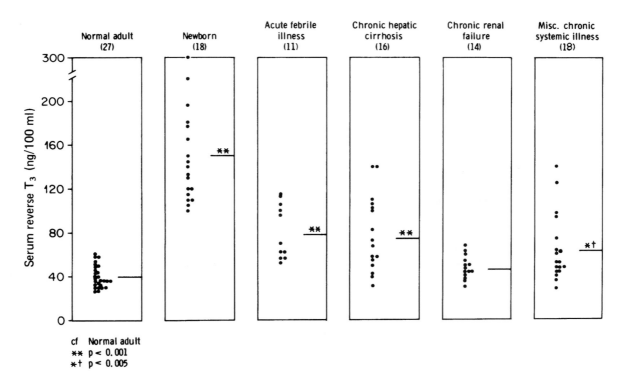

FIGURE 7-5. Serum rT_3 concentrations in newborn infants (cord serum) and in patients with various systemic illnesses. The horizontal lines indicate the mean values in each group. (Chopra IJ, Solomon DH, Chopra U, et al. Reciprocal changes in serum reverse T_3 [rT_3] and T_3 in systemic illnesses: evidence for independent path-ways of T_4 metabolism in adults. J Clin Endocrinol Metab 1975;41:1043)

Sources of Reverse Triiodothyronine

Reverse T_3 has been detected in rat and human thyroglobulin by both radioimmunoassay and chromatographic techniques, and its content has been estimated to be about 1% to 4.7% that of T_4.[30,31] This makes possible estimation of the rate of thyroidal rT_3 secretion by the method described for T_3. As measured by radioimmunoassay, the mean rT_3::T_4 ratio in normal human thyroid glands varies from 0.013 to 0.047. Thus, a normal secretion rate of 90 μg of T_4 daily would presumably be accompanied by rT_3 secretion of about 1.2 to 4.2 μg/d. This would account for 10% or less of the approximately 40 μg rT_3 normally produced each day. Complementary to these data are those that demonstrate virtually normal serum rT_3 concentrations in patients receiving replacement doses of T_4. These results strongly suggest that in humans, rT_3 is derived almost entirely from the peripheral deiodination of T_4; results leading to a similar conclusion have been obtained in fetal and adult sheep.[37] In humans, about 90% of T_3 disposal occurs by deiodination and the remaining 10% by biliary secretion and fecal excretion.

The rates of peripheral production of T_3 and rT_3 from T_4 can account for nearly all of the T_4 that undergoes deiodination. If removal of iodine atoms from T_4 occurs sequentially in the outer and inner ring, then only two products can result from removal of the first iodine—deiodination in the inner ring yielding rT_3, and deiodination in the outer ring yielding T_3. Studies with differentially labeled T_4 in rats indicate that deiodination of the inner and outer rings occurs at almost the same rate.[28,110] In humans, about 35% to 40% of the T_4 produced is deiodinated to yield T_3, and a little more, about 50%, to yield rT_3.[32] The evidence suggesting nearly equal extrathyroidal production of T_3 and rT_3 from T_4 in rats led to the suggestion that the initial deiodination of T_4 is by a random process that does not discriminate between the inner and outer rings.[28,110] More recent studies indicate that this near-equality was fortuitous and that T_4 is not metabolized by random deiodination. In sheep, as in humans, serum rT_3 concentrations are much higher and T_3 concentrations lower in the fetus than in the adult. These differences reflect similar differences in the measured production rates of the iodothyronines.[37] Because only a small proportion (about 3%) of rT_3 production can be attributed to direct thyroid secretion, in either fetus or adult, the very different production rates provide strong evidence that extrathyroidal deiodination is not random. Moreover, the reciprocal decrease in serum T_3 and increase in rT_3 concentrations that occurs in obese patients who undergo fasting, alluded to earlier, occurs not only in those with normally functioning thyroid tissue but in those receiving suppressive doses of T_4.[109] This finding excludes changes in the direct secretion of T_3 and rT_3 as the source of the changes in serum T_3 and rT_3 concentrations. In addition, kinetic studies have demonstrated a clear (about 50%) reduction (17% vs. 35%) in the rate of conversion of T_4 to T_3 during fasting, at a time when the rate of conversion of T_4 to rT_3 increased by about 50% (61% vs. 41%).[101] The daily production rate of T_3 also is reduced in catabolic situations in which serum T_3 concentrations are low (e.g., starvation, cirrhosis, and insulin-dependent diabetes mellitus). The daily production rate of rT_3 is normal in these situations, the rise in serum rT_3 concentrations resulting from decreased rT_3 catabolism. The ratio of the daily production rates of T_3 and T_4 (T_3::T_4) clearly is subnormal, whereas that of rT_3

and T_4 (rT_3::T_4) is either normal or moderately increased.[32,97,101,111] These findings also speak strongly for selective, rather than random, deiodination of T_4. Because the biologic activities of T_3 and rT_3 differ so greatly, starvation and the array of illnesses that lead to decreased serum T_3 and increased rT_3 concentrations divert peripheral T_4 metabolism from pathways leading to hormonal activation to those leading to hormonal inactivation.

Thyronine Derivatives Other Than Thyroxine and the Two Triiodothyronines

Besides T_4, T_3, and rT_3, several other T_0 derivatives are found in the circulation. These include three diiodothyronines (3,3'-T_2, 3,5-T_2, and 3',5'T_2), two monoiodothyronines (3'-T_1 and 3-T_1), two acetic acid analogues of T_4 (tetrac) and T_3 (triac),[36,38,112–120] and the sulfate and glucuronide conjugates of T_4, T_3, and rT_3. The serum concentrations, metabolic clearance rates, and daily production rates of many of these substances are shown in Table 7-1. Although small quantities of T_0 and the various iodothyronines other than T_4 and T_3 are detectable in thyroglobulin, thyroidal secretion probably contributes little to their serum concentrations, and the main source of all of these compounds is extrathyroidal deiodination of the more iodinated analogue. Tetrac and triac have not been found in thyroglobulin; they are probably entirely derived from extrathyroidal metabolism of T_4 and T_3, respectively. It is possible that some triac originates from extrathyroidal 5'monodeiodination of tetrac.[13] Only 1% to 2% of T_4 is metabolized normally to tetrac, whereas about 15% of T_3 may normally be metabolized by conversion to triac.[13,105,115,121] Up to 54% of the secreted iodothyronines are excreted in urine as T_0 or thyroacetic acid.[35,122]

There has been increased interest in the significance of glucuronide and sulfate conjugates of the iodothyronines.[13,117–120] This is related in part to the finding that sulfate conjugates of iodothyronines (e.g., T_3 sulfate [T_3S]) are subject to more active monodeiodination than the parent iodothyronines.[123] Highly sensitive and specific radioimmunoassays have been developed to measure serum levels of these conjugates of T_4, T_3, and rT_3.[117,118,120] Serum concentration of T_3S in normal man approximates 5.7 ng/dL (or 76 pmol/L, see Table 7-1), and its levels are increased in hyperthyroidism and in situations where tissue activity of 5'D-I is reduced (e.g., systemic illnesses, fetus, and newborn)[117] (Fig 7-6). Administration of sodium ipodate, a known potent inhibitor of 5'D-I, to hyperthyroid patients is associated with a marked increase in serum T_3S concentration. The mean serum concentration of T_4S in normal subjects approximates 1.6 ng/dL (or 19 pmol/L). Serum T_4S is not significantly altered in patients with hyperthyroidism, hypothyroidism, or systemic illnesses. It is, however, markedly elevated (~21 ng/dL) in the newborn cord blood serum.[120] The mean serum concentration of rT_3S in normal mean approximates 3.0 ng/dL (40 pmol/L). Serum rT_3S concentration is elevated in hyperthyroidism, in patients with systemic illnesses, and in the fetus and newborn, where the activity of 5'D-I is reduced in the tissues.[120] Curiously, serum levels of sulfoconjugates of T_3, T_4, or rT_3 are not elevated in pregnancy despite elevation of TBG, which avidly binds these compounds. The data suggest a markedly different metabolism of sulfoconjugates of iodothyronines in the mother and the fetus.[117–120]

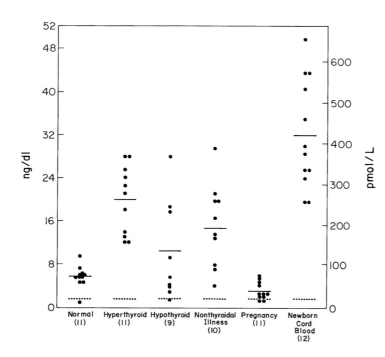

FIGURE 7-6. Serum T_3S concentration in normal subjects, hyperthyroid patients, hypothyroid patients, patients with nonthyroidal illness, cord blood of newborns, and pregnant women with a 15- to 31-week gestation. The results are expressed as ng/dL and pmol/L. The horizontal bars represent mean values. The dotted line represents the detection threshold of T_3S RIA. The numbers of subjects included in each group are indicated in parentheses. Each group can be compared with the normal group, $P<0.01$. (Chopra IJ, Wu SY, Chua Teco GN, et al. A radioimmunoassay for measurement of 3,5,3'-triiodothyronine sulfate: studies in thyroidal and nonthyroidal disease, pregnancy, and neonatal life. J Clin Endocrinol Metab 1992;75:189)

Only limited information is available on the kinetics of metabolism of sulfoconjugates of iodothyronines. Thus, it has been estimated that the metabolic clearance of T_3S in normal man approximates 135 L/d.[124] This information and that on its serum concentration suggests that the daily production rate of T_3S approximates 7.7 μg (10 nmoles)/d (see Table 7-1).[117,118] These data suggest that at least 20% of T_3 produced daily in normal man is metabolized via the sulfation pathway of metabolism. This is a minimal estimate, however, because the contribution of T_3S produced and metabolized in tissues without ever reaching the blood compartment remains unknown. Studies suggest that most of the nondeiodinative disposal of T_3 occurs through T_3S formation.[125]

Studies have also examined the biologic activity of T_3S in hypothyroid rats. T_3S is capable of thyromimetic effects, and its activity approximates about 20% that of T_3 in several tissue effects.[126] There is no information on the biologic activity of T_4S or rT_3S.

RELATIVE BIOLOGIC SIGNIFICANCE OF THYROID HORMONES

Because one third to one half of the T_4 that is secreted is converted to T_3, and because the calorigenic activity of T_3 is two to four times greater than that of T_4, conversion to T_3 is an important step in the action of T_4. Serum T_3 levels change little between doses in hypothyroid patients treated once daily with T_4, whereas those in patients treated with T_3 fluctuate widely.[110,127] Thus, the production of T_4 and its extrathyroidal conversion to T_3 provide a more constant source of T_3 than might be the case if T_3 were produced only by the thyroid. Furthermore, extrathyroidal T_3 production provides an additional level for regulation of biologic action of thyroid hormone.

The extent of T_4 conversion to T_3 has raised the question of whether circulating T_4 has any biologic activity by itself or whether it serves merely as a prohormone for T_3. T_4 action without intracellular conversion to T_3 is difficult to determine in vivo, and therefore a definite answer is lacking. Some evidence suggests that T_4 may itself be capable of hormonal action. For example, some clinically hypothyroid patients have elevated serum TSH, subnormal total and free T_4, but normal total and free T_3 concentrations.[127] These data suggest that in the absence of a normal level of T_4, a normal level of T_3 may not be adequate to sustain the euthyroid state and thus T_4 may have some hormonal activity.

Thyroid function test results in the newborn also are pertinent to the question of the hormonal activity of T_4. At birth, serum total and free T_3 concentrations are lower than those in adults and are comparable to those in many hypothyroid patients; serum total and free T_4 concentrations are similar to or higher than those in the adults; and serum TSH concentrations are slightly increased, but much less so than in hypothyroidism. If the normal newborn can be assumed to be euthyroid, these results suggest that fetal euthyroidism is probably maintained by T_4 and not by T_3. Although the presence of 5'D-II in brain[89,128] suggests the importance of T_3 in the fetal brain, thyromimetic effects observed in other tissues would appear related to T_4. Likewise, serum or tissue T_3 concentrations are low and T_4 concentrations are normal in apparently euthyroid adults with malnutrition and many nonthyroidal illnesses,[108,109,129–131] yet their serum TSH concentrations are usually normal. Moreover, during recovery, their serum T_3 concentrations may return to normal without appreciable changes in serum TSH.[108] An increase in serum TSH has, however, been noted during recovery from some systemic illnesses.[132,133] T_3 turnover studies have been conducted in some of these situations. In patients with cirrhosis and during starvation, like serum T_3, the daily turnover of T_3 may be reduced.[129,130,134] These data in clinically euthyroid people favor the concept that circulating T_4 is capable of hormonal action.

Studies of hypothyroid patients treated with replacement doses of T_3, who therefore have normal serum TSH levels, also provide evidence that supports a hormonal role for T_4. Serum T_3 levels in such patients given T_3 once daily range from normal to four times normal at various times of day. The mean serum T_3 concentration, calculated by integration of the curve of serum concentration against time, is about twice normal, as is the estimated daily turnover of T_3.[135] Serum T_3 concentrations may have to be maintained at two to three times normal to normalize serum TSH concentrations in hypothyroid patients.[127] These findings suggest that high levels of serum T_3 may be needed to maintain euthyroidism and to normalize serum TSH in hypothyroidism because serum T_4 is low.

Studies of inhabitants of endemic goiter regions also bear on the hormonal activity of circulating T_4. Many such subjects have subnormal serum T_4, high-normal or high T_3, and high TSH concentrations.[136–138] An analysis of the relation between thyroid hormones and TSH in these people revealed that their serum TSH concentrations were inversely correlated with their serum total T_4 as well as free T_4 concentrations[136] (Fig 7-7). On the other hand, serum TSH was not correlated with serum T_3 and was positively correlated with serum free T_3[136] (Fig 7-8). These results thus strengthen the notion that T_4 has hormonal activity.

Administration of iopanoic acid, a potent inhibitor of extrathyroidal conversion of T_4 to T_3, leads to no measurable change in thermogenesis, even though serum T_3 concentrations decline.[139] Studies in some other species also indicate that T_4 is an active hormone. Thus T_4 is as potent as or even more potent than T_3 in birds when judged by several criteria.[140] Similarly, rats

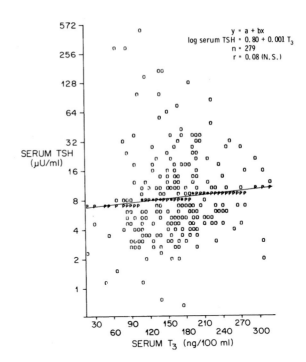

FIGURE 7-8. Relationship between serum T_3 and TSH concentrations in inhabitants of an endemic goiter region of New Guinea. (Chopra IJ, Hershman JM, Hornabrook RW. A study of serum thyroid hormone and thyrotropin levels in subjects from endemic goiter regions of New Guinea. J Clin Endocrinol Metab 1975;40:326)

given propylthiouracil die on exposure to cold at 4°C for 3 days, whereas those given T_4 in addition to propylthiouracil survive even though their serum T_3 levels are clearly subnormal.[141] T_4 has significant biologic activity in vitro as well. It increases intracellular accumulation of amino acids by embryonic chick bone,[142] inhibits phosphodiesterase activity in rat calvaria, liver, spleen, and kidney,[143–145] and stimulates erythropoiesis[145]; in some of these actions it is more potent than T_3.[143,145] T_4 also stimulates Na^+-K^+ adenosine triphosphatase (ATPase) in isolated rat kidney cells, with a potency comparable to that of T_3,[146] and the activity of calmodulin-dependent Ca^{2+} ATPase in human erythrocytes.[147] Several studies show that T_4 alters cytoskeletal organization in astrocytes by modulating actin polymerization and that this action of T_4 in turn regulates metabolism of 5'D-II.[148–152]

Administration of propylthiouracil to hypothyroid patients receiving a constant dose of T_4 results in a decrease in serum T_3, little or no change in serum T_4, and a modest increase in the serum TSH or an increase in serum TSH response to thyrotropin-releasing hormone.[153,154] Propylthiouracil decreases the rate of conversion of T_4 to T_3 as well as inhibiting T_4 and T_3 biosynthesis in the thyroid; the former action has been suggested to be the explanation for the anti-T_4 effects of propylthiouracil in rats.[155] The drug's ability to inhibit T_4 conversion to T_3 and its anti-T_4 biologic action were interpreted to indicate that T_3 may be the sole biologically active thyroid hormone.[155] Because several studies suggest that T_4 has biologic activity, the anti-T_4 effects of propylthiouracil may be caused not only by inhibition of conversion of T_4 to T_3 but by interference with cellular mechanisms of action of T_4. Unfortunately, the various mechanisms by which T_4 (and, for that matter, T_3) exerts tissue

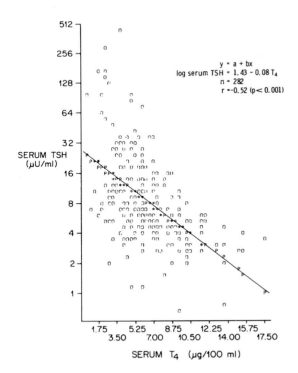

FIGURE 7-7. Relationship between serum T_4 and TSH concentrations in inhabitants of an endemic goiter region of New Guinea. (Chopra IJ, Hershman JM, Hornabrook RW. A study of serum thyroid hormone and thyrotropin levels in subjects from endemic goiter regions of New Guinea. J Clin Endocrinol Metab 1975;40:326)

effects are unclear. Low-capacity, high-affinity binding sites have been identified for T_3 in the nuclei of the kidney, liver, anterior pituitary, and other tissues[156,157]; the affinity of these sites for T_4 is about 1% that for T_3. The question whether binding to nuclei is the only mechanism whereby thyroid hormones exert biologic activity is unanswered at this time (see chap 9).

Some studies have emphasized the importance of in situ (local) conversion of T_4 to T_3 in suppression of TSH secretion in rat pituitary tissue.[158] It has been estimated that 40% to 50% of the T_3 in rat pituitary nuclei is derived from local conversion of T_4 to T_3. Intrapituitary T_3 production seems to be normal or supranormal in the fetus and in nonthyroidal illness in which serum TSH concentrations are normal despite low serum T_3 concentrations.[128,158,159] The suggestion that in situ conversion of T_4 to T_3 is an important determinant of TSH secretion is consistent with the findings of a strong negative correlation between serum T_4 and TSH in endemic goiter patients (see Fig 7-7).

Although the biologic significance of the conversion of T_4 to T_3, a more potent iodothyronine, can be appreciated, the physiologic function, if any, of the conversion of T_4 to rT_3, a relatively inert iodothyronine, is unclear. It has both thyroid agonist and antagonist activity in different systems. Considering the latter first, rT_3 inhibits the calorigenic action of T_4 and T_3 in rats and humans,[160,161] and it has been used to treat hyperthyroidism,[162] but massive doses are required, so the effect probably resulted from the antithyroid effects of the iodine released when rT_3 was metabolized. Reverse T_3 slows the rate of disappearance of T_4 from the serum in rats,[163] and it inhibits monodeiodination of T_4 to T_3 in vitro[164–167] and in the rat in vivo,[168] although not during short-term administration in humans in vivo. Reverse T_3 also inhibits the stimulation of epinephrine-induced lipolysis by T_3 in rat adipocytes.[169] As for thyroid agonist activity, rT_3 stimulates amino acid uptake by rat thymocytes and embryonic chick bone.[142] It also stimulates growth hormone secretion by GH1 cells[170] and the activity of hepatic L-T_3 aminotransferase, an enzyme that may be involved in inactivation of T_3.[171] Studies have also demonstrated that like T_4, rT_3 modifies actin polymerization and 5′-D-II activity in astrocytes.[149] Although some of these various effects require pharmacologic amounts of rT_3, they raise the possibility that rT_3 may not be just an inactivation product of T_4, but that it may contribute to the biologic action of T_4. There may or may not be high-affinity, low-capacity binding sites for rT_3 in nuclei of hepatic tissue.[172–174]

The conversions of T_4 to T_3 and rT_3 are probably physiologically regulated phenomena similar to those proposed for vitamin D_3. DeLuca and coworkers have described two parallel enzyme systems in the kidney that lead to the conversion of 25-hydroxyvitamin D_3 (25-OH-D_3) to either 1,25(OH)$_2$-D_3, which has considerable activity, or 24,25-(OH)$_2$-D_3, which has little activity.[175–177] When production of 1,25(OH)$_2$-D_3 is diminished, production of 24,25(OH)$_2$-D_3 usually is increased. In this respect, the findings, in normal newborn infants and in adults with nonthyroidal illnesses, of subnormal serum concentrations T_3 and T_3:·T_4 ratios and supranormal serum concentrations, rT_3 and rT_3:·T_4 ratios are similar.[31,95] The data on relative turnover rates of various iodothyronines and sources of rT_3 in adults with low T_3 and high rT_3 serum concentrations remain limited.[32] Studies in fetal sheep have demonstrated an increase in production rate of T_4 and, in relation to it, a decreased production rate of T_3 and a normal (not increased) production rate of rT_3. These results raise the possibility that in addition to T_3 and rT_3, there may be yet another pathway of metabolism of T_4 in the fetus.[37] This may comprise sulfoconjugation, deamination, or both. The situation appears to be similar, at least qualitatively, in adults with various nonthyroidal disorders in whom serum levels of iodothyronines are similar to those in the fetus.[32,124,125]

Iodothyronines other than T_4, T_3, and rT_3 also have been shown to have biologic activity.[140] Thus, tetrac and triac have about 11% and 21%, respectively, of the calorigenic activity of T_4. More notably, tetrac and triac are potent (10–20 × T_4) in stimulating tadpole metamorphosis. More recently, studies in humans demonstrated substantial hepatic and skeletal effects of triac without a major effect on the pituitary gland.[178] 3,3′-T_2 demonstrates about 25% to 70% and 3,5-T_2 about 40% of this activity of T_4, whereas 3′-T_1, 3-T_1, and T_0 are inactive.[140] Some diiodothyronines stimulate amino acid uptake by rat thymocytes[179]; 3,3′-T_2 is, like T_3, about three times more potent than T_4 in this action, whereas 3,5-T_2 and the two monoiodothyronines have only modest activity. 3,5-T_2 is active in a different assay system, however; it is nearly as active as T_3 in stimulation of lipolysis in rat adipose tissue.[180] 3′,5′-T_2, on the other hand, is an inhibitor of the conversion of T_4 to T_3 in rat liver or kidney homogenates.[164] As noted earlier, T_3S is about 20% as active as T_3 in several thyromimetic effects.[126] These data suggest that most iodothyronines have some biologic activity, but whether they are active in vivo remains uncertain.

References

1. Albert A, Keating FR. Metabolic studies with ^{131}I labeled thyroid compounds: distribution and excretion of radiodiiodotyrosine in human beings. J Clin Endocrinol Metab 1951;11:996
2. Meinhold H, Olbricht T, Schwatz-Porsche D. Turnover and urinary excretion of circulating diiodotyrosine. J Clin Endocrinol Metab 1987;64:794
3. McGirr EM, Hutchinson JH, Clement WE. Sporadic non-endemic goitrous cretinism: identification and significance of mono-iodotyrosine and diiodotyrosine in serum and urine. Lancet 1956;2:906
4. Stanbury JR, Kassinaar AAH, Meijer JW, Tepestre J. The occurrence of mono- and diiodotyrosine in the blood of a patient with congenital goiter. J Clin Endocrinol Metab 1955;15:1216
5. Stanbury JR. The metabolic errors in certain types of familial goiter. Recent Prog Horm Res 1963;19:547
6. Beale D, Whitehead JK. A preliminary investigation of the levels of 3-MIT and 3,5-DIT in human blood plasma using double isotope dilution technique. Clin Chim Acta 1960;5:150
7. Dimitriadou A, Turner PCR, Slater JDH, Fraser R. Iodotyrosine-like material in serum detected by analysis for [127]I but not [131]I. Biochem J 1962;82:20P
8. Faber J, Thomsen HF, Lumholtz IB, et al. Kinetic studies of thyroxine 3,5,3′-triiodothyronine, 3,3′,5′triiodothyronine, 3′,5′-diiodothyronine, 3,3′-diiodothyronine and 3′-monoiodothyronine in patients with liver cirrhosis. J Clin Endocrinol Metab 1981; 53:978
9. Weinert H, Masui H, Radichevich 1, Werner SC. Materials indistinguishable from iodotyrosines in normal human serum and human serum albumin. J Clin Invest 1967;46:1264
10. Werner SC, Block RJ, Mandl RH. Circulating iodoproteins in a nongoitrous adult with primary amenorrhoea, bony deformities and normal levels of serum precipitable iodine and thyroidal ^{131}I uptake. J Clin Endocrinol Metab 1957;17:1141
11. Nelson JC, Lewis JE. Radioimmunoassay of iodotyrosines. In: Abraham GE, ed. The handbook of radioimmunoassay. New York: Marcel Dekker, 1976:705

12. Meinhold H, Beckert A, Wenzel KW. Circulating diiodotyrosine: studies of its serum concentration, source, and turnover using radioimmunoassay after immunoextraction. J Clin Endocrinol Metab 1981;53:1171

13. Engler D, Burger AG. The deiodination of the iodothyronines and their derivatives in man. Endocr Rev 1984;5:151

14. Meinhold H, Gramm H-J, Meissner W, et al. Elevated serum diiodotyrosine (DIT) in severe infections and sepsis: DIT, a possible new marker of leukocyte activity. J Clin Endocrinol Metab 1991;72:945

15. McConahey WM, Keating FR Jr, Butt HR, Owen CA Jr. Comparison of certain laboratory tests in the diagnosis of Hashimoto's thyroiditis. J Clin Endocrinol Metab 1961;21:879

16. Roitt IM, Torrigiani G. Identification and estimation of undegraded thyroglobulin in human serum. Endocrinology 1967; 81:421

17. Torigiani G, Doniach D, Roitt IM. Serum thyroglobulin levels in healthy subjects and patients with thyroid disease. J Clin Endocrinol Metab 1969;29:305

18. Uller RP, Van Herle AJ, Chopra IJ. Comparison of alterations in circulating thyroglobulin, triiodothyronine and thyroxine in response to exogenous (bovine) and endogenous (human) thyrotropin. J Clin Endocrinol Metab 1973;37:741

19. Van Herle AJ, Uller RP. Elevated serum thyroglobulin: a marker of metastasis in differentiated thyroid carcinoma. J Clin Invest 1975;56:272

20. Van Herle AJ. Serum thyroglobulin measurement in the diagnosis and management of thyroid disease. Thyroid Today 1981;4:1

21. Daniel LM, Pratt OE, Roitt IM, Torrigiani G. The release of thyroglobulin from the thyroid gland into thyroid lymphatics: identification of thyroglobulin in the thyroid lymph and in the blood of monkeys by physical and immunological methods and its estimation by radioimmunoassay. Immunology 1967;12:489

22. Daniel LM. Pratt OE. Roitt IM, Torrigiani G. Thyroglobulin in the lymph draining from the thyroid gland and in the peripheral blood of rats. Q J Exp Physiol 1967;52:184

23. DeGroot LJ, Postel S, Litval J, Stanbury JB. Peptide-linked iodotyrosines and iodothyronines in the blood of patients with congenital goiter. J Clin Endocrinol Metab 1958;18:158

24. DeGroot LJ, Stanbury JB. The syndrome of congenital goiter with butanol-insoluble serum iodide. Am J Med 1959;27:586

25. Jonckheer MH, Karcher DM. Thyroid albumin: 1. Isolation and characterization. J Clin Endocrinol Metab 1971;32:7.

26. Otten J, Jonckheer M, Dumont JE. Thyroid albumin: II. In vitro synthesis of a thyroid albumin by normal human thyroid tissue. J Clin Endocrinol Metab 1971;32:18

27. Surks MI, Oppenheimer JH. Composition of nonextractable radioactivity formed after injection of labeled L-thyroxine and 3,5,3'-triiodo-L-thyronine in rats. Endocrinology 1970; 87:456

28. Surks MI, Oppenheimer JH. Metabolism of phenolic and tyrosyl-ring labeled L-thyroxine in human beings and rats. J Clin Endocrinol Metab 1971;33:616

29. Surks MI, Schwartz HL, Oppenheimer JH. Tissue iodoprotein formation during the peripheral metabolism of the thyroid hormone. J Clin Invest 1969;48:2168

30. Burman KD, Dimond RC, Wright FD, et al. A radioimmunoassay for 3,3',5'-L-triiodothyronine (reverse T$_3$): assessment of thyroid gland content and serum measurements in conditions of normal and altered thyroidal economy and following administration of thyrotropin releasing hormone (TRH) and thyrotropin (TSH). J Clin Endocrinol Metab 1977;44:660

31. Chopra IJ. A radioimmunoassay for measurement of 3,3',5'-triiodothyronine (reverse T$_3$). J Clin Invest 1974;54:583

32. Chopra IJ. An assessment of daily turnover and significance of thyroidal secretion of reverse T$_3$. J Clin Invest 1976;58:32

33. Chopra IJ, Fisher DA, Solomon DH, Beall GN. Thyroxine and triiodothyronine in the human thyroid. J Clin Endocrinol Metab 1973;36:311

34. Laurberg P. Thyroxine and 3,5,3'-triiodothyronine content of thyroglobulin in thyroid needle aspirates in hyperthyroidism and hypothyroidism. J Clin Endocrinol Metab 1987;64:969

35. Chopra IJ, Boado RJ, Geffner DL, Solomon DH. A radioimmunoassay for measurement of thyronine and its acetic acid analog in urine. J Clin Endocrinol Metab 1988;67:480

36. Chopra IJ. A radioimmunoassay of 3'-monoiodothyronine. J Clin Endocrinol Metab 1981;51:117

37. Chopra IJ, Sack J, Fisher DA. 3,3',5'-triiodothyronine (reverse T$_3$) in fetal and adult sheep: studies of metabolic clearance rate, production rate, serum binding and thyroidal content relative to thyroxine. Endocrinology 1975;97:1080

38. Geola F, Chopra IJ, Solomon DH, et al. Metabolic clearance and production rates of 3',5'-diiodothyronine (3',5'-T$_2$) and 3,3'-diiodothyronine (3,3'-T$_2$) in man. J Clin Endocrinol Metab 1979; 48:297

39. Taurog A, Chaikoff IL, Tong W. The nature of plasma iodine as revealed by filter paper partition chromatography. J Biol Chem 1950;184:99

40. Laidlaw JC. Nature of the circulating thyroid hormone. Nature 1949;164:927

41. Pileggi VJ, Segal J, Golub DJ. Determination of organic iodine compounds in serum: III. Iodotyrosines in normal human serum. J Clin Endocrinol Metab 1964;24:273

42. Ingbar SH. Observations concerning the binding of thyroid hormones by human serum prealbumin. J Clin Invest 1963; 42:143

43. Oppenheimer JH, Martinez M, Bernstein G. Determination of the maximal binding capacity and protein concentration of thyroxine-binding prealbumin. J Lab Clin Med 1966;67:500

44. Robbins J. Reverse flow electrophoresis: a method for determining the thyroxine binding capacity of serum protein. Arch Biochem Biophys 1956;63:461

45. Robbins J, Rall JE, Gorden P. The thyroid and iodine metabolism: nature of thyroxine-binding proteins. In: Bondy PK, Rosenberg LE, eds. Duncan's diseases of metabolism and endocrinology. 7th ed. Vol 2. Philadelphia: WB Saunders, 1974:1009

46. Sterling K. Thyroxine binding in serum. In: Hays RL, Goswitz FA, Murphy BEP, Anderson EB, eds. Radioisotopes in medicine: in vitro studies. Oak Ridge, TN: US Atomic Energy Commission, Division of Technical Information, 1968:293

47. Woeber KA, Ingbar SH. The contribution of thyroxine-binding pre-albumin to the binding of thyroxine in the human serum, as assessed by immunoadsorption. J Clin Invest 1968;47:1710

48. Gross J, Pitt-Rivers R. The identification of 3,5,3'triiodothyronine in human plasma. Lancet 1952;1:439

49. Cotton GE, Gorman CA, Mayberry WE. Suppression of thyrotropin (h-TSH) in serums of patients with myxedema of varying etiology treated with thyroid hormones. N Engl J Med 1971;285:529

50. Gross J, Pitt-Rivers R, Trotter WR. Effect of 3,5,3'L-triiodothyronine in myxedema. Lancet 1952;1:1044

51. Lerman J. The physiological activity of L-triiodothyronine. J Clin Endocrinol Metab 1953;13:1341

52. Hollander CS. On the nature of circulating thyroid hormones: clinical studies of triiodothyronine and thyroxine in serum using gas chromatographic methods. Trans Assoc Am Physicians 1968; 81:76

53. Nauman JA, Nauman A, Werner SC. Total and free triiodothyronine in human serum. J Clin Invest 1967;46:1346

54. Sterling K, Brenner MA, Newman ES. Determination of triiodothyronine concentration in human serum. J Clin Invest 1969;48:1150

55. Fisher DA, Dussault JH. Contribution of methodologic artifacts to the measurement of T$_3$ concentration in serum. J Clin Endocrinol Metab 1971;32:675

56. Chopra IJ, Ho RS, Lam R. An improved radioimmunoassay of triiodothyronine in serum: its application to clinical and physiological studies. J Lab Clin Med 1972;80:729

57. Chopra IJ, Solomon DH, Beall GN. Radioimmunoassay for measurement of triiodothyronine in human serum. J Clin Invest 1971;50:2033

57a. Larsen PR. Direct immunoassay of triiodothyronine in human serum. J Clin Invest 1972;51:1939

58. Faber J, Lumholtz IB, Kirkegaard C, Siersbaeck-Neilsen K, Friis T. Metabolic clearance and production rates of 3,3'-diiodothyronine, 3',5'-diiodothyronine and 3'-monoiodothyronine in hyper- and hypothyroidism. Clin Endocrinol (Oxf) 1982;16:199

59. Lieblich J, Utiger RD. Triiodothyronine radioimmunoassay. J Clin Invest 1972;51:157

60. Mitsuma T, Nihei N, Gershergorn MC, Hollander CS. Serum triiodothyronine: measurements in human serum by radioimmunoassay with corroboration by gas-liquid chromatography. J Clin Invest 1971;50:2679

61. Rubenstein HA, Butler VP Jr, Werner SC. Progressive decrease in serum triiodothyronine concentrations with human aging: radioimmunoassay following extraction of serum. J Clin Endocrinol Metab 1973;37:247

62. Dussault JH, Lam R, Fisher DA. The measurement of serum triiodothyronine by double column chromatography. J Lab Clin Med 1971;77:1039

63. Ekins RP, Brown BL, Ellis SM, Reith WS. The radioimmunoassay of serum triiodothyronine. In: Abstracts of the 6th International Thyroid Conference, Vienna, Austria, 1970

64. Sterling K, Milch PO. Thermal inactivation of thyroxine binding globulin for direct radioimmunoassay of triiodothyronine in serum. J Clin Endocrinol Metab 1974;38:866

65. Nicoloff JT, Low JC, Dussault JH, Fisher DA. Simultaneous measurement of thyroxine and triiodothyronine peripheral turnover kinetics in man. J Clin Invest 1972;51:473

66. Oppenheimer JH, Surks MI. Quantitative aspects of hormone production, distribution, metabolism and activity. In: Greer MA, Solomon DH, eds. Handbook of physiology. Sec 7. Endocrinology. Vol 3. Thyroid. Washington, DC: American Physiological Society, 1974:197

67. Cavalieri RR, Steinberg M, Searle GL. Metabolic clearance rate of L-triiodothyronine in man: a comparison of results by single injection and constant infusion methods. J Clin Endocrinol Metab 1971;33:624

68. Pitt-Rivers R, Stanbury JB, Rapp B. Conversion of thyroxine to 3,5,3'-triiodothyronine in vivo. J Clin Endocrinol Metab 1955; 15:616

69. Lassiter WC, Stanbury JB. The in vivo conversion of thyroxine to 3,5,3'-triiodothyronine. J Clin Endocrinol Metab 1958;18:903

70. Braverman LE, Ingbar SH, Sterling K. Conversion of thyroxine (T_4) to triiodothyronine (T_3) in athyrotic human subjects. J Clin Invest 1970;49:855

71. Chopra IJ, Solomon DH. Triiodothyronine in health and disease. In: Scow RO, Ebling FJG, Henderson IW, eds. Endocrinology. Amsterdam: Excerpta Medica, 1972:1163

72. Pittman CS, Chambers JB, Read VH. The extrathyroidal conversion rate of thyroxine to triiodothyronine in normal man. J Clin Invest 1971;50:1187

73. Erickson VJ, Cavalieri RR, Rosenberg LL. Phenolic and nonphenolic ring iodothyronine deiodinases from rat thyroid gland. Endocrinology 1981;108:1257

74. Galton VA. Iodothyronine 5'-deiodinase activity in the amphibian *Rana catesbeiana* tadpoles at different stages of the life cycle. Endocrinology 1988;122:1746

75. Galton VA, Hiebert A. Hepatic iodothyronine 5'deiodinase activity in *Rana catesbeiana* tadpoles at different stages of the life cycle. Endocrinology 1987;121:42

76. Galton VA, Hiebert A. The ontogeny of the enzyme systems for the 5'- and 5-deiodination of thyroid hormones in chick embryo liver. Endocrinology 1987;121:2604

77. McNabb FM, Lyons LJ, Hughes TE. Avian hepatic T_3 generation by 5'-monodeiodination: characterization of two enzymatic pathways and the effects of goitrogens. Comp Biochem Physiol [A] 1986; 85:249

78. Schwartz HL, Surks MI, Oppenheimer JH. Quantitation of extrathyroidal conversion of L-thyroxine to 3,5,3'-triiodothyronine in the rat. J Clin Invest 1971;50:1124

79. Oddie TH, Meade JH Jr, Fisher DA. An analysis of published data on thyroxine turnover in human subjects. J Clin Endocrinol Metab 1966;26:425

80. Van Middlesworth L. Metabolism and excretion of thyroid hormone. In: Greer MA, Solomon DH, eds. Handbook of physiology. Sec 7. Endocrinology. Vol 3. Thyroid. Washington, DC: American Physiological Society, 1974:215

81. Nagataki S, Uchimura H, Masuyama Y, et al. Triiodothyronine and thyroxine in thyroid glands of euthyroid Japanese subjects. J Clin Endocrinol Metab 1972;35:18

82. Abrams GM, Larsen PR. Triiodothyronine and thyroxine in the serum and thyroid glands of iodine deficient rats. J Clin Invest 1973;52:2522

83. Haibach H. Free iodothyronines in the rat thyroid gland. Endocrinology 1971;88:149

84. Laurberg P. Selective inhibition of the secretion of triiodothyronines from the perfused canine thyroid by propylthiouracil. Endocrinology 1978;103:900

85. Laurberg P. Iodothyronine secretion from perfused dog thyroid lobes after prolonged thyrotropin treatment in vivo. Endocrinology. 1981;109:1560

86. Wu SY, Reggio R, Florsheim W, Chopra IJ, Solomon DH. Stimulation of thyroidal iodothyronine 5'-monodeiodinase by long-acting thyroid stimulator (LATS). Acta Endocrinol (Copenh) 1987; 114:193

87. Chanoine JP, Braverman LE, Farwell AP, et al. The thyroid gland is a major source of circulating T_3 in the rat. J Clin Invest 1991; 87:2709

88. Chanoine JP, Safran M, Farwell AP, et al. Effects of selenium deficiency on thyroid hormone economy in rats. Endocrinology 1992;131:1787

89. Chanoine JP, Veronikis I, Alex S, et al. The postnatal serum 3,5,3'-triiodothyronine (T_3) surge in the rat is largely independent of extrathyroidal 5'-deiodination of thyroxine to T_3. Endocrinology 1993;133:2604

90. Roche J, Michael R, Nunez J. Sur la presence de la 3,3',5'-triiodothyronine dans le sang de rat. C R Soc Biol (Paris) 1956;105:20

91. Pittman HA, Brown RW, Register HB Jr. Biological activity of 3,3',5'-triiodo-DL-thyronine. Endocrinology 1962;70:79

92. Stasilli NR, Kroc RL, Meltzer R. Antigoitrogenic and calorigenic activities of thyroxine analogues in rats. Endocrinology 1959; 64:62

93. Dunn JT, Stanbury JB. The metabolism of 3,3',5'triiodothyronine in man. J Clin Endocrinol Metab 1958;18:713

94. Chopra IJ, Sack J, Fisher DA. Circulating 3,3'5'triiodothyronine (reverse T_3) in the human newborn. J Clin Invest 1975;55:1137

95. Chopra IJ, Solomon DH, Chopra U, et al. Reciprocal changes in serum reverse T_3 (rT_3) and T_3 in systemic illnesses: evidence for independent pathways of T_4 metabolism in adults. J Clin Endocrinol Metab 1975;41:1043

96. Spaulding SW, Chopra IJ, Sherwin RS, Lyall SS. Effect of caloric restriction and dietary composition on serum T_3 and reverse T_3 in man. J Clin Endocrinol Metab 1976;42:197

97. Eisenstein Z, Hagg S, Vagenakis AG, et al. Effect of starvation on the production and peripheral metabolism of 3,3',5-triiodothyronine in euthyroid obese subjects. J Clin Endocrinol Metab 1978;47:889

98. Gavin L, Castle J, McMahon F, et al. Extrathyroidal conversion of thyroxine to 3,3',5'-triiodothyronine (reverse T_3) and to 3,5,3'-triiodothyronine (T_3) in humans. J Clin Endocrinol Metab 1977; 44:733

99. Premchandra BN. Radioimmunoassay of reverse triiodothyronine. J Clin Endocrinol Metab 1978;47:746

100. Smallridge RC, Wartofsky L, Desjardins RE, et al. Metabolic clearance and production rates of 3,3′,5′triiodothyronine in hyperthyroid, euthyroid, and hypothyroid subjects. J Clin Endocrinol Metab 1978;47:345

101. Suda AK, Pittman CS, Shimizu T, et al. The production and metabolism of 3,5,3′-triiodothyronine and 3,3′,5′triiodothyronine in normal and fasting subjects. J Clin Endocrinol Metab 1978;47:1311

102. Chopra IJ, Wu SY, Nakamura Y, et al. Monodeiodination of 3,5,3′-triiodothyronine (T$_3$) and 3,3′,5′-triiodothyronine (reverse T$_3$) to 3,3′-diiodothyronine (T$_2$) in vitro. Endocrinology 1978; 102:1099

103. Chopra IJ. Crandall BF. Thyroid hormones and thyrotropin in amniotic fluid. N Engl J Med 1975;293:740

104. Chopra IJ. Kinetics of peripheral metabolism and production rates of T$_3$s. Monogr Endocrinol 1981;18:95

105. Chopra IJ, Solomon DH, Chopra U, et al. Pathways of metabolism of thyroid hormones. Recent Prog Horm Res 1978;34:521

106. Kaptein EM, Kaptein JS, Chang EI, Egodaxe PM, Nicoloff JT, Massy SG. Thyroxine transfer and distribution in critical nonthyroidal illnesses, chronic renal failure, and chronic ethanol abuse. J Clin Endocrinol Metab 1987;65:606

107. Kaptein EM, Quien-Verde H, Chooljian CJ, et al. The thyroid in end-stage renal disease. Medicine (Baltimore) 1988;67:187

108. Chopra IJ, Smith SR. Circulating thyroid hormones and thyrotropin in adult patients with protein-calorie malnutrition. J Clin Endocrinol Metab 1975;40:221

109. Vagenakis AG, Burger A, Portnay GI, et al. Diversion of peripheral thyroxine metabolism from activating to inactivating pathways during complete fasting. J Clin Endocrinol Metab 1975; 41:191

110. Surks MI, Schadlow AR, Oppenheimer JH. A new radioimmunoassay for plasma L-triiodothyronine: measurements in thyroid disease and in patients maintained on hormonal replacement. J Clin Invest 1972;51:3104

111. Pittman CS, Suda AK, Chambers JB Jr, et al. Abnormalities of thyroid hormone turnover in patients with diabetes mellitus before and after insulin therapy. J Clin Endocrinol Metab 1979;48:854

112. Burger A. Schulter M, Sakaloff C, et al. A radioimmunoassay (RIA) for serum tetraiodothyroacetic acid. Clin Res 1974;22:236

113. Crossley DN, Ramsden DB. Serum tetraiodothyroacetate (TA4) levels in normal healthy euthyroid individuals determined by gas chromatography-mass fragmentography (GC-MF). Clin Chim Acta 1979;94:267

114. Galeazzi RL, Burger AG. The metabolism of 3,3′diiodothyronine in man. J Clin Endocrinol Metab 1980;50:148

115. Gavin LA, Livermore BM, Cavalieri RR, et al. Serum concentration, metabolic clearance, and production rates of 3,5,3′-triiodothyroacetic acid in normal and athyrotic man. J Clin Endocrinol Metab 1980;51:529

116. Smallridge RC, Burman KD, Smith CE, et al. Metabolic clearance and production rates of 3′,5′-diiodothyronine in hyperthyroidism and hypothyroidism in man: comparison of infusions using radiolabeled versus unlabeled iodothyronines. J Clin Endocrinol Metab 1981 ;52:722

117. Chopra IJ, Wu SY, Chua Teco GN, et al. A radioimmunoassay for measurement of 3,5,3′-triiodothyronine sulfate: studies in thyroidal and nonthyroidal diseases, pregnancy, and neonatal life. J Clin Endocrinol Metab 1992;75:189

118. Chopra IJ, Santini F, Hurd RE, et al. A radioimmunoassay for measurement of thyroxine sulfate. J Clin Endocrinol Metab 1993; 76:145

119. Chopra IJ, Santini F, Wu SY, et al. The role of sulfation and desulfation in thyroid hormone metabolism. In: Wu SY, Visser TJ, eds. Thyroid hormone metabolism: molecular biology and alternate pathways. Boca Raton, FL: CRC Press, 1994:119

120. Wu SY, Huang WS, Polk D, et al. The development of a radioimmunoassay for reverse triiodothyronine sulfate in human serum and amniotic fluid. J Clin Endocrinol Metab 1993;76:1625

121. Pittman CS, Shimizu T, Burger A, Chambers JB Jr. The nondeiodinative pathways of thyroxine metabolism: 3,5,3′,5′-tetraiodothyroacetic acid turnover in normal and fasting human subjects. J Clin Endocrinol Metab 1980;50:712

122. Willets P, Crossley DN, Ramsden DB, Hoffenberg R. The role of thyronine in thyroid hormone metabolism. J Clin Endocrinol Metab 1979;49:658

123. Visser TJ, Mol JA, Otten MH. Rapid deiodination of triiodothyronine sulfate by rat liver microsomal fraction. Endocrinology 1983;112:1547

124. Lopresti JS, Mizuno L, Nimalsuriya A, et al. Characteristics of 3,5,3′-triiodothyronine sulfate metabolism in euthyroid man. J Clin Endocrinol Metab 1991;73:703

125. Lopresti JS, Nicoloff JT. 3,5,3′-Triiodothyronine (T$_3$) sulfate: a major metabolite in T$_3$ metabolism in man. J Clin Endocrinol Metab 1994;78:688

126. Santini F, Hurd RE, Lee B, Chopra IJ. Thyromimetic effects of 3,5,3′-triiodothyronine sulfate in hypothyroid rat. Endocrinology 1993;133:105

127. Chopra IJ, Solomon DH, Chua Teco GN. Thyroxine: just a prohormone or a hormone too? J Clin Endocrinol Metab 1973;36:1959

128. Cheron RG, Kaplan MM, Larsen PR. Divergent changes of thyroxine 5′-monodeiodination in rat pituitary and liver during maturation. Endocrinology 1980;106:1405

129. Nomura S, Pittman CS, Chambers JB Jr, et al. Reduced peripheral conversion of thyroxine to triiodothyronine in patients with hepatic cirrhosis. J Clin Invest 1975;80:643

130. Portnay GI, O'Brian JT, Bush J, et al. The effect of starvation on the concentration and binding of thyroxine and triiodothyronine in serum and on the response to TRH. J Clin Endocrinol Metab 1974;39:191

131. Arem R, Wiener GH, Daplan G, Kim HS, Reichlin SW, Kaplan MM. Reduced tissue thyroid hormone in fatal illness. Metabolism 1993;42:1102

132. Bacci V, Schussler GC, Kaplan TB. The relationship between serum triiodothyronine and thyrotropin during systemic illness. J Clin Endocrinol Metab 1982;45:1229

133. Hamblin PS, Dyer SA, Mohr VS, et al. Relationship between thyrotropin and thyroxine changes during recovery from severe hypothyroxinemia of critical illness. J Clin Endocrinol Metab 1986; 62:717

134. Portnay GI, O'Brian JT, Rudolph M, et al. Evidence of a probable decrease in T$_4$ to T$_3$ conversion during starvation in man. In: Abstracts of the 50th annual meeting of the American Thyroid Association, St. Louis, September 18–21, 1974:T-15

135. Surks MI, Schadlow AR, Stock JM, Oppenheimer JH. Determination of iodothyronine absorption and conversion of L-thyroxine (T$_4$) to L-triiodothyronine (T$_3$) using turnover rate techniques. J Clin Invest 1973;52:805

136. Chopra IJ, Hershman JM, Hornabrook RW. A study of serum thyroid hormone and thyrotropin levels in subjects from endemic goiter regions of New Guinea. J Clin Endocrinol Metab 1975; 40:326

137. DeLange F, Camus M, Ermans AM. Circulating thyroid hormones in endemic goiter. J Clin Endocrinol Metab 1972;34:891

138. Patel YC, Pharoah POD, Hornabrook RW, Hetzel BS. Serum triiodothyronine, thyroxine and thyroid stimulating hormone in endemic goiter: a comparison of goitrous and nongoitrous subjects in New Guinea. J Clin Endocrinol Metab 1973;37:783

139. Acheson KJ, Burger AG. A study of the relationship between thermogenesis and thyroid hormones. J Clin Endocrinol Metab 1980;51:84

140. Money WL, Kimaoka S, Rawson RW, Kroc RL. Comparative effects of thyroxine analogues in experimental animals. Ann NY Acad Sci 1960;86:512

141. Breuil AD. Galton VA. Thyroxine: studies concerning the intrinsic physiological activity. Acta Endocrinol (Copenh) 1978; 99:87

142. Adamson LF, Ingbar SH. Some properties of the stimulatory effect of thyroid hormones on amino acid transport by embryonic chick bone. Endocrinology 1967;81:1372

143. Marcus R. Cyclic nucleotide phosphodiesterase from bone: characterization of the enzyme and studies of inhibition by thyroid hormones. Endocrinology 1975;96:400

144. Marcus R, Lundquist C, Chopra IJ. In vitro inhibition of cyclic nucleotide phosphodiesterase (PDE) by thyroid hormones. Clin Res 1975;23:94A

145. Golde DW, Bersch N, Chopra IJ, Cline MJ. Potentiation of erythropoiesis in vitro by thyroid hormones. Br J Haematol 1977; 37:173

146. Blanchard RF, Davis PJ. Specific interaction of thyroid hormones with rat renal Na, K-ATPase in vitro. Clin Res 1979:27:248A

147. Davis FB, Davis PJ, Blas SB. Role of calmodulin in thyroid hormone stimulation in vitro of human erythrocyte Ca^{2+}-ATPase activity. J Clin Invest 1983;71:579

148. Farwell AP, Lynch RM, Okulicz WC, Comi AM, Leonard JL. The actin cytoskeleton mediates the hormonally regulated translocation of type II iodothyronine 5′-deiodinase in astrocytes. J Biol Chem 1990;265:18546

149. Siegrist-Kaiser CA, Juge AC, Tranter MP, Ekenbarger DM, Leonard JL. Thyroxine-dependent modulation of actin polymerization in cultured astrocytes: a novel, extranuclear action of thyroid hormone. J Biol Chem 1990;265:5296

150. Leonard JL, Siegrist-Kaiser CA, Zuckerman CJ. Regulation of type II iodothyronine 5′-deiodinase by thyroid hormone. Inhibition of actin polymerization blocks enzyme in activation in cAMP-stimulated glial cells. J Biol Chem 1990;265:940

151. Farwell AP, Leonard JL. Dissociation of actin polymerization and enzyme in activation in the hormonal regulation of type II iodothyronine 5′-deiodinase activity in astrocytes. Endocrinology 1992;131:721

152. Farwell AP, Dibenedetto DJ, Leonard JL. Thyroxine targets different pathways of internalization of type II iodothyronine 5′-deiodinase in astrocytes. J Biol Chem 1993:268:5055

153. Geffner DL, Azukizawa M, Hershman JM. Propylthiouracil blocks extrathyroidal conversion of thyroxine to triiodothyronine and augments TSH secretion in man. J Clin Invest 1975;55:224

154. Saberi M, Sterling FH, Utiger RD. Reduction in extrathyroidal triiodothyronine production by propylthiouracil in man. J Clin Invest 1975;55:338

155. Oppenheimer JH, Schwartz HL, Surks MI. Propylthiouracil inhibits the conversion of L-thyroxine to L-triiodothyronine: an explanation of the antithyroxine effect of propylthiouracil and evidence supporting the concept that triiodothyronine is the primary thyroid hormone. J Clin Invest 1972;51:2493

156. Oppenheimer JH, Koerner D, Schwartz HL, Surks MI. Specific nuclear triiodothyronine binding sites in rat liver and kidney. J Clin Endocrinol Metab 1972;35:330

157. Schadlow AR, Surks MI, Schwartz HL, Oppenheimer JH. Specific triiodothyronine sites in rat anterior pituitary. Science 1972;176:1252

158. Larsen PR, Silva JE, Kaplan M. Relationship between circulating and intracellular thyroid hormones: physiological and clinical implications. Endocr Rev 1981;2:87

159. Silva JE, Dick TE, Larsen PR. The contribution of local tissue thyroxine monodeiodination to the nuclear 3,5,3′-triiodothyronine in pituitary, liver and kidney of euthyroid rats. Endocrinology 1978; 103:1196

160. Pittman CS, Barker SB. Antithyroxine effects of some thyroxine analogues. Am J Physiol 1959;197:1271

161. Pittman JA, Tingley JO, Nickerson JF, Hill SR Jr. Antimetabolic activity of 3,3′,5′-triiodo-DL, thyronine in man. Metabolism 1960;9:293

162. Benua RS, Kumaoka S, Leeper RD, Rawson RW. The effect of DL-3,3′,5′-triiodothyronine in Graves' disease. J Clin Endocrinol Metab 1959;19:1344

163. Pittman CS, Shinohara M, Thrasher H, McGraw EF. Effect of thyroxine analogues on the peripheral metabolism of thyroxine: the half-life and pattern of elimination. Endocrinology 1964;74:611

164. Chopra IJ. Study of extrathyroidal conversion T_4 to T_3 in vitro. Endocrinology 1977;101:453

165. Han DC, Sato K, Fujii Y, et al. 3,3′,5′-Triiodothyronine inhibits ontogenetic development of iodothyronine-5′-deiodinase in the liver of neonatal mouse. Acta Endocrinol (Copenh) 1988; 119:181

166. Han DC, Sato K, Fujii Y, Tsushima T, Shizume K. 3,3′,5′-Triiodothyronine inhibits iodothyronine-5′deiodinating activity induced by 3,5,3′-triiodothyronine at equimolar concentration in cultured fetal mouse liver. Endocrinology 1986;119:1076

167. Larsen FC, Albright EC. Inhibition of L-thyroxine monodeiodination by thyroxine analogs. J Clin Invest 1961;40:1132

168. Coiro V, Harris A, Goodman HM, Vagenakis A, Braverman L. Effect of pharmacological quantities of infused 3,3′,5′-triiodothyronine on thyroxine monodeiodination to 3,5,3′-triiodothyronine. Endocrinology 1980;106:68

169. Hagg D, Poitz M, Ingbar SH. In vitro inhibitory effect of reverse triiodothyronine (rT_3) on lipolysis in rat adipocytes. In: Abstracts of 54th annual meeting of the American Thyroid Association, Portland, Oregon, September 13–16, 1978

170. Papavasiliou SS, Martial JA, Latham KR, et al. Thyroid hormone-like actions 3,3′,5′-L-triiodothyronine and 3,3′-diiodothyronine. J Clin Invest 1977;60:1230

171. Fishman M, Huang YP, Tergis DC, et al. Relation of tniiodothyronine and reverse triiodothyronine administration rats to hepatic L-triiodothyronine aminotransferase activity. Endocrinology 1977; 100:1055

172. Davis FB, Cutten AEC, Smith HC, Rashford VE, Waite KV, Eastman CJ. Deiodination of reverse 3,3′,5′-triiodothyronine by hepatic nuclear protein preparations. Endocrinology 1984; 115:600

173. Smith HC, Robinson SR, Eastman CJ. Binding of reverse T_3 to hepatic nuclear protein. Aust J Exp Biol Med Sci 1980;58:207

174. Wiersinga WM, Chopra IJ, Solomon DH. Specific nuclear binding sites triiodothyronine (T_3) and reverse triiodothyronine (rT_3) in rat and pork liver: similarities and discrepancies. Endocrinology 1982;110:2052

175. DeLuca HF. The kidney as endocrine organ for the production of 1,25-dihydroxyvitamin D_3, a calcium-mobilizing hormone. N Engl J Med 1973;289:359

176. Omdahl JL, DeLuca HF. Regulation of vitamin D metabolism and function. Physiol Rev 1973;53:327

177. Tanaka Y, DeLuca HF. Stimulation of 24,25-dihydroxyvitamin D_3 production by 1,25-di-hydroxyvitamin D_3. Science 1974; 183:1198

178. Sherman SI, Ladenson PW. Organ specific effects of tiractricol: a thyroid hormone analog with hepatic, not pituitary, superagonist effects. J Clin Endocrinol Metab 1992;75:901

179. Goldfine O, Smith GJ, Simmons GC, et al. Activities of thyroid hormones and related compounds in an in vitro thymocyte assay. J Biol Chem 1976;251:4233

180. Mandel LR. Kuehl FA. Lipolytic action of 3,3′,5-triiodo-L-thyronine. Biochem Biophys Res Commun 1967;28:13

181. Bianchi R, Zuccelli GL, Giannessi D, et al. Evaluation of triiodothyronine (T_3) kinetics in normal subjects, in hypothyroid, and hyperthyroid patients using specific antiserum for the determination of labeled T_3 in plasma. J Clin Endocrinol Metab 1978;46:203

182. Inada M, Kasagi K, Kurata S, et al. Estimation of thyroxine and triiodothyronine distribution and of conversion rate of thyroxine to triiodothyronine in man. J Clin Invest 1975;55:1337

183. Oppenheimer JH, Schwartz HL, Surks MI. Revised calculations of common parameters of iodothyronine metabolism and distribution by noncompartmental analysis. J Clin Endocrinol Metab 1975;41:1172

184. Green WL, Ingbar SH. The peripheral metabolism of tri- and tetraiodothyroacetic acids in man. J Clin Endocrinol Metab 1961; 21:1548

185. Ramsden DB, Crossley DN. Serum concentration of 3,5,3′,5′-tetraiodothyroacetate (T_4A) in subjects with hypo-, hyper- and euthyroidism. Acta Endocrinol (Copenh) 1986;112:192

Werner and Ingbar's The Thyroid, Seventh Edition,
edited by Lewis E. Braverman and Robert D. Utiger.
Lippincott–Raven Publishers, Philadelphia, © 1996

8

Intracellular Pathways of Iodothyronine Metabolism

Jack L. Leonard
Josef Koehrle

In 1915, Kendall[1] isolated the principal secretory product of the thyroid gland, thyroxine (T_4). Four decades later, triiodothyronine (T_3), an iodothyronine three to four times more potent than T_4 in eliciting metabolic responses,[2] was identified in thyroidal extracts.[3–5] Although initially it was thought that T_3 was exclusively of thyroidal origin,[4] in 1955 Pitt-Rivers and coworkers[6] proposed that in vivo conversion of T_4 to T_3 occurred in athyrotic humans; however, this was later retracted.[7] Two years later, the presence of T_3 in serum of athyrotic patients was reported,[8] but the conversion of T_4 to T_3 was not accepted until 1970, when the generation of T_3 from therapeutic doses of T_4 in athyrotic patients[9] and the conversion of T_4 to T_3 in normal humans[10] were demonstrated.

The discovery of other, lesser iodinated thyronines in thyroglobulin, such as $3,3',5'$-T_3 (reverse T_3 [rT_3]) and $3,3'$-T_2, stimulated the search for these compounds in vivo.[11] The identification of $3,3'$-T_2 in the plasma of hepatectomized dogs led to the suggestion that this iodothyronine was a metabolite of T_3, possibly a sulfated derivative. Both rT_3 and $3,3'$-T_2 were also found to be derived from T_4[12]; $3,3'$-T_2 and $3'$-T_1 from rT_3; and $3'$-T_1 from $3,3'$-T_2.[13] Both sulfoconjugated and glucuronoconjugated iodothyronines were also found in plasma and urine.[14] These early in vivo studies were limited by the lack of sensitive and specific methods to identify individual iodothyronines. Artifactual deiodination of the radiolabeled hormone(s) was a persistent technical problem that was solved only after the development of specifically labeled iodothyronines for kinetic investigations and sensitive radioimmunoassays. These techniques have now enabled us to provide a summary of the serum concentrations and production rates for individual iodothyronines (Table 8-1) in normal subjects. Thus, it is apparent that determination of the the *thyroid status* of an individual requires knowledge not only of the glandular production of T_4,

but of the intracellular metabolic transformations of this hormone in different tissues (Fig 8-1). The focus of this chapter is the physiology of $5'$- ($3'$-) (phenolic ring) and 5- (3-) (tyrosyl ring) deiodination, but the other pathways shown in Figure 8-2 are also be discussed briefly.

PATHWAYS OF SEQUENTIAL THYROXINE MONODEIODINATION

Soon after the first reports of T_4 to T_3 conversion in vivo, it was suggested that T_4 has little intrinsic metabolic activity. This proposal was based on the assumptions that (1) the T_3 generated in tissues exchanged readily with the entire T_3 pool, and (2) the removal of iodine from the phenolic and tyrosyl rings proceeded in a random fashion. Although early on it was generally accepted that the biologic responses of target tissues were ultimately determined by T_3 delivered from the serum,[15] it is now clear that these assumptions do not hold for individual target tissues.

There is compelling evidence that T_3 acts by binding to specific chromatin-bound receptors located in the cell nucleus.[16] These T_3 receptors belong to the c-*erb* A superfamily, which is a group of related protooncogenes that encode ligand-modulated transcription activation factors.[17–20] Members of this family bind small, hydrophobic molecules such as thyroid and steroid hormones, retinoids and vitamin D_3 (see chap 9). The concept of a direct correlation between plasma T_3 levels and initiation of thyroid hormone action mediated by hormone binding to its receptor[21] has been modified in light of the demonstration that individual target tissues generate T_3 for local use, and by the identification of multiple variants of the T_3 receptor.

TABLE 8-1.
Serum Concentrations and Turnover Kinetics of Iodothyronines as Derived from Thyroid Gland
Secretion and Intracellular T_4 Deiodination*

Iodothyronine	Serum Concentration (nmol/L)	Metabolic Clearance Rate (L/d)	Production Rate (nmol/d)	Conversion Rate (%)
Thyroxine (T_4)	80–106	1.19–1.32	104–126	—
Triiodothyronine (T_3)	1.40–2.64	19.5–28.9	40.4–61.8	35–48
Reverse triiodothyronine (rT_3)	0.15–0.40	82–157	22.8–54.9	40.3 ± 12.6
3,5-Diiodothyronine (3,5-T_2)	0.008–0.196	59–168	1.1–9.3	15 ± 5
3,3′-Diiodothyronine (3,3′-T_2)	0.018–0.324	560–1084	35–76	56 ($T_3 \rightarrow$ 3,3′-T_2) 40 (r$T_3 \rightarrow$ 3,3′-T_2)
3′,5′-Diiodothyronine (3′,5′-T_2)	0.012–0.137	159–354	10.9–48.4	29.1 ± 8.2
3-Monoiodothyronine (3-T_1)	?	?	?	?
3′-Monoiodothyronine (3′-T_1)	0.007–0.060	500 ± 135	29.7 ± 15.1	?
Thyronine (T_0)	?	?	15 (?)	?

Data are corrected for 70 kg of body weight.
For references and details, see Faber J. The metabolism of iodothyronines in health and disease with special reference to di-iodothyronines. Thesis, Medical Faculty University of Kopenhagen, Denmark, 1983, Laegeforeningens Forlag.

Thyroid-stimulating hormone (TSH; thyrotropin) secretion appears to be modulated by both T_4 and T_3, leading to the proposal that T_4 has intrinsic hormonal activity. Intrapituitary T_4-to-T_3 conversion is likely to participate in the T_4-dependent modulation of TSH synthesis and secretion,[22–25] possibly by thy- rotroph-specific deiodinating enzymes. This "locally produced" T_3 does not appear to exchange with the circulating T_3 pool,[24] providing support for the presence of nonexchangeable ("hidden") T_3 pools. Nonexchangeable, hidden pools may be found also for the other iodothyronines derived from T_4.[26–28]

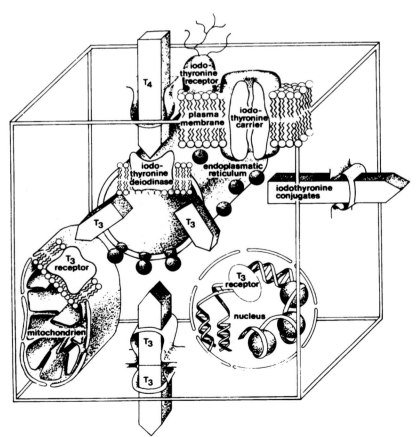

FIGURE 8-1. Model of cellular iodothyronine receptors, binding sites, and metabolic pathways. (Köhrle J, Brabant G, Hesch RD: Metabolism of thyroid hormones. Hormone Res 1987;26:58)

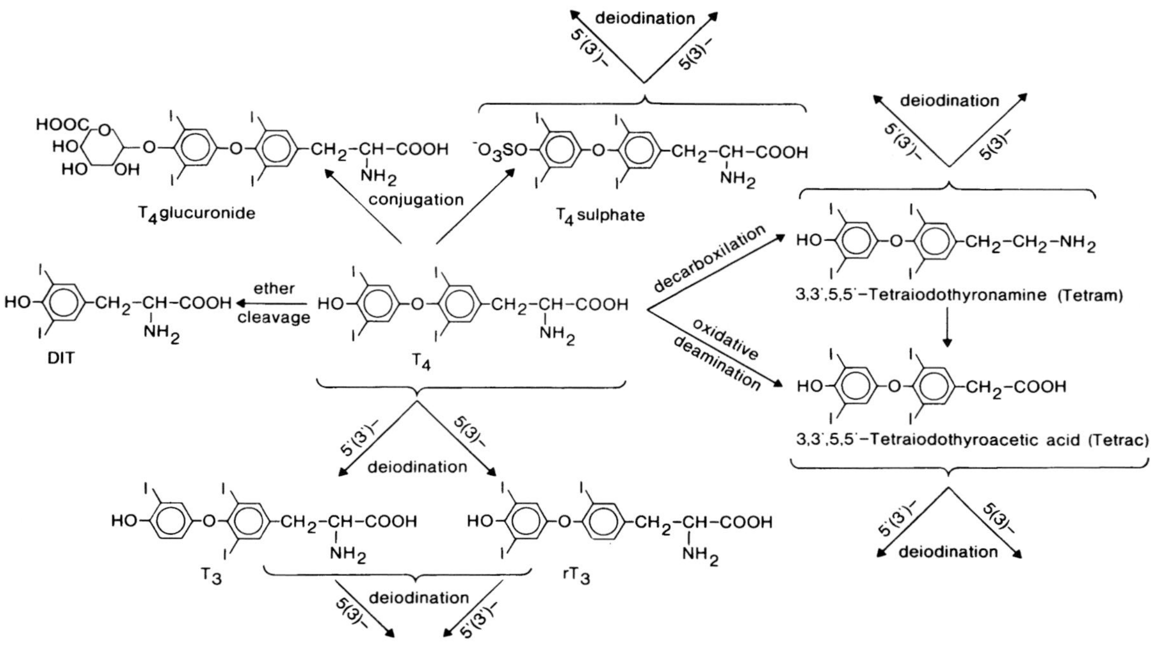

FIGURE 8-2. Pathways of thyroxine metabolism. (Köhrle J, Brabant G, Hesch RD: Metabolism of thyroid hormones. Hormone Res 1987;26:58)

Tissue-specific iodothyronine deiodinase isozymes produce a substantial fraction of the T_3 bound to nuclear receptors in pituitary, brain, and brown adipose tissue. Thus, target tissue generation of deiodination products of T_4, such as T_3, rT_3, $3,5$-T_2, and possibly other iodothyronines with hormonal action, is of particular interest in biosystems that do not freely exchange these bioactive molecules. The large reserves of protein-bound T_4 have renewed importance for intracellular thyroid hormone metabolism and action.

The deiodination of T_4 occurs by stepwise, sequential removal of iodine atoms from either the phenolic or tyrosyl ring. This deiodination cascade is shown in Figure 8-3. Both phenolic ring ($5'$- or $3'$-) and tyrosyl ring (5- or 3-) deiodination have now been demonstrated in vivo and in vitro. About 70% of the T_4 secreted daily is deiodinated to yield equal amounts of T_3 and rT_3. For T_3, 70% to 90% of the daily production originates from extrathyroidal deiodination from T_4, with the rest derived from the thyroid. From 95% to 98% of the rT_3 produced daily is generated by deiodination, and only a minute amount of rT_3 is derived from the thyroid. Subsequent deiodination of T_3 and rT_3 yields the three T_2s—$3,5$-T_2, $3,3'$-T_2, and $3',5'$-T_2. This combined daily production amounts to about two thirds of the total production of T_3 and rT_3. These data indicate that nondeiodinative pathways account for about one third of the metabolism of iodothyronines (see chap 7).

CLASSIFICATION OF IODOTHYRONINE DEIODINASE ISOZYMES

Two general types of deiodination reactions, *5'-deiodination* and *5-deiodination*, have been identified. These two pathways generate all of the iodothyronines shown in the deiodi-nation cascade, from the fully iodinated form (T_4) to the iodine-free thyronine molecule (T_0).

The basic characteristics of these enzymic reactions were established using tissue homogenates or subcellular particulate fractions from different species. The specific deiodinated metabolites were detected by specific radioimmunoassays, chromatographic analysis, or immunosequestration, and catalysis proved to depend on the protein concentration of the particulate fraction.[24,29–35] These deiodination reactions in mammals show a clear temperature optimum near 37°C, and the enzymes are heat labile.[32,36] The energy of activation and the Q_{10} factor of the reactions have not yet been determined. Some early work suggested that iodothyronine deiodination was activated by flavin mononucleotide, trypsin, heat, oxygen, and light, and was possibly mediated by a lipid peroxidation process catalyzed by ferrous ions and involving free radicals.[37] However, this hypothesis was based on the liberation of radioactive iodide from radiolabeled iodothyronine, and subsequent attempts to identify the iodothyronine metabolite proved fruitless.[37]

Phenolic Ring 5'- (3'-) Deiodination: Bioactivating Reaction

Removal of the $5'$- (or $3'$-) iodine atom from the phenolic ring of iodothyronines is designated *5'-deiodination*. The two phenolic ring iodine atoms are chemically equivalent owing to rotation around the diphenyl ether bond of the thyronine molecule. Iodine atoms present in the 5- or 3- positions, however, hinder this rotation and create a somewhat different chemical environment for the proximal $5'$- and the distal $3'$-iodine atoms. Because current methods do not distinguish which iodine atom is removed first, the terms *5'-deiodination* and *phenolic ring* deiodination are used synonymously. Removal of the remaining $3'$- iodine after $5'$-deiodination has

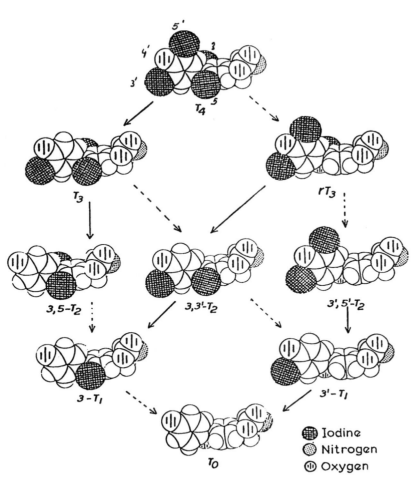

FIGURE 8-3. Pathways of the sequential monodeiodination cascade of thyroxine and other iodothyronines. Solid arrows illustrate 5'-deiodination routes, broken arrows 5-deiodination routes. (Köhrle J, Auf'mkolk M, Spanka M, Irmscher K, Cody V, Hesch RD: Iodothyronine deiodinase is inhibited by plant flavonoids. In: Cody V, Middleton E Jr, Harborne JB, eds. Progress in clinical and biological research. 1986;213:359)

also been demonstrated for both unconjugated and sulfoconjugated iodothyronines, and in one report for glucuronide conjugates. Because T_3 is obtained from the 5'-deiodination of T_4, 5'-deiodination bioactivates thyroid hormone. The addition of reduced thiols is absolutely required to measure 5'-deiodination in vitro if cytosolic fractions containing the still unknown thiol cofactor system are separated from the enzyme-containing membrane fraction.

Two isotypes of 5'-deiodinase (types I and II) have been identified by differences in (1) their substrate preference, (2) their degree of susceptibility to inhibition by 6-n-propyl-2-thiouracil (PTU), and (3) their response to physiologic perturbations. In the past, these isozymes were identified by operational definitions and not as specific polypeptides. The activities of the 5'-deiodinases are related to protein concentration, and are sensitive to proteases, time, and temperature; the deiodinase thus have all the characteristics of specific enzyme reactions.

Tyrosyl Ring 5- (3-) Deiodination: Bioinactivating Reaction

Removal of a single 5- (or 3-) iodine atom from the tyrosyl ring of iodothyronines is designated *5-deiodination*. In contrast to the 3'- and 5'- iodine atoms, which can be distinguished from each other, the 3- and 5- iodine atoms of T_4 are

chemically, energetically, and sterically equivalent. Enzymic 5-deiodination reactions are major routes for degradation of T_4, T_3, the diiodothyronines, and the monoiodothyronines.

The metabolites of T_4 generated by 5-deiodination reactions are devoid of calorigenic or thyromimetic potency; therefore this reaction has been designated a *bioinactivating* pathway. This reaction is key to the recycling of iodide and also yields rT_3, a competitive substrate for 5'-deiodination of T_4, and may represent an important pathway for the regulation of thyroid hormone metabolism and action.[38,39] Despite its importance in thyroid hormone economy, 5-deiodination has received much lower attention than 5'-deiodination and is less well characterized in vitro and in vivo.

At least three types of 5-deiodinating reactions are known. The type I 5'-deiodinase present in several tissues and species, as well as that found in transfected primate cells expressing the rat liver type I 5'-deiodinase cDNA, also catalyzes tyrosyl ring 5-deiodination, probably through some "wobble" in the active center that becomes apparent under certain in vitro incubation conditions.[39–41] Sulfation of the phenolic ring hydroxyl of iodothyronines also enhances 5-deiodination by several orders of magnitude, and therefore has profound effects on iodothyronine metabolism. A more specific 5-deiodinase has been demonstrated in brain, skin, and placenta, and this enzyme has catalytic properties that differ from the promiscuous liver enzyme. cDNAs from *Xenopus* and tadpole tails and rat skin have been cloned that code for selenocysteine-containing polypeptides catalyzing the 5-deiodination reaction and show homology to the cloned type I 5'-deiodinase cDNAs.[42–44] Conflicting data have been reported on the kinetic parameters, thiol requirements, and degree of PTU inhibition of the 5-deiodinases in the various tissues, suggesting the existence of several 5-deiodinase isozymes.

TYPE I 5'-DEIODINASE

Type I 5'-deiodinase is defined by its substrate specificity, the apparent Michaelis-Menten constant (K_m) for iodothyronines, and the ability of PTU and aurothioglucose (ATG) to inhibit catalysis. This isozyme catalyzes 5'-deiodination of T_4, yielding T_3, and of rT_3, yielding $3,3'-T_2$, as well as of diiodothyronines and monoiodothyronines with phenolic ring iodines. In intact cells, tissue homogenates, or subcellular membrane preparations, the apparent limiting K_m value for T_4 (0.5–2 μmol/L) is near that for rT_3 (0.1–0.5 μmol/L) and an order of magnitude lower that that for T_3 (10–20 μmol/L). Marked differences in the maximal velocities (V_{max}) for the different iodothyronines have been reported. Using the V_{max}/K_m ratio as an indicator of substrate preference reveals that rT_3 is the preferred substrate for type I 5'-deiodinase. Iodothyronines with a free or a sulfoconjugated phenolic hydroxyl serve as type I 5'-deiodinase substrates. 5'-Deiodination of glucuronide conjugates of T_4 and T_3 could be demonstrated at tracer substrate concentrations only by sensitive high-pressure liquid chromatography analysis after incubation of radiolabeled compounds with brain and liver microsomes of rats.[45] Sulfation of the 4'-hydroxyl of T_3 and $3,3'-T_2$, but not of rT_3, markedly increases the catalytic efficiency of type I 5'-deiodinase for these iodothyronines; 4'-sulfation blocks 5'-deiodination but favors the inactivating 5-deiodination.[41,46–48] These data suggest that type type I 5'-deiodinase plays an important role in the production of T_3, the elimination of sulfoconjugated T_3 and $3,3'-T_2$, and the disposal of rT_3 under normal conditions. Micromolar concentrations of PTU and ATG completely block type I 5'-deiodinase activity.[29,30,49]

Physicochemical Properties

Despite numerous studies during the last 25 years, only limited progress has been made in the purification of the type I 5'-deiodinase enzyme. One reason for this is that type I 5'-deiodinase is an intrinsic, membrane-bound enzyme, and catalytic activity is lost during solubilization unless ionic detergents (bile salts, CHAPS) or nonionic polyoxiethylene ether detergents (W1, Renex 690) are used.[50–57] Removal of detergent or membrane phospholipids (phosphatidyl-choline or -ethanolanine) results in the loss of catalytic activity.[51,55] Unfortunately, most commonly used detergents inhibit catalytic activity, presumably by disruption of essential phospholipid–protein interactions, by detergent-induced refolding of the protein, or by sequestration of the lipophilic iodothyronine substrates. Thus, purification strategies based on chromatographic fractionation of detergent-solubilized type I 5'-deiodinase from rat liver or kidney or from beef liver result in poor enrichment.

In spite of these difficulties, many of the physical properties of the enzyme polypeptides have been estimated. Detergent-solubilized, catalytically active type I 5'-deiodinase from liver, thyroid, kidney, or the porcine kidney cell line LLC-PK$_1$, has an M_r between 50 and 70 kd, sedimentation coefficients of 3.5 to 4.35, and a Stokes' radius of 32 to 37 Å. The isoelectric point of $(NH_{4})_2SO_4$-precipitated, partially delipidated enzyme is reported to be 9.33,[50,51,53–55] whereas that of the taurodeoxycholate/Nonidet P-40–solubilized enzyme is 6.11.[58] These differences in isoelectric point are likely to reflect the contribution of salts, detergents, and phospholipid to the overall charge of the enzyme. Type I 5'-deiodinase was partially purified using affinity chromatography; however, very low yields were obtained of the two major proteins with M_r of 56 and 25 kd.[54] Antibodies raised to specific regions of the rat type I 5'-deiodinase proved useful in Western blot analysis and radioimmunometric determination of the type I 5'-deiodinase protein.[57,59] Larger amounts of functional type I 5'-deiodinase protein will probably be available after successful establishment of eukaryotic expression systems capable of cotranslationally inserting the selenocysteine into the enzyme subunits. To date, none of the purification strategies attempted that combine detergent solubilization, precipitation, and conventional and affinity chromatographic steps have separated the type I 5'-deiodinase activity from 5-deiodinase activity in liver, suggesting that a single enzyme can catalyze both 5'- and 5-deiodination in vitro.[60] Attempts at purification of type I 5'-deiodinase from other tissues have not been reported.

Biochemical Characterization and Cloning

Studies have shown that type I 5'-deiodinase is a selenoenzyme and that the "hyperreactive cysteine," previously suggested as the essential active site residue, is likely to be a selenocysteine residue.[61–63] Type I 5'-deiodinase activity in liver and kidney, but not in thyroid homogenates from selenium-deficient rats, is less than 10% of that of homogenates from selenium-repleted animals, and selenium replacement restores type I 5'-deiodinase activity.[61,62,64,65] In vivo labeling of selenoproteins with [^{75}Se]selenite results in the appearance of a 27.8-kd protein in thyroid, liver, and kidney,[61,66,67] tissues expressing the highest type I 5'-deiodinase activity. Double-labeling studies of in vivo [^{75}Se]-labeled microsomal proteins with bromoacetyl [^{125}I]T$_4$ or bromoacetyl [^{125}I]rT$_3$ revealed comigration of the two isotopes in the type I 5'-deiodinase substrate-binding subunit,[61,62] and on peptide fingerprint analysis both radioisotopes are present in a 1:1 ratio in the fragments and in the intact 27-kd subunit.[61]

The subsequent cDNA cloning of rat and human type I 5'-deiodinase confirmed the size of the enzyme subunit and revealed the presence of an *opal* codon, UGA, in the mRNA, which is translated to selenocysteine in the presence of selenium-dependent eukaryotic translation factors.[63,68–70] The likelihood of the presence of this selenocysteine in the active site of type I 5'-deiodinase and the hyperreactivity of this nucleophile toward alkylating agents such as α-haloacids, suggests that a selenocysteine and not a cysteine residue is essential for effective catalytic activity in type I 5'-deiodinase. Such an unusual amino acid in the active site of type I 5'-deiodinase explains the peculiar reaction characteristics of the type I 5'-deiodinase active site toward alkylating reagents, which differ from those of conventional cysteine residues.

mic reticulum to plasma membrane is much lower in the kidney than it is in the liver, so that a plasma membrane localization of type I 5'-deiodinase is more easily established. It has been assigned to the basolateral plasma membrane of renal epithelial cells by copurification with Na$^+$,K$^+$ adenosine triphosphatase (ATPase) activity and by the failure of the enzyme to copurify with either 5'-nucleotidase or alkaline phosphatase, markers of the apical plasma membrane. An endoplasmic reticulum localization was excluded by comparing type I 5'-deiodinase activity with the well known marker enzymes of the organelle. In the kidney, type I 5'-deiodinase is restricted to the proximal convoluted tubule of the renal cortex, and no activity has been detected in glomeruli. Consis-

these enzymes.[175] On the other hand, 5-deiodinase was present in the endoplasmic reticulum based on a different subcellular fractionation strategy, indicating its probable origin from microsomal membranes.[176,178]

In the anterior pituitary, type I 5'-deiodinase is an intrinsic membrane protein; however, the subcellular distribution of this isozyme has not been studied. Rat pituitary tumor GH$_3$ cells contain type I 5'-deiodinase activity in the particulate fraction, but the subcellular location has not yet been assigned.[179] No data exist on the subcellular localization of the deiodinating enzymes in skeletal muscle, heart, thyroid, membranes of fetal tissues, or circulating blood cells, and limited information is available in skin and adipose tissue.

plotted, a set of lines that intersect on the I/v axis results[93] (see Fig 8-6C). These results lead to the conclusion that thiouracils are competitive inhibitors with respect to the cofactor thiols and uncompetitive inhibitors with respect to the iodothyronine substrate. Thus, a decrease in the concentration of cofactor produces an effect on the enzyme activity similar to that produced by addition of thiouracils; that is, the apparent K_m and V_{max} values decrease.[93]

Apart from regenerating the reduced selenocysteyl residue essential for catalysis, reduced thiols may also indirectly prevent oxidation-induced conformational changes leading to inactivation of the enzyme. Type I 5'-deiodinase activity is impaired by Hg, Ag, iodoacetic acid, N-ethylmaleimide, and mercury-containing compounds (e.g., p-chloro- or p-hydrox-~~ymercuribenzoic acid, merthiolate, and mercuhydrin), as well~~

uptake of the hormone, either by diffusion through the plasma membrane or by active or facilitated transport of the iodothyronine after binding to specific cell surface sites; and (4) transfer of the internalized iodothyronine to cytosol binding sites or nuclear receptors, initiating thyromimetic effects. The ability of target tissues to modify the biologic potency of iodothyronines by deiodination adds an important level of control to this cascade of thyroid hormone action. To unravel the sequence of events, it is necessary to know the subcellular distribution of the deiodinating enzymes.

The subcellular location of type I 5'-deiodinase is likely to differ from organ to organ. The enzyme is an integral membrane protein and the localization of the enzyme to a particular subcellular organelle is largely operational, depending on ~~the availability of biochemical markers, because immunohisto-~~

Principles of Determination of Type I 5'-Deiodinase Activity

Deiodination depends on protein, temperature, pH, and the time of incubation, and conditions for initial rate enzyme kinetics have been established.[24,36,39,46–48] Substrate or products are determined either by specific radioimmunologic or chromatographic methods.

Demonstration of a 1:1 stoichiometry ratio of iodide and iodothyronine production is a mandatory prerequisite both for specificity of the deiodination reaction and for exclusion of nonspecific dehalogenation. Unlike T_4, which can be deiodinated in both the phenolic and the tyrosyl ring, rT_3 is much less susceptible to tyrosyl ring deiodination at neutral pH. rT_3 has been shown to be an excellent competitive inhibitor of 5'-deiodination of T_4, and this property was exploited to develop a sensitive and rapid 5'-deiodinase assay.[91,94]

PH OPTIMUM

The pH optimum for 5'-deiodination differs from that of 5-deiodination for unconjugated iodothyronines.[38,180] Type I 5'-deiodinase activity is highest in a slightly acid to neutral pH (6.5–7.5), whereas 5-deiodinase activity proceeds more rapidly when the pH is higher than 8.0. It has been suggested that the pH optimum for the site of deiodination is primarily determined by the pK_a values of the 4'-OH group (Fig 8-7). Analysis of the pH optima for 5'- and 5-deiodination of various iodothyronines and their analogues clearly indicates that pH-dependent alterations of functional residues in the enzyme active site also contribute to the choice of which ring will be deiodinated.[46,181]

Several other amino acids appear to participate in catalysis by type I 5'-deiodinase. Histidine residues are located close to the substrate binding site and contribute in the type I 5'-deiodinase reaction, as judged by the rapid inactivation of the enzyme by the histidine-specific reagents, diethylpyrocarbonate or rose bengal.[182] Histidine residues are known to form ion pairs with nucleophilic side chains such as cysteines[183] or, presumably, selenocysteines, and pH-dependent changes in the dissociation state of a thiolate–imidazolium ion pair provide a plausible explanation for effects of pH on the reaction kinetics, substrate preference, and location of the iodide that is removed by type I 5'-deiodinase.[46] Because selenocysteine residues are more reactive nucleophiles than cysteine residues, an ion pair between histidine and a selenocysteine would also be consistent with the proposed reaction mechanism. Mutagenesis of the four histidine residues of rat type I 5'-deiodinase revealed that the loss of histidine 158 destroyed enzyme activity, and replacement of histidine 174 by either asparagine or

glutamine altered reactivity with the substrate and reduced inhibition by histidine-specific inhibitors. Mutations of the other two histidines had no effect of catalysis.[184]

LOW-K_M 5'-DEIODINASE

The presence of a low-K_m 5'-deiodinase enzyme in tissues has also been proposed.[108,185–187] This variant enzyme has been reported to be only modestly PTU sensitive and not to have the ping-pong reaction mechanism. Careful analysis of the reaction conditions used to demonstrate this variant 5'-deiodinase activity indicate that only the first half-reaction of type I 5'-deiodinase activity was measured (i.e., the initial rapid release of iodide by the reduced enzyme; see earlier discussion). Under these non–Michaelis-Menten reaction conditions, iodothyronine concentrations are almost equimolar to those estimated for type I 5'-deiodinase; because of the lack of true catalytic conditions, almost no inhibition of iodide release would be expected by PTU. Thus, these incubation conditions fail to fulfill the basic requirements for analysis of steady-state reaction kinetics.[40,188]

TYPE II 5'-DEIODINASE

The second 5'-deiodinase isoenzyme, known as type II 5'-deiodinase, was discovered in the early 1980s during analysis of the sources of intracellular T_3.[24,47,49,92,189–191] The type II enzyme has a preference for T_4 over rT_3, has K_m values in the low nanomolar range, follows a sequential mechanism of reaction, and is markedly resistant to inhibition by PTU (see Fig 8-5B). This isoenzyme also differs from type I 5'-deiodinase in tissue distribution and in regulation during development and various pathophysiologic conditions. Its tissue content and specific enzyme activities measured in vitro are significantly lower than those for type I 5'-deiodinase. Importantly, the type II 5'-deiodinase appears to generate T_3 for local use in organs such as pituitary, brain, and brown adipose tissue (Tables 8-3 and 8-4).

The adult brain, as well as a few other tissues such as spleen and testes, is widely considered to be unresponsive to thyroid hormones.[192] The brain contains abundant nuclear T_3 receptors, however, and analysis of the source of the T_3 bound to these receptors revealed that intracellular T_4-to-T_3 conversion was the primary source of this T_3.[24,47] (Fig 8-8). Using a dual-isotope technique, in vivo, with $[^{125}I]T_4$ as deiodinase substrate and $[^{131}I]T_3$ to control for serum contribution, intracellularly generated T_4-to-T_3 conversion was demonstrated in brain and pituitary.[24,92,190,191] This intracellular T_3 generation was not blocked by PTU concentrations sufficient to completely block liver and kidney type I 5'-deiodinase and at least

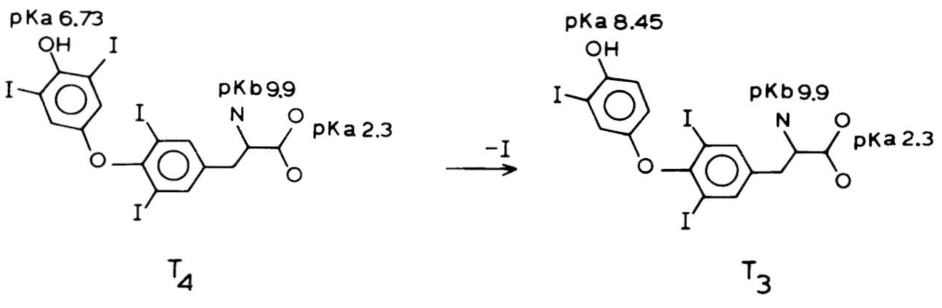

FIGURE 8-7. Schematic presentation of T_4 5'-deiodination resulting in T_3 production. Please observe alteration of the pK_a value of the 4'-hydroxy groups of iodothyronines. (Cody V. Triiodothyronine: molecular structure and function. In: Chopra IJ, ed. Triiodothyronines in health and disease. Berlin, Springer Verlag, 1981).

TABLE 8-3.
Summary of Properties of the Three Iodothyronine Deiodinase Isoenzymes

Property	Type I 5'-Deiodinase	Type II 5'-Deiodinase	5-Deiodinase
Reaction kinetics	Ping-pong	Sequential	Sequential
Substrate preference	$rT_3 > T_4 > T_3$	$T_4 > rT_3$	T_3(sulfate) $> T_4$
Substrate limiting K_m	0.5 μmol/L	1–2 nmol/L	5–20 μmol/L
In vitro cofactor limiting K_m	8 mmol/L DTT	28 mmol/L DTT	ca. 70 mmol/L DTT
Inhibitors			
Thiouracils	++++	±	–
Iopanoic acid	++++	++++	++++
Iodoacetate	++++	+	?
Flavonoids	++++	+++	+++
Halogenated aromates	++++		
Molecular weight	55,000, 27-kd subunit	200,000, 29-kd subunit	Unknown
Tissue distribution	Thyroid, kidney, liver, euthyroid central nervous system	Central nervous system, pituitary, brown adipose tissue	Almost every tissue
Subcellular location	Liver: endoplasmic reticulum; kidney: basolateral plasma membrane	Microsomal membranes	Microsomal membranes
Thyrotoxicosis	Increase	Decrease	Increase
Hypothyroidism	Decrease	Increase	Decrease
Low-T_3 syndromes	Decrease	No change	No change
Active site residues	Selenocysteine, histidine	Cysteine ?	?

80% of 5'-deiodination of rT_3 in pituitary and brain. Interestingly, thyroidectomy greatly increased this PTU-insensitive 5'-deiodinase activity in brain, whereas the 5'-deiodination of rT_3 was only marginally affected. These findings led to the characterization of type II 5'-deiodinase and established the specific reaction conditions that allowed simultaneous identification of both the type I and type II enzymes in the same tissue prepa-

rations. Deviation from these reaction conditions distorts the distinction between the two operationally defined enzymes and has led to some confusion over their identity.

Tissue Distribution

Type II 5'-deiodinase is restricted to fewer tissues than is type I 5'-deiodinase. The highest activities in euthyroid rats have been reported in the central nervous system, anterior pituitary, brown adipose tissue, and placenta.[24,49,92,189,193–196] The enzyme also has been found in the pineal gland, the harderian gland of rats and other rodents (a gland with unknown function located in the posteromedial aspect of the orbit), several pituitary tumor cell lines, NB41A3 neuroblastoma cells, and keratinocytes.[127,197–202] Similar to the cell-specific distribution of type I 5'-deiodinase in the kidney, type II 5'-deiodinase is not uniformly present in different cell types of these glands and organs. In the anterior pituitary of hypothyroid rats, somatotrophs and lactotrophs contain most of the type II 5'-deiodinase, followed by corticotrophs and gonadotrophs; the levels are lowest in the thyrotrophs.[193]

In the cerebral cortex, data from primary cultures suggest that neurons contain most of the type II 5'-deiodinase, although astrocytes may be stimulated to express the enzyme by elevation of intracellular cyclic adenosine monophosphate (cAMP) levels.[194,198,201–203] In euthyroid rat brain, type II 5'-deiodinase levels are low in the median eminence and throughout the limbic system. In hypothyroid rats, the hypothalamus, arcuate nucleus, and median eminence have high type II 5'-deiodinase levels, comparable to those in the anterior pituitary; in addition, intermediate activity was present in medial basal ganglia, and the paraventricular nucleus contained no detectable activity.[196]

TABLE 8-4.
Tissue-Specific Contribution of Local T_4 to T_3 Deiodination to Endogenous T_3 Levels in Intact Euthyroid Rats

Tissue	% Local T_3 Production	T_3 Content (ng/g wet weight)
Cerebral cortex	65.3 ± 7.2	1.68 ± 0.33
Cerebellum	51.3 ± 3.4	2.12 ± 0.65
Hypothalamus	32.3 ± 6.5	1.69 ± 0.24
Anterior pituitary	23.4 ± 4.7	5.67 ± 1.31
Thyroid gland	49.9 ± 11.9	ND
Brown adipose tissue	27.1 ± 8.7	1.01 ± 0.23
Heart	6.9 ± 4.0	1.29 ± 0.54
Skeletal muscle	4.4 ± 3.4	0.69 ± 0.10
Kidney	9.6 ± 5.0	6.58 ± 1.66
Liver	39.9 ± 10.6	4.50 ± 1.00
Other tissues	1–35	0.20–4.00
Plasma	—	0.44 ± 0.05

ND, not determined.
Data from van Doorn J, Roelfsema F, van der Heide D. Concentrations of thyroxine and 3,5,3'-triiodothyronine at 34 different sites in euthyroid rats as determined by an isotopic equilibrium technique. Endocrinology 1985;117:1201.

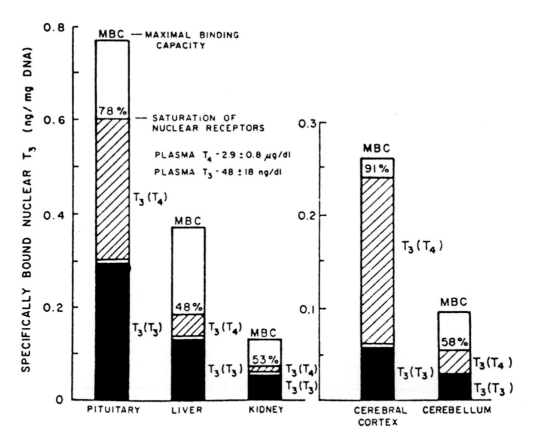

FIGURE 8-8. Sources of nuclear T_3 in anterior pituitary, liver, kidney, cerebral cortex, and cerebellum of euthyroid rats based on results of tracer distribution studies. The maximal T_3 binding capacity of nuclear receptors for each tissue as assessed by in vivo saturation analysis is indicated by the height of the bar. The component of nuclear T_3 deriving from either plasma T_3 [$T_3(T_3)$] or from intracellular T_4 5'-monodeiodination [$T_3(T_4)$] in each tissue is indicated by the coded area within each bar. (Larsen PR. Thyroid hormone metabolism in the central nervous system. Acta Med Austriaca 1988;15:4)

In placenta, type II 5'-deiodinase activity was lower in the chorionic membranes compared with the placental membranes, but was present in both human trophoblasts and decidual membranes.[49,117,129,136]

Subcellular Location

Similar to type I 5'-deiodinase, type II 5'-deiodinase is an integral component of cellular membranes, and soluble active enzyme preparations can be obtained only with ionic and some nonionic detergents. In the cerebral cortex, type II 5'-deiodinase cofractionates with the plasma membrane marker enzyme Na^+,K^+ ATPase, and it is found in fractions enriched in nerve terminal and dendritic plasma membranes.[175] Locally produced T_3 also has been found in partially purified synaptosomes, supporting the neuronal localization of type II 5'-deiodinase.[177,204] In cAMP-stimulated glial cells, type II 5'-deiodinase is localized in the plasma membrane fraction.[40] In bovine anterior pituitary, however, the enzyme copurified with glucose-6-phosphatase (but not with 5'-nucleotidase) and was assigned to the membranes of the endoplasmic reticulum.[205] Because of the low enzyme levels and limited amount of available tissue, the subcellular location of type II 5'-deiodinase is even more diffi-

cult to determine than that of the more abundant type I 5'-deiodinase, and specific antisera may be needed for detailed analysis in tissues expressing both enzymes.

Physicochemical Properties and Subunit Structure

As it is for type I 5'-deiodinase, bromoacetyl T_4 is a highly specific and selective affinity label for type II 5'-deiodinase. In cAMP-stimulated glial cells, a convenient homogenous cell source expressing between 2 and 10 pmol of enzyme activity per milligram of cell protein, this ligand labels a 29-kd intrinsic membrane protein that has all the properties of the substrate-binding subunit of type II 5'-deiodinase.[58,206] Using gel filtration, taurodeoxycholate-solubilized type II 5'-deiodinase has a calculated M_r value of 200 kd. It appears to be an asymmetric membrane protein with a sedimentation coefficient of 5.22, a frictional coefficient of 1.8, and a Stokes' radius of 4.97 nm. Comparative cyanogen bromide cleavage and proteolytic peptide map analysis of the affinity-labeled enzymes showed that the substrate-binding subunits of type I 5'-deiodinase and type II 5'-deiodinase were not identical.[58] These data clearly demonstrate that the two are separate enzymes, contrary to claims that the distinctions between them were artifactual. Neither substrate-binding subunit appears to be postranslationally glycosylated. No information is yet available on the nature of the other subunits of type II 5'-deiodinase.

Substrate Specificity

Substrate specificity is one of the primary criteria for the classification of iodothyronine deiodinases. Type II 5'-deiodinase has the highest affinity for T_4, with an apparent K_m value of 0.5 to 3 nmol/L, and a slightly higher K_m value for rT_3, in the range of 1 to 10 nmol/L when determined at 20 mmol/L DTT.[92] Limiting K_ms extrapolated from secondary replots of the kinetic data are in the same range, close to the substrate levels found in biologic fluids or cytosol (Fig 8-9). The V_{max} values of type II 5'-deiodinase for T_4 and rT_3 are 10 to 30 fmol of product formed per milligram of protein per minute, significantly lower than those for type I 5'-deiodinase, which reach up to 1 nmol product formed per milligram of protein per minute.[47,92] Type II 5'-deiodinase favors T_4 as the substrate (see Table 8-3).

Competition studies suggest that both T_4 and rT_3 are deiodinated by the same type II 5'-deiodinase enzyme. T_4 and rT_3 act as competitive ligands, and their mutual inhibitory constants are close to the limiting K_ms (see Fig 8-9A). No data are available on the stereoselectivity or the affinity of type II 5'-deiodinase for other iodothyronines or their analogues.

Cofactor Requirement and Reaction Mechanism

Type II 5'-deiodinase has an absolute requirement for reduced thiols (0.1–20 mmol/L) to maintain enzymic activity, and high concentrations of reduced thiols are required to measure maximal activity in vitro (see Fig 8-9B). This requirement has raised concern because of potential alterations of the redox state of the enzyme and of the stability of its intramolecular and intermolecular disulfide bridges, and because similarly high concentrations of reduced thiols prevent the formation of a stable PTU–type I 5'-deiodinase mixed disulfide and block the ability of PTU to inhibit type I 5'-deiodinase. No systematic studies have examined the structure–activity relationships for thiol stimulation of type II 5'-deiodinase and, similar to type I 5'-deiodinase, the physiologic cofactor remains to be identified.

Analysis of steady-state reaction kinetics has shown that type II 5'-deiodinase follows a sequential mechanism of reaction in all tissues in which it has been studied.[47,92,207] Double reciprocal plots of product formation against increasing T_4 or

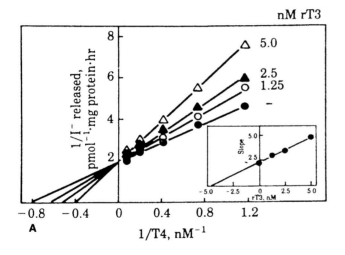
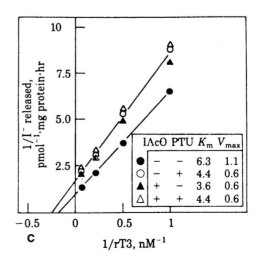
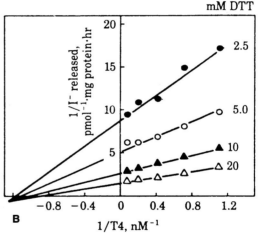

FIGURE 8-9. Kinetic analysis of type II 5'-deiodinase activity in rat brain cortex microsomes of hypothyroid rats. Lineweaver-Burke double reciprocal plots of the rate of type T_4 II 5'-deiodination as a function of T_4 concentration at 20 mmol/L DTT in the absence or presence of 1.25, 2.5, or 5 nmol/L rT_3 *(A)*; T_4 concentration at 2.5, 5, 10, or 20 mmol/L DTT) *(B)*; or rT_3 concentration at 20 mmol/L DTT with or without 1 mmol/L PTU after pretreatment of microsomes with or without 10 mmol/L iodoacetate (IAcO). The inserts show replots of ordinate intercepts for analysis of limiting kinetic parameters. (Visser TJ, Leonard JL, Kaplan MM, Larsen PR. Kinetic evidence suggesting two mechanisms for iodothyronine 5'- deiodinase in rat cerebral cortex. Proc Natl Acad Sci USA 1982; 79:5080)

rT_3 concentrations, done at several DTT concentrations, revealed a pattern of convergent lines. The same pattern was found when DTT concentrations were altered at several fixed T_4 or rT_3 concentrations. These results suggest that both iodothyronine and thiol must combine at the active site of the enzyme before deiodination takes place (see Fig 8-5B). Subsequent analysis showed that type II 5'-deiodinase lacks a hyperreactive nucleophilic selenocysteine residue found in the active center of type I 5'-deiodinase.[61,63,207] This finding suggests that no oxidized enzyme sulfenyl group would be available for the generation of a PTU–enzyme mixed disulfide and provides an explanation for the inability of PTU to inactivate type II 5'-deiodinase easily.

Principles of Determination of Type II 5'-Deiodinase Activity

Type II 5'-deiodinase activity is often determined together with the more abundant type I 5'-deiodinase activity in the same tissue preparation at T_4 concentrations in the nanomolar range and in the presence of sufficient PTU (1 mmol/L) to block completely any type I 5'-deiodinase activity. The production of T_3 or iodide from the substrate T_4 in the presence of PTU has been defined as type II 5'-deiodinase activity, whereas the difference in product formation in the absence and presence of PTU represents type I 5'-deiodinase activity.[92,188] This operational definition implies that alterations of these reaction conditions may blur the identification of the individual isoenzymes. An example of the consequences of altering reaction conditions is the identification of variant PTU-sensitive type II 5'-deiodinase isoenzymes.[185,186,208] Unfortunately, PTU impairment of type I 5'-deiodinase activity occurs only at suboptimal thiol concentrations, 1:1 ratios of enzyme to substrate, and incubation conditions that do not fulfill the requirements for measurements of initial-velocity reaction kinetics.

pH Optimum and Active Site Characteristics

The pH optimum for type II 5'-deiodinase is in the neutral to slightly acid range. No data are yet available to determine if the pH optimum reflects the dissociation of protons from the 4'-hydroxyl group of T_4 and rT_3, or if it is an intrinsic property of the functional amino acid residues in the active site of the enzyme. The fact that the substrate-binding subunit of type II 5'-deiodinase is readily alkylated by bromoacetyl T_4 and that incorporation of the affinity label is proportional to enzyme inactivation suggests that this isoenzyme contains a nucleophilic group, presumably a cysteine residue close to or directly in its active site.[206] However, the reactivity of this cysteine residue is at least two orders of magnitude lower than that of the selenocysteine residue present in the type I 5'-deiodinase isoenzyme, as judged by the much higher concentrations of α-haloacids required to inactivate type II 5'-deiodinase.[206,207] Type II 5'-deiodinase activity is reported to be diminished in the brain of selenium-deficient rats, and activity can be restored to normal by selenium replacement.[209] These changes in brain type II 5'-deiodinase are caused by the increase in circulating T_4 concentrations that are typically found in selenium-deficient rats, and not by direct selenium-dependent changes in the enzyme content per se.[184,210–212]

5-DEIODINASE

Tyrosyl Ring Deiodination

The tyrosyl ring deiodination of iodothyronines at the 5- or 3-position is one of the major routes for T_3 degradation and inactivation of T_4 (yielding rT_3). 5-Deiodination occurs in almost every tissue except the anterior pituitary, and high levels of activity are present in liver, brain, and placenta (see Table 8-3). At least two isoenzymes of 5-deiodinase appear to be present. Despite the importance of this inactivation pathway, only relatively recently has any information been obtained about this family of enzyme(s)—frequently referred to as *type III* deiodinases. This latter designation creates some confusion between these inactivating enzymes and the 5'-deiodinase isoenzyme classification.

Distribution, Subcellular Location, and Physicochemical Properties

High levels of 5-deiodinase activity are found in liver.[90,133,145,207] Several independent lines of evidence suggest that 5'- and 5-deiodination are catalyzed by a single enzyme (type I 5'-deiodinase) in this organ. Thus, the biochemical, biologic, and physiologic properties described for type I 5'-deiodinase appear to be valid for the 5-deiodinase reaction as well. 5-Deiodinase activity has been found to be highest in the endoplasmic reticulum of the parenchymal liver cells, and it is an intrinsic membrane protein oriented toward the liver cytosol.[54,133,142] Inhibitors of type I 5'-deiodinase also block 5-deiodination to a similar extent, if the 5-deiodinase reaction is done at the appropriate pH.[46,145] 5-Deiodinase and type I 5'-deiodinase also could not be physically separated during partial purification, suggesting that a single polypeptide catalyzes both reactions.[51,54]

The recent cloning of frog and neonatal rat skin 5-deiodinase showed that this enzyme was a member of the selenoenzyme family typified by type I 5'-deiodinase, and shared significant homology with this mammalian counterpart.[42,44] The cDNA encodes a polypeptide of approximately 30 kd that contains a single selenocysteine in a 30-amino acid core and shares greater than 70% identity with type I 5'-deiodinase. This polypeptide displays both 5-deiodinating and 5'-deiodinating activity, although the 5-deiodinating activity is at least an order of magnitude greater than the intrinsic 5'-deiodinating activity. The selenocysteine residue is essential for catalysis, and both PTU and ATG inhibit this reaction, although 10-fold greater concentrations are required to achieve similar inhibition of type I 5'-deiodinase.

pH Optimum

The phenomenon of "wobble" in the active site of deiodinating enzymes that allows deiodination at either the phenolic or the tyrosyl ring is not fully understood. 5-Deiodinase has a pH optimum in the alkaline range (8–8.5), and therefore 5-deiodination may be important when cell alkalinization occurs.[46,181] The only way to analyze selectively the 5-deiodination pathway in vitro is to use an alkaline pH mixture and to choose appropriate substrates, such as 3-T_1, 3,5-T_2, or T_3, which generate products that do not undergo 5'-deiodination. Interest in 5-deiodinase in rat liver increased when it was shown that 4'-sulfation, especially of T_4, T_3, and 3,3'-T_2, directed deiodination from the phenolic ring to the tyrosyl ring.[93,213-219] Sulfation of T_4, T_3, and 3,3'-T_2 decreases the limiting K_m values for 5-deiodinase and increases its V_{max} considerably. Therefore, the $V_{max}:K_m$ ratio, an indicator of catalytic efficiency, increases 50- to 200-fold, compared with the corresponding ratios for unconjugated iodothyronines.[219] Thus, alkalinization and sulfoconjugation are two means by which the thyromimetic potency of T_4 is lost.

Less comprehensive data are available for the apparent K_m value, and no clearcut structure–affinity relationships have been reported for 5-deiodinase. In vitro, T_4 and T_3 have K_m values of 10^{-5} to 10^{-6} mol/L, respectively, similar to those of 3,3'-T_2 and 3,5'-T_2. Owing to the rapid 5'-deiodination of rT_3, no reliable data have been reported for the apparent K_m and V_{max} values of the 5-deiodination of T_4.[143]

Kinetic Analysis Using Thyroxine Analogues

The biochemical properties of 5-deiodinase in rat liver have been analyzed using a T_4 analogue, *N*-acetyl,3,5-diiodo,3'-bromo,5'-nitro-L-thyronine (HB306). This T_4 analogue has several features that allow detailed analysis of the 5-deiodinase reaction. *N*-Acetylation increases substrate affinity to that of acetic acid derivatives owing to the absence of a positively charged functional side-chain group. The substitution of bromine for iodine in the phenolic ring is tolerated by 5-deiodinase with no loss in affinity, and bromine is not removed by 5'-deiodination. Likewise, a single N-substitution in either the phenolic or tyrosyl ring does not change the ligand-binding characteristics for the enzyme. Incubation of this T_4 analogue with liver microsomal membranes under routine incubation conditions yields the rT_3 analogue, *N*-acetyl,3-iodo,3'-bromo,5'-nitro-L-thyronine (HB338), which can be readily quantified because of its high cross-reactivity with rT_3 antisera. This rT_3 analogue is not further metabolized and may be useful for in vitro and in vivo studies of the regulatory role of rT_3.

Using HB306 as the substrate for 5-deiodinase, the alkaline pH optimum (8.5) was confirmed, and 5-deiodination of HB306 was inhibited by all established type I 5'-deiodinase inhibitors. The limiting K_m value for HB306 was 2 µmol/L, similar to that determined for T_4. The limiting K_m value for the thiol cofactor DTT, however, was two orders of magnitude (30 µmol/L) lower than reported previously, and the reaction mechanism and low thiol requirement are intrinsic properties of HB306 or represent true kinetic properties of 5-deiodinase.

Tissue-Specific 5-Deiodinases

True 5-deiodinases, which selectively deiodinate only the tyrosyl ring of iodothyronines, have been described but have not been well characterized. The central nervous system,

placenta, and several other tissues, such as skin and hepatocarcinoma cells, contain two different 5-deiodinase isoenzymes. Their subcellular location has not been established because of enzyme instability, but these enzymes appear to be intrinsic membrane proteins associated with microsomal membranes.

In placenta, 5-deiodinase activity is predominantly localized in cells of the chorionic membranes.[49,117,129,136,220] The high levels of rT_3 found in amniotic fluid may originate from this enzyme, a function that reduces delivery of T_4 (and T_3) from mother to fetus and that provides iodide to the fetal thyroid.

In the central nervous system, 5-deiodinase activity has been assigned to the astroglia[203,221,222] in neonatal rat brain. Unlike the frog 5-deiodinase, astroglial 5-deiodinase activity is induced in cells devoid of selenium, suggesting that the brain enzyme does not contain an essential selenocysteine residue.[223] It has a distinct perinatal developmental pattern in specific regions of the brain that follows glial cell proliferation.[224]

In cultured hepatocarcinoma cells, cultured chick embryonic heart, fetal membranes of sheep, rat, and chicken liver, and placental membranes of humans and rats, tyrosyl ring deiodination predominates over 5'-deiodination. This contrasts with results in freshly isolated tissues or adult cells.[24,36,129,166,225-228]

These observations strengthen the hypothesis that iodothyronine deiodination in undifferentiated (fetal) tissues and in organs unresponsive to thyroid hormone prevents the inappropriate accumulation of T_3. Thus, in fetal tissues, the minimal amounts of T_3 formed by 5'-deiodinase would be rapidly deiodinated to 3,3'-T_2, whereas the tyrosyl ring deiodination product of T_4, namely rT_3, would be relatively stable.[24,36,129,225,227] As maturation proceeds, 5'-deiodinase activity increases and 5-deiodinase activity decreases.[224] The stimulus for such a shift in iodothyronine metabolism is unknown; however, glucocorticoids, air breathing with a consequent shift to a more aerobic metabolism, and unidentified fetal factors are considered to be possible regulators.[225,229]

Substrate Specificity

The kinetic parameters for the naturally occurring iodothyronines indicate a preference for T_4 and rT_3, and limiting or apparent K_m values range from low nanomolar to micromolar.[176,222] Kinetic analysis is often complicated or even impossible if much 5'-deiodinase activity is present. Several attempts have been made to circumvent these methodologic problems (e.g., product sequestration by specific antisera and prevention of product deiodination by addition of excess alternative substrates for the competing reactions).[34,35,213]

Cofactor Requirement and Reaction Mechanism

In all tissues expressing 5-deiodinase, reduced dithiols are required for catalytic activity in vitro. The exact role of the reduced thiols is unclear, but kinetic analysis suggests that they are true cofactors and that the reaction mechanism is sequential.[230] Concentrations of reduced dithiols greater than 200 mmol/L inhibit catalysis, presumably by cleavage of structural disulfide bonds of the enzyme or other membrane pro-teins,[86,220,230] or by general alteration of protein or membrane conformation.

NONDEIODINATING METABOLISM OF IODOTHYRONINES

Ether Bond Cleavage

The physiologic significance of ether bond cleavage as a pathway of iodothyronine metabolism is controversial.[231–235] The extent of its contribution to overall T_4 metabolism can-not yet be quantified, and this process is observed mainly during T_4 degradation in leukocytes.[236] An increase in T_4 me-tabolism occurs in phagocytosing leukocytes. This increase results from enhanced cellular uptake and subsequent degra-dation of T_4, and is most evident during acute sepsis. The products of T_4 degradation are monoiodotyrosine and di-iodotyrosine, providing good evidence for ether bond cleav-age. The formation of diiodotyrosine by rat liver microsomes incubated in the presence of the catalase inhibitor aminotria-zole was reported, indicating that the reaction may be cat-alyzed by myeloperoxidase; PTU or cyanide block diio-dotyrosine formation.[231,235] An identical mechanism of ether bond cleavage was proposed for the leukocytes.[232] In the presence of H_2O_2 and myeloperoxidase, T_4 serves as the halogen donor, with the formation of a phenoxyl radical. Ex-cept possibly during severe infections, this ether bond cleav-age is probably of limited physiologic significance, although its activity under a variety of abnormal circumstances has not been tested. Very low serum diiodotyrosine levels were found in athyrotic patients receiving T_4 orally, and large oral doses of T_4 decreased circulating diiodotyrosine levels in normal subjects.[234] In critically ill patients with nonthyroidal disorders, significantly increased diiodotyrosine levels were found to be correlated with the presence and severity of bac-terial infections[235] (Fig 8-10).

The further metabolism of monoiodotyrosines and di-iodotyrosines occurs by unspecific dehalogenases, and these compounds are not substrates for the specific deiodinase enzymes.[86,237,238]

Metabolism of the Alanine Side Chain

In contrast to the deiodination of iodothyronines, only limited data are available on the characteristics of metabolic reactions affecting the alanine side chain. Specific enzymes have been characterized that catalyze the deamination, transamination, or decarboxylation of iodothyronines[239,240] (see Fig 8-2); how-ever, propionic acid, pyruvic acid, and acetic and formic acid derivatives of iodothyronines formed by oxidative deamina-tion have been found in vivo and in vitro.[240]

The production and metabolism of acetic derivatives of T_4 (tetrac) and T_3 (triac) have been studied in greater detail.[241] Serum levels of tetrac are similar to those of T_3, whereas levels of triac are much lower. Tetrac and triac both have thy-romimetic activity, which is lower than that of their precur-sors, regardless of whether calorigenic potency or suppression of thyrotropin-releasing hormone (TRH)-stimulated TSH se-cretion is used as the index of effectiveness.[242]

The short biologic half-life and a rapid metabolic clear-ance of these metabolites has been suggested as the reason for their lower thyromimetic activity. Taken together, these find-ings could explain the relative insignificance of these acetic acid derivatives, despite their high affinity for transthyretin and for the nuclear T_3 receptor.[96] Kinetic and turnover studies also indicate these acetic acid derivatives play a negligible role in physiologic and pathologic states in which thyroid hormone economy and metabolism are altered.[241] Triac has been used for the acute suppression of TSH in the syndrome of thyroid hormone resistance. because of its short half-life, cardiac and systemic side effects are limited, but the exact mechanism of its efficacy in TSH suppression mediated by the mutated T_3 re-ceptors in the thyrotrophs are unclear.[243]

The acetic acid derivatives, similar to sulfated iodothyro-nine conjugates, are readily deiodinated in vitro (discussed earlier) and in vivo, but this reaction also is of minor impor-tance in the overall degradation of thyroid hormone.[48,216,217] The in vivo occurrence of the decarboxylated metabolites of T_4 and T_3, 3,3',5,5'-tetraiodothyroethylamine (tetram), and 3,3',5-triiodothyroethylamine (triam; see Fig 8-1) has not been demonstrated. However, these derivatives may be of pharma-cologic interest because of their chemical similarity to bio-genic amines.[177,195,244]

Sulfoconjugation

Sulfoconjugation is an alternative pathway of thyroid hormone metabolism that is energy dependent and mediated by cytoso-lic phenol sulfotransferases in several tissues.[4,13,48] The sulfo-transferases of liver are normally involved in inactivation and detoxification reactions with a preference for lipophilic sub-strates.[14,245,246] Two alternate pathways of iodothyronine me-tabolism have been described[48,216]: one leads to activation of thyromimetic action by preferential deiodination of T_4 to T_3 at low substrate concentrations; the other leads to a sulfoconju-gation reaction of biologically active iodothyronines. Sulfation of iodothyronines facilitates rapid deiodination (see Table 8-2). This alternate pathway, shown in Figure 8-2, occurs with all substrates along the iodothyronine cascade starting with T_4, except for rT_3, which is the preferred substrate of type I 5'-deiodinase.[48] Teleologically, sulfation seems directed toward a further fine regulation of hepatic T_3 delivery to the organism and enables recirculation of the liberated trace element iodide.

Iodothyronines with two iodine atoms at the phenolic ring are preferentially conjugated with glucuronic acid, whereas iodothyronines that contain only one iodine atom in the phe-nolic ring are sulfated with the following preference: $3'-T_1 = 3,3'-T_2 > T_3 > rT_3 > T_4$.[48,166,228,245,247,248] T_3 sulfation has been demonstrated by human cytosolic liver phenol sulfotransferase (EC 2.8.2.1) with K_m values in the 100-μM range, considerably greater than those of type I 5'-deiodinase.[249] Whereas excretion of iodothyronine sulfates in bile, urine, and feces is a minor route for thyroid hormone elimination in humans, considerable amounts of iodothyronine sulfates are detectable in plasma and bile after inhibition of type I 5'-deiodinase by PTU in the rat.[48,213,214] Moreover, at a high substrate concentration (> 1 μM) in vitro, metabolism proceeds mainly by sulfation, whereas at lower concentrations (< 0.1 μM), sulfation is the rate-limiting step; no sulfates accumulate because of the rapid deiodination of the sulfated iodothyronines. Thus far, the cellular capacity

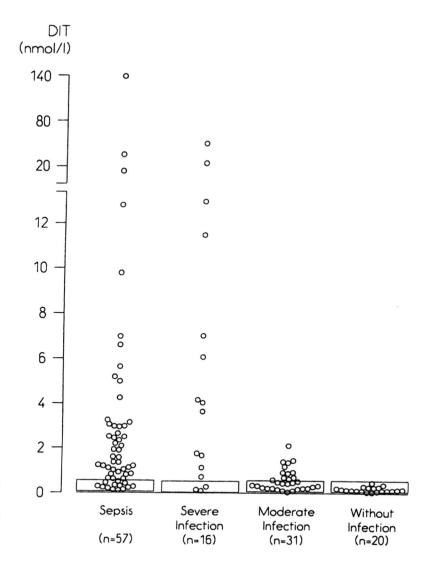

FIGURE 8-10. Serum concentrations of diiodotyrosine (DIT) in critical care patients. The rectangles indicate the normal range (0.02–0.55 nmol/L). (Meinhold H, Gramm HJ, Meissner W, Zimmermann J, Schwander J, Dennhardt R, Voigt K, Elevated serum diiodotyrosine (DIT) in severe infections and sepsis: DIT, a possible new marker of leukocyte activity. J Clin Endocrinol Metab 1991;72:945)

for conjugation could not be saturated, in contrast to enzymic monodeiodination.[166,228,250] In the human hepatocarcinoma cell line, HepG2, T_3 deiodination is reduced owing to deficient T_3 sulfation, which appears to be an obligatory step before hepatic deiodination of T_3.[251]

In the rat, serum T_3 sulfate levels are increased, enterohepatic cycling of T_3 sulfate is elevated, and the half-life of T_3 in the serum is longer under selenium deficiency because of the decreased type I 5′-deiodinase activity.[210] Under these conditions, sulfoconjugation might lead to greater availability of the active hormone. Sulfoconjugates of T_4, T_3, rT_3, and 3,3′-T_2 have been identified in human serum and amniotic fluid by specific radioimmunoassays.[252–257] Detailed analysis during pregnancy and in the amniotic fluid suggested that these conjugates are normal components of maternal and fetal serum and amniotic fluid, that their production and metabolism are regulated by the hormonal state, nonthyroidal illness, and drugs that suppress deiodinase activity, and that they might contribute to the fetal supply of maternal thyroid hormone.

Enzymic desulfation of the sulfate of T_3, but not of T_4-O-sulfate, occurs in microsomal membrane preparations of vari-

ous human or rat tissues, in intact rat hepatocytes, and the gut lumen. The importance of this reaction for thyroid hormone metabolism is unknown, but might be involved in regulating the receptor availability of thyroid hormone.[257–259]

Glucuronidation and O-Methylation

The 4′-OH-group of the phenolic ring of the iodothyronine is chemically activated by orthosubstitution with iodines, which also cause a steric hindrance of the metabolic action of enzymes catalyzing the conjugation of phenols. Thyroidectomized rats given [[131I]T_4 excrete O-methyl-[[131I]T_4 in the urine, but the enzymic O-methyl transfer to iodophenols catalyzed by a liver enzyme seems to be of marginal importance for iodothyronine metabolism in vivo.[260]

More attention must be paid to enzymic 4′-O-glucuronidation of iodothyronines, which renders these compounds more hydrophilic and thereby facilitates their excretion by bile, feces, and urine.[261] The identity of glucuronidase enzymes involved in iodothyronine metabolism remains obscure, but a substrate preference for iodothyronines with 3′,5′-diiodo-substitution (T_4, rT_3, 3′,5′-T_2) over those with only one (T_3, 3,3′-T_2, 3′T_1) or no iodine atoms in the phenolic ring (3,5-T_2, 3-T_1) has been suggested for rat hepatocytes.[228] Iodothyronine glucuronides are excreted in the bile and undergo further metabolism by intestinal bacteria, which partially liberate free iodothyronines, enabling enterohepatic circulation of iodothyronines.[48,217,247,262] In Gunn rats that have a defect in the gene coding for bilirubin and phenol uridine diphosphate (UDP)–glucuronyltransferase isozymes and WAG rats having a defect in the gene coding for androsterone UDP–glucuronyltransferase, rT_3 is more rapidly glucuronidated than T_4 and T_3. Furthermore, T_4 and rT_3 are glucuronidated by the bilirubin and phenol UDP-glucuronyltransferase isozymes, whereas T_3 is conjugated by androsterone UDP–glucuronyltransferase.[263] Compounds such as phenobarbital, 3-methylcholantrene, hexochlorobenzene, and drugs that induce hepatic conjugating enzymes in the liver also affect glucuronidation of thyroid hormones and the intestinal exchangeable thyroid hormone pool.[264,265]

TISSUE-SPECIFIC DISTRIBUTION AND PHYSIOLOGIC REGULATION OF DEIODINATION

In 1973, selective deficiency in serum T_3 with normal T_4 concentrations was described, and since then a large number of systemic diseases and other clinical situations have been associated with what is called the *low-T_3 syndrome*.[266] Later, the low serum T_3 levels were found to be accompanied by elevated rT_3 levels. Kinetic studies during total caloric deprivation or in patients with cirrhosis revealed that the production rates of T_3 and rT_3 were decreased and slightly increased, respectively.[267,268] These observations indicate that a variety of pathophysiologic states can selectively divert T_4 deiodination from T_3 generation to rT_3 formation. The exact nature of this apparent shift from phenolic ring to tyrosyl ring deiodination is not yet understood. Because the contribution of individual organs to iodothyronine metabolism varies considerably, most studies have focused on alterations in the deiodination of the main organs participating in T_4 deiodination. In general, many factors determine the T_4 deiodinating activity of an organ: (1) its size; (2) substrate delivery by the bloodstream; (3) binding of T_4 to serum proteins and their dissociation kinetics; (4) capillary transit time; (5) exposure and binding to, and transport through, cell membranes; (6) intracellular transport through cytosolic compartments and binding to microsomes; and (7) the overall activity of the deiodinating enzymes (see Table 8-4). Most of these factors cannot yet be quantified (Table 8-5) provides a partial list of these factors), but some data have been accumulated for the liver and a few other organs (see subchapter on nonthyroidal illness in chap 14).

The most comprehensive studies on the contribution of local T_4 deiodination to intracellular T_3 and rT_3 were done in rats by an isotope equilibrium technique and by constant infusion protocols.[26,114,269–273] These studies, done in a variety of physiologic conditions or after administration of drugs affecting thyroid hormone metabolism, revealed a complex pattern of tissue-specific regulation of iodothyronine metabolism.

Liver

The liver is the main metabolic organ in humans. Hepatic blood flow amounts to 1500 mL/min, so that about 30% of the cardiac output is directed to the liver. Its particular vasoarchitecture, with interendothelial gaps and incomplete basement membranes in the sinusoids, poses no barrier to the passage of protein-bound T_4 to hepatocytes.[274] Based on kinetic data, it is estimated that about 30% of the total extrathyroidal T_4 pool is in the liver in humans,[275] and the molar T_4:T_3 ratio in liver is 420:5. This contrasts with the extrahepatic intracellular compartments, in which the ratio of T_4 to T_3 is 100:5. Hepatocytes concentrate T_4, and equilibrium between serum and hepatocytes for T_4 is established within 3 hours in humans; for muscle, the equilibration time is about 24 hours. T_4 uptake by the liver is regulated by a complex kinetic system of fluxes influenced by the T_4-binding proteins in serum, that is, the free hormone fraction, transport through the membrane, and compartmentalization by intracellular binding proteins. The contribution of individual components to binding, uptake, and transport of thyroid hormone is still a matter of debate.[153,274,276–284]

Some kinetic parameters derived from rat experiments suggest possible directions of flux. It has been proposed that 98% of T_4 taken up unidirectionally by rat liver in vivo during one passage returns to the circulation unmetabolized[279], but if the residual 2% were metabolized to T_3, the fraction would be an important source of circulating T_3 because T_3 rapidly leaves the liver. Indeed, from studies done in perfused rat livers, it has been calculated that the liver could be responsible for roughly 40% of the whole-body deiodination of T_4.[154,181,285]

The total hepatic production of T_3 from T_4 is a function of (1) the size of the liver, (2) T_4 uptake, and (3) type I 5′-deiodinase activity. The liver size, that is, the mass of hepatocytes, is considerably reduced in patients with chronic liver diseases who have low serum T_3 levels, and hepatic T_4 uptake in fasting rats decreases in proportion to the fall in liver weight. The daily in vivo production rate of T_3 in intact rats was calculated to be 0.9 nmol; T_3 production by perfused rat livers, calculated by multiplying the endogenous liver T_4 content by the apparent T_4 to T_3 conversion, amounts to 0.65 nmol. Thus, 70% of the daily T_3 production could originate from the liver.[39,181] Because the maximal production rate of T_3 by type I 5′-deiodinase in perfused livers is more than 10-fold the daily production rate,[181] it seems that the in vivo capacity of type I 5′-deiodinase itself does not play the major role in limiting the production of T_3 from T_4. Other factors, such as the balance between 5′- and 5-deiodination and conjugation, are probably more important.[39,154,275,286]

The contribution of the liver to the production of other circulating iodothyronines is less clear. In rat liver perfusion studies, no rT_3 production could be demonstrated.[181,285] It was suggested that this was a result of the very high type I 5′-deiodinase activity and therefore rapid degradation of rT_3 to 3,3′-T_2.[181,285] The production of 3′,5′-T_2 by 5-deiodination of rT_3 has not yet been identified in intact liver. The production of rT_3 by 5-deiodination of T_4 in liver homogenates or microsomal fractions may be caused by (1) artificial conditions in vitro, in which the disintegration of liver cell membranes and loss of iodothyronine compartmentalization destroys cellular

TABLE 8-5.
Regulation of Deiodinase Isoenzymes

Factor	Cell Type/Tissue	Species	Type I 5'-Deiodinase	Type II 5'-Deiodinase	5-Deiodinase
Selenium	Liver, kidney	All	↑	nc ↓	nc
T_4/T_3	Liver, kidney, thyroid pituitary	All	↑	↓	↑
Thyrotropin	Thyroid	All	↑	nc	nc
Growth hormone/insulin-like growth factor I	Liver	Human, rat	↑	nc	
		Chicken	↓	↑	
Fibroblast growth factor	Thyroid/FRTL-5	Rat	↓		
	Astrocytes			↑	
Il-1β/Il-6	Liver	Rat	↓		
Tumor necrosis factor–α	Thyroid	Rat	↓ TSH effect		
	Liver		↑ nc		
Interferon-γ	FRTL-5	Rat	↓		
Somatostatin	Liver	Rat	↓		
E2*	Liver	Rat	↓		
	Pituitary	Rat	↑		
Dexamethasone	Liver, kidney cells	Rat	↑		
	Liver in vivo	Rat	↓		
CHO	Liver	All	↑	nc	
Fasting	Liver	All	↓	nc	
Cold	Liver	Swine ↑			
	BAT	Rodents		↑	

Estradiol or lack of testosterone.
nc, no change.

regulation; (2) access of products to nonphysiologic pathways; or (3) protection of metabolites from concurrent enzymatic degradation. In humans, who have higher circulating rT_3 concentrations, the situation may be different, but it appears that rT_3 in humans, dogs, and rats is of extrahepatic origin.[27,172] Thus, the liver appears to be an organ mainly responsible for meeting the demands of extrahepatic tissues for T_3 and for degrading the rT_3 produced by extrahepatic tissues. rT_3 delivered to the liver by the circulation could have a regulatory capacity with respect to hepatic T_3 production.[38,287] Clearance of rT_3 by liver and kidney type I 5'-deiodinase is similar to whole-body removal and is markedly inhibited by PTU.[172,288]

The biochemical and physiologic properties of rat and human liver type I 5'-deiodinase appear identical, and human liver type I 5'-deiodinase can produce up to 6 nmol/day T_3 at normal serum free T_4 concentrations.[93] Because T_4 accumulates in the parenchymal cells, and the free intracellular T_4 concentration may be higher than in serum, the higher free T_4 level in hepatocytes (20 pmol/L) allows the liver type I 5'-deiodinase to provide the total extrathyroidal human T_3 production of 36 nmol/day.[93] Similar calculations hold for rT_3, suggesting that type I 5'-deiodinase activity of human liver can account for disposal of all the rT_3 in serum.[48,93]

In the liver, T_4 deiodination occurs only in hepatocytes.[29,118,162–165,228,281] Isolated liver cells are especially suitable for the study of membrane effects[165] and iodothyronine transport.[153] T_4, T_3, and rT_3 are taken up by these cells by a high-affinity process (K_m ~10^{-9} mol/L) that is energy dependent.[128,159,274,278,279,281,289] The diminished uptake of T_4 and rT_3 caused by lowered cellular ATP content may contribute to altered substrate availability, with a subsequent change in deiodination. Both 5'- and 5-deiodination occur in these cells in vitro, but 5'-deiodination proceeds more rapidly, with an order of preference of $rT_3 > T_3 > T_4$. 5'-Deiodination and 5-deiodination reactions are equally inhibited by PTU in hepatocytes. T_4-to-T_3 conversion ranges from 0.1% to 0.8% in these preparations. Kinetic data on the enzymatic activity of 5'- and 5-deiodination in these cell preparations agree with those for microsomal membranes, and only T_4 deiodination occurs within the intact cells if no thiol cofactors are added, with release of only small amounts of T_3 and little or no rT_3 into the medium.[163,290] These results underline the need for the integrity of an organ in studies of the physiology of T_4 deiodination; they also indicate that isolated or cultured cells do not have the mechanisms for cell–cell communications that are found in an intact organ. T_4 metabolism by these cells is cell cycle dependent and developmentally expressed in the chicken liver.[225,291] This is even more the case for monkey hepatocarcinoma cell lines, in which 5-deiodinase activity predominates over that of 5'-deiodinase, and conjugation reactions also occur.

During caloric restriction, chronic obstructive pulmonary disease, chronic heart failure, and diabetes mellitus, increased levels of nonesterified fatty acids, the suspected "thyroid hormone binding inhibitors," may contribute to decreased T_4 uptake into hepatocytes and subsequently diminished 5'-deiodination of T_4 to T_3.[283,292] Furthermore, T_3 uptake is also decreased during caloric restriction, but no effects on T_3 deiodination were found.[293] Decreased concentrations of the 5'-deiodinase substrate-binding subunit[83] and diminished steady-state 5'-deiodinase mRNA levels were found during starvation and in diabetic rats.[294] In uremia, a furan fatty acid and indoxyl sulfate circulating in serum seem to be responsible for decreased thyroid hormone uptake and deiodination in the liver.[295] Decreased concentrations of albumin and increased levels of nonesterified fatty acids also contribute to decreased T_4 uptake into the liver in nonuremic, critically ill patients.[296]

Heart

Heart muscle differs metabolically from other muscle in many respects. Modest T_4-to-T_3 conversion (about 5%) occurs in isolated rat hearts perfused with high T_4 concentrations (50 µg/mL) during the initial perfusion phase.[297] Few in vitro observations[32,298–300] are available concerning rat or dog heart homogenates. In rat heart muscle, the formation of T_3 from T_4 is about 10% of that in liver. The contribution of the heart to the rapidly exchangeable pool of T_3 appears to be negligible, and local T_3 generation is minimal as judged by the contribution of this source to the saturation of nuclear receptors.[26,114,269–271] T_4 actively stimulates expression of atrial natriuretic peptide in cultured rat atrial myocytes, and PTU but not imidazole blocks this T_4 effect,[300] suggesting that type I 5'-deiodinase in rat atrium regulates T_3-dependent expression of atrial natriuretic peptide.

Other studies have failed to detect T_3 production in cardiac muscle, probably for methodologic reasons.[89] Cultured chick embryo heart cells contain abundant 5-deiodinase activity,[226] suggesting that cultured cells kept in a fetal state express mostly 5-deiodinase. More information about T_4-to-T_3 conversion by heart muscle should be forthcoming in view of the altered cardiac metabolism of T_3 that occurs after myocardial infarction and other nonthyroid illnesses, as well as the potent antiarrhythmic effects of amiodarone or its metabolites, which are potent inhibitors of type I 5'-deiodinase and also diminish thyroid hormone uptake.[265,301–306]

Thyroid

The human thyroid gland preferentially secretes T_3 compared with T_4, an indication of its capacity for T_4 deiodination.[307] Early perfusion studies of rat thyroids showed that, relative to T_4, the T_3 content of thyroid effluent was always higher that of thyroid hydrolysate.[308] This thyroidal T_4 deiodination was found to be independent of iodotyrosine deiodinase[308] and thyroid peroxidase.[309] In an elegant series of experiments in perfused dog thyroid glands, new insight into thyroid T_4 deiodination was obtained. In particular, both T_3 and rT_3 were found to be secreted in preference to T_4, and the relatively high T_4:T_3 ratios of thyroglobulin were not influenced by either acute or chronic TSH stimulation.[90,310,311] Further proof that the preferential secretion of locally formed T_3 (and rT_3) by the thyroid results from T_4 deiodination was derived from results indicating that PTU inhibited the preferential secretion of T_3 in iodine-deficient rats and that rT_3 secretion was less strongly inhibited.[52,87,135,312] T_4 deiodination in dogs, however,

differs from that in rats, and caution must be used when comparing data from different species.[39,313] 3,3'-T_2 is found in surprisingly similar concentrations in rat, dog, and human thyroids,[311] suggests intrathyroidal deiodination of T_3 and rT_3. In humans, the thyroid contributes about 20% of the T_3 and about 2% to 5% of the rT_3 produced daily; from 30% to 50% of the T_3 and more than half of the rT_3 that appears in the thyroid effluent are derived from local T_4 deiodination.[26,123]

The K_m value of type I 5'-deiodinase in dog thyroid tissue is 25 µmol/L, and that of 5-deiodinase is about 6 µmol/L; in the rat thyroid tissue, the K_m value for type I 5'-deiodinase under similar conditions is 3 µmol/L,[122] and in human thyroid tissue the K_m value is 4.5 µmol/L T_4. Thyroid tissue from patients with Graves' disease has a similar K_m value, but a higher V_{max} value than is found in normal thyroid tissue.[123] Nothing is known about the actual T_4 substrate concentrations at the site of thyroidal T_4 deiodination, but thyroid cells may be an ideal locale wherein T_4 deiodination may be regulated by the local T_4 concentration. Furthermore, experiments in hypophysectomized rats showed that replacement doses of T_4 did not restore thyroidal type I 5'-deiodinase activity, suggesting that the deiodinase was TSH dependent.[314] TSH may stimulate thyroidal T_4 deiodination directly through cAMP[122,123,314–317] or indirectly, as suggested by studies of T_4 metabolism in iodine-deficient hypothyroid rats.[318]

Thyroid tumors also contain type I 5'-deiodinase activity, whereas medullary carcinomas do not, suggesting a follicular but not a C-cell origin of enzyme activity.[87,123,130,319] Compared to normal thyroid tissue, expression of type I 5'-deiodinase is decreased in follicular thyroid carcinoma, in most papillary carcinomas, and undetectable in most anaplastic thyroid carcinomas.[132] This decrease is observed not only for enzyme activity, but for the type I 5'-deiodinase substrate-binding subunit and for steady-state mRNA levels, suggesting that expression of functional type I 5'-deiodinase is a sensitive marker for differentiated thyroid tissue.[39,132] This assumption was confirmed by the demonstration of abundant type I 5'-deiodinase activity in FRTL-5 cells,[319–323] a nontransformed rat thyroid cell line, in which TSH and T_3 synergistically induce type I 5'-deiodinase mRNA and enzyme expression. In contrast, human thyroid cell lines derived from follicular or anaplastic thyroid carcinomas express no or only minimal type I 5'-deiodinase activity and p27 substrate-binding subunit, even after TSH stimulation, a stimulus that increases thyroglobulin production in these cells through the cAMP second-messenger pathway.[39,324] In the follicular thyroid carcinoma cells FTC-133 and FTC-238, treatment with nanomolar concentrations of retinoids, well known differentiation agents, rapidly induced expression of functional type I 5'-deiodinase activity.[39,324] It remains to be shown that in vivo treatment of thyroid carcinoma with retinoids provides a strategy to stop the dedifferentiation process and to reexpress some differentiated thyrocyte functions such as type I 5'-deiodinase activity and iodide uptake.

These observations suggest that, apart from defects in thyroid hormone synthesis, the defective expression of type I 5'-deiodinase activity in thyroid carcinoma may contribute to the phenotype of thyroglobulin-positive follicular thyroid carcinomas that rarely present with hyperthyroidism.[325] Variable levels of type I 5'-deiodinase and 5-deiodinase activity have also been found in normal and other pathologic human thyroid glands. Thyroid tissue from some patients with autoimmune thyroiditis or follicular adenomas had low type I 5'-deiodinase activity, and a dissociation of type I 5'-deiodinase activity and serum TSH levels was found in toxic adenomas.[130]

Increased expression of type I 5'-deiodinase in hyperthyroidism may provide the molecular basis for some of the therapeutic effects of iodinated radiographic contrast agents such as ipodate and iopanoic acid.[326–328] The rapid and potent effect of these agents may be exerted by direct competitive inhibition of thyroid type I 5'-deiodinase and interaction with thyroid secretory function,[310] rather than their high iodine content (see effects of pharmacologic agents on thyroid hormone metabolism in chap 14). The demonstration of functional T_3 receptors in thyrocytes indicates that local generation and action of thyroid hormones at their site of synthesis requires tight metabolic and functional control.[329]

In the thyrocyte, type I 5'-deiodinase activity is modulated by cytokines and growth factors. Tumor necrosis factor-α (TNF-α) and interleukin-1β (IL-1β) inhibit the effects of TSH on the thyroid gland, but do not directly inhibit thyroid or liver type I 5'-deiodinase in vivo,[330,331] in contrast to the FRTL-5 cell culture model, where TNF-α, IL-1β, and γ-interferon decrease type I 5'-deiodinase activity.[332,333] Cytokines such as TNF-α and IL-1β inhibit the hypothylamus–pituitary–thyroid–periphery axis at several levels and alter food intake, which also decreases hepatic type I 5'-deiodinase activity in the rat. These complex interrelationships blur the picture of regulation of type I 5'-deiodinase even more.[333–336] The association of the low-T_3 syndrome or nonthyroidal illness with increased cytokine levels does not lead to direct inhibition of type I 5'-deiodinase per se and to decreased T_3 production in thyroid, liver, and kidney, but does lead to decreased thyroid hormone secretion or alterations in serum binding and cellular uptake.[335,337,338] The fact that these cytokines are produced and secreted in a paracrine or autocrine manner by the thyroid itself further complicates the analysis.[339,340] Similarly, both TNF-α and IL-1β follow a similar scenario to account for their association with elevated serum levels of IL-6 found during nonthyroidal illness.[341–344] IL-6 is synthesized by a variety of cells, either directly or secondary to stimulation by IL-1β. In contrast to the animal studies, infusion of recombinant human IL-6 did not alter circulating T_4 levels, but increased rT_3 and decreased T_3 and serum TSH levels in a way comparable to nonthyroidal illness, suggesting its role as one of the pathogenic factors of this syndrome.[343] Species differences with respect to the contribution of thyroidal type I 5'-deiodinase activity to T_3 secretion and circulating T_3 levels have been reported for the rat thyroid. Kinetic analysis of T_3 production in the neonatal and selenium-deficient rat indicated that, in contrast to the human, thyroidal type I 5'-deiodinase and T_3 secretion by the thyroid is the major contributor to circulating T_3 levels.[65,345]

Insulin and growth factors (insulin-like growth factor 1, acidic and basic fibroblast growth factor) also modulate type I 5'-deiodinase activity at the thyroid level and in the liver, but again, in vitro cell culture effects differ from in vivo observations.[346–349]

Anterior Pituitary Gland

Both rat and human pituitary glands and pituitary thyrotrophic tumors show specific pituitary T_4-to-T_3 deiodination.[25,190,207,350–352] Both growth hormone and TSH synthesis depend on intrapituitary T_4-to-T_3 conversion.[24] TRH increases pituitary type II 5'-deiodinase activity, an action that could counteract TRH-stimulated TSH secretion by a short-loop feedback. About 80% of the nuclear T_3 receptors in the pituitary gland are occupied, with half the nuclear T_3 being derived from serum T_3 and the other half from intrapituitary T_4 deiodination (see Fig 8-8). Type II 5'-deiodinase activity in the pituitary gland is decreased in hyperthyroidism and increased in hypothyroidism.[24] Early suggestions were that thyrotrophs would have the highest 5'-deiodinase activity because increased pituitary enzyme activity seemed to correspond to an increase in thyrotrophs. In subsequent studies, type II 5'-deiodinase activity was found to be highest in somatotrophs and lactotrophs, followed by gonadotrophs and thyrotrophs.[193] The possible adaptive advantages of these alterations of type II 5'-deiodinase are not understood, but markedly increased local T_3 production in thyrotrophs during hypothyroidism would lead to an unwanted suppression of TSH secretion, whereas increased T_3 production in hypothyroid somatotrophs may have advantages for T_3-dependent growth hormone (GH) and prolactin production.[193] The demonstration of functional type I 5'-deiodinase activity and its rapid stimulation by T_3 in anterior pituitaries of the rat indicates a role for this enzyme in the feedback regulation of pituitary hormone secretion and T_3-dependent gene expression.[25]

Rat GH_3 pituitary tumor cells contain type II 5'-deiodinase activity,[179] as do GH_4C_1 rat pituitary cells, which secrete both GH and prolactin. Type I 5'-deiodinase activity and its stimulation by T_3 has also been found in GH_3 pituitary tumor cells. Type II 5'-deiodinase activity in these cells is stimulated by at least two independent mechanisms, hypothyroid culture conditions and activation of protein kinase C by TRH or phorbol esters.[201] The role of TRH in the regulation of anterior pituitary type II 5'-deiodinase is still under debate. In rats, ablation of the hypothalamic paraventricular nucleus reduces the content of TRH in the median eminence and lowers serum TSH and T_4 concentrations, but does not affect type II 5'-deiodinase activity—in contrast to T_4, which lowers type II 5'-deiodinase activity.[195] Transplantation of the anterior pituitary to the renal capsule markedly decreases type II 5'-deiodinase activity and leads to an increase in type I 5'-deiodinase activity, suggesting that unidentified neuroendocrine factors are important in the control of expression of pituitary type II 5'-deiodinase activity.[353]

Variable expression of type II 5'-deiodinase activity, which can be blocked by iopanoic acid in vitro, has been demonstrated in human pituitary adenomas.[125] High enzyme levels were found in a thyrotroph adenoma, a corticotroph adenoma, two prolactinomas, and three somatotroph adenomas. Of five nonfunctioning tumors, type II 5'-deiodinase was undetectable in two and readily detected in three.

The content of T_4 and type II 5'-deiodinase in thyrotrophs probably occupies a key role in the hierarchy for the regulation of thyroid status. Surprisingly, no 5-deiodinase activity could be demonstrated in the anterior pituitary gland,[25,354] but an active thyroid hormone transport system has been characterized.[355,356] Posterior pituitary of the rat demonstrates activity of all three deiodinase isozymes.[25,354]

Brain

Thyroid hormones influence both the development and maturation of the central nervous system and are required throughout adult life for maintenance of normal central and peripheral nervous system activity. Because mature brain fails to increase its rate of oxygen consumption after exposure to thyroid hormone,[192] the nature of thyroid hormone action in the central nervous system is poorly understood. Since the demonstration of T_3 nuclear receptors[17-19,357] and the presence of T_3 derived from T_4 in the brain, the contribution of brain to thyroid hormone metabolism has become a subject of much interest. An estimate of T_4-to-T_3 deiodination in rat brain homogenates suggested that the rate of T_4 deiodination in brain is 40 to 80 times less than that in liver or kidney, which would mean that the brain contributes little to the rapidly exchangeable T_3 pool. However, local iodothyronine deiodinase activities in the brain exert important effects at the molecular as well as the functional levels. Both type II 5'-deiodinase and 5-deiodinase activities are present in cerebral cortical homogenates.[230] As in the pituitary gland, short-term hypothyroidism increases brain type II 5'-deiodinase activity, whereas in euthyroid and thyrotoxic states 5-deiodinase activity is predominant. rT_3 produced from T_4 by local 5-deiodination may participate in the regulation of local deiodination of T_4 to T_3.[358-360] The contributions of anatomically distinct regions of the nervous system to overall brain deiodination vary widely, the highest activity being found in the cortex and lesser amounts in the midbrain, pons, hypothalamus, and brain stem (Fig 8-11). Spinal cord and peripheral nerve tissue have little enzymatic activity.[224] The identity of the cell types that contain the deiodinases is uncertain, but both type I 5'-deiodinase and 5-deiodinase activity in rats is present mostly in glial cells, with little if any activity in neurons.[203,221,222] Although type II 5'-deiodinase is usually found in neurons, 5'-deiodinase activity can be induced in astrocytes by hydrocortisone and agents that stimulate intracellular production of cAMP.[194,203,222] Type II 5'-deiodinase activity is also expressed in mouse neuroblastoma cell lines.[118,198]

When 5-deiodinase activity was studied as T_3 tyrosyl ring deiodination in central nervous system tissues, the activity was higher in homogenates of normal tissue than in homogenates of hypothyroid tissue. Both the increase of fractional T_4-to-T_3 conversion in brain tissue from hypothyroid animals and the inhibition of T_3 degradation potentially defend the brain against intracellular deficiency of T_3 at the level of the nucleus. The kinetic behavior of brain deiodinases should be discussed cautiously because two separate thiol-dependent 5'-deiodinase isoenzymes are present in brain.[92] Their existence probably provides mechanisms for cell- or tissue-specific regulation of expression of thyroid hormone action. The type I 5'-deiodinase of liver, kidney, thyroid, and euthyroid pituitary and brain probably serves to deliver T_3 to the serum pool (see Fig 8-1), whereas brain type II 5'-deiodinase maintains an optimal T_3 content in the central nervous system.[24]

The developmental profiles of the brain deiodinase isoenzymes show patterns specific for each isoenzyme and every brain region. During and after the period of rapid growth of the developing brain, temporally related to neurite extension and the formation of myelin sheaths of neurons, type II 5'-deiodinase activity decreases and 5-deiodinase activity increases in the same brain region, suggesting progressive protection of already differentiated structures from exposure to excess thyromimetic activity.[224] The contribution of local 5'-deiodinase to regional T_3 production also changes

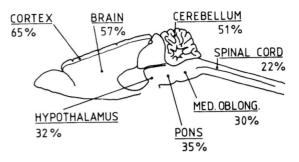

FIGURE 8-11. Contribution of local $T_4$5'-deiodination to the total concentration of T_3 in several regions of the central nervous system of the intact euthyroid rat. (van Doorn J, Roelfsema F, van der Heide D. Concentrations of thyroxine and 3,5,3' triiodothyronine at 34 different sites in euthyroid rats as determined by an isotopic equilibrium technique. Endocrinology 1985;117:1201)

during alterations of thyroidal status and after administration of drugs that interfere with thyroid hormone transport and metabolism.[4,26,114,269-271,361-363]

Hypothyroidism increases and thyrotoxicosis decreases the contribution of local T_3 production from T_4, compared with serum-derived T_3, in the cerebral cortex and cerebellum of rats. In the rat hypothalamus, where T_3 5-deiodinase activity is remarkably high, hypothyroidism enhances type II 5'-deiodinase activity in the arcuate nucleus and median eminence but not in the paraventricular nucleus, the site of the TRH-producing neurons.[196]

The regional uptake, metabolism, and local formation of iodothyronines has also been demonstrated after in vivo administration of radiolabeled iodothyronines to hypothyroid rats using thaw-mount film autoradiography.[177,204,364] Selective, saturable uptake and time-dependent retention of [125I]T_3-derived radioactivity in nerve cells (pyramidal cells of the hippocampus, granule cells of the dentate gyrus and cerebellar layer, and Purkinje cells) and choroid plexus has been demonstrated, and axonal transport has been proposed.[364] Inhibition of type II 5'-deiodinase with ipodate completely blocked labeling of the cerebellar granular layer after administration of [125I]T_4 but not [125I]T_3. In contrast, the distribution of [125I]rT_3 was not different from that of blood flow markers, and no specific regional labeling was found.[204] It is not yet clear if the specific retention of [125I]T_3 that is either systemically or locally derived from T_4 by type II 5'-deiodinase results from binding to nuclear T_3 receptors enriched in the granular layer of hypothyroid rats. More recently, the ability of the brain to deiodinate thyroid hormones has been extended to the developing human cerebral cortex,[116] and the catalytic activities present resemble those of the rodent brain.

Pineal and Harderian Glands

Type II 5'-deiodinase activity has been demonstrated in the pineal gland of rodents, Syrian hamsters, and ground squirrels and in rat and hamster harderian glands (a large tubuloalveolar gland located in the posteromedial aspect of the orbital cavity of many terrestrial species, especially those that have a nictitating membrane).[195,199,200,365-374] This type II 5'-deiodinase activity can be stimulated by thyroidectomy, and the increase can be prevented by administration of iopanoic acid. Significant diurnal variation in type II 5'-deiodinase activity was found, with a light–dark cycle entrained circadian rhythm coincident with but regulated differently than that of melatonin synthetic activity. The nocturnal increase in type II 5'-deiodinase activity is prevented by light exposure; repeated injections of isoproterenol to animals maintained in constant light mimicked the effect of darkness, whereas propranolol blocked the nocturnal increase. The β-adrenergic stimulation of type II 5'-deiodinase activity by sympathetic neural input also can be prevented by superior cervical ganglionectomy. A similar diurnal rhythm in type II 5'-deiodinase activity has also been found in pituitary tissue, in which it could be related to the circadian release pattern of TSH.[22] However, alterations of type II 5'-deiodinase activity have not been found in thyrotrophs.[195] In contrast, the diurnal pattern of serum T_3 is not TSH dependent but seems to be regulated by (dietary?) signals altering type I 5'-deiodinase activity in parenchymal tissues.[375] A circadian pattern of type II 5'-deiodinase also has been found in brown adipose tissue; in this tissue, regulation seems to occur by way of melatonin and α_1-adrenergic inputs.[367,376–382] Thus, neural networks can influence local production of T_3 by type II 5'-deiodinase in defined regions of the central nervous system and other tissues.

Brown Adipose Tissue

For discussion of the regulation of deiodination by this organ, see chapter 46.

Placenta

Phylogenic and ontogenic differences in maternoplacental thyroid hormone metabolism make it difficult to evaluate the contribution of the placenta to the overall deiodination of T_4.[229] Clear evidence for transplacental transfer of thyroid hormone from the mother to the fetus during early gestation has been presented,[383] although it appears that placental membranes present a partial barrier to thyroid hormones during later periods of gestation.[384–386] Rapid thyroid hormone degradation by human and rat placental membranes, both of which are derived from the ectoderm of the blastocyst, has been offered as a possible explanation for the limitation of transplacental hormone transport. There are only a few reports concerning the deiodinating activity of rodent and human placental membranes or cells, but deiodination requires the presence of reduced dithiols and is partially inhibited by PTU and iopanoic acid, and both 5'- and 5-deiodination reactions have been described.[9,117,126,129,136,171,387,388] It appears that the chorionic and amniotic membranes contain mainly a 5-deiodinase enzyme. The rT_3 formed by this enzyme is rather stable, which may explain the high rT_3 levels found in amniotic fluid. The formation of T_3 from T_4 by a placental type II 5'-deiodinase isozyme has also been reported.[49,126] Type II 5'-deiodinase activity was higher in human chorionic decidual membranes than in trophoblastic tissue or amnion. In rat placenta, basal zone activity was higher than that in placental labyrinth or amnion.[49] Therefore, the initial hypothesis that placental deiodination is directed mainly at degradation of T_4 and T_3 seems only partially substantiated.

Studies indicate that maternal T_4, but not T_3, plays a crucial role in protection of the fetal brain from T_3 deficiency under hypothyroid conditions in humans and in rodents during early and late pregnancy.[273,386,389,390] In particular, the fetal rat brain seems to be exclusively dependent on local T_3 production from T_4 by type II 5'-deiodinase.[26] Adaptive mechanisms of local T_3 production from T_4 by type II 5'-deiodinase are of essential importance during fetal brain development under conditions of iodine or selenium deficiency.[389,391–393] Placental 5-deiodinase, a phospholipid-requiring enzyme, differs from the other deiodinase isozymes[394–397] in that its activity is not affected by selenium deficiency in the pregnant rat, and fetal thyroid hormone levels (T_4, rT_3, and TSH) are not altered during selenium deficiency in the rat.[392]

Leukocytes, Lymphocytes, Erythrocytes, and Other Tissues

The possible role of leukocytes, lymphocytes, and erythrocytes in the metabolism of ligands transported in the blood is difficult to evaluate. All three cell types have been reported to degrade T_4 by various enzymatic reactions,[139,236,398,399] but only the generation of specific iodothyronines is considered here.

Leukocytes represent, as a whole, an organ with a weight of 1500 g. Of these, only 0.6% are circulating cells; about 60% are within the bone marrow and 40% are in peripheral tissues. Initial studies failed to demonstrate significant T_3 formation from T_4 by leukocytes, but subsequent work detected both T_3 and rT_3 generation by these cells.[139] The K_m value of the T_3-generating system is about 5 µmol/L T_4, similar to the K_m value in rat liver and kidney homogenates. The generation of rT_3 was only about half that of T_3, but PTU inhibits both reactions. Prior induction of phagocytosis inhibits both T_3 and rT_3 generation, whereas thyrotoxicosis increases T_3 formation. Although these observations suggest that leukocytes have an effective iodothyronine deiodinating enzyme, the contribution of T_3 and rT_3 from this source to circulating serum or tissue concentrations probably is small.

Erythrocytes do not deiodinate T_4.[398] In contrast, lymphocytes actively deiodinate T_4, presumably by type I 5'-deiodinase.[400,401] However, their contribution to total thyroid hormone metabolism is probably small.

Some type I 5'-deiodinase activity also has been detected in cultured human fibroblasts, keratinocytes, and white adipose tissue.[124,127,128,189,402] These tissues, together with muscle, may have considerable potential to contribute to extrathyroidal T_4 metabolism, but their quantitative role has not been assessed.

INHIBITORS OF IODOTHYRONINE DEIODINASE ISOENZYMES

Covalent Binding of Radiolabeled Thiourylenes to Type I 5'-Deiodinase

The binding of radiolabeled analogues of thiouracil ([^{35}S]PTU or 5-[^{125}I]-6-n-propyl-2-thiouracil) to microsomal or detergent-solubilized type I 5'-deiodinase in vitro provided experimental support for the proposed ping-pong reaction mechanism.[104,111,403] This binding is covalent and results from the formation of a selenosulfide bridge, as expected for the formation of a PTU–enzyme mixed selenosulfide.[111] Iodothyronine substrates facilitate the covalent binding of labeled PTU to the enzyme. The stimulation of covalent PTU binding to type I

5'-deiodinase by various iodothyronines parallels their affinity as substrates of the enzyme, and saturation of PTU binding with respect to substrate concentration can be achieved.

The binding behavior of PTU suggests that interference with the type I 5'-deiodinase reaction occurs only after the formation of the intermediate enzyme selenocysteinyl-iodide during deiodination. No enhancement of PTU binding by substrate occurs in the presence of agents that interfere with the intermediate by themselves forming transient or stable mixed disulfides with the intermediate enzyme–selenocysteinyl–iodide complex, for example, DTT, excess of unlabeled PTU, methylmercaptoimidazole (tapazole, MMI, or sulfite.[104,111] A preformed [^{35}S]PTU–enzyme mixed disulfide can be destroyed with release of [^{35}S]PTU by incubation with MMI or DTT.[111] Another important observation in this respect is that the binding of [^{35}S]PTU prevents the irreversible inactivation of type I 5'-deiodinase by agents such as iodoacetic acid that covalently block the essential reduced nucleophile[111]; iodothyronines, however, fail to protect type I 5'-deiodinase against inactivation by *N*-methylmaleimide, suggesting that the catalytic selenocysteinyl group of type I 5'-deiodinase is not sufficiently shielded by the substrate.[138] Similar to thiouracils, selenouracil derivatives are potent inhibitors of the selenoenzyme type I 5'-deiodinase, uncompetitive with respect to the iodothyronine substrates, and competitive with the in vitro cofactor DTT.[404] The formation of a rather stable enzyme–selenouracil diselenide might be the result of the high in vitro potency of this new class of inhibitors.

Iodothyronine Analogues That Are Not Substrates for Type I 5'-Deiodinase

Substitution of iodine by other halogen atoms (bromine, chlorine), a nitro group, or a hydroxyl group has been shown to alter the binding properties of these analogues to both receptors and transport proteins and to alter their biologic activity.[96] The introduction of bromine, which is less polarizable than iodine, induces a rather slight modification that is tolerated much better than the substitution of iodine by an NO_2 group, which is less polarizable than iodine but has a higher inductive effect, leading to acidification of the 4'-OH group (pK_a 4–5). Introduction of additional OH groups into the phenolic ring, which seem to fit into the iodine-binding pockets of the transport proteins, either acidifies the 4'-OH group, renders it more prone to oxidation (o-, p-substitution), or stabilizes it against radical-related reactions (m-substitution).

The most potent competitive inhibitors of type I 5'-deiodinase activity are acetic acid side-chain derivatives (acetic acid > *N*-acetyl-L-alanine > L-alanine), those with a tetrasubstitution pattern (e.g., 3,3',5-triiodo,5'-NO_2, or 5'-Br-thyroacetic acid), or the 3'-I,5'-NO_2-thyroacetic acid analogue of 3',5'-T_2.[405] A dinitrosubstitution in the 3',5' position decreased the inhibitory potency of all derivatives tested. Those results fit with the decreased affinity for binding to transport proteins of similarly substituted iodothyronines, and can be explained by the formation of strong intramolecular hydrogen bonds with the 4'-OH group.

The ligand-binding site of type I 5'-deiodinase of rat liver microsomes seems to exhibit marked similarities to the ligand-binding site of transthyretin.[46,85,96] Both proteins prefer as ligands 3,3',5,5'-tetrasubstituted iodothyronines with

negatively charged side chains of the tyrosyl ring. With few exceptions (e.g., rT_3), all potent ligands for transthyretin binding also have high affinity for type I 5'-deiodinase,[85] a phenomenon not fully understood because the ligand-binding site of transthyretin is formed by homopolymeric subunits that are not related to the type I 5'-deiodinase sequence (see chap 6).

The presence of iodine in the phenolic ring is not essential for effective inhibition of type I 5'-deiodinase activity; analogues that lack iodine substituents at the phenolic ring [2',4'-(OH)$_2$- or 3',4'-(OH)$_2$-3,5-12-T_2] also are potent type I 5'-deiodinase inhibitors in vitro. Therefore, not only bromine or nitro groups but also hydroxyl groups can replace iodine in the phenolic ring in the ligand-binding site interaction with type I 5'-deiodinase, as with other binding proteins.

A surprising conclusion from these studies was that type I 5'-deiodinase is not a general dehalogenase, because no removal of bromide in the corresponding analogues could be shown by various chromatographic procedures. Moreover, no evidence has yet been found for enzymic removal of iodide from the 3' position in analogues with a 3'-I,5'-NO_2 substitution, and no data are available as to whether iodide in the inner ring is liberated from these kinds of analogues.

Iodinated Radiographic Contrast Agents and Iodinated Aromatic Compounds

See chapter 14 for discussion.

Flavonoids

Polycyclic iodine-free or iodinated phenols or phenol-carboxylic acids (e.g., dicumarol, and the secondary plant metabolites rosmarinic acid, flavonoids, and auronoids) also are competitive inhibitors of type I 5'-deiodinase and 5-deiodinase activity. Even so, dicumarol has no effect on circulating iodothyronine concentrations (J. Leonard unpublished observation).

A remarkable observation in this context was the finding that those flavonoids and auronoids with rather rigid conformations resembling that of T_4 were very active as deiodinase inhibitors, whereas chalcones, which have a chemical constitution identical or similar to flavonoids but with a flexible conformation that is not fixed in a T_4-like conformation, did not interfere with deiodinase activity.[163,406–410] The inhibitory potency was increased by introduction of an iodine atom in the o-position of 4,4',6-(OH)$_3$-aurone. Surprisingly, a similar increase in inhibitory potency occurred in the case of the cofactor competitive effect of 5-iodo-PTU.[411] The structure–activity relationships and potency of naturally occurring or synthetic flavonoids and aurones were similar in rat liver microsomal membranes and in intact hepatocytes.[163]

In the rat, long-term administration of the synthetic flavonoid EMD 21388 inhibits T_3 formation in tissues expressing type I and also type II 5-deiodinase activity. Furthermore, serum thyroid hormone levels are reduced, thyroidal T_3 secretion is increased, and TSH levels are not increased.[412] T_4 transfer into tissues and T_4 elimination are increased. Although most tissues show diminished T_4 tissue contents, the T_4:T_3 tissue– plasma ratios were increased, indicating inhibition of both 5'-deiodinase isozymes.[412] As expected from in vitro binding studies, synthetic flavonoids also completely displace T_4 and T_3 from serum transthyretin in rats after in vivo administration.[413,414] The displacement from transthyretin occurs in minutes and leads to transient elevation of serum free hormone concentrations, followed by transient inhibition of TSH secretion.[413,415–418]

β-Adrenergic Antagonist and Agonist Drugs

See chapter 14 for discussion.

References

1. Kendall EC. The isolation in crystalline form of the compound containing iodine which occurs in the thyroid: its chemical nature and physiological activity. Trans Assoc Am Physicians 1915;30:420
2. Lerman J. The physiologic activity of L-triiodothyronine. J Clin Endocrinol Metab. 1953;13:1341
3. Gross J, Pitt-Rivers R. The identification of 3,5,3′-triiodothyronine in human plasma. Lancet 1952;1:439
4. Roche J, Lissitzky S, Michel R. Sur la triiodothyronine, produit intermediaire de la transformation de la diiodothyronine en thyroxine. CR Acad Sci (D) 1952;234:997
5. Roche J, Lissitzky S, Michel R. Sur la presence de triiodothyronine dans la thyroglobuline. CR Acad Sci (D) 1952; 234:1228
6. Pitt-Rivers R, Stanbury JB, Rapp B. Conversion of thyroxine to 3,5,3′-triiodothyronine in vivo. J Clin Endocrinol 1955;15:616
7. Lassiter WE, Stanbury JB. The in vivo conversion of thyroxine to triiodothyronine. J Clin Endocrinol Metab 1958;18:903
8. Pind K. Paper chromatographic determination of thyroid hormone (3,5,3′-triiodothyronine) in serum without radio-iodine. Acta Endocrinol 1957;26:263
9. Braverman LE, Ingbar SH, Sterling K. Conversion of thyroxine (T₄) to triiodothyronine (T₃) in athyreotic subjects. J Clin Invest 1970;49:855
10. Sterling K, Brenner MA, Newmann ES. Conversion of thyroxine to triiodothyronine in normal human subjects. Science 1970; 169:1099
11. Roche J, Michel R, Nunez J, Wolf W. Sur deux constitutants hormonaux nouveau du corps thyroide: la 3,3′-diiodothyronine et 3,3′,5′-triiodothyronine. Biochim Biophys Acta 1955;18:149
12. Flock EV, Bollman IL, Grindlay JH, Stobie GH. Partial deiodination of L-thyroxine. Endocrinology 1991;69:626
13. Flock EV, David C, Stobie GH, Owen CA. 3,3′,5′-triiodothyronine and 3,3′-diiodothyronine: partially deiodinated intermediates in the metabolism of the thyroid hormones. Endocrinology 1963;73:442
14. Flock EV, Bollman IL, Grindlay JH. Conjugates of triiodothyronine and its metabolites. Endocrinology 1960;67:419
15. Oppenheimer JH. Thyroid hormone action at the nuclear level. Ann Intern Med 1985;102:374
16. Oppenheimer JH, Schwartz HL, Surks MI, Koerner D, Dillmann WH. Nuclear receptors and the initiation of thyroid hormone action. Recent Prog Horm Res 1976;32:529
17. Evans RM. The steroid and thyroid hormone receptor superfamily. Science 1988;240:889
18. Sap J, Munoz A, Damm K, Goldberg Y, Ghysdael J, Leutz A, Beug H, Vennstroem B. The c-erb-A protein is a high affinity receptor for thyroid hormone. Nature 1986;324:635
19. Weinberger C, Thompson CC, Ong ES, Lebo R, Gruol DJ, Evans RM. The c-erb-A gene encodes a thyroid hormone receptor. Nature 1986;324:641
20. Yen PM, Chin WW. New advances in understanding the molecular mechanisms of thyroid hormone action. Trends Endocrinol Metab 1994;5:65
21. Bantle JP, Dillmann WH, Oppenheimer JH, Bingham C, Runger GC. Common clinical indices of thyroid hormone action: relationships to serum free 3,5,3′-triiodothyronine concentration and estimated nuclear occupancy. J Clin Endocrinol Metab 1980; 50:286
22. Brabant G, Brabant A, Ranft U, Ocran K, Köhrle J, Hesch RD, Von zur Mühlen A. Circadian and pulsatile thyrotropin secretion in euthyroid man under the influence of thyroid hormone and glucocorticoid administration. J Clin Endocrinol Metab 1987; 65:83
23. Emerson CH, Lew R, Braverman LE, DeVito WJ. Serum thyrotropin concentrations are more highly correlated with serum triiodothyronine concentrations than with serum thyroxine concentrations in thyroid hormone-infused thyroidectomized rats. Endocrinology 1989;124:2415
24. Larsen PR, Silva JE, Kaplan MM. Relationships between circulating and intracellular thyroid hormones: physiological and clinical implications. Endocr Rev 1981;2:87
25. Köhrle J, Schomburg L, Drescher S, Fekete E, Bauer K. Rapid stimulation of type I 5′-deiodinase in rat pituitaries by 3,3′,5-triiodo-L-thyronine. Mol Cell Endocrinol 1995;108:17
26. van Doorn J, Van der Heide D, Roelfsema F. Sources and quantity of 3,5,3′-triiodothyronine in several tissues of the rat. J Clin Invest 1983;72:1778
27. LoPresti JS, Anderson KP, Nicoloff JT. Does a hidden pool of reverse triiodothyronine (rT₃) production contribute to total thyroxine (T₄) disposal in high T₄ states in man. J Clin Endocrinol Metab 1990;70:1479
28. Obregon MJ, Roelfsema F, Morreale de Escobar G, Escobar del Rey F, Querido A. Exchange of triiodothyronine derived from thyroxine with circulating triiodothyronine as studied in the rat. Clin Endocrinol (Oxf) 1979;10:305
29. Hesch RD, Brunner G, Soeling HD. Conversion of thyroxine (T₄) and triiodothyronine (T₃) and the subcellular localisation of the converting enzyme. Clin Chim Acta 1975;59:209
30. Visser TJ, van der Does-Tobe I, Docter R, Hennemann G. Conversion of thyroxine into tri-iodothyronine by rat liver homogenate. Biochem J 1975;150:489
31. Borges M, Eisenstein Z, Burger AG, Ingbar SH. Immunosequestration: a new technique for studying peripheral iodothyronine metabolism in vitro. Endocrinology 1981;108:1665
32. Chopra IJ, Solomon DH, Chopra U, Wu SY, Fisher DA, Nakamura Y. Pathways of metabolism of thyroid hormones. Recent Prog Horm Res 1978.34:521
33. Imai Y, Yamauchi K, Nishikima M. A possible function of thiols, including glutathione, as cofactors of the conversion of thyroxine to 3,3′-5-triiodothyronine in rat liver microsomes. Endocrinol Jpn 1980;27:201
34. Kaminski T, Köhrle J, Ködding R, Hesch R-D. Autoregulation of 3,3′,5′-triiodothyronine production by rat liver microsomes. Acta Endocrinol 1981;98:240
35. Sato K, Robbins J. Glutathione deficiency induced by cysteine and/or methionine deprivation does not affect thyroid hormone deiodination in cultured rat hepatocytes and monkey carcinoma cells. Endocrinology 1981;109:117
36. Leonard JL, Rosenberg IN. Subcellular distribution of thyroxine 5′-deiodinase in the rat kidney: a plasma membrane location. Endocrinology 1978;103:274
37. Nakano M, Tsutsumi Y, Ushiima Y. Degradation of thyroxine by the microsomal particles from rat liver: I. Correlation between thyroxine degradation and lipid peroxides. Biochim Biophys Acta 1971;252:335
38. Höffken B, Ködding R, Hehrmann R, Von zur Mühlen A, Jüppner H, Hesch R-D. Regulation of thyroid hormone metabolism in rat liver fractions. Biochim Biophys Acta 1978;539:114
39. Köhrle J. Thyroid hormone deiodination in target tissues: a regulatory role for the trace element selenium? Exp Clin Endocrinol 1994;102:63
40. Leonard JL. Identification and structure analysis of iodothyronine deiodinases. In: Greer MA, ed. The thyroid gland. New York: Raven Press, 1991;285

41. Moreno M, Berry MJ, Horst C, Thoma R, Goglia F, Harney JW, Larsen PR, Visser TJ. Activation and inactivation of thyroid hormone by type I iodothyronine deiodinase. FEBS Lett 1994; 344:143

42. St. Germain DL, Schwartzman RA, Croteau W, Kanamori A, Wang Z, Brown DD, Galton VA. A thyroid hormone-regulated gene in *Xenopus laevis* encodes a type III iodothyronine 5-deiodinase. Proc Natl Acad Sci USA 1994;91:7767

43. Galton VA, Schneider MJ, Becker KB, Davey JC. The type III 5-deiodinase in *Rana catesbeiana* (RC) tadpoles is encoded by a thyroid hormone-responsive gene (abstract). Thyroid 1994;4:S-96

44. Croteau W, Whittemore SL, Schneider MJ, St. Germain DL. Cloning and expression of a cDNA for a mammalian type III iodothyronine deiodinase. J. Biochem 1994;270:16569

45. Hays MT, Cavalieri RR. Deiodination and deconjugation of the glucuronide conjugates of the thyroid hormones by rat liver and brain microsomes. Metabolism 1992;41:494

46. Köhrle J, Hesch RD. Biochemical Characteristics of iodothyronine monodeiodination by rat liver microsomes: the interaction between iodothyronine substrate analogues and the ligand binding site of iodothyronine deiodinase resembles that of the TBPA-iodothyronine ligand binding site. Horm Metab Res [Suppl] 1984;14:42

47. Leonard JL, Visser TJ. Biochemistry of deiodination. In: Hennemann G, ed. Thyroid hormone metabolism. New York: Marcel Dekker, 1986:189

48. Visser TJ. Role of sulfation in thyroid hormone metabolism. Chem Biol Interact 1994;92:293

49. Kaplan MM, Shaw EA. Type II iodothyronine 5'-deiodination by human and rat placenta in vitro. J Clin Endocrinol Metab 1984;59:253

50. Boye N, Frokiaer H, Kaltoft K, Laurberg P. Solid-phase iodothyronine-5'-deiodinase (5'-D) assays applied in production of monoclonal antibodies against 5'-D. J Endocrinol 1988;118:439

51. Fekkes D, van Overmeeren E, Hennemann G, Visser TJ. Solubilization and partial characterization of rat liver iodothyronine deiodinases. Biochim Biophys Acta 1980;613:41

52. Boye N, Laurberg P. Deiodination of T_4 to T_3 and rT_3 by microsomes from normal human thyroid tissue. Mol Cell Endocrinol 1984;37:295

53. Hummel BCW, Walfish PG. 5'-Iodothyronine deiodinase of rat liver: activity in microsomes prepared by various methods, solubilization by detergents and partial purification. Biochim Biophys Acta 1985;841:173

54. Mol JA, Berg TPv, Visser TJ. Partial purification of the microsomal rat liver iodothyronine deiodinase. Mol Cell Endocrinol 1988;55:149

55. Leonard JL, Rosenberg IN. Solubilization of a phospholipid-requiring enzyme, iodothyronine 5'-deiodinase, from rat kidney membranes. Biochim Biophys Acta 1981;659:205

56. Sakane S, Chopra IJ. Isolation of a hepatic iodothyronine 5'-monodeiodinase by nondenaturing agarose gel electrophoresis. Endocrinology 1990;127:2709

57. Santini F, Chopra IJ. A radioimmunoassay of rat type I iodothyronine 5'-monodeiodinase. Endocrinology 1992;131:2521

58. Safran M, Leonard JL. Comparison of the physicochemical properties of type I and type II iodothyronine 5'deiodinase. J Biol Chem 1991;266:3233

59. DePalo D, Kinlaw WB, Zhao C, Engelberg Kulka H, St. Germain DL. Effect of selenium deficiency on type I 5'-deiodinase. J Biol Chem 1994;269:16223

60. Nagasaka A, Yoshida S, Nakai A, Ohyama T, Iwase K, Ohtani S, Shinoda S, Masunaga R, Nakagawa H. DNA polymerase β in human thyroid of Graves' disease and thyroid tumors. Metabolism 1988;37:1051

61. Behne D, Kyriakopoulos A, Meinhold H, Köhrle J. Identification of type I iodothyronine 5'-deiodinase as a selenoenzyme. Biochem Biophys Res Commun 1990;173:1143

62. Arthur JR, Nicol F, Beckett GJ. Hepatic iodothyronine 5'-deiodinase: the role of selenium. Biochem J 1990;272:537

63. Berry MJ, Banu L, Larsen PR. Type I iodothyronine deiodinase is a selenocystein-containing enzyme. Nature 1991; 349:438

64. Meinhold H, Campos-Barros A, Behne D. Effects of selenium and iodine deficiency on iodothyronine deiodinases in brain, thyroid and peripheral tissue. Acta Med Austriaca 1992;19:8

65. Chanoine JP, Braverman LE, Farwell AP, Safran M, Alex S, Dubord S, Leonard JL. The thyroid gland is a major source of circulating T_3 in the rat. J Clin Invest 1993;91:2709

66. Behne D, Hilmert H, Scheid S, Gessner H, Elger W. Evidence for specific selenium target tissues and new biologically important selenoproteins. Biochim Biophys Acta 1988;966:12

67. Behne D, Scheid S, Kyriakopoulos A, Hilmert H. Subcellular distribution of selenoproteins in the liver of the rat. Biochim Biophys Acta 1990;1033:219

68. Berry MJ, Banu L, Chen YY, Mandel SJ, Kieffer JD, Harney JW, Larsen PR. Recognition of UGA as a selenocysteine codon in type I deiodinase requires sequences in the 3' untranslated region. Nature 1991;353:273

69. Mandel SJ, Berry MJ, Kieffer JD, Harney JW, Warne RL, Larsen PR. Cloning and in vitro expression of the human selenoproteins, type I iodothyronine deiodinase. J Clin Endocrinol Metab 1992;75:1133

70. Berry MJ, Banu L, J. W. Harney, and P. R. Larsen.1993. Functional characterization of the eukaryotic SECIS elements which direct selenocysteine insertion at UGA codons. EMBO J 12:3315-3322

71. Berry MJ, Kieffer JD, Harney JW, Larsen PR. Selenocysteine confers the biochemical properties characteristic of the type I iodothyronine deiodinase. J Biol Chem 1991;266:14155

72. Safran M, Farwell AP, Leonard JL. Evidence that type II 5'-deiodinase is not a selenoprotein. J Biol Chem 1991;266:13477

73. Berry MJ, Kieffer JD, Larsen PR. Evidence that cysteine, not selenocysteine, is in the catalytic site of type II iodothyronine deiodinase. Endocrinology 1991;129:550

74. Chaudiere J, Tappel AL. Interaction of gold (I) with the active site of selenium–glutathione peroxidase. J Inorg Biochem 1984; 20:31

75. Gross M, Oertel M, Köhrle J. Differential selenium-dependent expression of type I 5'-deiodinase and glutathione peroxidase in the porcine epithelial kidney cell line LLC-PK1. Biochem J 1995;306:851

76. Oertel M, Gross M, Rokos H, Kohrle J. Selenium-dependent regulation of type I 5'-deiodinase expression. Am J Clin Nutr 1993;57:313S

77. Beckett GJ, Beech S, Nicol F, Walker SW, Arthur JR. Species differences in thyroidal iodothyronine deiodinase expression and the effect of selenium deficiency on its activity. J Trace Elem Electrolytes Health Dis 1993;7:123

78. Schoenmakers CH, Pigmans IG, Poland A, Visser TJ. Impairment of the selenoenzyme type I iodothyronine deiodinase in C3H/He mice. Endocrinology 1993;132:357

79. DePalo D, Kinlaw WB, Zhao C, Engelberg-Kulka H, St. Germain DL. Effect of selenium deficiency on type I 5'-deiodinase. J Biol Chem 1994;269:16223

80. Köhrle J, Rasmussen U, Rokos H, Leonard JL, Hesch RD. Selective affinity labeling of a 27-kDa integral membrane protein in rat liver and kidney with N-Bromoacetyl derivatives of L-thyroxine and 3,5,3'-triiodothyronine. J Biol Chem 1990;265:6146

81. Köhrle J, Rasmussen UB, Ekenbarger DM, Alex S, Rokos H, Hesch RD, Leonard JL. Affinity labeling of rat liver and kidney

type I 5'-deiodinase: identification of the 27-kDa substrate binding subunit. J Biol Chem 1990;265:6155

82. Schoenmakers CHH, Pigmans IGAJ, Hawkins HC, Freedman RB, Visser TJ. Rat liver type I iodothyronine deiodinase is not identical to protein disulfide isomerase. Biochem Biophys Res Commun 1989;162:857

83. Safran M, Köhrle J, Braverman LE, Leonard JL. Effect of biological alterations of type I 5'deiodinase activity on affinity labeled membrane proteins in rat liver and kidney. Endocrinology 1990;126:826

84. Schoenmakers CHH, Pigmans IGAJ, Visser TJ. Species differences in liver type I iodothyronine deiodinase. Biochim Biophys Acta 1992;1121:160

85. Köhrle J, Auf'mkolk M, Rokos H, Hesch RD, Cody V. Rat liver iodothyronine monodeiodinase: evaluation of the iodothyronine binding site. J Biol Chem 1986;261:11613

86. Rosenberg IN, Goswami A. Purification and characterization of a flavoprotein from bovine thyroid with iodotyrosine deiodinase activity. J Biol Chem 1979;254:12318

87. Ishii H, Inada M, Tanaka K, Mashio Y, Naito K, Nishikawa M, Matsuzuka F, Kuma K, Imura H. Sequential deiodination of thyroxine in human thyroid gland. J Clin Endocrinol Metab 1982;55:890

88. Auf dem Brinke D, Hesch RD, Köhrle J. Re-examination of the subcellular localization of thyroxine-5'-deiodination in rat liver. Biochem J 1979;180:273

89. Kaplan MM, Utiger RD. Iodothyronine metabolism in rat liver homogenates. J Clin Invest 1978;61:459

90. Laurberg P, Boye N. Outer and inner ring monodeiodination of thyroxine by dog thyroid and liver: a comparative study using a particulate fraction. Endocrinology 1982;110:2124

91. Sato K, Robbins J. Thyroid hormone metabolism in cultured monkey hepatocarcinoma. J Biol Chem 1980;255:7347

92. Visser TJ, Leonard JL, Kaplan MM, Larsen PR. Kinetic evidence suggesting two mechanisms for iodothyronine-5'-deiodination in rat cerebral cortex. Proc Natl Acad Sci USA 1982;79:5080

93. Visser TJ, Kaptein E, Terpstra OT, Krenning EP. Deiodination of thyroid hormone by human liver. J Clin Endocrinol Metab 1988;67:17

94. Leonard JL, Rosenberg IN. Iodothyronine 5'-deiodinase from rat kidney: substrate specificity and the 5'-deiodination of reverse triiodothyronine. Endocrinology 1980;107:1376

95. Heinen E, Basler M, Herrmann J, Hafner D, Krüskemper HL. Enzyme kinetic and substrate binding-studies of the thyroxine to 3,3',5-triiodothyronine converting enzyme in rat liver microsomal fraction. Endocrinology 1980;107:1198

96. Cody V. Thyroid hormone interactions: molecular conformation, protein binding and hormone action. Endocr Rev 1980;61:163

97. Toyoda N, Harney JW, Berry MJ, Larsen PR. Identification of critical amino acids for 3,5,3'-triiodothyronine deiodination by human type 1 deiodinase based on comparative functional-structural analyses of the human, dog, and rat enzymes. J Biol Chem 1994;269:20329

98. Sorimachi K, Yasumura Y. High affinity of triiodothyronine (T_3) for nonphenolic ring deiodinase and high affinity for tetraiodothyroacetic acid (tetrac) for phenolic ring deiodinase in cultured monkey hepatocarcinoma cells and in rat liver homogenates. Endocrinol Jpn 1981;28:775

99. Visser TJ, van der Does-Tobe I, Docter R, Hennemann G. Subcellular localization of a rat liver enzyme converting thyroxine to triiodothyronine and possible involvement of essential thiol groups. Biochem J 1976;157:479

100. Balsam A, Ingbar SH. Observations on the factors that control the generation of triiodothyronine from thyroxine in rat liver and nature of the defect induced by fasting. J Clin Invest 1979;63:1145

101. Pardridge WM. On plasma protein-mediated transport of steroid and thyroid hormones: reply. Am J Physiol 1988;255:E224

102. Goswami A, Rosenberg IN. Stimulation of iodothyronine outer ring monodeiodinase by dihydrolipoamide. Endocrinology 1983;12:1180

103. Sawada K, Hummel BCW, Walfish PG. Cytosolic cofactors and dihydrolipoamide stimulate hepatic microsomal 5'-deiodination. Endocrinology 1985;117:1259

104. Yamada T, Chopra IJ, Kaplowitz N. Inhibition of rat heaptic thyroxine 5'-monodeiodinase by propylthiouracil: relation to site of interaction of thyroxine and glutathione. J Endocrinol Invest 1981;4:379

105. Gavin LA, McMahon FA, Moeller M. Dietary modification of thyroxine deiodination in rat liver is not mediated by hepatic sulfhydryls. J Clin Invest 1980;65:943

106. Gavin LA, McMahon FA, Moeller M. Carbohydrate in contrast to protein feeding increases the hepatic content of active thyroxine-5'-deiodinase in the rat. Endocrinology 1981;109:530

107. Sato K, Mimura H, Tomori N, Tsushima T, Shizume K. Modulating effect of glutathione disulfide on thyroxine-5'-deiodination by rat hepatocytes in primary culture: effect of glucose. Endocrinology 1983;113:878

108. Bhat GB, Iwase K, Hummel BCW, Walfish PG. Kinetic characteristics of a thioredoxin-activated rat hepatic and renal low-k_m iodothyronine 5'-deiodinase. Biochem J 1989;258:785

109. Iwase K, Hummel BCW, Walfish PG. Rat hepatic and renal 5'-deiodination of rT_3 during fasting: supportive role of intermediate M_r cytosolic non-glutathione thiol cofactor and NADPH. Metabolism 1989;38:230

110. Goswami A, Rosenberg IN. Thioredoxin stimulates enzymatic outer ring monodeiodination of reverse triiodothyronine. Endocrinology 1987;121:1937

111. Leonard JL, Rosenberg IN. Characterization of essential enzyme sulfhydryl groups of thyroxine 5'-deiodinase from rat kidney. Endocrinology 1980;106:444

112. Visser TJ. Mechanism of action of iodothyronine 5'-deiodinase. Biochim Biophys Acta 1979;569:302

113. Leonard JL, Visser TJ. Selective modification of the active center of renal iodothyronine 5'-deiodinase by iodoacetate. Biochim Biophys Acta 1984;787:122

114. van Doorn J, Roelfsema F, Van der Heide D. Concentrations of thyroxine and 3,5,3'-triiodothyronine at 34 different sites in euthyroid rats as determined by an isotopic equilibrium technique. Endocrinology 1985;117:1201

115. Tsukahara F, Nomoto T, Maeda M. Properties of 5'-deiodinase of 3,3',5'-triiodothyronine in rat skeletal muscle. Acta Endocrinol (Copenh) 1989;120:69

116. Karmarkar M, Prabarkaran D, Godbole MM. 5'-Monodeiodinase activity in developing human cerebral cortex. Am J Clin Nutr 1994;57(Suppl):291S

117. Banovac K, Bzik LI, Tislaric D, Sekso M. Conversion of thyroxine to triiodothyronine and reverse triiodothyronine in human placenta and fetal membranes. Horm Res 1980;12:253

118. Sterling K, Brenner MA, Saldhana VF. Conversion of thyroxine by cultured human cells. Science 1973;179:1000

119. Boye N. Thyroxine monodeiodination in normal human kidney tissue in vitro. Acta Endocrinol (Copenh) 1986;112:536

120. Harbottle R, Richardson SJ. Structural requirements of thiol compounds in the inhibition of iodothyronine 5'-deiodinase. Biochem J 1984;217:485

121. Hardy JJ, Thomas CL, Utiger RD. Characteristics of thyroxine 5'-deiodinase activity in human liver. Am J Med Sci 1986;292:193

122. Ishii H, Inada M, Tanaka K, Mashio Y, Naito K, Nishikawa M, Matsuzuka F, Kuma K, Imura H. Induction of outer and inner ring monodeiodinases in human thyroid gland by thyrotropin. J Clin Endocrinol Metab 1983;57:500

123. Ishii H, Inada M, Tanaka K, Mashio Y, Naito K, Nishikawa M, Imura H. Triiodothyronine generation from thyroxine in human

thyroid: enhanced conversion in Graves' thyroid tissue. J Clin Endocrinol Metab 1981;52:1211

124. Ishikawa S-E, Saito T, Kuzuya T. The effect of glucose deprivation or 2-deoxy-D-glucose on the monodeiodination of thyroxine in human fibroblasts in culture. J Clin Endocrinol Metab 1985;61:252

125. Itagaki Y, Yoshida K, Ikeda H, Kaise K, Kaise N, Yamamoto M, Sakurada T, Yoshinaga K. Thyroxine 5'-deiodinase in human anterior pituitary tumors. J Clin Endocrinol Metab 1990;71:340

126. Hidal JT, Kaplan MM. Characteristics of thyroxine 5'-deiodination in cultured human placental cells. J Clin Invest 1985;76:947

127. Kaplan MM, Pan C, Gordon PR, Lee JK, Gilchrest BA. Human epidermal keratinocytes in culture convert thyroxine to 3,5,3'-triiodothyronine by type II iodothyronine deiodination: a novel endocrine function of the skin. J Clin Endocrinol Metab 1988;66:815

128. Rao GS, Rao ML, Quednau HD, Greil W. Further evidence for the presence of thyroxine binding globulin-like protein in human breast adipose tissue: deiodination of thyroxine and triiodothyronine by the microsomal fraction. J Endocrinol Invest 1985;8:501

129. Roti E, Fang SL, Green K, Emerson CH, Braverman LE. Human placenta is an active site of thyroxine and 3,3',5-triiodotyrosyl ring deiodination. J Clin Endocrinol Metab 1981;53:498

130. Sugawara M, Lau R, Wasser HL, Nelson AM, Kuma K, Hershman JM. Thyroid T_4 5'-deiodinase activity in normal and abnormal human thyroid glands. Metabolism 1984;33:332

131. Yoshida K, Sakurada T, Kitaoka H, Fukazawa H, Kaise N, Kaise K, Yamamoto M, Suzuki M, Saito S, Yoshinaga K, Kimura S, Yamanaka M. Monodeiodination of thyroxine to 3,3'-5-triiodothyronine and 3,3',5'-triiodothyronine in human kidney homogenate. Fol Endocrinol Jpn 1982;58:199

132. Köhrle J, Oertel M, Hoang-Vu C, Schnieders F, Brabant G. Type I 5'-deiodinase: a marker for differentiated thyroid carcinoma? Exp Clin Endocrinol 1993;101(Suppl 3):60

133. Auf dem Brinke D, Köhrle J, Ködding R, Hesch RD. Subcellular localization of thyroxine-5-deiodinase in rat liver. J Endocrinol Invest 1980;3:73

134. Chiraseveenuprapund P, Buergi U, Goswami A, Rosenberg IN. Conversion of L-thyroxine to triiodothyronine in rat kidney homogenate. Endocrinology 1978;102:612

135. Erickson VJ, Cavalieri RR, Rosenberg LL. Phenolic and nonphenolic ring iodothyronine deiodinases from rat thyroid gland. Endocrinology 1981;108:1257

136. Roti E, Fang SL, Braverman LE, Emerson CH. Rat placenta is an active site of inner ring deiodination of thyroxine and 3,3',5-triiodothyronine. Endocrinology 1981;110:34

137. Sorimachi K, Niwa A, Yasumura Y. Phenolic ring deiodination in cultured rat hepatoma cells, and subcellular localization of deiodinase in cultured rat hepatoma, monkey hepatocarcinoma cells and normal rat liver homogenates. Biochim Biophys Acta 1980;630:469

138. Visser TJ, van Overmeeren-Kaptein E. Substrate requirement for inactivation of iodothyronine-5-deiodinase activity by thiouracil. Biochim Biophys Acta 1981;658:202

139. Woeber KA. L-triiodothyronine and L-reverse triiodothyronine generation in the human polymorphonuclear leukocyte. J Clin Invest 1978;62:577

140. Sato, K., Yamoto K, Takai T, Yoshida K. Thyroxine 5'-monodeiodinase activity in regenerating liver of triiodothyronine treated rats. J Biochem 1980;88:1595

141. Kaplan MM, Utiger RD. Iodothyronine metabolism in liver and kidney homogenates from hyperthyroid and hypothyroid rats. Endocrinology 1978;103:156

142. Fekkes D, van Overmeeren-Kaptein E, Docter R, Hennemann G, Visser TJ. Location of rat liver iodothyronine deiodinating enzymes in the endoplasmic reticulum. Biochim Biophys Acta 1979;587:12

143. Cavalieri RR, Gavin LA, Bui F. Conversion of thyroxine to 3,3',5'-triiodothyronine (reverse T_3) by a soluble enzyme of rat liver. Biochem Biophys Res Commun 1977;79:897

144. Maciel RMB, Ozawa Y, Chopra IJ. Subcellular localization of thyroxine and reverse triiodothyronine outer ring monodeiodinating activities. Endocrinology 1979;204:365

145. Fekkes D, Hennemann G, Visser TJ. Evidence for a single enzyme in rat liver catalyzing the deiodination of the tyrosyl and the phenolic ring of iodothyronines. Biochem J 1982;201:673

146. Boado RJ, Chopra IJ, Flink IL, Campbell DA. Enzyme binding-inhibiting assay for iodothyronine 5'-monodeiodinase (5'-MD) and its application to isolation of complementary deoxyribonucleic acid clones for the 5'-MD in rat liver. Endocrinology 1988;123:1264

147. Boado RJ, Campbell DA, Chopra IJ. Nucleotide sequence of rat liver iodothyronine 5'-monodeiodinase (5'-MD): its identity with the protein disulfide isomerase. Biochem Biophys Res Commun 1988;155:1297

148. Defer N, Dastague B, Sabatier MM, Thomopoulos P, Kruh J. Triiodothyronine binding proteins in rat liver cytosol. Biochem Biophys Res Commun 1975;67:995

149. Dillmann, W. H., Surks MI, Oppenheimer JH. Quantitative aspects of iodothyronine binding by cytosolic proteins of rat liver and kidney. Endocrinology 1974;95:492

150. Hamada S, Fukase M. Demonstration and some properties of cytosol-binding proteins for thyroxine and triiodothyronine in human liver. J Clin Endocrinol Metab 1976;42:302

151. Hashizume K, Kobayashi M, Miyamoto T, Yamauchi K. Dependence of the mitochondrial uptake of triiodothyronine (T_3) in rat kidney on cytosolic T_3-binding protein. Endocrinology 1986;119:1063

152. Obata T, Fukuda T, Willingham MC, Liang C-M, Cheng S-Y. A cytoplasmic thyroid hormone binding protein: characterization using monoclonal antibodies. Biochemistry 1989;28:617

153. De Jong M, Visser TJ, Bernard BF, Docter R, Vos RA, Hennemann G, Krenning EP. Transport and metabolism of iodothyronines in cultured human hepatocytes. J Clin Endocrinol Metab 1993; 77:139

154. Jennings AS, Ferguson DC, Utiger RD. Regulation of the conversion of thyroxine to triiodothyronine in the perfused rat liver. J Clin Invest 1979;64:1614

155. Ashizawa K, Kato H, McPhie P, Cheng S. Regulation of thyroid hormone binding to its cytosolic binding protein by L-α-alanine. Biochem Biophys Res Commun 1990;167:587

156. Bellabarba D, Bedard S, Lehoux J-G. Properties of triiodothyronine-binding proteins in liver cytosol of rat. Can J Physiol Pharmacol 1983;61:1035

157. Ishigaki S, Abramowicz MJ, Listowsky I. Glutathione-S-transferases are major cytosolic thyroid hormone binding proteins. Arch Biochem Biophys 1989;273:265

158. Mooradian AD, Schwartz HL, Mariash CN, Oppenheimer JH. Transcellular and transnuclear transport of 3,5,3'-triiodothyronine in isolated hepatocytes. Endocrinology 1985;117:2449

159. Pontecorvi A, Robbins J. The plasma membrane and thyroid hormone entry into cells. Trends Endocrinol Metab 1989;1:90

160. Lakshmanan M, Goncalves E, Pontecorvi A, Robbins J. Differential effect of a new thyromimetic on triiodothyronine transport into myoblasts and hepatoma and neuroblastoma cells. Biochim Biophys Acta 1993;1133:213

161. Aanderud S, Aarbakke J, Sundsfjord J. Metabolism of thyroid hormones in isolated rat hepatocytes: studies on the influences of carbamazepine and phenytoin. Acta Endocrinol 1983;104:479

162. Eelkman Rooda SJ, Van Loon MAC, Visser TJ. Metabolism of reverse triiodothyronine by isolated rat hepatocytes. J Clin Invest 1987;79:1740

163. Spanka M, Hesch R-D, Irmscher K, Köhrle J. 5'-Deiodination in rat hepatocytes: effects of specific flavonoid inhibitors. Endocrinology 1990;126:1660

164. Utiger RD. Triiodothyronine production by isolated rat hepatocytes: characterization and lack of glucoregulatory hormone effects. Horm Metab Res 1984;16:28

165. van Noorden CJ, Wiersinga WM, Touber JL. Propranolol inhibits the in vitro conversion of thyroxine into triiodothyronine by isolated rat liver parenchymal cells. Horm Metab Res 1979;11:166

166. Sorimachi K, Robbins J. Metabolism of thyroid hormones by cultured monkey hepatocarcinoma cells. J Biol Chem 1977; 252:4458

167. Leonard JL, Ekenbarger DM, Frank SJ, Farwell AP, Köhrle J. Localization of type I iodothyronine 5'deiodinase to the basolateral plasma membrane of rat kidney and LLC-PK1 renal cortical cells. J Biol Chem 1991;266:11262

168. Lee WS, Berry MJ, Hediger MA, Larsen PR. The type I iodothyronine 5'-deiodinase messenger ribonucleic acid is localized to the S3 segment of the rat kidney proximal tubule. Endocrinology 1993;132:2136

169. Heyma P, Larkins RG, Campbell DG. Inhibition by propranolol of 3,5,3'-triiodothyronine formation from thyroxine in isolated rat renal tubules: an effect independent of β-adrenergic blockade. Endocrinology 1980;106:1437

170. Faber J, Francis Thomsen H, Lumholtz IB, Kirkegaard C, Siersbaek-Nielsen K, Friis T. Kinetic studies of thyroxine, 3,5,3'-triiodothyronine, 3,3',5'-triiodothyronine, 3,3'-diiodothyronine and 3'-monoiodothyronine in patients with liver cirrhosis. J Clin Endocrinol Metab 1981;53:978

171. Faber J, Kirkegaard C, Jorgensen B, Kludt J. The hidden, nonexchangeable pool of 3,5,3'-triiodothyronine and 3,3',5'-triiodothyronine in man: Does it exist. Acta Endocrinol (Copenh) 1989;120:667

172. LoPresti JS, Eigen A, Kaptein E, Anderson KP, Spencer CA, Nicoloff JT. Alterations in 3,3',5'-triiodothyronine metabolism in response to propylthiouracil, dexamethasone, and thyroxine administration in man. J Clin Invest 1989;84:1650

173. Rogowski P, Faber J, Siersbaek-Nielsen K. Renal handling of 3,3',5'-triiodothyronine (reverse T_3) compared to thyroxine and 3,5,3'-triiodothyronine in different thyroid function states in man. Acta Endocrinol (Copenh) 1980;94:337

174. Adlkofer F, Schurek HJ, Sörje N. The renal clearance of thyroid hormones in the isolated rat kidney. Horm Metab Res 1980; 12:400

175. Leonard JL, Rennke H, Kaplan MM, Larsen PR. Subcellular distribution of iodothyronine 5'-deiodinase in cerebral cortex from hypothyroid rats. Biochim Biophys Acta 1982;718:109

176. Tanaka K, Inada M, Ishii H, et al. Inner ring monodeiodination of thyroxine and 3,3',5-L-triiodothyronine in rat brain. Endocrinology 1982;109:1619

177. Dratman MB, Crutchfield FL. Synaptosomal [^{125}I]triiodothyronine after intravenous [^{125}I]thyroxine. Am J Physiol 1979;253:E638

178. Tanaka K, Inada M, Mashio Y, et al. Characteristics of rT$_3$ 5-monodeiodination in rat brain: comparison with T$_4$ and T$_3$ monodeiodinations. Acta Endocrinol 1982;101:371

179. St. Germain DL. Metabolic effect of 3,3',5'-triiodothyronine in cultured growth hormone producing rat pituitary tumor cells: evidence for a unique mechanism of thyroid hormone action. J Clin Invest 198;76:890

180. Hüfner M, Grussendorf M. Investigations on the deiodination of thyroxine (T$_4$) to 3,3'-diiodothyronine (3,3'-T$_2$) in rat liver homogenate. Clin Chim Acta 1978;85:243

181. Köhrle J, Müller MJ, Ködding R, Seitz HJ, Hesch RD. pH Dependency of iodothyronine metabolism in isolated perfused rat liver. Biochem J 1982;202:669

182. Mol JA, Docter R, Hennemann G, Visser TJ. Modification of rat liver iodothyronine 5'-deiodinase activity with diethylpyrocarbonate and rose bengal: evidence for an active site histidine residue. Biochem Biophys Res Commun 1984;120:28

183. Tsai GS, Templeton DM, Wend AJ. Multifunctionality of lipoamide dehydrogenase: activities of chemically trapped monomeric and dimeric enzymes. Arch Biochem Biophys 1981; 206:77

184. Chanoine JP, Safran M, Farwell AP, Tranter P, Ekenbarger SM, Dubord S, Alex S. Selenium deficiency and type II 5'-deiodinase regulation in the euthyroid and hypothyroid rat. Endocrinology 1992;130:479

185. Boado RJ, Chopra IJ. A study of hepatic low K$_m$ iodothyronine 5'-monodeiodinase. Endocrinology 1989;124:2245

186. Goswami A, Rosenberg IN. Iodothyronine 5'-deiodinase in rat kidney microsomes. J Clin Invest 1984;74:2097

187. Sharifi J, St. Germain DL. The cDNA for the type I iodothyronine 5'-deiodinase encodes an enzyme manifesting both high K$_m$ and low K$_m$ activity. J Biol Chem 1992;267:12539

188. Silva JE, Mellen S, Larsen PR. Comparison of kidney and brown adipose tissue iodothyronine 5'-deiodinases. Endocrinology 1987;121:650

189. Leonard JL, Mellen SA, Larsen PR. Thyroxine 5'-deiodinase activity in brown adipose tissue. Endocrinology 1983;112:1153

190. Maeda M, Ingbar SH. Evidence that the 5'-monodeiodinases for thyroxine and 3,3',5-triiodothyronine in the rat pituitary are separate enzymes. Endocrinology 1984;114:747

191. Silva JE, Leonard JL, Crantz FR, Larsen PR. Evidence for two tissue-specific pathways for in vivo thyroxine 5'-deiodination in the rat. J Clin Invest 1982;69:1176

192. Kleinhaus N, Faber J, Kahana L, Schneer J, Scheinfeld M. Euthyroid hyperthyroxinemia due to a generalized 5'-deiodinase defect. J Clin Endocrinol Metab 1988;66:684

193. Koenig RJ, Leonard JL, Senator D, Rappaport N, Watson A, Larsen PR. Regulation of thyroxine 5'-deiodinase activity by 3,5,3'-triiodothyronine in cultured anterior pituitary cells. Endocrinology 1984;115:324

194. Leonard JL. Dibutyryl cAMP induction of type II 5'-deiodinase activity in rat brain astrocytes in culture. Biochem Biophys Res Commun 1988;151:1164

195. Murakami M, Tanaka K, Greer MA. There is a nyctohemeral rhythm of type II iodothyronine 5'-deiodinase activity in rat anterior pituitary. Endocrinology 1988;123:1631

196. Riskind PN, Kolodny JM, Larsen PR. The regional hypothalamic distribution of type II 5'-monodeiodinase in euthyroid and hypothyroid rats. Brain Res 1987;420:194

197. Gavin LA, Moller M, McMahon F, Gulli R, Cavalieri RR. Carbohydrate reactivation of thyroxine 5'-deiodinase (type II) in cultured mouse neuroblastoma cells is dependent upon new protein synthesis. Endocrinology 1989;124:635

198. Gavin LA, Moeller M, McMahon F, Gulli R, Cavalieri RR. Cyclic adenosine 3',5'-monophosphate and glucose stimulate thyroxine 5'-deiodinase type II in cultured mouse neuroblastoma cells. Metabolism 1990;39:474

199. Guerrero JM, Puig-Domingo M, Reiter R. Thyroxine 5'-deiodinase activity in pineal gland and frontal cortex: nighttime increase and the effect of either continuous light exposure or superior cervical ganglionectomy. Endocrinology 1988; 122:236

200. Guerrero JM, Puig-Domingo M, Vaughan GM, Reiter RJ. Characterization of type-II thyroxine 5'-deiodinase activity in rat harderian gland. Life Sci 1987;41:1179

201. Koenig RJ. Regulation of thyroxine 5'-deiodinase by thyroid hormones and activators of protein kinase C in GH4C1 cells. Endocrinology 1986;118:1491

202. St. Germain DL. Hormonal control of a low K$_m$ (type II) iodothyronine 5'-deiodinase in cultured NB41a3 mouse neuroblastoma cells. Endocrinology 1986;119:840

203. Leonard JL, Larsen PR. Thyroid hormone metabolism in primary cultures of fetal rat brain cells. Brain Res 1985;327:1

204. Dratman MB, Crutchfield FL. Thyroxine, triiodothyronine, and reverse triiodothyronine processing in the cerebellum: autoradiographic studies in adult rats. Endocrinology 1989;125:1723

205. Courtin F, Pelletier G, Walker P. Subcellular localization of thyroxine 5'-deiodinase activity in bovine anterior pituitary. Endocrinology 1985;117:2527

206. Farwell AP, Leonard JL. Identification of a 27-kDa protein with the properties of type II iodothyronine 5'-deiodinase in dibutyryl cyclic AMP-stimulated glial cells. J Biol Chem 1989; 264:20561

207. Visser TJ, Kaplan MM, Leonard JL, Larsen PR. Evidence for two pathways of iodothyronine 5'-deiodination in rat pituitary that differ in kinetics, propylthiouracil sensitivity, and response to hypothyroidism. J Clin Invest 1983;71:992

208. Goswami A, Rosenberg IN. Iodothyronine 5'-deiodinase in brown adipose tissue: thiol activation and propylthiouracil inhibition. Endocrinology 1986;119:916

209. Beckett GJ, MacDougall DA, Nicol F, Arthur JR. Inhibition of type I and type II iodothyronine deiodinase activity in rat liver, kidney and brain produced by selenium deficiency. Biochem J 1989;259:887

210. Chanoine JP, Safran M, Farwell AP, Dubord S, Alex S, Stone S, Arthur JR, Braverman LE, Leonard JL. Effects of selenium deficiency on thyroid hormone economy in rats. Endocrinology 1992;131:1787

211. Chanoine JP, Safran M, Farwell AP, et al. Selenium deficiency and type II 5'-deiodinase regulation in the euthyroid and hypothyroid rat: evidence of a direct effect of thyroxine. Endocrinology 1992;131:479

212. Chanoine JP, Safran M, Farwell AP, Dubord S, Alex S, Stone S, Arthur JR, Braverman LE, Leonard JL. Effects of selenium deficiency on thyroid hormone economy in rats. Endocrinology 1992;131:357

213. Eelkman Rooda SJ, Kaptein E, Rutgers M, Visser TJ. Increased plasma 3,5,3'-triiodothyronine sulfate in rats with inhibited type I iodothyronine deiodinase activity, as measured by radioimmunoassay. Endocrinology 1989;124:740

214. Eelkman Rooda SJ, Kaptein E, Visser TJ. Serum triiodothyronine sulfate in man measured by radioimmunoassay. J Clin Endocrinol Metab 1989;69:552

215. Mol JA, Visser TJ. Rapid and selective inner ring deiodination of thyroxine sulfate by rat liver deiodinase. Endocrinology 1985; 117:8

216. Otten MH, Hennemann G, Docter R, Visser TJ. Metabolism of 3,3'-diiodothyronine in rat hepatocytes. Endocrinology 1984; 115:887

217. Rutgers M, Heusdens FA, Visser TJ. Metabolism of triiodothyroacetic acid (TA$_3$) in rat liver: I. Deiodination of TA$_3$ and TA$_3$ sulfate by microsomes. Endocrinology 1989;125:424

218. Rutgers M, Heusdens FA, Bonthuis F, Visser TJ. Metabolism of triiodothyroacetic acid (TA$_3$) in rat liver: II. Deiodination and conjugation of TA$_3$ by rat hepatocytes and in rats in vivo. Endocrinology 1989;125:433

219. Visser TJ, van Buuren JCJ, Rutgers M, Eelkman Rooda SJ, De Herder WW. The role of sulfation in thyroid hormone metabolism. Trends Endocrinol Metab 1990;1:211

220. Fay M, Roti E, Fang SH, Wright G, Braverman LE, Emerson CH. The effects of propylthiouracil, iodothyronines, and other agents on thyroid hormone metabolism in human placenta. J Clin Endocrinol Metab 1984;58:280

221. Cavalieri RR, Gavin LA, Cole R, De Vellis J. Thyroid hormone deiodinases in purified primary glial cell cultures. Brain Res 1986;364:382

222. Courtin F, Chantoux F, Pierre M, Francon J. Induction of type II 5'-deiodinase activity by cyclic adenosine 3',5'-monophosphate in cultured rat astroglial cells. Endocrinology 1988; 123:1577

223. Ubl J, Murer H, Kolb H-A. Ion channels activated by osmotic and mechanical stress in membranes of opossum kidney cells. J Membr Biol 1988;104:223

224. Ködding R, Fuhrmann H, Von zur Mühlen A. Investigations on iodothyronine deiodinase activity in the maturing rat brain. Endocrinology 1986;118:1347

225. Borges M, LaBourene J, Ingbar SH. Changes in hepatic iodothyronine metabolism during ontogeny of the chick embryo. Endocrinology 1980;107:1751

226. Dickstein Y, Schwarz H, Gross J, Gordon A. The metabolism of T$_4$ and T$_3$ in cultured chick embryo heart cells. Mol Cell Endocrinol 1980;20:45

227. Harris ARC, Fang SL, Prosky J, Vagenakis AG, Braverman LE. Sex-related differences in outer ring monodeiodination of thyroxine and reverse T$_3$ in the adult rat. Endocrinology 1979; 104:645

228. Sato K, Robbins J. Thyroid hormone metabolism in primary cultured rat hepatocytes: effect of glucose, glucagon, and insulin. J Clin Invest 1981;68:475

229. Fisher DA, Dussault JW, Sack J, Chopra IJ. Ontogenesis of hypothalamus–pituitary–thyroid function and metabolism in man, sheep, and rat. Recent Prog Horm Res 1977;33:59

230. Kaplan MM, Visser TJ, Yaskoski K, Leonard JL. Characteristics of iodothyronine tyrosyl ring deiodination by rat cerebral cortical microsomes. Endocrinology 1983;112:35

231. Balsam A, Sexton F, Borges M, Ingbar SH. Formation of diiodotyrosine from thyroxine: ether-link cleavage, an alternate pathway of thyroxine metabolism. J Clin Invest 1983;72:1234

232. Burger AG, Engler D, Buergi U, Weissel M, Steiger G, Ingbar SH, Rosin RE, Babior BM. Ether link cleavage is the major pathway of iodothyronine metabolism in the phagocytosing human leukocyte and also occurs in vivo in the rat. J Clin Invest 1983;71:935

233. Meinhold H, Beckert A, Wenzel KW. Circulating diiodotyrosine: studies of its serum concentration, source, and turnover using radioimmunoassay after immunoextraction. J Clin Endocrinol Metab 1981;53:1171

234. Meinhold H, Olbricht T, Schwartz-Porsche T. Turnover and urinary excretion of diiodotyrosine. J Clin Endocrinol Metab 1987; 64:794

235. Meinhold H, Gramm H-J, Meissner W, Zimmermann J, Schwander J, Dennhardt R, Voigt K. Elevated serum diiodotyrosine (DIT) in severe infections and sepsis: DIT, a possible new marker of leukocyte activity. J Clin Endocrinol Metab 1991; 72:945

236. Klebanoff SJ, Green WL. Degradation of thyroid hormones by phagocytosing human leukocytes. J Clin Invest 1973;52:60

237. Lissitzky S, Roque M, Bevenet MT. Desiodation enzymatique de la thyroxine et de ses derives, I, II. Bull Soc Chim Biol 1961;43:727

238. Lissitzky S. Deiodination of iodotyrosines. In: Reinwein D, Klein E, eds. Diminished thyroid hormone formation: possible causes and clinical aspects. Merck International Thyroid Symposium, Hamburg, November 19–21, 1981. Stuttgart–New York: FK Schattauer Verlag, 1981:49

239. Fishman N, Huang YP, Tergis DC, Rivlin RS. Relation of triiodothyronine and reverse triiodothyronine administration in rats to hepatic L-triiodothyronine aminotransferase activity. Endocrinology 1977;100:1055

240. Visvanathan A, Shanmugasundaram KR. Alterations in L-triiodothyronine aminotransferase activity in hypothyroid rats: effects of administrations of iodobenzene and L-thyroxine. Indian J Exp Biol 1984;22:442

241. Pittman CS, Shimizu T, Burger A, Chambers JB Jr. The nondeiodinative pathways of thyroxine metabolism: 3,5,3',5'-tetraiodothyroacetic acid turnover in normal and fasting human subjects. J Clin Endocrinol Metab 1980;50:712

242. Bracco D, Morin O, Schutz Y, Liang H, Jequier E, Burger AG. Comparison of the metabolic and endocrine effects of 3,5,3'-triiodothyroacetic acid and thyroxine. J Clin Endocrinol Metab 1993;77:221

243. Refetoff S, Weiss RE, Usala SJ. The syndromes of resistance to thyroid hormone. Endocr Rev 1993;14:348

244. Cody V, Meyer T, Doehler KD, Hesch RD, Rokos H, Marko M. Molecular structure and biochemical activity of 3,5,3'-triiodothyronamine. Endocr Res 1984;10:91

245. Sekura RD, Sato K, Cahnmann HJ, Robbins J, Jacoby WB. Sulfate transfer to thyroid hormones and their analogs by hepatic aryl sulfotransferases. Endocrinology 1981;108:454

246. Anderson RJ, Babbitt LL, Liebentritt DK. Human liver triiodothyronine sulfotransferase: copurification with phenol sulfotransferases. Thyroid 19955:61

247. De Herder WW, Bonthuis F, Rutgers M, Otten MH, Hazenberg HP, Visser TJ. Effects of inhibition of type I iodothyronine deiodinase and phenol sulfotransferase on the biliary clearance of triiodothyronine in rats. Endocrinology 1988;122:153

248. Sorimachi K, Robbins J. Effects of propylthiouracil and methylmercaptoimidazole on metabolism of thyroid hormones by cultured monkey hepatocarcinoma cells. Horm Metab Res 1979; 11:39

249. Young W Jr. Human liver tyrosylsulfotransferase. Gastroenterology 1990;99:1072

250. Otten MH, Mol JA, Visser TJ. Sulfation preceding deiodination of iodothyronines in rat hepatocytes. Science 1983;221:81

251. van Stralen PG, Van der Hoek HJ, Docter R, De Jong M, Krenning EP, Lim CF, Hennemann G. Reduced T_3 deiodination by the human hepatoblastoma cell line HepG2 caused by deficient T_3 sulfation. Biochim Biophys Acta 1993;1157:114

252. Wu S-Y, Huang W-S, Polk DH, Fisher DA. Identification of thyroxine-sulfate (T_4S) in human serum and amniotic fluid by a novel T_4S radioimmunoassay. Thyroid 1992;2:101

253. Chopra IJ, Santini F, Hurd RE, Chua Teco GN. A radioimmunoassay for measurement of thyroxine sulfate. J Clin Endocrinol Metab 1993;76:145

254. Santini F, Cortelazzi S, Baggiani AM, Marconi AM, Beck-Peccoz P, Chopra IJ. A study of serum 3,5,3′-triiodothyronine sulfate concentration in normal and hypothyroid fetuses at various gestational stages. J Clin Endocrinol Metab 1993;76:1583

255. Wu S-Y, Huang W-S, Polk DH, Chen W-L, Reviczky A, Williams JI, Chopra IJ, Fisher DA. The development of a radioimmunoassay for reverse triiodothyronine sulfate in human serum and amniotic fluid. J Clin Endocrinol Metab 1993;76:1625

256. Wu S-Y, Polk DH, Chen W-L, Fisher DA, Huang W-S, Yee B. A 3,3′-diiodothyronine sulfate cross-reactive compound in serum from pregnant women. J Clin Endocrinol Metab 1994;78:1505

257. LoPresti J, Nicoloff JT. 3,5,3′-triiodothyronine (T_3) sulfate: a major metabolite in T_3 metabolism in man. J Clin Endocrinol Metab 1994;78:688

258. Kung M-P, Spaulding SW, Roth JA. Desulfation of 3,5,3′-triiodothyronine sulfate by microsomes from human and rat tissues. Endocrinology 1988;122:1195

259. Spaulding SW, Smith TJ, Hinkle PM, Davis FB, Kung M-P, Roth JA. Studies on the biological activity of triiodothyronine sulfate. J Clin Endocrinol Metab 1992;74:1062

260. Tomita K, Cha C-JM, Lardy HA. Enzymic O-methylation of iodinated phenols and thyroid hormones. J Biol Chem 1964; 239:1202

261. Visser TJ. Importance of deiodination and conjugation in the hepatic metabolism of thyroid hormone. In: Greer MA, ed. The thyroid gland. New York: Raven Press, 1991:255

262. Langer P, Földes O. Effect of adrenaline on biliary excretion of triiodothyronines in rats mediated by alpha$_1$-adrenoceptors and related to the inhibition of 5′-monodeiodination in liver. J Endocrinol Invest 1988;11:471

263. Visser TJ, Kaptein E, van Raaij JA, Joe CT, Ebner T, Burchell B. Multiple UDP-glucuronyltransferases for the glucuronidation of thyroid hormone with preference for 3,3′,5′-triiodothyronine (reverse T_3). FEBS Lett 1993;315:65

264. De Sandro V, Catinot R, Kriszt W, Cordier A, Richert L. Male rat hepatic UDP-glucuronosyltransferase activity toward thyroxine. Biochem Pharmacol 1992;43:1563

265. Curran PG, DeGroot LJ. The effect of hepatic enzyme-inducing drugs on thyroid hormones and the thyroid gland. Endocr Rev 1991;12:135

266. Wartofsky L, Burman KD. Alterations in thyroid function in patients with systemic illness: the "euthyroid sick syndrome." Endocr Rev 1993;3:164

267. Eisenstein Z, Hagg S, Vagenakis AG, Fang SL, Ransil B, Burger A, Balsam A, Braverman LE, Ingbar SH. Effect of starvation on the production and peripheral metabolism of 3,3′,5′-triiodothyronine in euthyroid obese subjects. J Clin Endocrinol Metab 1978; 47:889

268. Suda AK, Pittman CS, Shimizu T, Chambers IBJ. The production and metabolism of 3,5,3′-triiodothyronine and 3,3′,5′-triiodothyronine in normal and fasting subjects. J Clin Endocrinol Metab 1978;47:1311

269. van Doorn J, Roelfsema F, Van der Heide D. Contribution from local conversion of thyroxine to 3,5,3′-triiodothyronine to intracellular 3,5,3′-triiodothyronine in several organs in hypothyroid rats at isotope equilibrium. Acta Endocrinol (Copenh) 1982; 101:386

270. van Doorn J, Van der Heide D, Roelfsema F. The influence of partial food deprivations on the quantity and source of triiodothyronine in several tissues of athyreotic thyroxine-maintained rats. Endocrinology 1984;115:705

271. van Doorn J, Van der Heide D, Roelfsema F. The contribution of local thyroxine monodeiodination to intracellular 3,5,3′-triiodothyronine in several tissues of hyperthyroid rats at isotopic equilibrium. Endocrinology 1984;115:174

272. DiStefano JJ III, Jang M, Malone TK, Broutman M. Comprehensive kinetics of triiodothyronine production, distribution and metabolism in blood and tissue pools of the rat using optimized blood-sampling protocols. Endocrinology 1982; 110:198

273. Morreale de Escobar G, Calvo R, Escobar del Rey F, Obregon MJ. Thyroid hormones in tissues from fetal and adult rats. Endocrinology 1994;134:2410

274. Pardridge WM, Landaw EM. Plasma protein-mediated transport of steroid and thyroid hormones: further comment. Reply. Am J Physiol 1990;258:E396

275. Hennemann G. Thyroid hormone deiodination in healthy man. In: Hennemann G, ed. Thyroid hormone metabolism. New York: Marcel Dekker, 1986:277

276. Eckel J, Rao GS, Rao ML, Breuer H. Uptake of L-triiodothyronine by isolated rat liver cells. Biochem J 1979;182:473

277. Ekins RP, Edwards, PR. Plasma protein-mediated transport of steroid and thyroid hormones: a critique. Ann NY Acad Sci 1988;538:193

278. Ekins RP, Sinha AK, Pickard MR, Evans IM, Al Yatama F. Transport of thyroid hormones to target tissues. Acta Med Austriaca 1994;21(2):26

279. Mendel CM. The free hormone hypothesis: a physiologically based mathematical model. Endocr Rev 1989;10:232

280. Rao GS, Rao ML, Thilmann A, Quednau HD. Study of fluxes at low concentrations of L-tri-iodothyronine with rat liver cells and their plasma-membrane vesicles. Biochem J 1981;198:457

281. De Jong M, Docter R, Bernard BF, van der Heijden JT, Van Toor H, Krenning EP, Hennemann G. T_4 uptake into the perfused rat liver and liver T_4 uptake in humans are inhibited by fructose. Am J Physiol 1994;266:E768

282. Lim CF, Docter R, Krenning EP, Van Toor H, Bernard B, De Jong M, Hennemann G. Transport of thyroxine into cultured hepatocytes: effects of mild non-thyroidal illness and calorie restriction in obese subjects. Clin Endocrinol (Oxf) 1994;40:79

283. Lim CF, Docter R, Krenning EP, Van Toor H, Bernard B, De Jong M, Hennemann G. Transport of thyroxine into cultured hepatocytes: effects of mild non-thyroidal illness and calorie restriction in obese subjects. Clin Endocrinol (Oxf) 1994;40:79

284. De Jong M, Docter R, Bernard BF, Van der Heijden JTM, Van Toor H, Krenning E, Hennemann G. T_4 uptake into the perfused rat liver and liver T_4 uptake in humans are inhibited by fructose. Am J Physiol Endocrinol Metab 1994;29:E768

285. Müller MJ, Köhrle J, Hesch RD, Seitz HJ. Effect of cycloAMP on iodothyronine metabolism in the isolated perfused rat liver. Biochem Int 1982;5:495

286. Cheron RG, Kaplan MM, Larsen PR. Divergent changes of thyroxine-5'-monodeiodination in rat pituitary and liver during maturation. Endocrinology 1980;106:1405

287. Coiro V, Harris A, Goodman HM, Vagenakis A, Braverman L. Effect of pharmacological quantities of infused 3,3',5'-triiodothyronine on thyroxine monodeiodination to 3,5,3'-triiodothyronine. Endocrinology 1980;106:68

288. Bauer AGC, Wilson JHP, Lamberts SWJ, Docter R, Hennemann G, Visser TJ. Handling of iodothyronines by liver and kidney in patients with chronic liver disease. Acta Endocrinol (Copenh) 1987;116:339

289. Blondeau JP, Osty J, Francon J. Characterization of the thyroid hormone transport system of isolated hepatocytes. J Biol Chem 1988;263:2685

290. Gavin LA, Cavalieri RR, Moller M. Glucose and insulin reverse the effects of fasting on 3,5,3'-triiodothyronine neogenesis in primary cultures of rat hepatocytes. Endocrinology 1987; 121:858

291. Valverde R, Aceves C, Reyes E. Ontogenesis of iodothyronine deiodinase activities in brain and liver of the chick embryo. Endocrinology 1993;132:867

292. Suzuki Y, Nanno M, Gemma R, Yoshimi T. Plasma free fatty acids, inhibitor of extrathyroidal conversion of T_4 to T_3 and thyroid hormone binding inhibitor in patients with various nonthyroidal illnesses. Endocrinol Jpn 1992;39:445

293. De Jong M, Docter R, Van der Hoek HJ, Vos RA, Krenning EP, Hennemann G. Transport of 3,5,3'-triiodothyronine into the perfused rat liver and subsequent metabolism are inhibited by fasting. Endocrinology 1992;131:463

294. O'Mara B, Dittrich W, Lauterio TJ, St. Germain DL. Pretranslational regulation of type I 5'-deiodinase by thyroid hormones and in fasted and diabetic rats. Endocrinology 1994;133:1715

295. Lim CF, Bernard BF, De Jong M, Docter R, Krenning EP, Hennemann G. A furan fatty acid and indoxyl sulfate are the putative inhibitors of thyroxine hepatocyte transport in uremia. J Clin Endocrinol Metab 1993;76:318

296. Lim CF, Docter R, Visser TJ, Krenning EP, Bernard B, Van Toor H, De Jong M, Hennemann G. Inhibition of thyroxine transport into cultured rat hepatocytes by serum of nonuremic critically ill patients: effects of bilirubin and nonesterified fatty acids. J Clin Endocrinol Metab 76:1993;1165

297. Rabinovitz JL, Hercker ES. Thyroxine: conversion to triiodothyronine by isolated perfused rat hearts. Science 1971;1173:1242

298. Imai Y, Yamauchi K, Kitihara H, Nishikimi M. Correlation of T_4 to T_3 converting activity with T_3 concentration in rat tissue. Endocrinol Jpn 1981;28:271

299. Nauman JA, Kaminski T, Hertacynska-Cedro K. In vivo and in vitro effects of adrenaline on conversion of thyroxine to triiodothyronine and to reverse triiodothyronine in dog liver and heart. Eur J Clin Invest 1980;10:189

300. Mori Y, Nishikawa M, Matsubara H, Takagi T, Toyoda N, Oikawa S, Inada M. Stimulation of rat atrial natriuretic peptide (rANP) synthesis by triiodothyronine and thyroxine (T_4): T_4 as prohormone in synthesizing rANP. Endocrinology 1990;126:466

301. Burger AG, Dinichert D, Nicod P, Jenny M, Lemarchand-Beraud T, Valloton MB. Effect of amiodarone on serum triiodothyronine, reverse triiodothyronine, thyroxine and thyrotropin: a drug influencing peripheral metabolism of thyroid hormones. J Clin Invest 1976;58:255

302. Cavalieri RR, Pitt-Rivers R. The effects of drugs on the distribution and metabolism of thyroid hormones. Pharmacol Rev 1981; 33:55

303. Sogol PB, Hershman JH, Reed AW, Dillmann WH. The effects of amiodarone on serum thyroid hormones and hepatic thyroxine 5'-monodeiodination in rats. Endocrinology 1983;113:1464

304. Wenzel KW. Pharmacological interference with in vitro tests of thyroid function. Metabolism 1981;30:717

305. Zaninovich AA, Bosco SC, Fernandez-Pol AJ. Amiodarone does not affect the distribution and fractional turnover of triiodothyronine from the plasma pool, but only its generation from thyroxine in extrathyroidal tissues. J Clin Endocrinol Metab 1990; 70:1721

306. De Jong M, Docter R, Van der Hoek H, Krenning E, Van der Heide D, Quero C, Plaisier P, Vos R, Hennemann G. Different effects of amiodarone on transport of T_4 and T_3 into the perfused rat liver. Am J Physiol 1994;266:E44

307. Inoue K, Grimm Y, Greer MA. Quantitative studies on the iodinated components secreted by the rat thyroid gland as determined by in situ perfusion. Endocrinology 1967;81:946

308. Haibach H. Evidence for a thyroxine deiodinating mechanism in the rat different from iodotyrosine deiodinase. Endocrinology 1971;88:918

309. Galton VA, Ingbar SH. Role of peroxidase and catalase in the physiological deiodination of thyroxine. Endocrinology 1963; 73:596

310. Laurberg P. Multisite inhibition by ipodate of iodothyronine secretion from perfused dog thyroid lobes. Endocrinology 1985; 117:1639

311. Laurberg P. Iodothyronine secretion from perfused dog thyroid lobes after prolonged thyrotropin treatment in vivo. Endocrinology 1981;109:1560

312. St. Germain DL. Dual mechanism of regulation of type I iodothyronine 5'-deiodinase in the rat kidney, liver, and thyroid gland. J Clin Invest 1988;81:1476

313. Beech SG, Walker SW, Dorrance AM, Arthur JR, Nicol F, Lee D, Beckett GJ. The role of thyroidal type-I iodothyronine deiodinase in tri-iodothyronine production by human and sheep thyrocytes in primary culture. J Endocrinol 1993;136:361

314. Erickson VJ, Cavalieri RR, Rosenberg LL. Thyroxine-5'-deiodinase of rat thyroid, but not that of liver, is dependent on thyrotropin. Endocrinology 1982;111:434

315. Kubota K, Uchimura H, Mitsuhashi T, Chiu SC, Kuzuya N, Nagataki S. Effects of intrathyroidal metabolism of thyroxine on thyroid hormone secretion: increased degradation of thyroxine in mouse thyroids stimulated chronically with thyrotropin. Acta Endocrinol (Copenh) 1984;105:57

316. Wu S-Y. Thyrotropin-mediated induction of thyroidal iodothyronine monodeiodinases in the dog. Endocrinology 1983;112:417

317. Wu S-Y, Reggio R, Florsheim WH. Characterization of thyrotropin-induced increase in iodothyronine monodeiodinating activity in mice. Endocrinology 1985;116:901

318. Zimmerman GJ, Izumi M, Larsen PR. Isolation of labeled triiodothyronine from serum using affinity chromatography: application to the estimation of the peripheral T_4 to T_3 conversion in rats. Metabolism 1978;27:303

319. Campbell NR, Hasinoff BB, Stalts H, Rao B, Wong NC. Ferrous sulfate reduces thyroxine efficacy in patients with hypothyroidism. Ann Intern Med 1992;117:1010

320. Borges M, Ingbar SH, Silva JE. Iodothyronine deiodinase activities in FRTL-5 cells: predominance of type I 5'-deiodinase. Endocrinology 1990;126:3059

321. Toyoda N, Nishikawa M, Horimoto H, Yoshikawa N, Mori Y, Yoshimura M, Masaki H, Tanaka K, Inada M. Graves' immunoglobulin G stimulates iodothyronine 5'-deiodinating activity in FRTL-5 rat thyroid cells. J Clin Endocrinol Metab 1990; 70:1506

322. Toyoda N, Nishikawa M, Mori Y, Gondou A, Ogawa Y, Yonemoto T, Yoshimura M, Masaki H, Inada M. Thyrotropin and triiodothyronine regulate iodothyronine 5'-deiodinase messenger ribonucleic acid levels in FRTL-5 rat thyroid cells. Endocrinology 1992;131:389

323. Toyoda N, Nishikawa M, Horimoto M, Yoshikawa N, Mori Y, Yoshimura M, Masaki H, Tanaka K, Inada M. Synergistic effect of thyroid hormone and thyrotropin on iodothyronine 5'-deiodinase in FRTL-5 rat thyroid cells. Endocrinology 1990;127:1199

324. Schreck R, Schmutzler C, Schnieders F, Köhrle J. Retinoids stimulate type I iodothyronine 5'-deiodinase activity in human follicular thyroid carcinoma cell lines. J Clin Endocrinol Metab 1994; 79:791

325. Ottevanger PB, Hermus A, Smals AGH, Kloppenborg PWC. TSH-dependent production of T_4 and T_3 by metastases of thyroid carcinoma. Acta Endocrinol 1992;127:413

326. Shen D-C, Wu S-Y, Chopra IJ, Huang H-W, Shian L-R, Bian T-Y, Jeng C-Y, Solomon DH. Long term treatment of Graves' hyperthyroidism with sodium ipodate. J Clin Endocrinol Metab 1985;61:723

327. Wu S-Y, Chopra IJ, Solomon DH, Johnson DE. The effect of repeated administration of ipodate (Orographin) in hyperthyroidism. J Clin Endocrinol Metab 1978;47:1358

328. Capen CC. Pathophysiology of chemical injury of the thyroid gland. Toxicol Lett 1992;64–65(Spec No):381

329. Akiguchi I, Strauss K, Borges M, Silva JE, Moses AC. Thyroid hormone receptors and 3,5,3'-triiodothyronine biological effects in FRTL5 thyroid follicular cells. Endocrinology 1992;131:1279

330. Ozawa M, Sato K, Han DC, Kawakami M, Tsushima T, Shizume K. Effects of tumor necrosis factor-α/cachectin on thyroid hormone metabolism in mice. Endocrinology 1988;123:1461

331. Ongphiphadhanakul B, Fang SL, Tang KT, Patwardhan NA, Braverman LE. Tumor necrosis factor-alpha decreases thyrotropin-induced 5'-deiodinase activity in FRTL-5 thyroid cells. Eur J Endocrinol 1994;130:502

332. Pekary AE, Berg L, Santini F, Chopra IJ, Hershman JM. Cytokines modulate type I iodothyronine deiodinase mRNA levels and enzyme activity in FRTL-5 rat thyroid cells. Mol Cell Endocrinol 1994;101:R31

333. Fujii T, Sato K, Ozawa M, Kasono K, Imamura H, Kanaji Y, Tsushima T, Shizume K. Effect of interleukin-1 (IL-1) on thyroid hormone metabolism in mice: Stimulation by IL-1 of iodothyronine 5'-deiodinating activity (type I) in the liver. Endocrinology 1989;124:167

334. Pang X-P, Hershman JM, Mirell CJ, Pekary AE. Impairment of hypothalamic–pituitary–thyroid function in rats treated with human recombinant tumor necrosis factor-α (cachectin). Endocrinology 1989;125:76

335. Mooradian AD, Reed RL, Osterweil D, Schiffman R, Scuderi P. Decreased serum triiodothyronine is associated with increased concentrations of tumor necrosis factor. J Clin Endocrinol Metab 1990;71:1239

336. Dubuis J-M, Dayer J-M, Siegrist-Kaiser CA, Burger AG. Human recombinant interleukin-1β decreases plasma thyroid hormone and thyroid stimulating hormone levels in rats. Endocrinology 1988;123:2175

337. Hermus RM, Sweep CG, van der Meer MJ, Ross HA, Smals AG, Benraad TJ, Kloppenborg PW. Continuous infusion of interleukin-1 beta induces a nonthyroidal illness syndrome in the rat. Endocrinology 1992;131:2139

338. van Haasteren GA, van der Meer MJ, Hermus AR, Linkels E, Klootwijk W, Kaptein E, Van Toor H, Sweep CG, Visser TJ, De Greef WJ. Different effects of continuous infusion of interleukin-1 and interleukin-6 on the hypothalamic–hypophysial–thyroid axis. Endocrinology 1994;135:1336

339. Zheng RQH, Abney ER, Chu CG, Field M, Maini RN, Lamb JR, Feldmann M. Detection of in vivo production of tumour necrosis factor-alpha by human thyroid epithelial cells. Immunology 1992;75:456

340. Zerek Melen G, Zylinska K, Fryczak J, Mucha S, Stepien H. Influence of interleukin 1 and antihuman interleukin 1 receptor antibody on the growth and function of the thyroid gland in rats. Eur J Endocrinol 1994;131:531

341. van der Poll T, Romijn JA, Wiersinga WM, Sauerwein HP. Tumor necrosis factor: a putative mediator of sick euthyroid syndrome in man. J Clin Endocrinol Metab 1990;71:1567

342. Boelen A, Platvoet-ter Schiphorst MC, Wiersinga WM. Association between serum interleukin-6 and serum T_3 in non-thyroidal illness. J Clin Endocrinol Metab 1993;77:1695

343. Stouthard JM, van der Poll T, Endert E, Bakker PJ, Veenhof CH, Sauerwein HP, Romijn JA. Effects of acute and chronic interleukin-6 administration on thyroid hormone metabolism in humans. J Clin Endocrinol Metab 1994;79:1342

344. Hashimoto H, Igarashi N, Yachie A, Miyawaki T, Sato T. The relationship between serum levels of interleukin-6 and thyroid hormone in children with acute respiratory infection. J Clin Endocrinol Metab 1994;78:288

345. Chanoine J-P, Veronikis I, Alex S, Stone S, Fang SL, Leonard JL, Braverman LE. The postnatal serum 3,5,3'-triiodothyronine (T_3) surge in the rat is largely independent of extrathyroidal 5'-deiodination of thyroxine to T_3. Endocrinology 1993;133:2604

346. Jorgensen JO, Moller J, Skakkebaek NE, Weeke J, Christiansen JS. Thyroid function during growth hormone therapy. Horm Res 1992;38(Suppl 1):63

347. Geelhoed Duijvestijn PH, Roelfsema F, Schroder van der Elst JP, van Doorn J, Van der Heide D. Effect of administration of growth hormone on plasma and intracellular levels of thyroxine and tri-iodothyronine in thyroidectomized thyroxine-treated rats. J Endocrinol 1992;133:45

348. Tang KT, Braverman LE, DeVito WJ. Effects of fibroblast growth factor on type I 5'-deiodinase in FRTL-5 rat thyroid cells [see comments]. Endocrinology 1994;135:493

349. Chanoine JP, Stein GS, Braverman LE, Shalhoub V, Lian JB, Huber CA, DeVito WJ. Acidic fibroblast growth factor modulates gene expression in the rat thyroid in vivo. J. Cell Biochem 1992;50:392

350. Ford DH, Gross J. The metabolism of 131I-labeled thyroid hormones in the hypophysis and brain of the rabbit. Endocrinology 1958;62:416

351. Kaplan MM. Thyroxine 5'-monodeiodination in rat anterior pituitary homogenates. Endocrinology 1980;106:567

352. Maeda M, Ingbar SH. Effect of alterations in thyroid status on the metabolism of thyroxine and triiodothyronine by rat pituitary gland in vitro. J Clin Invest 1982;69:799

353. St. Germain DL, Adler R, Galton VA. Thyroxine 5'-deiodinase activity in anterior pituitary glands transplanted under the renal capsule in the rat. Endocrinology 1985;117:55

354. Tanaka K, Shimatsu A, Imura H. Iodothyronine 5-deiodinase in rat posterior pituitary. Biochem Biophys Res Commun 1992; 188:272

355. Everts ME, Docter R, van Buuren JC, Van Koetsveld PM, Hofland LJ, De Jong M, Krenning EP, Hennemann G. Evidence for carrier-mediated uptake of triiodothyronine in cultured anterior pituitary cells of euthyroid rats. Endocrinology 1993; 132:1278

356. Everts ME, Docter R, Moerings EP, Van Koetsveld PM, Visser TJ, De Jong M, Krenning EP, Hennemann G. Uptake of thyroxine in cultured anterior pituitary cells of euthyroid rats. Endocrinology 1994;134:2490

357. Strait KA, Schwartz HL, Perez-Castillo A, Oppenheimer JH. Relationship of c-erbA mRNA content to tissue triiodothyronine nuclear binding capacity and function in developing and adult rats. J Biol Chem 1990;265:10514

358. Silva JE, Leonard JL. Regulation of rat cerebrocortical and adenohypophyseal type II 5'deiodinase by thyroxine, triiodothyronine, reverse triiodothyronine. Endocrinology 1985;116:1627

359. Kaiser CA, Goumaz MO, Burger AG. In vivo inhibition of the 5'-deiodinase type II in brain cortex and pituitary by reverse triiodothyronine. Endocrinology 1986;119:762

360. Obregon M-J, Larsen PR, Silva JE. Plasma kinetics, tissue distribution, and cerebrocortical sources of reverse triiodothyronine in
the rat. Endocrinology 1985;116:2192

377. Obregon M-J, Mills I, Silva JE, Larsen PR. Catecholamine stimulation of iodothyronine 5'-deiodinase activity in rat dispersed
brown adipocytes. Endocrinology 1987;120:1069

Werner and Ingbar's The Thyroid, Seventh Edition,
edited by Lewis E. Braverman and Robert D. Utiger.
Lippincott–Raven Publishers, Philadelphia, © 1996

Section D
Thyroid Hormone Action

9

The Molecular Basis of Thyroid Hormone Actions

Jack H. Oppenheimer
Harold L. Schwartz
Kevin A. Strait

Students of the thyroid have demonstrated a long-standing interest in the mechanisms by which thyroid hormones exert their
diverse actions. In a review of this subject in 1964, 358 references on this topic were cited.[1] The multiple hypotheses advanced at that time, however, bear little resemblance to
contemporary thinking in this area. Earlier studies devoted
much attention to efforts to explain the presumed ability of thyroid hormones to uncouple mitochondrial oxidative phosphorylation. Support for this idea was based in large part on the
results of experiments in which isolated mitochondria were exposed to concentrations of thyroxine (T_4) far above the pathophysiologic range. Subsequently, however, it became clear that
under in vivo conditions even in rats rendered thyrotoxic by injection of supraphysiologic doses of triiodothyronine (T_3) oxidative phosphorylation was not uncoupled.[2]

Current views are that most thyroid hormone actions are
initiated by an interaction of T_3 with specific nuclear receptors. As discussed in detail below, these receptors are members of a large superfamily that includes receptors for steroid
hormones, vitamin D, and retinoic acid. Thyroid hormone receptors act largely as transcription factors. They function in
concert with a broad range of other nuclear proteins to modify
the expression of a diverse set of genes. Several investigative
groups, however, continue to explore the possibility that extranuclear processes may also contribute to the overall biologic actions of these hormones.

In this chapter we shall first review the general lines of
evidence that support the nuclear hypothesis and consider
several current proposals for operation of some extranuclear
pathways. We will review our current understanding of the
structure, function and distribution of the nuclear thyroid hormone receptors (TRs). We will discuss the thyroid response elements (TREs), the DNA sequences in target genes to which
the TRs bind. We will examine the factors which enable TRs to
dimerize with other members of the nuclear receptor superfamily and consider the growing evidence that the TRs also interact with other classes of transcription factors. Last, we will
attempt to relate the operation of initiating molecular mechanisms to the biologic action of thyroid hormone in selected
physiologic networks.

PROPOSED GENERAL MECHANISMS

Nuclear Pathways

We define a *hormone mechanism* as a cascade of molecular events initiated by an interaction of the active form of the hormone with specific subcellular sites that leads to a characteristic hormonal response. This definition skirts the possibility that transcellular transport of the hormone or metabolic transformation of the hormone could by themselves modulate hormonal expression. Our analysis assumes that the predominant, naturally occurring intracellular thyroid hormone is T_3, for which there is considerable evidence,[3] and that thyroxine (T_4) is largely a prohormone.

The hypothesis that thyroid hormone could stimulate transcription of mRNAs was first advanced 30 years ago.[2,4] This hypothesis was quite remarkable in as much as it was advanced at a time before mRNA could be directly measured. It was based on the observation that changes in the rate of incorporation of $[^{14}C]$-orotic acid into rapidly labeled nuclear RNA preceded increases in the rate of protein synthesis and mitochondrial oxygen consumption. However, subcellular fractionation studies failed to identify specific nuclear binding sites for T_3,[5,6] and it was proposed that thyroid hormone interacted with multiple subcellular sites and that thyroid hormone actions could not be explained exclusively by nuclear-initiated events.[7]

Specific nuclear binding sites for T_3 in rat liver and kidney were first recognized in 1972 by demonstrating the effects of graded doses of unlabeled T_3 on the subcellular distribution of tracer quantities of $[^{125}I]$-T_3.[8] Serial measurements of the specific activity of T_3 in serum permitted the calculation of the mass of T_3 specifically associated with nuclei, the affinity of such sites for T_3 and its analogues, and the total nuclear T_3 binding capacity in various tissues (Table 9-1).[9,10] In vitro determination of the binding capacity in whole nuclei and nuclear extracts yielded values very similar to those measured in whole animal studies.[11–14]

If these nuclear sites serve as the sole point of initiation of thyroid hormone action the biochemical effect of a given thyroid hormone analogue should correlate with the affinity of the receptors for that analogue after due account is taken of differences in the metabolism and distribution of the analogues. This expectation was realized when nuclear binding of some 40 thyroid hormone analogues was compared to their established biologic potency (Table 9-2).[14] The apparent discrepancy between the relatively high affinity of triiodothyroacetic acid for the nuclear receptors and its poor biologic potency can be explained by its rapid metabolic clearance.[15] Further, full occupancy of the receptors leads to a maximal biologic response.[16–18] However, the proportionality between occupancy and response is not generally linear.[18,19] In the case of hepatic malic enzyme, for instance, when the nuclear sites are one-half occupied, the level of malic enzyme mRNA or activity is only 10% of maximum. When the sites are 80% occupied, the steady state response is still only 20% of maximum. In the transition between 80% and 100% occupancy, the response increases from 20% to 100% of maximum. Clearly, this is not a linear relationship, but an amplified response instead. The degree of amplification varies with the specific target gene examined. The response of growth hormone accumulation in the rat anterior pituitary appears to be linear.[20] The nonlinearity of the response may reflect the complex interaction of the occupied receptor with other proteins involved in gene regulation. The cellular content of these proteins could itself be influenced by changing thyroidal status.

The nuclear hypothesis was validated further by studies of growth hormone–producing cells derived from rat pituitary tumors (GH and GC lines).[21] The results of these studies mirrored the in vivo studies cited earlier. The rate of production of growth hormone mRNA and protein was also limited by nuclear receptor occupancy by T_3. As in the in vivo studies, there was an excellent correlation between the binding of thyroid hormone analogues and the relative biologic potency of the analogue.

The identification of high affinity (ka 10^{10} to 10^{11}/L) T_3 nuclear binding sites with similar binding and physicochemical characteristics in the tissues of diverse species provided additional evidence for the role of these sites in the initiation of thyroid hormone action.[22] Direct and conclusive evidence supporting this thesis awaited the cloning of the receptor cDNA.[23,24]

TABLE 9-1.
Nuclear Binding Capacity and Fractional Occupancy of Nuclear Receptors in Euthyroid Adult Rat Tissues

Tissue	Binding Capacity (pmol/mg DNA)	Percentage of Saturation at Endogenous T_3 Concentrations
Liver	0.93	47
Brain	0.41	90
Heart	0.61	44
Spleen	0.03	50
Testis	0.003	Undetectable
Kidney	0.23	35
Anterior pituitary	1.21	80

(Oppenheimer JH, Schwartz HL, Surks MI. Tissue differences in the concentration of triiodothyronine nuclear binding sites in the rat: liver, kidney, pituitary, heart, brain, spleen, and testis. Endocrinology 1974;95:897; Crantz FR, Silva JE, Larsen PR. An analysis of the sources and quantity of 3,5,3' triiodothyronine specifically bound to nuclear receptors in rat cerebral cortex and cerebellum. Endocrinology 1982;110:367)

TABLE 9-2.
Relative Nuclear Binding Affinity and Biologic Activity of T_3 and Selected Analogues

Compound	Nuclear Binding (K_a/K_{T_3})	Relative Biologic Activity
L-T_3	1.0	1.0
D-T_3	0.6	0.5
Triiodothyroacetic acid	1.6	0.3
Isopropyl diiodothyronine	3.0	3.0
L-T_4	0.1	0.3
3,3′,5′-T_3 (reverse T_3)	0.001	0
Diiodothyronine	0.3	1.25
Diiodotyrosine	0	0
Monoiodotyrosine	0	0

(Data from references 14, 15, 259, and 260)

Proposed Non-nuclear Pathways

The evidence supporting a nuclear site of initiation does not negate the possibility of alternative mechanistic pathways. Given the opportunism of evolutionary processes, one would not be surprised if there were alternative extranuclear pathways for thyroid hormone action. An example of a widely accepted extranuclear effect of an iodothyronine is the negative regulation of type T_4-5′-deiodinase by T_4 (see chap 8). This process does not require new mRNA or protein synthesis.[25]

The physiologic relevance of any proposed in vitro model, whether nuclear or extranuclear, can only be established by a critical comparison with the operation of the process in vivo. A qualitatively similar biochemical result may be obtained in vivo and in vitro, but the specific mechanisms used in vivo may be totally unrelated to those responsible for the in vitro phenomenon. For example, in vitro addition of high concentrations of T_4 to mitochondrial preparations can directly stimulate the incorporation of labeled amino acids into mitochondrial protein[26,27] and, thus, simulate the effect of administering T_4 in vivo.[2] The similarity of the two systems, however, appears fortuitous. The in vitro effect is immediate and readily reversible when T_4 is removed from the mitochondria, whereas the in vivo process occurs only after many hours and is not dependent on the continued presence of T_4 in the mitochondria.[28]

MITOCHONDRIAL ACTION

The historic association of the thermogenic affects of thyroid hormone with the biochemistry of mitochondrial function undoubtedly accounts for the long-standing interest in the possibility of direct interactions of thyroid hormone and mitochondrial components. The initial reports indicated the existence of specific mitochondrial receptors for thyroid hormone and of rapid direct actions of the hormone in vitro on mitochondrial function, and the affinity of these mitochondrial sites for T_3, T_4, and their analogues corresponded to the reported relative thermogenic potencies of these compounds.[29,30] Unfortunately, there has since been a paucity of studies confirming these findings. Although two other groups[31,32] claim to have identified binding sites in isolated mitochondria, another[33] reported failure to do so. All attempts to demonstrate limited capacity, high affinity binding of thyroid hormone by mitochondria after in vivo injection of [^{125}I]-T_3,[8,34] or incubation of cells in culture with [^{125}I]-T_3[35,36] have failed. Nor have others detected any direct action of thyroid hormone on mitochondrial function in vitro.[37,38]

More recently, the mitochondrial component that might be the site of direct action of thyroid hormone on respiratory activity was suggested to be the adenine nucleotide (ADP/ATP) translocase.[39] However, appropriate controls for specificity of the hormone-protein interaction were not included. Although this protein is the most abundant mitochondrial protein, accounting for nearly 1% of total hepatic protein, there were only about 2000 mitochondrial T_3 binding sites per hepatocyte, and no T_3 binding sites were found in brain, spleen, or testis, a finding consistent with the known absence of thermogenic affect of thyroid hormone in these tissues.[40] Mitochondrial binding sites were apparently present in neonatal brain, but the early brain is no more thermogenically responsive to thyroid hormone than is the adult brain.[41] The reported absence of mitochondrial binding sites in the adult brain, testis, and spleen, is problematic, since the translocase is a fundamental component of the process of exchange of ADP for ATP in all mitochondria. Moreover, although the translocase is an inner membrane component, the bulk of hormone-binding sites in rat kidney mitochondria was in the outer membrane.[32]

There is other evidence arguing against both the rapid direct action of thyroid hormone on mitochondria and for a role of the ADP/ATP translocase in regulating thyroid hormone-induced thermogenesis. The mitochondrial respiratory rate did not change 15 minutes after injection of T_3 in rats.[38] In another study, ADP uptake by rat hepatic mitochondria did not change for at least 20 hours after injection of T_3.[37] Direct addition of hormone to mitochondria in vitro had no effect in either study. Furthermore, the translocase is only one of several factors, including cytochrome c and the F1-ATPase, that control the respiratory rate of mitochondria, and alterations in ADP/ATP translocase activity have only a minor effect on mitochondrial respiration.[42-44]

CELL MEMBRANE Ca^{2+}-ATPase

Incubation of human erythrocyte ghosts in vitro with thyroid hormone transiently increases Ca^{2+}-ATPase activity, with peak activity 60 minutes after the addition of hormone and loss of activity by 180 minutes.[45] In this system T_4 is somewhat more potent than T_3. Induction of enzyme activity is half-maximal at a concentration of about 10^{-12}M T_4 or T_3 and is maximal with 10^{-10}M hormone. Since the dissociation constant of binding of T_4 to the erythrocyte ghosts is approximately 2×10^{-10}M, it is unlikely that this interaction is the basis for the effect of the hormone on this enzyme, as the serum free T_4 concentration is 10^{-11}M. Thus, neither the site nor the mechanism of hormonal action in this system has been defined. One of the unexplained features of this model is the finding that analogues such as 3,5-diiodothyronine, mono- and diiodotyrosine, and tetrabromothyronine, virtually without effect in most assays of thyroid hormone action, were nearly equipotent with T_4 and T_3.[46] Tyrosine itself, at a concentration of 10^{-10}M, inhibited activity by about one-third. If plasma tyrosine

(10^{-6}M) acted in proportion to its concentration, erythrocyte Ca^{2+}-ATPase activity in vivo would be totally inhibited.

The profile of relative potencies of thyroid hormone analogues on the membrane Ca^{2+}-ATPase of rat thymocytes is very different,[47] in that the most potent compound was D-T_3 and reverse T_3, virtually inactive in all other systems, was as active as T_3. This profile of relative activities differs from that described for other metabolic functions in rat thymocytes, including glucose uptake, adenylate cyclase activity, and cAMP concentration. Moreover, the lowest effective concentration of T_3 (1pM) for induction of the Ca^{2+}-ATPase was 1000-fold lower than that required to induce the other thymocyte functions. Thus, it is unlikely that thyroid hormone regulation of the Ca^{2+}-ATPase is in any way related to the other actions of the hormone.

A critical test of this proposed action of thyroid hormone has not been carried out in laboratory animals. If a non-nuclear mechanism, independent of new mRNA or protein synthesis, is operative, then the cardiac sarcolemmal Ca^{2+}-ATPase should be activated very soon after injection of hormone.

GLUCOSE TRANSPORT

Thyroid hormones rapidly stimulate glucose uptake by rat thymocytes in vitro,[48–50] presumably by a direct effect on the plasma membrane, because the effect was not blocked by inhibitors of protein or mRNA synthesis. The minimum effective dose was 10^{-9}M T_3, a concentration about two orders of magnitude greater than the in vivo serum free T_3 concentration, and even 10^{-5}M T_3 failed to achieve maximal effects in vitro. Yet, administration to rats of as little as 1.5 nmol T_3/100 g body weight, which would raise the serum T_3 concentration only to the nanomolar (10^9M) range, caused maximum effects on thymocyte glucose uptake. In contrast, in several other tissues, including the heart, far smaller doses of T_3 (0.015–0.15 nmol/100 g body weight) induced maximum changes in glucose uptake while larger doses caused inhibition of uptake.[50] In contrast to these studies, thyroid hormone regulation of glucose uptake by cultured chick embryo cells was consistent with a nuclear site of action both with respect to the dose-response characteristics as well as the relative potency of hormonal analogues.[51]

In recent years, knowledge of the molecular basis of glucose transport across cell membranes has increased considerably.[52] Several specific transport proteins have been identified and their cDNAs cloned. One class of transporters, the so-called facultative glucose transporters, simply transfer glucose down its own gradient from plasma to cytosol. Thyroid hormone can regulate some of these transport proteins in several cell models and in rat tissues (see references 53 and 54 and the references therein). This hormonal regulation requires at least several hours of hormonal exposure and results from an increase in both the specific GLUT mRNA and protein. In studies of Sertoli cells in culture, the effect of T_3 on glucose uptake was limited to that period of cell development in which nuclear receptors are present, that is, cells from neonatal but not adult rats.[53] Further, the dose-response characteristics were consistent with an effect via nuclear receptors. Thus, in none of these reports was there evidence to support the concept of a rapid, direct effect of thyroid hormone independent of mRNA or protein synthesis.

TYPE II THYROXINE 5'-DEIODINASE ACTIVITY AND ACTIN POLYMERIZATION IN THE BRAIN

In the brain and pituitary, the bulk of intracellular T_3 is produced locally by 5'-monodeiodination of T_4, catalyzed by the type II T_4 5'-deiodinase. This enzyme differs from the type I deiodinase found in liver, kidney, and other tissues in its reaction kinetics, substrate specificities, and inhibitor sensitivity (reviewed in reference 55) (see chap 8). Cerebrocortical and pituitary type II T_4 5'-deiodinase is highly regulated in a manner designed to maintain intracellular T_3 concentrations within relatively narrow limits despite abrupt changes in thyroidal status. Brains of hypothyroid rats given only $^1/_{10}$ the normal daily replacement dose of T_4 contained near-normal concentrations of T_3.[56] Enzyme activity in the brain can increase up to fivefold within a day after thyroidectomy, and the increase is prevented by administration of T_4. Similarly, the high enzyme activity found in hypothyroid rats declines to normal within 4 hours after an injection of T_4. This regulation of brain T_4 5'-deiodinase activity involves a unique, non-nuclear site of hormone action. The relative potencies of T_4, T_3, and rT_3 in this reaction differ markedly from their affinities for the nuclear receptor; T_4 and rT_3 are both approximately 100 times more potent in causing a decrease in enzyme activity than is T_3. Inhibitors of transcription and translation do not block the effect of the hormones in down-regulating enzyme activity.[56] Alterations in the rate of disappearance of enzyme activity appear to fully account for the changes in steady-state T_4 5'-deiodinase activity.[25]

Studies of astrocytes in culture suggest that T_4 regulation of type II T_4 5'-deiodinase activity may be functionally related to the effect of the hormone on the organization of the cellular actin microskeleton.[57] In these cells, as in vivo, T_4 and rT_3 caused a reduction in T_4 5'-deiodinase activity due to an increased rate of degradation. The hormonal effect was not blocked by cycloheximide or actinomycin D but was disrupted by cytochalasin B, suggesting the process required an intact actin cytoskeleton. T_4 regulation of type II T_4 5'-deiodinase activity in these cells is probably related to the action of T_4 to maintain the cellular actin pool in a highly polymerized state, although it is not yet clear whether this mechanism is responsible for T_4 regulation of the enzyme in the brain in vivo.[58–61] Although polymerization of actin in the cerebellum of hypothyroid rats is reduced and normal concentrations were restored with T_4 treatment, this process required no less than 3 days, far more slowly than would be expected by non-nuclear mechanism.[62]

OTHER ACTIONS

There is growing interest in the potential clinical use of thyroid hormone as an inotropic and vasodilatory agent.[63] Since in many instances these effects were noted soon after T_3 administration, they could be mediated through non-nuclear mechanisms. Thus, thyroid hormone directly stimulates cardiac sarcolemmal and sarcoplasmic reticulum Ca^{2+}ATPase activity.[64] We have already discussed the proposed direct effect of thyroid hormone on plasma membrane Ca^{2+}ATPase and, as will be described later, the regulation of the sarcoplasmic reticulum Ca^{2+}ATPase is probably at a transcriptional level. Rapid effects of T_3 on Ca^{2+} channel activity have been noted[65,66] and T_3 has vasodilatory effects on vascular smooth muscle cells in culture[67] (see chap 38). In general, however, any immediate effects of T_3 observed clinically and experimentally require concentrations far above the physiologic range. Moreover, there is no firm correlation between the in vivo biologic effects of T_3 analogues and the effects exerted under in vitro circumstances.

In essence, there is at the time of this writing little evidence for extranuclear actions of thyroid hormone, with the exception of the negative regulation of type II T_4 5'-deiodinase activity by T_4. The diversity of approaches taken by investigators to study non-nuclear mechanisms may have impeded progress in this area. In the main, each laboratory interested in extranuclear mechanisms has focused on a distinctive model, thus limiting the opportunity for verification of experimental findings.

STRUCTURE AND DISTRIBUTION OF THYROID HORMONE RECEPTOR ISOFORMS

By the early 1980s the consensus was that there existed a single class of thyroid hormone (TR) receptors that was conserved among divergent species.[68] However, the cloning of multiple cDNAs encoding proteins with the characteristics of TRs brought about the realization that there is a family of TRs. The initial reports described the isolation of cDNA clones from libraries prepared from chick embryo and human placenta.[23,24] The encoded proteins had molecular weights of 50 to 55 kd and bound T_3 with high affinity. The molecular weights and the relative affinities of T_3, T_4, and other analogues were consistent with prior reports of the binding characteristics of the nuclear receptor. Both cDNAs were shown to code for cellular homologues (c-*erb* A) of the avian erythroblastosis virus, v-*erb* A. The substantial homology of the deduced amino acid sequences of the TRs with the previously reported steroid hormone receptors indicated that these proteins were members of a steroid-thyroid hormone receptor family.[69] Differences in the amino acid sequences encoded by these two cDNAs indicated that the receptors were products of separate genes (Fig 9-1). The gene coding for the human placental isoform has been designated β and is located on chromosome 3.[24] The chicken

receptor is designated α and its human homologue is on chromosome 17.[70] Alternate processing of the initial transcript yields two isoforms for the β receptor, designated TR-β1 and TR-β2, and two isoforms of the α receptor, designated TR-α1 and TR-α2. In retrospect, small differences in the molecular weights of the TRα and TRβ isoforms accounted for the results of earlier photoaffinity studies that had indicated heterogeneity in the size of nuclear T_3 binding proteins.[71]

cDNAs have been isolated from rat tissues that encode homologues of the human TR-β1 and the chicken TR-α1 receptors.[72,73] In addition, a second isoform of the β gene, TR-β2, has been cloned from the GH3 rat pituitary tumor,[74] a growth hormone-producing cell line. This protein, TR-β2, encoded by the β gene, is identical to TR-β1 except in the amino terminal region (Fig 9-1) and likely results from the differential function of an alternate promoter. TR-α1, -β1, and -β2 bind T_3 with high affinity and can, in the presence of T_3, transactivate reporter gene targets in transfection assays.

As indicated above the α gene also encodes multiple products. A cDNA was isolated from rat and human tissues[70,75,76] that is homologous to TR-α1 but differs from it at the carboxyl terminal. This second isoform, TR-α2, does not contain a 40 amino acid segment at the carboxyl terminus which is present in TR-α1, TR-β1, and TR-β2 and which is necessary for hormone binding (Fig 9-1). The two products of the α gene result from alternate splicing of the primary transcript. These proteins are identical for the first 370 amino acids. After that the sequences diverge and TR-α2 contains a 122-amino-acid sequence that replaces the critical ligand-binding region present in TR-α1. There are actually two closely related receptor variants of TR-α2 derived from the α gene, TR-α2vI and TR-α2vII.[77,78] TR-α1 is a true receptor in that it binds thyroid hormone and can transactivate reporter genes containing TREs in the promoter. In contrast, neither variant of TR-α2 can bind hormone or transactivate target genes. For this reason TR-α2 is designated as a receptor variant. The function of TR-α2 is still unknown. Studies in transient transfection assays suggest the possibility that TR-α2 may inhibit the action of the other TR isoforms.[79,80]

The T_3 receptor isoforms have substantial amino acid homology with the steroid hormone receptors.[81] Both are members of a large superfamily of receptors including the retinoic acid, vitamin D, and peroxisomal proliferator activators, as

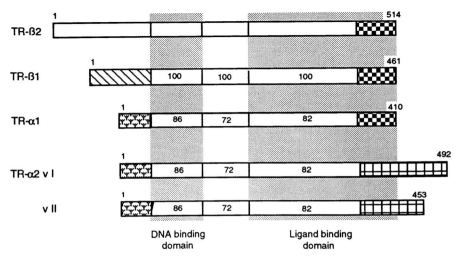

FIGURE 9-1. Structure of the thyroid hormone receptors. The numbers at the termini refer to the amino acid residue in each protein. The numbers within domains represent the degree of homology with the amino acid sequence of TR-β2. Similar patterns show areas of identity of amino acid sequence. (Schwartz HL, Strait KA, Oppenheimer JH. Molecular mechanisms of thyroid hormone action: a physiological perspective. In: Klee G, ed. Clinics in laboratory medicine: pathophysiology of thyroid disease. Philadelphia: WB Saunders, 1993:543)

well as a host of receptors or homologous proteins of un-known function known as orphan receptors. All proteins in this family contain multiple functional domains, including a DNA-binding domain and a carboxyl terminal ligand-binding region[82] (Fig 9-1). Near the amino terminus is a region of about 70 amino acids that can form two zinc finger motifs[83] (Fig 9-2). This segment, the DNA-binding domain, is well con-served and interacts with specific DNA segments, the hor-mone response elements (HRE) in the promoter regions of the target genes. Characteristic HREs have been identified for each hormone, but some overlap is possible. A short amino acid segment, designated the P box, in the base of the first of two zinc fingers in this domain serves to group members of the steroid-thyroid receptor family into two subgroups by their ability to recognize and bind to various HREs.[84,85] The first subgroup includes the TR, estrogen, retinoic acid, and vitamin D receptors, the second includes the androgen, mineralocorti-coid, and progesterone receptors. A short segment of the base of the second zinc finger, the D box, serves to distinguish among members of the subgroups by its specificity of binding to an even more restricted set of response elements. Com-pared with the structural conservation of the P box, the D box shows marked sequence divergence. This heterogeneity may play a role in recognition of specific characteristics of HREs ei-ther directly through interaction with the DNA sequence or by regulating the interaction of the receptors with other proteins that bind to the HRE.[85,86]

Whereas the steroid receptors have extended amino termi-nal regions that contain sequences involved in transactivation functions, the TR isoforms have rather short segments whose function is unclear. Removal of this segment of the steroid re-ceptors diminishes their functional capacity but appears to have no effect on TR function.[75,87] Following the DNA-binding seg-ment is a central element, the "hinge" region, the function of which is also not defined. The carboxyl terminal domain is crit-ical for both ligand binding and transactivation. Also within this region are segments that are involved in dimerization with other receptors and associated nuclear proteins. Starting in the hinge region and continuing into the carboxyl terminal domain there

is a series of nine heptad repeats that form a leucine zipper mo-tif that likely is involved in this dimerization function.[88] For both steroid and thyroid hormone receptors the transactivation func-tion of the receptors is linked to dimerization with other pro-teins. Mutations causing loss of this function result in loss of transactivation capacity.[89,90]

mRNAs for the TR isoforms are widely distributed among tissues and their concentrations vary widely.[91] The absolute quantities of the receptor mRNAs in various tissues of the rat are shown in Table 9-3.[92] In liver, TR-β1 mRNA accounted for about 80% of the total mRNA coding for T_3-binding isoforms, whereas in the brain TR-β1 and TR-α1 mRNAs were approxi-mately equal. TR-α2 mRNA was barely detectable in liver but represented almost 80% of the total TR mRNA in brain. Ini-tially, TR-β2 mRNA could only be found in the pituitary gland and cell lines derived from the pituitary,[74,93] but small quanti-ties of the mRNA for this isoform were recently detected in specific hypothalamic nuclei.[94] Thus, expression of these TR mRNAs is tissue-specific. Moreover, there is little direct rela-tionship between the concentrations of mRNAs for T_3-binding receptor isoforms and the total binding capacity (Table 9-3). These results indicate differences either in the efficiency of translation of individual mRNAs that result in variable produc-tion of receptor protein or variable rates of protein degrada-tion in different tissues.

The availability of antisera specific for each of the T_3-bind-ing TR isoforms allowed determination of the contribution of the individual TR to the total binding capacity in several rat tis-sues.[95,96] An antiserum prepared against a region of the car-boxyl terminus identical in TR-α1, -β1, and -β2 removed nearly all hormone-binding activity from nuclear extracts of liver, heart, brain, and kidney. Thus, it is unlikely that other receptor forms remain unidentified. As shown in Table 9-3, the contribu-tion of each of the TR isoforms to total binding capacity varied widely among adult rat tissues, and the protein:mRNA ratio for each isoform varied as much as tenfold among tissues.

Although TR-β2 mRNA could only be detected by North-ern analysis in rat pituitary tissue, immunohistochemical stud-ies indicate that the TR-β2 protein is widely distributed in rat brain.[97] Moreover, immunoprecipitation of nuclear extracts of liver, brain, kidney, and heart showed that 10% to 20% of the binding capacity in these tissues could be accounted for by TR-β2[96] (Table 9-3). TR-β2 mRNA was detected in these tissues using reverse transcription-polymerase chain reaction meth-ods. There is, therefore, in these tissues an enormous amplifi-cation of the protein:mRNA concentration ratio for this isoform. The mechanism of this phenomenon is not known. Treatment of GH cells in culture with T_3 leads to a 90% reduc-tion in the level of TR-β2 mRNA and a fall in total T_3 binding capacity.[74] In contrast, although administration of excess hor-mone to rats causes a marked fall in TR-β2 mRNA and a three-to fivefold rise in TR-β1 mRNA in the pituitary,[93] there is no detectable change in either the concentration of any of the TR isoform proteins or the total T_3 binding capacity.[98]

Consistent with earlier studies of the subcellular localiza-tion of T_3 binding, immunohistochemical analysis has shown the TRs to be concentrated in the nuclei of all target tis-sues.[96,99] TRs appear to be homogeneously distributed among liver and heart cells and in the nuclei of glomeruli and tubular epithelium in kidney, and they are present in neurons of the hippocampus and widely distributed among neurons in other

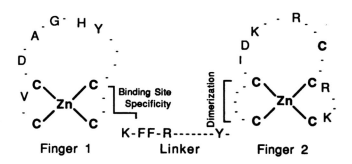

FIGURE 9-2. Structure of the two zinc fingers in the DNA-binding do-main of thyroid hormone receptors. Estrogen, glucocorticoid, and thy-roid hormone receptors are most similar in this domain. Amino acids common to the three receptors are shown, and the variable amino acids are shown as dashes. The region in the first zinc finger that dic-tates response element recognition is indicated (binding site speci-ficity), as is the region of the second zinc finger involved in dimer formation (dimerization). (From Williams GR, Brent GA. Thyroid hor-mone response elements. In: Weintraub BD, ed. Molecular endocrin-ology: basic concepts and clinical correlations. New York: Raven Press, 1995:217)

TABLE 9-3.
Concentrations of T_3-Receptor Protein and mRNA in Rat Tissues*

| Tissue | Binding Capacity (pmol/mg DNA) | | | | mRNA (fmol/mg DNA) | | | Protein:mRNA Ratio | |
	TOTAL	β_1	β_2	α_1	β_1	β_2	α_1	β_1	α_1
Liver	1.01	0.71	0.17	0.13	1.06	NM	0.23	669	565
Brain	0.66	0.19	0.07	0.40	4.20	NM	3.40	45	118
Kidney	0.25	0.10	0.04	0.10	2.80	NM	0.52	36	192
Heart	0.58	0.24	0.10	0.26	1.53	NM	0.56	157	464

NM, not measured.
*Concentrations of TR protein were calculated as the product of the fractional distribution of the TR protein determined by immunoprecipitation with specific antiserum and the total nuclear binding capacity.
(Schwartz HL, Lazar MA, Oppenheimer JH. Widespread distribution of immunoreactive thyroid hormone β2 receptor in the nuclei of extrapituitary rat tissues. J Biol Chem 1994;269:24777)

areas of the cerebrum. In the cerebellum, both granule cells and Purkinje cells contain nuclear TRs, with particularly high concentrations in the Purkinje cells. TRs are also present in oligodendroglia throughout both cerebrum and cerebellum.[100] These results are consistent with the many reports of the effect of altered thyroidal state on myelination in neonatal brain. Astrocytes appeared to be devoid of TRs, suggesting that the effects of T_3 on astrocyte development are indirect.[101]

ONTOGENY OF THYROID HORMONE RECEPTORS

Early studies of the ontogeny of the total nuclear binding capacity for T_3 in various tissues of rats showed marked differences in developmental patterns. Binding capacity in the liver was very low early in gestation and increased more than fivefold by 2 months of age.[102,103] In contrast, binding capacity was nearly as high as in fetal as in adult brain, it increased two- to threefold during the first week of life and then decreased.[41,104] Similarly, in sheep hepatic binding capacity was low early in gestation and rose continuously thereafter to a maximum at birth, whereas in the brain it was as high throughout gestation as in adult sheep, and it also increased transiently during the first week of life, the same as in rats.[105] In human fetuses, receptors are detectable in brain as early as 10 weeks and rise seven- to tenfold by the 16th week of gestation. Rats are an altricial species in which much of the development of both the thyroid hormone economy and central nervous system occurs postnatally, whereas sheep and humans are precocial. These results suggest that receptor numbers might play a role in regulation of the developmental process and the timing of tissue responsivity to thyroid hormone.

In rat brain, the mRNA for TR-α1 and TR-α2 have been identified throughout fetal life, but not TR-β1 or TR-β2 mRNA.[92] Consistent with these findings, immunoprecipitation of whole brain nuclear extracts[95] and immunocytochemical analysis of brain sections failed to detect TR-β1 or TR-β2 protein at gestational days 15, 17, or 19.[106] However, very low levels of TR-β1 may be present at this stage in development because weak in situ hybridization signals for TR-β1 mRNA can be detected in selected nuclei in fetal brain.[107] Thus, TR-α1 accounts for essentially all T_3 binding capacity in the fetal brain.[95] The TR-α1 mRNA rises transiently by about twofold

early in the postnatal period.[92] TR-α2 mRNA is present throughout both fetal and postnatal stages at a level tenfold greater than TR-α1 mRNA, a finding which suggests that processing of the α transcript is not altered during development. Quantitation of the TR-α2 protein has not been reported.

The level of TR-β1 mRNA in rat brain begins to rise about the time of birth and it increases 40-fold by postnatal day 10.[92] This rise is not dependent on T_3 because it also occurs in hypothyroid animals. Immunoprecipitation of nuclear extracts indicates that 20% to 30% of the total binding capacity in the adult brain is due to TR-β1.[95] The near-simultaneous rise in TR-β1 and T_3 suggest the operation of a coordinate system responsible for the dramatic developmental changes in brain during this period. These changes are also consistent with the hypothesis that TR-β1 and TR-α1 subserve distinctive functions.

In rat liver, mRNA for TR-α1, TR-α2, and TR-β1 can be detected as early as day 16 of gestation.[108] However, immunoprecipitation of nuclear extracts failed to detect the TR-β1 protein at this stage of development.[95] TR-α1 accounts for virtually all nuclear binding capacity in this tissue, as it does in brain throughout gestation. In the postnatal period, whereas TR-α1 protein remains constant, a rise in TR-β1 protein accounts entirely for the several-fold increase in total binding capacity. However, unlike TR-β1 in brain, the rise in TR-β1 protein does not result from changes in the level of the mRNA but from increased translational efficiency or increased stability of the protein.

The cloning of the TR genes in amphibia has allowed similar detailed studies of the expression of the TR isoforms during metamorphosis. In Xenopus, although TR-α and TR-β mRNA are not detected in oocytes, eggs, or embryos until after hatching, TR-α protein is detectable in the unfertilized oocyte,[109] presumably derived from maternal sources. The TR-α mRNA increases steadily from stage 38 throughout premetamorphosis and reaches a peak by early prometamorphosis at stage 56.[110] The TR-α mRNA remains elevated until climax and then decreases to about half the peak level in the frog liver. The expression of TR-α mRNA is independent of thyroid hormone since it is detectable even before establishment of the thyroid gland anlage. However, in some tissues, exogenous T_3 can cause small increases in expression of this isoform although the TR-α protein level is unaffected.[109] As in fetal rat brain and liver, the TR-α isoform accounts for nearly all the nuclear binding capacity in the early tadpole. In contrast, the expression pattern of TR-β mRNA closely follows that of secretion of thyroid hormone.[110] There is a small but steady increase of TR-β mRNA during premetamorphosis. From the beginning of prometamorphosis at stage 54 there is a rapid rise to a peak at climax, paralleling closely the serum concentrations of thyroid hormone. This is consistent with earlier studies demonstrating a rise in hepatic and tail nuclear binding capacity during this period.[111,112] In the head and tail, there is a steady rise in TR-α mRNA but no change in the α receptor protein. The TR-β levels increase to become the predominant isoform by the time of climax.[109]

Treatment of tadpoles with exogenous T_3 can increase TR-β mRNA expression many-fold even before premetamorphosis. This is the earliest response to T_3 and precedes any morphologic alterations by about 2 days.[110] Removal of the exogenous T_3 leads to loss of the TR-β mRNA and arrest of the morphologic changes that had begun. Tadpoles respond to T_3 with metamorphic changes only after the TR-β isoform is expressed. Curiously, the dependence of TR-β1 on a rise in serum T_3 in metamorphosizing tadpoles contrasts with the apparent lack of T_3 dependence in the rise of TR-β1 in neonatal rat brain tissue.[92]

Differential expression of the TR-α and -β isoforms also occurs in developing chicks. TR-α mRNA is ubiquitously expressed in the chick embryo from early stages of gestation.[113] The expression of TR-β is more restricted and appears to rise at the critical period of tissue development in brain, lung, and eye. In brain, TR-α mRNA is expressed widely early in embryogenesis; TR-β is not detected until about day 19.[114] In cerebellum, the TR-β expression begins after granule cell proliferation and migration are complete and correlates with the period of synapse formation between Purkinje cells and granule cells. TR-β mRNA appears to be restricted to the internal granular layer and the white matter, the latter suggesting that thyroid hormone stimulates myelogenesis in birds as well as in mammals. The TR-β gene is not expressed in nucleated erythrocytes in either amphibia[115] or chickens.[113]

Thus, TR-α is expressed widely and early, even before the appearance of thyroid hormone. TR-β is first expressed in brain as the thyroid hormone-dependent developmental processes unfold. This has led to the proposal that the TR-α may play a unique and possibly critical ligand-independent role in early development. This would be consistent with the absence of any known case of a naturally occurring mutant TR-α, whereas mutant TR-β1 has been identified in at least two hundred families with the syndrome of thyroid hormone resistance (see chap 90). Such a model suggests that TR-β acts as the primary transducing agent for hormonally regulated cellular differentiative processes. This suggestion is supported by evidence that T_3 blocks proliferation and induces differentiation in neuro-2A cells overexpressing TR-β1.[116] The hormone had no effect on cells overexpressing TR-α1.

INTERACTION OF THYROID HORMONE RECEPTORS WITH DNA

The ability of members of the steroid-thyroid receptor superfamily to regulate gene expression is at least in part dependent on the presence in the gene of specific hormone response elements (HREs). HREs are sequences of DNA that confer positive or negative influences on gene expression.[117,118] These regulatory sequences tend to be located near the start site of transcription in the 5′-upstream promoter region of genes, but occasionally are found in their 3′-untranslated or intronic regions. They function by providing a recognition site for the binding of specific transacting protein factors,[119] which results in either enhanced or suppressed DNA transcription. Most studies of how protein-DNA interactions influence the rate of transcription have been directed to two potential mechanisms.[120,121] One is direct interaction of the protein-DNA complex with the transcription initiation complex. In its simplest form, this model envisions direct binding of the receptor to a site close to the start site of transcription, allowing direct interaction of the TR protein with protein components of the initiation complex. A variant of this model is one in which the TR binding site is located at a distance from the transcription initiation complex. Under these circumstances regulation requires the folding of the DNA strand upon itself, allowing direct contact between the TR and the initiation complex. The second is an indirect influence of the T_3:TR complex on the transcriptional machinery by regulation of an intermediate protein. This intermediate protein would, in turn, interact with the transcription initiation complex. The finding that TRs can interact directly with TFIIB, a specific component of the transcription initiation complex,[122] tends to favor a direct action of the T_3:TR complex on transcription.

The typical gene contains several enhancer or silencer elements within its regulatory region. These elements bind a diverse group of transacting factors, some of which (e.g., SP-1 and NF-1) are present in multiple cell types and are involved in the transcription of many genes.[120,121] Other transacting factors, such as TRs and other members of the nuclear receptor superfamily, are cell-specific and developmentally regulated. This allows them to have very specific regulatory effects on a small subset of genes within defined cell types. The overall level of expression of a gene will thus be a reflection of the entire complement of transcription factors acting upon it and will be subject to change depending on the period of development, hormonal influences, and metabolic status.

Thyroid Hormone Response Elements

DNA sequences that specifically bind TR and confer positive thyroid hormone regulation upon a gene have been designated TREs, whereas sequences that confer negative regulation are referred to as negative TREs or nTREs (for a detailed review see reference 123). The minimal requirements for a sequence to be considered a TRE are that it bind TRs with high affinity and confer T_3 responsivity to a heterologous promoter. Assays of binding include the gel-shift or electrophoretic mobility shift assay[124] and the avidin-biotin complex assay.[125] Both assay systems measure the relative affinity with which the TR binds to the TRE. Footprinting and methylation interference analyses allow more precise determination of the particular bases that are contacted by the TR. The functional capacity of a potential TRE to confer T_3 responsivity is tested in transient transfection assays. The DNA sequence of interest is inserted upstream of a heterologous promoter that drives a reporter gene, such as chloramphenicol aminotransferase (CAT). This fusion construct is introduced into eukaryotic cells and incubated in the presence

TABLE 9-4.
Response Elements for Selected Thyroid Hormone–Responsive Genes

Gene	Sequence*	Position
POSITIVE TRES		
Rat growth hormone	A**AGGTAA**GATC**AGGGAC**G**TGACCG**C	−190 to −166
Rat myelin basic protein	**AGACCT**CGGCTG**AGGACA**CGGCGG	−186 to −163
Rat α myosin heavy chain	CTGG**AGGTGA**CAGG**AGGACA**AC**AGCCCT**GA	− 130 to −159
Rat malic enzyme	**AGGACG**TTGG**GGGTTA**GGGG**AGGACA**GTG	−287 to −260
Rat S14	TRE1: TACTT**GGGGCCTG**GCAGC	−2700 to −2683
	TRE2: GTCTA**GGGGCCTG**AGATG	−2797 to −2814
	TRE3: GGTCA**AGGGCCTG**GCCAG	−2616 to −2633
Pcp-2	**AGGCCT**TCTC**AGGTCA**GAGACC**AGGAGA**	−295 to −268
SERCA2	TRE1: GCGG**AGGCAA**GCC**AAGGACA**CCAG	−481 to −458
	TRE2: GCCG**CGACCG**CGTA**AGGTCG**GGCT	−310 to −287
	TRE3: CGCG**CGGCCT**CGATCC**GGGTTA**CTGG	−219 to −194
Synthetic TRE palindrome, based on rat growth hormone	TC**AGGTCATGACCT**GA	
NEGATIVE TRES		
Rat TSH β-subunit	AGTGCAAAGTA**AGGTAGGTCTCTACCC**GGC	+15 to +44
	TGAACAGAGTCT**GGGTCA**TCACAGCATTAAC	−22 to +4
	CGCCAGTGCAAAGTAAG	+11 to +27
Rat α-subunit	TGGGCTTA**AGGTGCAGGT**GGGAGCATGCAATTTGTATT	−74 to −38
Human TSH β-subunit	TTT**GGGTCACCA**CAGCATCTGC**TCACCA**ATGCAAAGTAAGGTAGGT	−3 to +43
	Domain 1 (+1 to +17) **GGGTCACCA**CAGCATCT	
	Domain 2 (+28 to +37) GCAAACTAAG	
Human α-subunit	GCAGG**TGAGGACTT**CA	−22 to −7
Mouse TSH β-subunit	TGAA**CGGAGA**GT**GGGTCA**TCACAGCA	−22 to +3
Human growth hormone	Multiple putative half sites in this region; whole region confers repression in transfections; regions bind in gel shifts; no accurate localization yet	+2021 to +2175

Bold letters indicate core consensus sequences. TRE, thyroid hormone response element. (A more complete list and all pertinent references are given in Williams GR, Brent GA. Thyroid hormone response elements. In: Weintraub BD, ed, Molecular endocrinology: basic concepts and clinical correlations. New York, Raven Press, 1995;217)

and absence of T_3 and the effect of T_3 on the reporter gene activity is measured. While these criteria will identify sequences with the *potential* for mediating T_3 regulation of gene expression, proof that this action occurs within the context of the native promoter requires a more detailed analysis of the promoter region of the particular gene.

The identification of a core consensus sequence for TREs is based on a comparison of the several TREs identified in T_3-responsive genes (Table 9-4). Based on the combination of transient transfection and mobility shift assays, the hexamer (A/G)GGT(C/A)A (alternate bases indicated in parentheses) represents the minimal TRE consensus sequence for binding of TRs.[126] The optimal TR binding motif may be an octamer consisting of the core hexamer with the 5′ addition of the two nucleotides TA to make the sequence TAAGGTCA.[127] Nevertheless, examination of all TREs identified to date indicates a marked degree of divergence from the core consensus sequence.[123] Whether these differences are reflected in differential responses to the hormone in vivo is not known.

Although a single hexameric sequence is sufficient for binding the TR as a monomer, it is insufficient to confer T_3 responsivity upon a gene. Analysis of the TRE sequences within the regulatory regions of target genes has demonstrated that the hexameric sequences are found in pairs.[128,129] This is similar to the reported structure of steroid hormone response elements,[130] which consist of pairs of hexamers in a palindromic configuration. Arranging two core TRE consensus sequences as a palindrome, AGGTCATGACCT, created a very potent synthetic TRE (TREpal)[125] (Fig 9-3). On the basis of these considerations, the single core hexamer sequence has been designated a "half-site." The arrangements of natural half-sites in target genes is, in fact, quite variable (Table 4). For the most part, they are found in one of three conformations: a palindrome similar to the TRE pal[125]; as a direct repeat of two hexameric sequences with a four-base separation of the half-sites[131]; or as an inverted repeat with a six-base spacing[132] (Fig 9-3). The importance of orientation and spacing will become apparent in the discussion of receptor dimerization.

The requirements for two half-sites initially led to the hypothesis that the TRs function as homodimers, analogous to the behavior of steroid hormone receptors.[130] Although experiments using the synthetic TREpal and the naturally occurring rat growth hormone TREs quickly confirmed the ability of the receptors to form homodimers, it soon became apparent that the action of TREs was more complicated. Unlike steroid hormone receptors, TREs could form heterodimers

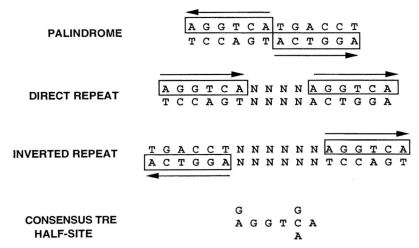

FIGURE 9-3. Conformation of thyroid response elements (TREs). The TREs shown are (top to bottom) a palindrome, a direct repeat +4 nucleotide spacer (N), and an inverted repeat +6N spacer. N is any nucleotide (A, G, C, or T). The conformations shown are idealized with respect to the constancy of the AGGTCA core sequence and the spacing of the half-sites. As discussed in the text, TREs have a great deal of diversity of sequence and conformation. (Adapted from Chin WW. Current concepts of thyroid hormone action: progress notes for the clinician. Thyroid Today 1992;15:1)

with other proteins.[133] Two early studies showed that proteins capable of stabilizing TR binding to TREs through dimerization were present in extracts of nuclear proteins. These were designated thyroid hormone receptor auxiliary proteins, or TRAPs.[134,135] TRAPs vary from tissue to tissue and include other members of the superfamily, particularly the retinoic acid and 9-cis retinoic acid receptors (RAR and RXR) (reviewed in reference 136).

Further complicating matters is the fact that the consensus sequence AGGTCA is also capable of binding both the retinoic acid and vitamin D receptors, and that the TREpal sequence can also function as a retinoic acid response element (RARE).[131] Thus, whereas steroid hormone response elements are relatively specific for their cognate receptors, TREs, RAREs, and vitamin D response elements do not by themselves have absolute specificity in their interactions with this group of receptors. Such specificity may be provided by the dimerization partner as a result of the orientation of the hexamer half-sites. Studies of the influence of nucleotide spacing between hexamer half-sites on the specificity of recognition by either TR, RAR, or vitamin D receptor revealed the following pattern: vitamin D bound and transactivated preferentially a direct repeat of AGGTCA separated by three bases (DR3), whereas TRs acted on the same repeat separated by four bases (DR4) and RARs on the repeat separated by five bases (DR5). These relationships are commonly referred to as the "3, 4, 5 rule" of transactivation. The subsequent identification of additional response elements demonstrates that TREs exist in a variety of configurations[123] (Table 9-4). Nevertheless, the general conclusion derived from these studies, that the capacity of receptors to form dimers on specific response elements and transactivate gene expression is influenced by the spacing of the half-sites, remains valid. In addition, certain nucleotides within this region may play a role in facilitating TR binding and transactivation.[137]

Negative Thyroid Hormone Response Elements

T_3 mediates TR repression as well as activation of gene expression. The ability of T_3 to produce both activation and repression of gene expression was documented in studies from the early 1980s of the effect of thyroidal status on 238 translation products of total rat hepatic mRNA.[138] Eighteen of the products

changed significantly; 11 increased and 7 decreased, suggesting that about 40% of the hepatic genes affected by T_3 were negatively regulated. These results occurring within the same tissue and possibly even in the same cell type reflect the ability of T_3 to regulate cellular processes in opposing directions.

To date, only a handful of negative thyroid hormone response elements (nTREs) have been tested in transfection studies and DNA binding assays (reviewed in 123). The best studied of the nTREs are those that inhibit transcription of the genes for the α- and β-subunits of thyrotropin (TSH) in the pituitary. The actual TR binding sequence among the identified elements varies considerably but tends to maintain roughly the same consensus motif of AGGTCA as the positive elements (Table 9-4), but there has yet to be described a definitive consensus sequence or structural requirement for the nTREs. What is clear is that the nTREs in many instances differ substantially from the positive TREs. For example, whereas all TREs require at least two half-sites to allow dimerization and transactivation, nTREs do not appear to share this requirement. Many contain only a single binding site for the TR.[139,140] When two potential binding sites are present within an nTRE element they may overlap and thus again lack dimerization capacity.[139,141] However, there is some evidence of protein-protein interaction even on these sequences. Dimerization was apparent on the nTRE in the mouse TSH-β gene that is arranged as a repeat sequence with no intervening bases (DR0).[142] A study of the nTRE for the epidermal growth factor (EGF) receptor gene[143] showed that high affinity binding of TR to this element required the presence of other nuclear proteins (TRAPs) and neither the TR nor the TRAP protein alone bound to the nTRE. Chemical cross-linking of the TR:TRAP complex suggested the presence of heterodimers. Interestingly, this TR-TRAP heterodimer bound to a seven-base pair sequence of DNA (GGGACTC) that resembles a single half-site.[143] Thus, the possibility exists that unlike the positive TREs that bind both proteins of the heterodimer directly, only one of the dimer partners may contact the nTRE DNA sequence analogous to monomer binding. Studies of the nTRE of the rat TSH-β gene also suggested only the presence of monomers.[139] Mutations of the nTRE that disrupted monomer binding also abolished the functional capacity of this nTRE.

The molecular mechanism by which binding of T_3 to the TR on an nTRE causes repression of transcription is no better defined than is the mechanism of positive regulation by this hormone. The idea of steric hindrance was first proposed as an explanation for transcriptional repression. This model was based on the finding that nTRE elements in the TSH-α and -β genes from several species were positioned very close to the start site of transcription, so that the T_3:receptor complex might interfere with the assembly of the transcription initiation complex or block polymerase II initiation and elongation and thus reduce the level of transcription. However, nTREs are position-independent, in that they can be placed upstream of the start site of transcription and still exert a negative influence on transcription.[139,140] Thus, nTRE repression appears to be more complex than a simple steric hindrance mechanism.

Repression by Unliganded Receptor

Unlike the steroid receptors, TRs bind to response elements in the absence of ligand. In transfection assays, the binding of unliganded TRs to TREs causes a decrease in the basal transcription rate of cotransfected genes.[144,145] The addition of T_3 causes not only relief of the inhibition but also induction of gene activity to levels well above the original baseline level. For an unliganded TR to have repressor activity the gene must have an intact TRE and the TR must have a functional dimerization domain.[146] Unliganded TR blocks formation of the preinitiation complex, thus repressing transcription[147]; addition of T_3 prevents this repression and allows formation of the transcriptional unit. However, if T_3 action were limited to this mechanism, it would only result in derepression and return of transcription rates to the original level. Yet in transfection assays T_3 causes true induction of expression to levels many-fold the basal value. Another mechanism must, therefore, be operative. The physiologic role of transcriptional repression remains speculative, since this has only been demonstrated for artificial gene constructs in transient transfection assays in the presence of excess receptor. This process could be tested, for example, in GH cells that have an endogenous complement of receptors and a target gene, GH. In the absence of T_3, GH mRNA levels should be higher in cells in which receptor levels have been reduced by tranfection of anti-sense probes than in control cells.

Dimerization of Receptors

Recognition that TR dimerization is an important determinant of both its specificity and transactivation potential has made this process the object of intensive investigation. Studies of TR binding to the rat GH promoter region have indicated the presence of a TRE sequence between −191 and −164 base pairs upstream of the start site of transcription in which the TRE hexamer half-sites are arranged as a direct repeat.[128,129] Further analysis revealed a potential palindrome-like sequence immediately 3′ to this repeat that is also functional in transfection assays.[125] Thus, the GH TRE appeared to be composed of three half-sites that form two overlapping TRE motifs. Gel-shift analysis of this region indicated that TRs are likely bound both as monomers and homodimers to this sequence.[148] Subsequent studies have showed that the dimer binding is indeed cooperative, the result of protein-protein interactions. The ability of the TRs to form dimers on the TREpal, DR4, and IR6 sequences demonstrates the structural flexibility of TRs. As earlier indicated, the ability to

form dimers is an absolute requirement for transactivation of positive TREs.[148]

On a molecular level, dimerization involves two regions of the receptor molecule. The primary interaction occurs via an association along a subregion of the T_3 binding domain comprised of nine heptad repeats.[149] These repeats form a structure within the protein analogous to a "leucine zipper" that is able to interact with a similar "zipper" structure in other receptor-related molecules to produce strong protein-protein binding. In addition, the D box of the second zinc finger may also play a role of dimerization.[85,150]

The interaction of TRs with other members of the nuclear receptor superfamily and other TRAPs indicate the possibility of a complex mechanism for producing a highly varied spectrum of regulatory responses among target genes. TRs dimerize with retinoic acid receptors (RAR),[88,151] but the biologic function of such dimers is not known. They apparently lose their specificity of binding to TREs and to retinoic acid response elements (RAREs). The retinoid X receptor (RXR), for which 9-cis retinoic acid is the primary ligand, can also form heterodimers with TRs, RARs, and vitamin D receptors (VDRs). Immunologic analyses suggest that RXRs may be the dominant TRAP in cultured cell lines[152] and rat tissues.[153] These heterodimers retain their ability to recognize and bind to natural response elements for whichever receptor, TR or RAR, is complexed with the RXR.[154] Heterodimers consisting of TR and RXR selectively bind to TREs, whereas dimers of RXR and RAR bind selectively to RAREs. The relative specificity and affinity of TR homodimers and heterodimers for various TREs is such that TR:RXR heterodimers have a several-fold higher affinity than do TR:RAR complexes and TR homodimers have by far the lowest affinity.[155]

Despite the presence of RXR as a heterodimer partner with TR on a DR4 sequence, its ligand 9 cis-retinoic acid is ineffective; it is T_3 that causes induction.[156] However, with a response element containing overlapping TRE and RXRE sequences, T_3 and 9 cis-retinoic acid acted in a synergistic fashion. Thus, for some genes RXR with its ligand may play a regulatory role as well as act as a TRAP. For others, it may only be required to be present as a TRAP to allow regulation by T_3.

The interaction of TR-RXR dimers with response elements has been examined using chimeric receptors in which the P box of the first zinc finger of the TR was replaced by the homologous sequence from the glucocorticoid receptor (GR). This results in a chimeric TR that binds only to the GRE consensus half-site. Modified TREs were then constructed in which the consensus GRE sequence was placed in the 5′ or 3′ position. Transactivation by T_3 and the affinity of binding of RXR:TR dimers were greatest when the TR bound to the 3′ half-site and the RXR to the 5′ half-site.[157,158] In a related study using the calbindin gene, orientation of VDR and TR proteins on the half-site sequences was critical in determining the specificity of the transcriptional response to the different ligands.[159] In a TR-VDR heterodimeric complex in which the TR was bound to the 3′ site, the complex functioned as a TR with no effect of vitamin D. However, if the positions were reversed and the VDR bound to the 3′ half-site, the element functioned as a VDRE and T_3 was ineffective.[159] These studies highlight two important aspects of TR-TRE function. First, the location of the TR in the 3′ site of a response element seems to confer T_3 responsiveness to that element. Second, the TR protein, besides acting as a ligand-dependent transcription factor, may also play a role as an auxiliary factor in the functions of other members of the superfamily.

TR also dimerizes with the peroxisomal proliferator activator receptor (PPAR) on a unique TRE with a DR2 structure. This heterodimer had no effect on TRE with a DR4 structure.[160] This ability to function with the PPAR on DR2 elements was restricted to the TR-β1 isoform,[160] and thus may help provide insight into potential functional differences among the TR isoforms.

TRs can also have negative influences on other transcription factors. The human epidermal growth factor gene contains overlapping TRE and SP-1 sites. Addition of SP-1 blocked the ability of TR to bind to the TRE sequence in this region,[161] and in transfection assays addition of T_3 blocked the ability of the SP-1 protein to activate transcription.[161] However, when constructs were prepared in which the TRE and SP-1 sites were separated, the interaction was synergistic. Thus, the way the TRE sequence relates to other response elements plays an important role in its regulatory abilities. TRs can also interact with other members of the superfamily in a negative manner to block transcription. For example, TRs can bind to the estrogen response element (ERE) without dimerizing with estrogen receptors (ER).[162,163] TR binding to the ERE inhibits the ability of the ER to transactivate by blocking access of the ER to the DNA element. TR can similarly inhibit the action of RAREs. These studies highlight a potential role for TRs as a negative regulator of transcriptional activation by other members of the superfamily. Not surprisingly, the reverse is also true, for while RXRs and RARs act as positive heterodimer partners for TRs, other members of the superfamily of nuclear receptors may have negative actions on TREs. A series of studies have shown that the COUP-TF protein blocks the ability of TRs to transactivate (reviewed in reference 164). The COUP-TF protein functions through heterodimerization with TRs.[165] These heterodimers occur on some but not all TREs, since the COUP-TF can bind to the TRE consensus sequence AGGTCA.[165] Dimerization between COUP-TF and TR was also shown in gel-shift assays by supershifting the complexes with antisera directed against the COUP-TF protein.[153] COUP-TF can antagonize the action of T_3 on a subset of TREs and thus result in the repression of selected T_3-responsive genes in tissues in which the COUP-TF is present.

An alternative mechanism for regulating TR activation of transcription of a gene containing a TRE was shown for the human placental lactogen B (hCS-B) gene.[166] There is a GHF1 element, close to the TRE, that is necessary for T_3 activation of hCS-B.[166] Neither the TRE nor the GHF1 sequence alone produced activation of a thymidine kinase promoter, whereas the combined element showed strong T_3 stimulation. The requirement for GHF1 was evident from the lack of T_3 induction in JEG-3 cells in which GHF1 is not expressed, and strong T_3 responses in GC cells in which GHF1 is present. Finally, synergy was not restricted to the interaction of T_3 with GHF1 but also occurred in combination with SP-1, NF-1, CP-1, and Oct-1 recognition sequences.[166] Therefore, this type of regulation may not be confined to the hCS B gene but instead may provide a general mechanism for allowing T_3 regulation only within the limits set by the presence of a secondary factor.

Although it is clear that TRs function as dimers, what has yet to be determined is whether homodimers, heterodimers, or a combination of both are the functional complex in vivo.

Besides the difference in affinity mentioned above, homo- and heterodimers have differential sensitivity to T_3. The presence of T_3 in DNA binding assays disrupts TR homodimer formation but does not affect heterodimers of TR and RXR.[167] This effect of T_3 appears to be TRE-dependent, with a loss of homodimerization on DR4, whereas homodimers on the TRE palindrome are not affected.[168] Studies examining the dimerization domain of the TRs may shed additional light on this area. Early data have shown the ninth heptad repeat of the dimerization domain of the TR is critical for heterodimerization but not homodimerization.[169] Mutations of this region cause a loss of heterodimerization capacity and of the capacity for ligand-independent repression of transactivation. Addition of T_3 restores the ability of these mutant receptors to heterodimerize and their ability to transactivate target genes.[169] Finally, the use of different antibodies directed against various regions of the TR indicate that heterodimerization causes a distinct conformational change in the receptor not present in the homodimer.[170] The ultimate role of homo- and heterodimerization in mediating transcriptional activation in vivo remains to be elucidated.

SPECIFIC GENE TARGETS FOR THYROID HORMONE

Many studies have attempted to define thyroid hormone action in a physiologic context. We have summarized those studies that describe thyroid hormone action on selected target genes known to respond to changes in the thyroid hormone status of the animal and we have attempted to integrate the available molecular and physiologic data in an effort to provide some tentative insights into the overall biologic role of thyroid hormone.

Growth Hormone

In adult rats, the synthesis and secretion of growth hormone (GH) is extremely sensitive to regulation by thyroid hormone.[171] In hypothyroid rats, GH is barely detectable in the pituitary and serum concentrations are very low.[20] In pituitary cell lines,[172] thyroid hormone induces an increase in the rate of transcription of the GH gene.[173–175] The cloning of the GH gene and use of the pituitary tumor GC and GH cell lines have allowed detailed studies of the cell-specific and hormone-dependent regulation of GH gene expression.[21] The rat GH gene was the first for which the thyroid hormone-inducible DNA sequences were defined.[126,176] This sequence, from −191 to −164 base pairs upstream of the transcription start site, consists of three hexameric half-sites arranged as a direct repeat with a four-base-pair gap and an imperfect palindrome. Each of these elements is necessary for full hormonal induction.[126] Mutational analysis indicates that TRs bind to all three sites as monomers, dimers, and oligomers in a manner suggesting cooperative binding. T_3 induction of the GH gene expression is highly correlated with the binding of TR to the TRE. The action of T_3 may be further modified by such cellular cofactors as the pituitary-specific transcription factor, Pit-1,[177] as well as other hormonal influences such as the retinoids.[178] Clearly, T_3 does not act in isolation but rather as part of a complex set of interacting regulatory factors.

T_3 control of the human GH gene is not as well defined. Serum GH concentrations in hypothyroid patients may be in the normal range, although some have a decrease in GH secretion in response to provocative stimuli[179,180] (see chap 68). Thyroid hormone also decreases the release of GH from primary cultures of human pituitary adenomas.[181] Moreover, thyroid hormone downregulates the expression of a transfected human GH gene while upregulating the expression of the endogenous rat GH gene.[182] Although sequences in the 5′-flanking region of the human GH gene bind TR with high affinity, these sequences are not sufficient to confer T_3-responsiveness to the GH promoter. The TRE responsible for the negative regulation of the human GH gene appears to be situated in the 3′-untranslated region, a novel position when compared with those of other TREs.[183]

Cardiac and Skeletal Muscle Genes

MYOSIN HEAVY CHAIN

Different myosin heavy chain isoforms are encoded by a closely related multigene family. The pattern of each isoform is developmental stage–specific in the heart and skeletal muscle. All the members of this gene family can be regulated by thyroid hormone,[184] and the same myosin heavy chain gene can be regulated in opposite directions depending on the tissue in which it is expressed. In rats in the first weeks of life thyroid hormone induces a change from neonatal to adult forms of the myosin gene, and an excess of hormone accelerates this process.[185] Conversely, embryonic forms are expressed in some muscles of adult hypothyroid rats.[184]

In the heart, two isoforms of myosin, myosin heavy chain α and β, are expressed. The expression of these genes in the cardiac ventricles is closely regulated by thyroid hormone.[186–188] In euthyroid adult rats, α-myosin predominates. Treatment with thyroid hormone increases the ratio of α to β, whereas in hypothyroid rats β myosin may represent more than 90% of the total myosin[189] (see chap 38). The fact that thyroid hormone also increases the cardiac work load raised the possibility that the effect on myosin heavy chain gene expression might not be direct but result from the hyperdynamic state. However, in the heterotopically transplanted heart, the effect of thyroid hormone on myosin expression was independent of work load.[190] More recently, TREs have been defined in the rat[78,191] and human[192] α-myosin genes. Despite the ability of T_3 to increase the expression of the human α gene in transfection assays, early reports suggested that myosin heavy chain gene expression in the human heart was unaffected by thyroid hormone. However, α-myosin mRNA levels were low in a patient with severe dilated cardiomyopathy and hypothyroidism and returned to normal when the patient was treated with thyroid hormone.[193]

SARCOPLASMIC RETICULUM Ca²⁺-ATPase

Cardiac function, including the velocity of contraction and diastolic relaxation time, is markedly affected by alterations in thyroidal state. Changes in the velocity of contraction are due to shifts in concentration of myosin heavy chain isoforms in ventricular muscle and the speed of relaxation is dependent on the velocity of sequestration of cytoplasmic Ca^{2+} in the sarcoplasmic reticulum (SR). Active Ca^{2+} uptake from the cytoplasm of the myocyte into the sarcoplasmic reticulum is mediated by isoforms of Ca^{2+}-ATPase (SERCA). The SERCA2 gene is expressed predominantly in slow-twitch skeletal muscle and cardiac muscle and to a much lesser degree in smooth muscle. SERCA1 is expressed almost exclusively in fast-twitch skeletal muscle. Calcium uptake into the sarcoplasmic reticulum and Ca^{2+}-dependent ATP hydrolysis are increased in hyperthyroid and decreased in hypothyroid animals,[194,195] and the levels of SERCA2 mRNA as well as the Ca^{2+}-ATPase protein are induced by thyroid hormone, suggesting a transcriptional mechanism of regulation.[196,197] The response of this gene to hormonal replacement in hypothyroid animals is relatively rapid: a detectable rise occurring within 2 hours after administration of T_3 to hypothyroid rats, and back to nearly normal—a threefold rise— by 5 hours.[196] This is a direct effect of thyroid hormone on this gene and not secondary to a hormone-induced increase in work load[190]; although total RNA did not change in the heterotopically transplanted heart in response to thyroid hormone, the SERCA2 mRNA was increased as it was in the host heart.[190] Three different thyroid hormone response elements have been identified in the promoter region of the SERCA2 gene, each capable of binding receptor and of responding to T_3 when cotransfected with TRs.[157] The most 5′ element is a homologue of a direct repeat with spacing of four nucleotides, whereas the others are inverted repeats of two half-sites with five and six nucleotide spacing. Despite these differences in spacing and orientation as well as variations in the character of binding receptor and RXR proteins, all three TREs conferred similar degrees of responsiveness to T_3 to a reporter gene in transfection assays. It is as yet not clear how these elements may interact in the endogenous promoter to transduce the hormonal signal.

Comparative studies of the response to altered thyroidal state of the SERCA2 and SERCA1 genes in striated muscle revealed that SERCA2 levels were reduced in slow soleus but increased in fast extensor digitorum longus muscle from hypothyroid rats.[198] However, whereas thyrotoxicosis leads to increased levels of this mRNA in heart, in both soleus and extensor muscles the SERCA2 mRNA levels were decreased. In contrast, the fast sarcoplasmic reticulum SERCA1 isoform was markedly increased above normal in soleus muscle of thyrotoxic animals but unaffected by thyroidal state in the extensor muscle. The TREs in the SERCA1 gene have as yet not been defined.

Lipogenic Enzymes

MALIC ENZYME

Hepatic malic enzyme was among the first models of thyroid hormone action. Early studies demonstrated that malic enzyme activity, together with that of other lipogenic enzymes, was directly related to thyroid hormone status, rising in thyrotoxic and falling in hypothyroid animals.[199] The 10- to 15-fold range of enzyme activities across this spectrum made this assay a useful one for the evaluation of thyroidal status and definition of the relationship between hormonal occupancy of the nuclear receptor and response of the enzyme. This relationship for GH was found to be linear, but for malic enzyme it was amplified, as described earlier.[20,200] These changes in enzyme activity result, at least in part, from alterations in transcription activity.[201,202] There may also be a T_3-induced slowing of the rate of degradation of the malic enzyme mRNA.[203] A functional TRE was identified in the 5'-flanking region of the gene, consisting of a complex sequence of three half-sites, similar to the rat GH gene.[204,205] The malic enzyme gene was among the first targets of thyroid hormone action proven to be affected by multiple interacting agents. It was long known that malic enzyme and the other lipogenic enzymes could be induced by high carbohydrate intake and reduced in the fasted state.[206] However, the response to carbohydrate feeding was markedly reduced in hypothyroid rats. Conversely, the effect of T_3 was attenuated in fasted rats and maximal in rats fed a high carbohydrate fat-free diet.[207] Further, there is a synergistic relationship between dietary and thyroidal stimuli, and the effect of both thyroid hormone and carbohydrate is at the nuclear level. However, it is not clear whether carbohydrate affects transcriptional rates or only causes a slowing of the degradation rate of the mRNA.[208,209]

Another characteristic of this gene is that despite its sensitivity to thyroid hormone and dietary manipulation in liver, heart, kidney, and white fat, it is highly expressed but hormonally unresponsive in brain,[41,210] even in the early neonatal period when thyroid hormone–dependent developmental processes are evolving. The mechanisms responsible for this refractory state are undefined but presumably involve tissue-specific factors interacting with particular elements within the regulatory sequences of the gene to block responsivity.

S14

S14 was first identified as a rapidly responding hepatic mRNA by the technique of two-dimensional gel electrophoresis of translation products of total mRNA. This mRNA was induced as much as 15-fold by thyroid hormone and reached 80% of its maximum level within 4 hours.[211] The cloning of the S14 cDNA[212] allowed detailed study of the integrated control of this gene. The gene consists of two exons separated by a single intron. The entire protein, Mr 17,010, is encoded in the 5'-exon. The levels of the nuclear precursor and the mature cytosolic mRNA increase within 10 and 20 minutes, respectively, after the administration of T_3 to hypothyroid rats.[213,214] This is the most rapid response to T_3 of any target gene studied to date. This gene is expressed and responsive to thyroid hormone only in the lipogenic tissues, liver, white fat, and mammary tissue of nursing dams.[215] Relatively little S14 mRNA is detectable in kidney, lung, or heart. Intragastric administration of sucrose to euthyroid but not hypothyroid rats also causes rapid increases in this mRNA,[216] and injection of T_3 restores the response of hypothyroid rats to sucrose. Conversely, the effect of T_3 is markedly blunted in starved rats.[217] A similar synergistic interaction occurred in cultured hepatocytes,[218] suggesting this regulation did not require the intervention of other dietary factors or hormones. Thus, there appears to be a direct and rapid interaction between carbohydrate and T_3 in the regulation of the S14 gene. Other evidence also suggests that S14 is in some manner related to lipogenesis. Levels of S14 mRNA are altered in parallel with the lipogenic enzymes, malic enzyme, and fatty acid synthetase, in a variety of physiologic and pathophysiologic states, including starvation, diabetes, and high carbohydrate feeding, and in suckling neonatal rat pups.[217]

Immunohistochemical studies suggest S14 protein is concentrated in hepatocyte nuclei.[219] Transfection of hepatocytes with S14 antisense oligonucleotides blocks the response of both S14 mRNA and S14 protein to carbohydrate,[220] and the response of malic enzyme mRNA to both T_3 and glucose was also markedly reduced. Thus, S14 may play a role in the nucleus to transduce hormonal and dietary signals in the regulation of lipogenesis.

Enhanced transcription plays a predominant role in the response of S14 to T_3.[221] This gene has three TREs unusually far upstream, approximately 2.7 kilobases (kb) from the start site of transcription.[222] Most response elements for steroid and thyroid hormones are located within 400 base pairs of the promoter. Each of the S14 TREs is independently capable of T_3-dependent activation of a reporter gene in transfection assays and of binding TRs.

Enhanced transcription has also been reported to result from sucrose gavage.[223] A carbohydrate response element (CHORE) has been identified between 1050 and 1600 base pairs 5' of the S14 promoter.[224,225] Sequences within this segment can confer responsivity to glucose when linked to a reporter gene in transfection systems. Deletion of this segment from the S14 5'-region results in the loss of response to glucose but not the response to T_3. In studies of the interaction of the CHORE and TRE in response to sugar and T_3, the unliganded TR almost completely abolished a response to high glucose, and the addition of T_3 induced a synergistic response with the sugar.[226] In the presence of sufficient T_3 and TR in the transfected cells the glucose response was maintained even after deletion of the CHORE from the reporter construct. Thus, the T_3:TR complex may interact with other as yet unidentified segments of the S14 promoter region to explain the synergistic interaction of T_3 and carbohydrate. Carbohydrate also may slow the degradation of the precursor nuclear RNA and increase the rate of processing to the mature mRNA.[227]

Thyrotropin

Early studies demonstrated a clear relationship between thyroid hormone effects on the TSH subunits and nuclear receptor occupancy by hormone. The acute inhibition of TSH secretion is directly related to saturation of pituitary T_3 receptors[228] and the effect of various analogues could be related to their affinity for the receptors.[229] In mice with TSH secreting tumors, the relation between receptor occupancy and transcriptional response was linear.[230] Lastly, the time course of altered gene transcription was closely linked to the binding of T_3 to nuclear receptors.[231]

Later studies focused on the regulation of each of the subunits, TSH-α and TSH-β, that constitute the TSH molecule and the expression of which is negatively regulated by thyroid hormone (see chap 11). T_3 causes a decrease in the synthesis rates of both subunits.[232,233] Cloning of the cDNAs for the TSH-β and TSH-α subunits has allowed detailed examination of the molecular mechanism of hormone regulation.[234] The levels of both TSH-β and TSH-α mRNA are markedly reduced after T_4 treatment of mice with thyrotropic tumors,[235] and the reductions begin within 1 hour after injection of T_3. Generally, the decrease in TSH-β mRNA is greater than that of the α-subunit mRNA regardless of the duration of T_3 treatment.[235,236] Even after 33 days of treatment the α-subunit mRNA was still about 20% of baseline, whereas TSH-β mRNA was undetectable.[235] The effects of T_4 treatment were similar in the pituitary of the mice bearing the tumors.

A

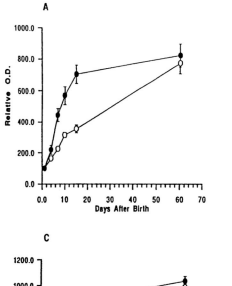

B

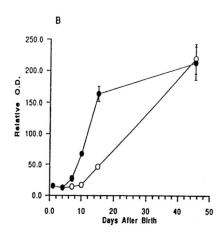

C

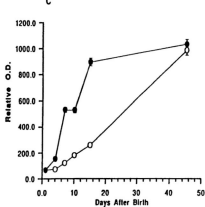

D

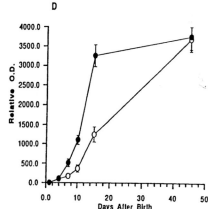

FIGURE 9-4. Ontogeny of expression of brain genes in response to T_3. Expression of mRNA for calbindin (*A*), IP3 receptor (*B*), *Pcp*-2 (*C*), and myelin basic protein. (*D*) in brain tissue of hypothyroid and T_3-treated hypothyroid rat pups. Levels of mRNA were determined by Northern blot analysis and expressed as optical density units (mean ± SE, n = 3 per point). Levels of the four mRNAs at neonatal day 15 in normal rat pups were: *A*, 723 ± 97; *B*, 171 ± 23; *C*, 883 ± 107; and *D*, 3320 ± 380 units. Open circles, hypothyroid pups; closed circles, hypothyroid pups treated with 0.1 μg T_3/day. (Strait KA, Zou L, Oppenheimer JH. β1 isoform-specific regulation of a triiodothyronine-induced gene during cerebellar development. Mol Endocrinol 1992;6:1874)

The locus of thyroid hormone action is at the level of transcription.[231,237] After T_3 injection to tumor-bearing mice, the transcription rate for TSH-β mRNA is decreased by 60% at 30 minutes and by 95% at 4 hours. The transcription rate for the α-subunit mRNA follows a similar time course, but the decline is only by 80%.[231] T_3 may reduce the half-life of TSH-β mRNA in pituitary cells by almost two-thirds but does not affect that of α-subunit mRNA.[238] Thus, the greater reduction in TSH-β mRNA after T_3 treatment may be a function of a reduction in transcription rate and an increase in turnover of the mRNA. As indicated earlier in this chapter, negative TREs (nTRE) have been identified in both the TSH-β and TSH-α-subunit genes (see Table 9-4).[123]

Brain Genes

The failure of thyroid hormone to influence the oxygen consumption in adult brain led to the widespread belief that this tissue may be totally unresponsive to thyroid hormone.[239] However, the demonstration that adult brain contains specific nuclear receptors for T_3,[41] together with multiple physiologic and clinical observations of alterations in brain function, has stimulated reconsideration of this conclusion. Nevertheless, at this time no studies have succeeded in identifying genes in the adult brain directly regulated by thyroid hormone.

In contrast, the importance of thyroid hormone in the developing brain has been widely recognized for several decades,[240,241] and alterations in the response of specific brain proteins to thyroid hormone are well documented (for reviews see references 242 and 243). However, the precise molecular mechanisms by which T_3 regulates the expression of target genes involved in brain development remain uncertain. In neonatal rats, hypothyroidism typically results in deficient myelinization. The gene coding for myelin basic protein, a component of myelin, has a TRE.[132,244] This TRE, situated −186 to −163 from the start site of transcription, is an inverted repeat with six nucleotides separating the half-sites.

Thyroid hormone stimulates differentiation of the cerebellum in neonatal rats.[241] Among other changes, hypothyroidism during the first 3 weeks of neonatal life results in marked reduction in the arborization of the cerebellar Purkinje cells, suggesting the existence of T_3-sensitive genes in Purkinje cells. Both oligodendrocytes, the cells responsible for the synthesis of myelin, and Purkinje cells show a strong signal for TR-β1 in immunohistochemical studies.[99,245] As discussed previously, a striking rise in the brain content of TR-β1 occurs about the same time that the level of brain T_3 increases in neonatal rats, thus raising the speculation that the TR-β1 isoform may play an important role in the structural changes that follow.

MYELIN BASIC PROTEIN AND Pcp-2

To assess the potential role of specific Purkinje cell–expressed genes, the effect of thyroid hormone deficiency on the developmental pattern of mRNAs in these cells was studied.[92,246] These were the IP3 receptor, calbindin, and *Pcp*-2 genes, the latter of which codes for a Purkinje cell protein of undefined function. The developmental patterns of the Purkinje cell-expressed genes were compared to that of the myelin basic protein gene that is expressed exclusively in oligodendrocytes.[247] The overall pattern of T_3 regulation of the expression of these genes in brain development is shown in Figure 9-4, which shows the time courses of specific mRNAs in neonatal rats made hypothyroid by the addition of methimazole to the diet of dams starting on the twelfth day of gestation and continued after birth so that the pups received the drug in the mother's milk. In hypothyroid pups also given T_3, the mRNA levels increased during the first 10–15 days of life from the low levels in the fetus to those of the adult. For each of the four genes the increase was more than sixfold; those patterns are similar to those in normal rat pups. In contrast, in the hypothyroid pups, there was a delay in this rise. By 45 days, however, the normal adult level was attained despite continued hypothyroidism. Thereafter, these genes were no longer subject to regulation by T_3.

Thus, there appear to be three developmental stages in the response of brain genes to thyroid hormone. During the first days after birth, there is a lag in responsiveness to thyroid hormone. During the second period, probably between postnatal days 4 and 20, the mRNA levels of target genes rise rapidly to a plateau. During the third period, although the genes appear fully expressed, such expression is independent of the circulating thyroid hormone concentration.

The response of the *Pcp*-2 gene has been characterized by transient transfection experiments. The native promoter is only minimally responsive to T_3 in transfection assays.[247] However, a TRE consisting of three half-sites has been identified (Table 9-4).[248] This 28-base-pair sequence can confer T_3 responsivity to heterologous promoters. When linked to the 68-base-pair segment immediately 3' to the TRE in the *Pcp*-2 promoter, responsivity is lost. This 68-base-pair segment can also blunt the T_3 response of other TREs.[249] These findings raise the possibility that a specific T_3 response silencer proteins bind to this 68 base region of the *Pcp*-2 gene and inhibit T_3 action during the fetal period and the first days of life.

The mechanistic details by which thyroid hormone serves to regulate the expression of brain genes are still unclear, and it is impossible to reach any global generalization on the basis of the data accumulated so far. Thus, T_3 may regulate some target genes indirectly by stimulating the formation of an intermediate protein that secondarily regulates the gene under study. For example, a growth factor, neurotrophin-3, synthesized in neighboring granule cells, could be responsible for Purkinje cell differentiation.[250] However, a more recent report failed to confirm this suggestion.[251] Under any circumstance, it is apparent that target genes in the developing brain are sensitive to T_3 only at specific times.

BIOLOGIC AND CLINICAL IMPLICATIONS

The apparent diversity of thyroid hormone effects in vertebrate species has been the subject of much speculation and wonder. Recent advances in our understanding of thyroid hormone initiating mechanisms provide some tantalizing clues that may allow us to see the thyroid hormone actions from new perspectives. The findings reviewed in this chapter indicate that T_3 is the preferred ligand for a set of closely related receptor isoforms that are widely distributed in the nuclei of tissues and are capable of interacting with a broad range of proteins anchored to the regulatory regions of target genes. However, the physicochemical properties of the receptors, interacting transcription factors, and DNA elements that permit such interactions are poorly understood. What is clear is that the structures of the TRs are closely related to that of a large superfamily of receptors that bind other small molecules, some of which have been conventionally designated as hormones, some as vitamins, and others as pharmacologically active substances such as peroxisomal proliferator activators.[69,130,160,252]

In some fashion as yet unspecified, T_3, by binding to its receptors, sets into motion a series of local molecular rearrangements. These involve homodimerization with other T_3 receptors, heterodimerization with other receptors, or interactions with structurally unrelated transcription factors. These molecular events activate or in some instances attenuate the transcriptional process and as a consequence alter the expression of target genes.

One of the important lessons to be learned from the profusion of data now available is the difficulty of making judgments about the molecular circuitry involved in the regulation of genes by thyroid hormone. The finding of a TRE-like sequence in the promoter region of a gene by itself does not establish that thyroid hormone initiates its action at that locus, nor does the failure to demonstrate thyroid regulation of a heterologous promoter rule out this possibility. Lack of compatibility between the putative TRE, the promoter used, and the cell line transfected could all obscure the regulatory role for the sequence. Moreover, even if all the tests are positive, one cannot be absolutely certain that the pathway identified is the only, or even the most important, pathway by which the hormone regulates the expression of the gene. Thus, it is entirely possible that there are multiple TREs further upstream or that thyroid hormone also stimulates an intermediate peptide inducer that then functions at a distinctive response element.

The disparate and apparently unrelated actions of thyroid hormone in multiple species and multiple physiologic domains remain unexplained. Comparative studies have identified T_4, T_3, and thyroid hormone receptors in lampreys, one of the earliest vertebrate species, as well as in freshwater fish.[22] The nuclear T_3 receptors in these species have the same general physicochemical characteristics as those in rats and humans. They have the same T_3-binding characteristics and analogue binding specificity. The functions of T_3 in these species are poorly understood but clearly differ from those in mammals. In fish, neither lipogenic enzymes nor oxygen consumption is stimulated by T_3. The metamorphosis of the aquatic tadpole to the terrestrial frog, however, has classically been used as a model of thyroid hormone–initiated development in poikilotherms.[253] Moreover, in tadpoles both TR-α and TR-β isoforms are present.[254] The spurt in serum T_3 and the accompanying rise in TR-β during metamorphosis are reminiscent of the pattern during brain development in rats.[92] It appears likely that the more recently differentiated species have preserved some of the regulatory functions of metamorphosis. The advent of the homeothermic species, birds and mammals, is associated with the first evidence of T_3-stimulated lipogenesis and thermogenesis.[22] Maintenance of a high basal level of thermogenesis may have necessitated the generation of sufficient adipose tissue to maintain a readily available energy source in the absence of an immediately available supply of food.[255] Thus, evolutionary pressures may have resulted in progressive acquisition of novel thyroid hormone–related functions and at the same time modified older functions. Such functional changes most likely occur as a consequence of the selection of spontaneous mutations in the regulatory regions of genes that provide survival advantage.

The newer concepts of thyroid action may also explain some anomalous clinical observations. Subjects ingesting a carbohydrate-restricted diet[256] and patients with nonthyroidal illness[257] have low serum T_3 concentrations but no symptoms and signs of hypothyroidism and no increase in serum TSH (see section on nonthyroidal illness in chap 14). Food restriction in rats may lead to reduced tissue TR levels.[258] The recent recognition that thyroid hormone effects are determined by complex interactions of the TRs with other transacting proteins in the regulatory regions of genes could explain such anomalies. A concomitant increase in the level of positively interacting receptors or their ligands might counterbalance the effect of the fall in TR in specific tissues. In the pituitary the opposite effects of the coordinate factors could prevent the rise in TSH secretion anticipated from the fall in serum T_3 concentrations. At the same time there might be in other tissues a similarly directed decrease in a coordinately regulated transacting factor that would magnify the biologic effect of a decrease in the T_3:TR complex. While such a formulation is clearly speculative, it serves to underscore the importance of defining the nature and nuclear content of the factors with which the T_3:TR complex interacts in regulating gene expression.

References

1. Wolf E, Wolf J. The mechanism of action of the thyroid hormones. In: Pitt-Rivers R, Trotter W, eds. The thyroid gland. London: Butterworths, 1964:237
2. Tata JR, Ernster L, Lindberg O, Arrhenius E, S P, Hedman R. The action of thyroid hormones at the cell level. Biochem J 1963; 86:408
3. Surks MI, Oppenheimer JH. Concentration of L-thyroxine and L-triiodothyrinine specifically bound to nuclear receptors in rat liver and kidney: quantitative evidence favoring a major role of T3 in thyroid hormone action. J Clin Invest 1977;60:508
4. Tata JR, Widnell CC. Ribonucleic acid synthesis during the early action of thyroid hormones. Biochem J 1966;98:604
5. Tata JR, Ernster L, Suranyi E. Interaction between thyroid hormones and cellular constituents. I. Binding to isolated sub-cellular particles and sub-particular fractions. Biochim Biophys Acta 1962;60:461
6. Tata JR, Ernster L, Suranyi EM. Interaction between thyroid hormones and cellular constituents. II. Intracellular distribution and the cell-sap effect. Biochim Biophys Acta 1962;60:480
7. Tata JR. How specific are nuclear "receptors" for thyroid hormone? Nature (London) 1975;257:18
8. Oppenheimer JH, Koerner D, Schwartz HL, Surks MI. Specific nuclear triiodothyronine binding sites in rat liver and kidney. J Clin Endocrinol Metab 1972;35:330
9. Oppenheimer JH, Schwartz HL, Surks MI. Tissue differences in the concentration of triiodothyronine nuclear binding sites in the rat: liver, kidney, pituitary, heart, brain, spleen, and testis. Endocrinology 1974;95:897
10. Oppenheimer JH, Koerner D, Surks MI, Schwartz HL. Limited binding capacity sites for L-triiodothyronine in rat liver nuclei: nuclear-cytoplasmic interrelationship, binding constants, and cross reactivity with L-thyroxine. J Clin Invest 1974;53:768
11. Surks MI, Koerner D, Dillmann W, Oppenheimer JH. Limited capacity binding sites for L-triiodothyronine (T3) in rat liver nuclei: localization to the chromatin and partial characterization of the T3-chromatin complex. J Biol Chem 1973;248:7066
12. Surks MI, Koerner DH, Oppenheimer JH. In vitro binding of L-triiodothyronine to receptors in rat liver nuclei: kinetics of binding, extraction properties, and lack of requirement for cytosol proteins. J Clin Invest 1975;55:50
13. Koerner D, Surks MI, Oppenheimer JH. In vitro demonstration of specific triiodothyronine binding sites in rat liver nuclei. J Clin Endocrinol Metab 1974;38:706
14. Koerner D, Schwartz HL, Surks MI, Oppenheimer JH, Jorgensen EC. Binding of selected iodothyronine analogues to receptor sites of isolated rat hepatic nuclei: high correlation between structural requirements for nuclear binding and biological activity. J Biol Chem 1975;250:6417
15. Goslings B, Schwartz HL, Dillman W, Surks MI, Oppenheimer JH. Comparison of the metabolism and distribution of 1-triiodothyronine and triiodothyroacetic acid in the rat: a possible explanation of differential hormonal potency. Endocrinology 1976;98:666
16. Oppenheimer JH, Schwartz HL, Surks MI. Nuclear binding capacity appears to limit the hepatic response to L-triiodothyronine (T3). Endocr Res Comm 1975;2:309
17. Oppenheimer JH, Silva E, Schwartz HL, Surks MI. Stimulation of hepatic mitochondrial alpha-glycerophosphate dehydrogenase and malic enzyme by L-triiodothyronine: Characteristics of the response with specific nuclear thyroid hormone binding sites fully saturated. J Clin Invest 1977;59:517
18. Oppenheimer JH, Coulombe P, Schwartz HL, Gutfeld N. Nonlinear (amplified) relationship between nuclear occupancy by triiodothyronine and the appearance rate of hepatic alpha-glycerophosphate dehydrogenase and malic enzyme. J Clin Invest 1978;61:987
19. Mariash CN, Kaiser FE, Schwartz HL, Towle HC, Oppenheimer JH. Synergism of thyroid hormone and high carbohydrate diet in the induction of lipogenic enzymes in the rat: mechanisms and implications. J Clin Invest 1980;65:1126
20. Coulombe P, Schwartz HL, Oppenheimer JH. Relationship between the accumulation of pituitary growth hormone and nuclear occupancy by triodothyronine in the rat. J Clin Invest 1978; 62:1020
21. Samuels HH. Identification and characterization of thyroid hormone receptors and action using cell culture techniques. In: Oppenheimer JH, Samuels HH, eds. Molecular basis of thyroid hormone action. New York: Academic Press, 1983:1
22. Weirich RT, Schwartz HL, Oppenheimer JH. An analysis of the interrelationship of nuclear and plasma triiodothyronine in the sea lamprey eel, lake trout, and the rat: evolutionary considerations. Endocrinology 1987;120:664
23. Sap J, Munoz A, Damm K, et al. The c-erb-A protein is a high affinity receptor for thyroid hormone. Nature 1986; 324:635
24. Weinberger C, Thompson CC, Ong ES, Lebo R, Gruol DJ, Evans RM. The c-erb-A gene encodes a thyroid hormone receptor. Nature 1986;324:641
25. Leonard JL, Silva JE, Kaplan MM, Mellen SA, Visser TJ, Larsen PR. Acute posttranscriptional regulation of cerebrocortical and pituitary iodothyronine 5′-deiodinases by thyroid hormone. Endocrinology 1984;114:998
26. Tapley DF, Cooper C. The effect of thyroxine and related compounds on oxidative phosphorylation. J Biol Chem 1956;222:341
27. Buchanan J, Tapley DF. Stimulation by thyroxine of amino acid incorporation into mitochondria. Endocrinology 1966;79:81
28. Gordon A, Surks MI, Oppenheimer JH. Thyroxine stimulation of amino acid incorporation into mitochondrial proteins: differences between in vivo and in vitro effects. Acta Endocrinol 1973;72:684

117. Diamond MI, Miner JN, Yoshinaga SK, Yamamoto KR. Transcription factor interactions: selectors of positive or negative regulation from a single DNA element. Science 1990;249:1266

118. Mitchell PJ, Tijan R. Transcriptional regulation in mammalian cells by sequence-specific DNA binding proteins. Science 1989;245:371

119. Schlief R. DNA binding by proteins. Science 1988;241:1182

120. Magasanik B. Gene regulation from sites near and far. New Biologist 1989;1:247

121. Ptashne M, Gan AAF. Activators and targets. Nature 1990;346:329

122. Baniahmad A, Ha I, Reinberg D, Tsai S, Tsai M-J, O'Malley BW. Interaction of human thyroid hormone receptor β with transcription factor TFIIB may mediate target gene derepression and activation by thyroid hormone. Proc Natl Acad Sci USA 1993;90:8832

123. Williams GR, Brent GA. Thyroid hormone response elements. In: Weintraub BD, ed. Molecular endocrinology: basic concepts and clinical correlations. New York: Raven Press, 1995:217

124. Garner MM, Revzin A. A gel electrophoresis method for quantifying the binding of proteins to specific DNA regions. Nucleic Acids Res 1981;9:3047

125. Glass CK, Franco R, Weinberger C, Albert VR, Evans RM, Rosenfeld MG. A c-erbA binding site in rat growth hormone gene mediates trans-activation by thyroid hormone. Nature 1987;329:738

126. Brent GA, Harney JW, Chen Y, Warne RL, Moore DD, Larsen PR. Mutations of the rat growth hormone promoter which increase and decrease response to thyroid hormone define a consensus thyroid hormone response element. Mol Endocrinol 1989;3:1996

127. Katz RW, Koenig RJ. Nonbiased identification of DNA sequences that bind thyroid hormone receptor alpha 1 with high affinity. J Biol Chem 1993;268:19392

128. Koenig RJ, Brent GA, Warne RL, Larsen PR, Moore DD. Thyroid hormone receptor binds to a site in the rat growth hormone promoter required for induction by thyroid hormone. Proc Natl Acad Sci USA 1987;84:5670

129. Samuels HH, Forman BM, Horowitz ZD, Ye ZS. Regulation of gene expression by thyroid hormone. J Clin Invest 1988;81:957

130. Beato M. Gene regulation by steroid hormones. Cell 1989;56:335

131. Umesono K, Murakami KK, Thompson CC, Evans RM. Direct repeats as selective response elements for the thyroid hormone, retinoic acid, and vitamin D3 receptors. Cell 1991;65:1255

132. Farsetti A, Robbins J, Nikodem V. Molecular basis of thyroid hormone regulation of myelin basic protein gene expression in rodent brain. J Biol Chem 1991;266:23226

133. Williams GR, Brent GA. Specificity of nuclear hormone receptor action: who conducts the orchestra. J Endocrinol 1992;135:191

134. Darling DS, Beebe JS, Burnside J, Winslow ER, Chin WW. 3,5,3'-triiodothyronine (T3) receptor-auxilliary protein (TRAP) binds DNA and forms heterodimers with the T3 receptor. Mol Endocrinol 1991;5:73

135. Murray MB, Towle HC. Identification of nuclear factors that enhance binding of the thyroid hormone receptor to a thyroid hormone response element. Mol Endocrinol 1989;3:1434

136. Rosen ED, O'Donnell AL, Koenig RJ. Protein-protein interactions involved erbA superfamily receptors: through the TRAP door. Mol Cell Endocrinol 1991;78:C83

137. Kim HS, Crone DE, Sprung CN, et al. Positive and negative thyroid hormone response elements are composed of strong and weak half-sites 10 nucleotides in length. Mol Endocrinol 1992;6:1489

138. Seelig SA, Liaw C, Towle HC, Oppenheimer JH. Thyroid hormone attenuates and augments hepatic gene expression at a pretranslational level. Proc Natl Acad Sci U S A 1981;78:4733

139. Carr FE, Kaseem LL, Wong NCWW. Thyroid hormone inhibits thyrotropin gene expression via a position-independent negative L-triiodothyronine-responsive element. J Biol Chem 1992;267:18689

140. Brent GA, Williams GR, Harney JW. Effects of varying the position of thyroid hormone reponse elements within the rat growth hormone promoter: implications for positive and negative regulation by 3.5.3'-triiodothyronine. Mol Endocrinol 1991;5:542

141. Darling DS, Burnside J, Chin WW. Binding of thyroid hormone receptors to the rat thyrotropin-beta gene. Mol Endocrinol 1989;3:1359

142. Naar AM, Boutin JM, Lipkin SM, et al. The orientation and spacing of core DNA-binding motifs dictate selective transcriptional responses to three nuclear receptors. Cell 1991;65:1267

143. Thompson KL, Santon JB, Shephard LB, Walton GM, Gill GN. A nuclear protein is required for thyroid hormone receptor binding to an inhibitory half-site in the epidermal growth factor receptor promoter. Mol Endocrinol 1992;6:627

144. Damm K, Thompson CC, Evans RM. Protein encoded by v-erb A functions as a thyroid-hormone receptor antagonist. Nature (London) 1989;339:593

145. Sap J, Munoz A, Schmitt J, Stunnenberg H, Vennstrom B. Repression of transcription mediated at a thyroid hormone response element by the v-erb-A oncogene product. Nature 1989; 340:242

146. Brent GA, Dunn MK, Harney JW, Gulick T, Larsen PR, Moore DD. Thyroid hormone aporeceptor represses T3-inducible promoters and blocks activation of the retinoic acid receptor. New Biologist 1989;1:329

147. Fondell J, Roy A, Roeder R. Unliganded thyroid hormone receptor inhibits formation of a functional preinitiation complex: implications for active repression. Genes Dev 1993;7:1400

148. Williams GR, Harney JW, Forman BM, Samuels HH, Brent GA. Oligometric binding of T3 receptor is required for maximal T3 response. J Biol Chem 1991;266:19636

149. Forman BM, Yang CR, Au M, Casanova J, Ghysdael J, Samuels HH. A domain containing a leucine zipper-like motif mediates novel in vivo interactions between the thyroid hormone and retinoic acid receptors. Mol Endocrinol 1989;3:1610

150. Luisis BF, Xu WX, Gtwinoski Z, Freedman LP, Yamamoto KR, Sigler PB. Crystallographic analysis of the interaction of the glucocorticoid receptor with DNA. Nature (London) 1991;352:497

151. Glass CK, Lipkin SM, Devary OV, Rosenfeld MG. Positive and negative regulation of gene transcription by a retinoic-thyroid hormone receptor heterodimer. Cell 1989;59:697

152. Leid M, Kastner P, Lyons R, et al. Purification, cloning, and RXR identify of the HeLa cell factor with which RAR or TR heterodimerizes to bind target sequences efficiently. Cell 1992; 68:377

153. Berrodin TJ, Marks MS, Ozato K, Linney E, Lazar MA. Heterodimerization among thyroid hormone receptor, retinoic acid receptor, retinoid X receptor, chicken ovalbumin upstream promoter transcription factor, and an endogenous liver protein. Mol Endocrinol 1992;6:1468

154. Hermann T, Hoffmann B, Zhang XK, Tran P, Pfahl M. Heterodimeric receptor complexes determine 3,5,3'-triiodothyronine and retinoid signaling specificities. Mol Endocrinol 1992; 6:1153

155. Wahlstrom GM, Sjoberg M, Andersson M, Nordstrom K, Vennstrom B. Binding characteristics of the thyroid hormone receptors homo- and heterodimers to consensus AGGTCA repeat motifs. Mol Endocrinol 1992;6:1013

156. Rosen ED, O'Donnell AL, Koenig RJ. Ligand-dependent synergy of thyroid hormone and retinoid X receptors. J Biol Chem 1992; 267:22010

157. Hartong R, Wang N, Kurokawa R, et al. Delineation of three different thyroid hormone-response elements in promoter of rat sarcoplasmic reticulum Ca²⁺ ATPase gene. J Biol Chem 1994; 269: 13021

158. Yen PM, Ikeda M, Wilcox EC, et al. Half-site arrangement of hybrid glucocorticoid and thyroid hormone response elements specifies thyroid hormone receptor complex binding to DNA and transcriptional activity. J Biol Chem 1994;269:12704

159. Schraeder M, Muller KM, Nayeri S, Kahlen JP, Carlberg C. Vitamin D3-thyroid hormone receptor heterodimer polarity directs ligand sensitivity of transactivation. Nature 1994; 370:382

160. Bogazzi F, Hudson LD, Nikodem VM. A novel heterodimerization partner for thyroid hormone receptor. J Biol Chem 1994;269:11683

161. Xu J, Thompson KL, Shephard LB, Hudson LG, Gill GN. T3 receptor suppression of Sp1-dependent transcription from the epidermal growth factor receptor promoter via overlapping DNA-binding sites. J Biol Chem 1993;268:16065

162. Glass CK, Holloway JM, Devary OJ, Rosenfeld MG. The thyroid hormone receptor binds with opposite transcriptional effects to a common sequence motif in thyroid hormone and estrogen response elements. Cell 1988;54:313

163. Graupner G, Zhang XK, Tzukerman M, Wills K, Hermann T, Pfahl M. Thyroid hormone receptors repress estrogen receptor activation of a TRE. Mol Endocrinol 1991;5:365

164. Pfahl M. Vertebrate receptors: molecular biology, dimerization and response elements. Cell Biol 1994;5:95

165. Cooney AJ, Tsai SY, O'Malley BW, Tsai M-J. Chicken ovalbumin upstream promoter transcription factor (COUP-TF) dimers bind to different GGTCA response elements, allowing COUP-TF to repress hormonal induction of vitamin D3, thyroid hormone and retinoic acid receptors. Mol Cell Biol 1992;12:4153

166. Voz ML, Peers B, Wiedig MJ, Jacquemin P, Belayew A, Martial JA. Transcriptional regulation by triiodothyronine requires synergistic action of the thyroid receptor with another trans-acting factor. Mol Cell Biol 1992;12:3991

167. Yen PM, Darling DS, Carter RL, Forgione M, Umeda PK, Chin WW. Triiodothyronine (T3) decreases binding to DNA by T3-receptor homodimers but not receptor auxiliary protein heterodimers. J Biol Chem 1992;267:3565

168. Miyamoto T, Suzuki S, DeGroot LJ. High affinity and specificity of dimeric binding of thyroid hormone receptors to DNA and their ligand-dependent dissociation. Mol Endocrinol 1993; 7:224

169. Au-Fliegner M, Helmer E, Casanova J, Raaka BM, Samuels HH. The conserved ninth C-terminal heptad in thyroid hormone and retinoic acid receptors mediates diverse responses by affecting heterodimer but not homodimer formation. Mol Cell Biol 1993;13:5725

170. Yen PM, Sugawara A, Forgione M, et al. Region-specific anti-thyroid hormone receptor (TR) antibodies detect changes in TR structure due to ligand-binding and dimerization. Mol Cell Endocrinol 1993;97:93

171. Hervas F, Morreale de Escobar G, Escobar Del Rey F. Rapid effects of single small doses of L-thyroxine and triiodo-L-thyronine on growth hormone as studied in the rat by radioimmunoassay. Endocrinology 1975;97:91

172. Samuels HH, Shapiro LE. Thyroid hormone stimulates de novo growth hormone synthesis in cultured GH₁ cells: evidence for the accumulation of a rate limiting RNA species in the induction process. Proc Natl Acad Sci USA 1976;73:3369

173. Martial JA, Seeburg PH, Guenzi D, Goodman HM, Baxter JD. Regulation of growth hormone gene expression: synergistic effects of thyroid and glucocorticoid hormones. J Biol Chem 1977; 74:4293

174. Seo H, Vassart G, Brocas H, Refetoff S. Triiodothyronine stimulates specifically growth hormone mRNA in rat pituitary cells. Proceedings of the Natl Acad Sci U S A 1977;74:2054

175. Nyborg JK, Nguyen AP, Spindle SR. Cyclic regulation of growth hormone gene transcription in vivo and in vitro. Endocrinology 1985;116:2361

176. Flug F, Copp RP, Casanova J, et al. cis-acting elements of the rat growth hormone gene which mediate basal and regulated expression by thyroid hormone. J Biol Chem 1987;262:6373

177. Schaufele F, West BL, Baxter JD. Synergistic activation of the rat growth hormone promoter by Pit-1 and the thyroid hormone receptor. Mol Endocrinol 1992;6:656

178. Garcia-Villalba P, Au-Fliegner M, Samuels H, Aranda A. Interaction of thyroid hormone and retinoic acid receptors on the regu-

lation of the rat growth hormone gene promoter. Biochem Biophys Res Commun 1993;191:580

179. Tolis G, Banovac K, Kleissl P, Martin JB, McKenzie JM. Episodic and TRH induced growth hormone release in primary hypothyroidism in man and the rat. Endocr Res Comm 1979;6:213

180. MacGillivray M, Aceto T Jr, Frohman L. Plasma growth hormone responses and growth retardation of hypothyroidism. Am J Dis Child 1968;115:273

181. Adams E, Brajkovich I, Mashiter K. Growth hormone and prolactin secretion by dispersed cell cultures of human pituitary adenomas: Long term effects of hydrocortisone, estradiol, insulin, 3,5,3'-triiodothyronine and thyroxine. J Clin Endocrinol Metab 1981;53:381

182. Cattini P, Anderson T, Baxter J, Mellon P, Eberhardt N. The human growth hormone gene is negatively regulated by triiodothyronine when transfected into rat pituitary tumor cells. J Biol Chem 1986;261:13367

183. Zhang W, Brooks R, Silversides D, et al. Negative thyroid hormone control of human growth hormone gene expression is mediated by 3'-untranslated/3'-flanking DNA. J Biol Chem 1992; 267:15056

184. Izumo S, Nadal-Ginard B, Mahdavi V. All members of the myosin heavy chain multigene family respond to thyroid hormone in a highly tissue specific manner. Science 1986;231:597

185. Gambke B, Lyons G, Haselgrove J, Kelly A, Rubenstein N. Thyroidal and neural control of myosin transitions during development of rat fast and slow muscles. FEBS Lett 1983;156:335

186. Sinha AM, Umeda PK, Kavinsky CJ, et al. Molecular cloning of mRNA sequences for cardiac α- and β-form myosin heavy chains: expression in ventricles of normal, hypothyroid, and thyrotoxic rabbits. Proc Natl Acad Sci U S A 1982;79:5847

187. Dillmann WH, Barrieux A, Neeley WE, Contreras P. Influence of thyroid hormone on the in vitro translational activity of specific mRNAs in the rat heart. J Biol Chem 1983;258:7738

188. Lompre AM, Nadal-Ginard B, Mahdavi V. Expression of the cardiac ventricular α- and β-myosin heavy chain genes is developmentally and hormonally regulated. J Biol Chem 1984; 259:6437

189. Everett AW, Clark WA, Chizzonite RA, Zak R. Change in the synthesis rates of α- and β-myosin heavy chains in rabbit heart after treatment with thyroid hormone. J Biol Chem 1983; 258:2421

190. Ojamaa K, Samarel AM, Kupfer JM, Hong C, Klein I. Thyroid hormone effects on cardiac gene expression independent of cardiac growth and protein synthesis. Am J Physiol 1992; 263:E534

191. Brent GA, Williams GR, Harney JW, et al. Capacity for cooperative binding of thyroid hormone (T3) receptor dimers defines wild type T3 response elements. Mol Endocrinol 1992;6:502

192. Flink IL, Morkin E. Interaction of thyroid hormone receptors with strong and weak cis-acting elements in the human a-myosin heavy chain gene promoter. J Biol Chem 1990;265:11233

193. Ladenson PW, Sherman SI, Baughman KL, Ray PE, Feldman AM. Reversible alterations in myocardial gene expression in a young man with dilated cardiomyopathy and hypothyroidism. Proc Natl Acad Sci USA 1992;89:5251

194. Suko J. The calcium pump of cardiac sarcoplasmic reticulum. functional alterations at different levels of thyroid state in rabbits. J Physiol 1973;228:563

195. Limas C. Calcium transport ATPase of cardiac sarcoplasmic reticulum in experimental hyperthyroidism. Am J Physiol 1978;235:H745

196. Rohrer D, Dillmann WH. Thyroid hormone markedly increases the mRNA coding for sarcoplasmic reticulum Ca²⁺-ATPase in the rat heart. J Biol Chem 1989;263:6941

197. Arai M, Otsu K, MacLennan D, Alpert N, Periasamy M. Effect of thyroid hormone on the expression of mRNA encoding sarcoplasmic reticulum proteins. Circ Res 1991;69:266

198. Sayen MR, Rohrer DK, Dillman WH. Thyroid hormone response of slow and fast sarcoplasmic reticulum Ca^{2+}ATPase mRNA in striated muscle. Mol Cell Endocrinol 1992;87:87

199. Bottger I, Kriegel H, Wieland O. Fluctuation of hepatic enzymes important in glucose metabolism in relation to thyroid function. Eur J Biochem 1970;13:253

200. Mariash CN, Kaiser F, Oppenheimer JH. Comparison of the response characteristics of four lipogenic enzymes to 3,5,3′ triiodothyronine administration: evidence for variable degrees of amplification of the nuclear -T3 signal. Endocrinology 1980;106:22

201. Dozin B, Magnuson MA, Nikodem VM. Thyroid hormone regulation of malic enzyme synthesis. J Biol Chem 1986;261:10290

202. Salati LM, Ma XJ, McCormick CC, Stapleton SR, Goodridge AG. Triiodothyronine stimulates and cyclic AMP inhibits transcription of the gene for malic enzyme in chick embryo hepatocytes in culture. J Biol Chem 1991;266:4010

203. Song M-KH, Dozin B, Grieco D, Rall JE, Nikodem VM. Transcriptional activation and stabilization of malic ennzyme mRNA precursor by thyroid hormone. J Biol Chem 1988;263:17970

204. Desvergen B. Functional characterization and receptor binding studies of the malic enzyme thyroid response element. J Biol Chem 1991;266:1008

205. Petty KJ, Desvergne B, Mitsuhashi T, Nikodem VM. Identification of a thyroid hormone response element in the malic enzyme gene. J Biol Chem 1990;265:7395

206. Gibson D, Lyons R, Scott D, Muto Y. Synthesis and degradation of the lipogenic enzymes of rat liver. Adv Enzyme Regul 1972; 10:187

207. Mariash CN, Oppenheimer JH. Thyroid hormone-carbohydrate interaction. In: Oppenheimer JH, Samuels HH, eds. Molecular basis of thyroid hormone action. New York: Academic Press, 1983:265

208. Dozin B, Rall JE, Nikodem VM. Tissue-specific control of rat malic enzyme activity and messenger RNA levels by a high carbohydrate diet. Proc Natl Acad Sci USA 1986;83:4705

209. Ma X-J, Salati L, Ash S, et al. Nutritional regulation and tissue-specific expression of the malic enzyme gene in chicken. J Biol Chem 1990;265:18435

210. Dozin B, Magnuson MA, Nikodem VM. Tissue-specific regulation of two functional malic enzyme mRNAs by triiodothyronine. Biochemistry 1985;24:5581

211. Seelig SA, Jump DB, Towle HC, et al. Paradoxical effects of cycloheximide on the ultra-rapid induction of two hepatic mRNA sequences by triiodothyronine (T3). Endocrinology 1982; 110:671

212. Liaw CW, Towle HC. Characterization of a thyroid hormone-responsive gene from rat. J Biol Chem 1984;259:7253

213. Narayan P, Liaw CW, Towle HC. Rapid induction of a specific nuclear mRNA precursor by thyroid hormone. Proc Natl Acad Sci USA 1984;81:4687

214. Jump DB, Narayan P, Towle HC, Oppenheimer JH. Rapid effects of triiodothyronine on hepatic gene expression: hybridization analysis of tissue specific T3-regulation of mRNA-S14. J Biol Chem 1984;259:2789

215. Jump DB, Oppenheimer JH. High basal expression and 3,5,3′-triiodothyronine regulation of messenger ribonucleic acid S14 in lipogenic tissues. Endocrinology 1985;117:2259

216. Mariash CN, Seelig S, Schwartz HL, Oppenheimer JH. Rapid synergistic interaction between thyroid hormone and carbohydrate on mRNA S14 induction. J Biol Chem 1986;261:9583

217. Carr FE, Bingham C, Oppenheimer JH, Kistner C, Mariash CN. Quantitative investigation of hepatic genomic response to hormonal and pathophysiological stimuli by multivariate analysis of two-dimensional mRNA activity profiles. Proc Natl Acad Sci USA 1984;81:974

218. Topliss DJ, Mariash CN, Seelig S, Carr FE, Oppenheimer JH. Effects of triiodothyronine and glucose on cultured rat hepatocyte gene expression. Endocrinology 1983;112:1868

219. Kinlaw WB. Unexpected nuclear localization and hepatic zonation of spot 14 (S14) protein revealed by anti-fusion protein antiserum. Thyroid 1992;2(Suppl1):S85

220. Kinlaw WB, Tron P, Harmon J, Mariash CN. "Spot 14" protein (lipomatrin) is a thyroid hormone-responsive component of nuclear matrix that promotes malic enzyme gene expression. Thyroid 1993;(Suppl1):T117

221. Jump DB. Rapid induction of rat liver S14 transcription by thyroid hormone. J Biol Chem 1989;264:4698

222. Zilz N, Murray M, Towle H. Identification of multiple thyroid hormone response elements located far upstream from the rat S_{14} promoter. J Biol Chem 1990;265:8131

223. Jump DB, Bell A, Santiago V. Thyroid hormone and dietary carbohydrate interact to regulate rat liver S14 gene transcription and chromatin structure. J Biol Chem 1990;265:3474

224. Jacoby DB, Zilz ND, Towle HC. Sequences within the 5′-flanking region of the S14 gene confer responsiveness to glucose in primary hepatocytes. J Biol Chem 1989;264:17623

225. Sudo Y, Goto Y, Mariash CN. Loacation of a glucose-dependent response region in the rat S14 promoter. Endocrinology 1993; 133:1221

226. Sudo Y, Mariash CN. The thyroid hormone receptor can unmask a glucose response in the S14 gene. Endocrinology 1993; 133:129

227. Burmeister LA, Mariash CN. Dietary sucrose enhances processing of mRNA-S14 nuclear precursor. J Biol Chem 1991;266:22905

228. Silva J, Larsen PR. Contributions of plasma triiodothyronine and local thyroxine monodeiodination to triiodothyronine to nuclear triiodothyronine receptor saturation in pituitary, liver and kidney of hypothyroid rats. Further evidence relating saturation of pituitary nuclear triiodothyrnine receptors and the acute inhibition of thyroid stimulating hormone release. J Clin Invest 1978; 61:1247

229. Gershengorn M. Thyroid hormone regulation of thyrotropin production and interaction with thyrotropin-releasing hormone in thryotropic cells in culture. In: Oppenheimer J, Samuels HH, eds. Molecular basis of thyroid hormone action. New York: Academic Press, 1983:387

230. Shupnik MA, Ardisson LJ, Meskell MJ, Bornstein J, Ridgway EC. Triiodothyronine (T3) regulation of thyrotropin subunit gene transcription is proportional to T3 nuclear receptor occupancy. Endocrinology 1986;118:367

231. Shupnik MA, Ridgway EC. Triiodothyronine rapidly decreases the transcription of the thyrotropin subunit genes in thyrotropic tumor explants. Endocrinology 1985;117:1940

232. Ross DS, Downing MF, Chin WW, Kieffer JD, Ridgway EC. Changes in tissue concentrations of thyrotropin, free, thyrotropin β and α subunits after thyroxin administration: comparison of mouse hypothyroid pituitary and thyrotropic tumors. Endocrinology 1983;112:2050

233. Weintraub BD, Stannard BS, Magner JA, et al. Glycosylation and posttranslational processing of thyroid-stimulating hormone: Clinical implications. Recent Prog Horm Res 1985;41:577

234. Shupnik MA, Ridgway EC, Chin WW. Molecular biology of thyrotropin. Endocr Rev 1989;10:459

235. Chin WW, Shupnik MA, Ross DS, Habener JF, Ridgway EC. Regulation of the α and thyrotropin β-subunit messenger ribonucleic acids by thyroid hormone. Endocrinology 1985; 116:873

236. Gurr JA, Kourides IA. Regulation of thyrotropin biosynthesis: discordant effect of thyroid hormone on α and β subunit mRNA levels. J Biol Chem 1982;258:10208

237. Gurr JA, Kourides IA. Thyroid hormone regulation of thyrotropin a and β subunit gene transcription. DNA 1985;4:301

238. Krane IM, Spindel ER, Chin WW. Thyroid hormone decreases the stability and the poly (A) tract length of rat thyrotropin β-subunit messenger RNA. Mol Endocrinol 1991;5:469

239. Barker SB, Klitgaard HM. Metabolism of tissues excised from thyroxine-injected rats. Am J Physiol 1952;170:81

240. Legrand J. Variations, as a function of age, of the response of the cerebellum to the morphogenetic action of the thyroid in rats. Arch D Anat Microsc et de Morphol Exp 1967;56:291

241. Legrand J. Thyroid hormone effects on growth and development. In: Hennemann G, ed. Thyroid hormone metabolism. New York: Marcel Dekker, 1986:503

242. Bernal J, Rodriguez-Pena A, Iniguez M, Ibarolla N, Munoz A. Influence of thyroid hormones on brain gene expresion. Acta Medica Austriaca 1992(Suppl 19);1:32

243. Nunez J, Couchie D, Aniello F, Bridoux A. Regulation by thyroid hormone of microtubule assembly and neuronal differentiation. Neurochem Res 1991;16:975

244. Farsetti A, Desvergne B, Hallenbeck P, Robbins J, Nokodem VM. Characterization of myelin basic protein thyroid hormone response element and its function in the context of native and heterologous promoter. J Biol Chem 1992;267:15784

245. Carlson DJ, Strait KA, Schwartz HL, Oppenheimer JH. Thyroid hormone receptor content in cultured astrocytes: β1 and α2 receptor in Type II astrocytes and absence of αl, α2, and β1 recepotors in Type I astrocytes. Thyroid 1992;(Suppl 1):S83

246. Nordquist DT, Kozak CA, Orr HT. cDNA cloning and characterization of three genes uniquely expressed in cerebellum by Purkinje cells. J Neurosci 1988;8:223

247. Strait KA, Zou L, Oppenheimer JH. β1 isoform-specific regulation of a triiodothyronine-induced gene during cerebellar development. Mol Endocrinol 1992;6:1874

248. Zou L, Hagen SG, Strait KA, Oppenheimer JH. Identification of thyroid hormone response elements in rodent Pcp-2, a developmentally regulated gene of cerebellar Purkinje cells. J Biol Chem 1994;269:13346

249. Adamson LF, Ingbar SH. Some properties of the stimulatory effect of thyroid hormones on amino acid transport by embryonic chick bone. Endocrinology 1967;81:1372

250. Lindholm D, Castern E, Tsouulfas P, et al. Neurotrophin-3 induced by triiodothyronine in cerebellar granule cells promotes Purkinje cell differentiation. J Cell Biol 1993;122:443

251. Alvarez-Dolado M, Iglesias T, Rodriguez-Pena A, Bernal J, Munoz A. Expression of neurotrophins and the trk family of neurotrophin receptors in normal and hypothyroid rat brain. Brain Res 1994;27:249

252. Green S, Chambon P. Nuclear receptors enhance our understanding of transcription regulation. Trends Genet 1988;4:309

253. Galton VA. Thyroid hormone action in amphibian metamorphosis. In: Oppenheimer JH, Samuels HH, eds. Molecular basis of thyroid hormone action. New York: Academic Press, 1983:445

254. Yaoita Y, Shi YB, Brown DD. The xenopus laevis alpha and beta thyroid hormone receptors. Proc Natl Acad Sci USA 1990; 87:7090

255. Oppenheimer JH, Schwartz HL, Lane JT, Thompson MP. Functional relationship of thyroid hormone-induced lipogenesis, lipolysis, and thermogenesis in the rat. J Clin Invest 1991; 87:125

256. Portnay GI, O'Brien JT, Bush J, et al. The effect of starvation on the concentration and binding of thyroxine and triiodothyronine in serum and in the response to TRH. J Clin Endocrinol Metab 1974;39:191

257. Bermudez F, Surks MI, Oppenheimer JH. High incidence of decreased serum triiodothyronine concentrations in patients with nonthyroidal disease. J Clin Enocrinol Metab 1975;41:27

258. Schussler G, Orland J. Fasting decreases triiodothyronine receptor capacity. Science 1978;199:686

259. Money W, Kumaoka S, Rawson R. Metabolic effects of thyroid hormones and their analogues. Comparative effects of thyroxine analogues in experimental animals. Ann NY Acad Sci 1960; 60:512

260. Westerfield WW, Richert DA, Ruegamer WR. New assay procedure for thyroxine analogs. Endocrinology 1965;77:802

Werner and Ingbar's The Thyroid, Seventh Edition,
edited by Lewis E. Braverman and Robert D. Utiger.
Lippincott–Raven Publishers, Philadelphia, © 1996

10

Thyroid Hormone Structure-Function Relationships

Vivian Cody

Studies of the thyroid hormones continue to provide new insights into the molecular events that control their biosynthesis, transport, and mechanism of action. Thyroid hormones are protein-bound during transport in the general circulation, at the cell membrane, and at the cell nucleus. Therefore, their molecular interactions with proteins are of paramount interest. Most recently emphasis has been focused on thyroid hormone-protein interactions of transthyretin (TTR), its retinol-binding protein complex, thyroxine-binding globulin, and the hormone-binding domain of the thyroid nuclear receptor.

The major product of the thyroid gland, thyroxine (T$_4$; 3',5',3,5-tetraiodo-L-thyronine) was first isolated by Kendall in 1914 (Fig. 10-1). Its correct composition, however, was not established until 1927, by Harrington and Barger.[2] Although thyroid hormones have been shown to elicit a multitude of biologic responses, the specific nature of their actions remains unclear. The impetus to synthesize and test many analogues stemmed from attempts to define those features essential for thyroxine-like activity.[3,4] A number of hypotheses have been proposed to relate various structural features of thyroid hormones to the expression of their biologic effects (Table 10-1). Among the proposals suggested, the following are considered of key importance: (1) the unique role of iodine, for both its steric and its electronic properties; (2) the diphenyl ether linkage in controlling conformation; and (3) the 4'-hydroxyl and side-chain composition for receptor binding. Investigation of these hypotheses has been carried out using such techniques as nuclear magnetic resonance (NMR), spectroscopy, and x-ray crystallography to elucidate their structure-activity relationships.

For example, it is well known that hypothyroidism is accompanied by high serum levels of low-density lipoprotein cholesterol and, potentially, an increased risk of atherosclerosis, whereas thyrotoxicosis is associated with decreased cholesterol levels. Thyroid hormones could not be used therapeutically to lower serum cholesterol because of their potential to induce cardiac side-effects. Thus, modification of the thyroid hormone molecule was carried out to produce analogues that could differentiate between liver-selective actions and cardiotoxic effects.[4] These studies revealed that introduction of specific arylmethyl groups at the 3'-position of T$_3$ resulted in analogues that are liver-selective, cardiac-sparing thyromimetic compounds.

STRUCTURE AND STEREOCHEMICAL CHARACTERISTICS

The thyronine nucleus constitutes the basic structural unit of thyroid hormones. By varying the degree of iodination, all known thyroid hormone structures can be derived (Fig. 10-2). Depending on the reference point, the molecule can be described as a substituted alanine amino acid or, in terms of the diphenyl ether moiety, with substituents in the 4'- and 1-positions (see Fig. 10-1).

The thyroid literature does not conform to the standard IUPAC nomenclature but uses instead the substituted diphenyl ether system. Because the thyronine nucleus has five single bonds (see Fig. 10-1), rotation about these bonds results in a number of conformations, many of which have been observed in the solid state.[5–7] This flexibility, quantitatively described by the magnitudes of these rotations, is controlled by (1) ring substitution effects, (2) ether bridge substitutions, (3) side-chain composition, and (4) hydrogen-bonding effects.

Diphenyl Ether Conformations

A major structural feature of the thyroid hormones is that the two phenyl rings are joined by a bridging ether oxygen with an angle of 120 degrees. Early in the study of the thyroid hormones, it became evident that these substances possessed

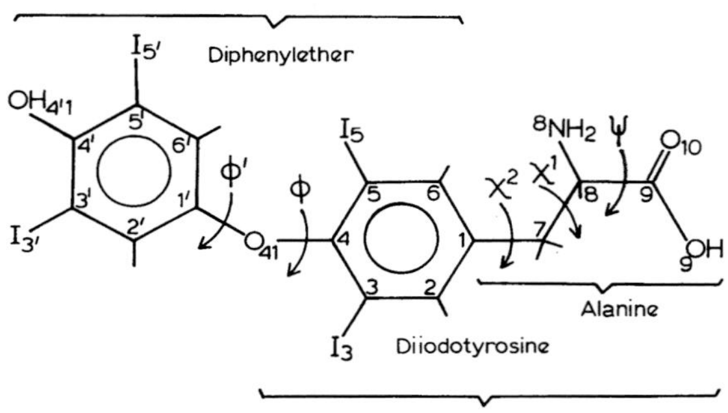

FIGURE 10-1. Thyroxine with torsion angles and molecular components. (Cody V. Thyroid hormone interactions: molecular conformation, protein binding, and hormone action. Endocrine Rev 1980;1:140)

special stereochemical characteristics and that their three-dimensional features must be considered. Examination of space-filling models of the thyroid hormones revealed that the bulky ortho iodine atoms near the ether bridge caused the two aromatic ring systems to be nearly perpendicular, and that these bulky groups hinder rotation about the phenyl ether bonds. Structural data for the thyroid hormones showed that the minimal steric interaction between the ortho tyrosyl iodine atoms and the phenolic ortho hydrogen atoms is maintained when one ring is coplanar with, and the other perpendicular to, the plane of the two ether bonds.[5] This gives rise to a skewed conformation of the hormone and the concept of preferred, if not somewhat rigid, orientations of the molecule (Fig. 10-3). These stereochemical properties also revealed that the 3'-iodine of the hormone 3,5,3'-triiodothyronine (T₃) possesses two positional isomers–distal and proximal–depending on whether the phenolic ring iodine atom is oriented away from or near the tyrosyl ring, respectively. Activity measurements of rigid analogues revealed that a distal T₃ conformation was the more active analogue.

Crystallographic analysis of thyroid hormones shows that a skewed diphenyl ether conformation is observed in the structures of all 3,5-disubstituted hormone analogues.[5–7] As mentioned, the bulk of the tyrosyl ring substituents forces the diphenyl ether to adopt a skewed conformation (i.e., $\Theta = 0$ degrees, $\Theta' = 90$ degrees), whereas removal of one of these substituents releases this constraint, permitting an anti-skewed conformation (i.e., the tyrosyl ring is perpendicular to, and bisecting, the phenolic ring; $\Theta = 90$ degrees and $\Theta' = 0$ degrees), as was observed in the crystal structure of 3',5',3-triiodothyronine[8] (rT₃; see Fig.10-3). T₄ cannot adopt an anti-skewed conformation since this would place the bulk of the tyrosyl ring iodine atom into the electron density of the phenolic ring. Therefore, the active hormones T₄ and T₃, as well as 3,5-T₂, can adopt only a skewed conformation, whereas those with at least one tyrosyl ring iodine can have either a skewed or anti-skewed conformation.[9]

All of the thyroid hormone-binding proteins have a requirement for a diphenyl ether moiety, since those derivatives of T₄ that contain only one ring or that have a biphenyl connection do not possess activity or binding affinity. The need for the bridging atom to be oxygen is not absolute. Studies of various oxygen bridge-substituted analogues (C-X-C, where X = CH_2, S) showed that the sulfur- and methylene-bridged analogues had substantial binding affinity and activity. Thus, one role of the oxygen bridge is to maintain the appropriate relative orientation of the iodophenyl substitutents.[10]

Side-Chain Conformation

The conformational space available to the thyroid hormone side-chain is defined by three torsion angles: χ^1, χ^2, and ψ, (see Fig. 10-1). From the set of all accessible conformations, only specific subsets are predicted to be energetically favored, and most of these have been observed.[5,7] Analysis of the side-chain conformational parameters of several thyroactive acid metabolites shows that the preferred orientation of the carbonyl function in the propionic acids is fully extended.[11] This is comparable to $\chi^1 = -60$ degrees in the amino acids. In the case of acetic acid structures, the carboxyl group is perpendicular ($\chi^1 = 90$ degrees), and depending on the deviation of this value from perpendicular, one of the oxygen atoms will come close to occupying the same space as the amine in the conformation with $\chi^1 = -60$ degrees and near one of the oxygen atoms in the amino acid when χ^1, = 180 degrees. These features play a role in differentiating the binding affinity of hormone analogues for their various hormone-binding proteins. For example, T₄ has

TABLE 10-1.
Relative Binding Affinities and Biologic Potencies of Selected Thyroid Hormone Analogues

Compound	TBG (%)	TTR (%)	Membrane (%)	Nuclear (%)	Potency * (%)
L-Thyroxine	100	39.3	96.6	12.5	18.1
D-Thyroxine	54.0	0.95	63.0	—	3.0
T₄-propionic acid	3.6	76.4	23.0	—	1.9
T₄-acetic acid	1.7	100.0	30.3	—	0.25
S-bridge T₄	63.0	—	—	—	—
CH₂-bridge T₄	35.0	—	—	2.6	—
L-T₃	9.0	1.4	100.0	100.0	100.0
rT₃	38.0	3.1	67.5	0.1	<0.1

*Potency is percentage of L-T₃
(Cody V. Thyroid hormone interactions: molecular conformation, protein binding, and hormone action. Endocr Rev 1980;1:140)

IODOTHYRONINE DEIODINATION

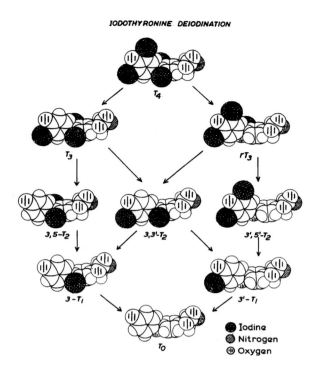

FIGURE 10-2. Spatial representation of thyroxine deiodination cascade. (Auf'mkolk M, Koehrle J, Hesch RD, Cody V. Inhibition of rat liver iodothyronine deiodinase: interactions of aurone with the iodothyronine deiodinase binding site. J Biol Chem 1986;261:11623)

the strongest binding affinity for thyroxine-binding globulin, whereas the metabolite tetraiodothyroacetic acid has the strongest binding affinity for TTR (see Table 10-1).

INTERMOLECULAR INTERACTIONS

In addition to understanding thyroid hormone molecular conformation, it is important to understand how these molecules interact with their environment. Under normal physiologic conditions, the amino acid is a zwitterion, the amine having a net positive charge and the carboxylic oxygens having a net negative charge. As a result of the differences in pK_a of the 4'-OH in T_3 and T_4 (8.47 and 6.73, respectively), the 4'-OH of T_4 is about 80% ionized at physiologic pH, whereas in T_3 it is about 10% ionized. Because many protein-substrate interactions are by way of receptor interactions, it is important to understand the nature of the hydrogen bonding in these structures. There are several potential sites for hydrogen bonding in T_4 (Fig. 10-4); the amine can act as a hydrogen bond donor, the carboxylic acid as an acceptor, and, depending on its environment, the 4'-OH can act as both a donor and acceptor. A study of the hydrogen bonding observed in the crystal structures of thyroid hormones shows that there is a high degree of directional specificity in the location of the hydrogen bond donors and acceptors.[6] One unique property of iodine is its polarizability, which is reflected in its predisposition to form short intermolecular contact distances of the type I...I and I...O in the crystal lattice.[12] The propensity for iodine to form such short intermolecular contacts may explain hormone-binding selectivity to the var-

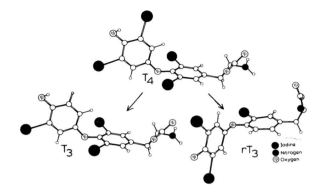

FIGURE 10-3. Deiodination products of thyroxine to skewed T_3 and anti-skewed rT_3. (Cody V, Koehrle J, Auf'mkolk M, Hesch RD. Structure-activity relationships of flavonoid deiodinase inhibitors and enzyme active site models. In: Cody V, Middleton E Jr, Harborne JB, eds. Plant flavonoids in biology and medicine: Biochemical, pharmaceutical and structure-activity relationships. New York: Alan R Liss, 1986:373)

ious thyroxine-binding proteins.

PROTEIN-BINDING INTERACTIONS

Structure-activity data show that thyroid hormone analogues have different binding affinities for TTR, depending on their substituent patterns (see Table 10-1). In addition, many pharmacologic agents and natural products such as plant flavonoids, nonsteroidal analgesic drugs, and inotropic bipyridines are strong competitors for T_4 binding to TTR with binding affinities much greater than T_4. Recent structure-activity correlations indicate that certain plant flavonoids that have long-standing use as folk remedies can exhibit various anti-hormonal properties, including inhibition of the enzyme iodothyronine deiodinase. These data further reveal that aurones are the most potent inhibitors of enzyme activity, and strong competitors for T_4 binding to TTR.[13] Computer graphic modeling of the binding interactions with TTR suggests that the best structural homology between thyroid hormones and flavonoids involves the phenolic ring of both classes of compound.[14,15] Studies of T_4 displacement from TTR further re-

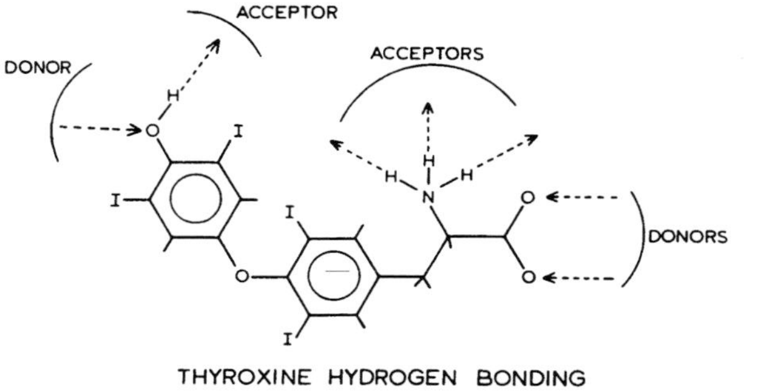

THYROXINE HYDROGEN BONDING

FIGURE 10-4. Thyroxine hydrogen bonding groups. (Cody V. Thyroid hormone interactions: molecular conformation, protein binding, and hormone action. Endocr Rev 1980;1:140)

vealed that a synthetic plant flavonoid, EMD 21388 (3-methyl-4', 6-dihydroxy-3', 5'-dibromo-flavone), is the strongest competitor for thyroxine binding to human TTR,[16,17] and showed that this T_4 antagonist alters the circulating total and percentage of free thyroid hormones and serum thyrotropin concentrations.[18]

To verify these structure-activity data, the crystal structures of a number of TTR-ligand complexes are under study.[19–23] All crystals of human TTR ligand complexes reported to date are isomorphous with the orthorhombic $P2_12_12$ cell reported previously for native TTR[24] and have two independent monomers in the asymmetric unit of the crystal lattice. Structural data for the TTR-T_4 complex[25,26] revealed that T_4 binds in a "forward" mode with its 4'-OH buried deep within the channel running through the tetrameric protein and has its amino acid side-chain near the channel entrance interacting with Lys-15 and Glu-54. The presence of a crystallographic twofold axis through the center of the binding domains requires that the ligand either possess molecular twofold symmetry or has a 50% statistical disorder. Since T_4 does not possess twofold symmetry, it must occupy this site with a statistical disorder.

Recently, the TTR-T_4 complex has been determined as a co-crystallized hormone complex.[23] These data show that T_4 binds deeper in the channel and displaces the bound water observed in the crystals soaked with T_4.[25] Although the orientation is similar, the hormone is rotated such that it shares common binding sites for the 3- and 3'-iodine atoms. These data verify that T_4 binding does not affect the main chain conformation significantly, but results in local rearrangements of

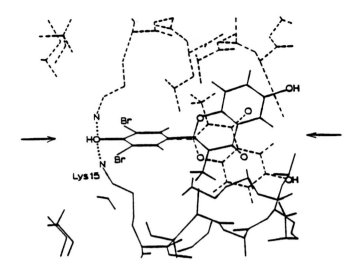

FIGURE 10-6. Representation of EMD 21388 in the "reverse" binding mode of human TTR. The close contact between the flavone 4'-OH and NZ of Lys-15 near the channel entrance is shown. (Cody V, Wojtczak A, Ciszak E, Luft JR. Differences in inhibitor and substrate binding in transthyretin crystal complexes. In: Gordon A, Gross J, Hennemann G, eds. Progress in thyroid research, Rotterdam: Balema, 1991:793)

residue side-chains in the binding channel.

The orientation of the weak binding metabolite, 3,3'-T_2[21] differs significantly from that of T_4. As shown (Fig. 10-5), it binds deeper in the channel than T_4, and in this orientation, 3,3'-T_2 occupies the binding domain in a completely different manner from T_4. The binding affinity of 3,3'-T_2, which is 100-fold lower than that of T_4, reflects the lack of the second pair of iodine atoms interacting in the channel.

Structural results show that the flavones bind to transthyretin in a manner different from T_4. Data for the structure of the hTTR-EMD 21388 complex reveals that bromoflavone binds deeper in the channel than T_4; the bromine atoms occupy symmetrical sites in a "forward" mode (Fig. 10-6), and in a "reverse" mode, with the bromophenolic ring near the channel entrance in TTR.[19] A bromoaurone analogue binds in a similar manner.[20] The observation of two alternative binding orientations for EMD 21388 may explain its greater binding affinity for TTR.[17] Similar results have been observed for TTR-thyroid hormone analogue complexes,[19,25] and NMR data on transthyretin indicate that thyroid hormones also may bind in more than one mode.[27]

Biochemical data for the competitive inhibition of T_4 binding by bipyridine inotropic agents revealed that the potent cardioactive positive inotrope milrinone, a 2-methyl-5-cyano-bipyridine, has a binding affinity 59% that of T_4, whereas its less potent parent inotrope, amrinone, the 5-amino-bipyridine analogue, was a weak competitor.[28,29] Structural results for the TTR-milrinone complex show the 5-cyano group binds in the same site as the 5'-iodo group of the hormone.[22] Modeling amrinone binding in the milrinone site reveals that the 5-amino group cannot participate in the same interactions as the 5-cyano group, thereby weakening its binding affinity.

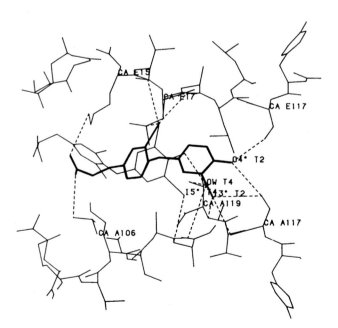

FIGURE 10-5. Position of T_4 (light line) and 3,3'-T_2 (thick line) bound in their respective TTR complexes. The one letter code symbols label the residues forming the binding site. (Wojtczak A, Luft JR, Cody V. Mechanism of molecular recognition: crystal structure of 3,3'diiodo-L-thyronine human transthyretin complex and mutant interactions. J Biol Chem 1992;267:353)

RAT TRANSTHYRETIN HORMONE-BINDING SITE INTERACTIONS

Sequence analysis shows that TTRs from various species are more than 85% identical to human.[30] In the case of rat TTR, there are 22 residues that differ in identity with the 127 residue monomer of the human sequence. Structural data for native and thyroxine-bound rat transthyretin show the crystals are tetragonal and crystallize in the space group $P4_32_12$ with a complete tetramer in the asymmetric unit of the lattice.[31] Although the overall structure of the rat tetramer is similar to the human tetramer, differences are observed in the loop regions near the dimer interface. Preliminary data for the rat TTR-T_4 complex reveal electron density in the binding domain, which is indicative of a single binding orientation for the hormone, despite the similarity of the rat TTR and human TTR complexes. In the rat complex, the hormone amino acid interacts with the side-chains of Lys-15 and Glu-54 from the same TTR monomer and its iodine atoms are bound in four unique hydrophobic pockets. This is the first observation of an unambiguous binding environment not complicated by the presence of crystallographically imposed symmetry constraints now present in all reported human structures. These data also provide the first opportunity to examine the hormone binding interactions in a unique environment. Comparison of the environment near the 22 residues in the rat sequence which differ from human will also permit evaluation of their influence on hormone-binding interactions and tetramer assembly.

References

1. Kendall EC. Thyroxine. American Chemical Society Monograph Series, No. 47. New York: Chemical Catalogue Company, 1929
2. Harrington Cr, Barger G. Chemistry of thyroxine. III. Constitution and synthesis of thyroxine. Biochem J 1927;21:169
3. Jorgensen EC, Stereochemistry of thyroxine and analogues. Mayo Clin Proc 1964;39:560
4. Leeson PD, Emmett JC, Shah VP, et al. Selective thyromimetics. Cardiac-sparing thyroid hormone analogues containing 3'-arylmethyl substituents. J Med Chem 1989;32:320
5. Cody V. Thyroid hormone interactions: molecular conformation, protein binding, and hormone action. Endocr Rev 1980;1:140
6. Cody V. Structure of thyroxine: role of thyroxine hydroxyl in protein binding. Acta Crystallogr 1981;B37:1685
7. Cody V. Triiodothyronine: molecular structure and biologic function. In: Chopra IJ, ed. Triiodothyronines in health and disease. New York: Springer-Verlag, 1981;15
8. Okabe N, Fujiwara T, Yamagata Y, Tomita K. The crystal structure of a major metabolite of thyroid hormone: 3',5',3-triiodo-L-thyronine. Biochim Biophys Acta 1982;717,179
9. Cody V, Koehrle J, Auf'mkolk M, Hesch RD. Structure-activity relationships of flavonoid deiodinase inhibitiors and enzyme active site models. In: Cody V, Middleton E Jr, Harborne JB, eds. Plant flavonoids in biology and medicine: biochemical, pharmaceutical and structure-activity relationships. New York: Alan R Liss, 1986;373
10. Cody V. Conformational effects of ether bridge substitution in thyroid hormone analogues. Endocr Res Commun 1982;9:55
11. Cody V. Thyroid hormone structure-activity relationships: molecular structure of 3,5,3'-triiodothyropropionic acid. Endocr Res 1988;14:165
12. Cody V, Murray-Rust P. Iodine...X(O,N,S) intermolecular contacts: models of thyroid hormone-protein binding interactions using information from the Cambridge Crystallogr Data Files. J Mol Struc 1984;112:189
13. Auf'mkolk M, Koehrle J, Hesch RD, Cody V. Inhibition of rat liver iodothyronine deiodinase: interactions of aurone with the iodothyronine deiodinase binding site. J Biol Chem 1986; 261:11623
14. Cody V, Luft JR, McCourt M, Irmscher K. Conformational analysis of flavonoids: crystal and molecular structure of 3',5'-dibromo-3-methyl-6,4'-dihydroxyflavone (1:2) triphenylphosphine oxide complex. Struc Chem 1991;2:601
15. Ciszak E, Cody V, Luft JR, Kempton RJ, Kesler BS. Flavonoid conformational analysis: comparison of the molecular structure of (z)-4,4',6-triacetoxyaurone and (z)-3',5'-dibromo-2,4,4',6-tetrahydroxyauronemonohydrate by crystallographic and molecular orbital methods. J Mole Struc (Theochem) 1991;251:345
16. Koehrle J, Fang SL, Yang Y, et al. Rapid effects of the flavonoid EMD 21388 on serum thyroid hormone binding and thyrotropin regulation in the rat. Endocrinology 1989;125:532
17. Rosen HN, Murrell JR, Liepnieks JJ, Benson, MD, Cody V, Moses AC. Threonine-for-alanine substitution at position 109 of transthyretin differentially alters TTR's affinity for iodothyronines. Endocrinology 1994;134:27
18. Safran M, Koehrle J, Braverman LE, Leonard JL. Effect of biological alternations of type I 5'-deiodinase activity on affinity labeled membrane proteins in rat liver and kidney. Endocrinology 1990;126:826
19. Cody V, Wojtczak A, Ciszak E, Luft JR. Differences in inhibitor and substrate binding in transthyretin crystal complexes. In: Gordon A, Gross J, Hennemann G, eds. Progress in thyroid research. Rotterdam: Balema, 1991:793
20. Ciszak E, Luft JR, Cody V. Crystal structure determination at 2.3A resolution of human transthyretin-3',5'-dibromo-2',4,4',6-tetrahydroxyaurone complex. Proc Natl Acad Sci U S A 1992; 89:6644
21. Wojtczak A, Luft JR, Cody V. Mechanism of molecular recognition: crystal structure of 3,3'-diiodo-L-thyronine human transthyretin complex and mutant interactions. J Biol Chem 1992;267:353
22. Wojtczak A, Luft JR, Cody V. Structural aspects of inotropic bipyridine binding: crystal structure determination to 1.9A of the human serum transthyretin-milrinone complex. J Biol Chem 1993;268:6202
23. Wojtczak A, Cody V, Luft JR, Pangborn W. Crystal structure determination to 2.0Å resolution of a co-crystallized complex of human transthyretin and thyroxine. Acta Crystallogr (submitted)
24. Blake CCF, Geisow MJ, Oatley SJ, Rerat B, Rerat C. Structure of prealbumin: secondary, tertiary and quaternary interactions determined by fourier refinement at 1.8A. J Mol Biol 1978; 121:339
25. Blake CCF, Oatley SJ. Protein-DNA and protein-hormone interactions in prealbumin: a model of the thyroid hormone nuclear receptor? Nature 1977;268:115
26. De LaPaz P, Burridge JM, Oatley SJ, Blake CCF. Multiple modes of binding thyroid hormones and other iodothyronines to human plasma transthyretin. In: Beddell CR, ed. The design of drugs to macromolecular targets. New York: Wiley & Sons, 1992:119
27. Reid DG, MacLachlan LK, Voyle M, Leeson PD. A proton and fluorine nuclear magnetic resonance and fluorescence study of the binding of some natural and synthetic thyromimetics to prealbumin (transthyretin). J Biol Chem 1989;264:2013
28. Mylotte KM, Cody V, Davis PJ, Davis FB, Blas SD, Schoenl M. Milrinone and thyroid hormone stimulate myocardial membrane Ca^{2+}-ATPase activity and share structural homologies. Proc Natl Acad Sci U S A 1985; 82: 7974
29. Davis PJ, Cody V, Davis FB, Warnick PR, Schoenl M, Edwards L. Milrinone, a non-iodinated bipyridine, competes with thyroid hormone for binding sites on human serum prealbumin (TBPA). Biochem Pharmacol 1987;36:3635
30. Sundelin J, Melhus H, Das S, Eriksson U, Lind P, Tragardh L, Peterson PA, Rask L. The primary structure of rabbit and rat prealbumin and a comparison with the ternary structure of human prealbumin. J Biol Chem 1985;260:6481
31. Wojtczak A, Cody V, Luft JR, Pangborn W. Crystal structure of rat transthyretin: the first observation of a unique tetramer. J Biol Chem (submitted)

Werner and Ingbar's The Thyroid, Seventh Edition,
edited by Lewis E. Braverman and Robert D. Utiger.
Lippincott–Raven Publishers, Philadelphia, © 1996

Section E
Factors That Control Thyroid Function

11

Thyrotropin

CHEMISTRY AND BIOSYNTHESIS OF THYROTROPIN

Fredric E. Wondisford
James A. Magner
Bruce D. Weintraub

CHEMISTRY

Pituitary thyrotropin or thyroid-stimulating hormone (TSH) is one of four related glycoprotein hormones synthesized either by the anterior lobe of the pituitary gland or by the placenta. TSH, pituitary luteinizing hormone (LH), follicle-stimulating hormone (FSH), and chorionic gonadotropin (CG) (isolated from pregnancy urine) consist of two noncovalently linked α- and β-subunits.[1,2] The amino acid sequence of the α-subunit is common to all four glycoprotein hormones within one mammalian species. However, the carbohydrate structure of the β-subunit may vary among the four hormones because of differences in a conformation induced by different β-subunits or because of various carbohydrate processing enzymes present in different cells of the pituitary and placenta.[3–5] The β-subunit has a different amino sequence in each hormone and carries the specific information relating to receptor binding and expression of hormonal activity. However, the free β-subunit is devoid of bioactivity and requires noncovalent combination with the common α to express such information.

Thyroid-stimulating activity has been extracted from virtually all mammalian pituitaries examined, as well as in those of lower vertebrates. The best chemical information has been derived from a study of bovine, porcine, and human TSH.[1] TSH preparations purified from pituitary glands by various chromatographic procedures contain heterogeneous but closely related components, which have variable biologic activity. Such components can be separated by gel electrophoresis, isoelectric focusing, or chromatofocusing. The molecular weights of these various components of mammalian TSH are in the range of 28,000 to 30,000 daltons. Differences in molecular weight are attributed to heterogeneity of the oligosaccharide chains, heterogeneity at amino termini, and the extent of amidation of glutamic and aspartic acid residues.

The linear sequence of the human α-subunit is shown in Figure 11-1A, together with the amino acid replacements found in the corresponding subunit from either bovine TSH or LH.[1] The human α-subunit contains an apoprotein core of 92 amino acid residues, while the bovine α-subunit contains 96. Amino terminal heterogeneity of α-subunits derived from different glycoprotein hormones probably is artifactual, since in vitro studies (see following) suggest that processing of the precursor protein yields a single product. The α-subunit contains 10 half-cystine residues, all of which are in disulfide linkage, as are those in the β-subunits. Knowledge of the specific location of the disulfide bonds in both subunits has been advanced recently after the successful x-ray crystallographic analysis of the closely related glycoprotein, hCG.[6,7]

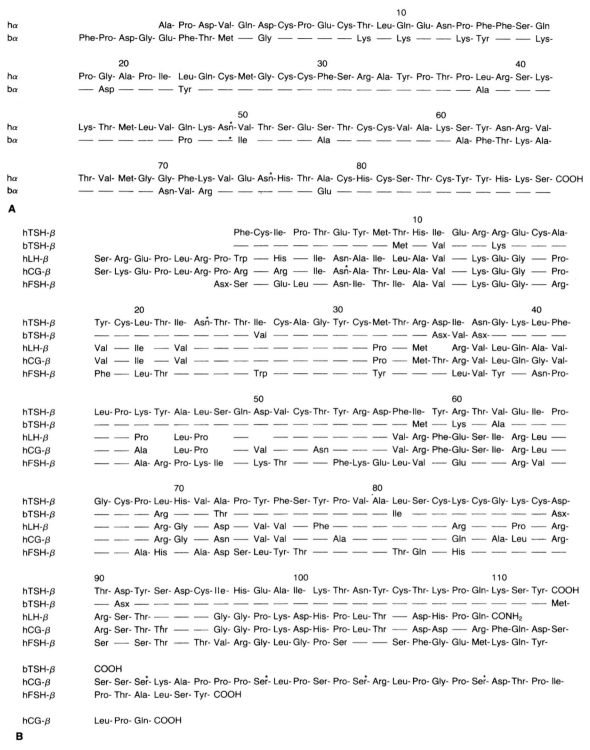

FIGURE 11-1. (*A*)Linear amino acid sequence of a human α chain compared with those of the bovine glyco-protein hormones. Dashes indicate residues identical with those shown for the human subunit. The sequence shown is that of hCG-α; hTSH-α begins with the valine at position 4. Asterisks indicate the positions of the carbohydrate groups. (*B*), Linear amino acid sequence of human TSH-β compared with that of bovine TSH-β and the β-subunits of the other human glycoprotein hormones. Dashes indicate identical residues; all glu-tamic-glutamine and aspartic-asparagine positions are not settled. Blank spaces are gaps inserted to align for maximum similarity. Asterisks indicate the position of the carbohydrate groups. (Pierce JG. Thyrotropin: chemistry. In: Ingbar S, Braverman L, eds. The thyroid. Philadelphia: JB Lippincott, 1986: 267)

The three-dimensional structure of TSH likely contains the curious cysteine knot motif and basic folding patterns found in hCG.

The linear amino acid sequence of human TSH-β is depicted in Figure 11-1*B* and compared with that of bovine TSH-β to show the extent of amino acid replacements between the two species, as well as with those of the β-subunits of the gonadotropins.[1] Human TSH-β dissociated from hormone prepared from human pituitaries has an apoprotein core of 112 amino acids, while bovine TSH-β has 113. However, the complementary DNA of bovine TSH-β predicts a protein of 118 amino acids, 5 more than present in the isolated protein. Similarly, both the gene as well as the complementary DNA of human TSH-β predict a protein of 118 amino acids. It is quite striking that when the linear sequences of various β-subunits are aligned to juxtapose half-cystine residues (12 total), many regions of similar or identical sequences are apparent. From such relationships and the fact that each subunit can recombine with a common α-subunit, it seems probable that three-dimensional structures of different β-subunits would be similar and the regions of interaction with the α-subunit would also be homologous. Indeed, there is evidence from chemical modification studies that the regions around residues 51–57 and 75–80 in the β structures are among those involved in interaction with the common α-subunit. Based on the similarities in sequences between the β chains, it is quite probable that they all evolved from a single gene precursor.

Both the α- and the β-subunits of TSH, as well as LH, FSH, and CH, contain covalently linked carbohydrate chains. For TSH, LH, and FSH such chains are all linked to asparagine residues (N-linked), while for the β-subunit of hCG there are additional linkages to serine residues (O-linked). Moreover, the free α-subunit which is secreted also contains an additional site of O-glycosylation.[8] In human TSH the sugar residues found are mannose, fucose, N-acetylglucosamine, galactose, N-acetylgalactosamine, and sialic acid. Moreover, TSH, like LH, contains an unusual sulfate group that terminates certain chains; such sulfation is found only to a small extent in FSH and not at all in CG.[3–5] The sugar residues are found in three oligosaccharide units, all of which are heterogeneous and whose specific structures may vary with the developmental and endocrine state (reviewed in references 8 and 9). Now that recombinant human TSH has been produced in large amounts (see following), the biologic properties of particular isoforms of TSH are being tested, and clinical use is being investigated.[10–15] Two oligosaccharide chains are found on the α-subunit and one on the β-subunit as indicated in Figures 11-1*A* and 11-1*B*.

THE GENES ENCODING THE SUBUNITS OF THYROTROPIN

Chromosome Localization

The gene encoding the common α-subunit of human chorionic gonadotropin (CG), follicle stimulating hormone (FSH), luteinizing hormone (LH), and thyroid stimulating hormone (TSH) and the genes encoding their respective β-subunits are all located on different chromosomes[16] (Table 11-1). The loca-

TABLE 11-1.
Chromosome Location and Number of Human Glycoprotein Subunit Genes

Gene	Chromosome	
	LOCALIZATION	NO.*
Common α	6	1
CGβ	19	7
FSHβ	11	1
LHβ	19	1
TSHβ	1	1

Genes or pseudogenes

tion of the common α-subunit and specific β-subunit on different chromosomes raises interesting questions about how their expression is coordinately regulated during the synthesis of each hormone. Moreover, the CGβ-subunit gene is the only β-subunit gene of this family that exists in more than one copy; and at least two of the seven copies on chromosome 19 are actively transcribed.

Structure of the Common α-Subunit Gene

The α-subunit gene has been isolated from a variety of species including cow,[17] mouse,[18] rat,[19] and human.[20] The organization of each gene is similar in that each contains four exons and three introns, and all are of approximately the same size. The human gene is 9.4 kilobases (kb) in length and contains three introns of 6.4 kb, 1.7 kb, 0.4 kb, respectively. Intron 1 is located between the 5′ untranslated region contained in exon 1 and 2; intron 2 interrupts the α-subunit peptide coding region in codon 6; and intron 3 is between codon 67 and 68 of the α-subunit peptide (see Fig. 11-1). In the rat and cow, intron 2 interrupts the peptide coding region within amino acid 10 and this results in a mature α-subunit peptide that is 4 amino acids longer than the human α-subunit peptide (96 amino acids versus 92 amino acids in human).

A single start of transcription has been found in each of these genes by mapping studies of pituitary RNA. Upstream of these start sites are consensus TATA boxes, thought to be important in correct and efficient transcription by RNA polymerase II.[21] In the human α-subunit gene, that TATA box is centered at −26 base pairs (bp) relative to the start of transcription.[20] In addition, there is a great degree of homology among these species in other 5′ flanking regions, including a palindromic sequence of TGACGTCA in the human α-subunit gene which confers cAMP responsiveness.[22,23] However, the palindrome is altered in the other species to TGATGTCA; and at least in the cow, this change appears to dramatically reduce its cAMP responsiveness.[24]

Structure of the Thyrotropin β-Subunit Gene

The TSH-β-subunit gene has been isolated from the rat,[25] human,[26–28] and mouse[29,30] species. The rat and human gene contain three exons while the mouse gene contains five exons. The two additional exons are 5′ untranslated regions which are unique to the mouse due to changes in its genomic sequence.[26] With this exception, the organization of these genes is quite similar in having the 5′ untranslated exons(s) separated from the TSH-β coding region by a large first intron (Fig. 11-1). The first exon of the human TSH-β gene is 37 bp and untranslated, while the second exon encodes the leader peptide and first 34 amino acids of the mature TSH-β peptide; the third exon contains the remaining coding region (amino acids 35–118) and 3′ untranslated sequences.

The start of transcription has been determined in the rat, mouse, and human TSH-β genes. Both the rat and mouse gene contain two transcriptional start sites approximately 40 bp apart as assessed by primer extension and/or S1 nuclease analysis of pituitary RNA.[25,29,30] Most transcription initiates from the downstream site (90%–99%); and both sites are preceded by consensus TATA box sequences. Transcription from the downstream site is dramatically increased in the hypothyroid state in both the rat and mouse TSH-β gene, while transcription from the upstream site is either unaffected or reduced by thyroid hormone.[25,29,30]

The human TSH-β gene contains only one transcriptional start in a location similar to that of the downstream site in the rat and mouse TSH-β genes.[26–28] This difference may be due to an alteration in the upstream TATA box (Fig. 11-2), which is changed from TATATAA in the rat and mouse gene to TGTATAA in the human gene. Samuels and colleagues[31] have suggested that an additional start site might exist in the human gene. However, based on RNA mapping studies done in one TSH-secreting adenoma, this site does not correspond to the upstream TATA box in the human TSH-β gene.

Familial Hypothyroidism Due to Thyrotropin β-Subunit Gene Abnormalities

Hayashizaki[32] and Dacou-Voutetakis[33] with their colleagues have described two kindreds with familial hypothyroidism due to mutations in the thyrotropin β-subunit gene. Two affected members of a Japanese family had a point mutation in exon 2 that changed a glycine amino acid to an arginine.[32] This mutation is in a region that is highly conserved among glycoprotein subunit genes (CAGY) and is thought to be important in sub-

unit combination (Fig. 11-3). In fact, this mutation was shown to result in a TSH-β-subunit that could not associate with the α-subunit and reduce a functional TSH heterodimer.

Two related Greek families have also been described[33] whose affected family members had a mutation in the 12th amino acid of the mature TSH-β polypeptide that alters the glutamic acid codon (GAA) to a premature stop codon (TAA). In these individuals, functional TSH heterodimer was also not synthesized. Both of these disorders are autosomal recessive in inheritance. A third Brazilian kindred has recently been described with central hypothyroidism due to a frame-shift deletion in codon 105 (C105V) of the TSH-β-subunit gene.[34] This mutation significantly reduces TSH secretion from the anterior pituitary gland but TSH levels are measurable in the serum. Based on the crystallographic structure of the related hormone, CG, this mutation interferes with a critical cystine bond between C105 and C19 that stabilizes the α-β heterodimer of TSH.[6] Thus, the spectrum of central hypothyroidism should be expanded to include patients with serum TSH levels that are inappropriate for their hypothyroid state. Finally, since the polymerase chain reaction can be used to determine the TSH-subunit gene structure in affected individuals with familial TSH deficiency, a prenatal diagnostic test would be available to screen at-risk pregnancies and allow the physician to initiate prompt thyroid hormone replacement therapy, if indicated.

PRETRANSLATIONAL REGULATION OF THYROTROPIN BIOSYNTHESIS

Thyroid Hormone

In a classic negative feedback system, thyroid hormone inhibits the synthesis of thyrotropin directly at the pituitary level and indirectly at the hypothalamic level by reducing the secretion of thyrotropin-releasing hormone (TRH).[35–38] In several animal models, thyroid hormone treatment results in a dramatic decrease in mRNA levels for the common α- and TSH-β-subunit genes.[35,36] However, the magnitude and rapidity of suppression varies between the subunits. In general, the TSH-β-subunit is suppressed more rapidly (50% inhibition at 4 hours) and to a greater extent (>95% suppression at 4 hours) than the common α-subunit. In addition, after prolonged T₃

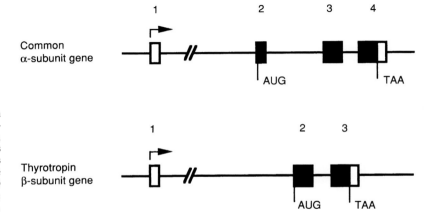

FIGURE 11-2. Schematic representation of the human TSH subunit genes. The human common α- and TSH-β-subunit genes have four and three exons (*numerals*), respectively, represented by boxes separated by itrons (*thin lines*). Coding exons are denoted by black boxes while untranslated regions are represented as white boxes. Translational start (AUG) and stop codons (TAA) are shown in their relative position below each gene; and the start of transcription is shown by a bent arrow.

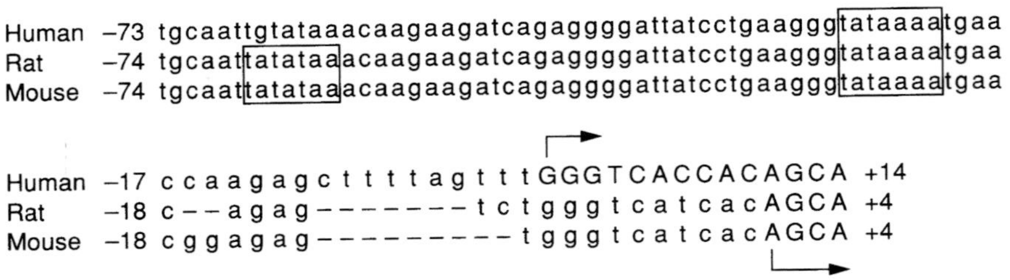

Human −73 tgcaattgtataaacaagaagatcagaggggattatcctgaagggtataaaatgaa
Rat −74 tgcaattatataaacaagaagatcagaggggattatcctgaagggtataaaatgaa
Mouse −74 tgcaattatataaacaagaagatcagaggggattatcctgaagggtataaaatgaa
Human −17 c c a a g a g c t t t t a g t t t GGGTCACCACAGCA +14
Rat −18 c − − a g a g − − − − − − − t c t g g g t c a t c a c AGCA +4
Mouse −18 c g g a g a g − − − − − − − − − t g g g t c a t c a c AGCA +4

FIGURE 11-3. Comparison of the human, rat, and mouse TSH-β-subunit 5′ flanking and first exon DNA sequences. The DNA sequences are aligned to maximize homology; and the 5′ flanking region and first exon sequences are in lowercase and uppercase letters, respectively. TATA boxes used in each species are boxed and the transcriptional start sites are denoted by a bent arrow. By convention 5′ flanking sequences are given negative numbers relative to the start of transcription.

treatment the TSH-β-subunit mRNA was undetectable while the α-subunit mRNA remained at approximately 25% of control levels.[35] Since these studies were performed in a mouse TSH-secreting tumor cell line, they strongly suggest that the mechanism of thyroid hormone inhibition of gene expression must be somewhat different between the subunits.

In addition to the expected suppression of TSH secretion by thyroid hormone, paradoxical increases in TSH secretion have been noted in the early stages of thyroid hormone replacement followed by suppression of TSH later on. Ridgway and coworkers[39] reported that subphysiologic T_3 treatment of hypothyroid patients increased the TSH response to TRH. This effect may be due to a generalized defect in protein synthesis, which is corrected by small doses of T_3, or to the fact that under some conditions TSH-subunit gene expression is stimulated by thyroid hormone, perhaps by a thyroid hormone stimulatory cis-acting element.

Shupnik and colleagues[35] first showed, using a transcriptional run on assay, that thyroid hormone inhibits TSH-subunit gene expression predominantly at the level of gene transcription. Changes in the rate of transcription preceded the observed decrease in subunit mRNA levels but were otherwise similar to the changes in steady state mRNA levels. These data suggest that thyroid hormone, bound to its receptor, binds to cis-acting elements on the common α and TSH-β genes and alters their transcriptional rates.

The proto-oncogene c-*erb*A is the nuclear thyroid hormone receptor and is present in several distinct isoforms.[40–42] In addition, cis-acting elements, which bind the thyroid hormone-receptor complex, are responsible for thyroid hormone inhibition of gene expression and have been identified near the transcriptional start site in the common α- and TSH-β-subunit genes.[43–48] Figure 11-4 shows the location of these elements in the human α- and TSH-β-subunit genes. In the human α gene, the thyroid hormone inhibitory element has been localized to a region from −100 to +4 bp using transient DNA transfection assays.[47] The thyroid hormone receptor has been shown to bind to DNA sequence from −22 to −7 bp (boxed sequences), which contains a region homologous to a positive thyroid hormone response element in the rat GH gene known to bind the thyroid hormone receptor.[49] Recent evidence suggests that a second response element located more 5′ to the originally described element may mediate thyroid hormone inhibition of the common α-subunit.[50] Unlike the α-subunit gene, the thyroid hormone response element of the human TSH gene has been functionally localized to DNA sequences from +3 to +37 bp, entirely within the first exon of the gene.[44] Two thyroid hormone binding sites have also been identified in this element (boxed sequences) and both are necessary to produce thyroid hormone inhibition.

Detailed study of the thyroid hormone inhibitory element in the human TSH-β-subunit genes has revealed unique properties of this element in comparison to thyroid hormone stimulatory elements. First, this element is a "composite element" binding both thyroid hormone receptors and the transcription factor AP-1.[51–53] Binding of AP-1 to this element antagonizes thyroid hormone inhibition, and this may be responsible for a change in set-point regulation of the TSH-β gene mediated by TRH.[51,52] Second, this element does not bind the retinoid X receptor (RXR); and unlike stimulating thyroid hormone response elements, RXR antagonizes thyroid hormone receptor binding to this element.[54] Finally, the mechanism of thyroid hormone inhibition is distinct from thyroid hormone stimulation as evidence by thyroid hormone receptor mutations that can dissociate these functions.[55] These data indicate that unique transcriptional proteins may mediate thyroid hormone stimulation versus inhibition.

Steroid Hormones

Regulation of TSH-subunit gene expression by steroid hormones, including glucocorticoids, estrogen, and testosterone, has been studied by several investigators. In man, pharmacologic doses of dexamethasone decrease plasma TSH levels[56]; and dexamethasone has been used to treat patients with TSH-secreting pituitary adenomas.[57] However, Ross and cowork-

+12
+29
+105
ATC GAA AGG AGA
Ile Glu Arg Arg
ATC TAA AGG AGA
Ile *
TGT GCT GGA TAT
Cys Ala Gly Tyr
TGT GCT AGA TAT
Cys Ala Arg Tyr
TAC TGT ACC AAA
Tyr Cys Thr Lys
TAC GTA CCA AAC
Tyr Val Pro Asn
Wild type
Mutant

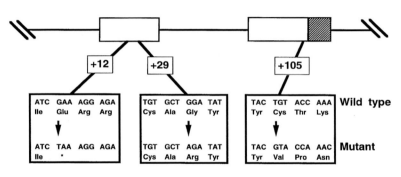

FIGURE 11-4. Point mutations of the human TSH-β gene in patients with familial TSH deficiency. Three-point mutations in the human TSH-β-subunit gene have been described (see text). Two mutations occur in exon 2, and are found in exon 3 and predict either a truncated TSH-β-subunit or one with an amino acid change in the CAGY region.

ers[58] have reported that while dexamethasone in thyrotropic tumor-bearing mice reduced plasma TSH levels, it did not significantly change TSH-subunit mRNA levels. Therefore, dexamethasone may exert its effect on TSH-subunit biosynthesis at a translational or posttranslational level.

In animals and man, estrogen administration does not appear to alter basal or TRH-stimulated TSH levels in the euthyroid state.[59,60] In the hypothyroid rat, however, pharmacologic doses of estradiol appear to augment the effect of thyroid hormone replacement to suppress TSH-α and -β mRNA levels.[60] Since there appears to be some overlap in the cis-acting elements that mediate thyroid hormone and estrogen responses,[61] these studies suggest that pharmacologic doses of estrogen may alter TSH-subunit gene expression through the same or a similar response element as thyroid hormone.

Finally, the effect of testosterone on TSH secretion in humans is unclear. In animal models, however, testosterone appears to have effects similar to estrogen; and this may in part be explained by peripheral conversion of testosterone to estrogen.[61] In summary, steroid hormones do not appear to be major regulators of TSH secretion under normal conditions but may play a role during some pathologic conditions such as hypothyroidism.

Thyrotropin-Releasing Hormone (TRH)

TRH is the major positive regulator of TRH secretion in humans. In animal models, TRH stimulates the transcriptional activity of the TSH-subunit genes three- to fivefold.[62] The stimulatory effect of TRH is augmented in the hypothyroid state and this may, in part, be explained by an alteration in TRH receptor number by thyroid hormone[63] or an alteration in thyroid hormone receptor number by TRH.[64] Alternatively, there may be an interaction between the mechanism of TSH induction and thyroid hormone repression of common α- and TSH-β-subunit gene expression.

In the human TSH-β gene, cis-acting elements that mediate TRH induction are located between −128 and +8 bp.[65] One element is located between −128 and −91 bp and the second element is located from −28 to +8 and includes the TATA box and transcription initiation site. On the other hand, Carr[66] and Shupnik[67] and colleagues have localized TRH induction in the rat TSH-β gene upstream of −204 bp. The reason for the discrepancies in localization studies between the rat and human gene are unknown; the DNA sequences that mediate TRH induction in the human gene are unknown, but the DNA sequences that mediate TRH induction in the human gene are identical to those in the rat TSH-β gene. The upstream element in humans and equivalent region in the rat binds the pituitary-specific transcription factor, Pit-1,[68] and mediates both TRH and cAMP responsiveness of this gene through changes in the state of this protein.[69] Additionally, mutations of the Pit-1 gene have been described in man.[70,71] These patients suffer from a selective loss of somatotroph, lactotroph, and thyrotroph function (combined pituitary hormone deficiency). In some families, only TRH-stimulated expression of TSH and/or prolactin is affected but basal expression of these hormones is maintained, further implicating Pit-1 in the TRH signaling pathway. In the somatotroph and lactotroph, Pit-1 bound to this element is also responsible for cell-specific expression of the prolactin and growth hormone gene.

cAMP

Elevation of intracellular cAMP levels have been shown to increase expression of the common α- and TSH-β-subunit genes. The hypothalamic factor, arginine vasopressin (AVP), is a potent stimulator of TSH release from the thyrotroph.[72] AVP stimulates TSH-subunit gene expression via an increase in cAMP levels; however, it is unclear at present whether the vasopressin receptor in pituitary thyrotrophs is coupled to adenylate cyclase. In the human TSH-β gene, DNA sequences that mediate cAMP induction are located predominantly between −128 and −28 bp of the 5′ flanking region.[65] This region does not contain DNA sequences homologous to the cAMP-responsive element that binds the transacting factor, cAMP-response DNA-binding protein termed CREB,[73] and that mediates induction of the common α-subunit gene. In contrast, Pit-1 via changes in its phosphorylation state mediates cAMP induction of gene expression.[69,74] Convergence of the protein kinase A and C pathways allows for phosphorylation and activation of this protein.

Dopamine

Dopamine rapidly decreases basal and TRH-stimulated TSH secretion in man by approximately 50%.[75] In rat pituitary cells 15 minutes of dopamine treatment decreased TSH-subunit gene transcription by about 50%, and a maximal effect of 75% inhibition was observed after 30 minutes of treatment.[62] Dopamine may act to decrease intracellular cAMP levels and thus interfere with cAMP-mediated stimulation of cAMP TSH-subunit gene expression. Interestingly, dopamine may exert some tonic control of TSH secretion since dopamine antagonists have been shown to increase serum TSH levels in hypothyroid individuals.[76]

Summary of Pretranslation Regulation of the Human Common α- and TSH-β-Subunit Gene Expression

Figure 11-5 is a schematic representation of a thyrotroph and the regulatory pathways that appear to be important in modifying TSH-subunit gene expression. Thyroid hormone is the major negative regulator of TSH-subunit gene expression; dopamine and somatostatin are less important negative regulatory hormones. Thyroid hormone inhibits gene expression by binding to DNA cis-acting elements, via a nuclear thyroid hormone receptor and presumably interacts with the transcription initiation complex. Somatostatin and presumably dopamine reduce intracellular cAMP levels, via an inhibitory guanyl nucleotide binding protein (G), and thus reduce TSH-subunit gene expression.

TRH is the major positive regulator of TSH-subunit gene expression and acts through a guanyl nucleotide binding protein to activate phospholipase C (PLC). Phospholipase C hydrolyzes phosphatidylinositol 4,5-bisphosphate (PIP2) to diacylglycerol (DAG) and inositol 1,4,5 triphosphate (IP$_3$). DAG activates protein kinase C which, in turn, phosphorylates and presumably activates transacting nuclear factors responsible for TSH-subunit gene expression. IP$_3$ releases Ca^{2+} from intracellular pools and raises intracellular Ca^{2+} levels. Another positive regulator of TSH-subunit gene expression is vaso-

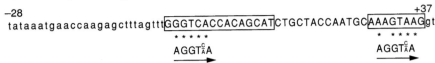

Human common α-subunit gene

–30   +10

    gtataaaa gcaggtgaggactt cattaactGCAGTTACTG
             * * * * * * * * *
             AGGT AT ACC T
                  C   G
                  A   T
                 →   ←

Human TSH β-subunit gene

–28   +37

    tataaatgaaccaagagctttagttt GGGTCACCACAGCAT CTGCTACCAATGC AAAGTAAG gt
                               * * * * *   * * * * *
                               AGGT A   AGGT A
                                   C   C
                                 →   →

FIGURE 11-5. Thyroid hormone inhibitory elements in the human common α- and TSH-β subunit genes. Shown are the 5′ flanking and first exon sequences of the human common a- and TSH-β subunit genes. DNA sequences that bind the thyroid hormone receptor are boxed in either gene, and below each sequence is the consensus binding site (6 pb) for the thyroid hormone receptor proposed by Brent et al.[49] Nucleotides that match the consensus are indicated by asterisks and the relative direction of the element is shown by an arrow.

pressin, which may act via a stimulatory guanyl nucleotide binding protein (G$_s$) to increase intracellular cAMP levels. cAMP then activates protein kinase A (PKA) and cellular proteins are phosphorylated. One such protein is CREB, the cAMP-response DNA-binding protein that has been shown to activate common α-subunit gene transcription. Still unclear are the roles of Ca^{2+} in regulating TSH-subunit gene expression and of cAMP in mediating some of TRH effects on gene expression.

POSTTRANSLATIONAL PROCESSING OF TSH

In Vitro Translation of TSH-α and -β Messenger RNA

The posttranslational processing of TSH was initially studied in cell-free translation systems, which were important to defin-

ing the initial translation products, termed *presubunits.*[77-82] Such pre-α and pre-β-subunits contained the subunit apoproteins as well as aminoterminal leader or signal peptides necessary for translocation across the membrane of the endoplasmic reticulum (Fig. 11-6).

TSH-α messenger RNA was extracted from mouse thyrotropic tumors and translated in wheat germ or reticulocyte lysate cell-free systems that were devoid of enzymes necessary for the proteolytic cleavage of polypeptide precursors or glycosylation.[77-81] The major cell-free translation product, pre-α-subunit, had an apparent molecular weight of 14,000 to 17,000 daltons, depending on the conditions of the gel electrophoresis. Even though it did not contain carbohydrate, its molecular weight was about 3000 daltons greater than the apoprotein portion of the standard α-subunit, suggesting the presence of a signal peptide.

Detection of the TSH-β-subunit precursor, pre-β, in cell-free translation mixtures of mouse tumor mRNA also was

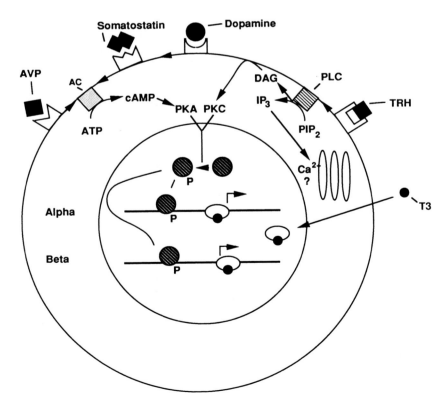

FIGURE 11-6. Overview of the regulation of TSH-subunit biosynthesis in the thyrotroph. The regulatory pathways of TSH-subunit biosynthesis are illustrated in this figure and described in the text. AC, adenylyl cyclase; DAG, diacylglycerol; IP$_3$, inositol 1,4,5 triphosphate; PIP$_2$, phosphatidylinositol 4,5-biphosphate; PKA, protein kinase A; PKC, protein kinase C; PLC, phospholipase C; T$_3$, triiodothyronine; cross-hatched circle, nuclear protein; cross-hatched circle with P, phosphorylated nuclear protein; white oval with overlapping black circle, nuclear thyroid hormone receptor occupied by T$_3$

achieved.[79,80,82] This proved to be more difficult than detection of pre-α, since smaller amounts of the β-precursor were present, and use of an antiserum directed at determinants in the primary structure of reduced, denatured, carboxymethyl TSH-β-subunit was necessary. Gel electrophoresis of the β-precursor disclosed an apparent molecular weight of 15,000, or 2500 daltons greater than the apoprotein portion of standard TSH-β-subunit, consistent with the presence of a signal peptide.

Biosynthesis of TSH in Intact Cells

Studies employing cell-free mRNA translation were important to defining the initial precursor forms of TSH-subunits because these forms are rapidly processed in vivo. Studies of TSH biosynthesis in intact cells, however, were necessary to elucidate the steps of posttranslational processing of TSH, including the glycosylation and combination of TSH-subunits, and the subsequent processing of the oligosaccharides.[83-88]

Following incubation of mouse thyrotropic tumor tissue (derived from a pituitary adenoma containing a pure population of thyrotrophs) with ^{35}S-methionine for 10 minutes, most α-subunits were of molecular weight of 18,000 daltons, while a few were 21,000 daltons.[83-87] When the pulse incubation was followed by chase incubations, the 18,000-dalton form of α-subunit was progressively converted to the 21,000-dalton form. Treatment with endoglycosidase H converted both the 18,000- and 21,000-dalton molecular weight forms of α-subunit to an 11,000-dalton form, consistent with the weight of the apoprotein portion of standard α-subunit. This suggested that the 11,000-dalton, 18,000-dalton, and the 21,000-dalton forms of the α-subunit have 0, 1, and 2 asparagine-linked oligosaccharide chains, respectively.

^{35}S-methionine-labeled β-subunits accumulated as an 18,000-dalton form that was converted to an 11,000-dalton form after endoglycosidase H treatment. Thus, it appeared that the 11,000- and 18,000-dalton forms had 0 and 1 asparagine-linked oligosaccharide units, respectively.[85,86] Approximately 20% of the β-subunits had combined with excess α-subunits after a 20-minute pulse incubation. Analyses of subcellular fractionations disclosed that combination of α- and β-subunits began in the rough endoplasmic reticulum (RER), and that combining subunits had high-mannose, endoglycosidase H–sensitive oligosaccharides.[87,89,90] TSH-subunit precursors were processed slowly to forms with mature complex oligosaccharides that were resistant to endoglycosidase H. TSH and excess free α-subunits, but no free β-subunits, were released into the medium after a 60 to 240-minute chase, and most had endoglycosidase H–resistant oligosaccharide chains.

The free α-subunits that were secreted had a slightly higher molecular weight than the form of α-subunit that combined with β-subunits, and this had been noted in studies of glycoprotein hormones other than TSH as well. Parsons and coworkers[91] reported in 1983 that the free α-subunit derived from bovine pituitaries is glycosylated at an additional site: the threonine at position 43. This residue is located in a domain of the α-subunit believed to contact the β-subunit during heterodimer formation.[1,2] Apparently, free α-subunits bearing this O-linked oligosaccharide are no longer able to bind β-subunits, but the physiologic significance of such noncombining forms of α is unclear.

Processing of High-Mannose Precursor Oligosaccharides

TSH-subunits are cotranslationally glycosylated with oligosaccharides containing three glucose and nine mannose residues, termed *high mannose precursors* (Figs. 11-7 and 11-8). In 1970 Behrens and Leloir[92] demonstrated that hepatocytes contain lipid-linked oligosaccharides that serve as intermediates in glycoprotein biosynthesis. The oligosaccharide (glucose)$_3$ (mannose)$_9$ (N-acetylglucosamine)$_2$, abbreviated Glc$_3$Man$_9$GlcNAc$_2$, is preassembled in rough endoplasmic reticulum linked by phosphates at the reducing terminus to a long organic molecule containing approximately 20 polyprene units, the dolichol phosphate carrier. Asparagine residues in nascent peptides destined to become glycosylated in an N-linked fashion are present in the sequence: asparagine—(X)—serine or asparagine—(X)—threonine, where X is any amino acid. There is a cotranslational en bloc transfer of the oligosaccharide from the dolichol carrier to the asparagine in the nascent chain. Two glucose residues are then quickly trimmed by a glucosidase followed by a slower cleavage of the third glucose by another glucosidase. Mannose residues are then progressively cleaved by two mannosidases until a three-unit "core" remains, followed by addition of GlcNAc and other sugars by specific glycosyltransferases to form complex oligosaccharides. For the pituitary glycoprotein hormones, TSH and LH, such complex oligosaccharides may terminate in either sulfate or sialic acid residues and yield heterogeneous forms with one sulfate (S$_1$), two sulfates (S$_2$), one sialic acid (N$_1$), two sialic acids (N$_2$), three sialic acids (N$_3$), or one sulfate and one sialic acid (S-N). The proposed pathway for such carbohydrate chain synthesis is depicted in Figure 11-8.

Tunicamycin is a drug that inhibits the formation of the oligosaccharide-dolichol carrier precursors and thereby prevents glycosylation of asparagine residues in nascent proteins. In doses of 1 to 5 μg/mL, tunicamycin caused the appearance of new forms of TSH α- and β-subunits of about 11,000 to 12,000 daltons.[85-87] These species incorporated ^{35}S-methionine but not ^{3}H-glucosamine, confirming that they were not glycosylated. These nonglycosylated TSH-subunits were subject to intracellular aggregation and proteolytic degradation, probably because the nascent peptides had not folded properly, and correct internal disulfide bonding had not been achieved.[87,93]

Processing of the high-mannose oligosaccharides of the TSH-subunits is relatively slow compared to other glycoproteins.[84-87,94-96] The rate of trimming of a mannose residue from Man$_9$GlcNAc$_2$ to produce Man$_8$GlcNAc$_8$ units appeared to be much faster for free α-subunits than for TSH. Also, differential processing of α- versus β-subunits of the TSH heterodimer was noted; after a 60-minute incubation with ^{3}H-mannose, the α-subunits of heterodimers had both Man$_9$GlcNAc$_2$ and Man$_8$GlcNAc$_2$ oligosaccharides present, whereas the β-subunits of heterodimers had predominantly Man$_9$GlcNAc$_2$ units.[89]

The structures of high mannose oligosaccharides at the individual glycosylation sites of mouse TSH have been determined by Miura and colleagues.[97] Man$_9$GlcNAc$_2$ and Man$_8$GlcNAc$_2$ units predominated early at each site, but the processing of high mannose oligosaccharides differed at each glycosylation site. These differences were attributed to local conformational differences that affected the interaction of the TSH-subunits with the cellular processing enzymes.

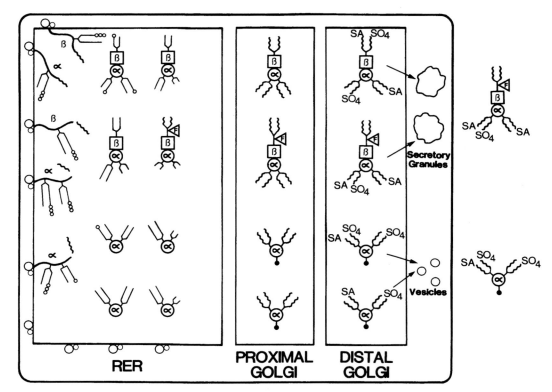

FIGURE 11-7. Model of TSH biosynthesis depicting the RER (rough endoplasmatic reticulum), proximal Golgi, distal Golgi, secretory granules, secretory vesicles, and secreted products of a thyrotroph cell. The cell secretes intact and excess free α-subunit. Circles and squares represent α- and β-subunits of TSH, respectively. In the RER there is contranslational cleavage of signal peptides (*wavy lines*), and glycosylation of asparagine residues in the α- and β-subunit nascent peptide chains. The α-subunit receives two high mannose carbohydrate units while the β-subunit receives one. The oligosaccharides added en bloc generally contain three glucose residues (*small circles*); two glucose residues are rapidly trimmed, followed by trimming of the final glucose residue. Excess α-subunits are present in the RER, and combination of α- and β-subunits begins in the RER while subunits still contain high mannose oligosaccharides (Y). Mannose residues are trimmed from oligosaccharides at different asparagine sites at slightly different rates. In active thyrotrophs, a few Golgi enzymes may be active in the RER resulting in core fucosylation (*F in triangle*) or other "Golgi" processing steps occurring at an unusually early site in the secretory pathway.

In the proximal Golgi, galactose, N-acetylgalactosamine, or other sugars are added to the asparagine-linked oligosaccharides (*zigzag lines*) to yield endoglycosidase H-resistant forms of subunits. Excess α-subunits are O-glycosylated (*solid circles*). In the distal Golgi, sulfate (SO_4) and/or sialic acid (SA) residues are added. TSH heterodimers enter a regulated pathway of secretory granules, whereas excess α-subunits enter a more constitutive pathway of secretory vesicles. Finally, fully processed TSH and α-subunits containing heterogeneous oligosaccharide structures are secreted.

Terminal Sulfation and Sialylation of Complex Oligosaccharides

The presence of an unusual terminal substituent on TSH oligosaccharides had been suggested by studies showing that TSH, unlike CG, was partially resistant to neuraminidase digestion. Subsequently Parsons and Pierce[98] detected the presence of sulfate on certain complex oligosaccharides of bovine TSH and LH α-subunits as well as human LH, but not hCG. They postulated that the negatively charged sulfate may play some functional role comparable to that of the negatively charged sialic acid. Hortin and coworkers[99] demonstrated the metabolic incorporation of ^{35}S-sulfate into the oligosaccharides of the α- and β-subunits of bovine LH while Anumula and Bahl[100] obtained similar results using ovine LH. Gesundheit and colleagues[101] showed that mouse TSH-subunits could

be metabolically labeled with sulfate and sialic acid. They also showed differential sulfation of TSH-α and β-subunits, as well as the fact that the sulfate moieties were entirely linked to carbohydrate chains.[102]

Baenziger and his associates first demonstrated that the sulfate moiety in TSH and LH oligosaccharides is covalently linked to N-acetylgalactosamine residues, in contrast to the usual terminal structure of complex oligosaccharides where sialic acid is bound to galactose residues.[3–5,103] Subsequently these workers have partially characterized an N-acetylgalactosaminidase-transferase in bovine pituitary membranes that specifically recognizes the β-subunits of TSH and LH, as well as the common α-subunit.[104] There are amino acid sequences in the linear structure of the subunits that allow specific recognition by this enzyme.[105] A pituitary sulfotransferase, specific for the oligosaccharide sequence GalNac-GlcNAc-Man, is responsible for trans-

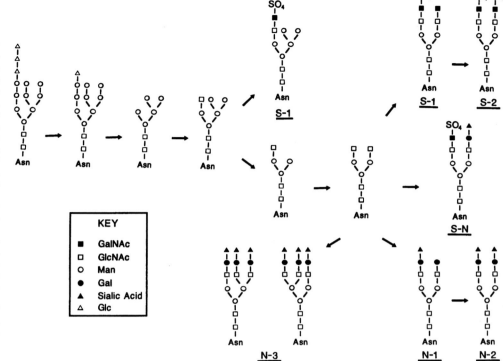

FIGURE 11-8. Pathway for biosynthesis of sulfated and sialylated Asn-linked oligosaccharides. Asn residues are glycosylated with high mannose units containing three glucose residues. Two glucose residues are then rapidly trimmed, followed by removal of the final glucose and then several mannose residues; N-acetylglucosamine residues are then added to the three core mannoses. A key branch point is the addition of Gal vs. GalNAc residues; Gal residues may then have sialic acid attached, whereas GalNAc residues may become sulfated. S-1, S-2, or S-3, number of sulfates; N-1, N-2, or N-3, number of sialic acid residues present; S-N, an oligosaccharide with one antenna capped with sulfate and the other with sialic acid. (Baenziger JU, Green ED. Pituitary glycoprotein hormone oligosaccharides: structure, synthesis and function of the asparagine-like oligosaccharides on lutropin, follitropin and thyrotropin. Biochem Biophys Acta 1988; 947:287)

fer of the sulfate moiety to the oligosaccharide and does not require subunit peptide determinants for recognition. This enzyme, like the GalNAc-transferase is absent from the placenta, which explains why only pituitary glycoprotein hormones contain the unusual GalNAc-sulfate terminal residues. Sulfotransferase activity has been observed in Golgi-derived membranes from bovine and mouse pituitary tissue, and it has been shown that the subcellular site of sulfation of mouse TSH and free α-subunits is in the Golgi apparatus.[106,107] A hepatic receptor specific for SO^4-GalNAc has been described.[108]

The structures and distributions of heterogeneous forms of sulfated and sialyated oligosaccharides on TSH as well as various other glycoprotein hormones have been determined.[8,9,102,109] In general such studies have employed characterization of biosynthetically or chemically labeled oligosaccharides released from subunits by the use of specific endoglycosidases and subsequently characterized by anion exchange high performance liquid chromatography. Green and Baenziger have extensively characterized the complex oligosaccharide structures for a variety of glycoprotein hormones purified from bovine or human pituitary tissues.[3,4] These workers found that for bovine TSH, 48% of the oligosaccharides contained 2 sulfate residues, 32% 1 sulfate, 18% neutral, and 2% contained 1 sulfate and 1 sialic acid; no complex oligosaccharides contained sialic acid residues exclusively. In contrast, the complex oligosaccharide structure of human TSH was somewhat different: 25% contained 1 sulfate, 21% 1 sulfate and 1 sialic acid, 18% neutral, 12% 2 sialic acids and 5% 1 sialic acid residue. The distributions of sulfated and sialyated oligosaccharides of bovine, ovine, and human gonadotropins also were reported, and each glycoprotein hormone had a unique spectrum of sulfated and sialyated

oligosaccharides. Using similar methods, Gyves[110,111] and DeCherney[112] with coworkers found that secreted forms of rat and mouse TSH had somewhat different distributions of sialyated and sulfated oligosaccharides, and that there were major differences between the α- and β-subunits. As described next, such heterogeneous forms of complex oligosaccharides were further modified depending on the developmental and endocrine status of the animal.

In addition to terminal sulfation and sialylation, TSH oligosaccharides contain variable amounts of fucose linked to the innermost N-acetylglucosamine residue.[109] In general the β-subunit of TSH contains about twice as much fucose as α-subunit.[101,113] Although fucosylation is normally thought to occur primarily in the Golgi apparatus, Magner and associates have demonstrated that in pituitaries from hypothyroid mice a major proportion of fucosylation occurs in the rough endoplasmic reticulum.[114] Intravenous infusion of TRH into normal persons causes the acute release of TSH isoforms that are more highly fucosylated than the basal TSH,[115] but a further increase in TSH fucosylation is not observed after TRH administration to patients with thyrotropic pituitary tumors.[116]

DEVELOPMENTAL AND ENDOCRINE REGULATION OF TSH GLYCOSYLATION

Ronin and colleagues first demonstrated that high mannose oligosaccharides of TSH were differentially processed in mouse pituitary glands depending on the thyroidal state of the animal or after treatment with TRH.[96] Gesundheit and associates showed that complex oligosaccharides on TSH secreted from hypothyroid mouse pituitary glands could be altered by treatment with TRH.[117] After in vitro TRH administration there was increased secretion of TSH enriched in biantennary complex oligosaccharides as opposed to more complicated triantennary forms. Interestingly, this effect was closely coupled to hormone secretion, and intracellular forms of TSH did not show modulation of carbohydrate structure. In vivo studies by Taylor and coworkers using rats with hypothalamic or thyroidal hypothyroidism also found alterations in TSH oligosaccharide structure using lectin analysis of TSH glycopeptides.[118–121] These workers found that animals with paraventricular nuclear lesions of the hypothalamus resulting in endogenous TRH deficiency showed TSH with fewer biantennary structures compared to normal controls. In contrast, thyroidectomized animals showed secretion of TSH with more complex triantennary structures. After in vivo administration of TRH animals with hypothalamic hypothyroidism showed an increase in multiantennary structures approaching those of normal animals. The differences between in vitro and in vivo TRH administration on TSH carbohydrate structure may relate to the fact that static administration of TRH in culture produces a different pattern of glycosylation from the presumably endogenous pulsatile pattern of TRH in vivo. Technical or other factors may explain differing results.[122] Gyves and colleagues described the pattern of sulfated and sialylated oligosaccharides of secreted rat TSH in fetal and neonatal animals during maturation of the pituitary thyroid axis.[110,123] During neonatal development there were increased amounts of sialylated compared to sulfated oligosaccharides, as well as an increase in all forms of complex oligosaccharides containing three or more negatively charged terminal moieties. These effects, presumably related to increased endogenous TRH secretion, may have implications for the understanding of the unique physiology of TSH in the neonatal period.

Using anion exchange HPLC, Gyves and others[111] and DeCherney and coworkers[12] have characterized changes in the carbohydrate structure of TSH from hypothyroid rats in the neonatal as well as in adult animals. In the neonatal period hypothyroidism of even a few days' or weeks' duration resulted in major increases in the sialylated compared to sulfated oligosaccharides. This effect, which was observed in both the α- and β-subunits, was particularly striking in the latter. Moreover, β-subunit showed a major increase in forms containing three or more charged oligosaccharide units. Similar increases in the proportion of sialylated compared to sulfated oligosaccharides have been noticed in adult animals. However, in contrast to the neonatal period, adult rats did not show major changes until after a longer period of hypothyroidism.

Using lectin analysis of TSH in human serum, Miura and associates also demonstrated different degrees of sialylation of TSH in sera of euthyroid, primary and central hypothyroid subjects,[124] findings that were confirmed and extended by Papandreou and colleagues.[125,126] Moreover, Lee and coworkers have reported that patients with severe nonthyroidal illness secrete forms of TSH with altered binding to concanavalin-A, suggesting increased amounts of multiantennary complex chains.[127]

Gesundheit and coworkers reported that TSH in α-subunits secreted by an aggressive pituitary adenoma demonstrated more bisecting and multiantennary oligosaccharide units than those from a less aggressive tumor.[128] Oligosaccharide heterogeneity of TSH and free α-subunits secreted by

TSH-producing pituitary tumors has now been well documented.[129–131] The somatostatin analogue octreotide often lowers TSH secretion by such tumors[132] and also may change the qualitative nature of the TSH that is secreted.[133]

All of the above studies have clearly demonstrated that the complex carbohydrate structure of TSH can be regulated by a variety of developmental and endocrine factors, as well as in neoplasia. It thus seems likely that the majority of changes previously noted in studies of TSH heterogeneity by isoelectric focusing or chromatofocusing relate to such changes in carbohydrate structure.[134–138] However, as pointed out previously, a certain degree of heterogeneity in purified pituitary preparations may relate to proteolytic cleavages either at the amino- or carboxy-terminus of TSH subunits, as well as to the amidation of glutamic and aspartic acid residues. Although the functional role of changes in TSH carbohydrated structure have not been completely elucidated, it is very clear that certain of these changes in carbohydrate structure are associated with changes in TSH in vitro biologic activity or in metabolic clearance rate.

Only recently have studies been performed to elucidate the underlying cellular mechanisms responsible for the physiologic modulation of TSH oligosaccharide structures. Helton and Magner employed in situ hybridization and demonstrated that, when mice received propylthiouracil and became hypothyroid, the thyrotrophs developed increased levels of mRNAs for α-2,6 sialyltransferase, β-1,4 galactosyltransferase and α-mannosidase II.[139,140] These increased mRNA levels may have resulted from increased gene transcription or from message stabilization.

BIOACTIVITY AND METABOLIC CLEARANCE OF TSH

Heterogeneous forms of TSH may show different degrees of biologic activity in a variety of in vivo and in vitro bioassays (reviewed in references 8 and 9). Such differences in activity are primarily due to differences in carbohydrate composition, as noted previously. The earliest in vivo bioassays were related to the ability of TSH to elicit a release of labeled iodine from the thyroid into guinea pig or mouse blood. Subsequently a variety of sensitive in vitro bioassays were developed, including measurement of labeled iodine release from prelabeled guinea pig thyroid slices, intact mouse thyroid glands, and measurements of cyclic AMP accumulation or adenylyl cyclase activity in thyroid membranes or intact cells.[141] Moreover, a very sensitive cytochemical bioassay has been developed, which is technically demanding and has only been applied in a few centers. The development of the rat FRTL-5 thyroid cell line has provided a convenient TSH bioassay system. Moreover, a variety of endpoints can be studied, including cAMP production, iodine trapping, and stimulation of cell growth. Unfortunately, except for the cytochemical bioassay, even such new in vitro methods still require purification and concentration of TSH from crude serum before assay, and recovery of immunoactive TSH is not always complete.[142–145] Recombinant human TSH isoforms available in larger quantities have recently expanded our understanding of the relationship between TSH oligosaccharide structure, particularly sialylation, and bioactivity.[11]

The role of the complex oligosaccharide moieties in TSH action also has been determined by studies in which chemical or enzymatic deglycosylation was used to remove complex side-chains. Initial studies employed preparations of bovine or human TSH treated in anhydrous hydrogen fluoride or trifluoromethane sulfonic acid.[146-148] Although deglycosylated TSH showed similar receptor binding properties compared to the native hormone, it showed markedly decreased biologic activity both in vitro and in vivo. Moreover, the deglycosylated hormone was shown to be a competitive antagonist for the native hormone.[147] However, it had not been unequivocally established that the loss of biologic activity after chemical deglycosylation was due only to carbohydrate removal rather than to other changes such as alteration of the conformation of the polypeptide chains. Thus it was important to re-examine the effect of deglycosylation using newly available endoglycosidases. As mentioned above, exoglycosidase treatment of TSH was not effective because most carbohydrate chains terminated in sulfate, for which no specific sulfatase has yet been purified. Using enzymatic deglycosylation by endoglycosidase F, Thotakura and colleagues demonstrated that the receptor binding activity of enzymatically deglycosylated TSH was minimally affected by carbohydrate removal, yet the in vitro bioactivity was greatly reduced.[148] More recent studies have confirmed the link between TSH oligosaccharide structure and bioactivity, and they have established that the oligosaccharides of the α-subunit are particularly important for bioactivity.[149-156]

Early workers had shown that a variety of TSH isohormones separated by isoelectric focusing had different bioactivities, but the chemical basis of these differences remained unclear. Joshi and Weintraub demonstrated that diverse forms of mouse TSH with different carbohydrate composition based on interaction with lectin columns showed different biologic:immunologic ratios.[157] Menezes-Ferreira and coworkers showed that in vitro treatment of rat pituitary glands with TRH led to secretion of TSH with increased bioactivity.[158] Since other studies described above have demonstrated that TRH treatment alters TSH carbohydrate structure, it seems reasonable to conclude that such altered bioactivity is related to changes in carbohydrate. Faglia and associates[159] as well as Beck-Peccoz and colleagues[142] have proved that serum TSH from certain patients with central hypothyroidism displayed decreased biologic:immunologic ratios in both a cytochemical bioassay as well as an adenylyl cyclase stimulating assay. When some of these patients were treated chronically with TRH, the biologic:immunologic ratios increased and resulted clinically in increased serum thyroid hormone levels.[142] Again, such changes in bioactivity may be related to the change in carbohydrate structure demonstrated by lectin binding studies mentioned above. Dahlberg and colleagues have noted increased biologic:immunologic ratios in certain patients with primary hypothyroidism, as well as a general correlation between the degree of hypothyroidism and the elevation of the ratio.[144] Moreover, increased biologic:immunologic ratios have been observed in hyper- or euthyroid patients with TSH-producing tumors[143,145] and the bioactivity has decreased towards normal after pituitary surgery.[143] In certain cases dissociations have been noticed between the cAMP response and the iodide-trapping response for certain forms of TSH secreted by pituitary tumors.[143] Isoforms of thyrotropin having enhanced bioactivity are secreted by patients who are resistant to thyroid hormone.[160]

However, a change in the biologic:immunologic ratio of thyrotropin in serum does not necessarily prove an alteration in the intrinsic bioactivity of the hormone.[141,161] It is possible that the immunologic activity of the ratio may also vary, although most polyclonal antisera are relatively insensitive to minimal structural modification, including near-total chemical or enzymatic deglycosylation. Such altered immunoactivity may be more of a problem with certain monoclonal antibodies developed to very specific epitopes which are now used in newer sandwich immunoassays. However, immunoactivity has been the most widely available technique to estimate the mass of the hormone in crude human sera and it is not usually feasible to purify the hormone from serum to estimate mass by more rigorous chemical methods. However, for purified hormone in which the mass can be determined rigorously by amino acid analysis, such bioactivity studies are free from these caveats.

In addition to the role of oligosaccharides in TSH bioactivity in vitro, other studies have also shown that they affect the metabolic clearance rate in vivo. Early studies of the metabolic clearance rate of human TSH showed that the specific half-time of disappearance depended on the thyroid state of the patient—being slower in hypothyroid individuals and faster in hyperthyroid individuals.[162] Moreover, when the clearance of human TSH was studied in the dog, the kidney was found to be the major organ of clearance.[163] Similarly, studies of rat TSH clearance have shown the kidney as the major organ of clearance, with the thyroid being the organ of secondary importance, and virtually no clearance related to the liver, which clears asialoglycoproteins containing terminal galactose residues.[164] Constant and Weintraub showed that after chemical deglycosylation the clearance of rat TSH was increased.[164] Moreover, TSH from hypothyroid rat pituitaries or rat sera displayed a slower metabolic clearance rate even when injected into euthyroid rats. These studies suggested that, in addition to the metabolic status of the animal in which the clearance studies were performed, the thyroid status of the animal from which the TSH was derived was also important. Presumably, the slower metabolic clearance rate in hypothyroid rats related to its increased sialylation as discussed earlier in direct studies of TSH carbohydrate structure.[111,112,124] Studies of recombinant human TSH have proven that sialylation is an important determinant of the hormone's metabolic clearance rate and in vivo bioactivity.[11] These studies strongly suggest that thyroid-induced changes in TSH carbohydrate structure can alter the metabolic clearance rate and thus the in vivo bioactivity in addition to changes previously described on intrinsic bioactivity.

THREE-DIMENSIONAL CONFORMATION OF THYROTROPIN

During the early 1990s a number of workers using computer modeling, site-directed mutagenesis of the α-subunit and/or antibodies or synthetic peptides attempted to make inferences about the three-dimensional conformation of TSH, the subunit contact domains, and the receptor binding domains of the two subunits.[165–178] A great advance occurred in 1994, when the crystallographic structure of hCG was determined.[6,7] It is likely that the general conformation of TSH will be similar to that of hCG, although the specific differences will be extremely important to determine in the future. The hCG structure has allowed the correct disulfide bonds within the subunits to be determined, crucial information for a meaningful model to be constructed. Peculiar features of the hCG structure include a curious cystine knot motif, and the existence of a "seatbelt" binding the two subunits: the carboxy-terminal tail of the β-subunit loops around the α-subunit and then is tethered to another region of the β-subunit by a disulfide bond. The folding of the α- and the β-subunits are similar. Both subunits have an elongated shape with a high ratio of protein surface to hydrophobic core. One of the α-subunit oligosaccharides known to be more important for signal transduction, the oligosaccharide at Asn-52, lies near α-subunit and β-subunit residues believed to be vital for receptor binding. However, it must be emphasized that in addition to differences between hCG and TSH amino acids, differences in glycosylation may also affect structure. Finally, TSH may undergo a conformational change when bound to its receptor. Thus, ultimately TSH and its receptor must be separately crystallized and then cocrystallized.

RECOMBINANT HUMAN THYROTROPIN

Recombinant human TSH has been produced after transfection of the common α-subunit gene as well as the specific human TSH-β-subunit gene into human embryonic kidney cells or Chinese hamster ovary cells.[10,11,179–181] The carbohydrate compositional analysis of recombinant TSH showed it to be more highly sialylated than standard pituitary TSH and also contained no N-acetylgalactosamine which implied the absence of terminal sulfate moieties, both of which are present in pituitary TSH.[11,166] The absence of N-acetylgalactosamine and sulfate was expected, since only the pituitary was shown to contain the specific enzymes for transfer of these moieties to carbohydrate chains. The recombinant human TSH showed a maximum stimulatory activity similar to that of pituitary TSH in two different in vitro bioassays.[180] However, the recombinant preparation showed slightly less potency as judged by the concentration required for half-maximal response. This decreased potency was clearly related to the increased sialic acid content, because after neuraminidase treatment the activity of the preparation was restored toward normal. The recombinant human TSH also had a twofold slower metabolic clearance rate than pituitary TSH, which resulted in a greater than tenfold higher serum concentration at 3 hours as compared to pituitary TSH after intravenous injection.[180] The slower metabolic clearance rate was again related to the increased sialic acid content, since after neuraminidase treatment the clearance rate was considerably greater. These studies indicate that recombinant human TSH, like TSH from rodents[111,112] or humans[124] with primary hypothyroidism, contains a higher degree of sialylation than standard pituitary TSH, which results in a slower metabolic clearance rate and a higher serum concentration.

In recent years, it has been possible to produce recombinant human TSH in large quantities from both large commercial[10] as well as smaller laboratory bioreactors.[11] Unlike natural human TSH derived from a large number of human pituitaries obtained at autopsy, recombinant TSH is more homogeneous and free of other contaminating pituitary hormones and growth factors as well as artifactual proteolytic cleavage products. Heterogeneity of the recombinant hormone has been shown to be primarily related to six to nine different isoforms differing in the number of terminal sialic acid residues present in the carbohydrate chains.[11] Such material has provided valuable new insights into structure-function relationships of TSH as well as the role of each sugar moiety in hormone action.[11,154]

Recombinant TSH is also valuable clinically and has provided a new diagnostic agent for the stimulation of radioactive iodide uptake and thyroglobulin secretion in patients with thyroid cancer. Preliminary phase 1 and 2 clinical trials have shown that this agent, which can be given while patients are euthyroid on replacement or suppressive therapy, produces thyroid and whole body scans apparently equivalent to those achieved after 2 weeks of hypothyroidism.[15] A larger and more definitive phase 3 trial has been completed and the data from this trial are currently being analyzed.

References

1. Pierce JG. Thyrotropin: Chemistry. In: Ingbar S, Braverman L, eds. The thyroid. Philadelphia: JB Lippincott, 1986:267
2. Pierce JG, Parsons TF. Glycoprotein hormones: structure and function. Annu Rev Biochem 1981;50:465
3. Green ED, Baenziger JU. Asparagine-linked oligosaccharides on lutropin, follitropin, and thyrotropin. I. structural elucidation of the sulfated and sialylated oligosaccharides on bovine, ovine, and human pituitary glycoprotein hormones. J Biol Chem 1988;263:25
4. Green ED, Baenziger JU. Asparagine-linked oligosaccharides on lutropin, follitropin, and thyrotropin. II. Distributions of sulfated and sialylated oligosaccharides on bovine, ovine, and human pituitary glycoprotein hormones. J Biol Chem 1988;263:36
5. Green ED, Gruenebaum J, Bielinska M, Baenziger JU, Boime I. Sulfation of lutropin oligosaccharides with a cell-free system. Proc Natl Acad Sci U S A 1984;81:5320
6. Lapthorn AJ, Harris DC, Littlejohn A, et al. Crystal structure of human chorionic gonadotropin. Nature 1994;369:455
7. Wu H, Lustbader JW, Liu Y, Canfield RE, Hendrickson WA. Structure of human chorionic gonadotropin at 2.6Å resolution from MAD analysis of the selenomethionyl protein. Structure 1994;2:545
8. Magner JA. Thyroid-stimulating hormone: biosynthesis, cell biology, and bioactivity. Endocrinol Rev 1990;11:354
9. Magner JA. Biosynthesis, cell biology, and bioactivity of thyroid-stimulating hormone: update 1994. Endocrinol Rev Mono 1994;3:55
10. Cole ES, Lee K, Lauziere K, et al. Recombinant human thyroid stimulating hormone: development of a biotechnology product for detection of metastatic lesions of thyroid carcinoma. Biotechnology 1993;11:1014
11. Szkudlinski MW, Thotakura NR, Bucc I, et al. Purification and characterization of recombinant human thyrotropin (TSH) isoforms produced by Chinese hamster ovary cells: the role of sialylation and sulfation in TSH bioactivity. Endocrinology 1993; 133:1490
12. Huber GK, Fong P, Concepcion ES, Davies TF. Recombinant human thyroid-stimulating hormone: initial bioactivity assessment

using human fetal thyroid cells. J Clin Endocrinol Metab 1991;72:1328

13. Kashiwai T, Ichihara K, Endo Y, Tamaki H, Amino N, Miyai K. Immunological and biological characteristics of recombinant human thyrotropin. J Immunol Methods 1991;143:25

14. Braverman LE, Pratt BM, Ebner S, Longcope C. Recombinant human thyrotropin stimulates thyroid function and radioactive iodine uptake in the rhesus monkey. J Clin Endocrinol Metab 1992;74:1135

15. Meier CA, Braverman LE, Ebner SA, et al. Diagnostic use of recombinant human thyrotropin in patients with thyroid carcinoma. J Clin Endocrinol Metab 1994;78:188

16. Dracopoli NC, Retting WJ, Whitfield GK, et al. Assignment of the gene for the β subunit of thyroid stimulating hormone to the short arm of human chromosome 1. Proc Natl Acad Sci U S A 1986;83:1822

17. Goodwin RG, Moncman CL, Rottman FM, Nilson JH. Characterization and nucleotide sequence of the gene for the common α subunit of the bovine pituitary glycoprotein hormones. Nucleic Acids Res 1983;11:6873

18. Gordon DF, Wood WM, Ridgway EC. Organization and nucleotide sequence of the mouse α subunit gene of the pituitary glycoprotein hormones. DNA 1988;7:679

19. Burnside J, Buckland PR, Chin WW. Isolation and characterization of the gene encoding the α subunit of the rat pituitary glycoprotein hormones. Gene 1988;70:67

20. Fiddes JC, Goodman HM. The gene encoding the common alpha subunit of the four human glycoprotein hormones. J Mol Appl Genet 1981;1:3

21. Breathnach R, Chambon P. Organization and expression of eucaryotic split genes coding for proteins. Annu Rev Biochem 1981;50:349

22. Deutsch PJ, Jameson JL, Habener JF. Cyclic AMP responsiveness of human gonadotropin a gene transcription is directed by a repeated 10-bp enhancer. J Biol Chem 1987;262:12169

23. Silver BJ, Bokar JA, Virgin JB, Vallen EA, Milsted A, Nilson JH. Cyclin AMP regulation of the human glycoprotein hormone α subunit is mediated by an 18-bp element. Proc Natl Acad Sci U S A 1987;84:2198

24. Bokar JA, Keri RA, Farmerie TA, et al. Expression of the glycoprotein hormone α subunit gene in the placenta requires a functional cyclic AMP response element, whereas a different cis-acting element mediates pituitary-specific expression. Mol Cell Biol 1989;9:5113

25. Carr FE, Heed LR, Chin WW. Isolation and characterization of the rat thyrotropin β subunit gene: differential regulation of two transcriptional start sites by thyroid hormone. J Biol Chem 1987;262:981

26. Wondisford FE, Radovick S, Moates JM, Usala SJ, Weintraub BD. Isolation and characterization of the human thyrotropin β subunit gene. J Biol Chem 1988;262:12538

27. Guidon PT, Whitfield GK, Porti D, Kourides IA. The human thyrotropin β subunit gene differs in 5′ structure from murine TSHβ genes. DNA 1988;7:691

28. Tatsumi K, Hayashizaki Y, Hiraoka Y, Miyai K, Matsubara K. The structure of the human thyrotropin β subunit gene. 1988;73:489

29. Wolf D, Kourides IA, Gurr JA. Expression the gene for the β subunit of mouse thyrotropin results in multiple mRNAs differing in their 5′ untranslated region. J Biol Chem 1987;262:16596

30. Gordon DF, Wood WM, Ridgway EC. Organization and nucleotide sequence of −16 gene encoding the β subunit of murine thyrotropin. DNA 1988;7:17

31. Samuels MH, Wood WM, Gordon DF, Kleinschmidt-DeMasters BK, Lillehei K, Ridgway EC. Clinical and molecular studies of a thyrotropin-secreting pituitary adenoma. J Clin Endocrin Metab 1989;68:1211

32. Hayashizaki Y, Hiraoka Y, Endo Y, Miyai K, Matsubara K. Thyroid-stimulating hormone (TSH) deficiency caused by a single base substitution in the CAGYC region of the β subunit. EMBO J 1989;8:2291

33. Dacou-Voutetakis C, Feltquate DM, Drakopoulou M, Kourides IA, Dracopoli NC. Familiar hypothyroidism caused by a nonsense mutation in the thyroid-stimulating hormone β subunit gene. Am J Hum Genet 1990;16:988

34. Rajan SG, Kommareddi S, Nations M, et al. Familial hypothyroidism caused by a frameshift mutation in the thyrotropin beta-subunit gene: evidence for a bioinactive molecule. 66th Annual Meeting of the American Thyroid Association, Rochester, MN, 1992

35. Shupnik MA, Chin WW, Habener JF, Ridgway EC. Transcriptional regulation of the thyrotropin subunit genes by thyroid hormone. J Biol Chem 1985;260:2900

36. Gurr JA, Kourides IA. Thyroid hormone regulation of thyrotropin α and β subunit gene transcription. DNA 1985;4:301

37. Segerson TP, Kauer J, Wolfe HC, et al. Thyroid hormone regulates TRH biosynthesis in the paraventricular nucleus of the rat hypothalamus. Science 1987;238:78

38. Taylor T, Wondisford FE, Blaine T, Weintraub BD. The paraventricular nucleus of the hypothalamus has a major role in thyroid hormone feedback regulation of thyrotropin synthesis and secretion. Endocrinology 1990;126:317

39. Ridgway EC, Kourides IA, Chin WW, Cooper DS, Maloof F. Augmentation of pituitary thyrotropin response to TRH during subphysiological tri-iodothyronine therapy in hypothyroidism. Clin Endocrinol (Oxf) 1979;10:343

40. Weinberger C, Thompson CC, Ong ES, Lebo R, Gruol DJ, Evans RM. The c-erbA gene encodes a thyroid hormone receptor. Nature 1986;324:641

41. Sap J, Munoz A, Damm K, et al. The c-cibA protein is a high affinity receptor for thyroid hormone. Nature 1986;324:635

42. Lazar MA. Thyroid hormone receptors: multiple forms, multiple possibilities. Endocr Rev 1993;14:84

43. Carr FE, Burnside J, Chin WW. Thyroid hormones regulate rat thyrotropin β gene promoter activity expressed in GH3 cells. Mol Endocrinol 1989;3:709

44. Wondisford FE, Farr EA, Radovick S, et al. Thyroid hormone inhibition of human thyrotropin b subunit gene expression is mediated by a cis-acting element located in the first exon. J Biol Chem 1989;264:14601

45. Wood WM, Kao MY, Gordon DF, Ridgway EC. Thyroid hormone regulates the mouse thyrotropin β subunit gene promoter in transfected primary thyrotropes. J Biol Chem 1989;264:14840

46. Burnside J, Darling DS, Carr FE, Chin WW. Thyroid hormone regulation of the rat glycoprotein hormone a subunit gene promoter activity. J Biol Chem 1989; 264:6886

47. Chatterjee VKK, Lee J, Rentoumis A, Jameson JL. Negative regulation of the thyroid hormone-stimulating hormone α gene by thyroid hormone:receptor interaction adjacent to the TATA box. J Biol Chem 1989;86:9114

48. Balfour NJ, Franklyn JA, Gurr JA, Sheppard MC. Multiple DNA elements determine basal and thyroid hormone regulated expression of the human glycoprotein α subunit gene in pituitary cells. J Mol Endocrinol 1990;4:187

49. Brent GA, Harney JW, Chen Y, Warne RL, Moore DD, Larsen PR. Mutations of the rat growth hormone promoter which increase and decrease response to thyroid hormone define a consensus thyroid hormone response element. Mol Endocrinol 1989; 3:1996

50. Pennathur S, Madison LD, Kay TWH, Jameson JL. Localization of promoter sequences required for thyrotropin-releasing hormone and thyroid hormone responsiveness of the glycoprotein hormone α-gene in primary cultures of rat pituitary cells. Mol Endocrin 1993;7:797

51. Wondisford FE, Steinfelder HJ, Nations M, Radovick R. AP-1 antagonizes thyroid hormone receptor action on the thyrotropin β-subunit gene. J Biol Chem 1993;268:4,2749

52. Kim MK, McClaskey JH, Bodenner DL, Weintraub BD. An AP-1-like factor and the pituitary-specification Pit-1 are both necessary to mediate hormonal induction of human thyrotropin beta gene expression. J Biol Chem 1993;268:4,23366

53. Pfahl M. Nuclear receptor/AP-1 interaction. Endocr Rev 14;5:651

54. Cohen O, Hegarty MK, Wondisford FE. Retinoid X receptors inhibit binding and function of thyroid hormone receptors on a negative thyroid hormone response element. American Thyroid Association Annual Meeting, Tampa, FL, 1993

55. Flynn TR, Hollenberg AN, Cohen O, Menke JB, Usala SJ, Tollin S, Hegarty MK. A novel C-terminal domain in the thyroid hormone receptor selectively mediates thyroid hormone inhibition. J Biol Chem 1994;269:32713

56. Re RN, Kourides IA, Ridgway EC. The effect of glucocorticoid administration on human pituitary secretion of thyrotropin and prolactin. J Clin Endocrinol Metab 1976;43:338

57. Smallridge RC. Thyrotropin-secreting pituitary tumors. In: Molitch ME, ed. Endocrinology and metabolism clinics of North America. Philadelphia: WB Saunders Co, 1987:765

58. Ross DS, Ellis MF, Milbury P, Ridgway EC. A comparison of changes in plasma thyrotropin β and α subunits, and mouse thyrotropic tumor thyrotropin β and α subunit mRNA concentrations after in vivo dexamethasone or T3 administration. Metabolism 1987;36:799

59. Spitz IM, Zylber-Horan EA, Trestian S. The thyrotropin (TSH) profile in isolated gonadotropin deficiency: a model to evaluate the effect of sex steroids on TSH secretion. J Clin Endocrinol Metab 1983;57:415

60. Ahlquist JAO, Franklyn JA, Wood DF, et al. Hormonal regulation of thyrotropin synthesis and secretion. Horm Metab Res 1987; 517:86

61. Glass CK, Holloway JM, Devary OV, Rosenfeld MG. The thyroid hormone receptor binds with opposite transcriptional effects to a common sequence motif in thyroid hormone and estrogen response elements. Cell 1988;54:313

62. Shupnik MA, Greenspan SL, Ridgway EC. Transcriptional regulation of thyrotropin subunit genes by thyrotropin-releasing hormone and dopamine in pituitary cell culture. J Biol Chem 1986; 261:12675

63. Perrone MH, Hinkle PM. Regulation of pituitary receptors for thyrotropin-releasing hormone by thyroid hormones. J Biol Chem 1978;253:5168

64. Kaji H, Hinkle PM. Regulation of thyroid hormone receptors and responses by thyrotropin-releasing hormone in GH4C cells. Endocrinology 1987;121:1697

65. Weintraub BD, Wondisford FE, Farr EA, et al. Pre-translational and post-translational regulation of TSH synthesis in normal and neoplastic thyrotrophs. Horm Res 1989;32:22

66. Carr FE, Shupnik MA, Burnside J, Chin WW. Thyrotropin-releasing hormone stimulates the activity of the rat thyrotropin β subunit gene promoter transfected into pituitary cell. Mol Endocrinol 1989;3:717

67. Shupnik MA, Rosenzweig BA, Showers MO. Interactions of thyrotropin-releasing hormone, phorbol ester, and forskolin-sensitive regions of the rat thyrotropin-β gene. Mol Endocrinol 1990; 4:829

68. Nelson C, Albert VR, Elsholtz HP, Lu LIW, Rosenfeld MG. Activation of cell-specific expression of rat growth hormone and [prolactin] genes by a common transcription factor. Science 1988; 239:1400

69. Steinfelder HJ, Radovick S, Wondisford FE. Hormonal regulation of the thyrotropin β-subunit gene by phosphorylation of the pituitary-specific transcription factor Pit-1. Proc Natl Acad Sci U S A 1992;89:5942

70. Radovick S, Nations M, Du Y, Berg LA, Weintraub BD, Wondisford FE. A mutation in the POU-homeodomain of Pit-1 responsible for combined pituitary hormone deficiency. Science 1992; 257:1115

71. Pfaffle RW, DiMattia GE, Parks JS, et al. Mutation of the POU-specific domain of Pit-1 and hypopituitarism without pituitary hypoplasia. Science 1992;257:1118

72. Lumpkin MD, Samson WK, McCann SM. Arginine vasopressin as a thyrotropin releasing hormone. Science 1987;235:1070

73. Hoeffler JP, Meyer TE, Yun Y, Jameson JL, Habener JF. Cyclic AMP-responsive DNA-binding protein structure based on a cloned placental cDNA. Science 1988; 242:1430

74. Steinfelder HF, Radovick S, Mroczynski MA, et al. Role of a pituitary-specific transcription factor (pit-1/GHF-1) or a closely related protein in cAMP regulation of human thyrotropin-β subunit gene expression. J Clin Invest 1992;89:409

75. Cooper DS, Klibanski A, Ridgway EC. Dopaminergic modulation of TSH and its subunits; in vivo and in vitro studies. Clin Endocrinol (Oxf) 1983;18:265

76. Scanlon WF, Weightman DR, Shale DJ, et al. Dopamine is a physiological regulator of thyrotropin secretion in man. Clin Endocrinol (Oxf) 1979;10:7

77. Chin WW, Habener JF, Kieffer JD, Maloof F. Cell-free translation of the messenger RNA coding for the α subunit of thyroid-stimulating hormone. J Biol Chem 1978;253:7985

78. Giudice LC, Waxdal MJ, Weintraub BD. Comparison of bovine and mouse pituitary glycoprotein hormone pre-α subunits synthesized in vitro. Proc Natl Acad Sci U S A 1979;76:4798

79. Giudice LC, Weintraub BD. Evidence for conformational differences between precursor and processed forms of TSH-β subunit. J Biol Chem 1979;254:12679

80. Kourides IA, Vamvakopoulos NC, Maniatis GM. mRNA-directed biosynthesis of α- and β-subunits of thyrotropin. J Biol Chem 1979;254:11106

81. Kourides IA, Weintraub BD. mRNA directed biosynthesis of α-subunit of thyrotropin: translation in cell-free and whole-cell systems. Proc Natl Acad Sci USA 1979;76:298

82. Vamvakopoulos NC, Kourides IA. Identification of separate mRNAs coding for the α- and β-subunits of thyrotropin. Proc Natl Acad Sci U S A 1979;76:3809

83. Chin WW, Maloof F, Habener JF. Thyroid-stimulating hormone biosynthesis. J Biol Chem 1981;256:3059

84. Weintraub BD, Stannard BS. Precursor-product relationships in the biosynthesis and secretion of thyrotropin and its subunits by mouse thyrotropic tumor cells. FEBS Lett 1978;92:303

85. Weintraub BD, Stannard BS, Linnekin D, Marshall M. Relationship of glycosylation to de novo thyroid-stimulating hormone biosynthesis and secretion by mouse pituitary tumor cells. J Biol Chem 1980;255:5715

86. Weintraub BD, Stannard BSD, Magner JA, et al. Glycosylation and post-translational processing of thyroid-stimulating hormone: clinical implications. Recent Prog Horm Res 1985;41:577

87. Weintraub BD, Stannard BS, Meyers L. Glycosylation of thyroid-stimulating hormone in pituitary tumor cells. Influence of high-mannose oligosaccharide units on subunit aggregation, combination and intracellular degradation. Endocrinology 1983; 112:1331

88. Weintraub BD, Wondisford FE, Farr EA, et al. Pre-translational and post-translational regulation of TSH synthesis in normal and neoplastic thyrotrophs. Horm Res 1989;32:22

89. Magner JA, Papagiannes E. Structures of high-mannose oligosaccharides of mouse thyrotropin: differential processing of α- versus β-subunits of the heterodimer. Endocrinology 1987;120:10

90. Magner JA, Weintraub BD. Thyroid-stimulating hormone subunit processing and combination in microsomal subfractions of mouse pituitary tumor. J Biol Chem 1982;257:6709

91. Parsons TF, Bloomfield GA, Pierce JG. Purification of an alternative form of the α-subunit of the glycoprotein hormones from bovine pituitaries and identification of its O-linked oligosaccharides. J Biol Chem 1983;258:240

92. Behrens NH, Leloir LF. Dolichol monophosphate glucose: an intermediate in glucose transfer in liver. Proc Natl Acad Sci U S A 1970;66:153

93. Strickland TW, Pierce JG. The α-subunit of pituitary glycoprotein hormones: formation of three-dimensional structure during cell-free biosynthesis. J Biol Chem 1983;258:55927

94. Weintraub BD, Stannard BS, Myers L. Glycosylation of thyroid-stimulating hormone in pituitary tumor cells: Influence of high mannose oligosaccharide units on subunit aggregation, combination, and intracellular degradation. Endocrinology 1983; 112:1331

95. Ronin C, Stannard BS, Rosenbloom IL, Magner JA, Weintraub BD. Glycosylation and processing of high-mannose oligosaccharides of thyroid-stimulating hormone subunits: comparison to nonsecretory cell glycoproteins. Biochemistry 1984 ;23:4503

96. Ronin C, Stannard BS, Weintraub BD. Differential processing and regulation of thyroid-stimulating hormone subunit carbohydrate chains in thyrotropic tumors and in normal and hypothyroid pituitaries. Biochemistry 1985;24:562

97. Miura Y, Perkel VS, Magner JA. Rates of processing of the high mannose oligosaccharide units at the three glycosylation sites of mouse thyrotropin and the two sites of free α-subunits. Endocrinology 1988;123:1296

98. Parsons TF, Pierce JG. Oligosaccharide moieties of glycoprotein hormones: bovine lutropin resists enzymatic deglycosylation because of terminal O-sulfated N-acetylhexosamines. Proc Natl Acad Sci U S A 1980;77:7089

99. Hortin G, Natowicz M, Pierce J, Baenziger J, Parsons T, Boime I. Metabolic labeling of lutropin with [^{35}S]sulfate. Proc Natl Acad Sci U S A 1981;78:7468

100. Anumula KR, Bahl OP. Biosynthesis of lutropin in ovine pituitary slices: incorporation of [^{35}S]sulfate in carbohydrate units. Arch Biochem Biophys 1993;220:645

101. Gesundheit N, Magner JA, Chen T, Weintraub BD. Differential sulfation and sialylation of secreted mouse thyrotropin (TSH) subunits: regulation by TSH-releasing hormone. Endocrinology 1986;119:455

102. Gesundheit N, Gyves PW, DeCherney GS, Stannard BS, Winston RL, Weintraub BD. Characterization and charge distribution of the asparagine-linked oligosaccharides on secreted mouse thyrotropin and free α-subunits. Endocrinology 1989;124:2967

103. Baenziger JU, Green ED. Pituitary glycoprotein hormone oligosaccharides: structure, synthesis and function of the asparagine-linked oligsaccharides on lutropin, follitropin and thyrotropin. Biochem Biophys Acta 1988;947:287

104. Smith PL, Baenziger JU. A pituitary N-acetylgalactosamine transferase that specifically recognizes glycoprotein hormones. Science 1988;242:930

105. Baenziger JU. Protein-specific glycosyltransferases: How and why they do it! FASEB J 1994;8:1019

106. Magner JA. Assay of sulfotransferase in subcellular fractions of hypothyroid mouse pituitary and liver tissue. Biochem Med Metab Biol 1989;41:81

107. Magner JA, Papagiannes E. The subcellular sites of sulfation of mouse thyrotropin and free alpha subunits: studies employing subcellular fractionation and inhibitors of the intracellular translocation of proteins. Endocr Res 1987;13:337

108. Flete D, Srivastava V, Hindsgaul O, Baenziger JU. A hepatic reticuloendothelial cell receptor specific for SO$_4$-4 Gal-NAcβ1,4 Glc-

109. Hiyama J, Weisshaar G, Renwick AG. The asparagine-linked oligosaccharides at individual glycosylation sites in human thyrotrophin. Glycobiology 1992;2:401

110. Gyves PW, Gesundheit N, Stannard BS, DeCherney GS, Weintraub BD. Alterations in the glycosylation of secreted thyrotropin during ontogenesis: analysis of sialylated and sulfated oligosaccharides. J Biol Chem 1989;264:6104

111. Gyves PW, Gesundheit N, Thotakura NR, Stannard BS, DeCherney GS, Weintraub BD. Changes in the sialylation and sulfation of secreted thyrotropin in congenital hypothyroidism. Proc Natl Acad Sci U S A 1990;87:3792

112. DeCherney GS, Gesundheit N, Gyves PW, Showalter CR, Weintraub BD. Alterations in the sialylation and sulfation of secreted mouse thyrotropin in primary hypothyroidism. Biochem Biophys Res Commun 1989;159:755

113. Magner JA, Papagiannes E. Studies of double-labeled mouse thyrotropin and free α-subunits to estimate relative fucose content. Proc Soc Exp Biol Med 1986;83:237

114. Magner JA, Novak W, Papagiannes E. Subcellular localization of fucose incorporation into mouse thyrotropin and free α-subunits: studies employing subcellular fractionation and inhibitors of the intracellular translocation of proteins. Endocrinology 1986;119:1315

115. Magner JA, Kane J, Chou ET. Intravenous thyrotropin (TSH)-releasing hormone releases human TSH that is structurally different than basal TSH. J Clin Endocrinol Metab 1992;74:1306

116. Magner JA, Kane J. Binding of thyrotropin to lentil lectin is unchanged by thyrotropin-releasing hormone administration in three patients with thyrotropin-producing pituitary adenomas. Endocr Res 1992;18:163

117. Gesundheit N, Fink DL, Silverman LA, Weintraub BD. Effect of thyrotropin-releasing hormone on the carbohydrate structure of secreted mouse thyrotropin: analysis by lectin affinity chromatography. J Biol Chem 1987;262:5197

118. Taylor T, Gesundheit N, Gyves PW, Jacobowitz DM, Weintraub BD. Hypothalamic hypothyroidism caused by lesions in rat paraventricular nuclei alters the carbohydrate structure of secreted thyrotropin. Endocrinology 1988;122:283

119. Taylor T, Gesundheit N, Weintraub BD. Effects of in vivo bolus versus continuous TRH administration on TSH secretion, biosynthesis, and glycosylation in normal and hypothyroid rats. Mol Cell Endocrinol 1986;46:253

120. Taylor T, Weintraub BD. Altered thyrotropin (TSH) carbohydrate structures in hypothalamic hypothyroidism created by paraventricular nuclear lesions are corrected by in vivo TSH-releasing hormone. Endocrinology 1989;125:2198

121. Taylor T, Wondisford FE, Blaine T, Weintraub BD. The paraventricular nucleus of the hypothalamus has a major role in thyroid feedback regulation of thyrotropin synthesis and secretion. Endocrinology 1990;126:317

122. Magner JA, Miura Y, Rubin D, Kane J. Structure of high-mannose and complex oligosaccharides of mouse TSH and free alpha subunits after in vitro incubation of thyrotropic tissue with TRH. Endocr Res 1992;18:175

123. Gyves PW, Gesundheit N, Taylor T, Butler J, Weintraub BD. Changes in thyrotropin (TSH) carbohydrate structure and response to TSH-releasing hormone during postnatal ontogeny: analysis by concanavalin A chromatography. Endocrinology 1987;121:133

124. Miura Y, Perkel VS, Papenberg KA, Johnson MJ, Magner JA. Concanavalin-A lentil and ricin affinity binding characteristics of human thyrotropin: differences in the sialylation of thyrotropin in

NAcβ,2 Man α that mediates rapid clearance of lutropin. Cell 1991;67:1103

sera of euthyroid, primary and central hypothyroid patients. J Clin Endocrinol Metab 1989;69:985

125. Papandreou M-J, Persani L, Asteria C, Ronin C, Beck-Peccoz P. Variable carbohydrate structures of circulating thyrotropin as studied by lectin affinity chromatography in different clinical conditions. J Clin Endocrinol Metab 1993;77:393

126. Papandreou M-J, Asteria C, Pettersson K, Ronin C, Beck-Peccoz P. Concanavalin A affinity chromatography of human serum gonadotropins: evidence for changes of carbohydrate structure in different clinical conditions. J Clin Endocrinol Metab 1993; 76:1008

127. Lee HL, Suhl J, Pekary AE, Hershman JM. Secretion of thyrotropin with reduced concanavalin-A-binding activity in patients with severe nonthyroidal illness. J Clin Endocrinol Metab 1987;65:942

128. Gesundheit N, Petrick PA, Taylor T, Oldfield EH, Weintraub BD. Comparison of a pituitary TSH-secreting micro- versus macroadenoma. In: Medeiros-Neto G, Gaitan E, eds. Frontiers in thyroidology. New York:Plenum, 1986:259

129. Magner JA, Klibanski A, Fein H, et al. Ricin and lentil lectin-affinity chromatography reveals oligosaccharide heterogeneity of thyrotropin secreted by 12 human pituitary tumors. Metabolism 1992;41:1009

130. Magner JA. TSH-mediated hyperthyroidism. Endocrinologist 1993;3:289

131. Sergi I, Medri G, Papandreou M-J, Gunz G, Jaquet P, Ronin C. Polymorphism of thyrotropin and alpha subunit in human pituitary adenomas. J Endocrinol Invest 1993;16:45

132. Chanson P, Weintraub BD, Harris AG. Octreotide therapy for thyroid-stimulating hormone-secreting pituitary adenomas: a follow-up of 52 patients. Ann Intern Med 1993;119:236

133. Francis TB, Smallridge RC, Kane J, Magner JA. Octreotide changes serum thyrotropin (TSH) glycoisomer distribution as assessed by lectin chromatography in a TSH macroadenoma patient. J Clin Endocrinol Metab 1993;77:183

134. Mori M, Kobayashi I, Kobayashi S. Thyrotropin-releasing hormone does not accumulate glycosylated thyrotropin, but changes heterogeneous forms of thyrotropin within the rat anterior pituitary gland. J Endocrinol 1986;109:227

135. Mori M, Murakami M, Iriuchijima T, et al. Alteration by thyrotropin-releasing hormone of heterogeneous components associated with thyrotropin biosynthesis in the rat anterior pituitary gland. J Endocrinol 1984;103:165

136. Mori M, Ohshima K, Fukuda H, Kobayashi I, Wakabayashi K. Changes in the multiple components of rat pituitary TSH and TSH β-subunit following thyroidectomy. Acta Endocrinol 1984;105:49

137. Yora T, Matsuzaki S, Kondo Y, Ui N. Changes in the contents of multiple components of rat pituitary thyrotropin in altered thyroid states. Endocrinology 1979;104:1682

138. Pickles AJ, Peers N, Robertson WR, Lambert A. Microheterogeneity of thyroid-stimulating hormone from the pituitaries of euthyroid, hypothyroid and hyperthyroid rats. J Mol Endocrinol 1992;9:245

139. Helton TE, Magner JA. Sialyltransferase messenger ribonucleic acid increases in thyrotrophs of hypothyroid mice: an in situ hybridization study. Endocrinology 1994;134:2347

140. Helton TE, Magner JA. β-1,4-galactosyltransferase and α-mannosidase-II messenger ribonucleic acid levels increase with different kinetics in thyrotrophs of hypothyroid mice. Endocrinology 1994;135:1980

141. Gorden P, Weintraub BD. Radioreceptor and other functional hormone assays. In: Wilson JD, Foster DF, eds. Williams' textbook of endocrinology. 8th ed. Philadelphia: WB Saunders, 1992:1647

142. Beck-Peccoz, Amr S, Menezes-Ferreira MM, Faglia G, Weintraub BD. Decreased receptor binding of biologically inactive thyrotropin in central hypothyroidism: effect of treatment with thyrotropin-releasing hormone. N Engl J Med 1985;312:1085

143. Beck-Peccoz P, Piscitelli G, Amr S, et al. Endocrine, biochemical and morphological studies of pituitary adenoma secreting growth hormone, thyrotropin (TSH), and α-subunit: evidence for secretion of TSH with increased bioactivity. J Clin Endocrinol Metab 1986;62:704

144. Dahlberg PA, Petrick PA, Nissim M, Menezes-Ferreira MM, Weintraub BD. Intrinsic bioactivity of thyrotropin in human serum is inversely correlated with thyroid hormone concentrations: application of a new bioassay using the FRTL-5 rat thyroid cell strain. J Clin Invest 1987;79:1388

145. Nissim M, Lee KO, Petrick PA, Dahlberg PA, Weintraub BD. A sensitive thyrotropin (TSH) bioassay based on iodide uptake in rat FRTL-5 thyroid cells: comparison with the adenosine 3′, 5′-monophosphate response to human serum TSH and enzymatically deglycosylated bovine and human TSH. Endocrinology 1987;121:1278

146. Amir SM, Kubota K, Tramontano D, Ingbar SH, Keutmann HT. The carbohydrate moiety of bovine thyrotropin is essential for full bioactivity but not for receptor recognition. Endocrinology 1987;120:345

147. Amr S, Menezes-Ferreira MM, Shimohigashi Y, Chen HC, Nisula B, Weintraub BD. Activities of deglycosylated thyrotropin at the thyroid membrane receptor adenylate cyclase system. J Endocrinol Invest 1986;8:537

148. Thotakura NR, LiCalzi L, Weintraub BD. The role of carbohydrate in thyrotropin action assessed by a novel method of enzymatic deglycosylation. J Biol Chem 1990;265:11527

149. Endo Y, Tetsumoto T, Nagasaki H, et al. The distinct roles of α- and β-subunits of human thyrotropin in the receptor-binding and postreceptor events. Endocrinology 1990;127:149

150. Pickles AJ, Peers N, Robertson WR, Lambert A. Different isoforms of human pituitary thyroid-stimulating hormone have different relative biological activities. J Mol Endocrinol 192;9:251

151. Sergi I, Papandreou M-J, Madri G, Canonne C, Verrier B, Ronin C. Immunoreaction and bioactive isoforms of human thyrotropin. Endocrinology 1991;128:3259

152. Papandreou M-J, Sergi I, Gabriella M, et al. Differential effect of glycosylation on the expression of antigenic and bioactive domains in human thyrotropin. Mol Cell Endocrinol 1991;78:137

153. Thotakura NR, Desai RK, Szkudlinksi MW, Weintraub BD. The role of the oligosaccharide chains of thyrotropin α- and β-subunits in hormone action. Endocrinology 1992;131:82

154. Thotakura NR, Szkudlinski MW, Weintraub BD. Structure-function studies of oligosaccharides of recombinant human thyrotrophin by sequential deglycosylation and resialylation. Glycobiology 1994;4:525

155. Medri G, Sergi I, Papandreou M-J, Beck-Peccoz P, Verrier B, Ronin C. Dual activity of human pituitary thyrotrophin isoforms on thyroid cell growth. J Mol Endocrinol 1994;13:187

156. Beck-Peccoz P, Persani L. Variable biological activity of thyroid-stimulating hormone. Acta Endocrinol (Copenh) 1994;131:331

157. Joshi LR, Weintraub BD. Naturally occurring forms of thyrotropin with low bioactivity and altered carbohydrate content act as competitive antagonists to more bioactive forms. Endocrinology 1983;113:2145

158. Menezes-Ferreira MM, Petrick PA, Weintraub BD. Regulation of thyrotropin (TSH) bioactivity by TSH-releasing hormone and thyroid hormone. Endocrinology 1986;118:2125

159. Faglia G, Bittensky L, Pinchera A, et al. Thyrotropin secretion in patients with central hypothyroidism: evidence for reduced biological activity of immunoreactive thyrotropin. J Clin Endocrinol Metab 1979;48:989

160. Persani L, Asteria C, Tonacchera M, Vitti P, Chatterjee VKK, Beck-Peccoz P. Evidence for the secretion of thyrotropin with enhanced

bioactivity in syndromes of thyroid hormone resistance. J Clin Endocrinol Metab 1994;78:1034

161. Chappel S. Editorial: Biological to immunological ratios: Reevaluation of a concept. J Clin Endocrinol Metab 1990;70:1494
162. Ridgway EC, Weintraub BD, Maloof F. Metabolic clearance and production rates of human thyrotropin. J Clin Invest 1974;53:895
163. Ridgway EC, Singer FR, Weintraub BD. Lorenz L, Maloof F. Metabolism of human thyrotropin in the dog. Endocrinology 1974;95:1181
164. Constant RB, Weintraub BD. Differences in the metabolic clearance of pituitary and serum thyrotropin (TSH) derived from euthyroid and hypothyroid rats: effects of chemical deglycosylation of pituitary TSH. Endocrinology 1986;119:2720
165. Reichert Jr LE, Dattatreyamurty B, Grasso P, Santa-Coloma TA. Structure-function relationships of the glycoprotein hormones and their receptors. Trends Pharmacol Sci 1991;12:199
166. Papandreou M-J, Darbon H, Ronin C. Polymorphisme biologique et domaines fonctionnels des dormones glycoproteiques hypophusaires. Ann Endocrinol (Paris) 1991;52:254
167. Combarnous Y. Molecular basis of the specificity of binding of glycoprotein hormones to their receptors. Endocr Rev 1992;13:670
168. Keutmann HT. Receptor-binding regions in human glycoprotein hormones. Mol Cell Endocrinol 1992;186:C1
169. Reed DK, Ryan RJ, McCormick DJ. Residues in the subunit of human choriotropin that are important for interaction with the lutropin receptor. J Biol Chem 1991;266:14251
170. Leinung MC, Reed DK, McCormick DJ, Ryan RJ, Morris JC. Further characterization of the receptor-binding region of the thyroid-stimulating hormone α-subunit: A comprehensive synthetic peptide study of the α-subunit 26–46 sequence. Biochemistry 1991;88:9707
171. Bielinska M, Boime I. Site-directed mutagenesis defines a domain in the gonadotropin α-subunit required for assembly with the chorionic gonadotropin β-subunit. Mol Endocrinol 1992;6:267
172. Liu C, Roth KE, Shepard BAL, Shaffer JB, Dias JA. Site-directed alanine mutagenesis of Phe33, Arg35, and Arg42-Ser43-Lys44 in the human gonadotropin α-subunit. J Biol Chem 1993;268:21613
173. Xia H, Chen F, Puett D. A region in the human glycoprotein hormone α-subunit important in holoprotein formation and receptor binding. Endocrinology 1994;134:1768
174. Chen F, Wang Y, Puett D. The carboxy-terminal region of the glycoprotein hormone α-subunit: Contributions to receptor binding and signaling in human chorionic gonadotropin. Mol Endocrinol 1992;6:914
175. Yoo J, Zeng H, Ji I, Murdoch WJ, Ji TH. COOH-terminal amino acids of the α-subunit play common and different roles in human choriogonadotropin and follitropin. J Biol Chem 1993; 28:13034
176. Morris JC, McCormick DJ, Ryan RJ. Inhibition of thyrotropin binding to receptor by synthetic human thyrotropin β peptides. J Biol Chem 1990;265:1881
177. Leinung MC, Bergert ER, McCormick DJ, Morris JC. Synthetic analogs of the carboxyl-terminus of β-thyrotropin: The importance of basic amino acids in receptor binding activity. Biochemistry 1992;31:10094
178. Freeman SL, McCormick DJ, Ryan RJ, Morris JC. Inhibition of TSH bioactivity by synthetic TSH beta peptides. Endocr Res 1992;18:1
179. Wondisford FE, Usala SJ, DeCherney SG, et al. Cloning of the human thyrotropin beta subunit gene and transient expression of biologically active human thyrotropin after gene transfection. Mol Endocrinol 1988;2:32
180. Thotakura NR, Desai RK, Bates LG, Cole ES, Pratt BM, Weintraub BD. Biological activity and metabolic clearance of a recombinant human thyrotropin produced in Chinese hamster ovary cells. Endocrinology 1991;128:341
181. Watanabe S, Hayashizaki Y, Endo Y, et al. Production of human thyroid-stimulating hormone in Chinese hamster ovary cells. Biochem Biophys Res Commun 1989;149:1149

MECHANISM OF ACTION OF THYROTROPIN AND OTHER THYROID GROWTH FACTORS

Basil Rapoport
Stephen W. Spaulding

Thyrotropin (TSH) is the primary factor that regulates thyroid follicular cell (thyrocyte) function and, ultimately, thyroid hormone secretion. Thyrocyte proliferation and thyroid size are also dependent on TSH. The functional and proliferative responses of the thyrocytes to TSH are either dampened or enhanced by the organic iodine content of the cell, a process called *iodine autoregulation*.[1] All actions of TSH follow its binding to the TSH receptor, which transduces signals via multiple intracellular pathways that influence many aspects of thyrocyte function (reviewed in reference 2). Because of its importance in regulating thyrocyte metabolism, the TSH receptor plays an important role in the pathogenesis of some diseases of the thyroid, in particular, Graves' disease and certain thyroid tumors.

The existence of the TSH receptor was first recognized in 1966.[3] Subsequently, the availability of radiolabeled TSH led to the direct demonstration of TSH binding to thyrocyte membranes.[4] TSH receptors are localized primarily on the basal surface of the cell.[5] Binding of TSH to its receptor activates the adenylyl-cyclase–cAMP–protein kinase A pathway[6,7] and also, with an importance less well defined, the Ca^{++}–protein kinase C pathway.[8,9]

MOLECULAR CLONING OF THE TSH RECEPTOR

Information on the structure of the TSH receptor is fundamental to understanding the mechanism by which the receptor is activated by TSH. Efforts at TSH receptor purification using biochemical approaches failed, probably because of receptor instability and its very low concentration in thyroid tissue. Instead, the TSH receptor was studied by indirect approaches, the most informative of which were the analysis of the kinetics of TSH binding and covalent cross-linking of radiolabeled TSH. Purification of the luteinizing hormone/chorionic gonadotropin (LH/CG) receptor and development of monoclonal antibodies to this receptor enabled the molecular cloning in 1989 of the cDNA for the rat and pig LH/CG receptors,[10,11] followed shortly thereafter by the molecular cloning of TSH receptor cDNA from dogs,[12] humans,[13–16] and rats.[17]

Studies of recombinant TSH receptors have dispelled a number of long-held conceptions. For example, until recently, two forms of TSH receptor were believed to exist in thyroid tissue, one of high affinity and one of low affinity for TSH.[18] The high affinity binding site was clearly important physiologically,[19] and the low affinity site was also believed to mediate TSH action (reviewed in reference 20), or to be of pathophysiologic importance in autoimmune thyroid disease.[21] It is now clear that the low affinity TSH binding site is an artifact (reviewed in reference 22). Another misconception (reviewed in reference 20) was that the TSH receptor consists of two components, one a glycoprotein and the other a ganglioside. The glycoprotein component was reported to bind the β-subunit of TSH, and the ganglioside component to mediate signal transduction after interacting with the α-subunit of TSH. Although gangliosides may play a role in post-receptor events involved in signal transduction, the molecular cloning of the TSH receptor as a single polypeptide chain undermines the concept of a ganglioside as an integral part of the receptor.

STRUCTURE OF THE TSH RECEPTOR

The human,[13-16] dog,[12] and rat[17] TSH receptor cDNAs have a single open reading frame encoding a protein of 764 amino acids. Although the exact length of the signal peptide is uncertain, the best estimate[15] is 21 amino acid residues. After cleavage of the signal peptide, the protein backbone of the TSH receptor is, therefore, 743 amino acids in length with a calculated molecular weight of 84.5 kd. The recent generation of monoclonal antibodies to the TSH receptor has permitted an estimation of the extent of TSH receptor glycosylation, namely 15 to 20 kd of carbohydrate moieties.[5,23] Therefore, the holoreceptor is approximately 100 kd in size.

The mature TSH receptor (without signal peptide) contains a heavily glycosylated amino-terminal extracellular region of 397 amino acids and a carboxyl-terminal region of 344 amino acids (Fig. 11-9). The carboxyl-terminal region is divided into a 264 amino acid segment that spans the plasma membrane seven times, as well as a cytoplasmic tail of 82 amino acids. Three loops in the membrane-spanning segment contribute to the extracellular component. This structure makes the receptor a member of the large family of receptors coupled to guanine nucleotide regulatory (G) proteins.

Early studies, involving chemical or photoaffinity cross-linking of radiolabeled TSH to thyroid membranes (reviewed in reference 24), indicated that TSH binds to a 50 kd extracellular fragment (A subunit) of the receptor that is linked by disulfide bonds to a membrane-associated B subunit. These results have been corroborated since the cloning of the TSH receptor. The cloning of the TSH receptor has also answered the important question of whether or not the TSH receptor subunits, like the subunits of TSH, are encoded by two different genes (see chap 11). The functional expression of the TSH receptor from a single mRNA species indicates a single gene origin.[13-15]

The generation of two subunits from a single polypeptide chain indicates that the TSH receptor undergoes proteolytic cleavage. The approximate site of cleavage can be deduced from stoichiometric information. First, the TSH receptor A subunit (~50-54 kd) is smaller than the calculated size of the extracellular region of the receptor (~60-64 kd; 397 amino acids plus 15-20 kd of carbohydrate). Therefore, cleavage must occur within the extracellular region, upstream of its insertion

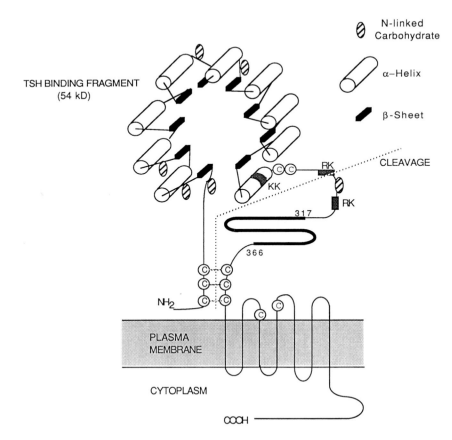

FIGURE 11-9. Schematic representation of the three-dimensional structure of the TSH receptor, modified in the context of the first data on the three-dimensional structure of a protein (porcine ribonuclease inhibitor) with leucine-rich repeats. The basic amino acid clusters at amino acids 261–262, 287–293, and 310–313 in the extracellular region of the TSH receptor are annotated as KK or RK and are indicated by the hatched segments. Disulfide bonds are shown between the highly conserved clusters of cysteine residues (C). The thick black segment represents amino acid residues 317–366, which can be deleted without altering the size of the fragment that remains cross-linked to TSH. Proteolytic cleavage would release (after reduction) a fragment upstream of the dotted line. In this hypothetic example, a region adjacent to the middle cluster of basic amino acids is depicted as the cleavage site. (Chazenbalk GD, Rapoport B. Cleavage of the thyrotropin receptor does not occur at a classical subtilisin-related proprotein convertase endoproteolytic site. J Biol Chem 1994; 269:32209)

into the plasma membrane. Second, cross-linking of TSH to mutated, recombinant TSH receptor variants indicates that the cleavage site is proximate to amino acid residue 317 (all amino acid numbering includes the 21 residue signal peptide).[25] There are three clusters of positively charged amino acids (arginines and lysines) between amino acid residues 261 and 313 that could be endoproteolytic sites, but none appear to represent the TSH receptor cleavage site.[26]

The stage of TSH receptor maturation at which cleavage occurs is not known. Cleavage could occur within the endoplasmic reticulum or Golgi apparatus within the cell, or on the cell surface, before or after TSH binding. Evidence that a portion of TSH receptor molecules on the cell surface are in the uncleaved state[25,27,28] has not been confirmed.[5,26]

TSH BINDING TO THE EXTRACELLULAR REGION OF THE TSH RECEPTOR

Consistent with the large size of TSH, the extracellular region of the TSH receptor is one of the largest in the entire family of G protein-coupled receptors. This region comprises three distinct segments. A middle segment containing 9 leucine-rich repeat motifs (amino acid residues 58–277) is relatively homologous (~50%) to the LH/CG and follicle-stimulating hormone (FSH) receptors. The smaller segments adjacent to this region (amino acid residues 22–57 and 278–418) are less conserved (~35% homology) and contain two additional segments or insertions (amino acid residues 38–45 and 317–366) when compared with the LH/CG receptor. The segments on either side of the leucine-rich region contain numerous cysteine residues.

This information suggests a circular configuration for the extracellular region of the receptor in which the amino- and carboxyl-termini of the receptor, apposed through disulfide bonding, are likely to comprise at least part of the TSH binding site.[25] Although this model is controversial, the three-dimensional structure of a member of the family of proteins with leucine-rich repeats (porcine ribonuclease inhibitor)[29] supports the concept that the extracellular domain of the TSH receptor is shaped like the air filter on an automobile, with the amino- and carboxy-termini in apposition (see Fig. 11-9).

The molecular cloning of the TSH receptor has led to many studies attempting to define the precise amino acids in the extracellular region of the molecule that compose the TSH binding site. The approaches used have included site-directed mutagenesis to create deletions or nonhomologous amino acid substitutions in unique, potentially important regions of the TSH receptor, binding of TSH to synthetic peptides corresponding to selected regions of the TSH receptor, and substitution of portions of the extracellular domain of the TSH receptor with homologous regions of the closely related LH/CG receptor to form TSH-LH/CG chimeric molecules.

Much of the data obtained by the first two approaches (reviewed in references 2, 22, and 30) is conflicting because of the flaws inherent in mutagenesis and peptide studies, namely nonspecific disruption of three-dimensional structure and low affinity interactions, respectively. Nevertheless, the amino terminus of the extracellular region probably contains, at least in part, the TSH binding site. Deletion of the unique 50 amino acid segment (residues 317–365) near the carboxyl terminus of the extracellular region has no effect on TSH binding, thereby excluding this region from the TSH binding site.[31]

The chimeric molecule approach involving homologous amino acid substitutions between related molecules has provided more definitive information (reviewed in references 2 and 22). All regions of the extracellular region of the receptor can be substituted on an individual basis without the loss of high affinity TSH binding.[32] This redundancy indicates that TSH binds to multiple, discontinuous segments of the receptor that are brought into apposition by folding of the protein into its complex three-dimensional structure.

A corollary is that the TSH binding site on the receptor is highly dependent on its three-dimensional conformation. Therefore, only if LH/CG receptor segment substitution can both diminish TSH binding affinity and cause a reciprocal increase in CG binding can part of the TSH binding site be definitively localized. Loss of TSH binding alone could be an allosteric effect on the conformation of the TSH binding site resulting from substitutions, even though homologous, that are introduced at a distant site. The one segment of the TSH binding site defined by this approach is amino acid residues 201–211 within the leucine-rich repeat area.[33] TSH receptor autoantibodies bind to the receptor with similar properties to those described for TSH (reviewed in[2,22,34]). The binding site for these autoantibodies overlaps with, but is not identical to, the TSH binding site.[35]

The contribution of the three extracellular loops formed by the membrane-spanning portion of the receptor to high affinity TSH binding remains to be established. Deletion of these loops[36] or substitution with the corresponding region of the LH/CG receptor[34] does not affect high affinity TSH binding. The importance of the carbohydrate moieties in TSH receptor function is uncertain. Clearly, adequate glycosylation is required for normal processing of the receptor and its expression on the surface of the thyrocyte.[37] Data regarding the role of the asparagine-linked glycosylation site at amino acid residue 113 in TSH binding are conflicting,[37,38] but glycosylation of the closely related LH/CG receptor does not appear to be necessary for ligand binding. On the other hand, the nonglycosylated TSH receptors generated in bacteria[39,40] and the inadequately glycosylated receptors produced in insect cells with baculovirus vectors[23,41,42] are mostly insoluble. Attempts to refold these proteins so as to restore physiologic high affinity TSH binding have been unsuccessful.[43]

GENOMIC STRUCTURE OF THE TSH RECEPTOR GENE

The human TSH receptor gene spans more than 60 kilobases (kb)[44] and is located on chromosome 14q31.[45,46] The mouse TSH receptor gene is on chromosome 2.[17] Nine exons code for the large extracellular region of the TSH receptor. A much larger 10th exon, relatively conserved in the family of G protein-coupled receptors, codes for the entire transmembrane and cytoplasmic domains.[44] All of the introns in the TSH receptor are in phase 2, meaning that the splice junction occurs between the second and third bases of each codon.[44]

The glycoprotein hormone receptors, including the TSH receptor, have evolved by the integration of a multi-exon component at the 5′-end of an ancestral gene represented by exon 10. Many members of the family of G protein-coupled receptors with seven membrane-spanning segments, such as the adrenergic receptors with very small extracellular regions, lack introns and contain little more than this prototypic exon 10. TSH receptor exons 2–8 code for the leucine-rich repeat areas described earlier. These segments represent the region with greatest homology among the glycoprotein hormone receptors, whereas exons 1 and 9, coding for the extreme ends of the TSH receptor extracellular domain, have less homology.

TSH RECEPTOR GENE EXPRESSION

The major mRNA transcripts for the TSH receptor are approximately 4 kb in length, but smaller transcripts also exist. A 1.2-kb TSH receptor mRNA variant has recently been characterized. This variant comprises the first 8 exons of the TSH receptor gene followed by a short unidentified segment, presumably part of an intron, and a poly (A) tail.[47,48] This transcript is of particular interest because it would code for a receptor lacking the transmembrane region and could, therefore, be secreted into the extracellular fluid. A variant TSH receptor mRNA species has been described in dogs in which the region coding for amino acids 61–86 is deleted.[49] This deletion corresponds to the leucine-rich glycoprotein repeat coded for by exon 3.[44] Whether these transcripts generate any proteins and what is their pathophysiologic importance are not known.

The TSH receptor gene is expressed not only in thyrocytes but also in extrathyroidal tissue, most notably in adipocytes,[50,51] consistent with the earlier demonstration of TSH binding to these cells.[52,53] The TSH receptor gene may also be expressed in retro-orbital tissue, of possible importance in the ophthalmopathy of Graves' disease, as well as in fibroblasts and lymphocytes (reviewed in reference 30). If TSH receptor mRNA is transcribed in orbital tissue, the cell type(s) in which this occurs is not clearly defined.

Although TSH has major effects on the level of expression of mRNA species for many thyroid cell genes, it has little effect on TSH receptor mRNA levels, at least in human and dog thyrocytes (reviewed in reference 2). In cultured rat thyrocytes, TSH initially increases, then decreases, TSH receptor mRNA levels, primarily through an effect on mRNA transcription.[54]

SIGNAL TRANSDUCTION BY THE TSH RECEPTOR

As with all members of the G protein-coupled receptor family with seven membrane-spanning regions, the cytoplasmic regions of the TSH receptor are important in conducting a cascade of signals into the interior of the cell. Based on the known three-dimensional structure of other receptors, the seven TSH receptor transmembrane segments, linked by three cytoplasmic and three extracellular loops, are likely to form a cylindrical structure imbedded within the plasma membrane. In the case of receptors with very small ligands, such as those for adrenergic hormones, the extracellular component of the receptor is very small and the ligand enters the lipid bilayer and binds to

residues within the transmembrane cylinder. Ligand binding is then believed to cause conformational changes in the cytoplasmic segments of the receptor, which lead to activation of the membrane-associated guanine nucleotide-binding proteins G_s (adenylyl cyclase pathway) and G_q (phospholipase C pathway).[55] The mechanism of signal transduction by TSH, a large ligand, after binding to the large extracellular region of the TSH receptor is likely to be more complex. Transduction of an intracellular signal by the TSH receptor may involve an extracellular step before activation of the cytoplasmic segments of the receptor. Thus, certain mutations introduced into the extracellular region of the TSH receptor can diminish or abolish the transduction of a signal without altering high-affinity TSH binding to the receptor.[56] An important, unresolved question is whether conformational changes consequent to TSH binding make part of the extracellular region of the receptor, TSH, or both, "dip" into the pocket formed by the transmembrane loops, or indirectly cause a conformational change in this pocket. Because of the importance of the reaction of cytoplasmic segments of the receptor with G proteins, there has been an intensive search for the precise amino acids in these cytoplasmic segments which are responsible for intracellular signal transduction.

From mutagenesis studies, it appears that portions of the second cytoplasmic loop (amino acids 528–537) play a role in transducing a cAMP signal.[57,58] The carboxyl terminus of the third cytoplasmic loop (amino acids 617–625) and the amino terminus of the cytoplasmic tail (amino acids 683–708) are also important in this regard.[57] Alanine 623 in this region appears to be particularly important for transmission of a cAMP, but not a phosphatidyl inositol, signal.[59] There are conflicting data with respect to the importance of the first cytoplasmic loop (amino acid residues 441–450) in adenylyl cyclase activation.[57,60] In interpreting the relative effects of TSH receptor mutations on the two major pathways, it is important to recognize that the unmutated (wild-type) receptor is far more sensitive to TSH in the transduction of an adenylyl cyclase than a phosphatidyl inositol signal.

An important advance has been the identification of TSH receptor mutations in some autonomously functioning thyroid adenomas (see also chap 32). This association was prompted by the discovery that replacement of alanine 293 in the α_{1b}-adrenergic receptor with any other amino acid results in a receptor that is activated in the absence of ligand.[61] Ala 293 in the α_{1b}-adrenergic receptor corresponds to Ala 623 in the TSH receptor. Several thyroid adenomas proved to have mutations at Ala 623 in the TSH receptor, as well as at closely adjacent sites.[62] Such mutations, not present in nonfunctioning thyroid adenomas or carcinomas,[63] cause constitutive activation of the TSH receptor.[62]

The mutations in these thyroid adenomas arise by somatic mutation. In contrast, germline mutations in membrane-spanning segments of the TSH (Val509Ala and Cys672Tyr) have recently been found to underlie a rare form of nonautoimmune familial hyperthyroidism with autosomal dominant inheritance.[64] An important question is the frequency of TSH receptor mutations in thyroid adenomas and other thyroid diseases. Distinction must be made in future studies between nonfunctional TSH receptor polymorphisms and mutations of pathogenetic importance.

TSH RECEPTOR DESENSITIZATION

Hormonal regulation of tissue activity is influenced both by the amount of hormone binding to the tissue and by changes in the sensitivity of the tissue response after hormone binding. Reduction in tissue response, or densitization, is a general phenomenon involving many hormones and hormone-responsive tissues. Desensitization may be homologous (hormone-specific) or heterologous (one hormone inducing desensitization to other hormones). In the case of the thyrocyte, prior TSH stimulation leads to a 30% to 70% decrease in the subsequent cAMP response to TSH stimulation.[65,66] TSH desensitization involves decreased coupling of the TSH receptor with G_s,[67] whereas both the functional activity of G_s and the adenylyl cyclase catalytic unit are unaffected.[67] Because chronic TSH stimulation in vivo results in thyroid overactivity and goiter, TSH desensitization must involve a decreased response to a particular level of stimulation, not an absent response.

The mechanism underlying TSH desensitization is not known. It is not caused by TSH receptor down-regulation,[68,69] which is a reduction in the number of receptors on the cell surface. Functional TSH desensitization occurs within 2 hours of TSH stimulation and is near maximal within 4 to 6 hours in dog, human, and FRTL-5 rat thyroid cells.[68–71] In contrast, TSH receptor down-regulation occurred only after considerably longer periods of TSH stimulation.[72,73]

A putative desensitization protein in thyrocytes may play a role in this process,[68,74] as may TSH-mediated ADP-ribosylation of an unknown substrate.[70,75] Knowledge of the molecular structure of the TSH receptor should permit further elucidation of the TSH desensitization mechanism, including identification of the putative desensitization protein. One candidate for a desensitization protein would be a thyroid arrestin-like protein. Arrestin is a protein that reduces coupling to G_s in the prototype receptor in this family, rhodopsin.[76,77] A similar mechanism has been suggested for β-adrenergic receptor desensitization after phosphorylation by β-adrenergic receptor kinase.[78] A unique arrestin has been isolated from thyrocytes,[79] but its role in TSH desensitization is not known.

Iodide reduces the adenylyl cyclase response to a constant level of TSH stimulation.[80,81] Inhibitors of iodide organification such as methimazole prevent this effect. These two criteria establish iodide-induced desensitization of adenylyl cyclase activation by TSH as one of the many examples of iodine autoregulation [1] (see chap 13). Although iodine and TSH desensitization resemble one another in terms of the ultimate cAMP response to TSH stimulation, their mechanisms are quite different. Unlike TSH desensitization, iodine desensitization does not involve the TSH receptor itself or G_s. The constraint on adenylyl cyclase activation by TSH occurs at a more distal site, probably at the adenylyl cyclase molecule.[82] The inhibitory form of organic iodine responsible for iodine desensitization has not been identified.

INTERACTION OF GONADOTROPINS WITH THE TSH RECEPTOR

High concentrations of CG can bind to and activate the TSH receptor. Such a mechanism has been implicated in the thyrotoxi-cosis in patients with hydatidiform mole or choriocarcinoma (see chap 33). In human thyrocytes, CG also stimulates the phosphatidyl inositol pathway to a far greater extent relative to the adenylyl cyclase pathway, than does TSH.[83]

INTRACELLULAR ACTIONS OF THYROTROPIN

Several different second messenger pathways regulate most thyroid functions. This redundancy in regulatory pathways has permitted evolutionary divergence in how a homeostatic effect will be accomplished. Most of the functions affected by TSH are modulated in the same direction by activating cAMP and protein kinase A, and this pathway is best understood. However some functions are mimicked by increasing the level of intracellular Ca^{++} or by activating protein kinase C. Furthermore, there may be synergism or antagonism among these pathways, and there are probably additional interactions with arachidonate metabolites and other pathways.

A single pulse of TSH rapidly causes formation of colloid droplets in thyrocytes, releases hormone, and depletes thyroglobulin stores. If TSH is injected for several days, however, the droplets disappear, hormone release diminishes, and thyroglobulin reaccumulates.[84] Not all thyrocytes in a gland display the same TSH responsiveness: neighboring cells interact both via factors on their surfaces and via secretion of factors that affect only nearby cells. Although thyrocytes in culture have provided much information concerning how second messengers mediate TSH actions, important interactions may be missing and the response of certain pathways can be altered. For example, in FRTL-5 cells, TSH can be ten thousand times more potent in raising cAMP levels than in activating the Ca^{++}/phosphoinositol pathway, yet if a purine receptor is activated, both pathways then respond within the same range of TSH concentrations.[85]

Overview of the Protein Kinase A Pathway

Forskolin or membrane-permeable analogues of cAMP activate cAMP-dependent protein kinases and mimic many actions of TSH. There are two types of protein kinase A; both are tetrameric enzymes but they differ according to the type of cAMP-binding regulatory subunit dimer they contain (reviewed in reference 86). By binding cooperatively to two sites on each regulatory subunit, cAMP molecules activate protein kinase A holoenzymes, causing each to release its catalytic subunit. TSH increases cAMP levels and kinase activity within minutes.[87] Once the catalytic subunits have been released, they can phosphorylate substrate proteins until the hormonal stimulus stops, then phosphodiesterases (which are also hormonally regulated) reduce the level of cAMP. As the regulatory subunits lose their cAMP they rebind the catalytic subunits. When the subunits are bound together as holoenzymes, they are more resistant to proteolysis than when dissociated, so prolonged elevation of cAMP can foster proteolysis of protein kinase A subunits, and thus reduce the cells' responsiveness to cAMP. Hormones also change the level of expression of protein kinase A subunits; for example, adding TSH to growth factor–starved FRTL-5 cells increases the level of regulatory subunit mRNA within 30 minutes, and the level of protein within 6 hours.[88] The major difference between the regulatory subunits of protein kinase A is that type II subunit dimers can bind to anchoring proteins in subcellular organelles, whereas type I dimers do not. The type II holoenzyme therefore preferentially phosphorylates substrates that neighbor these anchoring sites, but the catalytic subunit from any holoenzyme can diffuse throughout the cell and phosphorylate many substrates.

Regulation of Gene Expression by Protein Kinase A

One class of nuclear substrates for protein kinase A are the CRE-binding proteins (CREBs). Several are expressed in the thyroid.[89] These proteins bind to a consensus DNA sequence in the promoter of cAMP-responsive genes, called the cAMP response element, or CRE. They are members of a large family of leucine zipper (b-ZIP) DNA binding proteins (such as c-jun and c-fos) that regulate transcription of many genes. One important example is AP-1, the dimer of c-jun with c-fos, that binds to a DNA sequence in the promoter of genes that respond to tetraphorbol acetate (TPA), called the *TPA-response element,* which is very closely related to the CRE sequence. Both TPA and activators of protein kinase A rapidly affect transcription of many b-ZIP early genes including ICER, a CRE-repressor, but the transcription of CREB remains constant.[90] Protein kinase A phosphorylates CREB within minutes, enhancing its ability to form dimers with other b-ZIP proteins. The increase in the level of phosphorylated CREB shifts the balance of heterodimers and alters expression of genes involved in thyroid growth and function—thus, when a dominant negative CREB mutant that binds and inactivates endogenous CREBs was expressed in FRTL-5 cells, it slowed their growth and inhibited TSH-stimulated iodide uptake.[89] CREB-PO_4 also binds to a protein called *CREB binding protein* (CBP) that interacts with the transcription factor TFIIB to recruit RNA polymerase II to the genes containing the CREB-PO_4/CBP/TFIIB complex.[91] Another nuclear site of action of TSH is on chromatin structure: HMG 14, a protein associated with transcriptionally active chromatin, undergoes rapid cAMP-dependent phosphorylation, altering its interactions with nucleosomes.[92]

TSH and forskolin and TPA alter the transcription of many genes within minutes to hours.[93] TSH also alters the expression of its own receptor, of G-proteins, of various other hormone or autocrine factors and their receptors, of factors involved in protein synthesis and processing, of enzymes involved in energy metabolism, and of tissue-specific genes like thyroglobulin and thyroperoxidase.

Regulating TSH-Responsiveness at the Level of TSH Receptor Expression

CHANGES IN THE TSH RECEPTOR MEDIATED BY THE PROTEIN KINASE A PATHWAY

TSH briefly increases expression of the TSH receptor in TSH-starved FRTL-5 cells, but then TSH-R expression falls.[94]

The promoter of the rat TSH receptor gene contains a CRE-like sequence, but contains other b-ZIP response elements and a TTF-1 response element as well (see following). Cells must be synthesizing protein before TSH or cAMP can decrease TSH receptor gene expression: if cycloheximide is present, TSH or cAMP merely increases receptor expression. Thus, protein kinase A must phosphorylate stable protein(s) that promote(s) TSH receptor gene transcription until TSH has acted long enough to alter the synthesis of protein(s) that then decrease(s) the transcription of the TSH receptor gene.[94] TTF-1 is a protein found in thyroid nuclei that is needed for cells to express thyroid-specific genes such as thyroglobulin, thyroperoxidase, and the TSH receptor itself. When the protein kinase A catalytic subunit is overexpressed, TTF-1 activity initially increases along with the formation of the TSH receptor promoter/TTF-1 complex and the expression of the TSH receptor gene in TSH-starved FRTL-5 cells.[95] However, after exposure to TSH for 2 hours, the expression of TTF-1 declines, along with TTF-1/TSH receptor promoter complexes and TSH receptor expression.[95]

CHANGES IN THE TSH RECEPTOR MEDIATED BY CA^{++} AND/OR PROTEIN KINASE C PATHWAYS

In addition to activating adenylyl cyclase, TSH can liberate diacylglycerol (DAG) from membrane lipids to activate protein kinase C, and can liberate inositol phosphates to increase intracellular Ca^{++} concentrations. Two agents have been used widely to explore the actions of these pathways: the phorbol ester TPA, which activates protein kinase C, and the ionophore A43187, which increases intracellular levels of ionized calcium.

If dogs are injected with TSH for 4 weeks, their serum T_3 and T_4 concentrations initially rise but then fall below normal, and their thyroid glands display diminished sensitivity to TSH or forskolin when tested in vitro.[96] When dog thyrocytes are treated with TSH in vitro, the level of TSH receptor mRNA increases slightly up to 20 hours,[97] but adenylyl cyclase responsiveness falls over this period.[98] TSH receptor mRNA levels return to baseline after exposure to TSH for 24 hours, whereas the effect of forskolin is different: exposure to forskolin for 48 hours increases both the TSH binding and the cAMP response to TSH. Clearly the inhibitory actions of long-term exposure to TSH are not being mediated by cAMP levels in this model.[97] TPA, in contrast, mimics the inhibitory action of TSH by decreasing TSH binding and adenylyl cyclase responsiveness, but the protein kinase C inhibitor H-7 blocks only the actions of TPA, not those of TSH or carbachol.[98] (Both carbachol and TSH raise Ca^{++} concentrations in these cells and diminish the adenylyl cyclase response to TSH, but do not affect TSH binding.[99]) Thus, the decrease in TSH responsiveness in dog thyrocytes does not always parallel the change in TSH binding, which can be mimicked by activating protein kinase C.

The Ca^{++} ionophore A23187 raises intracellular Ca^{++} concentrations and decreases TSH receptor expression in rat FRTL-5 cells.[100] Adding the Ca^{++} chelator EGTA blocks the ability of both TSH and A23187 to decrease TSH receptor expression. Adding EGTA does not affect the ability of TSH to increase cAMP levels, however, so the Ca^{++}-mediated decrease in TSH receptors does not appear to involve cAMP, despite the role played by cAMP in regulating TSH receptors outlined earlier.[100] Unlike the dog model, TPA does not affect TSH receptors in rats,[101] so protein kinase C does not appear to be involved at this level, even though TPA does inhibit the actions of TSH on cAMP production and DNA synthesis in FRTL-5 cells.[102]

MODELS WITHOUT A DECREASE IN TSH RESPONSIVENESS OR RECEPTOR EXPRESSION

Chronic stimulation by TSH does not always decrease TSH receptor levels or TSH responsiveness. In guinea pigs, for example, constant infusion of TSH (1 U/day) for a week increases thyroid weight, TSH receptor content, and adenylyl cyclase response per gland.[103] When cultured human thyrocytes are exposed to TSH or forskolin for a day, the level of TSH-receptor mRNA doubled but returned to baseline shortly thereafter.[97,104]

Regulation of TSH Responsiveness at the Level of G-Proteins

The TSH receptor activates adenylyl cyclase and phospholipase C by different G-proteins.[55] Thyrocytes have receptors for many agents in addition to TSH that act through various G-protein heterotrimers on the same transducing enzymes and second messenger pathways. By changing levels or activities G-protein subunits can modulate TSH responsiveness.

RAT THYROID CELL LINES

If FRTL-5 cells are grown without TSH for 12 hours, their responsiveness to TSH increases. Adding 1,25 $(OH)_2$-vitamin D blocks this increased responsiveness because it increases the level of the inhibitory G-protein subunit, $G_{I-2\alpha}$; the level of stimulatory subunit $G_s\alpha$ is unaffected.[105] In the WRT rat thyroid cell line, G_s is important for TSH action, since microinjecting an antibody to G_s blocks both TSH-mediated gene expression and mitosis.[106] (Vitamin D also affects cAMP responsiveness in FRTL-5 cells by selectively increasing protein kinase A type II regulatory subunit levels[107] and by decreasing TSH receptor number.[105])

PIG THYROID CULTURE MODELS

Pig thyroid follicles must be cultured with low levels of TSH or else they lose adenylyl cyclase responsiveness. The presence of TSH raises the level of the stimulatory G-protein subunit $G_s\alpha$ threefold, and this effect is mimicked by forskolin, indicating it is cAMP-mediated. A high level of TSH, in contrast, blocks the increase in adenylyl cyclase responsiveness to TSH, whereas high levels of forskolin do not.[108] Since large doses of TSH increase protein kinase C in thyrocyte membranes, the desensitization may involve activation of this enzyme.[109] TPA by itself has no effect on the synthesis of $G_s\alpha$-subunit, but when added with TSH or forskolin for 2 days, TPA abolishes their effects on $G_s\alpha$. (TPA had no effect on the level of the inhibitory G-protein $G_I\alpha$.[110]) Thus, activation of protein kinase C could be involved in the decrease in TSH responsiveness after a high dose of TSH, while TSH in turn can modify the response to TPA.[109,111]

TSH and Arachidonate Metabolism

TSH releases arachidonate from membrane lipids in FRTL-5 cells. Both phospholipase C and phospholipase A_2, which are activated by distinct G-proteins, have been implicated in the production of arachidonic acid in these cells.[112] As levels of eicosanoid metabolites of arachidonate change in the thyroid, they affect many of the second messenger pathways that mediate the actions of TSH.

Iodine Metabolism and the TSH Receptor

Several actions of TSH on iodide metabolism are mimicked by activating the Ca^{++} and protein kinase C pathways, whereas the protein kinase A pathway antagonizes these effects. Although higher doses of TSH are generally required to change the total cellular levels of Ca^{++} or diacylglycerol than are required to raise cAMP levels, local effects may occur at lower doses, and additive or synergistic effects may occur when the Ca^{++} and protein kinase C pathways are activated simultaneously or sequentially.

ACTIONS OF TSH ON IODIDE EFFLUX

TSH causes a rapid efflux of iodide from thyrocytes by pathways that do not require protein synthesis. In FRTL-5 cells, high doses of TSH stimulate iodide efflux and increase free Ca^{++} concentrations, an action reproduced by A23817 but not by agonists of protein kinase A.[113] ATP also increases the Ca^{++} concentration and causes iodide efflux, whereas the calcium chelator BAPTA blocks the increase in Ca^{++} but not the response to ATP.[114] Melittin, which activates phospholipase A_2, also causes iodide efflux,[115] whereas inhibitors of phospholipase C, phospholipase A_2, lipoxygenase, and epoxygenase all inhibit iodide efflux from these cells.[114,115]

When pig thyrocytes are grown as a continuous tight monolayer, they become polarized. Adding TSH to the basal medium stimulates iodide efflux through the apical membrane. In marked contrast to FRTL-5 cells, however, this effect of TSH is mimicked by agonists of protein kinase A, whereas A23187 (and TPA) are inactive.[116]

ACTIONS OF TSH ON IODIDE UPTAKE

Although isolated thyrocytes can transport iodide, the organized structure of the thyroid follicle is essential for efficient thyroid hormone synthesis. The follicular structure permits the vectorial uptake of iodide across the basolateral membrane and its efflux across the apical membrane (see chap 4). The TSH-mediated increase in iodide uptake requires the synthesis of RNA and protein and is accompanied by sodium influx and energy consumption.[117] The crucial importance of follicular structure on thyroid responses is illustrated by the pathways involved in iodine organification in three different dog thyroid preparations. TPA, norepinephrine, and carbechol stimulate iodide organification in dog thyroid slices and also isolated follicles, but these agents actually inhibit organification in isolated dog thyrocytes.[118] TSH, in contrast, is stimulatory in all three preparations.

In FRTL-5 cells, TSH and agonists of protein kinase A increase iodide uptake, whereas the ionophore A23187 blocks their effect.[113] Therefore, free Ca^{++} has divergent actions on io-dide metabolism in FRTL-5 cells, stimulating iodide efflux (as described earlier) but blocking uptake.

ACTIONS OF TSH ON IODINE ORGANIFICATION

Once iodide has been transported into thyroid cells, it must be converted to a high energy state in order to be organ-ified, a process that involves the generation of H_2O_2, which in turn involves the oxidization of glucose and NADPH. TSH rapidly increases NAD kinase activity in guinea pig thyroid segments and subsequently increases microsomal reoxidation of NADPH as well.[119]

Actions of TSH on the Uptake and Phosphorylation of Glucose

TSH affects thyroidal carbohydrate metabolism at numer-ous points, beginning with the uptake of glucose: TSH induces transcription of a glucose transport gene (Glut-1) in FRTL-5 within hours, an action mimicked by agonists of protein kinase A.[120] After the cell takes up glucose, it must phosphorylate it; TSH/cAMP increases hexokinase I gene expression.[121]

Actions of TSH on [1-C]-Glucose Oxidation and H_2O_2 Generation

TSH has a biphasic effect on [C-1]-glucose oxidation in human thyroid slices: low doses of TSH inhibit this response, while high doses enhance it.[122] Cyclic AMP inhibits [C-1]-glu-cose oxidation and probably mediates the low-dose effect of TSH, while the Ca^{++}/protein kinase C pathways mediate the stimulatory effect of TSH in calf[123] and human thyroid slices.[124] The Ca^{++} and protein kinase C pathways also imitate the stim-ulatory action of TSH on H_2O_2 generation. Agonists of protein kinase A inhibit H_2O_2 generation in bovine[123] and human thy-roid slices,[122] but in dog thyroid slices they have a positive ac-tion.[124] Porcine thyrocytes have only a weak H_2O_2 response to TSH, and agonists of protein kinase A have no effect, yet TPA is a potent stimulator.[125] In FRTL-5 cells, TSH stimulates H_2O_2 production, an effect mimicked by agonists of both protein ki-nase A and C in TSH-deficient medium.[125] The purinergic ago-nist PIA inhibits the cAMP response of TSH but potentiates the action of TSH on H_2O_2 production.[126] These examples illus-trate how, for a given response, a second messenger pathway can be stimulatory in one species, ineffective in a second, and antagonistic in a third.

Actions of TSH on Thyroperoxidase

Thyroperoxidase (TPO) activity is necessary for organify-ing iodine. TSH/cAMP rapidly increases the expression of the TPO gene in human,[127] dog,[97,128] and FRTL-5 cells,[129] whereas TPA reduces TPO expression (TPA increases H_2O_2 generation in human thyroid slices[122] but inhibits TPO gene expression in human thyrocytes[127]).

Although the rat TPO promoter lacks a classic CRE,[130] it can confer cAMP responsiveness on a reporter gene.[129] One factor that regulates TPO is TTF-2, a thyroid-specific nuclear protein that binds to and activates transcription of the TPO promoter. In TSH/insulin-starved FRTL-5 cells, TTF-2 binding to the TPO promoter is induced by TSH/cAMP but is inhibited by TPA and A23187.[129]

Iodide Autoregulation and TSH Responsiveness

In the presence of a high concentration of iodide, thyroid cells produce an unidentified organified iodide intermediate that inhibits the cAMP response to TSH, but iodide also in-hibits some actions of agonists of protein kinase A as well as of TPA and A23187, indicating iodine intermediate(s) also act beyond cAMP generation.[131] Iodide can actually potentiate the mitogenic action of TSH on FRTL-5 cells at a dose too low to affect cAMP levels,[132] but how the second messengers are in-volved in mitogenesis is not known.

Autocrine, Paracrine, and Endocrine Factors and TSH Responsiveness

TSH increases the production of or sensitivity to a variety of auto-, juxta-, and endocrine factors, depending on species, io-dine content, and the hormonal milieu. These factors act via some of the G-proteins and second messengers that also medi-ate the responses to TSH, and thus can influence its action. For example, when a purinergic receptor is activated, it inhibits both the cAMP and arachidonate responses to TSH in FRTL-5 cells.[133]

THYROID HORMONES

Thyroid cells contain thyroid hormone receptors (TRs), so thyroid hormone could function as a regulator of thyroid func-tion. Both TR-α and TR-β isoforms have been found in FRTL-5 cells, and the level of the TR-α1 appears to be TSH-depen-dent.[134,135] This receptor binds to the rat TSH receptor pro-moter and inhibits its activity, suggesting one possible mechanism for short-loop feedback.[136]

TYPE I THYROXINE-5'-DEIODINASE

Type I T_4 5'-deiodinase activity may be involved in the thy-roidal production of T_3 in certain species (the activity is present in human, mouse, guinea pig, and rat thyroids, but not in cattle, sheep, goats, rabbits, or pigs[137]). Both TSH and T_3 stimulate the expression of the type I T_4-5'-deiodinase gene in FRTL-5 cells.[138] The induction of this deiodinase by TSH or cAMP is inhibited by cycloheximide but the induction by T_3 is not, indicating that T_3 acts through factor(s) already present and does not require new protein synthesis.[134]

EPIDERMAL GROWTH FACTOR AND ITS RECEPTORS

TSH increases epidermal growth factor (EGF) binding to its receptors,[139] which also serve as the receptors for factors such as transforming growth factor-α, activating the receptors' intrinsic tyrosine kinase (this can even occur in FRTL-5 cells, which lack the high affinity cooperative EGF receptor binding sites found in most thyroid cells[140]). EGF promotes thyrocyte growth under some conditions, but in the mature thyroid it in-hibits thyrocyte function.[141] In mice, the serum concentration of thyroid hormone affects the thyroidal content of immunore-active EGF and its mRNA directly, whereas the serum thyroid hormone concentration is inversely related to the serum con-centration of EGF.[142,143] Thus, the thyroidal content of EGF could behave in vivo as a short-loop feedback inhibitor of thy-roid function in mice.[142,143]

INSULIN-LIKE GROWTH FACTORS AND THEIR RECEPTORS

TSH can stimulate the release of insulin-like growth factor-I (IGF-I) from human, sheep, and pig thyrocytes, and of IGF-II from sheep and FRTL-5 cells.[144,145] IGFs are mitogenic in many thyroid cell cultures, and pretreatment with TSH or agonists of protein kinase A potentiates the mitogenic response to IGF-I.[73,146] An IGF-like substance must be present in the medium before TSH can decrease the expression of the TSH receptor gene in FRTL-5 cells.[94] TSH pretreatment promotes transient autophosphorylation of the IGF-I receptor, an action inhibited by agonists of both protein kinase A and C.[147] IGF-I causes prolonged Ca^{++} influx, which appears to be required for DNA synthesis; the Ca^{++} channel agonist BAYK 8644 mimics the effect of IGF-I on DNA synthesis.[148] However, the tyrosine kinase antagonist genistein blocks DNA synthesis without affecting the Ca^{++} response,[148] another example of the complexity of the second messenger pathways and mitogenesis.

ADRENERGIC AGENTS AND RECEPTORS

Different thyroid cells have different complements of α- and β-adrenergic receptors, dramatically altering how adenylyl cyclase, phospholipase A_2, phospholipase C, cytosolic Ca^{++}, and arachidonate release will respond to a given agonist. In rats with low serum TSH concentrations, β-adrenergic agonists raise cAMP concentrations and stimulate colloid droplet formation, iodide efflux, and hormone release,[149,150] whereas superior cervical ganglionectomy reduces intrathyroidal catecholamines and promotes goitrogenesis.[151] Beta-adrenergic agonists also raise cAMP concentrations in primary cultures of rat thyrocytes, while α-agonists inhibit the cAMP responses. FRTL-5 cells are diametrically opposite, showing no cAMP response to β-agonists,[152] an example of how different this immortalized line is in its second messenger responses, compared with rat thyrocytes in vitro.[152] When a β-adrenergic receptor is transfected into FRTL-5 cells[153] or when it appears as a spontaneous mutant,[154] however, the β-agonist isoproterenol is then able to stimulate cAMP production, iodide uptake, and cell growth.[153,154] TSH increases the level of α1b-receptors in TSH-starved FRTL-5 cells, and α_{1b}-adrenergic receptor mRNA rises tenfold, presumably through the CRE in this gene's promoter.[155]

PURINERGIC RECEPTORS

Thyrocytes contain receptors for various purinergic agents, such as ATP, GTP, and adenosine (ATP is released from sympathetic and parasympathetic neurons present in thyroid tissue). In FRTL-5 cells, the purinergic agonist phenylisopropyl-adenosine (PIA) mimics several actions of TSH: releasing Ca^{++}, activating phospholipases C and A_2, releasing arachidonic acid, and enhancing TSH-mediated H_2O_2 generation.[85] The purinergic agonist PIA blocks the adenylyl cyclase response to TSH or forskolin but enhances α-adrenergic responses in FRTL-5 cells.[156] However, PIA did not affect either adenylyl cyclase responses or H_2O_2 generation in pig thyrocytes, whereas ATP was weakly active, again demonstrating how different the responses are between species.[126]

CONCLUSION

TSH receptor homologues in different species have different G-protein specificity and use different signaling mechanisms.[157] The search for an all-encompassing diagram establishing the way each second messenger pathway mediates the effects of TSH has been unsuccessful and it is unlikely that TSH acts via the same pathways in all species. Redundant regulatory systems permit interspecies variability and permits thyrocytes from different species to respond in different ways. The challenge is now to learn how different species use different backup systems to produce equivalent homeostatic results in vivo.

References

1. Ingbar SH. Autoregulation of the thyroid. Response to iodide excess and depletion. Mayo Clin Proc 1972;47:814
2. Vassart G, Dumont JE. The thyrotropin receptor and the regulation of thyrocyte function and growth. Endocr Rev 1992;13:596
3. Pastan I, Roth J, Macchia V. Binding of hormone to tissue: the first step in polypeptide hormone action. Proc Natl Acad Sci U S A 1966;56:1802
4. Manley SW, Bourke JR, Hawker RW. Reversible binding of labelled and non-labelled thyrotrophin by intact thyroid tissue in vitro. J Endocrinol 1972;55:555
5. Loosfelt H, Pichon C, Jolivet A, et al. Two-subunit structure of the human thyrotropin receptor. Proc Natl Acad Sci U S A 1992;895:3765
6. Yamashita K, Field JB. Preparation of thyroid plasma membranes containing a TSH-responsive adenyl cyclase. Biochem Biophys Res Comm 1970;40:171
7. Wolff J, Jones AB. The purification of bovine thyroid plasma membranes and the properties of membrane-bound adenyl cyclase. J Biol Chem 1971;246:3939
8. Philip NJ, Grollman EF. Thyrotropin and norepinephrine stimulate the metabolism of phosphoinositides in FRTL-5 thyroid cells. FEBS Lett 1986;202:193
9. Laurent E, Mockel J, Van Sande J, Graff I, Dumont JE. Dual activation by thyrotropin of the phospholipase C and cAMP cascades in human thyroid. Mol Cell Endocrinol 1987;520:273
10. McFarland KC, Sprengel R, Phillips HS, et al. Lutropin-choriogonadotropin receptor: an unusual member of the G protein-coupled receptor family. Science 1989;245:494
11. Loosfelt H, Misrahi M, Atger M, et al. Cloning and sequencing of porcine LH-hCG receptor cDNA: variants lacking transmembrane domain. Science 1989;245:525
12. Parmentier M, Libert F, Maenhaut C, et al. Molecular cloning of the thyrotropin receptor. Science 1989;246:1620
13. Nagayama Y, Kaufman KD, Seto P, Rapoport B. Molecular cloning, sequence and functional expression of the cDNA for the human thyrotropin receptor. Biochem Biophys Res Comm 1989;165:1184
14. Libert F, Lefort A, Gerard C, et al. Cloning, sequencing and expression of the human thyrotropin (TSH) receptor: evidence for binding of autoantibodies. Biochem Biophys Res Comm 1989;165:1250
15. Misrahi M, Loosfelt H, Atger M, Sar S, Guiochon-Mantel A, Milgrom E. Cloning, sequencing and expression of human TSH receptor. Biochem Biophys Res Comm 1990;166:394
16. Frazier AL, Robbins LS, Stork PJ, Sprengel R, Segaloff DL, Cone RD. Isolation of TSH and LH/CG receptor cDNAs from human thyroid: regulation by tissue specific splicing. Mol Endocrinol 1990;90:1264
17. Akamizu T, Ikuyama S, Saji M, et al. Cloning, chromosomal assignment, and regulation of the rat thyrotropin receptor: expres-

sion of the gene is regulated by thyrotropin, agents that increase cAMP levels, and thyroid autoantibodies. Proc Natl Acad Sci U S A 1990;87:5677

18. Goldfine ID, Amir SM, Ingbar SH, Tucker G. The interaction of radioiodinated thyrotropin with plasma membrane. Biochim Biophys Acta 1976;448:45

19. Pekonen F, Weintraub BD. Thyrotropin receptors on bovine thyroid membranes: two types with different affinities and specificities. Endocrinology 1979;105:352

20. Kohn LD, Aloj SM, Tombaccini D, et al. The thyrotropin receptor. In: Litwack G, ed. Biochemical actions of hormones. Vol. XII. Academic Press, 1985:457–512

21. Weiss M, Ingbar SH, Winblad S, Kasper DL. Demonstration of a saturable binding site for thyrotropin in Yersinia enterocolitica. Science 1983;219:1331

22. Nagayama Y, Rapoport B. The thyrotropin receptor twenty five years after its discovery: new insights following its molecular cloning. Mol Endocrinol 1992;6:145

23. Huang GC, Page MJ, Nicholson LB, Collison KS, McGregor AM, Banga JP. The thyrotropin hormone receptor of Graves' disease: overexpression of the extracellular domain in insect cells using recombinant baculovirus, immunoaffinity purification and analysis of autoantibody binding. J Mol Endocrinol 1993;10:127

24. Rees Smith B, McLachlan SM, Furmaniak J. Autoantibodies to the thyrotropin receptor. Endocr Rev 1988;9:106

25. Russo D, Chazenbalk GD, Nagayama Y, Wadsworth HL, Seto P, Rapoport B. A new structural model for the thyrotropin receptor as determined by covalent crosslinking of thyrotropin to the recombinant receptor in intact cells: evidence for a single polypeptide chain. Mol Endocrinol 1991;5:1607

26. Chazenbalk GD, Rapoport B. Cleavage of the thyrotropin receptor does not occur at a classical subtilisin-related proprotein covertase endoproteolytic site. J Biol Chem 1994;269:32209

27. Russo D, Nagayama Y, Chazenbalk GD, Wadsworth HL, Rapoport B. Role of amino acids 261–418 in proteolytic cleavage of the extracellular region of the human thyrotropin receptor. Endocrinology 1992;130:2135

28. Endo T, Ikeda M, Ohmori M, Anzai E, Haraguchi K, Onaya T. Single subunit structure of the human thyrotropin receptor. Biochem Biophys Res Comm 1992;187:887

29. Kobe B, Deisenhofer J. Crystal structure of porcine ribonuclease inhibitor, a protein with leucine-rich repeats. Nature 1993; 366:751

30. Nagayama Y, Nagataki S. The thyrotropin receptor: its gene expression and structure-function relationships. Thyroid Today 1994;17:1

31. Wadsworth HL, Chazenbalk GD, Nagayama Y, Russo D, Rapoport B. An insertion in the human thyrotropin receptor critical for high affinity hormone binding. Science 1990;249:1423

32. Nagayama Y, Wadsworth HL, Chazenbalk GD, Russo D, Seto P, Rapoport B. Thyrotropin-luteinizing hormone/chorionic gonadotropin receptor extracellular domain chimeras as probes for TSH receptor function. Proc Natl Acad Sci U S A 1991;88:902

33. Nagayama Y, Russo D, Wadsworth HL, Chazenbalk GD, Rapoport B. Eleven amino acids (Lys-201 to Lys-211) and 9 amino acids (Gly-222 to Leu-230) in the human thyrotropin receptor are involved in ligand binding. J Biol Chem 1991;266: 14926

34. Nagayama Y, Takeshita A, Luo W, Ashizawa K, Yokoyama N, Nagataki S. High affinity binding of thyrotropin (TSH) and thyroid-stimulating autoantibody for the TSH receptor extracellular domain. Thyroid 1994;4:155

35. Nagayama Y, Wadsworth HL, Russo D, Chazenbalk GD, Rapoport B. Binding domains of stimulatory and inhibitory thyrotropin (TSH) receptor autoantibodies determined with chimeric TSH-lutropin/chorionic gonadotropin receptors. J Clin Invest 1991;88:336

36. Shi Y, Zou M, Parhar RS, Farid NR. High-affinity binding of thyrotropin to the extracellular domain of its receptor transfected in Chinese hamster ovary cells. Thyroid 1993;3:129

37. Russo D, Chazenbalk GD, Nagayama Y, Wadsworth HL, Rapoport B. Site-directed mutagenesis of the human thyrotropin receptor: Role of asparagine-linked oligosaccharides in the expression of a functional receptor. Mol Endocrinol 1991;5:29

38. Kosugi J, Akamizu T, Mori T. Possible differences in glycosylation of the thyrotropin receptor among species. Biochem Biophys Res Comm 1994;200:1207

39. Takai O, Desai RK, Seetharamaiah GS, et al. Prokaryotic expression of the thyrotropin receptor and identification of an immunogenic region of the protein using synthetic peptides. Biochem Biophys Res Comm 1991;179:319

40. Huang GC, Collison KS, McGregor AM, Banga JP. Expression of a human thyrotropin receptor fragment in Escherichia coli and its interaction with the hormone and autoantibodies from patients with Graves' disease. J Mol Endocrinol 1992;8:137

41. Seetharamaiah GS, Desai RK, Dallas JS, Tahara K, Kohn LD, Prabhakar BS. Induction of TSH binding inhibitory immunoglobulins with the extracellular domain of human thyrotropin receptor produced using baculovirus expression system. Autoimmunity 1993;14:315

42. Chazenbalk GD, Rapoport B. Expression of the extracellular region of the thyrotropin receptor in a baculovirus vector using a promoter active earlier than the polyhedrin promoter. Implications for the expression of functional, highly glycosylated proteins. J Biol Chem 1995;270:1543

43. Seetharamaiah GS, Kurosky A, Desai RK, Dallas JS, Prabhakar BS. A recombinant extracellular domain of the thyrotropin (TSH) receptor binds TSH in the absence of membranes. Endocrinology 1994;134:549

44. Gross B, Misrahi M, Sar S, Milgrom E. Composite structure of the human thyrotropin receptor gene. Biochem Biophys Res Comm 1991;177:679

45. Libert F, Passage E, Lefort A, Vassart G, Mattei M-G. Localization of human thyrotropin receptor gene to chromosome region 14q31 by in situ hybridization. Cytogenet Cell Genet 1990;54:82

46. Rousseau-Merck MF, Misrahi M, Loosfelt H, Atger M, Milgrom E, Berger R. Assignment of the human thyroid stimulating hormone receptor (TSHR) gene to chromosome 14q31. Genomics 1990; 8:233

47. Graves PN, Tomer Y, Davies TF. Cloning and sequencing of a 1.3 kb variant of human thyrotropin receptor mRNA lacking the transmembrane domain. Biochem Biophys Res Comm 1992;187:1135

48. Takeshita A, Nagayama Y, Fujiyama K, et al. Molecular cloning and sequencing of an alternatively spliced form of the human thyrotropin receptor transcript. Biochem Biophys Res Comm 1992;188:1214

49. Libert F, Parmentier M, Maenhaut C, et al. Molecular cloning of a dog thyrotropin (TSH) receptor variant. Mol Cell Endocrinol 1990;68:R15

50. Roselli-Rehfuss L, Robbins LS, Cone RD. Thyrotropin receptor messenger ribonucleic acid is expressed in most brown and white adipose tissues in the guinea pig. Endocrinology 1992;130:1857

51. Endo T, Ohno M, Kotani S, Gunji K, Onaya T. Thyrotropin receptor in non-thyroid tissue. Biochem Biophys Res Comm 1993; 190:774

52. Davies TF, Teng CS, McLachlan SM, Smith BR, Hall R. Thyrotropin receptors in adipose tissue, retro-orbital tissue and lymphocytes. Mol Cell Endocrinol 1978;9:303

53. Gill DL, Marshall NJ, Ekins RP. Binding of thyrotropin to receptors in fat tissue. Mol Cell Endocrinol 1978;10:89

54. Ikuyama S, Shimura H, Hoeffler JP, Kohn LD. Role of the cyclic adenosine 3',5'-monophosphate response element in efficient

expression of the rat thyrotropin receptor promoter. Mol Endocrinol 1992;6:1701

55. Allgeier A, Offermanns S, Van Sande J, Spicher K, Schultz G, Dumont JE. The human thyrotropin receptor activates G-proteins Gs and Gq/11. J Biol Chem 1994;269:13733

56. Nagayama Y, Rapoport B. Role of the carboxyl-terminal half of the extracellular domain of the human thyrotropin receptor in signal transduction. Endocrinology 1992;131:548

57. Chazenbalk GD, Nagayama Y, Russo D, Wadsworth HL, Rapoport B. Functional analysis of the cytoplasmic domains of the human thyrotropin receptor by site-directed mutagenesis. J Biol Chem 1990;265:20970

58. Kosugi S, Kohn LD, Akamizu T, Mori T. The middle portion in the second cytoplasmic loop of the thyrotropin receptor plays a crucial role in adenylate cyclase activation. Mol Endocrinol 1994;8:498

59. Kosugi S, Okajima F, Ban T, Hidaka A, Shenker A, Kohn LD. Mutation of alanine 623 in the third cytoplasmic loop of the rat thyrotropin (TSH) receptor results in a loss in the phosphoinositide but not cAMP signal induced by TSH and receptor autoantibodies. J Biol Chem 1992;267:24153

60. Kosugi S, Mori T. The first cytoplasmic loop of the thyrotropin receptor is important for phosphoinositide signaling but not for agonist-induced adenylate cyclase activation. FEBS Lett 1994;341:162

61. Kjelsberg MA, Cotecchia S, Ostrowski J, Caron MG, Lefkowitz RJ. Constitutive activation of the alpha 1B-adrenergic receptor by all amino acid substitutions at a single site. Evidence for a region which constrains receptor activation. J Biol Chem 1992;267:1430

62. Parma J, Duprez L, Van Sande J, et al. Somatic mutations in the thyrotropin receptor gene cause hyperfunctioning thyroid adenomas. Nature 1993;365:649

63. Matsuo K, Friedman E, Gejman P, Fagin JA. The thyrotropin receptor (TSH-R) is not an oncogene for thyroid tumors: structural studies of the TSH-R and the alpha-subunit of Gs in human thyroid neoplasms. J Clin Endocrinol Metab 1993;76:1446

64. Duprez L, Parma J, Van Sande J, et al. Germline mutations in the thyrotropin receptor gene cause non-autoimmune autosomal dominant hyperthyroidism. Nature Genet 1994;7:396

65. Rapoport B. Dog thyroid cells in monolayer tissue culture: adenosine 3′,5′-cyclic monophosphate response to thyrotropic hormone. Endocrinology 1976;98:1189

66. Shuman SJ, Zor U, Chayoth R, Field JB. Exposure of thyroid slices to thyroid-stimulating hormone induces refractoriness of the cyclic AMP system to subsequent hormone stimulation. J Clin Invest 1976;57:1132

67. Rapoport B, Filetti S, Takai N, Seto P. Studies on the desensitization of the cyclic AMP response to thyrotropin in thyroid tissue. FEBS Lett 1982;146:23

68. Rapoport B, Adams RJ. Induction of refractoriness to thyrotropin stimulation in cultured thyroid cells. J Biol Chem 1976;251:6653

69. Foti D, Catalfamo R, Russo D, Costante G, Filetti S. Lack of relationship between cAMP desensitization and TSH receptor downregulation in the rat thyroid cell line FRTL-5. J Endocrinol Invest 1991;14:213

70. Filetti S, Takai NA, Rapoport B. Prevention of nicotinamide of desensitization to thyrotropin stimulation in cultured human thyroid cells. J Biol Chem 1981;256:1072

71. Hirayu H, Magnusson RP, Rapoport B. Studies on the mechanism of desensitization of the cyclic AMP response to TSH stimulation in a cloned rat thyroid cell line. Mol Cell Endocrinol 1985;42:21

72. Takasu N, Charrier B, Mauchamp J, Lissitzky S. Modulation of adenylate cyclase/cyclic AMP response by thyrotropin and prostaglandin E2 in cultured thyroid cells.1.Negative regulation. Eur J Biochem 1978;90:131

73. Tramontano D, Ingbar SH. Properties and regulation of the thyrotropin receptor in the FRTL5 rat thyroid cell line. Endocrinology 1986;118:1945

74. Filetti S, Rapoport B. Inhibitors of specific aminoacyl-tRNA synthetases prevent thyrotropin-induced desensitization in cultured human thyroid cells. J Biol Chem 1982;257:1342

75. Filetti S, Rapoport B. Hormonal stimulation of eucaryotic cell ADP-ribosylation. Effect of thyrotropin on thyroid cells. J Clin Invest 1981;68:461

76. Kühn H, Hall S, Wilden U. Light-induced binding of 48-kd protein to photoreceptor membranes is highly enhanced by phosphorylation of rhodopsin. FEBS Lett 1984;176:473

77. Wilden U, Hall S, Kühn H. Phosphodiesterase activation by photoexcited rhodopsin is quenced when rhodopsin is phosphorylated and binds the intrinsic 48-kd protein of rod outer segments. Proc Natl Acad Sci U S A 1986;83:1174

78. Lohse MJ, Benovic JL, Codina J, Caron MG, Lefkowitz RJ. β-Arrestin: a protein that regulates β-adrenergic receptor function. Science 1990;248:1547

79. Rapoport B, Kaufman KD, Chazenbalk GD. Cloning of a member of the arrestin family from a human thyroid cDNA library. Mol Cell Endocrinol 1992;84:R39

80. Van Sande J, Grenier G, Willems C, Dumont JE. Inhibition by iodide of the activation of the thyroid cyclic 3′,5′-AMP system. Endocrinology 1975;96:781

81. Rapoport B, West MN, Ingbar SH. Inhibitory effect of dietary iodine on the thyroid adenylate cyclase response to thyrotropin in the hypophysectomized rat. J Clin Invest 1975;56:516

82. Filetti S, Rapoport B. Evidence that organic iodine attenuates the adenosine 3′,5′-monophosphate response to thyrotropin stimulation in thyroid tissue by action at or near the adenylate cyclase catalytic unit. Endocrinology 1983;113:1608

83. Kraiem Z, Sadeh O, Blithe DL, Nisula BC. Human chorionic gonadotropin stimulates thyroid hormone secretion, iodide uptake, organification, and adenosine 3′,5′-monophosphate formation in cultured human thyrocytes. J Clin Endocrinol Metab 1994;790:595

84. Gerber H, Studer H, Conti A, Engler H, Kohler H, Haeberli A. Reaccumulation of thyroglobulin and colloid in rat and mouse thyroid follicles during intense thyrotropin stimulation. J Clin Invest 1981;68:1338

85. Sho K, Okajima F, Majid MA, Kondo Y. Reciprocal modulation of thyrotropin actions by P1-purinergic agonists in FRTL-5 thyroid cells. J Biol Chem 1991;266:12180

86. Spaulding SW. The ways in which hormones change cyclic adenosine 3′,5′-monophosphate-dependent protein kinase subunits, and how such changes affect cell behavior. Endocr Rev 1993;14:632

87. Spaulding SW, Burrow GN. TSH regulation of cAMP-dependent protein kinase activity in the thyroid. Biochem Biophys Res Comm 1974;59:386

88. Tortora G, Pepe S, Cirafici AM, et al. Thyroid-stimulating hormone-regulated growth and cell cycle distribution of thyroid cells involve type I isozyme of cyclic AMP-dependent protein kinase. Cell Growth Differentiation 1993;4:359

89. Woloshin PI, Walton KM, Rehfuss RP, Goodman RH, Cone RD. 3′,5′-cyclic adenosine monophosphate-regulated enhancer binding (CREB) activity is required for normal growth and differentiated phenotype in the FRTL5 thyroid follicular cell line. Mol Endocrinol 1992;6:1725

90. Lalli E, Sassone-Corsi P. Signal transduction and gene regulation: the nuclear response to cAMP. J Bio Chem 1994;269:17359

91. Kwok RPS, Lundblad JR, Chrivia JC, et al. Nuclear protein CBP is a coactivator for the transcription factor CREB. Nature 1994;370:223

92. Spaulding SW, Fucile NW, Bofinger DP, Sheflin LG. Cyclic adenosine 3′,5′-monophosphate-dependent phosphorylation of HMG 14 inhibits its interactions with nucleosomes. Mol Endocrinol 1991;5:42

93. Colletta G, Cirafici AM. TSH is able to induce cell cycle-related gene expresion in rat thyroid cell. Biochem Biophys Res Comm 1992;183:265

94. Saji M, Akamizu T, Sanchez M, Obici S, Avvedimento E, Gottesman ME. Regulation of thyrotropin receptor gene expression in rat FRTL-5 thyroid cells. Endocrinology 1992;130:520

95. Shimura H, Okajima F, Ikuyama S, et al. Thyroid-specific expression and cyclic adenosine 3′,5′-monophosphate autoregulation of the thyrotropin receptor gene involves thyroid transcription factor-1. Mol Endocrinol 1994;8:1049

96. Laurberg P. Paradoxically subnormal serum T_4 and T_3 in dogs after prolonged excessive TSH stimulation of the thyroid caused by post-cAMP refractoriness of thyroid hormone secretion. Metabolism 1989;38:265

97. Maenhaut C, Brabant G, Vassart G, Dumont JE. *In vitro* and *in vivo* regulation of thyrotropin receptor mRNA levels in dog and human thyroid cells. J Biol Chem 1992;267:3000

98. Deery WJ, Rani CSS. Protein kinase C activation mimics but does not mediate thyrotropin-induced desensitization of adenylyl cyclase in cultured dog thyroid cells. Endocrinology 1991;128:2967

99. Pasquali D, Rani CSS, Deery WJ. Carbachol-induced decrease in thyroid cell adenylyl cyclase activity is independent of calcium and phosphodiesterase activation. Mol Pharmacol 1991;41:163

100. Saji M, Ikuyama S, Akamizu T, Kohn LD. Increases in cytosolic Ca^{++} down regulate thyrotropin receptor gene expression by a mechanism different from the cAMP signal. Biochem Biophys Res Comm 1991;176:94

101. Akamizu T, Ikuyama S, Saji M, et al. Cloning, chromosomal assignment, and regulation of the rat thyrotropin receptor: expression of the gene is regulated by thyrotropin, agents that increase cAMP levels, and thyroid autoantibodies. Proc Natl Acad Sci U S A 1990;87:5677

102. Lombardi A, Veneziani BM, Tramontano D, Ingbar SH. Independent and interactive effects of tetradecanoyl phorbol acetate on growth and differentiated function of FRTL5 cells. Endocrinology 1988;123:1544

103. Davies TF. Positive regulation of the guinea pig thyrotropin receptor. Endocrinology 1985;117:201

104. Huber GK, Concepcion ES, Graves PN, Davies TF. Positive regulation of human thyrotropin receptor mRNA by thyrotropin. J Clin Endocrinol Metab 1991;72:1394

105. Berg JP, Sandvik JA, Ree AH, et al. 1,25-Dihydroxyvitamin D_3 attenuates adenylyl cyclase activity in rat thyroid cells: reduction of thyrotropin receptor number and increase in guanine nucleotide-binding protein $G_{i-2}\alpha$. Endocrinology 1994;135:595.

106. Meinkoth JL, Goldsmith PK, Spiegel AM, Feramisco JR, Burrow GN. Inhibition of thyrotropin-induced DNA synthesis in thyroid follicular cells by microinjection of an antibody to the stimulatory G protein of adenylate cyclase, G_s. J Biol Chem 1992;267:13239

107. Berg JP, Ree AH, Sandvik JA, et al. 1,25-Dihydroxyvitamin D_3 alters the effect of cAMP in thyroid cells by increasing the regulatory subunit type II beta of the cAMP-dependent protein kinase. J Biol Chem 1994;269:32233

108. Saunier B, Dib K, Delemer B, Jacquemin C, Correze C. Cyclic AMP regulation of G_s protein. J Biol Chem 1990;265:19942

109. Ginsberg J, Murray PG, Parent, Wong K. Translocation of protein kinase C in porcine thyroid cells following exposure to thyrotropin. FEBS Lett 1988;226:223

110. Dib K, Delemer B, Jamali AE, Haye B, Jacquemin C, Correze C. 12-O-tetradecanoyl-phorbol-13-acetate (TPA) counteracts the cAMP up-regulation of the expression of the stimulatory guanine nucleotide binding protein ($Gs\alpha$) and $Gs\alpha$ messenger RNA in cultured pig thyroid cells. Mol Cell Endocrinol 1994;99:229

111. Haye B, Aublin JL, Champion S, Lambert B, Jacquemin C. Tetradecanoyl phorbol-13-acetate counteracts the responsiveness of cultured thyroid cells to thyrotropin. Biochem Pharmacol 1985;34:3795

112. Burch RM, Luini A, Axelrod J. Phospholipase A_2 and phospholipase C are activated by distinct GTP-binding proteins in response to α_1-adrenergic stimulation in FRTL-5 thyroid cells. Proc Nat Acad Sci U S A 1986;83:7201

113. Bidey SP, Tomlinson S. Differential modulation by Ca^{2+} of iodide transport processes in a cultured rat thyroid cell strain. J Endocrinol 1987;112:51

114. Smallridge RC, Gist ID. P_2 purinergic stimulation of iodide efflux in FRTL-5 rat thyroid cells involves parallel activation of PLC and PLA_2. Am J Physiol 1994;267:E323

115. Marcocci C, Luini A, Santisteban P, Grollman EF. Norepinephrine and thyrotropin stimulation of iodide efflux in FRTL-5 thyroid cells involves metabolites of arachidonic acid and is associated with the iodination of thyroglobulin. Endocrinology 1987; 120:1127

116. Nilsson M, Bjorkman U, Ekholm R, Ericson LE. Polarized efflux of iodide in porcine thyrocytes occurs via a cAMP-regulated iodide channel in the apical plasma membrane. Acta Endocrinol 1992;126:67

117. Weiss SJ, Philp NJ, Ambesi-Impiombato FS, Grollman EF. Thyrotropin-stimulated iodide transport mediated by adenosine 3′,5′-monophosphate and dependent on protein synthesis. Endocrinology 1984;114:1099

118. Rani CSS, Field JB. Comparison of effects of thyrotropin, phorbol esters, norepinephrine, and carbachol on iodide organification in dog thyroid slices, follicles and cultured cells. Endocrinology 1988;122:1915

119. Perrild H, Loveridge N, Reader SCJ, Robertson WR. Acute stimulation of thyroidal NAD+ kinase, NADPH reoxidation, and peroxidase activities by physiological concentrations of thyroid stimulating hormone acting *in vitro:* a quantitative cytochemical study. Endocrinology 1988;123:2499

120. Hosaka Y, Tawata M, Kurihara A, Ohtaka M, Endo T, Onaya T. The regulation of two distinct glucose transporter (GLUT1 and GLUT4) gene expressions in cultured rat thyroid cells by thyrotropin. Endocrinology 1992;131:159

121. Yokomori N, Tawata M, Hosaka Y, Onaya T. Transcriptional rregulation of hexokinase I mRNA levels by TSH in cultured rat thyroid FRTL5 cells. Life Sci 1992;52:1613

122. Corvilain B, Laurent E, Lecomte M, Vansande J, Dumont JE. Role of the cyclic adenosine 3′,5′-monophosphate and the phosphatidylinositol-Ca^{2+} cascades in mediating the effects of thyrotropin and iodide on hormone synthesis and secretion in human thyroid slices. J Clin Endocrinol Metab 1994;79:152

123. Lippes HA, Spaulding SW. Peroxide formation and glucose oxidation in calf thyroid slices: regulation by protein kinase-C and cytosolic free calcium. Endocrinology 1986;118:1306

124. Corvilain B, Van Sande J, Laurent E, Dumont JE. The H_2O_2-generating system modulates protein iodination and the activity of the pentose phosphate pathway in dog thyroid. Endocrinology 1991;128:779

125. Bjorkman U, Ekholm R. Hydrogen peroxide generation and its regulation in FRTL-5 and porcine thyroid cells. Endocrinology 1992;130:393

126. Bjorkman U, Ekholm R. Effect of P_1-purinergic agonist on thyrotropin stimulation of H_2O_2 generation in FRTL-5 and porcine thyroid cells. Eur J Endocrinol 1994;130:180

127. Collison KS, Banga JP, Barnett PS, Kung AWC, McGregor AM. Activation of the thyroid peroxidase gene in human thyroid cells: Effect of thyrotrophin, forskolin and phorbol ester. J Mol Endocrinol 1989;3:1

128. Pohl V, Abramowicz M, Vassart G, Dumont JE, Roger PP. Thyroperoxidase mRNA in quiescent and proliferating thyroid epithelial cells: expression and subcellular localization studied by in situ hybridization. Eur J Cell Biol 1993;62:94

129. Aza-Blanc P, DiLauro R, Santisteban P. Identification of a cis-regulatory element and a thyroid-specific nuclear factor mediating the hormonal regulation of rat thyroid peroxidase promoter activity. Mol Endocrinol 1993;93:1297

130. Damante G, DiLauro R. Thyroid-specific gene expression. Biochem Biophys Acta 1994;1218:255

131. Tseng FY, Rani CSS, Field JB. Effect of iodide on glucose oxidation and ^{32}P incorporation into phospholipids stimulated by different agents in dog thyroid slices. Endocrinology 1989;124:1450

132. Tramontano D, Veneziani BM, Lombardi A, Villone G, Ingbar SH. Iodine inhibits the proliferation of rat thyroid cells in culture. Endocrinology 1989;125:984

133. Nazarea M, Okajima F, Kondo Y. P_2-purinergic activation of phosphoinositide turnover is potentiated by A_1-receptor stimulation in thyroid cells. Eur J Pharm [Mol Pharm Sec] 1991;206:47

134. Akiguchi I, Strauss K, Borges M, Silva JE, Moses AC. Thyroid hormone receptors and 3,5,3'-triiodothyronine biological effects in FRTL5 thyroid follicular cells. Endocrinology 1992;131:1279

135. Kamikubo K, Nayfeh SN, Chae CB. Differential regulation of multiple c-*erbA* expression by thyrotropin, insulin and insulin-like growth factor I in rat thyroid FRTL-5 cells. Mol Cell Endocrinol 1992;84:219

136. Saiardi A, Falasca P, Civitareale D. The thyroid hormone inhibits the thyrotropin receptor promoter activity: evidence for a short loop regulation. Biochem Biophys Res Comm 1994;205:230

137. Beech SG, Walker SW, Dorrance AM, et al. The role of thyroidal type-I iodothyronine deiodinase in tri-iodothyronine production by human and sheep thyrocytes in primary culture. J Endocrinol 1993;136:361

138. Toyoda N, Nishikawa M, Mori Y, et al. Thyrotropin and tri-iodothyronine regulate iodothyronine 5'-deiodinase messenger ribonucleic acid levels in FRTL-5 rat thyroid cells. Endocrinology 1992;132:389

139. Tseng YCL, Burman KD, Lahiri S, D'Avis J, Wartofsky L. Thyrotropin modulation of epidermal growth factor (EGF) binding to receptors on cultured thyroid cells. Thyroid 1992;2:181

140. Sugawa H, Beniko M, Imura H, Moril T. Characterization of epidermal growth factor receptor in a rat thyroid cellline, FRTL-5. Biochem Biophy Res Comm 193:390

141. Ozawa S, Spaulding SW. Epidermal growth factor inhibits radioiodine uptake but stimulates deoxyribonucleic acid synthesis in newborn rat thyroids grown in nude mice. Endocrinology 1990;127:604

142. Ozawa S, Sheflin LG, Spaulding SW. Thyroxine increases epidermal growth factor levels in the mouse thyroid *in vivo*. Endocrinology 1991;128:1396

143. Sheflin LG, Fucile NW, Ozawa S, Spaulding SW. Thyroxine increases the levels of epidermal growth factor messenger ribonucleic acid (EGF mRNA) in the thyroid *in vivo*, as revealed by quantitative reverse transcription polymerase chain reaction with an internal control EGF mRNA. Endocrinology 1993;132:2319

144. Eggo MC, Sheppard MC. Autocrine growth factors produced in the thyroid. Mol Cell Endocrinol 1994;100:97

145. Bachrach LK, Eggo MC, Hintz RL, Burrow GN. Insulin-like growth factors in sheep thyroid cells: action, receptors and production. Biochem Biophys Res Commun 1988;1454:861

146. Takahasi SI, Conti M, Prokop C, VanWyk JJ, Earp III HS. Thyrotropin and insulin-like growth factor I regulation of thyrosine phosphorylation in FRTL-5 cells. J Biol Chem 1991;266:7834

147. Condorelli G, Formisano P, Miele C, Beguinot F. Thyrotropin regulates autophosphorylation and kinase activity of both the insulin and the insulin-like growth factor-I receptors in FRTL5 cells. Endocrinology 1992;130:1615

148. Takano T, Takada K, Tada H, Nishiyama S, Amino N. Genistein, a tyrosine kinase inhibitor, blocks the cell cycle progression but not Ca^{2+} influx induced by bay K8644 in FRTL-5 cells. Biochem Biophys Res Comm 1993;190:801

149. Bjorkman U, Ekholm R, Ericson LE. Effects of thyrotropin on thyroglobulin exocytosis and iodination in the rat thyroid. Endocrinology 1978;102:460

150. Melander A, Ranklev E, Sundler F, Westgren U. Beta$_2$-adrenergic stimulation of thyroid hormone secretion. Endocrinology 1975;97:332

151. Pisarev MA, Cardinali DP, Juvenal GJ, Vacas MI, Bartontini M, Boado RJ. Role of the sympathetic nervous system in the control of the goitrogenic response in the rat. Endocrinology 1981;109:2202

152. Brandi ML, Rotella CM, Zonefrati R, Toccafondi R, Aloj SM. Loss of adrenergic regulation of cAMP production in the FRTL-5 cell line. Acta Endocrinol 1986;111:54

153. Tzuzaki S, Cone RD, Frazier AL, Moses AC. The interaction of signal transduction pathways in FRTL5 thyroid follicular cells: Studies with stable expression of β2-adrenergic receptors. Endocrinology 1991;128:1359

154. Endo T, Shimura H, Saito T, Onaya T. Cloning of malignantly transformed rat thyroid (FRTL) cells with thyrotropin receptors, and their growth inhibition by 3',5'-cyclic adenosine monophosphate. Endocrinology 1990;126:1492

155. Kanasaki M, Matsubara H, Murasawa S, Masaki H, Nio Y, Inada M. cAMP responsive element-mediated regulation of the gene transcription of the α1B adrenergic receptor by thyrotropin. J Clin Invest 1994;94:2245

156. Okajima F, Sato K, Sho K, Kondo Y. Stimulation of adenosine receptor enhances α1-adrenergic receptor-mediated activation of phospholipase C and Ca^{2+} mobilization in a pertussis toxin-sensitive manner in FRTL-5 thyroid cells. FEBS Lett 1989;248:145

157. Jockers R, Linder ME, Hohenegger M, et al. Species difference in the G protein selectivity of the human and bovine A_1-adenosine receptor. J Biol Chem 1994;269:32077

Werner and Ingbar's The Thyroid, Seventh Edition,
edited by Lewis E. Braverman and Robert D. Utiger.
Lippincott–Raven Publishers, Philadelphia, © 1996

12

Regulation of Thyrotropin Secretion

Maurice F. Scanlon
Anthony D. Toft

Thyrotropin (thyroid-stimulating hormone; TSH) is responsible for normal thyroid function. It is synthesized and secreted by basophilic cells (thyrotrophs) in the anterior pituitary gland. Its secretion is controlled in part by the brain via thyrotropin-releasing hormone (TRH) and other molecules. The role of the brain in the control of thyroid function has been appreciated for many years; it was believed initially that overactivity of the pituitary gland as a consequence of stress or emotional trauma was a common cause of thyrotoxicosis. Although we now know that this is not the case, data accruing from the emerging discipline of neuroendocrine immunology may well reveal mechanisms by which stress or emotional trauma precipitate or enhance immunologic episodes that lead to autoimmune hyperthyroidism (Graves' disease) in predisposed patients.

The hypothalamus exerts stimulatory control over thyroid function through the mediation of TSH because hypothyroidism occurs if the hypothalamus is lesioned or diseased or if the pituitary stalk is transected. This stimulatory hypothalamic control is exerted by TRH, a small tripeptide that is produced by hypothalamic neurons and transported along their axons to specialized nerve terminals in the median eminence of the hypothalamus, where it is released into hypophyseal portal blood. It is then carried directly to the anterior pituitary gland. The other major component of the hypothalamic-pituitary-thyroid axis is the powerful inhibitory action of circulating thyroid hormones. This inhibition is exerted primarily on the thyrotrophs but also to a lesser extent on the TRH-producing neurons of the hypothalamus (Fig 12-1). In addition, a variety of secondary modulators exert lesser control over TSH secretion, the net result of which is the maintenance of a steady output of TSH and therefore of thyroid hormones. The important secondary modulators are somatostatin and dopamine, both of which inhibit the function of the thy-

rotrophs, and α-adrenergic pathways, which are, in general, stimulatory. Other modulators of thyroid function include glucocorticoid hormones, various cytokines, and other inflammatory mediators.

CONTROL OF TSH RELEASE

The maintenance of euthyroidism is dependent on complex and highly tuned interactions between thyroid hormones and a hierarchical system of neuropeptides and neurotransmitters.[1] Although the dominant hypothalamic control over TSH is stimulatory by way of TRH, thyroid hormones exert a powerful, dose-related, negative-feedback control over TSH synthesis and release; the direct pituitary action of thyroid hormones on the suppression of basal and TRH-stimulated TSH release has been demonstrated clearly in many studies.

Role of Thyroid Hormones

After acute administration of a single pharmacologic dose of triiodothyronine (T_3) in rats, there is rapid suppression of serum TSH to 10% of pretreatment concentrations within 5 hours after T_3 administration. Thereafter, further TSH suppression occurs more slowly and only after chronic treatment with T_3.[2,3] The rapid phase of TSH suppression is paralleled by an increase in nuclear T_3 content, and serum TSH concentrations rise as nuclear T_3 levels decline.[4,5] There is also an inverse relationship between nuclear T_3 receptor occupancy and serum TSH concentrations after acute administration of T_3.[6] About half of pituitary nuclear T_3 is derived from the intracellular 5'-monodeiodination of thyroxine (T_4),[6] which is a greater fraction than in other tissues; this monodeiodination may be the

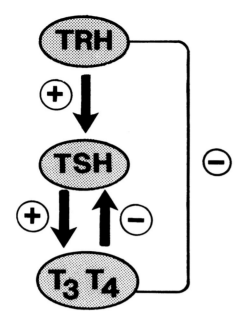

FIGURE 12-1. Schematic representation of the primary system for regulation of hypothalamic-pituitary-thyroid function. The fundamental actions are hypothalamic stimulation of thyrotroph function balanced by the powerful negative-feedback inhibition exerted by thyroid hormones. ⊕, stimulation; ⊖, inhibition.

mechanism by which the thyrotrophs respond to changes in serum T_4 concentrations.

The major actions of thyroid hormones are to regulate gene expression after binding to specific nuclear receptors.[7,8] Thyroid hormone receptors are structurally related to the viral oncogene v-*erb* A and, together with steroid, vitamin D and retinoic acid receptors, form a family of receptor proteins with important structural similarities (see chap 9). Several cDNAs that encode different thyroid hormone receptors (α and β) have been described. Binding of T_3 to a site on the carboxyl-terminal end of the receptor activates the receptor so that the T_3-receptor complex binds to specific nucleotide sequences on target genes.[9] Within the thyrotrophs, the activated T_3 receptors inhibit transcription of the α-subunit and TSH-β-subunit genes in proportion to nuclear T_3-receptor occupancy.

Role of TRH

Although the existence of TRH was first suggested 45 years ago,[10] it was not until 30 years ago that an extract of porcine hypothalami with TSH-releasing properties was isolated.[11] Elucidation of the structure and subsequent synthesis of porcine[12] and ovine[13] TRH established its nature as the weakly basic tripeptide pyro-Glu-His-Pro-amide (Fig 12-2). Synthetic TRH has biologic activity identical to that of the natural material and, like other hypothalamic regulatory peptides, has no phylogenic specificity. The importance of TRH in the maintenance of normal thyroid function is now well established; in addition, TRH has several other actions on the anterior pituitary (see later). It is also widely distributed throughout the extrahypothalamic brain, spinal cord, pituitary gland, and other body tissues, where it probably has important neuromodulatory and paracrine roles.

SYNTHESIS AND METABOLISM OF TRH

TRH, like other, more complex peptides, is derived from posttranslational cleavage of a larger precursor molecule.[14–16] Investigation of the synthesis of TRH proved difficult for many years, in part because antibodies to this small peptide did not cross-react with precursor molecules. However, antibodies to a peptide sequence present in the pro-TRH molecule, deduced from cloned amphibian skin cDNA,[17] cross-react with neuronal perikarya in the parvicellular division of the paraventricular nucleus of the hypothalamus and in the raphe complex of the medulla oblongata of rats.[14] Similar antibodies have been used to characterize the mammalian (rat) pro-TRH hormone, and both TRH and pro-TRH have been found in neurons of the paraventricular nucleus, whereas only TRH is present in axon terminals in the median eminence.[14,16] The cDNA sequence of the rat TRH precursor encodes a protein with a molecular size of 29,000 daltons that contains five copies of the sequence Gln-His-Pro-Gly.[18] Rat pro-TRH is processed at paired basic residues to a family of peptides that include TRH and flanking and intervening sequences. These peptides may prove to exert important intracellular or extracellular actions,[19,20] in particular prepro-TRH-(160-169), which stimulates TSH gene expression.[21,22] There may be preferential processing of pro-TRH to produce different peptides in different brain regions.[16]

TRH is rapidly degraded in tissues and serum to TRH free acid, the stable, cyclized metabolite, histidyl-proline-diketopiperazine (His-Pro-DKP), and its constituent amino acids.[23,24] TRH is hydrolyzed at the pyro-Glu-His bond by a particular enzyme, pyroglutamyl aminopeptidase, which is present in synaptosomal and anterior pituitary membrane preparations.[25,26] This enzyme is similar to the serum-degrading enzyme[27] in that it has great specificity for TRH.[28] His-Pro-DKP has several pharmacologic actions; TRH may be a prohormone for this molecule, but it may arise independently in some tissues.[29,30] The plasma half-life of TRH is short, ranging from about 2 minutes in thyrotoxic animals to 6 minutes in hypothyroid animals; the differences reflect in part the effects of thyroid status on the serum-degrading enzyme.[31] The half-life is similarly short in humans. The activity of the anterior pituitary TRH-degrading enzyme is rapidly and potently stimulated by thyroid hormones, whereas brain-degrading activity is unaffected.[32,33] This is entirely appropriate to the differing roles of TRH within the pituitary and brain; the potency of the thyroid hormone effect on the degradation of TRH by anterior pituitary membranes indicates that this may be an important regulatory mechanism.

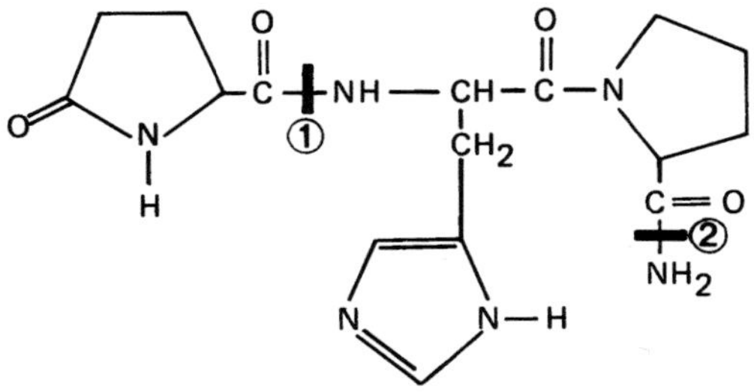

FIGURE 12-2. Structure of TRH, pyroglutamyl-histidylprolinamide. Metabolic degradation occurs at site 1 by way of membrane-bound pyroglutamyl aminopeptidase and at site 2 by way of TRH deamidase.

HYPOTHALAMIC AND PITUITARY DISTRIBUTION AND ACTIONS OF TRH AND ITS METABOLITES

Immunoreactive TRH is widely distributed in the hypothalamus, particularly high concentrations being found in the median eminence and in the nuclei of the so-called thyrotrophic area of the paraventricular nuclei.[1] Lesions of the paraventricular nuclei reduce circulating TSH concentrations and prevent the increase in serum TSH that occurs in primary hypothyroidism.[34] TRH and pro-TRH perikarya are present in the parvicellular division of this nucleus,[14,35] which is the major site of origin of the immunoreactive TRH in the median eminence as opposed to other brain regions such as the tractus solitarius.[36] The TRH gene is also expressed in anterior pituitary tissue,[37,38] and TRH-positive nerve fibers are present in posterior pituitary tissue.[35] However, lesions of the paraventricular nuclei reduce the content of TRH in both anterior and posterior pituitary tissue, indicating that the hypothalamus is a source of some of the immunoreactive TRH in these areas.

The best defined physiologic actions of TRH concern its role in the control of anterior pituitary function. Although first recognized because of its effects on the release of TSH, TRH was soon found to have several other physiologic and pathophysiologic actions on anterior pituitary hormone secretion.

EFFECTS OF TRH ON TSH SECRETION

The dominant stimulatory role of the hypothalamus in the control of TSH synthesis and release is mediated by TRH. TRH has a direct dose-related action on TSH release both in vivo and in vitro,[1] and decreased TSH release and hypothyroidism occur after hypothalamic-pituitary dissociation and hypothalamic lesions and disease. TRH is present in hypophyseal portal blood at physiologically relevant concentrations[39] and administration of antibodies to TRH to animals can cause hypothyroidism. Intravenous administration of 15 to 500 µg of TRH to normal humans causes a dose-related release of TSH from the pituitary. In normal subjects given TRH intravenously serum TSH concentrations increase within 2 to 5 minutes, are maximal at 20 to 30 minutes, and return to basal levels by 2 to 3 hours. An increase in thyroid secretion follows, the peak serum T_3 and T_4 concentrations occurring about 3 and 8 hours, respectively, after TRH administration. In addition to stimulating TSH release, TRH also stimulates TSH synthesis by promoting transcription and translation of the TSH subunit genes, an action that involves calcium influx and activation of protein kinase C[40–45] and is modulated by cAMP and the pituitary-specific transcription factor, Pit-1.[46–48]

TRH plays an important role in the posttranslational processing of the oligosaccharide moieties of TSH and hence exerts an important influence on the biologic activity of the TSH that is secreted.[49] Full glycosylation of TSH is required for complete biologic activity (see section on chemistry and biosynthesis of thyrotropin in chap 11). This provides an explanation for the clinical observation that some patients with central hypothyroidism and slightly elevated basal serum TSH concentrations secrete TSH with reduced biologic activity that increases after TRH administration. It is likely that alterations in both hypothalamic TRH secretion and in the response of thyrotrophs to TRH contribute to the variable biologic activity of the TSH secreted by patients with different thyroid disorders[50,51] and those with TSH-secreting pituitary adenomas[52,53] (see chap 31).

INTERACTIONS BETWEEN TRH AND THYROID HORMONES

TRH acts in concert with hypothalamic somatostatin and dopamine to regulate TSH synthesis and release, and its stimulatory effect is counterbalanced by the direct pituitary inhibition of TSH synthesis and secretion by thyroid hormones. In this process, local intrapituitary conversion of T_4 to T_3 is particularly important.

In addition to their direct inhibitory actions on TSH-subunit gene expression and TSH release, thyroid hormones also modulate the expression of the TRH-receptor gene.[54] The number of TRH receptors on thyrotrophs increases in hypothyroidism and can be reduced by thyroid hormone replacement.[55,56] Conversely, in pituitary tumor (GH_4C_1) cells, TRH causes a dose-related reduction in T_3-receptor gene expression,[57] receptor number, and T_3 responsiveness,[58] which may represent a further site of feedback interaction between T_3 and TRH at the level of the pituitary.

In addition to their ability to inhibit TSH secretion, thyroid hormones exert powerful effects on hypothalamic function. The levels of TRH mRNA in the paraventricular nuclei increase in hypothyroidism and are reduced by thyroid hormone treatment.[59,60] Furthermore, rats with bilateral lesions of the paraventricular nuclei do not have the normal rise of serum TSH and TSH-subunit mRNA after induction of primary hypothyroidism,[61] an effect that presumably reflects depletion of TRH. These results indicate that the paraventricular nuclei are a target for the action of thyroid hormones in the control of TRH gene expression and release,[61–64] providing an additional mechanism for thyroidal regulation of TSH secretion.

EFFECTS OF TRH ON OTHER ANTERIOR PITUITARY HORMONES

TRH is a potent stimulator of prolactin (PRL) release and may play a physiologic role in mediating certain PRL responses, such as the response to suckling in rats, but it does not appear that TRH has any important role in the control of PRL secretion in humans.[65] Although often assumed, there is no firm evidence to indicate that the hyperprolactinemia that is found in up to 30% of patients with primary hypothyroidism is due to increased TRH secretion (see chap 68). There also is no evidence of a physiologic role of His-Pro-DKP[66] or any TRH metabolites in the control of PRL release in humans.

The actions of TRH on growth hormone (GH) release are complex, but in normal subjects GH release does not occur after TRH administration. In contrast, patients with several disorders including acromegaly and diabetes mellitus may have increases in serum GH in response to TRH administration. It seems likely that many, if not all, of these serum GH responses to TRH are a consequence of functional or structural dissociation between the hypothalamus and the anterior pituitary somatotrophs, perhaps operating through reduced somatostatin activity. In normal subjects, TRH has no demonstrable effects on ACTH release, but a rise in serum ACTH concentrations occurs after TRH administration in some patients with Cushing's disease or Nelson's syndrome.[67] Exogenous TRH can also stimulate vasopressin secretion,[68] which suggests a possible function for the TRH neurons with axons that enter the posterior pituitary gland.

MECHANISMS OF NEUROENDOCRINE ACTIONS OF TRH

In TSH-secreting tumors in mice and in GH$_3$ cells (another pituitary tumor cell line), TRH can reduce the number of its own receptors after chronic exposure.[69,70] This finding has not been confirmed for normal anterior pituitary cells, and it is not known whether it has any physiologic relevance in normal animals. TRH administration does, however, cause marked desensitization of hormonal responses.[71] This secretory refractoriness probably occurs at a site beyond the TRH receptor and, because it occurs in vitro, cannot be fully explained by the increase in serum T$_3$ and T$_4$ concentrations that accompanies TRH administration in vivo.

Human and rodent TRH receptors are structurally similar and belong to the family of seven transmembrane domain, G-protein coupled receptors.[72] Much of the work on the secondary message events involved in TRH action has been performed on GH$_3$ cells and mouse thyrotrophic tumor cells. TRH stimulates the activity of phospholipase C, which causes rapid hydrolysis of phosphatidyl-inositol 4,5-bisphosphate to inositol 1,4,5-bisphosphate and 1,2-diacylglycerol.[73,74] The latter in turn activates intracellular protein kinase C. Protein kinase C may participate in an intracellular feedback system to limit receptor-mediated hydrolysis of inositol phospholipids (Fig 12-3). This system may underlie the desensitization of hormonal responses to chronic TRH administration, because staurosporine, a potent inhibitor of protein kinase C, can prevent TRH-induced refractoriness of inositol phospholipid hydrolysis in rat anterior pituitary tissue.[75]

TRH causes an immediate, rapid increase in intracellular free calcium (which decays rapidly), which is followed by an extended plateau of elevated intracellular free calcium. This biphasic action correlates with secretory activity, electrical changes, and the induction of calcium fluxes in GH$_3$ cells.[74] The first phase reflects increased calcium release from intracellular stores, whereas the second phase represents calcium influx from the extracellular space. The biphasic pattern of TSH and intracellular free calcium responses to maximal doses of TRH in mouse thyrotrophic tumor cells is determined by the number of TRH receptors; down-regulation of TRH receptors abolishes the early secretory burst of TSH release and the rise in intracellular free calcium.[76]

TRH increases cAMP levels in pituitary tissue, but the increase probably is secondary to stimulation of phosphatidylinositol turnover by TRH.[77] In different brain regions, TRH selectively stimulates either cAMP generation or phosphatidylinositol turnover.[78] These results indicate that TRH receptors in different sites are functionally linked to different intracellular pathways.

Role of Somatostatin

Somatostatin, which is the major physiologic inhibitor of GH secretion, was initially isolated and characterized from ovine hypothalamus on the basis of its ability to inhibit GH release from anterior pituitary tissue. In addition, somatostatin is an inhibitor of TSH secretion in both animals and humans. Somatostatin-producing hypothalamic neurons are found mainly in the anterior periventricular region. About half the somatostatin in the median eminence arises from the preoptic region, and the remainder arises from the suprachiasmatic and retrochiasmatic regions. A lower density of somatostatin-producing neurons is present in the ventromedial and arcuate nuclei and also in the lateral hypothalamus.[79] Somatostatin is also widely distributed throughout the extrahypothalamic nervous

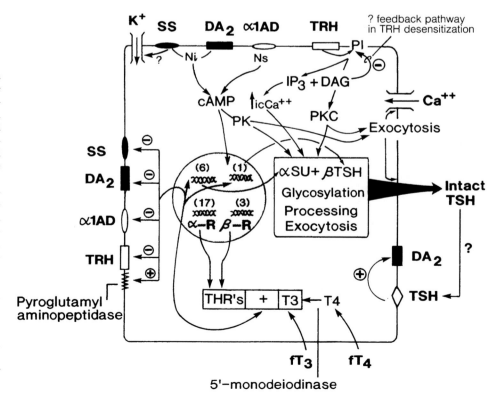

FIGURE 12-3. Schematic representation of some important interactions in the thyrotroph cell. Thyroid hormones reduce the biologic actions of somatostatin (SS), dopamine (DA), epinephrine, and TRH. This is due to a reduction in number rather than affinity of DA$_2$, TRH, and α_1-adrenergic (α1AD) receptors, and the same may well apply to SS receptors. These actions and the stimulation of pyroglutamyl aminopeptidase by T$_3$ are probably due to binding of the activated thyroid hormone receptor (THR) to relevant parts of the genome. Diacylglycerol (DAG) may participate in feedback inhibition of the functional response to TRH receptor agonism, causing apparent TRH desensitization. TRH and α1AD agonism exert additive effects on TSH release, indicating separate intracellular pathways. The numbers in parentheses indicate the chromosomal location of the genes for the α and β thyroid hormone receptors (R) and the α-subunits and β-subunits of TSH.

system and other body tissues, where it exerts a wide array of inhibitory actions. It is secreted in two principal forms: a 14-amino-acid peptide (somatostatin-14; Fig 12-4) and an N-terminal extended peptide (somatostatin-28). Its precursor, preprosomatostatin, is a 116-amino acid peptide[80,81] that undergoes differential posttranslational processing in different tissues to yield varying amounts of the 14- and 28-amino acid forms of the hormone. Each of these forms is secreted into hypophyseal portal blood in physiologically relevant concentrations.[82] The structure of the gene that encodes somatostatin in both humans[81] and rats[83] is now known.

During studies on the effects of somatostatin on other anterior pituitary hormones, it was found to inhibit basal and TRH-stimulated TSH release from cultured rat anterior pituitary cells,[84] and that the effect was greater in the presence of low thyroid hormone concentrations.[85] This led to the proposal that TSH release was regulated by the hypothalamus through a dual control system—stimulation by TRH and inhibition by somatostatin—analogous to that demonstrated for GH regulation.[84] The physiologic relevance of this proposal was established in studies using antiserum directed against somatostatin. Incubation of anterior pituitary cells with anti-somatostatin serum causes increased secretion of TSH (as well as GH), and administration of antiserum to rats increases basal serum TSH concentrations and the serum TSH responses to both cold stress and TRH.[86,87] In humans, somatostatin administration reduces the elevated serum TSH concentrations in patients with primary hypothyroidism, reduces the serum TSH response to TRH, abolishes the nocturnal elevation in TSH secretion, and prevents TSH release after administration of dopamine antagonist drugs. Somatostatin-14 and -28 exert equipotent effects on TSH release.[88] Furthermore, GH administration in humans decreases basal and TRH-stimulated TSH secretion,[89] probably owing to direct stimulatory effects of GH on hypothalamic somatostatin release.[90] In patients with pituitary disease, TSH secretory status correlates inversely with GH secretory status.[91] Despite these potent acute inhibitory effects of somatostatin on TSH secretion in humans, long-term treatment with somatostatin or the long-acting analogue, octreotide, does not cause hypothyroidism,[92] presumably because the great sensitivity of the thyrotrophs to any decrease in serum thyroid hormone concentrations overrides the inhibitory effect of somatostatin in the long term.

Somatostatin binds to several distinct types of specific, high-affinity receptors in the anterior pituitary and brain[93–95]; in the anterior pituitary, one of the types is expressed only in the presence of 17 β-estradiol.[96] The receptor subtypes differ in binding specifities, molecular weight, and linkage to adenylyl cyclase. The somatostatin receptor is negatively coupled to adenylyl cyclase through the inhibitory subunit of the guanine nucleotide regulatory protein, conventionally termed G_I or N_I (see Fig 12-3), a mechanism that mediates at least some of the inhibitory actions of this neuropeptide.[97] However, somatostatin may also act independently of cAMP by inducing hyper-polarization of membranes through modulation of voltage-dependent potassium channels,[98] leading to reduced calcium influx and a fall in intracellular calcium levels.[99]

Role of Neurotransmitters

An extensive network of neurotransmitter neurons terminates on the cell bodies of the hypophysiotropic neurons and within the interstitial spaces of the median eminence, where they regulate neuropeptide release into hypophyseal portal blood. In addition, dopamine (and possibly other neurotransmitters) is released directly into hypophyseal portal blood and exerts direct actions on anterior pituitary cells, particularly as the major physiologic inhibitor of prolactin release, but to a lesser extent as a physiologic inhibitor of TSH release.

Because of the specialized anatomic arrangements within the hypothalamus, each of the hypophysiotropic neuronal systems that regulate TSH secretion (TRH, somatostatin, and dopamine) are influenced by networks of other neurons that project from several brain regions.[100] Without these projections, basal TSH secretion (in rats and presumably in humans) and feedback regulation by thyroid hormones is relatively normal, suggesting that basal TRH secretion is regulated by intrinsic hypothalamic function. In contrast, circadian rhythms of TSH and pituitary-thyroid changes in response to stress and cold exposure (in lower animals) are mediated by nerve pathways that project to the medial basal hypothalamus.[101]

The principal systems that influence tuberoinfundibular neurons contain a bioamine neurotransmitter (dopamine, serotonin, histamine, or epinephrine), although several other neuropeptides and amino acid neurotransmitters may play a role. Virtually all the dopaminergic, noradrenergic, and serotoninergic pathways that project to the hypothalamus arise from groups of nuclei located in the midbrain.[102] Two dopaminergic systems exist within the hypothalamus: one, entirely intrinsic to the hypothalamus, arises in the arcuate nuclei, and the other projects from the midbrain. Histaminergic pathways are intrinsic to the hypothalamus, whereas adrenergic pathways arise from cell groups in the midbrain, although an intrinsic hypothalamic noradrenergic system also may exist. Opioid and γ-aminobutyric acid systems are mainly intrinsic to the hypothalamus. Cholinergic systems appear to play little part in the neuroregulation of TSH secretion.[103]

In view of the complexity of these interacting neuronal networks, it is hardly surprising that neuropharmacologic attempts to dissect the relative contributions of different neurotransmitter systems to the neuroregulation of TSH secretion have proved difficult. Furthermore, certain pathways have been studied extensively in rats yet hardly at all in humans, and the lack of availability of specific neuropeptide antagonists has limited study of the direct physiologic relevance of many of these molecules. Despite these problems consensus views have developed about the roles of several neurotransmitter pathways.

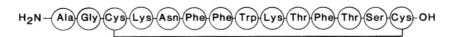

FIGURE 12-4. Structure of somatostatin-14. Somatostatin-28 is a 14-amino acid, N-terminal extension of this peptide.

CATECHOLAMINERGIC PATHWAYS

Studies using central neurotransmitter agonist and antagonist drugs have indicated the existence of stimulatory α-noradrenergic and inhibitory dopaminergic pathways in the control of TSH secretion in rats[104] (see Fig 12-3). α-Adrenergic agonists injected sytemically or into the third ventricle stimulate TSH release, and α-adrenergic antagonists or catecholamine-depleting drugs block TSH responses to cold.[103] More precisely, it appears that α_2 pathways are stimulatory, whereas α_1 pathways are inhibitory,[105] particularly in hypothyroid animals.[106] It has been assumed from such in vivo studies that these neurotransmitter effects are mediated by the appropriate modulation of the release of TRH or somatostatin, or both, into hypophyseal portal blood. A clear example of this is that the acute TSH release that follows cold stress in rats can be abolished by pretreatment with either anti-TRH antibodies or α-adrenergic antagonists, suggesting that adrenergically stimulated TRH release mediates this effect.[1]

The results of in vitro studies using rat hypothalamic tissue, however, are not in keeping with this attractive and simple hypothesis. For example, dopamine and dopamine-agonist drugs stimulate both TRH and somatostatin release from rat hypothalamus, acting through the DA_2 class of dopamine receptors.[107,108] This may reflect a general action of DA_2 receptors to mediate enhanced neuropeptide release at the level of the median eminence, in contrast to the usual inhibitory action of DA_2 agonists at the level of the anterior pituitary.

Although little precise knowledge exists about central mechanisms, it is clear that dopamine and epinephrine exert opposing actions on TSH release directly at the anterior pituitary level. Furthermore, both these molecules are present in rat hypophyseal portal blood in higher concentrations than in peripheral blood and in concentrations that could exert physiologic actions on the thyrotrophs.[109,110] Dopamine inhibits TSH release from rat[111] and bovine[112] anterior pituitary cells in a dose-related, stereospecific way, and there is striking parallelism between the inhibition of TSH and PRL by dopamine and dopamine-agonist drugs.[113] As with PRL, this inhibitory action on TSH release is mediated by DA_2 receptors[113] that are negatively coupled to adenylyl cyclase (see Fig 12-3). TSH release by thyrotroph cells from hypothyroid animals is more sensitive to the inhibitory effects of dopamine, which may reflect increased DA_2 receptor number rather than affinity.[114] In contrast, the sensitivity of PRL to the inhibitory effects of dopamine is reduced in lactotroph cells from hypothyroid animals,[114,115] a phenomenon that may contribute to the hyperprolactinemia that occurs in some patients with primary hypothyroidism.

Evidence from in vitro studies using rat anterior pituitary cells suggests that TSH may specifically regulate its own release through the induction of DA_2 receptors on the thyrotroph cells.[116] These data indicate a mechanism for the ultrashort-loop feedback control of TSH secretion that is dependent on the functional integrity of the hypothalamic-pituitary axis and consequent catecholamine supply (see Fig 12-3).

In addition to its acute inhibitory effects on TSH secretion in vitro, dopamine also decreases the levels of α-subunit and TSH-β-subunit mRNAs and gene transcription by up to 75% in cultured anterior pituitary cells from hypothyroid rats. These effects occur within a few minutes and can be reversed by activation of adenylyl cyclase with forskolin.[42] Similar actions of dopamine have been described in relation to PRL gene expression (Fig 12-5).

In contrast to dopamine, adrenergic activation stimulates TSH release by cultured rat and bovine anterior pituitary cells in a dose-related stereospecific fashion. This effect is mediated by high-affinity α_1-adrenoreceptors,[117–119] and both α_1-adrenoreceptors and α_1-receptor-mediated TSH release are reduced in cells from hypothyroid animals.[120] Quantitatively, the adrenergic release of TSH is almost equivalent to that induced by TRH[117]; together, at maximal dosage, these two agents have additive effects on TSH release, indicating activation of separate intracellular pathways. It is likely that dopamine and epinephrine exert their direct actions on the thyrotrophs by opposing actions on cAMP generation, with DA_2 receptors being negatively linked to adenylyl cyclase and α_1-adrenoreceptors being positively linked.

In humans, it is well established that dopamine has a physiologic inhibitory role in the control of TSH release, and some data suggest a stimulatory α-adrenergic pathway. In contrast to the situation in animals, evidence for direct effects of dopaminergic and adrenergic manipulation on TSH release by normal human pituitary cells is lacking. Data from the use of dopamine, dopamine agonists, and specific dopamine-receptor antagonist drugs such as domperidone, which does not penetrate the blood-brain barrier to any appreciable extent, suggest that dopamine-induced decreases in TSH secretion are a direct pituitary or median eminence action mediated by the DA_2 class of dopamine receptor.[121–123]

The dopaminergic inhibition of TSH release varies according to sex, thyroid status, time of day, and PRL secretory status. TSH release after endogenous dopamine disinhibition with dopamine-receptor-blocking drugs, such as metoclopramide and domperidone, is greater in women than in men.[123] It is assumed that estrogens determine this effect, but the mechanism of action is unknown. The dopaminergic inhibition of TSH release, like the stimulation of TSH release by TRH, is also greater in patients with mild or subclinical hypothyroidism than in normal subjects or severely hypothyroid patients.[124] The mechanisms that underlie this biphasic relationship between the dopaminergic inhibition of TSH release and thyroid status are not known, but data from in vitro stud-

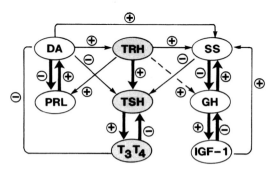

FIGURE 12-5. Schematic representation of the complex interactions that can occur between primary and secondary modulators of thyrotroph function. This scheme represents a summary of the data available from in vivo and in vitro studies in animals and in humans. DA, dopamine; SS, somatostatin; IGF-1, insulin-like growth factor-1. ⊕ stimulation; ⊖, inhibition.

ies of anterior pituitary cells from hypothyroid rats suggest an increase in dopamine-receptor capacity rather than affinity.[114] Also, the concentration of dopamine in hypophyseal portal blood of thyroidectomized rats is greater than that of sham-operated rats; this is due to increased activity of tyrosine hydroxylase in the median eminence, an effect that can be reversed by thyroid hormone replacement.[125,126] In addition to its effects on the release of TSH, dopamine also inhibits the release of α-subunit and TSH-β-subunit, the greatest effect occurring in patients with primary hypothyroidism.[65,127]

Only limited data are available on the adrenergic control of TSH release in humans. α-Adrenergic blockade with phentolamine, which does not readily cross the blood-brain barrier, or with thymoxamine, which does, inhibits the serum TSH response to TRH[128] and reduces but does not abolish the nocturnal rise in TSH secretion.[129] Overall, these data suggest a small stimulatory role for endogenous adrenergic pathways in TSH control in humans. However, adrenergic activation with epinephrine or α-amphetamine and β-adrenoreceptor blockade with propranolol do not influence the serum TSH response to TRH.[130,131] The catecholaminergic control of TSH secretion appears to act as a fine-tuning mechanism rather than being of primary importance. This is not to say that the effects of catecholamines are so small as to be without consequence. For example, acute dopaminergic blockade in humans releases enough TSH to elicit subsequent release of thyroid hormones. As with somatostatin-agonist analogues, however, chronic administration of catecholaminergic drugs does not lead to long-term alterations in thyroid status, reflecting the action of compensatory mechanisms to maintain TSH secretion and euthyroidism.

OTHER NEUROTRANSMITTER PATHWAYS, NEUROPEPTIDES, AND CYTOKINES

The role of the serotoninergic system in the control of TSH release in animals and humans is unclear, both stimulatory and inhibitory actions having been described.[103,132] Opioid pathways appear to play an important role in the inhibitory control of TSH secretion in rats. Opioid peptides decrease basal TSH secretion and their action can be blocked by the specific antagonist naloxone,[133] which also blocks the stress-induced fall in TSH secretion.[134] In humans, however, endogenous opioids may have a stimulatory effect on TSH secretion, especially during the nocturnal TSH surge.[135] A variety of other neuropeptides including neurotensin, vasoactive intestinal polypeptide, bombesin, vasopressin, oxytocin, substance P, and cholecystokinin can produce small alterations in TSH secretion both in vitro and in vivo in animals, but the lack of suitable specific antagonist drugs has not allowed adequate physiologic studies to be undertaken. These molecules should be added to the list of agents that can affect TSH secretion, but their physiologic relevance is uncertain.

Tumor necrosis factor (TNF; cachectin) is a peptide produced by macrophages that acts as an inflammatory mediator and can cause many of the clinical phenomena that accompany severe systemic illness. Interleukin-1 (IL-1) is a cytokine produced by many cells, including monocytes, that stimulates B- and T-lymphocytes to produce a range of other cytokines and lymphokines. Both TNF and IL-1β inhibit TSH secretion in rats and mice,[136–138] and IL-1β causes a relative and inappro-

priate reduction in TRH gene expression in the paraventricular nucleus in the face of low thyroid hormone concentrations.[139]

These molecules each produce a biochemical pattern similar to that which occurs in patients with acute nonthyroidal illness[140,141] and they also activate the hypothalamic-pituitary-adrenal axis,[142–144] probably via stimulation of the release of hypothalamic corticotropin-releasing hormone.[145] This family of molecules plays a crucial role in mediating and coordinating the thyroidal and adrenal responses to nonthyroidal illness (see section on nonthyroidal illness in chap 14). IL-1β is produced by rat anterior pituitary cells, and its release from them can be stimulated by bacterial lipopolysaccharide. It colocalizes with TSH in thyrotroph cells.[146] Presumably IL-1β subserves an important autocrine or paracrine role in anterior pituitary control, as has also been suggested for the IL-1–dependent cytokine IL-6, which is also produced by rat anterior pituitary cells,[147] particularly folliculostellate cells.[148]

ALTERATIONS IN SECRETORY PATTERNS OF TSH

Alterations in TSH secretion may be manifested in the pattern and degree of change in basal TSH secretion or in the pattern and degree of serum TSH responses to TRH or dopamine-receptor blockade.

Circadian and Ultradian Changes in Serum TSH

A clear circadian variation is evident in serum TSH concentrations. In most humans, serum TSH concentrations begin to rise several hours before the onset of sleep, reaching maximal concentrations between 2300 and 0400 hours and declining gradually thereafter, with the lowest concentrations occurring at about 1100 hours (Fig 12-6). The concentrations during the nocturnal surge are sometimes slightly above the normal range reported by most clinical laboratories. Sleep itself modulates TSH secretion, by reducing pulse amplitude rather than frequency,[149,150] but the underlying mechanisms are not clear. Furthermore, a seasonal variation in TSH secretion has been described in patients with primary hypothyroidism receiving T_4 therapy; some of these patients have higher basal serum TSH concentrations in the winter than in the summer.[151] This may be a consequence of temperature effects on the peripheral metabolism of thyroid hormones, but such a difference was not found in euthyroid subjects.[152] Although there is some evidence that estrogens can enhance and androgens reduce serum TSH responses to TRH,[153,154] no sex-related difference in amplitude or frequency of circadian TSH changes has been found.[152]

TSH is secreted in a pulsatile manner with increases in pulse amplitude and frequency at night.[149,155–158] Patients with severe primary hypothyroidism have increased pulse amplitude throughout the day but loss of the usual nocturnal increase in pulse amplitude. The pulses of TSH-α-subunit and the gonadotropins are concordant, consistent with the operation of a common hypothalamic pulse generator.[159]

The circadian and pulsatile changes in TSH secretion are not secondary to peripheral factors, such as changes in serum T_4 and T_3 concentrations, hemoconcentration, or changes in

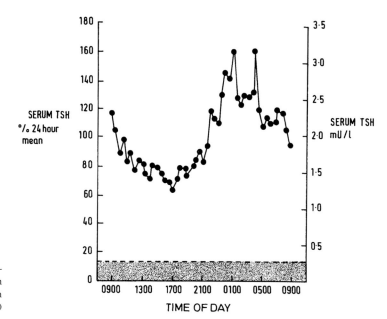

FIGURE 12-6. Circadian variation in mean serum TSH concentrations in seven normal subjects. (Modified from Caron PJ, Nieman LK, Rose SR, Nisula BC. Deficient nocturnal surge of thyrotropin in central hypothyroidism. J Clin Endocrinol Metab 1986;62:960)

cortisol secretion,[160] although the latter may modulate TSH rhythms. Furthermore, circadian changes in serum TSH concentrations can be detected in some patients with mild thyrotoxicosis,[161] suggesting that central mechanisms can override to some extent the powerful negative-feedback effects of thyroid hormones at the pituitary level.

Basal serum TSH concentrations rise slightly after serum cortisol concentrations are lowered by 11β-hydroxylase inhibition with metyrapone,[162] suggesting that cortisol exerts a small inhibitory influence on TSH secretion. Furthermore, pharmacologic doses of glucocorticoids acutely inhibit basal TSH secretion and abolish the circadian variation in serum TSH concentrations.[152,163,164] This mechanism may well explain the reduction in basal and TRH-stimulated serum TSH concentrations and in circadian TSH changes that occur in patients with depression,[165,166] after major surgery,[167] and in nonthyroidal illness. Total abolition of the circadian rhythm of cortisol with metyrapone, however, did not cause disruption of overall circadian TSH changes, although a small but significant decrease did occur in the acrophase and amplitude of the TSH profile.[168]

The central mechanisms that underlie TSH pulsatility and rhythmicity are unknown. Pulsatile TRH release does not appear to be involved in TSH pulse frequency although it may influence amplitude.[169] Pulsatility is probably mediated in part by signals from the suprachiasmatic nuclei of the hypothalamus. These nuclei are paired structures situated just above the optic chiasm that initiate intrinsic circadian rhythmicity, the timing of which can be influenced by nonvisual nerve impulses arising in the retina.[170] Although both dopamine and dopamine agonists acutely abolish the circadian change in TSH secretion,[152,171] endogenous dopaminergic pathways probably do not play a role in determining the circadian changes in TSH secretion. The nocturnal increase in TSH secretion is not due to a decline in dopaminergic inhibition because dopaminergic inhibition of TSH release is greater at night than during the day.[158,172,173]

Dopamine is, however, a determinant of TSH pulse amplitude (but not frequency).[158] It appears that dopamine acts as a fine-tuning control to dampen TSH pulsatility, presumably to maintain basal TSH concentrations and hence thyroid function in as steady a state as possible. Why the serum TSH response to dopamine blockade is greater at night than during the day is not known. It is unlikely to be due to increased central dopaminergic activity, since the serum PRL response to dopamine blockade is the same during the day and night.[160]

Similarly, α-adrenergic pathways do not play a primary role in determining TSH circadian rhythmicity, since α-adrenergic blockade with thymoxamine, which penetrates the blood-brain barrier, did not affect the circadian pattern of TSH secretion, although serum TSH concentrations decreased slightly throughout the entire period of study.[129] Serotonin, although present in high concentrations in the suprachiasmatic nucleus, does not play any major role in circadian TSH secretion in humans,[174] nor does the pineal hormone melatonin,[175] which in animals exerts an inhibitory effect on hypothalamic-pituitary-thyroid function.[176] TSH may regulate its own secretion through an increase in dopamine receptors at the level of the thyrotrophs,[116] a finding that could explain the higher serum TSH and unaltered serum PRL responses to dopamine blockade at the time of greatest TSH secretion.[160] A further possible contributor to the changes in circadian TSH secretion in rats is the diurnal variation in the activity of anterior pituitary T_4-5'-deiodinase in this species.[177]

Effects of Temperature, Age, and Calorie Restriction

TEMPERATURE

Cold exposure in rats causes an acute rise in serum TSH concentrations that is accompanied by an increase in hypothalamic TRH gene expression and increased TRH release.[178,179] A similar phenomenon occurs in human neonates, but is unusual in adults; when it does occur the increase is very small. The cold-induced effect in rats can be abolished by either passive immunization with anti-TRH antibodies or α-adrenergic blockade, indicating that adrenergic release of hypothalamic TRH mediates the phenomenon[1,103,124] (Fig 12-7). Lesions that affect the temperature-regulating center of the preoptic nucleus of the hypothalamus abolish the serum TSH response to cold stress but do not cause hypothyroidism.[103]

AGING

Aging itself causes a slight decrease in TSH secretion, due to a resetting of the threshold of TSH inhibition by thyroid hormones as a result of increased pituitary conversion of T_4 to T_3, increased T_4 uptake by thyrotrophs, or decreased T_4 and T_3 clearance.[180] In one study of healthy elderly subjects 5% had low basal serum TSH concentrations and those same subjects had a reduced serum TSH response to TRH.[181] In addition, TSH pulse amplitude was reduced, with preservation of the frequency of pulsatility and the overall pattern of circadian change.[182] These data should introduce caution into the use of TSH assays alone in the assessment of thyroid function in the elderly. The underlying mechanism is unclear, but the change in TSH secretion may reflect an adaptive mechanism to the reduced need for thyroid hormones in the elderly.[182]

CALORIC RESTRICTION

Caloric restriction causes a small decrease in basal and TRH-stimulated serum TSH concentrations despite a decline in serum T_3 concentrations.[183,184] This is associated with reduced hypothalamic TRH gene expression in rats.[185,186] The components of the decrease in TSH secretion in humans are a reduction in the daytime serum TSH concentration and in the nocturnal increase in TSH secretion, with an overall decrease

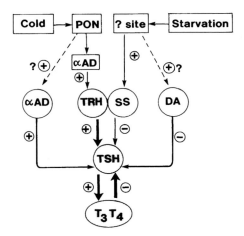

FIGURE 12-7. Schematic representation of probable pathways involved in secondary alterations in hypothalamic-pituitary-thyroid function in response to temperature and caloric restriction. PON represents the temperature-sensitive region of the preoptic nucleus of the hypothalamus. The hypothalamic site for integration of the metabolic signals resulting from caloric restriction is unknown. ⊕, stimulation; ⊖, inhibition.

in TSH pulse amplitude.[187] In the more extreme clinical setting of anorexia nervosa, the reduced basal and stimulated serum TSH concentrations may be a consequence of increased serum cortisol concentrations. Passive immunization with somatostatin antibodies abolishes the starvation-induced decline in TSH secretion in rats,[188] indicating a mediating role of hypothalamic somatostatinergic pathways secondary to unknown metabolic signals (see Fig 12-7). There is no evidence of increased dopaminergic inhibition of TSH secretion during caloric restriction,[189,190] and TRH administration does not reverse the acute decline in serum TSH concentrations during fasting.[191]

Effects of Stress, Nonthyroidal Illness, and Neuropsychiatric Disorders

STRESS

In rats stress causes an acute decline in serum TSH concentrations. In humans, surgical stress causes both transient acute lowering of serum TSH[192,193] and a longer-term abolition of the nocturnal increase in serum TSH.[167] This occurs despite a fall in serum free T_3 concentrations, whereas serum free T_4 concentrations do not change.[167,194] In animals, both opioids and dopamine may play a role in this stress phenomenon, whereas in humans glucocorticoids and dopamine have been implicated.[134,167,193] As with the effects of caloric restriction, these stress phenomena bear some resemblance to the altered neuroregulation of TSH that can occur in nonthyroidal illness and in certain neuropsychiatric disorders (see section on nonthyroidal illness in chap 14). Although basal serum TSH concentrations are usually normal in patients with both acute and chronic nonthyroidal illness, they may be either low or slightly raised.[195,196] In addition to the frequent use of pharmacologic agents such as glucocorticoids and dopamine that acutely inhibit TSH secretion,[196,197] intrinsic central suppression of thyrotroph function is common, as illustrated by the abolition of the nocturnal increase in serum TSH concentrations in up to 60% of acutely ill patients in the presence of low serum free T_3 concentrations.[198] However, true central hypothyroidism is rare in these patients, who usually but not always have normal serum free T_4 concentrations.[198,199]

NONTHYROIDAL ILLNESS

It seems clear that, in addition to peripheral alterations in thyroid hormone economy usually manifest as low serum free T_3, high reverse T_3, and normal free T_4 concentrations, there is central suppression of thyrotroph function in patients with severe nonthyroidal illness, for example, heart failure, infection, diabetes mellitus,[200,201] or chronic renal failure.[202] The precise initiating signals and underlying mechanisms are unknown, although alterations in opioidergic, dopaminergic, and somatostatinergic activity may each contribute. In addition, peripheral, glucocorticoid-mediated inhibitory feedback probably plays an important role, particularly in acutely ill patients.[203] Finally, activation of the cytokine pathways involving tumor necrosis factor-α and IL-1β, each of which inhibit TSH and stimulate ACTH release in animals,[136,137] may be a crucial mediating event in the coordination of the thyroidal and adrenal responses to stress and nonthyroidal illness (Fig 12-8).

Abnormalities in TSH secretion also occur in patients with anorexia nervosa and endogenous depression. A common abnormality is a reduced serum TSH response to TRH.[189,204] Even more common is loss of the nocturnal increase in TSH secretion,[165] which together with the low serum free thyroid hormone, ferritin, and sex hormone-binding globulin concentrations may indicate central hypothyroidism. Once again, the mechanisms are unclear. Dopamine is not involved in central TSH suppression in anorexia nervosa;[189] both serum cortisol and body temperature changes have been implicated in depression.[165,166]

Without doubt, the debate will continue about whether central hypothyroidism exists in patients with stress, severe nonthyroidal illness, depression, or anorexia nervosa. It is of interest, therefore, that thyroid hormone treatment of patients with nonthyroidal illness is of no benefit or may even be detrimental.[205] In contrast, thyroid hormone administration may enhance the therapeutic benefits of tricyclic antidepressant drug therapy in depression.[206]

SERUM TSH CONCENTRATIONS IN PATIENTS WITH THYROID DISEASE

Measurement of Serum TSH

The radioimmunoassays for serum TSH in the 1970s had poor sensitivity (1 mU/L) and specificity. Hence, basal measurements did not discriminate between euthyroid and thyrotoxic patients, and distinguishing between them required a TRH test. The introduction of monoclonal antibodies and the development of labeled antibody immunometric assays (IMA) for the measurement of TSH in the 1980s increased the sensitivity tenfold or more, allowing reliable classification of patients as euthyroid or thyrotoxic and rendering the TRH test obsolete.[207] Strategies for assessment of thyroid function were completely altered and measurement of serum TSH concentrations became the most cost-effective first-line test[208] (see also chap 18).

Many commercial IMA methods for measurement of TSH are available, and the manufacturers have caused some confusion in their descriptions of assay sensitivity, using terms such as "highly sensitive," "super-sensitive," and "ultra-sensitive." Their claims for sensitivity (or detection limit) were usually based on what is known as "analytical sensitivity," defined as the concentration of TSH corresponding to the mean + 2.5 SD of the signal response.[209] Such a calculation overestimates the sensitivity of the routine assay. The interassay precision profile provides a more accurate estimate of sensitivity for routine use. The American Thyroid Association has recommended the concept of "functional sensitivity," defined as the serum TSH concentration corresponding to an interassay coefficient of variation of 20% on the precision profile obtained from multiple assays, preferably using different batches of reagents.[210–212]

Although it might be anticipated that most of the IMAs would perform well, this is not the case, because the sensitivity of the same commercial kit in different laboratories can vary by as much as 100-fold.[213] Figure 12-9 shows serum TSH concentrations using an assay with a functional sensitivity of 0.01 mU/L in a large number of patients with thyroid disease or nonthyroidal illness.[214] Although there is complete separation of euthyroid and thyrotoxic patients, serum TSH concentrations are detectable (>0.01 mU/L) in some patients with thyrotoxicosis, indicating graded suppression of thyrotroph secretion. In contrast, serum TSH concentrations are undetectable in a substantial proportion of patients with nonthyroidal illness or those receiving T_4 therapy, indicating that there can be little benefit in developing increasingly sensitive assays for clinical purposes.

Thyrotoxicosis

With the exception of the entity of thyrotoxicosis caused by inappropriate TSH secretion, serum TSH concentrations are low or undetectable in patients with thyrotoxicosis, irrespective of the cause, owing to the increased negative feedback of thyroid hormones on the thyrotrophs (Table 12-1). After treatment with an antithyroid drug, thyroidectomy, or radioactive iodine (^{131}I), serum TSH concentrations remain low or undetectable in patients with thyrotoxicosis, irrespective of the cause, for 4 to 6 weeks after serum T_4 and T_3 concentrations have fallen to the normal or even the hypothyroid range. This seemingly anomalous behavior reflects the delay in recovery of synthesis and secretion of TSH by the previously suppressed thyrotrophs.[215,216] During this period of recovery of thyrotroph function, a low serum T_4 concentration is the best predictor of impending clinical hypothyroidism.[217] The same sequence of events occurs after the withdrawal of suppressive doses of T_4.[218]

Hypothyroidism that occurs within 6 months after thyroidectomy (or occasionally ^{131}I therapy) in patients with Graves' hyperthyroidism may be temporary (Fig 12-10),[219,220] even though serum TSH concentrations may be in excess of 100 mU/L 3 to 4 months after the operation. The serum TSH concentration may remain high for several years, until the thyroid remnant undergoes hyperplasia and hypertrophy and its function increases, as a result of not only the high serum TSH concentration but sometimes also the continued presence of thyroid-stimulating antibodies.[221,222]

The most common finding after ablative treatment of hyperthyroidism is subclinical hypothyroidism, the term used to describe a euthyroid patient with the combination of normal

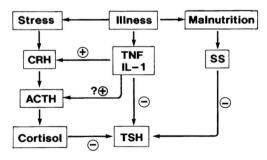

FIGURE 12-8. Proposed interaction between some of the pathways mediating changes in TSH secretion in response to stress, illness, and caloric restriction in humans. Some animal data indicate that stress-related TSH inhibition may be mediated by opioidergic and dopaminergic pathways. ⊕, stimulation; ⊖, inhibition.

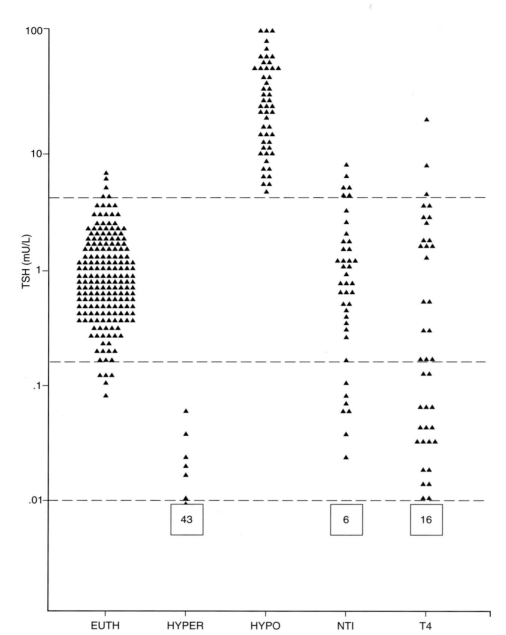

FIGURE 12-9. Serum TSH concentrations in normal subjects (EUTH), thyrotoxic patients (HYPER), hypothyroid patients (HYPO), patients with nonthyroidal illness (NTI), and T_4-treated hypothyroid patients (T4). The numbers in the boxes are the numbers of patients with each condition who had serum TSH concentrations less than 0.01 mU/L.

serum T_3 and T_4 and raised TSH concentrations, that may persist unchanged for many years (see chap 87).

Primary Hypothyroidism

Serum TSH concentrations usually are in excess of 20 mU/L in patients with overt symptomatic primary hypothyroidism (see Fig 12-9), whereas concentrations between 5 and 20 mU/L normally are associated with serum thyroid hormone concentrations in the lower part of their respective normal ranges. Markedly elevated values of 500 mU/L or more usually are found only in patients—usually children and young adults—with severe, long-standing hypothyroidism; otherwise, little relation exists between serum TSH concentrations and the clinical findings. Basal serum TSH concentrations are unchanged by fasting in patients with severe or moderate hypothyroidism; patients with slightly elevated serum TSH concentrations (5 to 10 mU/L), however, may have some decline.[183] It follows that mild degrees of hypothyroidism might be overlooked in critically ill and malnourished patients.

After initiation of T_4 therapy, serum TSH concentrations fall slowly in relation to the increase in serum T_4. For example, in a hypothyroid patient with a basal serum TSH concentration of 100 or 200 mU/L, treatment with T_4 in a dose of 100 μg/d for 4 to 8 weeks is required to restore serum TSH to normal or near-normal, whereas serum T_4 concentrations return to the normal range within a few days.[223] This differential response is useful in identifying poorly compliant patients, in whom it is

TABLE 12-1.
Alterations in Control of TSH Secretion in Disease States

	Basal TSH Secretion	Nocturnal TSH Secretion	Serum TSH Response to TRH	Response to Dopamine Antagonism	Serum Free T₃	Serum Free T₄
PRIMARY THYROID DISEASE						
Thyrotoxicosis	↓	↓	↓	↓	↑	↑
Uni- or multinodular goiter*	N or ↓	?	N or ↓	?	N or ↑	N or ↑
Stimulatory TSH-receptor* antibodies (Graves' disease)	N or ↓	N or ↓	N or ↓	N or ↓	N	N
Thyroxine treatment*	N or ↓	N or ↓	N or ↓	N or ↓	N	N
After treatment of thyrotoxicosis*	N or ↓	N or ↓	N or ↓	?	N	N
Hypothyroidism	↑	↑	↑	↑	↓	↓
NONTHYROIDAL ILLNESS						
Acute and chronic illness	N or ↓	N or ↓	N or ↓	?	↓	N or ↓
Critical illness	N or ↓	N or ↓	N or ↓	?	↓	N or ↓
PREGNANCY (EARLY)*	N or ↓	?	?	?	N	N or ↓
PITUITARY DISEASES						
Acromegaly²	N or ↓	?	N or ↓	↓, N or ↑	N or ↓	N or ↓
Cushing's disease	N or ↓	N or ↓	N or ↓	?	N or ↓	N or ↓
Microprolactinoma	N or ↑	N or ↑	N or ↓	↑	N	N
Macroprolactinoma	N or ↓	?	N or ↓	N or ↓	N or ↓	N or ↓
Gonadotropinomas	N or ↓	?	N or ↓	?	N or ↓	N or ↓
Inappropriate TSH Secretion						
Adenoma	↑	?	↓	↓	↑	↑
Non-adenoma	↑	?	N or ↑	↑	↑	↑
Nonsecretory adenoma	N or ↓	?	N or	N or ↓	N or ↓	N or ↓
HYPOTHALAMIC DISEASE	N, ↑, or ↓	?	N, ↑, or ↓	?	N or ↓	N or ↓
Idiopathic GH deficiency	N	?	N or ↑	?	N	N
NEUROPSYCHIATRIC DISORDERS						
Endogenous depression	N	N or ↓	N or ↓	?	N or ↓	N
Anorexia nervosa	N or ↓	?	N or ↓	N or ↓	↓	N or ↓
ENDOCRINE/METABOLIC DISORDERS						
Caloric restriction	N or ↓	↓	N or ↓	N or ↓	↓	N or ↓
Hypercortisolism	N	N or ↓	N or ↓	?	N or ↓	N or ↓
Primary adrenal insufficiency	N or ↑	?	N or ↑	?	N or ↓	N or ↓
Acute stress (e.g., surgery)	N or ↓	N or ↓	?	?	↓	N
DRUGS						
Dopamine and agonists (acute)	↓	↓	↓		N	N
Adrenergic antagonists (acute)	?	↓	↓		N	N
Somatostatin (acute)	↓	↓	↓	↓	N	N
Dopamine antagonists (acute)	↑	↑	?		N	N
Glucocorticoids	↓	↓	↓	?	N	N
Phenytoin	N	?	N or ↓	?	N or ↓	N or ↓
Carbamazepine	N	?	?	?	N or ↓	N or ↓

N, normal; ↓ decreased; ↑ increased.
*Low serum TSH due to increase in concentration of thyroid hormones within the normal range (i.e. subclinical thyrotoxicosis).
†Acromegalic patients with hyperprolactinemia and a mixed mammosomatotroph tumor may have an increased serum TSH response to dopamine antagonism.

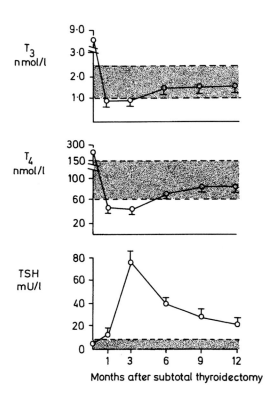

FIGURE 12-10. Mean (± SE) serum total T_3 and T_4 and TSH concentrations in 20 patients with temporary hypothyroidism after subtotal thyroidectomy for hyperthyroidism caused by Graves' disease. The normal ranges are indicated by the dashed lines. To convert serum T_3 and T_4 values to nmol/L, divide by 0.015 and 12.9, respectively. (Modified from Toft AD, Irvine WJ, Sinclair I, McIntosh D, Seth J, Cameron EHD. Thyroid function after surgical treatment with propanolol before operation. N Engl J Med 1978;298:643)

not uncommon to record both raised serum T_4 and TSH concentrations as a result of regular, or even excessive, ingestion of T_4 only for the few days before the clinic visit.

The aim of T_4 replacement therapy is to restore euthyroidism, but controversy exists about whether the adequacy of treatment should be assessed clinically[224] or biochemically and, if the latter, whether subnormal serum TSH concentrations are a sign of overtreatment. The latter is an important issue, because in a recent study serum TSH concentrations were low in 60% of a large group of T_4-treated patients.[225] The secretion of TSH is sensitive to very small changes in serum T_4 and T_3 concentrations,[226] but is the pituitary unique in this respect among target organs? On the one hand, evidence from rats suggests that more of the T_3 occupying nuclear receptors in the pituitary is derived from intrapituitary monodeiodination of T_4 and less from the circulation than in other organs such as liver and kidney.[227] If the same were true in humans, thyrotroph suppression would not necessarily be accompanied by excess thyroid hormone action in other target organs, and therefore the induction of subclinical thyrotoxicosis by treatment with T_4 would be of no clinical importance.[228] However, doses of T_4 that suppress TSH secretion have more widespread effects, such as changes in nocturnal heart rate, left ventricular wall thickness, systolic time intervals, urinary sodium excretion, liver and muscle enzyme activity, red cell

sodium concentrations, and serum lipid concentrations, similar to, but less marked than, those found in overt thyrotoxicosis[229–231] (see chap 88). There is also evidence that a low serum TSH concentration, for whatever reason, is a risk factor for the development of atrial fibrillation.[232] The greatest concern, however, is with bone, because significant decreases in bone density at various sites have been found in some but by no means all studies of pre- and postmenopausal women receiving long-term T_4 therapy in doses sufficient to lower TSH secretion to below the normal range,[231] although there is no evidence of an increased rate of fracture.[233]

Some would question the relevance of many of these changes in target organ function in patients who are asymptomatic, the more so when a retrospective study has failed to demonstrate an increase in morbidity or mortality in T_4-treated patients with low serum TSH concentrations as compared with those with normal serum TSH concentrations.[225] There is also the clinical observation that some patients prefer taking a daily dose of thyroxine of 50 μg in excess of that required to normalize serum TSH response to TRH.[234] In addition, many of the above studies have been relatively short-term and there is some evidence of tissue adaptation to thyroid hormone excess.[235]

However sound the advice of the American Thyroid Association for the management of primary hypothyroidism, that "the goal of therapy is to restore most patients to the euthyroid state and to normalize serum T_4 and TSH concentrations,"[236] there will be some patients for whom well-being is only restored by a dose sufficient to suppress serum TSH. As long as serum T_4 is only marginally elevated it is difficult to believe that such patients are at substantial risk of osteoporosis in the long term (see chap 77 for additional discussion of the treatment of hypothyroidism).

Other Thyroid Diseases

Most euthyroid patients with a diffuse, a uninodular, or a multinodular goiter, or thyroid carcinoma have serum TSH concentrations in the normal range. However, patients with a variety of other thyroid diseases who are clinically euthyroid and have serum T_3 and T_4 concentrations within the normal range frequently have abnormal serum TSH concentrations. These patients are increasingly identified when serum TSH assay is the first-line test of thyroid function. The conditions associated with a low or undetectable serum TSH concentration, in the absence of thyrotoxicosis, are listed in Table 12-1.[29,198,215,216,228,237–244]

Raised serum TSH concentrations in the presence of normal serum T_3 and T_4 concentrations (subclinical hypothyroidism) may be found in the following circumstances: chronic autoimmune thyroiditis[245]; endemic goiter[246]; thyroid dyshomonogenesis[247]; lithium carbonate therapy[248]; iodine-containing medications, usually as an expectorant or as the antiarrhythmic drug amiodarone, in a patient with preexisting thyroid disease[249]; those who received neck irradiation for diseases such as lymphoma or laryngeal cancer[250,251]; previous treatment with [131]I[252]; subtotal thyroidectomy[253]; or antithyroid drugs.[239] In all these conditions, raised serum TSH concentrations may remain unchanged for many years, but the elevation is an indication of the possible development of overt hypothyroidism. There is little evidence that restoration of the serum TSH concentration to normal is of benefit,[231] unless the aim is goiter shrinkage, when sufficient T_4 should be given to suppress TSH secretion. Clinicians who favor therapy will be most influenced by the knowledge that between 25% and 50% of such patients feel better while taking T_4,[254,255] and by the fact that the annual rate of evolution from subclinical to overt hypothyroidism is approximately 5% to 20%[245,256–258] (Table 12-2) (see also chap 87).

Serum TSH concentrations may be temporarily elevated in the hypothyroid phase of subacute thyroiditis,[259] silent thyroiditis,[260] or postpartum thyroiditis[261]; in neonates, because of the transplacental passage of maternal TSH-receptor blocking antibodies[262]; and after treatment of thyrotoxicosis with ^{131}I or by subtotal thyroidectomy, as described previously.

SERUM TSH CONCENTRATIONS IN HYPOTHALAMIC-PITUITARY DISEASE

In most patients with pituitary disease (with the exception of hyperprolactinemia), basal serum TSH concentrations and serum TSH responses to TRH are normal or reduced; an absent serum TSH response to TRH is suggestive of a pituitary lesion (see Table 12-1; also see chap 59). Occasional patients with pituitary tumors have a delayed serum TSH response to TRH, which is associated frequently with mild hyperprolactinemia and may be due to stalk compression.[263] Factors other than tumor size alone may determine the degree of serum TSH responsiveness to TRH; among patients with pituitary disease, those with GH deficiency have greater serum TSH responses to TRH than do those with normal GH reserve.[91]

In hypothalamic disease of any etiology, the serum TSH response to TRH may be normal, suppressed, or delayed, with peak serum TSH concentrations being achieved 60 minutes after TRH administration. In some hypothyroid patients with hypothalamic disease, basal serum TSH concentrations may be slightly elevated; in this instance, excess TSH-β-subunit and intact TSH with reduced biologic activity may be secreted. This situation can be reversed by TRH administration.

In patients with hyperprolactinemia due to a prolactinoma, thyroid status depends on the size of the tumor. Patients with prolactin-secreting macroadenomas may have impaired serum TSH responses to both TRH and dopamine antagonism[263] or, less commonly, overt clinical and biochemical hypothyroidism. Patients with microprolactinomas, however, are almost invariably clinically and biochemically euthyroid. Their basal serum TSH concentrations may be slightly elevated (although still within the normal range) both in the morning and in the evening, indicating slightly exaggerated circadian TSH secretion.[264] Characteristically, the serum TSH response to dopamine receptor blockade is exaggerated,[264,265] in contrast to patients with either puerperal or stalk-compression hyperprolactinemia, in whom the serum TSH response is usually reduced.[263,266] Occasional patients with prolactin-secreting microadenomas have exaggerated serum TSH responses to TRH.[263] It is thought that autonomous PRL production leads to increased hypothalamic dopamine turnover and release into the hypophyseal portal circulation, causing increased dopaminergic inhibition of TSH release with consequent exaggerated responses to dopamine antagonism. The precise mechanism that underlies the slight elevation in basal and TRH-stimulated serum TSH concentrations is unknown, but this is presumably a consequence of some compensatory mechanism operating in the face of the increased dopaminergic inhibition of TSH release. Such compensation must occur because central hypothyroidism is not a feature of microprolactinomas.

Clinically important disorders of the hypothalamic-pituitary-thyroid axis are uncommon in patients with either Cushing's disease or acromegaly, although impaired serum TSH responses to TRH are common. In the former case, this probably results from the high serum cortisol concentrations; similar findings occur during treatment with pharmacologic doses of glucocorticoids.[156] In acromegaly, the impaired serum TSH response to TRH is probably caused by GH- or insulin-like growth factor I-induced increases in hypothalamic somatostatin release,[91,267] although direct evidence for this in humans is lacking. Central hypothyroidism is rare in either clinical situation and is usually associated with large tumors. Occasional patients with acromegaly also have TSH-induced hyperthyroidism caused by either a mixed (dimorphous) GH- and TSH-secreting pituitary tumor or a single cell type (monomorphous) secreting both GH and TSH (see chap 31).

Finally, some patients with acromegaly have exaggerated serum TSH responses to dopamine antagonism.[268,269] They are patients with coexistent hyperprolactinemia who may well have mixed GH- and PRL-secreting tumors.

Inappropriate secretion of TSH is diagnosed in patients in whom basal or TRH-stimulated TSH release is inappropriately elevated in the presence of increased serum free T_4 and T_3 concentrations.[270] Clearly, the sensitivity of the thyrotrophs to the negative-feedback action of thyroid hormones is reduced in these patients. TSH hypersecretion accounts for less than 0.2% of all cases of thyrotoxicosis. It usually results from a TSH-secreting pituitary macroadenoma, although some patients have microadenomas and others have no detectable pituitary abnormality. The tumors also secrete increased amounts of α-subunit and, on occasion, other pituitary hormones (see above and chap 31). Serum TSH concentrations vary widely in these patients, suggesting that the hormone secreted varies in biologic activity. In general terms, patients with TSH-secreting pituitary

TABLE 12-2.
Mean (± SE) Serum Total T_4 and TSH Concentrations in 69 Patients with Subclinical Hypothyroidism as a Result of Treatment with ^{131}I for Graves' Hyperthyroidism*

Year	Serum T_4 (nmol/L)	Serum TSH (mU/L)	Percentage Developing Overt Hypothyroidism Each Year
0	88 ± 1	25.0 ± 2.0	–
1	84 ± 1	22.6 ± 1.8	5
2	84 ± 1	21.6 ± 2.0	5
3	75 ± 3	26.6 ± 2.6	2
4	80 ± 3	24.9 ± 2.9	6
5	75 ± 2	27.3 ± 4.1	3

*Patients were treated 6 to 18 years earlier and followed for 5 years. The annual incidence of the development of overt hypothyroidism is similar to that described in patients with subclinical hypothyroidism resulting from autoimmune thyroid disease. To convert serum T_4 values to μg/dL, divide by 12.9.

adenomas have little serum TSH response to functional stimuli and elevated serum α-subunit concentrations and α-subunit/intact TSH molar ratios. In contrast, those patients with no evidence of tumor have serum TSH responses to both TRH and dopamine-antagonist administration and normal serum α-subunit concentrations; some of these patients have mutations in the β_2 form of the nuclear T_3 receptor.

TSH hypersecretion also occurs in the familial syndrome of generalized resistance to thyroid hormones. These patients may be either euthyroid or hypothyroid in the presence of elevated serum T_4 and T_3 concentrations; most if not all the patients have mutations in the thyroid hormone receptor (see chap 90).

References

1. Jackson IMD. Thyrotropin releasing hormone. N Engl J Med 1982;306:145
2. Surks L, Oppenheimer JH. Incomplete suppression of thyrotropin secretion after single injection of large L-triiodothyronine doses into hypothyroid rats. Endocrinology 1976; 99:1432
3. Surks MI, Lifschitz BM. Biphasic thyrotropin suppression in euthyroid and hypothyroid rats. Endocrinology 1977;101:769
4. Silva JF, Larsen PR. Pituitary nuclear 3,5,3′triiodothyronine and thyrotropin secretion; an explanation for the effect of thyroxine. Science 1977;198:617
5. Silva JE, Dick TE, Larsen PR. The contribution of local tissue thyroxine monodeiodination to the nuclear 3,5,3′triiodothyronine in pituitary, liver and kidney of euthyroid rats. Endocrinology 1978;103:1196
6. Silva JE, Larsen PR. Contributions of plasma triiodothyronine and local thyroxine monodeiodination to triiodothyronine to nuclear triiodothyronine receptor saturation in pituitary, liver and kidney of hypothyroid rats. J Clin Invest 1978;61:1247
7. Oppenheimer JH, Schwartz HL, Mariash CN, Kinlaw WB, Wong NCW, Freake HC. Advances in our understanding of thyroid hormone action at the cellular level. Endocr Rev 1987;8:288
8. Samuels HH, Forman BM, Horowitz ZD, Ye Z-S. Regulation of gene expression by thyroid hormone. J Clin Invest 1988;81:957
9. Evans RM. The steroid and thyroid hormone receptor super family. Science 1988;240:889
10. Greer MA. Evidence of hypothalamic control of the pituitary release of thyrotrophin. Proc Soc Exp Biol Med 1951;77:603
11. Schally AV, Bowers CY, Redding TW, Barrett JF. Isolation of thyrotropin releasing factor (TRF) from porcine hypothalamus. Biochem Biophys Res Commun 1966;25:165
12. Folkers K, Enzman F, Boler J, Bowers CY, Schally AV. Discovery of modification of the synthetic tripeptide sequence of the thyrotropin releasing hormone having activity. Biochem Biophys Res Commun 1969;37:123
13. Burgus R, Dunn TF, Desiderio D, Ward DN, Vale W, Guillemin R. Characterisation of the hypothalamic hypophysiotropic TSH-releasing factor (TRF) of ovine origin. Nature 1970;226:321
14. Jackson IMD, Wu P, Lechan RM. Immunohistochemical localisation in the rat brain of the precursor for thyrotropin-releasing hormone. Science 1985;229:1097
15. McKelvy JF. Thyrotropin-releasing hormone synthesis. In: Griffiths EC, Bennett GW, eds. Thyrotropin-releasing hormone. New York: Raven Press, 1983:51
16. Lechan RM, Wu P, Jackson IMD, et al. Thyrotropin releasing hormone precursor: characterisation in rat brain. Science 1986;231:159
17. Richter K, Kawashima E, Egger R, Kreil G. Biosynthesis of thyrotropin releasing hormone in the skin of xenopus laevis: partial sequence of the precursor deduced from cloned cDNA. EMBO J 1984;3:617
18. Jackson IMD. Controversies in TRH biosynthesis and strategies towards the identification of a TRH precursor. Ann NY Acad Sci 1989;553:7
19. Wu P. Identification and characterization of TRH-precursor peptides. Ann NY Acad Sci 1989;553:60
20. Wu P, Jackson IM. Post-translational processing of thyrotropin-releasing hormone precursor in rat brain: identification of 3 novel peptides derived from pro-TRH. Brain Res 1988;456:22
21. Carr FE, Fein HG, Fisher CU, Wessendorf MW, Smallridge RC. A cryptic peptide (160–169) of thyrotropin-releasing hormone prohormone demonstrates biological activity in vivo and in vitro. Endocrinology 1992;131:2653
22. Carr FE, Reid AH, Wessendorf MW. A cryptic peptide from the preprothyrotropin-releasing hormone precursor stimulates thyrotropin gene expression. Endocrinology 1993;133:809
23. Jackson IMD, Papapetrou PD, Reichlin S. Metabolic clearance of thyrotropin-releasing hormone in the rat in hypothyroid and hyperthyroid states: comparison with serum degradation in vitro. Endocrinology 1979;104:1292
24. Yanagisawa T, Prasad C, Peterkofsky A. The subcellular and organ distribution and natural form of histidyl-proline-diketopiperazine in rat brain determined by a specific radioimmunoassay. J Biol Chem 1980;255:10290
25. Garat B, Miranda J, Charli J-L, Joseph-Bravo P. Presence of a membrane bound pyroglutamyl aminopeptidase degrading thyrotropin releasing hormone in rat brain. Neuropeptides 1985;6:27
26. O'Connor B, O'Cuinn G. Localization of a narrow-specificity thyroliberin hydrolyzing pyroglutamate aminopeptidase in synaptosomal membranes of guinea-pig brain. Eur J Biochem 1984;144:271
27. Bauer K, Nowak P, Kleinkauf H. Specificity of a serum peptidase hydrolyzing thyroliberin at pyroglutamyl-histidine base. Eur J Biochem 1981;118:173
28. O'Connor B, O'Cuinn G. Purification of and kinetic studies on a narrow specificity synaptosomal membrane pyroglutamate aminopeptidase from guinea pig brain. Eur J Biochem 1985;150:47
29. Lamberton RP, Lechan RM, Jackson IMD. Ontogeny of thyrotropin releasing hormone (TRH) and histidyl proline diketopiperazine (His-Pro-DKP) in the rat CNS and pancreas. Endocrinology 1984;115:2100
30. Lechan RM, Jackson IMD. Thyrotropin-releasing hormone but not histidyl-proline-diketopiperazine is depleted from rat spinal cord following 5,7 dihydroxytryptamine treatment. Brain Res 1985;326:152
31. Bauer K. Regulation of degradation of thyrotropin releasing hormone by thyroid hormones. Nature 1976;259:591
32. Bauer K. Adenohypophyseal degradation of thyrotropin releasing hormone regulated by thyroid hormones. Nature 1987;330:375
33. Ponce G, Charli J-L, Pasten JA, Aceves C, Joseph-Bravo P. Tissue-specific regulation of pyroglutamate amino-peptidase II activity by thyroid hormones. Neuroendocrinology 1988;48:211
34. Taylor T, Wondisford FE, Blaine T, Weintraub BD. The paraventricular nucleus of the hypothalamus has a major role in thyroid hormone feedback regulation of thyrotropin synthesis and secretion. Endocrinology 1990;126:317
35. Lechan RM, Jackson IMD. Immunohistochemical localisation of thyrotropin-releasing hormone in the rat hypothalamus and pituitary. Endocrinology 1982;111:55
36. Siaud P, Tapia-Arancibia L, Szafarczyk A, Alonso G. Increase of thyrotropin-releasing hormone immunoreactivity in the nucleus of the solitary tract following bilateral lesions of the hypothalamic paraventricular nuclei. Neurosci Lett 1987;79:47
37. Bruhn TO, Rondeel JM, Bolduc TG, Jackson IM. Thyrotropin-releasing hormone (TRH) gene expression in the anterior pituitary. I. Presence of pro-TRH messenger ribonucleic acid and pro-TRH-derived peptide in a sub-population of somatotrophs. Endocrinology 1994;134:815

38. Croissandeau G, Grouselle D, Li JY, Roche M, Peillon F, Le Dafniet M. Hypothyroidism increases TRH and TRH precursor levels in rat anterior pituitary. Biochem Biophys Res Comm 1994;201:1248

39. Sheward WJ, Harmar AJ, Fraser HM, Fink G. TRH in rat pituitary stalk blood and hypothalamus. Studies with high performance liquid chromatography. Endocrinology 1983;113:1865

40. Carr FE, Shupnik MA, Burnside J, Chin WW. Thyrotropin-releasing hormone stimulates the activity of the rat thyrotropin β-subunit gene promoter transfected into pituitary cells. Mol Endocrinol 1989;3:717

41. Murakami M, Mori M, Kato Y, Kobayashi I. Hypothalamic thyrotropin-releasing hormone regulates pituitary thyrotropin beta- and alpha-subunit mRNA levels in the rat. Neuroendocrinology 1991;53:276

42. Shupnik MA, Greenspan SL, Ridgway EC. Transcriptional regulation of thyrotropin subunit genes by thyrotropin-releasing hormone and dopamine in pituitary cell culture. J Biol Chem 1986;261:12675

43. Shupnik MA, Rosenzweig BA, Friend KE, Mason ME. Thyrotropin (TSH)-releasing hormone-responsive elements in the rat TSH beta gene have distinct biological and nuclear protein-binding properties. Mol Endocrinol 1992;6:43

44. Carr FE, Galloway RJ, Reid AH, et al. Thyrotropin-releasing hormone regulation of thyrotropin beta-subunit gene expression involves intracellular calcium and protein kinase C. Biochemistry 1991;30:3721

45. Haisenleder DJ, Yasin M, Yasin A, Marshall JC. Regulation of prolactin, thyrotropin subunit, and gonadotropin subunit gene expression by pulsatile or continuous calcium signals. Endocrinology 1993;133:2055

46. Kim DS, Ahn SK, Yoon JH, et al. Involvement of a cAMP-responsive DNA element in mediating TRH responsiveness of the human thyrotropin alpha-subunit gene. Mol Endocrinol 1994;8:528

47. Mason ME, Friend KE, Copper J, Shupnik MA. Pit-1/GHF-1 binds to TRH-sensitive regions of the rat thyrotropin beta gene. Biochemistry 1993;32:8932

48. Steinfelder HJ, Radovick S, Wondisford FE. Hormonal regulation of the pituitary-specific transcription factor Pit-1. Proc Natl Acad Sci USA 1992;89:5942

49. Magner JA. Thyroid-stimulating hormone: biosynthesis, cell biology and bioactivity. Endocr Rev 1990;11:354

50. De Cherney GS, Gesundheit N, Gyves PW, Showalter CR, Weintraub BD. Alterations in the sialylation and sulfation of secreted mouse thyrotropin in primary hypothyroidism. Biochem Biophys Res Commun 1989;159:755

51. Miura Y, Perkel VS, Papenberg KA, Johnson MJ, Magner JA. Concanavalin-A, lentil and ricin affinity binding characteristics of human thyrotropin: differences in the sialylation of thyrotropin in sera of euthyroid, primary, and central hypothyroid patients. J Clin Endocrinol Metab 1989;69:985

52. Beck-Peccoz P, Piscitelli G, Amir S, et al. Endocrine, biochemical and morphological studies of a pituitary adenoma secreting growth hormone, thyrotropin (TSH) and α-subunit: evidence for secretion of TSH with increased bioactivity. J Clin Endocrinol Metab 1986;62:704

53. Gesundheit N, Petrick PA, Nissim M, et al. Thyrotropin-secreting pituitary adenomas: clinical and bio-chemical heterogeneity. Ann Intern Med 1989;111:827

54. Yamada M, Monden T, Satoh T, Iizuka M, Murakami M, Iriuchijima T, Mori M. Differential regulation of thyrotropin-releasing hormone receptor mRNA levels by thyroid hormone in vivo and in vitro (GH3 cells). Biochem Biophys Res Commun 1992;184:367

55. De Lean A, Ferland L, Drouin J, et al. Modulation of pituitary thyrotrophin releasing hormone receptor levels by oestrogens and thyroid hormones. Endocrinology 1977;100:1496

56. Hinkle PM, Perrone MH, Schonbrunn A. Mechanism of thyroid hormone inhibition of thyrotropin-releasing hormone action. Endocrinology 1981;108:199

57. Jones KE, Chin WW. Differential regulation of thyroid hormone receptor messenger ribonucleic acid levels by thyrotropin-releasing hormone. Endocrinology 1991;128:1763

58. Kaji H, Hinkle PM. Regulation of thyroid hormone receptors and responses by thyrotropin-releasing hormone in GH_4C_1 cells. Endocrinology 1987;121:1697

59. Koller KJ, Wolff RS, Warden MK, Zoeller RT. Thyroid hormones regulate levels of thyrotropin-releasing hormone mRNA in the paraventricular nucleus. Proc Natl Acad Sci USA 1987;84:7329

60. Segerson TP, Kauer J, Wolfe HC, et al. Thyroid hormone regulates TRH biosynthesis in the paraventricular nucleus of the rat hypothalamus. Science 1987;238:78

61. Taylor T, Wondisford FE, Blaine T, Weintraub BD. The paraventricular nucleus of the hypothalamus has a major role in thyroid hormone feedback regulation of thyrotropin synthesis and secretion. Endocrinology 1990;126:317

62. Kakucska I, Rand W, Lechan RM. Thyrotropin-releasing hormone gene expression in the hypothalamic paraventricular nucleus is dependent upon feedback regulation by both triiodothyronine and thyroxine. Endocrinology 1992;130:2845

63. Greer MA, Sato N, Wang X, Greer SE, McAdams S. Evidence that the major physiological role of TRH in the hypothalamic paraventricular nuclei may be to regulate the set-point for thyroid hormone negative feedback on the pituitary thyrotroph. Neuroendocrinology 1993;57:569

64. Rondeel JM, de Greef WJ, Klootwijk W, Visser TJ. Effects of hypothyroidism on hypothalamic release of thyrotropin-releasing hormone in rats. Endocrinology 1992;130:651

65. Peters JR, Foord SM, Dieguez C, Scanlon MF. TSH neuroregulation and alterations in disease states. Clin Endocrinol Metab 1983;12:669

66. Peters JR, Foord SM, Dieguez C, Salvador J, Hall R, Scanlon MF. Lack of effect of the TRH related dipeptide histidyl-proline-diketopiperazine on TSH and PRL secretion in normal subjects, in patients with microprolactinomas and in primary hypothyroidism. Clin Endocrinol 1985;23:289

67. Krieger DT, Luria M. Plasma ACTH and cortisol responses to TRH, vasopressin or hypoglycemia in Cushing's disease and Nelson's syndrome. J Clin Endocrinol Metab 1977;44:361

68. Sowers JR, Hershman JM, Skowsky WR, Carlson HE. Effects of TRH on serum arginine vasopressin in euthyroid and hypothyroid subjects. Horm Res 1976;7:232

69. Gershengorn MC. Bihormonal regulation of the thyrotropin-releasing hormone receptor in mouse pituitary thyrotropic tumour cells in culture. J Clin Invest 1978;62:937

70. Hinkle PM, Tashjian AH. Thyrotropin-releasing hormone regulates the number of its own receptors in the GH_3 strain of pituitary cells in culture. Biochemistry 1975;14:3845

71. Sheppard MC, Shennan KJ. Desensitisation of rat anterior pituitary gland to thyrotrophin releasing hormone. J Endocrinol 1984;101:101

72. Duthie SM, Taylor PL, Anderson L, Cook J, Eidne KA. Cloning and functional characterisation of the human TRH receptor. Mol Cell Endocrinol 1993;95:R11

73. Drummond AH. Inositol lipid metabolism and signal transduction in clonal pituitary cells. J Exp Biol 1986;124:337

74. Gershengorn MC. Thyrotropin-releasing hormone action: mechanism of calcium-mediated stimulation of prolactin secretion. Recent Prog Horm Res 1985;41:607

75. Iriuchijima T, Mori M. Inhibition by staurosporine of TRH-induced refractoriness of inositol phospholipid hydrolysis by rat anterior pituitaries. J Endocrinol 1990;124:75

76. Winikov I, Gershengorn MC. Receptor density determines secretory response patterns mediated by inositol lipid-derived

second messengers. Comparison of thyrotropin-releasing hormone and carbamylcholine actions in thyroid-stimulating hormone-secreting mouse pituitary tumor cells. J Biol Chem 1989;264:9438

77. Gershengorn MC, Rebecchi MJ, Geras E, Arevalo CO. Thyrotropin-releasing hormone (TRH) action in mouse thyrotropic tumour cells in culture. Evidence against a role for adenosine, 3,5′-monophosphate as a mediator of TRH-stimulated thyrotropin release. Endocrinology 1980;107:665

78. Iriuchijima T, Mori M. Regional dissociation of cyclic AMP and inositol phosphate formation in response to thyrotropin-releasing hormone in the rat brain. J Neurochem 1989;52:1944

79. Halasz B. A 1985 view of the hypothalamic control of the anterior pituitary. In: Muller EE, MacLeod RM, eds. Neuroendocrine perspectives. Vol 5. Amsterdam: Elsevier, 1986:1

80. Goodman RH, Aron DC, Roos BA. Rat-preprosomatostatin: structure and processing by microsomal membranes. J Biol Chem 1983:258:5570

81. Shen L-P, Pictet RL, Rutter WJ. Human somatostatin. I. Sequence of the cDNA. Proc Natl Acad Sci USA 1982;79:4575

82. Millar RP, Sheward RJ, Wegener I, Fink G. Somatostatin 28 is a hormonally active peptide secreted into hypophysial portal vessel blood. Brain Res 1983;260:334

83. Montminy MR, Goodman RH, Horovitch SJ, et al. Primary structure of the gene encoding rat pre-prosomatostatin. Proc Natl Acad Sci USA 1984;81:3337

84. Vale W, Brazeau P, Rivier C, et al. Somatostatin. Recent Prog Horm Res 1975;31:365

85. Lamberts SWJ, Zuyderwijk J, den Holder F, van Koetsveld P, Hofland L. Studies on the conditions determining the inhibitory effect of somatostatin on adrenocorticotropin, prolactin and thyrotropin release by cultured rat pituitary cells. Neuroendocrinology 1989;50:44

86. Arimura A, Schally AV. Increase in basal and thyrotropin-releasing hormone stimulated secretion of thyrotropin by passive immunization with antiserum to somatostatin. Endocrinology 1976;98:1069

87. Ferland L, Labrie F, Jobin M, et al. Physiological role of somatostatin in the control of growth hormone and thyrotropin secretion. Biochem Biophys Res Commun 1976;68:149

88. Rodriguez-Arnao MD, Gomez-Pan A, Rainbow SJ, et al. Effects of prosomatostatin on growth hormone and prolactin response to arginine in man. Comparison with somatostatin. Lancet 1981;1:353

89. Lippe BM, Van Herle AJ, Lafranchi SH, et al. Reversible hypothyroidism in growth-hormone deficient children treated with growth hormone. J Clin Endocrinol Metab 1975;40:143

90. Berelowitz M, Firestone SL, Frohman LA. Effects of growth hormone excess and deficiency on hypothalamic somatostatin content and release and on tissue somatostatin distribution. Endocrinology 1981;109:714

91. Cobb WE, Reichlin S, Jackson IMD. Growth hormone secretory status is a determinant of the thyrotropin response to thyrotropin-releasing hormone in euthyroid patients with hypothalamic pituitary disease. J Clin Endocrinol Metab 1981;52:324

92. Page MD, Millward ME, Hourihan M, Hall R, Scanlon MF. Long-term treatment of acromegaly with a long-acting analogue of somatostatin, octreotide. Q J Med 1990;74:189

93. Gonzalez BJ, Leroux P, Bodenant C, Laquerriere A, Coy DH, Vaudry H. Ontogeny of somatostatin receptors in the rat brain: biochemical and autoradiographic study. Neuroscience 1989;29:629

94. Kimura N. Developmental change and molecular properties of somatostatin receptors in the rat cerebral cortex. Biochem Biophys Res Commun 1989;160:72

95. Srikant CD, Patel YC. Somatostatin receptors in the rat adrenal cortex: characterisation and comparison with brain and pituitary receptors. Endocrinology 1985;116:1717

96. Kimura N, Hayafuji C, Kimura N. Characterization of 17-β-estradiol-dependent and -independent somatostatin receptor subtypes in rat anterior pituitary. J Biol Chem 1989;264:7033

97. Enjalbert A. Multiple transduction mechanisms of dopamine, somatostatin and angiotensin II receptors in anterior pituitary cells. Horm Res 1989;31:6

98. Nabekura J, Mizuno Y, Oomura Y. Inhibitory effect of somatostatin on vagal motoneurons in the rat brain stem in vitro. Am J Physiol 1989;256:C155

99. Nilsson T, Arkhammar P, Rorsman P, Berggren P-O. Suppression of insulin release by galanin and somatostatin is mediated by a G-protein. An effect involving repolarization and reduction in cytoplasmic free Ca+ concentration. J Biol Chem 1989;264:973

100. Hokfelt T, Elde R, Fuxe K, et al. Aminergic and peptidergic pathways in the nervous system with special reference to the hypothalamus. In: Reichlin S, Baldessarini RJ, Martin JB, eds. The hypothalamus. New York: Raven Press, 1978:69

101. Fukuda H, Greer MA. The effect of basal hypothalamic deafferentiation in the nycthemeral rhythm of plasma TSH. Endocrinology 1975;97:749

102. Cuello AC. Immunocytochemical studies of the distribution of neurotransmitters and related substances in CNS. Handbook Psychopharmacol 1978;9:69

103. Morley JE. Neuroendocrine control of thyrotropin secretion. Endocr Rev 1981;2:396

104. Krulich L, Giachetti A, Marchlewska KOJ, et al. On the role of the central noradrenergic and dopaminergic systems in the regulation of TSH secretion in the rat. Endocrinology 1977;100:496

105. Krulich L. Neurotransmitter control of thyrotropin secretion. Neuroendocrinology 1982;35:139

106. Mannisto PT, Ranta T. Neurotransmitter control of thyrotropin secretion in hypothyroid rats. Acta Endocrinol 1978;89:100

107. Lewis BM, Dieguez C, Lewis MD, Scanlon MF. Dopamine stimulates release of thyrotrophin-releasing hormone from perfused intact rat hypothalamus via hypothalamic D$_2$ receptors. J Endocrinol 1987;115:419

108. Lewis BM, Dieguez C, Ham J, et al. Effects of glucose on TRH, GHRH, somatostatin and LHRH release from rat hypothalamus *in vitro*. J Neuroendocrinol 1989;1:437

109. Ben-Jonathan N, Oliver C, Weiner HJ, Mical RS, Porter JC. Dopamine in hypophyseal portal plasma of the rat during the estrous cycle and throughout pregnancy. Endocrinology 1977;100:452

110. Johnston CA, Gibbs DM, Negro-Vilar A. High concentrations of epinephrine derived from a central source and of 5-hydroxyindole-3-acetic acid in hypophysial portal plasma. Endocrinology 1983;113:819

111. Foord SM, Peters JR, Scanlon MF, Rees Smith B, Hall R. Dopaminergic control of TSH secretion in isolated rat pituitary cells. FEBS Lett 1980;121:257

112. Cooper DS, Klibanski A, Ridgway EC. Dopaminergic modulation of TSH and its subunits: in vivo and in vitro studies. Clin Endocrinol 1983;18:265

113. Foord SM, Peters JR, Dieguez C, Scanlon MF, Hall R. Dopamine receptors on intact anterior pituitary cells in culture: functional association with the inhibition of prolactin and thyrotropin. Endocrinology 1983;112:1567

114. Foord SM, Peters JR, Dieguez C, et al. Hypothyroid pituitary cells in culture: an analysis of TSH and PRL responses to dopamine and dopamine receptor binding. Endocrinology 1984;115:407

115. Foord SM, Peters JR, Dieguez C, Lewis MD, Lewis BM, Hall R, Scanlon MF. In: Lightman S, Everitt B, eds. Neuroendocrinology. London: Blackwell Scientific Publications, 1986:450

116. Foord SM, Peters JR, Dieguez C, Shewring AG, Hall R, Scanlon MF. TSH regulates thyrotroph responsiveness to dopamine in vitro. Endocrinology 1985;118:1319

117. Dieguez C, Foord SM, Peters JR, Hall R, Scanlon MF. Interactions among epinephrine, thyrotropin (TSH)-releasing hormone, dopamine and somatostatin in the control of TSH secretion in vitro. Endocrinology 1984;114:957

118. Klibanski A, Milbury PE, Chin WW, Ridgway EC. Direct adrenergic stimulation of the release of thyrotropin and its subunits from the thyrotrope in vitro. Endocrinology 1983;113:1244

119. Peters JR, Foord SM, Dieguez C, Scanlon MF, Hall R. α_1- Adrenoreceptors on intact rat anterior pituitary cells: correlation with adrenergic stimulation of thyrotropin release. Endocrinology 1983; 113:133

120. Dieguez C, Foord SM, Peters JR, Hall R, Scanlon MF. α_1-Adrenoreceptors and α_1-adrenoreceptor-mediated thyrotropin release in cultures of euthyroid and hypothyroid rat anterior pituitary cells. Endocrinology 1985;117:624

121. Burrow GN, May PB, Spaulding SW, Donabedian RK. TRH and dopamine interactions affecting pituitary hormone secretion. J Clin Endocrinol Metab 1977;45:65

122. Scanlon MF, Mora B, Shale DJ, et al. Evidence for dopaminergic control of thyrotrophin (TSH) secretion in man. Lancet 1977;2:421

123. Scanlon MF, Weightman DR, Shale DJ, et al. Dopamine is a physiological regulator of thyrotrophin (TSH) secretion in man. Clin Endocrinol 1979;10:7

124. Scanlon MF, Lewis M, Weightman DR, Chan V, Hall R. The neuroregulation of human thyrotropin secretion. In: Martini L, Ganong WF, eds. Frontiers in neuroendocrinology. New York: Raven Press, 1980:333

125. Reymond MJ, Benotto W, Lemarchand-Beraud T. The secretory activity of the tuberoinfundibular dopaminergic neurons is modulated by the thyroid status in the adult rat: consequence of prolactin secretion. Neuroendocrinology 1987;46:62

126. Wang PS, Gonzalez HA, Reymond MJ, Porter JC. Mass and in situ molar activity of tyrosine hydroxylase in the median eminence. Neuroendocrinology 1989;49:659

127. Scanlon MF, Chan V, Heath M, et al. Dopaminergic control of thyrotropin, alpha-subunit and prolactin in euthyroidism and hypothyroidism: dissociated responses to dopamine receptor blockade with metoclopramide in euthyroid and hypothyroid subjects. J Clin Endocrinol Metab 1981;53:360

128. Zgliczynski S, Kaniewski M. Evidence for α-adrenergic receptor mediated TSH release in men. Acta Endocrinol 1980;95:172

129. Valcavi R, Dieguez C, Azzarito C, Artioli C, Portioli I, Scanlon MF. Alpha-adrenorceptor blockade with thymoxamine reduces basal thyrotrophin levels but does not influence circadian thyrotrophin changes in man. J Endocrinol 1987;115:187

130. Little KY, Garbutt JC, Mayo JP, Mason G. Lack of acute α-amphetamine effects on thyrotropin release. Neuroendocrinology 1988;48:304

131. Rogol AD, Reeves GD, Varma MM, Blizzard RM. Thyroid stimulating hormone and prolactin response to thyrotropin-releasing hormone during infusion of epinephrine and propanolol in man. Neuroendocrinology 1979;29:413

132. Smythe GA, Bradshaw JE, Cai WY, Symons RG. Hypothalamic serotoninergic stimulation of thyrotropin secretion and related brain-hormone and drug interactions in the rat. Endocrinology 1982;111:1181

133. Scharp B, Morley JE, Carlson HE, et al. The role of opiates and endogenous opioid peptides in the regulation of rat TSH secretion. Brain Res 1981;219:335

134. Judd AM, Hedge GA. The role of opioid peptides in controlling thyroid stimulating hormone release. Life Sci 1982;31:2529

135. Samuels MH, Kramer P, Wilson D, Sexton G. Effects of naloxone infusions on pulsatile thyrotropin secretion. J Clin Endocrinol Metab 1994;78:1249

136. Dubuis JM, Dayer JM, Siegrist-Kaiser CA, Burger AG. Human recombinant interleukin-1β decreases plasma thyroid hormone and thyroid stimulating hormone levels in rats. Endocrinology 1988;123:2175

137. Ozawa M, Sato K, Han DC, Kawakami M, Tsushima T, Shizume K. Effects of tumor necrosis factor-α/cachectin on thyroid hormone metabolism in mice. Endocrinology 1988;123:1461

138. Pang XP, Hershman JM, Mirell CJ, Pekary AE. Impairment of hypothalamic-pituitary-thyroid function in rats treated with human recombinant tumour necrosis factor-α (cachectin). Endocrinology 1989;125:76

139. Kakucska I, Romero LI, Clark BD, Rondeel JM, Qi Y, Alex S, Emerson CH, Lechan RM. Suppression of thyrotropin-releasing hormone gene expression by interleukin-1-beta in the rat: implications for nonthyroidal illness. Neuroendocrinology 1994;59:129

140. Hermus RM, Sweep CG, van der Meer MJ, et al. Continuous infusion of interleukin-1 beta induces a nonthyroidal illness syndrome in the rat. Endocrinology 1992;131:2139

141. Pang XP, Yoshimura M, Hershman JM. Suppression of rat thyrotroph and thyroid cell function by tumor necrosis factor-alpha. Thyroid 1993;3:325

142. Bernton EW, Beach JE, Holaday JW, et al. Release of multiple hormones by a direct action of interleukin-1 on pituitary cells. Science 1987;238:519

143. Besedovsky H, Del Rey A, Sorkin E, et al. Immunoregulatory feedback between interleukin-1 and glucocorticoid hormones. Science 1986;233:652

144. Woloski BM, Smith EM, Meyer WJ III, Fuller GM, Blalock JE. Corticotropin-releasing activity of monokines. Science 1985;230:1037

145. Sapolsky R, Rivier C, Yamamoto G, et al. Interleukin-1 stimulates the secretion of hypothalamic corticotropin-releasing factor. Science 1987;238:522

146. Koenig JI, Snow K, Clark BD, et al. Intrinsic pituitary interleukin-1 beta is induced by bacterial lipopolysaccharide. Endocrinology 1990;126:3053

147. Spangelo BL, MacLeod RM, Isaacson PC. Production of interleukin-6 by anterior pituitary cells in vitro. Endocrinology 1990;126:582

148. Vankelecom H, Carmeliet P, Van Damme J, Billian A, Denef C. Production of interleukin-6 by folliculo-stellate cells of the anterior pituitary gland in a histiotype cell aggregate culture system. Neuroendocrinology 1989;49:102

149. Brabant G, Frank K, Ranft U, et al. Physiological regulation of circadian and pulsatile thyrotropin secretion in normal man and woman. J Clin Endocrinol Metab 1990;70:403

150. Parker DC, Rossman LG, Pekary AE, Hershman JM. Effect of 64-hour sleep deprivation on the circadian waveform of thyrotropin (TSH): further evidence of sleep-related inhibition of TSH release. J Clin Endocrinol Metab 1987;64:157

151. Konno N, Morikawa K. Seasonal variation of serum thyrotropin concentration and thyrotropin response to thyrotropin-releasing hormone in patients with primary hypothyroidism on constant replacement dosage of thyroxine. J Clin Endocrinol Metab 1982;54:1118

152. Brabant G, Ocran K, Ranft U, von zur Muhlen A, Hesch RD. Physiological regulation of thyrotropin. Biochimie 1989;71:293

153. LeRoith D, Liel Y, Sack J, et al. The TSH response to TRH is exaggerated in primary testicular failure and normal in the male castrate. Acta Endocrinol 1981;97:103

154. Spitz IM, Zylber-Haran EA, Trestian S. The thyrotropin (TSH) profile in isolated gonadotropin deficiency: a model to evaluate the effect of sex steroids on TSH secretion. J Clin Endocrinol Metab 1983;57:415

155. Brabant G, Ranft U, Ocran K, Hesch RD, von zur Muhlen A. Thyrotropin: an episodically secreted hormone. Acta Endocrinol 1986;112:315

156. Brabant G, Brabant A, Ranft U, et al. Circadian and pulsatile thyrotropin secretion in euthyroid man under the influence of thyroid hormone and glucocorticoid administration. J Clin Endocrinol Metab 1987;65:83

157. Greenspan SL, Klibanski A, Schoenfeld D, Ridgway EC. Pulsatile secretion of thyrotropin in man. J Clin Endocrinol Metab 1986;63:661

158. Rossmanith WG, Mortola JF, Laughlin GA, Yen SS. Dopaminergic control of circadian and pulsatile pituitary thyrotropin release in women. J Clin Endocrinol Metab 1988;67:560

159. Samuels MH, Veldhuis JD, Henry P, Ridgway EC. Pathophysiology of pulsatile and copulsatile release of thyroid-stimulating hormone, luteinising hormone, follicle-stimulating hormone and α-subunit. J Clin Endocrinol Metab 1990;71:425

160. Salvador J, Dieguez C, Scanlon MF. The circadian rhythms of thyrotropin and prolactin secretion. Chronobiol Int 1988;5:85

161. Evans PJ, Weeks I, Jones MK, Woodhead JS, Scanlon MF. The circadian variation of thyrotropin in patients with primary thyroidal disease. Clin Endocrinol 1986;24:343

162. Re RN, Kourides IA, Ridgway EC, Weintraub BD, Maloof F. The effect of glucocorticoid administration on human pituitary secretion of thyrotropin and prolactin. J Clin Endocrinol Metab 1976;43:338

163. Otsuki M, Dakoda M, Baba S. Influence of glucocorticoids on TRH-induced TSH response in man. J Clin Endocrinol Metab 1973;36:95

164. Sowers JR, Carlson HE, Brautbar N, Hershman JM. Effect of dexamethasone on prolactin and TSH responses to TRH and metoclopramide in man. J Clin Endocrinol Metab 1977;44:237

165. Bartalena L, Placidi GF, Martino E, et al. Nocturnal serum thyrotropin (TSH) surge and the TSH response to TSH-releasing hormone: dissociated behaviour in untreated depressives. J Clin Endocrinol Metab 1990;71:650

166. Souetre E, Salvati E, Wehr TA, Sack DA, Krebs B, Darcourt G. Twenty-four hour profiles of body temperature and plasma TSH in bipolar patients during depression and during remission and in normal control subjects. Am J Psychiatry 1988;145:1133

167. Bartalena L, Martino E, Brandi LS, et al. Lack of nocturnal serum thyrotropin surge after surgery. J Clin Endocrinol Metab 1990;70:293

168. Salvador J, Wilson DW, Harris PE, et al. Relationships between the circadian rhythms of TSH, prolactin and cortisol in surgically treated microprolactinoma patients. Clin Endocrinol 1985;22:265

169. Samuels MH, Henry P, Luther M, Ridgway EC. Pulsatile TSH secretion during 48-hour continuous TRH infusions. Thyroid 1993;3:201

170. Moore RY. Organization and function of a nervous system circadian oscillator. Fed Proc 1983;42:2783

171. Sowers JR, Catania RA, Hershman JM. Evidence for dopaminergic control of circadian variations in thyrotropin secretion. J Clin Endocrinol Metab 1982;54:673

172. Perez Lopez F, Gonzalez Moreno CM, Abos MD, Andonegui JA, Corvo RH. Pituitary responses to a dopamine antagonist at different times of the day in normal women. Acta Endocrinol 1982;100:481

173. Scanlon MF, Weetman AP, Lewis M, et al. Dopaminergic modulation of circadian thyrotropin rhythms and thyroid hormone levels in euthyroid subjects. J Clin Endocrinol Metab 1980;51:1251

174. O'Malley BP, Jennings PE, Cook N, Barnett DB, Rosenthal FD. The role of serotonin in the control of TSH and prolactin release in euthyroid subjects as assessed by the administration of ketanserin (5-HT2) antagonist) and zimelidine (5-HT re-uptake inhibitor). Psychoneuroendocrinology 1984;9:13

175. Strassman RJ, Peake GT, Qualls CR, Lisansky EJ. Lack of an acute modulatory effect of melatonin on human nocturnal thyrotropin and cortisol secretion. Neuroendocrinology 1988;48:387

176. Gordon J, Morley JE, Hershman JM. Melatonin and the thyroid. Horm Metab Res 1980;12:71

177. Murakami M, Tanaka K, Greer MA. There is a nyctohemeral rhythm of type II iodothyronine 5'-deiodinase activity in rat anterior pituitary. Endocrinology 1988;123:1631

178. Rage F, Lazaro JB, Benyassi A, Arancibia S, Tapia-Arancibia L. Rapid changes in somatostatin and TRH mRNA in whole rat hypothalamus in response to acute cold exposure. J Neuroendocrinol 1994;6:19

179. Zoeller RT, Kabeer N, Alberts HE. Cold exposure elevates cellular levels of messenger ribonucleic acid encoding thyrotropin-releasing hormone in paraventricular nucleus despite elevated levels of thyroid hormones. Endocrinology 1990;127:2955

180. Lewis GF, Alessi CA, Imperial JG, Refetoff S. Low serum free thyroxine index in ambulating elderly is due to a resetting of the threshold of thyrotropin feedback suppression. J Clin Endocrinol Metab 1991;73:843

181. Finucane P, Rudra T, Church H, et al. Thyroid function tests in elderly patients with and without an acute illness. Age Ageing 1989;18:398

182. Van Coeverden A, Laurent E, DeCoster C, et al. Decreased basal and stimulated thyrotropin secretion in healthy elderly men. J Clin Endocrinol Metab 1989;69:177

183. Borst GC, Osburne RC, O'Brian JT, Georges LP, Burman KD. Fasting decreases thyrotropin responsiveness to thyrotropin-releasing hormone: a potential cause of misinterpretation of thyroid function tests in the critically ill. J Clin Endocrinol Metab 1983;57:380

184. Vinik AI, Kalk WJ, McLaren H, Henrick S, Pimstone BL. Fasting blunts the TSH response to synthetic thyrotropin-releasing hormone (TRH). J Clin Endocinol Metab 1975;40:509

185. Blake NG, Eckland DJ, Foster OJ, Lightman SL. Inhibition of hypothalamic thyrotropin-releasing hormone messenger ribonucleic acid during food deprivation. Endocrinology 1991;129:2714

186. Shi ZX, Levy A, Lightman SL. The effect of dietary protein on thyrotropin-releasing hormone and thyrotropin gene expression. Brain Res 1993;606:1

187. Romijn JA, Adriaanse R, Brabant G, Prank K, Endert E, Wiersinga WM. Pulsatile secretion of thyrotropin during fasting: a decrease of thyrotropin pulse amplitude. J Clin Endocrinol Metab 1990;70:1631

188. Hugues JN, Enjalbert A, Moyse E, et al. Differential effects of passive immunization with somatostatin antiserum on adenohypophysial hormone secretions in starved rats. J Endocrinol 1986;109:169

189. Mora B, Hassanyeh F, Schapira K, et al. Calorie restriction, thyroid status and inhibitory dopaminergic control of thyrotrophin secretion in man. In: Stockigt JR, Nagataki S, eds. Proceedings of Australian Academy of Science. Thyroid Research VIII. Proceedings of the VIIIth International Thyroid Congress, Sydney, Australia, 1980:59

190. Rojdmark S. Are fasting-induced effects on thyrotropin and prolactin secretion mediated by dopamine? J Clin Endocrinol Metab 1983;56:1262

191. Spencer CA, Lum SMC, Wilber JF, Kaptein EM, Nicoloff JT. Dynamics of serum thyrotropin and thyroid hormone changes in fasting. J Clin Endocrinol Metab 1983;56:883

192. Kehlet H, Klauber PV, Weeke J. Thyrotropin, free and total triiodothyronine, and thyroxine in serum during surgery. Clin Endocrinol 1979;10:131

193. Zalaga GP, Chernow B, Smallridge RC, et al. A longitudinal evaluation of thyroid function in critically ill surgical patients. Ann Surg 1985;201:456

194. Wartofsky L, Burman KD. Alterations in thyroid function in patients with systemic illness: the "euthyroid sick syndrome." Endocr Rev 1982;3:164

195. Hamblin PS, Dyer SA, Mohr VS, et al. Relationship between thyrotropin and thyroxine changes during recovery from severe hypothyroxinemia of critical illness. J Clin Endocrinol Metab 1986;62:717

196. Wehman RE, Gregerman RI, Burns WH, Saral R, Santos GW. Suppression of thyrotropin in the low-thyroxine state of severe nonthyroidal illness. N Engl J Med 1985;312:546

197. Vierhapper H, Laggner A, Waldhausl W, Grubeck-Loebenstein B, Kleinberger G. Impaired section of TSH in critically ill patients with "low-T4 syndrome." Acta Endocrinol 1982;101:542

198. Romijn JA, Wiersinga WM. Decreased nocturnal surge of thyrotropin in nonthyroidal illness. J Clin Endocrinol Metab 1990;70:35

199. Faber K. Kirkegaard C, Rasmussen B, Westh H, Busch-Sorensen M, Jensen IW. Pituitary-thyroid axis in critical illness. J Clin Endocrinol Metab 1987;65:315

200. Kabadi UM. Impaired pituitary thyrotroph function in uncontrolled type II diabetes mellitus: normalization on recovery. J Clin Endocrinol Metab 1984;59:521

201. Small M, Cohen HN, McLean JA, Beastall GH, McCuish AC. Impaired thyrotropin secretion following the administration of thyrotropin-releasing hormone in type II diabetes mellitus. Postgrad Med J 1986;62:445

202. Pokroy N, Epstein S, Hendricks S, Pimstone B. Thyrotropin response to intravenous thyrotropin releasing hormone in patients with hepatic and renal disease. Horm Metab Res 1974:6:132

203. Delitala G, Tomasi P, Virdis R. Prolactin, growth hormone and thyrotropin-thyroid hormone secretion during stress states in man. Baillieres Clin Endocrinol Metab 1987;1:391

204. Loosen PT. Thyroid function in affective disorders and alcoholism. Endocrinol Metab Clin North Am 1988;17:55

205. Brent GA, Hershman JM. Thyroxine therapy in patients with severe nonthyroidal illness and low serum thyroxine concentration. J Clin Endocrinol Metab 1986;63:1

206. Joffe RT, Sokolov STH, Singer WT. Thyroid hormone treatment of depression. Thyroid 1995;5:235

207. Seth J, Kellett HA, Caldwell G, et al. A sensitive immunoradiometric assay for serum thyroid stimulating hormone: a replacement for the thyrotrophin-releasing hormone test? BMJ 1984;289:1334

208. Caldwell G, Kellett HA, Gow SM, et al. A new strategy for thyroid function testing. Lancet 1985;1:1117

209. Rodbard D. Statistical estimation of the minimal detectable concentration ("sensitivity") by radioligand assay. Ann Biochem 1978;90:1

210. Hay ID, Bayer MF, Kaplan MM, Klee GG, Larsen PR, Spencer CA. American Thyroid Association assessment of current free thyroid hormone and thyrotropin measurements and guidelines for future clinical assays. Clin Chem 1991;37:2002

211. McConway MG, Chapman RS, Beastall GH, et al. How sensitive are immunoassays for thyrotropin? Clin Chem 1989;35:289

212. Spencer CA. Thyroid profiling for the 1990s. FT$_4$ estimate or sensitive TSH measurement? J Clin Immunoassay 1989:12:82

213. Nicoloff JT, Spencer CA. The use and misuse of the sensitive thyrotropin assays. J Clin Endocrinol Metab 1990:71:553

214. Wilkinson E, Rae PWH, Thomson KJT, Toft AD, Spencer CA, Beckett GJ. Chemiluminescent third-generation assay (Amerlite TSH-30) of thyroid-stimulating hormone in serum or plasma assessed. Clin Chem 1993;39:2166

215. Toft AD, Irvine WJ, Hunter WM, Ratcliffe JG, Seth J. Anomalous plasma TSH levels in patients developing hypothyroidism in the early months after ^{131}I therapy for thyrotoxicosis. J Clin Endocrinol Metab 1974;39:607

216. Toft AD, Irvine WJ, Sinclair I, McIntosh D, Seth J, Cameron EHD. Thyroid function after surgical treatment of thyrotoxicosis: a report of 100 cases treated with propranolol before operation. N Engl J Med 1978;298:643

217. Toft AD, Seth J, Hunter WM, Irvine WJ. Plasma thyrotrophin and serum thyroxine in patients becoming hypothyroid in the early months after iodine-131. Lancet 1974;1:704

218. Vagenakis AG, Braverman LE, Azizi F, et al. Recovery of pituitary thyrotropic function after withdrawal of prolonged thyroid-suppression therapy. N Engl J Med 1975;293:681

219. Sawers JSA, Toft AD, Irvine WJ, Brown NS, Seth J. Transient hypothyroidism after iodine-131 treatment of thyrotoxicosis. J Clin Endocrinol Metab 1980;50:226

220. Toft AD, Irvine WJ, McIntosh D, Seth J, Cameron EHD, Lidgard GP. Temporary hypothyroidism after surgical treatment of thyrotoxicosis. Lancet 1976;2:817

221. Toft AD, Kellett HA, Sawers JSA et al. What is the significance of raised plasma TSH levels after thyroid surgery? Scot Med J 1982;27:216

222. Hardisty CA, Talbot CH, Munro DS. The effect of partial thyroidectomy for Graves' disease on serum long-acting thyroid stimulator protector (LATS-P). Clin Endocrinol 1980;14:181

223. Cotton GE, Gorman CA, Mayberry WE. Suppression of thyrotropin (h-TSH) in serums of patients with myxoedema of varying etiology treated with thyroid hormones. N Engl J Med 1971;285:529

224. Fraser WD, Biggart EM O'Reilly DS, et al. Are biochemical tests of thyroid function of any value in monitoring patients receiving thyroxine replacement? BMJ 1986;293:808

225. Leese GP, Jung RT, Guthrie C, et al. Morbidity in patients on L-thyroxine: comparison of those with a normal TSH to those with a suppressed TSH. Clin Endocrinol 1992;37:500

226. Snyder PJ, Utiger RD. Inhibition of thyrotropin response to thyrotropin-releasing hormone by small quantities of thyroid hormones. J Clin Invest 1972;51:2077

227. Visser TJ, Kaplan MM, Leonard JL, Larsen PR. Evidence for two pathways of iodothyronine 5'-deiodination in rat pituitary that differ in kinetics, propylthiouracil sensitivity, and response to hypothyroidism. J Clin Invest 1983;71:992

228. Evered D, Young ET, Ormston BJ, et al. Treatment of hypothyroidism: a reappraisal of thyroxine therapy. BMJ 1973;3:131

229. Biondi B, Fazio S, Carella C, et al. Cardiac effects of long term thyrotropin-suppression therapy with Levothyroxine. J Clin Endocrinol Metab 1993;77:334

230. Franklyn JA, Daykin J, Betteridge J, et al. Thyroxine replacement therapy and circulating lipid concentrations. Clin Endocrinol 1993;38:453

231. Toft AD. Thyroxine therapy. N Engl J Med 1994;331:174

232. Sawin CT, Geller A, Wolf PA, et al. Low serum thyrotropin concentrations as a risk factor for atrial fibrillation in older persons. N Engl J Med 1994;331:1249

233. Solomon BL, Wartofsky L, Burman KD. Prevalence of fractures in postmenopausal women with thyroid disease. Thyroid 1993;3:17

234. Carr D, McLeod DT, Parry G, et al. Fine adjustment of thyroxine replacement dosage: comparison of the thyrotrophin-releasing hormone test using a sensitive thyrotrophin assay with measurement of free thyroid hormones and clinical assessment. Clin Endocrinol 1988;28:325

235. Nystrom E, Lundberg P-A, Petersen K, et al. Evidence for a slow tissue adaptation to circulating thyroxine in patients with chronic L-thyroxine treatment. Clin Endocrinol 1989;31:143

236. Surks MI, Chopra J, Mariash CN, et al. American Thyroid Association guidelines for the use of laboratory tests in thyroid disorders. JAMA 1990;263:1529

237. Ehrmann DA, Weinberg M, Sarne DH. Limitations to the use of a sensitive assay for serum thyrotropin in the assessment of thyroid status. Arch Intern Med 1989;149:369

238. Gow SM, Kellett HA, Seth J, Sweeting VM, Toft AD, Beckett GJ. Limitations of new thyroid function tests in pregnancy. Clin Chim Acta 1985;152:325

239. Irvine WJ, Gray RS, Toft AD, Seth J, Lidgard GP, Cameron EHD. Spectrum of thyroid function in patients remaining in remission after antithyroid drug therapy for thyrotoxicosis. Lancet 1977;2:179

240. Lamberg B-A, Helenius T, Liewendahl K. Assessment of thyroxine suppression in thyroid carcinoma patients with a sensitive immunoradiometric assay. Clin Endocrinol 1986;25:259

241. Morgans ME, Thompson BD, Whitehouse SA. Sporadic nontoxic goitre: an investigation of the hypothalamic-pituitary-thyroid axis. Clin Endocrinol 1978;8:101

242. Mori T, Imura H, Bito S, et al. Clinical usefulness of a highly sensitive enzyme-immunoassay of TSH. Clin Endocrinol 1987;27:1

243. Ormston BJ, Garry R, Cryer RJ, Besser GM, Hall R. Thyrotropin-releasing hormone as a thyroid function test. Lancet 1971;2:10

244. Piketty ML, Talbot JN, Askienazy S, Milhaud G. Clinical significance of a low concentration of thyrotropin: five immunometric "kit" assays compared. Clin Chem 1987:33:1237

245. Tunbridge WMG, Brewis M, French JM, et al. Natural history of autoimmune thyroiditis. BMJ 1981;1:258

246. Chopra IJ, Hershman JM, Hornabrook RW. Serum thyroid hormone and thyrotropin levels from endemic goitre regions of New Guinea. J Clin Endocrinol Metab 1975;40:326

247. Fisher DA, Klein AH. Thyroid development and disorders of thyroid function in the newborn. N Engl J Med 1981;304:702

248. Emerson CH, Dyson WL, Utiger RD. Serum thyrotropin and thyroxine concentrations in patients receiving lithium carbonate. J Clin Endocrinol Metab 1973;36:338

249. Braverman LE, Ingbar SH, Vagenakis AG, et al. Enhanced susceptibility to iodine myxoedema in patients with Hashimoto's disease. J Clin Endocrinol Metab 1971;32:515

250. Fuks Z, Glatstein E, Marsa GW, et al. Long-term effects of external radiation on the pituitary and thyroid glands. Cancer 1976;37:1152

251. Schimpff SC, Diggs CH, Wiswell JG, et al. Radiation-related thyroid dysfunction: implications for the treatment of Hodgkin's disease. Ann Intern Med 1980;92:91

252. Toft AD, Irvine WJ, Hunter WM, Seth J. Plasma TSH and serum T$_4$ levels in long-term follow-up of patients treated with ^{131}I for thyrotoxicosis. BMJ 1974;3:152

253. Evered D, Young ET, Tunbridge WMG, et al. Thyroid function after subtotal thyroidectomy for hyperthyroidism. BMJ 1975;1:25

254. Cooper DS, Halpern R, Wood LC, et al. L-thyroxine therapy in subclinical hypothyroidism: a double blind placebo-controlled trial. Ann Intern Med 1984;101:18

255. Nystrom E, Caidahl K, Fager G, et al. A double-blind cross-over 12-month study of L-thyroxine treatment of women with "subclinical" hypothyroidism. Clin Endocrinol 1988;29:63

256. Lundstrom B, Gillquist J. The importance of elevated TSH in serum after subtotal thyroidectomy for hyperthyroidism: a five year follow-up study. Acta Chir Scand 1981;147:645

257. Rosenthal MJ, Hunt WC, Garry PJ, et al. Thyroid failure in the elderly. Microsomal antibodies as discriminant for therapy. JAMA 1987;258:209

258. Toft AD, Irvine WJ, Seth J, Cameron EHD. How often should patients be reviewed after treatment with iodine-131 for thyrotoxicosis. BMJ 1978;2:1115

259. Himsworth RL. Hyperthyroidism with a low iodine uptake. Clin Endocrinol Metab 1985;14:397

260. McConnon JK. Thirty-five cases of transient hyperthyroidism. Can Med Assoc J 1984;130:1159

261. Fung HYM, Kologlu M, Collison K, et al. Postpartum thyroid dysfunction in Mid-Glamorgan. BMJ 1988;96:241

262. Iseki M, Shimizu M, Oikawa T, et al. Sequential serum measurements of thyrotropin binding inhibitor immunoglobulin G in transient familial neonatal hypothyroidism. J Clin Endocrinol Metab 1983;57:384

263. Scanlon MF, Peters JR, Salvador J, et al. The preoperative and postoperative investigation of TSH and prolactin release in the management of patients with hyperprolactinaemia due to prolactinomas and nonfunctional pituitary tumours: relationship to adenoma size at surgery. Clin Endocrinol 1985;24:435

264. Scanlon MF, Rodriguez-Arnao MD, McGregor AM, et al. Altered dopaminergic regulation of thyrotrophin release in patients with prolactinomas: comparison with other tests of hypothalamic-pituitary function. Clin Endocrinol 1981;14:133

265. Massara F, Camanni F, Martra M, Dolfin GC, Muller EE, Molinatti GM. Reciprocal pattern of the TSH and PRL responses to dopamine receptor blockade in women with physiological or pathological hyperprolactinaemia. Clin Endocrinol 1983; 18:103

266. Rodriguez-Arnao MD, Weightman DR, Hall R, Scanlon MF, Camporro JM, Gomez-Pan A. Reduced dopaminergic inhibition of thyrotrophin release in states of physiological hyperprolactinaemia. Clin Endocrinol 1982;17:15

267. Berelowitz M, Szabo M, Frohman LA, et al. Somatomedin-C mediates growth hormone negative feedback by effects on both the hypothalamus and the pituitary. Science 1981;212:1279

268. Masturzo P, De Maria A, Murialdo G, Bonura ML, Zauli C, Polleri AP. Benserazide effects on growth hormone, prolactin and thyrotropin in normal and acromegalic man. J Clin Endocrinol Metab 1985;61:378

269. Prescott RWG, Weightman D, Kendall-Taylor P, Johnston DG. Differential TSH and PRL responses to dopamine receptor blockade in acromegaly. Clin Endocrinol 1984;21:369

270. Weintraub BD, Gershengorn MC, Kourides IA, Fein H. Inappropriate secretion of thyroid-stimulating hormone. Ann Intern Med 1981;95:339

Werner and Ingbar's The Thyroid, Seventh Edition,
edited by Lewis E. Braverman and Robert D. Utiger.
Lippincott–Raven Publishers, Philadelphia, © 1996

13

Other Factors Regulating Thyroid Function

Autoregulation: Effects of Iodide

Shigenobu Nagataki
Naokata Yokoyama

Iodine has been central to any consideration of thyroid physiology since the last century, and the concept of autoregulation of iodine metabolism was established several decades ago. Autoregulation was originally defined as the regulation of thyroidal iodine metabolism independent of thyrotropin (TSH) or other external stimulators, and the major autoregulatory factor was considered to be excess iodide. This chapter examines this process, which has been the subject of several reviews.[1,2]

In humans, autoregulation results in the maintenance of normal thyroid secretion despite wide variations in dietary iodide intake. Although the intake of iodide varies from 50 μg/day to several milligrams per day in iodine-sufficient areas, serum thyroid hormone concentrations as well as serum TSH concentrations are remarkably constant in these areas. Even in mildly iodine-deficient areas, many subjects are euthyroid and have normal serum thyroid hormone and TSH concentrations. In patients with hyperthyroidism, excess iodide ameliorates the symptoms and signs of thyrotoxicosis and decreases serum thyroid hormone concentrations. This antithyroid effect of excess iodide disappears, however, with continuous administration and thyrotoxicosis reappears (via escape or adaptation).

In animal thyroid tissue, acute inhibition of thyroidal iodine organification by excess iodide, escape from the acute inhibitory effect of excess iodide, and changes of thyroid radioiodine uptake in hypophysectomized animals in response to variations in dietary iodide intake are representative examples of autoregulation. The acute inhibitory effect of excess iodide (Wolff-Chaikoff effect) is temporary and escape occurs despite continuous administration of iodide. Escape also occurs in hypophysectomized animals, indicating that it is not dependent on changes in TSH secretion. When hypophysectomized rats are fed a low

iodine diet, thyroidal radioactive iodine uptake increases; this increase is abolished by intake of excess iodide.

Glandular organic iodine content and iodide-transport activity are inversely related, even in hypophysectomized rats.[3] In hypophysectomized rats the weight of the thyroid and its uptake of radioactive iodine were higher if the rats had been iodine depleted before hypophysectomy, and administering TSH to these same two groups produced a greater effect in the iodine-depleted rats.[4]

The concept of autoregulation was established when the only methods of investigation were the dynamics of radioactive iodine metabolism, chromatography of iodoamino acids, electrophoresis of serum thyroid hormone-binding proteins, and measurements of serum protein-bound iodine and bioactive TSH concentrations.

IODIDE AUTOREGULATION IN ANIMALS

Acute Inhibitory Effects of Excess Iodide

The acute inhibitory effects of excess iodide were first demonstrated about 40 years ago.[5,6] In rats injected with 100 μg of iodide containing a tracer quantity of radioiodine, serum iodide concentrations decreased rapidly with time; thyroidal iodine organification was inhibited as long as serum iodide concentrations were above 20 to 30 μg/dL. When serum iodide decreased below this range, organification of newly accumulated iodine began to occur. This inhibition of thyroidal iodine organification in response to an acute increase of serum iodide concentrations is commonly called the *Wolff-Chaikoff effect*.

Escape from Acute Iodide Inhibition

When a high serum iodide concentration (100–200 μg/dL) is maintained by repeated administration of iodide, the inhibitory effect disappears and thyroidal iodine organification increases.[7] This is called *escape* from the Wolff-Chaikoff effect. Studies of the mechanism of escape suggested that it occurs because of impairment in the ability of the thyroid to concentrate sufficient iodine to inhibit thyroidal iodine organification.[8,9] Escape from the acute inhibitory effect of iodide explains why hypothyroidism or goiter does not occur in humans or animals maintained on high doses of iodide for a long time (see later); however, the mechanism of the decrease in iodide transport activity in response to chronic excess iodide is unknown.

Effects of Moderate Doses of Iodide

The acute response to iodide loading is associated not only with rejection of large iodide loads but also with qualitative alterations in hormonal biosynthesis.[10] Even during the acute Wolff-Chaikoff effect, a small amount of organic iodine is formed in thyroid tissue, but the newly-formed organic iodine consists mostly of monoiodotyrosine (MIT) and diiodotyrosine (DIT), and very little thyroxine (T_4) or triiodothyronine (T_3) can be detected. The thyroid, however, concentrates substantial proportions of iodide when serum iodide concentrations are only moderately increased.[11] (Fig. 13–1) shows the results of studies in which rats were given graded doses of iodide (2.5–250 μg) and a tracer dose of radioiodine 30 minutes before being killed and then studied for the incorporation of radioiodine into several thyroidal components. Two phases of response could be distinguished. The percentage of thyroidal radioiodine as inorganic iodide increased and the percentage of ^{131}I amino acids as T_4 and T_3 decreased with increasing iodide doses above 50 μg. The ratio of labeled MIT/DIT also increased. As for the total quantity of newly formed organic iodine, the changes in total organification were biphasic, increasing as the iodide dose increased to 50 μg and then decreasing. T_4 and T_3 formation decreased more abruptly than did total organification.

Definition of Excess Iodide

From the results mentioned previously, the effects of excess iodide can be divided into the following four categories.[1] First, relatively low doses of iodide do not change the proportionate metabolism of iodine. In this range, the percentage uptake

and incorporation of radioactive iodine into iodinated amino acids are unaltered. The total accumulation and incorporation of stable iodide into T_4 and T_3 increase with and remain proportional to the dose of stable iodide administered. Second, moderate doses of iodide decrease the percentage uptake of administered iodide, the proportion of newly formed organic iodine, and the proportion of T_4 and T_3 among the newly formed iodinated amino acids, but they increase the absolute rate of organic iodination and T_4 and T_3 synthesis. Third, large doses of iodide decrease both the percentage of incorporation of administered iodine and the absolute rate of organic iodine formation (Wolff-Chaikoff effect). Fourth, very large doses of iodide acutely saturate the mechanism for iodide transport.

Balance Between Uptake of Iodide and Release of Thyroid Hormones

When excess iodide is given chronically, iodide transport decreases, and the effect of a large dose of iodide changes to that of a moderate dose. Therefore, the absolute rates of organification and of T_4 and T_3 synthesis increase. For example, adapted thyroid glands contain 2.5 times as much iodide in the organic form and 2.5 times as much T_4 and T_3 as do "unadapted" thyroid glands, but the thyroidal content and the release of T_4 and T_3 are similar in "adapted" and control rats.[1] The explanation for this balance between uptake and release may be that the thyroid in adapted rats uses mainly serum iodide to produce hormone, and reuse of intrathyroidally generated iodide is decreased, whereas control rats use both iodide from the serum and intrathyroidally generated iodide.[1]

IODIDE AUTOREGULATION IN HUMANS

Acute Inhibitory Effect and Escape from the Acute Effect

When the iodide dose reaches a certain level (more than 1 mg/d) in humans, thyroidal uptake of tracer doses of radioiodine decreases, and the administration of perchlorate or thio-

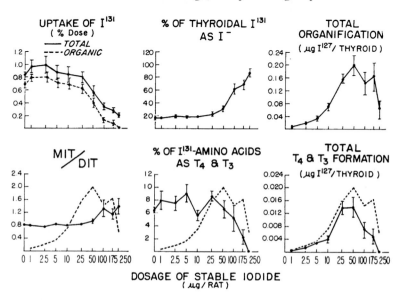

FIGURE 13-1. Effects of graded doses of iodide administered 30 minutes before killing on the thyroidal metabolism of iodine in rats. The results shown are the mean ± SE (in brackets) of values obtained in five rats. For reference purposes, the curve of total organic iodination is shown as a dashed line in the lower three panels. (Adapted from Nagataki S, Ingbar SH. Relation between qualitative and quantitative alterations in thyroid hormone synthesis induced by varying doses of iodide. Endocrinology 1964;74:731)

cyanate results in discharge of radioiodine from the thyroid, indicating a proportionate decrease in organification of thyroidal iodide. There is no evidence, however, that overall organification is actually decreased by excess iodide; that is, there is no evidence for an acute Wolff-Chaikoff effect in humans. The discharge of iodine means only that it has accumulated in excess of the thyroid's ability to organify it. If a large dose is given, the thyroid radioiodine uptake is so low that the absolute iodine uptake cannot be calculated. Hence, it is not possible to demonstrate either a Wolff-Chaikoff effect or escape from it.

In contrast, in patients with hyperthyroidism caused by Graves' disease, acute administration of iodide decreases serum T_4 and T_3 concentrations and ameliorates thyrotoxicosis. The acute effect is, however, due to inhibition of hormone release, and as discussed later there is little evidence that the Wolff-Chaikoff effect occurs in these patients.

Effects of Moderate Doses of Iodide

The response of human thyroid tissue to excess iodide is similar to that in rats. Acute administration of small or moderate amounts of iodide does not change the percentage thyroid uptake of concomitantly administered radioiodine, leading to a linear increase in absolute iodine uptake. With progressively larger doses of iodide, thyroid radioiodine uptake decreases, but the absolute iodine uptake calculated from thyroid radioiodine and serum or urinary iodide values increases.[1]

During chronic iodide administration, thyroid radioiodine uptake decreases, but the absolute iodine uptake increases as the intake of iodide increases; serum T_4 and T_3 concentrations are not affected.[12] In patients with Graves' hyperthyroidism, the absolute iodine uptake increases several-fold during iodide treatment. In one study, thyroid radioiodine uptake 24 hours after injection averaged 20% of the dose, despite daily administration of 10 mg of iodide, and the proportion of inorganic radioiodine was only about 14% of total thyroidal content of radioiodine.[13] Thus, thyroidal organic iodine formation in Graves' hyperthyroidism is increased by iodide treatment despite a significant decrease in T_4 and T_3 secretion. Furthermore, thyroidal organic iodine formation did not change after escape from inhibition of hormone release when serum T_4 and T_3 concentrations had increased to their pretreatment concentrations. The dissociation between thyroidal organic iodine formation and T_4 and T_3 release in these patients is another unexplained feature of autoregulation.

Pituitary-Thyroid Responses to Excess Iodide in Normal Subjects

Autoregulation was originally defined as the regulation of thyroidal iodine metabolism independent of TSH, and when the concept was established serum TSH was measured by bioassay. However, the development of sensitive assays for serum TSH and free T_4 and T_3 concentrations has made it possible to determine the changes in serum concentrations of these hormones within the normal range.[14]

Serum TSH responses to thyrotropin-releasing hormone (TRH) are increased in normal subjects given moderate to large doses of iodide, indicative of a small antithyroid ef-

fect.[14,15] Serum TSH and thyroglobulin (T_g) concentrations increase slightly, mostly within the normal range, and thyroid gland size increases in normal subjects given iodide for several weeks (Fig 13-2).[16] In addition, the administration of as little as 0.75 to 1.5 mg iodide daily to normal subjects leads to unsustained increases in serum TSH concentrations and serum TSH responses to TRH.[17,18]

These results indicate that moderate doses of iodide have antithyroid actions, even if the action is sufficient to decrease serum free T_4 concentrations by only about 25%. Thus, many phenomena of autoregulation may, in fact, be dependent on TSH, and the definition of autoregulation may have to be reconsidered, because serum TSH concentrations are significantly increased by excess iodide at least in normal human subjects.

INTRACELLULAR EFFECTS OF EXCESS IODIDE

There are other regulators of thyroid secretion in addition to TSH. They include growth factors, neurotransmitters, and cytokines, which may affect thyroid membrane signal transduction; and T_4 and T_3, corticosteroids, estrogen, vitamin D_3, and retinoic acid, which may activate nuclear receptors in thyroid tissue. These regulators exert their functions not only in endocrine but also in paracrine and autocrine ways. It is likely that iodide regulates thyroid function at least in part through these regulators. The effects of excess iodide are discussed in the section on the effects of excess iodide in Chapter 14, but some recent findings that may relate to autoregulation are discussed here.

Signal Transduction

Iodide inhibits the increase in adenylyl cyclase activity in response to TSH.[19–25] This inhibition is not accompanied by decreased binding of TSH to thyroid cell membranes.[26] In FRTL-5 cells, iodide causes dose-dependent inhibition of TSH-stimulated thymidine incorporation into DNA, and also the increase of thymidine incorporation into DNA stimulated by dibutyryl cAMP, forskolin, thyroid-stimulating antibodies, insulin, insulin-like growth factor-I, and tetradecanoyl phorbol acetate. These results indicate that iodide inhibits the growth of thyroid cells at multiple loci related to both cAMP-dependent and cAMP-independent pathways. These inhibitory effects are abolished by methimazole and ethionamide.[27–29]

In contrast to FRTL-5 cells, a high dose of iodide markedly increases c-*myc* mRNA concentrations, labeled thymidine incorporation, and mitotic activity in primary suspension cultures of porcine thyroid cells that, unlike FRTL-5 cells, are capable of organifying iodide.[30] Moreover, the stimulatory effect of iodide is reduced in the presence of forskolin, suggesting that an organic form of iodide stimulates thyroid cell growth and that the stimulatory pathway is independent of exogenous polypeptide growth factors.[30] The different responses to iodide in FRTL-5 cells and porcine cells are probably due to differences in the characteristics of the two types of cells, since TSH is not a growth factor for human or porcine thyroid cells in vitro.[31]

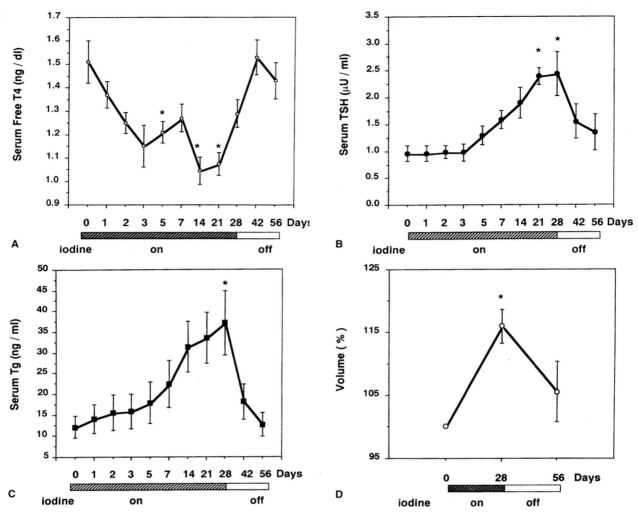

FIGURE 13-2. Serum free T$_4$ (*A*), TSH (*B*), and Tg (*C*) concentrations and thyroid volume (*D*) serum measured by ultrasonography before, during, and after administration of 27 mg of iodine daily in 10 normal subjects. To convert free T$_4$ values to nmol/L, multiply by 12.9. Asterisks indicate where *P* <0.05 vs. value before iodide administration. (Adapted from Namba H, Yamashita S, Kimura H, et al. Evidence of thyroid volume increase in normal subjects receiving excess iodide. J Clin Endocrinol Metab 1993;76:605)

Protein Synthesis

Iodide-induced suppression of iodide transport in cat thyroid slices is inhibited by the addition of cycloheximide or puromycin. Two-dimensional column chromatography of iodoproteins of control and cycloheximide-treated tissue suggests that the iodide-induced effects are associated with reduced iodination of an 8- to 10-kd soluble component of the thyroid gland.[32] Iodide decreases amino acid transport in dog thyroid cells in primary culture. The effect is abolished by methimazole, and iodide does not inhibit amino acid transport in cells lacking a mechanism for iodide organification.[33]

Organic Iodinated Compounds

Iodinated lipids, including iodinated derivatives of arachidonic acid or purified iodolactone, inhibit radioactive uptake, basal and TSH-induced organification of radioiodine, and uri-

dine incorporation into total RNA in calf thyroid slices.[34,35] These iodinated lipids decrease the action of iodine on thyroid growth and cAMP production in rat thyroid tissue in vitro. They also inhibit growth of FRTL-5 cells, an effect that is not abolished by methimazole.[36] In isolated porcine thyroid follicles, iodolactone inhibits, dose-dependently, epidermal growth factor–induced thyroid cell growth, which also is not abolished by methimazole. Basal as well as TSH-induced cAMP formation, however, are not changed by iodolactone.[37] Iodotyrosines (MIT or DIT) inhibit iodide transport and cAMP generation in the presence of TSH in porcine thyroid cell cultures, suggesting that iodotyrosines can serve as a negative control factor for thyroid hormone formation.[38]

Growth Factors

Insulin-like growth factor-I (IGF-I) and transforming growth factor-β (TGF-β) are both produced by thyroid follicular cells, and the inhibitory action of TGF-β on follicular cell growth may involve a decrease in the thyroidal production of IGF-I. Furthermore, the attenuating action of iodide on cell growth may in part reflect increased production of TGF-β.[39,40] Iodide induces TGF-β1 mRNA in sheep thyroid cells,[41] and TGF-β inhibits TSH-induced DNA synthesis and iodide uptake and DNA synthesis induced by IGF-I in FRTL-5 rat thyroid cells.[42]

In human thyroid cells, iodide increases thyroidal TGF-β1 mRNA expression, and TGF-β1 almost completely abolishes cAMP-induced stimulation of iodide uptake and thyroid peroxidase synthesis.[43,44] These results emphasize the potentially major role of TGF-β1 as a local modulator of thyroid functions.

Thyroid Expression of HLA Molecules and Other Proteins

Iodide markedly decreased HLA class I molecule RNA concentrations in both TSH-treated and untreated FRTL-5 cells. The effect of iodide on class I gene expression reflects iodide autoregulation and does not require TSH-induced iodide transport. Understanding the basis for iodide regulation of class I gene expression and the relationship of the action of iodide to the inhibitory effect of methimazole on class I gene transcription may contribute to understanding of the mechanism of iodide autoregulation as well as methimazole action.[45] The increase in Tg mRNA induced by methimazole is inhibited by iodide in FRTL-5 rat thyroid cells.[46] Incubation with iodide decreases the cellular content of thyroid peroxidase (TPO) and TPO gene expression in primary cultures of human thyroid cells[47] and TPO activity in porcine thyroid cells in primary culture.[48]

MECHANISM OF AUTOREGULATION

Acute Inhibitory Effect

Despite the numerous reports on the effects of excess iodide on thyroid tissue, little is known about the mechanism of autoregulation. Various effects of excess iodide are abolished by thiocyanate or by methimazole.[9,30] For example, methimazole inhibits the effects of excess iodide on expression of the mRNAs for c-*myc*[30] and TGF-β1.[33,40] It also inhibits the effects of iodide on amino acid transport,[33] cell toxicity (necrosis),[49] and inhibition of H_2O_2 production,[50] but not the expression of HLA class I molecules by excess iodide.[45] Hence, production of one or more organic iodine compounds has been proposed to be important in autoregulation.[3,27–30,33–35,51–55]

In the acute inhibitory effect of excess iodide, inhibition of organification of intrathyroidal iodide is the fundamental phenomenon. TPO-catalyzed iodination requires the peroxidase, an acceptor (protein or free tyrosine), iodide, and H_2O_2. It was originally proposed that the acute inhibitory effect of excess iodide was due to formation of I_2 in preference to iodination of protein.[56]

In dog thyroid slices, H_2O_2 generation is stimulated by TSH and by carbamylcholine. The action of carbamylcholine is mimicked by ionomycin and by phorbol myristate ester, suggesting that the action is mediated by signals generated by the Ca^{2+}-phosphatidyl-inositol cascade. Preincubation of dog thyroid slices with excess iodide greatly inhibits iodide organification and H_2O_2 generation stimulated by TSH and by carbamylcholine. While inhibition of H_2O_2 generation may be the cause of the acute inhibitory effect, the nature of the organic iodine compound that inhibits H_2O_2 generation is unknown.[53] Monoamine oxidase (MAO) in the thyroid has been postulated to play a role in the biosynthesis of thyroid hormone because of its ability to generate hydrogen peroxide, but a MAO inhibitor was found to inhibit thyroid iodide transport in rats.[57]

Iodide-induced cell toxicity requires the oxidation of iodide catalyzed by TPO in the presence of H_2O_2. The necrotizing effect could result from the synthesis of an organic iodo compound. In this hypothesis, toxicity could be due to the overproduction of the molecule involved in the mechanism of iodine-induced autoregulation.[49]

Iodinated phospholipids and iodinated derivatives of arachidonic acid or iodolactone inhibit organification of iodide in both calf thyroid slices and homogenates, whereas arachidonic acid has no such effect.[34,35] It is possible that iodinated arachidonic acid plays an important role in the acute inhibitory effect of excess iodide.

Mechanism of Adaptation

ACUTE INHIBITION

Decreased iodide transport is an important mechanism in the adaptation to or escape from the acute inhibitory effect of iodide. Iodinated arachidonic acid or iodolactone is one of the iodinated compounds that is proposed to reduce iodide transport.[34,35] Iodinated arachidonic acid may decrease iodide transport, but it is hard to see how the same substance could inhibit organification of iodide on the one hand and mediate the adaptation by which organification of iodide increases in response to chronic iodide administration on the other hand. However, the changes in iodide transport in response to excess iodide could be due mainly to changes in sodium transport and not to the production of an organic iodine compound.[58,59]

CHRONIC EXCESS IODIDE

The amounts of iodide taken up by the thyroid and incorporated into iodoamino acids and iodothyronines differ greatly according to dietary iodide intake, but the amount of T_4 and T_3 released from the thyroid is remarkably constant in both humans and animals. Inhibition of hormone release by iodide is a well-known phenomenon in Graves' disease and other forms of hyperthyroidism, and the inhibitory effect of excess iodide on thyroid hormone secretion has been demonstrated in sheep thyroid cell cultures.[1] Preferential inhibition of hormone secretion, however, cannot explain the balance between hormone formation and hormone release unless thyroid tissue has an almost infinite capacity to store thyroid hormones.

The acute Wolff-Chaikoff effect, escape from this effect, and increased thyroidal iodide uptake in hypophysectomized rats fed a low-iodine diet are the typical autoregulations in animals. In contrast, constant hormone release regardless of the amount of iodide taken up by the thyroid and inhibition of hormone release from the thyroid by iodide are the important autoregulatory effects in humans. It is still not clear, however, whether these types of autoregulation share the same mechanism or are due to different mechanisms.

Most recent studies of autoregulation have been performed in vitro using thyroid slices, primary cell cultures, and cell lines from different species. Although they clearly showed the effects of iodine on certain functions, the results are not compatible with the mechanism of autoregulation defined from in vivo studies.[55,60,61]

Species Differences

Differences among species in thyroid sensitivity to the inhibitory effect of iodide and escape from the acute inhibitory effect of iodide have been demonstrated in many studies. The rarity in humans of hypothyroidism and goiter despite exposure of many patients to excess iodide suggests that the human thyroid can easily escape from the inhibitory effect of iodide. This also explains the difficulty in producing iodide goiter in rats. In contrast to humans and rats, long-term iodide feeding leads to colloid goiter in mice despite functional adaptation to iodide excess. Iodide feeding to hens leads to colloid goiter in their chicks, and guinea pigs treated with excess iodide show signs of histologic activation of the thyroid.[1] These variations in iodide effects in different species make it difficult to propose a uniform mechanism for autoregulation.

References

1. Nagataki S. Effect of excess quantities of iodide. Handbook Physiol 1974;3:329
2. Pisarev MA. Thyroid autoregulation. J Endocrinol Invest 1985;8:475
3. Halmi NS. Thyroidal iodide transport. Vitam Horm 1961;19:133
4. Halmi NS, Spirtos BN. Analysis of the modifying effect of dietary iodine levels on the thyroidal response of hypophysectomized rats to thyrotropin. Endocrinology 1955;56:157
5. Morton ME, Chaikoff IL, Rosenfeld S. Inhibiting effect of inorganic iodide on the formation in vitro of thyroxine and diiodotyrosine by surviving thyroid tissue. J Biol Chem 1944;154:381
6. Wolff J, Chaikoff IL. Plasma inorganic iodide as a homeostatic regulator of thyroid function. J Biol Chem 1948;174:555
7. Wolff J, Chaikoff IL, Goldberg RC, Meier JR. The temporary nature of the inhibitory action of excess iodide on organic iodine synthesis in the normal thyroid. Endocrinology 1949;45:504
8. Braverman LE, Ingbar SH. Changes in thyroidal function during adaptation to large doses of iodide. J Clin Invest 1963;42:1216
9. Raben MS. The paradoxical effects of thiocyanate and of thyrotropin on the organic binding of iodine by the thyroid in the presence of large amounts of iodide. Endocrinology 1949;45:296
10. Galton VA, Pitt-Rivers R. The effect of excessive iodine on the thyroid of the rat. Endocrinology 1959;64:835
11. Nagataki S, Ingbar SH. Relation between qualitative and quantitative alterations in thyroid hormone synthesis induced by varying doses of iodide. Endocrinology 1964;74:731
12. Nagataki S, Shizume K, Nakao K. Thyroid function in chronic excess iodide ingestion: comparison of thyroidal absolute iodine uptake and degradation of thyroxine in euthyroid Japanese subjects. J Clin Endocrinol Metab 1967;27:638
13. Nagataki S, Shizume K, Nakao K. Effect of iodide on thyroidal iodine turnover in hyperthyroid subjects. J Clin Endocrinol Metab 1970;30:469
14. Nagataki S. Autoregulation of thyroid function by iodide. In: Delange F, Dunn JT, Glinoer D, eds. Iodine deficiency in Europe: A continuing concern. New York: Plenum Press, 1993:43
15. Ikeda H, Nagataki S. Augmentation of thyrotropin responses to thyrotropin-releasing hormone following inorganic iodide. Endocrinol Japon 1976;23:431
16. Namba H, Yamashita S, Kimura H, et al. Evidence of thyroid volume increase in normal subjects receiving excess iodide. J Clin Endocrinol Metab 1993;76:605
17. Gardner DF, Centor RM, Utiger RD. Effects of low dose oral iodide supplementation on thyroid function in normal men. Clin Endocrinol 1988;28:283
18. Chow CC, Phillips DIW, Lazarus JH, Parkes AB. Effect of low dose iodide supplementation on thyroid function in potentially susceptible subjects: are dietary iodide levels in Britain acceptable? Clin Endocrinol 1991;34:413
19. Cochaux P, Van Sande J, Swillens S, Dumont JE. Iodide-induced inhibition of adenylate cyclase activity in horse and dog thyroid. Eur J Biochem 1987;170:435
20. Rapoport B, West MN, Ingbar SH. Inhibitory effect of dietary iodine on the thyroid adenylate cyclase response to thyrotropin in the hypophysectomized rat. J Clin Invest 1975;56:516
21. Uchimura H, Chiu SC, Kuzuya N, Ikeda H, Ito K, Nagataki S. Effect of iodine enrichment in vitro on the adenylate cyclase-adenosine 3′,5′monophosphate system in thyroid glands from normal subjects and patients with Graves' disease. J Clin Endocrinol Metab 1980;50:1066
22. Van Sande J, Dumont JE. Effects of thyrotropin, prostaglandin E1 and iodide on cyclic 3′,5′-AMP concentration in dog thyroid slices. Biochim Biophys Acta 1973;313:320
23. Van Sande J, Grenier G, Willems C, Dumont JE. Inhibition by iodide of the activation of the thyroid cyclic 3′,5′-AMP system. Endocrinology 1975;96:781
24. Van Sande J, Lefort A, Beebe S, et al. Pairs of cyclic AMP analogs, that are specifically synergistic for type I and type II cAMP-dependent protein kinase, mimic thyrotropin effects on the function, differentiation expression and mitogenesis of dog thyroid cells. Eur J Biochem 1989;183:699
25. Yamada T, Takasu N. Effects of excess iodide on thyroid hormone synthesis and release. In: Hall R, Kobberling J, eds. Thyroid disorders associated with iodine deficiencies and excess. New York: Raven Press, 1985:319
26. Uchimura H, Amir SM, Ingbar SH. Failure of organic iodine enrichment to influence the binding of bovine thyrotropin to rat thyroid tissue. Endocrinology 1979;104:1207
27. Becks GP, Eggo MC, Burrow GN. Organic iodine inhibits deoxyribonucleic acid synthesis and growth in FRTL-5 thyroid cells. Endocrinology 1988;123:545
28. Saji M, Isozaki O, Tsushima T, et al. The inhibitory effect of iodide on growth of rat thyroid (FRTL-5) cells. Acta Endocrinol (Copenh) 1988;119:145
29. Tramontano D, Veneziani BM, Lombardi A, Villone G, Ingbar SH. Iodine inhibits the proliferation of rat thyroid cells in culture. Endocrinology 1989;125:984
30. Heldin NE, Karlsson FA, Westermark B. A growth stimulatory effect of iodide is suggested by its effect on c-*myc* messenger ribonucleic acid levels, [3H] thymidine incorporation, and mitotic activity of porcine follicular cells in suspension culture. Endocrinology 1987;121:757
31. Westermark K, Karlsson FA, Westermark B. Epidermal growth factor modulates thyroid growth and function in culture. Endocrinology 1983;112:1680
32. Sherwin JR, Prince DJ. Autoregulation of thyroid iodide transport: evidence for the mediation of protein synthesis in iodide-induced suppression of iodide transport. Endocrinology 1986;119:2553
33. Filetti S, Rapoport B. Autoregulation by iodine of thyroid protein synthesis: influence of iodine on amino acid transport in cultured thyroid cells. Endocrinology 1984;114:1379

34. Chazenbalk GD, Pisarev MA, Krawiec L, Juvenal GJ, Burton G, Valsecchi RM. In vitro inhibitory effects of an iodinated derivative of arachidonic acid on calf thyroid. Acta Physiol Pharmacol Latinoam 1984;34:367

35. Chazenbalk GD, Valsecchi RM, Krawiec L, et al. Thyroid autoregulation: inhibitory effects of iodinated derivatives of arachidonic acid on iodine metabolism. Prostaglandins 1988;36:163

36. Pisarev MA, Bocanera LV, Chester HA, et al. Effect of iodoarachidonates on thyroid FRTL-5 cells growth. Horm Metab Res 1992;24:558

37. Dugrillion A, Bechtner G, Uedelhoven WM, Weber PC, Gartner R. Evidence that an iodolactone mediates the inhibitory effect of iodide on thyroid cell proliferation but not an adenosine 3′,5′-monophosphate formation. Endocrinology 1990;127:337

38. Nasu M, Sugawara M. Exogenous free iodotyrosine inhibits iodide transport through the sequential intracellular events. Eur J Endocrinol 1994;130:601

39. Beere HM, Soden J, Tomlinson S, Bidey SP. Insulin-like growth factor-I production and action in porcine thyroid follicular cells in monolayer: regulation by transforming growth factor-β. J Endocrinol 1991;130:3

40. Cowin AJ, Davis JRE, Bidey SP. Transforming growth factor-β 1 production in porcine thyroid follicular cells: regulation by intrathyroidal organic iodine. J Mol Endocrinol 1992;9:197

41. Yuasa R, Eggo MC, Meinkoth J, Dillmann WH, Burrow GN. Iodide induces transforming growth factor beta$_1$ (TGF-β 1) mRNA in sheep thyroid cells. Thyroid 1992;2:141

42. Pang X-P, Park M, Hershman JM. Transforming growth factor-β blocks protein kinase-A-mediated iodide transport and protein kinase-C-mediated DNA synthesis in FRTL-5 rat thyroid cells. Endocrinology 1992;131:45

43. Cowin AJ, Bidey SP. Transforming growth factor-β 1 synthesis in human thyroid follicular cells: differential effects of iodide and plasminogen on the production of latent and active peptide forms. J Endocrinol 1994;141:183

44. Taton M, Lamy F, Roger PP, Dumont JE. General inhibition by transforming growth factor β 1 of thyrotropin and cAMP responses in human thyroid cells in primary culture. Mol Cel Endocrinol 1993;95:13

45. Saji M, Moriarty J, Ban T, Singer DS, Kohn LD. Major histocompatibility complex class I gene expression in rat thyroid cells is regulated by hormones, methimazole, and iodide as well as interferon. J Clin Endocrinol Metab 1992;75:871

46. Isozaki O, Tsushima T, Emoto N, et al. Methimazole regulation of thyroglobulin biosynthesis and gene transcription in rat FRTL-5 thyroid cells. Endocrinology 1991;128:3113

47. Yokoyama N, Tominaga T, Eishima K, Izumi M. Effect of iodide on human thyroid peroxidase in thyroid cells. In: Gordon A, Gross J, Hennemann G, eds. Progress in thyroid research. Rotterdam: Balkema, 1991:483

48. Kasai K, Yamaguchi F, Hosoya T, et al. Effects of inorganic iodide, epidermal growth factor and phorbol ester on hormone synthesis by porcine thyroid follicles cultured in suspension. Life Sci 1992;51:1095

49. Many MC, Mestdagh C, Van Den Hove MF, Denef JF. *In vitro* study of acute toxic effects of high iodide doses in human thyroid follicles. Endocrinology 1992;131:621

50. Corvilain B, Van Sande J, Laurent E, Dumont JE. The H_2O_2-generating system modulates protein iodination and the activity of the pentose phosphate pathway in dog thyroid. Endocrinology 1991;128:779

51. Becks GP, Eggo MC, Burrow GN. Regulation of differentiated thyroid function by iodide: preferential inhibitory effect of excess iodide on thyroid hormone secretion in sheep thyroid cell cultures. Endocrinology 1987;120:2569

52. Burke G. Effects of iodide on thyroid stimulation. J Clin Endocrinol 1970;30:76

53. Corvilain B, Van Sande J, Dumont JE. Inhibition by iodide of iodide binding to proteins: The "Wolff-Chaikoff" effect is caused by inhibition of H_2O_2 generation. Biochem Biophys Res Commun 1988;154:1287

54. Grollman E, Smolar A, Ommaya A, Tombaccini D, Santisteban P. Iodine suppression of iodine uptake in FRTL-5 thyroid cells. Endocrinology 1986;118:2477

55. Price DJ, Sherwin JR. Autoregulation of iodide transport in the rabbit: Absence of autoregulation in fetal tissue and comparison of maternal and fetal thyroid iodination products. Endocrinology 1986;119:2547

56. Taurog A. Thyroid peroxidase and thyroxine biosynthesis. Recent Prog Horm Res 1970;26:189

57. Cabanillas AM. Masini-Repiso AM, Costamagna ME, Pellizas C, Coleoni AH. Thyroid iodide transport is reduced by administration of monoamine oxdase A inhibitors to rats. J Endocrinol 1994;143:303

58. Saito K, Yamamoto K, Nagayama I, Uemura J, Kuzuya T. Effect of internally loaded iodide, thiocyanate, and perchlorate on sodium-dependent iodide uptake by phospholipid vesicles reconstituted with thyroid plasma membranes: iodide counterflow mediated by the iodide transport carrier. J Biochem 1989;105:790

59. Saito K, Yamamoto K, Nagayama I, Uemura J, Kuzuya T. Preservation of sodium-dependent iodide transport activity by methimazole and mercaptoethanol in phospholipid vesicles containing thyroid plasma membranes: with evidence of difference in the action of perchlorate and thiocyanate. Endocrinol Japon 1989;36:325

60. Penel C, Rognoni JB, Bastiani P. Thyroid autoregulation: impact on thyroid structure and function in rats. Am J Physiol 1987;253:E165

61. Takasu N, Honda Y, Kawaoi A, Shimizu Y, Yamada T. Effects of iodide on thyroid follicle structure and electrophysiological potentials of culture thyroid cells. Endocrinology 1985;117:71

AUTONOMIC NERVOUS CONTROL: ADRENERGIC, CHOLINERGIC, AND PEPTIDERGIC REGULATION

Torsten Grunditz
Frank Sundler

It is well established that thyroid-stimulating hormone (TSH or thyrotropin) from the anterior pituitary and iodide play the key roles in the physiologic regulation of the thyroid gland.[1] Thyroid function may also be influenced by various neurotransmitters, including catecholamines, acetylcholine, and peptides.[2–4] The effects and interrelations of these neurotransmitters or transmitter candidates are complex not only because of their multitude and possible interactions both reciprocally and with TSH but also because some of these transmitters may be co-produced and co-released from the same neuron. This chapter briefly reviews the evidence supporting an adrenergic, cholinergic, and peptidergic neuronal regulation of thyroid function. In addition, some aspects are given concerning interactions between these neurotransmitters.

ADRENERGIC REGULATION

Shortly after hyperthyroidism was first described, the proposal was made that it might be caused by overactivity of the cervical sympathetic nerves.[5,6] The discovery of epinephrine was followed by the observation that this catecholamine can produce several of the phenomena that characterize hyperthyroidism. Pathologic changes in cervical sympathetic structures were observed in hyperthyroid patients, and efforts were made to cure the disease by division or removal of cervical sympathetic nerves. Although this therapeutic approach was abandoned long ago, current therapy for hyperthyroidism includes antiadrenergic drugs. Such use is based, however, on the assumption that antiadrenergic drugs interfere with the excess adrenergic effects of thyrotoxicosis and not with the secretion or production of thyroid hormone.[5,6]

Several studies have suggested that thyroid function can be enhanced under conditions associated with increased sympathetic nervous activity.[5-7] Similarly, studies on the effects of exogenous catecholamines on thyroid function have yielded contradictory results. Both stimulatory and inhibitory effects have been recorded, and it has also been argued that the influence of catecholamines on the thyroid is restricted to effects on thyroid blood flow.[5,6,8-10] Several possible explanations for such diverse results concern the impact of the sympathetic-adrenergic system on thyroid function. One explanation is that the number and distribution of sympathetic nerve fibers, particularly those reaching the follicles, display a great interspecies variation. Whereas interfollicular sympathetic nerve endings are numerous in several mammals such as mice, hamsters, sheep, and humans, they are sparse in the thyroids of other species such as rats, dogs, and pigs.[11] Moreover, as studied in rats, the number of interfollicular sympathetic nerve fibers declines with increasing age.

Complex interactions occur between catecholamines, TSH, and thyroid hormone.[1,5,6,12] Catecholamines can induce secretion of thyroid hormone, but this effect is not necessarily disclosed by measurements of the plasma levels of thyroid hormone because catecholamines can also enhance its clearance. In addition, catecholamines may affect the secretion of TSH, and catecholamine-induced changes in thyroid blood flow may alter the distribution of TSH to the thyroid and the outflow of thyroid hormone from the gland. More importantly, exogenous catecholamines and TSH can exert either additive or mutually antagonistic effects on thyroid hormone secretion, depending on the timing of their administration relative to one another and on the prevailing state of thyroid activity.[5,6]

Fluorescence histochemistry of thyroid tissue specimens treated with formaldehyde vapor reveals the presence of catecholamines. By this technique, it has been established that numerous adrenergic nerve terminals exist in thyroid tissue of several mammals, including normal humans. More recently the catecholamine-forming enzymes tyrosine hydroxylase and dopamine-β-hydroxylase have been used as immunocytochemical markers for adrenergic nerves.[4,13,14] Adrenergic nerves are present not only in a network around vessels but also between and around follicles. Since they disappear after surgical or chemical sympathectomy, they are most likely sympathetic, postganglionic, norepinephrine-containing nerve terminals. It has been documented that the interfollicular sympathetic nerve terminals have a close relation to the follicular cells as well as to capillaries and arterioles.[4,5,6,13] There is thus a morphologic basis for a direct nonvascular influence of sympathetic stimuli on the follicular cells. In addition, sympathetic stimuli may influence thyroid function indirectly through effects on the microcirculation of the gland.[8,9]

Accumulating evidence indicates that sympathetic stimuli indeed influence thyroid activity by effects within the thyroid as studied in mice and humans.[5,6,12] In mice, in which TSH secretion is eliminated, electrical sympathetic stimulation or drug-induced release of norepinephrine or other catecholamines induces secretion of thyroid hormone, as reflected by both electron and light microscopic signs of endocytosis of thyroglobulin, migration of lysosomes toward the engulfed thyroglobulin, and the release of thyroid radioiodine into the plasma.[5,6] Most importantly, the secretory response to unilateral sympathetic nerve stimulation is restricted to those portions of the thyroid that are innervated by the stimulated nerve. The effect is probably evoked by a direct action of norepinephrine released from nerve endings within the gland. The sympathetic-adrenergic activation of thyroid hormone secretion most likely results from a direct action on follicular cells rather than from an influence on thyroid microcirculation.[5,6] In humans, studies of normal thyroid tissue suggest that norepinephrine can induce the secretion of thyroid hormone in vitro, as reflected by colloid droplet formation and migration of lysosomes.[12] In addition, epinephrine, norepinephrine, and isoproterenol stimulate cAMP accumulation in isolated human thyroid cells.[12] Finally, there is unequivocal evidence that catecholamines can directly stimulate thyroid follicular cells, enhance the incorporation of iodine, and enhance the synthesis of thyroid hormone in isolated calf thyroid cells.[15]

Both TSH and catecholamines stimulate adenylate cyclase in follicular cells, and the effect of each in stimulating hormone secretion is mimicked by the dibutyryl derivative of cAMP.[1,5,6,12] Moreover, both in vivo and in vitro studies indicate that the thyroid-stimulating effect of catecholamines is abolished by drugs that block adrenergic receptors. The effect of TSH, on the other hand, is not blocked by these agents, but it is inhibited by polyphloretin phosphate, a drug that does not diminish the effect of catecholamines.[6] The in vivo effect of dibutyryl-cAMP is blocked neither by adrenergic receptor blockers nor by polyphloretin phosphate.[6] From these findings, it seems logical to conclude that TSH and catecholamines interact with different receptors on the follicular cell membrane, but both then activate adenylate cyclase and increase the formation of cAMP, which in turn mediates their common action on the release of thyroid hormone.

In vitro studies of thyroid tissue from humans and dogs indicate that catecholamines stimulate thyroid activity by an action on β-adrenoceptors, whereas α_1-adrenergic activation exerts an inhibitory influence.[5,6,12] In addition, TSH-induced thyroid hormone secretion may be inhibited by an α_1-adrenergic mechanism. Also an α_2-adrenergic inhibitory mechanism has been described.[16] In vivo studies in mice have shown that β-adrenergic activation evokes secretion of thyroid hormone, and evidence classifies this effect as a β_2-adrenergic mechanism.[5,6] This pattern of β_2-adrenergic stimulation and α_1-adrenergic inhibition fits well with classic concepts; however, not only β- but also α-adrenergic activation can evoke secretion of thyroid hormone in vivo.[5,6] Moreover, catecholamine stimulation of thyroid hormone biosynthesis in isolated calf thyroid cells seems to be mediated by α-adrenergic receptors.[15]

Although there is evidence in favor of a sympathetic influence on thyroid activity in mice and in humans, this need not imply that this mechanism has major physiologic or clinical importance. To what extent is the secretion of thyroid hormone altered in the euthyroid animal exposed to withdrawal or an increase of sympathetic nervous activity? In mice with intact TSH secretion, sympathectomy evokes a moderate, brief reduction in thyroid hormone secretion.[5,6]

In humans treated with the sympathomimetic drug amphetamine for mental diseases, the plasma levels of both triiodothyronine (T_3) and tetraiodothyronine (T_4) increase in parallel with the increase in amphetamine levels.[5,6] Because the plasma TSH levels do not increase and because catecholamines increase rather than reduce the clearance of thyroid hormone, it seems likely that amphetamine stimulates the secretion of thyroid hormone, probably through release of norepinephrine from intrathyroid nerve endings.

In conclusion, in humans, as well as in certain other mammalian species, there is morphologic and functional evidence for a direct influence of sympathetic stimuli on thyroid activity. The tonic sympathetic influence may be of minor importance, but the existence of a direct pathway between the sympathetic nervous system and the thyroid constitutes a means for rapid adaptation of thyroid hormone secretion to certain stimuli.

CHOLINERGIC REGULATION

The existence of a sympathetic-adrenergic regulation of thyroid activity suggests that there might also be a parasympathetic-cholinergic influence having the opposite effect, and there are reports favoring this concept. Histochemical studies have revealed numerous intrathyroidal acetylcholinesterase (AChE) positive, presumably cholinergic, nerve fibers not only around blood vessels but also around follicles (Fig. 13-3).[17–19] This type of neuronal distribution is similar to that of adrenergic nerves, and the frequency of cholinergic nerves appears to be at least as great as that of adrenergic nerves in the species examined.

The close spatial relationship between cholinergic nerves and follicle cells implies that cholinergic stimuli may have a direct effect on hormone secretion from these cells. There is also experimental evidence of such an influence.[18–23] The acetylcholine (ACh) analogue carbamylcholine (CCh) reduces thyroid hormone secretion from the dog thyroid in vitro and the mouse thyroid in vivo.[18,19,23] This effect is counteracted by atropine. Moreover, atropine enhances the secretory response to TSH.[18] In addition, both CCh and ACh themselves increase the accumulation of cyclic GMP in human and canine thyroid tissue.[19,20] This effect is blocked by atropine, a muscarinic receptor antagonist, but not by d-tubocurarine, a nicotinic receptor antagonist.[18] Thus, morphologic and biochemical evidence indicates that the parasympathetic nervous system has an inhibitory effect on thyroid activity in humans and other mammals, in opposition to the stimulatory influence of the sympathetic nervous system. The cholinergic effect seems to be mediated by muscarinic receptors in the follicular cells.

PEPTIDERGIC REGULATION

Several regulatory peptides may function as both neuronal and humoral messengers.[14,24–27] All divisions of the peripheral nervous system contain neuropeptides. Sympathetic-adrenergic nerves, particularly those supplying blood vessels, contain neuropeptide Y (NPY).[14,27] Parasympathetic postganglionic cholinergic nerves contain vasoactive intestinal peptide (VIP) and NPY.[4,13,24,26] In addition, primary sensory neurons, notably the unmyelinated nociceptive C fiber type neurons, contain substance P (SP) and calcitonin gene-related peptide (CGRP).[4,13] These peptides have been demonstrated in neuronal elements within the thyroid gland (Figs. 13-4 and 13-5).[4,13]

VIP-containing nerve fibers are found both around blood vessels and close to the follicular cells in the thyroid of numerous species, including humans.[4,13,28,29] In the murine thyroid,

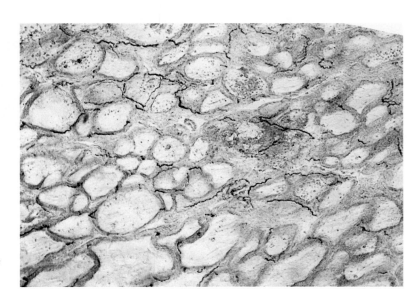

FIGURE 13-3. Dog thyroid. Numerous acetylcholinesterase positive, presumably cholinergic, nerve fibers among the follicles. (×175).

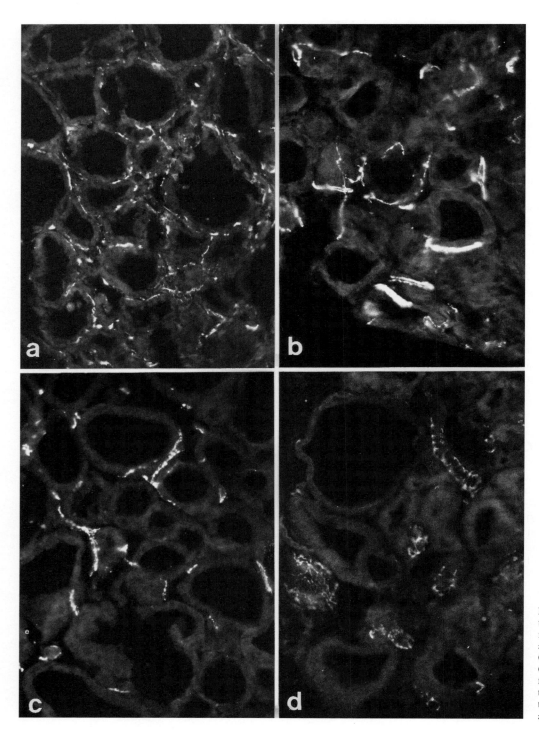

FIGURE 13-4. Rat thyroid. Vasoactive intestinal peptide (VIP)–immunoreactive nerve fibers are visible around blood vessels and follicles (*a*) and forming nerve bundles (*b*). (*c*) Substance P—containing nerve fibers between the follicles in rat thyroid. (*d*) Neuropeptide Y—containing nerve fibers predominate around blood vessels in rat thyroid.

VIP has been found to occur in cell bodies within a local parasympathetic ganglia.[13,28,29] Exogenous VIP stimulates thyroid hormone secretion in vivo [28–30]; like that of TSH and catecholamines, the action of VIP is mediated by an adenylate cyclic-cAMP system.[20,28,31,32] VIP has a dose-dependent stimulatory effect on cAMP accumulation in human cultured follicular cells, and it stimulates T_4 release from human thyroid slices.[20,28,32] The effect of VIP is additive to that of TSH and is probably evoked by activation of distinct receptors.[20,28,32] The

VIP response is unaffected by α- and β-adrenergic receptor blockade[2,30,31] but may be inhibited by a cholinergic agent.[20,32] An interaction between VIP and cholinergic agonists is of particular interest, since VIP is a constituent of cholinergic nerves. VIP may increase the inhibitory threshold dose of carbachol on thyroid hormone secretion.[20] VIP has been found to increase thyroid blood flow[8,9,21,33,34] and enhance iodide uptake.[35]

Subsequently, other peptides have been demonstrated within thyroid nerve fibers. Among them are NPY, peptide his-

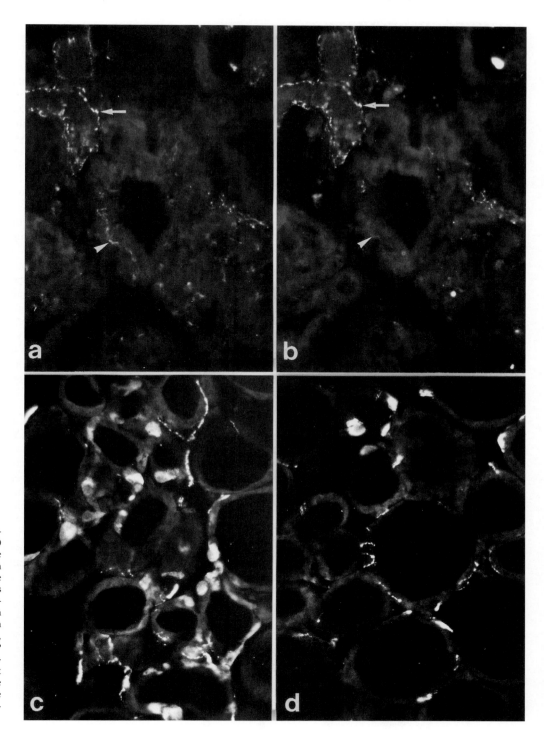

FIGURE 13-5. Rat thyroid. Double immunostaining for NPY (*a*) and DBH (*b*) reveals coexistence of NPY and DBH in a population of nerve fibers (*arrows*). One NPY-immunoreactive fiber lacks DBH (*arrowheads*). (*c*) CGRP-immunoreactive nerve fibers in nerve bundles running between follicles in rat thyroid. In addition, numerous C cells display CGRP immunofluorescence. (*d*) CGRP-immunoreactive nerve fibers in rat thyroid are seen to penetrate the basal membrane of the follicle cell; they appear to reach the follicle lumen.

tidine-isoleucine (PHI), galanin, SP, neurokinin A (NKA), CGRP, and cholecystokinin.[4,13,29] Nerve fibers that store peptides are distributed fairly uniformly in thyroid tissue, usually around blood vessels and between follicles. There is a pronounced interspecies variation also in the density of intrathyroidal peptidergic nerves, and there is an apparent decline in their density with increasing age, as is the case for sympathetic-adrenergic interfollicular nerves. Occasionally, single delicate fibers seem to penetrate the basal membrane, passing between follicular cells, at times apparently reaching the follicular lumen. The peptide-containing nerve fibers often form networks around arteries; they are more rarely found around veins.[4,13,29] This indicates that peptides may be involved in the regulation of local blood flow and thyroid hormone secretion. Recent in vivo studies in rats have revealed that neuropeptides (VIP, PHI, SP, and NPY) are involved in the regulation of thyroid microcirculation but have no effects on thyroid hormone release.[8–10,21,33,34]

NITRINERGIC REGULATION

A recent study by Syed and colleagues,[36] using the NADPH-diaphorase technique to demonstrate nitric oxide synthase activity, revealed neuronal staining in the thyroid of chickens and mice. Nitrinergic nerve fibers were mainly localized around blood vessels, although single fibers were closely associated with follicle cells. Nitrinergic nerve cell bodies were seen in the thyroid ganglion of the mouse and as single cell bodies within the chicken thyroid gland.

Nitric oxide is a potent activator of soluble guanylate cyclase in the thyroid as studied in vitro.[37] A role for nitrinergic nerves in thyroid physiology is quite possible, both indirectly by participating in the regulation of blood flow and directly by controlling the follicle cells.

COEXISTENCE OF NEUROMESSENGERS

Peptides may be found together with classic transmitters within the same neuron, and a neuron may also contain more than one peptide.[24,25] This may be anticipated when two coexisting peptides arise from a larger common peptide precursor. However, there are also neurons that seem to produce peptides that do not share a common precursor.[24,25]

VIP and PHI have a common precursor, and so have SP and NKA.[4,13] This explains the coexistence of each of these pairs of peptide in individual thyroid nerve fibers.[4,13] The peptides probably are stored within the same vesicles and are released together after nerve stimulation. Neuropeptides that arise from separate precursors but seem to coexist in thyroid nerve fibers are NPY with VIP/PHI and CGRP with SP/NKA.[4,13] The coreleased messengers may interact closely in evoking a certain response, but thay may also have completely different effects exerted through separate receptors. For instance, one transmitter may evoke an immediate response, while another may have a long-term trophic effect. NPY coexists with the classic neurotransmitter norepinephrine within thyroid nerves.[4,13] Although the former alters neither basal nor norepinephrine-induced thyroid hormone secretion, it seems to augment the vasoconstriction evoked by norepinephrine.[8,10,34] NPY also coexists with VIP in some nonadrenergic thyroid

nerve fibers, and may enhance VIP-induced thyroid hormone secretion.[4,13,29] SP and CGRP coexist in primary sensory neurons of the C (unmyelinated) type; such fibers are numerous within the thyroid as studied in the rat.[4,13] There are also CGRP-containing nerve fibers that contain no SP. Some CGRP/SP-containing fibers even contain galanin.[4,13] Of these three neuropeptides, only CGRP influences thyroid hormone secretion in that it may enhance the secretory response to VIP.[4,13] Further, SP raises cAMP and increases the release of thyroid hormone as studied in vitro.[38]

Several ganglia in the cervical region have been found to project to the thyroid gland, which indicates an extensive and complex innervation pattern (Fig. 13-6).[4,7,13] The activity of the thyroid may be modulated by many ganglia of presumed sympathetic, parasympathetic, and sensory nature. The sympathetic nerves originate in the superior and stellate ganglia, whereas the parasympathetic nerve fibers derive from the vagal (nodose and local) ganglia. The sensory innervation has three sources: the jugular ganglion, the cervical dorsal root ganglia, and the trigeminal ganglion. Each of the neuronal systems seems to contain multiple potential messengers, including an impressive list of neuropeptides. As judged by the distribution pattern of nerve fibers in the thyroid and the known effects of the various messengers, diverse roles for the nerve supply in the regulation of local blood flow and of thyroid hormone synthesis and secretion are likely.[4,10,13,29,33,34]

ENDOCRINE-PARACRINE THYROID PEPTIDES

In addition to the follicular cells that produce iodothyronines, the thyroid contains another endocrine cell system, the C cells. The close anatomic relation between C cells and follicular cells in the mammalian thyroid has fostered the idea of a functional interaction between these two endocrine cell populations. There is no firm evidence of a direct influence of thyroid hormone on C-cell activity, nor of the C-cell constituents calcitonin, CGRP, somatostatin, and gastrin-releasing peptide on thyroid function.[39] However, a peptide similar to or identical with helodermin (originally isolated from the salivary gland venom of the lizard *Heloderma suspectum*) is present in thy-

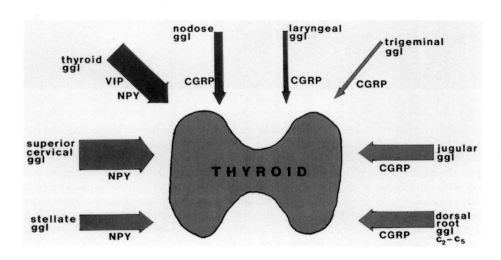

FIGURE 13-6. The various ganglia that supply the thyroid gland are provisionally classified as sympathetic (the superior cervical and stellate ganglia), parasympathetic (the thyroid, nodose, and laryngeal ganglia), and sensory (the trigeminal, jugular, and dorsal root ganglia). The scheme illustrates the contributions made by NPY-, VIP-, and CGRP-containing neurones in the different ganglia to the thyroid innervation. The magnitude of each contribution, as studied in the rat, is reflected in the thickness of the arrows.

roid C cells in several species and stimulates thyroid hormone secretion.[39] It has sequence homologies with peptides of the VIP-secretin family, and it has VIP-like actions in several biologic systems.[39] The thyroid secretory response to helodermin is longer lasting and more pronounced than the response to VIP,[39] but in contrast to the latter, it does not augment TSH-induced thyroid hormone release.[39] Nevertheless, the structural similarity between VIP and helodermin implies that these two peptides may act on the same receptor. These findings support the possibility that a C-cell peptide may be involved in the regulation of thyroid hormone secretion and that this may be mediated by a paracrine mechanism.

References

1. Dumont JE, Takeuchi A, Lamy F, et al. Thyroid control: an example of a complex cell regulation network. Adv Cyclic Nucleotide Protein Phophorylation Res 1981;14:479

2. Green ST, Singh J. Petersén OH. Control of cyclic nucleotide metabolism by non-cholinergic, non-adrenergic nerves in rat thyroid gland. Nature 1982;296:751

3. Green ST. Intrathyroidal autonomic nerves can directly influence hormone release from rat thyroid follicles: a study in vitro employing electrical field stimulation and intracellular microelectrodes. Cli Sci 1987;72:233

4. Grunditz T, Sundler F, Håkanson R, Uddman, R. Regulatory peptides in the thyroid gland. Avd Exp Med Biol 1989; 261:121

5. Melander A, Ericsson LE, Sundler F. Sympathetic regulation of thyroid hormone secretion. Life Sci 1974; 14:237

6. Melander A, Ericson LE, Sundler F, Westgren U. Intrathyroidal amines in the regulation of thyroid activity. Rev Physiol 1975;73:39

7. Romeo HE, Boado RJ, Cardinali DP. Role of the sympathetic nervous system in the control of thyroid compensatory growth of normal and hypophysectomized rats. Neuroendocrinology 1985;40:309

8. Dey M, Michalkiewicz M, Huffman L, Hedge GA. NPY is not a primary mediator of the acute thyroid blood flow response to sympathetic nerve stimulation. Am J Physiol 1993;265:E24

9. Dey M, Michalkiewicz M, Huffman L, Hedge GA. Sympathetic thyroidal vasoconstriction is not blocked by a neuropeptide Y antagonists or antiserum. Peptides 1993;14:1179

10. Michalkiewicz M, Huffman LJ, Dey M, Hedge GA. Endogenous neuropeptide Y regulates thyroid blood flow. Am J Physiol 1993;264:E699

11. Melander A, Sundler F, Westgren U. Sympathetic innervation of the thyroid: variation with species and age. Endocrinology 1975;96:102

12. Toccafondi RS, Brandi IL, Rotella CM, Zonefrati R. Studies of catecholamine effect on cyclic AMP in human cultured thyroid cells: their interaction with thyrotropin receptor. Acta Endocrinol (Copenh) 1983;102:62

13. Grunditz T, Håkanson R, Sundler F, Uddman R. Neuronal pathways to the rat thyroid gland revealed by retrograde tracing and immunocytochemistry. Neuroscience 1988;24:321

14. Sundler F, Håkanson R, Ekblad E, Uddman R, Wahlestedt C. Neuropeptide Y in the peripheral adrenergic and enteric nervous systems. Int Rev Cytol 1986;102:243

15. Maayan ML, Ingbar SH. Epinephrine: Effect on uptake of iodine by dispered cells of calf thyroid glands. Science 1968;162:124

16. Muraki T, Nakaki T, Kato R. Predominance of α_2-adrenoceptors in porcine thyroid: biochemical and pharmacological correlations. Endocrinology 1984;114:1645

17. Amenta F, Caporuscio D, Ferrante F, Porcelli F, Zomparelli M. Cholinergic nerves in the thyroid gland. Cell Tissue Res 1978;195:367

18. Melander A, Sundler F. Presence and influence of cholinergic nerves in the mouse thyroid. Endocrinology 1979;105:7

19. Van Sande J, Dumont JE, Melander A, Sundler F. Presence and influence of cholinergic nerves in the human thyroid. J Clin Endocrinol Metab 1980;51:500

20. Brandi ML, Tanini A, Toccafondi R. Interaction of VIPergic and cholinergic receptors in human thyroid cell. Peptides 1987;8:893

21. Ito H, Matsuda K, Sato A, Tohgi H. Cholinergic and VIPergic vasodilator actions of parasympathetic nerves on the thyroid blood flow in rats. Jap J Physiol 1987;37:1005

22. Unger JP, Ketelbant J, Erneux J, Mockel J, Dumont JE. Mechanism of cholinergic inhibition of dog thyroid secretion in vitro. Endocrinology 1984;114:1266

23. Van Sande J, Erneux C, Dumont J. Negative control of TSH action by iodide and acetylcholine: mechanism of action in intact thyroid cells. J Cyclic Nucleotide Res 1977;3:335

24. Håkanson R, Böttcher G, Ekblad E, Grunditz T, Sundler F. Functional implications of messenger coexpression in neurons and endocrine cells. In: Schwartz TW, Hilsted LH, Rehfeld JF, eds. Neuropeptides and their receptors. Copenhagen: Munksgaard, 1990:211

25. Lundberg JM, Martling CR, Hökfelt T. Airways, oral cavity and salivary glands: classical transmitters and peptides in sensory and autonomic motor neurons. In: Björklund A, Hökfelt T, eds. Handbook of chemical neuroanatomy. Vol 6: The peripheral nervous system. Amsterdam, Elsevier, 1988:391

26. Sundler F, Ekblad E, Grunditz T, Håkanson R, Luts A, Uddman R. NPY in peripheral non-adrenergic neurons. In: Mutt V, Hökfelt T, Fuxe K, eds. Neuropeptide Y. New York: Raven Press, 1989:93

27. Wahlestedt C, Edvinsson L, Ekblad E, Håkanson R. Neuropeptide Y potentiates noradrenaline-evoked vasoconstriction: mode of action. J Pharm Exp Ther 1985;234:735

28. Ahrén B, Alumets J, Ericsson M, et al. VIP occurs in intrathyroidal nerves and stimulates thyroid hormone secretion. Nature 1980;287:343

29. Grunditz T, Ekman R, Håkanson R, Sundler F, Uddman R. Neuropeptide Y and vasoactive intestinal peptide coexist in rat thyroid nerve fibers emanating from the thyroid ganglion. Regul Peptides 1988;23:193

30. Ahrén B, Håkanson R, Rerup C. VIP-stimulated thyroid hormone secretion: effects of other neuropeptides and α- and β-adrenoceptor blockade. Acta Physiol Scand 1982;114:471

31. Brandi ML, Toccafondi R. Neuropeptidergic control of cyclic AMP accumulation in human thyroid cell. Peptides 1985;6:641

32. Toccafondi RS, Brandi ML, Melander A. Vasoactive intestinal peptide stimulation of human thyroid cell function. J Clin Endocrinol Metab 1984;58:157

33. Huffman L, Hedge GA. Effects of vasoactive intestinal peptide on thyroid blood flow and circulating thyroid hormone levels in the rat. Endocrinology 1986;118:550

34. Huffman L, Hedge GA. Neuropeptide control of thyroid blood flow and hormone secretion. Life Sci 1986;39:2143

35. Pietrzyk Z, Michalkiewicz M, Huffman LJ, Hedge GA. Vasoactive intestinal peptide enhances thyroidal iodide uptake during dietary iodine deficiency. Endocrine Res 1992;18:2131

36. Syed MA, Leong S-K, Chan A-S. Localization of NADPH-diaphorase reactivity in the chick and mouse thyroid gland. Thyroid 1994;4:475

37. Esteves RZ, van Sande J, Dumont JE. Nitric oxide as a signal in thyroid. Mol Cell Endocrinol 1992;90:R1

38. Yamashita K, Koide Y, Aiyoshi Y. Effects of substance P on thyroidal cyclic AMP levels and thyroid hormone release from canine thyroid slices. Life Sci 1983;32:2163

39. Grunditz T, Persson P, Håkanson R, et al. Helodermin-like peptides in thyroid C cells: stimulation of thyroid hormone secretion and suppression of calcium incorporation into bone. Proc Natl Acad Sci USA 1989;86:1357

Werner and Ingbar's The Thyroid, Seventh Edition,
edited by Lewis E. Braverman and Robert D. Utiger.
Lippincott–Raven Publishers, Philadelphia, © 1996

14

Intrinsic and Extrinsic Variables

AGE AND PHYSIOLOGIC VARIABLES

Steven R. Gambert

EFFECTS OF AGE

Basal Metabolic Rate and Tissue Responsiveness to Thyroid Hormone

Basal or resting metabolic rate, as measured by oxygen consumption, declines as a function of increasing age. This change correlates with a decline in muscle mass.[1] Although these findings alter the interpretation of the decline in basal metabolic rate with age, they do not put to rest the idea that cells may become less responsive to thyroid hormone with age.

In rats, there is a linear decline in minimal oxygen consumption with increasing age, even after corrections for changes in muscle mass. (Minimal oxygen consumption is the oxygen consumption per unit of fat-free body weight under barbiturate anesthesia; additional corrections are made for variations in core body temperature.) Because older rats also have less of an increment in minimal oxygen consumption than young rats in response to exogenous thyroxine (T_4), the notion that tissue hypothyroidism occurs in aging rats was suggested.[2] This age-related finding was attributed to a specific nonthyrotropin (TSH) pituitary component that remains unidentified. In contrast, in another study, senescent rats were more sensitive to pharmacologic doses of T_4 than younger rats, as measured by increases in whole body oxygen consumption and nitrogen excretion.[3]

Na^+,K^+-ATPase is an enzyme whose activity changes in parallel with oxygen expenditure as a function of thyroid status and is thought to be responsible for some of the calorigenic action of thyroid hormone. Measurements of Na^+,K^+-ATPase activity in liver and renal cortical tissue from euthyroid, hypothyroid, and thyrotoxic rats of increasing age revealed not only a lower absolute level of Na^+,K^+-ATPase activity in older rats than younger rats, but the increment of enzyme activity after triiodothyronine (T_3) administration declined with age as well.[4] A similar age-related decline in the responsiveness of cellular Na^+,K^+-ATPase activity to T_3 stimulation in vitro was found in mononuclear cells from normal human subjects.[5]

Whether this apparent change in responsiveness to thyroid hormone is in any way responsible for the altered clinical manifestations of thyrotoxicosis in elderly persons is unknown. Because there are no age-related changes in T_3 receptors, at least in human mononuclear cells,[6] some alteration in postreceptor function would have to be postulated as the most likely explanation for this clinical phenomenon.

Anatomy of the Thyroid

The normal thyroid gland decreases in size with age in both humans and experimental animals.[7–10] It also becomes more fibrotic, contains more mononuclear cell infiltrates, and shows follicular atrophy.[11] Microscopic nodules are commonly noted in senescent thyroid glands. Occult carcinomas occur with increasing frequency with age, especially in Japanese people.

Influence of Growth and Development

The fetal thyroid gland produces increasing amounts of T_4 throughout gestation, so that at term, serum T_4 concentrations in newborn infants are similar to those in their mothers.[12,13] Until midgestation serum T_3 concentrations are virtually undetectable. Although they begin to rise near term, cord serum T_3 concentrations are about one-third of those of the mother.[12,14,15] The fetal thyroid is sensitive to excess iodine, so infants of mothers who ingest large amounts of iodide may have a congenital goiter.[16] Serum thyroxine-binding globulin (TBG) concentrations in the newborn are about 1.5 times those of adults but somewhat less than those in maternal serum at the time of delivery.[15] This increase in fetal serum TBG likely results from maternally derived estrogen. Studies of T_4 binding in cord serum have demonstrated that it has greater binding capacity than can be explained by its concentration of TBG.[17,18] Because newborn infants have lower serum concentrations of transthyretin (TTR) than their mothers,[19] some other factor is likely responsible for the differences in overall T_4 binding.

Serum reverse T_3 (rT_3) concentrations are considerably higher in newborn infants than in adults. This rT_3 is thought to be derived from placental and peripheral deiodination of T_4; little comes from the thyroid.[20]

After delivery, serum T_4 and T_3 concentrations rapidly increase, and serum rT_3 concentrations decline. The former increases are due to a transient postnatal increase in TSH secretion and increased extrathyroidal T_4 conversion to T_3. The decline in serum rT_3 reflects the absence of its placental source. These and other changes in pituitary-thyroid function in fetuses and neonates are discussed in more detail in chapter 84.

There are minor changes in thyroid hormone economy during childhood. Serum TTR concentrations remain low until adolescence, when they increase.[21] Serum TBG concentrations remain higher than in adults,[22] although the concentrations decline gradually during childhood and adolescence.[21,23] Serum total T_4 concentrations, paralleling the changes in TBG, fall throughout childhood until about age 14 to 15 years. Serum T_3 also decreases and rT_3 increases slightly.[24] A small decrease in serum free T_4 concentration has been reported during adolescence; free T_3 concentrations in children are similar to those in adults.[21,25] The half-life of T_4 lengthens from 5 days in children aged 3 to 9 years to 6 days in children aged 10 to 16 years.[26]

Influence of Maturation

In normal subjects, serum total and free T_4 and T_3 concentrations change little during adult life.[27,28] In fact, no changes in serum protein-bound iodine concentrations were found in adults into late life.[29,30] Serum TBG and TTR concentrations also change little during adult life. The half-life of T_4, however, continues to increase, the mean value being 6.7 days in adults aged 23 to 36 years.[26]

Influence of Senescence

Senescence affects almost all cellular and organ systems. Nevertheless, if one carefully excludes illness as a variable, it is surprising how little change occurs in serum T_4 or T_3 concentrations in elderly people. In most studies, no changes in either serum total or free T_4 concentrations were found throughout life,[22,27,28,31–33] but in a few, a slight decrease after the seventh decade was recorded.[31,34–36] The half-life of T_4, however, increases to 9.3 days in adults aged 80 to 90 years,[26] implying there is less thyroidal production of T_4 with increasing age.

A small decline in serum T_3 concentrations with age has been found in a few studies, but the decline is more likely attributable to mild nonthyroidal illness than age itself.[37,38] Advanced age is not thought to affect binding protein production to any great extent, although a rise in serum TBG and fall in TTR in the aged was found in one study.[39]

In a study of 41 healthy centenarians (age range 100–110 years), the prevalence of subclinical hypothyroidism (defined as high serum TSH and normal serum T_4 concentrations) was 7.3%. Although there was no age-related change in median serum free T_4, the median serum free T_3 and TSH concentrations were inversely correlated with age as compared with two groups of healthy persons aged 65 to 80 and 20 to 64 years, with a significant difference noted for the oldest group; serum rT_3 concentrations were higher in the group of centenarians. The authors concluded that thyroid function was well preserved until the eighth decade of life in normal subjects, with a decline in serum free T_3 at the later stages of life due to a defect in 5'-monodiiodinase activity and possibly decreased TSH secretion.[40]

This latter phenomenon was also suggested by authors of a study of healthy elderly subjects in whom the nocturnal increase in TSH secretion was blunted,[41] suggesting a resetting of the pituitary threshold of TSH feedback suppression leading to a decrease in TSH secretion for a given concentration of circulating thyroid hormone.[42]

Hypothalamic-Pituitary Function and Age

In a study of 344 relatively healthy people over 60 years of age, serum TSH concentrations were more than 10 μU/mL in 5.9%. Of these latter subjects, almost half had low serum T_4 and free T_4 index values. An additional 14.4% had lesser elevations in serum TSH, none of whom had low serum T_4 or free T_4 index values.[43] Among elderly subjects in general, most who have elevated serum TSH concentrations have antithyroid autoantibodies, suggesting that their elevated serum TSH values are due to subclinical chronic autoimmune thyroiditis rather than aging itself.

Pituitary TSH content does not change with age in humans.[27,32] Likewise, TSH secretion changes little, if care is taken to exclude patients with minor degrees of thyroid disease as noted above. Indeed, TSH secretion may decline slightly; the slower clearance of T_4 and T_3 in older persons implies less TSH is needed to maintain thyroid secretion. Serum TSH concentrations were lower in the group of centenarians mentioned above.[40]

The results of studies of the serum TSH response to thyrotropin-releasing hormone (TRH) in elderly people are conflicting. A progressive decline with age was reported in elderly men[44] but not elderly women.[45,46] In another study, an age-related decline in TRH responsiveness was found in aged women but not in aged men;[47] in a third study, TRH responsiveness was increased in aged subjects of both sexes.[27] In men aged 30 to 96 years given a continuous TRH infusion, instead of bolus TRH administration as was used in the previously mentioned studies, the serum TSH response was biphasic, and neither phase was affected by age.[32] The serum T_4 response to the TSH secreted after bolus TRH administration is not altered by age, although the serum T_3 response may decrease.[45] Administration of large doses of exogenous TSH has been reported to increase serum T_4 to a lesser extent in older subjects than in younger subjects.[48,49]

Deiodination of T_4 and T_3 by Peripheral Tissues

The rate of disposal (clearance) of T_4 decreases with increasing age in both men and women.[26,36,38,50,51] This decrease is consonant with the age-related decrease in thyroid radioiodide accumulation and maintenance of stable serum T_4 concentrations throughout life. The decrease in T_4 clearance is thought to result from decreases in both the fractional turnover rate and distribution space of T_4.[26,52,53] The decrease in clearance is responsible for the lower requirement for exogenous T_4 in elderly as compared with younger hypothyroid patients.[54] The rate of T_3 clearance has also been reported to decline with advancing age.[36]

Clinical Aspects of Thyroid Disease in the Elderly

Thyroid physiology and function demonstrate key principles of geriatric medicine. For example, normal aging is associated with physiologic changes; certain diseases are more common during later life; and many diseases present atypically or nonspecifically in elderly persons.[55,56] The frequency of thyrotoxicosis and hypothyroidism in elderly people is as high as 2% and 10%,[57] respectively.

In general, the signs and symptoms of hypothyroidism do not change with age (after linear growth ceases in adolescence). The presence of other age-prevalent diseases and manifestations of normal aging, however, may make it extremely difficult to recognize this often slowly progressive disorder in elderly people. For this reason, many have advocated routine screening for hypothyroidism using serum TSH assays among the elderly.

Thyrotoxicosis, on the other hand, may present atypically in the elderly. About 15% of all thyrotoxic patients are over age 60, and the frequency of toxic nodular goiter as the cause of thyrotoxicosis is increased. Among patients with Graves' disease, the frequency of goiter and ophthalmopathy is lower in the elderly. The major clinical manifestations of thyrotoxicosis in the elderly are anorexia, cardiovascular dysfunction, and weight loss; tremor, irritability, and heat intolerance are less common than in younger patients.

Subclinical hypothyroidism is common in older persons, more so in women than in men, between 4% and 14% of persons over the age of 60 being affected.[43,57,58] Patients with subclinical hypothyroidism have few symptoms but may have some neuropsychological or electrocardiographic manifestations of hypothyroidism.[59] T_4 treatment for persons with subclinical hypothyroidism tends to improve left ventricular function,[59–61] performance on psychometric testing,[59] and symptoms of constipation.[62] The clinical manifestations and management of subclinical hypothyroidism are discussed in detail in chapter 87.

Although much less common than subclinical hypothyroidism, subclinical thyrotoxicosis (low serum TSH and normal serum T_4) appears to be common during later life.[63] Among persons 60 years of age and older, a low serum TSH concentration has been associated with a threefold higher risk for the development of atrial fibrillation in the subsequent decade[64] and also with increased bone resorption[65] (see chap 88).

INFLUENCE OF SEX AND GONADAL HORMONES AND PREGNANCY

Thyroid function is similar in normal women and men.[66–68] Although serum TBG concentrations are slightly higher and serum TTR concentrations are slightly lower in women than in men,[69] their serum total and free T_4 and T_3 concentrations are similar, as are their serum TSH concentrations and thyroid radioiodine uptake values. Infants given large doses of estrogen have accelerated thyroid radioiodine release,[70] but it is not different in women and men despite their different serum sex hormone concentrations. Estrogens do acutely inhibit the rate of hormone release from the thyroid in adults,[71] which may explain the occasional improvement in thyrotoxicosis during estrogen therapy.

Sex differences have been reported in the serum TSH response to TRH administration. Young and middle-aged women have slightly greater serum TSH responses to TRH, given either orally or intravenously, than do men of similar age.[28,45,72,73] The serum TSH response to TRH also varies slightly during the menstrual cycle; TSH release is greater in the preovulatory phase, and the postovulatory phase response is similar to the response in men.[73]

The variations in thyroid function that occur during pregnancy largely reflect associated changes in sex steroid production. Throughout pregnancy, however, maternal thyroid function remains normal. There is a 50% to 75% increase in serum T_4 and T_3 concentrations in the first trimester of pregnancy due to a twofold increase in TBG binding capacity caused by increased estrogen production.[74] This increase persists until 6 weeks postpartum. Serum free T_4 and T_3 concentrations remain within the normal range during most of pregnancy, but rise transiently to near or just above the upper limit of normal near the end of the first trimester.[75] This rise is caused by the week thyroid-stimulating action of chorionic gonadotropin, which peaks at that time. Serum TSH concentrations decline transiently at the same time, to near or just below the lower limit of normal, but otherwise are similar to those of nonpregnant persons during pregnancy.[76,77]

Effects of Progestational Agents, Androgens, and Anabolic Steroids

Although exogenous androgen administration does not affect thyroid gland function directly,[78,79] androgens such as testosterone and methyltestosterone do decrease serum TBG and total T_4 concentrations.[19,78,80] A similar effect follows the administration of several anabolic steroids, including nandrolone and norethandrolone[79,81,82]; the latter also stimulates TTR synthesis.[83] Androgenic and anabolic steroids increase the fractional rate of turnover of T_4 but have little if any effect on the total daily disposal rate of T_4.

Although most progestational agents do not affect thyroid function, those with androgenic properties, such as 17-α-ethinyl-19-nortestosterone (norethindrone), increase TTR production.[81]

Effects of Adrenocortical Hormones

Glucocorticoids inhibit thyroid hormone activity. Large doses of cortisone decrease radioiodide accumulation by the thyroid gland after both acute and chronic administration.[84] This decrease is accompanied by an increase in renal radioiodide clearance and decreases in thyroid iodide clearance and fractional release of iodide from the thyroid gland.[85] Serum total T_4 concentrations may decrease because glucocorticoids decrease TBG[86] and TTR production. Glucocorticoids also inhibit the peripheral conversion of T_4 to T_3. Serum concentrations of T_3 decline about 20% to 40% after administration of large doses of dexamethasone. This effect persists for the duration of dexamethasone administration and is accompanied by a rise in serum rT_3.[53,87]

Although glucocorticoids have no effect on TSH action on the thyroid gland,[88] they inhibit TSH secretion, particularly the nocturnal surge of TSH secretion in normal subjects. They also inhibit TSH secretion in patients with primary hypothyroidism. This is the mechanism by which glucocorticoids exert their inhibitory effects on thyroid radioiodine metabolism. There is a transient rebound above the prior baseline after glucocorticoids are discontinued, and withdrawal of glucocorticoid therapy in patients with Addison's disease may be followed by transient TSH hypersecretion.[89] These reciprocal relationships have led to the notion that the circadian rhythm of TSH secretion is linked inversely to that of ACTH and cortisol.[90,91]

Glucocorticoids also result in blunted serum TSH responses to TRH administration.[92] Such diminished responses have been reported both in subjects receiving a relatively low dose (20–50 mg/d cortisol equivalent) for 7 to 25 months and those receiving a relatively high dose (80–180 mg/d) for 1 to 4 months.

Thus, glucocorticoids have effects on TSH secretion, serum thyroid hormone binding, and extrathyroidal T_3 production. Their net effect, when given chronically, is to decrease serum total and free T_4 and T_3 concentrations slightly, but major decreases are undoubtedly prevented by the increase in TSH secretion that occurs when serum T_4 and T_3 concentrations decline appreciably.

References

1. Tzankoff SP, Norris AH. Effect of muscle mass decrease on age-related BMR changes. J Appl Physiol 1977;43:1001
2. Denkla WD. Role of the pituitary and thyroid glands in the decline of minimal O_2 consumption with age. J Clin Invest 1974;53:572
3. Frolkis VV, Verzhakovskaya NV, Valueva GV. The thyroid and age. Exp Gerontol 1973;8:285
4. Gambert SR, Ingbar SH, Hagen TC. Interaction of age and thyroid hormone status on Na+-K+ATPase in rat renal cortex and liver. Endocrinology 1981;108:27
5. Gambert SR. Effect of age on basal and 3,5,3′ triiodothyronine (T_3) stimulated human mononuclear cell sodium-potassium adenosine-triphosphatase (Nap+-K+ATPase) activity. Horm Metab Res 1986;18:649
6. Gambert SR, Tsitouras PD. Effect of age on nuclear triiodothyronine receptors in circulating human lymphocytes. Age 1983;6:76
7. Bourne GH. Aging changes in the endocrines. In: Gitman L, ed. Endocrines and aging. Springfield, IL: Charles C Thomas, 1967:66
8. Haensley WE, Getty R. Age changes in the weight of the thyroid glands of swine from birth to eight years. Exp Gerontol 1970;5:203
9. Irvine RE. Thyroid disease in old age. In: Brocklehurst JC, ed. Textbook of geriatric medicine and gerontology. London: Churchill Livingstone, 1973:435
10. Pittman JA Jr. The thyroid and aging. J Am Geriatr Soc 1962;10:10
11. Garner HS, Bernick S. Effect of age upon the thyroid gland and pituitary thyrotrophs of the rat. J Gerontol 1975;30:137
12. Fisher DA, Dussault JH, Hobel CJ, et al. Serum and thyroid gland triiodothyronine in the human fetus. J Clin Endocrinol Metab 1973;36:397
13. Pickering DE. Maternal thyroid hormone in the developing fetus. Am J Dis Child 1964;107:567
14. Abuid J, Stinson DA, Larsen PR. Serum triiodothyronine and thyroxine in the neonate and the acute increases in these hormones following delivery. J Clin Invest 1973;52:1195
15. Erenberg A, Phelps DL, Lam R, et al. Total and free thyroid hormone concentrations in the neonatal period. Pediatrics 1974;53:211
16. Ayromlooi J. Congenital goiter due to maternal ingestion of iodides. Obstet Gynecol 1972;39:818
17. Pickering DE. Maternal thyroid hormone in the developing fetus. Am J Dis Child 1964;107:567
18. Spafford NR, Carr EA, Lowrey GR, et al. I 131-labeled triiodothyronine erythrocyte uptake of mothers and newborn infants. Am J Dis Child 1960;100:844
19. De Nayer P, Malvaux P, Van Den Schrieck HG, et al. Free thyroxine in maternal and cord blood. J Clin Endocrinol Metab 1966;26:233
20. Bernard B, Oddie TH, Klein AH, et al. Oscillations in reverse triiodothyronine levels in serum of healthy infants aged 0 to 130 hours. J Clin Endocrinol Metab 1979;48:790
21. Malvaux P, De Nayer P, Beckers C, et al. Serum free thyroxine and thyroxine binding proteins in male adolescents. J Clin Endocrinol Metab 1966;26:459
22. Braverman LE, Dawber NA, Ingbar SH. Observations concerning the binding of thyroid hormones in sera of normal subjects of varying ages. J Clin Invest 1966;45:1273
23. Starr P, Nicoloff J. Comparison of serum protein-bound iodine and thyroxine-binding globulin saturation capacity values in Negro and white school children: ethnic difference. Acta Endocrinol 1967;56:577
24. Florsheim WH, Faircloth MA. Effect of oral ovulation inhibitors on serum protein-bound iodine and thyroxine binding proteins. Proc Soc Exp Biol Med 1964;117:56
25. Boyd AE, Sanchez-Franco F. Changes in the prolactin response to thyrotropin-releasing hormone (TRH) during the menstrual cycle of normal women. J Clin Endocrinol Metab 1977;44:985
26. Gregerman RI, Gaffney GW, Shock NW. Thyroxine turnover in euthyroid man with special reference to changes with age. J Clin Invest 1962;41:2065
27. Ohara H, Kobayashi T, Shiraishi M, et al. Thyroid function of the aged as viewed from the pituitary-thyroid system. Endocrinol Jpn 1974;21:377
28. Wenzel KW, Meinhold H, Herpich M, et al. TRH-Stimulationstest mit alters und geschlechtsabhangigem TSH-Anstieg bei Normalpersonen. Klin Wochenschr 1974;52:721
29. Gaffney GW, Gregerman RI, Shock NW. Relationship of age to the thyroidal accumulation, renal excretion and distribution of radioiodide in euthyroid man. J Clin Endocrinol Metab 1962;22:784
30. Osathanondh R, Chopra IJ, Tulchinsky D. Effects of dexamethasone on fetal and maternal thyroxine, triiodothyronine, reverse triiodothyronine, and thyrotropin levels. J Clin Endocrinol Metab 1978;47:1236
31. Hansen JM, Skovsted L, Siersbaek-Nielsen K. Age-dependent changes in iodine metabolism and thyroid function. Acta Endocrinol 1975;79:60
32. Harman SM, Wehmann RE, Blackman MR. Pituitary-thyroid hormone economy in healthy aging men: basal indices of thyroid function and thyrotropin responses to constant infusions of thyrotropin releasing hormone. J Clin Endocrinol Metab 1984;58:320
33. Oliner L, Kohlenbrenner RM, Fields T, et al. Thyroid function studies in children: normal values for thyroid I 131 uptake and PBI 131 levels up to the age of 18. J Clin Endocrinol Metab 1957;17:61

34. Bermudez F, Surks MI, Oppenheimer JH. High incidence of decreased serum triiodothyronine concentration in patients with nonthyroidal disease. J Clin Endocrinol Metab 1975;41:27

35. Hermann J, Rusche HJ, Kroll HJ, et al. Free triiodothyronine (T_3) and thyroxine (T_4) serum levels in old age. Horm Metab Res 1974;6:239

36. Wenzel KW, Horn WR. Triiodothyronine (T_3) and thyroxine (T_4) kinetics in aged men. In: Robbins J, Braverman LE, eds. Thyroid research. Amsterdam: Excerpta Medica, 1976:270

37. Henneman HA, Reineke EP, Griffin SA. The thyroid secretion rate of sheep as affected by season, age, breed, pregnancy, and lactation. J Anim Sci 1955;14:419

38. Nishikawa M, Inada M, Naito K, et al. Age-related changes of serum 3,3'-diiodothyronine, 3',5'-diiodothyronine, and 3,5-diiodothyronine concentrations in man. J Clin Endocrinol Metab 1981;52:517

39. Hesch RD, Gatz J, Juppner H, et al. TBG-dependency of age-related variations of thyroxine and triiodothyronine. Horm Metab Res 1977;9:141

40. Mariotti S, Barbesino G, Caturegli P, et al. Complex alteration of thyroid function in healthy centenarians. J Clin Endocrinol Metab 1993;1130

41. Van Coevorden A, Laurent E, Decoster C, et al. Decreased basal and stimulated thyrotropin secretion in healthy elderly men. J Clin Endocrinol Metab 1989;69:177

42. Lewis GF, Alessi CA, Imperial JG, Refetoff S. Low serum free thyroxine index in ambulatory elderly is due to a setting of the threshold of thyrotropin feedback suppression. J Clin Endocrinol Metab 1991;73:843

43. Sawin CT, Chopra D, Azizi F, et al. The aging thyroid: increased prevalence of elevated serum thyrotropin levels in the elderly. JAMA 1979;242:247

44. Snyder PJ, Utiger RD. Response to thyrotropin releasing hormone (TRH) in normal man. J Clin Endocrinol Metab 1972;34:380

45. Azizi F, Vagenakis AG, Portnay GI, et al. Pituitary-thyroid responsiveness to intramuscular thyrotropin-releasing hormone based on analyses of serum thyroxine, triiodothyronine and thyrotropin concentrations. N Engl J Med 1975;292:273

46. Snyder PJ, Utiger RD. Thyrotropin response of thyrotropin releasing hormone in normal females over forty. J Clin Endocrinol Metab 1972;34:1096

47. Sowers JA, Catania RA, Hershman JM. Evidence for dopaminergic control of circadian variation in thyrotropin secretion. J Clin Endocrinol Metab 1982;54:673

48. Einhorn J. Studies on the effect of thyrotropic hormone on thyroid function in man. Acta Radiol 1958;suppl 160:107

49. Lederer J, Bataille JP. Senescence et fonction thyroidienne. Ann Endocrinol 1969;30:598

50. Anbar M, Guttmann S, Rodan G, et al. The determination of the rate of deiodination of thyroxine in human subjects. J Clin Invest 1965;44:1986

51. Oddie TH, Meade JH Jr, Fisher DA. An analysis of published data on thyroxine turnover in human subjects. J Clin Endocrinol Metab 1966;26:425

52. Inada M, Koshiyama K, Torizuka K, et al. Clinical studies of the metabolism of 131I-labeled L-thyroxine. J Clin Endocrinol Metab 1964;24:775

53. Ingbar SH, Freinkel N. The influence of ACTH, cortisone and hydrocortisone on the distribution and peripheral metabolism of thyroxine. J Clin Invest 1955;34:1375

54. Rosenbaum RL, Barzel US. Levothyroxine replacement dose for primary hypothyroidism decreases with age. Ann Intern Med 1982;96:53

55. Atkinson RL, Dahms, WT, Fisher DA, et al. Occult thyroid disease in an elderly population. J Gerontol 1978;33:372

56. Gambert SR, Tsitouras PD. Effect of age on thyroid hormone physiology and function. J Am Geriatr Soc 1985;33:360

57. Bagchi N, Brown TR, Parish RF. Thyroid dysfunction in adults over age 55 years: a study in an urban US community. Arch Intern Med 1990;150:785

58. Sawin CT, Castelli WP, Hershman JM, et al. The aging thyroid: thyroid deficiency in the Framingham study. Arch Intern Med 1985;145:1386

59. Nystrom E, Caidahl K, Fager G, et al. A double-blind crossover 12-month study of L-thyroxine treatment of women with subclinical hypothyroidism. Clin Endocrinol 1988;29:63

60. Bell GM, Todd WTA, Forfar JC, et al. End-organ responses to thyroxine therapy in subclinical hypothyroidism. Clin Endocrinol 1985;22:83

61. Cooper DS, Halpern R, Wood LC, et al. L-thyroxine therapy in subclinical hypothyroidism. A double-blind, placebo-controlled trial. Ann Intern Med 1984;101:18

62. Rahman Q, Haboubi NY, Hudson PR, et al. The effect of thyroxine on small intestinal motility in the elderly. Clin Endocrinol 1991;35:443

63. Figge J, Leinung M, Goodman AD, et al. The clinical evaluation of patients with subclinical hyperthyroidism and free triiodothyronine (free T_3) toxicosis. Am J Med 1994;96:229

64. Sawin CT, Geller A, Wolf PA, et al. Low serum thyrotropin concentrations as a risk factor for atrial fibrillation in older persons. N Engl J Med 1994;331:1249

65. Ross DS, Neer RM, Ridgway EC, Daniels GH. Subclinical hyperthyroidism and reduced bone density as a possible result of prolonged suppression of the pituitary thyroid-axis with L-thyroxine. Am J Med 1987;82:1167

66. Gregerman RI. Estimation of thyroxine secretion rate in the rat by the radioactive thyroxine turnover technique: influences of age, sex, and exposure to cold. Endocrinology 1963;72:382

67. Oddie TH, Fisher DA. Protein-bound iodine level during childhood and adolescence. J Clin Endocrinol Metab 1967;27:89

68. Pipes GW, Bauman TR, Brooks JR, et al. Effect of season, sex, and breed on the thyroxine secretion rate of beef cattle and a comparison with dairy cattle. J Anim Sci 1963;22:476

69. Braverman LE, Foster AE, Ingbar SH. Sex-related difference in the binding in serum of thyroid hormones. J Clin Endocrinol Metab 1967;27:227

70. Fisher DA, Oddie TH. Thyroxine secretion rate during infancy: effect of estrogen. J Clin Endocrinol Metab 1963;23:811

71. Gross HA, Appleman MD Jr, Nicoloff JT. Effect of biologically active steroids on thyroid function in man. J Clin Endocrinol Metab 1975;33:242

72. Noel GD, Dimond RC, Wartofsky L, et al. Studies of prolactin and TSH secretion by continuous infusion of small amounts of thyrotropin-releasing hormone (TRH). J Clin Endocrinol Metab 1974;39:6

73. Sanchez-Franco F, Garcia MD, Cacicedo L, et al. Influence of sex phase of the menstrual cycle on the thyrotropin (TSH) response to thyrotropin-releasing hormone (TRH). J Clin Endocrinol Metab 1973;37:736

74. Hotelling DR, Sherwood LM. The effect of pregnancy on circulating triiodothyronine. J Clin Endocrinol Metab 1971;33:783

75. Harada A, Hershman JM, Reed AW, et al. Comparison of thyroid stimulators and thyroid hormone concentrations in the sera of pregnant women. J Clin Endocrinol Metab 1979;48:793

76. Guillaume J, Schussler GC, Goldman J, et al. Components of the total serum thyroxine during pregnancy. High serum free thyroxine and blunted thyrotropin (TSH) response to TSH-releasing hormone in the first trimester. J Clin Endocrinol Metab 1985;60:678

77. Glinoer D, De Nayer P, Bourdoux P, et al. Regulation of maternal thyroid during pregnancy. J Clin Endocrinol Metab 1990;71:276

78. Federman DD, Robbins J, Rall JE. Effects of methyl testosterone on thyroid function, thyroxine metabolism, and thyroxine-binding protein. J Clin Invest 1958;37:1024

79. Feldman EB, Carter AC. Endocrinologic and metabolic effects of 17-alpha-methyl-19-nortestosterone in women. J Clin Endocrinol Metab 1960;20:842

80. Keitel HC, Sherer MG. Marked depression of the plasma protein-bound iodine concentration in the absence of clinical hypothyroidism during testosterone medication. J Clin Endocrinol Metab 1957;17:854

81. Braverman LE, Ingbar SH. Effects of norethandrolone on the transport in serum and peripheral turnover of thyroxine. J Clin Endocrinol Metab 1967;27:389

82. Braverman LE, Socolow EL, Woeber KA, et al. Effect of norethandrolone on the metabolism of 125 I-labeled thyroxine-binding prealbumin. J Clin Endocrinol Metab 1968;28:831

83. Dussault JH, Hobel CJ, DiStefano JJ, et al. Triiodothyronine turnover in maternal and fetal sheep. Endocrinology 1972;90:1301

84. Berson SA, Yalow RS. The effect of cortisone on the iodine accumulating function of the thyroid gland in euthyroid subjects. J Clin Endocrinol Metab 1952;12:407

85. Visser TJ, Lamberts SWJ. Regulation of TSH secretion and thyroid function in Cushing's disease. Acta Endocrinol 1981;96:480

86. Oppenheimer JH, Werner SC. Effect of prednisone on thyroxine-binding proteins. J Clin Endocrinol Metab 1966;26:715

87. Kumar RS, Musa BU, Appleton WG, et al. Effect of prednisone on thyroxine distribution. J Clin Endocrinol Metab 1968;28:1335

88. Bruck K, Baun E, Schwennicke HP. Cold-adaptive modifications in man induced by repeated short-term cold-exposures and during a 10-day and night cold exposure. Pflugers Arch 1976; 363:125

89. Nicoloff JT, Fisher DA, Appleman MD. The role of glucocorticoids in the regulation of thyroid function in man. J Clin Invest 1979;49:1922

90. Custro N, Scaglione R. Circadian rhythm of TSH in adult men and women. Acta Endocrinol 1980;95:465

91. Sowers JA, Catania RA, Hershman JM. Evidence for dopaminergic control of circadian variation in thyrotropin secretion. J Clin Endocrinol Metab 1982;54:673

92. Otsuki M, Dakoda M, Baba S. Influence of glucocorticoids on TRF-induced TSH response in man. J Clin Endocrinol Metab 1975;36:95

Environmental Influences on Thyroid Hormone Regulation

H. Lester Reed*

The environment in which people live and work can be defined as a complex of climatic, terrestrial, and biotic factors that act on an organism to determine its form and survival. Accumulating evidence over the last two decades now supports the concept that human physiology acclimates to changing environmental factors, such as temperature,[1,2] photoperiod,[3] altitude,[4] gravity,[5,6] season,[7–13] and time zone.[14] These extrinsic influences on iodothyronine homeostasis may be character-

---
*The opinion or assertions contained herein are the private views of the author and are not to be construed as official or as reflecting the views of the Department of the Army or the Department of Defense.

ized as *direct* and include cold[15–17] and warm[18] temperature, photoperiod,[3] altitude,[19] microgravity,[20] or more *interactive* to include exercise,[21] sleep,[22,23] nutrition,[24] age,[25] pregnancy,[26] illness,[27,28] depression,[29] and toxic exposure.[30] Under usual circumstances individuals cannot completely isolate themselves from many of the direct factors such as temperature,[31] photoperiod,[3,14] and altitude.[19,32]

Unfortunately, much of the existing information regarding mammalian adaptation involves small rodents. Although detailed studies are possible using these animals, they often lack similarity to human beings with respect to such basic homeostatic mechanisms as thermal regulation.[17,33] Therefore, this review includes studies using human subjects and will only cite alternate animal models when no other data are available.

The present review does not address whether the human thyroidal responses to environmental changes of temperature, altitude, gravity, exercise, sleep, and changing seasons are adaptive or maladaptive for well-being and thus ultimately affect survival. Such a subject must, of course, include tissue-specific responses that are generally unknown for human beings and therefore is beyond the scope of this overview. Complementary topics that are covered elsewhere include the regulation of thyroid hormone economy by nutrition,[24] illness,[27,28] age,[25] pregnancy,[26] sympathetic nervous system activity, dietary selenium and iodine, and toxins.[30]

EFFECTS OF ENVIRONMENTAL TEMPERATURE

Cold

PHYSIOLOGIC COLD ADAPTATION

Human subjects, when tested during a cold air tolerance test,[1,16,34] show physiologic cold adaptation after repeated exposure to either cold water or air.[34] These characteristics include a fall in skin and rectal temperature,[16] the threshold temperature needed to stimulate shivering, and the blood pressure response with cold air.[34] Such findings are collectively called hypothermic cold adaptation.[1]

THYROID HORMONE RESPONSES TO BRIEF COLD CLIMATE CHAMBER EXPOSURES

Circulating iodothyronines and thyrotrophin (TSH) do not change dramatically in adults during a 30-minute to 2-hour cold air challenge when they have not been previously exposed to cold (cold naive).[17] A recent report suggests that after correcting for changes in plasma volume, free triiodothyronine (FT_3) and thyroxine (FT_4) declined after 115 minutes of cold air exposure without changes in total T_3 (TT_3), total T_4 (TT_4), or TSH.[16] Neonates, however, unlike adults, have substantial thermogenic brown adipose tissue, and, in contrast to adults, show an increase in TSH during cold air exposure.[17]

THYROID HORMONE RESPONSES TO REPEATED COLD CLIMATE CHAMBER EXPOSURES

Subjects undergoing multiple[15,16,35] (−20 to 8°C) or extended (12°C) air exposure for 12 to 14 days show changes in both thyroid hormone kinetic and static values. Ingbar and

Bass reported in seminude men exposed to cold (11–16°C) for 12 to 14 days that organic iodide production more than doubled and radiolabeled T_4 degradation increased.[17] We have recently reported that in a group of 16 men exposed to cold air (4°C) for 30 minutes, twice a day for 8 weeks,[15] the T_3 plasma clearance rate (PCR) and T_3 plasma appearance rate (PAR) increased by approximately 18% after 14 days of the protocol and maintained this elevation over the next 6 weeks of cold exposure. All of these men displayed similar increases in T_3 PCR and PAR and all developed hypothermic cold adaptation, even though half the subjects received oral T_3 to suppress TSH and FT_4 by about 50%.[15] After 40 exposures of the legs to cold (4°C) water for between 5 to 60 minutes each, over a period of 30 days, a 115-minute cold air test showed both cold adaptation physiology and decreases in serum TT_3 when contrasted with paired cold-naive conditions.[16] This decrease is at variance with shorter cold air tests[34] and in general agreement with longer cold air tests[35,36] (Table 14-1). Solter and colleagues divided factory workers into temperature-graded categories of intermittent exposure for about 3.5 hours to severe cold (−40°C to −20°C) or continuous moderate exposure (−10–8°C) for 8 h/d.[35] In both groups the TT_3 declined about 10% with cold exposure while only with the most severe temperature did TT_4 decrease about 16%. Basally before the daily exposure, Ti_4 was decreased also only in the severely cold-exposed group when compared to controls. In contrast, the FT_4 and FT_3 were generally elevated over controls and did not change much with cold exposure.[35] Specific occupational controls and study protocol, subject gender, lack of volume status correction, and free hormone analogue assay differences may account for the discrepancy in FT_4 and FT_3 values when compared to other studies.[16,34,36] The study also reported reverse T_3 (rT_3) to follow the same pattern as the TT_3 and TT_4 decline, thus arguing against the notion that the decline in T_3[16,17,34,35] is from a decrease in PAR or inhibition of 5'-deiodinase (5'-DI) type I activity as seen with fasting[24,37] or illness.[27] This hormone pattern might reflect alterations in protein binding, an increased T_3 PCR,[15] or increased distribution volume (V_d).[38]

THYROID HORMONE RESPONSES TO COLD CLIMATE ENVIRONMENTAL FIELD STUDIES

Early field studies have been thoroughly reviewed by Fregly[17]; some show increases in serum T_4 and T_3 with cold challenge tests of polar residents and others show increased T_3 in poorly housed natives of Japan.[17] These findings are in contrast to more recent publications describing polar residents[36,38–41] or occupational exposure[35] (see Table 14-1) and may have been confounded by sleep deprivation,[22] dietary changes,[24] and plasma volume shifts[16] that are not addressed.

Extended residence in Antarctica and other high latitude environments is associated with exposures to extremes of photoperiod, low relative humidity, social isolation, and low temperatures. We have reported that individuals living in these conditions for approximately 5 months develop hypothermic cold adaptation[36] although only the hands and face may be di-

---

TABLE 14-1.
Effects of Cold on Thyroid Hormones*

Cold Exposure	Initial Exposure	Multiple Exposures	Multiple Exposures	Field Exposures	Field Exposures	Field Exposures (~d)
Testing	0–4°C	0–4°C	20–24°C	−10–8°C	20–24°C	20–24°C
Conditions	Chamber	Chamber	Ambient	Chamber	Ambient	Ambient
TT_3	≈	≈/↓	≈	≈/↓	≈/↓	5–30
FT_3	↓	↓	≈/↓	≈/↓	≈/↓ (↑ 35,39)	30–60 5–60
TT_4	≈	≈	≈	≈	↓	60–140
FT_4	≈/↓	≈/↓	≈	≈/(↑35)	≈/↓ (↑39)	60–140 5–60
TBG	≈	≈	≈	≈	≈/↑	60–120
TSH	≈	≈	≈	≈	↑	70–140
T_3 PAR	NA	NA	↑	NA	↑↑	14–30
T_3 PCR	NA	NA	↑	NA	↑↑	14–30
$T_3 V_d$	NA	NA	≈	NA	↑↑	70–140
T_4 PAR	NA	↑	NA	NA	≈	—
Adapted	No	Yes	Yes	Yes	Yes	10–14
References	16, 34	16, 17, 34	15, 16, 34	35, 36	35, 38, 39, 40, 41	16, 17, 39, 40, 41, 73

*The total (TT_4), free (FT_4) T_4, T_3 (TT_3, FT_3), thyroxine-binding globulin (TBG), thyrotropin (TSH), T_3 plasma appearance rate (PAR), plasma clearance rate (PCR), distribution volume (V_d), and T_4 PAR are listed. Studies in a cold air challenge test, described as Chamber, or those carried out at thermoneutral temperatures, listed as Ambient, are categorized in the table. Subjects are described as never exposed to experimental cold testing (Initial), with repeated exposures to cold air in an environmental chamber (Multiple), or after cold exposure from their occupation or geographic relocation (Field). The general direction of the change is summarized as increased (↑), decreased (↓), no change (≈), or not available (NA). The comparisons of the changes are between conditions of either before and after the chamber studies, before and after the geographic relocation, or between cold-exposed and non–cold-exposed occupations. The possible time course is listed for the changes noted in the Field Ambient category to develop, the presence or absence of hypothermic cold adaptation is provided (Adapted), and the pooled references are indicated.

rectly exposed to outdoor temperatures.[31] Furthermore, energy intake is increased about 40% without a change in body weight when compared to measurements taken before deployment to Antarctica.[31,36,38,41] Because much of the 24-hour energy expenditure depends on skeletal muscle[42] and the T_3 pools are concentrated here, we focused our attention on T_3.[15] A decline in both serum FT_3 and body temperature is weakly correlated after extended Antarctic residence.[36] Additionally, the serum TSH response to TSH-releasing hormone (TRH) is augmented by about 50%,[41] yet it retains its sensitivity to oral T_3.[41] The unstimulated TSH increases logarithmically 30% to 50% above baseline after 2 to 4 months in Antarctica.[40] These changes in static measures are associated with more than a doubling in the T_3 V_d, PAR, and PCR.[38] Small changes in T_4 kinetics suggest a 17% decline in the T_4 V_d without an increase in the T_4 PAR.[38] A recent study confirmed a small decline in FT_4 (about 6%) and TT_4 (about 8%) during 10 serial monthly measurements in Antarctica.[40] We interpret these findings as a primary change in T_3 kinetics and distribution, initiating a chain of effects that replaces in an equal molar fashion about 17% of the T_4 pool with T_3 and thus more than doubling the T_3 pool[38]; hence the term polar T_3 syndrome.[16,36,38] The acquired increased T_3 PCR and cold adaptation seem independent[15] of low serum FT_4 and TSH, while the TSH response[41] that subsequently occurs[40] is insufficient to return FT_4 to basal concentrations.[40]

Military troops operating in circumpolar locations who are involved in physical exercise with marginal nutritional intake and partial sleep deprivation have declines in TT_3 and TT_4 regardless of their housing conditions.[39,43] The FT_4 may increase after 1 to 10 days[39,39a] but FT_3 and FT_4 decline after 60 days.[43] T_3 PCR and V_d are increased, and TSH is insufficient after 60 days to return FT_4 to predeployment concentrations.[40,43] The values and kinetics of T_3 and T_4 sulfur conjugates are unknown in this setting. Multifactorial influences such as undernutrition, sleep deprivation, and exercise possibly interact to produce an element of hypothyroxinemia that does not inhibit either the T_3 kinetic changes of cold exposure[15] or development of cold adaptation.[16,34]

POSSIBLE CELLULAR MECHANISMS

Recently, the human nuclear T_3 receptor maximum binding capacity has been reported to increase three- to fivefold when the circulating FT_4 concentrations are decreased during multiple cold exposures.[44] These findings support an interrelationship between small declines in circulating FT_4 during cold exposure and the possible expansion of T_3 V_d.[16,38,40] Human cytosolic T_3-binding proteins that show retained binding with cold[45] may help differentiate hormone delivery to tissue-specific sites during hypothermic cold adaptation.

Heat

PHYSIOLOGIC AND THYROID HORMONE RESPONSES TO HEAT EXPOSURE

Human physiologic adaptation to heat involves an expansion of the plasma compartment, increased rate of sweat loss, and changes in aldosterone, which have been well described.[2] In contrast to cold exposure, the human hypothalamic-pituitary-tissue axis during exposure to heat has been studied much less.

Thyroidal uptake of ^{131}I is decreased in warm environments[46] although some of this decrement may be accounted for by an expanded extracellular volume. Heat-naive subjects exposed to 60 minutes of 35°C air show an elevation in rectal temperature, a fall in TT_3, and an increase in rT_3 without changes in TT_4, suggesting a decrease in 5′-DI activity.[18] More recently, Saini and colleagues reported that although the nocturnal surge of TSH seems to be attenuated at 35°C, it was not statistically different, whereas 24-hour elevations in plasma renin activity (PRA) occurred during the 6 days of heat exposure.[2] The specific role of changing energy intake on peripheral T_3 metabolism during heat and cold adaptation is unknown for human beings.

EFFECTS OF ALTITUDE AND HYPOXIA

Individuals either residing at or being transported to high altitudes of 2315,[32] 3000,[47] 3500,[19] 3810,[48] 4300,[49,50] 5400,[51] and 6300[51] meters are exposed to graded changes in low partial pressures of oxygen, hypobaric conditions, cold temperatures, low relative humidity, increased ultraviolet radiation, high winds, and often excessive physical exertion during altitude acclimation.[4] Some studies have tried to isolate these factors by using hypobaric chamber experiments[19,47,48] and others have evaluated field conditions.[50–52]

Simulated Altitude in Environmental Chambers

Intermittent (4–8 h/d) exposure to simulated altitude in thermoneutral hypobaric environmental chambers has been reported.[19,47,48] These reports show that elevations of 3500 meters increase serum TT_4 and TT_3 concentrations[19] and thyroidal ^{131}I uptake[48] without changes in thyroxine-binding globulin (TBG).[19] Additionally, in these chamber studies, T_4 administration and subsequent TSH suppression do not appear to negate this increase in T_4 and T_3[19] (Table 14-2).

Altitude Field Studies

In a 5-day study in which subjects were transported rapidly to 2315 meters, they showed a mild hypoxic response of increased serum erythropoietin concentration; FT_4, FT_3, and TSH values remained unchanged.[32] Field studies conducted at higher elevations of 4300 meters[49,50] and 5400 to 6300 meters[51] showed elevations in serum TT_4, FT_4, and TT_3 without changes in FT_3, which are in general agreement with chamber studies.[19,48] A decreased peripheral T_4 conversion from undernutrition and excessive exercise[53] may modify the FT_3 response.[51] Changes in TBG are found in some[51] but not all[19] reports. Thyroidal ^{131}I uptake[49] and T_4 degradation[50] are increased at 4300 meters. At 5000 meters, serum TSH and a TRH challenge test of TSH are elevated over preascent responses[51] in contrast to that observed at lower elevations.[19] Changes in plasma volume and binding proteins cannot account for all the reported hormone elevation,[19] and some authors speculate a decrease in extravascular binding may occur.[52] The discordant responses of FT_4 and TSH at high altitudes support the concept that the hypothalamic-pituitary feedback of FT_4 may be altered near 5400 meters.[51] Possibilities to describe these findings would include an inhibition

TABLE 14-2.
Effects of Altitude on Thyroid Function*

	Altitude (m)					
	2315–3045	3500	3810	4300	5400	6300
TT_3	≈	↑(17%–80%)	NA	NA	↑(16%)	↑(12%)
FT_3	NA	NA	NA	NA	≈	≈
TT_4	≈	↑(70%–128%)	NA	↑(PAR)	↑(27%)	↑(44%)
FT_4	NA	NA	NA	NA	↑(28%)	↑(28%)
$T_4{:}T_3$	≈	↑	NA	NA	↑	↑
TSH	≈	≈	NA	NA	↑(69%)	↑(50%)
TSH_{TRH}	NA	NA	NA	NA	NA	↑(~60%)
TBG	NA	≈	NA	NA	↑(23%)	↑(19%)
$RAIU_{24h}$	NA	NA	↑(80%–100%)	↑(50%)	NA	NA
References	32, 47	19	48	49, 50	51	51

*The thyroid hormone responses to altitude that are derived from hypobaric chamber studies and field conditions are listed. The abbreviations in this table are the same as those used in the text and in Table 14-1. In addition, the $T_4{:}T_3$ ratio, TSH response to a TRH stimulus (TSH_{TRH}), and 24-hour thyroidal radioiodine uptake ($RAIU_{24h}$) are listed.

of pituitary 5′-D type II activity, as well as possible peripheral contributions by decreased activity of 5′-DI from exercise-mediated undernutrition.[53,54]

EFFECTS OF MICROGRAVITY AND EXAGGERATED GRAVITY

Acceleration is a special physiologic stimulus that results in impaired cerebral blood flow when the inertial vector is in a head-to-foot direction ($+G_z$).[55] A human centrifuge can isolate this stimulus from other aviation-related conditions such as hypoxia and microgravity.[5,55] Serum TSH does not change with about 1 minute of 1 to 6 G_z stress.[55] This degree of G_z stimulus decreases plasma volume[55] and is accompanied by an increase in PRA and serum T_4 without changes in T_3.[5]

Microgravity is encountered routinely on space shuttle flights,[6] and a G stress of between 1 and 3 has been documented for Apollo flights during re-entry into the earth's atmosphere.[20] Flights lasting between 8 and 13 days with microgravity, hyperoxia, and re-entry G exposures are associated with an elevated serum TT_4 and FT_4 index. These elevated values, obtained 2 hours after an ocean landing, do not appear to result from a decreased plasma volume, and they gradually returned to preflight concentrations over 14 days.[20] More information is needed to better understand the thyroidal influences from the combinations of microgravity and excess gravitation encountered during routine space travel.[6]

EFFECTS OF EXERCISE

Physical training is associated with a rapid net energy expenditure[56] that results in a negative energy balance unless nutrient intake is increased.[53] The threshold for developing the low T_3 syndrome of undernutrition has been recently documented in a series of elaborate studies.[53] Four-day energy expenditures with small deficits in energy availability will lower FT_3 about 9% and, with further negative energy balance, will show an increase in FT_4 by 11% and in rT_3 by 22%. This situation is similar to brief periods of energy restriction without exercise where small decreases in energy intake will reduce serum T_3,[24] although the exact role of 5′-DI when exercise and undernutrition interact is unclear.[21,24,37,53,54] Strenuous 7-day weight training protocols in men are associated with declines in T_4, T_3, and TSH, as well as a declining trend in FT_4.[57]

During a 6-week aerobic training session using male subjects, T_3 PAR increased about 10%, PCR increased about 9%, and body weight did not change.[21] In contrast, T_4 degradation rate was decreased about 9% during this training and FT_4 tended to decline by about 7%, but did not reach a level of significance. These results are at variance with an earlier study that showed an increase in T_4 degradation when athletes were compared to sedentary controls.[58] Unfortunately, because the earlier study was carried out for only 48 hours, the duration was insufficient for accurate kinetic estimates.[58] Recently, male athletes were found to have a 30% increase in T_3 PAR, PCR, and V_d with no difference in serum TT_3, TT_4, and TSH when compared to sedentary controls[59] (Table 14-3).

Serum values of thyroid hormones have been used in a serial fashion to examine acute effects of exercise,[56] and static values have been used for contrasting groups of athletic and sedentary men[59,60] and women.[54] During 3.5 hours of bicycle exercise, T_3 will decrease and rT_3 will rise, a change that is blunted with glucose infusion.[56] Athletic men do not show dramatic changes in T_4, T_3, or TSH,[59,60] whereas women, depending on their menstrual and gonadal status, have decreases in TT_4, FT_4, TT_3, and FT_3 when compared with gender-specific sedentary controls.[54] TSH stimulation by TRH is not different in trained men,[60] but may be blunted in women with hypothalamic-pituitary-ovarian dysfunction who chronically engage in high-volume athletic training.[54]

TABLE 14-3.
Effects of Exercise and Nutrition on Thyroid Hormones*

	↑ Energy Intake†	↓ Energy Intake‡	Exercise and ↓ Energy Intake	Exercise and Balanced Energy Intake§
TT_3	↑ (≈)	↓↓	↓	≈(↓)
FT_3	↑	↓↓	↓	≈(↓)
rT_3	↓ (↓)	↑ (↑)	↑	≈(↓)
TT_4	≈(≈)	≈(≈/↓)	↑	≈(↓)
FT_4	NA(≈)	↑(↑)	↑	≈(↓)
TSH	≈(≈)	≈(↓)	≈	≈(↓)
T_3PAR	↑	↓↓	NA	↑
T_3PCR	↑	↓	NA	↑
T_3V_d	↑	NA	NA	↑
T_4PAR	≈	≈/↓	NA	↓
T_4PCR	≈	≈/↓	NA	≈
rT_3PCR	↑↑	↓↓	NA	NA
Weight	↑	↓	↓	≈
References	24	24, 37	53	21, 54, 59

*The abbreviations are similar to those in Table 14-1 and 14-2. In addition, indicators within parentheses identify special situations
†Extended overnutrition for 3–7 months
‡Extended fasting for 14 days
§Amenorrheic athletic women

Exercise is therefore associated with increased energy requirements that, if unsatisfied, reduce serum T_3 and elevate rT_3 possibly through decreased peripheral 5'-DI activity. However, the increased energy requirements during metabolic balance are associated with increased T_3 PAR and PCR that are similar, but not identical, to overfeeding studies[24] (see Table 14-3). Furthermore, hypothalamic-pituitary-thyroid axis changes with excessive exercise may be found in amenorrheic women without comparable data for hypogonadal men.

EFFECTS OF PHOTOPERIOD, SLEEP, AND CIRCADIAN RHYTHMS

The circadian pattern of TSH appears as a combination of the ultradian rhythm[61] and influences such as sleep,[22,23] photoperiod,[3] and serum T_4 and T_3.[62] This circadian TSH oscillation is linked closely with the body temperature rhythm[3] and regulated in part by TRH.[63] Body temperature is symmetrically out of phase with TSH where the peak TSH and trough temperature occur at 2400 to 0400 hours and the trough TSH and peak body temperature occur at 1400 to 1600 hours.[3] The nocturnal surge in TSH is about 70%[3,28,61] over the 24-hour mean, whereas the ratio of T_3:T_4 has a nocturnal rise of 8%.[64] Furthermore, the changing T_3:T_4 ratio is eliminated by fasting and unaltered by T_4 administration sufficient to suppress TSH, suggesting a peripheral mechanism for this rhythm unrelated to TSH.[64] The TSH and body temperature rhythm can be reset by a pulse of light (5000 lux)[3] and sleep can suppress the circadian peak TSH value by 25% to 30%.[22] Both total and partial sleep deprivation will elevate TSH, TT_4, FT_4,

and TT_3, although the patterns are slightly different with the degree of deprivation.[22,23]

EFFECTS OF CIRCANNUAL RHYTHMS

Midlatitude residents who are exposed to changing patterns of light and temperature demonstrate physiologic and endocrine seasonal rhythms for cerebral[8] and myocardial infarct,[8] blood pressure,[10] serum cholesterol,[7] calcium metabolism,[11] growth hormone profiles,[12] female gonadal hormones,[13] and mood disorder.[65]

TSH Seasonal Rhythm in Hypothyroid and Euthyroid Subjects

The TSH response to TRH increases during the winter in hypothyroid patients taking a fixed dose of replacement T_4.[9,66] In early studies, euthyroid subjects have not been reported to show increased serum TSH or TRH-stimulated TSH during the winter season.[17] Likewise, in another study where pooled groups were used, the intersubject variation was large and no seasonal difference in TSH was found.[67] However, when 24-hour circadian patterns were studied in the same elderly (77 ± 7 years) euthyroid females during each of four seasonal samplings, the serum TSH displayed a clear circannual pattern, but this was not seen in men near the same age.[68] Only recently has this issue been clarified with a study of 8310 euthyroid subjects, stratified by age and gender.[69] In this study, Italian men and women, greater than 41 years of age, showed a circannual cosinor TSH peak in December that increased about

30% over the trough summer measure. Subjects under age 41, however, showed no circannual TSH pattern.[69]

T_4 and T_3 Seasonal Rhythm in Euthyroid and Hypothyroid Subjects

It is unknown whether these circannual patterns of TSH are a primary response of the hypothalamic-pituitary axis to changing light and temperature or whether they reflect small declines in serum total[9] and FT_4 as seen in patients on fixed T_4 replacement[9,66] or in normal subjects transported to polar regions.[36,38,40] Early investigations of T_3 and T_4 describe a serum T_3 elevation, urinary T_3 elevation,[70] or no change in serum T_3 during the winter months,[17] with little change in T_4 during the same time and no circannual pattern of FT_4.[69] These observations suggested to Fregly a possible increased peripheral conversion of T_4 in winter.[17] Our own preliminary kinetic studies suggest that T_3 PCR and PAR increase by about 30% from summer troughs to winter peaks, even though the serum TT_3, TT_4, FT_3, and FT_4 values remain nearly unchanged during these seasons.[71]

Circannual Changes of Thyroidal Size and Iodine Content

The intrathyroidal iodine content studied in Belgian subjects, using x-ray fluorescence, has a cosinor peak in April and a trough in September.[72] The approximate 40% increase in these subjects' thyroidal iodine during April was not thought to be from differences in dietary iodine between winter and summer.[72] Thyroidal size in euthyroid Danish men measured with serial ultrasounds increased by about 23% from summer to winter without a change in serum T_4, T_3, and TSH levels.[73] In a later publication[67] these same Danish subjects[73] were reported to have reduced serum thyroglobulin in winter when their gland size was enlarged over the summer measures.[67] The interpretation of this observation is uncertain and a better understanding will require further studies.

References

1. Bittel J. The different types of general cold adaptation in man. Int J Sports Med 1992;13:S172
2. Saini J, Brandenberger G, Libert JP, Follenius M. Nocturnal pituitary hormone and renin profiles during chronic heat exposure. J Appl Physiol 1993;75:294
3. Allan JS, Czeisler CA. Persistence of the circadian thyrotropin rhythm under constant conditions and after light-induced shifts of circadian phase. J Clin Endocrinol Metab 1994;79:508
4. West JB. Human physiology at extreme altitudes on Mount Everest. Science 1984;223:784
5. Vangelova KK, Zlatev RZ, Changes in some biochemical and physiological indexes after hypergravity. Rev Environ Health 1994;10:33
6. Stein TP, Schluter MD. Excretion of IL-6 by astronauts during spaceflight. Am J Physiol 1994;266:E448
7. Gordon DJ, Trost DC, Hyde J, et al. Seasonal cholesterol cycles: the lipid research clinics coronary primary prevention trial placebo group. Circulation 1987;76:1224
8. Keatinge WR, Coleshaw SR, Holmes J. Changes in seasonal mortalities with improvement in home heating in England and Wales from 1964 to 1984. J Biometeorol 1989;33:71
9. Konno N, Morikawa K. Seasonal variation of serum thyrotropin concentration and thyrotropin response to thyrotropin-releasing hormone in patients with primary hypothyroidism on constant replacement dose of thyroxine. J Clin Endocrinol Metab 1982;54:1118
10. Tanaka S, Konno A, Hashimoto A, et al. The influence of cold temperature on the progression of hypertension: an epidemiological study. J Hypertension 1989;7(suppl 1):S49
11. Dawson-Hughes B, Dallal GE, Krall EA, et al. Effect of vitamin D supplementation on wintertime and overall bone loss in healthy postmenopausal women. Ann Intern Med 1991;115:505
12. Malarkey WB, Hall JC, Pearl DK, et al. The influence of academic stress and season on 24-hour concentrations of growth hormone and prolactin. J Clin Endocrinol Metab 1991;73:1089
13. Ronkainen H, Pakarinen A, Kirkinen P, Kauppila A. Physical exercise-induced changes and season-associated differences in the pituitary-ovarian function of runners and joggers. J Clin Endocrinol Metab 1985;60:416
14. Petrie K, Conaglen JV, Thompson L, Chamberlain K. Effect of melatonin on jet lag after long haul flights. Br Med J 1989;298:705
15. Reed HL, D'Alesandro MM, Kowalski KR, Homer LD. Multiple cold air exposures change oral triiodothyronine kinetics in normal men. Am J Physiol 1992;263:E85
16. Savourey G, Caravel J, Barnavol B, Bittel JHM. Thyroid hormone changes in a cold air environment after local cold acclimation. J Appl Physiol 1994;76:1963
17. Fregly MJ. Activity of the hypothalamic-pituitary-thyroid axis during exposure to cold. Pharmacol Ther 1989;41:85
18. Epstein Y, Udassin R, Sack J. Serum 3,5,3'-triiodothyronine and 3,3',5'-triiodothyronine concentrations during acute heat load. J Clin Endocrinol Metab 1979;49:677
19. Sawhney RC, Malhotra AS. Thyroid function in sojourners and acclimatised low landers at high altitude in man. Horm Metab Res 1991;23:81
20. Sheinfeld M, Leach CS, Johnson PC. Plasma thyroxine changes of the Apollo Crewmen. Aviat Space Environ Med 1975;46:47
21. Balsam A, Leppo LE. Effect of physical training on the metabolism of thyroid hormones in man. J Appl Physiol 1975;38:212
22. Baumgartner A, Dietzel M, Saletu B, et al. Influence of partial sleep deprivation on the secretion of thyrotropin, thyroid hormones, growth hormone, prolactin, luteinizing hormone, follicular stimulating hormone, and estradiol in healthy women. Psychiatry Res 1993;48:153
23. Parker DC, Rossman LG, Pekary AE, Hershman JM. Effect of 64-hour sleep deprivation on the circadian waveform of thyrotropin (TSH): further evidence of sleep-related inhibition of TSH release. J Clin Endocrinol Metab 1987;64:157
24. Danforth E, Burger AG. The impact of nutrition on thyroid hormone physiology and action. Annu Rev Nutr 1989;9:201
25. Greenspan SL, Klibanski A, Rowe JW, Elahi D. Age-related alterations in pulsatile secretion of TSH: role of dopaminergic regulation. Am J Physiol 1991;260:E486
26. Burrow GN, Fisher DA, Larsen PR. Maternal and fetal thyroid function. N Engl J Med 1994;331:1072
27. Kaptein EM, Robinson WJ, Grieb DA, Nicoloff JT. Peripheral serum thyroxine, triiodothyronine and reverse triiodothyronine kinetics in the low thyroxine state of acute nonthyroidal illnesses. A noncompartmental analysis. J Clin Invest 1982;69:526
28. Romijn JA, Wiersinga WM. Decreased nocturnal surge of thyrotropin in nonthyroidal illness. J Clin Endocrinol Metab 1990;70:35
29. Bartalena L, Placidi GF, Martino E, et al. Nocturnal serum thyrotropin (TSH) surge and the TSH response to TSH-releasing hormone: dissociated behavior in untreated depressives. J Clin Endocrinol Metab 1990;71:650
30. Safran M, Paul TL, Roti E, Braverman LE. Environmental factors affecting autoimmune thyroid disease. Endocrinol Metab Clin N Am 1987;16:327
31. Campbell IT. Nutrition in adverse environments. 2. Energy balance under polar conditions. Hum Nutr Appl Nutr 1982;36A:165

32. Hanns-Christian G, Kirsch K, Röcker L, Schobersberger W. Time course of erythropoietin, triiodothyronine, thyroxine, and thyroid stimulating hormone at 2,315 m. J Appl Physiol 1994;76:1068

33. Silva JE, Larsen PR. Potential of brown adipose tissue type II thyroxine 5'-deiodinase as a local and systemic source of triiodothyronine in rats. J Clin Invest 1985;76:2296

34. Hesslink RL, D'Alesandro MM, Armstrong DW, Reed HL. Human cold air habituation is independent of thyroxine and thyrotropin. J Appl Physiol 1992;72:2134

35. Solter M, Brkic K, Petek M, et al. Thyroid hormone economy in response to extreme cold exposure in healthy factory workers. J Clin Endocrinol Metab 1989;68:168

36. Reed HL, Brice D, Shakir KM, et al. Decreased free fraction of thyroid hormones after prolonged Antarctic residence. J Appl Physiol 1990;69:1467

37. LoPresti JS, Gray D, Nicoloff JT. Influence of fasting and refeeding on 3,3',5'-triiodothyronine metabolism in man. J Clin Endocrinol Metab 1991;72:130

38. Reed HL, Silverman ED, Shakir KM, et al. Changes in serum triiodothyronine (T_3) kinetics after prolonged antarctic residence: the polar T_3 syndrome. J Clin Endocrinol Metab 1990;70:965

39. Hackney AC, Hodgdon JA. Thyroid hormone changes during military field operations: effects of cold exposure in the Arctic. Aviat Space Environ Med 1992;63:606

39a. Hackney AC, Hodgon JA, Hesslink R, Trygg K. Thyroid hormone responses to military winter exercises in the Arctic region. Arcti Med Res 1995;54:82

40. Harford RR, Reed HL, Morris MT, et al. Relationship between changes in serum thyrotropin and total and lipoprotein cholesterol with prolonged Antarctic residence. Metabolism 1993;42:1159

41. Reed HL, Ferreiro JA, Shakir KM, et al. Pituitary and peripheral hormone responses to T_3 administration during Antarctic residence. Am J Physiol 1988;254:E733

42. Zurol F, Larson K, Bogardus C, Ravussin E. Skeletal muscle metabolism is a major determinant of resting energy expenditure. J Clin Invest 1990;86:1423

43. Kowalski K, Reed L, Lopez A, et al. Changes in energy intake and triiodothyronine (T_3) kinetics with extended Arctic winter operations (abstract). FASEB J 1991;4:A393

44. D'Alesandro MM, Malik M, Reed HL, Homer LD. Changes in triiodothyronine (T_3) mononuclear leukocyte receptor kinetics after T_3 administration and multiple cold air exposures. Receptor 1994;4:259

45. Fanjul AN, Farias RN. Novel cold-sensitive cytosolic 3,5,3'-triiodo-L-thyronine-binding proteins in human red blood cell. J Biol Chem 1991;266:16145

46. Lewitus Z, Hasenfrantz J, Toor M, et al. [131]I uptake studies under hot climatic conditions. J Clin Endocrinol Metab 1964;24:1084

47. Vaernes RJ, Owe JO, Myking O. Central nervous reactions to a 6.5-hour altitude exposure at 3048 meters. Aviat Space Environ Med 1984;55:921

48. Rawal SB, Singh MV, Tyagi AK, Chaudhuri BN. Thyroidal handling of radioiodine in sea level residents exposed to hypobaric hypoxia. Eur J Nucl Med 1993;20:16

49. Moncola F, Guerra-García R, Subauste C, et al. Endocrine studies at high altitude. I. Thyroid function in sea level natives exposed for two weeks to altitude of 4300 meters. J Clin Endocrinol Metab 1966;26:1237

50. Surks MI, Beckwitt HJ, Chidsey CA. Changes in plasma thyroxine concentration and metabolism, catecholamine excretion and basal oxygen consumption in man during acute exposure to high altitude. J Clin Endocrinol Metab 1967;27:789

51. Mordes JP, Blume FD, Boyer S, et al. High-altitude pituitary-thyroid dysfunction on Mount Everest. N Engl J Med 1983;308:1135

52. Rastogi GK, Malhotra MS, Srivastava MC, et al. Study of the pituitary-thyroid functions at high altitude in man. J Clin Endocrinol Metab 1977;44:447

53. Loucks AB, Heath EM. Induction of low-T_3 syndrome in exercising women occurs at a threshold of energy availability. Am J Physiol 1994;266:R817

54. Loucks AB, Laughlin GA, Mortola JF, et al. Hypothalamic-pituitary-thyroidal function in eumenorrheic and amenorrheic athletes. J Clin Endocrinol Metab 1992;75:514

55. Mills FJ, Marks V. Human endocrine responses to acceleration stress. Aviat Space Environ Med 1982;53:537

56. O'Connell M, Robbins DC, Horton ES, et al. Changes in serum concentrations of 3,3',5'-triiodothyronine and 3,5,3'-triiodothyronine during prolonged moderate exercise. J Clin Endocrinol Metab 1979;49:242

57. Pakarinen A, Häkkinen K, Alen M. Serum thyroid hormones, thyrotropin and thyroxine binding globulin in elite athletes during very intense strength training of one week. J Sports Med Phys Fitness 1991;31:142

58. Irvine CHG. Effects of exercise on thyroxine degradation in athletes and non-athletes. J Clin Endocrinol Metab 1968;28:942

59. Rone JK, Dons RF, Reed HL. The effect of endurance training on serum triiodothyronine kinetics in man: physical conditioning marked by enhanced thyroid hormone metabolism. Clin Endocrinol (Oxf) 1992;37:325

60. Smallridge RC, Whorton NE, Burman KD, Ferguson EW. Effects of exercise and physical fitness on the pituitary-thyroid axis and on prolactin secretion in male runners. Metabolism 1985;34:949

61. Samuels MH, Veldhuis JD, Henry P, Ridgway EC. Pathophysiology of pulsatile and copulsatile release of thyroid-stimulating hormone, luteinizing hormone, follicle-stimulating hormone, and α-subunit. J Clin Endocrinol Metab 1990;71:425

62. Brabant G, Brabant A, Ranft U, et al. Circadian and pulsatile thyrotropin secretion in euthyroid man under the influence of thyroid hormone and glucocorticoid administration. J Clin Endocrinol Metab 1987;65:83

63. Brabant G, Prank K, Hoang-Vu C, et al. Hypothalamic regulation of pulsatile thyrotropin secretion. J Clin Endocrinol Metab 1991;72:145

64. Nimalasuriya A, Spencer CA, Lin SC, et al. Studies on the diurnal pattern of serum 3,5,3'-triiodothyronine. J Clin Endocrinol Metab 1986;62:153

65. Wehr TA, Rosenthal NE. Seasonality and affective illness. Am J Psychiatry 1989;146:829

66. Hamada N, Ohno M, Morii H, et al. Is it necessary to adjust the replacement dose of thyroid hormone to the season in patients with hypothyroidism? Metabolism 1984;33:215

67. Feldt-Rasmussen U, Hegedüs L, Perrild H, et al. Relationship between serum thyroglobulin, thyroid volume and serum TSH in healthy non-goitrous subjects and the relationship to seasonal variations in iodine intake. Thyroidology 1989;3:115

68. Nicolau GY, Lakatua D, Sackett-Lundeen L, Haus E. Circadian and circannual rhythms of hormonal variables in elderly men and women. Chronobiol Int 1984;1:301

69. Simoni M, Velardo A, Montanini V, et al. Circannual rhythm of plasma thyrotropin in middle-aged and old euthyroid subjects. Hormone Res 1990;33:184

70. Rastogi GK, Sawhney RC. Thyroid function in changing weather in a subtropical region. Metabolism 1976;25:903

71. Reed HL, D'Alesandro MM, Kowalski KR, et al. Circannual cycling of triiodothyronine kinetics in normal subjects (abstract). Program and Abstracts Book of the Endocrine Society. 73rd Annual Meeting 1991;341:1244

72. Jonckheer M, Coomans D, Broeckaert I, et al. Seasonal variation of stable intrathyroidal iodine in nontoxic goiter disclosed by x-ray fluorescence. J Endocrinol Invest 1982;5:27

73. Hegedüs L, Rasmussen N, Knudsen N. Seasonal variation in thyroid size in healthy males. Horm Metab Res 1987;19:391

ANTITHYROID COMPOUNDS

William L. Green

A variety of compounds can inhibit thyroid hormone synthesis in vivo at doses that do not have major adverse effects on other organ systems. When given to animals or human beings, they are "goitrogens," that is, their administration can lead to decreased levels of circulating thyroid hormones, resulting in activation of thyroid-stimulating hormone (TSH) secretion and hence to thyroid enlargement or goiter. When the blockade of synthesis is incomplete, secretion of hormone by the TSH-stimulated gland may be sufficient to maintain eumetabolism. When the block is more severe, compensation fails and goiter is accompanied by hypothyroidism. Antithyroid compounds can be classified according to which step in hormone synthesis and secretion they affect. As Table 14-4 indicates, agents are available that will inhibit each of the steps in thyroidal iodine metabolism outlined in chapter 4 and the subchapter below and that can mimic several of the inborn errors in hormone synthesis described in chapter 56.

Other agents can affect thyroid function indirectly by producing changes in the peripheral metabolism of the thyroid hormones or antagonizing their action; examples are also given in Table 14-4. Although these peripheral effects are not a common cause of clinical goiter, they have been of great physiologic interest and may complicate the treatment of hypothyroidism.

Several goitrogens have proved effective in the treatment of hyperthyroidism; their clinical use is discussed in chapter 53. Antithyroid actions may also result from drugs used for other therapeutic indications or from some environmental toxins, and these will be mentioned. Iodide, because of the special interest in its effects, is the subject of a separate section of this chapter.

In rodents, chronic administration of antithyroid agents can lead not only to hyperplasia but also to thyroid tumors,[1,2] and these compounds appear in some lists of possible carcinogens. However, the weight of evidence is that the tumorigenic stimulus is chronic TSH stimulation, because tumors can also result from iodine deficiency, and can be prevented by thyroid hormone treatment.[2,3] Finally, human beings seem less susceptible to this mechanism of tumor formation; although iodine deficiency goiter is relatively common, it is not epidemiologically related to thyroid cancer.[1,3]

The subject of environmental goitrogenesis has been recently reviewed,[4] and there are several reviews of drug effects on thyroid hormone metabolism.[3,5,6]

COMPLEX ANIONS

Iodide is actively transported in the thyroid gland, and normal thyroid tissue can maintain iodide concentrations much higher than those in plasma. The same active transport mechanism will accept other monovalent anions whose partial molal ionic volume is similar to that of iodide.[7] Thus, perchlorate (ClO_4^-), pertechnetate (TcO_4^-), perrhenate (ReO_4^-), and tetrafluorobo-

---

TABLE 14-4.
Antithyroid Compounds

Process Affected	Examples of Inhibitors
INTRATHYROID IODINE METABOLISM	
Active transport of iodide	Complex anions: ClO_4^-, TcO_4^-, thiocyanate
Iodination of thyroglobulin	Thionamides: propylthiouracil, methimazole, carbimazole
	Thiocyanate
	Aniline derivatives: sulfonamides
	Substituted phenols: resorcinol
	Iodide
Coupling reaction	Thionamides, other inhibitors of iodinations
	Minocycline
	Lithium salts
Hormone release	Iodide
	Lithium salts
Iodotyrosine deiodination	Nitrotyrosines
PERIPHERAL HORMONE DISPOSAL	
Iodothyronine deiodination	Thiouracil derivatives
	Oral cholecystographic agents
	Amiodarone
Hormone excretion or inactivation	Inducers of hepatic drug-metabolizing enzymes: phenobarbital, phenytoin, carbamazepine, rifampicin
Hormone action	?Phenytoin
	Amiodarone

rate (BF_4^-) can be concentrated by the thyroid and are competitive inhibitors of iodide transport; unlike iodide, these anions do not undergo significant metabolic transformation in the gland. These properties have made TcO_4^-, labeled with the short-lived gamma-emitting isotope ^{99m}Tc, a useful agent for studying thyroid function in human beings; the uptake of $^{99m}TcO_4^-$ indicates the activity of the iodide transport mechanism, and distribution of the isotope on scintiscan localizes functioning thyroid tissue.[8,9] These anions also competitively inhibit the active transport of iodide. The order of affinity for the iodide-concentrating mechanism is as follows[7]:

$$TcO_4^- > ClO_4^- > ReO_4^- > BF_4^- > I^-.$$

Presumably this order reflects affinity for a carrier. It was once postulated that the carrier is an anion-binding phospholipid,[10] but it has long been clear that transport of ions and small molecules across cell membranes is mediated by intrinsic membrane proteins.[11] Because iodide transport depends on maintenance of an extracellular/intracellular Na^+ gradient by the Na^+/K^+ ATPase, a model system for I^- accumulation has been proposed in which I^- is cotransported with Na^+ by a membrane carrier.[12] There is now considerable evidence for the Na^+/I^- symport model, but the putative symporter protein has not been fully characterized.[11,13]

When iodine intake is normal or low, these anions can inhibit iodine accumulation so markedly that goiter and hypothyroidism result. When iodine intake is high, however, sufficient iodide can enter the gland by simple diffusion to permit normal rates of hormone synthesis. ClO_4^- is an effective agent in the treatment of clinical hyperthyroidism, but it has not been widely used because of reports of serious toxic reactions, especially aplastic anemia.[14] However, the drug has proven effective in treating the hyperthyroidism that occasionally occurs in patients receiving the iodine-rich antiarrhythmic agent, amiodarone. A major obstacle to effective treatment of this condition is high intrathyroidal iodide levels that may persist for months after discontinuing amiodarone but that can be lowered by ClO_4^-. In one study, the combination of ClO_4^- and methimazole (MMI) was much more effective than MMI alone; the doses of ClO_4^- used, 1 g or less daily, have not been associated with serious side effects.[15] Amiodarone treatment may also cause hypothyroidism; the hypothesis that this also is secondary to high intrathyroidal iodide levels is supported by reports that hypothyroidism is relieved by treatment with perchlorate.[16] The effects of amiodarone on thyroid function and the peripheral metabolism of the thyroid hormones are discussed in detail in following subchapters.

Iodide concentrated in the thyroid is in equilibrium with extracellular iodide, and there is a net loss of iodide from the thyroid when transport is blocked. Normally, organification of transported iodide is so rapid that the thyroid inorganic iodide pool is small, and relatively little iodide leaves the gland when ClO_4^- is administered. Conversely, a large loss of thyroid iodide after ClO_4^- administration implies that organification is inefficient, owing to an inherent defect or to an inhibitor of iodinations. In clinical diagnosis, the "perchlorate discharge test," which assesses whether previously accumulated radioiodine is rapidly lost from the gland when ClO_4^- is given, can be used to determine whether inefficiency of iodide organification is present.[17] The sensitivity of the test is increased if a

potassium iodide supplement is given with the radioiodine tracer.[18,19]

THIOCYANATE

Thiocyanate (SCN^-) is also a potent inhibitor of iodide transport and has a molecular size similar to that of other transport inhibitors.[7,10] However, it differs in several respects from the complex anions already discussed. First, it is not concentrated by thyroid tissue.[20] Second, it has a more marked effect on iodide efflux in vivo,[21] and in plasma membranes in vitro,[22] where it engages in countertransport with iodide.[23] Third, it is actively metabolized by thyroid tissue.[24,25] Fourth, SCN^- is an inhibitor of organic iodinations at concentrations only slightly greater than those that inhibit iodide transport.[26,27] It has been proposed that SCN^-, in addition to inhibiting iodide transport, is a competitive substrate for the thyroid peroxidase (TPO), explaining both its biotransformation and its ability to inhibit iodination. Indeed, SCN^- can substitute for iodide in two iodide-catalyzed reactions of TPO: the oxidation of thionamides, discussed below, and the coupling of iodotyrosines to form iodothyronines.[28,29]

Thiocyanate is normally present in body fluids, and cigarette smoking can increase its concentration, via detoxification of the cyanide in smoke, to levels potentially capable of affecting the thyroid.[27,30] There is increased goiter incidence in smokers, without depression of serum thyroid hormone levels or elevations of TSH.[31,32] However, smokers with subclinical evidence of decreased hypothyroidism have higher serum TSH levels and evidence of peripheral thyroid hormone action than nonsmokers.[32a] Smoking during pregnancy may affect the fetal thyroid; cord serum thiocyanate levels correlate both with maternal smoking habits and with thyroid volume/birthweight ratios.[33] The effects of smoking on the thyroid were recently reviewed.[34] Thiocyanate is a metabolite of nitroprusside, and one case of hypothyroidism associated with prolonged nitroprusside therapy and increased SCN^- levels has been reported.[35] In a series of patients receiving nitroprusside, high SCN^- levels, which were particularly likely to occur in patients with renal failure, were associated with low thyroxine (T_4) levels.[36]

Thiocyanate is a metabolic product of glucosinolates, compounds that are found in various vegetable foods, such as cabbage, broccoli, turnips, and rapeseed. Also, the so-called cyanogenic glucosides, found in cassava, lima beans, and sweet potatoes, can be a source of cyanide that is detoxified to thiocyanate. The goitrogenic potential of thiocyanate and of these foods has recently been discussed at length[37]; cassava ingestion resulting in high serum SCN^- levels may be a factor in at least one goiter endemic, in Zaire.[38]

THIONAMIDES

A family of compounds that share the thionamide grouping, S4CN4 inhibit the organification of iodide. The most potent are thioureylenes, defined by the grouping below:

$$S=C\left\langle \begin{array}{l} N= \\ N= \end{array} \right.$$

Examples are shown in Figure 14-1. Propylthiouracil (PTU), MMI, and carbimazole are often used in the treatment of hyperthyroidism. Goitrin is of special interest, because it was first isolated from plants of the genus *Brassicae* (rutabaga, turnip, cabbage), and thus is a naturally occurring goitrogen.[39] A goiter endemic in Finland has been attributed to the presence of goitrin in milk.[40] Antithyroid activity has also been reported for two widely used drugs that contain thionamide groupings, ethionamide and 6-mercaptopurine.[41–43] None of the foregoing agents inhibits iodide transport, and their administration results in accumulation of perchlorate-dischargeable iodide. In rats, graded doses of PTU affect each step in hormone synthesis beyond iodide transport, the order of susceptibility being the coupling of iodotyrosines to form iodothyronines (most susceptible); then iodination of monoiodotyrosine to form diiodotyrosine; then iodination of tyrosine to form monoiodotyrosine.[44] Selective inhibition of coupling by PTU has also been demonstrated in cell-free preparations of thyroid tissue in vitro.[45] This dose-response sequence may characterize most agents that inhibit organic iodinations and may explain why some hyperthyroid patients become euthyroid during treatment with PTU even though radioiodine uptake by the thyroid remains high. Presumably, the high uptake in these cases chiefly reflects synthesis of iodotyrosines, iodothyronine synthesis being normal because of partial inhibition of the coupling reaction.[46]

The biochemical mechanism for the inhibitory actions of the thionamides has been explored by several investigators. Major contributions have been made by Taurog, who reviews this area in chapter 4. In brief, binding of iodine to tyrosyl residues in thyroglobulin and the coupling of iodotyrosyl residues to form iodothyronines are catalyzed by TPO, and the thionamide drugs are inhibitors of these peroxidatic reactions. Thionamide drugs can be metabolized by peroxidases; iodide (or SCN^-; see above) is required for these reactions, in which disulfides and further oxidation products are formed.[47,48] It has been proposed that thionamide oxidation is coupled to reduction of the "active iodine" once presumed to be the iodinium ion, I^+, but recently said to be a free radical[49] formed by peroxidation of iodide, a reduction that prevents binding of the iodine to tyrosine.[28,47] Formation of a charge

transfer complex between thionamide and iodine may be involved.[50] This provides a mechanism for reversible inhibition of iodinations; by appropriate adjustment of the concentrations of peroxide, iodide, and thionamide, conditions can be created in which inhibition of iodinations persists only until the thionamide has been degraded. However, in the absence of iodide, or at low iodide/thionamide ratios, the thionamide can react directly with the enzyme and cause irreversible inhibition or inactivation;[47,50] one postulated sequence is S-oxygenation of the inhibitor followed by covalent binding to the enzyme's prosthetic heme group.[51] The situation in man has not been studied directly, and it is uncertain whether the usual dosage regimens for PTU and MMI result in reversible inhibition or in inactivation of the human TPO.

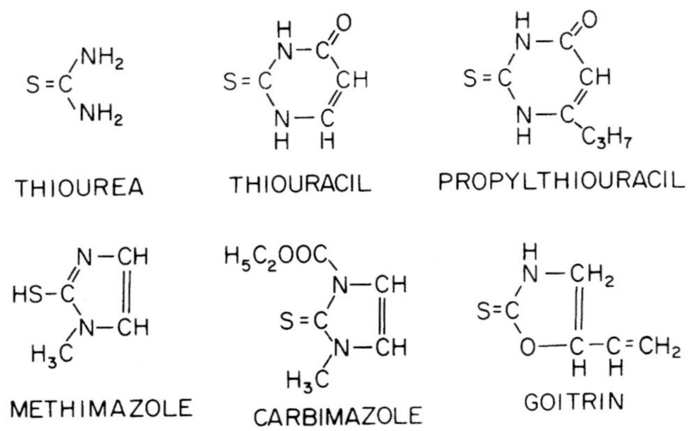

Although it can be regarded as the parent compound for other thioureylenes, thiourea differs from PTU and other related thionamides in several respects. It does not inhibit guaiacol oxidation, one standard assay for peroxidase, and does not cause inactivation of TPO. Its ability to inhibit organic iodinations, then, is due primarily to the reversible mechanism, reduction of active iodine, discussed above. Also, unlike the cyclic thioureylenes, which are metabolized to inactive products by peroxidases, thiourea is converted, via disulfide formation and decomposition, to cyanamide, NH_2CN, a compound that can inhibit peroxidase directly, and that has been shown to have goitrogenic properties in vivo.[52,53] Cyanamide also has disulfiram-like properties, and has been used to treat chronic alcoholism. In one therapeutic trial, it had no effect on thyroid function in euthyroid subjects, but did cause hypothyroidism in one subject with reduced thyroid function.[54]

Thionamides have several other actions. Their important effects on the coupling reaction are discussed below. Some thionamides, such as thiouracil and PTU, but not MMI, inhibit the deiodination of thyroid hormones. There have been several studies of effects on thyroglobulin synthesis, with a confusing set of findings. One group finds that MMI stimulates formation of both thyroglobulin and its mRNA, and that this effect is inhibited by PTU[55]; another finds that MMI and PTU have similar stimulatory effects on thyroglobulin and its mRNA.[56] A third group finds no effect of either drug on thyroglobulin synthesis in vivo or in vitro.[57]

Thionamide drugs may also have an immunosuppressive action. When used to treat the thyrotoxicosis of Graves' disease, they not only control thyroid hypersecretion by their antithyroid action, but may also cause a fall in the circulating levels of thyroid-stimulating immunoglobulins.[58] After a course of antithyroid treatment, many patients with Graves' disease have a prolonged remission, which some have attributed to a direct effect of the drugs on the immune system.[59,60] Others believe that any changes seen in the autoimmune process are the immunologic consequences of amelioration of thyrotoxicosis.[61] This is discussed more fully in chapters 30 and 53.

ANILINE DERIVATIVES AND RELATED COMPOUNDS

The common feature of aniline derivatives is a *para*-substituted aminobenzene structure. The group includes sulfonamides, para-aminobenzoic acid, para-aminosalicylic acid, and

FIGURE 14-1. Thionimide structures. Propylthiouracil, methimazole, and carbimazole are used in the treatment of hyperthyroidism; goitrin has been isolated from certain plants.

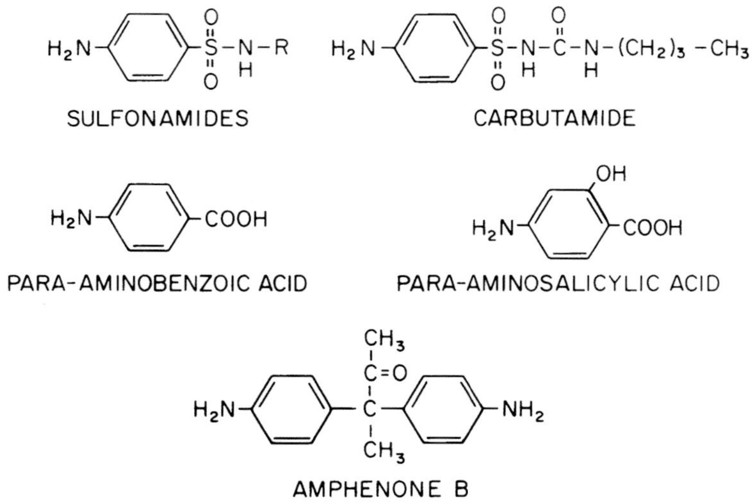

FIGURE 14-2. The structures of aniline derivatives with antithyroid actions.

amphenone (Fig 14-2). The importance of the amino group is illustrated by the effects of sulfonylureas, drugs used to treat diabetes mellitus. Carbutamide (no longer used clinically) has definite antithyroid activity, whereas tolbutamide, in which a methyl group replaces the amino group, has little or no antithyroid effect.[62] The antithyroid activity of aminoglutethimide, an inhibitor of adrenal steroid and estrogen synthesis, may be due to its similarity to these drugs.[63–65] Compounds in this class are generally less potent than the thioureylenes but have qualitatively similar actions; that is, they inhibit the coupling reaction as well as iodination of thyroglobulin.[62,64–66] Sulfonamides do differ from thionamides in some respects. The shapes of the dose-response curves for inhibition of iodination in vitro differ, thionamides showing a steeper slope,[45] and sulfonamides cause chiefly a reversible inhibition of TPO-mediated hormone formation.[67] In addition, the antithyroid potency of the sulfonamides, but not of the thionamides, is markedly potentiated by iodide.[66,68,69] This raises the possibility that the two classes of compounds interact differently with TPO, even though the end result, a decline in iodinations, is the same.

None of these compounds has proved useful in the treatment of hyperthyroidism. The usual doses of sulfonamides used to treat infections, or of sulfonylureas used to treat diabetes, are too low to have important antithyroid effects. Primates may be particularly resistant to the antithyroid action of sulfonamides.[70] Para-aminosalicylic acid, which has been used in high doses for long periods in the treatment of tuberculosis, has occasionally caused goiter.

SUBSTITUTED PHENOLS

The antithyroid activity of resorcinol was first noted when prolonged application of the drug to varicose ulcers led to hypothyroidism and goiter.[71] Subsequent studies revealed that many phenolic compounds have antithyroid activity.[72,73] The most potent are aromatic compounds with hydroxyl groups *meta* to one another; examples are shown in Figure 14-3. Among compounds with a single hydroxyl group, salicylate is

inactive, and para-hydroxybenzoate has moderate potency; antithyroid activity is not potentiated by iodide.[73] These compounds are also peroxidase inhibitors; in vitro resorcinol is more potent than MMI[45,74] or PTU,[75] and, like thionamides, causes irreversible inhibition of TPO.[76] There is an extensive review of this family of compounds by Lindsay and Gaitan,[77] who note that resorcinol and allied compounds are found in cigarette smoke and in the waste water from coal conversion processes, and may also arise from degradation of humic substances and flavonoids. Thus polyhydroxyphenols contaminating water or food supplies are a potential cause of goiter, and may be a factor in goiter endemics in Colombia and Kentucky.[78]

OTHER INHIBITORS OF IODINATIONS

Dihydroxypyridines and *3-hydroxypyridine* inhibit iodinations by TPO in vitro with potency similar to PTU[75] and can produce goiter in rodents.[79] 3,4-Dihydroxypyridine is a metabolite of the amino acid mimosine. It is produced in the rumen of cattle grazing on mimosine-rich legumes and high blood levels are associated with goiter.

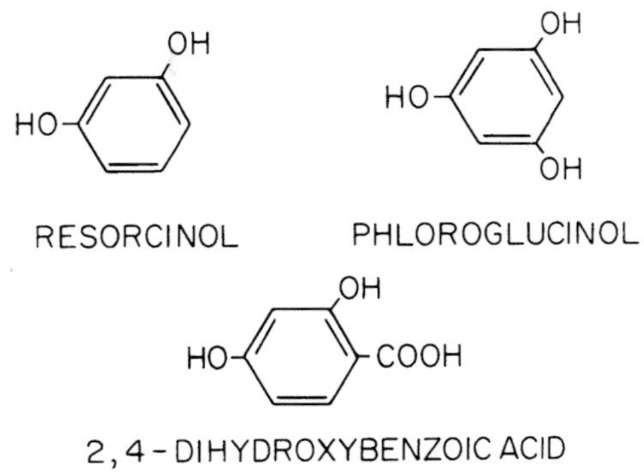

FIGURE 14-3. The structures of substituted phenols with antithyroid actions.

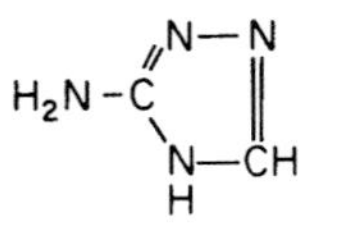

FIGURE 14-4. The structures of other inhibitors of iodide oxidation and organification.

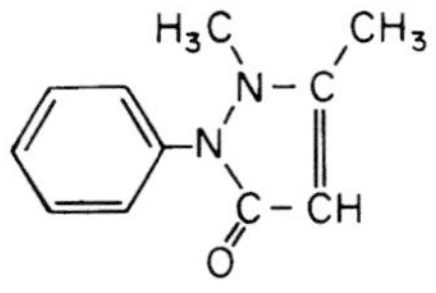

Aminotriazole (Fig 14-4) inhibits thyroid iodine uptake, produces goiter in vivo, and is a potent peroxidase inhibitor in vitro.[45,80,81] *Tricyanoaminopropene*, another goitrogen in laboratory animals, has been successfully used to ameliorate hyperthyroidism in patients.[82] It is a substrate for chloroperoxidase, forming chlorinated products[28]; an analogous mechanism, iodination of tricyanoaminopropene by TPO, is a possible explanation of antithyroid action.

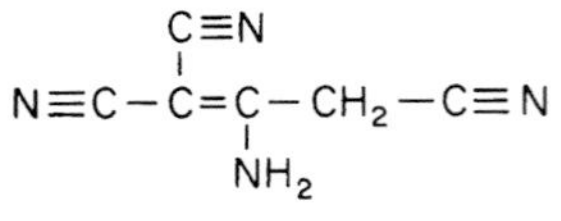

Antipyrine (phenazone) has attracted special interest because its iodinated derivative, iodopyrine, causes goiter. In rats, antipyrine alone is a weak goitrogen but can act synergistically with iodine to produce major inhibition of iodinations,[83] resembling sulfonamides in this respect. *Phenylbutazone*, chemically similar to phenazone, and *oxyphenbutazone* are also weak antithyroid agents.[84,85] The chemical basis for the antithyroid action of these compounds in uncertain, but both are rapidly metabolized to substituted phenols in vivo.[86] The activity of *dipyrone*, another related compound, on rat TPO has been studied, with the conclusion that it competes with tyrosine for I[+], thus resembling thiourea.[87] *Pyrazole*, an inhibitor of hepatic alcohol dehydrogenase that is also chemically related to phenazone, decreases serum thyroid hormone levels and increases TSH concentrations in rats, and causes thyroid necrosis when administered in high doses; its precise mode of action is unknown.[88]

INHIBITION OF THE COUPLING REACTION

Propylthiouracil is a more potent inhibitor of the coupling reaction than of organic iodinations. The other inhibitors of iodinations that have been tested behave similarly; selective inhibition of iodination, with no effect on coupling, has not been reported. Evidence indicates that the mechanism for iodinations differs from that for coupling, even though both require the same enzyme and are susceptible to inhibition by the same group of compounds.

Like other peroxidases, TPO exists in different forms.[89] One form, analogous to cytochrome c peroxidase compound I, catalyzes iodination of thyroglobulin. Another form, analogous to cytochrome c peroxidase compound II, catalyzes coupling. Formation of TPO-compound II is facilitated by diiodotyrosine. In the scheme proposed by Taurog,[47] it is an interaction with TPO-compound II that leads to irreversible inhibition of the peroxidase; this should directly prevent coupling. With low levels of thionamide and high levels of iodide, iodinations by TPO-compound I could continue. This affords an explanation for the greater sensitivity of coupling to thionamide inhibition. Very recently, Taurog and Dorris have reported new findings showing that coupling with TPO may involve the porphyrin π-cation radical form of compound I and that in very similar peroxidases, coupling is better mediated by this radical form.[47a]

To test for inhibition of coupling, a common procedure is to analyze the iodoamino acid residues in thyroglobulin and to determine the iodothyronine/iodotyrosine ratio. This ratio is a function of the total iodine content of thyroglobulin and can be lowered by severe iodine deficiency.[90–92] In the presence of moderate iodine deficiency, administration of perchlorate, by further decreasing entry of iodine into the gland, can produce a marked lowering of iodothyronine/iodotyrosine ratios that is reversed by iodide salts.[92] A similar decline in the rate of iodothyronine formation by iodine-deficient rats, reversible by iodide administration, can be produced by nitrotyrosine,[93] an inhibitor of iodotyrosine deiodination, which aggravates iodine deficiency, as discussed later. There has been a suggestion that thioureylenes inhibit coupling indirectly by this mechanism, that is, by inducing the production of poorly iodinated thyroglobulin. However, thioureylenes inhibit coupling in iodine-rich thyroglobulin,[94] and there seems no doubt that they can have a direct effect on the coupling reaction.

The demonstrable differences between iodination and coupling reactions raise the possibility that an agent incapable of inhibiting iodotyrosine formation could inhibit coupling, perhaps interfering with the role of diiodotyrosine or with binding of TPO to one of the sites on thyroglobulin where coupling is initiated. Selective inhibition of the coupling reaction and thyroid enlargement have been reported in rats given minocycline, a tetracycline derivative.[95] Minocycline also causes a blackening of the rat thyroid, which can be prevented by PTU treatment[96]; the pigment may be a product of minocycline peroxidation.[97] Minocycline treatment can also lead to black thyroid in man.[98] In detailed investigations of these phenomena, Dorris and Taurog have very recently demonstrated that minocycline is a potent inhibitor of both TPO catalyzed iodination and coupling.[98a]

Lithium salts may also inhibit coupling,[99–101] but their major effect is thought to be inhibition of hormone secretion, discussed in the next section.

INHIBITION OF HORMONE SECRETION: LITHIUM SALTS

For many years, the only agent known to inhibit secretion of thyroid hormone was iodide; this phenomenon is discussed in chapter 13 and a subchapter below. However, after the introduction of lithium carbonate for the treatment of manic and depressive states and the recognition that lithium occasionally produces hypothyroidism and goiter, it was shown that lithium has a striking inhibitory effect on thyroid hormone release in animals[100] and human beings.[102] Studies in vitro have shown that lithium inhibits the colloid droplet formation stimulated by cyclic adenosine monophosphate, a critical step in hormone secretion.[103]

If the only effect of lithium on the thyroid is inhibition of release, and hormone synthesis continues at a normal rate, hormone stores should increase until a normal amount is secreted despite a decreased fractional rate of secretion. In studies involving rats, such compensation seems to occur, so that the animals remain euthyroid and have only moderate thyroid enlargement with increased thyroid iodine stores[100]; a similar adaptation must occur in the majority of lithium-treated subjects, who remain euthyroid. This leaves the occasional cases of goiter and hypothyroidism, and the frequent occurrence of modest TSH elevations,[104,105] unexplained. Also, lithium alone has been an effective treatment for hyperthyroidism,[106,107] and restoration of euthyroidism must require a fall in rates of hormone synthesis as well as in secretion rates. The early observation that lithium inhibits the coupling reaction, with little or no effect on earlier steps in hormonogenesis,[99–101] may be the best explanation for these observations. The increased radioiodine uptake noted in some subjects[101,108,109] would represent a compensation for the decreased coupling, while hyperthyroid subjects, with fixed rates of iodine uptake, would have a fall in iodothyronine synthesis. The occasional individual who develops goiter or hypothyroidism presumably has some limitation in thyroid reserve, and many have antithyroid antibodies, suggesting autoimmune thyroid disease. Here there is yet another interesting finding; prospective testing for changes in thyroid function and autoantibodies has revealed that an increase in the titer of antibodies may accompany the development of hypothyroidism.[110,111] This has led to the postulate that lithium is an immunostimulant.[112] Presumably this action would still require a susceptible person, in whom the biochemical and immunologic actions of the drug synergize to produce clinical disease. Finally, the incidence of hyperthyroid Graves' disease is increased in lithium-treated patients[113]; this could be another outcome of lithium's immunostimulant effect.

INHIBITION OF IODOTYROSINE DEIODINATION

Secretion of thyroid hormone requires the proteolysis of thyroglobulin, which releases free iodotyrosines as well as the hormonally active iodothyronines (see chap 4). Normally, the iodotyrosines are deiodinated, liberating iodide that is again available for hormone synthesis. At usual levels of iodine intake, iodotyrosine deiodination is essential to iodide conservation; patients with a congenital inability to deiodinate iodotyrosines ("dehalogenase defect") lose large amounts of organic iodine (iodotyrosines and iodotyrosine metabolites) in the urine and may develop goiter and hypothyroidism. If iodide supplements are given, hypothyroidism can be corrected, further evidence that iodine waste is the proximate cause of decreased hormone synthesis. By analogy to the dehalogenase defect, pharmacologic inhibition of iodotyrosine deiodination should provide another mechanism of goitrogenesis. Nitrotyrosines are potent inhibitors of iodotyrosine deiodination and have the expected effect on thyroid function; that is, they cause iodotyrosines to be secreted by the thyroid and iodotyrosine metabolites to appear

in the urine.[114] When iodine intake is low, a fall in serum T_4, increase in serum TSH, and thyroid enlargement result; the goitrogenic effect is reversed by a high iodine intake.[115]

INHIBITORS OF IODOTHYRONINE DEIODINATION

Because T_4 is the major secretory product of the normal thyroid, and triiodothyronine (T_3) is the compound with greatest affinity for nuclear thyroid hormone receptors, inhibition of the conversion of T_4 to T_3 is a potential cause of hypothyroidism, TSH secretion, and goiter. However, even though many drugs can inhibit deiodinases responsible for T_3 formation, this mechanism is not an important cause of goiter because inhibition is incomplete. The expected consequences of sustained, partial inhibition of 5′-deiodination of T_4 would be an initial fall in serum and tissue T_3 levels, leading to feedback stimulation of TSH secretion, followed by a rise in T_4 levels until a new steady state is reached with a normal level of TSH and a high T_4:T_3 ratio. Serum levels of reverse T_3, because its clearance depends chiefly on 5′-deiodination, should rise. In subjects treated with the known deiodinase inhibitors propranolol,[116] oral cholecystographic agents,[117] and amiodarone,[118] the data are generally compatible with this interpretation, that is, they have increased serum T_4 and reverse T_3, normal to low serum T_3, and normal serum TSH concentrations. A recent symposium dealt with many aspects of hormone metabolism[119] including drug effects.[6] The effects of drugs on 5′-deiodinases are discussed in detail in the following subchapter and chapter 8.

INDUCERS OF HEPATIC DRUG-METABOLIZING ENZYMES

Many compounds induce the synthesis of hepatic enzymes that metabolize drugs; in some cases the induced enzymes, such as glucuronyl transferases, act on thyroid hormones and increase the rate at which they are conjugated and excreted in bile. If hormone wastage is severe, the feedback mechanism may cause TSH secretion and goiter. Effects of this type have been shown for several carcinogens, pesticides and environmental toxins, including 3,4-benzpyrene, chlordane, various isomers of DDD and DDT, and polychlorinated biphenyl and other polyhalogenated hydrocarbons.[120–123] In addition, several drugs commonly used in medical practice have similar actions; these include phenobarbital, the anticonvulsants phenytoin and carbamazepine, and an antituberculous drug, rifampin. This topic was recently reviewed[3] and is discussed further in the following subchapter.

In rats, phenobarbital accelerates T_4 disposal[124]; the most important mechanism is increased formation of T_4 glucuronide secondary to increased glucuronyl transferase activity.[125] A fall in serum T_4 and a rise in TSH result, but both return toward normal with time, as thyroidal hypertrophy and increased hormone secretion compensate for the defect. In normal subjects, phenobarbital does not consistently influence either circulating thyroid hormone levels nor thyroid size.[126] This reflects the relatively weak enzyme-inducing activity of usual clinical doses. When combined with another inducer, antipyrine, a fall in T_4 did follow.[127]

Phenytoin (diphenylhydantoin or Dilantin) and carbamazepine (Tegretol), in doses used to treat epilepsy, and rifampin, during treatment of tuberculosis, are potent inducers of hepatic microsomal oxygenases.[3,126–130] Chronic administration results in a fall in both total and free T_4 concentrations in serum[3,126–128,130–136] reflecting the increase in T_4's metabolic clearance rate[126,137,138] produced, presumably, by increased glucuronidation and biliary-fecal excretion. Despite the fall in T_4, serum TSH remains normal. The failure of TSH to rise could simply mean that near normal amounts of T_3 are reaching pituitary receptors. The effect of these drugs on T_3 disposal and serum T_3 levels is much less than their effects on T_4.[126,138,139] Also, with lower T_4 levels the rate of T_3 formation in the pituitary may increase, a phenomenon well documented in laboratory animals.[140] Slight or transient increases in serum TSH may occur; this would explain the increased thyroid size observed during chronic treatment with these drugs.[130,133] However, some investigators, noting patients whose TSH is normal despite definite depression of both free T_4 and free T_3 in serum, have postulated that these drugs have a direct effect on TSH secretion[126,131,132]; this is discussed below.

In any case, most patients receiving these drugs show no clinical signs of hypothyroidism and have euthyroid TSH levels. Patients taking carbamazepine have normal resting metabolic rates[141] and systolic time intervals,[142] confirming euthyroidism. A problem can arise, though, in hypothyroid patients receiving thyroid hormone therapy, who may need higher doses of T_4 to compensate for the increased rate of T_4 disposal. This has been documented in hypothyroid patients receiving phenytoin,[138,143] rifampin,[144] carbamazepine,[145] and phenobarbital.[146] Also, a T_4 dose that is appropriate when combined with one of these drugs may become excessive when the drug is discontinued. In one report, a woman being treated with a barbiturate remained euthyroid despite taking large doses of T_4, but became thyrotoxic when the barbiturate was discontinued.[147]

In patients with hyperthyroidism, drug-induced acceleration of hormone disposal could be beneficial. In one study, phenobarbital treatment led to a lowering of T_4 levels and clinical improvement in a group of thyrotoxic patients.[146]

DRUGS THAT INTERACT WITH HORMONE RECEPTORS

Older studies give evidence that reverse T_3 and other analogues antagonize certain effects of T_3, presumably by competing for binding to receptors, but large doses were required.[148,149] However, in recent years many compounds have been tested for their ability to interfere with T_3 binding to receptors and with specific receptor-mediated processes, with some apparently positive results.

Some drugs that induce hepatic enzymes and accelerate T_4 disposal may also antagonize TSH secretion. Both phenobarbital[150] and phenytoin inhibit TSH secretion in rats.[151,152] Phenytoin has been studied further and has been shown to interfere with binding of T_3 to pituitary receptors, supporting the theory that it is a weak thyroid hormone agonist.[129,153] However, the combination of binding to T_3 receptors and T_3-like actions has been more difficult to show in other tissues.

In liver, for example, phenytoin displaces T_3 from nuclear binding but does not stimulate synthesis of T_3-responsive enzymes.[134] Until its action is better defined, phenytoin's position as a receptor antagonist (i.e., an antithyroid compound) or agonist will be uncertain.

Amiodarone is used to treat both ventricular and supraventricular cardiac arrhythmias. Its most serious side effects vis-a-vis the thyroid are the occasional occurrence of hypothyroidism and hyperthyroidism. Both complications relate to the high iodine content of amiodarone and the drug's ability to induce thyroiditis, and are discussed in later subsections. Amiodarone is also an inhibitor of T_4 deiodination and causes changes in serum levels of thyroid hormones that are discussed above and in the following subsection. There may, however, be yet another way in which amiodarone interacts with thyroid hormones. The cardiac status of patients during amiodarone treatment mimics that seen in hypothyroidism; in both circumstances there are bradycardia, lengthened repolarization time, increased effective refractory period, increased threshold for ventricular fibrillation, a shortened duration of the action potential in Purkinje fibers, and a decreased number of β-adrenergic receptors.[154] Thyroid hormones can reverse some of the effects of amiodarone on cardiac conduction[155,156] and on myosin synthesis,[157] and amiodarone antagonizes the beneficial effects of T_3 treatment in thyroidectomized rats.[158] The drug is a potent inhibitor of the conversion of T_4 to T_3, but other deiodinase inhibitors do not duplicate these actions of amiodarone.[159–161] Thus, deiodinase inhibition is an unlikely mechanism for amiodarone's hypothyroid-like effects, and the possibility that amiodarone might be a T_3 antagonist at the receptor level was considered. Indeed, desethylamiodarone, a major metabolite, blocks T_3 binding to solubilized nuclear receptors from rat liver, human lymphocyte, and bovine heart,[162] as well as to the rat β-1 receptor protein[163] Amiodarone also competes with T_3 for binding to pituitary receptors, and, as would be expected of a T_3 antagonist, stimulates TSH release.[164]

Still other compounds have been shown to displace T_3 from binding to nuclear receptors; these include nonsteroidal anti-inflammatory agents (NSAIDs),[165] free fatty acids,[166,167] and oral cholecystographic agents.[168–170] However, in a recent study, the ability of these types of drugs to displace T_3 from binding to nuclear extracts was compared to their effect on T_3-stimulated secretion of sex hormone-binding globulin (SHBG) by Hep-G2 cells. Free fatty acids, NSAIDs, and bromosulphthalein all displaced T_3 from nuclear binding but did not influence SHBG secretion.[171] The tentative conclusion would be that studies of receptor binding in vitro may be misleading, and must be correlated with findings in more complete systems. The rapid advances in our knowledge of the structure and mode of action of thyroid hormone receptors should facilitate further investigation of this mode of drug action.

References

1. Capen CC. Pathophysiology of chemical injury of the thyroid gland. Toxicol Lett 1992;64-65:381
2. Kanno J, Matsuoka C, Furuta K, et al. Tumor promoting effect of goitrogens on the rat thyroid. Toxicol Pathol 1990; 18:239

3. Curran PG, DeGroot LJ. The effect of hepatic enzyme-inducing drugs on thyroid hormone and the thyroid gland. Endocr Rev 1991;12:135

4. Gaitan E. Environmental goitrogenesis. Boca Raton, FL: CRC Press, 1989:250

5. Cavalieri RR, Pitt-Rivers R. The effects of drugs on the distribution and metabolism of thyroid hormones. Pharmacol Rev 1981;33:55

6. Green WL. Effect of drugs on thyroid hormone metabolism. In: Wu SY, Hershman JM, eds. Thyroid hormone metabolism. Oxford: Blackwell, 1990:239

7. Wolff J. Transport of iodide and other anions in the thyroid gland. Physiol Rev 1964;44:45

8. Andros G, Harper PV, Lathrop KA, McCardle RJ. Pertechnetate-99m localization in man with applications to thyroid scanning and the study of thyroid physiology. J Clin Endocrinol Metab 1965;25:1067

9. Kusic Z, Becker DV, Saenger EL, et al. Comparison of technetium-99m and iodine-123 imaging of thyroid nodules: correlation with pathologic findings. J Nucl Med 1990;31:393

10. Bastomsky CH. Thyroid iodide transport. In: Greer MA, Solomon DH, eds. Handbook of physiology. Vol III. Thyroid. Washington, DC: American Physiological Society, 1973:81

11. Carrasco N. Iodide transport in the thyroid gland. Biochim Biophys Acta 1993;1154:65

12. Bagchi N, Fawcett DM. Role of sodium ion in active transport of iodide of cultured thyroid cells. Biochim Biophys Acta 1973;318:235

13. Vilijn KF, Carrasco N. Expression of the thyroid sodium/iodide symporter in *Xenopus laevis* oocytes. J Biol Chem 1989;264:11901

14. Barzilai D, Sheinfeld M. Fatal complications following use of potassium perchlorate in thyrotoxicosis: report of two cases and a review of the literature. Isr J Med Sci 1966;2:453

15. Martino E, Aghini-Lombardi F, Mariotti S, et al. Treatment of amiodarone-associated thyrotoxicosis by simultaneous administration of potassium perchlorate and methimazole. J Endocrinol Invest 1986;9:201

16. van Dam EW, Prummel MF, Wiersinga WM, Nikkels RE. Treatment of amiodarone-induced hypothyroidism with potassium perchlorate. Neth J Med 1993;42:21

17. Gray HW, Hooper LA, Greig WR. An evaluation of the twenty-minute perchlorate discharge test. J Clin Endocrinol Metab 1973;37:351

18. Friis J. The perchlorate discharge test with and without supplement of potassium iodide. J Endocrinol Invest 1987;10:581

19. Creagh FM, Parkes AB, Lee A, et al. The iodide perchlorate discharge test in women with previous post-partum thyroiditis: relationship to sonographic appearance and thyroid function. Clin Endocrinol 1994;40:765

20. Maloof F, Soodak M. The inhibition of the metabolism of thiocyanate in the thyroid of the rat. Endocrinology 1959;65:106

21. Scranton JR, Nissen WM, Halmi NS. The kinetics of the inhibition of thyroidal iodide accumulation by thiocyanate: a reexamination. Endocrinology 1969;85:603

22. Saito K, Yamamoto K, Takai T, Yoshida S. Inhibition of iodide accumulation by perchlorate and thiocyanate in a model of the thyroid iodide transport system. Acta Endocrinol 1983;104:456

23. Saito K, Yamamoto K, Nagayama I, et al. Effect of internally loaded iodide, thiocyanate, and perchlorate on sodium-dependent iodide uptake by phospholipid vesicles reconstituted with thyroid plasma membranes: iodide counterflow mediated by the iodide transport carrier. J Biochem (Tokyo) 1989;105:790

24. Maloof F, Soodak M. Oxidation of thiocyanate, another index of thyroid function. Endocrinology 1966;78:1198

25. Ohtaki S, Rosenberg IN. Prompt stimulation by TSH of thyroid oxidation of thiocyanate. Endocrinology 1971;88:566

26. Greer MA, Stott AK, Milne KA. Effect of thiocyanate, perchlorate and other anions on thyroidal iodine metabolism. Endocrinology 1966;79:237

27. Fukayama H, Nasu M, Murakami S, Sugawara M. Examination of antithyroid effects of smoking products in cultured thyroid follicles: only thiocyanate is a potent antithyroid agent. Acta Endocrinol 1992;127:520

28. Morris DR, Hager LP. Mechanism of the inhibition of enzymatic halogenation by antithyroid agents. J Biol Chem 1966;241:3582

29. Virion A, Dème D, Pommier J, Nunez J. Opposite effects of thiocyanate on tyrosine iodination and thyroid hormone synthesis. Eur J Biochem 1980;112:1

30. Karakaya A, Tunçel N, Alptuna G, et al. Influence of cigarette smoking on thyroid hormone levels. Hum Toxicol 1987;6:507

31. Christensen SB, Ericsson UB, Janzon L, et al. Influence of cigarette smoking on goiter formation, thyroglobulin, and thyroid hormone levels in women. J Clin Endocrinol Metab 1984;58:615

32. Hegedüs L, Karstrup S, Veiergang D, et al. High frequency of goitre in cigarette smokers. Clin Endocrinol 1985;22:287

32a. Miller B, Zulewski H, Huber P, et al. Impaired action of thyroid hormone associated with smoking in women with hypothyroidism. N Eng J Med 1995;333:964.

33. Chanoine JP, Toppet V, Bourdoux P, et al. Smoking during pregnancy: a significant cause of neonatal thyroid enlargement. Br J Obstet Gynaecol 1991;98:65

34. Bertelsen JB, Hegedüs L. Cigarette smoking and the thyroid. Thyroid 1994;4:327

35. Nourok DS, Glassock RJ, Solomon DH, Maxwell MH. Hypothyroidism following prolonged sodium nitroprusside therapy. Am J Med Sci 1964;284:129

36. Bödigheimer K, Nowak F, Schoenborn W. Pharmacokinetics and thyrotoxicity of the sodium nitroprusside metabolite thiocyanate. Dtsch Med Wochenschr 1979;104:939

37. Ermans AM, Bourdoux P. Antithyroid sulfurated compounds. In: Gaitan E, ed. Environmental goitrogenesis. Boca Raton, FL: CRC Press, 1989:15

38. Delange F. Cassava and the thyroid. In: Gaitan E, ed. Environmental goitrogenesis. Boca Raton, FL: CRC Press, 1989:173

39. Greer MA. Isolation from rutabaga seed of progoitrin, the precursor of the naturally occurring antithyroid compound, goitrin (L-5-vinyl-2-thiooxazolidone). J Am Chem Soc 1956;78:1260

40. Gaitan E. Epidemiological aspects of environmental goitrogenesis. In: Gaitan E, ed. Environmental goitrogenesis. Boca Raton, FL: CRC Press, 1989:161

41. Drucker D, Eggo MC, Salit IE, Burrow GN. Ethionamide-induced goitrous hypothyroidism. Ann Intern Med 1984;100:837

42. Jubiz W, Nolan G. The effects of 6-mercaptopurine (6-MP) on the thyroid gland. Endocrinology 1974;94:1583

43. Moulding T, Fraser R. Hypothyroidism related to ethionamide. Am Rev Respir Dis 1970;101:90

44. Richards JB, Ingbar SH. The effects of propylthiouracil and perchlorate on the biogenesis of thyroid hormone. Endocrinology 1959;65:198

45. Taurog A. Thyroid peroxidase and thyroxine biosynthesis. Recent Prog Horm Res 1970;26:189

46. Nagataki S, Uchimura H, Matsuzaki F, Masuyama Y. Comparison of the triiodothyronine suppression test by the twenty-minute and the twenty-four hour thyroidal ^{131}I uptake in patients receiving thioamide drugs. J Clin Endocrinol Metab 1974;38:255

47. Taurog A, Dorris ML, Guziec FS Jr, Uetrecht JP. Metabolism of ^{35}S- and ^{14}C-labeled propylthiouracil in a model in vitro system containing thyroid peroxidase. Endocrinology 1989;124:3030

47a. Taurog A, Dorris ML. Analysis of thyroid peroxidase-catalyzed iodinator and coupling mechanisms. Program 11th International Thyroid Congress. Toronto, Canada, Sept. 10–15, 1995; Thyroid 1995;5:S67

48. Taurog A, Dorris ML, Guziec FS Jr. Metabolism of ^{35}S- and ^{14}C-labeled 1-methyl-2-mercaptoimidazole in vitro and in vivo. Endocrinology 1989;124:30

49. Verma S, Kumar GP, Laloraya M, Singh A. Activation of iodine into a free-radical intermediate by superoxide: a physiologically significant step in the iodination of tyrosine. Biochem Biophys Res Commun 1990;170:1026

50. Raby C, Lagorce JF, Jambut-Absil AC, et al. The mechanism of action of synthetic antithyroid drugs: iodine complexation during oxidation of iodide. Endocrinology 1990;126:1683

51. Doerge DR, Decker CJ, Takazawa RS. Chemical and enzymatic oxidation of benzimidazoline-2-thiones: a dichotomy in the mechanism of peroxidase inhibition. Biochemistry 1993;32:58

52. Davidson B, Soodak M, Strout HV, et al. Thiourea and cyanamide as inhibitors of thyroid peroxidase: the role of iodide. Endocrinology 1979;104:1979

53. Kramer AW Jr, Dambach G, Pridgen WA. The effects of calcium carbimide and thyroid powder on thyroid morphology and feed efficiency in rats. Toxicol Appl Pharmacol 1967;11:432

54. Peachey JE, Annis HM, Bornstein ER, et al. Calcium carbimide in alcoholism treatment. Part 2: medical findings of a short-term, placebo-controlled, double-blind clinical trial. British Journal of Addiction 1989;84:1359

55. Isozaki O, Tsushima T, Emoto N, et al. Methimazole regulation of thyroglobulin biosynthesis and gene transcription in rat FRTL-5 thyroid cells. Endocrinology 1991;128:3113

56. Leer LM, Cammenga M, De Vijlder IJ. Methimazole and propylthiouracil increase thyroglobulin gene expression in FRTL-5 cells. Mol Cell Endocrinol 1991;82:R25

57. Moura EG, Pazos-Moura CC, Dorns ML, Taurog A. Lack of effect of propylthiouracil and methylmercaptoimidazole on thyroglobulin biosynthesis. Proc Soc Exp Biol Med 1990;194:48

58. Wilson R, McKillop JH, Pearson C, et al. Differential immunosuppressive action of carbimazole and propylthiouracil. Clin Exp Immunol 1988;73:312

59. Weetman AP. The immunomodulatory effects of antithyroid drugs. Thyroid 1994;4:145

60. Weetman AP, McGregor M. Autoimmune thyroid diseases: further developments in our understanding. Endocr Rev 1994;15:788

61. Volpé R. Evidence that the immunosuppressive effects of antithyroid drugs are mediated through actions on the thyroid cell, modulating thyrocyte-immunocyte signaling: a review. Thyroid 1994;4:217

62. Tranquada RE, Solomon DH, Brown J, Greene R. The effect of oral hypoglycemic agents on thyroid function in the rat. Endocrinology 1960;67:293

63. Brown CG, Fowler KL, Nicholls PJ, Atterwill C. Assessment of thyrotoxicity using in vitro cell culture systems. Food Chem Toxicol 1986;24:557

64. Rallison ML, Kumagai LF, Tyler FH. Goitrous hypothyroidism induced by amino-glutethimide, anticonvulsant drug. J Clin Endocrinol Metab 1967;27:265

65. Studer H, Kohler H, Bürgi H, et al. Goiters with high radioiodine uptake and other characteristics of iodine deficiency in rats chronically treated with aminoglutethimide. Endocrinology 1970;87:905

66. Milne K, Greer MA. Comparison of the effects of propylthiouracil and sulfadiazine on thyroidal biosynthesis and the manner in which they are influenced by supplemental iodide. Endocrinology 1962;71:580

67. Doerge DR, Decker CJ. Inhibition of peroxidase-catalyzed reactions by arylamines: mechanism for the anti-thyroid action of sulfamethazine. Chem Res Toxicol 1994;7:164

68. Brown J, Solomon DH. Mechanism of antithyroid effects of a sulfonylurea in the rat. Endocrinology 1958;63:473

69. MacKenzie CG. Differentiation of the antithyroid action of thiouracil, thiourea and PABA from sulfonamides by iodide administration. Endocrinology 1947;40:137

70. Takayama S, Aihara K, Onodera T, Akimoto T. Antithyroid effects of propylthiouracil and sulfamonomethoxine in rats and monkeys. Toxicol Appl Pharmacol 1986;82:191

71. Bull GM, Fraser R. Myxoedema from resorcinol ointment applied to leg ulcers. Lancet 1950;1:851

72. Arnott DG, Doniach I. The effects of compounds allied to resorcinol upon the uptake of radioactive iodine (^{131}I) by thyroid of the rat. Biochem J 1952;50:473

73. Woeber KA, Ingbar SH. Antithyroid effect of noncalorigenic congeners of salicylate, with observations on the influence of serum proteins on the potency of antithyroid agents. Endocrinology 1965;76:584

74. Rosenberg IN. The antithyroid activity of some compounds that inhibit peroxidase. Science 1952;116:503

75. Lindsay RH, Hill JB, Gaitan E, et al. Antithyroid effects of coal-derived pollutants. J Toxicol Environ Health 1992;37:467

76. Divi RL, Doerge DR. Mechanism-based inactivation of lactoperoxidase and thyroid peroxidase by resorcinol derivatives. Biochemistry 1994;33:9668

77. Lindsay RH, Gaitan E. Polyhydroxyphenols and phenol derivatives. In: Gaitan E, ed. Environmental goitrogenesis. Boca Raton, FL: CRC Press, 1989:73

78. Gaitan E, Lindsay RH, Cooksey RC. Goiter endemias attributed to chemical and bacterial pollution of water supplies. In: Gaitan E, ed. Environmental goitrogenesis. Boca Raton, FL: CRC Press, 1989:207

79. Lindsay RH. Hydroxypyridines. In: Gaitan E, ed. Environmental goitrogenesis. Boca Raton, FL: CRC Press, Inc., 1989:97

80. Alexander NM. Iodide peroxidase in rat thyroid and salivary glands and its inhibition by antithyroid compounds. J Biol Chem 1959;234:1530

81. Alexander NM. Antithyroid action of 3-amino-1,2,4-triazole. J Biol Chem 1959;234:148

82. Ingbar SH. The action of 1,1,3-tricyano-2-amino-1-propene (U-9189) on the thyroid gland of the rat and its effects in human thyrotoxicosis. J Clin Endocrinol Metab 1961;21:128

83. Pasternak DP, Socolow EL, Ingbar SH. Synergistic interaction of phenazone and iodide on thyroid hormone biosynthesis in the rat. Endocrinology 1969;84:769

84. Abiodun MO, Bird R, Havard CWH, Sood NK. The effects of phenylbutazone on thyroid function. Acta Endocrinol 1973;72:257

85. Lane RJM, Clark F, McCollum JK. Oxyphenbutazone-induced goitre. Postgr Med J 1977;53:93

86. Gilman AG, Rall TW, Nies AS, Taylor, P eds. The pharmacological basis of therapeutics. 8th ed. New York: Pergamon Press, 1990:654

87. Varela V, del Valle Paz C, Houssay AB, Targovnik HM. Inhibitory action of dipyrone on rat thyroid peroxidase and lactoperoxidase activities. Acta Physiol Pharmacol Ther Latinoam 1985;35:259

88. Szabo S, Horvath E, Kovacs K, Larsen PR. Pyrazole-induced thyroid necrosis: a distinct organ lesion. Science 1978;199:1209

89. Virion A, Courtin F, Dème D, et al. Spectral characteristics and catalytic properties of thyroid peroxidase-H_2O_2 compounds in the iodination and coupling reactions. Arch Biochem Biophys 1985;242:41

90. DeCrombrugghe B, Edelhoch H, Beckers C, DeVisscher M. Thyroglobulin from human goiters: effects of iodination on sedimentation and iodoamino acid synthesis. J Biol Chem 1967;242:5681

91. Ermans AM, Kinthaert J, Camus M. Defective intrathyroidal iodine metabolism in non-toxic goiter: inadequate iodination of thyroglobulin. J Clin Endocrinol Metab 1968;28:1307

92. Inoue K, Taurog A. Acute and chronic effects of iodide on thyroid radioiodine metabolism in iodine-deficient rats. Endocrinology 1968;83:279

93. Green WL. Induction of a coupling defect in rats during inhibition of tyrosine dehalogenase. Endocrinology 1976;98:10

94. Engler H, Taurog A, Dorris ML. Preferential inhibition of thyroxine and 3,5,3'-triiodothyronine formation by propylthiouracil and methylmercaptoimidazole in thyroid peroxidase-catalyzed iodination of thyroglobulin. Endocrinology 1982;110:190

95. Saito K, Jujio T, Hashizume I, et al. Studies on goitrogenic action of minocycline and related compounds. Endocrinology 1972;90:1192

96. Kurosumi M, Fujita H. Fine structural aspects of the black thyroid induced by minocycline, and the effects of a low iodine diet, propylthiouracil, thyroxine tablet and TSH, on the black discoloration of the rat thyroid. Virchows Arch B Cell Pathol Incl Mol Pathol 1985;48:219

97. Tajima K, Miyagawa J, Nakajima H, et al. Morphological and biochemical studies on minocycline-induced black thyroid in rats. Toxicol Appl Pharmacol 1985;81:393

98a. Dorris ML, Taurog A. Role of thyroid peroxidase minocycline-induced black pigmentation of the thyroid: antithyroid effects of minocycline. Program 11th International Thyroid Congress, Toronto, Canada, Sept. 10–15, 1995; Thyroid 1995;5:S107

98. Pastolero GC, Asa SL. Drug-related pigmentation of the thyroid associated with papillary carcinoma. Arch Pathol Lab Med 1994;118:79

99. Bagchi N, Brown TR, Mack RE. Studies of the mechanism of inhibition of thyroid function by lithium. Biochim Biophys Acta 1978;542:163

100. Berens SC, Bernstein RS, Robbins J, Wolff J. Antithyroid effects of lithium. J Clin Invest 1970;49:1357

101. Burrow GN, Burke WR, Himmelhoch JM, et al. Effect of lithium on thyroid function. J Clin Endocrinol Metab 1971;32:647

102. Spaulding SW, Burrow GN, Bermudez F, Himmelhoch JM. The inhibitory effect of lithium on thyroid hormone release in both euthyroid and thyrotoxic patients. J Clin Endocrinol Metab 1972;35:905

103. Williams JA, Berens SC, Wolff J. Thyroid secretion in vitro: inhibition of TSH and dibutyryl cyclic-AMP stimulated ^{131}I release by Li. Endocrinology 1971;88:1385

104. Emerson CH, Dyson WL, Utiger RD. Serum thyrotropin and thyroxine concentrations in patients receiving lithium carbonate. J Clin Endocrinol Metab 1973;36:338

105. Vincent A, Baruch P, Vincent P. Early onset of lithium-associated hypothyroidism. J Psychiatry Neurosci 1993;18:74

106. Kristensen O, Andersen HH, Pallisgaard G. Lithium carbonate in the treatment of thyrotoxicosis: a controlled trial. Lancet 1976;1:603

107. Lazarus JH, Richards AR, Addison GM, Owen GM. Treatment of thyrotoxicosis with lithium carbonate. Lancet 1974;2:1160

108. Rogers MP, Whybrow PC. Clinical hypothyroidism occurring during lithium treatment: two case histories and a review of thyroid function in 19 patients. Am J Psychiatry 1971;128:158

109. Sedvall G, Jönsson B, Petterson U. Evidence of an altered thyroid function in man during treatment with lithium carbonate. Acta Psychiatr Scand 1969;(suppl)207:59

110. Calabrese JR, Gulledge AD, Hahn K. Autoimmune thyroiditis in manic-depressive patients treated with lithium. Am J Psychiatry 1985;142:1318

111. Myers DH, Carter RA, Burns BH, et al. A prospective study of the effects of lithium on thyroid function and on the prevalence of antithyroid antibodies. Psychol Med 1985;15:55

112. Wilson R, McKillop JH, Crocket GT, et al. The effect of lithium therapy on parameters thought to be involved in the development of autoimmune thyroid disease. Clin Endocrinol 1991;34:357

113. Barclay ML, Brownlie BE, Turner JG, Wells JE. Lithium associated thyrotoxicosis: a report of 14 cases, with statistical analysis of incidence. Clin Endocrinol 1994;40:759

114. Green WL. Inhibition of thyroidal iodotyrosine deiodination by tyrosine analogues. Endocrinology 1968;83:336

115. Green WL. Effects of 3-nitro-L-tyrosine on thyroid function in the rat: an experimental model for the dehalogenase defect. J Clin Invest 1971;50:2474

116. Cooper DS, Daniels GH, Ladenson PW, Ridgway EC. Hyperthyroxinemia in patients treated with high-dose propranolol. Am J Med 1982;73:867

117. Suzuki H, Kadena N, Takeuchi K, Nakagawa S. Effects of three-day oral cholecystography on serum iodothyronines and TSH concentrations: comparison of the effects among some cholecystographic agents and the effects of iopanoic acid on the pituitary-thyroid axis. Acta Endocrinol 1978;92:477

118. Nademanee K, Singh BN, Callahan B, et al. Amiodarone, thyroid hormone indexes, and altered thyroid function: long-term serial effects in patients with cardiac arrhythmias. Am J Cardiol 1986;58:981

119. Wu SY, Hershman JM, eds. Thyroid hormone metabolism. Oxford: Blackwell, 1990

120. Barsano CP. Polyhalogenated and polycyclic aromatic hydrocarbons. In: Gaitan E, ed. Environmental goitrogenesis. Boca Raton, FL: CRC Press, 1989:115

121. Fregly MJ, Waters IW, Straw JA. Effect of isomers of DDD on thyroid and adrenal function in rats. Can J Physiol Pharmacol 1968;46:59

122. Goldstein JA, Taurog A. Enhanced biliary excretion of thyroxine glucuronide in rats pretreated with benzpyrene. Biochem Pharmacol 1968;17:1049

123. Hurst JG, Newcomer WS, Morrison JA. Some effects of DDT, toxaphene, and polychlorinated biphenyl on thyroid function in Bobwhite quail. Poult Sci 1974;53:125

124. Oppenheimer JH, Bernstein G, Surks MI. Increased thyroxine turnover and thyroidal function after stimulation of hepatocellular binding of thyroxine by phenobarbital. J Clin Invest 1968;47:1399

125. McClain RM, Levin AA, Posch R, Downing JC. The effect of phenobarbital on the metabolism and excretion of thyroxine in rats. Toxicol Appl Pharmacol 1989;99:216

126. Ohnhaus EE, Bürgi H, Burger A, Studer H. The effect of antipyrine, phenobarbitol and rifampicin on thyroid hormone metabolism in man. Eur J Clin Invest 1981;11:381

127. Ohnhaus EE, Studer H. A link between liver microsomal enzyme activity and thyroid hormone metabolism in man. Br J Clin Pharmacol 1983;15:71

128. Connell JM, Rapeport WG, Gordon S, Brodie MJ. Changes in circulating thyroid hormones during short-term hepatic enzyme induction with carbamazepine. Eur J Clin Pharmacol 1984;26:453

129. Smith PJ, Surks MI. 5,5'-Diphenylhydantoin (Dilantin) decreases cytosol and specific nuclear 3,5,3'-triiodothyronine binding in rat anterior pituitary in vivo and in cultured GC cells. Endocrinology 1984;115:283

130. Christensen HR, Simonsen K, Hegedüs L, et al. Influence of rifampicin on thyroid gland volume, thyroid hormones and antipyrine metabolism. Acta Endocrinol 1989;121:406

131. Evans PJ, Woodhead JS, Weeks I, Scanlon MF. Circulating TSH levels measured with an immunochemiluminometric assay in patients taking drugs interfering with biochemical thyroid status. Clin Endocrinol 1987;26:717

132. Liewendahl K, Tikanoja S, Helenius T, Majuri H. Free thyroxine and free triiodothyronine as measured by equilibrium dialysis and analog radioimmunoassay in serum of patients taking phenytoin and carbamazepine. Clin Chem 1985;31:1993

133. Hegedüs L, Hansen JM, Lühdorf K, et al. Increased frequency of goitre in epileptic patients on long-term phenytoin or carbamazepine treatment. Clin Endocrinol 1985;23:423

134. Smith PJ, Surks MI. Multiple effects of 5,5'-diphenylhydantoin on the thyroid hormone system. Endocr Rev 1984;5:514

135. Rozza L, Marcolla A, Ferrari G. Endocrine function changes in young males during long-term antiepileptic therapy with phenobarbitone and carbamazepine. Ital J Neuro Sci 1987;8:331

136. Isojarvi JI, Pakarinen AJ, Myllyla VV. Thyroid function with antiepileptic drugs. Epilepsia 1992;33:142

137. Larsen PR, Atkinson AJ, Wellman HN, Goldsmith RE. The effect of diphenylhydantoin on thyroxine metabolism in man. J Clin Invest 1970;49:1266

138. Faber J, Lumholtz IB, Kirkegaard C. The effects of phenytoin (diphenylhydantoin) on the extrathyroidal turnover of thyroxine, 3,5,3'-triiodothyronine, 3,3'5'-triiodothyronine, and 3',5'-diiodothyronine in man. J Clin Endocrinol Metab 1985;61:1093

139. Finke C, Juge C, Goumaz M, et al. Effects of rifampicin on the peripheral turnover kinetics of thyroid hormones in mice in men. J Endocrinol Invest 1987;10:157

140. Chanoine JP, Safran M, Farwell AP, et al. Selenium deficiency and type II 5'-deiodinase regulation in the euthyroid and hypothyroid rat: evidence of a direct effect of thyroxine. Endocrinology 1992;130:479

141. Herman R, Obarzanek E, Mikalauskas KM, et al. The effects of carbamazepine on resting metabolic rate and thyroid function in depressed patients. Biol Psychiatry 1991;29:779

142. Isojarvi JI, Airaksinen KE, Repo M, et al. Carbamazepine, serum thyroid hormones and myocardial function in epileptic patients. J Neurol Neurosurg Psychiatry 1993;56:710

143. Blackshear JL, Schultz AL, Napier JS, Stuart DD. Thyroxine replacement requirements in hypothyroid patients receiving phenytoin. Ann Intern Med 1983;99:341

144. Isley WL. Effect of rifampin therapy on thyroid function tests in a hypothyroid patient on replacement L-thyroxine. Ann Intern Med 1987;107:517

145. DeLuca F, Arrigo T, Pandullo E, et al. Changes in thyroid function tests induced by 2 month carbamazepine treatment in L-thyroxine-substituted hypothyroid children. Eur J Pediatr 1986;145:77

146. Cavalieri RR, Sung LC, Becker CE. Effects of phenobarbital on thyroxine and triiodothyronine kinetics in Grave's disease. J Clin Endocrinol Metab 1973;37:308

147. Hoffbrand BI. Barbiturate/thyroid-hormone interaction. Lancet 1979;2:903

148. Pittman CS, Barker SB. Antithyroxine effects of some thyroxine analogues. Am J Physiol 1959;197:1271

149. Pittman JA, Brown RW, Beschi RJ, Smitherman TC. Selectivity of action of 3,3',5'-triiodothyronine. Endocrinology 1970;86:1451

150. Theodoropoulos TJ, Zolman JC. Effects of phenobarbital on hypothalamic-pituitary-thyroid axis in the rat. Am J Med Sci 1989;297:224

151. Surks MI, Ordene KW, Mann DN, Kumara-Siri MH. Diphenylhydantoin inhibits the thyrotropin response to thyrotropin-releasing hormone in man and rat. J Clin Endocrinol Metab 1983;56:940

152. Theodoropoulos T, Fang S-L, Azizi F, et al. Effect of diphenylhydantoin on hypothalamic-pituitary-thyroid function in the rat. Am J Physiol 1980;239(Endocrinol Metab 2):E468

153. Franklyn JA, Davis JRE, Ramsden DB, Sheppard MC. Phenytoin and thyroid hormone action. J Endocrinol 1985;104:201

154. Singh BN, Venkatesh N, Nademanee K, et al. The historical development, cellular electrophysiology and pharmacology of amiodarone. Prog Cardiovasc Dis 1989;31:249

155. Patterson E, Shlafer M, Walden KM, et al. Changes in cardiac muscle function and biochemistry produced by long-term amiodarone and amiodarone + triiodothyronine administration in the rabbit. Pharmacology 1987;35:130

156. Patterson E, Walden KM, Khazaeli MB, et al. Cardiac electrophysiologic effects of acute and chronic amiodarone administration in the isolated perfused rabbit heart: altered thyroid hormone metabolism. J Pharmacol Exp Ther 1986;239:179

157. Franklyn JA, Green NK, Gammage MD, et al. Regulation of α- and β-myosin heavy chain messenger RNAs in the rat my-ocardium by amiodarone and by thyroid status. Clin Sci 1989;76:463

158. Paradis P, Lambert C, Rouleau J. Amiodarone antagonizes the effects of T_3 at the receptor level: an additional mechanism for its in vivo hypothyroid-like effects. Can J Physiol Pharmacol 1991;69:865

159. Lindenmeyer M, Sporri S, Staübli M, Studer H. Does amiodarone affect heart rate by inhibiting the intracellular generation of triiodothyronine from thyroxine? Br J Pharmacol 1984;82:275

160. Meese R, Smitherman TC, Croft CH, et al. Effect of peripheral thyroid hormone metabolism on cardiac arrhythmias. Am J Cardiol 1985;55:849

161. Staübli M, Studer H. The effects of amiodarone on the electrocardiogram of the guinea-pig are not explained by interaction with thyroid hormone metabolism alone. Br J Pharmacol 1986;88:405

162. Latham KR, Sellitti DF, Goldstein RE. Interaction of amiodarone and desethylamiodarone with solubilized nuclear thyroid hormone receptors. J Am Coll Cardiol 1987;9:872

163. Bakker O, van Beeren HC, Wiersinga WM. Desethylamiodarone is a noncompetitive inhibitor of the binding of thyroid hormone to the thyroid hormone beta 1-receptor protein. Endocrinology 1994;134:1665

164. Franklyn JA, Davis JR, Gammage MD, et al. Amiodarone and thyroid hormone action. Clin Endocrinol 1985;22:257

165. Topliss DJ, Hamblin PS, Kolliniatis I, et al. Furosemide, fenclofenac, diclofenac, mefenamic acid and meclofenamic acid inhibit specific T_3 binding in isolated rat hepatic nuclei. J Endocrinol Invest 1988;11:355

166. Inoue A, Yamamoto N, Morisawa Y, et al. Unesterified long-chain fatty acids inhibit thyroid hormone binding to the nuclear receptor: solubilized receptor and the receptor in cultured cells. Eur J Biochem 1989;183:565

167. Wiersinga WM, Chopra IJ, Chua Teco GN. Inhibition of nuclear T_3 binding by fatty acids. Metabolism 1988;37:996

168. Burman KD, Lukes YG, Latham KR, Wartofsky L. Ipodate and 8-anilino-1-naphthalene sulfonic acid block receptor binding of T_3 in rat liver. Horm Metab Res 1980;12:685

169. DeGroot LJ, Rue PA. Roentgenographic contrast agents inhibit triiodothyronine binding to nuclear receptors in vitro. J Clin Endocrinol Metab 1979;49:538

170. Eil C, Chestnut RY. The effects of radiographic contrast agents and other compounds on the nuclear binding of L-[^{125}I]triiodothyronine in dispersed human skin fibroblasts. J Clin Endocrinol Metab 1985;60:548

171. Barlow JW, Curtis AJ, Raggatt LE, et al. Drug competition for intracellular triiodothyronine-binding sites. Eur J Endocrinol 1994;130:417

EFFECTS OF PHARMACOLOGIC AGENTS ON THYROID HORMONE HOMEOSTASIS

Christoph A. Meier
Albert G. Burger

Pharmacologic agents may influence thyroid hormone homeostasis at four different levels (Fig 14-5). First, they may alter the synthesis and secretion of thyroid hormones. Second, they may change the serum concentrations of thyroid hormones by altering either the level of binding proteins or by competing for their hormone-binding sites. Third, drugs may modify the cellular uptake and metabolism of thyroid hormones. Lastly, pharmacologic agents may interfere with hormone action at the target tissue level. Although most drug-induced changes in

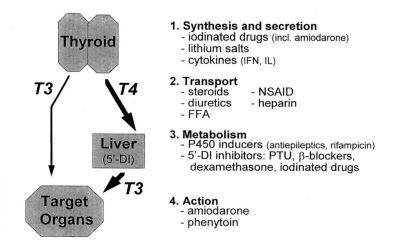

1. Synthesis and secretion
- iodinated drugs (incl. amiodarone)
- lithium salts
- cytokines (IFN, IL)

2. Transport
- steroids   - NSAID
- diuretics   - heparin
- FFA

3. Metabolism
- P450 inducers (antiepileptics, rifampicin)
- 5'-DI inhibitors: PTU, β-blockers, dexamethasone, iodinated drugs

4. Action
- amiodarone
- phenytoin

FIGURE 14-5. Drugs may perturb thyroid hormone homeostasis at different levels. Some drugs, such as amiodarone and phenytoin, have several mechanisms of interaction. IFN, interferon; IL, interleukin; FFA, free fatty acids; NSAID, nonsteroidal antiinflammatory drugs; 5'-DI, 5'-monodeiodinase type I; PTU, prophylthiouracil.

thyroid hormone homeostasis are transient, they may render the interpretation of thyroid function tests difficult. With improvements in the quality of routine measurements of serum free thyroid hormone and thyroid-stimulating hormone (TSH; thyrotropin) concentrations, the latter difficulties have decreased in importance. New drugs, however, particularly the cytokines, are finding a place as therapeutic agents and they can affect not only the function of the thyroid gland but also the peripheral metabolism of thyroid hormones.[1]

ALTERATIONS IN THYROID HORMONE SECRETION

Hormone secretion can be either increased or decreased in response to iodinated drugs, such as radiographic contrast media and amiodarone. Although the inhibitory effect of iodine on thyroidal hormone synthesis and secretion is usually spontaneously reversible after several days, TSH and free thyroxine (T_4) levels may transiently change for 1 to 2 weeks after an acute iodine load. Long-standing iodine-induced hyper- and hypothyroidism occur less frequently and are discussed in detail elsewhere in this chapter. Similarly, the pharmacologic actions of antithyroid drugs are described elsewhere in this chapter and in another chapter (see chap 53).

Pharmacologic agents, such as amiodarone, lithium, and cytokines, may cause thyroid dysfunction by various mechanisms. Amiodarone in particular induces clinically overt hyper- and hypothyroidism. Although amiodarone-induced hyperthyroidism is particularly prevalent (10%) in iodine-deficient regions and in patients with underlying thyroid disease, such as nodular autonomy or Graves' disease, its pathogenesis is heterogeneous, because in a substantial proportion the thyroid was found to be normal before treatment.[2,3] Bartalena and colleagues have proposed two types of amiodarone-induced thyrotoxicosis: a first type (type I), which is compatible with classical iodine-induced increase and release of thyroid hormones in patients with preexisting thyroid abnormalities and with a normal or elevated radioiodine uptake despite the iodine contamination,[4] and a second type (type II), which resembles subacute destructive thyroiditis with excess hormone release in patients with no history of prior thyroid disease,

possibly due to a direct cytotoxic effect of amiodarone.[5–8] The latter form is characterized by a low 24-hour thyroidal radioactive iodine uptake and elevated interleukin-6 serum levels, the latter reflecting a thyroid destructive process.[9] Amiodarone-induced thyroid gland dysfunction, including thyrotoxicosis and hypothyroidism, is discussed in detail elsewhere in this chapter. The other inhibitory effects of amiodarone on thyroid hormone action and on the peripheral deiodination of the thyroid hormones are discussed in detail below.

Lithium, used in the treatment of bipolar depression, is associated with subclinical and overt hypothyroidism in up to 34% and 15% of patients, respectively, and can appear abruptly even after many years of treatment. Therefore, the patient should be regularly examined for symptoms and signs of thyroid dysfunction and thyroid function tests should be performed once or twice a year.[10] The inhibitory effects of lithium occur at multiple sites and this is discussed in detail in the preceding subchapter.

Several cytokines were shown to alter thyroid hormone secretion and metabolism. Administration of interferons, interleukins, and granulocyte-macrophage colony-stimulating factor has been associated with a high frequency of transient hypo- and hyperthyroidism during treatment.[11–15] Although these cytokines may elicit either the appearance or an increase in thyroid autoantibody titers, these changes are not always associated with thyroid dysfunction, which may conversely also occur in the absence of antibodies, possibly through direct effects on the thyroid gland as discussed below. It is nevertheless advisable that patients scheduled to receive cytokine treatments be screened for thyroid antibodies because antibody-positive patients may be at higher risk to develop thyroid dysfunction. Interferons, interleukin-1, and tumor necrosis factor α inhibit iodine organification and hormone release and modulate thyroglobulin production and thyrocyte growth.[16–19] In contrast to interferon-α and interleukin-2, interferon-γ increases the expression of the major histocompatibility complex class II molecules on the cell surface, which is thought to be a crucial event in the initiation of autoimmune diseases.[20,21] Interleukin-2 is used experimentally in the immunotherapy of cancer, which results in transient thyroid dysfunctions in 15% to 40% of the patients.[13] Hypo- and hyperthyroidism were observed, but the occurrence of transient hyperthyroidism followed by a hypothyroid phase, compatible with silent thyroiditis, has also been reported.[22–24] Thyroid function normalizes sometimes during but always after stopping cytokine treatment.

ALTERATIONS IN THYROID HORMONE TRANSPORT

Alterations in Concentrations of Thyroid Hormone-Binding Proteins

In human beings, approximately 0.02% of the circulating T_4 and about 0.1% of circulating T_3 is free, hence the serum total T_4 and T_3 concentrations are equivalent to the concentrations of bound T_4 and T_3.[29] The bound hormones represent a circulating reservoir and are usually not directly accessible to the tissues. Little evidence suggests that substantial amounts of protein-bound T_4 or T_3 can be taken up by cells.[29,30] There may be some exceptions to this rule. For example, the choroid plexus synthesizes and secretes transthyretin into the cerebrospinal fluid. This represents a transport mechanism for T_4. In addition, glial cells have specific receptors for transthyretin, so there may be uptake of T_4 bound to protein into these cells.[31–33] For most tissues, however, the circulating free T_4 and T_3 concentrations determine delivery of T_4 and T_3 and are considered responsible for the cellular effects of thyroid hormones.

Further details on the physiology and abnormalities of the thyroid hormone-binding proteins and the clinical understanding of these perturbations in thyroid hormone transport are discussed in detail in chapters 6, 7, and 18 and elsewhere in this chapter.

Drugs That Compete With T_4 and T_3 Binding Sites on Serum Thyroid Hormone-Binding Proteins

Many drugs inhibit the binding of T_4 and T_3 to their binding sites on serum transport proteins in vitro.[34,35] These effects require high concentrations of such drugs, and the effects are therefore not frequently observed in vivo. The following paragraphs describe the effects of drugs that result in in vivo alteration of serum thyroid hormone levels. When such alterations occur, serum total T_4 and T_3 concentrations decline, but the free hormone concentrations do not.

NONSTEROIDAL ANTI-INFLAMMATORY DRUGS

Salicylates are important drugs in this category because of their widespread use in clinical medicine. Salicylates inhibit T_4 and T_3 binding to both TBG and transthyretin, resulting in the changes in serum T_4 and T_3 concentrations.[36,37] Other nonsteroidal anti-inflammatory drugs also displace T_4 from its binding sites, in particular fenclofenac, but this drug is no longer available in most countries.[38]

DIURETICS

Furosemide has been reported to inhibit T_4 binding.[39] The effect does not occur with oral doses of less than 100 mg but is found consistently with very large intravenous doses of furosemide.

FLAVONS

These naturally occurring substances are structurally similar to thyroid hormones. A synthetic flavonoid (EMD 21388) has been designed to optimize its competitive effect for thyroid hormone-binding and in rats EMD has proven to be a potent displacing agent of T_4 from transthyretin. Its effect on T_3 is less marked. EMD does not compete for T_4 binding to TBG. The flavonoid-induced alterations of free hormone levels in the rat affect TSH-feedback regulation, tissue transfer, and elimination of thyroid hormones. EMD is in addition an inhibitor of 5'-monodeiodination. These findings support the idea that naturally occurring flavonoids may have similar but less dramatic effects on thyroid function than EMD.[33,40–42]

HEPARIN AND FATTY ACIDS

Although the addition of heparin to serum does not increase serum free T_4 levels, some reports document transient rises of free T_4 levels in vivo, particularly when equilibrium dialysis was used for its measurement.[43,44] In most of these studies, crude heparin preparations were used and more recent reports on this subject with highly purified heparin preparations are lacking. Nevertheless, large doses of heparin affect the distribution of T_4 between plasma and its rapidly exchangeable tissue pools so as to increase the former and decrease the latter.[45,46] These changes are of no clinical consequence because heparin-treated patients are euthyroid. The underlying pathogenesis of heparin effect is thought to be due to lipoprotein lipase activation both in vivo and in vitro, hydrolyzing triglycerides to free fatty acids (FFA). This is increased when samples are repeatedly frozen and thawed. To be effective serum FFA levels have to exceed 2.5 to 3 mEq/L. In vivo, such concentrations occur rarely. They may be encountered during hemodialysis and intravenous hyperalimentation, particularly if serum albumin levels are decreased and if the patient is treated with heparin.[44] It is claimed that newer analogue methods for measuring serum free T_4 or T_3 concentrations are unaffected by heparin-lipase-FFA effects.

ALTERATIONS OF THYROID HORMONE ACTION IN TISSUES

Drugs can not only alter hormone availability by means of changes in the free serum concentration, but also by modulating the cellular uptake, metabolism, and nuclear actions of thyroid hormone.

Thyroid Hormone Uptake

The inhibition of thyroid hormone uptake by drugs may occur at the intestinal level, thereby leading to decreased serum hormone levels, or in other target tissues, potentially resulting in cellular hypothyroidism despite normal serum levels. However, the physiologic relevance of thyroid hormone transport systems is still controversial.[47–49]

RESORPTION

Several drugs are known to markedly reduce the absorption of T_4 from the gut, such as cholestyramine, diphenylhydantoin, propranolol, aluminum hydroxide, ferrous sulfate-activated charcoal, and sucralfate.[50-52] Although normally 80% of a 1000-mg dose of T_4 is absorbed within 6 hours, this value drops to 23% when sucralfate is taken simultaneously, resulting in lower T_4 and higher TSH serum levels.[53] This problem can be circumvented by separating the intake of both drugs by 8 hours. The malabsorption of T_4 in the presence of sucralfate may be due to either the formation of an insoluble complex or an inhibition of hormone transport by intestinal cells.

CELLULAR UPTAKE

Amiodarone is the best characterized drug inhibiting cellular thyroid hormone uptake. A selective decrease in hepatic T_4 transport was demonstrated in hepatocytes and perfused rat liver and an impaired T_3 uptake was observed in an anterior pituitary cell line.[54,55] In addition, amiodarone inhibits thyroid hormone deiodination and its binding to nuclear receptors as described below. Benzodiazepines were also shown to inhibit cellular L-T_3 uptake, possibly due to their conformational similarity with this hormone, allowing an interaction with the hepatic iodothyronine membrane transporter at similar sites as the endogenous ligand.[56] Interestingly, the hepatic and muscular L-T_3 uptake seems to be a calcium-dependent process as has been inferred from the profound inhibition of hormone uptake by various calcium channel blockers, such as nifedipine, verapamil, and diltiazem.[57] Finally, furosemide and some nonsteroidal anti-inflammatory drugs were shown to compete for cytosolic T_3-binding sites in cultured cells.[58] However, whether the in vitro observations for these various drugs are quantitatively relevant in vivo remains to be demonstrated.

Drugs That Alter the Intracellular Metabolism of Iodothyronines

DRUGS THAT INDUCE HEPATIC MIXED-FUNCTION OXYGENASES

Many lipophilic drugs are made water soluble by oxidation and conjugation in the liver before their elimination from the body.[59] The enzymes responsible for the oxidative processes are the mixed-function oxygenases, and their activity can be augmented by a number of drugs. Prominent among such agents are the antiepileptic agents phenytoin (DPH), phenobarbital, carbamazepine, and the antituberculous drug rifampicin.

Antiepileptic Agents. It has been known for 30 years that the administration of phenytoin causes alterations in serum thyroid hormone levels.[51,60-63] Similar effects are seen with carbamazepine. Like phenytoin and carbamazepine, phenobarbital induces hepatic mixed-function oxygenases, but its effects on serum thyroid hormone levels are minimal. It may, however, potentiate the effects of the other antiepileptic agents when used in combination with them.[64]

Phenytoin is of particular interest because its effects are not limited to the induction of hepatic drug metabolism. Early in vitro studies had indicated that phenytoin displaced T_4 and T_3 from the binding site of TBG. However, the in vivo serum concentrations do not reach such levels and, therefore, this effect is insignificant. This is also documented by the fact that the percent free fractions of T_4 and T_3 that would be directly affected by a displacing drug are normal in such patients. Nevertheless, the serum total and free T_4 levels are clearly decreased in euthyroid phenytoin-treated patients, whereas in most reports the total and free T_3 concentrations are unchanged or even slightly increased. The decreased serum T_4 levels are not typical of the other drugs inducing the mixed-function oxygenases, which do not change serum levels of total and free T_4 and suggest more complex functions of phenytoin. For instance, it has been reported that phenytoin decreases serum TSH levels and inhibits the TSH response to 500 μg thyrotropin-releasing hormone (TRH) intravenously.[65,66] These findings and others have led to the hypothesis that phenytoin may interfere with cellular uptake and may have agonistic nuclear effects.[67,68] However, because in euthyroid subjects serum TSH levels are in the normal range, hypothyroidism is almost certainly not present. However, newer studies with highly sensitive TSH measurements have not yet been reported. However, serum TSH levels increase in T_4-substituted hypothyroid subjects. This can in part be explained by a decrease in intestinal absorption of T_4.[51] Because the metabolic clearance rate and the hepatic metabolism of T_4 increase in patients treated with phenytoin, it is likely that in normal subjects thyroidal secretion increases to compensate for the hepatic losses and hypothyroid subjects need increased doses of T_4.[69]

Rifampicin. Although the effects of phenytoin and the other antiepileptic drugs have received the most attention, the antituberculosis agent rifampicin is one of the most potent inducers of hepatic mixed-function oxygenases. Significant decreases in serum total and free T_4 and reverse T_3 (rT_3) concentrations have been described by some but not others. Serum T_3 concentrations tend to increase slightly. Rifampicin acts like phenytoin on intracellular thyroid hormone metabolism, but no evidence indicates that it inhibits T_4 and T_3 binding to serum-binding proteins.[70-73] T_4 kinetic data show that rifampicin increases the plasma clearance rate of T_4; in normal subjects, T_4 secretion increases to compensate for the moderate increase in T_4 clearance, T_4 to T_3 conversion does not change, and T_3 production is normal. That thyroid secretion increases is also suggested by the increase in thyroid volume that occurs during rifampin treatment.[74] Therefore, in hypothyroid T_4-substituted subjects, serum TSH levels must be monitored. One L-T_4 treated hypothyroid patient developed marked hypothyroidism during rifampicin treatment.[75]

Both phenytoin and rifampicin have little effect on T_3 metabolism. This is shown more clearly in experimental rat models using the most potent inducer of mixed function oxygenases, nafenopin.[76] This drug greatly increases the metabolic clearance rate of T_4 and its hepatic disposal without changing the T_3 kinetics in these rats. This difference is best explained by the fact that glucuronidation of T_4 is specifically increased, whereas T_3 is preferentially a substrate for sulfation, which is not increased by the induction of mixed-function oxygenases.[77]

In summary, drugs that enhance the activity of the hepatic mixed-function oxygenases result in a decrease in serum total T_4 concentrations. This is due primarily to an acceleration of the hepatic metabolism of T_4 and results in a decrease in its plasma half-life or, more specifically, in an increase in its metabolic clearance rate. In euthyroid subjects there is also a slight increase in T_4 production with the consequence that serum T_3 levels do not change or tend to increase even slightly. Basal serum TSH concentrations increase slightly but not significantly. These findings suggest that the function of the pituitary-thyroid axis can compensate in euthyroid patients, and this is in accordance with the clinical impression of euthyroidism in these subjects. However, in T_4-substituted athyrotic patients the T_4 dose often needs to be adjusted.

DRUGS THAT INHIBIT THE MONODEIODINATION OF T_4

Monodeiodination is a process that involves the sequential removal of iodine atoms from T_4 and is the most important metabolic pathway of this iodothyronine.[78-80] This topic is discussed in detail in chapter 8. Monodeiodination of the outer, phenolic ring of iodothyronines is different from that of the inner ring. Outer-ring monodeiodination is responsible not only for the conversion of T_4 to T_3 but also for the degradation of rT_3 and any other iodothyronine with iodine atoms in the outer ring. At least two enzymes are known to catalyze this reaction, one present primarily in liver, kidney, heart, muscle, and thyroid, called 5'-deiodinase type I, the other predominating in brain cortex, cerebellum, anterior pituitary, and placenta, called 5'-deiodinase type II. 5'-Monodeiodinase type I is a selenoprotein. Its activity is reduced in hypothyroidism and catabolic states and can be inhibited by several drugs (see below), propylthiouracil (PTU) being the specific inhibitor of this enzyme.

5'-Deiodinase type II has a different tissue distribution and its regulation is opposite to 5'-deiodinase type I. For example its activity is reduced in hyperthyroidism and increased in hypothyroidism. It is not affected by catabolic states and so far the only known specific inhibitors are T_4, rT_3, and $3',5'-T_2$. It can be inhibited by iodinated contrast agents (see below), but these agents are not specific inhibitors because they do not directly block the catalytic site. PTU cannot inhibit this enzyme and this property is used for determining its specific activity.[81]

Only one enzyme deiodination has been demonstrated for inner ring, 5'-deiodinase type III. It is a selenoprotein that can be found in brain, subcutis, and placenta. Because the enzyme has recently been cloned, knowledge about its regulation is actively being studied.[82]

Drugs inhibiting monodeiodination can be divided into two groups, those that are iodinated and those that are not. The iodinated drugs are more potent in vivo and inhibit 5'-monodeiodinase types I and II and less so 5-monodeiodinase type III activities; the noniodinated drugs inhibit mainly 5'-monodeiodinase type I activity. Both types of compounds exert their effects predominantly on the process of 5'-deiodination, and this results in a decrease in serum T_3 concentrations. Concentrations of rT_3 are increased to a variable extent by the action of these agents. Because they decrease 5'-deiodination of rT_3, its metabolism is slowed. Production of rT_3 remains unchanged because inner ring monodeiodination of T_4 is not, or only minimally, affected. Dexamethasone may even increase its production.[83]

Noniodinated Drugs

The most important drugs in the noniodinated class are PTU, the synthetic glucocorticoid dexamethasone, and the β-receptor antagonist propranolol.

Propylthiouracil. PTU is one of the antithyroid drugs used for the treatment of hyperthyroidism and, in addition, the only known specific inhibitor of this enzyme. It was the first drug shown to inhibit the conversion of T_4 to T_3 in peripheral tissues but is not the most potent.[84] When it is administered in doses of 450 to 600 mg/d to T_4-treated hypothyroid patients, serum T_3 concentrations fall by 25% to 30% within 48 hours and remain at this level as long as PTU is given.[85] Basal serum TSH concentrations rise slightly, and the serum TSH response to TRH is augmented. In untreated euthyroid subjects, serum rT_3 concentrations increase initially but tend to decline slowly if the drug is continued.[86,87] All values return to pretreatment levels when the drug is discontinued. Therapeutically, this effect is exploited in the treatment of iodine-induced hyperthyroidism where antithyroid drugs are often poor inhibitors of thyroid hormone synthesis and where this additional action is most welcome. A PTU analogue, anilino thiouracil, has been demonstrated in rats to inhibit 5'-deiodinase type I, but it does not affect thyroid hormonogenesis.[88]

Dexamethasone. Dexamethasone has multiple effects on thyroid physiology in human beings. Large doses given acutely or moderate doses administered for a prolonged period suppress the secretion of TSH by the anterior pituitary in euthyroid and hypothyroid individuals, and therefore decrease thyroid hormone secretion.[89,90] In addition, large doses of dexamethasone decrease serum T_3 concentrations in normal subjects and in hypothyroid patients receiving T_4 therapy.[91,92] This latter effect is predominantly due to an inhibitory action on 5'-monodeiodination.[93,94] Recent kinetic data on the in vivo effects of dexamethasone, however, are not identical to those of PTU; dexamethasone increases serum rT_3 levels by increasing rT_3 production, whereas PTU increases rT_3 by decreasing its plasma clearance.[83] In patients with hyperthyroidism caused by Graves' disease, large doses of dexamethasone decrease serum concentrations of T_4.[95] This is due to a decrease in T_4 secretion, whether by a direct thyroidal effect or by decreasing thyroid-stimulating immunogobulin production is not known. Other glucocorticoids in comparable doses have some of these same effects, but none have been studied as extensively as dexamethasone. Clinically the effect of dexamethasone on thyroid hormone metabolism has little or no therapeutic indication but its anti-inflammatory effect is useful in a subset of patients with amiodarone-induced hyperthyroidism (see above and a subsection of this chapter).

These in vivo findings are supported by the observations that treatment of rats for 5 days with dexamethasone reduces the rate of T_4 to T_3 conversion and the rate of rT_3 degradation in vitro in liver homogenates of these animals.[96] In contrast to other potent inhibitors of the 5'-deiodination reaction, however, the addition of dexamethasone to rat liver homogenates in vitro has no effect on the rate of T_4 to T_3 conversion.[97]

Propranolol. β-Receptor antagonists are useful agents in the symptomatic treatment of thyrotoxicosis (see chap 53).

These agents reduce the pulse rate, tremor, anxiety, and hyperreflexia, and they are particularly useful in the treatment of thyrotoxic crisis[98–104] (see chap 51). The mechanisms by which decreased sympathetic nervous system activity alleviates these symptoms and signs are far from clear, however. Studies in thyrotoxic patients have shown that propranolol has no demonstrable effect on thyroid iodine release or T_4 turnover.[105] Propranolol must be given in moderate to high doses to euthyroid or hyperthyroid subjects to induce a modest reduction in serum free T_3 concentrations and a small increase in rT_3 concentrations. Serum TSH levels are not affected by these hormonal changes. This action of propranolol on T_4 metabolism in vivo is not shared by the β-receptor antagonists metoprolol or atenolol and the mixed β- and α-receptor antagonist labetalol.[102,106] These drugs are nevertheless effective in the relief of the symptomatology of hyperthyroidism.

The effects of propranolol on the extrathyroidal metabolism of T_4, T_3, and rT_3 have been evaluated by noncompartmental kinetic methods.[52] The results indicate that the reduction in serum T_3 is mainly due to a reduction in its generation from T_4. The increase in serum rT_3 is largely due to reduction in its metabolic clearance rate, and its generation rate from T_4 is unchanged. The disposal rate of T_4 is reduced, suggesting that its bioavailability to tissues is reduced by the drug.

In vitro studies have shown that the racemic form of propranolol, and other β-adrenergic antagonists[106] inhibit T_4 conversion to T_3 and rT_3 degradation in rat liver homogenates, isolated intact liver cells, and renal tubules. The latter results suggested that the major site of action of propranolol might be at the cell membrane.[107–109] Generation of T_3 from T_4 in isolated rat renal tubules is significantly inhibited not only by DL-propranolol but also by the D- and L-isomers of propranolol. Because D-propranolol is devoid of β-receptor antagonist properties, DL-propranolol is thought to affect T_4 5′-monodeiodination by its ability to stabilize cell membranes. This latter action is akin to that exerted by quinidine, and, indeed, quinidine also inhibits T_4 5′-deiodination in this system. Alternatively, there is evidence for a specific uptake mechanism for T_4 and T_3 by some tissues; propranolol could block this transport system,[47,48] although the effect of propranolol did not appear to be due to an alteration in the cellular uptake of T_4 by the renal tubules.

In summary, propranolol, as well as other β-receptor antagonists, alleviates the peripheral manifestations of thyrotoxicosis. This clinical benefit far exceeds the modest reduction in serum T_3 concentrations caused by the drug, and other related drugs produce the same clinical benefits without altering serum T_3 concentrations. These results indicate that the clinical benefits of β-receptor antagonists are not related to their ability to inhibit T_4 to T_3 conversion.

Iodinated Drugs

Drugs considered in this section include the iodinated radiographic contrast agents and the antiarrhythmic drug, amiodarone.

All iodinated agents affect thyroid function by their large iodine content. Some of these compounds, all of which are lipid soluble and are used for cholecystography, namely iopanoic acid, sodium ipodate, and tyropanoate, also inhibit T_4 5′-monodeiodination.[110,111] Their in vivo effects have been studied in normal subjects and are qualitatively similar. When given to normal subjects, they significantly increase serum free T_4 and rT_3 and decrease serum free T_3 concentrations.[110] However, the extent of the changes varies from one compound to another. In contrast to these lipid-soluble substances, water-soluble contrast agents such as those used for arteriography and venography do not affect monodeiodination.

In patients without thyroid dysfunction, most changes of serum thyroid hormone levels are due to alterations in their metabolism. This can be illustrated in normal subjects receiving 200 μg T_4 daily in whom serum TSH levels were suppressed. Iopanoic acid caused highly significant increases in serum total and free T_4 and rT_3 levels and produced similar decreases in serum T_3 concentrations as in normal subjects not receiving T_4 (Fig 14-6). The rise in serum T_4 concentrations is mainly a reflection of a decreased disposal rate (see Fig 14-6). In addition, kinetic studies have shown that these drugs can acutely discharge T_4 from hepatic (and possibly renal) storage sites.[112] For example, in normal subjects who received an intravenous injection of ^{125}I-T_4, tyropanoate and, to a lesser extent, ipodate, led to a 50% to 60% reduction in hepatic radioactivity within 4 hours. This fall in hepatic radioactivity was accompanied by a 57% to 70% increase in serum radioactivity as well as an increase in serum T_4 concentrations. As a result of these changes, the plasma clearance rate of T_4 decreased. These changes are, however, not only limited to the peripheral metabolism, because in euthyroid subjects, changes in thyroid secretion also occur during the readaptation of thyroid homeostasis. There is an initial rise in serum TSH concentration. This is likely due to a dual effect of these inhibitors, which inhibit 5′-monodeiodinase type II as well as 5′-monodeiodinase type I activity. Serum TSH levels subsequently return to normal.

In addition to the radiographic contrast agents, the antiarrhythmic agent, amiodarone (2-n-butyl-3,4′-diethylaminoethoxy-3′,5′-diiodobenzoylbenzofurane; 75 mg iodine per 200 mg active substance) is known to markedly interfere with thyroid function. Besides thyroid dysfunction, discussed above and in a subsection of this chapter, it induces in every euthyroid subject alterations in thyroid hormone metabolism that are due to the specific ability of the drug to inhibit T_4 5′-monodeiodination.[113–115] The changes in serum T_4, T_3, rT_3, and TSH concentrations are similar to those produced by the iodinated radiographic contrast agents, and the magnitude of these alterations is dose dependent. In normal volunteers given 400 mg amiodarone (150 mg organic iodine) for 3 weeks, serum total and free T_4 concentrations increased, again due to a decrease in the T_4 metabolic clearance rate. The results of kinetic studies suggest decreased transfer of T_4 from the plasma pool to the rapidly exchangeable tissue pools, such as the liver.[116] The T_3 plasma clearance rate tended to be only slightly decreased.[117] Therefore, the decreased serum T_3 levels mainly reflect the decreased conversion of T_4 to T_3. The effect of thyroidal secretion is probably twofold. Initially the large iodine excess is likely to decrease thyroidal secretion, as has been shown to occur with a saturated solution of potassium iodide.[118] After the first 2 weeks, the thyroid escapes form this inhibition and under the drive of an increased TSH secretion, T_4 production tends to increase. This has been demonstrated to occur for iopanoic acid, which has similar effects on thyroid hormone metabolism as amio-

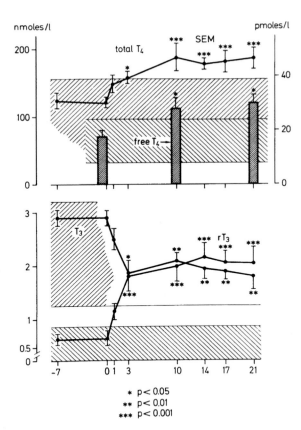

FIGURE 14-6. Effect of iopanoic acid (Telepaque) on mean (± SE) serum thyroid hormone levels in four normal subjects maintained on 0.2 µg L-T$_4$ per day. The number of days are indicated on the abscissa. Iopanoic acid (2 g) was administered on days 0, 7, and 14. (*Upper panel*) Total T$_4$ (●—●) and free T$_4$ (*hatched bars*) concentrations rapidly increased above the normal range (▨ = normal range for total T$_4$; ▨ = normal range for free T$_4$). (*Lower panel*) Iopanoic acid induced significant decreases in serum T$_3$ and significant increases in reverse T$_3$ (rT$_3$) concentrations (▨ = normal range for total T$_3$; ▨ = normal range for rT$_3$). (Data adapted from Burgi H, Wimpfheimer C, Burger AG, Zaunbauer W, Roesler H, LeMarchand-Beraud T. Changes of circulating thyroxine, triiodothyronine and reverse triiodothyronine after radiographic contrast agents. J Clin Endocrinol Metab 1976;43:1203)

darone. However, T$_4$ secretion does not increase sufficiently to restore serum T$_3$ levels to pretreatment levels. This suggests that the inhibition of intrapituitary conversion is less affected than in the periphery. These effects have attracted much attention and it has been postulated that some of the excellent antiarrhythmic effects of this drug might be due to a hypothyroid state of the heart. Experiments in rats largely support this hypothesis even though in these studies only tissue T$_3$ content and not the actual saturation of the T$_3$ receptor with T$_3$ was measured.[119] In addition, it is thought that amiodarone and/or its main metabolite, desethyl amiodarone, may be a weak antagonist of thyroid hormone action.[120] However, clinical studies do not support the hypothesis that the antiarrhythmic effect of amiodarone is due to decreased T$_3$ production and there is also no evidence that the action of T$_3$ is decreased in these patients.[121–123]

In clinical practice, amiodarone is used for long-term treatment. After several weeks of treatment with a moderate dose

(200 or 100 mg/d), serum thyroid hormone levels tend to remain within the normal limits, even though serum free T$_4$ levels are higher and serum T$_3$, free T$_3$, and TSH levels are lower than before treatment. In some patients, however, particularly those treated with larger doses of amiodarone, serum free T$_4$ levels can be as high as in moderate hyperthyroidism.[115] When T$_4$ kinetic parameters are compared in chronically treated subjects with normal TSH levels with those of hyperthyroid Graves' disease patients, striking differences are found. Thus, the T$_4$ production rate of the amiodarone-treated group is significantly lower than that of the hyperthyroid group, and the disappearance of injected ^{125}I-T$_4$ is significantly delayed (Fig 14-7). These findings demonstrate that, despite increased total and free serum T$_4$ concentrations, T$_4$ kinetics in amiodarone-treated patients more closely approximate those of euthyroid subjects. In addition, these patients have normal serum T$_3$ or free T$_3$ levels. These studies were performed before the introduction of highly sensitive TSH measurements and it is possible that some of these patients had a decreased serum TSH level (<0.1 mU/L). Often, these patients have no obvious clinical stigmata of hyperthyroidism and possibly the peripheral tissues are not frankly hyperthyroid. Nevertheless, the suppressed serum TSH (<0.1 mU/L) suggests the escape of thyroidal secretion from the normal feedback control mechanism.

Clinical Use of Iodinated Inhibitors of Monodeiodination

These agents have been used successfully in the treatment of severe forms of Graves' disease and toxic multinodular goiter.[124–126] Most studies have used the more rapidly cleared ipodate that decreases serum T$_3$ levels to within the normal range in a short period of time (2–6 days).[127,128] Serum T$_4$ levels decrease more slowly than with potassium iodide treatment, probably reflecting the decrease in T$_4$ plasma clearance rate induced by ipodate. The therapeutic use of these agents is mainly restricted to preoperative treatment; during long-term treatment escape from the iodide inhibition of thyroidal secretion often occurs.[129] Another rare indication

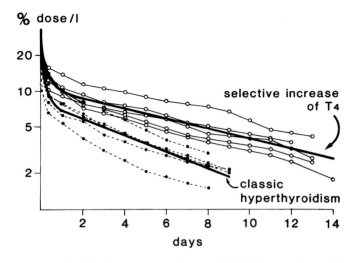

FIGURE 14-7. The disappearance of serum ^{125}I-T$_4$ in four patients with classic hyperthyroidism (–●–) and in five patients treated with amiodarone who had selective increases in serum total and free T$_4$ concentrations (–○–). The mean values are represented as solid lines.

may be self-limited neonatal hyperthyroidism (see chap 86) or thyrotoxicosis factitia.[130] Even amiodarone has been proposed for this purpose, but its long half-life makes this unwise.[131,132]

In summary, the lipid-soluble radiographic contrast agents and amiodarone induce alterations in thyroid hormone levels by actions on the peripheral tissues, on thyroidal secretion, and probably also on the pituitary gland. These actions result in elevations in serum T_4 and rT_3 concentrations, transient increases in TSH concentrations, and decreases in T_3 concentrations. These findings may be explained by inhibition of T_4 and rT_3 5′-monodeiodination in many tissues (liver, kidney, brain) and in the thyrotrophs, and by the liberation of T_4 (and rT_3) from hepatic and renal storage pools. In contrast to their effects in normal patients, in hyperthyroid patients these agents cause a decrease in serum T_4 concentrations as well as a marked decrease in serum T_3 levels. In addition, these agents, particularly amiodarone, are prone to induce thyroid dysfunction that is particularly difficult to treat.

Effects on Nuclear Hormone Action

Amiodarone decreases thyroid hormone synthesis, secretion, and deiodination. In addition, desethylamiodarone, the major metabolite of this iodinated benzofurane derivative, is a noncompetitive inhibitor of T_3 binding to *Escherichia coli* expressed β_1-T_3 receptor protein with an IC50 of 2×10^{-5} M and preferential binding to unoccupied receptors.[120] This observation might explain the decreased nuclear receptor T_3-binding capacity in the myocardium of amiodarone-treated rats, as well as the antagonistic effect of amiodarone treatment on the expression of pituitary growth hormone expression and cardiac β-adrenoreceptor density.[54,133–136] No data exist in human studies to support the notion of selective target tissue resistance to T_3 in amiodarone-treated patients. Although an elevation of serum TSH levels during amiodarone treatment has been described in patients on a constant replacement dose of T_4, this finding is most compatible with an amiodarone-induced decrease in pituitary and peripheral deiodination. However, a contribution from decreased cellular uptake and nuclear action cannot be excluded.[137,138] In contrast, phenytoin, in addition to its effects on thyroid hormone metabolism described above, has been considered as a partial thyroid hormone agonist, although these early studies await confirmation by more direct methods using the cloned thyroid hormone receptor proteins.[65,66]

References

1. Dubuis JM, Dayer JM, Siegrist-Kaiser CA, Burger AG. Human recombinant interleukin-1b decreases plasma thyroid hormone and thyroid stimulating hormone levels in rats. Endocrinology 1988;123:2175
2. Martino E, Safran M, Aghini-Lombardi F, et al. Environmental iodine intake and thyroid dysfunction during chronic amiodarone therapy. Ann Intern Med 1984;101:28
3. Trip MD, Wiersinga W, Plomb TA. Incidence, predictability, and pathogenesis of amiodarone-induced thyrotoxicosis and hypothyroidism. Am J Med 1991;91:507
4. Martino E, Bartalena L, Mariotti S, et al. Radioactive iodine thyroid uptake in patients with amiodarone-iodine-induced thyroid dysfunction. Acta Endocrinol (Copenh) 1988;119:167
5. Roti E, Minelli R, Gardini E, et al. Thyrotoxicosis followed by hypothyroidism in patients treated with amiodarone. A possible consequence of a destructive process in the thyroid. Arch Intern Med 1993;153:886
6. Smyrk TC, Goellner JR, Brennan MD, Carney JA. Pathology of the thyroid in amiodarone-induced thyrotoxicosis. Am J Surg Pathol 1987;11:197
7. Bartalena L, Grasso L, Brogioni S, et al. Serum interleukin-6 in amiodarone-induced thyrotoxicosis. J Clin Endocrinol Metab 1994;78:423
8. Chiovato L, Martino E, Tonacchera M, et al. Studies on the in vitro cytotoxic effect of amiodarone. Endocrinology 1994;134:2277
9. Bartalena L, Brogioni S, Grasso L, et al. Interleukin-6: a arker of thyroid-destructive processes? J Clin Endocrinol Metab 1994; 79:1424
10. Davies PH, Franklyn JA. The effects of drugs on tests of thyroid function. Eur J Clin Pharmacol 1991;40:439
11. Burman P, Titterman TH, Orberg K, Karlsson FA. Thyroid autoimmunity in patients on long term therapy with leukocyte-derived interferon. J Clin Endocrinol Metab 1986;63:1086
12. Reichlin S. Neuroendocrine-immune interactions. N Engl J Med 1993;329:1246
13. Atkins MB, Mier JW, Parkinson DR, et al. Hypothyroidism after treatment with interleukin-2 and lymphokine-activated killer cells. N Engl J Med 1988;318:1557
14. Hoekman K, von Blomberg-van der Flier BME, Wagstaff J, et al. Reversible thyroid dysfunction during treatment with GM-CSF. Lancet 1991;338:541
15. Van Hoff ME, Howell A. Risk of thyroid dysfunction during treatment with G-CSF. Lancet 1992;340:1169
16. Sato K, Satoh T, Shizume K, et al. Inhibition of ^{125}I organification and thyroid hormone release by interleukin-1, tumor necrosis factor-alpha, and interferon-gamma in human thyrocytes in suspension culture. J Clin Endocrinol Metab 1990;70:1735
17. Mooradian AD, Reed RL, Osterweil D, et al. Decreased serum T_3 is associated with increased concentrations of tumor necrosis factor. J Clin Endocrinol Metab 1990;71:1239
18. Chopra IJ, Sakane S, Teco GNC. A study of the serum concentration of tumor necrosis factor-α in thyroidal and nonthyroidal illnesses. J Clin Endocrinol Metab 1991;72:1113
19. Yamazaki K, Kanaji Y, Shizume K, et al. Reversible inhibition by interferons alpha and beta of ^{125}I incorporation and thyroid hormone release by human thyroid follicles in vitro. J Clin Endocrinol Metab 1993;77:1439
20. Kraiem Z, Sobel E, Sadeh O, et al. Effects of gamma-interferon on DR antigen expression, growth, 3,5,3′- triiodothyronine secretion, iodide uptake, and cyclic adenosine 3′,5′-monophosphate accumulation in cultured human thyroid cells. J Clin Endocrinol Metab 1990;71:817
21. Kasuga Y, Matsubayashi S, Akasu F, et al. Effects of recombinant human interleukin-2 and tumor necrosis factor-alpha with or without interferon-gamma on human thyroid tissues from patients with Graves' disease and from normal subjects xenografted into nude mice. J Clin Endocrinol Metab 1991;72:1296
22. Schwartzentruber DJ, White DE, Zweig MH, et al. Thyroid dysfunction associated with immunotherapy for patients with cancer. Cancer 1991;68:2384
23. Vialettes B, Guillerand MA, Viens P, et al. Incidence rate and risk factors for thyroid dysfunction during recombinant interleukin-2 therapy in advanced malignancies. Acta Endocrinol (Copenh) 1993;129:31
24. Vassilopoulou-Sellin R, Sella A, Dexeus FH, et al. Acute thyroid dysfunction (thyroiditis) after therapy with interleukin-2. Horm Metab Res 1992;24:434
25. Robbins J, Cheng SY, Gershengorn MC, et al. Thyroxine transport proteins in plasma. Molecular properties and biosynthesis.

In: Greep RO, ed. Recent progress in hormone research. New York, Academic Press, 1978;84:477

26. Benvenga S, Cahnmann HJ, Gregg RE, Robbins J. Characterization of the binding of thyroxine to high density lipoproteins and apolipoproteins A-I. J Clin Endocrinol Metab 1989;68:1067

27. Benvenga S, Cahnmann HJ, Robbins J. Localization of the thyroxine binding sites in apolipoprotein B-100 of human low density lipoproteins. Endocrinology 1990;127:2241

28. Benvenga S, Cahnmann HJ, Robbins J. Characterization of thyroid hormone binding to apolipoprotein-E: localization of the binding site in the exon 3-coded domain. Endocrinology 1993; 133:1300

29. Mendel CM. The free hormone hypothesis: a physiologically based mathematical model. Endocr Rev 1989;10:232

30. Mendel CM, Cavalieri RR, Weisiger RA. Uptake of thyroxine by the perfused rat liver: implications for the free hormone hypothesis. Am J Physiol 1988;255:E110

31. Divino CM, Schussler GC. Receptor-mediated uptake and internalization of transthyretin. J Biol Chem 1990;265:1425

32. Harms PJ, Tu GF, Richardson SJ, et al. Transthyretin (prealbumin) gene expression in choroid plexus is strongly conserved during evolution of vertebrates. Comp Biochem Physiol 1991; 99:239

33. Chanoine JP, Alex S, Fang SL, et al. Role of transthyretin in the transport of thyroxine from the blood to the choroid plexus, the cerebrospinal fluid, and the brain. Endocrinology 1992;130:933

34. Wenzel KW. Pharmacological interference with in vitro tests of thyroid function. Metabolism 1981;30:717

35. Cavalieri RR. Effects of drugs on human thyroid hormone metabolism. In: Hennemann G, ed. Thyroid hormone metabolism. New York and Basel: Marcel Dekker, 1986:359

36. Ratcliffe WA, Hazelton RA, Thompson JA. Effect of fenclofenac on thyroid-function tests. Lancet 1980;1:432

37. Baranetsky NG, Chertow BS, Webb MD, et al. Combined phenytoin and salicylate effects on thyroid function tests. Arch Int Pharmacodyn Ther 1986;284:166

38. Humphrey MJ, Capper SJ, Kurtz AB. Fenclofenac and thyroid hormone concentrations. Lancet 1980;1:487

39. Lim CF, Bai Y, Topliss DJ, et al. Drug and fatty acid effects on serum thyroid hormone binding. J Clin Endocrinol Metab 1988;67:682

40. Spanka M, Hesch RD, Irmscher K, Kohrle J. 5'-Deiodination in rat hepatocytes: effects of specific flavonoid inhibitors. Endocrinology 1990;126:1660

41. Lueprasitsakul W, Alex S, Fang SL, et al. Flavonoid administration immediately displaces thyroxine (T_4) from serum transthyretin, increases serum free T_4, and decreases serum thyrotropin in the rat. Endocrinology 1990;126:2890

42. Abend SL, Fang SL, Alex S, et al. Rapid alteration in circulating free thyroxine modulates pituitary type II 5' deiodinase and basal thyrotropin secretion in the rat. J Clin Invest 1991; 88:898

43. Wang YS, Hershman JM, Smith V, Pekary AE. Effect of heparin on free thyroxine as measured by equilibrium dialysis and ultrafiltration. Clin Chem 1986;32:700

44. Mendel CM, Frost PH, Kunitake ST, Cavalieri RR. Mechanism of the heparin-induced increase in the concentration of free thyroxine in plasma. J Clin Endocrinol Metab 1987;65:1259

45. Saeed-Uz-Zafar M, Miller JM, Breneman GM, Mansour J. Observations on the effect of heparin on free and total thyroxine. J Clin Endocrinol Metab 1971;32:633

46. Schwartz HL, Schadlow AR, Faierman D, et al. Heparin administration appears to decrease cellular binding of thyroxine. J Clin Endocrinol Metab 1973;36:598

47. Krenning, EP, Docter R. Plasma membrane transport of thyroid hormone. In Hennemann G, ed. Thyroid hormone metabolism. New York and Basel: Marcel Dekker, 1986:107

48. Pontecorvi A, Robbins J. The plasma membrane and thyroid hormone entry into cells. Trends Endocrinol Metab 1989;1:90

49. Dejong M, Visser TJ, Bernard BF, et al. Transport and metabolism of iodothyronines in cultured human hepatocytes. J Clin Endocrinol Metab 1993;77:139

50. Northcutt RC, Stiel JN, Hollifield JW, Stant EG. The influence of cholestyramine on thyroxine absorption. JAMA 1969;208:1857

51. Faber J, Lumholtz IB, Kirkegaard C, et al. The effects of phenytoin (diphenylhydantoin) on the extrathyroidal turnover of thyroxine, 3,5,3'-triiodothyronine, 3,3',5'- triiodothyronine, and 3',5'-diiodothyronine in man. J Clin Endocrinol Metab 1985;61:1093

52. Lumholtz IB, Siersbaek-Nielsen K, Faber J, et al. Effect of propanolol on extrathyroidal metabolism of thyroxine and 3,3',5-triiodothyronine evaluated by noncompartmental kinetics. J Clin Endocrinol Metab 1978;47:587

53. Sherman SI, Tielens ET, Ladenson PW. Sucralfate causes malabsorption of L-thyroxine. Am J Med 1994;96:531

54. Norman MF, Lavin TN. Antagonism of thyroid hormone action by amiodarone in rat pituitary tumor cells. J Clin Invest 1989; 83:306

55. de Jong M, Docter R, Van der Hoek H, et al. Different effects of amiodarone on transport of T_4 and T_3 into the perfused rat liver. Am J Physiol 1994;266:E44

56. Kragie L, Forrester ML, Cody V, Mccourt M. Computer-assisted molecular modeling of benzodiazepine and thyromimetic inhibitors of the HepG2 iodothyronine membrane transporter. Mol Endocrinol 1994;8:382

57. Topliss DJ, Scholz GH, Kolliniatis E, et al. Influence of calmodulin antagonists and calcium channel blockers on triiodothyronine uptake by rat hepatoma and myoblast cell lines. Metabolism 1993;42:376

58. Barlow JW, Curtis AJ, Raggatt LE, et al. Drug competition for intracellular triiodothyronine-binding sites. Eur J Endocrinol 1994; 130:417

59. Brosen K. Recent developments in hepatic drug oxidation. Implications for clinical pharmacokinetics. Clin Pharmacokinet 1990;18:220

60. Yeo PP, Bates D, Howe JG, et al. Anticonvulsants and thyroid function. Br Med J 1978;1:1581

61. Cavalieri RR, Gavin LA, Wallace A, et al. Serum thyroxine, free T_4, triiodothyronine, and reverse-T_3 in diphenylhydantoin-treated patients. Metabolism 1979;28:1161

62. Kozlowski BW, Taylor ML, Baer MT, et al. Anticonvulsant medication use and circulating levels of total thyroxine, retinol binding protein, and vitamin A in children with delayed cognitive development. Am J Clin Nutr 1987;46:360

63. Larkin JG, Macphee GJ, Beastall GH, Brodie MJ. Thyroid hormone concentrations in epileptic patients. Eur J Clin Pharmacol 1989;36:213

64. Rootwelt K, Ganes T, Johannessen SI. Effect of carbamazepine, phenytoin and phenobarbitone on serum levels of thyroid hormones and thyrotropin in humans. Scand J Clin Lab Invest 1978;38:731

65. Surks MI, Ordene KW, Mann DN, Kumara-Siri MH. Diphenylhydantoin inhibits the thyrotropin response to thyrotropin-releasing hormone in man and rat. J Clin Endocrinol Metab 1983; 56:940

66. Smith PJ, Surks MI. Multiple effects of 5,5'-diphenylhydantoin on the thyroid hormone system. Endocr Rev 1984;5:514

67. Zemel LR, Biezunski DR, Shapiro LE, Surks MI. 5,5'-Diphenylhydantoin decreases the entry of 3,5,3'-triiodo-L- thyronine but not L-thyroxine in cultured GH-producing cells. Acta Endocrinol 1988;117:392

68. Gingrich SA, Smith PJ, Shapiro LE, Surks MI. 5,5'-Diphenylhydantoin (phenytoin) attenuates the action of 3,5,3'- triiodo-L-thyronine in cultured GC cells. Endocrinology 1985;116:2306

69. Surks MI. Hypothyroidism and phenytoin (letter). Ann Intern Med 1985;102:871

70. Ohnhaus EE, Studer H. The effect of different doses of rifampicin on thyroid hormone metabolism (proceedings). Br J Clin Pharmacol 1980;9:285

71. Ohnhaus EE, Burgi H, Burger A, Studer H. The effect of antipyrine, phenobarbitol and rifampicin on thyroid hormone metabolism in man. Eur J Clin Invest 1981;11:381.

72. Ohnhaus EE, Studer H. A link between liver microsomal enzyme activity and thyroid hormone metabolism in man. Br J Clin Pharmacol 1983;15:71

73. Finke C, Juge C, Goumaz M, et al. Effects of rifampicin on the peripheral turnover kinetics of thyroid hormones in mice and in men. J Endocrinol Invest 1987;10:157

74. Christensen HR, Simonsen K, Hegedus L, et al. Influence of rifampicin on thyroid gland volume, thyroid hormones, and antipyrine metabolism. Acta Endocrinol (Copenh) 1989; 121:406

75. Isley WL. Effect of rifampin therapy on thyroid function tests in a hypothyroid patient on replacement L-thyroxine. Ann Intern Med 1987;107:517

76. Kaiser CA, Seydoux J, Giacobino JP, et al. Increased plasma clearance rate of thyroxine despite decreased 5'-monodeiodination: study with a peroxisome proliferator in the rat. Endocrinology 1988;122:1087

77. Visser TJ, Joop C, van Buuren J, et al. The role of sulfatation in thyroid hormone metabolism. Trends Endocrinol Metab 1990;2:211

78. Engler D, Burger AG. The deiodination of the iodothyronines and of their derivatives in man. Endocr Rev 1984;5:151

79. Leonard JL, Visser TJ. Biochemistry of deiodination. In: Hennemann G, ed. Thyroid hormone metabolism. New York and Basel: Marcel Dekker, 1986:189

80. Danforth E, Burger AG. The impact of nutrition on thyroid hormone physiology and action. Annu Rev Nutr 1989;9:201

81. Visser TJ, Leonard JL, Kaplan MM, Larsen PR. Different pathways of iodothyronine 5'-deiodination in rat cerebral cortex. Biochem Biophys Res Commun 1981;101:1297

82. St Germain DL, Schwartzman RA, Croteau W, et al. A thyroid hormone-regulated gene in *Xenopus laevis* encodes a type III iodothyronine 5-deiodinase. Proc Natl Acad Sci U S A 1994;91:7767

83. LoPresti JS, Eigen A, Kaptein E, et al. Alteration in 3,3',5'-triiodothyronine metabolism in response to propylthiouracil, dexamethasone, and thyroxine administration in man. J Clin Invest 1989;84:1650

84. Geffner DL, Azukizawa M, Hershman JM. Propylthiouracil blocks extrathyroidal conversion of thyroxine to triiodothyronine and augments thyrotropin secretion in man. J Clin Invest 1975;55:224

85. Saberi M, Sterling FH, Utiger RD. Reduction in extrathyroidal triiodothyronine production by propylthiouracil in man. J Clin Invest 1975;55:218

86. Kaplan MM, Schimmel M, Utiger RD. Changes in serum 3,3',5'-triiodothyronine (reverse T_3) concentrations with altered thyroid hormone secretion and metabolism. J Clin Endocrinol Metab 1977;45:447

87. Westgren U, Melander A, Wahlin E, Lindgren J. Divergent effects of 6-propylthiouracil on 3,3',5'-triiodothyronine (rT_3) serum levels and in man. Acta Endocrinol (Copenh) 1977;85:345

88. Nogimori T, Braverman LE, Taurog A, et al. A new class of propylthiouracil analogs: comparison of 5'-deiodinase inhibition and antithyroid activity. Endocrinology 1986;118:1598

89. Wilber JF, Utiger RD. The effect of glucocorticoids on thyrotropin secretion. J Clin Invest 1969;48:2096

90. Nicoloff JT, Fisher DA, Appleman MD Jr. The role of glucocorticoids in the regulation of thyroid function in man. J Clin Invest 1970;49:1922

91. Duick DA, Warren DW, Nicoloff JT, et al. Effect of single-dose dexamethasone on the concentration of serum triiodothyronine in man. J Clin Endocrinol Metab 1974;39:1151

92. DeGroot LJ, Hoye K. Dexamethasone suppression of serum T_3 and T_4. J Clin Endocrinol Metab 1976;42:976

93. Chopra IJ, Williams DE, Orgiazzi J, Solomon DH. Opposite effects of dexamethasone on serum concentrations of 3,3',5'-triiodothyronine (reverse T_3) and 3,3',5-triiodothyronine (T_3). J Clin Endocrinol Metab 1975;41:911

94. Burr WA, Ramsden DB, Griffiths RS, et al. Effect of a single dose of dexamethasone on serum concentrations of thyroid hormones. Lancet 1976;2:58

95. Williams DE, Chopra IJ, Orgiazzi J, Solomon DH. Acute effects of corticosteroids on thyroid activity in Graves' disease. J Clin Endocrinol Metab 1975;41:354

96. Kaplan MM, Utiger RD. Iodothyronine metabolism in rat liver homogenates. J Clin Invest 1978;61:459

97. Cavalieri RR, Castle JN, McMahon FA. Effects of dexamethasone on kinetics and distribution of triiodothyronine in the rat. Endocrinology 1984;114:215

98. Verhoeven RP, Visser TJ, Docter R, et al. Plasma thyroxine, 3,3',5-triiodothyronine and 3,3',5'-triiodothyronine during beta-adrenergic blockade in hyperthyroidism. J Clin Endocrinol Metab 1977;44:1002

99. Lotti G, Delitala G, Devilla L, et al. Reduction of plasma triiodothyronine (T_3) induced by propranolol. Clin Endocrinol (Oxf) 1977;6:405

100. Saunders J, Hall SEH, Crowther A, Sonksen PH. The effect of propranolol on thyroid hormones and oxygen consumption in thyrotoxicosis. Clin Endocrinol 1978;9:67

101. Kallner G, Ljunggren JG, Tryselius M. The effect of propranolol on serum levels of T_4, T_3 and reverse-T_3 in hyperthyroidism. Acta Med Scand 1978;204:35

102. Murchison LE, How J, Bewsher PD. Comparison of propranolol and metoprolol in the management of hyperthyroidism. Br J Clin Pharmacol 1979;8:581

103. Feely J, Isles TE, Ratcliffe WA, Crooks J. Propranolol, triiodothyronine, reverse triiodothyronine and thyroid disease. Clin Endocrinol (Oxf) 1979;10:531

104. Faber J, Friis T, Kirkegaard C, et al. Serum T_4, T_3 and reverse T_3 during treatment with propranolol in hyperthyroidism, L-T_4 treated myxedema and in normal man. Horm Metab Res 1979;11:34

105. Wartofsky L, Dimond RC, Noel GL, et al. Failure of propranolol to alter thyroid iodine release, thyroxine turnover, or the TSH and PRL responses to thyrotropin-releasing hormone in patients with thyrotoxicosis. J Clin Endocrinol Metab 1975;41:485

106. Shulkin BL, Peele ME, Utiger RD. Beta-adrenergic antagonist inhibition of hepatic 3,5,3'-triiodothyronine production. Endocrinology 1984;115:858

107. Heyma P, Larkins RG, Stockigt JR, Campbell DG. The formation of tri-iodothyronine and reverse tri-iodothyronine from thyroxine in isolated rat renal tubules. Clin Sci Mol Med Suppl 1978; 55:567

108. Heyma P, Larkins RG, Higginbotham L, Ng KW. D-propanolol and DL-propanolol both decrease conversion of L-thyroxine to L-triiodothyronine. Br Med J 1980;281:24

109. Heyma P, Larkins RG, Campbell DG. Inhibition by propanolol of 3,5,3'-triiodothyronine formation from thyroxine in isolated rat renal tubules: an effect independent of beta-adrenergic blockade. Endocrinology 1980;106:1437

110. Burgi H, Wimpfheimer C, Burger A, et al. Changes of circulating thyroxine, triiodothyronine and reverse triiodothyronine after radiographic contrast agents. J Clin Endocrinol Metab 1976;43:1203

111. Suzuki H, Kadena N, Takeuchi K, Nakagawa S. Effects of three-day oral cholecystography on serum iodothyronines and TSH concentrations: comparison of the effects among some cholecystographic agents and the effects of iopanoic acid on the pituitary-thyroid axis. Acta Endocrinol (Copenh) 1979;92:477

112. Felicetta JV, Green WL, Nelp WB. Inhibition of hepatic binding of thyroxine by cholecystographic agents. J Clin Invest 1980;65:1032

113. Burger A, Dinichert D, Nicod P, et al. Effect of amiodarone on serum triiodothyronine, reverse triiodothyronine, thyroxin, and thyrotropin. A drug influencing peripheral metabolism of thyroid hormones. J Clin Invest 1976;58:255

114. Melmed S, Nademanee K, Reed AW, et al. Hyperthyroxinemia with bradycardia and normal thyrotropin secretion after chronic amiodarone administration. J Clin Endocrinol Metab 1981;53:997

115. Lambert MJ, Burger AG, Galeazzi RL, Engler D. Are selective increases in serum thyroxine (T_4) due to iodinated contrast agents. J Clin Endocrinol Metab 1982;55:1058

116. Kaptein EM, Egodage PM, Hoopes MT, Burger AG. Amiodarone alters thyroxine transfer and distribution in humans. Metabolism 1988;37:1107

117. Zaninovich AA, Bosco SC, Fernandez-Pol AJ. Amiodarone does not affect the distribution and fractional turnover of triiodothyronine from the plasma pool, but only its generation from thyroxine in extrathyroidal tissues. J Clin Endocrinol Metab 1990;70:1721

118. Vagenakis AG, Downs P, Braverman LE, et al. Control of thyroid hormone secretion in normal subjects receiving iodides. J Clin Invest 1973;52:528

119. Schroder van der Elst JP, Van der Heide D. Thyroxine, 3,5,3'-triiodothyronine, and 3,3',5'-triiodothyronine concentrations in several tissues of the rat: effects of amiodarone and desethylamiodarone on thyroid hormone metabolism (corrected) (published erratum appears in Endocrinology 1991 Jan;128:393). Endocrinology 1990;127:1656

120. Bakker O, van Beeren HC, Wiersinga WM. Desethylamiodarone is a noncompetitive inhibitor of the binding of thyroid hormone to the thyroid hormone beta 1-receptor protein. Endocrinology 1994;134:1665

121. Polikar R, Goy JJ, Schlapfer J, et al. Effect of oral triiodothyronine during amiodarone treatment for ventricular premature complexes. Am J Cardiol 1986;58:987

122. Polikar R, Goy JJ, Schlapfer J, et al. Effect of oral T_3 during amiodarone treatment for ventricular premature complexes. Am J Cardiol 1986;58:987

123. Lambert M, Burger AG, de Nayer P, Beckers C. Decreased TSH response to TRH induced by amiodarone. Acta Endocrinol 1988;118:449

124. Wu SY, Chopra IJ, Solomon DH, Bennett LR. Changes in circulating iodothyronines in euthyroid and hyperthyroid subjects given ipodate (Oragrafin), an agent for oral cholecystography. J Clin Endocrinol Metab 1978;46:691

125. Wu SY, Chopra IJ, Solomon DH, Johnson DE. The effect of repeated administration of ipodate (Oragrafin) in hyperthyroidism. J Clin Endocrinol Metab 1978;47:1358

126. Karpman BA, Rapoport B, Filetti S, Fisher DA. Treatment of neonatal hyperthyroidism due to Graves' disease with sodium ipodate. J Clin Endocrinol Metab 1987;64:119

127. Roti E, Robuschi G, Gardini E, et al. Comparison of methimazole, methimazole and sodium ipodate, and methimazole and saturated solution of potassium iodide in the early treatment of hyperthyroid Graves' disease. Clin Endocrinol (Oxf) 1988;28:305

128. Berghout A, Wiersinga WM, Brummelkamp WH. Sodium ipodate in the preparation of Graves' hyperthyroid patients for thyroidectomy. Horm Res 1989;31:256

129. Martino E, Balzano S, Bartalena L, et al. Therapy of Graves' disease with sodium ipodate is associated with a high recurrence rate of hyperthyroidism. J Endocrinol Invest 1991;14:847

130. Cohen JH, Ingbar SH, Braverman LE. Thyrotoxicosis due to ingestion of excess thyroid hormone. Endocr Rev 1994;10:364

131. Van Reeth O, Unger J. Effects of amiodarone on serum T_3 and T_4 concentrations in hyperthyroid patients treated with propylthiouracil. Thyroid 1991;1:301

132. Van Reeth O, Decoster C, Unger J. Effect of amiodarone on serum T_4 and T_3 levels in hyperthyroid patients treated with methimazole. Eur J Clin Pharmacol 1987;32:223

133. Gotzsche LBH, Orskov H. Cardiac triiodothyronine nuclear receptor binding capacities in amiodarone-treated, hypo- and hyperthyroid rats. Eur J Endocrinol 1994;130:281

134. Paradis P, Lambert C, Rouleau J. Amiodarone antagonizes the effects of T_3 at the receptor level: an additional mechanism for its in vivo hypothyroid-like effects. Can J Physiol Pharmacol 1991;69:865

135. Perret G, Yin YL, Nicolas P, et al. Amiodarone decreases cardiac beta-adrenoceptors through an antagonistic effect on 3,5,3' triiodothyronine. J Cardiovasc Pharmacol 1992;19:473

136. Gotzsche LBH. Beta-adrenergic receptors, voltage-operated Ca^{2+}-channels, nuclear triiodothyronine receptors and triiodothyronine concentration in pig myocardium after long-term low-dose amiodarone treatment. Acta Endocrinol (Copenh) 1993;129:337

137. Figge HL, Figge J. The effects of amiodarone on thyroid hormone function: a review of the physiology and clinical manifestations. J Clin Pharmacol 1990;30:588

138. Figge J, Dluhy RG. Amiodarone-induced elevation of thyroid stimulating hormone in patients receiving levothyroxine for primary hypothyroidism. Ann Intern Med 1990;113:553

NONTHYROIDAL ILLNESSES

John T. Nicoloff
Jonathan S. LoPresti

Many, if not all, nonthyroidal systemic illnesses are associated with alterations in serum thyroid hormone concentrations in patients with no apparent intrinsic thyroid disease.[1-3] Most commonly, these assume the form of either a low T_3 state, in which serum total and free triiodothyronine (T_3) concentrations are decreased while serum thyroxine (T_4) and free T_4 concentrations remain normal, or a low T_3/T_4 state, in which both serum T_4 and T_3 concentrations are decreased. This latter pattern is characteristically associated with more severe life-threatening illnesses. Despite these low serum thyroid hormone concentrations, however, there is usually little clinical evidence of hypothyroidism. Further, serum thyrotropin (TSH) concentrations generally remain normal despite the reduction in serum T_3 and sometimes T_4 concentrations. The patients, therefore, are not generally considered to be thyroid hormone deficient in a classic sense, but instead to have altered thyroid hormone metabolism and be euthyroid. The term *euthyroid sick syndrome* is often used to describe this condition, but there is no single biochemical syndrome and the assumption that the patients are euthyroid—at least in all tissues—may be incorrect.

The types of illnesses responsible for these abnormalities in thyroid function vary widely and include infectious disease, sepsis, surgery, trauma, chronic degenerative and chronic diseases, and metabolic disorders, such as diabetes mellitus, undernutrition, and fasting.[4-12] Moreover, these illnesses not only result in abnormal thyroid function but often are associated with a wide array of other endocrine alterations, including reductions in serum insulin-like growth factor I (IGF-I), IGF-I binding protein-3, gonadotropin, and sex hormone concentrations as well as increases in serum ACTH and cortisol concentrations.[13–15] These endocrine responses to illness appear to be orchestrated by another group of hormonal signals originating from the immune system, collectively referred to as *cytokines*, as shown in Figure 14-8.[16]

Cytokines are medium-sized polypeptide hormones primarily secreted by the mononuclear cells of the immune system (macrophages, monocytes, and lymphocytes) that have an array of systemic and local actions characteristic of illness, including the ability to cause fever, prostration, and inflammation as well as to initiate tissue repair. Based on their molecular structure, three general classes of cytokines are recognized: interleukins (IL-1, IL-2, IL-3, etc), interferons (α and γ), and tumor necrosis factor (TNF). Experimental administration of these cytokines (IL-1, IL-2, IL-6, and TNF) to patients or laboratory animals[17–20] results in most of the features of systemic illness described above.[17–21] However, the cascade of cytokine responses in naturally occurring illnesses is varied and depends on the inciting agent as well as the intrinsic immune status of the host. Cytokine responses are also modified by feedback regulation of their production,[16] and cytokine-induced ACTH and cortisol secretion exerts inhibitory actions on cytokine production at multiple stages in the cascade.[23] By this mechanism, the ACTH and cortisol response plays an important role in determining the overall inflammatory and injury reaction. With respect to thyroid function in illness, the administration of cortisol or synthetic glucocorticoids can induce most if not all of the biochemical alterations characteristic of the low T_3 state.[24] Additionally, cytokines are capable of directly altering the synthesis of thyrotropin-releasing hormone (TRH) and the secretion of TSH and of the thyroid gland in experimental animals.[26] Taken together, the alterations of thyroid function in nonthyroidal illnesses should not be viewed as an isolated event, but rather as a part of a complex integrated phenomenon involving multiple aspects of the endocrine and immunologic systems.

In the clinical realm, it is important for the physician to distinguish between the changes in serum thyroid hormone concentrations resulting from nonthyroidal illnesses from those due to thyroid gland dysfunction. This may be particularly difficult in patients with severe illnesses, in whom serum T_3, T_4, and TSH concentrations may all be low, mimicking the biochemical findings of central hypothyroidism. This chapter focuses on the typical as well as the variant patterns of the abnormalities in thyroid function associated with nonthyroidal illnesses, speculates on their pathogenesis, and discusses how they may be differentiated from those caused by intrinsic thyroid disease.

LOW T_3 STATE

The most common abnormality in patients with nonthyroidal illness is a decrease in extrathyroidal T_3 production resulting in low serum total and free T_3 concentrations; serum T_4 and TSH concentrations are normal. This pattern is usually referred to as the low T_3 state and is found in 25% to 50% of hospitalized patients.[27] The magnitude of the fall in serum T_3 concentrations depends on the severity of the underlying illness (Fig 14-9). For patients with alcoholic cirrhosis or human immunodeficiency virus (HIV) infection, this decline may also serve as an important prognostic indicator of clinical outcome.[28,29] The biochemical changes characteristic of the low T_3 state also are caused by a variety of catabolic conditions including uncontrolled diabetes mellitus, glucocorticoid therapy, calorically restricted or ketogenic diets, and fasting.[10,12,30,31]

As noted above, the fall in serum T_3 concentrations results from decreased extrathyroidal T_3 production from T_4.[32,33] Normally, about 80% of circulating T_3 is produced in peripheral tissues by 5'-deiodination of T_4, while the remainder is directly secreted by the thyroid gland (see chaps 7 and 8). The evidence that peripheral tissue 5'-deiodinase enzyme activity is reduced in human beings is based on kinetic studies using radiolabeled T_3 and T_4 rather than by direct assessment. Further, there is some uncertainty about which peripheral tissue T_4 5'-deiodinase systems (type I or type II) or even organs or

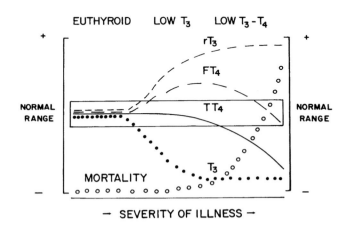

FIGURE 14-9. A schematic representation of the changes in serum thyroid hormone values with increasing severity of nonthyroidal illness. The mortality rate increases rapidly among patients with low serum total T_4 (TT_4) and free T_4 (FT_4) concentrations. (From Nicoloff JT. Abnormal endocrine measurements in nonendocrine chronic illness. In: Hurst JW, ed. Medicine for the practicing physician. 2nd ed. Stoneham, MA: Butterworths, 1991:574)

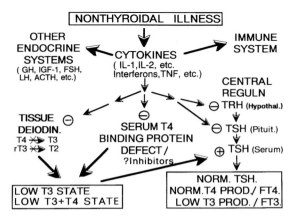

FIGURE 14-8. A schematic diagram of the possible role of the cytokine system in initiating both the immunologic and endocrine responses to nonthyroidal illnesses.

tissues are primarily responsible for generating circulating T_3 (see chap 8).

This issue regarding the mechanism(s) responsible for the low T_3 state is further compounded by the appearance of an apparent accounting gap or discrepancy in T_4 disposal products that occurs as the low T_3 state of nonthyroidal illness develops (Fig 14-10).[32,33] Normally, most T_4 is metabolized by conversion to T_3 or its biologically inactive isomer, reverse T_3 (rT_3). As the low T_3 state develops, net outer-ring (5′) deiodination of T_4 declines, as indicated by the reduction in serum T_3 concentrations and blood T_3 production rates.[32,33] Although serum rT_3 concentrations increase, this rise results from impaired rT_3 clearance as a consequence of the decreased 5′-deiodinase activity associated with illness, rather than from increased production from T_4.[34] Because T_3 production declines but rT_3 and T_4 production does not change, the disposal of some T_4 is unaccounted for. In other words, some T_4 is diverted from conversion to T_3 into other metabolic pathways. The source and character of these products of T_4 metabolism have not been fully characterized, but one likely pathway involves the formation of T_3 sulfate (T_3S). T_3S is a hormonally inactive metabolite of T_3 normally formed in many tissues through the action of thyronine sulfotransferases.[35,37] Up to one-half of T_3 disposal normally occurs by this route.[38,39] Recently, elevations in serum T_3S concentrations have been described in patients with nonthyroidal illnesses, consistent with an increase in T_3S formation.[40] Some of this increased T_3S formation, however, may be at the expense of the circulating serum T_3 concentration, if this process occurs in those tissues where T_4 to T_3 conversion is taking place. In other words, T_3S formation may, in part, represent a mechanism for shunting T_3 away from the circulation, thereby lowering the serum T_3 concentration.

Another pathway may involve the formation of triiodothyroacetic acid (T_3AC). T_3AC is a naturally occurring metabolite of T_3 that is formed by deamination of the alanine side-chain of T_3 by the action of T_3-aminotransferases or oxidative decarboxylases located in a variety of tissues.[41,42] Although exogenously administered T_3AC has much less thyromimetric activity than T_3, it binds avidly to T_3 nuclear receptors;[43,44] this disparity between systemic and nuclear activity of T_3AC is explained by more rapid clearance of T_3AC from the circulation as compared with T_3.[45,46] If produced locally, however, it could contribute to thyroid hormone action in an autocrine manner. Conceivably, such localized autocrine actions of T_3AC might explain both the lack of clinical features of hypothyroidism as well as the maintenance of nor-

mal serum TSH concentrations in patients with low serum T_3 concentrations. It is also possible that T_3 produced from T_4 in nonthyroidal illness could be sequestered or compartmentalized intracellularly. However, direct analysis of tissue T_3 content from patients dying of nonthyroidal illnesses does not support such a T_3-sequestration hypothesis because their tissue T_3 concentrations are reduced in proportion to the decrease in serum T_3 concentrations.[47]

Regardless of the exact alterations in T_4 and T_3 metabolism that occur in the low T_3 state, the central question is whether the low serum T_3 concentrations result in decreased thyroid hormone actions in tissues (e.g., hypothyroidism). Perhaps the best answer to this question comes from the studies of fasting in normal subjects. Within 2 days after the initiation of fasting, urinary nitrogen excretion increases, reflecting increased mobilization of body protein stores to provide substrate for gluconeogenesis[48]; nitrogen excretion then progressively falls because there is a switch from glucose to fatty acids as the primary fuel. Serum T_3 concentrations begin to fall in 36 hours and reach their nadir as urinary nitrogen excretion decreases. When T_3 is administered to maintain serum T_3 concentrations at prefasting values, however, urinary nitrogen excretion is further increased.[48,49] In contrast, a calorie-restricted diet designed to maintain protein balance (600 to 800 kcal/d of carbohydrate or protein) does not acutely result in a low T_3 state, but a similar dietary intake limited to fat does.[30,31] Further, individual variations in the magnitude of the initial fall in serum T_3 with caloric restriction may predict the subsequent nitrogen-sparing efficiency; the greater the initial fall in serum T_3, the greater the subsequent level of nitrogen conservation.[50] All these results support the concept that the low T_3 state results in a mild form of thyroid deficiency that limits the breakdown of skeletal muscle for gluconeogenesis. The observation that some patients suffering from prolonged caloric deprivation, such as those with anorexia nervosa,[51] may have some clinical features of hypothyroidism, such as delayed tendon reflexes, supports this interpretation. However, such a functional hypothyroid state does not occur in all tissues because serum TSH concentrations do not increase (Fig 14-11).

Conversely, after refeeding of undernourished subjects or administering insulin and glucose to patients with severe hyperglycemia, serum T_3 concentrations promptly increase.[10,52] However, if the premorbid weight is not fully restored, serum T_3 values do not return completely to normal.[51] Carbohydrate overfeeding to normal subjects increases both peripheral tissue T_4 conversion to T_3 and serum T_3 concentrations.[53] These

NORMAL

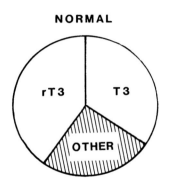

FASTING OR NTI

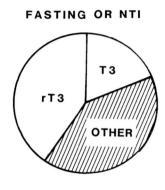

FIGURE 14-10. Diagrams showing the relative proportions of different products of metabolism of T_4 in a normal subject (*left*) and in a patient who is fasting or has a nonthyroidal illness (NTI) (*right*).

changes in response to refeeding and overnutrition are also accompanied by an array of other hormonal responses including increases in serum insulin, sex steroid, and IGF-I concentrations and in sympathetic nervous system outflow.[54–56] The specific pattern of these complex hormonal responses also may be important in determining the whether the weight gained is lean body tissue or fat.[57,58]

The metabolic impact and adaptive importance of the low T_3 state, as it occurs in patients with nonthyroidal illness, is less well understood than for responses induced by alterations in nutritional intake. Decreases in peripheral thyroid hormone action secondary to low serum T_3 concentrations could mitigate the catabolic effects of illness by fostering protein conservation and by providing substrates for the repair of injured tissue by autocrine mechanisms. Unfortunately, it has been difficult to test this hypothesis because of the varied character of systemic illnesses and nutritional intake in sick people. In tumor-bearing rats, which have many of the features of nonthyroidal illness that occur in patients, the activity of some thyroid-sensitive enzymes (α-glycerolphosphate dehydrogenase) is increased and that of others (malic enzyme) is depressed.[59,60] Apparently, these divergent end-organ responses result from the influence of multiple factors acting at a posttranscriptional level. A similar divergence occurs in fasted rats.[61] However, administration of T_3 to fasted rats does not alter the loss of nitrogen[62] as it does in human.[48,49] This latter finding raises the question as to whether fasted or tumor-bearing rats are appropriate models for humans. Thus, the question of the metabolic impact of the low T_3 state in patients with nonthyroidal illnesses remains unsettled.

Adding additional interest to the question of the thyroid status of patients with nonthyroidal illness are studies showing that supra-physiologic doses of T_3 given intravenously may improve cardiac performance and possibly survival in patients undergoing open-heart surgical procedures.[63,64] Because of the rapidity of action, less than 5 minutes, these findings raise the possibility of non–nuclear-mediated thyroid hormone action (see chap 9).

LOW T_3/T_4 STATE

In addition to low serum T_3 concentrations, very sick patients may have decreased serum T_4 concentrations, as shown in Figure 14-9. The time required for the transition from a normal well condition to a low T_3/T_4 state is related to the type and severity of the illness. It may require days or even weeks if progression is gradual, but can occur within hours after major trauma, sepsis, or shock.[7] Among patients studied in intensive care units, the decline in serum total T_4 concentration correlates closely with prognosis, as reflected by the mortality rate during hospitalization[65,66] (see Fig 14-9). In fact, the prognostic value of low serum T_4 concentrations alone is similar to that of more complex multifactorial prognostic indicators such as the Apache II index.[67]

Why should low serum T_4 concentrations be related to mortality? The reason is not that the patients are hypothyroid, because T_4 production rates and serum free T_4 concentrations are usually normal[68] and exogenous T_4 administration does not favorably influence the eventual clinical outcome.[69] The answer may lie in the mechanism(s) that cause the defect in T_4 binding to thyroxine-binding globulin (TBG) in the low,T_3/T_4 state. A substance released from injured tissues that inhibits T_4 binding to TBG may be responsible for this T_4-binding defect[70,71] because serum immunoreactive TBG concentrations are initially normal.[68] In some studies, this inhibitor substance had the characteristics of an unsaturated fatty acid, such as oleic acid;[72,73] it also may impair hepatic T_4 5′- deiodinase activity[74] and reduce the phagocytic activity of leukocytes,[75] thereby providing an explanation for the poor prognosis in the low T_3/T_4 state. The importance, or even the presence, of such a putative inhibitor has not been confirmed.[71] Alternatively, the TBG-binding defect may be the result of an acquired structural alteration that reduces the affinity of TBG for T_4.[76] This altered TBG is called slow TBG because its electrophoretic migration is retarded. In summary, the pathogenetic role of a T_4-binding inhibitor or an altered TBG as causative agents in the low T_3/T_4 state remains an open question.

Changes in hepatic uptake and metabolism of T_3, T_4, and rT_3 also have been proposed as a possible mechanism(s) for some of the changes in peripheral thyroid hormone metabolism in fasting and nonthyroidal illnesses.[77] Studies in isolated hepatocytes and perfused liver preparations indicate that a variety of naturally occurring compounds may impair plasma membrane transport, thereby reducing the uptake and metabolism of these thyronines by the liver. Such transport inhibitors may include fatty acids,[78] bilirubin,[78] hippuric acid,[79] and indoxyl sulfate.[79] However, like the situation with T_4-binding inhibition, it has been difficult to rationalize the importance of inhibition of thyroid hormone transport into cells in the pathogenic process in vivo.

SERUM FREE THYROID HORMONE MEASUREMENTS

The measurement of serum free T_4 in patients with nonthyroidal illnesses who have the low T_3/T_4 pattern has been a subject of considerable controversy and confusion (see chap 18). In these patients, serum free T_4 values estimated by the

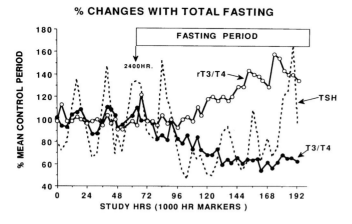

FIGURE 14-11. The relative changes in serum TSH concentrations and serum rT_3/T_4 and T_3/T_4 ratios before and during a voluntary fast in normal men. The falling serum T_3 (T_3/T_4) and TSH and the rise in serum rT (rT_3/T_4) values occur at different times after the start of the fast. (Adapted from Spencer CA, Lum SM, Wilber JF, Kaptein EM, Nicoloff JT. Dynamics of serum thyrotropin and thyroid hormone changes in fasting. J Clin Endocrinol Metab 1983;56:883)

free T_4 index determination (the product of serum total T_4 and THBR [T_3-uptake] measurements) are often in the hypothyroid range, especially in patients with very low serum total T_4 concentrations.[80] In contrast, serum free T_4 concentrations measured by equilibrium dialysis or ultrafiltration are usually normal or even increased.[81–83] These latter results are more likely correct because they correspond with the normal or near-normal T_4 production rate in the few patients in whom it has been measured.[68] However, the T_4-binding defect of the low T_3/T_4 state does result in a marked increase in T_4 clearance and shortened T_4 half-life.[68] In fact, the T_4 clearance rate is similar to that in healthy subjects with congenital deficiency or absence of serum TBG.[68] However, compartmental analysis of T_4 tracer disappearance curves reveals that the binding defect is exclusively extracellular (serum) in patients with TBG deficiency, whereas it is both intra- and extracellular in those with nonthyroidal illnesses.[68] In fact, the defect in intracellular T_4 binding (hepatic) appears to be even greater than that in serum. These in vivo findings independently support the possible existence of either a T_4-binding or transport inhibitor phenomenon in these patients.

Although dialysis or ultrafiltration methods provide accurate assessments of serum free T_4 concentrations, they are too complex and costly for routine clinical use. Efforts to develop more accurate, rapid, simple, and inexpensive methods for measuring serum free T_4 in patients with the low T_3/T_4 state have proven difficult. However, several commercially available assays are now available that provide fairly accurate values for serum free T_4 in patients with the low T_3/T_4 state (see chap 18). Issues relating to the measurement of serum free T_3 values are somewhat less ambiguous than for free T_4 because there is consensus that both serum T_3 concentrations and T_3 production rates are reduced in patients with nonthyroidal illnesses.[32,33]

TSH REGULATION OF TSH SECRETION

About 15% of patients admitted to a hospital for nonthyroidal illnesses have abnormal serum TSH concentrations (two-thirds low and one-third high)[84] (Fig 14-12). Most of the values are only slightly abnormal, but about 2% to 3% of the patients have serum TSH concentrations that are as low as the values in patients with overt thyrotoxicosis (<0.01 mU/L) or as high as in patients with overt hypothyroidism (>20 mU/L).[84] In general, serum TSH concentrations are low during the early phases of illness and become normal 2 to 5 days later as the patient recovers. The high concentrations, when they occur, follow in a day or so and also are transient; they represent the rebound of TSH secretion from its earlier suppression.[84] However, more persistent suppression of serum TSH concentrations may occur in patients receiving high-dose glucocorticoid or dopamine therapy,[86–88] and in some patients the recovery-related elevations in serum TSH may last for a week or more.[84]

The causes of the transient alterations in serum TSH concentrations in association with nonthyroidal illnesses are poorly understood. Low serum TSH concentrations are common in patients receiving pharmacologic doses of glucocorticoids (Figs 14-13 and 14-14). Glucocorticoids also produce this effect primarily by inhibiting endogenous TRH secretion[86]; conversely, acute withdrawal of glucocorticoid therapy results in a transient increase in TSH secretion.[89] Glucocorticoids reduce the pulsatility of TSH secretion,[86] a change that also is common in patients with nonthyroidal illness not receiving glucocorticoids. Because glucocorticoids not only inhibit TSH secretion but also cause the low low T_3 state, endogenous cortisol secretion likely plays an important role in the pathogenesis of many of the abnormalities that occur in patients with nonthyroidal illness. However, in contrast to spontaneous illnesses, glucocorticoid administration to healthy subjects elevates serum rT_3 concentrations primarily by increasing rT_3 production rather than by reducing its clearance.[90] Further, inhibition of endogenous cortisol production does not prevent the low T_3 state associated with fasting.[91] Thus, an alteration in endogenous cortisol secretion is not likely to be the sole factor mediating the changes in thyroid function in nonthyroidal illnesses.

The results of TRH stimulation testing in patients with nonthyroidal illness are often abnormal.[92] Although a few patients have exaggerated serum TSH responses to TRH, most have blunted responses.[68,92] As in normal subjects, the serum TSH responses to TRH in patients with nonthyroidal illness are proportional to the basal serum TSH concentrations[93] (see Fig 14-13). TRH stimulation testing in patients with nonthyroidal illness, therefore, provides no additional information to that afforded by an accurate measurement of the basal serum TSH concentration alone.

SPECIFIC TYPES OF NONTHYROIDAL ILLNESS

Most systemic illnesses and metabolic derangements result in a reasonably predictable pattern of alterations in thyroid hormone metabolism and TSH secretion, as shown in Figures 14-9, 14-11, and 14-12. There are, however, distinctively different response patterns in patients with certain pathologic states depending on the primary organ of involvement and the underlying nature of the disease. Listed below are the conditions most often associated with such variant patterns.

Liver Disease

Acute inflammation of the liver, as occurs in acute viral hepatitis, often is associated with substantial elevations in serum total T_4 and T_3 concentrations.[94] These increases, however, are not the result of increased T_4 secretion but rather of elevated serum TBG concentrations, resulting from either release of stored TBG or increased TBG synthesis and secretion.[95] However, as liver failure develops, serum T_3 and later serum T_4 concentrations decrease.[94]

HIV Infection

During the asymptomatic phases of HIV infection, the patients tend to have modest elevations in serum T_3, T_4, and TBG concentrations and low serum rT_3 concentrations.[96,97] Patients who have substantial weight loss often have similar values although low serum T_3 concentrations would be expected.[98] Whether this failure of serum T_3 concentrations to fall in response to weight

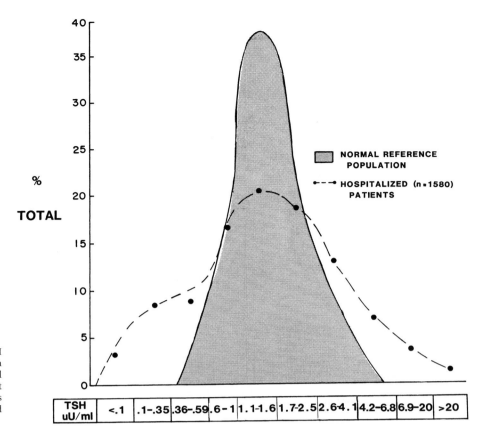

FIGURE 14-12. Distribution of serum TSH concentrations in normal subjects and in 1580 patients hospitalized for nonthyroidal illnesses. (Spencer CA, Eigen A, Shen D, et al. Sensitive TSH tests: specificity limitations for screening thyroid disease in hospitalized patients. Clin Chem 1987;33:1392)

loss contributes to the wasting that occurs in these patients is not known.[99,100] Serum TSH concentrations remain within the normal range, but they are often in the upper portion of that range.[97] As the HIV infection progresses these alterations tend to become more prominent until acquired immunodeficiency syndrome-defining illnesses, such as pneumocystis pneumonia, occur, when a typical low T_3 state usually develops.[29,96] The cause(s) of the alterations in the asymptomatic phases of HIV infection is unknown but may be related to changes in the cytokine signaling pattern associated with the disease.

Renal Disease

Although patients with renal disease often have low serum T_3 concentrations, they characteristically have normal rather than elevated serum rT_3 concentrations.[101] This failure of serum rT_3 to increase does not appear to be related to the degree of the renal impairment.[102] Serum rT_3 concentrations do not increase in these patients because rT_3 uptake into the liver is increased.[101] The increased hepatic rT_3 uptake may be caused by a circulating factor, possibly furanoic acid[79] or parathyroid hormone.[103] Whatever the cause, this finding points to the independence of factors regulating rT_3 and T_3 metabolism in some nonthyroidal illnesses.

Pregnancy

Pregnant women have increased serum TBG concentrations because of increased estrogen secretion, which alters TBG gly-

cosylation so that the half-life of TBG in serum is prolonged.[104] Serum free T_4, T_3, and rT_3 concentrations remain within the normal range throughout pregnancy[105] (see chap 89). Whether the low T_3 state develops during systemic illness or metabolic disorders in pregnant women is unknown. Glucocorticoids, in doses that ordinarily decrease serum T_3 concentrations, do not have this effect when administered to pregnant women.[106] Transplacental passage of glucocorticoids increases the normally low serum total T_3 concentrations in the fetus, possibly by increasing fetal tissue maturation and therefore increasing T_4 5'-deiodinase activity.[106]

Psychiatric Disorders

Transient abnormalities in serum TSH and thyroid hormone concentrations occur in 5% to 30% of patients hospitalized for treatment of acute psychiatric disorders.[107,108] The most common abnormalities are isolated elevations in serum total and free T_4 concentrations. Serum T_3 concentrations are usually normal, as are serum TSH concentrations, but the latter may be either slightly high or slightly low. The most plausible explanation for these findings is a transient increase in TRH-stimulated TSH secretion that in turn stimulates thyroidal T_4 secretion.[109] The low serum TSH concentration in some patients presumably reflects the transient nature of the increases in TRH (and TSH) secretion and the resultant negative feedback action of increased serum free T_4 concentrations on TSH release. Whatever the cause, serum T_4, T_3, and TSH concentrations usually become normal 1 to 2 weeks

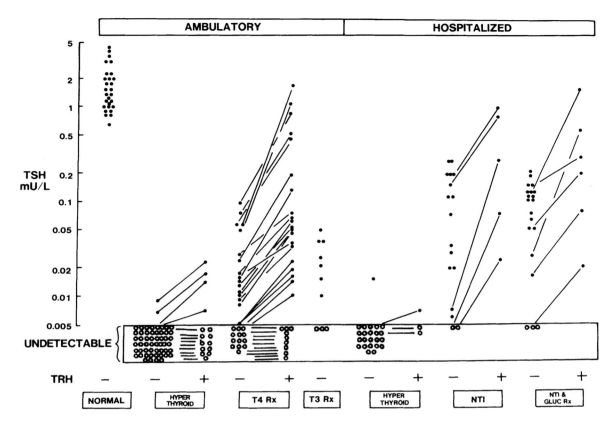

FIGURE 14-13. Basal and peak TRH-stimulated serum TSH concentrations in ambulatory and hospitalized patients. The serum TSH assay used in these studies had a sensitivity of 0.005 mU/L. The hospitalized patients with nonthyroidal illness (NTI) were selected from those patients who had serum TSH values below 0.1 mU/L in Figure 14-12. (From Spencer CA, LoPresti JS, Guttler RB, Eigen AC, Shen D, Nicoloff JT. Applications of a new chemiluminescent thyrotropin assay to subnormal measurement. J Clin Endocrinol Metab 1990;70:453; The Endocrine Society)

later. Thus, it is prudent to defer evaluation of thyroid status in these patients.

DIFFERENTIAL DIAGNOSIS

When and how to evaluate a patient with nonthyroidal illness for the presence of intrinsic thyroid disease can be a diagnostic challenge, particularly for hospitalized patients with medical or psychiatric illnesses. One approach is simply to defer thyroid testing until the acute nonthyroidal illness subsides or stabilizes. However, delay may not be feasible when there are questions regarding the presence of clinically important thyroid dysfunction. These questions usually arise when the patient has not responded appropriately to therapy for the nonthyroidal illness or when there are clinical manifestations of thyroid disease, such as goiter, tachycardia or bradycardia, atrial fibrillation, congestive heart failure, an altered state of consciousness, hyper- or hypothermia, or abnormal tendon reflexes.

Combined measurements of serum TSH and free T_4 are the most useful and cost-effective means of evaluating thyroid function in sick patients. If both serum TSH and free T_4 values are normal, it can reasonably be concluded that the patient is euthyroid or at least does not have a clinically important dis-

order of thyroid function. On the other hand, if the serum TSH value is either slightly low (0.1–0.5 mU/L) or high (5–20 mU/L) and the serum free T_4 value is normal, the most likely diagnosis is nonthyroidal illness. These isolated alterations in serum TSH concentrations occur in about 15% of hospitalized patients (see Fig 14-12) and reflect the inherent lability of TSH secretion in response to either the development or recovery from illness.[84,85]

About 2% to 3% of hospitalized patients have serum TSH concentrations that are more severely suppressed (<0.1 mU/L) or elevated (>20 mU/L), in which case underlying thyroid dysfunction is more likely, as shown in Figure 14-14.[84] It becomes even more likely if there is a reciprocal change in the serum free T_4 concentration and there are clinical manifestations of thyroid dysfunction. If the change in serum TSH concentration is an isolated finding, most patients subsequently prove not to have thyroid disease.

The availability of a more sensitive TSH assay may be of particular assistance because most patients with serum TSH values less than 0.1 mU/L as a result of nonthyroidal illness have detectable values when using this type of assay, for example, their serum TSH concentration will be greater than 0.01 mU/L.[110] If such a highly sensitive TSH assay is not available, a TRH test can be done; a detectable serum TSH value (>0.1

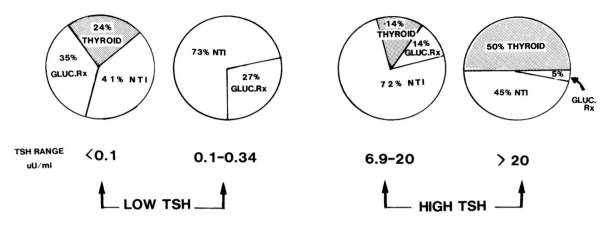

FIGURE 14-14. The proportions of patients with thyroid disease (Thyroid), nonthyroidal illness (NTI), and receiving glucocorticoid therapy (Gluc.Rx) among a large group of hospitalized patients subdivided according to four ranges of serum TSH concentrations. (From Spencer CA. Clinical utility and cost-effectiveness of sensitive thyrotropin assays in ambulatory and hospitalized patients. Mayo Clin Proc 1988;63:1214)

mU/L) after TRH stimulation would indirectly indicate that the basal serum TSH value was not as low (<0.01 mU/L) as in most thyrotoxic patients. No TRH stimulation test results, however, can exclude central hypothyroidism in a patient with nonthyroidal illness who has low serum TSH and free T_4 concentrations. Because the changes in serum TSH values associated with nonthyroidal illnesses are transient, repeated measurements are useful in patients in whom there is difficulty in establishing the diagnosis. The values usually become normal, or even slightly high for a few days, in patients with nonthyroidal illness as they recover from that illness, but are persistently low in patients with thyrotoxicosis or persistently high in those with primary hypothyroidism. An exception is patients receiving prolonged dopamine infusions or high-dose glucocorticoid therapy, in whom persistently low serum TSH concentrations are expected from the therapy. Furthermore, in patients with primary hypothyroidism, serum TSH concentrations can be reduced to normal by those drugs.

SUMMARY AND CONCLUSIONS

Alterations in thyroid hormone values in patients with nonthyroidal illnesses represent one component of the broad endocrine-immunologic response to illness (see Fig 14-8). Although the magnitude of the changes in pituitary and thyroid function varies depending on the severity of the underlying illness and the premorbid health status of the patient, reductions in serum total and free T_3 concentrations represent its most constant feature. Development of a low T_3 state during fasting or caloric deficiency may be a protective mechanism designed to limit mobilization of lean body tissue for gluconeogenesis. This mechanism of protein conservation likely applies to the low T_3 state of nonthyroidal illness as well. Indeed, the increased loss of protein stores commonly encountered during the early phases of HIV infection may, in part, be best explained by the failure of these patients to develop such an adaptive low T_3 state.[96–99] This view is also consistent with the enhanced protein catabolism that occurs when serum T_3 concentrations are raised to normal by T_3 administration in fasted

euthyroid subjects.[48,49] Thus, it would seem reasonable to conclude that the low T_3 state of nonthyroidal illness most likely represents a form of adaptive hypothyroidism.

This concept of adaptive hypothyroidism may, however, be too simplistic. First, serum TSH concentrations are usually normal, or even transiently low, rather than being elevated as one would expect if hypothyroidism were present. Second, there is a general absence of clinical features of hypothyroidism in these patients, and enzyme markers of thyroid hormone action measured in the tissues of animals with nonthyroidal illness do not indicate that thyroid hormone deficiency is present. Lastly, the rapid growth rate during fetal life when a low T_3 state is present is incompatible with a state of hypothyroidism.[111] It should be noted, however, that this low T_3 state of fetal life may account for the low level of gluconeogenesis at this stage of life. The latter observations indicate that the low T_3 state is unlikely to represent a condition of universal hypothyroidism but rather a special state in which thyroid status may vary from one tissue to another.

Only limited information is available on the mechanism(s) responsible for this variable thyroid action in different tissues of patients with nonthyroidal illnesses. The study of alternate routes of T_3 metabolism affords one such possibility; local inactivation (T_3S) or activation (T_3AC) of T_3 may occur at the end-organ, modifying autocrine and paracrine hormone actions. The activity of these alternate pathways of T_3 metabolism is probably increased in patients with nonthyroidal illness and during fasting,[112,113] but definite proof is not available. Other explanations include modifications in the action of T_3 in different tissues, leading to variable thyroid tissue responses.[114] Substantial evidence exists that these various cellular mechanisms play a role in determining eventual thyroid hormone action. However, a coherent understanding of the multiplicity of events responsible for producing the alterations in thyroid hormone production, transport, and action in patients with nonthyroidal illness does not exist. Therefore, we must conclude that the low T_3 and low T_3/T_4 states of nonthyroidal illness represent an adaptive phenotype for which we only have a rudimentary understanding of either their cause or effect.

References

1. Wartofsky L, Burman KD. Alterations in thyroid function in patients with systemic illnesses: the "euthyroid sick syndrome." Endocr Rev 1982;3:164

2. Tibaldi JM, Surks MI. Effect of nonthyroidal illness on thyroid function. Med Clin North Am 1985;69:899

3. Docter R, Krenning EP, deJong M, Hennemann G. The sick euthyroid syndrome: changes in thyroid hormone serum parameters and hormone metabolism. Clin Endocrinol 1993;39:499

4. Lutz JH, Gregerman RF, Spaulding SW, et al. Thyroxine binding proteins, free thyroxine and thyroxine turnover interrelationships during acute infectious illness in man. J Clin Endocrinol Metab 1972;35:230

5. Talwar KK, Sawhney RC, Rastogi RK. Serum levels of thyrotropin, thyroid hormones and their response to thyrotropin releasing hormone in infective febrile illness. J Clin Endocrinol Metab 1977;44:398

6. Brandt MR, Skovsted L, Kehlet H, Hansen JM. Rapid decrease in plasma triiodothyronine during surgery and epidural anesthesia independent of afferent neurogenic stimuli and cortisol. Lancet 1976;2:1333

7. Vitek V, Shatney CH. Thyroid hormone alterations in patients with shock and injury. Injury 1987;18:336

8. Phillips RH, Valente WA, Caplan ES, et al. Circulating thyroid hormone changes in acute trauma: prognostic implications for clinical outcome. J Trauma 1984;24:116

9. Chopra IJ, Solomon DH, Chopra U, et al. Alterations in circulating thyroid hormones and thyrotropin in hepatic cirrhosis: evidence for euthyroidism despite subnormal serum triiodothyronine. J Clin Endocrinol Metab 1974;39:501

10. Alexander CM, Kaptein EM, Lum SMC, et al. Pattern of recovery of thyroid hormone indices associated with treatment of diabetes mellitus. J Clin Endocrinol Metab 1982;54:362

11. Chopra IJ, Smith SR. Circulating thyroid hormones and thyrotropin in adult patients with protein-calorie malnutrition. J Clin Endocrinol Metab 1975;40:221

12. Spencer CA, Lum SMC, Wilber JF, et al. Dynamics of serum thyrotropin and thyroid hormone changes in fasting. J Clin Endocrinol Metab 1983;56:883

13. Moller S, Juul A, Becker U, et al. Concentrations, release, and disposal of insulin-like growth factor (IGF)-binding proteins (IGFBP), IGF-1, and growth hormone in different vascular beds in patients with cirrhosis. J Clin Endocrinol Metab 1995; 80:1148

14. Spratt DI, Gigas ST, Beitins I, et al. Both hyper and hypogonadotropic hypogonadism occur transiently in acute illness: bio and immunoactive gonadotropins. J Clin Endocrinol Metab 1992; 74:1562

15. Parker LN, Levin ER, Lifrak ET. Evidence for adrenocortical adaptation to severe illness. J Clin Endocrinol Metab 1985;60:947

16. Whicher JT, Evans SW. Cytokines in disease. Clin Chem 1990; 26:1269

17. Van der Poll T, Van Zee KJ, Endert E, et al. Interleukin-1 receptor blockade does not affect endotoxin-induced changes in plasma thyroid hormone and thyrotropin concentrations in man. J Clin Endocrinol Metab 1995;80:1341

18. Dubuis JM, Dayer JM, Siegrist-Kaiser CA, Burger AG. Human recombinant interleukin I-β decreases plasma thyroid hormone and thyroid stimulating hormone levels in rats. Endocrinology 1988;123:2175

19. Atkins MB, Mier JW, Parkinson DR, et al. Hypothyroidism after treatment with interleukin-2 and lymphokine-activated killer cells. N Engl J Med 1988;318:1557

20. Stouthard JML, van der Poll T, Endert E, et al. Effects of acute and chronic interleukin-6 administration on thyroid hormone metabolism in humans. J Clin Endocrinol Metab 1994;79:1342

21. Van der Poll T, Romijn JA, Wiersinga WM, Sauerwein HP. Tumor necrosis factor: a putative mediator of the sick euthyroid syndrome in man. J Clin Endocrinol Metab 1990;71:1567

22. Ozawa M, Sato K, Han DC, et al. Effects of tumor necrosis factor-alpha/cachectin on thyroid hormone metabolism in mice. Endocrinology 1988;123:1461

23. Munck A, Luyre PM. Glucocorticoids and immune function. In: Adler R, Felton DL, Cohen N, eds. Psychoneuroendocrinology. New York: Academic Press, 1989:132

24. Chopra IJ, Williams DE, Orgiazzi J, Solomon DH. Opposite effects of dexamethasone on serum concentrations of 3,3',5'-triiodothyronine (reverse T_3) and 3,3',5-triiodothyronine (T_3). J Clin Endocrinol Metab 1975;41:911

25. Kakuscka I, Romero LI, Clark BD, et al. Suppression of thyrotropin-releasing hormone gene expression by interleukin-1-beta in the rat: implications for nonthyroidal illness. Neuroendocrinology 1994;59:129

26. Pang X-P, Hershman JM, Mirell CJ, Pekary EA. Impairment of hypothalamic-pituitary-thyroid function in rats treated with human recombinant tumor necrosis factor-α (cachectin). Endocrinology 1989;125:76

27. Bermudez F, Surks MI, Oppenheimer JI. High incidence of decreased serum triiodothyronine concentration in patients with nonthyroidal disease. J Clin Endocrinol Metab 1975;41:27

28. Walfish PG, Orrego H, Israel Y, Blake J, Kalant H. Serum triiodothyronine and other clinical and laboratory indices of alcoholic liver disease. Ann Intern Med 1979;91:13.

29. Fried JC, LoPresti JS, Micon M, et al. Serum triiodothyronine values. Prognostic indicators of acute mortality due to *Pneumocystis carinii* pneumonia associated with acquired immunodeficiency syndrome. Arch Intern Med 1990;150:406

30. O'Brian JT, Bybee DE, Burman KD, et al. Thyroid hormone homeostasis in states of relative caloric deprivation. Metabolism 1980;29:721

31. Otten MH, Hennemann G, Docter R, Visser TJ. The role of dietary fat in peripheral thyroid hormone metabolism. Metabolism 1980;29:930

32. Kaptein EM, Robinson WJ, Grieb DA, Nicoloff JT. Peripheral serum thyroxine, triiodothyronine, and reverse triiodothyronine kinetics in the low thyroxine state of acute nonthyroidal illness. J Clin Invest 1982;69:526

33. Faber J, Francis-Thomsen H, Lumholtz IB, et al. Kinetic studies of thyroxine, 3,5,3'-triiodothyronine, 3,3',5'-triiodothyronine, 3',5'-diiodothyronine, 3,3'-diiodothyronine and 3'-monoiodo- thyronine in patients with liver cirrhosis. J Clin Endocrinol Metab 1981;53:978

34. LoPresti JS, Gray D, Nicoloff JT. Influence of fasting and refeeding on reverse T_3 metabolism (rT_3) in man. J Clin Endocrinol Metab 1991;72:130

35. Young WF, Gorman CA, Weinshilboum RM. Triiodothyronine: a substrate for thermostabile and thermolabile forms of human phenol sulfotransferase. Endocrinology 1988;122:1816

36. LoPresti JS, Mizuno L, Nimalysuria A, et al. Characteristics of 3,5,3'-triiodothyronine sulfate metabolism in euthyroid man. J Clin Endocrinol Metab 1991;73:703

37. Spaulding SW, Smith TJ, Hinkle PM, et al. Studies on the biological activity of triiodothyronine sulfate. J Clin Endocrinol Metab 1992;74:1062

38. Engler D, Merkelbach U, Steiger G, Burger AG. The monodeiodination of triiodothyronine and reverse triiodothyronine in man: a quantitative evaluation of the pathway by the use of turnover rate techniques. J Clin Endocrinol Metab 1984;58:49

39. LoPresti JS, Nicoloff JT. 3,5,3'-triiodothyronine sulfate (T_3): major metabolite in T_3 metabolism in man. J Clin Endocrinol Metab 1994;78:688

40. Chopra IJS, Wu SY, Teco GN, Santini F. A radioimmunoassay for measurement of 3,5,3'-triiodothyronine sulfate: Studies in thy-

roidal and nonthyroidal diseases, pregnancy and neonatal life. J Clin Endocrinol Metab 1992;75:189

41. Fishman N, Huang YP, Tergis DC, Rivlin RS. Relation of triiodothyronine and reverse triiodothyronine administration in rats on hepatic L-triiodothyronine aminotransferase activity. Endocrinology 1977;100:1055

42. Siergrist-Kaiser CA, Bubloz C, Burger AG. Studies on L-amino acid oxidase, a renal enzyme converting 3,5,3′-triiodothyronine (T3) to 3,5,3′-triiodothyroacetic acid (triac). Program of the 75th Annual Meeting of the Endocrine Society, 1993;812:253. Abstract

43. Bracco D, Morin O, Schutz Y, et al. Comparison of the metabolic and endocrine effects of 3,5,3′-triiodothyroacetic acid and thyroxine. J Clin Endocrinol Metab 1993;77:221

44. Lazar MA, Chin WW. Nuclear thyroid hormone receptors. J Clin Invest 1990;86:1777

45. Menegay C, Juge C, Burger AG. Pharmacokinetics of 3,5,3-triiodothyroacetic acid and its effects on serum TSH levels. Acta Endocrinologica 1989;121:651

46. Dlott RS, Nicoloff JT, LoPresti JS. Does triiodothyroacetic acid (T$_3$AC) formation mediate the low T$_3$ state (LT$_3$S) in man? Program of the 74th Annual Meeting of the Endocrine Society 1992;338:136. Abstract

47. Arem R, Wiener GJ, Kaplan SG, et al. Reduced tissue thyroid hormone levels in fatal illness. Metabolism 1993;42:1102

48. Gardner DR, Kaplan MM, Stanley CA, Utiger RD. Effect of triiodothyronine replacement on the metabolic and pituitary responses to starvation. N Engl J Med 1979;300:579

49. Burman KD, Wartofsky L, Dinterman RE, et al. The effect of T$_3$ and reverse T$_3$ administration on muscle protein catabolism during fasting as measured by 3-methylhistidine excretion. Metabolism 1979;28:805

50. Fisler JS, Kaptein EM, Drenick EJ, Nicoloff JT, Yoshimura NN, Swendseid ME. Metabolic and hormonal factors as predictors of nitrogen retention in obese men consuming very low calorie diets. Metabolism 1985;34:101

51. Croxson MS, Ibbertson HK. Low serum triiodothyronine (T$_3$) and hypothyroidism in anorexia nervosa. J Clin Endocrinol Metab 1977;44:167

52. Scriba PC, Bauer M, Emmert D, et al. Effect of obesity, total fasting and re-alimentation on L-thyroxine (T$_4$), 3,5,3′-triiodothyronine (T$_3$), 3,3′,5′-triiodothyronine (rT$_3$), thyroxine binding globulin (TBG), cortisol, thyrotropin, cortisol binding globulin (CBG), transferrin, α$_2$-haptoglobin and complement C3 in serum. Acta Endocrinol 1979;91:629

53. Danforth E Jr, Horton ES, O'Connell M, et al. Dietary-induced alterations in thyroid hormone metabolism during overnutrition. J Clin Invest 1979;64:1336

54. Palmblad JL, Levi A, Burger A, et al. Effect of total energy withdrawal (fasting) on levels of growth hormone, thyrotropin, cortisol, adrenaline, noradrenaline, T$_4$, T$_3$, and rT$_3$ in healthy males. Acta Med Scand 1977;201:15

55. Cameron JL, Weltzin TE, McConaha C, et al. Slowing the pulsatile luteinizing hormone secretion in man after forty eight hours of fasting. J Clin Endocrinol Metab 1991;73:35

56. Bang P, Brismar K, Rosenfeld RG, Hall K. Fasting affects serum insulin-like growth factors (IGFs) and IGF-binding proteins differently in patients with noninsulin-dependent diabetes mellitus versus healthy nonobese and obese subjects. J Clin Endocrinol Metab 1994;78:960

57. Young UR, Baker HWG, Lui G, Seeman E. Body composition and muscle strength in healthy men receiving testosterone enanthate for contraception. J Clin Endocrinol Metab 1993;77:1028

58. Rudman D, Feller AG, Nagray HS, et al. Effects of human growth hormone in men over 60 years old. N Engl J Med 1990;323:1

59. Tibaldi JM, Surks MI. Animal models of nonthyroidal disease. Endocr Rev 1985;6:87

60. Tibaldi J, Surks MI. Response of hepatic mitochondrial α-glycerophosphate dehydrogenase and malic enzyme to constant infusion of L-triiodothyronine in rats bearing the Walker 256 carcinoma: evidence for divergent post-receptor regulation of thyroid hormone response. J Clin Invest 1984;74:705

61. Oppenheimer JH, Schwartz HL. Factors determining the level of activity of 3,5,3′-triiodothyronine-responsive hepatic enzymes in the starved rat. Endocrinology 1980;107:1460

62. Schwartz HL, Lancer SR, Oppenheimer JH. Thyroid hormones influence starvation-induced protein loss in the rat: possible role of thyroid hormones in the generation of labile protein. Endocrinology 1980;107:1684

63. Novitsky D, Cooper DKC, Swanepoel A. Inotropic effect of triiodothyronine (T$_3$) in low cardiac output following cardioplegic arrest and cardiopulmonary bypass: an initial experience in patients undergoing open heart surgery. Eur J Cardiothoracic Surg 1989;3:140

64. Novitsky D, Cooper DKC, Barton CI, et al. Triiodothyronine as an inotropic agent after open heart surgery. J Thorac Cardiovasc Surg 1989;98:972

65. Slag MF, Morley JE, Elson MK, et al. Hypothyroxinemia in critically ill patients as a predictor of high mortality. JAMA 1981;245:43

66. Kaptein EM, Weiner JM, Robinson WJ, et al. Relationship of altered thyroid hormone indices to survival in nonthyroidal illness. Clin Endocrinol 1982;16:565

67. Kaufman DA, Dlott R, Townsend R, et al. Indices of thyroid function as predictors of outcome in critically ill patients. Clin Res 1988;36:101A

68. Kaptein EM, Grieb DA, Spencer CA, et al. Thyroxine metabolism in the low T$_4$ state of critical nonthyroidal illness. J Clin Endocrinol Metab 1981;53:764

69. Brent GA, Hershman JM. Thyroxine therapy in patients with severe nonthyroidal illness and low serum thyroxine concentration. J Clin Endocrinol Metab 1986;63:1

70. Oppenheimer JH, Schwartz HL, Mariash CN, Kaiser FE. Evidence for a factor in the sera of patient with nonthyroidal disease which inhibits iodothyronine binding by solid matrices, serum proteins and rat hepatocytes. J Clin Endocrinol Metab 1982;54:757

71. Chopra IJ, Huang T-S, Hurd RE, et al. A competitive ligand binding assay for measurement of thyroid hormone-binding inhibitor in serum and tissues. J Clin Endocrinol Metab 1984;58:619

72. Chopra IJ, Huang T-S, Solomon DH, et al. The role of thyroxine (T$_4$)-binding serum proteins in oleic acid-induced increase in free T$_4$ in nonthyroidal illness. J Clin Endocrinol Metab 1986;63:776

73. Haynes IG, Lockett SJ, Farmer MJ, et al. Is oleic acid the thyroxine binding inhibitor in the serum of ill patients? Clin Endocrinol 1989;31:25

74. Chopra IJ, Huang T-S, Beredo A, et al. Evidence for an inhibitor of extrathyroidal conversion of thyroxine to 3,5,3′-triiodothyronine in sera of patients with nonthyroidal illnesses. J Clin Endocrinol Metab 1985;60:666

75. Huang TS, Hurd RE, Chopra IJ, et al. Inhibition of phagocytosis and chemiluminesence in human leukocytes by a lipid soluble factor in normal tissue. Infect Immun 1984;46:544

76. Reilly CP, Welby ML. Slow thyroxine binding globulin in the pathogenesis of increased dialyzable fraction of thyroxine in nonthyroidal illness. J Clin Endocrinol Metab 1983;57:15

77. Lim CF, Docter R, Krenning EP, et al. Four inhibitors of liver T$_4$ uptake in nonthyroidal illness. Thyroid 1992;2S:87

78. Lim CF, Docter R, Visser TJ, et al. Inhibition of thyroxine transport into cultured rat hepatocytes by serum of non-uremic critically ill patients, bilirubin and non-esterified fatty acids. J Clin Endocrinol Metab 1993;76:1165

79. Lim CF, Bernard BF, de Jong M, et al. A furan fatty acid and indoxyl sulfate are the putative inhibitors of thyroxine hepatocyte transport in uremia. J Clin Endocrinol Metab 1993;76:318

80. Kaptein EM, MacIntyre SS, Weiner JM, et al. Free thyroxine estimates in nonthyroidal illness: comparison of eight methods. J Clin Endocrinol Metab 1981;52:1073

81. Nelson JC, Weiss RM. The effect of serum dilution on free thyroxine (T_4) concentration in the low T_4 syndrome of nonthyroidal illness. J Clin Endocrinol Metab 1985;61:239

82. Faber J, Kirkegaard C, Rasmussen B, et al. Pituitary-thyroid axis in critical illness. J Clin Endocrinol Metab 1987;65:315

83. Surks MI, Huprat KH, Pan C, Shapiro LE. Normal free thyroxine in critical nonthyroidal illnesses measured by ultrafiltration of undiluted serum and equilibrium dialysis. J Clin Endocrinol Metab 1988;67:1031

84. Spencer CA, Eigen A, Shen D, et al. Specificity of sensitive assays of thyrotropin (TSH) used to screen for thyroid disease in hospitalized patients. Clin Chem 1987;33:1391

85. Hamblin PS, Dyer SA, Mohr VS, et al. Relationship between thyrotropin and thyroxine changes during recovery from severe hypothyroxinemia of illness. J Clin Endocrinol Metab 1986;62:717

86. Brabant G, Brabant A, Ranft U, et al. Circadian and pulsatile thyrotropin secretion in euthyroid man under the influence of thyroid hormone and glucocorticoid administration. J Clin Endocrinol Metab 1987;65:83

87. Samuels MH, Luther M, Ridgway EC. Effect of hydrocortisone on pulsatile pituitary glycoprotein secretion. J Clin Endocrinol Metab 1994;78:211

88. Kaptein EM, Spencer CA, Kamiel MB, Nicoloff JT. Prolonged dopamine administration and thyroid hormone economy in normal and critically ill subjects. J Clin Endocrinol Metab 1980; 51:387

89. LoPresti JS, Dlott RS, Nicoloff JT. Dexamethasone (DEX): an important in vivo regulator of triac (TA_3) production in man. Thyroid 1991;1(suppl1):S38

90. LoPresti JS, Eigen A, Kaptein E, et al. Alterations in 3,3',5'-triiodothyronine metabolism in response to propylthiouracil, dexamethasone, and thyroxine administration in man. J Clin Invest 1989;84:1650

91. Croxson MS, Hall TD, Kletsky OA, Jacamillo JE, Nicoloff JT. Decreased serum thyrotropin induced by fasting. J Clin Endocrinol Metab 1977;45:560

92. Sumita S, Ujike Y, Namilsi A, et al. Suppression of the thyrotropin response to thyrotropin-releasing hormone and its association with severity of critical illness. Crit Care Med 1994;22:1603

93. Spencer CA, Schwarzbein D, Guttler RB, Lopresti JS, Nicoloff JT. Thyrotropin (TRH)-releasing hormone stimulation test responses employing third and fourth generation TSH assays. J Clin Endocrinol Metab 1993;76:494

94. Yamanaka T, Ido K, Kimura K, Saito T. Serum levels of thyroid hormones in liver disease. Clin Chim Acta 1980; 101:45

95. Schussler GC, Schaffner F, Korn F. Increased serum thyroid hormone binding and decreased free hormone in chronic active liver disease. N Engl J Med 1978;299:510

96. LoPresti JS, Fried JC, Spencer CA, Nicoloff JT. Unique alterations of thyroid hormone indices in the acquired immunodeficiency syndrome. Ann Intern Med 1989;110:970

97. Hommes MJT, Romijn JA, Endert E, et al. Hypothyroid-like regulation of the pituitary thyroid axis in stable human immunodeficiency virus infection. Metabolism 1993;42:556

98. Coodley GO, Loveless MO, Nelson HD, Coodley MK. Endocrine function in the HIV wasting syndrome. J Acquir Immune Defic Syndr 1994;7:46

99. Hommes MJT, Romijn JA, Goodfried MH, et al. Increased resting energy expenditure in human immunodeficiency virus-infected men. Metabolism 1990;39:1186

100. Grunfeld C, Pang M, Shimizu L, et al. Resting energy expenditure, caloric intake, and short-term weight change in human immunodeficiency virus infection and the acquired immunodeficiency syndrome. Am J Clin Nutr 1992;55:455

101. Kaptein EM, Feinstein EI, Nicoloff JT, Massry SG. Serum reverse triiodothyronine and thyroxine kinetics in patients with chronic renal failure. J Clin Endocrinol Metab 1983;57:181

102. Feinstein EI, Kaptein EM, Nicoloff JT, Massry SG. Thyroid function in patients with nephrotic syndrome and normal renal function. Am J Nephrol 1982;2:70

103. Kaptein EM, Massry SG, Quion-Verde H, et al. Serum thyroid hormone indexes in patients with primary hyperparathyroidism. Arch Intern Med 1984;1448:313

104. Ain KB, Mau Y, Refetoff S. Reduced clearance rate of thyroxine binding globulin (TBG) with increased sialylation: a mechanism for estrogen-induced elevations of serum TBG concentration. J Clin Endocrinol Metab 1987;65:689

105. Glinoer D, DeNayer P, Bourdoux P, et al. Regulation of maternal thyroid function during pregnancy. J Clin Endocrinol Metab 1990;71:276

106. Osathanondh R, Chopra IJ, Tulchinsky D. Effects of dexamethasone on fetal and maternal thyroxine, triiodothyronine, and reverse triiodothyronine and thyrotropin levels. J Clin Endocrinol Metab 1978;47:1236

107. Hein MD, Jackson IMD. Thyroid function in psychiatric illness. Gen Hosp Psychiatry 1990;12:232

108. Warner MD, Nader S, Griffin M, et al. Routine thyroid screening in psychiatric patients. Depression 1993;1:143

109. Roca BP, Blackman MR, Ackerly MB, et al. Thyroid hormone elevations during acute psychiatric illness: relationship to severity and distinction from hyperthyroidism. Endocr Res 1990;16:415

110. Spencer CA, LoPresti JS, Patel A, et al. Applications of a new chemiluminometric thyrotropin assay to subnormal measurement. J Clin Endocrinol Metab 1990;70:453

111. Fisher DA, Klein AH. Thyroid development and disorders of thyroid function in newborn. N Engl J Med 1981;304:702

112. LoPresti JS, Dlott RS. Augmented conversion of T_3 to triac (T_3AC) is the major regulator of the low T_3 state in fasting man. Thyroid 1992;2(suppl1):S39

113. LoPresti JS, Dlott R, VanderVelden D, Nicoloff JT. Triac's role in the production of the low T_3 state of fasting in man. Clin Res 1993;41:239A

114. Oppenheimer JH, Schwartz HL, Mariash CN, et al. Advances in our understanding of thyroid hormone action at the cellular level. Endocr Rev 1987;8:288

IODINE DEFICIENCY

François M. Delange
André-Marie Ermans

Iodine is a trace element present in the human body in minute amounts (15–20 mg, i.e., 0.02×10^{-3} % of body weight). Its only confirmed role is in the synthesis of thyroid hormones. Consequently, iodine deficiency, if severe enough, will impair thyroid hormonogenesis.

The dietary allowances of iodine recommended by the Food and Nutrition Board of the US National Research Council[1] are 150 μg/d for adolescents and adults (175 μg/d and 200 μg/d for pregnant and lactating women, respectively), 70 to 120 μg/d for children aged 1 to 10 years, 50 μg/d for infants aged 6 to 12 months, and 40 μg/d for infants 6 months of age or younger, which represents about 8 μg/kg, 5 μg/dL milk and 7 μg/100 Kcal. A reevaluation of the iodine requirements in young infants based on iodine balance studies showed that, at least in conditions of marginally low intake as observed in Europe, the recommended dietary allowance (RDA) for infants aged less than 1 year should be increased to 90 μg/d.[2] It has been suggested that an intake of about 200 μg/d is associated with the lowest serum level of thyroid-stimulating hormone (TSH; thyrotropin) in adults and, consequently, represents the optimal intake.[3]

When the physiologic requirements of iodine are not met in a given population, a series of functional and developmental abnormalities occur (Table 14-5), including thyroid function abnormalities and, when iodine deficiency is severe, endemic goiter and cretinism,[4,5] decreased fertility rate, and increased perinatal death and infant mortality.[6] These complications, which constitute a hindrance to the development of the affected populations, are grouped under the general heading of iodine deficiency disorders, IDD.[7]

Broad geographic areas exist in which the population's daily intake of iodine is below the RDA and in which the population is affected by IDD.[8,9] These areas usually are mountainous because the soils lowest in iodine are those that were covered longest by the quaternary glaciers. When these glaciers melted, most of the iodine leached out of the ground beneath.[10] The most important goitrous areas in the world today include the Himalayas and the Andes. Iodine deficiency also occurs in lowlands far from the oceans, such as in the central parts of Africa or, to a lesser extent, of Europe.

Based on the most recent evaluation, IDD currently represent a significant public health problem for 1572 million people (28.9% of the world population) in 110 countries (Table 14-6); 655 million are affected by goiter.[11] Twenty million are believed to be significantly mentally handicapped as a result of iodine deficiency,[9] which, therefore, is the most prevalent preventable cause of impaired intellectual development in the world today.

Although the disorders that result from iodine deficiency are preventable by appropriate iodine supplementation, they continue to occur because of various socioeconomic, cultural, and political limitations to adequate iodine supplementation programs.[12]

This chapter reviews our present knowledge of thyroid disorders induced by iodine deficiency. Endemic cretinism and endemic mental retardation are discussed in chapters 57 and 67. As indicated in Table 14-7, three different degrees of severity of IDD have been considered: mild, moderate, and severe. Although the basic mechanisms of adaptation to iodine deficiency are similar in the three degrees, severe IDD complicated by cretinism, as seen typically in remote areas in preindustrialized countries, and mild to moderate IDD, as seen typically in Europe are considered separately. In the three degrees of severity of IDD, special emphasis is placed on the pediatric aspects of adaptation to iodine deficiency. Neonates and young infants constitute the target population for the effects of iodine deficiency because, from a public health viewpoint, the most important complications of iodine deficiency are irreversible brain damage and mental retardation, which result from iodine deficiency and thyroid failure during fetal and early postnatal life.[9] Extensive reviews with exhaustive bibliographies are available on endemic goiter and the other disorders induced by iodine deficiency,[4,5,8,13–16] including the pediatric aspects.[17,18]

SEVERE IODINE DEFICIENCY DISORDERS

Epidemiology

The following definitions were proposed by the Pan American Health Organization (PAHO) for public health studies conducted in the field.[19]

GOITER. A thyroid gland whose lateral lobes have a volume greater than the terminal phalanges of the thumbs of the person examined is considered *goitrous*. In these conditions, the thyroid is enlarged by a factor of 4 to 5.

TABLE 14-5.
Spectrum of Iodine Deficiency Disorders

FETUS

Abortions

Stillbirths

Increased perinatal and infant mortality

Endemic cretinism

   Neurologic
      Mental deficiency
      Deaf-mutism
      Spastic diplegia
      Squint

   Myxedematous
      Mental deficiency
      Hypothyroidism
      Dwarfism

NEONATE

Goiter

Overt or subclinical hypothyroidism

INFANT, CHILD

Goiter

ADOLESCENT

Juvenile hypothyroidism

Impaired mental and physical development

ADULT

Goiter and its complications

Hypothyroidism

Endemic mental retardation

Decreased fertility rate

Adapted from Hetzel BS. Iodine deficiency disorders (IDD) and their eradication. Lancet 1983;ii:1126.

TABLE 14-6.
Population Living in Areas at Risk of Iodine Deficiency Disorders and Affected by Goiter*

WHO Regions	Population (millions)	Population at Risk of IDD		Population Affected by Goiter	
		MILLIONS	%	MILLIONS	%
Africa	550	181	32.8	86	15.6
Americas	727	168	23.1	63	8.7
Eastern Mediterranean	406	173	42.6	93	22.9
Europe	847	141	16.7	97	11.4
Southeast Asia	1355	486	35.9	176	13.0
Western Pacific	1553	423	27.2	141	9.0
TOTAL	5438	1572	28.9	655	12.0

*Includes areas where the total goiter rate in school-aged children is equal to or greater than 5%.
(Modified from Micronutrient Deficiency Information System. Global prevalence of iodine deficiency disorders. MDIS Working Paper n-1. Geneva: World Health Organization, 1993:1.)

The following stages classify goiter according to the size of the thyroid gland:

Stage 0: no goiter
Stage Ia: goiter detectable only by palpation and not visible when the neck is fully extended
Stage Ib: goiter palpable and visible only when the neck is fully extended; includes nodular glands, even if not goitrous
Stage II: goiter visible with the neck in normal position; palpation not needed for diagnosis
Stage III: very large goiter that can be recognized at a considerable distance

The total goiter rate is the prevalence of stages I, II, and III; the visible goiter rate is the prevalence of stages II and III.

This classification can be simplified (WHO/UNICEF/IC-CIDD* consultation on IDD indicators, unpublished) into:

Grade 0: no palpable or visible goiter
Grade 1: a mass in the neck that is consistent with an enlarged thyroid that is palpable but not visible when the neck is in the neutral position. It also moves upward in the neck as the subject swallows.
Grade 2: a swelling in the neck that is visible when the neck is in a neutral position and is consistent with an enlarged thyroid when the neck is palpated

These clinical classifications are appropriate for field surveys in remote areas where no other methods are available. However, the use of transportable ultrasonographic equipment in field studies has shown that in such studies, the clinical assessment of thyroid size is imprecise for small goiters, especially in small children.[20] In these conditions, the distinction between grade 0 and grade 1 is difficult and, consequently, the total goiter rate can be incorrect. Therefore, the frequency distribution of thyroid volume measured by ultrasonography is highly recommended,[21] especially in endemic areas where the visible goiter rate is low.

*International Council for Control of Iodine Deficiency Disorders

ENDEMIC GOITER. According to PAHO,[19] an area is arbitrarily defined as endemic with respect to goiter if more than 10% of the children aged 6 to 12 years are found to be goitrous. The figure 10% was chosen because a higher prevalence usually implies an environmental factor, while a prevalence of several percent is common even when all known environmental factors are controlled. The recent WHO/UNICEF/ICCIDD consultation on IDD indicators proposed to decrease the threshold of prevalence of goiter from 10% to 5%.

Goiter endemia should be described not only by the frequency of goiter but also by the severity of iodine deficiency. Table 14-7 indicates the present recommendations for classification of goiter endemias based on public health surveys.

The PAHO definitions are deliberately less severe and less elaborate than the criteria used in clinical endocrinology to avoid overestimation of an epidemiologic situation and to facilitate comparison of epidemiologic results obtained in different parts of the world by health workers who are not necessarily endocrinologists.

In epidemiologic surveys, the most rigorous method for evaluating the prevalence of goiter consists of examination of the entire population of a likely area. This is occasionally difficult to organize, especially in urban areas. Many surveys are limited, therefore, to particular age groups, most typically to children in school.[22]

Goiter prevalence is critically influenced by age and sex (Fig 14-15). In severe endemias the disease appears very early. Its prevalence increases sharply and attains a peak value during puberty and childbearing age. From the age of 10, the prevalence is higher in girls than in boys. In both sexes, goiter prevalence decreases during adulthood, but the decline is sharper in men than in women. A similar pattern is seen for the frequency of visible or nodular goiters.

Etiology

IODINE DEFICIENCY

Low dietary supply of iodine is the main factor responsible for the development of endemic goiter.[4,5,8,9,13–16,23] When

TABLE 14-7.
Classification of Goiter Endemias by Severity

Variables	Target Population	Mild IDD	Moderate IDD	Severe IDD
Prevalence of goiter, % (Grade > 0)	SAC	5–19.9	20–29.9	>30
Frequency of thyroid volume > 97th centile by ultrasound, %	SAC	5–9.9	10–19.9	>20
Median urinary iodine level, μg/dL	SAC	5–9.9	2–4.9	<2
Median breast milk, iodine level, μg/dL	Lactating women, day 5	3.5–5	2–3.5	<2
Median urinary iodine level, μg/dL	Newborns	3.5–5	1.5–3	<1.5
Frequency of TSH > 5 mU/L whole blood, %	Newborns	3–19.9	20–39.9	>40
Median Tg ng/mL	C/A	10–19.9	20–39.9	>40

IDD, *iodine deficiency disorders;* SAC, *school-aged children;* C/A, *children and adults;* Tg, *thyroglobulin.*
Adapted from references 114, 144, and 145.

iodine supplementation is introduced appropriately in an endemic area, goiter incidence is always markedly reduced. The persistence of a significant prevalence of goiter despite iodine prophylaxis suggests the additional role of a naturally occurring goitrogen.[24]

Goiter develops in iodine-deficient environments in populations that consume locally grown foods. The iodine content of most foodstuffs is generally low; the highest content is found in fish and, to a lesser extent, in milk, eggs, and meat.[25,26] Very low iodine content is usually found in fruits and vegetables. Iodine concentration in foodstuffs varies greatly depending on the country, season, and method of cooking. The iodine content of drinking water is too low to serve as a consistent contributor to the iodine supply.[16]

A rigorous assessment of the iodine content of foods is extremely difficult for methodologic reasons.[25] Iodine balance studies have shown that adults are in equilibrium with their iodine environment and that the fecal excretion of iodine is usually negligible (5 μg/d).[27] Therefore, most estimates of the dietary supply of iodine are based on the measurement of the excretion of iodine in urine. In nonendemic areas the daily urinary excretion of iodine is at least 100 μg/d. In endemic areas it is usually much lower and varies from 45 to 3 μg/d (see reviews in references 5, 8, 9, 13–16, 23). Complete 24-hour collection of urine is often difficult to achieve in field investigations. An alternative procedure is the measurement of the ratio between the concentrations of iodine and creatinine in casual urine samples[28,29] or even just the concentration of iodine provided that the observation covers at least 50 to 100 randomly selected urine samples.[30]

The etiologic role of iodine deficiency in endemic goiter also has been demonstrated by an enormous amount of experimental work in animals.[23] In several regions, it has been possible to demonstrate geographic superimposition of human endemic goiter and enzootic goiter.[14,16,23,31–33]

The correction of iodine deficiency usually is followed by the disappearance of endemic goiter (see treatment and prophylaxis).

OTHER GOITROGENIC FACTORS

Iodine deficiency is not the sole cause of endemic goiter. Indeed, the disease has been found in regions where there is no iodine deficiency[34–36] or even iodine excess.[37,38] Conversely, in other regions with an extremely severe iodine deficiency, endemic goiter is not observed.[24,39–41] These data strongly suggest that some goitrogenic factors in the diet or environment, other than iodine deficiency, could play a criti-

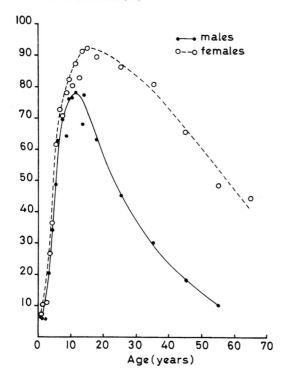

Prevalence of Goiter (%)

males
females

Age (years)

FIGURE 14-15. Pattern of goiter prevalence in relation to age and sex in the inhabitants of Idjwi Island endemic goiter area, Zaire. (Modified from Delange[98])

cal role in the etiology of the disease.[24,42–46] Table 14-8 summarizes data from goiter endemias in which such environmental goitrogenic factors have been demonstrated.

Natural goitrogens were first found in vegetables of the genus *Brassica*[45] (the Cruciferae family), which possesses goitrogenic properties in animals. Their antithyroid action is related to the presence of thioglucosides, which, after digestion, release thiocyanate and isothiocyanate.[44,47,48] A particular thioglucoside, goitrin (L-5-vinyl-2 thiooxazolidone) is present in certain Cruciferae growing as weeds in pastures in Finland and Tasmania.[34,48] Goitrin has potent thionamide-like properties.[14,47] Goitrin in human beings could probably be ingested from milk.[45,49]

Another important group of naturally occurring goitrogens is the cyanoglucosides, which have been found in several staples (cassava, maize, bamboo shoots, sweet potatoes, lima beans).[42,43,46,47] After ingestion, these glucosides release cyanide, which is detoxified by conversion to thiocyanate, a powerful goitrogenic agent that acts acutely by inhibiting thyroid iodide transport and, at higher doses, competes with iodide in the organification processes.[50–52]

Cassava (manioc), one of the basic foodstuffs in tropical areas, has definite goitrogenic properties in rats.[43,53] Its role in the etiology of endemic goiter, in association with iodine deficiency, has been clearly demonstrated in Africa[42,43,54–56] and confirmed in Malaysia[57] and Brazil.[58] The chronic consumption of poorly detoxified cassava induces in the inhabitants of these areas a marked increase in the serum concentration of thiocyanate that, in association with iodine deficiency, results in impairment of thyroid function characterized by low serum thyroxine (T_4) and elevated TSH concentrations and in the development of goiter.[54] Improvement of the detoxification of

TABLE 14-8.
Goiter Endemias Attributed to Goitrogens in Food and to Chemical and Bacterial Pollution of the Water-Exposure Pathway

Locality	Source	Vehicle	Active Principle
EUROPE			
Finland	Grass and weeds	Milk	L-5-vinyl-2-thiooxazolidone (goitrin)
England (Sheffield area)	Grass	Milk	—
Spain (Navarro)	Grass	Milk	Thiocyanate
Spain (Avila)	Walnuts		—
Ex-Czechoslovakia (Bohemia-Moravia)	Grass (*Brassica* sp)	Milk	Goitrin
Ex-Yugoslavia (Krk Island)	Grass (*Brassica* sp)	Milk	Goitrin
Greece	*Escherichia coli*	Water	Thyroid antibodies (?)
NORTH AMERICA			
West Virginia	*Escherichia coli*	Water	—
Eastern Kentucky	Coals and gram-negative bacteria	Water	Phenolic and phthalate ester derivates (?)
SOUTH AMERICA			
Colombia	Shales and coals, humic substances, and gram-negative bacteria	Water	Resorcinol, phthalate ester derivates and disulfides
Venezuela	Various rocks and soils	Water	Lithium
Chile	Pinon nuts		—
Brazil	Palmtree fruit (Babassu)		Phenolic derivates (?)
AFRICA			
Nigeria	Cassava		Thionamide-like goitrogen
Zaire	Cassava		Cyanogenic glucoside (linamarin → thiocyanate)
Sudan	Millet		Flavonoids and thiocyanate
ASIA			
Lebanon	Onions, garlic		—
Japan	Seaweeds		Iodide and polyhydroxyphenols (?)
Malaysia	Cassava		Linamarin → thiocyanate
China	Seaweeds		Iodide
OCEANIA			
Tasmania	Grass and weeds		Isothiocyanate (cheilorine)

Data from references 14, 24, and 58.

cassava results in normalization of serum thiocyanate and thyroid function.[59]

The determining factor involved in the goitrogenic action of cassava is the balance between the dietary supplies of iodine and thiocyanate. Goiter develops when the urinary iodine/thiocyanate ratio, used as an index of this balance, decreases below a critical threshold of about 3 μg iodine per mg thiocyanate.[42] This can occur when thiocyanate is elevated in the presence of overt iodine deficiency or even in the presence of an almost normal iodine supply when thiocyanate overload is important.[60] Experimentally, acute thiocyanate overload inhibits thyroidal uptake of ^{131}I, but chronic administration of cassava or of small doses of thiocyanate in iodine-deficient rats does not decrease thyroidal uptake of ^{131}I despite elevated concentrations of thiocyanate. A marked inhibition of the thyroidal pump may be detected, however, in the same animals if iodine organification is blocked by propylthiouracil.[47,50] These findings agree with previous observations that a moderate increase of the thiocyanate concentration markedly accelerates the exit rate of iodide from the gland but does not affect unidirectional iodide clearance.[61] These observations account both for the clinical observation of a very high thyroidal uptake of radioiodine in iodine-deficient subjects with abnormally high thiocyanate serum levels and for the fact that iodine supplementation completely reverses the goitrogenic influence of cassava.

Pathophysiology: Adaptation of Thyroid Function to Iodine Deficiency

Endemic goiter is an adaptive disease that develops in response to an insufficient supply of dietary iodine. This classic concept was established in 1954 by Stanbury and colleagues[4] and has been confirmed since by enormous numbers of clinical and experimental observations.[8,13–16,23,32,62]

When iodine intake is abnormally low, adequate secretion of thyroid hormones may still be achieved by marked modifications of thyroid activity. These adaptive processes include stimulation of the trapping mechanism as well as of the subsequent steps of the intrathyroidal metabolism of iodine leading to preferential synthesis and secretion of T_3. They are triggered and maintained by increased secretion of TSH. The morphologic consequence of prolonged thyrotropic stimulation is the development of goiter. Teleologically, however, large goiters may no longer be considered as adaptive processes in view of their decreased ability to synthesize thyroid hormones.

INCREASED STIMULATION BY TSH

Elevated serum TSH levels have been reported repeatedly but not systematically in individuals with chronic iodine deficiency.[63–67] Moreover, within a given area, striking and large variations in serum TSH levels are observed in adults independently of the presence or absence of goiter.[63,64,66] The lack of systematic correlation between goiter and TSH levels suggests that differences in the duration of elevated TSH levels and in thyroid responsiveness to TSH, as well as other factors (e.g., growth hormone, epidermal and fibroblast factors, insulin, cortisone, cyclic guanosine monophosphate, or

other intrathyroidal mechanisms) may determine whether goiter develops.[68]

INCREASE IN IODIDE TRAPPING

The fundamental mechanism by which the thyroid gland adapts to an insufficient iodine supply is to increase the trapping of iodide. This results in the accumulation within the gland of a larger percentage of the ingested exogenous iodide and a more efficient reuse of iodide directly released by the thyroid or generated by the degradation of thyroid hormones.[4,26,32] The increased iodide trapping is the result of both TSH-independent augmentation of membrane iodide trapping and TSH stimulation of the iodide pump.[69]

For any adequate adjustment of iodide supply to the thyroid, iodide trapping must fulfill two conditions. First, it must reduce the amount of iodine excreted in the urine to a level corresponding to the level of iodine intake, this condition being required to preserve preexisting iodine stores. Second, it must ensure the accumulation in the thyroid of definite amounts of iodide per day (about 100 μg). This latter parameter is extremely important because it quantitatively controls all further steps of intrathyroid iodine metabolism, including the secretion rate of the thyroid hormones. Two examples of adjustment of iodide trapping are given in Figure 14-16, the first for a presumably normal subject (iodine supply: 100 μg/d) and the second for a goitrous subject living in an endemic area (iodine supply: 20 μg/d). In the normal subject, renewal of the extrathyroid iodide compartment (ei) is 200 μg/d, half of which originates from iodine intake (In) and the other half from peripheral degradation of the thyroid hormones (D). Thyroid iodide clearance (Clt) is adjusted to 30 mL/min and thus equals renal iodide clearance (Clr). The fraction of the iodide compartment taken up by the thyroid gland (U) is given by the following equation: U = Clt /(Clt + Clr). The amount of iodide taken up by the gland (A) and excreted in urine (E) per day are thus, respectively, IU and I (1 − U). In a normal subject: U = 30/(30 + 30) = 0.5, and A and E are both 100 μg/d (200 μg × 0.5). In a patient with goiter, renewal of the extrathyroid iodide compartment (ei) is only 120 μg/d, reflecting the reduction of iodide intake (20 μg/d). Thyroid clearance is adjusted to 155 mL/min, and the resulting value of U is 155/(155 + 30) = 0.83, A being equal to 120 μg × 0.83 = 100 μg and E = 120 μg × 0.17 = 20 μg.

Thus, despite a drastic reduction in the iodide supply, renal iodide excretion does not exceed iodine intake, and adequate amounts of iodine are accumulated in the gland. It is obvious that this oversimplified scheme accounts neither for the qualitative changes of thyroid secretion nor for the iodide spillage observed in endemic goiter.[70] The fraction of extrathyroid iodide taken up by the gland (U) thus appears as the main determining factor of the distribution of both exogenous and endogenous iodide. The U fraction does not, however, give a reliable estimate of the true modification of the trapping mechanism. As shown in Figure 14-16, the adaptation from a normal iodine supply to a poor one enhances the value of U from 50% to 83%, that is by a factor of 1.7. This situation is achieved only by a tremendous augmentation of the thyroid clearance, which passes from 30 to 150 mL/min, an increase by a factor of 5.7.

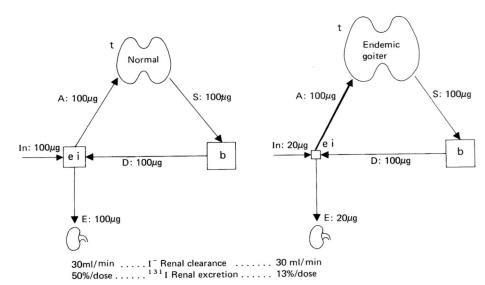

30ml/min . . . . . I⁻ Thyroidal clearance 155ml/min
50%/dose . . . . . . ¹³¹I Thyroid uptake 87%/dose

30ml/min . . . . . I⁻ Renal clearance . . . . 30 ml/min
50%/dose . . . . . . ¹³¹I Renal excretion 13%/dose

FIGURE 14-16. Kinetics of iodide in a normal subject (*left*) and in a goitrous subject living in an iodine-deficient area (*right*). Respective iodine intakes (In) are 100 μg and 20 μg/d. The three iodine compartments are intrathyroid iodine (t), hormonal ("bound") extrathyroid iodine (b), and extrathyroid iodide (ei). Transfer rates of iodine are expressed in micrograms per day; ei, renewal of extrathyroid iodide originating from intake and from hormonal degradation (D); A, accumulation rate within the thyroid; S, secretion rate; E, urinary excretion rate. Iodine-131 thyroid uptake (U) is the fraction of ¹³¹I tracer accumulated in the thyroid and 1-U, the fraction of ¹³¹I excreted in urine. Thyroid and renal clearances of iodide are expressed in milliliters per minute. The schema is based on the three compartments model of iodine metabolism proposed by Riggs.[155]

For practical purposes, U is given with a good approximation by the usual ¹³¹I thyroid uptake. Absolute iodine uptake (A) is generally estimated from the daily renal excretion of iodide (E) according to the formula: $A = EU/(1 - U)$. This equation is based on the assumption that the distribution of extrathyroid stable iodide during 24 hours is the same as the distribution of a single tracer dose of ¹³¹I.[4] The ratio between thyroid accumulation and renal excretion is the same for ¹²⁷I and ¹³¹I-iodide; therefore, the equation from which the formula mentioned earlier is derived: $A/E = U (1 - U)$.

Increased thyroid uptake of ¹³¹I and reduction of urinary iodine excretion are the main characteristic markers of a goiter endemia caused by iodine deficiency. A clearcut inverse relationship between both parameters was demonstrated in 1954,[4] has been confirmed in a large number of goiter endemias,[23] and is further illustrated in Figure 14-17. The figure indicates that as soon as the iodine supply decreases below the physiologic requirement of 100 μg/d iodine in adults, there is an increase in the thyroid uptake of radioiodine, indicating an increase in the clearance rate of iodide by the thyroid.

In these conditions, despite a decrease in the serum concentration of iodide, the absolute uptake of iodide by the thyroid remains normal[26] and the organic iodine content of the thyroid remains within the limits of normal (i.e., 10–20 mg), as long as the iodine intake remains above a threshold of about 50 μg/d. Below this critical level of iodine intake, despite a further increase of thyroid clearance, the absolute uptake of iodide diminishes and the iodine content of the thyroid decreases. Goiter, the visible consequence of iodine deficiency by public health standards, starts to develop only when the iodine intake is still lower, although for low iodine intake, the prevalence of goiter markedly varies from one area to another.

Because of the relationship between thyroidal uptake and urinary iodine excretion, it has been suggested that the estimation of urinary ¹²⁷I excretion, and therefore of the io-

dine intake, could be directly deduced, with considerable accuracy, from the value of the ¹³¹I thyroid uptake.[71]

MODIFICATIONS OF INTRATHYROID IODINE METABOLISM

In experimental conditions, increased TSH stimulation induced by iodine deficiency provokes a marked acceleration of all steps of intrathyroid iodine metabolism with a consequently faster turnover of this compartment and an increase of its heterogeneity.[72] A similar pattern is observed in endemic goiter but only in a restricted number of subjects, generally children and adolescents.[73] In most goitrous subjects, on the contrary, ¹³¹I distribution reveals a slow-release pattern: plasma protein-bound ¹³¹I is as low as in subjects with normal thyroid uptake living in nongoitrous areas and the biologic half-life of thyroid ¹³¹I is long. These observations would paradoxically suggest that in these highly stimulated glands, intrathyroid iodine would be turning over at a subnormal rate. A possible explanation of this finding[72] is that the glands with apparently slow secretion could have access to a large endogenous source of stable iodine not in equilibrium with the compartment labeled by the exogenous tracer. This unlabeled iodine could dilute the tracer and render the fast turnover undetectable by isotope studies.

Studies in the rat show that thyroid hyperplasia induced by iodine deficiency is associated with an altered pattern of tracer iodine distribution in the gland, characterized by an increase in poorly iodinated compounds, monoiodotyrosine (MIT) and triiodothyronine (T₃), and a decrease in diiodotyrosine (DIT) and T₄.[32,72,74,75] Figure 14-18 indicates that the increases of the MIT:DIT and T₃:T₄ ratios are closely related to the degree of iodine depletion of the gland. Table 14-9 confirms these findings by showing that in iodine depleted glands of iodine deficient rats, there is a dramatic reduction of thyroid T₄ and a markedly increased T₃:T₄ ratio.

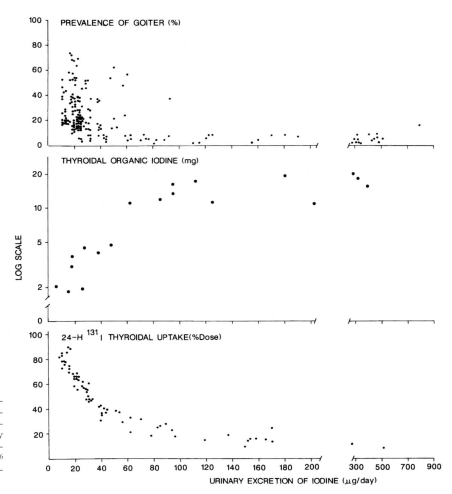

FIGURE 14-17. Relationship between the daily urinary excretion of iodine and the prevalence of goiter, the hormonal iodine content of the thyroid (exchangeable organic iodine pool Qg determined by kinetic studies) and thyroidal uptake of radioiodine. (Compiled from Schaefer and colleagues,[156] Delange and colleagues,[157] and Tovar and colleagues.[158])

Corresponding information in human endemic goiter is more limited. In large human goiters, iodine concentration is markedly reduced and the MIT:DIT ratio is increased.[73,76,77] There is also, as in sporadic goiter, an increased DIT:T_4 ratio suggesting reduced efficiency of the coupling reaction.[78]

The main features of intrathyroid metabolism in endemic goiter appear to be as follows.[62,72] Because of a large iodine pool within the thyroid not in equilibrium with the compartment labeled by the exogenous tracer, the iodination level of the large amounts of thyroglobulin accumulated within the colloid remains low. The subsequent abnormal configuration of thyroglobulin is responsible for reduced efficiency of iodothyronines synthesis. Only a small fraction of the large iodine stores is, therefore, actually moving along the normal pathway of hormone synthesis and secretion, while a considerable percentage seems to be wasted, accounting for the tremendous heterogeneity of endemic goiter from the morphologic, functional, and biochemical points of view.

TSH STIMULATION AND ALTERATIONS IN CIRCULATING THYROID HORMONES

The pattern of circulating thyroid hormones in clinically euthyroid adults in areas of severe iodine deficiency is characterized by low serum T_4, elevated TSH, and normal or supranormal T_3[63,64,66,67,79,80] (Table 14-10). The mechanisms responsible for this pattern are unclear but may include thyroidal secretion of T_4 and T_3 in the proportion in which they exist within the gland,[72,74,75] preferential secretion of T_3[81] or increased peripheral conversion of T_4 to T_3. The shift to increased T_3 secretion and serum T_3:T_4 ratios may play an important role in the adaptation to iodine deficiency because T_3 possesses about four times the metabolic potency of T_4 but requires only 75% as much iodine for synthesis.[81] It is only under conditions of extreme thyroid failure, as are found in myxedematous endemic cretinism (see chap 57), that both serum T_4 and T_3 are particularly low and serum TSH is dramatically elevated. In less severe goiter endemias, serum T_4 and T_3 levels are only slightly modified or remain normal. In these conditions, basal TSH and TSH response to the intravenous injection of thyrotropin-releasing hormone (TRH) is often exaggerated, indicating an increase in the pituitary TSH reserve,[82] a condition often reported as subclinical hypothyroidism.[83]

In severe endemic goiter, an inverse relationship exists between serum T_4 and TSH, but this correlation is not found for serum T_3, which is the most active thyroid hormone.[72] This paradoxical finding is explained, in part, by the fact that the direct effect of T_4 on TSH suppression results from intrapitu-

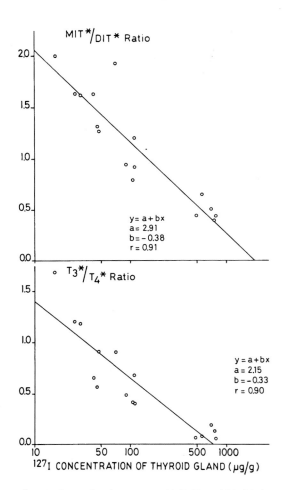

FIGURE 14-18. Relationship between MIT*/DIT* and T_3*/T_4* ratios in the hydrolysates of rat thyroids and corresponding concentrations of ^{127}I iodine in the thyroid tissue. Each point corresponds to the mean value of five animals. Rats were fed a Remington diet for 15 to 20 days with, in some groups, an iodine supplement of 5 μg/d. Asterisk indicates radioactive compound.

itary T_4 to T_3 conversion and the subsequent binding of T_3 to the nucleus of the thyrotrophs while, in other tissues, the largest part of intracellular T_3 originates from circulating T_3.[84] These findings account for the observation in endemic goiter that normal serum T_3 levels enable a patient to maintain an overall euthyroid status, but pituitary stimulation persists as long as the serum T_4 level is depressed.

In endemic goiter, the serum concentration of T_4-binding globulin (TBG) is normal unless there is decreased TBG synthesis due to the concomitant presence of protein malnutrition.[85] The serum concentration of thyroglobulin is markedly elevated.[86–89] Serum thyroglobulin correlates with serum TSH and is not higher in goitrous than in nongoitrous subjects. Finally, the incidence of antithyroglobulin and antimicrosomal antibodies (anti-TPO) is very low[89,90] but may increase after iodine prophylaxis.[90]

Morphologic Changes

Morphologic modifications observed in patients with endemic goiter are mainly nodular enlargement of the gland with striking macroscopic and microscopic heterogeneity.[16,91] Diffuse enlargement is rarely found in severe endemic goiter and then only in young subjects. At this stage, the characteristic hyperplastic picture induced experimentally by iodine deficiency may be observed: parenchyma is abundant, follicular epithelium is high with papillary infolding, and colloid is rare. A later stage is the formation of small nodules that dissect the entire thyroid tissue with nodules of different size and consistency. At this time, histologically, the major part of the gland is occupied by extremely distended vesicles with a flattened epithelium filled with colloid. A few patches of thyroid follicles, on the contrary, show a typical pattern of stimulation.

CLINICAL ASPECTS AND DIAGNOSIS

The physical symptoms of endemic goiter do not differ from those found in nontoxic sporadic goiter; the differential diagnosis is established mainly by epidemiologic criteria. In individual patients, all types of thyroid enlargement may be observed, from the small, solitary thyroid nodule without any appreciable hyperplasia of the rest of the gland, to a huge, multinodular goiter. Complications are those described for sporadic goiter. The most common are deviation and compression of the trachea, venous distention, the development of a collateral venous circulation on the chest, and thyroid hormone insufficiency. Evidence of hypothyroidism is often difficult to demonstrate on clinical grounds and from biologic data because the serum T_4 concentration is often low, the TSH concentration elevated, and the ^{131}I thyroid uptake elevated (>50% at 24 hours) in clinically euthyroid subjects living in goitrous areas. Scintigraphy of the thyroid emphasizes the marked heterogeneity of the goiters and frequently shows cold or hot nodules.

TABLE 14-9.
Weight, Iodine Content, and Iodoamino Acid Distribution in the Thyroid and in the Serum of Control and Iodine-Deficient Adult Rats

Variables	Control Rats (n = 12)	Iodine-Deficient Rats (n = 10)
THYROID		
Weight (mg/100 g)	4.1 ± 0.7	12 ± 3
Iodine content (ng/mg thyroid wt)	880 ± 180	21 ± 30
MI*T:DI*T ratio	0.42 ± 0.07	2.0 ± 0.3
T_3*:T_4* ratio	0.12 ± 0.01	1.8 ± 0.9
T_3:T_4 ratio (molar)	0.12 ± 0.03	1.01 ± 0.90
SERUM		
T_4 (μg/dL)	4.2 ± 0.6	<0.5
T_3 (ng/dL)	44 ± 9	43 ± 6

*Results are given as mean ± SD, calculated from the percentages of ^{125}I found in each iodocompound in thyroid hydrolysates, 24 hours after injection of ^{125}I. Abrams GM, Larsen PR. Triiodothyronine and thyroxine in the serum and thyroid glands of iodine-deficient rats. J Clin Invest 1973;52:2522.

TABLE 14-10.
Comparison of Epidemiologic and Biochemical Data Exploring Thyroid Function in Brussels and in the Idjwi Island and Ubangi Endemic Goiter Areas of Zaire

Variables	Belgium	Zaire
Daily urinary excretion of iodine (μg/d)	51.2 ± 5.8 (38)	15.5 ± 1.3 (243)
Prevalence of goiter (%)	3	76.8
Serum concentration of:		
T_4 (μg/dL)	8.1 ± 0.1 (125)	4.9 ± 0.2 (358)
T_3 (ng/dL)	144 ± 3 (124)	166 ± 3 (299)
TSH (μU/mL)	1.7 ± 1.1 (255)	18.6 ± 2.1 (365)
PB ^{131}I 24 h (% dose/L)	0.06 ± 0.01 (27)	0.17 ± 0.02 (105)
Thyroidal uptake of ^{131}I 24 h (% dose)	46.4 ± 1.1 (255)	65.2 ± 0.9 (167)
Thyroid organic iodine exchangeable pool (mg)	15.8 ± 3.5 (12)	1.6 ± 0.2 (30)

Results given as mean ± SE. The number of patients is given in parentheses. The differences between the two groups are highly significant (P < 0.0001) for all variables.
Data from references 17, 42, 79, and 146–148.

The presence of hard thyroid nodules may suggest the diagnosis of thyroid cancer. An increase in the absolute number of thyroid cancers in endemic goiter remains controversial;[92–94] however, the mortality rate by thyroid cancer is definitely increased because of delayed diagnosis due to the frequency of enlarged thyroids in the population and because the relative frequency of aggressive thyroid cancer, such as follicular and anaplastic carcinomas and sarcomas, is higher than in nonendemic areas.[93]

Pediatric Aspects of Adaptation to Iodine Deficiency

SEQUENTIAL DEVELOPMENT OF THE MECHANISMS OF ADAPTATION TO IODINE DEFICIENCY DURING GROWTH: PATHOGENESIS OF ENDEMIC GOITER

The view that endemic goiter constitutes the most efficient mechanism of adaptation to iodine deficiency is based, with a few exceptions,[39,95–97] on information obtained only from adults. Therefore, in an attempt to define the metabolic history of endemic goiter, a study was conducted[98] on the time course, as a function of age from 3 to 22 years, of the changes in thyroid function in goitrous and nongoitrous inhabitants of the Idjwi Island endemic goiter area in Zaire (Fig 14-19). Thyroid uptake of radioiodine reached its maximum value in the earliest years of life and then declined progressively until adulthood. Uptake was systematically higher in goitrous than in nongoitrous patients. The thyroid exchangeable hormonal iodine pool increased progressively with age. The value was about 0.5 mg iodine in young infants; it increased progressively with age but reached only 2.5 mg in adults, which is four to ten times lower than in adults in nonendemic areas. Conversely, the renewal rate of intrathyroidal radioactive iodine (apparent secretion rate, $K'4$) decreased drastically with age.

The study demonstrates that the acceleration of the main steps of iodine kinetics is much more marked in childhood and adolescence than in adulthood, and it progressively decreases during growth. Similar studies conducted in the area of Idjwi Island with a similar degree of iodine deficiency but without goiter showed that in this area 1) radioiodine uptake also was increased but to a lesser extent, 2) iodine stores in the thyroid were much lower, and 3) the plasma protein-bound iodine was higher. These data suggest that goiter is by no means the optimal mechanism of adaptation to environmental goitrogens but constitutes a rather unfavorable side effect of such a mechanism.

AGE-RELATED MODIFICATIONS OF TSH REGULATION

By studying the time course, as a function of age, of the serum concentrations of TSH, T_4, and T_3 in clinically euthyroid subjects residing in a severe endemic goiter area in the Ubangi region in Zaire, it was shown (Fig 14-20) that, unexpectedly, the highest values of serum TSH were observed in the youngest infants despite the fact that they also had the highest T_4 values.[99] For a given value of T_4, the level of TSH was about twice as high in the 4- to 15-year-old group than in the 16- to 20-year-old group (Fig 14-21). These variations of the TSH:T_4 ratio as a function of age are poorly understood and could reflect the increase in the iodine stores within the thyroid as a function of age. They also could be explained by modifications with age of the turnover rate of T_4[100] or by modifications in thyroid gland sensitivity to TSH, including progressive development of thyroid autonomy.[101]

THYROID FUNCTION IN EARLY LIFE

One of the major achievements of recent years has been the results obtained by systematic screening for congenital hypothyroidism in the neonates in iodine-deficient areas.[18] The studies have shown that in such areas the alterations of thyroid function in neonates are much more frequent and severe than in adults. A large number of neonates and young infants exhibit the biochemical features of thyroid failure found in Western countries only in permanent sporadic congenital hypothyroidism.

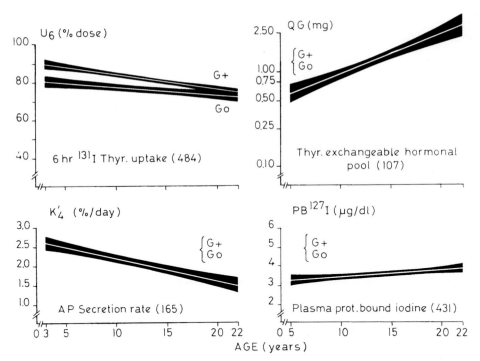

FIGURE 14-19. Changes with age of the 6-hour thyroidal uptake of radioiodine (U_6), the thyroidal iodine exchangeable hormonal pool (QG), the apparent secretion rate of radioiodine by the thyroid ($K'4$), and the serum concentration of protein-bound iodine (PBI) in goitrous (G+) and nongoitrous (Go) inhabitants of the Idjwi Island endemic goiter area, Zaire. Values recorded as mean and SE. The number of patients is shown in parentheses. (From Delange[17])

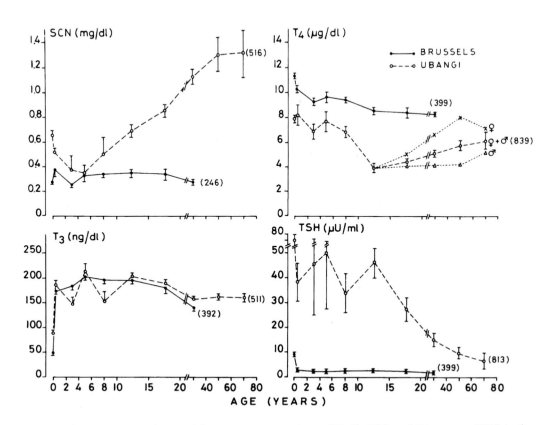

FIGURE 14-20. Changes with age of the serum concentrations of T_4, T_3, TSH, and thiocyanate (SCN) in the Ubangi endemic goiter area, Zaire (o) and in Brussels (•). Values recorded as mean ± SE. The number of patients is shown in parentheses. (From Delange[17])

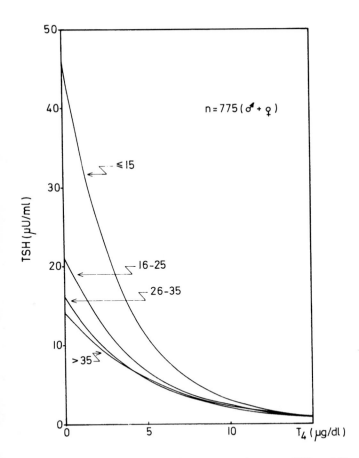

FIGURE 14-21. Computed correlation curves between TSH and T_4 serum concentrations in 840 inhabitants of the Ubangi endemic goiter area (Zaire). The curves are derived from the linear inverse correlations ($P < 0.001$) between log TSH and T_4 in four age groups (<15, 16–25, 26–35 and >35 years) (From Bourdoux and Ermans[99])

The most extreme situation has been reported from Zaire,[102–104] where thyroid failure in neonates results from the combined action of iodine deficiency and thiocyanate overload during late fetal life (see chap 57). In this area (Fig 14-22), cord serum TSH and T_4 levels in unselected newborns were variable and were frequently outside the normal range. Eleven percent of the neonates had both a cord serum TSH value above 100 μU/mL and a cord serum T_4 concentration below 40 nmol/L, indicating severe congenital hypothyroidism according to the criteria used in Western countries, where the incidence of the condition is only 0.025%. A similar frequency of biochemical hypothyroidism has been found in the same area in young infants,[105] indicating that the findings in neonates were not due to nonspecific factors, such as the stress of delivery. The picture of congenital hypothyroidism was only transient in some infants but remained unchanged in others.[17]

The abnormalities of neonatal thyroid function were prevented by correcting iodine deficiency in mothers before or during pregnancy [104,106] (see Fig 14-22). It has been suggested that permanent congenital hypothyroidism in severe endemic goiter that starts during the perinatal period is responsible for the development of myxedematous endemic cretinism and that

transient hypothyroidism that occurs during the critical period of brain development is responsible for the endemic mental retardation frequently observed in clinically euthyroid children in severely affected areas[17] (see also chaps 57 and 67).

A similar frequency of congenital hypothyroidism in severe endemic goiter has been reported from the Himalayas in Northern India, Nepal, and Bhutan.[107] Alterations of thyroid function in neonates have been subsequently reported from other less severe endemic areas, even when thyroid function in adults was normal.[108] The alterations are characterized by a shift of the frequency distributions of neonatal TSH and T_4 toward elevated and low values, respectively.

MILD TO MODERATE IODINE DEFICIENCY DISORDERS: THE SITUATION IN EUROPE

Epidemiology

Endemic goiter, occasionally complicated by endemic cretinism, had been reported in Europe up to the turn of the twentieth century, especially from remote, isolated, mountainous areas in central parts of the continent including Switzerland, Austria, Northern Italy, Bulgaria, and Poland.[109–111] The problem of IDD has been entirely eradicated in Switzerland due to the implementation and monitoring of a program of salt iodization.[112] Probably because of the impact on the medical world of this remarkable program, IDD seems to be no longer considered a significant public health problem in Europe during the last five decades.

However, reevaluation of the problem in the late 1980s under the sponsorship of the European Thyroid Association clearly indicated that, with the exception of some of the Scandinavian countries, Austria, and Switzerland, most of the European countries or at least certain areas of these countries, were still iodine deficient, especially in the southern part of the continent.[113] Shortly thereafter, it was shown that differences in the iodine supplies in the adult populations of several countries or areas were accompanied by parallel differences in the iodine content of breast milk and of neonatal urine[114] (Table 14-11). The status of iodine nutrition was reevaluated in 1992 in all European countries, including the eastern part of the continent.[111] The results are summarized in Figure 14-23. Iodine deficiency was controlled in only five countries, namely Austria, Finland, Norway, Sweden, and Switzerland. Iodine deficiency was marginal or present mainly in "microfoci" (pockets of goiter) in Belgium, the Czech and Slovak republics, Denmark, France, Hungary, Ireland, Portugal, and the United Kingdom. IDD have recurred after transitory resolution in Croatia, the Netherlands, and possibly some Eastern Europe countries. Finally, iodine deficiency persisted and varied from moderate to severe in all the other European countries, namely Bulgaria, the Commonwealth of Independent States (CIS), Germany, Greece, Italy, Poland, Romania, Spain, and Turkey. In some of these countries, such as Bulgaria and Romania, the prevalence of goiter in schoolchildren varied from 16% to 81% and the median urinary iodine concentrations were as low as 2 μg/dL, that is, similar to the most severely affected areas in Central Africa.[42]

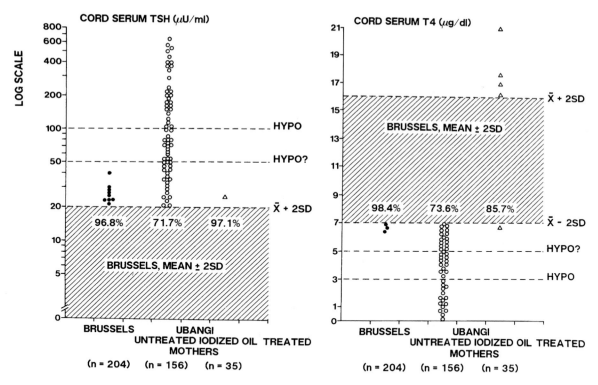

FIGURE 14-22. Comparison of the distribution of the serum concentrations of TSH and T$_4$ in cord blood in Brussels and in newborns in the Ubangi endemic goiter area in Zaire born to untreated mothers or to mothers treated with one single injection of iodized oil during pregnancy. The number of newborns is shown in parentheses. The dotted lines correspond to the values considered as suggestive (hypo?) or characteristic (hypo) of permanent sporadic congenital hypothyroidism in the neonatal thyroid screening program of Brussels. (Modified from Delange and coworkers[17] and Ermans and colleagues[159])

Public Health Consequences

The state of mild to severe iodine deficiency persisting in many European countries or regions has important consequences from a public health standpoint, including the intellectual development of infants and children. As an example, Table 14-12 summarizes the situation in Belgium where the consequences of mild IDD on the main target groups (i.e., pregnant and lactating women, neonates and young infants) have been extensively investigated.

More generally speaking, the consequences of iodine deficiency in Europe can be summarized as follows.

ADULTS. The frequency of simple goiter is elevated in many countries and the cost of therapy of thyroid problems resulting from iodine deficiency in the adult population is enormous. For example, the cost for the diagnosis and treatment of goiter due to iodine deficiency in Germany in 1986 was estimated at $700 million,[115] yet prevention by iodized salt would cost only 2 to 8 US cents per person, per year.[116] Thyroid uptake of radioiodine varies markedly from one European country to another and is inversely related to the iodine intake.[117] Elevated thyroid uptake due to iodine deficiency aggravates the risk of thyroid irradiation and development of thyroid cancer in case of a nuclear accident.[118] The best prophylaxis of radioiodine fallout from nuclear accidents is to increase the basal intake of iodine of the population.[119]

Thyroid function is usually normal in adults in Europe. In contrast, it is frequently altered in pregnant women. During pregnancy, the gland undergoes stimulatory events due to the synergic effects of three mechanisms: direct stimulation by human chorionic gonadotropin, stimulation through the usual feedback mechanism via the increase in TBG and the lowering of free hormone concentrations, and additional loss of iodide through increased renal clearance of iodide and to the fetoplacental unit.[120] It has been shown that, at least in conditions of borderline iodine intake as seen in Belgium (50–70 μg/d), pregnancy is accompanied by a progressive decrease of serum free T$_4$ and consequently by an increase in serum TSH. This state of chronic TSH hyperstimulation results in the development of goiter in about 10% of the pregnant women and in a progressive increase in the serum concentration of thyroglobulin.[120] Goiter can persist after pregnancy in a significant number of women.[121] Pregnancy, especially in conditions of borderline iodine intake, at least partly explains the higher frequency of thyroid problems in women than in men.

The consequences of marginal iodine deficiency during pregnancy in Belgium on thyroid function of the neonate include even more elevated serum levels of TSH and thyroglobulin in cord blood than in the mothers and a slight enlargement of the thyroid gland. The role played by iodine deficiency in these changes is demonstrated by the fact that they are prevented by iodine supplementation of the mothers during pregnancy[122] and that they do not occur in iodine-re-

TABLE 14-11.
Comparison of the Results Obtained in European Countries for Urinary Iodine Excretion in
Adults and for the Iodine Content of Breast Milk and of Urine of Infants on Day 5 of Life.

			Iodine Concentration (μg/dL)	
Country or Region	**Urinary Excretion of Iodine in Adults (μg/d)**	**City**	**BREAST MILK (MEAN ± SE)***	**URINE FROM INFANTS ON DAY 5 (MEDIAN)**
The Netherlands	88–140	Rotterdam		16.2 (64)
Finland	238–270	Helsinki		11.2 (39)
Sweden	91–140	Stockholm	9.3 (60)	11.0 (52)
Sicily (nonendemic area)	113	Catania		7.1 (14)
Switzerland	126–141	Zürich		6.2 (62)
Spain	89	Madrid	7.7 ± 0.9 (69)	
France	55–126	Paris	8.2 ± 0.5 (68)	
		Lille		5.8 (82)
Belgium	51	Brussels	9.5 ± 0.6 (91)	4.8 (196)
Italy	37	Rome		4.7 (114)
Germany				
North	35	Berlin		2.8 (87)
South	20	Freiburg	2.5 (41)	1.2 (41)
South	16	Iena	1.2 ± 0.1 (55)	0.8 (54)
Sicily (endemic area)	22	San Angelo	2.7 ± 0.3 (59)	

The number of determinations is shown in parentheses.
Adapted from Delange F, Bürgi H. Iodine deficiency disorders in Europe. Bull WHO 1989;67:317.

plete areas in Europe such as some parts of The Netherlands.[123]

ADOLESCENTS AND CHILDREN. Euthyroid pubertal goiter is especially frequent in adolescents and occasionally requires therapy with L-T$_4$ or iodide.

Even in Europe, clinically euthyroid schoolchildren born and living in an iodine-deficient environment exhibit subtle or even overt neuropsychointellectual deficits as compared to controls living in the same ethnic, demographic, nutritional and socioeconomic system, except that they are not exposed to iodine deficiency (Table 14-13). These deficits are of the same nature, although less marked, than those found in schoolchildren in areas with severe iodine deficiency and endemic mental retardation (see chaps 57 and 67). These deficits could result, as demonstrated in severe endemic goiter, from transient thyroid failure occurring during fetal or early postnatal life, that is, during the critical period of brain development (see chaps 57 and 67).

NEONATES. The most important and frequent alterations of thyroid function due to iodine deficiency in Europe occur in neonates and young infants.

The frequency of transient primary hypothyroidism is almost eight times higher in Europe than in North America.[124] The syndrome is characterized by postnatally acquired primary hypothyroidism lasting for a few weeks and requiring substitutive therapy.[125] The risk of transient hypothyroidism in the neonates increases with the degree of prematurity.[126] The specific role played by iodine deficiency in the etiology of this type of hy-

pothyroidism is demonstrated by the disappearance of transient neonatal thyroid failure in Belgian preterms since they were systematically supplemented with 30 μg potassium iodide/d.

As shown in Figure 14-24, there is an inverse relationship between the urinary iodine concentration in newborn populations in Europe used as an index of their status of iodine nutrition and the frequency of serum TSH above 50 μU/mL at day 5, at the time of screening for congenital hypothyroidism, that is, the recall rate when congenital hypothyroidism is suspected.[15] Consequently, neonatal thyroid screening appears as a particularly sensitive index of the presence and action of goitrogenic substances in the environment[127] and can be used as a monitoring tool in the evaluation of the effects of iodine prophylaxis of a population.[128]

The reason for the particular sensitivity of the newborn, especially of the preterm infant, to the effects of iodine deficiency appears from the data summarized in Table 14-14. In Toronto, where the iodine intake is elevated, the iodine content of the thyroid in full-term infants is 300 μg. In Brussels, with a borderline iodine intake, the iodine content of the thyroid is 82 μg and in Leipzig, which was severely iodine deficient, the content is only 43 μg. Table 14-14 also shows that the turnover rate of intrathyroidal iodine is markedly accelerated in iodine-deficient neonates. Therefore, thyroid failure is more likely to occur. These neonatal data contrast with adult data that have shown that the iodine stores of the thyroid are not affected by iodine deficiency unless severe iodine deficiency is present (see Fig 14-17).

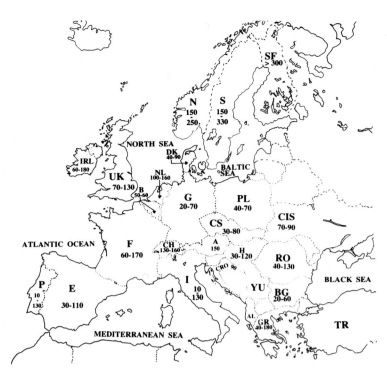

FIGURE 14-23. Evaluation of iodine intake in Europe (μg/d) at 1992. Range of the values observed during regional or national surveys. The figures correspond to the measurement of the daily urinary excretion of iodine or to the extrapolation to one liter of urine per day when the results were expressed as iodine concentrations or iodine/creatinine ratios. N, Norway; S, Sweden; SF, Finland; DK, Denmark; IRL, Ireland; UK, United Kingdom; B, Belgium; NL, The Netherlands; G, Germany; PL, Poland; CS, Former Czechoslovakia; CIS, The Commonwealth of Independent States; F, France; CH, Switzerland; A, Austria; H, Hungary; RO, Romania; P, Portugal; E, Spain; I, Italy; CRO, Croatia; BG, Bulgaria; GR, Greece; AL, Albania; TR, Turkey. (From Delange[15])

TREATMENT AND PROPHYLAXIS OF IODINE DEFICIENCY DISORDERS

Prolonged administration of iodide or of thyroid hormones has been found highly effective in reducing the size of endemic goiter.[129] Surgical treatment is often justified in large goiters with pressure symptoms. Nevertheless, such types of treatment are, in practice, impossible to apply to a general population in view of the epidemiologic size of the problem and the general lack of adequate medical infrastructure in the most severely affected

TABLE 14-12.
Functional Consequences of Mild Iodine Deficiency in Europe: the Case of Belgium

Age Groups	Recommended Iodine Intake (μg/d)	Actual Iodine Intake (μg/d)	Consequences
Adults	150	51–60	Elevated thyroidal uptake of radioiodine
			Increased risk in case of nuclear accident
Pregnant women	200	<100 in 90% of the cases	Increased thyroid stimulation
			Development of goiter with only partial recovery after pregnancy
			Prevention of these anomalies by iodine supplementation
Adolescents	150	30–50	"Puberty" simple goiter
Children	90–120	<90 in 90% of the cases	Potential risk for brain and intellectual development
Neonates and infants	90	Deficient in 79% of the cases	Elevated serum TSH and Tg at birth (cord blood)
			Elevated TSH at screening for congenital hypothyroidism; high recall rate and frequency of false-positive results
			Increased risk of transient hypothyroidism in the premature infant

Adapted from Delange F. Iodine deficiency in Europe. Thyroid International 1994;3:1.

TABLE 14-13.
Neuropsychointellectual Deficits in Infants and Schoolchildren in Conditions of Mild to Moderate Iodine Deficiency in Europe

Regions	Tests	Findings	References
Spain	Locally adapted: Bayley, McCarthy, Cattell	Lower psychomotor and mental development than controls	Bleichrodt et al, 1989[150]
Italy			
Sicily	Bender-Gestalt	Low perceptual integrative motor ability; neuromuscular and neurosensorial abnormalities	Vermigglio et al, 1990[151]
Tuscany	Wechsler Raven	Low verbal IQ, perception, motor and attentive functions	Fenzi et al, 1990[152]
Tuscany	Wisc; reaction time	Low velocity of motor response to visual stimuli	Vitti et al, 1992[153]

populations. The most logical approach is the introduction of iodine prophylaxis. The public health aspects of iodine prophylaxis, including the planning and monitoring of prophylactic campaigns, the technical aspects of production and distribution of iodized salt and the other methods of iodine prophylaxis, and the cost-benefit evaluation of iodine prophylaxis are discussed in detail elsewhere.[5,8,9,31,130–132]

For almost 80 years, iodized salt has been used as the simplest and most effective way of providing extra iodine in the diet.[130–132] Iodine is most often added in the form of potassium iodide but iodate is preferred in humid regions, owing to its greater stability. The first large-scale successful campaign to prevent endemic goiter by iodized salt was carried out in the United States in 1917.[133] Later epidemiologic surveys demonstrated the successful result of this program.[131] The effectiveness of the method was confirmed by a number of similar campaigns in Switzerland, India, Mexico, Guatemala, Greece, Argentina, Finland, and the former Czechoslovakia.[5,9,11,12,14] These programs resulted in not only a dramatic reduction in the prevalence of goiter but also progressive disappearance of endemic cretinism.

The recommended levels of iodine supplementation vary widely. In the United States, 1 part iodide is added to 10,000 parts salt. In other countries, the ratio is 1:100,000. If salt consumption of 5 g/d is presumed, the extra iodine supply would vary therefore from 500 μg to 50 μg/d. A reasonable recommendation is 1:20,000 to 50,000.[130,132] Iodide has been used as a supplement in bread in Holland and in Tasmania but wide variations in the amount of bread consumption make this a less than satisfactory technique.[132] Iodination of water has been successfully used in some areas with adequate water supply and control of the iodination process.[134–136] Iodination of irrigation water has been successfully used in China.[137]

In many developing countries with severe problems of endemic goiter, iodination of salt, bread, or water has failed to prevent or eradicate the disease because various socioeconomic, climatic, or geographic conditions made systematic iodine supplementation difficult or even impossible, such as when iodized salt did not reach the endemic areas or when house salt was not available.[131,132] In such conditions, prophylaxis and therapy can be achieved extremely effectively by the

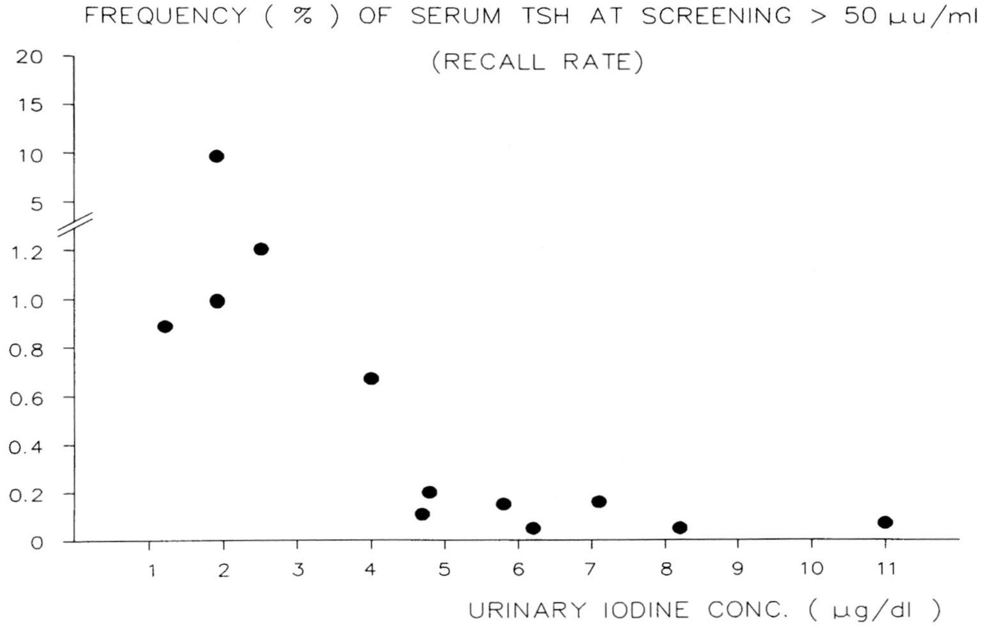

FIGURE 14-24. Relationship between the urinary iodine concentration and the recall rate at the time of screening for congenital hypothyroidism in newborn populations in Europe. Each point results from the analysis of 50 to 200 urine samples and from 20,000 to 300,000 screening tests. (From Delange[15])

TABLE 14-14.
Relation Between the Iodine Content of Urine in Adults and Neonates Used as an Index of Iodine Supply and Thyroid Weight, Iodine Content, and Estimated Turnover Rate of Thyroidal Iodine

City	Adults: Urinary Excretion of Iodine (μg/d)	Neonates: Iodine Concentration in Urine			Neonates: Thyroids	
		MEDIAN (μg/dL)	VALUES BELOW 5 μG/dL (%)	WEIGHT (g)*†	IODINE CONTENT (μg)*	ESTIMATED TURNOVER RATE‡ (%/d)
Toronto	600–800	14.8 (81)	11.9	1.00 ± 0.12 (13)	292 ± 47	17
Brussels	51	4.8 (196)‖	53.2	0.76 ± 0.25 (4)	81 ± 9§	62
Leipzig	16	1.6 (70)‖	97.2	3.27 ± 0.39 (10)§	43 ± 6§	125

Results given as mean ± SE.
†*The number of patients is shown in parentheses.*
‡*Based on a requirement of T_4 of 50 μg/d in neonates in three areas with markedly different iodine intake.*
§*Levels of significance as compared with Toronto, P < 0.01.*
‖*Levels of significance as compared with Toronto, P < 0.001.*
Adapted from Delange F, Walfish P, Willgerodt H, et al. Reduction of the iodine stores of the thyroid in iodine deficient newborns. (Abstract) Horm Res 1989;31:75.

administration of large quantities of iodine in the form of slowly resorbable iodized oil given by intramuscular injections or orally.[131,138,139] The method is inexpensive and can be easily implemented through local health services using existing facilities or by small teams. The method is most convenient for isolated communities beyond the reach of commercial channels.

In the light of studies of the injection of iodized oil completed in various countries,[9,131,138,139] it appears necessary to inject the entire population from birth to 45 years of age for females and from birth to 20 years of age for males. For psychological reasons, however, this sex distinction is not always applied.[12] The long-term effectiveness and safety of this procedure have been extensively documented for at least 7 years in adults and for 2 to 3 years in young children. The usual dose for intramuscular injections of iodized oil is 1 mL (480 mg iodine) for subjects 1 year of age and older and 0.5 mL for infants under 1 year of age.

Administering iodized oil orally has the advantage of avoiding injections, but its duration of action is definitely shorter and more variable from one subject to another, depending on the absorption of iodine through the gastrointestinal tract.[138,139] An oral dose of 1 mL (480 mg) to 2 mL (960 mg) provides adequate iodine for 1 year after a single administration in adults.[139] Preliminary studies suggesting that smaller doses (0.1–0.25 mL) may be equally effective, at least for 1 year,[140] were not confirmed.[141]

The principal complication of iodine prophylaxis is the occurrence of thyrotoxicosis.[132] This complication was first noticed in the early days after the introduction of iodide supplementation. An increased incidence of thyrotoxicosis was observed in Tasmania after bread iodination in 1966 and was most evident in the older age groups.[142] It was attributed to the presence of autonomous nodules or underlying Graves' disease. Patients with thyrotoxicosis were occasionally reported after administration of iodized oil in Ecuador, Peru, and Argentina but not in New Guinea and Zaire.[132] In all reports, the disease was mild and easily managed. The question may arise whether this development of thyrotoxicosis is to be considered as a complication of iodine prophylaxis or an unavoidable consequence of the normalization of the iodine intake. Even in nongoitrous areas, it has been shown that the shift from a low-normal iodine intake (100 μg/d) to a high-normal intake (500 μg/day) may induce clearcut thyrotoxicosis in euthyroid subjects with autonomous thyroid nodules.[143] A 25-year experience actually showed that long-term correction of iodine deficiency not only abolishes endemic goiter, endemic cretinism, and endemic mental retardation but also ultimately reduces the incidence of hyperthyroidism.[143a] The large amount of information now available worldwide clearly establishes that the occurrence of thyrotoxicosis is exceptionnal and does not negate the enormous benefit that follows the introduction of iodine prophylaxis in endemic goiter regions.

References

1. Food and Nutrition Board. Committee on Dietary Allowances. US National Research Council. Iodine. In: Recommended dietary allowances, 10th ed. Washington, DC: National Academy Press Publishers, 1989:213
2. Delange F. Requirements of iodine in humans. In: Delange F, Dunn JT, Glinoer D, eds. Iodine deficiency in Europe. A continuing concern. New York: Plenum Press, 1993:5
3. Moulopoulos DS, Koutras DA, Mantzos J, et al. The relation of serum T_4 and TSH with the urinary iodine excretion. J Endocrinol Invest 1988;11:437
4. Stanbury JB, Brownell GL, Riggs DS, et al. Endemic goiter. The adaptation of man to iodine deficiency. Cambridge: Harvard University Press, 1954:1
5. Stanbury JB, Hetzel BS. Endemic goiter and cretinism: iodine nutrition in health and disease. New York: John Wiley & Sons, 1980:1
6. McMichael AJ, Potter JD, Hetzel BS. Iodine deficiency, thyroid function and reproductive failure. In: Stanbury JB, Hetzel BS, eds. Endemic goiter and endemic cretinism. Iodine nutrition in health and disease. New York: John Wiley & Sons, 1980:445

7. Hetzel BS. Iodine deficiency disorders (IDD) and their eradication. Lancet 1983;ii:1126

8. Hetzel BS, Dunn JT, Stanbury JB. The prevention and control of iodine deficiency disorders. Amsterdam: Elsevier, 1987:1

9. Hetzel BS, Pandav CS. S.O.S. for a billion. The conquest of iodine deficiency disorders. Dehli: Oxford University Press, 1994:1

10. Koutras DA, Matovinovic J, Vought R. The ecology of iodine. In: Stanbury JB, Hetzel BS, eds. Endemic goiter and endemic cretinism. New York: John Wiley & Sons, 1980:185

11. Micronutrient Deficiency Information System. Global prevalence of iodine deficiency disorders. MDIS working paper no. 1. Geneva: WHO-Nutrition Unit Publishers, 1993:1

12. Thilly CH, Hetzel BS. An assessment of prophylactic programs: social, political, cultural and economic issues. In: Stanbury JB, Hetzel BS, eds. Endemic goiter and endemic cretinism. New York: John Wiley & Sons, 1980:475

13. Boyages SC. Iodine deficiency disorders. J Clin Endocrinol Metab 1993;77:587

14. Delange F, Ermans AM. Endemic goiter and cretinism. Naturally occurring goitrogens. Pharmacol Ther 1976;1:57

15. Delange F. The disorders induced by iodine deficiency. Thyroid 1994;4:107

16. Matovinovic J. Endemic goiter and cretinism at the dawn of the third millennium. Annu Rev Nutr 1983;3:341

17. Delange F. Adaptation to iodine deficiency during growth: etiopathogenesis of endemic goiter and cretinism. In: Delange F, Fisher D, Malvaux P, eds. Pediatric thyroidology. Basel: S. Karger, 1985:295

18. Delange F. Iodine nutrition and congenital hypothyroidism. In: Delange F, Fisher DA, Glinoer D, eds. Research in congenital hypothyroidism. New York: Plenum Press, 1989:173

19. Delange F, Bastani S, Benmiloud M, et al. Definitions of endemic goiter and cretinism, classification of goiter size and severity of endemias, and survey techniques. In: Dunn JT, Pretell E, Daza CH, Viteri FE, eds. Towards the eradication of endemic goiter, cretinism and iodine deficiency. PAHO Sc publ no. 502. Washington, DC: Pan American Health Organization, 1986:373

20. Gutekunst R, Smolarek H, Hasenpusch V, et al. Goitre epidemiology, thyroid volume, iodine excretion, thyroglobulin and thyrotropin in Germany and Sweden. Acta Endocrinol (Kbh) 1986;112:494

21. Gutekunst R, Martin-Teichert H. Requirements for goiter surveys and the determination of thyroid size. In: Delange F, Dunn JT, Glinoer D, eds. Iodine deficiency in Europe. A continuing concern. New York: Plenum Press, 1993:109

22. Thilly CH, Delange F, Stanbury JB. Epidemiologic surveys in endemic goiter and cretinism. In: Stanbury JB, Hetzel BS, eds. Endemic goiter and endemic cretinism. Iodine nutrition in health and disease. New York: John Wiley & Sons, 1980:157

23. Beckers C, Delange F. Etiology of endemic goiter. Iodine deficiency. In: Stanbury JB, Hetzel BS, eds. Endemic goiter and endemic cretinism. New York: John Wiley & Sons, 1980:199

24. Gaitan E. Environmental goitrogenesis. Boca Raton, FL: CRC Press, 1989:1

25. Koutras DA, Papapetrou PD, Yataganas X, Malamos B. Dietary sources of iodine in areas with and without iodine-deficiency goiter. Am J Clin Nutr 1970;23:870

26. Wayne EJ, Koutras DA, Alexander WD. Clinical aspects of iodine metabolism. Oxford: Blackwell, 1964:1

27. Malamos B, Koutras DA, Marketos SG, et al. Endemic goiter in Greece: an iodine balance study in the field. J Clin Endocrinol Metab 1967;27:1372

28. Follis RH. Patterns of urinary iodine excretion in goitrous and nongoitrous areas. Am J Clin Nutr 1964;14:253

29. Jolin T, Escobar del Rey F. Evaluation of iodine/creatinine ratios of casual samples as indices of daily urinary iodine output during field studies. J Clin Endocrinol Metab 1965;25:540

30. Bourdoux P, Thilly C, Delange F, Ermans AM. A new look at old concepts in laboratory evaluation of endemic goiter. In: Dunn JT, Pretell E, Daza CH, Viteri FE, eds. Towards the eradication of endemic goiter, cretinism and iodine deficiency. PAHO Sc publ no. 502. Washington, DC: Pan American Health Organization, 1986:115

31. Hetzel BS, Potter BJ, Dulberg EM. The iodine deficiency disorders: nature, pathogenesis and epidemiology. World Rev Nutr Diet 1990;62:59

32. Studer H, Greer MA. The regulation of thyroid function in iodine deficiency. Bern: Hans Huber, 1968:1

33. Orts S, Dustin P, Delange F. Goitrous enzootic in the wild rat with a geographical distribution similar to endemic human goitre. Acta Endocrinol (Kbh) 1971;66:193

34. Clements FW, Wishart JW. A thyroid-blocking agent in the etiology of endemic goiter. Metabolism 1956;5:623

35. Costa A, Cottino F. Research on iodine metabolism in endemic goitre in Piedmont. Metabolism 1963;12:35

36. Peltola P, Virtanen A. Effect of the prophylactic use of iodine on the thyroid of cattle in the endemic goitre in Finland. Ann Med Intern Fenn (Helsinki) 1954;43:209

37. Ma Tai, Yu Z-H, Lu T-Z, et al. High-iodide endemic goiter. Chin Med J 1982;95:692

38. Suzuki H, Higuchi T, Sawa K, et al. "Endemic coast goitre" in Hokkaido, Japan. Acta Endocrinol (Kbh) 1965;50:161

39. Choufoer JC, Van Rhijn M, Kassenaar AAH, Querido A. Endemic goiter in Western New Guinea. Iodine metabolism in goitrous and non-goitrous subjects. J Clin Endocrinol Metab 1963;23:1203

40. Delange F, Thilly C, Ermans AM. Iodine deficiency, a permissive condition in the development of endemic goiter. J Clin Endocrinol Metab 1968;28:114

41. Roche M, Perinetti H, Barbeito A. Urinary excretion of stable iodine in a small group of isolated Venezuelan Indians. J Clin Endocrinol Metab 1961;21:1009

42. Delange F, Iteke FB, Ermans AM. Nutritional factors involved in the goitrogenic action of cassava. Ottawa: International Development Research Centre, 1982:1

43. Ermans AM, Mbulamoko NM, Delange F, Ahluwalia R. Role of cassava in the etiology of endemic goitre and cretinism. Ottawa: International Development Research Centre, 1980:1

44. Langer P, Greer MA. Antithyroid substances and naturally occurring goitrogens. Basel: S. Karger, 1977:1

45. Podoba J, Langer P. Naturally occurring goitrogens and thyroid function. Bratislava: Publishing House of the Slovak Academy of Sciences, 1964:1

46. Van Etten CH. Goitrogens. In: Liener IE, ed. Toxic constituents of plant foodstuffs. New York: Academic Press, 1969:103

47. Ermans AM, Bourdoux P. Antithyroid sulfurated compounds. In: Gaitan E, ed. Environmental goitrogenesis. Boca Raton, FL: CRC Press, 1989:15

48. Gmelin R, Virtanen AI. The enzymic formation of thiocyanate (SCN−) from a precursor(s) in *Brassica* species. Acta Chem Scand 1960;14:507

49. Gibson HB, Howeler JF, Clements FW. Seasonal epidemics of endemic goitre in Tasmania. Med J Aust 1960;1:875

50. Ermans AM, Kinthaert J, Van Der Velden, Bourdoux P. Studies of the antithyroid effects of cassava and of thiocyanate in rats. In: Ermans AM, Mbulamoko NM, Delange F, Ahluwalia R, eds. Role of cassava in the etiology of endemic goitre and cretinism. Ottawa: International Development Research Centre, 1980:93

51. Wolff J. Transport of iodide and other anions in the thyroid gland. Physiol Rev 1964;44:45

52. Wollman SH. Inhibition by thiocyanate of accumulation of radioiodine by thyroid gland. Am J Physiol 1962;203:517

53. Ekpechi OL. Pathogenesis of endemic goitre in Eastern Nigeria. Br J Nutr 1967;21:537

54. Bourdoux P, Delange F, Gérard M, et al. Evidence that cassava ingestion increases thiocyanate formation: a possible etiologic factor in endemic goiter. J Clin Endocrinol Metab 1978;46:613

55. Delange F. Cassava and the thyroid. In: Gaitan E, ed. Boca Raton, FL: CRC Press, 1989:173

56. Delange F, Ermans AM. Role of a dietary goitrogen in the etiology of endemic goiter in Idjwi Island. Am J Clin Nutr 1971; 24:1354

57. Maberly GF, Eastman CJ, Waite KV, et al. The role of cassava in endemic goitre in Sarawak, Malaysia. In: Ui N, Torizuka K, Nagataki S, Miayi K, eds. Current problems in thyroid research. Amsterdam: Excerpta Medica, 1983:341

58. Gaitan E, Cooksey RC, Legan J, et al. Antithyroid effects in vivo and in vitro of babassu and mandioca: a staple food in goiter areas in Brazil. Eur J Endocrinol 1994;131:138

59. Bourdoux P, Seghers P, Mafuta M, et al. Cassava products: HCN content and detoxification processes. In: Delange F, Iteke FB, Ermans AM, eds. Nutritional factors involved in the goitrogenic action of cassava. Ottawa: International Development Research Centre, 1982:51

60. Delange F, Vigneri R, Trimarchi F, et al. Etiological factors of endemic goiter in North-Eastern Sicily. J Endocrinol Invest 1978; 2:137

61. Scranton JR, Nissen WM, Halmi NS. The kinetics of the inhibition of thyroidal iodide accumulation by thiocyanate: a reexamination. Endocrinology 1969;85:603

62. Studer H, Kohler H, Bürgi H. Iodine deficiency. In: Greer MA, Solomon DH, eds. Handbook of physiology. Sect 7. Endocrinology. Vol III. Thyroid. Washington, DC: American Physiology Society, 1974:303

63. Chopra IJ, Hershman JM, Hornabrook RW. Serum thyroid hormone and thyrotrophin levels in subjects from endemic goiter regions of New Guinea. J Clin Endocrinol Metab 1975; 40:326

64. Delange F, Hershman JM, Ermans AM. Relationship between the serum thyrotropin level, the prevalence of goiter and the pattern of iodine metabolism in Idjwi Island. J Clin Endocrinol Metab 1971;33:261

65. Henneman G, Djokomoeljanto R, Docter R, et al. The relationship between serum protein-bound iodine levels and urinary iodine excretion and serum thyrotropin concentrations in subjects from an endemic goitre area in Central Java. Acta Endocrinol (Kbh) 1978;88:474

66. Patel YC, Pharoah POD, Hornabrook RW, Hetzel BS. Serum triiodothyronine, thyroxine and thyroid-stimulating hormone in endemic goiter: a comparison of goitrous and nongoitrous subjects in New Guinea. J Clin Endocrinol Metab 1973;37:783

67. Pharoah POD, Lawton NF, Ellis SM, et al. The role of triiodothyronine (T_3) in the maintenance of euthyroidism in endemic goitre. Clin Endocrinol 1973;2:193

68. Dumont JE, Lamy F, Roger P, et al. Physiological and pathological regulation of thyroid cell proliferation and differentiation by thyrotropin and other factors. Physiol Rev 1992;72:667

69. Dumont JE, Vassart G, Refetoff S. Thyroid disorders. In: Scriver CR, Beaudet AL, Fly WS, Valle D, eds. The metabolic basis of inherited diseases, 6th ed., Vol 2. New York: McGraw-Hill, 1989:1843

70. Ermans AM, Dumont JE, Bastenie PA. Thyroid function in a goitrous endemic. II. Nonhormonal iodine escape from the goitrous gland. J Clin Endocrinol Metab 1963;23:550

71. Oddie TH, Fisher DA, McConahey WM, Thompson CS. Iodine intake in the United States: a reassessment. J Clin Endocrinol Metab 1970;30:659

72. Ermans AM. Etiopathogenesis of endemic goiter. In: Stanbury JB, Hetzel BS, eds. Endemic goiter and endemic cretinism. New York: John Wiley & Sons, 1983:287

73. Ermans AM, Dumont JE, Bastenie PA. Thyroid function in a goiter endemic. I. Impairment of hormone synthesis and secretion in the goitrous gland. J Clin Endocrinol Metab 1963;23:539

74. Abrams GM, Larsen PR. Triiodothyronine and thyroxine in the serum and thyroid glands of iodine-deficient rats. J Clin Invest 1973;52:2522

75. Lamas L, Morreale de Escobar G. Iodoaminoacid distribution in the thyroid of rats on different iodine intakes and with normal plasma protein bound iodine. Acta Endocrinol (Kbh) 1972;69:473

76. Ermans AM, Bastenie PA, Galperin H, et al. Endemic goiter in the Uele region. II. Synthesis and secretion of thyroid hormones. J Clin Endocrinol Metab 1961;21:996

77. De Crombrugghe B, Edelhoch H, Beckers C, de Visscher M. Thyroglobulin from human goiters: effects of iodination on sedimentation and iodoamino acid synthesis. J Biol Chem 1967;242:5681

78. Ermans AM, Kinthaert J, Camus M. Defective intrathyroidal iodine metabolism in nontoxic goiter: inadequate iodination of thyroglobulin. J Clin Endocrinol Metab 1968;28:1307

79. Delange F, Camus M, Ermans AM. Circulating thyroid hormones in endemic goiter. J Clin Endocrinol Metab 1972;34:891

80. Kochupillai N, Karmakar MG, Weightman D, et al. Pituitary-thyroid axis in Himalayan endemic goitre. Lancet 1973;i:1021

81. Greer MA, Grimm Y, Studer H. Qualitative changes in the secretion of thyroid hormones induced by iodine deficiency. Endocrinology 1968;83:1193

82. Medeiros-Neto GA, Imai Y, Kataoka K, Hollander CS. Thyroid function studies in endemic goiter and endemic cretinism. In: Robbins J, Braverman LE, eds. Thyroid research. Amsterdam: Excerpta Medica, 1976:497

83. Evered DC, Ormston BJ, Smith PA, et al. Grades of hypothyroidism. Br Med J 1973;i:657

84. Silva JE, Dick TE, Larsen PR. The contribution of local tissue thyroxine monodeiodination to the nuclear 3,5,3' triiodothyronine in pituitary, liver and kidney of euthyroid rats. Endocrinology 1978;103:1196

85. Ingenbleek Y, Luypaert B, De Nayer Ph. Nutritional status and endemic goitre. Lancet 1980;i:388

86. Fenzi GF, Ceccarelli C, Macchia E, et al. Reciprocal changes of serum thyroglobulin and TSH in residents of a moderate endemic goitre area. Clin Endocrinol 1985;23:115

87. Hershman JM, Due DT, Sharp B, et al. Endemic goiter in Vietnam. J Clin Endocrinol Metab 1983;57:243

88. Pezzino V, Vigneri R, Squatrito S, et al. Increased serum thyroglobulin levels in patients with nontoxic goiter. J Clin Endocrinol Metab 1978;46:653

89. Van Herle AJ, Chopra IJ, Hershman JM, Hornabrook RW. Serum thyroglobulin in inhabitants of an endemic region of New Guinea. J Clin Endocrinol Metab 1976;43:512

90. Boukis MA, Koutras DA, Souvatzoglou A, et al. Thyroid hormone and immunological studies in endemic goiter. J Clin Endocrinol Metab 1983;57:859

91. Studer H, Peter HJ, Gerber H. Natural heterogeneity of thyroid cells: the basis for understanding thyroid function and nodular goiter growth. Endocrinol Rev 1989;10:125

92. Harach HR, Escalante DA, Onativia A, et al. Thyroid carcinoma and thyroiditis in an endemic goitre region before and after iodine prophylaxis. Acta Endocrinol (Kbh) 1985;108:55

93. Riccabona G. Thyroid cancer and endemic goiter. In: Stanbury JB, Hetzel BD, eds. Endemic goiter and endemic cretinism. New York: John Wiley & Sons, 1980:333

94. Wahner HW, Cuello C, Correa P, et al. Thyroid carcinoma in an endemic goiter area, Cali, Columbia. Am J Med 1966;40:58

95. De Visscher M, Beckers C, Van den Schrieck HG, et al. Endemic goiter in the Uele region (Republic of Congo). I. General aspects and functional studies. J Clin Endocrinol Metab 1961;21:175

96. Maisterrena JA, Tovar E, Cancino A, Serrano O. Nutrition and endemic goiter in Mexico. J Clin Endocrinol Metab 1964;24:166

97. Wahner HW, Gaitan E. Thyroid function in adolescents from the goiter endemic of the Cauca Valley, Columbia. In: Stanbury JB, ed. Endemic goiter. PAHO Sc publ no. 193. Washington, DC: Pan American Health Organization, 1969:291

98. Delange F. Endemic goitre and thyroid function in Central Africa. Monographs in Pediatrics, Vol 2. Basel: S. Karger, 1974:1

99. Bourdoux P, Ermans AM. Factors influencing the levels of circulating T_4, T_3 and TSH in human beings submitted to severe iodine deficiency (abstract). Ann Endocrinol 1981;42:40a

100. Malvaux P. Thyroid function during the neonatal period, infancy and childhood. In: Delange F, Fisher DA, Malvaux P, eds. Pediatric thyroidology. Basel: S. Karger, 1985:33

101. Bachtarzi H, Benmiloud M. TSH-regulation and goitrogenesis in severe iodine deficiency. Acta Endocrinol (Kbh) 1983;103:21

102. Delange F, Thilly C, Camus M, et al. Evidence for fetal hypothyroidism in severe endemic goiter. In: Robbins J, Braverman LE, eds. Thyroid research. Amsterdam: Excerpta Medica, 1976:493

103. Delange F, Thilly C, Bourdoux P, et al. Influence of dietary goitrogens during pregnancy in humans on thyroid function of the newborn. In: Delange F, Iteke FB, Ermans AM, eds. Nutritional factors involved in the goitrogenic action of cassava. Ottawa: International Development Research Centre, 1982:40

104. Thilly CH, Delange F, Lagasse R, et al. Fetal hypothyroidism and maternal thyroid status in severe endemic goiter. J Clin Endocrinol Metab 1978;47:354

105. Courtois P, Delange F, Bourdoux P, Ermans AM. Significance of neonatal thyroid screening tests in severe endemic goiter (abstract no. 81). Ann Endocrinol 1982;43:51a

106. Thilly C, Vanderpas J, Bourdoux P, et al. Prevention of myxedematous cretinism with iodized oil during pregnancy. In: Ui N, Torizuka K, Nagataki S, Miyai K, eds. Current problems in thyroid research. Amsterdam: Excerpta Medica, 1983:386

107. Kochupillai N, Pandav CS. Neonatal chemical hypothyroidism in iodine-deficient environments. In: Hetzel BS, Dunn JT, Stanbury JB, eds. The prevention and control of iodine deficiency disorders. Amsterdam: Elsevier, 1987:85

108. Sava L, Delange F, Belfiore A, et al. Transient impairment of thyroid function in newborn from an area of endemic goiter. J Clin Endocrinol Metab 1984;59:90

109. Koutras DA. Europe and the Middle East. In: Stanbury JB, Hetzel BS, eds. Endemic goiter and endemic cretinism. New York: John Wiley & Sons, 1980:79

110. Langer P. Eastern and Southeast Europe. In: Stanbury JB, Hetzel BS, eds. Endemic goiter and endemic cretinism. New York: John Wiley & Sons, 1980:141

111. Delange F, Dunn JT, Glinoer D. Iodine deficiency in Europe. A continuing concern. New York: Plenum Press, 1993:1

112. Bürgi H, Supersaxo Z, Selz B. Iodine deficiency diseases in Switzerland one hundred years after Theodor Kocher's survey: a historical review with some new goitre prevalence data. Acta Endocrinol (Kbh) 1990;123:577

113. Gutekunst R, Scriba PC. Goiter and iodine deficiency in Europe. The European Thyroid Association report as updated in 1988. J Endocrinol Invest 1989;12:209

114. Delange F, Heidemann P, Bourdoux P, et al. Regional variations of iodine nutrition and thyroid function during the neonatal period in Europe. Biol Neonate 1986;49:322

115. Pfannenstiel P. The costs of continuing iodine deficiency in the Federal Republic of Germany. IDD Newsletter 1989;5:7.

116. Mannar VMG. The iodization of salt for the elimination of iodine deficiency disorders. In: Hetzel BS, Pandav CS, eds. S.O.S. for a billion. The conquest of iodine deficiency disorders. Dehli: Oxford University Press, 1994:89

117. Thilly CH, Vanderpas JB, Bebe N, et al. Iodine deficiency, other trace elements and goitrogenic factors in the etiopathogeny of iodine deficiency disorders (IDD). Biol Trace Elem Res 1992;32:229

118. Delange F. Iodine nutrition and risk of thyroid irradiation from nuclear accidents. In: Rubery E, Smales E, eds. Iodine prophylaxis following nuclear accidents. Oxford: Pergamon Press, 1990:45

119. Ermans AM. Dietary iodine supply and radioiodine uptake: the case for generalized iodine prophylaxis. In: Delange F, Dunn JT, Glinoer D, eds. Iodine deficiency in Europe. A continuing concern. New York: Plenum Press, 1993:237

120. Glinoer D, De Nayer P, Bourdoux P, et al. Regulation of maternal thyroid during pregnancy. J Clin Endocrinol Metab 1990;71:276

121. Glinoer D, Lemone M, Bourdoux P, et al. Partial reversibility during late postpartum of thyroid abnormalities associated with pregnancy. J Clin Endocrinol Metab 1992;74:453

122. Glinoer D, De Nayer P, Delange F, et al. A randomized trial for the treatment of excessive thyroidal stimulation in pregnancy: maternal and neonatal effects. J Clin Endocrinol Metab 1995;80:258

123. Berghout A, Endert E, Ross A, et al. Thyroid function and thyroid size in normal pregnant women living in an iodine replete area. Clin Endocrinol 1994;41:375

124. Burrow GN, Dussault JH. Neonatal thyroid screening. New York: Raven Press, 1980:1

125. Delange F, Dodion J, Wolter R, et al. Transient hypothyroidism in the newborn infant. J Pediatr 1978;92:974

126. Delange F, Dalhem A, Bourdoux P, et al. Increased risk of primary hypothyroidism in preterm infants. J Pediatr 1984;105:462

127. Delange F, Bourdoux P, Ermans AM. Neonatal thyroid screening used as an index of an extraphysiological supply of iodine. In: Hall R, Köbberling J, eds. Thyroid disorders associated with iodine deficiency and excess. New York: Raven Press, 1985:273

128. Nordenberg G, Sullivan K, Maberly G, et al. Congenital hypothyroid screening programs and the sensitive thyrotropin assay: strategies for the surveillance of iodine deficiency disorders. In: Delange F, Dunn JT, Glinoer D, eds. Iodine deficiency in Europe. A continuing concern. New York: Plenum Press, 1993:211

129. Riccabona G. Treatment of the individual patient with endemic goiter. In: Stanbury JB, Hetzel BS, eds. Endemic goiter and endemic cretinism. New York: John Wiley & Sons, 1980:351

130. DeMayer EM, Lowenstein FW, Thilly CH. The control of endemic goitre. Geneva: World Health Organization, 1979:1

131. Matovinovic J. Recent results in goiter prophylaxis. In: Stanbury JB, Hetzel BS, eds. Endemic goiter and endemic cretinism. New York: John Wiley & Sons, 1980:589

132. Stanbury JB, Ermans AM, Hetzel BS, et al. Endemic goitre and cretinism: public health significance and prevention. WHO Chronicle 1974;28:220

133. Marine D, Kimball OP. Prevention of simple goiter in man. Arch Intern Med 1920;25:661

134. Maberly GF, Eastman CJ, Corcoran JM. Effect of iodination of a village water-supply on goitre size and thyroid function. Lancet 1981;ii:1270

135. Squatrito S, Vigneri R, Runello F, et al. Prevention and treatment of endemic iodine-deficiency goiter by iodination of a municipal water supply. J Clin Endocrinol Metab 1986;63:368

136. Fisch A, Pichard E, Prazuck T, et al. A new approach to combatting iodine deficiency in developing countries: the controlled release of iodine in water by a silicone elastomer. Am J Publ Health 1993;83:540

137. Cao XY, Jiang XM, Kareem A, et al. Iodination of irrigation water as a method of supplying iodine to a severely iodine-deficient population in Xinjiang, China. Lancet 1994;344:107

138. Hetzel BS, Thilly CH, Fierro-Benitez R, et al. Iodized oil in the prevention of endemic goiter and cretinism. In: Stanbury JB, Hetzel BS, eds. Endemic goiter and endemic cretinism. New York: John Wiley & Sons, 1980:513

139. Dunn JT. Iodized oil in the treatment and prophylaxis of IDD. In: Hetzel BS, Dunn J, Stanbury J, eds. The prevention and control of iodine deficiency disorders. Amsterdam: Elsevier, 1987:127

140. Tonglet R, Bourdoux P, Minga T, et al. Efficacy of low oral doses of iodized oil in the control of iodine deficiency in Zaire. New Engl J Med 1992;326:236

141. Benmiloud M, Chaouki ML, Gutekunst R, et al. Oral iodized oil for correcting iodine deficiency: optimal dosing and outcome indicator selection. J Clin Endocrinol Metab 1994;79:20

142. Connolly RJ, Vidor GI, Stewart JC. Increase in thyrotoxicosis in endemic goitre area after iodation of bread. Lancet 1970;i:500

143. Ermans AM, Camus M. Modifications of thyroid function induced by chronic administration of iodide in the presence of "autonomous" thyroid tissue. Acta Endocrinol (Kbh) 1972;70:463

143a. Baltisberger BL, Minder CE, Bürgi H. Decrease of incidence of toxic nodular goiter in a region of Switzerland after full correction of mild iron deficiency. Eur J Endocrinol 1995;132:546

144. Delange F, Bürgi H. Iodine deficiency disorders in Europe. Bull WHO 1989;67:317

145. Dunn JT, Van Der Haar F. A practical guide to the correction of iodine deficiency. Wageningen: International Council for the Control of Iodine Deficiency Disorders, 1990:1

146. Ermans AM, Kinthaert J, Delcroix D, Collard J. Metabolism of intrathyroidal iodine in normal men. J Clin Endocrinol Metab 1968;28:169

147. Dumont JE, Ermans AM, Bastenie PA. Thyroidal function in a goiter endemic. IV. Hypothyroidism and endemic cretinism. J Clin Endocrinol Metab 1963;23:325

148. Camus M, Ermans AM, Bastenie PA. Alterations of iodine metabolism in asymptomatic thyroiditis. Metabolism 1968;17:1064

149. Delange F. Iodine deficiency in Europe. Thyroid International 1994;3:1

150. Bleichrodt N, Escobar del Rey F, Morreale de Escobar G, et al. Iodine deficiency. Implications for mental and psychomotor development in children. In: De Long GR, Robbins J, Condliffe G, eds. Iodine and the brain. New York: Plenum Press, 1989:269

151. Vermiglio F, Sidoti M, Finocchiaro MD, et al. Defective neuromotor and cognitive ability in iodine-deficient schoolchildren of an endemic goiter region in Sicily. J Clin Endocrinol Metab 1990;70:379

152. Fenzi GF, Giusti LF, Aghini-Lombardi F, et al. Neuropsychological assessment in schoolchildren from an area of moderate iodine deficiency. J Endocrinol Invest 1990;13:427

153. Vitti P, Aghini-Lombardi F, Antonangeli L, et al. Mild iodine deficiency in fetal/neonatal life and neuropsychological performances. Acta Medica Austriaca 1992;19:57

154. Delange F, Walfish P, Willgerodt H, et al. Reduction of the iodine stores of the thyroid in iodine deficient newborns (abstract). Horm Res 1989;31:75

155. Riggs DS. Quantitative aspects of iodine metabolism in man. Pharmacol Rev 1952;4:284

156. Schaefer AE. Status of salt iodization in PAHO member countries. In: Dunn JT, Medeiros-Neto GA, eds. Endemic goiter and cretinism: continuing threats to world health. PAHO Sc Publ no. 292. Washington, DC: Pan American Health Organization, 1974:242

157. Delange F, Bourdoux P, Chanoine JP, Ermans AM. Physiopathology of iodine nutrition during pregnancy, lactation and early postnatal life. In: Berger H, ed. Vitamins and minerals in pregnancy and lactation. Nestlé Nutrition Workshop Series Vol 16. New York: Raven Press, 1988:205

158. Tovar E, Maisterrena JA, Chavez A. Iodine nutrition levels of schoolchildren in rural Mexico. In: Stanbury JB, ed. Endemic goiter. PAHO Sc publ no. 193. Washington, DC: Pan American Health Organization, 1969:411

159. Ermans AM, Bourdoux P, Lagasse R, et al. Congenital hypothyroidism in developing countries. In: Burrow GN, Dussault JH, eds. Neonatal thyroid screening. New York: Raven Press, 1980:61

160. Indications for assessing iodine deficiancy disorders and their control through salt iodization. Geneva: World Health Organization, 1994

EFFECT OF EXCESS IODIDE: CLINICAL ASPECTS

Elio Roti

Apostolos G. Vagenakis

An adequate supply of dietary iodine is essential for the synthesis of the thyroid hormones. Iodine deficiency results in endemic goiter in many geographic areas, including continental Western Europe; in many other regions, however, dietary iodine intake has increased, such as in the United States, Great Britain, and Scandinavia. This increase in dietary iodine intake is mainly due to iodination of salt or bread, the addition of iodide-containing substances to food as preservatives, and improved farming conditions. As a result of this increase, in some communities the daily iodine intake exceeds the recommended daily requirement of 150 μg. In the United States, the average iodine intake is approximately 150 to 250 μg/d and varies from region to region.

Strong evidence indicates that excess iodide can induce thyroid dysfunction, and these iodine-induced abnormalities in thyroid function are the subject of this subchapter.

NORMAL RESPONSE TO IODINE EXCESS

In animals and human beings, the thyroid gland has intrinsic autoregulatory mechanisms to effectively handle excess iodine intake. The acute, transient inhibitory effect of iodine excess on iodide organification, the Wolff-Chaikoff effect, and the escape phenomenon are discussed in chapter 13. The well-known but less understood effect of iodine on the release of thyroxine (T_4) and triiodothyronine (T_3) from the thyroid have been prospectively studied in human beings. When normal subjects were given approximately 40 to 150 mg iodide for 1 to 3 weeks, a small but significant decrease in the serum concentrations of T_4 and T_3 occurred, with a small but significant compensatory rise in the serum thyroid-stimulating hormone (TSH; thyrotropin) concentration and an increased TSH response to thyrotropin-releasing hormone (TRH).[1-3] These alterations were all within the normal range for each parameter. In another study, daily mouth rinsing with polyvinylpyrrolidone iodine for 6 months for gingivitis resulted in the absorption of about 3 mg iodide daily and small but significant increases in the serum TSH concentration.[4] After iodide withdrawal, all values returned to baseline levels. In contrast to these findings, the acute increase of serum iodide concentrations, approximately 90-fold above baseline values, following endoscopic retrograde cholangiopancreaticography with iopamidol, a non-ionic contrast agent, was not followed by significant changes of serum TSH, free T_4, and free T_3 concentrations.[5]

Smaller quantities of iodide (1500 and 4500 µg/d) administered to normal subjects who resided in iodine-replete areas resulted in significant decreases in serum T_4 and free T_4 but not in serum T_3 concentrations. Serum TSH concentration increased, as did the serum TSH response to TRH. The smallest quantity of iodine that did not affect thyroid function was 500 µg/d.[6] In other studies, however, this small quantity of iodine enhanced the TSH response to TRH[7] and in a few patients also increased the basal serum TSH concentration above the normal range. Thus,[8] iodine supplement of about 500 µg/d above the normal diet in iodine-sufficient areas might cause subtle changes in thyroid function.

These subtle changes of thyroid function during iodide administration are accompanied by a small increase of thyroid volume determined by echography[9] and by a decrement of thyroid blood flow evaluated by echocolor Doppler.[10] The latter finding, however, was not related to serum TSH changes.

SOURCES OF EXCESS IODINE

Various drugs and food preservatives contain a large quantity of iodide that is either absorbed directly or released after metabolism of the drug. Many vitamin preparations are supplemented with about 150 µg iodine, a quantity that is considered to be the physiologic daily requirement. Iodophors contain large quantities of iodine and are used as udder antiseptics in the dairy industry, resulting in contamination of the milk with iodine. Iodine is also concentrated by the mammary gland and secreted into the milk and, therefore, may influence thyroid function in the newborn fed cow's milk. Many iodine-rich products, such as kelp, are available in nature food stores. In some areas of Japan, bread is made exclusively from seaweed, exposing the population to large quantities of iodine.

Iodides are present in high concentration in various proprietary and prescribed expectorants, including iodinated glycerol, although iodine has been removed from this latter medication, Organidin, in the United States. Another potential source of excess iodine is the use of contrast media in radiologic studies. Preparations used for computed tomography, arteriography, or pyelography are cleared from the plasma relatively quickly, but the iodine released during these procedures affects thyroid function. However, a dye commonly used for arteriography, meglumine ioxaglate (Hexabrix), did not affect serum T_4, T_3, or free T_4 index up to 56 days after catheterization but serum TSH was not measured.[11] Drugs used in the past for myelography, uterosalpingography, or bronchography were lipid soluble and cleared slowly, main-

taining high plasma inorganic iodine concentrations for years. The newer water-soluble iodine-containing preparations, such as metrizamide, have markedly reduced this problem. A partial list of medications and other preparations containing large quantities of iodine is given in Table 14-15.

IODIDE-INDUCED HYPOTHYROIDISM OR GOITER

In certain susceptible people, the thyroid cannot escape from the transient inhibitory effect of iodine on the organification mechanism. As a result, hypothyroidism may result after prolonged iodine administration. The hypothyroidism is usually transient, and thyroid function returns to normal after iodide withdrawal. Although the exact frequency of iodide goiter and hypothyroidism, or both, in subjects with apparently normal underlying thyroid function is not known, they are probably uncommon; in patients with underlying thyroid dysfunction, however, they are common (Table 14-16). Iodide goiter may be seen with or without hypothyroidism. Most patients who develop iodide goiter have received iodides for years. The mechanism by which the inhibitory effect of iodide is sustained in these susceptible people is not clear.

In the Absence of Apparent Thyroid Disease

NORMAL SUBJECTS

Iodide-induced goiter occurs in about 10% of the population of Hokkaido, a Japanese island. The inhabitants of this island, particularly the fishermen and their families, consume large quantities of an iodine-rich seaweed called kombu. It has been estimated that the quantity of iodide ingested daily may exceed 200 mg. Despite goiter, hypothyroidism is rare. Endemic iodide goiter has also been observed in 64% of children residing in a village located in central China.[12] These children drank water containing 462 µg iodine per liter. No increased prevalence of lymphocytic thyroiditis was found in these patients with goiter. Thyroid autoantibodies as well as immunoglobulins that inhibited TSH binding were negative. Thyroid growth-stimulating immunoglobulins were found in 60% of goitrous children but were absent in children without goiter who resided in an area with increased iodine concentrations in the drinking water.[13] This finding remains to be confirmed.

An increased prevalence of hypothyroidism (12.1%), defined by serum TSH concentrations higher than 5 mU/L, was observed in Japanese subjects with an iodide concentration in the morning urine greater than 75 µmol/L; in subjects with normal iodide excretion the prevalence of hypothyroidism was only 2.3%.[14] When the iodine intake was restricted, the increased serum TSH concentrations returned to normal in patients with negative antithyroid antibodies but not in those with positive antibodies.[15] Histologic examination of the thyroid of patients with iodine-induced hypothyroidism revealed the presence of lymphocytic infiltration in only half the specimens examined. In the other specimens hyperplastic changes in the follicles with papillary folding, cuboidal or

TABLE 14-15.
Commonly Used Iodine-Containing Drugs

Drugs	Iodine Content
ORAL OR LOCAL	
Amiodarone	75 mg/tab
Benziodarone*	49 mg/100-mg tab
Calcium iodide (eg, Calcidrine syrup)	26 mg/mL
Diiodohydroxyquin (eg, Yodoxin)	134 mg/tab
Echothiophate iodide ophthalmic solution (eg, Phospholine)	5–41 µg/drop
Hydriodic acid syrup	13–15 mg/mL
Iodochlorhydroxyquin (eg, Entero-Vioform)	104 mg/tab
Iodine-containing vitamins	0.15 mg/tab
Iodinated glycerol (eg, Organidin,† Iophen)	15 mg/tab
	25 mg/mL
Idoxuridine ophthalmic solution (eg, Herplex)	18 µg/drop
Isopropamide iodide (eg, Darbid, Combid)	1.8 mg/tab
Kelp	0.15 mg/tab
KI (eg, Quadrinal)	145 mg/tab
	24 mg/mL
Lugol's solution	6.3 mg/drop
Niacinamide hydroiodide + KI (eg, Iodo-Niacin)	115 mg/tab
Ponaris nasal emollient	5 mg/0.8 mL
SSKI	38 mg/drop
PARENTERAL PREPARATIONS	
Sodium iodide, 10% solution	85 mg/mL
TOPICAL ANTISEPTICS	
Diiodohydroxyquin cream (eg, Vytone)	6 mg/g
Iodine tincture	40 mg/mL
Iodochlorhydroxyquin cream (eg, Vioform)	12 mg/g
Iodoform gauze (eg, NuGauze)	4.8 mg/100 mg gauze
Povidone iodine (eg, Betadine)	10 mg/mL
RADIOLOGY CONTRAST AGENTS	
Diatrizoate meglumine sodium (eg, Renografin-76)	370 mg/mL
Iodized oil	380 mg/mL
Iopanoic acid (eg, Telepaque)	333 mg/tab
Ipodate (eg, Oragrafin)	308 mg/cap
Iothalamate (eg, Angio-Conray)	480 mg/mL
Metrizamide (eg, Amipaque)	483 mg/mL before dilution

*Not FDA approved.
†Iodine was removed from Organidin and Tuss Organidin in 1995.
Adapted from Braverman LE. Iodide-induced thyroid disease. In: Ingbar SH, Braverman LE, eds. Werner's the thyroid, ed 5. Philadelphia: JB Lippincott, 1986:734.

columnar change of cells with clear and vesicular cytoplasm, and markedly reduced colloid in the distended follicles were observed. These changes were reversible after iodine withdrawal.[16] These findings suggest that iodide-induced hypothyroidism might, indeed, appear even in subjects with no underlying thyroid disease.

An interesting finding has been observed in patients who develop goiter and hypothyroidism while receiving iodides.

Usually, serum T_4 and T_3 concentrations are low or low normal and serum TSH is increased. The thyroid radioactive iodine uptake would be expected to be very low in these patients; however, about 30% of patients with iodide goiter or hypothyroidism may have readily detectable, normal, or high thyroid radioactive iodine uptakes.[17] Similar findings have been observed in patients who developed iodine-induced hypothyroidism after amiodarone administration.[18,19]

TABLE 14-16.
Iodine-Induced Hypothyroidism or Goiter

UNDERLYING THYROID DISEASE

Hashimoto's thyroiditis

Euthyroid patients previously treated for Graves' disease by ^{131}I, thyroidectomy, or antithyroid drugs

Subclinical hypothyroidism, especially in the elderly

After transient postpartum thyroiditis

After subacute, painful thyroiditis

After hemithyroidectomy for benign nodules

Euthyroid patients with a previous episode of amiodarone-induced destructive thyrotoxicosis

NO UNDERLYING THYROID DISEASE

Cystic fibrosis

Chronic lung disease (Hashimoto's thyroiditis was not ruled out)

Chronic nonthyroidal illness (rare)

Elderly subjects

IODINE PLUS OTHER POTENTIAL GOITROGENS

Sulfisoxazole: cystic fibrosis

Lithium

Sulfadiazine (?)

FETUS AND NEONATE, MOSTLY PRETERM

Secondary to transplacental passage of iodine and exposure of newborn infants to topical or parenteral iodine-rich substances

Adapted from Braverman LE. Iodide-induced thyroid disease. In: Ingbar SH, Braverman LE, eds. Werner's the thyroid, ed 5. Philadelphia: JB Lippincott. 1986:734.

PERINATAL PERIOD

Iodides readily cross the placenta and are concentrated by the fetal thyroid. Large quantities of iodide administered to pregnant women resulted in goiter in the newborn, probably because the fetal thyroid is inordinately sensitive to the inhibitory effect of iodide.[20] Whether the inhibitory effect is exerted on the organification mechanism or on the release of thyroid hormones, or both, is not clear. Studies in the rat strongly suggest that the inhibitory effects are exerted in utero as well as in the late neonatal period, which corresponds to the last few weeks of term human fetal life.[21] Iodides are actively transported by breast tissue and secreted into the milk, and the administration of iodides to the nursing mother could result in iodine-induced hypothyroidism and goiter in the infant.

The thyroid of the fetus and newborn can be exposed to iodine from various routes. Vaginal douching with iodine-containing solutions in nonpregnant women results in a small increase in the serum TSH concentration.[22] In contrast, in nonpregnant women vaginal disinfection with povidone-iodine vaginal pessaries and obstetric cream does not affect serum iodine concentrations and thyroid function.[23,24] Transient hypothyroidism of the newborn, as indicated by an elevation of the serum TSH, has been reported to follow the application of vaginal solutions of povidone-iodine and in a few cases after povidone-iodine cream application,[25] during

the last trimester and during labor,[20,25] or topical application of povidone-iodine to the skin of the newborns. The latter appears to be more common in premature, low-birthweight infants. Serum TSH concentrations above 20 mU/L occurred in 25% of the cases, promptly normalizing after the iodine-containing antiseptic was discontinued.[26] Very recently, the injection of small amounts of an iodinated contrast dye through nonradiopaque silastic catheters in premature infants induced hypothyroidism in some.[26a] Iodine contamination is the major cause of transient neonatal hypothyroidism,[27] being responsible for 3% of recalls at screening for congenital hypothyroidism in comparison with 0.1% in control subjects.[28] It is possible, therefore, that iodides are responsible for most cases of transient hypothyroidism during neonatal life. Because these reports emanate primarily from continental Europe where mild iodine deficiency is present, it is possible that iodine deficiency might predispose the fetal and neonatal thyroid to the inhibitory effect of iodine. In contrast to the above studies, Momotani and colleagues[29] reported that only 2 of 35 newborns, whose mothers had been treated with 6 to 40 mg iodine daily from 11 to 37 weeks of gestation for Graves' disease, had elevated cord serum TSH concentrations. It is possible that the lack of fetal iodine-induced hypothyroidism in these newborns was due to the concomitant presence of autoimmune thyroid hyperfunction in the fetuses as well as in the mothers and the high ambient iodine intake in Japan.

Drugs containing iodine may also induce hypothyroidism in the fetus. A case of congenital goiter has been described in a neonate whose mother was treated with amiodarone during pregnancy.[30]

CHRONIC NONTHYROIDAL ILLNESS

Patients with chronic nonthyroidal illness usually are not susceptible to the inhibitory effect of iodide despite the multiplicity of thyroid dysfunction observed. However, certain diseases that affect the thyroid gland may predispose the patient to iodide-induced thyroid dysfunction.

Iodine-induced hypothyroidism has been reported to occur in patients with a variety of chronic lung diseases, including asthma, treated for a prolonged period of time with iodine-containing expectorants; however, underlying Hashimoto's thyroiditis predisposing these patients to the inhibitory effect of iodide was not ruled out (see references 1 and 2).

Children with cystic fibrosis, especially those treated with sulfisoxazole, are particularly susceptible to iodine-induced hypothyroidism.[31] No apparent thyroid dysfunction was found in these patients although accumulation of lipofuscin has been observed in the thyroids of patients with cystic fibrosis. The significance of the latter finding is unclear because lipofuscin is found in the thyroid of mice fed large quantities of iodides. The effect of chronic iodide administration on healthy children has not been evaluated, however, although chronic amiodarone administration may induce hypothyroidism in as many as 20% of children treated with this drug.[32]

In children and adults suffering from thalassemia major and requiring chronic blood transfusion therapy, iodide administration (60 mg daily) resulted in subclinical hypothyroidism (TSH > 5 mU/L) in 60% of these patients. TSH returned to basal levels 2 to 3 weeks after iodide withdrawal.

It appears that thyroid hemosiderosis renders the thyroids of these patients susceptible to the inhibitory effects of iodide.[33]

Patients with chronic renal failure frequently exhibit thyroid dysfunction, including thyroid enlargement and abnormal thyroid function tests. Part of these abnormalities are due to chronic disease, although iodides have been suspected as a potential pathogen because they are used as antiseptics in these patients. In one study, however, no relation of thyroid abnormalities to iodine retention after application of iodide-containing antiseptics was found.[34] More recently, iodine-induced hypothyroidism was diagnosed in 3.2% of patients on chronic dialysis treatment.[35] In these patients the thyroid was enlarged, thyroid radioactive uptake was normal or elevated, the iodine-perchlorate discharge test was positive, and no lymphocytic infiltration was present at cytologic examination. After restriction of the iodine intake, 83% of patients with renal dysfunction and increased serum TSH concentrations normalized their thyroid function tests.[36]

The use of mucolytic expectorants containing iodinated glycerol is particularly frequent in elderly subjects, although this problem may abate in the United States because iodine has been removed from Organidin. The occurrence of mild hypothyroidism after iodinated glycerol administration has been observed in an elderly patient with a previous episode of severe hypothyroidism induced by potassium-iodide administration and also in subjects without known underlying thyroid disorders.[37] In these subjects, the abnormalities of thyroid function resolved spontaneously after therapy was withdrawn.

In the Presence of Underlying Thyroid Disease

CHRONIC LYMPHOCYTIC THYROIDITIS

Patients with Hashimoto's thyroiditis often develop hypothyroidism due to thyroid destruction by the autoimmune process and the presence of TSH-blocking antibodies. In about 60% of patients, an abnormal iodide-perchlorate discharge test suggests a defect in the intrathyroidal organic binding of iodine. Administration of pharmacologic quantities of iodide (180 mg/d) resulted in hypothyroidism in more than 60% of the patients in one study. The iodide-perchlorate discharge test was positive in patients who developed iodide-hypothyroidism and negative in those who did not (see references 1 and 2 for review). The failure of the thyroid to escape from the inhibitory effect of iodide is probably due to a persistent Wolff-Chaikoff effect and not to the inhibition of the release of T_4 and T_3 from the thyroid. Direct measurement of intrathyroidal thyroid hormone content, however, has not been carried out. In Bio-Breeding/Worcester (BB/Wor) rats, which are genetically susceptible to chronic lymphocytic thyroiditis, pharmacologic quantities of iodine surprisingly do not consistently induce hypothyroidism, and no demonstrable abnormality in intrathyroidal organification of iodine was found.[38] In those BB/Wor sublines with the most extensive lymphocytic thyroiditis, however, iodine administration does induce hypothyroidism.[39] It is not known whether susceptible patients with Hashimoto's thyroiditis exposed to a moderately increased iodine intake develop hypothyroidism, although preliminary results suggest that the administration of 1.5 mg iodide daily for 3

months in patients with Hashimoto's thyroiditis does not induce hypothyroidism.[40] A few patients with primary hypothyroidism due to lymphocytic thyroiditis and an elevated alimentary iodine intake became euthyroid when the iodine intake was restricted.[41] It is possible that this phenomenon may occur in Japanese patients with Hashimoto's thyroiditis and transient hypothyroidism.[42]

Contradictory results have been reported in two other studies. When small quantities of iodide were given chronically to four patients with Hashimoto's disease who resided in an area of sufficient iodine intake, no apparent effect on thyroid function was observed,[4] whereas a transient increase in serum T_4 and T_3 concentrations was seen in patients residing in an area of low ambient iodine intake.[43]

GRAVES' DISEASE

Before the discovery of antithyroid drugs, the sole medical treatment of Graves' disease was the chronic administration of large quantities of iodide. Most patients were reasonably well controlled on this regimen, but hyperthyroidism recurred in some patients, and a few patients developed reversible hypothyroidism. When patients with Graves' disease treated with ^{131}I were given iodides (250 mg/d) 1 to 2 weeks after ^{131}I therapy, 60% developed transient hypothyroidism during iodine administration. Euthyroid patients treated years earlier either with ^{131}I or thyroidectomy also developed hypothyroidism during the administration of pharmacologic quantities of iodine. The hypothyroidism was transient, and thyroid function returned to normal after iodide withdrawal. All patients who developed hypothyroidism on iodides had a positive iodide-perchlorate discharge test (see references 1 and 2 for review).

In euthyroid subjects previously treated with antithyroid drugs for Graves' disease, the chronic administration of 10 drops of a saturated solution of potassium iodide (SSKI) induced an increase in basal or TRH-stimulated serum TSH concentrations irrespective of the iodide-perchlorate discharge test results.[44] Basal and TRH-stimulated serum TSH concentrations returned to normal 60 days after SSKI withdrawal.

AFTER POSTPARTUM THYROIDITIS

Women euthyroid after a previous episode of postpartum thyroid dysfunction are prone to iodine-induced hypothyroidism. In 9 of 11 women, the administration of 300 mg iodine daily for 3 months induced hypothyroidism and, in some, goiter. As observed in other thyroid diseases prone to develop iodine-induced hypothyroidism, a positive iodide-perchlorate discharge test was common.[45] Two months after the iodine was withdrawn, thyroid function returned to normal.[45] Consonant with those observations are findings suggesting that small doses of iodides administered to patients expected to develop postpartum thyroiditis may intensify rather than ameliorate the disease.[46]

POSTSUBACUTE THYROIDITIS

The chronic administration of large quantities of iodine (300 mg/d) to euthyroid patients long after an episode of painful, subacute thyroiditis resulted in a significant increase in the serum TSH concentrations in 10 of 18 subjects. Most of these patients had a slight increase in serum TSH concentration, but 2 had values higher than 50 mU/L and developed a goiter. A positive iodide-perchlorate discharge test was highly predictive of the occurrence of iodide-induced hypothyroidism.[47] Persistent autoimmunity was found up to 39 months after the onset of subacute thyroiditis.[48] The serum of these patients was negative for antithyroglobulin and antimicrosomal antibodies. The nature of the thyroid antigens reacting with serum antibodies in these patients has not been clearly defined, but the antigens were contained in the 2000-g supernatant of crude thyroid extract. These findings may explain the subtle thyroid defects frequently observed in these patients and their sensitivity to iodide excess.

POSTHEMITHYROIDECTOMY FOR BENIGN NODULES

Patients undergoing hemithyroidectomy for benign thyroid nodules are also susceptible to hypothyroidism when pharmacologic quantities of iodides are administered for a prolonged period.[49] No underlying defect in thyroid hormone synthesis could be detected. Similar effects were observed in hemithyroidectomized BB/Wor rats prone to develop lymphocytic thyroiditis.[50] This suggests that the hyperfunctioning thyroid remnant is unable to adapt to iodide excess. The question exists whether the thyroid gland of a patient with a thyroid nodule should be considered normal.

SYNERGISM WITH OTHER DRUGS

Several drugs exert mild inhibitory effects on the intrathyroidal organification of iodine, and, when administered alone, do not have appreciable antithyroid activity. When these drugs are administered with excess iodide, however, or when alimentary iodine intake is greatly elevated, hypothyroidism or goiter may ensue.

Lithium is frequently used in the treatment of manic-depressive psychosis. Lithium has multiple effects on thyroid function, including inhibition of thyroid hormone release and inhibition of organification of iodine as judged by positive iodide-perchlorate discharge tests, and may induce goiter or hypothyroidism, especially in patients with Hashimoto's thyroiditis. Iodide-induced hypothyroidism has been reported in a patient receiving lithium.

The sulfonamides, sulfadiazine and sulfisoxazole, are mild inhibitors of thyroid hormone synthesis. Sulfisoxazole enhanced the inhibitory effects of iodide on hormone synthesis in patients with cystic fibrosis, resulting in goiter in many and mild hypothyroidism in some patients.[31] The sulfonylurea hypoglycemic drugs, although potential goitrogens, had no significant inhibitory effect on iodine metabolism in patients, even when these drugs were administered with iodine-containing substances.

IODIDE-INDUCED HYPERTHYROIDISM

Iodide-induced hyperthyroidism is not a single etiologic entity. Since the initial description by Coindet in 1821[51] and the subsequent definition by Breuer and Kocher in 1904, iodine-induced hyperthyroidism has been reported in patients with a variety of underlying thyroid diseases. As shown in Table 14-17 iodide-

---

TABLE 14-17.
Iodine-Induced Hyperthyroidism

Iodine supplementation for endemic iodine-deficiency goiter

Iodine administration to patients with euthyroid Graves' disease, especially those in remission after antithyroid drug therapy

Nontoxic nodular goiter

Autonomous nodule

Nontoxic diffuse goiter

Iodine administration to patients with no recognized underlying thyroid disease, especially in areas of mild to moderate iodine deficiency

Adapted from Braverman LE. Iodide-induced thyroid disease. In: Ingbar SH, Braverman LE, eds. Werner's the thyroid, ed 5. Philadelphia: JB Lippincott, 1986:734.

---

induced hyperthyroidism may occur in patients with iodine deficiency goiter, in euthyroid Graves' disease patients after antithyroid drug therapy, in patients with multinodular goiters who reside in areas of iodine sufficiency or deficiency, and in people with no evidence of underlying thyroid disease.[1,2,52,53]

Iodide-Induced Hyperthyroidism in Endemic Iodine-Deficient Areas

Widespread iodination of salt and bread or administration of iodized oil has almost eliminated endemic goiter in many countries. The incidence of iodide-induced hyperthyroidism in areas previously considered iodine deficient varied from no incidence in Austria to 7% in Sweden after iodination programs. The incidence of iodide-induced hyperthyroidism in an endemic goiter area has been estimated to be up to 1.7%.[54] The natural course of the disease was mild, and it resolved spontaneously.

Most patients who developed hyperthyroidism had multinodular thyroid disease. Eighty-five percent of the cases of iodide-induced hyperthyroidism occurred in patients with long-standing multinodular goiters. The risk of developing hyperthyroidism is particularly high in these patients. Most are euthyroid before iodine administration, but they may have nonsuppressible radioactive iodine uptakes and low or undetectable serum TSH values and the serum TSH may fail to respond to TRH. Approximately 20% of patients with multinodular goiters in Greece have either abnormal suppression of the radioactive iodine uptake or undetectable serum TSH that fails to respond to TRH (A.G. Vagenakis, unpublished observations). These patients are at risk to develop iodide-induced hyperthyroidism. Similar results have been reported from central Europe.[55] Recently, single oral doses of 200, 400, and 800 mg iodine administered to adult goitrous subjects residing in the Sudan induced four cases of hyperthyroidism. However, in the three groups of subjects, serum TSH concentrations below 0.1 mU/L were present in 5.9% to 16.7% of the cases 12 months after iodine administration.[55a] Similar data have been reported 2 years after iodized salt distribution in Zaire. Among 190 adult subjects with nodular goiter, 14 subjects (7.4%) developed severe thyrotoxicosis, and 2 patients required antithyroid drug treatment.[55b]

It appears, therefore, that masked thyroid autonomy becomes evident when iodine repletion permits the autonomous tissue to synthesize and release excess quantities of thyroid hormone. The importance of thyroid autonomy for the development of iodide-induced hyperthyroidism is strengthened by a report of iodide-induced hyperthyroidism in a woman with a multinodular goiter treated with suppressive doses of T_4 and simultaneously exposed to high quantities of iodide.[56] Attempts have been made to associate these events to thyroid autoimmunity, but the results are conflicting. Long-acting thyroid stimulator (LATS) or LATS protector was found in some patients but not in others.[54] In a recent study, no change in the incidence of thyroid autoantibodies was found after oral iodized oil administration.[57]

These observations suggest that the increased incidence of hyperthyroidism in endemic areas after iodide exposure was due to an increased supply of iodine to patients with underlying macro- or micronodular disease with autonomous thyroid nodules or, in a few instances, underlying latent Graves' disease. This is consonant with studies from Belgium and Greece[58,59] in which the administration of small quantities of iodide (0.5 mg/d) to patients with autonomous nodules induced frank hyperthyroidism. It is interesting to note that among 147 patients reported in the literature who developed sporadic hyperthyroidism without a preexisting thyroid abnormality, 137 cases occurred in areas with urinary iodine excretion of 40 to 80 μg/d or iodine intake of less than 50 μg/d.[52] It is evident, therefore, that the remarkably greater incidence of iodine-induced hyperthyroidism in Europe than in the United Kingdom, United States, and Japan is at least partially due to the iodine deficiency that occurs in Europe in contrast to the latter three countries, where iodine intake is sufficient.

Iodine-Induced Hyperthyroidism in Iodine-Sufficient Areas

In nonendemic euthyroid goiter areas, the incidence of iodine-induced hyperthyroidism is low. The goiter prevalence in the United States is about 3.1%, and it is surprising that only a few cases have been reported since the initial report from Boston,[60] where four of eight patients with goiter developed severe iodine-induced hyperthyroidism after administration of 180 mg iodide daily for several weeks. Although suppression scans or TRH stimulation tests were not carried out before the administration of iodide, it is likely that the susceptible patients had nonsuppressible thyroids. Many apparently euthyroid patients with multinodular goiters who reside in iodine-replete areas may have abnormal suppression tests. Iodine-induced hyperthyroidism has also been reported in other patients residing in the United States.[52,61]

Iodine-induced hyperthyroidism has also been reported in 7 of 28 elderly subjects residing in Australia[62] and in Germany,[63] after non-ionic contrast radiography. These subjects did not have positive anti-thyroid peroxidase (TPO) antibodies and a thyroid scan revealed the presence of a multinodular goiter. Thus, elderly subjects who have an increased prevalence of nodular goiter are prone to develop iodine-induced hyperthyroidism.

The large difference in the rate of occurrence of iodide-induced hyperthyroidism between iodine-deficient and iodine-replete areas is difficult to explain. It is possible that people with increased iodine intake are "resistant" to iodine-induced hyperthyroidism because the sensitivity of the autoregulatory mechanism has changed, rendering the thyroid better able to handle the excessive quantities of iodide.

A characteristic of iodine-induced hyperthyroidism in patients with multinodular goiter is its transient although, at times, protracted course. The thyrotoxicosis is more severe after iodide withdrawal due to the abrupt, uninhibited release of preformed T_4 and T_3 from the thyroid. Serum T_4 is invariably increased, and serum T_3 is usually but not always elevated. Serum TSH is undetectable, and there is no response to TRH. Radioactive iodine uptake is low but occasionally may be normal or increased. Due to the large store of preformed hormone in the thyroid, therapy is more difficult (see section on amiodarone-induced thyroid disease).

Latent Graves' Disease

Antithyroid drug therapy for Graves' disease reduces thyroidal iodine content, and the thyroid is iodine depleted. Overt hyperthyroidism can develop only if sufficient iodine is available. It has been reported that a small increase in dietary iodine from either iodide ingestion or thyroid hormone administration increases the frequency of recurrence of hyperthyroidism after antithyroid drug therapy. The difference in remission rates between the United States and Europe and the preference of American thyroidologists to treat Graves' disease with radioactive iodine instead of antithyroid drugs is attributed, at least in part, to the higher recurrence rate of Graves' disease in the United States due to adequate iodine intake.[64] It is evident, therefore, that large quantities of iodides administered to patients with latent Graves' disease may result in frank hyperthyroidism.

Consonant with this view are recent observations in Graves' disease patients treated with antithyroid drugs. In one study,[65] simultaneous administration of methimazole and ipodate reduced the effectiveness of the antithyroid drug. In another study, iodide administration to patients rendered euthyroid after antithyroid drug therapy was accompanied by frank hyperthyroidism in some and with an absent TSH response to TRH in others.[44] Excess iodide administered to hyperthyroid patients with Graves' disease significantly increased thyrotropin receptor antibody, suggesting that this phenomenon was responsible for iodine-induced thyroid dysfunction in predisposed subjects.[66]

Unusual episodes of iodine-induced hyperthyroidism have been observed in a few patients suffering from severe burns treated with povidone iodine[67] and in a patient who had metastatic thyroid carcinoma.[68] In a patient with a TSH-producing pituitary tumor with mild hyperthyroidism, accidental exposure to high iodine intake resulted in severe hyperthyroidism, which was ameliorated after iodine withdrawal (A.G. Vagenakis, unpublished observation).

AMIODARONE-INDUCED THYROID DISEASE

Amiodarone, a benzofuranic derivative containing 75 mg iodine per 200-mg tablet, is widely used for the long-term treatment of cardiac arrhythmias. About 9 mg iodine is released daily during the metabolism of the drug (300-mg dose), which is prolonged with a half-life of at least 100 days. Beyond its effects on the heart, amiodarone is a potent inhibitor of type I 5'-deiodinase, may inhibit pituitary TSH secretion, and is frequently associated with iodide-induced thyroid dysfunction. Amiodarone-induced hyperthyroidism occurs in about l0% of patients residing in iodine-deficient areas.[52,69] In the United States, amiodarone-induced hypothyroidism is more common, occurring in up to 20% of patients, whereas hyperthyroidism is far less common. These differences are attributed to increased ambient iodine intake in the United States preceding the administration of the drug.[69,70]

The etiology of amiodarone-induced hypothyroidism can be partially explained by the excess iodide released during the metabolism of the drug. Measurements of intrathyroid iodine content by radiographic fluorescence revealed increased iodine content in patients who developed hypothyroidism.[43] Evidence for the essential role of iodine in the pathogenesis of amiodarone-associated hypothyroidism stems from the observation that administration of potassium perchlorate, which prevents thyroid iodine uptake and enhances the release of inorganic iodide from the thyroid, restored the patients to euthyroidism. Hypothyroidism returned on withdrawal of potassium perchlorate.[71] Iodine-induced hypothyroidism is also related to the presence of thyroid autoimmunity. Circulating antithyroid antibodies are common in patients who develop hypothyroidism during amiodarone treatment.[69,70] Hypothyroidism is easy to diagnose because an elevated serum TSH is invariably present. L-T$_4$ treatment is indicated and does not require interruption of amiodarone therapy. However, in a single patient with amiodarone-induced hypothyroidism the continuation of amiodarone treatment induced destructive thyrotoxicosis.[72]

Amiodarone-induced thyrotoxicosis results from two different mechanisms. The iodine released during the metabolism of the drug is responsible for the thyrotoxicosis in most cases. Predisposing factors included micro- and macronodular goiter, which are common in older patients who most often require amiodarone. Thyroid autoimmunity has also been incriminated as a predisposing factor and antithyroid antibodies have been found in some patients[73] but not in others.[74] In an interesting study, the prevalence of serum thyroid-stimulating antibodies and TSH-binding inhibiting antibodies was similar to that seen in patients with spontaneous hyperthyroidism.[74] Amiodarone may also induce destructive thyroiditis resulting in thyrotoxicosis as suggested by clinical, histologic, and in vitro studies.[75–77] The clinical and laboratory characteristics of amiodarone-induced thyrotoxicosis are presented in Table 14-18.

The evaluation of thyroid function is difficult in patients receiving amiodarone therapy. Serum T$_4$ may be elevated, serum T$_3$ decreased, and TSH occasionally undetectable in a euthyroid subject receiving the drug. Hyperthyroidism is best confirmed by an elevation of serum T$_3$ and free T$_3$ concentrations as well as by an increase in sex hormone-binding globulin.[78] The distinction between iodine-induced hyperthyroidism (type I) and destructive thyrotoxicosis (type II) may be achieved by measurement of serum interleukin-6, which is invariably elevated in the destructive form[79] and by fine-needle biopsy, which shows cytologic findings consistent with thyroiditis.[76] The thyroid radioiodine uptake is always low in the destructive form and is often low in iodine-induced thyrotoxicosis but may be normal or rarelSy elevated. In the latter, ^{131}I therapy is an alternative.

Distinction of the two forms is important for determining the most efficacious form of therapy. Amiodarone should almost always be discontinued. Large doses of antithyroid drugs are recommended for iodine-induced hyperthyroidism. If this treatment fails, potassium perchlorate (250 mg TID) should be added.[80,81] The latter drug blocks the thyroid iodide trap, thereby decreasing the intrathyroidal iodide content.

In patients with destructive thyrotoxicosis, administration of large doses of corticosteroids is rapidly effective.[76,82] Surgery has been successfully used for the treatment of amiodarone-induced thyrotoxicosis.[83]

After recovering from amiodarone-induced destructive thyrotoxicosis, patients may develop permanent hypothyroidism[72,76] as a result of fibrosis of the gland.[84] In a recent study,[85] the iodine-perchlorate discharge test was positive in 60% of euthyroid patients who had recovered from amiodarone-induced destructive thyrotoxicosis. The chronic administration of 300 mg iodide daily to these patients induced a marked increase in basal and TRH-stimulated serum TSH concentrations, which returned to normal after iodide withdrawal.

In view of the high incidence of thyroid dysfunction, amiodarone should be administered with caution to patients with preexisting goiter or a history of thyroid disease. Examination and thyroid function tests, including antithyroglobulin and anti-TPO thyroid antibodies, are indicated every 6 months.

IODINE AS A PATHOGEN

Animal studies suggest that iodine administration has an important role in the development of autoimmune thyroid disease. Spontaneous lymphocytic infiltration of the thyroid has been observed in hamsters, beagles, NOD mice, Buffalo rats, BB/Wor rats, and obese strain chickens.[86] Spontaneous lymphocytic thyroiditis occurs in about 30% of 90-day-old rats who also develop spontaneous insulin-dependent diabetes mellitus (BB/Wor rat).[38,87] The administration of iodine in their drinking water (0.05% sodium iodide) from 30 to 90 days strikingly increased the prevalence of lymphocytic thyroiditis to approximately 75% or more.[38] Excess iodine administration to strains of rats that do not develop spontaneous thyroiditis does not induce histologic changes in the thyroid. Excess iodine administration also induces lymphocytic thyroiditis in obese-strain chickens[88] and Buffalo rats.[89]

The mechanism by which iodine excess increases the occurrence of autoimmune thyroiditis may be due to the enhanced immunogenicity of iodine-rich thyroglobulin, as demonstrated in the obese-strain chickens.[90] Conversely, immunization of the BB/Wor rat with iodine-poor thyroglobulin did not induce thyroiditis.[91] However, as demonstrated in obese-strain chickens, iodine excess induced thyroid infiltration only in predisposed animals[92] and the greatest effect was observed when iodine was given to the embryos.[93] Furthermore, an essential requirement for the development of iodine-induced thyroiditis is the uptake and metabolism of iodine within the gland.[93] Other mechanisms for the development of iodine-induced thyroiditis, such as cellular damage due to elevated oxygen free radicals, direct cytotoxic effects of iodine or autoregulation of the MHC class I have been proposed.[92,94,95a]

TABLE 14-18.
Features of Amiodarone-Induced Thyrotoxicosis

	Iodine-Induced Thyrotoxicosis (Type I)	Destructive Thyroxicosis (Type II)
Underlying thyroid abnormality	Yes	No
Thyroidal RAIU	Low, normal or elevated	Low
Serum IL-6 concentrations	Slightly elevated	Markedly elevated
Cytologic findings	?	Abundant colloid, hystiocytes, vacuolated cells
Pathogenic mechanism	Excessive thyroid hormone synthesis	Excessive thyroid hormone release (destructive thyroiditis)
Response to thionamides	Poor	No
Response to perchlorate	Yes	No
Response to glucocorticoids	?	Yes
Subsequent hypothyroidism	Unlikely	Possible
Effect of excess iodine administration following the thyrotoxic phase	Likely iodine-reinduced hyperthyroidism	Possible iodine-induced hypothyroidism

Modified from Bartalena L et al.[79]

In contrast to the present view that excess iodine increases the occurence of autoimmune thyroiditis, it has been recently reported that iodine deficiency in Wistar rats led to goiter formation with signs of lymphocytic infiltration.[95]

The relationship of iodine intake to the occurrence of Hashimoto's thyroiditis in patients is controversial. Some studies[96,97] have strongly suggested that increased iodine intake is associated with an increased incidence of Hashimoto's thyroiditis and antithyroid antibodies, especially when supplemental iodine is introduced in the treatment of endemic, iodine-deficient goiter. In elderly women residing in an area of adequate iodine intake, the prevalence of positive antimicrosomal antibodies was far higher than in subjects living in an area of mild iodine deficiency.[86] In contrast, other studies did not find a relation between iodine-intake and the prevalence of thyroid autoimmunity.[7,54]

The mechanism by which iodine interacts with the immune system is unknown. In the presence of iodine, the production of immunoglobulin G from human peripheral blood lymphocytes was increased after stimulation with pokeweed mitogen. These studies suggest that factors other than iodine, such as HLA type or unknown environmental influences, contribute to the development of Hashimoto's thyroiditis.

New evidence is emerging concerning the role of iodine in modulating the effects of growth factors in the thyroid. Transforming growth factor-β, a well-known inhibitor of cell growth, is substantially decreased in multinodular goiters and iodine induced its production.[98] Finally, pharmacologic concentrations of iodine inhibit, in part, the in vitro growth of FRTL-5 cells but not of thyroid follicular cells obtained from autonomously growing hyperthyroid feline multinodular goiters, suggesting that the inhibitory action of iodide on thyroid cell growth is a constitutive trait of each thyrocyte.[99]

Several clinical implications are involved in the rise in dietary iodine levels. As mentioned earlier, iodide-induced hyperthyroidism is likely to become more common, particularly in iodine-deficient areas. In Great Britain, iodine intake has tripled during the past 30 years, and the incidence of hyperthyroidism due to toxic multinodular goiter correlates closely with the previous prevalence of endemic goiter.[100] A seasonal increase of hyperthyroidism was observed in Great Britain, which was suggested to be related to increased iodine intake through milk consumption.[101] However, in New Zealand no relationship has been observed between the iodine content in milk, the mean 24-hour urinary iodine excretion, and the seasonal incidence of thyrotoxicosis.[102]

Another possible consequence of iodine supplement is that Graves' disease may become more difficult to control with antithyroid drugs. The presence of iodine deficiency is associated with a higher remission rate after treatment with antithyroid drugs. The response to thionamide drugs is rapid in Graves' disease patients who reside in iodine-deficient areas and the dose required to control the disease is smaller.[103] For example, 80% of patients with Graves' disease residing in Greece, an area of moderate iodine deficiency, can be controlled with as little as 5 mg carbimazole daily.

The increase in dietary iodine has also resulted in a decrease in the thyroid radioactive iodine uptake and a corresponding increase in the dose of radioactive iodine required to control hyperthyroidism. In Cardiff, Wales, the required dose was 267 MBq in 1967 and increased to 465 MBq in 1982. The results of surgery are also influenced by the ambient iodine intake. The incidence of hyperthyroidism after thyroid surgery for Graves' disease in an area of high iodine intake was five times higher and hypothyroidism five times lower than in areas where the iodine intake is low.[100]

References

1. Braverman LE. Iodine and the thyroid: 33 years of study. Thyroid 1994;4:351
2. Vagenakis AG, Braverman LE. Adverse effects of iodides on thyroid function. Med Clin North Am 1975;59:1075
3. LeMar HJ, Georgitis WJ, McDermott MT. Thyroid adaption to chronic tetraglycine hydroperiodide water purification tablet use. J Clin Endocrinol Metab 1995;80:220
4. Ader AW, Paul TL, Reinhardt W, et al. Effect of mouth rinsing with two polyvinylpyrrolidone-iodine mixtures on iodine absorption and thyroid function. J Clin Endocrinol Metab 1988;66:632

5. Mann K, Rendl J, Busley R, et al. Systemic iodine absorption during endoscopic application of radiographic contrast agents for endoscopic retrograde cholangiopancreaticography. Eur J Endocrinol 1994;130:498

6. Paul T, Meyers B, Witorsch RJ, et al. The effect of small increases in dietary iodine on thyroid function in euthyroid subjects. Metabolism 1988;37:14

7. Gardner DF, Centor RM, Utiger RD. Effect of low dose oral iodide supplementation on thyroid function in normal men. Clin Endocrinol 1988;28:283

8. Chow CC, Phillips DIW, Lazarus JH, Parker AB. Effect of low iodide supplementation on thyroid function in potentially susceptible subjects: are dietary iodide levels in Britain acceptable? Clin Endocrinol 1991;34:413

9. Namba H, Yamashita S, Kimura H, et al. Evidence of thyroid volume increase in normal subjects receiving excess iodide. J Clin Endocrinol Metab 1993;76:605

10. Arntzenius AB, Smit LJ, Schipper J, et al. Inverse relation between iodine intake and thyroid blood flow: color Doppler flow imaging in euthyroid humans. J Clin Endocrinol Metab 1991;73:1051

11. Grainger RG, Pennington GW. A study of the effect of sodium/meglumine ioxaglate (Hexabrix) on thyroid function. Br J Radiol 1981;54:768

12. Li M, Liew DR, Qu CY, et al. Endemic goitre in Central China caused by excessive iodine intake. Lancet 1987;2:257

13. Boyages S, Bloot A, Glen F, et al. Thyroid autoimmunity in endemic goitre caused by excessive iodine intake. Clin Endocrinol 1989;31:453

14. Konno N, Makita H, Yuri K, et al. Association between dietary iodine intake and prevalence of subclinical hypothyroidism in the coastal regions of Japan. J Clin Endocrinol Metab 1994; 78:393

15. Konno N, Yuri K, Taguchi H, et al. Screening for thyroid diseases in an iodine sufficient area with sensitive thyrotrophin assays, and serum thyroid autoantibody and urinary iodide determinations. Clin Endocrinol 1993;38:273

16. Mizukami Y, Michigishi T, Nonomura A, et al. Iodine-induced hypothyroidism: a clinical and histological study of 28 patients. J Clin Endocrinol Metab 1993;76:466

17. Wolff J. Iodine goiter and pharmacologic effects of excess iodide. Am J Med 1969;47:101

18. Martino E, Bartalena L, Mariotti S, et al. Radioactive iodine thyroid uptake in patients with amiodarone-iodine-induced thyroid dysfunction. Acta Endocrinol (Copenh) 1988;119:167

19. Wiersinga WM, Touber KL, Trip MD, et al. Uninhibited thyroidal uptake of radioiodine despite iodine excess in amiodarone-induced hyperthyroidism. J Clin Endocrinol Metab 1986;63:485

20. Roti E, Gnudi A, Braverman LE. The placental transport synthesis and metabolism of hormones and drugs which affect thyroid function. Endocr Rev 1987;4:131

21. Theodoropoulos T, Braverman LE, Vagenakis AG. Iodine-induced hypothyroidism: a potential hazard during perinatal life. Science 1979;205:502

22. Safran M, Braverman LE. Effect of chronic douching with polyvinylpyrrolidone. Obstet Gynecol 1982;60:35

23. Darwish NA, Shaarawy M. Effect of treatment with povidone-iodide vaginal pessaries on thyroid function. Postgrad Med J 1993;69:S39

24. Sakakura K, Iwata Y, Hayashi S. Study on the usefulness of povidone-iodine obstetric cream with special reference to the effect on thyroid functions of mothers and the newborn. Postgrad Med J 1993;69:S49

25. Novaes M Jr, Biancalana MM, Garcia SA, et al. Elevation of cord blood TSH concentration in newborn infants of mothers exposed to acute povidone iodine during delivery. J Endocrinol Invest 1994;17:805

26. Smerdely P, Lim A, Boyages SC, et al. Topical iodine-containing antiseptics and neonatal hypothyroidism in very-low-birth-weight infants. Lancet 1989;2:661

26a. Ares S, Pastor I, Quero J, Morreale de Escobar G. Thyroid complications including overt hypothyroidism, related to the use of non-radiopaque silastic catheters for parenteral feeding in prematures requiring injection of small amounts of an iodinated contrast medium. Acta Paediatr 1995;84:579

27. L'Allemand D, Gruters AJ, Beyer P, Weber B. Iodine in contrast agents and skin disinfectants is the major cause for hypothyroidism in premature infants during intensive care. Horm Res 1988;28:42

28. Chanoine JP, Boulvain M, Bourdoux P, et al. Increase recall rate at screening for congenital hypothyroidism in breast fed infants born to iodine overloaded mothers. Arch Dis Child 1988;63:1027

29. Momotani N, Hisaoka T, Noh J, et al. Effects of iodine on thyroid status of fetus versus mother in treatment of Graves' disease complicated by pregnancy. J Clin Endocrinol Metab 1992;75:738

30. De Wolf D, De Schepper J, Verhaaren H, Deneyer M, Smitz J, Sacre-Smits L. Congenital hypothyroid goiter and amiodarone. Acta Paediatr Scand 1988;77:616

31. Azizi F, Bentley D, Vagenakis A, et al. Abnormal thyroid function and response to iodides in patients with cystic fibrosis. Trans Assoc Am Physicians 1974;87:111

32. Costigan DC, Holland FJ, Daneman D, et al. Amiodarone therapy effects on childhood thyroid function. Pediatrics 1986;77:703

33. Alexandrides T, Pagoni C, Georgopoulos N, et al. Subclinical hypothyroidism in patients with β-thalassemia major and normal thyroid function after iodine treatment. Washington, DC: Program Endocrine Society, 77th Annual Meeting 1995:215

34. Gardner DF, Mars DR, Thomas RG, et al. Iodide retention and thyroid dysfunction in patients with hemodialysis and continuous ambulatory peritoneal dialysis. Am J Kidney Dis 1986;7:471

35. Tacheda S, Michigishi T, Takazakura E. Iodine-induced hypothyroidism in patients on regular dialysis treatment. Nephron 1993;65:51

36. Sato K, Okamura K, Yoshinari M, et al. Reversible primary hypothyroidism and elevated serum iodine level in patients with renal dysfunction. Acta Endocrinol (Copenh) 1992;126:253

37. Drinka PJ, Nolten WE. Effects of iodinated glycerol on thyroid function: studies in elderly nursing home residents. J Am Geriatr Soc 1988;36:911

38. Allen EM, Appel MC, Braverman LE. The effect of iodide ingestion on the development of spontaneous lymphocytic thyroiditis in the diabetes-prone BB/W rat. Endocrinology 1986;118:1977

39. Rajatanavin R, Reinhardt W, Alex S, et al. Variable prevalence of lymphocytic thyroiditis among diabetes-prone sublines of BB/Wor rats. Endocrinology 1991;128:153

40. Paul T, Reinhardt W, Meyers B, et al. Small increases in dietary iodine intake do not induce hypothyroidism in euthyroid patients with Hashimoto's thyroiditis. Clin Res 1987;35:400A

41. Tajiri J, Higashi K, Morita M, et al. Studies of hypothyroidism in patients with high iodine intake. J Clin Endocrinol Metab 1986;63:412

42. Takasu N, Yamada T, Takasu M, et al. Disappearance of thyrotropin-blocking antibodies and spontaneous recovery from hypothyroidism in autoimmune thyroiditis. N Eng J Med 1992;326:513

43. Fragu P, Schlumberger M, Tubiana M. Thyroid iodine content and serum thyroid hormone levels in autoimmune thyroiditis: effect of iodide supplementation. J Nucl Med 1985;26:133

44. Roti E, Gardini E, Minelli R, et al. Effects of chronic iodine administration on thyroid status in euthyroid subjects previously treated with antithyroid drugs for Graves' hyperthyroidism. J Clin Endocrinol Metab 1993;76:928

45. Roti E, Minelli R, Gardini E, et al. Impaired intrathyroidal iodine organification and iodine-induced hypothyroidism in euthyroid women with a previous episode of postpartum thyroiditis. J Clin Endocrinol Metab 1991;73:958

46. Kampe 0, Jansson R, Karlsson FA. Effects of L-thyroxine and iodide on the development of autoimmune post-partum thyroiditis. J Clin Endocrinol Metab 1990;70:1014

47. Roti E, Minelli R. Gardini E, et al. Iodine induced hypothyroidism in euthyroid subjects with a previous episode of subacute thyroiditis. J Clin Endocrinol Metab 1990;70:1581

48. Weetman AP, Smallridge RC, Nutman TB, et al. Persistent thyroid autoimmunity after subacute thyroiditis. J Clin Lab Immunol 1987;23:1

49. Clark OH, Cavalieri RR, Moser C, ME, et al. Iodide-induced hypothyroidism in patients after thyroid resection. Eur J Clin Invest 1990;20,573

50. Allen EM, Appel MC, Braverman LE. Iodine-induced thyroiditis and hypothyroidism in the hemithyroidectomized BB/W rat. Endocrinology 1987;121:481

51. Coindet JF. Nouvelles recherches sur les effects de l'iode, et sur les precautious a suivre dans le traitement de goitre par le nouveau remede. Bibl Univ Sci Belles Lettres Arts 1821;16:140

52. Fradkin JE, Wolff J. Iodide-induced thyrotoxicosis. Medicine 1983:62:1

53. McGregor AM, Weetman AP, Ratanachaiyavong S, et al. In: Hall R, Kobberling J, ed. Thyroid disorders associated with iodine deficiency and excess. Serono Symposia Series. New York: Raven Press, 1985:209

54. Martins ML, Lima N, Knobel M, Medeiros-Neto G. Natural course of iodine-induced thyrotoxicosis (JodBasedow) in endemic goiter area: a 5 year follow up. J Endocrinol Invest 1989;12:329

55. Kutzin H, Modler C, Buschsieweke U. Iodine kinetics in facultative hyperthyroidism. J Mol Med 1980;4:75

55a. Elnagar B, Eltom M, Karlsson FA, Ermans AM, Gebre-Medhin M, Bourdoux PP. The effects of different doses of oral iodized oil on goiter size, urinary iodine, and thyroid related hormones. J Clin Endocrinol Metab 1995;80:891

55b. Ermans AM, Gullo D, Mugisho SG, et al. Iodine supplementation must be monitored at the population level in iodine deficient areas (abstract) Thyroid 1995;5(suppl 1):5/37

56. Reith PE, Granner DK. Iodine-induced thyrotoxicosis in a woman with a multinodular goiter taking levothyroxine. Arch Intern Med 1985;145:355

57. Lazarus JH, Parkes AB, John R, N'Diaye M, G Prysor-Jones S. Endemic goitre in Senegal—thyroid function etiological factors and treatment with oral iodized oil. Acta Endocrinol (Copenh) 1992;126:149

58. Ermans AM, Camus M. Modifications of thyroid function induced by chronic administration of iodide in the presence of "autonomous" thyroid tissue. Acta Endocrinol (Copenh) 1972;70:463

59. Livadas DP, Koutras PA, Souvatzoglou A, et al. The toxic effects of small iodine supplements in patients with autonomous thyroid nodules. Clin Endocrinol 1977;7:121

60. Vagenakis AG, Wang CA, Burger A, et al. Iodide induced thyrotoxicosis in Boston. N Engl J Med 1972;287:523

61. Rajatanavin R, Safran M, Stoller W, et al. Five patients with iodine-induced hyperthyroidism. Am J Med 1984;77:378

62. Martin FIR, Brian WT, Colman PG, Deam DR. Iodine-induced hyperthyroidism due to nonionic contrast radiography in the elderly. Am J Med 1993;95:78

63. Steidle B. Iodine-induced hyperthyroidism after contrast media. Animal experimental and clinical studies. In: Taenzer V, Wend S (eds). Recent developments in non-ionic contrast media. New York: Thieme 1989:6

64. Solomon BL, Evanl JE, Burman KD, et al. Remission rates with antithyroid drug therapy: continuing influence of iodine uptake? Arch Intern Med 1987;107:510

65. Roti E, Gardini E, Minelli R, et al. Sodium ipodate and methimazole in the long-term treatment of hyperthyroid Graves' disease. Metabolism 1993;42:403

66. Wilson R, McKillop JH, Thomson JA. The effect of preoperative potassium iodide therapy on antibody production. Acta Endocrinol (Copenh) 1990;123:531

67. Rath TH, Meissl G, Weissel M. Induction of hyperthyroidism in burn patients treated topically with povidone-iodine. Burns 1988;14:320

68. Yoshinari M, Tokuyama T, Okamura K, et al. Iodide-induced thyrotoxicosis in a thyroidectomized patient with metastatic thyroid carcinoma. Cancer 1988;61:1674

69. Lombardi A, Martino E, Braverman LE. Amiodarone and the thyroid. Thyroid Today 1990;23:2

70. Martino E, Aghini-Lombardi F, Mariotti S, et al. Amiodarone iodine-induced hypothyroidism risk factors and follow up in 28 cases. Clin Endocrinol 1987;26:227

71. Martino E, Mariotti S, Aghini-Lombardi F, et al. Short-term administration of potassium perchlorate restores euthyroidism in amiodarone iodine-induced hypothyroidism. J Clin Endocrinol Metab 1988;63:1233

72. Minelli R, Gardini E, Bianconi L, et al. Subclinical hypothyroidism, overt thyrotoxicosis and subclinical hypothyroidism: the subsequent phases of thyroid function in a patient chronically treated with amiodarone. J Endocrinol Invest 1992;15:853

73. Monteiro E, Galvao-Teles A, Santos ML, et al. Antithyroidal antibodies as an early marker for thyroid disease induced by amiodarone. Br Med J 1986;292:227

74. Safran M, Martino E, Aghini-Lombardi F, et al. Effect of amiodarone on circulating antithyroid antibodies. Br Med J 1988;297:456

75. Chiovato L, Martino E, Tonacchera M, et al. Studies on the in vitro cytotoxic effect of amiodarone. Endocrinology 1994;134:2277

76. Roti E , Minelli R, Gardini E, et al. Thyrotoxicosis followed by hypothyroidism in patients treated with amiodarone. Arch Intern Med 1993;153:886

77. Smyrk TC, Goellner JR, Brennan MD, Carnej JA. Pathology of the thyroid in amiodarone-associated thyrotoxicosis. Am J Surg Pathol 1987;11:197

78. Bambini G, Aghini-Lombardi F, Rosner W, et al. Sex hormone-binding globulin in amiodarone-treated patients: a marker for tissue thyrotoxicosis. Arch Intern Med 1987;147:1781

79. Bartalena L, Grasso L, Brogioni S, et al. Serum interleukin-6 in amiodarone-induced thyrotoxicosis. J Clin Endocrinol Metab 1994;78:423

80. Martino E, Aghini-Lombardi F, Mariotti S, et al. Treatment of amiodarone associated hyperthyroidism by simultaneous administration of potassium perchlorate and methimazole. J Endocrinol Invest 1986:9:201

81. Reichert LJ, Derooy HA. Treatment of amiodarone induced hyperthyroidism with potassium perchlorate and methimazole during amiodarone treatment. Br Med J 1989;298:1547

82. Brousolle C, Ducotett X, Martin C, et al. Rapid effectiveness of prednisone and thionamides combined therapy in severe amiodarone iodine-induced thyrotoxicosis: comparison of two groups of patients with apparently normal thyroid glands. J Endocrinol Invest 1989;12:37

83. Farwell AP, Abend SL, Huang SK, et al. Thyroidectomy for amiodarone-induced thyrotoxicosis. JAMA 1990;263:1526

84. Roti E, Bianconi L, De Chiara F, et al. Thyroid ultrasonography in patients with a previous episode of amiodarone induced thyrotoxicosis. J Endocrinol Invest 1994;17:259

85. Roti E, Minelli R, Gardini E, et al. Iodine-induced subclinical hypothyroidism in euthyroid subjects with a previous episode of amiodarone-induced thyrotoxicosis. J Clin Endocrinol Metab 1992;75:1273

86. Safran M, Paul TL, Roti E, Braverman LE. Environmental factors affecting autoimmune thyroid disease. Endocrinol Metab Clin North Am 1987;16:32779

87. Braverman LE, Paul T, Reinhardt W, et al. Effect of iodine intake and methimazole on lymphocytic thyroiditis in the BB/Wor rat. Acta Endocrinol (suppl) (Copenh) 1987;281:70

88. Bagchi N, Brown TR, Urdanivia E. Induction of autoimmune thyroiditis in chickens by dietary iodide. Science 1985;230:3258

89. Allen EM, Braverman LE. The effect of iodine on lymphocytic thyroiditis in the thymectomized Buffalo rat. Endocrinology 1990;127:1613

90. Sundick RS, Herdgen DM, Brown TR, Bagchi N. The incorporation of dietary iodine into thyroglobulin increases its immunogenicity. Endocrinology 1987;120:2078

91. Ebner SA, Lueprasitsakul W, Alex S, et al. Iodine content of rat thyroglobulin affects its antigenicity in inducing lymphocytic thyroiditis in the BB/Wor rat. Autoimmunity 1992;13:209

92. Bagchi N, Brown TR, Anand P, Sundick RS. Early cellular events in the thyroid after exposure to iodine. Thyroid 1994;4(suppl 1):S34

93. Brown TR, Sundick RS, Dhar A, et al. Uptake and metabolism of iodine is crucial for the development of thyroiditis in obese strain chickens. J Clin Invest 1991;88:106

94. Li M, Boyages SC. Iodine induced lymphocytic thyroiditis in the BB/W rat: evidence of direct toxic effects of iodide on thyroid subcellular structure. Autoimmunity 1994;18:31

95. Mooij P, deWit HJ, Bloot AM, et al. Iodine deficiency induces thyroid autoimmune reactivity in Wistar rats. Endocrinology 1993;133:1197

95a. Taniguchi SL, Giuliani C, Saji MS, et al. Transcriptional regulation of major histocompatibility (MHC) class I gene expression in thyroid cells by iodide involves enhancer A and transcription factor NF-KB. 77th Annual Meeting Endocrine Society (Abstr) 1995:77

96. Boukis MA, Koutras DA, Souvatzoglou A, et al. Thyroid hormone and immunologic studies in endemic goiter. J Clin Endocrinol Metab 1983;57:4

97. Harach HR, Escalante DA, Onativia A, et al. Thyroid carcinoma and thyroiditis in an endemic goiter region before and after iodine prophylaxis. Acta Endocrinol (Copenh) 1985;108:55

98. Grubeck-Loebenstein B, Buchan G, Sadegi R, et al. Transforming growth factor beta regulates thyroid growth: role in the pathogenesis of non toxic goiter. J Clin Invest 1989;83:764

99. Aeschimann S, Gerber H, Von Grunigen C, et al. The degree of inhibition of thyroid follicular cell proliferation by iodide is a highly individual characteristic of each cell and differs profoundly in vitro and in vivo. Eur J Endocrinol 1994; 130:595

100. Philips DIW, Lazarus JH, Hall R. Iodine metabolism and the thyroid. J Endocrinol 1988;119:361

101. Philips DIW, Nelson M, Barker DJP, et al. Iodine in milk and the incidence of thyrotoxicosis in England. Clin Endocrinol 1988;28:61

102. Ford HC, Johnson LA, Feek CM, Newton JD. Iodine intake and seasonal incidence thyrotoxicosis in New Zealand. Clin Endocrinol 1991;34:179

103. Azizi F. Environmental iodine intake affects the response to methimazole in patients with diffuse toxic goiter. J Clin Endocrinol Metab 1985;61:374

TWO

Laboratory Assessment of Thyroid Function

Werner and Ingbar's The Thyroid, Seventh Edition,
edited by Lewis E. Braverman and Robert D. Utiger.
Lippincott–Raven Publishers, Philadelphia, © 1996

Section A
Radioisotopes and Direct Tests of Thyroid

15

Radiation Physics

Jonathan M. Links

Many radioactive substances are useful in the study of thyroid physiology, the diagnosis of thyroid dysfunction, and the treatment of patients with thyrotoxicosis or thyroid carcinoma. The appropriate use of radioactive materials for such purposes requires knowledge of the characteristics of radionuclides, particularly isotopes of iodine, and an understanding of radiation biology and safety. This chapter focuses on the basic structure of the atom, the properties of the radionuclides that are important to endocrinologists, the instrumentation used to measure radioactivity, and the principles of radiation dosimetry and safety.

ATOMIC STRUCTURE

The atom is composed of a dense central nucleus surrounded by a cloud of orbiting electrons (Fig 15-1). The nucleus consists of protons and neutrons, which together are called nucleons. The number of nucleons in a nucleus is its mass number A. The number of protons in a nucleus is its atomic number Z, which defines the element (and thus its chemical properties). The number of neutrons in a nucleus is its neutron number N.

Any nuclear species is called a nuclide. Nuclides are typically denoted by either $^A_Z X$ or X-A, where X is the element. Nuclides of the same Z but different N and A are called isotopes. Nuclides of the same A but different Z and N are called isobars. Nuclides of the same N but different Z and A are called isotones.

The nucleus of an atom is surrounded by shells, or orbits, and subshells of electrons, each electron having a mass about 1/1835 that of a proton. The most important electron shell is the innermost orbit, the K shell. The two electrons making up the K shell are tightly bound to the nucleus, while each successive shell's (L, M, N, and so on) electrons are less tightly bound. For example, to displace an electron from the K shell requires a minimum energy of 13.6 electron volts (eV), compared with 0.85 eV for the N shell. An electron volt is the energy acquired by an electron accelerated across a potential of 1 volt.

The mass of a nucleus or atom is given in units of atomic mass units (amu). One amu is equal to one-twelfth the mass of a neutral carbon 12 atom. One amu equals 1.66×10^{-24} g. If all the masses of the constituent nucleons of a nucleus are added together, the sum of these masses is greater than the actual mass of the nucleus. The difference in mass represents the amount of energy (from $E = mc^2$) that binds the constituents of the nucleus together. This energy is called the binding energy of the nucleus. The ratio of the binding energy of any nuclide to its mass number A (which represents the number of nucleons in the nucleus) is the binding energy per nucleon.

RADIOACTIVITY

Radioactive decay results from the tendency of nuclides to reach a state as energetically stable as possible, that is, one in

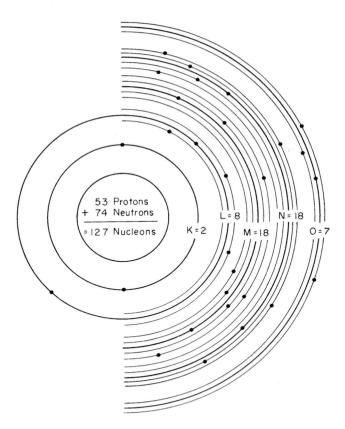

FIGURE 15-1. Iodine–127 atom, which has a nucleus containing 74 neutrons and 53 protons, is surrounded by 5 shells of electrons.

which the binding energy per nucleon is as high as possible. In the process of radioactive decay, the binding energy per nucleon increases, and radiation is emitted that carries off the excess energy. Because the process of radioactive decay is exoergic (energy is given off rather than consumed), radioactive decay occurs spontaneously.

The rate of radioactive decay can be expressed by:

$$-dN/dt = \lambda N$$

where λ is the probability of decay per unit time per atom (the decay constant) and N is the number of radioactive atoms present. The minus sign indicates that N is decreasing with time. Rearranging and integrating this equation yields the radioactive decay law:

$$N = N_0 e^{-\lambda t}$$

where N is the number of nuclei present at time t that have not yet decayed, and N_0 is the initial number of radioactive nuclei at t = 0. The number of disintegrations per unit time ($-dN/dt$) is equal to λN and is called the activity A. It is measured in units of curies (Ci), where 1 Ci equals 3.7×10^{10} radioactive atoms decaying (disintegrations) per second. (The Ci was originally defined as the activity of 1 g of radium.) The SI unit for radioactivity is the becquerel (Bq), where 1 Bq equals 1 disintegration per second; 1 mCi is equivalent to 37 MBq. Substituting $A = \lambda N$ into the radioactive decay law above yields:

$$A = A_0 e^{-\lambda t}$$

The time for A (or N) to decrease to A/2 (or N/2) is called the half-life ($T_{1/2}$). The relationship between the half-life and decay constant for any radionuclide is given by:

$$\lambda = 0.693/T_{1/2}$$

TYPES OF RADIOACTIVE DECAY

Radioactive decay occurs by the expulsion of particulate or electromagnetic radiation from the nucleus of an unstable atom. In the process, the components of the nucleus are usually rearranged to form a new nuclide. There are several modes of radioactive decay.

Alpha Decay. A mode of decay available to some nuclides with high mass number is alpha decay. An alpha particle is emitted, with energy characteristic of a given radionuclide. The alpha particle has two protons and two electrons; it is in fact a helium nucleus. Alpha particles have extremely short ranges in tissue; radionuclides that decay by alpha emission are infrequently used by endocrinologists.

Beta Decay. There are two types of beta decay. The most common type of beta decay results from the spontaneous transformation of a nuclear neutron into a proton. The resultant beta particle (β^-) is an electron, and carries a negative charge. Radionuclides that are naturally neutron rich or are manufactured in a nuclear reactor undergo this type of beta decay. The second type of beta decay arises from the spontaneous transformation of a nuclear proton into a neutron. The particle emitted is a positron (an antimatter electron, β^+). Positron decay occurs in nuclides that are relatively rich in protons compared with neutrons.

Both types of beta emissions have a continuous spectrum of kinetic energy, with a maximum value characteristic of the particular radionuclide: for example, iodine-122, β^+, 3.1 MeV; and iodine-131, β^-, 0.606 MeV. Beta particles are absorbed in tissues within a few millimeters of their origin; for example, iodine-131, 2.2 mm. The energy absorbed by tissue is proportional to the energy of the beta emission.

Electron Capture. All proton-rich nuclides are capable of transforming a nuclear proton into a neutron by capturing an orbiting electron. This results in a nuclide with the atomic number reduced by one unit and an electron shell with a vacancy. An electron from a higher energy level immediately fills the vacancy, and the excess energy is emitted as a characteristic x-ray (see later discussion). In electron capture, the K shell is most often robbed of an electron, yielding a characteristic K-shell x-ray.

Isomeric Transition. Isomeric transition is a process whereby one nuclide decays to a nuclide of the same mass and atomic number but lower quantum energy. The excess energy is emitted as a gamma ray. Examples of radionuclides that undergo this type of decay are iodine-121m and technetium-99m. Here, the 'm' stands for metastable, denoting an elevated energy state with a finite lifetime.

Internal Conversion. A gamma ray ejected from the nucleus may not escape the electron shells surrounding the nucleus. When it does not, its energy can be transferred to one of the orbital electrons, usually in the K shell, and that electron is ejected from the atom. The energy of the conversion electron is equal to the energy of the gamma ray minus the electron's binding energy. This process of internal conversion leaves a vacancy in the electron shell that is immediately filled by an electron from a more distant shell, and characteristic radiation is given off in the process.

Characteristic Radiation. If an electron is ejected from an atom, there is a vacancy in that orbit. Those orbits closest to the nucleus have the highest electron binding energies. The innermost orbit (the K shell) is the energetically most favorable shell for an electron (i.e., that shell has the highest electron-binding energy). An electron from an outer orbit will spontaneously fill a vacancy in an inner orbit. In doing so, that electron has increased its binding energy. The excess energy is given off in the form of an x-ray, whose energy is equal to the difference in binding energies between the two orbits. This difference is characteristic of the particular element.

Auger Electrons. During rearrangement of electrons in orbits, which would otherwise produce x-rays, the energy is sometimes transferred to another electron, termed an Auger electron, which is ejected from the atom. The energy of the Auger electron is equal to the energy of the x-ray minus the electron's binding energy.

NATURE AND PROPERTIES OF RADIATION

Radiation transfers energy to electrons in the material the radiation traverses. If the energy transferred is greater than the binding energy of the electron in the atom, it is ejected, and the atom is ionized. Any excess energy transferred to the electron over and above the binding energy is carried off by the ejected electron as kinetic energy. If the energy transferred to an electron is insufficient to completely eject it from the atom, the electron is raised to a more outer orbit, and the atom is said to be in an excited state.

The alpha, beta, and positron together are called particulate radiation. They transfer energy to the atoms of the materials they are passing through by inelastic collisional energy transfer and radiative transfer (producing Bremsstrahlung). In an inelastic collision, the particle collides with an orbiting electron, transferring some of its energy. In radiative transfer, the particle is decelerated as it encounters the electromagnetic field of a nearby nucleus. The deceleration results in a loss of energy, which is given off as an x-ray, termed Bremsstrahlung.

An alpha particulate is more apt to interact and transfer energy to the material than is a beta particle or a positron because of its greater mass and charge. Thus, for a given energy particle, an alpha transfers all of its kinetic energy over a shorter distance than a beta or a positron; it is said to have a shorter range in tissue. Furthermore, a given type and energy particle tends to have a well-defined, reproducible range in tissue.

Linear energy transfer is the energy transferred by particulate radiation to the material it is passing through per unit length; higher linear energy transfer radiation tends to produce more biologic consequences. Specific ionization is the number of ion pairs formed per unit length; linear energy transfer and specific ionization are related to each other by the average amount of energy required to form one ion pair, which is a characteristic of the material.

Gamma rays and x-rays are electromagnetic radiation. They interact with matter in different ways than particulate radiation because electromagnetic radiation has no rest mass and no charge. Electromagnetic radiation is apt to travel relatively large distances in material without interacting. Electromagnetic radiation has no well-defined range in a given material; its effective range is orders of magnitude larger than that for particulate radiation of the same energy.

The three main mechanisms by which electromagnetic radiation transfers energy to electrons are photoelectric effect, Compton scatter, and pair production. In the photoelectric effect, the radiation interacts with the electromagnetic field of the nucleus of atoms in the tissue; in the process, the radiation's energy is transferred to an electron in the atom (usually a K-shell electron). The electron is ejected, ionizing the atom, with kinetic energy equal to the incoming radiation's energy minus the electron-binding energy. In Compton scatter, the radiation collides with an unbound electron, and both are scattered in different directions. The amount of energy transferred to the electron depends on scatter angle; the greater the angle by which the incoming radiation is scattered, the greater the fraction transferred to the electron. In pair production, the incoming radiation interacts with the atom, and a positron-electron pair appears in its place. Because the mass equivalent to the positron-electron pair is 1.02 MeV (from $E = mc^2$), electromagnetic radiation with less than this energy cannot interact by pair production. Energy in excess of 1.02 MeV is given as kinetic energy to the positron-electron pair.

The intensity of x-rays or gamma rays after passing through some material is given by:

$$I = I_0 e^{-\mu x}$$

where I is the intensity of electromagnetic radiation passing through a thickness x of the material given an initial intensity I_0. μ is the linear attenuation coefficient, which describes the attenuating ability per unit distance of a given material; it is a function of both the material and the energy of the impinging electromagnetic radiation.

RADIONUCLIDES OF IMPORTANCE FOR STUDYING THYROID STRUCTURE AND FUNCTION

Iodine is unique among the halogens in that it is mandatory for thyroid homeostasis. As a consequence, the thyroid has a natural avidity for iodine, as well as for several other ions of similar size and charge, such as pertechnetate and perchlorate. The requirement for iodine allows its various isotopes to be used in studying the structure and function of the gland. The radionuclides in most common use for evaluating the thyroid are the various isotopes of iodine, technetium-99m, and thallium-201. 241-Americium is sometimes, but rarely, used (see later discussion). Of these, the isotopes of iodine are the most useful for in vitro testing, and iodine and technetium for in vivo studies.

The selection of a radionuclide for in vivo use should be made on the basis of its potential for providing the necessary information to resolve a specific clinical question that cannot be answered by an in vitro test, or for achieving a desired therapeutic goal with the least amount of irradiation, inconvenience, or cost to the patient. Radionuclides used in tracer studies that use external detection, such as thyroid imaging, should be chosen to provide a high rate of photon emissions of proper energy to allow effective detection and precise spatial localization. To minimize radiation exposure to the patient, the rate of physical decay should be matched to the physiologic function under study. In radiation therapy with radioiodine, it is desirable to have a nuclide that emits a high percentage of locally absorbed particles and a low percentage of poorly absorbed radiations that may result in irradiation to the rest of the body. Consequently the best radionuclides for therapy may not be the best for diagnostic tests.

ISOTOPES OF IODINE

The currently available isotopes of iodine are produced by irradiation in nuclear reactors, cyclotron-charged particle irradiation, or separation from nuclear fission products. The isotopes of iodine of greatest use in the thyroid area are listed in Table 15-1, along with some of their important properties.

Iodine-131. ^{131}I is widely used for the diagnosis and therapy of thyroid disorders. This isotope is used for in vitro and in vivo testing by virtue of its gamma ray emissions, and in therapy owing to its beta particle emissions. The half-life is 8.05 days, with a maximum beta energy of 0.606 MeV and gamma photon of 364 keV. Its decay scheme is shown in Figure 15-2. At one time, ^{131}I was used in all the standard in vivo radioiodine tests of function and morphology, for example, thyroid uptake (from 30 minutes to 72 hours), efficiency of thyroid organification (perchlorate discharge test), and imaging. It is not ideal for these purposes because of its high level of beta emissions. The average absorbed beta dose in soft tissue is 9.63 rad/d/μCi/g.[1] The dose of ^{131}I required for a standard thyroid uptake measurement is 2 to 20 μCi and for imaging, 25 to 200 μCi. The minimum concentration of the iso-

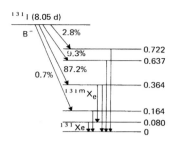

FIGURE 15-2. Decay scheme for ^{131}I.

tope required for adequate counting or imaging should be used. This amount is directly dependent on the sensitivity and resolution capability of the detecting equipment.

Iodine-125. ^{125}I is the most frequently used isotope for in vitro thyroid testing. The half-life is 60.2 days, and there are no beta emissions. Its decay scheme is shown in Figure 15-3. Its principal gamma photon is 35.4 keV. The long half-life and lower rate of self-irradiation result in long shelf life of ^{125}I compounds, making it a nearly ideal isotope for in vitro thyroid studies that require labeled hormones or proteins. For in vivo thyroid studies, particularly imaging, ^{125}I is never used because of its low-energy gamma photon. The long half-life is useful in long-term animal studies. For example, an animal can be placed in isotopic equilibrium; that is, it can be fed ^{125}I-labeled sodium iodine until the specific activity of the diet and the animal become equal. This permits the iodine content to be accurately determined in the living animal or in a sample from the animal without direct chemical measurement. The sensitivity of this method is equal to that of the chemical methods of iodine determination. ^{125}I also can be used to produce autoradiographs of good quality (see later discussion) because the low-energy Auger electrons emitted from K-shell electron capture react with the film emulsion to produce minute silver grains that are demonstrable at both the light and electron microscopic level.

Iodine-123. ^{123}I is, for most purposes, an ideal isotope for in vivo diagnostic studies of thyroid function and structure.

TABLE 15-1.
Biomedically Useful Isotopes of Iodine

Mass Number	Half-Life	Decay: Percentage Abundance, Mode of Decay, Maximum Energy (MeV)	Principal x- or Gamma Photons, keV (% Abundance)
121	2.12 h	91% electron capture, 9% β + (1.2)	28, 212 (90%), others
123	13.3 h	100% electron capture	28, 159 (83%)
125	60.2 d	100% electron capture	28, 35 (7%)
127	stable		
128	25.0 min	7.4% electron capture, 93.6% β − (2.1)	28, 441 (14%), others
129	1.60×10^7 y	β − (0.15)	28, 40 (9%)
130	12.3 h	β − (1.04)	419, (35%), 358 (99%), 669 (100%), 743 (87%), 1150 (12%)
131	8.05 d	β − (0.606)	28, 80 (3%), 284 (5%), 364 (82%), others
132	2.26 h	β − (2.12)	520 (20%), 670 (144%), 773 (89%), others
133	20.3 h	β − (1.27)	530 (90%)

Data from the Radiological Health Handbook, Washington, DC, US Dept HEW, 1970.

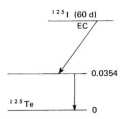

FIGURE 15-3. Decay scheme for ^{125}I.

The half-life is 13.3 hours, with a 28-keV x-ray and a 159-keV gamma photon in essentially equal quantities, and no beta emissions (Fig 15-4). The ratio of detectable photons to radiation dose is high, and the short half-life is suitable for routine uptake measurements and imaging. A precise thyroid uptake measurement can be performed 20 minutes after an intravenous dose, or 1 to 24 hours after an oral dose.[2] High-resolution imaging is possible with the 159-keV photon as early as 20 to 30 minutes after a large dose of the isotope. With 100 to 300 μCi doses given orally, images superior in resolution to those afforded by ^{99m}Tc or ^{131}I can be obtained at 6 hours after administration, the absorbed radiation dose being about 1/85 that for an ^{131}I study. High-purity ^{123}I can be produced from a cyclotron and is available for clinical use in many locales. However, in vivo imaging more often is performed with ^{99m}Tc because of its lower radiation dose and cost (see later discussion).

Other Isotopes of Iodine. The other isotopes of iodine are not in general use but may be useful in selected situations. For instance, ^{121}I has a half-life of 2.1 hours and a peak gamma energy of 0.212 keV, making it a suitable agent for imaging. The radiation dose per millicurie is less than that for ^{132}I but greater than that for ^{123}I; its major disadvantage is that the study laboratory must be close to the isotope source.

Iodine-128 (half-life of 25 minutes) has potential use for activation analysis. When iodine-127 (stable iodine) is exposed to a neutron flux by thermal neutron irradiation, a neutron can enter an I-127 nucleus, changing the atom to ^{128}I. The total quantity of ^{128}I produced is in proportion to the quantity of I-127 present. Consequently, small amounts of stable iodine can be quantitated in tissues and fluids.[3]

Iodine-129 (half-life of 1.6×10^7 years) is useful in animal tracer studies in which extreme analytical sensitivity is required or in which the radiation dose must be minimized. Animals can be placed in isotopic equilibrium with this isotope and samples can be analyzed by neutron activation to ^{130}I. With this technique, the sensitivity of iodine detection can be increased as much as a thousandfold over other chemical methods for analyzing iodine-containing compounds. In addition, ^{129}I has been used as an internal standard in the neutron activation method for the in vivo measurement of total thyroid iodine.

I^{130} (half-life of 12.5 hours) is produced by thermal neutron activation of ^{129}I. Like ^{123}I, its half-life closely matches the time of measurement in several thyroid tests. Its major disadvantages are its weak emission energies and the greater radiation dose from its beta emissions. On the other hand, ^{130}I is less expensive than ^{123}I and may, therefore, be useful when repeated studies are necessary in evaluating thyroid responses to various agents.

Iodine-132 (half-life of 2.3 hours) is obtained from a generator wherein tellurium-132 (^{132}Te; half-life of 3.2 days), a fission product of uranium-235, decays to ^{132}I. Transient equilibrium of the two nuclides is quickly reached, 43% of the maximum possible ^{132}I activity being attained after 2 hours, and maximum activity after about 12 hours. ^{132}I can be separated by distillation from the ^{132}Te two or three times daily. Because of its short half-life, ^{132}I has a substantially lower total radiation dose per millicurie than ^{131}I does; however, owing to its beta emissions, the radiation dose is greater than is the case with ^{123}I. Because of its short half-life, ^{132}I has been used in tests on children and pregnant women, and in tests that must be repeated at short intervals. The rapid decay makes it unsuitable for certain tests of thyroid function, such as a 24-hour uptake measurement. It can be used to assess the thyroid's avidity for iodine by measuring the neck/thigh ratio 2 hours after an oral dose.

Iodine-133 (half-life of 20.8 hours) has been used in the therapy of hyperthyroidism. It is essentially as effective as ^{131}I, with somewhat less total body irradiation. ^{133}I is separable from the fission products of uranium. From this source, about 85% of the total radioactivity is ^{133}I at the time of use. With decay, the relative amounts of other isotopes of iodine increase.

Technetium-99m

Technetium-99m is a useful radionuclide for studying thyroid structure and function because its emissions are favorable for in vivo imaging and because it is readily available from a generator system. It is eluted from a molybdenum-99Tc-99m generator either as sodium pertechnetate or as pertechnic acid, depending on whether the eluting solution is sodium chloride or hydrochloric acid. The life of the generator is determined by the half-life of the parent nuclide, 99 molybdenum (half-life of 67 hours).

The half-life of ^{99m}Tc is 6 hours, 99% of emissions being 140-keV gamma photons, with no beta emissions (Fig 15-5). The energy deposited in situ is low and, when coupled with the short half-life, provides a very low radiation dose to the subject. The thyroid dose is about 0.1 rad/mCi compared with about 1 rad/μCi for ^{132}I, a factor of 10^4 less.

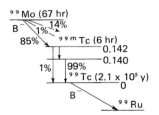

FIGURE 15-5. Decay scheme for ^{99m}Tc.

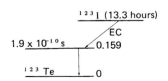

FIGURE 15-4. Decay scheme for ^{123}I.

Although ^{99m}Tc is actively trapped in the thyroid by the same mechanism as iodine, it does not undergo organification, the next step in hormonogenesis. The radionuclide achieves maximum accumulation in the thyroid in an average of 17.8 minutes, with a range of 5 to 30 minutes. High-resolution thyroid imaging is obtainable with ^{99m}Tc, as with ^{123}I, because the short half-life and the low radiation allow larger mCi amounts of radionuclide to be administered. Hence, better images are obtained with ^{99m}Tc than with ^{131}I. This difference is particularly useful in patients with a hypofunctioning gland. In fact, ^{99m}Tc frequently is the radionuclide of choice for imaging, although some institutions prefer the slightly better image quality and "functional specificity" of ^{123}I.[4]

Thallium-201

^{201}Thallium (^{201}Tl) has been used in conjunction with technetium in in vivo imaging of the thyroid, particularly in the setting of a tumor that suppresses function (and thus technetium uptake) in the contralateral lobe. ^{201}Tl decays by electron capture, with a half-life of 3.04 days. The principal emissions of interest for in vivo imaging are 68- to 80-keV K-shell characteristic x-rays and a 167-keV gamma ray. For imaging, thallium is given as thallous chloride (the same form used for nuclear medicine imaging of myocardial perfusion). The mechanism of thallium uptake by the thyroid is poorly understood, but involves a combination of blood flow moderated by mediated transport.

Americium-241

Jacobson first described the determination of thyroid iodine content by activation analysis in 1953; however, only since the development of a high-resolution semiconductor detector has there been a potential for in vivo fluorescent imaging.[5] An emitter of 60-keV gamma rays, ^{241}Am is used as an external source for the excitation of glandular ^{127}I. This photoelectric interaction produces characteristic 28.5-keV x-rays that are detectable with a high-resolution semiconductor detector oriented at zero degrees to the exciting source.

The advantages of fluorescent imaging are low radiation dose to the thyroid (about 15 millirad), with no whole body irradiation, high-resolution structural images, and the capability of imaging patients with an iodide load or those receiving suppressive doses of thyroid hormone. Unfortunately, the technique has never become technically feasible for most diagnostic nuclear medicine laboratories.

MEASUREMENT OF RADIOACTIVITY

Both in vivo and in vitro measurements of radioactivity are useful in studying the thyroid; these are covered in detail in chapters 17 and 18. In vivo measurements include the use of nonimaging probes to determine thyroid uptake of radioiodine and Anger scintillation cameras to image the thyroid. The most common in vitro applications are analytic chemical techniques, such as radioimmunoassays, for measuring thyroid hormones, although nonradioactive assays have become more common over the past few years.

BASIC APPROACHES TO RADIATION DETECTION

Two main types of detectors have been used for in vivo and in vitro measurements: gas-filled detectors and scintillation detectors. The basic approach of a gas-filled detector is quite simple: radiation is sensed by detecting the ionization of gas molecules produced by deposition of energy during radiation's passage through the gas-filled detector. In essence, a gas-filled detector is a container of gas with two electrodes, one positive (the anode) and one negative (the cathode). When ionizing radiation produces ion pairs in the gas, the resulting free electrons are attracted to the anode, and the positively charged gas molecule ions are attracted to the cathode. This bulk movement of charge produces an electrical signal from the detector. Commonly used gases include helium, neon, argon, hydrogen, and air. Gases that have a high affinity for electrons, such as oxygen or halogens, are not used because these would compete with the anode for the free electrons.

There are three main types of gas-filled detectors: ionization chambers, proportional counters, and Geiger-Mueller tubes. Although in practice many factors determine which type a given detector represents, in theory the type is given by the value of the applied voltage across the electrodes in the detector. In general, a gas-filled detector gives one electrical pulse for every alpha, beta, x-ray, or gamma ray it detects, with the size of the pulse determined by the number of ion pairs collected at the electrodes. The number of ion pairs collected is the product of the number produced in the gas (which is proportional to the amount of energy deposited in the gas), and the fraction of ion pairs collected.

A complete detection system consists of the gas-filled detector itself, a high-voltage power supply, a preamplifier (used to shape the pulses to increase count rate capability), an amplifier (used to linearly increase the size of the pulses), and a read-out device, consisting of either a scaler (used to actually count the pulses) and a timer (used to control the duration of counting), or a rate meter. Since it is possible for noise to arise in the electronics that count the pulses, a discriminator is used to eliminate the noise pulses, which are typically of lower amplitude. This discriminator, which is located in the preamplifier or amplifier, is an electronic threshold that only allows pulses above a certain size to pass on to be counted.

The scintillation detector is more sensitive for electromagnetic radiation than is the gas-filled detector. This type of detector is based on the property of certain crystals to emit light photons (scintillate) after deposition of energy in the crystal by ionizing radiation. The most commonly used scintillation crystal in nuclear instrumentation is sodium iodide. This crystal absorbs moisture from the air, it is hygroscopic and is therefore hermetically sealed in an aluminum can. Because the aluminum absorbs alphas and betas, sodium iodide detectors are generally used only for detection of x-rays and gamma rays.

The scintillation photons are converted to an electrical signal through the use of a photomultiplier tube, which is optically coupled with the crystal. The output of the photomultiplier tube is directed into a preamplifier circuit, which forms and shapes a pulse that is then further amplified by a linear amplifier from a few millivolts to a few volts.

The size or height of each pulse from the photomultiplier tube is proportional to the energy deposited in the crystal by ionizing radiation. As with gas-filled detectors, the number of pulses coming from the detector per unit time is related to the activity of the source. Scintillation spectrometry, or pulse-height analysis, refers to the use of a scintillation counting system to obtain an energy spectrum from a radioactive source. This energy spectrum is a graph of pulse height (which is proportional to energy) on the x-axis versus the number of pulses with a given pulse height on the y-axis. This spectrum is a function of the energies of the x-rays or gamma rays emitted by the source, and the interactions of these radiations in the crystal.

One special spectrometry technique is liquid scintillation counting. This technique is used to assess the activity of small sources of beta emitters, such as tritium (^{3}H) or carbon-14. In liquid scintillation counting, the radioactive samples are dissolved in a liquid that scintillates, called a cocktail. This liquid scintillation cocktail is put into a vial and coupled to a photomultiplier tube.

Two major problems in liquid scintillation counting are noise and quenching. Because the pulses from liquid scintillation counting systems are very small, electronic noise pulses may be of the same magnitude as the desired pulses. It is common to cool the entire counting system by putting it in a refrigerator to reduce noise from stray electrical signals that originate in the electronics as electrons that are "freed" from atoms by heat. Quenching refers to any undesirable reduction in light output from the scintillation cocktail. The three main types of quenching are: chemical quenching, which is caused by the presence of materials in the cocktail that interfere with the transfer of energy from the solvent to the fluor or from the primary fluor to the secondary fluor; color quenching, which is the result of any colored material in the cocktail that absorbs light from the primary or secondary fluor; and optical quenching, from condensation, fingerprints, or dirt on the vial containing the cocktail.

FACTORS AFFECTING COUNT RATE

In practice, the observed count rate from a detector is typically less than the actual disintegration or decay rate of the radioactive source. First, after the deposition of energy in the detector, a finite amount of time is required for the electrical signal to be produced. For example, when energy is deposited in a gas-filled detector by an alpha, beta, x-ray, or gamma ray, it takes a certain amount of time for the ions and electrons to travel to the electrodes. During this time, the detector is either not responsive or only partially responsive to the deposition of additional energy. The resolving time represents how long it takes to "count" a given event. Thus, in theory its inverse yields the maximum count rate capability of the detector. The second factor is the efficiency of the detector itself. Not every alpha, beta, x-ray, or gamma ray that passes through the detector will deposit energy in the detector material. If no energy is deposited, obviously no pulse will be generated. Gas-filled detectors can approach 100% efficiency for most alphas and betas that enter the detector, but are only about 1% efficient for x-rays and gamma rays. Scintillation detectors are completely inefficient for particulate radiation (because of the aluminum can), but are very efficient for electromagnetic radiation. The third factor is called geometry and takes into account the inverse square law. The greater the distance between the source and the detector, the lower the observed count rate. The count rate is changed by the square of the change in distance (e.g., if the distance is doubled, the count rate is reduced by a factor of four). Geometry also takes into account the front cross-sectional area of the detector. The larger the surface area of the detector facing the source, the more radioactive emissions that will intersect the detector, and the higher the count rate. Efficiency and geometry are often combined into a single term called sensitivity. This term reflects the fraction of radioactive emissions from the source that is ultimately detected. The fourth factor is attenuation of the radioactive emissions, either self-attenuation in the source itself, or attenuation in the medium between the source and the detector, as alluded to above. In either case, radioactive emissions from the source are "removed" from the beam before they can strike the detector, thus lowering the observed count rate. One final factor is the statistical nature of radioactive decay.

In Vivo Measurement

In vivo measurements, as described in chapter 17, most often make use of scintillation detectors. Typically, a 2-inch diameter cylindrical crystal is coupled to an appropriate photomultiplier tube and attached to counting electronics, forming a "thyroid uptake probe system." A collimator attached to the front of the crystal is used to permit measurements to be limited to a restricted field of view. Collimators are blocks or cylinders of lead, cast with a single hole or a geometric array of holes. The collimator allows those x-rays or gamma photons traveling in an appropriate direction (i.e., those that can pass through the holes without being absorbed in the lead) to interact with the crystal. There are several types of collimators: converging, diverging, pinhole, and parallel hole. Converging collimators have a single tapered hole, or an array of tapered holes, that focus at a point at some distance in front of the collimator. Diverging collimators are upside-down converging collimators with a tapered hole or array of holes that diverge from a hypothetical point behind the crystal. Pinhole collimators are thick, tapered collimators with a single pinhole in the center. Parallel-hole collimators consist of an untapered hole or array of parallel (straight) holes.

The simplest in vivo measurement is the determination of thyroid uptake of radioiodine with a single, collimated sodium iodide crystal. A collimator with a single hole provides the most uniform detection response across the thyroid. The front opening of the collimator should subtend a solid angle just large enough to enable the detector to see the whole gland (Fig 15-6). The most common thyroid uptake procedure is to estimate the uptake at 20 to 30 minutes after an intravenous tracer dose or at 1, 2, 4, 6, and 24 hours after an oral tracer dose of radioiodine. This method is sufficiently accurate for routine uptakes performed 1 hour or more after the dose is administered; because of high background levels, earlier uptakes are prone to large errors.

The principal sources of error in external quantitation are the variation in the size and shape of the thyroid, the variation

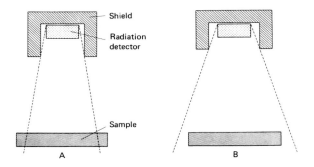

FIGURE 15-6. Shielding of a nonimaging probe for radioiodine uptake measurements in the thyroid. (*A*) Excess. (*B*) Correct collimation.

in the depth of the gland in the neck, and the radioactivity in other parts of the body (extrathyroid activity). The variable depth of the thyroid gland within the neck causes variable attenuation (absorption and scatter) of radioactive emissions from the thyroid. This error is greatest in the case of low-energy isotopes such as ^{125}I. The estimated errors for the three most commonly used isotopes are shown in Table 15-2. Methods of correcting for the thickness of tissues overlying the thyroid have been devised to increase the precision of thyroid uptake measurement. One method measures the ratio of Compton to photopeak activity to derive a correction factor.[6] Another method of measuring the thyroid iodine uptake with greater precision is to make measurements over the gland at two precisely determined distances. These measurements, when compared with a standard curve obtained with a phantom, give a count ratio that is a measure of thyroid depth. When this value is known, one can correct the uptake value for gland depth.[7]

In vivo images of the thyroid gland can provide structural details of the gland's shape, size, location, and function. In the past, imaging was performed with either a rectilinear scanner or an Anger scintillation camera (named for its inventor, Hal Anger of Donner Laboratory, University of California, Berkeley). Rectilinear scanners are no longer available; the scintillation camera is the most widely used imaging instrument in

nuclear medicine. The scintillation camera consists of a lead collimator, a 10- to 24-inch-diameter sodium iodide scintillation crystal (either circular or rectangular in shape), an array of photomultiplier tubes on the crystal, a positioning logic network, a pulse-height analyzer, a scaler-timer, and a cathode ray tube display or computer.

Scintillation cameras have an array of 19 to 91 photomultiplier tubes optically coupled to the back of the scintillation crystal. The outputs of the photomultiplier tubes go to a positioning logic network, which assigns an X,Y coordinate for every scintillation event (i.e., x-ray or gamma ray interaction) in the crystal. When a scintillation event occurs, each photomultiplier tube produces an output current pulse. The amplitude of the pulse from a given photomultiplier tube is directly proportional to the amount of light (number of scintillation photons) its photocathode has received. Therefore, those photomultiplier tubes closest to the scintillation event have the largest output pulses. By combining the pulses from each photomultiplier tube through a resistor or capacitor network, an X,Y coordinate can be generated.

A signal proportional to the total energy deposited in the crystal during a photon interaction is used by the pulse-height analyzer to discriminate against scattered photons. Photons interact predominantly by photoelectric effect or Compton scattering. Photons emerging from a patient, therefore, either have all their energy (i.e., they did not interact with the patient) or have some reduced amount of energy (i.e., they underwent Compton scattering within the patient). Because the collimator allows only those photons traveling in predetermined directions to interact in the crystal, a line drawn from the scintillation event in the crystal through the collimator pinhole is presumed to intersect the site of origin of the photon (i.e., the radioactive atom it came from) in the patient. If the photon has been scattered, a line drawn through its direction of flight does not intersect its site of origin, only the site of the Compton interaction. The desired goal of the scintillation camera is to create a picture that portrays the biodistribution of radioactivity (i.e., sites and numbers of radioactive atoms) within the patient. Therefore, it is not desirable to have these scattered photons contributing toward the final image. The pulse-height

TABLE 15-2.
Estimated Error of Radioiodine Uptake Measurements Due to Variation of Thyroid Depth

	Estimated Thyroid Depth (cm)*								
	>3.5	3.5	3.0	2.6	2.1	1.8	1.5	1.2	<1.2
Percentage of patients having this depth[6] (mean thyroid depth, 2.6 cm)	1.9	3.8	9.4	32.1	17.0	13.2	11.3	7.2	3.8
Expected deviation from standard (%)†									
^{125}I (28 keV)‡	−40.9	−21.3	0	+33.3		−51.1	+86.7		+126.7
^{123}I (159 keV)‡	−208.0	−10.4	0	+16.7		+25.0	+35.4		+47.9
^{131}I (364 keV)‡	−19.9	−8.8	0	+12.1		+21.0	+30.4		+40.0

Distance between the surface of the neck and the center of activity of each thyroid lobe.
†The mean depth (2.6 cm) is used as the standard. The expected deviation represents the error in the uptake measurement if the mean depth is assumed.
‡Photon energy.

analyzer can be used to reject these photons by adjusting its window so that only full-energy photons are accepted and contribute to the final picture. Without the pulse-height analyzer, the final image would be blurred.

The scaler-timer controls the on-off cycle of the camera. The camera may be set up to "take a picture" for a predetermined time interval, or until a predetermined amount of radioactivity has been detected ("counted").

In older cameras, the X,Y coordinates are used to drive a cathode ray tube display, which produces a picture of the distribution of radioactivity within the patient. The coordinates are used to position a finely focused dot of light on the cathode ray tube face. A collection of these light dots over time produces the image. Because it takes a period of time for a complete picture to be obtained, some sort of integration medium must be used to record the image. The most frequently used media are various types of photographic film. A photographic camera is mounted on the cathode ray tube, and the shutter is left open during the entire image acquisition period. The film is developed in the usual way, and a photograph of the distribution of radioactivity is obtained. Alternatively, data from the Anger camera can be fed into a digital computer for further analysis; all modern Anger cameras are integrated with computer systems. For example, thyroid uptake of radioiodine or ^{99m}Tc may be determined by outlining the thyroid on the computer image, thereby excluding extrathyroid activity from the neck and salivary glands.[8,9]

In the past, thyroid imaging was always performed with a pinhole collimator, which provides magnification. This magnification was necessary to obtain images of sufficiently high resolution. With advances in both camera and collimator technology, it has now become acceptable to use low-energy high-resolution parallel-hole collimators for thyroid imaging. This is fortunate because parallel-hole collimators are the most commonly used collimators in nuclear medicine studies, while pinhole collimators are used almost exclusively for thyroid imaging. In today's busy nuclear medicine department, where a scintillation camera may be required to perform many different types of studies during the day, it is not desirable to have to take the time to change collimators between different patient studies. In general, the purchase and use of a pinhole collimator is typically only justified when using older equipment.

The newest form of imaging is single-photon emission computed tomography (often referred to as SPECT). In its most common implementation, an Anger camera is rotated 360° around the subject, acquiring planar "projection" views at 64 to 128 equiangular views. For these images, a parallel-hole collimator, rather than a pinhole collimator, is used. These views are used by a computer to reconstruct transverse, sagittal, and coronal tomographic slices through the thyroid.[10] These tomographic images, because they eliminate the contribution of overlying and underlying activity, can provide more diagnostically useful images of the distribution of ^{99m}Tc or ^{123}I within the thyroid. Furthermore, the data can be quantified to yield estimates of thyroid volume.

In Vitro Measurement

Radioiodine can be identified and quantified in solutions, in precipitates, on chromatographic strips, or in bits of tissue.

Scintillation spectrometry systems are generally used to determine which radionuclides (and their amounts) are present in a mixed sample, or to determine how much activity of a known radionuclide is present in a sample. To assay the amount of radioactivity in a test tube, a well counter is commonly used. This counter consists of a cylindrical lead-shielded sodium iodide detector 1 to 3 inches in diameter, containing a hole passing through the lead and partway through the crystal, which permits the insertion of a test tube containing the radioactive sample. Because the crystal surrounds the test tube on all sides except the top, the counting geometry is very close to optimum.

Microscopic imaging can be accomplished by autoradiography. This technique is useful for determining the distribution of radioiodine at a cellular or subcellular level. In this procedure, a photographic emulsion is placed in close contact with a section of thyroid tissue containing either ^{131}I or, for better spatial resolution, ^{125}I. The extent of blackening of the emulsion after development is proportional to the concentration of the radioactivity in the corresponding region of the tissue.

Radioiodine can be used in a variety of analytic chemical techniques for measuring blood and tissue iodine and iodine-containing compounds. Compounds that contain the isotopes of iodine, primarily ^{125}I, are widely used as reagents in the following techniques for assessing thyroid function: competitive protein-binding assays, radioimmunoassays, and assays by equilibrium dialysis or electrophoresis. These methods are used to measure serum total and free thyroxine and triiodothyronine and the products of their metabolism, thyroglobulin, thyroid microsomal (thyroid peroxidase) and thyroglobulin antibodies, thyroxine-binding globulin, and thyrotropin.

As alluded to above, activation analysis is a sensitive, accurate, and simple method for determining the quantity of iodine in biologic samples. A 25-minute irradiation of stable ^{127}I induces one-half the maximum ^{128}I radioactivity in the sample. On removal of the sample from the reactor, the ^{128}I is separated from other radionuclides by distillation and precipitation, and the amount of radioactivity is assayed. Standards containing known quantities of iodine are irradiated together with the unknown, and a comparison is made between the ^{128}I activity of the sample and the standards. From these data, the amount of ^{127}I in the original sample can be calculated.

RADIATION DOSIMETRY

Particulate or electromagnetic radiations interact with tissue, causing ionization, electron excitation to outer orbits, or the production of active free radicals. These processes result in varying degrees of tissue damage. The extent of injury may range from cell death to the production of tumors, or the cell may completely recover.

The energy of particulate or electromagnetic radiation determines the number of ionizations it produces, and the nature of the radiation determines the spatial distribution of the induced ionizations. For example, when ^{131}I irradiates the human thyroid, most of the beta radiation, but only about 10% of the gamma ray energy, is absorbed within the organ (Fig 15-7). Alpha particles produce a very short, very dense ionization zone. Beta particles follow an irregular path that is both less

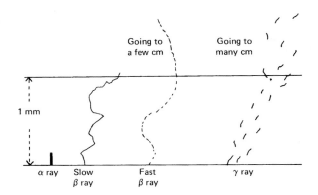

FIGURE 15-7. Schematic representation of relative distribution of ions produced by α, β, and γ rays.

densely ionizing and longer the greater the particle energy. X-ray and gamma ray ionizations are produced by secondary electrons produced in the tissue by photoelectric effect or Compton scattering. Some of these particles pass through the tissue, whereas others do not. It is the latter particles that provide the greatest amount of absorbed tissue dose.

Several quantities can be used to express the amount of radiation present or the energy transferred from the radiation to some material. The term exposure strictly only applies to electromagnetic radiation. The unit of exposure is the roentgen (R) and represents the number of ion pairs produced in a specific volume of air. The SI unit for exposure is coulombs per kg of air (C/kg); 1 C/kg = 3876 R.

The unit of absorbed dose is the rad, which is defined as the absorption of 100 ergs per gram. Note that this unit refers to an energy-deposition concentration rather than a total amount of energy. The SI unit for absorbed dose is the gray (Gy); 1 Gy = 100 rads.

It is often useful to be able to measure exposure but express the results as dose to an individual in that radiation field. Because of the way in which the roentgen and rad are defined, a relationship between exposure in air and dose in air may be easily derived: 1 R = 0.87 rad. To compute the dose to a material other than air, the f-factor is used as a conversion:

$$f = 0.87 \frac{\mu/_\rho \text{material}}{\mu/_\rho \text{air}}$$

and D = f × E.

To account for the cellular and subcellular differences in energy deposition pattern (which depends on the radiation's linear energy transfer), which affect biologic consequences, doses are frequently expressed as dose equivalents. The dose equivalent is given by the absorbed dose multiplied by a quality factor, which describes the ability of a given radiation to produce a certain biologic effect relative to x-rays. Quality factors range from 1 (for x-rays, electrons, and positrons of any specific ionization) to over 20 (for high-linear energy transfer alphas). The conventional unit for dose equivalent is the rem; the SI unit is the Sievert (Sv); 1 Sv = 100 rem.

For the purpose of relating exposure to risk, an extension of the dose equivalent is used to express dose as that which would have been received if the whole body had been irradiated uniformly. The effective dose equivalent is obtained as the sum of dose equivalents to different organs or body tissues weighted in such a fashion as to provide a value proportional to radiation-induced somatic and genetic risk even when the body is not uniformly irradiated.

To accurately calculate the dose of radiation to be delivered to the target (thyroid) and nontarget (other glands and whole body) tissues requires a knowledge of the mode of decay of the nuclide to be used, the target tissue uptake and distribution of the nuclide, the effective $T_{1/2}$ of the radioactivity, and the weight and geometry of the gland. The effective $T_{1/2}$ of a radionuclide combines the decay $T_{1/2}$ (physical $T_{1/2}$) and the $T_{1/2}$ of the secretion of the radionuclide by the gland (biologic $T_{1/2}$):

$$\text{effective } T_{1/2} \frac{\text{physical } T_{1/2} \times \text{biological } T_{1/2}}{\text{physical } T_{1/2} + \text{biological } T_{1/2}}$$

The biologic $T_{1/2}$ of iodine in a normal person is about 60 days (or 1440 hours), with a decrease to about 20 days (or 480 hours) in thyrotoxicosis. Knowledge of the half-time of uptake of radioiodine by the gland is also required. The biologic uptake $T_{1/2}$ is about 5 hours in most normal people, but it may be as short as 1.5 hours in a patient with thyrotoxicosis.

Although the mode of radioactive decay for a given radionuclide is always known, and the thyroid uptake and retention of the radionuclide can be individually determined, the weight, geometry, and radionuclide distribution within the gland cannot always be accurately determined by current techniques. As a result, there are several formulas for estimating the dose of radiation delivered to the thyroid. Clinically, one formula proves to be no better than another. In fact, many clinicians do not use a formula but estimate the dose based on physical examination and clinical evaluation. As an example of one approach, the weight of the thyroid in grams (M), the fractional uptake (U) of the administered activity (A), and the effective $T_{1/2}$ of that radionuclide in the gland are used as follows:

$$\text{dose (rad)} = (\text{effective} T_{1/2} - \text{uptake} T_{1/2}) \times A \times U \times K/M$$

The physical constant (K) in this formula depends on gland weight and the fraction of particulate and photon energy deposited within the gland. It also contains factors for converting the units of energy deposited per gram into rads. The K values for the more important isotopes of iodine are listed in Table 15-3.

The error in this method of dose calculation arises from the problems noted above and is further compounded by the erroneous assumption that the radionuclide is uniformly distributed within the gland. Dose calculations by this formula or other formulas must be used with caution, acknowledging the attendant inaccuracies; nonetheless, these efforts offer some general guidelines to safer and perhaps more effective use of radionuclides in research and diagnosis. In terms of therapy for thyrotoxicosis, there is no convincing evidence that such detailed calculations result in less incidence of recurrence or hypothyroidism than the choice of a dose based purely on clinical parameters.

DOSE GUIDELINES

The only effect observed within the thyroid 10 months after a thyroid dose of 1600 rad is a decreased capacity of the tissue to multiply in response to drug or hormonal stimulation.[11] In diagnostic tests, absorbed doses are well below this level. For example, 5 to 25 μCi doses of ^{131}I are more than adequate for most diagnostic tests, and deposit about 5 to 25 rad in the thyroid.

During the first several hours after administration of radioiodine, high local concentrations accumulate in the stomach, gastrointestinal tract, kidney, bladder, and salivary glands, and, to a potentially significant but far lesser degree, in the ovaries, testes, bone marrow, and liver. The areas of high concentration may receive several times the amount of radiation delivered to the whole body and may demonstrate distinct radiation effects when larger doses of radioiodine are used. For example, an occasional patient experiences a dry mouth, usually temporary, from salivary gland irradiation produced by the use of therapeutic doses of radioiodine. The estimated radiation dose per microcurie of administered isotope for several important tissues in average-sized adults is shown for the important isotopes of iodine in Table 15-3. Because tissue may recover from the effects of radiation, the net effect of divided doses is not the same as when the total dose is given at one time. Furthermore, the second dose may have a different distribution than the first as a result of the physiologic effects of the initial dose.

Consideration of whole body irradiation also is important. The radiation dose to the entire body depends on the size of the patient and the rate at which radioactivity is cleared from the blood. The whole body dose from the administration of 1 mCi of ^{131}I is about 0.45 rad. Whole body dose becomes particularly important when large doses are used in cancer therapy. With repeated large doses, whole body irradiation may seriously damage the bone marrow. In addition, toxic effects may occur. Radiation should always be considered potentially harmful and should never be used unless definite patient benefit is expected. This applies to diagnostic as well as therapeutic uses. Potential hazards to patients receiving radioiodine are outlined in Table 15-4.

RADIATION SAFETY

Care must be taken to minimize the radiation exposure of those who work with or administer radioactive iodine. Permissible occupational doses are limited to 5 rem/y. People under age 18 are not permitted to receive occupational exposures. Surgeons handling thyroid glands that have been labeled either with ^{131}I or with other radionuclides should minimize their contact with the radioactive gland. Iodine can be absorbed through the pulmonary alveolocapillary interface and the skin; in time, laboratory workers can acquire a significant dose to the thyroid. With the proper handling of radionuclides, this problem is not serious, but it is wise to check the thyroids of personnel on a routine basis.

Another group that requires protective precautions are those exposed to radioactive patients, that is, nurses, family, and friends. The Nuclear Regulatory Commission (NRC) requires hospitalization for any patient whose body either 1) contains 30 mCi or more of a radionuclide or 2) produces a dose rate greater than 5 mrem/h at 1 m. For example, a patient who has been given 30 mCi of ^{131}I produces a gamma ray exposure rate of about 8 mR/h at a distance of 1 m from the body. When the total body content of radioactivity drops below this figure, the patient may be allowed again to urinate into the usual sewage system and may be discharged from the hospital. To determine when this level of radioactivity has been reached, the amount of radioiodine in a 24-hour urine sample is measured and subtracted from the amount initially administered to the patient. With a suitable correction for decay, the remaining radioactivity can be determined. Although there is wide variation from patient to patient depending on the mass of functional metastases taking up the radionuclide and renal function, most patients receiving a dose of 100 mCi of ^{131}I are able to go home within 48 hours.

Regulations of the NRC require that records be kept about the receipt and disposal of all radioactive materials. The amount of radioactivity that can be disposed of daily into sanitary sewers depends on the volume of dilution in the sewers and must, therefore, be determined separately for each installation. The burning of radioactive wastes is also subject to regulation. With the exception of [129]I, the isotopes of iodine can be disposed of by other means. Because of their long half-life, [129]I wastes should be handled as low level radioactive waste.

A license to both obtain and use radioactive material is required. There are several types of licenses, ranging from the

TABLE 15-3.
Radiation Dose Constant and Dosages Delivered to Several Organ Systems in Euthyroid Patient*

Isotope	Dose Constant (K)	Organ System (Absorbed Dose, mrad/μCi Administered)†						
		THYROID	STOMACH WALL	SALIVARY GLANDS	OVARIES	TESTES	BONE MARROW	TOTAL BODY
[123]I	0.13	13.0	0.2	0.7	0.03	0.012	0.03	0.03
[125]I	0.11	790.0	0.3	0.4	0.04	0.024	0.12	0.49
[131]I	0.68	1300.0	1.4	0.7	0.14	0.088	0.26	0.71
[132]I	2.01	13.0	1.1	0.6	0.13	0.074	0.09	0.11

*Absorbed-dose values may vary as much as 50%.
†Average adult organ size and 25% uptake in the thyroid.
Wellman HN. Anger RT Jr. Radioiodine dosimetry and the use of radioiodines other than ^{131}I in thyroid diagnosis.
Semin Nucl Med 1971;1:356; values from MIRD/Dose Estimate Report no. 5. J Nucl Med 1975;16:857

TABLE 15-4.
Potential Hazards to Patients Receiving Radioiodine*

Average Dose	Potential Hazard		
	MINIMAL	MODERATE	HIGH
Diagnostic tests	—	—	—
Hyperthyroidism therapy	Dry mouth (temporary) Sore throat (temporary) Blood changes (transient) Genetic damage	Hypothyroidism (temporary)†	Hypothyroidism (permanent)†
Thyroid ablation	Blood changes (transient) Genetic damage	Dry mouth (temporary) Sore throat (temporary) Nausea (temporary)	Hypothyroidism (permanent)
Thyroid cancer therapy (repeated doses)	Blood changes (permanent) Hair loss (with skull metastases) Amenorrhea (permanent) Sterility	Dry mouth (temporary) Nausea (temporary) Blood changes (transient) Amenorrhea (temporary) Genetic damage Radiation fibrosis (in areas of uptake)	Hypothyroidism (permanent)

Radioiodine should not be given during pregnancy or lactation.
†In toxic diffuse goiter.

general license issued to an individual physician for the use of limited quantities of certain radionuclides to broad medical licenses issued to institutions. License information can be obtained from the NRC or from state agencies where the state has assumed licensing and regulation responsibilities.

References

1. Greenfield MA, Lane RG. Radioisotope dosimetry. In: Blahd WH, ed. Nuclear medicine. New York: McGraw-Hill, 1971:101
2. Rhodes BA, Wagner HN Jr, Gerrard M. Iodine-123: development and usefulness of a new radiopharmaceutical. Isot Radiat Tech 1967;4:275
3. Smith EM, Mozley JM, Wagner HN Jr. Determination of protein-bound iodine (PBI) in human plasma by thermal neutron activation analysis. J Nucl Med 1964;5:828
4. Kusic Z, Becker DV, Saenger EL, et al. Comparison of technetium-99m and iodine-123 imaging of thyroid nodules: correlation with pathologic findings. J Nucl Med 1990;31:393
5. Hoffer PB, Bernstein J, Gottschalk A. Fluorescent techniques in thyroid imaging. Semin Nucl Med 1971;1:379
6. Wellman HN, Kerjiakes JG, Yeager TB, et al. A sensitive technique for measuring thyroidal uptake of iodine-131. J Nucl Med 1967;9:86
7. Schulz AG, Rollo FD. A method for measurement of radioiodine uptake which corrects for thyroid depth. J Nucl Med 1970;11:600
8. Hurley PJ, Maisey MN, Natarajan TK, Wagner HN Jr. A computerized system for rapid evaluation of thyroid function. J Clin Endocrinol Metab 1972;34:354
9. Maisey MN, Natarajan TK, Hurley PJ, Wagner HN Jr. Validation of a rapid computerized method of measuring Tc-99m pertechnetate uptake for routine assessment of thyroid structure and function. J Clin Endocrinol Metab 1973;36:317
10. Chen JJS, LaFrance ND, Allo MD, et al. Single photon emission computed tomography of the thyroid. J Clin Endocrinol Metab 1988;66:1240
11. Greig WR, Boyle JA, Buchanan WW, Fulton S. Clinical and radiobiological observations on latent effects of x-irradiation on the thyroid gland. J Clin Endocrinol Metab 1965;24:1009

Werner and Ingbar's The Thyroid, Seventh Edition,
edited by Lewis E. Braverman and Robert D. Utiger.
Lippincott–Raven Publishers, Philadelphia, © 1996

16

Biologic Effects of Radioiodines on the Human Thyroid Gland

Harry R. Maxon

Eugene L. Saenger

This chapter evaluates the potential of radioiodines to induce clinically important changes in the human thyroid gland. Unfortunately, many of these changes such as benign thyroid neoplasms, thyroid cancers, and hypothyroidism that may be caused by irradiation are indistinguishable from those that occur spontaneously. Therefore, we are left with limited human data, usually based on relatively large therapeutic administrations of radioiodine to patients with thyroid disease, on diagnostic administrations to patients suspected of having thyroid disease, or on individuals incidentally exposed to nuclear fallout. The use of data from these limited epidemiologic studies to estimate the effects of radioiodine on individuals must include an understanding of multiple, often ill-defined factors such as the impact of dose rate and dose distribution; limitations of dose calculations; effects of gender, age at exposure, and predisposing genetic or environmental factors; the impact of varying methods of surveillance; and the problem of variable durations of follow-up.

In this chapter, we concentrate on the biologic effects of radioiodines (^{123}I, ^{125}I, ^{129}I, ^{131}I, ^{132}I, ^{133}I, and ^{135}I) on the human thyroid gland. Chapters or sections of chapters 15, 28, 53, and 80 are relevant to this discussion, and the reader is referred to them.

RADIOBIOLOGIC MODEL FOR THYROID EFFECTS—MINIMUM INDUCTION PERIOD

In all studies of radiation effects in which the subjects have been examined for some endpoint after radiation exposure, there has been some period of time, referred to as the minimum induction or latent period, between the radiation exposure and the detection of the first clinical abnormality in the subject. This period may vary from a matter of hours in the case of acute radiation thyroiditis to years in the case of thyroid neoplasms. In the case of thyroid cancers, limited follow-up may result in artifactual shortening of the estimated mean time from exposure to the development of the cancer,[1] whereas prolongation of the interval between early clinical evidence of the development of the cancer and its ultimate confirmation in surgery may overestimate the minimum induction period.[2] Although the minimum induction period for solid cancers generally has been considered to be between 5 and 15 years,[3] our analysis[4] of combined data from Beach and Dolphin[5] and from Raventos and Winship[6] indicated that the mean time of appearance of thyroid cancers after external radiation of 660 individuals in childhood was 10.5 years with two standard deviation limits of 3.6 to 30.8 years.

IMPACT OF DOSE RATE AND DOSE DISTRIBUTION

External x- or gamma irradiation delivers the entire radiation dose over a matter of seconds to minutes with uniform penetration of the radiation throughout the thyroid gland. Internal emitters such as the radioiodines must be ingested or inhaled, absorbed, cleared from the circulation by the thyroid epithelial cell, and incorporated in the thyroid follicle where they will remain for some finite period of time while undergoing radioactive decay.

Once localized in the gland, the distribution of radiation dose from radioiodines to the thyroid will depend on the type and energy of the emissions and the distribution of iodine within the follicle. As seen in Table 16-1, 73% to 96% of the total radiation dose from radioiodines will be due to particulate radiation. However, the mean range of particles in the thyroid is highly variable, being much shorter for non-beta emitters such as ^{123}I and ^{125}I than for beta emitters such as ^{131}I, [132]I, [133]I, and [135]I. VanBest[7] evaluated average thyroid epithelial cell doses for various radioiodines, including ^{125}I and [131]I. The ratios between the average follicular cell dose and the average thyroidal gland dose were closer to unity for [131]I (0.8), than for [125]I (0.5). Within the normal human thyroid gland, follicular sizes may range between 0.01 and 0.9 mm and average 0.2 mm.[8,9] Based on the mean ranges of the dominant particulate radiations in the thyroid from iodine isotopes, nonuniformity of dose would be greatest with ^{125}I, would be modest with ^{131}I, and would be negligible with [132]I, [133]I, and [135]I.

The effect of dose rate from radioiodines in the thyroid gland also appears to be a major factor in determining their biologic effects.[10–12] For example, there are large differences in dose rate between ^{131}I and [125]I (see Table 16-1), the ratio being about 7:1.

The total dose delivered also is important. The shape of the radiation dose-response curve is not well established for internal emitters but, based on external radiation data, most likely consists of a linear quadratic response. Although a linear model may best define dose response over the total dose range of 50 to 600 rad, it most likely will overestimate effects at doses below 50 rad and will underestimate effects at doses above 600 rad. Nevertheless, in general, there is an increase in radiobiologic effect as the total radiation dose increases. When the total dose is such that the thyroid gland is completely sterilized or destroyed, then functional effects dominate over the induction of neoplasms.[4]

As can be seen in Table 16-1, when one considers the uniformity of dose distribution as reflected in the mean range of particulate radiation in the thyroid, the average dose rate, and the total dose delivered, one can anticipate that, for the same activities of radioiodine in the thyroid, very little biologic effect will be seen from ^{123}I, that ^{125}I and ^{131}I probably will have similar biologic effects on the function of the thyroid gland, and that [132]I, [133]I, and [135]I will be similar in effect to external radiation.

EXPERIENCE WITH SPECIFIC RADIOIODINE ISOTOPES

Iodine-129

Iodine-129 is derived primarily from nuclear fuel activities, and any [129]I released to the environment was considered initially to potentially result in thyroid gland irradiation. However, in contrast to other radioiodines, [129]I has a very low specific activity of 0.17 µCi/mg iodine so that there are relatively few radioactive iodine atoms as compared with nonradioactive iodine atoms in [129]I from reactors. The restricted capacity of the normal human thyroid to store a maximum of about 12 mg of iodine additionally limits any potential hazards to the thyroid from [129]I release.[4] Even in rats exposed to higher specific activity, purified [129]I in amounts calculated to deliver 1 rad/d to the thyroid with a total thyroidal dose of 660 rad at median lifetime, no thyroidal effects were found by Book.[13] The absence of effects was attributed to the very low dose rate of [129]I. Thus, [129]I does not seem to pose a meaningful threat to the human thyroid.

Iodine-123

Iodine-123 is widely used in diagnostic nuclear medicine. Based on the mean range of its particulate radiation in the thyroid (see Table 16-1), it would be expected to have a microscopic dose distribution similar to ^{125}I with a much lower total dose related to its very short half-life and relatively low dose rate. No specific biologic data indicate that ^{123}I in currently approved medical uses will cause adverse thyroidal effects, and it is not anticipated that ^{123}I poses any appreciable threat to the human thyroid in the ranges of administered activities currently used in diagnostic nuclear medicine.

Iodine-125

Iodine-125 is used extensively in radioassay techniques in clinical and research laboratories, but it has been used only rarely for the in vivo diagnosis or treatment of thyroid disorders in man.

Holm and colleagues[14] evaluated 1111 patients who had received an average of 50 µCi of ^{125}I and 2 µCi of ^{131}I for diag-

TABLE 16-1.
Dose, Dose Rate, and Dose Distribution for Radioiodines in the Human Thyroid Gland

Radionuclide	% of Dose Due to Particulate Radiation	Effective Half-Life in the Thyroid (hs)	Mean Range (mm) of Particles in the Thyroid	Total Dose From 1 mCi in the Thyroid (rad)	Average Dose Rate (rad/h) for Delivery of 10 rad From 1 mCi of Activity in the Thyroid Gland
[123]I	77	13	0.1	76	3.7
[125]I	73	866	0.01	3747	3.0
[131]I	94	177	0.4	5627	22
[132]I	90	2.3	1.7	199	59
[133]I	96	20	1.3	1335	46
[135]I	90	6.7	1.1	434	45

Modified from Maxon HR, Thomas SR, Book SA, et al. Induction of thyroid cancer by ionizing radiation. In: National Council on Radiation Protection and Measurements, Report 80. Washington, DC:1985.

nostic studies. The average age of these subjects at the time of administration of the radioiodines was 44 years, and women outnumbered men by a ratio of 5:1. Seventy-seven percent of the patients received one, 17% received two, and 6% received three or more administrations of the radioiodines. Forty-four percent were being evaluated for suspected thyroid tumors, and 56% were being evaluated for other reasons. A follow-up time of at least 5 years was required for inclusion in the study, and the average follow-up time was approximately 20 years. Two of the 1111 subjects developed thyroid cancers. The calculated standardized incidence ratio (SIR) for thyroid cancer was 2.47 (95% confidence interval = 0.30–8.92), calculated as the ratio between observed cancers in the irradiated cohort and the expected numbers of cancers in a theoretical control group adjusted for age, gender, and calendar year specific cancer incidence rates obtained from the Swedish Cancer Register. If the lower bound of the 95% confidence interval for the SIR is greater than 1, then the SIR is considered to be significant. Thus, there was no evidence of a statistically significant increase in risk of thyroid cancer following diagnostic ^{125}I administrations in these patients.

Radioiodine-125 has been used therapeutically in two large trials in man.[15,16] The combined results indicate that 138 of 418 subjects treated for thyrotoxicosis with an average administered activity of 13.8 mCi ^{125}I had become hypothyroid at a mean follow-up time of 47 months. Based on our subsequent work,[17] we calculated that a similar mean administered activity of 13.8 mCi of ^{131}I would have resulted in 136 cases of clinical hypothyroidism in these same 418 subjects. Thus, at these relatively high levels of administered activity, both ^{125}I and ^{131}I would appear to be equally effective in inducing hypothyroidism.[4,17]

MIXTURES OF SHORT-LIVED RADIOIODINE ISOTOPES IN RADIOACTIVE FALLOUT

On March 1, 1954, the United States undertook an aboveground nuclear weapon test in the Marshall Islands known as Operation Castle Bravo. Persons living on Rongelap Island, Rongelap Atoll; Sifo Island, Ailingnae Atoll; and Utirik Island, Utirik Atoll were exposed accidentally to acute radioactive fallout. Beginning on March 8, 1954, medical surveillance was instituted. In 1992, Conard[18] reported on the follow-up of these people through 1987. In addition, extensive reevaluations of their thyroid dosimetry had been completed in 1985 by Lessard and colleagues.[19] The average total thyroidal doses were 2100 rad on Rongelap Island, 670 rad on Sifo Island, and 280 rad on Utirik Island. Seventy-five to 80% of the total thyroidal dose was due to short-lived radioiodine mixtures, 5% to 16% of the total dose was due to external radiation, and only 8% to 17% of the total thyroid dose was due to [131]I. The 253 irradiated subjects were compared with 227 Marshallese who had been followed consecutively in the same manner and who were considered to be a nonexposed control group.[18] Although there has been some debate regarding whether the control group might in fact have had some low-dose exposure to fallout,[20] Conard[18] concluded that the incidence of thyroid nodules in the control group was similar to those in other world

populations. In any event, the Marshallese data clearly indicate that mixtures of highly energetic short-lived radioiodine isotopes in atomic fallout can result in a significant increase in both benign and malignant thyroid nodules. The earliest thyroid cancer observed in the irradiated population was diagnosed approximately 8 years after the fallout occurred. These observations confirm the postulate that short-lived, relatively high-energy isotopes of iodine have an effect similar to that of external gamma radiation on the human thyroid.[4]

In addition to the Marshallese, 4818 children living in Utah, Nevada, and Arizona also were exposed to atomic fallout subsequent to nuclear weapons testing at Nevada test sites from 1951 through 1957.[21] A total of 74 tests occurred, and the subsequent fallout, consisting primarily of a mixture of ^{131}I and [133]I, resulted in a median thyroid dose of 2.5 rad with a mean thyroid dose of 9.8 rad. Seventy-three percent of the dose came from milk, 10% from vegetables, 13% from external radiation due to fallout on the ground, and 3% from inhalation. A total of 217 children in the irradiated population received estimated thyroidal doses of greater than 40 rad, with an average thyroidal dose of 60 rad, and the patients with the highest doses appear to have had a more marked exposure to early fallout, at which time [133]I would have been dominant. Although Stevens and colleagues[21] state that ^{131}I was a "major contributor" to total thyroidal dose, data from 4 randomly-selected individuals reported in detail in their paper indicate that approximately 45% of the dose from milk was due to ^{131}I and 55% to [133]I. Those 4 patients had calculated total thyroidal doses of 24, 107, 133, and 139 rad. A subgroup of 2473 people who had been irradiated in childhood from the fallout were included in their long-term follow-up from 1965 through 1986. In the exposed group of 1055 people receiving 5 rad or more to the thyroid, they found 3 with thyroid cancer (0.28%) as compared with 5 with thyroid cancer in 1418 "control" subjects (0.35%) who received 0 to 4 rad to the thyroid. Nine benign thyroid neoplasms were found in the group receiving 5 rad or more, and two benign thyroid neoplasms were found in the control group. Although the prevalence of both benign and malignant thyroid neoplasms in the irradiated group was not significantly different from that in the control group, when all thyroid neoplasms were considered, there was a suggestive trend in relative risk as the thyroidal dose increased ($P = 0.02$). No other relationships between radiation dose and thyroid disorders were noted.

On April 26, 1986, reactor number 4 at Chernobyl in the Soviet Union broke down. The resulting radioactive plume passed first over the Gomel region of Belarus, then the Brest and Grodno regions of Belarus, and finally over three remaining contaminated regions in Belarus and Minsk City[22] before dispersing elsewhere. Approximately 30 to 40 million curies of short-lived radioiodine isotopes were released from the reactor along with 12 to 21 million curies of ^{131}I and other nonradioiodine contaminants.[23,24]

Soviet estimates suggested that the concentrations of ^{131}I in milk might range from 0.02 to 10.0 µCi/L. VanMiddlesworth[24] calculated an average value of 1.4 µCi/L, which would result in approximately 200 rad to the thyroid of a child who continued to drink fresh milk. Clearly, the doses to the thyroids of the exposed children are not well established but could range as high as 1400 to 1500 rad from ^{131}I in addition to external radiation from fallout deposited on the ground. There was most likely a significant additional dose from short-lived radioiodines, particularly in the areas initially crossed by the plume. It is logical to assume that the highest level of short-lived iodine isotopes and external fallout occurred in Gomel, with the next highest levels being in Brest and Grodno, and the least levels occurring in the other three regions from Belarus that were reported along with Minsk City.

Unfortunately, the areas affected in Belarus and Ukraine also are areas of known iodine deficiency, and dietary iodine supplements had been stopped in 1981 for reasons that are not clear.[23,25] No stable iodine for thyroidal blocking became available until well after the initial plume had passed.[23] The physiology of radiogenic thyroid cancer has been reviewed extensively in the 1990 BEIR V report:[26] data from rats suggest that amplification of radiation-mutated clones under the mitogenic stimulation of thyroid-stimulating hormone in the presence of iodine deficiency may result in a very high initiation of neoplastic growth. In addition, Perkel and colleagues[27] studied 572 individuals who were members of 286 sibling pairs who had received childhood external radiation treatment in Chicago and for whom long-term follow-up information was available. For all thyroid neoplasms, both benign and malignant, within-family concordance was significant. When thyroid cancers were considered alone, the results were suggestive but not definitive. They concluded that, in addition to the known increased risk of radiation-induced thyroid cancer associated with female gender, younger age, and radiation exposure in higher doses, it was likely that there are independent familial risk factors for developing thyroid neoplasms after radiation exposure. They were unable to determine whether these are genetic or environmental. Thus, factors such as the very young age of the children in Belarus and Ukraine at irradiation and endemic iodine deficiency as well as other genetic or environmental factors might well have played a role in the consequences of fallout in Belarus and Ukraine.

During the first 4 years following the accident at Chernobyl, there was a steady, low rate of thyroid cancer per year in Belarus.[22,23] In 1990, which would be 5 years after the accident, there was a dramatic increase in all regions that became even more pronounced in 1991 and 1992 (Table 16-2). From a background rate in the first 4 years after the accident of approximately 4 thyroid cancers per year, there was an increase to 29 cancers in 1990, 55 in 1991, and a projected total of 60 thyroid cancers for calendar year 1992. Approximately 93% of

the cancers have been papillary, and 6% have been follicular. Local invasion beyond the thyroid capsule has been noted in 45% of the cases, and multifocality within the thyroid gland has been noted in 42%. All of the childhood thyroid cancer cases reported from Belarus occurred in children less than 15 years of age at exposure. At the time of the diagnosis of thyroid cancer, 6 children were 4 years of age or younger, 75 were between the ages of 5 and 9, and 66 were between the ages of 10 and 14 years. The findings in Belarus are entirely consistent with an expected response following exposure predominantly to short-lived radioiodines and to external radiation from fallout in Gomel, with a lower component of short-lived radioiodines in Brest and Grodno, and predominantly ^{131}I, and possibly ^{133}I in the other regions of Belarus.

Kiev, Ukraine, in the former Soviet Union, also was exposed to fallout, but apparently the fallout did not arrive there until 4 days after the accident, at which time ^{131}I was the dominant radioiodine involved.[28] The resulting average thyroid doses in children were correspondingly smaller, ranging from 1.8 rad in persons aged 12 to 15 years up to 10.4 rad in persons aged 3 years or less at exposure. Kiev also is an area of iodine deficiency with endemic goiter, and an apparent increase in thyroid cancers in children exposed to fallout has been noted.[29] In both Belarus and Ukraine the thyroid cancers in children have been aggressive with a high prevalence of lung metastases.[30]

CLINICAL EFFECTS OF ^{131}I ON THE HUMAN THYROID—ACUTE RADIATION THYROIDITIS

Acute radiation thyroiditis describes an acute condition occurring within 2 weeks after exposure of the thyroid to ^{131}I and characterized by symptoms of inflammation and eventual necrosis of some or all cells in the thyroid.[17] The symptoms usually are mild and are related to local pain and tenderness over the gland.[31–33] However, on occasion, significant systemic symptoms have been associated with massive release of stored thyroid hormone,[33,34] and this syndrome may require treatment with anti-inflammatory drugs and β blockers. It generally resolves within 2 to 4 weeks.

In 1956, Beierwaltes and Johnson[31] reported that acute radiation thyroiditis could be found in 4% to 5% of patients with thyrotoxicosis treated with ^{131}I. However, the symptoms were

TABLE 16-2.
Thyroid Cancers in Children Exposed to Radioactive Fallout in Belarus

Region of Belarus	Average Cases per Year, 1986–1989	1990	1991	9 months in 1992
Gomel	1.5	14	38	25
Brest and Grodno	1.8	6	7	14
Three other regions and Minsk City	1.0	9	10	6

Modified from Kazakov VS, Demidchik EP, Astakhova LN. Thyroid cancer after Chernobyl (letter). Nature 1992;359:21; Baverstock K, Egloff B, Pinchera A, et al (letter). Nature 1992;359:21; and Bertin M, Laccemand J. Augmentation des cancers de la thyroide de l'enfant en Belarus. Ann Endocrinol (Paris) 1992;53:173.

so mild that the patients usually had to be questioned carefully to establish their presence. More significant symptoms of worsening thyrotoxicosis were considered to be unlikely below single oral administrations of about 13 mCi of ^{131}I, which, by our calculation, would result in approximately 17,000 to 18,000 rad to the thyroid, assuming a mean 45-g thyroid weight with a mean 24-hour thyroidal radioiodine uptake of 65% and an effective half-life of ^{131}I in the thyroid gland of 6 days.

Segal and colleagues[36] evaluated 65 euthyroid patients with severe ischemic heart disease who were treated with thyroid ablative administrations of ^{131}I to relieve the cardiac symptoms. Three of the 65 patients (4.6%) died shortly after therapy with acute radiation thyroiditis thought to be a contributing factor. Assuming a 20-g thyroidal weight and a 6-day effective half-life of ^{131}I, we calculate that the radiation doses to the thyroids of their patients were between 70,000 and 125,000 rad. Clinically evident acute radiation thyroiditis did not develop in any of their patients who received calculated radiation doses of less than 32,000 rad. Obviously, these dose estimates were first-order approximations only.

Our own data from the University of Cincinnati[17] obtained from patients treated with ^{131}I to ablate residual thyroid tissue after thyroidectomy for thyroid cancer indicated that 90% of the patients experienced acute radiation thyroiditis at thyroid radiation doses of more than 200,000 rad. The resulting symptoms were severe and required supportive therapy in about 4% of our patients.

On the basis of these observations, clinically significant acute radiation thyroiditis would seem to be unlikely at thyroid radiation doses below 20,000 rad from [131]I. Acute radiation thyroiditis is estimated to develop in an additional 5% of exposed individuals for each 10,000-rad increment above the 20,000-rad threshold.

HYPOTHYROIDISM AFTER EXPOSURE OF THE HUMAN THYROID TO RADIOIODINE

Much of the existing human experience with ^{131}I is obtained from treatment of patients with thyrotoxicosis. These data are confounded by the fact that Graves' disease accounts for a large proportion of the thyrotoxic patients and is itself an autoimmune disease associated with an underlying spontaneous rate of development of hypothyroidism calculated by us to be approximately 0.7%/y based on our analysis[17] of data from the National Cooperative Thyrotoxicosis Treatment Follow-up Study.[37] In support of this hypothesis are the long-term follow-up data of Wood and Maloff[38] on adult patients treated with iodides alone for Graves' disease. They found that 2 of 15 such patients had become clinically hypothyroid by 20 years after iodide therapy, suggesting again that the incidence of hypothyroidism in patients with Graves' disease treated without surgery or ^{131}I is about 0.7%/y, almost certainly due to progression of an autoimmune destructive process.

The data from the National Cooperative Thyrotoxicosis Treatment Follow-up Study[37] included approximately 6000 patients who were treated with one administration of [131]I. The cumulative probability of becoming hypothyroid was related to the amount of ^{131}I retained by the thyroid gland in terms of

microcuries per estimated gram of initial thyroid weight (Fig 16-1). An analysis of the slopes of the curves shown in Figure 16-1 revealed that there was not a statistical difference in any of the slopes beyond 5 years, at which time optimal numbers of patients for evaluating the prevalence of hypothyroidism were still included.[17] A cumulative probability of 3.5% (0.7%/y × 5 years) for spontaneous hypothyroidism in Graves' disease was subtracted from the ^{131}I cumulative probability dose-response curves at this 5-year period to result in an estimate of the probability of hypothyroidism from ^{131}I exposure alone.[17] The results (Fig 16-2) demonstrated a strong linear correlation between radiation dose to the thyroid from ^{131}I and the probability of developing hypothyroidism above a lower dose limit of approximately 2500 rad, the lowest dose for which data were available. In performing these dose calculations, we assumed an average effective half-life of ^{131}I in the thyroid gland of 6 days. Although the effective half-life of ^{131}I in the thyroid in Graves' disease may vary between approximately 2 and 8 days in individuals, the mean values appear to be in the range of 5.2 to 5.9 days.[39]

Euthyroid adult patients were treated occasionally with ^{131}I for cardiac disease in the past. Assuming a 20-g thyroid gland with a 6-day effective half-life of ^{131}I, we were able to calculate that 80% of 28 such patients treated by the late Dr. Earl Chapman were clinically hypothyroid 5 years after therapy with a mean thyroidal dose of 32,000 rad from [131]I.[17] Similar calculations were performed by us on separate data from Segal and colleagues[36] and Goolden and Davey[40] on the ablation of normal thyroid tissue with ^{131}I in a larger series of patients. Their data indicate that overt hypothyroidism could be obtained within the first year after ^{131}I therapy, but that it always required at least 27,000 rad of radiation delivered from the [131]I.

In 1983, we were able to demonstrate a radiation dose response in the ablation of residual thyroid tissue after surgery for thyroid cancer.[41] We found that 22 of 23 patients had successful ablation when they received 30,000 rad or more to their thyroid remnants, whereas only 3 of 7 patients whose remnants received less than 30,000 rad responded. In a somewhat smaller study using different methodology, Flower and colleagues[42] demonstrated similar results. We subsequently prospectively evaluated the efficacy of using dosimetric criteria to project outcome in a separate group of patients with thyroid cancer.[43] Seventy patients received ^{131}I ablative therapy for thyroid remnants after their initial surgery for thyroid cancer. The administered activities were calculated to deliver at least 30,000 rad to the thyroid remnants and averaged 86.8 mCi (range 25.8–246.3 mCi). Ablation was considered to be successful when there was no visual evidence of uptake in the thyroid bed and when the percent instantaneous uptake in the neck was less than 0.1% on follow-up about 1 year later. Eighty-one percent of patients and 86% of foci of residual thyroid tissue responded to the initial treatment. There was no apparent gain from using progressively increasing radiation doses above 30,000 rad. These combined data indicate a clear relationship between the radiation dose delivered to the human thyroid by ^{131}I and the development of hypothyroidism, with approximately 80% of nonthyrotoxic patients exposed to 30,000 rad developing thyroid ablation and hypothyroidism.

In contrast, the dose-response curve appears to be shifted in patients with Graves' disease. Our calculations from data

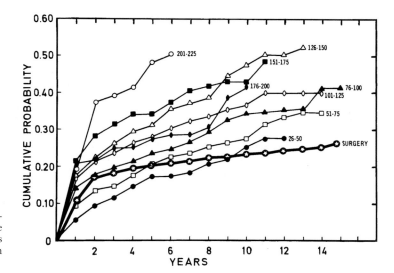

FIGURE 16-1. Probability of becoming hypothyroid after a single treatment with ^{131}I for Graves' disease. The numbers on the curves represent the administered activity of ^{131}I in microcuries per gram of thyroid tissue. (From Becker and colleagues[37] with permission.)

presented by Sofa and Skillern[44] indicate that at an approximate mean thyroid dose of 16,000 rad, 90% of 229 patients treated with ^{131}I for thyrotoxic Graves' disease had developed hypothyroidism 1 year later. At Kyoto University Hospital in Japan, Konishi and colleagues[45] evaluated 762 patients with thyrotoxic Graves' disease treated with ^{131}I between 1956 and 1985. All patients were followed for at least 5 years, and the mean follow-up time was 8.3 years. The targeted thyroidal radiation dose was 5000 to 6000 rad. At 5 years, they noted that 24% of their patients were hypothyroid, a finding that is consistent with earlier data reported by Becker and coworkers.[37] In addition, they were able to divide their patients into those receiving relatively low administered activities of less than 50 μCi ^{131}I per gram and relatively higher administered activities resulting in 75 to 100 μCi ^{131}I per gram, subsequently calculated by us to represent groups treated with approximately 4000 and 8000 rad to the thyroid, respectively. The rates of hypothyroidism at 5 and 10 years of follow-up were 14% and 27% in the "low-dose" group

and 25% and 36% in the "high-dose" group. Thus, their data also indicate a dose-response relationship. On comparing these dose-response data from Graves' disease patients with those derived above for "normal" thyroid tissue in patients without thyrotoxicosis, it would appear that the radiosensitivity of the Graves' disease gland is significantly greater than the radiosensitivity of normal thyroid tissue, probably by a factor of about 2.

The Marshallese were exposed to atomic fallout with resultant thyroid doses that were largely due to short-lived radioiodines and to external radiation. On the whole, only about 10% (range 8–17%) of their total thyroidal dose was due to [131]I. Conard[46] has reported the most recent data on hypothyroidism in the Marshallese. On the island of Rongelap, where the average total thyroidal dose was 2100 rad, 13 of 67 subjects (19%) followed for 27 years after exposure developed hypothyroidism. On Sifo island, where the average thyroidal dose was 670 rad, 1 of 19 (5%) subjects became hypothyroid, and on Utirik, where the mean thyroidal dose was 280 rad, 1

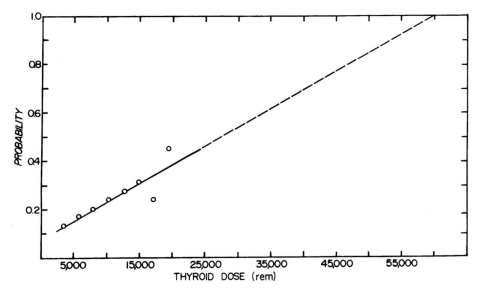

FIGURE 16-2. Probability of hypothyroidism 5 years after exposure of normal thyroidal tissue to [131]I. (From Maxon and colleagues[17] with permission.)

of 164 (0.6%) individuals developed hypothyroidism. In the unexposed control population, 2 of 600 (0.3%) individuals had developed hypothyroidism. Thus, in these individuals whose thyroidal doses were about 75% to 80% due to short-lived radioiodines and 5% to 16% due to external radiation with the remainder being due to ^{131}I, there also is an apparent dose response for hypothyroidism.

In unpublished data communicated to us in 1975 by Hamilton and Tompkins,[17] preliminary results of a follow-up survey of subjects regarded as having normal thyroid glands after diagnostic ^{131}I tests at ages of less than 16 years and followed for an average of 14 years thereafter indicated that 8 of 297 (2.7%) individuals receiving an average thyroidal dose of about 380 rad subsequently developed hypothyroidism, whereas there were no cases of hypothyroidism in 146 children who had a mean thyroidal dose of about 18 rad.

In the most recent follow-up of children exposed to atomic fallout in Utah, Arizona, and Nevada, Stevens and colleagues[21] reported a phase two diagnostic follow-up of 2829 subjects during the years 1985 to 1987. Laboratory testing was performed in 413 of the 730 subjects suspected of having a thyroid abnormality, and 33 confirmed cases of hypothyroidism were diagnosed on the basis of low serum thyroxine or elevated serum TSH values. Twenty-four confirmed cases of hypothyroidism were found in 1790 subjects exposed to fallout in Utah and Nevada (1.3%) as compared to 9 of 1039 (0.9%) subjects living in Arizona. Multiple analyses of the likelihood of developing hypothyroidism showed no apparent differences ($P = 0.7$) by age, gender, state of residence, and thyroidal radiation dose. The mean thyroidal dose in this population was 9.8 rad with a median thyroidal dose of 2.5 rad and a maximum thyroidal dose of 461 rad. Therefore, at these relatively low mean thyroidal doses of approximately 10 rad, there was no evidence of a significantly increased likelihood of hypothyroidism even after almost 30 years of follow-up.

In summary, although there is a linear increase in the chance of developing hypothyroidism as radiation doses increase from several hundred rad up to more than 30,000 rad, hypothyroidism from ^{131}I seems unlikely at doses below 10 to 20 rad. Graves' disease patients seem to have twice the chance of developing hypothyroidism per rad from ^{131}I, probably reflecting potentiating interactions between their underlying autoimmune disorder and the radiation.

DEVELOPMENT OF THYROID NEOPLASMS AFTER EXPOSURE OF THE THYROID TO THERAPEUTIC [131]I

In 1974, Dobyns and colleagues[47] reported that 86 of 16,042 patients with Graves' disease who did not have palpable nodules at the time of radioiodine therapy subsequently were operated and found to have nodules. Nine of the 86 nodules were thyroid cancer and 77 were benign. In an additional 494 of the 16,042 patients, palpable nodules were found at some time after radioiodine therapy, but surgery had not been carried out. Assuming that the distribution of benign and malignant neoplasms in these unoperated patients would be the same as it was in the smaller group subjected to surgery, we

would predict that 519 of 16,042 patients (3.2%) might have developed benign thyroid neoplasms and that 61 of 16,042 (0.4%) patients might have developed thyroid cancer. We subsequently estimated that the mean thyroidal radiation dose in patients treated with ^{131}I was approximately 9000 rad.[17] The average follow-up was approximately 8 years.

In addition to the patients who received ^{131}I therapy at some point in their treatment, Dobyns and colleagues[47] also reported that 1553 of 10,014 (15.5%) of patients who had primary surgical treatment for thyrotoxic Graves' disease had palpable thyroid nodules. In 9 patients (0.6%) the palpable nodules subsequently were proved to be thyroid cancer, and the remainder were benign. Applying these overall prevalence figures to the 16,042 patients with Graves' disease who received ^{131}I therapy, one might predict a total of 2487 nodules as compared with the 580 nodules actually found. Based on their incomplete observations, it would appear that ^{131}I therapy had a protective effect against the development of benign nodules but might be associated with a slight increase in the long-term chances of developing thyroid cancer. An extended 21-year follow-up of patients in the National Cooperative Thyrotoxicosis Treatment Follow-up Study recently has been completed, but, as of this writing, the data have not been analyzed fully.

Konishi and colleagues[45] reported follow-up on 762 patients treated at Kyoto University Hospital in Japan with ^{131}I for Graves' disease between 1956 and 1985. The average age at treatment was 37.4 years, and the average follow-up time was 8.3 years. None were followed for less than 5 years. The average administered activity of ^{131}I was 7.3 mCi. Seven nodules were found to have developed in 762 subjects (0.9%), and all were benign. The average time of appearance of the nodules was 14 years following initial ^{131}I therapy.

Anno and colleagues[48] reported on 11,500 patients treated with ^{131}I in Japan between 1953 and 1966 for thyrotoxicosis. A total of 4204 of these patients were followed for an average of 6.7 years after a median administration of 7.8 mCi of [131]I. They observed three thyroid cancers in 3332 women who had been treated versus an expected 0.8 cancer in this same group, based on their general neoplastic registry data.

In Germany, Globel and colleagues[49] found 4 patients with thyroid cancers among 1183 patients after ^{131}I therapy for thyrotoxicosis. The average follow-up time was about 17 years, and the administered activities of ^{131}I ranged from 0.5 to 5.4 mCi. Based on data reported elsewhere in that paper, one would expect 7 patients with thyroid cancers in this same group.

Holm and colleagues[50] evaluated cancer risk after the ^{131}I treatment of 10,522 patients with thyrotoxicosis in Sweden, and the average follow-up was 15 years. The mean administered activity was 9.7 mCi in patients with thyrotoxic Graves' disease (51%) and 18.9 mCi in patients with toxic nodular goiter (42%). Six thyroid cancers were observed in patients with Graves' disease and 10 in patients with toxic nodular goiter. Comparisons were made using record linkage with the Swedish cancer register for the period 1958 to 1985. Analysis of the results revealed an SIR for thyroid cancer of 0.81 (95% confidence interval 0.30–1.76) in Graves' disease and of 1.74 (95% confidence interval 0.84–3.20) in toxic nodular goiter.

In addition to the large series noted above, Tezelman and colleagues[51] reviewed their experience at the University of California, San Francisco (7 cases) and 29 isolated case reports since 1966 of thyroid cancer after ^{131}I therapy for thyrotoxicosis. The causes of thyrotoxicosis included Graves' disease, solitary adenoma, and multinodular goiter. Administered activities of ^{131}I ranged from 1.25 to 180 mCi. No data were presented to indicate the sizes of the thyrotoxic populations from which the cancer cases were drawn.

These data from thyrotoxic patients treated with relatively large therapeutic activities of ^{131}I do not indicate a definite increase in the likelihood of developing subsequent thyroid neoplasms due to the radioiodine alone. However, more extensive follow-up of populations that include control patients with thyrotoxicosis who were not treated with ^{131}I clearly is needed. It is hoped that within the next year such additional data will be forthcoming from the National Cooperative Thyrotoxicosis Treatment Follow-up Study in the United States.

THYROID NEOPLASMS DEVELOPING AFTER EXPOSURE TO DIAGNOSTIC ADMINISTERED ACTIVITIES OF [131]I

Globel and colleagues[49] obtained follow-up on 13,896 mostly adult patients who received diagnostic amounts of ^{131}I between 1954 and 1979. The average follow-up time was 17 years. The average administered activity was 54 µCi of ^{131}I per diagnostic test. Shore[52] subsequently calculated that the average thyroidal dose in these patients was approximately 1000 rad. Eighty-three thyroid cancers were found as compared with an expected number of 80 thyroid cancers. There was no observed increase in the risk of thyroid cancer as the number of diagnostic exposures to ^{131}I increased.

Holm and colleagues[14] evaluated 35,074 patients who underwent diagnostic radioiodine studies between 1951 and 1969. All had a follow-up of at least 5 years, and the mean follow-up time was 20 years. No patients were included who had received any external radiation therapy to the head and neck or any type of radionuclide therapy. The average age of the patients at the time of the diagnostic exposures was 44 years. Thirty-four thyroid cancers were found in a subgroup of patients (31%) who were evaluated for suspected neoplasms by scans using an average of 71 µCi [131]I. The resultant SIR for thyroid cancer was 2.77 (95% confidence interval 1.92–3.87). They postulated that this might be due in part to selection of the patients with a higher a priori risk of thyroid cancer and in part to more sensitive medical surveillance in this group. All of the significant increase in thyroid cancers in the subgroup originally tested for suspected thyroid neoplasms occurred during years 5 through 9 or after more than 20 years of follow-up, whereas a true radiation effect would have been anticipated to be continuous over time.[52] When they examined the remainder of their patients who received an average administered activity of 45 µCi of ^{131}I, they found only 16 thyroid cancers resulting in an SIR of 0.62 (95% confidence interval 0.35–1.00).

Hamilton and coworkers[53] and Chiacchierini[54] obtained data comparing 3500 children who received diagnostic ^{131}I with 2600 age-, gender-, and race-matched control subjects. The average follow-up was 27 years. Thyroidal doses were estimated to range from between less than 10 to 2000 rad. Five or more years after exposure, there was no significant difference between the thyroid cancer rates in the two groups. Four

thyroid cancers were detected in the radioiodine-exposed group and one among controls, although cancer registry data would suggest that about 3.7 cancers should have been found in the ^{131}I group.[52]

Based on these limited observations, there is no definite evidence of an increased risk of benign or malignant thyroid neoplasms after diagnostic or therapeutic administrations of [131]I. However, the data at low thyroid dose levels are extremely limited, and the data at high therapeutic dose levels are confounded by the fact that at those higher levels thyroid destruction may be the predominant factor. For example, Sikov[55] evaluated the effects of ^{131}I on rats exposed prenatally, as newborns, as weanlings, or as adults using administered activities calculated to deliver 40 rad, 425 rad, or 3400 rad to the thyroid. He found an excess of radiation-associated follicular neoplasms that increased with radiation dose at the two lower dose levels in all groups. Interestingly, the incidence of follicular neoplasms continued to increase at the higher dose level in those exposed during the prenatal or newborn periods but decreased in the weanling and adult exposed groups as a result of marked parenchymal cell destruction.

CONCLUSION

Because of the ability of the thyroid gland to concentrate radioiodine, it is uniquely susceptible to the biologic effects resulting from such exposures. Depending on the particular radioisotope in question, widely variable dose rates and dose distributions may be obtained. These, along with the age of the subject, the total radiation dose delivered to the thyroid, and possibly genetic or environmental factors will have a profound effect on outcome. The results may range from no discernible clinical effects to metabolically important processes such as acute radiation thyroiditis and hypothyroidism and to the induction of both benign and malignant neoplasms. Because the rate of cell division in the normal thyroid is so slow, sublethal radiation effects such as the induction of neoplasms may take many years to become clinically apparent. This is particularly true for adults exposed to low doses at low dose rates. To date, none of the irradiated human populations have been followed to the completion of their life spans, surveillance techniques have been highly variable, and the dosimetry has in many instances been only a crude first-order approximation. Nevertheless, radiation dose-response relationships are evident for many of the clinical effects of radioiodine on the thyroid that must be considered when one is evaluating potential outcomes of radioiodine exposures. Although the human data indicate clearly that ^{131}I is less effective on a rad-for-rad basis in inducing biologic effects in the thyroid than is external radiation delivered at a high dose rate and with uniform distribution, that is not to say that there are no potential biologic effects of ^{131}I, even in the induction of neoplasms. The hazards of short-lived iodine isotopes from atomic fallout are evident from the reported data on the Marshallese; the Americans living in Utah, Arizona, and Nevada; and individuals in Belarus and Ukraine. It is important that thyroidologists distinguish between the variable likelihoods and magnitudes of potential effects of exposure to the different radioiodine isotopes on the human thyroid gland when advising their patients.

References

1. Shore RE. Radiation and host factors in human thyroid tumors following thymus irradiation. Health Phys 1980;38:451

2. Winship T, Rosvoll RV. Thyroid carcinoma in childhood: final report on a 20-year study. Clin Proc Child Hosp Nat Med Cent 1970;26:327

3. Land CE. Estimating cancer risks from low doses of ionizing radiation. Science 1980;209:1197

4. Maxon HR, Thomas SR, Book SA, et al. Induction of thyroid cancer by ionizing radiation. In: National Council on Radiation Protection and Measurements, Report 80. Washington, DC: 1985

5. Beach SA, Dolphin GW. A study of the relationship between X-ray dose delivered to the thyroids of children and the subsequent development of malignant tumors. Phys Med Biol 1962; 6:583

6. Raventos SA, Winship T. The latent interval for thyroid cancer following irradiation. Radiology 1964;83:501

7. VanBest JA. Dose calculations for ^{123}I, ^{124}I, ^{125}I, and ^{131}I in the thyroid gland of the mouse, rat and man and comparison with thyroid function for mice and rats. Phys Med Biol 1981;26:1035

8. Gillespie FC, Orr JS, Greig WR. Microscopic dose distribution from ^{125}I in the toxic thyroid gland and its relation to therapy. Br J Radiol 1970;43:40

9. Maximow AA, Bloom W. Textbook of histology. Philadelphia: WB Saunders, 1957:304

10. Anspaugh LR. Special problems of thyroid dosimetry: considerations of ^{131}I as a function of gross size and inhomogeneous distribution. Report No. UCRL-12492. US Atomic Energy Commission. Livermore: Lawrence Livermore National Laboratory, 1965

11. Walinder G, Sjoden AM. Effects of irradiation on thyroid growth in mouse fetuses and goitrogen challenged adult mice. Acta Radiol Ther Phys Biol 1971;10:579

12. Malone JF. The radiation biology of the thyroid. Current Topics in Radiation Research Quarterly 1975;10:263

13. Book SA. Iodine-129 uptake and effects of lifetime feeding in rats. Health Phys 1983;45:61

14. Holm L-E, Wiklund KE, Lundell GE, et al. Thyroid cancer after diagnostic doses of ^{131}I: a retrospective cohort study. J Natl Cancer Inst 1988;80:1132

15. McDougall IR, Greig WR. ^{125}I therapy in Graves' disease: long-term results in 355 patients. Ann Intern Med 1976;85:720

16. Weidinger P, Johnson PM, Werner SC. Five years' experience with ^{125}I therapy of Graves' disease. Lancet 1974;II:74

17. Maxon HR, Thomas SR, Saenger EL, et al. Ionizing irradiation and the induction of clinically significant disease in the human thyroid gland. Am J Med 1977;63:967

18. Conard RA. Fallout: the experiences of a medical team in the care of a Marshallese population accidentally exposed to fallout radiation. BNL 46444-Medical Department. Upton, NY: Brookhaven National Laboratories, 1992

19. Lessard E, Miltenberger R, Conard R, et al. Thyroid absorbed dose for people at Rongelap, Utirik, and Sifo on March 1, 1954. BNL 51882. Upton, NY: Brookhaven National Laboratory, 1985

20. Hamilton TE, vanBelle G, Logorfo JF. Thyroid neoplasia in Marshall Islanders exposed to nuclear fallout. JAMA 1987;258:629

21. Stevens W, Till JE, Thomas DC, et al. Assessment of leukemia and thyroid disease in relation to fallout in Utah: report of a cohort study of thyroid disease and radioactive fallout from the Nevada test site. Salt Lake City: University of Utah Press, 1992

22. Kazakov VS, Demidchik EP, Astakhova LN. Thyroid cancer after Chernobyl (letter). Nature 1992;359:21; and Baverstock K, Egloff B, Pinchera A, et al (letter). Nature 1992;359:21

23. Bertin M, Laccemand J. Augmentation des cancers de la thyroide de l'enfant en Belarus. Ann Endocrinol (Paris) 1992;53:173

24. VanMiddlesworth L. Effects of radiation on the thyroid gland. Adv Intern Med 1989;34:265

25. Ashizawa K, Yamashita S, Mishikawa T, et al. Childhood thyroid diseases around Chernobyl. Thyroid 1995;5(suppl 1):S227

26. NAS/NRC: National Academy of Sciences/National Research Council. Health effects of exposure to low levels of ionizing radiation. BEIR V Committee on the Biological Effects of Ionizing Radiations. Washington, DC: National Academy Press, 1990

27. Perkel VS, Gail MH, Lubin J, et al. Radiation-induced thyroid neoplasms: evidence for familial susceptibility factors. J Clin Endocrinol Metab 1988;66:1316

28. Likhtarev IA, Gulko GM, Kairo IA, et al. Thyroid doses resulting from the Ukraine Chernobyl accident—Part I: dose estimates for the population of Kiev. Health Phys 1994;66:137

29. Oleynic VA, Cheban AK. Thyroid cancer in children of Ukraine from 1981 to 1992. In: Robbins J, ed. Treatment of thyroid cancer in childhood. Monograph DOE/EH-0406. Bethesda, MD: National Institutes of Health, 1994:45

30. Delbot T, Leenhardt L, Moutet A, et al. Management of thyroid cancer following the Chernobyl accident. [Abstract] Thyroid 1995;5 (suppl 1):S30

31. Beierwaltes WH, Johnson PC. Hyperthyroidism treated with radioiodine; seven-year experience. Arch Intern Med 1956;97:393

32. Werner SC, Ingbar SH. The thyroid. 3rd ed. New York: Harper and Row, 1971:703

33. DeGroot LJ, Stanbury JB. The thyroid and its diseases. New York: John Wiley & Sons, 1971:335

34. Shafer RB, Nuttall FQ. Thyroid crisis induced by radioactive iodine. J Nucl Med 1971;12:262

35. Krishnamurthy GT, Blahd WH. Case reports. Hyperthyroidism in the presence of panhypopituitarism. Thyroid crisis and hypothyroidism following radioiodine treatment. West J Med 1974; 120:491

36. Segal RL, Silver S, Yohalem SB, et al. Use of radioactive iodine in the treatment of angina pectoris. Am J Cardiol 1958;1:671

37. Becker DV, McConahey WM, Dobyns BM, et al. The results of the thyrotoxicosis therapy follow-up study. In: Fellinger K, Hofer R, eds. Further advances in thyroid research. Vol 1. Vienna: G Gistel und Cie, 1971:603

38. Wood LC, Maloof F. Thyroid failure after potassium iodide treatment of diffuse toxic goiter. Trans Assoc Am Physicians 1975; 88:235

39. Maxon HR, Thomas SR, Chen I-W. The role of nuclear medicine in the treatment of hyperthyroidism and well differentiated thyroid adenocarcinoma. Clin Nucl Med 1981;6:87

40. Goolden AW, Davey JB. The ablation of normal thyroid tissue with ^{131}I. Br J Radiol 1963;36:340

41. Maxon HR, Thomas SR, Hertzberg VS, et al. Relation between effective radiation dose and outcome of radioiodine therapy for thyroid cancer. N Engl J Med 1983;309:937

42. Flower MA, Schlesinger T, Hinton PJ, et al. Radiation dose assessment in radioiodine therapy. 2. Practical implementation using quantitative scanning and PET, with initial results on thyroid carcinoma. Radiother Oncol 1989;15:345

43. Maxon HR, Englaro EE, Hertzberg VS, et al. Radioiodine-131 therapy for well differentiated thyroid cancer—a quantitative radiation dosimetric approach: outcome and validation in 85 patients. J Nucl Med 1992;33:1132

44. Sofa AM, Skillern PG. Treatment of hyperthyroidism with a large initial dose of sodium iodide I-131. Arch Intern Med 1975; 135:673

45. Konishi J, Iida Y, Kasagi K, et al. Radiation therapy for Graves' disease in Japan. In: Nagataki S, ed. Radiation and the thyroid. Amsterdam: Excerpta Medica, 1989:68

46. Conard RA. Late radiation effects in Marshall Islanders exposed to fallout 28 years ago. In: Boice JD Jr, Fraumeni JF Jr, eds. Radiation carcinogenesis: epidemiology and biological significance. New York: Raven Press, 1984:57

47. Dobyns BM, Sheline GE, Workman JG, et al. Malignant and benign neoplasms of the thyroid in patients treated for hyperthyroidism: a report of the Cooperative Thyrotoxicosis Study. J Clin Endocrinol Metab 1974;38:976

48. Anno Y, Takeshita A, Iwamoto M. Medical use of radioisotopes in Japan, especially for treating hyperthyroidism and evaluation of the consequent radiation risk. Gann Monograph. Tokyo: Marvzen Press, 1970:241

49. Globel B, Globel H, Oberhausen E. Epidemiologic studies on patients with ^{131}I diagnostic and therapy. In: Kaul A, Neider R, Pensko J, et al, eds. Proceedings of the 6th International Congress on Radiation-Risk-Protection. Köln, Germany: Fachuerbandfur Strahienschutz ev, 1984:565

50. Holm L-E, Hall P, Wiklund K, et al. Cancer risk after ^{131}I therapy for hyperthyroidism. J Natl Cancer Inst 1991;83:1072

51. Tezelman S, Grossman RF, Siperstein AE, et al. Radioiodine-associated thyroid cancers. World J Surg 1994;18:522

52. Shore RF. Issues and epidemiologic evidence regarding radiation-induced thyroid cancer. Radiat Res 1992;131:98

53. Hamilton PM, Chiacchierini R, Kaczmare K. A follow-up of persons who had ^{131}I and other diagnostic procedures during childhood and adolescence. FDA 89-8276. Rockville, MD: CDRH-Food and Drug Administration, 1989:37

54. Chiacchierini RP. Iodine-131 exposures and neoplasia (abstract). Radiat Res 1990;124:359

55. Sikov MR. Tumor development following internal exposures to radionuclides during the perinatal period. In: Napalkov NP, Rice JM, Tomatis L, Yamasaki H, eds. Perinatal and multigeneration carcinogenesis. Lyon: International Agency for Research on Cancer, 1989:403

Werner and Ingbar's The Thyroid, Seventh Edition,
edited by Lewis E. Braverman and Robert D. Utiger.
Lippincott–Raven Publishers, Philadelphia, © 1996

17

In Vivo Isotopic Tests and Imaging

Ralph R. Cavalieri
I. Ross McDougall

QUANTITATIVE IN VIVO RADIOISOTOPIC TESTS

The measurement of the uptake of radioiodine by the thyroid (RAI-U), first introduced in human beings in the late 1930s, remained a primary test of thyroid function for several decades.[1] In recent years sensitive and specific in vitro tests have eclipsed the RAI-U and other in vivo tests of thyroid gland activity. Nevertheless, in some clinical situations these tests provide invaluable diagnostic information.

Radionuclides: Physical Properties of Clinical Importance

IODINE-123

Of the several radioactive isotopes of iodine, ^{123}I is the best suited for in vivo measurement of thyroid uptake and for imaging the gland. The short half-life (13 hours) and the absence of beta emission of ^{123}I account for the relatively low radiation exposure to the thyroid from this radionuclide, so that a dose of 300 μCi of ^{123}I (a commonly prescribed dose for imaging the thyroid) gives the same radiation exposure to the gland as 3 μCi of ^{131}I (Table 17-1). The energy of the gamma photon (159 keV) makes ^{123}I nearly ideal for imaging of the gland with modern gamma cameras. Imaging can be performed up to 24 hours after the dose. Use of a high-energy proton accelerator with natural iodine as the target has resulted in an ^{123}I product that contains less than 1% ^{125}I and no other impurities, such as ^{124}I.[2] Nevertheless, because the concentration of longer-lived isotopic contaminants builds up as the ^{123}I decays, it is recommended that ^{123}I be administered on the day of delivery, particularly when used for in vivo testing of children.[3]

Iodine-123 has become the isotope of choice for uptake determination in diagnostic testing of patients with thyrotoxicosis.[4]

IODINE-131

The principal diagnostic application of ^{131}I is in total body scanning for metastatic deposits of thyroid carcinoma. The high energy of the gamma emissions of ^{131}I makes this isotope less suited to modern gamma cameras, so the quality of images is not as good as that obtained with ^{123}I or ^{99m}Tc, but the 8-day half-life of ^{131}I permits scanning of the patient for many days after administration of a tracer dose.

TECHNETIUM-99M

Although not a radioiodine, ^{99m}Tc in the form of pertechnetate (TcO_4^-) is useful in imaging the thyroid and in a limited way in assessing thyroid gland function.[5] Because the pertechnetate ion has the same charge and (when its hydration shell is included) a similar size as iodide, it is trapped by the thyroid iodide-concentrating mechanism but is not incorporated into organic form. The physical half-life of ^{99m}Tc (6 hours), short residence time, and absence of beta emission are responsible for the low radiation exposure to the thyroid and the whole body. The gamma energy of this radionuclide (140 keV) renders it nearly ideal for imaging with modern scintillation cameras. Because ^{99m}Tc is available virtually around the clock in nearly all nuclear medicine laboratories and can be given in millicurie doses with low radiation exposure to the patient, ^{99m}Tc-pertechnetate is widely used for imaging the gland and in some laboratories for assessing the activity of the thyroid iodide trap, as discussed below.

TABLE 17-1.
Radionuclides Used for in Vivo Thyroid Studies

Radionuclide	Half-life	Principal Gamma Energy (MeV)	Radiation Exposure to Thyroid (cGy/mCi)*	Usual Dose Range (mCi)	Comment
^{123}I	13 h	0.159	13.0	0.1–0.4	Nearly ideal for uptake and imaging
^{124}I	4.2 d	0.511	890.0	—	Positron emitter (not in routine use)
^{125}I	60 d	0.035	790.0	—	Used only for in vitro tests
^{131}I	8 d	0.364	1,300.0	0.005–0.01 (uptake) 2–10 (imaging)	Used mainly for imaging thyroid cancer
^{99m}Tc	6 h	0.14	0.13	2–5	Widely available; excellent imaging agent

Radiation exposures (in centigray per millicurie administered) for radioiodines were calculated using the following assumptions: thyroid gland weight = 20 g (normal adult); maximal uptake = 25% of dose; half-time of uptake = 5 h; biologic half-life in gland = 65 d. The radiation exposure to the gland in infants and children is several-fold higher than in adults. The value for ^{123}I assumes no contamination with other radioiodines. The exposure calculations for radioiodines came from: MIRD: Dose Estimate Report No. 5 (J Nucl Med 1975;16:857) and those for ^{99m}Tc from: MIRD: Dose Estimate Report No. 8 (J Nucl Med 1977;17:74).

OTHER RADIONUCLIDES

Because of its long half-life (60 days) and its low-energy photon emissions, ^{125}I is rarely used for in vivo testing, except for intraoperative localization (see below). However, ^{125}I is widely used in diagnostic radioassays. In view of its widespread use in research laboratories (usually as a radiotracer of proteins), there is a potential for radiation exposure to the thyroid from accidentally internalized ^{125}I (see Table 17-1). The positron emitter, ^{124}I (half-life of 4.2 days), produces high-resolution images of the thyroid using positron emission tomography (PET). Because of the high cost of ^{124}I, the relatively high radiation exposure from this isotope, and the widespread availability of single photon emission computed tomography (SPECT; using ^{123}I or ^{99m}Tc) and limited number of PET facilities, ^{124}I is rarely used clinically. Thallium-201 (half-life of 73 hours), as thallous chloride, and the newer radiopharmaceutical agent, ^{99m}Tc-sestamibi, have been used for the localization of metastases from thyroid carcinoma. The advantages and limitations of these imaging agents in various thyroid disorders are discussed below.

THYROID UPTAKE OF RADIOIODINE (RAI-U)

Indications and Principle

Table 17-2 lists the major clinical indications for RAI-U testing. This list does not include investigational uses, such as kinetic studies of iodine metabolism.

The procedure involves the oral administration of a tracer dose of radioiodide followed by quantitation by external counting of the thyroid gland content of the tracer at given times after administration. RAI-U measures the fraction of the extrathyroidal iodide pool taken up by the thyroid in a given interval of time. Because the size of the iodide pool is not known without independent measurement, the RAI-U does not by itself provide the absolute amount of iodide taken up. The RAI-U is a function of several rates: the activity of the thyroid iodide-trapping mechanism, the rate of organic binding of the iodine within the gland, and the rate of release of iodine in all forms from the gland. When measured during the initial 4 to 6 hours after the dose, the thyroid content of radioiodine reflects mainly the rates of trapping and organification; at 24 hours and later times the "uptake" reflects these functions and the rate of release of radioiodine from the gland.

In the hyperthyroid individual with a small intrathyroid pool of iodine and rapid fractional turnover rate, the RAI-U at an early time (e.g., at 4 or 6 hours) is typically elevated but a late uptake (24 hours) may fall within the normal range. This "rapid turnover" pattern is observed in a small subgroup of hyperthyroid patients (see below). For this reason measurement of RAI-U at least at an early time (within 6 hours postdose) is recommended when the test is done for the diagnosis of hyperthyroidism.

Because the RAI-U is expressed as a percentage of the administered dose of radioiodine present in the gland at a given time, changes in the size of the extracellular pool of iodide affect the results. Other things being equal, an expansion of the iodide pool is associated with a decrease in the normal values

TABLE 17-2.
Clinical Indications for Thyroid Uptake Testing

Confirm the diagnosis of hyperthyroidism, when necessary

Distinguish other causes of thyrotoxicosis from hyperthyroidism

Provide data needed for calculation of a therapeutic dose of ^{131}I

Determine whether the thyroid is autonomously functioning (often combined with imaging of the gland)

Detect intrathyroid defects in organification (with perchlorate)

Determine whether a thyroid nodule is functioning

Estimate the volume of functioning thyroid

Determine whether a cervical or mediastinal mass contains functioning thyroid tissue

Determine whether functioning metastases from thyroid cancer are present and amenable to treatment with ^{131}I for RAI-U. In normal individuals, exposure to excessive iodine loads, especially if sustained for a period of days or weeks, leads to a reduction in RAI-U by virtue of complex physiologic adjustments in thyroid gland activity. (See chap 13 for a discussion of these mechanisms.)

Techniques and Results

RADIOIODINE UPTAKE

At the time the test is scheduled the patient or the referring physician is asked to provide information regarding current medications, recent radiographs with contrast agents, health foods and over-the-counter preparations that contain iodine, and menstrual history. Pregnancy and breast-feeding are contraindications to in vivo testing with radionuclides. The patient reports to the laboratory in the morning of the test. If measurement of uptake is planned within 4 hours of the oral dose of radioiodine, the patient is instructed to take no solid food from midnight until 2 hours after the dose. If there is a history of a recent nuclear medicine procedure, a preliminary "background" count over the neck is advised before administration of the radioiodine dose. In most laboratories ^{123}I is given in the form of a capsule, which is more convenient than the liquid form. However, dissolution of the capsule may be delayed for an hour or two in some patients, making early uptake measurements less reliable than later measurements (see below). The usual dose ranges of radionuclides for uptake testing and for imaging are listed in Table 17-1.

A dose standard is prepared before the dose is given to the patient. The same capsule that is to be given to the patient is inserted into a tissue-equivalent lucite neck phantom and counted with the same scintillation detector and geometry that is used in counting the patient. If the dose is in liquid form, an accurately measured aliquot is used as the standard. It is important to use the International Atomic Energy Agency (IAEA) "Standard Neck Phantom" to correct for tissue attenuation of the gamma photons from radioiodine.[6] Because the gamma energy of ^{123}I is lower than that of ^{131}I, extreme variations in the size of the thyroid and in thickness of the neck lead to greater errors in RAI-U with ^{123}I than with [131]I. Methods of correction for variable tissue attenuation in patients with very large goiters or thick necks have been proposed.[7] The usual type of scintillation counting equipment includes a detector, which consists of a 2-inch sodium iodide crystal housed in lead shield and fitted with a flat-field collimator, a spectrometer (pulse-height analyzer), and scaler. The spectrometer is set usually with a 20% window centered on the peak energy of the radioiodine (159 keV in the case of ^{123}I).[8] Commercially available thyroid uptake units often feature a dedicated computer that automatically calculates uptake from the counting rate of the dose standard and of the patient. Whatever type of equipment is used, a stable high-voltage power supply and spectrometer are essential. One potential source of error is voltage variation resulting in a shift in the gamma energy window, so periodic quality control checks are important to ascertain uniform efficiency of the counting equipment.[9] The distance from the detector to the patient's neck must be the same as the distance from the detector to the neck phantom.

Correction for neck "background," that is, radioactivity in the neck outside of the thyroid, is estimated in many laboratories by counting over the midthigh at the same detector-to-skin distance as that used for neck counting. Alternatively, a background neck count is taken with a 2×2-inch lead shield suspended over the neck to cover the thyroid. Whichever method is used to correct for extrathyroidal neck counts, this correction is especially important when measuring uptake at early times (<6 hours postdose).

$$\text{Thyroid Uptake (\%)} = \frac{(\text{Net CPM over Neck} - \text{Net CPM over Thigh}) \times 100}{\text{Net CPM over Dose Std} \times R \times F}$$

where Net CPM are counts/min minus room background, R is the ratio of dose administered to dose in the standard, and F is the factor that corrects for physical decay of the isotope between the time of counting the dose standard and the patient.

The normal range of thyroid uptake values varies from one region to another and from time to time. It is essential that each laboratory establish its own reference values. In the laboratory of one of the authors (RRC) the normal ranges are 2% to 12% at 2 hours, 5% to 15% at 6 hours, and 8% to 35% at 24 hours. The lower limit is less well defined than the upper limit because of variable iodine intake in euthyroid individuals.

Variations on the RAI-U

NECK/THIGH RATIO

This is a simple index that is useful in confirming the thyroid uptake determination at early times postdose and that does not require additional patient measurements. The counting rate over the (unshielded) neck divided by the counting rate over the midthigh (N:T ratio), both counts done at 2 hours postdose of radioiodine, was shown many years ago to correlate well with thyroid iodide clearance.[10]

$$\text{Neck/Thigh Ratio (at time t)} = \text{CPM over Neck(t)/CPM over Thigh(t)}$$

where both neck and thigh counts are obtained at the same time, t, postdose. Both counts are gross counts, uncorrected for room background. The N:T ratio can be performed at any time up to 6 hours postdose, but it is not useful at later times because of the low thigh counts after 6 hours. Of course, each laboratory must determine its own normal range for a given time. In the experience of one of the authors (RRC), the upper limit of normal for the N:T ratio at 2 hours is 4.2 and at 6 hours is 42. There is no lower limit of normal. If the N:T ratio is determined at the same time as the thyroid uptake measurement, no additional patient measurements need to be made. We have found that a plot of the N:T ratio versus the 6-hour RAI-U is hyperbolic, with the N:T ratio rising faster than the RAI-U as one goes from the euthyroid to the hyperthyroid state, so the N:T ratio in the hyperthyroid patient typically is more markedly elevated than is the RAI-U. This is understandable because the thyroid (neck) counts increase at the expense of the extrathyroid (thigh) counts. The N:T ratio offers two other advantages: it is a quality control check on the measurement of the dose standard, and it is independent of variations in the rate and extent of absorption of the dose of radioiodine.

UPTAKE OF ⁹⁹ᵐTC-PERTECHNETATE

Some laboratories where ⁹⁹ᵐTc-pertechnetate is used routinely for thyroid imaging use this agent also to estimate thyroid uptake, that is, thyroid trapping activity. The thyroid uptake of pertechnetate is normally rapid, but because it is not organified and retained, peak activity in the gland is reached at 20 to 30 minutes after intravenous administration of the dose.[5,11–13] At this time extrathyroid activity is high, so correction for background in the neck is essential. This correction is made in any of several ways (see above). Thigh counting offers a reasonable method, but due to rapid changes in circulating ⁹⁹ᵐTc concentration, simultaneous counting of neck and thigh is required.[14] Alternatively, sufficiently accurate determination of ⁹⁹ᵐTc uptake by the thyroid can be done by using a scintillation camera and defining one region of interest to include the gland and another to include a nearby background region in the neck (avoiding salivary glands).[11,13,15,16] Of course, a dose standard must be counted in a neck phantom. In normal individuals the peak thyroid uptake of ⁹⁹ᵐTc ranges from 0.2% to 3.5% of the dose.[11,12,16] Some have found the N:T ratio using ⁹⁹ᵐTc at 15 minutes postdose intravenously to be useful in the diagnosis of hyperthyroidism in children[15] and in adults.[14] The advantages of the use of ⁹⁹ᵐTc-pertechnetate and the 15-minute N:T ratio are the ready availability of this radiopharmaceutical, its low radiation exposure to the patient (as little as 10–20 μCi is sufficient), and the lack of a need to prepare and measure a dose standard. The normal values for N:T ratio must of course be determined by each laboratory because variations in type of counting equipment and in geometry of counting will affect the results.

FACTORS INFLUENCING RADIOIODINE UPTAKE TESTS

The environmental factors, diseases, and drugs that influence the RAI-U are listed in Table 17-3. In the following discussion it is worth keeping in mind that these factors generally alter both the N:T ratio and the percent uptake value in a parallel manner, and with few exceptions early uptake values are affected as well as late (24 hours) uptake results. The thyroid uptake of ⁹⁹ᵐTc-pertechnetate is affected in a similar manner.

Iodine

The most important single factor determining RAI-U is the iodine intake. Day-to-day fluctuations in dietary iodine, provided the load of excess iodine is less than 1 mg and not sustained, have no noticeable effect on RAI-U, particularly in North America, where the typical daily intake is 0.3 to 0.7 mg.[17] In areas of the world where iodine intake is much lower, close to the recommended minimum of 0.07 mg/d, small increments (0.5–1.0 mg) in excess of this level lead to a significant reduction of RAI-U. There are geographic variations in dietary iodine even within North America. It is necessary, therefore, that the reference range for the thyroid uptake test and any of its variations be determined within each locale. Because changes occur from time to time in the practice of adding iodine in one form or another to certain foods, such as bread and cereals, it is also important to check the reference range at periodic intervals.

TABLE 17-3.
Factors That Influence Thyroid Radioiodine Uptake

CAUSING *INCREASED* UPTAKE

Hyperthyroidism
Iodine deficiency
Pregnancy (normal)
Hydatidiform mole; choriocarcinoma
Recovery phase of subacute or other destructive thyroiditis
Rebound after suppression of TSH
Rebound phase after withdrawal of iodine or other antithyroid drugs (if TSH is elevated)
Lithium administration
Excessive excretion of thyroid hormone
Chronic thyroiditis (if TSH is elevated)
Inborn errors of thyroid hormonogenesis

CAUSING *DECREASED* UPTAKE

Primary hypothyroidism (athyreotic or atrophic type)
Status postthyroidectomy, postradioiodine, or postradiotherapy
Central hypothyroidism (secondary or tertiary type)
Thyroid hormone administration
Destructive (eg, subacute) thyroiditis (active phase)
Lymphocytic painless thyroiditis (postpartum or sporadic)
Renal failure with iodide retention
Iodine excess (See chap 14)
Drugs other than those containing iodine:
  Thionamides (decrease in later phases of uptake)
  Aromatic compounds (sulfonamides, PAS)
  Monovalent anions (perchlorate, thiocyanate)
  Glucocorticoids (in large doses, acutely)
  Salicylates (in large doses, more than 5 g/d)
  Drugs having minor effect: phenylbutazone, resorcinol, aminoglutethimide, sulfonylureas

Exposure to larger amounts of iodine (10 mg or more), particularly if exposure is prolonged for days, predictably leads to a progressive reduction in RAI-U. The immediate effect is one of dilution of the tracer dose in an expanded extrathyroidal iodide pool and saturation of the thyroid iodide trap, but within a few days, physiologic mechanisms are called into play to reduce the activity of the thyroid trap and subsequent steps of iodine metabolism within the gland (see chap 13). For a given increment in iodine intake and the more prolonged the exposure, the greater the reduction in RAI-U. Sternthal and coworkers found that a single oral dose of 30 mg iodide, administered to normal adults at the same time as a tracer dose of ¹²³I, resulted in a lowering of the 24-hour thyroid uptake of ¹²³I to 1.5% of the dose.[18] The same authors found that only 15 mg iodine, given daily for 12 days, gave a similar reduction in RAI-U as the larger single dose.[18] With an increase in the delay between the time of administration of the radioiodine dose and the time the dose of stable iodine is given, there is a progressive decrease in the effect on the RAI-U because radioiodine already taken up and organified cannot be discharged from the thyroid with excess iodine.[19] This fact has relevance for any program designed to protect individuals who work with radioiodine and members of the public living in the vicinity of nuclear reactors.[20]

A list of iodine-containing agents is presented in chapter 14. The most frequent source of excess iodine among patients undergoing diagnostic testing is radiographic contrast agents, which contain gram quantities of stable iodine in each dose administered. The iodide released in vivo from these agents is responsible for the suppression of thyroid RAI-U. The duration of the effect varies with the nature of the contrast agent, the quantity administered, and the patient's thyroid and renal functional status. The more frequently used radiographic agents are water soluble and excreted by the kidneys. These contrast agents reduce RAI-U typically for periods of 3 to 4 weeks in individuals with normal thyroid and renal function, but the effect may last longer in patients with reduced renal clearance. The effect of lipid-soluble contrast agents persists for months. In hyperthyroid patients the effect of radiographic contrast agents on thyroid uptake of radioiodine may be of shorter duration due to the great avidity of the thyroid for iodine in most of these patients. In patients who develop iodine- induced hypothyroidism (with elevated serum thyrotropin [TSH]), the RAI-U is usually low during the period when iodine is being administered but often shows a rebound to elevated levels after the discontinuation of iodine.[21] Similarly, individuals with iodine-induced hyperthyroidism may show normal or depressed thyroid uptake values during exposure to excess iodine and a rebound in uptake to elevated levels after removal of the iodine.

Among drugs that contain iodine, amiodarone, which contains 37% iodine, has long-lasting effects due to the prolonged half-life of this drug in the body of the order of months. Amiodarone-induced hypothyroidism, which is more common in regions where iodine intake is high (e.g., in the United States), is associated with a low thyroid uptake, as would be expected. Individuals with hyperthyroidism induced by amiodarone, a complication encountered more commonly in Europe than in the United States, may have a normal or elevated RAI-U.[22,23] (See chap 14 for further details of the topic.)

Administration of thyroid hormones, by suppressing TSH secretion, reduces RAI-U in patients whose thyroid glands are not autonomously functioning. Thyroxine (T_4), given in replacement doses, has a somewhat longer lasting effect (4–5 weeks) after withdrawal of the hormone than triiodothyronine (T_3), which in physiologic doses suppresses uptake for about 2 weeks. However, when either hormone is given in supraphysiologic doses the suppressive effect on TSH and on thyroid uptake may last much longer, for example, for 2 months or more after withdrawal of the hormone.[24]

Iodine Deficiency

Although some progress has been made in prevention of the most serious effects of extreme iodine deficiency in many parts of the world, in some regions the intake of this vital element remains less than adequate. The thyroid gland responds to iodine deficiency by increasing the efficiency of the thyroid iodide trap and thus euthyroidism is maintained (see chap 14). Even in regions where iodine intake is adequate among the general population, an occasional individual is encountered in whom restrictions or idiosyncrasies in diet may be associated with a borderline or frankly low intake of iodine. In such cases the RAI-U will be elevated compared to the uptake in the population with an adequate iodine intake. In the evaluation of patients with abnormally high uptake values (relative to that in the normal population), it is important to obtain a dietary history. Measurement of the 24-hour urinary (stable) iodine excretion may be helpful in establishing a low iodine intake as the cause of the "high" thyroid uptake. An inverse correlation between thyroid trapping function, as assessed by ^{99m}Tc uptake, and the urinary excretion of iodine has been observed in an endemic goiter region.[25] Similarly, when excess iodine is suspected as the cause of low uptake, measurement of urinary iodine may be useful. However, because urinary excretion reflects current rather than prior dietary intake, this measurement may be misleading.

Drugs Other Than Those That Contain Iodine

A variety of drugs affect iodine metabolism in the thyroid. The effect of a particular agent on the thyroid uptake depends on the mechanism of action of the drug. The commonly used antithyroid drugs of the thionamide class (propylthiouracil, methimazole, carbimazole) inhibit the steps leading to thyroid hormone synthesis subsequent to iodide trapping. As a consequence these agents have a greater effect on late uptake than on early (i.e., 2-hour) uptake values. Sulfonamides, *p*-aminosalicylic acid, resorcinol, and sulfonylureas (in large doses) have an effect on thyroid iodine metabolism similar to the action of thionamides but in general are less potent. In contrast, perchlorate (used in some countries as an antithyroid agent) and thiocyanate (no longer used clinically) inhibit the thyroid iodide trap and thereby diminish both early and late uptake values. Lithium has a unique action on the thyroid: this drug inhibits the release of thyroid hormone but not the transport of iodide or its organification, with the result that RAI-U is unimpaired and may in fact be elevated due to prolonged retention of radioiodine in the gland.[26] After discontinuation of any agent that inhibits thyroid function there may be a transient rebound in RAI-U because the elevated TSH outlasts for a time the effect of the inhibitor.

Results in Hyperthyroid States

In most patients with hyperthyroidism of Graves' disease the RAI-U is elevated. Because the residence time in the gland is usually abnormally short (biologic $T_{1/2}$ of 30 days or less in contrast to the normal 90 days), the early uptake measurements tend to be increased to a greater degree than the 24-hour value. Indeed, in a small proportion of these patients the 24-hour uptake may fall within the normal range, but the uptake in the 2- to 6-hour interval postdose is more often above normal. The prevalence of cases with a small, rapidly turning over intrathyroidal iodine pool varies depending on how these are defined, but as many as 15% of thyrotoxic patients may show this phenomenon.[27] In addition, age has an effect on the RAI-U in hyperthyroid individuals. Using a normal range established in their own laboratory, Caplan and colleagues studied untreated cases of Graves' disease in patients of various ages and found the 24-hour uptake within the normal range in 15% of patients under age 65 and in 27% of those over 65 years of age.[28] More recently, a study of thyrotoxic patients over age 75, most of whom had Graves' disease, revealed that the 24-hour RAI-U was within the normal range in 5 of 18 patients tested.[29] Even when measured at early times postdose, the RAI-U may be normal in a significant number of elderly hyperthyroid individuals; these tend to be Graves' patients with normal-size thyroids (unpublished observation).

In general, patients with toxic nodular goiter, either due to a single hyperfunctioning adenoma or to a toxic multinodular goiter, have lower radioiodine uptake values than do patients with Graves' disease. The 24-hour RAI-U was normal in nearly two-thirds of patients with toxic nodular goiter.[28,30,31] Part of this difference between the two conditions may be due to the fact that patients with toxic nodular goiter are on average older than those with Graves' disease.

Despite the limited sensitivity of the test, particularly in the elderly, the positive predictive value of an elevated thyroid uptake is high and helps to confirm the diagnosis in a patient in whom clinical and in vitro laboratory data suggest hyperthyroidism.

Thyrotoxicosis Not Due to Hyperthyroidism

Thyrotoxicosis, defined as an excess of circulating free thyroid hormones, is in most cases due to excessive activity of the thyroid gland, but there are other causes of the thyrotoxic state. These include destructive thyroiditides (subacute thyroiditis, "silent" thyroiditis, postpartum thyroiditis) and thyrotoxicosis factitia. In each of these instances the RAI-U may provide the important clue that leads to the correct diagnosis because the RAI-U is typically extremely low in these patients.[32,33]

Effects of Age and Gender

Thyroid uptake values are not significantly different in children and in adults,[34] but there is a slight decrease in euthyroid values with advancing age.[35] Other factors, particularly iodine intake, have a more marked effect on RAI-U, masking any influence of age. There are no significant differences between RAI-U values for male or female subjects.[36]

Effects of Nonthyroid Illness

Probably the most common reason for a decreased RAI-U in hospitalized patients is the administration of radiographic contrast dyes. However, abnormalities in thyroid function tests are frequently abnormal in patients who have no clinical evidence of thyroid dysfunction. Although it has not been studied as extensively as in vitro tests of thyroid function, RAI-U may be abnormally low in patients with severe systemic nonthyroid illness to the degree that their serum TSH concentration is diminished. The lowest levels of serum TSH are seen in patients given large doses of glucocorticoids or dopamine, and one would expect the RAI-U to be low in these cases. An increase in renal iodide excretion induced by glucocorticoids may be an additional factor in reducing RAI-U as a result of the competition for iodide between the thyroid and the kidneys. In moderate to severe renal insufficiency the urinary excretion of iodide is diminished.

The extracellular iodide pool is usually expanded in such patients and RAI-U is reduced but not to the same extent as renal clearance, so early thyroid uptake and measures of thyroid iodide clearance (e.g., N:T ratio) are only mildly decreased. Because the radioiodide tracer remains in the circulation longer than normal in renal insufficiency, the maximum uptake in the thyroid is attained later than usual (i.e., 48 hours rather than 24 hours), but this rarely poses a diagnostic problem.

TESTS FOR INTRATHYROID DEFECTS IN IODINE METABOLISM

The transport of iodide into the thyroid is normally the rate-limiting step in iodine metabolism in the gland. Any of the subsequent steps in the process of hormonogenesis, including oxidation and organic binding of iodine to tyrosine residues of thyroglobulin catalyzed by thyroid peroxidase and coupling of iodotyrosines to form the hormones, may be impaired by genetic defects, by disease (e.g., thyroiditis), or by thionamide drugs. The most common defect in thyroid hormonogenesis involves the organification step. This abnormality can be detected in vivo by the perchlorate discharge test. The standard procedure involves a measurement of the thyroid uptake of radioiodine at 2 and 3 hours postdose, followed by the oral administration of a solution of 1 g potassium perchlorate (adult dose) and continued measurement of the thyroid content of radioiodine for an additional 1 to 2 hours. A decrease in thyroid radioiodine content of more than 10% of the value obtained immediately before the perchlorate is a positive test and indicates a defect in organification of trapped iodide. The extent of perchlorate-induced "washout" of thyroidal radioiodide reflects the severity of the organification block. In addition to its use in the detection of genetic abnormalities of thyroid hormonogenesis, this test has been used to study the duration of action of methimazole in patients.[37]

A modification of the perchlorate discharge test that provides increased sensitivity involves giving a small dose (0.5 mg) of stable iodine (as KI) with the radioiodine tracer. A discharge of more than 20% of the thyroidal radioiodine content following administration of the perchlorate (at 2 or 3 hours after radioiodine) indicates impaired organification. A positive iodide-perchlorate test has been found in patients with chronic autoimmune thyroiditis[38,39] and in many patients with untreated hyperthyroidism, probably indicating an abnormal sensitivity of the gland to the Wolff-Chaikoff effect.[40]

SPECIAL IN VIVO TESTS

Methods were developed years ago for quantitation of various phases of iodine metabolism in patients and are still used in clinical investigation, but these are rarely used today for diagnostic purposes. These methods include thyroid iodide clearance (which usually requires measurements of circulating radioiodide concentration as well as measurement of thyroid gland activity), absolute thyroid iodide uptake, thyroid iodine secretion rate, plasma protein-bound radioiodine concentration, and in vivo kinetics studies of thyroid hormone distribution and metabolism.

THYROID SCINTIGRAPHY

Thyroid scintigraphy allows the physician to determine function and structure of thyroid tissue. Scintigraphy can determine whether midline masses contain thyroid and whether solitary or multiple nodules are functional or not. It can demonstrate whether metastases from thyroid cancer concentrate iodine and would be amenable to treatment with radioiodine. The discussion below reviews the choice of radiopharmaceutical, instrumentation, and normal findings before describing scintigraphy in specific pathologic situations. The importance of careful clinical examination for correlation with scintigraphy, and on occasion, in place of scintigraphy, is stressed.

TECHNIQUES

Choice of Radiopharmaceutical

The two commonly used radiopharmaceuticals for standard imaging are ^{123}I and ^{99m}Tc as pertechnetate (TcO$_4$) (see Table 17-1). The usual dose of ^{123}I for imaging is 200 to 400 μCi orally. It is not necessary for the patient to be fasted, but it is necessary for a review of medications, foodstuffs, and sources of iodine to be excluded before administering the dose. A comprehensive list of iodine-containing medications is shown in chapter 14. ^{123}I is trapped by functioning thyroid, organified, and retained. Iodine is trapped by other tissues including salivary glands, choroid plexus, gastric parietal cells, and parietal cells in a Meckel's diverticulum and lactating mammary tissue. With the exception of iodine lost in milk, the remainder is recycled in the extracellular iodide pool. The radioiodine not retained in the thyroid is excreted by the kidneys. Uptakes in these sites must be considered when scintigrams are interpreted.

Technetium-99m is given by intravenous injection. The dose used varies considerably and ranges from 1 to 10 mCi. In general, if the clinician suspects that the uptake will be low a higher dose can be given. This radiopharmaceutical is trapped by follicular cells but not organified. Therefore, imaging should be done early before there is leakage out of the thyroid. The standard time is 20 minutes, but imaging can be started seconds after the injection in hyperfunctioning glands. Because of the high photon flux, it is possible to do dynamic imaging of the entry of pertechnetate into the thyroid.[41] This has limited clinical usefulness but has been used to provide instantaneous diagnosis of Graves' hyperthyroidism in a delirious patient.[42] There is usually more background activity on pertechnetate scan because the thyroidal uptake is lower and because imaging is done sooner after administration of the isotope. Pertechnetate is also trapped by the tissues that trap iodine, as listed previously. Because of secretion of ^{99m}Tc into saliva, radioisotope in the esophagus superimposed on the thyroid can cause confusion with interpretation. It is advisable that the patient drink water immediately before scintigraphy to obviate this problem.

Iodine-131 has an important role in scintigraphy of patients with differentiated thyroid cancer who have had surgical treatment. This radionuclide emits beta particles, which are valuable for treatment, plus a gamma photon that can be imaged. The photon energy is higher than desirable for conventional nuclear imaging devices and the resolution of the images are of modest quality. However, ^{131}I can determine where therapy will localize and to quantitate the uptake in lesions.

Other Radionuclides and Radiopharmaceuticals

Several other tracers have limited value in evaluating specific aspects of thyroid disease. Because most of these isotopes are used in patients with thyroid cancer, they are discussed later.

IMAGING TECHNIQUES

Gamma Camera

Routine thyroid imaging is conducted using a gamma camera fitted with a pinhole collimator. The aperture is usually 2 to 5 mm and inserts of different dimensions are available.

The pinhole is about 20 to 25 cm from the detector head and the conical collimator constructed with lead or dense metal. The collimator and detector function like a box camera. The image is "inverted" and magnified by the ratio of the length of the collimator/distance from pinhole to thyroid. Because of the magnification, this collimator does not give a linear representation of tissues at different depths. As a result, the scintiscan is not absolutely identical to the true structure. Nevertheless, the resolution is good, the time for imaging reasonable, and ^{99m}Tc, ^{123}I, and ^{131}I can be imaged. A minimum of 100,000 counts should be obtained for scintiscans of ^{99m}Tc and 30,000 to 50,000 counts for ^{123}I scans. An anterior image is standard and oblique images can easily be obtained[44] to further delineate the thyroid architecture.[43] It is important that a clinician examine the patient at the time of scintigraphy to determine the site of abnormalities such as nodules and use a radioactive marker held over or adjacent to the lesions. The marker(s) is superimposed on the scan at these sites. Therefore, what is seen on scan and what is noted clinically are correlated, avoiding imaging pitfalls.[45]

Rectilinear Scanner

The rectilinear scanner has a probe with a sodium iodide crystal and a focused collimator that moves back and forth over the area of interest. It builds up the image in lines with dots representing radioactive incidents. The distribution of radioactivity in the patient is translated into an image that is the integration of these dots. Areas with more radioactivity appear dark, and those with less appear light. This difference is accentuated by the fact that the dots increase in intensity as the count rate increases. The image is life size. However, resolution is inferior to gamma camera images. In addition, the instrument is inflexible and oblique views cannot be obtained. Vendors of nuclear medicine equipment do not make rectilinear scanners and parts and service are scarce.

Overall, pinhole images are superior to rectilinear images in higher sensitivity (97% versus 69%), specificity (90% versus 86%), and overall accuracy (94% versus 77%).[46] In addition, the time for imaging is less.

Single Photon Emission Computed Tomography

This technique produces various tomographic and three-dimensional images. Images of organs including the thyroid are acquired by rotating the head of the gamma camera through 6° steps up to 180° to 360°. Any of the radiopharmaceuticals discussed above can be imaged by SPECT and the equipment is readily available. The data collected are reconstructed using a computer and transverse, sagittal, or coronal images produced. Chen and colleagues[47] demonstrated that SPECT was superior to planar imaging in defining functional anatomy in two patients with multinodular goiter and tracheal compression. A second study showed good correlation of SPECT with planar imaging in four patients with hypofunctioning nodules. However, in five patients with palpable nodules and normal planar scintigrams, SPECT showed that one nodule was hypofunctional, one hyperfunctional, and three equivocal.[48] In most cases it is unlikely that SPECT will add much to clinical examination. Volume measurements can be made with precision and this might help in calculation of the therapeutic dose of ^{131}I for Graves' hyperthyroidism and thyroid cancer.[49] Chen and colleagues[47] found volume determined by SPECT was 108 ± 7% of true weight in surgically removed glands. SPECT can demonstrate deeply positioned small lesions such as metastases in lung or liver. Its role in detecting metastases is described below in the section on ^{201}Tl.

Positron Emission Tomography (PET)

Positrons are positive electrons that when emitted from a radionuclide interact with an electron. These two particles annihilate one another and their mass is conserved as energy in the form of two gamma photons of 511-keV energy, which are emitted at an angle of 180°. For positron imaging of the thyroid, ^{124}I is used and images obtained by reconstructing data obtained by coincidence counting from a ring or rings of collimators positioned round the area of interest in the patient. This technique is experimental and most clinical nuclear medicine laboratories do not have a positron camera. The radionuclides are short lived and their availability often requires a dedicated cyclotron. Reports demonstrate that the technique provides excellent resolution and that the distribution of radioiodine judged by planar imaging to be uniform is in fact inhomogeneous.[50] The contrast in activity between lesion and surrounding tissue is better than that obtained by conventional imaging. The images do not allow benign nodules to be differentiated from malignant nodules. Studies evaluating the ratio of uptake in the nodule, compared to normal thyroid, might help.[51] Thyroid volume can be calculated with precision using positron scintigraphy. F-18 deoxyglucose is a positron emitter that has demonstrated nonfunctioning metastases in a small number of patients. This approach has to be compared with other more commonly available and used radiopharmaceuticals that are discussed later.

Intraoperative Scintigraphy

This technique allows surgeons to detect small remnants of functioning thyroid at the time of operation. It is not widely used. One technique involves giving the patient 500 μCi ^{125}I a day before operation. No thyroid medications are prescribed. A small handheld cadmium telluride detector picks up radioactive counts that can be read from a dose meter or by sound. Lennquist and colleagues[52] studied 64 patients and found counts in 43 of 64 patients undergoing total thyroidectomy. In 33 of the 43 patients the source of the counts could be removed. The investigators concluded that the test helps prove that all functioning thyroid is removed, making the need for postoperative radioiodine less and interpretation of TSH levels simpler. The rationale for this approach is not convincing for the average patient, but the test could have limited value in selected patients. These probes can also be used to detect sites of uptake of cancer-seeking radiopharmaceuticals such as ^{111}In-octreotide or ^{99m}Tc-sestamibi, which are discussed later. ^{125}I cannot be used for scintigraphy with a gamma camera because its photon energies are too low.

Fluorescent Scanning

This imaging technique does not involve the use of radionuclides and no material has to be administered to the patient. The test is based on the principle of directing photons whose energies are greater than the binding energy of inner (K) shell electrons of iodine. The incident photon causes the K-shell electron to be ejected from its orbit thus creating a "gap" that is filled by an outer (L) shell electron moving into the vacancy. The difference in binding energy between the L and K shells is emitted as a characteristic x-ray (fluorescence), which has an energy of 28.5 keV. The energy of the fluorescent x-rays is sufficiently high to be imaged and because the number of x-ray emissions is proportional to the amount of iodine in the thyroid, quantitative measurements can be made by comparing patient counts with those from known standards. The most frequently used source of photons is Americium (^{241}Am), which emits gamma photons of 59.6 keV. The test provides qualitative and quantitative data of the distribution of natural, nonradioactive ^{127}I in the thyroid.[53]

The spatial resolution of the scan is not as good as that of images using ^{123}I or ^{99m}Tc. Because no systemic radiation is used, fluorescent scanning can be done when imaging is necessary during pregnancy or lactation.

The thyroidal iodine content in normal subjects in the United States ranges from 5 to 15 mg. Lower values are found in primary hypothyroidism. In untreated Graves' disease the mean value in one study was 36.5 mg.[54] The iodine content of the thyroid in hyperthyroidism can be normal (Cavalieri, unpublished observations). As the dietary iodine falls so does the thyroidal iodine, and the normal range in France is 2.5 to 7.5 mg. High values are found in patients who have had iodine contrast or have been treated with iodine-rich medications such as amiodarone.

Because malignant nodules have less uptake of radioiodine than surrounding normal tissue as judged by autoradiography, it was hoped that fluorescent imaging would differentiate thyroid cancers from nonmalignant lesions. Patton and Sandler[54] calculated the ratio of iodine in a nodule with that in the opposite lobe and when the result was less than 0.6 they correctly identified 37 of 38 cancers. Unfortunately, ratios in 41 of 112 benign nodules fell into the same range. Thus, the test has poor discriminative value.

The radiation to patients from fluorescent scanning is about 20 to 40 mrad to the thyroid and there is no systemic radiation. The equipment is not universally available and despite the safety of the procedure and its ability to quantitate iodine content, it has not gained wide acceptance because it seldom adds new information to that available from clinical examination and biochemical tests.

Transmission Scanning

This form of scan is obtained by placing a source of radiation behind the patient who is positioned in front of the gamma camera. ^{99m}Tc or ^{57}Co are potential sources of radiation. Emitted photons are attenuated by tissues in proportion to their density. An outline of the patient is obtained and there is less attenuation by the thorax because of the lungs. This is a "poor man's" radiograph. It can be used to provide anatomic landmarks that can be superimposed on radioiodine scintiscans, which demonstrate functioning metastases without adequate localizing information.

NORMAL THYROID SCINTISCAN

The lobes of the gland appear as pear-shaped homogeneous structures as shown in Figure 17-1. The long axis is approximately 5 cm and the widest transverse diameter about 2 to 3 cm. A slight degree of asymmetry is common and the right lobe is larger more often. Detailed measurements of dimensions and methods of determining volume are in practice not important.[55-58] Many variations have been described[59] and knowledge of these is important in interpreting abnormalities. Visualization of the pyramidal lobe, which is the inferior vestige of the thy-

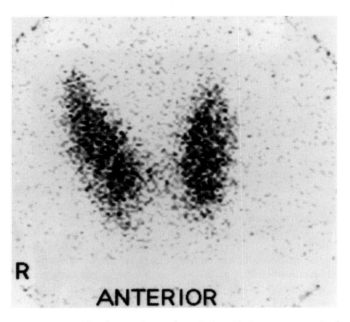

FIGURE 17-1. This figure shows normal thyroid. Image was made 6 hours after an oral dose of 200 μCi ^{123}I. The lobes are symmetric and the isthmus is not well visualized. Patient had mild symptoms suggestive of hyperthyroidism but no signs. Thyroid was not palpable. Free T$_4$ and TSH levels were normal.

roglossal tract, is more frequent in Graves' disease and Hashimoto's thyroiditis. Levy and colleagues[60] observed pyramidal lobes in 29 of 46 hyperthyroid patients with Graves' disease, but in only 4 of 51 euthyroid subjects, although others have found a higher percentage in normal patients.[61] The pyramidal lobe can arise from the medial aspect of either lobe or the isthmus and its shape can be pyramidal, linear, oval, or beaded. When patients are imaged after thyroidectomy for thyroid cancer, the pyramidal lobe, if left, can be misinterpreted as a lymph node metastasis.[62] There is a tendency for the thyroid to become more inferior with advancing age.

PATHOPHYSIOLOGY

Abnormal Descent and Development

Failure of the thyroid to migrate to its normal cervical position can result in functioning thyroid at any point from the foramen cecum at the base of the tongue to the pyramidal lobe. In a patient with suspected lingual thyroid an ^{123}I scintiscan would quickly establish the diagnosis without need for biopsy.[63] Apart from goiter, cysts in the thyroglossal duct are the most common midline lesions.[64] However, maldescended thyroid is common and its management is different from a thyroglossal cyst. Thyroglossal cysts seldom contain sufficient follicular tissue to be imaged.[65] Therefore, in a patient with a midline anterior neck mass an ^{123}I scintiscan will usually clarify the diagnosis. Ectopic thyroid is seen on scan, whereas thyroglossal cyst is not. Very rarely ectopic thyroid is found inferior to the cervical thyroid, even in the heart.[66] In these cases its discovery and identification are usually fortuitous, and when thyroid histology is documented, it is important to ensure that the tissue is benign and ectopic rather than malignant. Rare cases have been diagnosed scintigraphically.

Hemiagenesis with absence of a lobe or lobe and isthmus is rare. Hamburger and Hamburger[67] found 4 from 7000 scintigrams. In general, patients having scintigraphy have a reason for the test. Therefore, the true incidence could be different. The left lobe is absent four times as often as the right[68,69] and women are about three times more likely to have this developmental defect.[69] Many of these patients are hyperthyroid or have a palpable abnormality in the lobe, which brings them to medical attention. The main differential diagnosis is a functioning nodule with suppression of normal thyroid. The scintigraphic appearance of hemiagenesis, where only a lobe is missing, is characteristic and unlikely to be mistaken for a hot nodule. The thyroid looks like a "hockey stick."[69] When both a lobe and isthmus are absent, the remaining lobe can be confused with functioning nodule, especially when the patient is hyperthyroid. Methods of showing absence versus suppression of a lobe include using ultrasonography,[70] thallium (^{201}Tl),[71] ^{99m}Tc-sestamibi[72]; shielding the site of ^{123}I uptake with a lead shield and imaging longer[73]; or giving parenteral TSH and repeating the ^{123}I scintigram.

Hyperthyroidism

In Graves' disease the gland is diffusely enlarged and there is increased uptake of ^{123}I; consequently there is little or no background activity. Just as there are variations in the appearance

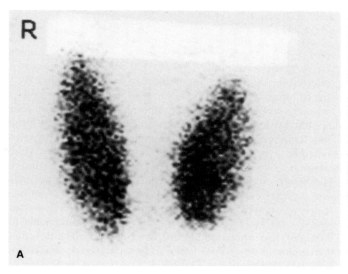

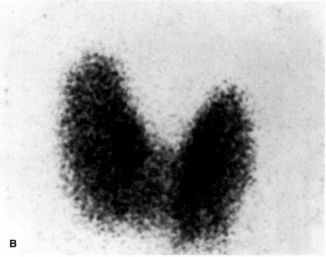

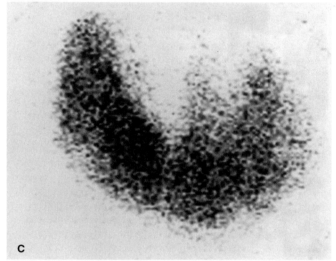

FIGURE 17-2. All scintiscans are from three patients with Graves' hyperthyroidism. They were made 4, 6, and 24 hours after 200 μCi ^{123}I. (*A*) Shows the thyroid lobes are enlarged, the isthmus is imaged, and there is almost no background activity. (*B*) Shows a similar appearance but the isthmus was not visualized. (*C*) Shows a larger gland with both right and left lobes and isthmus demonstrating increased uptake that measured 65% at 24 hours. There is also a pyramidal lobe arising from the medial aspect of the left lobe; this is found most frequently in autoimmune thyroid disease, especially Graves' disease. In each patient the uptake was considerably elevated (60-80%).

of the normal thyroid, likewise the shape of the gland in Graves' hyperthyroidism can vary considerably. Figure 17-2 shows the range of findings. Does the scintiscan help with diagnosis and management? In most patients with a clinically apparent diffusely enlarged thyroid an uptake measurement is sufficient.[74] A number of syndromes are associated with biochemical and clinical thyrotoxicosis but with low uptake of radioiodine. Figure 17-3 shows an example. However, in this situation an uptake measurement is often adequate. Occasionally a patient who has recently been treated for hyperthyroidism with ^{131}I is referred for another scintigraphic study, such as a bone or heart scan. It should be remembered that the high-energy photons will interfere with these investigations.[75]

Solitary Thyroid Nodule

Scintigraphy has been used in evaluating thyroid nodules for the following reasons. First, functioning nodules, especially those showing increased uptake in relation to normal thyroid, have a low probability of being malignant. Secondly, based on

autoradiographic studies, thyroid cancers concentrate less radioiodine (1/100) than normal tissue. Therefore, cancers should appear hypofunctioning or cold on scintiscan. However, most benign nodules are also cold. In addition, not all cancers are cold. Figure 17-4 shows a typical hyperfunctioning nodule in a patient with mild hyperthyroidism. The remainder of the gland is "suppressed." Figure 17-5 shows a typical nonfunctioning nodule. In both situations it is important to prove that the palpable lesion corresponds with the nodule on scintiscan. In some functioning nodules there can be central degeneration that produces a cold region within the hot nodule. This does not indicate malignancy. This has been likened to an "owl's eye" (Fig 17-6). It is generally accepted that the most cost-effective method of evaluating a solitary thyroid nodule in a euthyroid patient is fine-needle aspiration biopsy.[76–78]

A palpable nodule implies a greater thickness than surrounding tissue. Therefore, if it appears to have equal activity to adjacent tissue, the palpable lesion is probably hypofunctional, or nonfunctional, rather than normofunctional. Terminology has been inconsistent, and whether a nodule is classified hy-

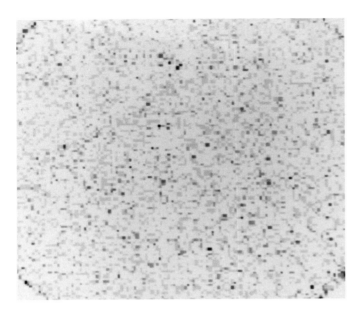

FIGURE 17-3. Scintiscan 24 hours after 200 μCi ^{123}I in a 21-year-old man who was clinically and biochemically hyperthyroid. The scan finding plus low 24-hour uptake are consistent with various thyroiditides, exogenous thyroid hormone, or excess iodine. The patient had prior neck irradiation for Hodgkin's disease and had no neck pain; he had a syndrome like silent thyroiditis, which has also been described after external radiation.

pofunctional or not can reflect the judgment of the interpreter. In addition, a small nonfunctional nodule covered by normal thyroid tissue can appear normofunctional due entirely to emissions from overlying tissue. A small nodule overlying normal thyroid can also appear normofunctional on anterior image due to gamma emissions passing through the nodule. The half-value for ^{123}I in tissues is about 6 cm, which means that there has to be 6 cm of nonfunctioning tissue in front of the source to reduce the counts by 50%. The half-value for ^{99m}Tc is 5 cm.

What proportion of hypofunctional nodules are malignant? In a comprehensive study, Ashcraft and Van Herle[76] determined this by first reviewing published reports in which all patients went to operation irrespective of scan findings. A cold nodule was present in 84%, a hot nodule in 5%, and the remainder were classified as hypo/normofunctioning. Sixteen percent of the cold nodules, 4% of the hot nodules, and 9% of the interme-

diate nodules were malignant. Secondly, they analyzed 17 publications in which there was some selection used in the decision to operate. Twenty percent of patients with cold nodules had cancer, but there were factors leading to selection of patients for surgery because only 1399 of 3720 with cold nodules were referred for operation. One percent of hot nodules and 8% of hypo/normofunctioning nodules were malignant. However, it was not always possible to determine if the cancer corresponded to the scintigraphic abnormality. Neither was it possible to determine how often oblique views were used and whether hypo/normofunctioning nodules would have been classified differently with modern equipment, ^{123}I as the radionuclide, additional views, or a different observer. Nevertheless, several important conclusions can be drawn. One, most palpable nodules are hypofunctional or nonfunctional on scintiscan. Two, most nodules, whether hypo- or nonfunctional, are benign. Three, hot nodules are not common and are seldom malignant. In an analysis using ^{99m}Tc scintigraphy, similar findings were observed.[78]

It has to be accepted that there is likely to be some selection of patients with a nodule who are referred for scintigraphy. This probably accounts for the higher percentage of patients found to have cancer compared with series in which fine-needle aspiration is used as the primary investigation.

Comparison of ^{123}I and ^{99m}Tc in the Same Patient

There are numerous reports of a nodule showing disparate scintigraphic appearance on radioiodine and ^{99m}Tc scintiscans. The more frequent discrepancy is a nodule that appears hot on ^{99m}Tc but cold on ^{123}I scintiscan. Because radioiodine is trapped and organified, whereas ^{99m}Tc is only trapped, discrepancies can be explained. A significant proportion of nodules showing this pattern are follicular cancers. Erjavec and colleagues[79] studied 58 patients with both radionuclides and found disparate results in 18 patients, 12 with follicular cancer, 2 with papillary cancers and 4 with benign lesions. It is recommended that a radioiodine study be done whenever a hot nodule is noted with pertechnetate.[80] Turner and Spencer[81] reviewed the literature and determined that this would occur in about 1 of 30 studies. Reverse disparity can also be found, that is, a nodule cold on ^{99m}Tc scan is hot on radioiodine scan and, therefore, unlikely to be malignant. The Task Force on Short-lived Radionuclides for

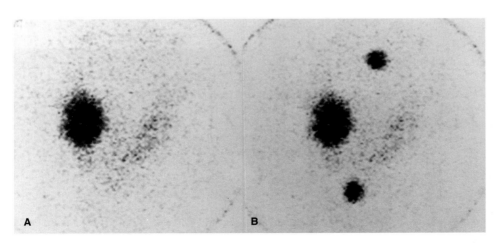

FIGURE 17-4. (*A*) A functioning "hot" nodule in right upper pole of thyroid made 3 hours after 200 μCi ^{123}I. The remainder of the thyroid shows reduced uptake. This patient had a palpable right-sided nodule; she was mildly hyperthyroid and serum TSH was low. (*B*) Same image with markers over the thyroid cartilage and suprasternal notch.

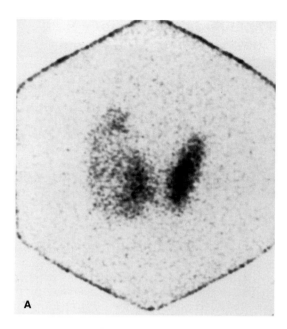 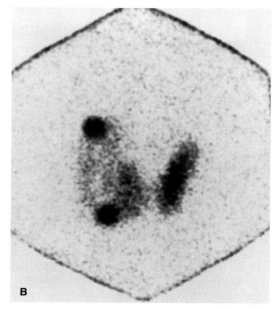

FIGURE 17-5. (*A*) Thyroid scintiscan in a woman with a right side thyroid nodule. The nodule shows reduced uptake ("cold" nodule) on ^{123}I scan. (*B*) Markers at the upper and lower pole of the nodule demonstrate that the palpable lesion corresponded with the nonfunctioning area. Fine-needle aspiration biopsy showed the nodule was benign. However, because of sudden growth of the lesion it was excised and proven pathologically to be benign.

Medical Applications[82] concluded that ^{99m}Tc is a suitable substitute for radioiodine for thyroid imaging but that it may be necessary to reimage the thyroid with radioiodine when the pertechnetate images demonstrate no abnormality corresponding to a palpable nodule(s), the pertechnetate images demonstrate a hyperfunctioning nodule(s) without suppression of extranodular thyroid tissue, and the pertechnetate concentration is low and image contrast unsatisfactory. Pertechnetate is a less satisfactory substitute for radioiodine in the evaluation of aberrant thyroid tissue and is not useful in the management of thyroid cancer.

In another study comparing ^{99m}Tc with ^{123}I, disparate findings were noted in 5% to 8% of cases.[83] Discrepancies were more often found with benign lesions but only 4% of the total group were found to have cancer. Senior experienced physicians prefer radioiodine because of "slightly better overall quality."

In summary, a nodule that is functioning on ^{99m}Tc imaging should be reimaged with [123]I. [123]I scintiscans have better thyroid/background characteristics. Thus, we favor the use of ^{123}I acknowledging the wide use of pertechnetate, its availability, and economic advantage. Nevertheless, physicians conducting thyroid scintigraphy in the evaluation of nodules should be conversant with these facts.

Thyroid Cancer in a Hot Nodule

The term "hot nodule" refers to a nodule that contains proportionally more radioiodine than surrounding thyroid when scintigraphy is done several hours after administration of the radionuclide. Disparity between ^{123}I and ^{99m}Tc has already been discussed. When the results of several series are combined the chance of a hot nodule being malignant is 0% to 1%.[84,85] However, there are documented cases including some in patients who were hyperthyroid due to the malignant lesion.[86,87] In these

reports it is clear that the palpable lesion corresponds with the scintigraphic hot nodule and that the hot nodule was the malignant lesion. The reports of Nagai and coworkers[87] of three cases and Sandler and colleagues[88] of a single case are well referenced and good sources for the interested reader. From scintigraphy alone, it is not possible to differentiate the rare thyroid cancer in

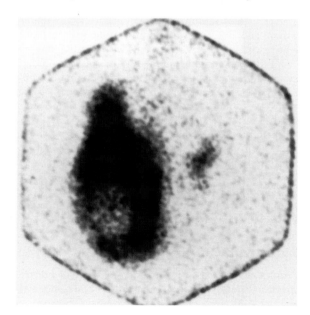

FIGURE 17-6. Large functioning nodule in right lobe of thyroid. Scintiscan was made 6 hours after 200 µCi ^{123}I, in patient who had a palpable right-sided nodule and a low serum TSH. The hot nodule shows a cold area in the lower pole; this appearance has been compared to an owl's eye. There is a small area of uptake in the right lobe, which is mostly "suppressed." The patient had surgery, which showed the nodule, including the cold area, was benign.

a hot nodule from a benign lesion. Prior external radiation, young age of the patient, and radioiodine uptake in lymph nodes in the neck would increase the possibility of cancer.

Multinodular Goiter

There are several causes of multinodular goiter including Hashimoto's thyroiditis, iodine deficiency, goitrogens, autoimmune disease unrelated to Graves' or Hashimoto's disease, and idiopathic. With the increase in immigration into the United States of citizens from areas of low or marginal dietary iodine intake, nodular goiter is a more frequent clinical finding. Scintigraphy with ^{123}I can demonstrate whether nodules are functioning or not. Using an analysis of the clinical findings and thyroid hormone and TSH measurements, the clinician can determine if the goiter is a nontoxic or a toxic nodular goiter. RAI-U measurement is important to determine whether radioiodine therapy is appropriate. The 24-hour uptake is usually in the range of 20% to 45%, which may overlap with normal. In some patients with mild hyperthyroidism, usually associated with T_3 toxicosis, the thyroid iodide trapping can even be low, thus making radioiodine therapy impracticable.

Substernal Goiter

Multinodular goiter as it enlarges has a tendency to move inferiorly due to fascial planes favoring this route. This may be due to gravity, but when the inferior edge of the gland enters the thoracic inlet the reduced pressure on inspiration is said to accelerate the migration. The finding can be apparent clinically, when the inferior part of a goiter cannot be determined because it is behind the manubrium, or it is noted serendipitously on a chest roentgenogram or computed tomography (CT) scan as an anterior mediastinal mass. In some patients, the CT scan appearance is typical and no additional tests are required.[89] When there is doubt, one way of proving the presence of functional thyroid tissue is by ^{123}I scintiscan. Because the scan is done with the patient lying supine and the neck extended, the imaged goiter may be more cephalad than determined clinically when the patient is seated. This probably accounts for the fact that many substernal goiters can be successfully removed using a standard cervical surgical approach.[90] ^{99m}Tc-pertechnetate should not be used in suspected substernal goiter because radioactivity remains within the blood pool of the great vessels and heart. In addition, the low pertechnetate uptake in the thyroid (1–3%) makes delineation difficult or impossible. Anterior mediastinal lesions noted on chest radiograph should first be evaluated by ^{123}I scintigram before CT scan because the contrast agent invariably delays radioiodine studies.

Hypothyroidism

In an adult with clinical and laboratory evidence of primary hypothyroidism, there is seldom a reason to obtain either an uptake or scintigram. In neonatal hypothyroidism, the scan can be of value to determine whether the infant has ectopic thyroid or is athyrotic. The absence of a thyroid can be used to stress to the parents the need for life-long thyroid hormone replacement in their child. Uptake and scan plus measurement of radionuclide in saliva can help define whether there is a defect in transport of iodine as the cause of neonatal hypothyroidism.

Whole Body Scintigraphy for Thyroid Cancer

This procedure is done in selected patients after surgical treatment of differentiated thyroid cancer. The scan is used to define whether there is residual thyroid or local or distant metastases. The result of the scan helps in the decision to treat with ^{131}I and, if so, what dose would be appropriate. Although there are differences of opinion about several aspects of the procedure, the general concepts are important. First, exogenous thyroid medication should be discontinued, levothyroxine (L-T$_4$) for 4 to 6 weeks[91] and levotriiodothyronine (L-T$_3$), because of its shorter half-life, should be withdrawn for at least 10 days.[92] Thyroid hormone is discontinued so that the serum TSH rises and stimulates residual thyroid tissue. Many centers recommend that serum TSH values of greater than 35 µU/mL are necessary before the ^{131}I scintigram is carried out. Recombinant human TSH (rhTSH) may reduce the need for thyroid hormone withdrawal prior to scan as discussed below. If L-T$_3$ is substituted for L-T$_4$ in preparation for scintigraphy, it is necessary for the L-T$_3$ to be given for 4 weeks to allow the L-T$_4$ to be metabolized. L-T$_3$ is then discontinued for approximately 10 days, a serum TSH obtained, and if markedly elevated, the scan is carried out. Another method of potentially increasing the radioiodine uptake in lesions is to lower the plasma inorganic iodine. Radiographic contrast, iodine-containing medications, and red dyes should be avoided. Most diets low in iodine are unpalatable, complex, and not easy to prepare.[93] One diet that is relatively simple and lowers excretion of urinary iodide to 50 µg/d recommends no iodized or sea salt, eggs, milk and dairy products, seafood, bread containing iodate conditioners, and restaurant meals for 2 weeks before scintigraphy.[94] The diet is continued for several more days after radioiodine treatment is given. A low iodine diet has been developed for patients who have to be tube fed.[95] Additional steps to lower plasma inorganic iodine such as diuretics, although supported by experimental data,[96] are seldom used. There is no controlled study showing that this improves image quality, detection of lesions, or response to radioiodine therapy. Endogenous TSH is superior to exogenous bovine TSH.[97] In addition, repeated exposure to bovine TSH causes a high incidence of allergic reactions.[98] In view of the side effects associated with bovine TSH, this product is rarely, if ever, used and is no longer available for human use. The availability of rhTSH may make it possible to conduct testing without discontinuing thyroid medications. rhTSH has been investigated in a controlled study[99] in which patients were scanned after two injections of rhTSH, then after a standard protocol with discontinuing thyroid hormone. The conditions of dietary iodine and dose of ^{131}I were constant. The scans were read in a blinded fashion. It was concluded that the scans after discontinuing thyroid hormone gave slightly better data in 14% of the patients studied. rhTSH was well tolerated and the quality of life was far better compared to withdrawal of thyroid hormone. Ongoing studies have confirmed the efficacy of rhTSH and the agent should be available for general use in the near future.

The radionuclide used for imaging is ^{131}I. Its half-life allows imaging at 48 to 72 hours. There is considerable debate about what dose of ^{131}I should be used. Some use 1 or 2 mCi; others advise 5 or even 10 mCi and some even more. There is evidence that about 10% of lesions are seen better with larger doses and some additional lesions detected. This has been documented by comparing diagnostic scans with those made after treatment where the dose can range from 30 to 200 mCi. Figure 17-7 shows whole body scans in the same patient, *A* after thyroidectomy using 2 mCi ^{131}I, *B* after a therapeutic dose of ^{131}I, and *C* 1 year later after 2 mCi [131]I. The scans are not entirely comparable because the therapy scan is made with the patient off thyroid hormone longer and frequently there is a longer delay between administration of the therapeutic dose and the second scan. Thus, some have advised using a therapeutic dose for diagnostic purposes, but this policy will lead to treatment of some patients who do not need therapy. Recently, there has been growing evidence that the larger the diagnostic dose of ^{131}I, the less likely subsequent therapy will be taken up by functioning lesions. This has been termed "stunning" of the lesion. Park and colleagues[100] found that 2 of 5 patients given 3 mCi ^{131}I, 2 of 3 given 5 mCi, and 16 of 18 given 10 mCi had this effect. We recommend a 1- to 2-mCi dose of [131]I.

Iodine-123, which is used for routine thyroid scintigraphy, appears to be of less value in whole body scintigraphy for thyroid cancer. Maxon and colleagues[101] demonstrated that even very large doses of ^{123}I gave less information than conventional doses of [131]I. It seems appropriate, in light of the data on "stunning," to revisit the use of [123]I. The low dose to the thyroid would be of considerable advantage, provided there was no diminution in information.

Anterior and posterior whole body scintigrams are made and spot views of the neck with uptake measurements give the most comprehensive evaluation. Normally, there is uptake in residual thyroid, salivary glands, stomach, and gut. The majority

of radioiodine is excreted through the kidneys (the percentage of renal excretion is inverse to that trapped by the thyroid). At the time of imaging, 48 to 72 hours after administration of ^{131}I, the kidneys are not imaged, although the bladder sometimes is. The uptake of radioiodine is usually greatest in normal residual thyroid. Metastases in lymph nodes, lung, bone, and other organs are imaged provided the volume of residual thyroid is small. Figure 17-8*A* shows uptake in the neck consistent with metastases in lymph nodes after 2 mCi [131]I. Figure 17-8*B* shows the same region after the therapy dose demonstrating more lesions; Figure 17-8*C* is a follow-up scan a year later, which shows no abnormality. Pulmonary lesions can be microscopic and diffuse or macroscopic and focal. Figure 17-9*A* demonstrates diffuse pulmonary plus right cervical nodal functioning metastases. Figure 17-9*B* is the follow-up whole body scan approximately 1 year after treatment with 150 mCi [131]I. Figure 17-10 shows whole body scans after 2 and 200 mCi, respectively, in a patient with disseminated follicular cancer. In this patient, both scintiscans show similar distribution of diagnostic and therapeutic radionuclide. Scintigraphy is done to determine extent of disease and unsuspected lesions, which influence subsequent management, can be detected. The converse is sometimes found, namely failure of known lesions to be imaged. In this situation the clinician should make sure exogenous thyroid was stopped for sufficient time, that iodine intake was low, and that no radiographic contrast was given. When these are excluded, there remain a small proportion of lesions (approximately 10%) that fail to take up radioiodine and are considered false negatives. In that situation, measurement of

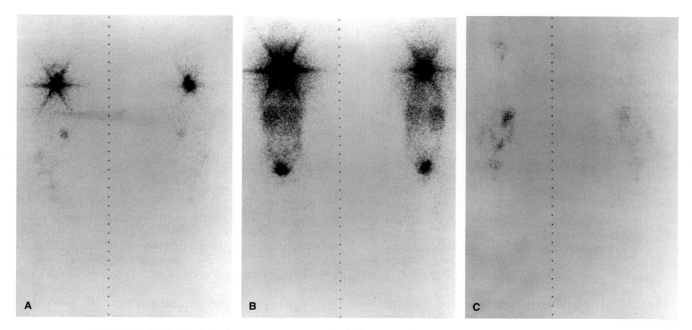

FIGURE 17-7. (*A*) Whole body scan in a patient who had near total thyroidectomy for papillary cancer. The scan was obtained 48 hours after 2 mCi [131]I. The patient had stopped levothyroxine for 4 weeks. There is intense uptake in the region of the thyroid (4%) and there is uptake in the stomach and intestines, which is normal. (*B*) Whole body scan in the same patient 7 days after a therapy dose of 100 mCi [131]I. There is intense uptake in the thyroid, with a "star" effect, due to the high-energy photons breaking through the thinner lead septa of the collimator. This scan also shows diffuse uptake in the liver, which was not seen on prior diagnostic scan. This was due to the liver metabolizing radioiodinated thyroid hormones secreted by the functioning thyroid tissue. (*C*) Follow-up diagnostic scan made about 1 year later after a 2-mCi dose of [131]I. This shows a trace of uptake in cervical area (< 0.1%) but similar uptake in the abdomen, which is considered normal.

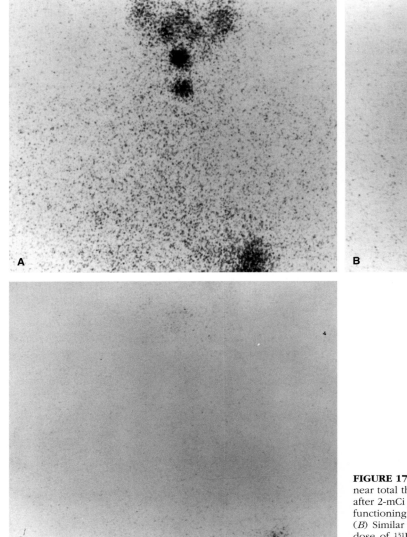

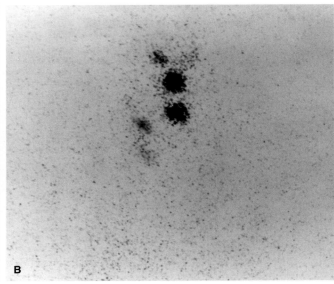

FIGURE 17-8. (*A*) Spot view of neck and chest in a woman who had near total thyroidectomy for thyroid cancer. Scintiscan made 48 hours after 2-mCi dose of [131]I. There are two areas of uptake consistent with functioning metastases, plus normal uptake in mouth and stomach. (*B*) Similar spot view in the same patient 7 days after a therapeutic dose of ^{131}I shows more functioning metastases. (*C*) Scan made approximately 1 year later shows no abnormality.

serum thyroglobulin may confirm the presence of functioning tissue and the radiopharmaceuticals described below have an important role.

False-positive results have been described in organs that normally accumulate iodine. An important cause is contamination of the patient or clothes with radioactive secretions, such as urine, saliva, or mucus.[102] Norby and coworkers[103] stress that uptake in the nasal mucosa is normal and they found uptake greater than background in 20 of 21 patients scanned 72 hours after 5 mCi ^{131}I, and in 15 patients the uptake was spherical. Uptake of ^{131}I has been described in inflammatory lung disease,[104] Meckel's diverticulum,[105] renal cyst,[106] and sweat.[107] Apart from the first, all of these are sites where iodine could be expected. Therefore, when the scintigram is interpreted, the distribution of iodine must be considered. In addition, there are reports of uptake in other sites such as tracheostomy,[108] and in benign and malignant nonthyroidal tumors. These include bronchogenic,[109] stomach, and ovary. Sometimes the liver is seen on scan and this is discussed in more detail below. Several references provide comprehensive lists of potential false-positive whole body ^{131}I scintiscans, many of which are listed in Table 17-4.[103,110,111] Figure 17-11 shows a false-positive scan in the region of the left hip, which was due to a contaminated handkerchief. Figure 17-12 shows a spot view of the neck and chest with uptake in right cervical nodes plus diffuse uptake in the breasts, which could be confused for pulmonary metastases. This patient had recently stopped nursing.

Scintigraphy after therapeutic doses of ^{131}I often shows additional lesions not seen on the prior diagnostic scan.[112,113] For example Spies and coworkers[114] found significant new information in 12 of 39 patients. The diagnostic dose of ^{131}I was 5 mCi and the average therapy dose was 121 mCi. Diagnostic scans were made at 48 to 72 hours, the therapeutic dose scanned after an average of 2.4 days, although the "therapeutic" scan was completed on average 5.4 days after the diagnostic one. Similar findings have been reported by others.[115] When the patient is

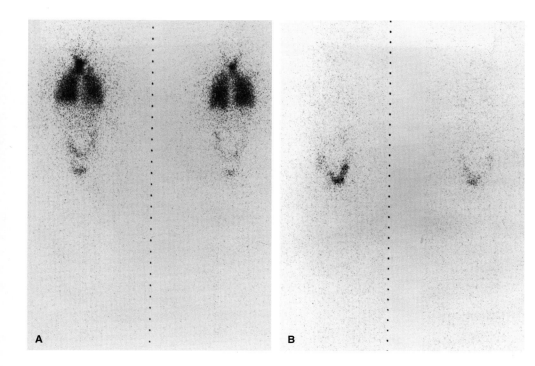

FIGURE 17-9. (*A*) Anterior and posterior whole body scans 3 days after 2 mCi [131]I. There is abnormal uptake in the right cervical region, plus diffuse uptake in both lungs, due to diffuse pulmonary metastases. The patient was treated with 150 mCi [131]I. (*B*) Follow-up scintiscan in the same projections approximately 1 year later. The metastases are no longer imaged and the patient has done well clinically.

scanned 5 to 7 days after administration of a therapeutic dose of ^{131}I, homogeneous uptake can be seen in the liver. This is not indicative of metastases but is due to concentration of radioactive thyroid hormones in the liver. Rosenbaum and colleagues[116] found diffuse hepatic uptake in 12 of 23 of posttreatment scans but in only 5 of 38 diagnostic scans. A positive correlation of liver visualization and the dose of ^{131}I prescribed was documented in another study.[117] There are probably three important facts that lead to this finding: 1) sufficient functioning thyroid to make radioactive hormones; 2) enough radioiodine to allow those hormones to be imaged in the liver; and 3) enough time for the radioiodine to be incorporated into thyroid hormones, the hormones released, and subsequently concentrated in the liver. This is shown in Figure 17-8. In contrast, focal lesions in the liver that concentrate radioiodine are likely to be metastases.

Similarly, functioning thyroid tissue producing radioiodinated thyroid hormone could be detected by sensitive in vitro measurement of T_4-bound [131]I. Hays and McDougall[118] compared this measurement made on serum drawn at the time of whole body scintigraphy (48–72 hours) and compared it to the whole body scintiscan and serum thyroglobulin in 20 patients with differentiated thyroid cancer. There was complete agreement between ^{131}I-T_4 and ^{131}I scan. Thyroglobulin was undetectable in 3 patients who had small identifiable remnants of presumably normal thyroid. Because of the concordance of the blood test with the ^{131}I scan and because the scan provides anatomic and functional information, the latter alone is recommended.

Measurements of serum thyroglobulin at the time of scintigraphy or when the patient is taking L-T_4 provide important correlative information along with the results of scintigraphy. This is discussed in more detail in chapters 20 and 80. However, it has been suggested that the serum thyroglobulin should not replace the scan and that both tests are indicated.[119]

Other Radionuclides and Radiopharmaceuticals

THALLIUM

Thallium-201 belongs to group IIIA metals but is distributed and handled in vivo like potassium. [201]Tl is taken into cells by the Na-K pump, which is dependent on ATP. The explanation of why Tl+ (in practice ^{201}Tl), which is a very large atom with different properties than K+, should be handled in vivo like potassium is explained by their hydrated nuclei having almost identical radii.[120] [201]Tl as thallous chloride has been used widely in clinical practice to determine myocardial perfusion.[121] It has a half-life of 73 hours and emits x-ray photons of 69 to 80 keV, from its daughter mercury-201. After exercise, about 4% of ^{201}Tl is taken into viable myocardial cells.[122] It is also taken up by liver, salivary glands, testes, bowel (in particular if active), kidneys, eyes, and thyroid.[123,124] These organs are seen on whole body scintigraphy. [201]Tl is concentrated in various thyroid disorders including cancers (papillary, follicular, medullary, or anaplastic), subacute and chronic lymphocytic thyroiditis, and Graves' disease. Therefore, it is not specific as an imaging agent for thyroid cancer. An extensive review of lesions that accumulate ^{201}Tl has been published by Krasnow and colleagues.[125] The time course of uptake of ^{201}Tl in cancers is the same as myocardial uptake, with maximal tumor/background ratios at 8 to 20 minutes after intravenous injection.[124] From that time there is "washout" from the lesions. Therefore, imaging should be started 10 to 15 minutes after injection.[124] Anterior and posterior whole body images are made using a gamma camera. Figure 17-13 shows an abnormal ^{201}Tl scintiscan with uptake in cervical lymph nodes in a patient with metastatic thyroid cancer.

There is substantial literature concerning the results of ^{201}Tl scintigraphy for thyroid cancer. The data are not consistent.

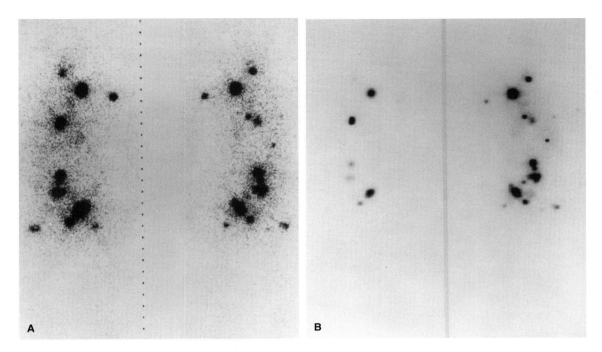

FIGURE 17-10. (*A*) Anterior and posterior images 72 hours after 2 mCI ^{131}I in a patient with metastatic follicular thyroid cancer. Multiple widespread lesions concentrate [131]I. (*B*) Appearance 7 days after 200 mCi [131]I. The distribution of lesions is similar to the diagnostic scan. However, there appears to be less background because the settings of the gamma camera had to be adjusted because the lesions would have produced a "burned-out" appearance.

Hoefnagel and associates[126] studied 326 patients of whom 291 had differentiated thyroid cancer. They found a sensitivity of 94% and specificity of 97%. However, in the same patients, ^{131}I combined with thyroglobulin measurements had a sensitivity and specificity of 92%. [201]Tl imaging, although often correct, did not add much new information. When all three tests were done, all known lesions were discovered. Brendel and coworkers[127] found the sensitivity to be low at 45%. One reason for the low sensitivity was failure to detect skeletal metastases. These authors advise against using ^{201}Tl as the only agent for follow-up. Iida and colleagues[128] used a combination of ^{201}Tl and serum thyroglobulin for follow-up of patients who had surgery for differentiated thyroid cancer. In 55 with positive ^{201}Tl scintiscan, 51 had recurrent disease and 80 of 94 who had a negative ^{201}Tl scan had no evidence of recurrence. One-half of the 14 false-negative results were detected by an elevated thyroglobulin measurement. The sensitivity of ^{201}Tl in the study of Sorge-Van Boxel and colleagues[129] was only 55%. [131]I whole body diagnostic scan, ^{131}I therapy scan, serum thyroglobulin at the time of ^{131}I scintigraphy, and ^{201}Tl scan were evaluated. Thyroglobulin alone was the best test and the combination of this plus ^{131}I scan produced a sensitivity of 100% and specificity of 98%. [201]Tl scan plus thyroglobulin had results of 97% and 91%, respectively.

What is the role of ^{201}Tl scintigraphy in thyroid cancer? It is not a diagnostic test for primary thyroid cancer. It has a role in follow-up of patients who have had surgery and or radioiodine therapy to determine whether there is residual or recurrent cancer. From the data presented above it is apparent that there is no universal opinion of the sensitivity and specificity of the test. In patients with clinical or laboratory evidence of recurrent disease and negative ^{131}I scintigraphy, ^{201}Tl whole body scintigraphy might define the abnormal site. This information can potentially aid in management but clearly ^{131}I therapy is not an option. It was hoped that, because it is not necessary to discontinue L-T$_4$ before ^{201}Tl scintigraphy, this test would be pivotal in determining which patients would have to have ^{131}I scans. The data do not support that thesis.

As described in the section on hot nodules, ^{201}Tl provides a method of demonstrating suppressed "normal" thyroid tissue.

^{99m}*Tc-Sestamibi*

Technetium-99m sestamibi was developed as a technetium radiopharmaceutical for imaging the myocardium. Like ^{201}Tl, it is concentrated by thyroid tissue, including thyroid cancers, and other cancers, especially breast cancer. The procedure involves intravenous injection of 20 to 25 mCi ^{99m}Tc-sestamibi followed by anterior and posterior whole body images after a delay of 10 to 20 minutes (Fig 17-14). Its role for thyroid imaging is, therefore, similar to [201]Tl. It can demonstrate suppressed thyroid tissue. ^{99m}Tc-sestamibi can also be used to detect cancer when the ^{131}I scan is negative but the suspicion of cancer is high. This has been demonstrated in metastatic Hurthle cell cancer. Yen and colleagues[130] studied 22 patients who had elevated thyroglobulin measurements. Four had positive ^{131}I, 15 positive ^{201}Tl, and 18 positive sestamibi scans, respectively (18%, 68%, and 82%). Figure 17-15 shows a spot view of the legs in a patient who had metastatic Hurthle cell cancer in that site. The sensitivities and specificities of ^{201}Tl and ^{99m}Tc-sestamibi are similar. Which should be used and

TABLE 17-4.
Normal and Abnormal Distribution of Radioiodine
That Can be Misinterpreted as Metastatic Cancer on
Whole-Body Scan

Physiologic	Pathologic
Salivary glands	Dacrocystitis
Nasopharynx	Warthin's tumor
Gastrointestinal tract	Artificial eye
Urinary tract	Sinusitis
Sweat	Tracheostomy
	Inflammatory lung disease
	Adenocarcinoma of lung
Liver on delayed scan	Squamous cancer of lung
	Undifferentiated lung cancer
	Thymus
	Breast
	Gallbladder
	Pleuropericardial cyst
	Struma cordis
Contamination with saliva or urine	Renal cyst
	Ectopic kidney
	Gastric pull-up
	Meckel's diverticulum
	Struma ovarii
	Cystadenoma of ovary
	Adenocarcinoma of stomach
	Meningioma
	Hiatal hernia
	Contamination with sputum
	Zenker's diverticulum

For comprehensive review, see references 103, 110, and 111.

when? Because both tests are expensive, they should be used when the result provides new, clinically relevant information. 99mTc-sestamibi images have better resolution and are easier to interpret. However, there is a considerable amount of this radiopharmaceutical concentrated in the liver and abdomen. 201Tl would be preferred if that area was the main suspected site of disease.

99mTc-Pertechnetate

Technetium-99m pertechnetate should not be used for whole body scintigraphy for detecting metastases from thyroid carcinoma. In one small study, only three abnormal sites were detected with 99mTc compared with 33 with 131I.[131] Khammash and colleagues[132] compared 99mTc with 131I in 66 patients. In 48 patients both studies were negative and of the remainder, 5 patients had false-negative 99mTc results. They also found one negative 131I study that was positive on 99mTc. Because the diagnostic radioiodine study is obtained not only to define extent of disease but to determine the role of radioiodine therapy and because 99mTc fails to detect lesions and cannot be used to plan therapy, 99mTc is not recommended.

111In-Octreotide

In 1994, the United States Food and Drug Administration (FDA) approved the use of 111In-octreotide. This radiopharmaceutical had already been evaluated and used extensively in Europe.[133] The agent is an analogue of somatostatin, which can be used for in vivo imaging of somatostatin receptors. Originally the agent was labeled with radionuclides of iodine. More recently its structure has been altered slightly and 111In used as the radioactive tracer. For thyroid imaging its major role is to detect residual or metastatic medullary cancer, which is discussed below.[134] In-octreotide has been used to image lymphoma, neuroblastoma, pheochromocytoma, and the enlarged muscles in the orbits of patients with Graves' eye disease.[133]

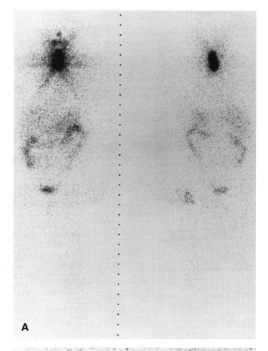

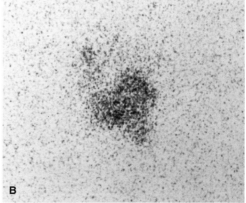

FIGURE 17-11. (*A*) Whole body scintiscans 7 days after 100 mCi 131I. There is an intense uptake in the cervical region, plus normal excretion through the gut and faint uptake in the liver. On the posterior view there is abnormality in the region of the left hip. This was not seen on the prior diagnostic scintiscan and does not appear "anatomic." This should raise the question of an artefact. (*B*) The cause was found to be contamination of his handkerchief; the patient had a very bad upper respiratory infection.

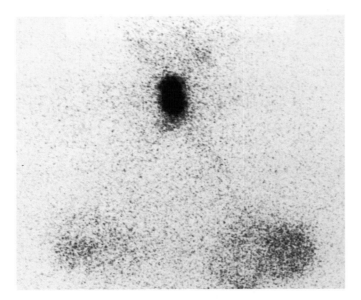

FIGURE 17-12. Scintiscan demonstrates neck and chest 72 hours after 2 mCi ^{131}I in a woman with papillary cancer who has had nearly total thyroidectomy. There is uptake in the right cervical region, plus diffuse uptake in the breasts. She had discontinued nursing several days previously. The importance of ensuring patients who receive diagnostic or therapeutic doses of radioiodine are not nursing is stressed. In addition, this distribution could possibly be mistaken for pulmonary metastases.

Gallium-67

Gallium is a group IIIA metal that has been used as a tumor-seeking radiopharmaceutical and one that localizes in inflammation. ^{67}Ga-citrate is administered intravenously in a dose of 3 to 10 mCi. Imaging for inflammation can be conducted as early as 6 hours, but for cancer a delay of 48 to 72 hours is advised. There are reports of its uptake in thyroid cancer, usually anaplastic and lymphoma.[134] However, ^{67}Ga is not recommended for differentiating benign from malignant thyroid nodules. In one study of 136 patients with rapidly enlarging neck masses that were cold on radioiodine scintigraphy, there was intense ^{67}Ga uptake in 17 of 20 anaplastic cancers, all 35 lymphomas, but essentially none of 19 differentiated adenocarcinomas.[135] The data show that ^{67}Ga is not sensitive enough to be used to determine the presence of primary cancer or the extent of metastatic differentiated thyroid cancer. Because the clinical features in anaplastic cancer and lymphoma are seldom subtle and tissue diagnosis necessary, ^{67}Ga is not advised for routine use. In addition, ^{67}Ga is concentrated by a range of nonthyroidal cancers including lung, breast, both Hodgkin's and non-Hodgkin's lymphomas, hepatoma, and bone.

There are reports of ^{67}Ga uptake in chronic lymphocytic,[136] subacute, and silent thyroiditis[137]; Graves' disease[138]; and amiodarone-induced hyperthyroidism.[139] In most of these reports, the ^{67}Ga scan was ordered for a nonspecific reason, such as fever and intense uptake in the thyroid pointed to the cause.[140] There are, however, few a priori indications for doing this study with the exception of staging lymphoma.

In patients with specific symptoms such as bone pain a routine ^{99m}Tc-diphosphonate bone scan can help. However, skeletal lesions from metastatic thyroid cancer can be subtle and in one study the sensitivity of this test was low.[141] Because there are several radionuclides (^{99m}Tc, ^{99m}Tc-dimercaptosuccinate [DMSA], ^{99m}Tc-sestamibi, ^{201}Tl, ^{67}Ga, ^{123}I, ^{131}I, [124]I), which could be used alone or in combination in a single patient, it is frequently beneficial to "coregister" the images. Thus, the exact relation of the agents can be compared. There is considerable interest in coregistration of all relevant images in a patient (e.g., ultrasound, magnetic resonance imaging [MRI], and nuclear). This will provide the advantage of functional nuclear studies to be superimposed on the precise resolution of the other procedures.

IMAGING STUDIES FOR MEDULLARY CANCER

A number of scintigraphic techniques have a limited role in searching for medullary cancer in patients who have elevated calcitonin levels after total thyroidectomy. These tests should be considered along with other imaging methods such as ultrasound, CT, and MRI when there is an elevated calcitonin but no obvious source. The parafollicular cells do not trap or concentrate iodine. Therefore, radioiodine scintigraphy for metastases is useless. One report describing uptake in metastatic pulmonary lesions is misleading and undoubtedly the functioning tissue was metastatic follicular rather than medullary cancer.[142] [201]Tl discussed above for imaging differentiated thyroid cancer also localizes in recurrent[143] and extrathyroidal medullary cancer lesions[144] and 11 of 12 lesions

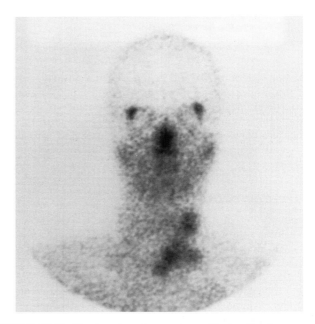

FIGURE 17-13. Head and neck scan immediately after intravenous dose of 2 mCi ^{201}Tl in a patient with papillary cancer who has had surgical thyroidectomy. [131]I scan was negative, but the serum thyroglobulin level was elevated. [201]Tl scintiscan shows abnormal uptake in left cervical nodes.

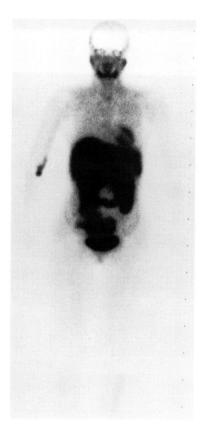

FIGURE 17-14. Whole body anterior scintiscan made 15 minutes after an intravenous injection of ^{99m}Tc sestamibi. The patient had two surgeries and ^{131}I treatment for metastatic papillary thyroid cancer. Follow-up ^{131}I scan was negative; however, serum thyroglobulin level was elevated. The scan shows normal distribution of sestamibi in the liver, intestines, myocardium, and salivary glands. In addition, there is a small area of abnormal uptake in the region of the substernal notch. At surgery nodes containing metastatic papillary thyroid cancer were removed. Serum thyroglobulin is now undetectable.

were detected in a comparative study of ^{201}Tl and other agents described below.[145] Several publications show that ^{99m}Tc-pentavalent dimercaptosuccinate (^{99m}Tc-DMSA) can image medullary cancers.[146,147] The radiopharmaceutical is not widely available. Neck and chest plus whole body images are made 2 hours after intravenous injection of the radiopharmaceutical. There is a difference of opinion of the value of the test. Hilditch and coworkers[148] found a high proportion of false-negative results, whereas other investigators detected recurrent disease early and at a time the lesion was small.[149,150] The number of patients studied is small and the results in a larger number of patients hopefully will clarify the differences. There has been development in production of rhenium 186 and rhenium 188-labeled DMSA. These are beta emitters that could be used for therapy.[151]

Iodine 131-metaiodobenzylguanidine (^{131}I-MIBG), used mainly to detect pheochromocytoma, does concentrate in some medullary cancers but because of low sensitivity this is not a useful screening test.[152–155] Several of the reports were in patients who were being studied for pheochromocytoma and in

whom abnormal uptake in the neck or mediastinum showed the coexistent medullary cancer. This radiopharmaceutical has also recently been approved by the FDA. If there is intense uptake of ^{131}I-MIBG in unresectable medullary cancer, consideration can be given for therapy with a larger dose.[155]

Krenning and colleagues have published their extensive experience with ^{111}In-octreotide in more than 1000 patients.[133] This series included 17 patients with medullary cancer and metastases were correctly diagnosed in 11.[134] One patient with residual disease in the thyroid and 7 with liver metastases (1 patient with disease in both sites) were not diagnosed. They advise combining a standard liver scan with the OctreoScan in patients suspected of having liver metastases. Figure 17-16 shows ^{111}In-octreotide and ^{99m}Tc-sestamibi scans in a patient with medullary cancer.

Radiolabeled monoclonal antibodies have not yet reached the point where they can be recommended for routine clinical use.[156]

THYROID SCINTIGRAPHY IN WOMEN WHO ARE PREGNANT OR BREAST-FEEDING

Thyroid disease is common in women of childbearing age. In general, patients who are pregnant should not be given radionuclides of iodine because these cross the placenta. If there is a clinical situation that can only be resolved by an in vivo study, the smallest dose of ^{123}I that will provide the answer should be used. Likewise if the patient is nursing, tests with radiopharmaceuticals, in particular radioiodine, should not be used because these are secreted in the milk and ingested by the baby, whose thyroid is small (about 1 g at birth) and traps avidly. Ingestion of 1 μCi ^{131}I will deliver 16 to 21 rad to the thyroid in this circumstance. The maximum permissible dose to the thyroid is 150 mrad and ingestion of ^{131}I should be limited to 0.001 μCi. Ingestion of 1 μCi ^{123}I is calculated to deliver about 1 rad to the thyroid and the dose to the infant should be less than 0.15 μCi. These data show that if the mother is treated with ^{131}I she should not nurse the baby. Even a tracer of ^{131}I (5–10 μCi) necessitates stopping breast-feeding for 8 weeks. When ^{123}I is used, nursing should be stopped for at least 2 days and a measured sample of milk counted in a well counter and compared with a known control. The amount of radioiodine in this volume should be multiplied by the daily milk volume to determine the total ^{123}I secreted each day. The literature on this topic is limited[57,158] and additional carefully obtained data, with measurements made over time, would be of considerable value. Mountford and Coakely[159] recommend that the following questions be answered before administering radioactivity to a woman who is breast-feeding:

1. Is the study essential?
2. Is there an alternative nonradionuclide procedure?
3. Is there an alternative radiopharmaceutical that yields lower radiation dose to the infant?
4. Can the desired result be obtained with less than the usual administered activity?
5. What is the possibility of a repeat investigation?

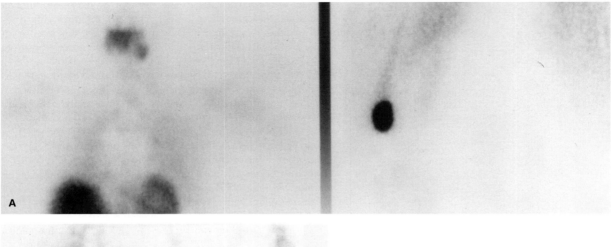

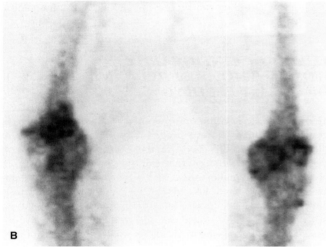

FIGURE 17-15. Spot view of the thighs and knees about 1 hour after intravenous injection of 25 mCi ^{99m}Tc sestamibi in a woman with metastatic Hurthle cell cancer. She had undergone several surgical treatments for locally invasive and regional metastatic disease. Whole body ^{131}I, ^{201}Tl, and ^{99m}Tc MDP bone scans did not show evidence of metastases, but serum thyroglobulin values were very high. The sestamibi scan surprisingly showed a distal femoral metastasis, which was confirmed by other non-nuclear imaging tests and treated by external radiation.

PHARMACOLOGIC INTERVENTIONS

Suppression Tests: T3 Suppression

This test is seldom used in practice, except to determine whether the thyroid is indeed suppressed when the patient is receiving exogenous TSH suppressing doses of L-T$_4$ to decrease the size of a nodular or diffuse goiter. The rationale for suppression tests is to determine if thyroid function, such as uptake or scintigraphic appearance, is altered when the patient is given exogenous thyroid. Normal tissue suppresses, whereas autonomous tissue such as in Graves' disease or in a hot nodule do not. The test was used most often in the past to determine if patients with equivocal symptoms and signs and borderline in vitro high test results had hyperthyroidism. With current in vitro tests (free hormone and ultrasensitive TSH measurements) separation of normal from abnormal is clear. There are several protocols. The Werner test involved measurement of the 24-hour radioiodine uptake,[160,161] followed by the administration of T$_3$ in a dose of 25 µg three times daily for 8 days, followed by a repeat uptake. Charkes and colleagues[162] used the same daily dose of T$_3$ but found that 4 days was sufficient. In 29 of 30 normal individuals, the second uptake measurement showed a decline of more than 30%. An even shorter test used 150 µg T$_3$ daily for 2 days and uptake in normal subjects fell by 50%.[163]

Thyrotropin Stimulation Test

This TSH test was introduced to differentiate hypothyroidism from primary thyroid disease from central hypothyroidism and it should no longer be used for this purpose. TSH has also been used to increase radioiodine uptake into metastatic thyroid cancer but also is no longer used because of the potential side effects from exogenous bovine TSH and the relative simplicity of obtaining a rise in endogenous TSH by stopping whatever thyroid preparation the patient is taking for an appropriate time (see above). Bovine TSH has been used in the past to differentiate a hot nodule with suppression of adjacent normal tissue from hemiagenesis. In the former, the suppressed tissue will be imaged. Because there are other simpler methods of determining this such as ultrasound, imaging after bovine TSH stimulation should not be done. Bovine TSH has been used to diagnose thyrotoxicosis factitia.[164] However, a low thyroglobulin in addition to a low uptake plus clinical and biochemical thyrotoxicosis provide the necessary information. In addition to allergic reactions to bovine TSH,[98] there are reports of rapid swelling of the thyroid.[165]

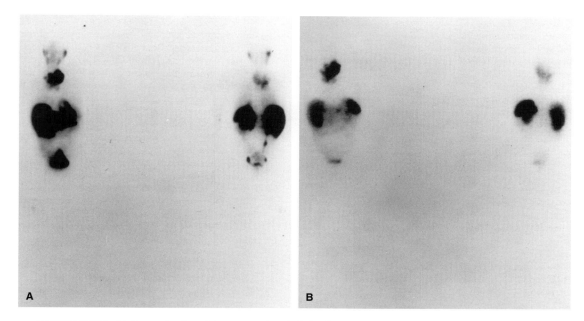

FIGURE 17-16. (*A*) Example of an ^{111}In-octreotide whole body scan in a patient who had surgery for proven medullary cancer of thyroid. The scan shows abnormal uptake in low cervical/mediastinal nodes. Imaging is usually recommended 4 and 24 hours after intravenous injection of 3 to 6 mCi ^{111}In-octreotide. (*B*) Whole body ^{99m}Tc sestamibi scan in the same patient shows a similar mediastinal abnormality. Note the different distributions of the radiopharmaceuticals. (Scan provided by Dr. Daniel Navarro, Oakland Kaiser Permanente Hospital, Oakland, CA)

The safety and the future availability of rhTSH may result in the reintroduction of the use of TSH in some of the above-described clinical situations and as a means of stimulating radioiodine uptake in patients with toxic or nontoxic goiter in whom basal radioiodine is not elevated and in whom ^{131}I therapy is desirable.

References

1. Chapman E. History of the discovery and early use of radioactive iodine. JAMA 1983;250:2042
2. Paras P, Hamilton D, Evans C, et al. Iodine-123 assay using a radionuclide calibrator. Int J Nuc Med Biol 1983;10:111
3. Zeissman H, Fahey F, Gochoco J. Impact of radiocontaminants in commercially available iodine-123: dosimetric evaluation. J Nucl Med 1986;27:428
4. Solomon B, Glinoer D, Lagasse R, Wartofsky L. Current trends in the management of Graves' disease. J Clin Endocrinol Metab 1990;70:1518
5. Burke G, Halko A, Silverstein G, Hilligoss M. Comparative thyroid uptake studies with ^{131}I and [99m]Tc. J Clin Endocrinol Metab 1972;34:630
6. Vahjen G, Lange R, Merola T. Thyroid uptake neck phantoms are not created equal. J Nucl Med 1992;33:304
7. Martin P, Rollo F. Estimation of thyroid depth and correction for I-123 measurements. J Nucl Med 1977;18:919
8. Chervu S, Chervu L, Goodum P, Blaufox M. Thyroid uptake measurements with [123]I: problems and pitfalls: concise communication. J Nucl Med 1982;23:667
9. Hine G, Williams J. Thyroid radioiodine uptake measurement. In: Hine G, ed. Instrumentation in nuclear medicine. Vol 1. New York: Academic Press, 1967:327
10. Pochin E. Investigation of thyroid function and disease with radioactive iodine. Lancet 1950;2:41
11. Atkins HL, JF, Klopper JF. Measurement of thyroidal technetium uptake with the gamma camera and computer system. AJR Am J Roentgenol 1973;118:831
12. Hays M, Wesselossky B. Simultaneous measurement of thyroid trapping ([99m]TcO$_4^-$) and binding (^{131}I): clinical and experimental studies in man. J Nucl Med 1973;14:785
13. Higgins H, Ball D, Eastham S. 20-min ^{99m}Tc thyroid uptake: a simplified method using the gamma camera. J Nucl Med 1973;14:907
14. Schneider P. Simple, rapid thyroid function testing with ^{99m}Tc-pertechnetate thyroid uptake and neck/thigh ratio. Am J Roentgenol 1979;132:249
15. Duck S, Sty J. Technetium thyroid uptake ratios in pediatric Graves' disease. J Pediatr 1985;107:905
16. Hurley P, Maisey M, Natarajan T, Wagner HJ. A computerized system for rapid evaluation of thyroid function. J Clin Endocrinol Metab 1972;34:354
17. Robertson J, Nolan N, Wahner H, McConahey W. Thyroid radioiodine uptakes and scans in euthyroid patients. Mayo Clin Proc 1975;50:79
18. Sternthal E, Lipworth L, Stanley B, et al. Suppression of thyroid radioiodine uptake by various doses of stable iodide. N Engl J Med 1980;303:1083
19. Lengemann F, Thompson J. Prophylactic and therapeutic measures for radioiodine contamination: a review. Health Phys 1963;9:1391
20. Becker D, Braverman L, Dunn J, et al. The use of iodine as a thyroidal blocking agent in the event of a reactor accident. JAMA 1984;252:659
21. Wolff J. Iodide goiter and the pharmacologic effects of excess iodide. Am J Med 1969;47:101
22. Wiersinga W, Touber J, Trip M, van Royen E. Uninhibited thyroidal uptake of radioiodine despite iodine excess in amiodarone-induced hypothyroidism. J Clin Endocrinol Metab 1986;63:485

23. Martino E, Bartalena L, Mariotti S. Radioactive iodine thyroid uptake in patients with amiodarone-iodine-induced thyroid dysfunction. Acta Endocrinol (Copenh) 1988;119:167

24. Roti E, Minelli R, Gardini E, Braverman L. The use and misuse of thyroid hormone. Endocr Rev 1993;14:401

25. Bahre M, Hilgers R, Lindemann C, Emrich D. Physiologic aspects of the thyroid trapping function and its suppression in iodine deficiency using ^{99m}Tc pertechnetate. Acta Endocrinol (Copenh) 1987;115:175

26. Sedvall G, Jonsson B, Petterson U. Evidence of an altered thyroid function in man during treatment with lithium carbonate. Acta Psychiatr Scand 1969;297(suppl):59

27. Barandes M, Hurley J, Becker D. Implications of rapid intrathyroidal iodine turnover for ^{131}I therapy: the small pool syndrome. J Nucl Med 1973;14:379

28. Caplan R, Glasser J, Davis K, et al. Thyroid function tests in elderly hyperthyroid patients. J Am Geriatr Soc 1978;26:116

29. Tibaldi J, Barzel U, Albin J, Surks M. Thyrotoxicosis in the very old. Am J Med 1986;81:619

30. Hamburger J, Hamburger S. Diagnosis and management of large toxic multinodular goiters. J Nucl Med 1985;26:888

31. Hooper P, Caplan R. Thyroid uptake of radioactive iodine in hyperthyroidism. JAMA 1977;238:411

32. McDougall I. The importance of obtaining thyroid uptake measurement in patients with hyperthyroidism. Nucl Med Commun 1990;11:73

33. Cavalieri R, Gerard S. Unusual types of thyrotoxicosis. Adv Intern Med 1991;36:271

34. Oliner L, Kohlenbrener R, Fields T, Kunstadter R. Thyroid function studies in children: normal values for thyroidal ^{131}I uptake and PB^{131}I levels up to the age of 18. J Clin Endocrinol Metab 1957;17:61

35. Gaffney G, Gregerman R, Shock N. Relationship of age to the thyroidal accumulation, renal excretion and distribution of radioiodide in euthyroid man. J Clin Endocrinol Metab 1962;22:784

36. Oddie T, Myhill J, Pernique F, Fisher D. Effect of age and sex on the radioiodine uptake in euthyroid subjects. J Clin Endocrinol Metab 1968;28:776

37. McCruden D, Hilditch T, Connell J, et al. Duration of antithyroid action of methimazole estimated with an intravenous perchlorate discharge test. Clin Endocrinol (Oxf) 1987;26:33

38. Takeuchi K, Suzuki K, Horiuchi Y, Mashimo K. Significance of iodide-perchlorate discharge test for detection of iodine organification defect of the thyroid. J Clin Endocrinol Metab 1970;31:144

39. Greer MA, Stot AK, Milne KA. Effect of thiocyanate, perchlorate and other anions on thyroidal iodine metabolism. Endocrinology 1966;79:237

40. Roti E, Minelli R, Gardini E, et al. The iodine perchlorate discharge test before and after one year of methimazole treatment of hyperthyroidism of Graves' disease. J Clin Endocrinol Metab 1994;78:795

41. Black MB. ^{99m}Tc pertechnetate flow study for evaluation of cold thyroid nodules. Radiology 1972;102:705

42. Goldfarb CR, Varma C, Roginsky M. Diagnosis in delirium: prompt confirmation of thyroid storm. Clin Nucl Med 1980;5:66

43. Smith ML, Wraight EP. Oblique views in thyroid imaging. Clin Radiol 1989;40:505

44. Karelitz JR, Richards JB. Necessity of oblique views in evaluating the functional status of a thyroid nodule. J Nucl Med 1974;15:782

45. Hamburger JI. Diagnostic methods in management of thyroid patients: a practical approach. Southfield, MI: 1985:17

46. Sostre S, Ashare AB, Quinones JD, et al. Thyroid scintigraphy: pinhole images versus rectilinear scans. Radiology 1978; 129:759

47. Chen JJS, LaFrance ND, Allo MD, et al. Single photon emission computed tomography of the thyroid. J Clin Endocrinol Metab 1988;66:1240

48. Chen JJS, LaFrance ND, Rippin R, et al. Iodine-123 SPECT of the thyroid in multinodular goiter. J Nucl Med 1988;29:110

49. Webb S, Flower MA, Ott RJ, et al. Single photon emission computed tomography imaging and volume estimation of the thyroid using fan-beam geometry. Br J Radiol 1986;59:951

50. Flower MA, Irvine AT, Ott RJ, et al. Thyroid imaging using positron emission tomography—a comparison with ultrasound imaging and conventional imaging in thyrotoxicosis. Br J Radiol 1990;63:325

51. Adler LP, Bloom AD. Positron emission tomography of thyroid masses. Thyroid 1993;3:195

52. Lennquist S, Persliden J, Smeds S. The value of intraoperative scintigraphy as a routine procedure in thyroid carcinoma. World J Surg 1988;12:586

53. Hoffer PB, Gottschalk A. Fluorescent thyroid scanning. Scanning without radioisotopes: initial clinical results. Radiology 1971; 99:117

54. Patton JA, Sandler MP. X-ray fluorescent scanning. In: Sandler MP, Patton JA, Partain CL, eds. Thyroid and parathyroid imaging. East Norwalk, CT: Appleton-Century-Crofts, 1986:247

55. Du Cret RP, Choi RE, Roe SJ, et al. Improved prediction of thyroid lobar mass from parameters obtained by routine thyroid scintigraphy. Clin Nucl Med 1987;12:436

56. Krasnai I, Foldes J, Farkas G, et al. Determination of euthyroid mass. Nucl Med Commun 1985;6:169

57. Renda F, Holmes RA, North WA, Wagner HN Jr. Characteristics of thyroid scans in normals, hyperthyroidism and nodular goiter. J Nucl Med 1968;9:156

58. Spencer RP, Waldman R. Size and positional relationships between thyroid lobes in the adult as determined by scintillation scanning. J Nucl Med 1965;6:53

59. Hurley PJ, Strauss HW, Pavoni P, et al. The scintillation camera with pinhole collimator in thyroid imaging. Radiology 1971;101:133

60. Levy HA, Sziklas JJ, Rosenberg RJ, Spencer RP. Incidence of a pyramidal lobe on thyroid scans. Clin Nucl Med 1987; 12:560

61. Siraj QH, Aleem N, Inam-Ur-Rehman A, et al. The pyramidal lobe: a scintigraphic assessment. Clin Nucl Med 1989;10:685

62. Sternberg JL. Sublingual pyramidal lobe: complications of subtotal thyroidectomy for Graves' disease. Clin Nucl Med 1986; 11:766

63. Katz AD, Zager WJ. The lingual thyroid. Arch Surg 1971; 102:582

64. Knight PJ, Hamoudi AB, Vassy LE. The diagnosis and treatment of midline neck masses in children. Surgery 1983;93:603

65. Noyek AM, Friedberg J. Thyroglossal duct and ectopic thyroid disorders. Otolaryn Clin N Am 1981;14:187

66. Rieser GD, Ober KP, Cowan RJ, Cordell AR. Radioiodine imaging of struma cordis. Clin Nucl Med 1988;13:421

67. Hamburger JI, Hamburger SW. Thyroid hemiagenesis. Arch Surg 1970;100:319

68. Avramides A, Vichayanrat A, Solomon N, Carter AC. Thyroid hemiagenesis. Clin Nucl Med 1977;9:310

69. Melnick JC, Stemkowski PE. Thyroid hemiagenesis (hockey stick sign): a review of the world literature and a report of four cases. J Clin Endocrinol Metab 1981;52:247

70. Cornelius EA. Combined nuclear medicine and ultrasound studies in the evaluation of suppressed thyroid tissue. Clin Nucl Med 1983;8:8

71. Corstens F, Huysmans D, Kloppenberg P. Thallium-201 scintigraphy of the suppressed thyroid: an alternative for iodine-123 scanning after TSH. J Nucl Med 1988;29:1360

72. Ramanathan P, Patel RB, Subrahmanyan N, et al. Visualization of suppressed thyroid tissue by technetium-99m-tertiary butyl isonitrile: an alternative to post-TSH stimulation scanning. J Nucl Med 1990;31:1163

73. Rizzi G, Argiro G, Gentile L, et al. Use of the ^{99m}Tc scintiscan with lead-shield on the hot nodule in the diagnosis of adenomatous adenoma. Nucl Med Commun 1987;8:217

74. Ripley SD, Freitas JE, Nagle CE. Is thyroid scintigraphy really necessary before I-131 therapy of hyperthyroidism? Concise communication. J Nucl Med 1984;25:664

75. Vaccaro RM, Sorek M, Wulkan A, Pugliese P. Therapeutic radioiodine interference with subsequent diagnostic imaging. Clin Nucl Med 1994;19:829

76. Ashcraft MW, Van Herle AJ. Management of thyroid nodules. II. Scanning techniques, thyroid suppressive therapy, and fine needle aspiration. Head Neck Surg 1981;3:296

77. Gharib H, Goellner JR. Fine-needle aspiration of the thyroid. Ann Intern Med 1993;118:282

78. Mazzaferri EL. Management of a solitary thyroid nodule. N Engl J Med 1993;328:553

79. Erjavec M, Movrin T, Auersperg M, Golough R. Comparative accumulation of ^{99m}Tc and ^{131}I in thyroid nodules: case report. J Nucl Med 1977;18:346

80. Dos Remedios LV, Weber PM, Jasko IA. Thyroid scintiphotography in 1,000 patients: rational use of ^{99m}Tc and ^{131}I compounds. J Nucl Med 1971;12:1360

81. Turner JW, Spencer RP. Thyroid carcinoma presenting as a pertechnetate "hot" nodule, but without ^{131}I uptake: case report. J Nucl Med 1976;17:22

82. Task Force on Short-lived Radionuclides for Medical Applications. Evaluation of diseases of the thyroid with the in vivo use of radionuclides. J Nucl Med 1978;19:107

83. Kusic Z, Becker DV, Saenger EL, et al. Comparison of technetium-99m and iodine-123 imaging of thyroid nodules: correlation with pathologic findings. J Nucl Med 1990;31:393

84. Landgarten S, Spencer RP. A study of the natural history of "hot" nodule. Yale J Biol Med 1973;46:259

85. Livadas DP, Kotoulas OB, Bouropoulos V, et al. The coexistence of thyroid malignancy with autonomous hot nodules of the thyroid. Clin Nucl Med 1977;2:350

86. Ghose MK, Genuth SM, Abellera RM, et al. Functioning primary thyroid carcinoma and metastases producing hyperthyroidism. J Clin Endocrinol Metab 1971;33:639

87. Nagai GR, Pitts WC, Basso L, et al. Scintigraphic hot nodules and thyroid cancer. Clin Nucl Med 1987;12:123

88. Sandler MP, Fellmeth B, Salhany KE, Patton JA. Thyroid carcinoma masquerading as a solitary benign hyperfunctioning nodule. Clin Nucl Med 1988;13:410

89. Bashist B, Ellis K, Gold RP. Computed tomography and intrathoracic goiters. AJR Am J Roentgenol 1983;140:455

90. Sand ME, Laws HL, McElvein RB. Substernal and intrathoracic goiter: reconsideration of surgical approach. Am Surg 1983;49:196

91. Beierwaltes WH. Radioiodide in the therapy of thyroid carcinoma. In: Spencer RP, ed. Therapy in nuclear medicine. New York: Grune & Stratton, 1978:101

92. Hilts SV, Hellman D, Anderson J, et al. Serial TSH determination after T$_3$ withdrawal or thyroidectomy in the therapy of thyroid carcinoma. J Nucl Med 1979;20:928

93. Maxon HR, Thomas SR, Washburn LC, Hinnefeld JD. High-activity I-123 for the diagnostic evaluation of patients with thyroid cancer (abstract). J Nucl Med 1993;34:42P

94. Lakshmanan M, Schaffer A, Robbins J, et al. A simplified low iodine diet in I-131 scanning and therapy of thyroid carcinoma. Clin Nucl Med 1988;13:866

95. Ain KB, Dewitt PA, Gardner TG, Berryman SW. Low-iodine tube-feeding diet for iodine-131 scanning and therapy. Clin Nucl Med 1994;19:504-507

96. Barakat RM, Ingbar SH. The effect of acute iodide depletion on thyroid function in man. J Clin Invest 1965;44:1117

97. Hershman JM, Edwards L. Serum thyrotropin (TSH) levels after thyroid ablation compared with TSH levels after exogenous bovine TSH: implications for I-131 treatment of thyroid carcinoma. J Clin Endocrinol 1972;34:814

98. Krishnamurthy GT. Human reaction to bovine TSH. Concise communication. J Nucl Med 1978;19:284

99. Meier CA, Braverman LE, Ebner, et al. Diagnostic use of recombinant human thyrotropin in patients with thyroid carcinoma (phase I/II study). J Clin Endocrinol Metabol 1992;74:1135

100. Park H-M, Perkins OW, Edmondson JW, et al. Influence of diagnostic radioiodines on the uptake of ablative dose of iodine-131. Thyroid 1994;4:49-54

101. Maxon HR, Boehringer TA, Drilling J, et al. Low iodine diet in I-131 ablation of thyroid remnants. Clin Nucl Med 1983; 8:123

102. Greenler DP, Klein HA. The scope of false-positive iodine-131 images for thyroid carcinoma. Clin Nucl Med 1989;14:111

103. Norby EH, Neutze J, Van Nostrand D, et al. Nasal radioiodine activity: a prospective study of frequency, intensity, and pattern. J Nucl Med 1990;31:52

104. Hoschl R, Choy DH-L, Gandevia B. Iodine-131 uptake in inflammatory lung disease: a pitfall in treatment of thyroid carcinoma. J Nucl Med 1988;29:701

105. Caplan RH, Gunderson GA, Abellera RM, Kisken WA. Uptake of iodine-131 by a Meckel's diverticulum mimicking metastatic thyroid cancer. Clin Nucl Med 1987;12:760

106. Brachman MB, Rothman BJ, Ramanna L. False-positive iodine-131 body scan caused by a large renal cyst. Clin Nucl Med 1988;13:416

107. Camponovo EJ, Goyer PF, Silverman ED, et al. Axillary iodine-131 accumulation due to perspiration. Clin Nucl Med 1989;14:762

108. Ain KB, Shih W-J. False-positive I-131 uptake at a tracheostomy site: discernment with Tl-201 imaging. Clin Nucl Med 1994; 19:619

109. Acosta J, Chitkara R, Kahn F, et al. Radioactive iodine uptake by a large cell undifferentiated bronchogenic carcinoma. Clin Nucl Med 1982;7:368

110. Bakheet SM, Hammami MM. False-positive radioiodine whole-body scan in thyroid cancer patients due to unrelated pathology. Clin Nucl Med 1994;19:325

111. McDougall IR. Whole body scintigraphy with radioiodine. A comprehensive list of false-positives with some examples. Clin Nucl Med 1995;20:868

112. Halpern SE, Preisman R, Hagan PL. Scanning dose and the detection of thyroid metastases. J Nucl Med 1979;20:1099

113. Nemec J, Rohling S, Zamrazil V, et al. Comparison of the distribution of diagnostic and thyroablative I-131 in the evaluation of differentiated thyroid cancers. J Nucl Med 1979;20:92

114. Spies WG, Wojtowitcz CH, Spies SM, et al. Value of post-therapy whole-body I-131 imaging in the evaluation of patients with thyroid carcinoma having undergone high-dose I-131 therapy. Clin Nucl Med 1989;14:793

115. Pacini F, Lippi L, Formica M, et al. Therapeutic doses of iodine-131 reveal undiagnosed metastases in thyroid cancer patients with detectable serum-thyroglobulin levels. J Nucl Med 1987;28:1888

116. Rosenbaum RC, Johnston GS, Valente WA. Frequency of hepatic visualization during I-131 imaging for metastatic thyroid carcinoma. Clin Nucl Med 1988;13:657

117. Zeissman HA, Bahar H, Fahey FH, Dubiansky V. Hepatic visualization on iodine-131 whole-body thyroid cancer scans. J Nucl Med 1987;28:1408

118. Hays MT, McDougall IR. Circulating ^{131}I thyroxine and thyroid cancer. Thyroid 1994;4:195

119. Ronga G, Fiorentino A, Paserio E, et al. Can iodine-131 whole body scan be replaced by thyroglobulin measurement in the post-surgical follow-up of differentiated thyroid carcinoma. J Nucl Med 1990;31:1766

120. Mullins LJ, Moore RD. The movement of thallium ions in muscle. J Gen Physiol 1960;43:759

121. Berman DS, Kiat H, Maddahi J, Shah PK. Radionuclide imaging of myocardial perfusion and viability in assessment of acute myocardial infarction. Am J Cardiol 1989;64:9B

122. Leppo JA . Dipyridamole-thallium imaging: the lazy man's stress test. J Nucl Med 1989;30:281

123. Atkins HL, Budinger TF, Lebowitz E, et al. Thallium-201 for medical use. Part 3: human distribution and physical imaging properties. J Nucl Med 1977;18:133

124. Sehweil AM, McKillop JM, Ziada J, et al. The optimum time for tumor imaging with thallium-201. Eur J Nucl Med 1988;13:527

125. Krasnow AZ, Collier BD, Isitman AT, et al. The clinical significance of unusual sites of thallium-201 uptake. Semin Nucl Med 1988;18:350

126. Hoefnagel CA, Delprat CC, Marcuse HR, Vijlder JJM. Role of thallium-201 total-body scintigraphy in follow-up of thyroid carcinoma. J Nucl Med 1986;27:1854

127. Brendel AJ, Guyot M, Jeandot R, et al. Thallium-201 imaging in the follow-up of differentiated thyroid carcinoma. J Nucl Med 1988;29:1515

128. Iida Y, Hidaka A, Hatabu H, et al. Follow-up study of postoperative patients with thyroid cancer by thallium-201 scintigraphy and serum thyroglobulin measurement. J Nucl Med 1991;32:2098

129. Sorge-Van Boxel RAJ, Van Eck-Smit BLF, Goslings BM. Comparison of serum thyroglobulin, ^{131}I and ^{201}Tl scintigraphy in the postoperative follow-up of differentiated thyroid cancer. Nucl Med Commun 1993;14:365

130. Yen T-C, Lin H-D, Lee C-H, et al. The role of technetium-99m sestamibi whole-body scans in diagnosing metastatic Hurthle cell carcinoma of the thyroid gland after total thyroidectomy: a comparison with iodine-131 and thallium-201 whole-body scans. Eur J Nucl Med 1994;21:980

131. Campbell CM, Khafagi FA. Insensitivity of Tc-99m pertechnetate for detecting metastases of differentiated thyroid carcinoma. Clin Nucl Med 1990;15:1

132. Khammash NF, Halkar RK, Abdel-Dayem HM. The use of technetium-99m pertechnetate in postoperative thyroid carcinoma. A comparative study with iodine-131. Clin Nucl Med 1988;13:17

133. Krenning EP, Kwekkeboom DJ, Bakkar WH, et al. Somatostatin receptor scintigraphy with [^{111}In-DTPA-D-Phe1]- and [^{123}I-Tyr3]-octreotide: the Rotterdam experience with more than 1000 patients. Eur J Nucl Med 1993;20:716

134. Kwekkeboom DJ, Reubi JC, Lamberts SWJ, et al. In vivo somatostatin receptor imaging in medullary thyroid carcinoma. J Clin Endocrinol Metab 1993;76:1413

135. Higashi T, Ito K, Mimura T, et al. Clinical evaluation of ^{67}Ga in the diagnosis of anaplastic carcinoma and lymphoma of the thyroid. Radiology 1981;141:491

136. Moreno AJ, Brown JM, Spicer MJ, et al. Thyroid localization of Ga-67 citrate. Semin Nucl Med 1985;15:224

137. Sanders LR, Moreno AJ, Pittman DL, et al. Painless giant cell thyroiditis diagnosed by fine needle aspiration and associated with intense thyroidal uptake of gallium. Am J Med 1986;80:971

138. Allard JC, Lee VW, Franklin P. Thyroid uptake of gallium in Graves' disease. Clin Nucl Med 1988;13:663

139. Ling MCC, Dake MD, Okerlund MD. Gallium uptake in the thyroid gland in amiodarone-induced hyperthyroidism. Clin Nucl Med 1988;13:258

140. White WB, Spencer RP, Sziklas JJ, Rosenberg RJ. Incidental finding of intense thyroid radiogallium activity during febrile illness. Clin Nucl Med 1985;10:71

141. Castillo LA, Yeh SDJ, Leeper RD, Benua RS. Bone scans in bone metastases from functioning thyroid carcinoma. Clin Nucl Med 1980;5:200

142. Spencer RP, Garg V, Raisz LG, et al. Radioiodine uptake and turnover in a pseudo-medullary thyroid carcinoma. J Nucl Med 1982;23:1006

143. Arnstein NB, Juni JE, Sisson JC, et al. Recurrent medullary carcinoma of the thyroid demonstrated by thallium-201 scintigraphy. J Nucl Med 1986;27:1564

144. Parthasary KL, Shimaoka K, Bakshi SP, et al. Radiotracer uptake in medullary cancer of the thyroid. Clin Nucl Med 1980;5:45

145. Hoefnagel CA, Delprat CC, Zanin D, et al. New radionuclide tracers for the diagnosis and therapy of medullary thyroid cancer. Clin Nucl Med 1988;13:159

146. Miyauchi A, Endo K, Ohta H, et al. [99m]Tc (V) dimercaptosuccinic acid scintigraphy for medullary thyroid carcinoma. World J Surg 1986;10:640

147. Ohta H, Yamamoto K, Endo K, et al. A new imaging agent for medullary carcinoma of the thyroid. J Nucl Med 1984;25:323

148. Hilditch TE, Murray T, Connell JMC, et al. Imaging with pentavalent [^{99m}Tc]DMSA in patients with medullary cancer of the thyroid. J Nucl Med 1988;29:1746

149. Clarke SEM, Lazarus CR, Wraight P, et al. Pentavalent [^{99m}Tc]DMSA, [^{131}I]MIBG and [^{99m}Tc]MDP—an evaluation of three imaging techniques in patients with medullary carcinoma of the thyroid. J Nucl Med 1988;29:33

150. Mojiminiyi OA, Udelsman R, Shepstone BJ, et al. More on [^{99m}Tc](V)DMSA scintigraphy in patients with medullary carcinoma of the thyroid. J Nucl Med 1989;30:1420

151. Singh J, Reghebi K, Lazarus CR, et al. Studies on the preparation and isometric composition of [186]Re and [188]Re-pentavalent rhenium dimercaptosuccinic acid complex. Nucl Med Commun 1993;14:197

152. Endo K, Shiomi K, Kasagi K, et al. Imaging of medullary thyroid cancer with ^{131}I-MIBG. Lancet 1984;ii:1273

153. Keeling CA, Basso LV. Iodine-131 MIBG uptake in metastatic medullary carcinoma of the thyroid. Clin Nucl Med 1988;13:260

154. Laflamme L, Taillefer R, Duranceau A, et al. Medullary thyroid carcinoma: localization of a mediastinal metastasis with I-131 MIBG. Clin Nucl Med 1988;13:577

155. Sone T, Kununaga M, Otsuka S, et al. Metastatic medullary thyroid cancer: localization with iodine-131 meta-iodobenzyl-guanidine. J Nucl Med 1985;26:604

156. Guilloteau D, Baulieu J-L, Besnard J-C. Medullary-thyroid-carcinoma imaging in an animal model: use of radiolabeled anticalcitonin F(ab<pg> and meta-iodobenzylguanidine. Eur J Nucl Med 1985;11:198

157. Romney BM, Nickoloff EL. Diagnostic nuclear medicine and the nursing mother. Appl Radiol 1987;May:51

158. Romney BM, Nickoloff EL, Esser PD, Alderson PO. Radionuclide administration to nursing mothers: mathematically derived guidelines. Radiology 1986;160:549

159. Mountford PJ, Coakley AJ. A review of the secretion of radioactivity in human breast milk: data, quantitative analysis and recommendations. Nucl Med Commun 1989;10:15

160. Werner SC. Response to triiodothyronine as an index of persistence of disease in the thyroid remnant of patients in remission from hyperthyroidism. J Clin Invest 1956;35:57

161. Werner SC, Spooner M. A new and simple test for hyperthyroidism employing L-triiodothyronine and the 24 hour ^{131}I uptake method. Bull N Y Acad Med 1955;31:137

162. Charkes ND, Cantor RE, Goluboff B. A three day, double isotope, L-triiodothyronine suppression test of thyroid autonomy. J Nucl Med 1967;8:627

163. Dresner S, Schneeberg NL. Rapid radioiodine suppression test using triiodothyronine. J Clin Endocrinol Metab 1958; 18:797

164. Gorman CA, Wahner HW, Tauxe WN. Metabolic malingerers. Am J Med 1970;48:708

165. Charkes ND. Thyroid and whole-body imaging In: Ingbar SH, Braverman LE, eds. Werner's the thyroid: a fundamental and clinical text, 5th ed. Philadelphia: JB Lippincott, 1986:458

Werner and Ingbar's The Thyroid, Seventh Edition,
edited by Lewis E. Braverman and Robert D. Utiger.
Lippincott–Raven Publishers, Philadelphia, © 1996

18

Serum Thyrotropin and Thyroid Hormone Measurements and Assessment of Thyroid Hormone Transport

Jan R. Stockigt

In the past 5 years, as thyrotropin (TSH) assays of greater sensitivity have come into widespread use, important changes have occurred in the strategy of thyroid function testing. It is now possible to distinguish not only between normal and low serum TSH concentrations but also between the very low concentrations typical of thyrotoxicosis and low TSH concentrations due to other causes. Proliferation of assays for serum free thyroxine (T_4) has continued, with a trend for these to replace the dual measurements of total hormone and an index of binding.

As with all new diagnostic methods,[1] the potential for false-positive or false-negative serum free T_4 and TSH results may not become known for several years, until the full diversity of the nondiseased population is appreciated. Assessment of specificity must include studies of patients with a full range of incidental illnesses and those taking many medications.

THE TSH-FREE T_4 RELATIONSHIP

If a sensitive serum TSH assay is used together with a valid serum free T_4 estimate, a sensitive and specific assessment of thyroid status can usually be made from the general relation between the two hormones (Fig 18-1). Serum TSH is best shown on a logarithmic scale because its response to changes in serum free T_4 is markedly amplified. Because of negative feedback, typical disease-related changes lead to diagonal deviations from the normal relationship between serum TSH and free T_4. The figure emphasizes the distinction between primary target gland failure (high serum TSH, low free T_4: A), failure of TSH secretion (both low: B), autonomous or abnormally stimulated target gland function (high serum free T_4, low TSH: C), and primary excess of TSH or thyroid hormone resistance (both high: D). If serum TSH and free T_4 changes are considered in terms of their feedback correlation, it is possible to identify unusual deviations from normal in which some other factor has disturbed this relationship, or the sample was collected in non–steady-state conditions (see later discussion). Serum free T_4 rather than triiodothyronine (T_3) is shown in Figure 18-1 because it is the major circulating determinant of TSH secretion (see chap 12). However, T_3 also has an important direct inhibitory effect on TSH secretion.[2]

Small changes in serum T_4 and T_3 concentrations, within the normal range, alter serum TSH in individual subjects,[3,4] indicating that tropic and target hormones are inversely related across the normal ranges as well as in disease states. In Figure 18-1, normality is defined by a circle or ellipse, rather than the square or rectangle that would befit reference ranges of two unrelated variables. Hence, some results fall outside the normal reference area for the T_4-TSH relation, without the values being clearly abnormal for either.

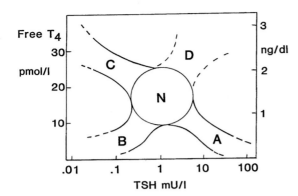

FIGURE 18-1. The relationship between serum TSH and free T$_4$ concentrations in normal subjects (N) and patients with various abnormalities of thyroid function: A, primary hypothyroidism; B, central (secondary) hypothyroidism; C, thyrotoxicosis (excluding TSH-induced thyrotoxicosis). Results in area D are uncommon but suggest a possible methodologic artefact, an unrecognized binding abnormality, generalized thyroid hormone resistance, or TSH-induced thyrotoxicosis. Findings that fall in the undefined areas suggest that an additional factor may be modifying the feedback relationship or that samples have been taken in non–steady-state conditions. Serum free T$_4$ is shown on a linear scale, whereas the scale for serum TSH is logarithmic.

Diagnostic Assumptions

The schema outlined in Figure 18-1 allows precise diagnosis of thyroid dysfunction to be made from a single serum sample, dependent on the following assumptions (Table 18-1):

1. The sample is taken in steady-state conditions. Common deviations from the steady state are related to short-term pulsatile or diurnal fluctuations in hormone secretion, responses to treatment, and spontaneous evolution of disease. Examples of the latter are the fluctuations that occur in patients with subacute thyroiditis and postpartum thyroid dysfunction during the evolution of their illness[5,6] (see chaps 34 and 89). Discrepancies also occur in the early phases of treatment for both thyrotoxicosis and hypothyroidism and during recovery from the hypothyroxinemia of severe illness.[7] In considering these discrepancies, it is worth noting that serum TSH tends to deviate more rapidly from the steady state because it has a much shorter half-life in the circulation than either serum T$_4$ or T$_3$.

2. The active hormone concentration has been accurately measured. TSH and iodothyronine assays make comparative, rather than absolute, measurements of hormone concentrations, based on the assumption that sample and assay standard differ only in their concentration of analyte. Any other difference between a serum sample and assay standards may influence the assay value, as, for example, with dissimilar protein binding of tracer or possible nonspecific interference with enzymatic, fluorescent, or chemiluminescent detection systems.[8,9]

    If the biologic activity of circulating immunoreactive TSH is increased or decreased, the normal relationship between measured serum TSH and free T$_4$ may be altered (Table 18-2). Secreted immunoreactive TSH is heterogeneous, due to differences in its three oligosaccharide side chains.[10] In hypothalamic hypothyroidism, the secreted TSH may have decreased bioactivity, whereas it may be enhanced in thyroid hormone resistance and primary hypothyroidism[10] (see chap 11).

3. Tissue responses are proportional to the active hormone concentration. In most patients, there is a close correlation between the active hormone concentration and clinical features, but in generalized thyroid hormone resistance, high serum free T$_4$ and T$_3$ concentrations are required to maintain the euthyroid state.[11,12] In the absence of a sensitive, specific index of thyroid hormone action in tissues other than the pituitary, clinical assessment remains crucial for assessing the peripheral effects of thyroid hormone excess or deficiency. The onset and offset of thyroid hormone action is slow, so that tissue responses may lag behind changes in serum free T$_4$ and T$_3$ concentrations. Some medications (e.g., amiodarone and phenytoin) may modify expression of thyroid hormone action.

4. The analytic method can reliably distinguish low from normal values. Assay precision inevitably deteriorates as the limit of detection is approached; this characteristic is crucial in evaluating new TSH assays. In general, the lower working limit of a TSH assay should be defined in terms of its between-assay reproducibility, defined as functional sensitivity, rather than as the analytical sensitivity of individual assays (see below).

5. Normal reference ranges apply to the study subject. Age-related variations, associated illness, nutritional changes, and various medications may cause assay results to fall outside the normal reference ranges shown in Table 18-3, as defined in normal subjects. TSH reference ranges need to be calculated after logarithmic transformation to define properly the lower normal limit (see below).

6. The tropic-target hormone relationship is normal. As summarized in Table 18-2, numerous factors can disturb the relationship between serum free T$_4$ and immunoreactive TSH. After prolonged thyrotoxicosis, TSH secretion may remain low for several weeks or even months after serum free T$_4$ concentration becomes normal.[13] Conversely, in some children with chronic hypothyroidism, TSH hypersecretion may persist, albeit at a lower level, during T$_4$ therapy.[14] The issue of an individual setpoint for the feedback link between serum free T$_4$ and TSH is discussed below.

ASSAY CHOICE AND APPLICATION

For definitive diagnosis, assessment of both serum TSH and free T$_4$ is required, but a more limited approach can be used for initial case finding and follow-up. In the interests of cost effectiveness, evaluation of thyroid status may often begin with an assay for either serum TSH or free T$_4$, followed by further algorithm-based assessment if the initial result is abnormal. As an initial test, serum total T$_4$ measurements give an unacceptable rate of abnormal results, due to the fre-

TABLE 18-1.
Major Assumptions in the Laboratory Assessment of Thyroid Function

Assumption	Exceptions or Limitations
Steady-state conditions	Fluctuating hormone secretion
	Response to therapy
	Evolution of disease
	Transient effects of medications
Accurate estimate of active hormone concentration	Changes in serum binding:
	Thyroxine-binding globulin
	Albumin
	Transthyretin (thyroxine-binding prealbumin)
	Autoantibodies to T_4 or T_3
	Effects of circulating inhibitors
	TSH of altered biologic activity
	Nonspecific differences between sample and assay standards
Tissue response proportional to hormone concentrations	Delayed offset or onset of thyroid hormone action
	Hormone-resistance syndromes
	Some drug effects (eg, amiodarone, phenytoin)
Adequate assay sensitivity	Poor precision at limits of detection
Reference ranges apply to the study subject	Influence of age
	Associated illness
	Nutrition
	Medications
Normal tropic-target hormone relationship	See Table 18-2

quency of abnormalities in serum thyroid hormone-binding proteins.

Four distinct clinical situations in which evaluation of thyroid function is done can be considered: testing of unselected populations for case finding or screening, testing of untreated patients who have clinical features that suggest thyroid disease, assessment of the response to treatment for thyroid dysfunction, and evaluation of patients in whom associated illnesses or drug therapy are likely to complicate clinical and laboratory assessment or whose initial results are atypical or unclear.

Screening and Case Finding

Compared with the clear benefit of thyroid screening in newborn infants (see section on neonatal screening in chap 85), the cost benefit of routine thyroid testing in adults is much less certain.[15] The results of relevant studies have varied depending on the population studied, choice of test, and definitions of overt and subclinical disease. In neither unselected healthy persons nor patients seeking medical care does it appear justified to measure serum TSH or T_4 routinely, although 2% to 7% of women over age 40 years may have slightly elevated serum TSH concentrations[15–17] (see chap 26). The case for routine assessment of thyroid status is strongest in elderly women who have any symptoms that could be consistent with hypothyroidism.[15] Among hospitalized patients, the large majority of abnormal results are due to nonthyroidal illness or medications.[16] Because the incidence of thyroid disease is much lower than its prevalence, there is no justification for regular, periodic laboratory reassessment.[15]

Most persons found to have either high or low serum TSH values in screening or case-finding studies have subclinical disease. That is, they have no clinical manifestations of

TABLE 18-2.
Alterations in the Normal Relation Between Serum Free T_4 and TSH Concentrations

Alternative thyroid stimulators
   Immunoglobulins
   Chorionic gonadotropin
TSH isoforms with altered biologic activity
Pulsatile TSH secretion
Medications
   T_4, T_3, thyroid extract or triiodothyroacetic acid
   Dopamine
   Glucocorticoids
   Amiodarone
Severe nonthyroidal illness
Recent thyrotoxicosis
Long-standing hypothyroidism
Selective T_3 secretion
Variable individual setpoint
Iodine deficiency [141]
Overfeeding, caloric deprivation[142,143]
Thyrotropin receptor mutations[144]

TABLE 18-3.
Typical Reference Ranges for Serum Thyroid Hormones and TSH in Humans*

| Hormone | Reference Ranges | | Variations Unrelated to Thyroid Disease |
	METRIC	SI UNIT	
Thyroxine (T_4)	4–11 µg/dL	60–140 nmol/L	Binding protein changes, binding competitors
Free T_4	0.7–2.1 ng/dL	10–25 pmol/L	Methodologic factors, pregnancy
Triiodothyronine (T_3)	75–175 ng/dL	1.1–2.7 nmol/L†	Binding protein changes, binding competitors, age-related changes, nutrition, illness, surgery, drugs
Free T_3	0.2–6.5 ng/dL	3–8 pmol/L†	Methodologic factors and influences on total T_3
Reverse T_3	15–45 ng/dL	0.2–0.7 nmol/L	Nutrition, illness, surgery, drugs
TSH	0.3–4.0 mU/L‡	~1–15 pmol/L§	Diurnal variation, pulse secretion, age-related changes, drugs
TSH α-subunit	<0.2 µg/dL	<100 pmol/L	Postmenopausal woman, hypogonadism
THBR‖	80%–115%	80%–115%	Hereditary variations, pregnancy, medications

These ranges should be determined for the particular methods used in each laboratory; the neonatal period is excluded.
Higher values in childhood.[64]
§Assumes biologic potency of 7–15 U/mg.
‡IRMA (immunoradiometric assay) values; RIA (radioimmunoassay) values may be higher.
‖Calculated as resin divided by serum counts in relation to a reference serum.
THBR; thyroid hormone-binding ratio.

thyroid dysfunction and normal serum free T_4 and T_3 concentrations. The importance of subclinical hypothyroidism and subclinical thyrotoxicosis is discussed in chapters 87 and 88, respectively.

Regardless of which initial test is used, assessment of thyroid status has a high priority in patients at increased risk of having thyroid dysfunction, as for example in those with goiter, those treated previously for thyrotoxicosis or receiving lithium or amiodarone, and patients with associated autoimmune disease or connective tissue diseases or a history of neck or whole body irradiation.

Untreated Patients

In untreated ambulatory patients, a normal serum TSH concentration has high negative predictive value in ruling out thyroid disease.[16] If serum TSH is abnormal, serum free T_4 concentration must also be measured before treatment is given. Diagnostic strategies have been evaluated in which serum T_4 measurements are done routinely only if the serum TSH is abnormal,[17,18] unless pituitary disease is suspected. Long-term assessment of this approach will need to balance cost savings against potentially serious adverse outcomes, for example, if thyrotoxicosis is missed because of spuriously normal serum TSH values (see below), or central hypothyroidism is missed on the basis of normal serum TSH values.[10]

The following groups of patients will be incompletely or incorrectly assessed if either serum TSH or free T_4 alone is measured.

- Patients with subclinical hypothyroidism[19,20] (high serum TSH, normal free T_4), in whom replacement therapy may be beneficial
- Those with subclinical thyrotoxicosis[20,21] (low serum TSH, normal free T_4), in whom treatment with an antithyroid drug or thyroid ablation may be beneficial

- Those being treated for thyrotoxicosis, in whom suppression of TSH secretion may persist for weeks or months after normalization of serum T_4 and T_3[13]
- Those with central (secondary or hypothyrotropic) hypothyroidism (low serum free T_4, low or normal TSH), who should be evaluated for adrenal insufficiency before T_4 therapy is initiated
- Those with binding abnormalities such as familial dysalbuminemic hyperthyroxinemia (FDH)[22] or T_4- or T_3-binding autoantibodies,[23] in whom some serum free T_4 estimates are invalid (see below)
- Those with thyroid hormone resistance with high serum T_4 and T_3 concentrations and normal or high serum TSH concentrations,[11,12] who are often not recognized until after inappropriate treatment has been given
- Those with thyrotoxicosis caused by excess TSH secretion caused by a pituitary tumor[24] or selective pituitary resistance to thyroid hormone[25]

Notwithstanding the widespread acceptance of serum TSH as a single initial test, some still advocate an estimate of free T_4 as the best initial test for suspected thyrotoxicosis.[26]

Assessment of the Response to Treatment

In the testing of ambulatory patients with known thyroid disease, the use of serum TSH alone can also be considered. In a study of 460 ambulatory patients attending a thyroid clinic, hypothyroid patients taking T_4 for either replacement or suppression seldom needed a serum free T_4 measurement if the serum TSH was greater than 0.05 mU/L, although at lower values, the magnitude of hyperthyroxinemia did influence management.[27] In contrast, in patients with newly diagnosed thyrotoxicosis, measurements of serum free T_4 or free T_3, or both, were necessary in addition to serum TSH not only to establish the degree of hormone excess but also to evaluate the response to treatment. This study included few new cases of hypothyroidism, in whom serum T_4 measurement also would be required to establish the degree of hormone deficiency. In patients with thyroiditis and pituitary-hypothalamic disease, combined assessment was required.[27]

In evaluating patients receiving T_4 therapy, some have suggested that hormone measurements add little to a clinical assessment made by experts,[28] but there is justification for periodic serum TSH assessment to avoid subtle tissue effects of thyroid hormone excess or deficiency.[29,30] A serum TSH value in the low-normal range is probably the best single indicator of appropriate dosage and is certainly of more use than a serum free T_4 value alone, which may be increased without clinical features of thyrotoxicosis[31] and may vary slightly depending on the time interval between dose and sampling.[32] In some situations (e.g., patients with ischemic heart disease and hypothyroidism), the appropriate dose of T_4 should be based on clinical judgment rather than laboratory findings (see chap 77).

Difficult Diagnostic Situations

The prevalence of abnormal serum T_4 or TSH values in patients with acute medical[16,33] or psychiatric illness is high,[34] but there is controversy as to the value of thyroid function testing in these situations because most of the abnormalities do not indicate the presence of thyroid disease.[16,33,34] Although some advocate widespread or routine testing in acutely ill patients because of the potential importance of intercurrent thyroid disease and the difficulty in assessing clinical features of thyroid dysfunction,[33] others suggest that testing should not be done without some clinical indication.[16] If frequent or routine testing is to be done, some advocate the serum T_4 index as the initial test,[33] whereas others favor serum TSH;[35] in either case, an abnormal result should be followed by assessment of both by the best available methods. Although the combination of low serum T_4 and low TSH concentrations indicates a poor prognosis in critically ill patients,[36,37] there is no evidence that these findings can usefully influence management decisions.

In patients hospitalized for acute illness, one or more of the assumptions outlined above may not be justified, for example, when there are wide fluctuations from the steady state.[7] Serum TSH values frequently are subnormal in the absence of thyrotoxicosis[38,39] and serum free T_4 estimates are subject to multiple interfering influences, depending often on the particular method used (see later discussion and section on nonthyroidal illness in chap 14). Dual assessment clearly is necessary to identify the serum free T_4-TSH combinations that indicate true thyroid dysfunction (see Fig 18-1). When a patient has both thyroid dysfunction and a severe nonthyroidal illness, assessment becomes especially difficult[40] because the effects of the illness, medications, or changes in nutrition can alter the expected changes in serum free T_4 or TSH. Only clinical reevaluation and repeated sampling may resolve the dilemma.

MEASUREMENT OF SERUM TSH CONCENTRATIONS

Thyrotropin, a 28- to 30-kd glycoprotein composed of two subunits, is secreted by the thyrotropic cells of the anterior pituitary in negative feedback relation to the serum free T_4 and T_3 concentrations, acting in concert with thyrotropin-releasing hormone (TRH) and other signals of central nervous origin (see chaps 11 and 12).

In normal subjects, serum TSH concentrations vary as a result of both pulsatile and diurnal secretion, with mean maximum concentrations of approximately 3 mU/L at about 2400 hours and mean nadir values of about 1 mU/L at about 1600 hours; there is no significant sex difference.[41] Most TSH pulses occur at night and are accentuated by sleep deprivation and suppressed during sleep after sleep withdrawal.[41] The nocturnal increase in TSH secretion is lost in critical illness[42] and after surgery.[43] Patients with overt or subclinical thyrotoxicosis and those receiving T_4 therapy who have very low serum TSH concentrations have no detectable nocturnal peak.[44] Because TSH secretion is pulsatile, with an amplitude of 20% to 50% around the mean,[41] it can be difficult to decide in follow-up studies, particularly in patients with subclinical hypothyroidism, whether serial changes in TSH are relevant, because a change of up to 30% to 40% could reflect random variation rather than progression of disease.

Reference values between 0800 and 2100 hours for serum immunoreactive TSH assays generally are in the range of 0.3 to 4 mU/L (see Table 18-3), with higher values in the immediate neonatal period when there is a surge of TSH secretion.[45] Values in old age are more variable, but in one study the geometric mean and 95% confidence limits for serum TSH were similar in middle-aged and elderly subjects.[46] The TSH reference range should be evaluated logarithmically to achieve an accurate estimate of the lower normal limit. If reference ranges are based on untransformed data, the mean values are higher and the lower normal limit is less precise[46] (Fig 18-2).

Serum Free T_4-TSH Setpoint

There may be individual variations in the feedback link between serum free T_4 and TSH. Some healthy elderly subjects have normal serum TSH concentrations despite having low serum free T_4 index values, attributed to resetting of the threshold for TSH inhibition.[47] The results of studies of monozygotic and dizygotic twin pairs also suggest that genetic factors influence the serum concentrations of total and free T_4 within the normal range,[48] which raises the possibility that the TSH setpoint for a particular serum free T_4 or free T_3 concentration is a definable personal or familial characteristic. In a study in which normal subjects were given incremental doses of T_3, there were significant individual variations in setpoint of the pituitary-thyroid axis that were independent of age and sex.[49]

Assay Methodology

The early serum TSH radioimmunoassays had a sensitivity limit of 0.5 to 1 mU/L, which was not sufficient to distinguish

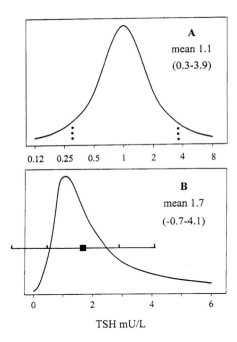

FIGURE 18-2. Typical serum TSH values in normal subjects. (*A*) Logarithmic transformation shows a normal distribution with a 95% confidence limit of 0.3 to 3.9 mU/L. (*B*) Without logarithmic transformation, the same results show a skewed distribution with a higher mean value and an imprecise, or apparently negative, lower limit of normal, when estimated as mean minus 2 SD.

low from normal values.[50] The introduction of immunometric assays that use two antibodies against different epitopes on the subunits of TSH has resulted in much improved sensitivity and specificity.[50] These techniques allow measurement of serum TSH concentrations below 0.1 mU/L, so that the lowest concentrations in normal subjects can be clearly distinguished from those found in patients with thyrotoxicosis.

In immunometric assays, the TSH serves as a bridge between the two antibodies. One antibody is usually linked to a solid phase, while the second antibody is labeled with an isotope or enzyme, or a fluorescent or chemiluminescent reagent. Some isoforms of circulating TSH that are recognized by radioimmunoassays do not have both epitopes for recognition by immunometric assays so that the values are 20% to 30% lower than those measured by radioimmunoassay.[51] This difference is much less after TRH stimulation because the newly secreted TSH more closely resembles the pituitary standard used in the assays.[51]

In contrast to radioimmunoassays, immunometric assays are noncompetitive, that is, the signal is *directly* proportional to the analyte concentration. Nevertheless, they are still comparative and depend on identity between sample and assay standard in all measured characteristics other than TSH concentration.

Sensitivity and Assay Classification

Several factors in addition to the inherent sensitivity of the dose-response curve become important when clinical decisions are based on values close to the limits of detection. They include between-assay reproducibility or precision profile, choice and consistency of zero matrix, possible appearance of nonspecific interference during sample storage, and the method of calculating reference ranges from normal data.

Analytical sensitivity can be defined from the dose-response characteristics of a single assay by expressing sensitivity (the limit of detection) as two or three standard deviations above the zero point, but practical experience demonstrates that this estimate is often too optimistic.[52] For example, a serum TSH value reported as 0.15 mU/L may appear accurate within a particular assay, but between-assay variation could lead to undetectable or near-normal values in subsequent assays of the same sample. Hence, a definition of functional sensitivity in terms of the between-assay coefficient of variation is preferable. A 20% between-assay coefficient of variation is becoming accepted as the criterion of functional sensitivity.[39,51] Based on this definition, TSH assays are now commonly designated as first, second or third generation, depending on whether their limit of functional sensitivity is in the range 1.0 to 2.0, 0.1 to 0.2, or 0.01 to 0.02 mU/L. Manufacturers' estimates of functional sensitivity are often not confirmed in clinical application,[52] and assay performance may vary markedly between laboratories, despite apparently identical reagents and instrumentation.[52] Hence, laboratories should make their own assessment by evaluation of the between-assay precision profile in the subnormal range.

Serum TSH Values in Nonthyroidal Illness

Third-generation TSH assays are sufficiently sensitive to distinguish the very low serum TSH values in most thyrotoxic patients from the subnormal but somewhat higher values in some patients with nonthyroidal illness.[38,39,53] Among a group of patients with low serum TSH values (<0.1 mU/L), almost all thyrotoxic patients had values less than 0.01 mU/L, whereas most critically ill euthyroid patients had values between 0.01 and 0.1 mU/L[39] (Fig 18-3). In another study, however, about 4% of patients with nonthyroidal illness had values below the functional sensitivity of a third-generation assay.[54]

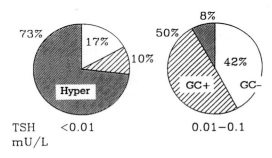

FIGURE 18-3. Specificity for thyrotoxicosis of a third-generation serum TSH assay in hospitalized patients with serum TSH concentrations less than 0.1 mU/L who had either proven thyrotoxicosis (Hyper) or nonthyroidal illness, with or without glucocorticoid treatment (GC+ or GC-). Serum TSH values less than 0.01 mU/L were 73% specific for thyrotoxicosis, whereas values in the range of 0.01 to 0.1 mU/L indicated thyrotoxicosis in only 8% (Data from Spencer CA, et al[39]; figure modified from Kaptein EM[53].) .

Serum TSH Values During T_4 Therapy

The availability of third-generation TSH assays has refined some therapeutic objectives. When the aim of T_4 suppressive therapy is regression of benign thyroid tissue, it may be adequate to give sufficient T_4 to reduce serum TSH to 0.1 to 0.3 mU/L.[55] However, in patients with thyroid carcinoma, further TSH suppression may be appropriate, although the benefit of higher T_4 dosage remains unproven[55] (see chap 80).

Subclinical Thyrotoxicosis

Clearly detectable serum TSH values below the lower limit of normal (i.e., 0.05–0.3 mU/L) are found in 4% to 5% of men and women over age 60 years.[56] Few of these subjects developed frank thyrotoxicosis within 1 year, and in many, serum TSH returned to normal.[56] The 10-year risk of atrial fibrillation was not increased in men and women over age 60 years who had initial serum TSH values in the range 0.1 to 0.4 mU/L, although this risk was increased threefold in subjects whose serum TSH concentrations were initially less than 0.1 mU/L.[57]

Nonspecific Interference

Although immunometric TSH assays offer much greater sensitivity than was possible previously, there can be problems with nonspecific interference. An important assay artifact can occur in immunometric methods that use mouse monoclonal antibodies, if an antimouse immunoglobulin in the test serum allows the formation of a false bridge between the solid phase and the signal antibodies, thereby generating a spuriously high assay value[58] (Fig 18-4). Inclusion of nonspecific mouse immunoglobulin in the assay blocks this effect.[59]

In a study in which serum TSH was measured by six different third-generation assays in 63 patients with thyrotoxicosis, all patients had low values in a least one assay, but 11 had reproducible serum TSH values greater than 0.1 mU/L in one or more assays.[60] These detectable concentrations did not increase in response to TRH and could not be eliminated by addition of mouse serum in the assay. Such anomalous values may be more frequent if serum samples are not refrigerated.[52] The finding of what appear to be nonspecific effects of serum from some thyrotoxic patients is an important drawback to the use of serum TSH assay as a sole initial test.

INDICATIONS FOR TRH TESTING

The development of high-sensitivity TSH assays has nearly eliminated the need for TRH testing in clinical practice. In patients with intact hypothalamic-pituitary function, TRH testing has no diagnostic advantage over accurate measurement of the basal serum TSH concentration.[61] Nevertheless, measurement of serum TSH 20 to 30 minutes after intravenous injection of 200 to 500 µg TRH is still useful for some purposes:

- To assess patients whose basal serum TSH values are out of context, to identify assay artifacts. For example,

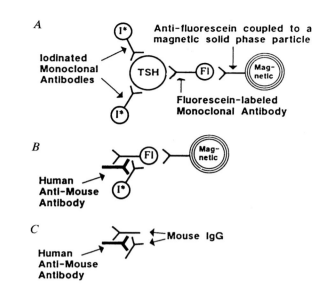

FIGURE 18-4. Proposed mechanism for falsely elevated serum TSH concentrations in an immunoradiometric TSH assay that uses mouse monoclonal antibodies, due to the presence of antibodies to mouse immunoglobulin in the patient's serum. (*A*) Normal assay conditions in which TSH forms a bridge between two monoclonal antibodies; the signal antibody in this assay is linked to fluorescein, which is identified by binding to antifluorescein linked to a magnetic particle. (*B*) Human antimouse antibodies allow the formation of a false bridge that imitates the presence of TSH. (*C*) Prevention of interference by addition of normal mouse immunoglobulin. (From Kahn BB, Weintraub BD, Csako G, Zweig MH. Factitious elevation of thyrotropin in a new ultra sensitive assay; implications for the use of monoclonal antibodies in "sandwich" immunoassay. J Clin Endocrinol Metab 1988;66:526)

a detectable serum TSH concentration that is unresponsive to TRH in a thyrotoxic patient suggests either nonspecific assay interference,[51,58,60] or pituitary-dependent thyrotoxicosis.

- To define apparent cases of thyroid hormone resistance or pituitary-dependent thyrotoxicosis. Most patients with thyrotoxicosis caused by TSH-secreting pituitary tumors have no increase in serum TSH in response to TRH.[24] In contrast, patients who have no tumor and those with thyroid hormone resistance usually have an increase in serum TSH in response to TRH[11,12] (see chap 31).

- To identify central hypothyroidism in a patient with a borderline-low serum free T_4 value and a normal serum TSH. In such a patient, the serum response to TRH may be impaired or abnormally prolonged in its time course.[62]

ASSAYS FOR SERUM TSH α-SUBUNIT

Most patients with TSH-secreting pituitary tumors have increased serum α-subunit concentrations.[24,63] The values also may be elevated in postmenopausal women and in hypogonadal men[63] because both thyrotrophs and gonadotrophs secrete this subunit.

ASSAYS FOR SERUM TOTAL IODOTHYRONINE CONCENTRATIONS

Since the early 1970s, serum total T_4 and T_3 concentrations have been measured by radioimmunoassay and, more recently, related nonisotopic methods. Serum total T_4 and T_3 values reflect not only hormone production but also the serum concentrations of thyroid hormone-binding proteins. When protein binding is increased, serum total T_4 and T_3 concentrations are usually increased but serum free T_4 and T_3 concentrations are not. Typical normal reference ranges are shown in Table 18-3. Serum total and free T_4 and T_3 concentrations are slightly higher in children,[64] but they are similar in young middle-aged and elderly adults[46] (see section on age-related changes in chap 14).

For assays of T_4 and T_3 in unextracted serum, it is necessary to include a reagent that blocks T_4 and T_3 binding to serum proteins without markedly inhibiting antibody binding. The reagent most widely used in 8-anilinonaphthalene sulfonic acid (0.5–1 mmol/L) although it can cause fluorescence quenching in some systems; an alternative is phenoxynaphthalenesulfonic acid.[65] To obtain satisfactory discrimination in assays that have two key cut-off points (hypothyroid-normal and normal-thyrotoxic), it is essential that serum volume and reagent concentrations be adjusted to achieve optimal dose-response characteristics.

ESTIMATION OF SERUM FREE T_4 AND FREE T_3 CONCENTRATIONS

Many approaches have been used to estimate serum free T_4 and T_3 concentrations, with vigorous discussion about the theoretical basis, practical utility, and validity of these methods.[66,67] Although almost all serum free T_4 methods correct for minor or moderate variations in serum T_4-binding globulin (TBG) concentration, many give inaccurate results with extreme variations of serum TBG, dysalbuminemia, endogenous T_4 antibodies and circulating competitors of T_4 binding, and in severe nonthyroidal illness.

Serum free T_4 is commonly estimated by separation of free from bound T_4 by a semipermeable membrane in equilibrium dialysis or ultrafiltration, by the ability of free T_4 to inhibit binding between T_4 tracer and solid phase antibody, or by partition of tracer T_4 between serum proteins and a nonspecific solid-phase matrix (e.g., resin-binding ratio).

A distinction should be made between the methods that measure the T_4 *concentration* in a fraction of serum and those that calculate the free *fraction* from the distribution of labeled T_4 between the bound and unbound phases, using the free fraction together with the total T_4 value to calculate the free T_4 concentration. Of the former, two-step methods that separate a fraction of the free T_4 pool from the binding proteins before the T_4 assay is performed are generally least prone to artifacts. The principle of such a free T_4 method, based on back-titration of unoccupied solid phase antibody with labeled T_4 after washing of the solid phase, is shown in Figure 18–5. In contrast, many of the one-step methods that attempt to measure free T_4 in the presence of binding proteins become invalid

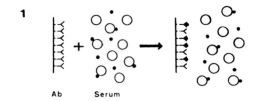

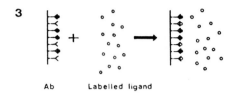

FIGURE 18-5. Summary of a two-step serum free T_4 immunoassay. After incubation of serum or standard with the solid-phase T_4 antibody, the serum is removed and the antibody washed, followed by incubation with labeled T_4. (Reproduced with permission from Ekins.[66] © The Endocrine Society)

whenever the sample and standard differ in their binding of assay tracer.[66,67]

No current method conveniently measures the free T_4 concentration in undisturbed, undiluted serum under in vivo conditions. Although equilibrium dialysis is widely considered the best method for free T_4 measurement, it is also subject to methodologic errors. As a reference method, ultrafiltration may be preferable to equilibrium dialysis, especially when the possible effects of binding competitors are assessed.[68,69]

Important factors that influence serum free T_4 methods are:

1. **Radiochemical purity** is crucial whenever a labeled compound is used as a marker for the natural compound. In some reference systems, for example, equilibrium dialysis or ultrafiltration of undiluted serum, as little as 0.1% free ^{125}I can lead to a 5- to 10-fold overestimate of the free T_4 fraction. For this reason, authentic ^{125}I-T_4 must be isolated from each sample after dialysis by a procedure such as magnesium chloride precipitation[70] or chromatography.[69]

2. **Protein-tracer interactions.** The labeled analogues of T_4 that are used as tracers in some free T_4 assays interact with serum proteins, particularly albumin.[67,71] If the labeled analogue is protein bound to a greater extent in the sample serum than in the standard serum, less tracer is available to compete for the assay antibody, giving a falsely high free T_4 estimate, as in FDH[71] and with T_4-binding immunoglobulins.[72] Conversely, if binding of labeled analogue is less in the sample than in the standard serum, for example, lower albumin concentration in the sample serum, or

increased occupancy of albumin by other ligands such as nonesterified fatty acids, the results are falsely low.[66]

3. Dilution effects and protein dependence. Mass action dictates that dissociation of a bound ligand occurs with progressive sample dilution, so that the free concentration should decrease little with dilution until the reservoir of bound ligand becomes depleted. In theory, the free concentration begins to fall steeply when about 20% of bound ligand has dissociated.[66] In human serum, this occurs at a dilution of about 1:1000 for T_4 and about 1:100 for T_3. In practice, many commercial assays yield much lower than predicted free T_4 concentrations with progressive dilution. This protein dependence of free hormone estimates[73] reflects the extent to which the method samples or depletes the reservoir of bound T_4 (or T_3).

4. Binding competitors. Few free T_4 assays properly reflect the effect of binding competitors, which are usually less protein-bound than T_4 itself. With progressive dilution, the free concentration of competitor usually declines long before the free T_4 concentration declines. The hormone-displacing effect of a dialyzable competitor will then be underestimated, the error being greatest in assays with the highest sample dilution. To avoid this artifact, ultrafiltration of undiluted serum is the optimal method, although a direct dialysis technique using 0.2 mL undiluted serum and 2.4 mL buffer[74] gives valid results comparable with ultrafiltration in patients with nonthyroidal illness or with addition of salicylate.[68]

5. Assay sensitivity may be the limiting factor in direct immunoassays of free T_4 that has been isolated by dialysis or ultrafiltration. Such assays require a specific antibody of high affinity to achieve acceptable precision.[74]

6. Temperature dependence. It is self-evident that in vivo hormone secretion is geared to the serum free T_4 concentration at 37°C, but most assays are equilibrated at room temperature. This may lead to biased results in serum samples with anomalous TBG concentrations because of temperature-dependent differences in T_4 dissociation between samples and standards.[67,75]

Evaluation of Serum Free T_4 Methods

Some free T_4 methods have been marketed before they have been rigorously assessed. Adequate evaluation requires that the method should be tested with progressive serum dilutions.[66,67] The effect of serum from patients with all known binding protein abnormalities and the effect of agents that compete for hormone-binding sites on serum proteins should also be tested. When such an evaluation was made of a non-isotopic method that depends on the ability of serum free T_4 to inhibit binding between a horseradish peroxidase-labeled anti-T_4 monoclonal antibody and a T_3-coated solid phase,[76] serum free T_4 estimates were comparable between 1:5 and 1:100 serum dilution and gave valid estimates in individuals with FDH. In critically ill patients the results were similar to values obtained by equilibrium dialysis and were not influenced by modest increases in serum nonesterified fatty acid concentrations.[76]

Thyroid Hormone-Binding Ratio or T_3-Resin Uptake

A special example of a two-step method is the time-honored serum free T_4 index, computed from the serum total T_4 value and the thyroid hormone-binding ratio (THBR).[77] The latter test estimates the number of unoccupied serum protein-binding sites, based on the distribution of ^{125}I-T_3 between a solid phase absorbent (usually a resin) and serum-binding proteins (Fig 18-6). The THBR value, which is calculated as the ratio of the solid-phase radioactivity in the test serum to that of a pool of serum from normal subjects, is multiplied by the serum total T_4 (or T_3) concentration to yield the free T_4 (or free T_3) index. The results are still sometimes directly expressed simply as the percentage of ^{125}I-T_3 bound to the resin in the presence of the test serum. ^{125}I-T_3 is used rather than ^{125}I-T_4, because its higher free fraction gives a more convenient index of changes in the occupancy of binding proteins. Proper use of the THBR requires the calculation to be made as resin/serum rather than resin/total counts, to improve the correction for very high and very low serum TBG concentrations.[77] Measurements of serum total T_4 and a separate index of binding have the advantage that they can define whether an abnormal serum free T_4 estimate is due to abnormal hormone production or abnormal protein binding. Most serum free T_4 methods do not give this information.

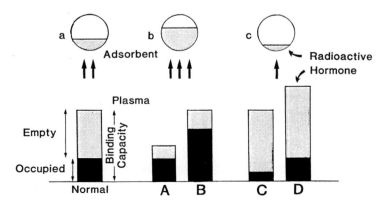

FIGURE 18-6. Principle of the thyroid hormone-binding ratio (THBR) or T_3-resin uptake test. Radioactive hormone (^{125}I-T_3) added to the serum distributes between the unoccupied T_4-binding sites in the serum sample (or standard) and an absorbent (usually a resin). The binding of ^{125}I-T_3 to the absorbent is increased (b) if the number of unoccupied binding sites is decreased, due either to a low binding protein concentration (A) or an increased total hormone concentration (B). The binding of ^{125}I-T_3 to the absorbent is decreased if the number of unoccupied binding sites is increased, due either to a low hormone concentration (C) or a high binding protein concentration (D). The serum free hormone estimate is calculated as a function of absorbed counts and total hormone concentration.

As an alternative to the serum free T_4 index, the ratio between serum total T_4 and immunoreactive TBG can be used to correct total T_4 for abnormal binding.[78] This approach is obsolete because it fails to compensate for TBG variants with reduced T_4 affinity (see below) or for abnormal albumin binding, and takes no account of competitors that may occupy T_4 binding sites.

Serum Free T_4 Estimates in Nonthyroidal Illness

Methodologic artifacts and discrepancies have blurred our understanding of the complex changes in serum free T_4 that occur in patients with nonthyroidal illness. The two-step methods that have been critically validated give the lowest prevalence of falsely low serum free T_4 values.[53] However, high serum free T_4 estimates by these methods are much less likely to be due to true thyrotoxicosis than to putative factor(s) that may inhibit T_4 binding[53] (see below).

Indications for Serum Total or Free T_3 Measurement

The relationships between serum T_3 and T_4 are summarized in Table 18-4. In practice, serum T_3 measurements are indicated:

- In patients with suspected thyrotoxicosis in whom serum T_4 is normal and serum TSH is low, to distinguish T_3 thyrotoxicosis from subclinical thyrotoxicosis
- During antithyroid drug therapy to identify patients who have persistent serum T_3 excess, despite normal or low serum T_4 values[79]
- For diagnosis of amiodarone-induced thyrotoxicosis, which should not be based on T_4 excess because of the occurrence of euthyroid hyperthyroxinemia in many amiodarone-treated patients[80] (see sections on

effects of pharmacologic agents and effect of excess iodide in chap 14)

Serum T_3 values may also be useful:

- For estimation of the serum $T_3:T_4$ ratio. A high ratio (>0.024 on a molar basis or >20 calculated as ng/μg) that persists during antithyroid drug treatment may indicate that patients with hyperthyroid Graves' disease are unlikely to achieve remission.[81] This ratio usually is lower in patients with iodide-induced thyrotoxicosis[82] or thyrotoxicosis caused by thyroiditis[83] than in those with thyrotoxicosis caused by Graves' disease.
- To detect early recurrence of thyrotoxicosis after cessation of antithyroid therapy
- To establish the extent of active hormone excess during high-dose replacement or suppressive therapy with T_4[55] or when an intentional T_4 overdose has been taken

Owing to its short half-life in serum, measurement of serum T_3 is not useful in assessing the effectiveness of treatment with T_3; the serum concentration is highly dependent on the interval between dosage and sampling.[84] As with T_4, serum total T_3 concentrations are influenced by alterations in binding proteins. Standard corrections applied to serum total T_4 values to derive a free T_4 estimate can be used to derive a free T_3 estimate as well.

Low serum T_3 concentrations have little specificity or sensitivity for the diagnosis of hypothyroidism. Many patients with nonthyroidal illness have low values, and some hypothyroid patients have normal values.

SERUM THYROID HORMONE CONCENTRATIONS IN ANIMAL SPECIES

Serum total T_4 concentrations vary widely between species. This variation is largely due to differences in binding

TABLE 18-4.
Relation Between Serum Total T_4 and T_3 Concentrations in Various Disorders*

Serum T_3 Concentration	Serum T_4 Concentration		
	LOW	NORMAL	HIGH
High	Iodine deficiency T_3 treatment Antithyroid drug therapy	T_3-thyrotoxicosis T_3-binding autoantibodies	Thyrotoxicosis of any cause Excess T_4 ingestion Thyroid hormone resistance Thyroxine-binding globulin excess
Normal	Iodine deficiency T_3 treatment Hypothyroidism		T_4 treatment Euthyroid hyperthyroxinemia Thyrotoxicosis with acute or moderate nonthyroidal illness T_4 binding autoantibodies
Low	Severe hypothyroidism Thyroxine-binding globulin deficiency Drugs Severe nonthyroidal illness	Acute and chronic non-thyroidal illness Drugs Fetal life Restricted nutrition	Thyrotoxicosis with severe nonthyroidal illness

Excluding short-term changes related to commencement or cessation of antithyroid drug or thyroid hormone replacement therapy.

TABLE 18-5.
Euthyroid Hyperthyroxinemia

A. High serum total T_4, normal free T_4

   Increase in binding protein affinity or concentration

      Thyroxine-binding globulin
         Hereditary
         Pregnancy
         Liver diseases[145]
         Drugs
            Estrogen, heroin, methadone, clofibrate, 5-fluorouracil, perphenazine
      Transthyretin
         Hereditary*
         Pancreatic neuroendocrine tumors[146]
      Albumin
         Familial dysalbuminemic hyperthyroxinemia (FDH)*
      T_4 antibody-associated hyperthyroxinemia

B. High serum total T_4, high free T_4

   Thyroid hormone resistance

   Severe nonthyroidal illness (small proportion)

   Altered hormone synthesis, release, or clearance
      Oral cholecystographic contrast agents
      Amiodarone
      Propranolol (high doses)[147]

   Thyroxine therapy

   Thyroid stimulation
      Hyperemesis gravidarum[148]
      Acute psychiatric illness?
      Amphetamines?[149]

C. Normal serum total T_4, high free T_4

   Severe nonthyroidal illness (small proportion)

   Drug competitors

   Heparin (in vitro effect)

D. Miscellaneous

   Extrathyroidal T_4 5'-deiodinase defect?

   Cell/membrane transport abnormality?

   High altitude[150]

   Hyponatremia[151]

Changes in binding affinity of the protein.

---

proteins,[85] so that serum free T_4 concentrations vary less.[86] Few serum free T_4 assays have been validated for animal use, and serum-based assay standards developed for human use may not be appropriate for assays of animal serum.

Assays for human TSH are not useful in other species. Although the TSH of some primates is weakly reactive in some radioimmunoassays for human TSH,[87] immunometric assays are more specific. Hence, diagnosis of thyroid dysfunction in animals largely depends on serum total or free T_4 measurements. Because reference ranges vary widely, it is advisable to include samples from normal animals whenever a heterologous assay is used. The recent report of an assay for canine TSH[88] will greatly improve diagnostic sensitivity and specificity for this species.

EUTHYROID HYPERTHYROXINEMIA AND EUTHYROID HYPOTHYROXINEMIA

These terms describe situations in which serum total or free T_4 concentrations are abnormal without evidence of thyroid dysfunction, usually in association with normal serum TSH concentrations. Such findings occur with binding-protein abnormalities, medications, associated illness, and, in the case of hyperthyroxinemia, in the hormone resistance syndromes (Table 18-5). The changes may be transient or persistent and may be associated with high, normal, or low serum T_3 concentrations.

These variations usually reflect true in vivo changes in serum T_4 concentrations. However, they may also be caused by assay artifacts such as tracer misclassification in assay separation methods[71,72] or in vitro generation of binding competitors during dialysis for free hormone estimation.[89]

Changes in Binding Proteins

Molecular changes in TBG, transthyretin (TTR), or albumin can be associated with altered serum concentrations of these binding proteins, or may increase or decrease their affinity for T_4 and T_3[22] (see chap 6). Of 15 known X-linked TBG variations,[90] three cause complete TBG deficiency, and at least three other types are associated with reduced affinity for T_4 with subnormal serum TBG concentrations.[91] Diminished TBG binding is especially prevalent in some ethnic groups,[91] as for example among Australian aborigines up to 30% of whom have low serum total T_4 concentrations associated with subnormal serum TBG concentrations. This TBG is abnormally heat labile in vitro.[91,92] In general, various serum free T_4 methods, as well as binding corrections based on THBR measurements, give a valid correction for TBG abnormalities, whether hereditary or acquired.

The albumin variant responsible for FDH, due to an Arg-His substitution at position 218,[93] has a markedly increased affinity for T_4 and numerous T_4 analogue tracers, resulting in spuriously high serum free T_4 estimates with these tracers.[66,67,71] In FDH, serum total T_4 and free T_4 index values and free T_4 measured by analogue-based methods give results suggestive of thyrotoxicosis, whereas serum total T_3, free T_3, and TSH values, and free T_4 measured by most two-step methods or equilibrium dialysis, are normal.[67,71] Of the 12 known variants in TTR structure, 3 have increased affinity for T_4, and therefore may result in euthyroid hyperthyroxinemia,[94] while 5 have decreased affinity. The TTR variants associated with hyperthyroxinemia do not appear to give spuriously high serum free T_4 values by one-step methods.[95]

Iodothyronine-Binding Autoantibodies

The circulating T_3- or T_4-binding autoantibodies sometimes associated with high titers of antithyroglobulin antibodies in serum can cause methodologic artifacts in both total and free T_4 and free T_3 measurements.[23,72] Depending on the separation method used, tracer T_4 or T_3 bound to the endogenous antibody will be falsely classified as bound in adsorption methods or free in double antibody methods, leading respectively to falsely low or falsely high serum total T_4 or T_3 values.[23] Assay after ethanol extraction of serum will establish the true total hormone concentration. In some patients, these antibodies are sufficiently potent to increase T_3 or T_4 binding in vivo markedly, with consequent elevation in serum total T_4 or T_3 concentrations, but serum free T_4 or T_3 concentrations are normal.[23] If hypothyroidism is present, high serum TSH concentrations can be associated with spuriously high serum total or free T_4 or T_3 concentrations.[96] Labeled analogues of T_4 used for free T_4 estimation commonly bind to these antibodies, leading to spuriously high serum free T_4 results.[72]

T_4 Therapy

Mild hyperthyroxinemia, both total and free, with normal serum TSH and T_3 concentrations is common in patients receiving T_4 replacement therapy,[2,31] with a small variation depending on the time interval between T_4 ingestion and blood sampling.[32]

Psychiatric Illness

An unusual variety of euthyroid hyperthyroxinemia occurs in some patients hospitalized with acute psychiatric illness.[34] Serum T_4 is increased, but serum T_3 is less frequently elevated; serum TSH is generally normal or slightly high.[97] These abnormalities, presumed to be due to central activation of the hypothalamic-pituitary-thyroid axis, usually resolve in several weeks.

Other Causes

High serum total and free T_4 concentrations have been described in a small proportion of patients with acute medical illness,[33] but findings often depend on the particular T_4 method that is used.[53]

There are reports of individuals or kindreds who are euthyroid with persistently high serum free T_4 concentrations with no apparent cause. Impaired T_4 entry into cells[98] or defective peripheral conversion of T_4 to T_3[99] has been suggested, but conclusive proof for either defect is lacking.

Hypothyroxinemia

The complex changes that can lead to lowering of serum total T_4 concentrations in patients with nonthyroidal illness are still poorly understood (see section on nonthyroidal illness in chap 14). Inhibition of TSH secretion, decreased production of binding proteins, and accelerated T_4 clearance, possibly related to inhibition of serum protein binding by competitors, may be key factors. The role of the latter is unresolved, however, because of methodologic difficulties in detecting the effect of competitors in standard free T_4 assays and because of incomplete documentation of possible drug effects,[100] especially heparin[89] (see below). The presence of binding inhibitors has been inferred on the basis of anomalous dilution-related changes in apparent T_4 affinity in serum,[101] but drugs that affect binding would have the same effect.

Triiodothyronine or other thyromimetic compounds such as triiodothyroacetic acid (Triac), inhibit TSH and, therefore, T_4 secretion. Serum T_4 concentrations may be low in the face of normal or even elevated serum T_3 concentrations, in pa-

tients with iodine deficiency,[102] and in situations of partial thyroid failure in which organification of iodide is impaired.[103]

Diagnostic Approach

An approach to the problem of anomalous serum T_4 values can be summarized as follows:

- Clinical reevaluation, with particular attention to long-term features suggestive of thyroid disease and to the medication history (see below)
- Measurement of serum TSH by a third-generation method to identify conclusively the degree of TSH suppression
- Measurement of the serum T_3 concentration with appropriate binding correction
- An authentic estimate of serum free T_4, avoiding one-step methods known to give spurious results in euthyroid hyperthyroxinemia
- Follow-up to establish whether the abnormality is transient or persistent
- Search for evidence of unusual binding abnormalities or hormone resistance in the propositus and family members (see below)

IDENTIFICATION OF SPECIFIC BINDING ABNORMALITIES

An altered ratio between serum total and free T_4 concentrations suggests a binding abnormality but does not establish which binding protein is involved. Such information is valuable in particular patients, families, or ethnic groups to emphasize the possibility of diagnostic misclassification. The following methods have been used to characterize specific variants:

1. Electrophoretic techniques, followed by autoradiography of ^{125}I-T_4, can be used to compare the distribution of labeled hormone in serum from affected and normal subjects (Fig 18-7). Such techniques tend to give unreliable quantitation of T_4 binding to various proteins, because of tracer redistribution during electrophoresis.
2. Kinetic binding studies of isolated proteins have defined numerous hereditary and acquired alterations in binding proteins. After defining the affinity and capacity of the abnormal site for various iodothyronines, as well as its sensitivity to buffer reagents and competitors, simpler comparative tests can be developed.
3. Comparative assays of binding involve adjustment of hormone concentration and serum dilution so as to accentuate a particular class of binding site. The abnormal high-capacity binding sites of FDH- and TTR-associated hyperthyroxinemia can be identified when serum, diluted 1:100 in phosphate buffer, is incubated with ^{125}I-T_4 and 5-, 50-, and 1000-fold amounts of unlabeled T_4, followed by charcoal separation at 4°C (Fig 18-8). The presence of FDH- or TTR-associated hyperthyroxinemia is identified by lower charcoal counts (i.e., greater protein binding) in the abnormal serum. At 50-fold T_4 excess, high TBG concentrations

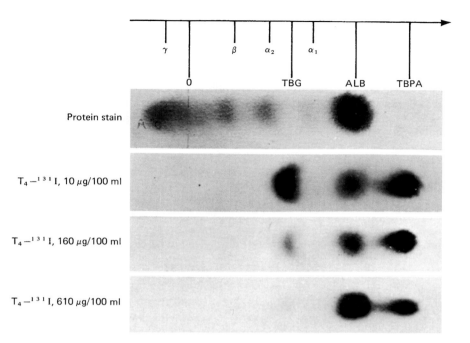

FIGURE 18-7. Distribution of ^{125}I-T$_4$ added to normal human serum in vitro in the presence of varying quantities of unlabeled T$_4$ after electrophoresis in glycine-acetate buffer of pH 8.6. The top panel shows the strip stained for protein. The three lower panels are autoradiographs of ^{131}I-T$_4$ in the presence of increasing concentrations of added unlabeled T$_4$. As the T$_4$ concentration increases, the high-affinity, low-capacity binding sites of TBG become saturated and ^{131}I-T$_4$ is increasingly bound to the lower-affinity, higher-capacity sites on transthyretin (TBPA) and albumin (ALB).

are saturated; at 1000-fold T$_4$, the abnormal albumin characteristic of FDH shows unique persistence of increased T$_4$ binding.[104] Abnormal immunoglobulin binding of T$_3$ or T$_4$ can be simply identified by increased precipitation of tracer after addition of 20% polyethylene glycol.[23,104]

4. Molecular characterization of the binding protein[90,91,93] (see chap 6)

DRUG EFFECTS ON MEASUREMENTS OF SERUM T$_4$ AND TSH

The effects of drugs on the pituitary-thyroid axis are considered in detail in chapter 14. This discussion emphasizes effects on diagnostic tests and on the relationship between serum TSH and free T$_4$. In general, drugs do not directly influence assays for TSH or iodothyronines, although possible interference with novel detection systems requires continuing vigilance.

The time course of drug effects on diagnostic tests depends on the pharmacokinetics of the drug itself. For example, lipid-soluble, iodine-rich drugs such as amiodarone and oral cholecystographic contrast agents have long-lasting effects because they may remain in the tissues for months, whereas a rapidly cleared inhibitor of serum binding will have only a transient effect.[105]

Effects on Serum TSH

Dopamine infusions in critically ill patients cause profound transient lowering of serum TSH concentrations, associated with lowering of serum T$_3$ and T$_4$.[106] Glucocorticoids[107] and phenytoin[108] also inhibit TSH secretion, so that serum TSH

concentrations may be abnormally low for the prevailing serum free T$_4$ concentration. Conversely, serum TSH concentrations may be inappropriately high in the face of glucocorticoid deficiency.[109] Bromocriptine lowers serum TSH concentrations in patients with primary hypothyroidism, al-

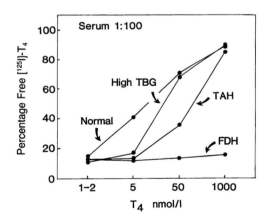

FIGURE 18-8. Effect of a progressive increase in the concentration of unlabeled T$_4$ on dextran-charcoal uptake of ^{125}I-T$_4$ in serum from a normal subject and patients with TBG excess, transthyretin-associated hyperthyroxinemia (TAH), and familial dysalbuminemic hyperthyroxinemia (FDH). The serum samples were diluted 1:100 in phosphate buffer, 0.04 mol/L, pH 7.4, giving an endogenous T$_4$ concentration of 1 to 2 nmol/L. When total T$_4$ is 50-fold in excess of normal, all TBG sites are saturated. At 1000-fold T$_4$ excess, serum from patients with FDH shows unique persistence of increased T$_4$ binding, consistent with an increased affinity for T$_4$ binding to albumin, which has a high capacity for T$_4$. Transthyretin has a binding capacity intermediate between that of TBG and albumin. Inhibition of binding is shown by an increase in the percentage of free ^{125}I-T$_4$. Each point is the mean of the results in four or more subjects.

though this effect is probably not sufficient to cause diagnostic misclassification.[110]

Amiodarone has complex effects on TSH secretion. Its major metabolite competes for T_3 binding to thyroid hormone receptors,[111] which may account for the fact that serum TSH concentrations tend to rise slightly in amiodarone-treated patients[112] and that serum TSH concentrations are higher in amiodarone-treated patients than in T_4-treated patients who have the same serum free T_4 and free T_3 concentrations.[113] However, a decrease in serum TSH has been reported in partially treated hypothyroid patients given amiodarone, suggesting that it also may act as a T_3 agonist in some circumstances.[114]

An important interaction occurs when a drug associated with central suppression of TSH, such as dopamine, is given together with an inhibitor of serum T_4 binding, such as furosemide.[115] The combined effects of accelerated T_4 clearance and inhibition of TSH secretion can lead to profound hypothyroxinemia (Fig 18-9).

Effects on Thyroid Hormone Synthesis and Release

Lithium has multiple effects on thyroid hormones, its predominant action being to impair hormone release from the thyroid.[116] Glucocorticoids acutely inhibit iodide uptake,[117] probably due to inhibition of TSH release. They also decrease serum T_3 and T_4 concentrations in patients with thyro-

toxicosis caused by Graves' disease,[118] an effect due either to direct inhibition of hormone secretion or decreased production of thyroid-stimulating autoantibodies. Iodine-rich compounds such as radiographic contrast media and amiodarone, as well as some cough medications and topical antiseptics, can markedly increase the pool of intrathyroidal iodine. An iodide load may induce either hypothyroidism or thyrotoxicosis, depending on the amount of iodine and the preexisting state of the gland (see section on effect of excess iodine in chapter 14).

Altered Serum Concentrations of Binding Proteins

Oral estrogens or pregnancy increase serum TBG concentrations primarily by increasing the glycosylation of TBG, which slows TBG clearance.[119] Serum total T_4 concentrations are increased, although most values remain within the normal range, but serum free T_4 concentrations are normal. This effect does not occur with transdermal estrogens.[120] Other drugs that can cause small increases in serum TBG concentrations include tamoxifen, heroin, methadone, clofibrate, perphenazine, and 5-fluorouracil.[113,121] Conversely, androgens decrease serum TBG concentrations,[122] as do glucocorticoids,[123] although serum total T_4 concentrations usually are not below normal. In contrast, serum TTR concentrations are increased by glucocorticoids[123] and androgens.[122] Only a small proportion of T_4 and T_3 normally is

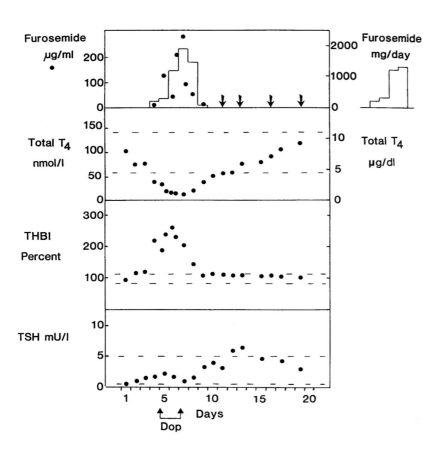

FIGURE 18-9. The effect of high intravenous doses of furosemide (5–100 mg/h) on indexes of thyroid function in a critically ill patient with transient oliguric renal failure, showing duration of drug therapy and serum drug concentration, serum total T_4 concentration, thyroid hormone binding index (THBI), and TSH concentration. THBI was measured as T_3-resin uptake. Dopamine infusion (DOP) (1–3 μg/kg/min) was given from 0300 on day 5 to 0930 on day 7. The broken lines show the limits of the respective reference ranges. The arrows in the top panel represent undetectable serum furosemide concentrations (< 5 μg/mL). High-dose furosemide therapy together with dopamine infusion was associated with profound hypothyroxinemia; note the rise in serum TSH and return of serum T_4 to normal after cessation of both drugs. (Adapted from Stockigt JR, Lim CF, Barlow JW, et al. High concentrations of furosemide inhibit plasma binding of thyroxine. J Clin Endocrinol Metab 1984;59:62)

albumin bound, so changes in serum albumin concentrations have negligible direct effects on serum T_4 and T_3 concentrations.

Occupancy of Binding Proteins

The nonsteroidal anti-inflammatory drugs fenclofenac,[124] mefenamic acid, and meclofenamic acid,[125] aspirin and its analogues,[126] and the loop diuretic furosemide[115] compete with T_4 for binding to TBG. The effect in vivo depends on the total drug concentration and free fraction as well as affinity for the T_4-binding site.[127] Therapeutic doses of salsalate (salicyl salicylic acid) lower serum total T_4 by 40% and serum total T_3 by 30%; naproxen and diclofenac lower serum T_3 but not T_4; serum TSH is not altered.[128]

The effects of competitors differ for samples taken shortly after drug ingestion and under steady-state conditions, depending on the pharmacokinetics of the drug. For example, a long-acting drug such as fenclofenac initially increases the serum free T_4 concentration, leading to transient inhibition of TSH secretion[124] and increased T_4 clearance, and eventually to a new steady state associated with normal serum free and lower total T_4 concentrations (Fig 18-10). In contrast, furosemide, which has a short half-life, causes transient changes in T_4 binding, depending on the interval between drug ingestion and blood sampling.[105]

No commonly used assay for serum free T_4 and free T_3 is completely reliable in detecting the presence of circulating inhibitors of serum binding. Sample dilution, particularly dilution of competitor into the buffer compartment in dialysis

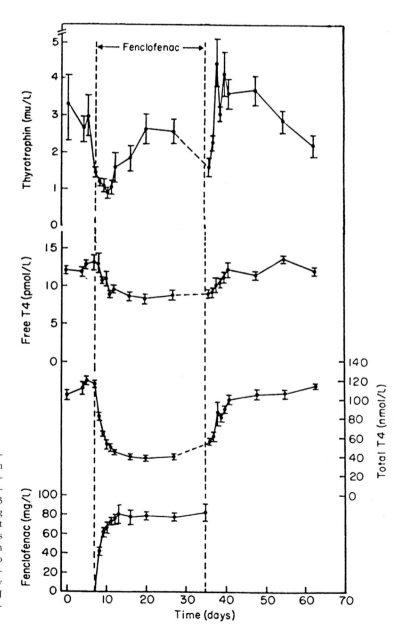

FIGURE 18-10. The effect of treatment for 28 days with fenclofenac, 500 mg twice daily by mouth, on mean (± SE) serum TSH, free T_4, total T_4, and drug concentrations in normal subjects. Serum TSH decreased to a nadir after 2 to 4 days of treatment, rose during continued treatment, and reached a peak 3 to 5 days after fenclofenac was discontinued, before returning to the pretreatment concentration. During the drug treatment period, serum total T_4 decreased to a new steady state at less than 50% of its pretreatment value. The small decrease in serum free T_4 may result from a dilution-related artefact. To convert serum free T_4 values to nanograms per deciliter and total T_4 values to micrograms per deciliter, multiply each by 12.87. (Composite figure from Kurtz AB, Capper SJ, Clifford J et al. The effect of fenclofenac on thyroid function. Clin Endocrinol (Oxf) 1981;15:117)

systems, depletes the serum free drug concentration, leading to marked underestimates of inhibitory potency[129] (see above). Conversely, addition of competitors in vitro to prediluted serum will lead to overestimation of their potency because the free competitor concentration will be artificially high at low albumin concentrations.[129,130]

The effect of heparin to increase serum free T_4 is an interesting in vitro phenomenon that does not reflect changes in circulating free T_4.[89] An increased free T_4 fraction has been found in serum obtained from heparin-treated patients,[131] despite the fact that heparin is a very weak inhibitor of T_4 binding to TBG and TTR in vitro.[131] This increase in free T_4 fraction is due to in vitro generation of nonesterified fatty acids during incubation for equilibrium dialysis,[89] as a result of heparin-induced lipase activity. The recent suggestion that this effect may also occur with doses of heparin as low as 10 units may account for some reports of apparent increases in serum free T_4 in hospitalized or dialyzed subjects.[132]

Tissue Distribution

Iodinated cholecystographic contrast agents cause net efflux of T_4 from a tissue pool, presumably the liver, leading to an acute increase in serum T_4 after their ingestion.[133]

Effects on Iodothyronine Metabolism

Numerous drugs inhibit the outer ring monodeiodination of T_4 to T_3 by type 1 $T_4$5'-deiodinase (see chap 8). They include amiodarone, cholecystographic contrast agents, glucocorticoids, propylthiouracil, and some β-adrenergic antagonists (see section on effects on pharmacologic agents on thyroid hormone metabolism in chap 14).

Apart from the influence of drugs on deiodinative metabolism, phenytoin, phenobarbital, carbamazepine, and rifampicin increase nondeiodinative metabolism of T_4.[108,134] In a study of epileptic patients, phenytoin and carbamazepine, but not valproate, decreased serum total and free T_4 concentrations slightly, but serum TSH concentrations did not increase.[134]

Modified Tissue Effects of Thyroid Hormone

As well as influencing peripheral thyroid hormone metabolism, an amiodarone derivative[111] and phenytoin[108] bind to nuclear T_3 receptors, where they could act as antagonists or partial agonists. Their complex effects on TSH secretion, possibly by direct interaction with T_3 receptors, remain a cause of diagnostic difficulty.

Altered Efficacy of Ingested T_4

In T_4-treated hypothyroid patients, serum total and free T_4 concentrations can be influenced by numerous medications. Cholestyramine,[135] soybean formulations,[136] sucralfate,[137] ferrous sulfate,[138] and aluminum hydroxide can impair T_4 absorption[139] (see chap 77). In T_4-treated hypothyroid women with breast cancer, androgen therapy in the form of fluoxymesterone was associated with a sustained increase in serum free T_4 concentrations necessitating a reduction of T_4 dosage in some patients that was attributed to decreased serum TBG concentrations.[140]

CLINICALLY CONCORDANT AND DISCORDANT LABORATORY FINDINGS

When laboratory results are correlated with clinical findings, the relation may be either concordant or discordant. A concordant result that confirms thyrotoxicosis (i.e., high serum free T_4 and low TSH concentrations) establishes neither the cause of the thyrotoxicosis nor its clinical severity, which is best assessed by clinical evaluation. Careful clinical examination of the eyes and the thyroid gland and, if necessary, additional investigations, such as measurement of thyroid autoantibodies and radionuclide scanning or uptake tests, should establish the exact cause of the thyrotoxicosis.

If the laboratory results and clinical picture are discordant, a distinction needs to be made between a previously unsuspected diagnosis, subclinical disease, anomalous assay results, and a discrepancy caused by specific or nonspecific assay interference. If repeat analyses confirm the abnormality, consideration of the assumptions in Table 18-1 may give a clue to the discrepancy. If the discordance remains unresolved, a therapeutic trial is unlikely to be helpful; continued observation is preferable. The growing trend toward automation of thyroid function testing does not in any way diminish the need for critical clinical evaluation of assay results.

References

1. Ransohoff DF, Feinstein AR. Problems of spectrum and bias in evaluating the efficacy of diagnostic tests. N Engl J Med 1978; 299:926
2. Fish LH, Schwartz HL, Cavanaugh J, et al. Replacement dose, metabolism, and bioavailability of levothyroxine in the treatment of hypothyroidism. N Engl J Med 1987;316:764
3. Snyder PJ, Utiger RD. Inhibition of thyrotropin response to thyrotropin-releasing hormone by small quantities of thyroid hormones. J Clin Invest 1972;51:2077
4. Vagenakis AG, Rapoport B, Azizi F, et al. Hyperresponse to thyrotropin-releasing hormone accompanying small decreases in serum thyroid hormone concentrations. J Clin Invest 1974; 54:913
5. Volpe R. Subacute (de Quervain's) thyroiditis. Clin Endocrinol Metab 1979;8:81
6. Amino N, Mori H, Iwatani Y, et al. High prevalence of transient post-partum thyrotoxicosis and hypothyroidism. N Engl J Med 1982;306:849
7. Hamblin PS, Dyer SA, Mohr VS, et al. Relationship between thyrotropin and thyroxine changes during recovery from severe hypothyroxinemia of critical illness. J Clin Endocrinol Metab 1986;62:717
8. Law LK, Cheung CK, Swaminathan R. Falsely high thyroxine results by fluorescence polarization in sera with high background fluorescence. Clin Chem 1988;34:1918
9. Ritter D, Stott R, Grant N, Nahm NH. Endogenous antibodies that interfere with thyroxine fluorescence polarization assay but not with radioimmunoassay or EMIT. Clin Chem 1993;39:508
10. Beck-Peccoz P, Persani L. Variable biological activity of thyroid-stimulating hormone. Eur J Endocrinol 1994;131:331
11. Smallridge RC, Parker RA, Wiggs EA, et al. Thyroid hormone resistance in a large kindred: physiologic, biochemical, pharmacologic, and neuropsychologic studies. Am J Med 1989;86:289

12. Refetoff S, Weiss RE, Usala SJ. The syndromes of resistance to thyroid hormone. Endocr Rev 1993;14:348

13. Fischer HRA, Hackeng WHL, Schopman W, Silberbusch J. Analysis of factors in hyperthyroidism, which determine the duration of suppressive treatment before recovery of thyroid stimulating hormone secretion. Clin Endocrinol 1982;16:575

14. Sato T, Suzuki Y, Taketani T, et al. Age-related change in pituitary threshold for TSH release during thyroxine replacement therapy for cretinism. J Clin Endocrinol Metab 1977;44:553

15. Helfand M, Crapo LM. Screening for thyroid disease. Ann Intern Med 1990;112:840

16. Rae P, Farrar J, Beckett G, Toft A. Assessment of thyroid status in elderly people. BMJ 1993;307:177

17. Martino E, Bambini G. Bartalena L, et al. Human serum thyrotropin measurement by ultrasensitive immunoradiometric assay as a first-line test in the evaluation of thyroid function. Clin Endocrinol 1986;24:141

18. Eggertsen R, Petersen K, Lundberg P-A, et al. Screening for thyroid disease in a primary care unit with a thyroid stimulating hormone assay with a low detection limit. BMJ 1988;297:1586

19. Cooper DS. Subclinical hypothyroidism. JAMA 1987;258:246

20. Jayme JJ, Ladenson PW. Subclinical thyroid dysfunction in the elderly. Trends Endocrinol Metab 1994;5:79

21. Studer H, Ramelli F. Simple goiter and its variants: euthyroid and hyperthyroid multinodular goiters. Endocr Rev 1982;3:40

22. Bartalena L. Recent achievements in studies of thyroid hormone binding proteins. Endocr Rev 1990;11:47

23. Sakata S, Nakamura S, Miura K. Autoantibodies against thyroid hormones or iodothyronine. Ann Intern Med 1985;103:579

24. Gesundheit N, Petrick PA, Nissim M, et al. Thyrotropin-secreting pituitary adenomas: clinical and biochemical heterogeneity. Ann Intern Med 1989;111:827

25. Beck-Peccoz P, Chatterjee VKK. The variable clinical phenotype in thyroid hormone resistance syndrome. Thyroid 1994;4:225

26. Helfand M, Schmittner J. Screening for thyroid dysfunction: which test is best? JAMA 1993;270:2297

27. Ross DS, Daniels GH, Gouveia D. The use and limitations of a chemiluminescent TSH assay as a single thyroid function test in an outpatient endocrine clinic. J Clin Endocrinol Metab 1990; 71:764

28. Fraser WD, Biggart EM, O'Reilly DStJ, et al. Are biochemical tests of thyroid function of any value in monitoring patients receiving thyroxine replacement? BMJ 1986;293:808

29. Toft AD. Thyroxine replacement treatment: clinical judgment or biochemical control? BMJ 1985;291:233

30. Leese GP, Jung RT, Guthrie C, et al. Morbidity in patients on L-thyroxine: a comparison of those with a normal TSH to those with a suppressed TSH. Clin Endocrinol 1992;37:500

31. Pearce CJ, Himsworth RL. Total and free thyroid hormone concentrations in patients receiving maintenance replacement treatment with thyroxine. BMJ 1984;288:693

32. Ain KB, Pucino F, Shiver TM, Banks SM. Thyroid hormone levels affected by time of blood sampling in thyroxine-treated patients. Thyroid 1993;3:81

33. DeGroot LJ, Mayor G. Admission screening by thyroid function tests in an acute general care teaching hospital. Am J Med 1992;93:558

34. Hein MD, Jackson IMD. Thyroid function in psychiatric illness. Gen Hosp Psychiatry 1990;12:232

35. Ross DS. Screening thyroid function tests in an acute care hospital. Am J Med 1994;96:393

36. Kaptein EM, Weiner JM, Robinson WJ, et al. Relationship of altered thyroid hormone indices to survival in non-thyroidal illnesses. Clin Endocrinol 1982;16:565

37. Vexiau P, Perez-Castiglioni P, Socie G, et al. The 'euthyroid sick syndrome': incidence, risk factors and prognostic value soon af-ter allogeneic bone marrow transplantation. Br J Haematol 1993; 85:778

38. Spencer CA. Clinical utility and cost-effectiveness of sensitive thyrotropin assays in ambulatory and hospitalized patients. Mayo Clin Proc 1988;63:1214

39. Spencer CA, LoPresti JS, Patel A, et al. Applications of a new chemiluminometric thyrotropin assay to subnormal measurement. J Clin Endocrinol Metab 1990;70:453

40. Lum SMC, Kaptein EM, Nicoloff JT. Influence of nonthyroidal illnesses on serum thyroid hormone indices in hyperthyroidism. West J Med 1983;128:670

41. Brabant G, Prank K, Ranft U, et al. Physiological regulation of circadian and pulsatile thyrotropin secretion in normal man and woman. J Clin Endocrinol Metab 1990;70:403

42. Romijn JA, Wiersinga WM. Decreased nocturnal surge of thyrotropin in nonthyroidal illness. J Clin Endocrinol Metab 1990; 70:35

43. Bartalena L, Martino E, Brandi LS, et al. Lack of nocturnal serum thyrotropin surge after surgery. J Clin Endocrinol Metab 1990; 70:293

44. Bartalena L, Martino E, Falcon M, et al. Evaluation of the nocturnal serum thyrotropin (TSH) surge, as assessed by TSH ultrasensitive assay, in patients receiving long term L-thyroxine suppression therapy in patients with various thyroid disorders. J Clin Endocrinol Metab 1987;65:1265

45. Fisher DA, Klein AH. Thyroid development and disorder of thyroid function in the newborn. N Engl J Med 1981;304:702

46. Hershman JM, Pekary AE, Berg L, et al. Serum thyrotropin and thyroid hormone levels in elderly and middle-aged euthyroid persons. J Am Geriatr Soc 1993;41:823

47. Lewis GF, Alessi CA, Imperial JG, Refetoff S. Low serum free thyroxine index in ambulating elderly is due to a resetting of the threshold of thyrotropin feedback suppression. J Clin Endocrinol Metab 1991;73:843

48. Meikle AW, Stringham JD, Woodward MG, Nelson JC. Hereditary and environmental influences on the variation of thyroid hormone in normal male twins. J Clin Endocrinol Metab 1988; 66:588

49. Meier CA, Maisey MN, Lowry A, Müller J, Smith MA. Interindividual differences in the pituitary-thyroid axis influence the interpretation of thyroid function tests. Clin Endocrinol 1993;39:101

50. Nicoloff JT, Spencer CA. The use and misuse of the sensitive TSH assays. J Clin Endocrinol Metab 1990;71:553

51. Wilkinson E, Rae PW, Thomson KJ, et al. Chemiluminescent third-generation assay of TSH in serum or plasma assessed. Clin Chem 1993;39:2167

52. Spencer CA, Takeuchi M, Kazarosyan M, et al. Inter-laboratory intermethod differences in functional sensitivity of immunometric assays of thyrotropin (TSH) and impact on reliability of measurement of subnormal concentrations of TSH. Clin Chem 1995; 41:367

53. Kaptein EM. Thyroid in vitro testing in non-thyroidal illness. Exp Clin Endocrinol 1994;102(suppl 2):92

54. Franklyn JA, Black EG, Betteridge J, Sheppard MC. Comparison of second and third generation methods for measurement of serum thyrotropin in patients with overt hyperthyroidism, patients receiving thyroxine therapy, and those with nonthyroidal illness. J Clin Endocrinol Metab 1994;78:1368

55. Bartalena L, Pinchera A. Levothyroxine suppressive therapy: harmful and useless or harmless and useful? J Endocrinol Invest 1994;17:675

56. Parle JV, Franklyn JA, Cross KW, et al. Prevalence and follow-up of abnormal thyrotropin (TSH) concentrations in the elderly in the United Kingdom. Clin Endocrinol 1991;34:77

57. Sawin CT, Geller A, Wolf PA, et al. Low serum thyrotropin concentrations as a risk factor for arterial fibrillation in older persons. N Engl J Med 1994;331:1249

58. Kahn BB, Weintraub BD, Csako G, Zweig MH. Factitious elevation of thyrotropin in a new ultrasensitive assay: implications for the use of monoclonal antibodies in "sandwich" immunoassay. J Clin Endocrinol Metab 1988;66:526

59. Csako G, Weintraub BD, Zweig MH. The potency of immunoglobulin G fragments for inhibition on interference caused by antiimmunoglobulin antibodies in a monoclonal immunoradiometric assay for thyrotropin. Clin Chem 1988;34:1481

60. Laurberg P. Persistent problems with the specificity of immunometric TSH assays. Thyroid 1993;3:279

61. Spencer CA, Schwarzbein D, Guttler RB, et al. Thyrotropin (TSH)-releasing hormone stimulation test responses employing third and fourth generation TSH assays. J Clin Endocrinol Metab 1993;76:494

62. Peters JR, Foord SM, Dieguez C, Scanlon MF. TSH neuroregulation and alterations in disease states. Clin Endocrinol Metab 1983;12:669

63. Smallridge RC. Thyrotropin-secreting pituitary tumors. Endocrinol Metab Clin North Am 1987;16:765

64. Westgren U, Burger A, Ingemansson S, et al. Blood levels of 3,5,3′-triiodothyronine and thyroxine: differences between children, adults and elderly subjects. Acta Med Scand 1976;200:493

65. Grenner G, Ingbar S, Meneghini FA, et al. Multilayer fluorescent immunoassay technique. Clin Chem 1989;35:1865

66. Ekins R. Measurement of free hormones in blood. Endocr Rev 1990;11:5

67. Ekins R. The free hormone hypothesis and measurement of free hormones. Clin Chem 1992;38:1289

68. Faber J, Waetjen I, Siersbaek-Nielsen K. Free thyroxine measured in undiluted serum by dialysis and ultrafiltration: effects of non-thyroidal illness, and an acute load of salicylate or heparin. Clin Chim Acta 1993;223:159

69. Surks MI, Hupart KH, Chao P, Shapiro LE. Normal free thyroxine in critical nonthyroidal illnesses measured by ultrafiltration of undiluted serum and equilibrium dialysis. J Clin Endocrinol Metab 1988;67:1031

70. Sterling K, Brenner MA. Free thyroxine in human serum: simplified measurement with aid of magnesium precipitation. J Clin Invest 1966;45:153

71. Stockigt JR, DeGaris M, Csicsmann J, et al. Limitations of a new free thyroxine assay (Amerlex Free T$_4$). Clin Endocrinol 1981;15:313

72. Beck-Peccoz P, Romelli PB, Cattaneo MG, et al. Evaluation of free T$_4$ methods in the presence of iodothyronine autoantibodies. J Clin Endocrinol Metab 1984;58:736

73. Nelson JC, Weiss RM, Wilcox RB. Underestimates of serum free thyroxine (T$_4$) concentrations by free T$_4$ immunoassays. J Clin Endocrinol Metab 1994;79:76

74. Nelson JC, Tomei RT. Direct determination of free thyroxin in undiluted serum by equilibrium dialysis/radioimmunoassay. Clin Chem 1988;34:1737

75. van der Sluijs Veer G, Vermes I, Bonte HA, Hoorn RKJ. Temperature effects on free-thyroxine measurements: analytical and clinical consequences. Clin Chem 1992;38:1327

76. Docter R, van Toor H, Krenning EP, et al. Free thyroxine assessed with three assays in sera of patients with nonthyroidal illness and of subjects with abnormal concentrations of thyroxine-binding proteins. Clin Chem 1993;39:1668

77. Larsen PR. Alexander NM, Chopra IJ, et al. Revised nomenclature for tests of thyroid hormones and thyroid-related proteins in serum. J Clin Endocrinol Metab 1987;64:1089

78. Burr WA, Evans SE, Lee J. The ratio of thyroxine to thyroxine-binding globulin in the assessment of thyroid function. Clin Endocrinol 1979;11:333

79. Takamatsu J, Sugawara M, Kuma K, et al. Ratio of serum triiodothyronine to thyroxine and the prognosis of triiodothyronine-predominant Graves' disease. Ann Intern Med 1984;100:372

80. Borowski GD, Garofano CD, Rose LI, et al. Effect of long-term amiodarone therapy on thyroid hormone levels and thyroid function. Am J Med 1985;78:443

81. Takamatsu J, Kuma K, Mozai T. Serum triiodothyronine to thyroxine ratio: a newly recognized predictor of the outcome of hyperthyroidism due to Graves' disease. J Clin Endocrinol Metab 1986;62:980

82. Sobrinho LG, Limbert ES, Santos MA. Thyroxine toxicosis in patients with iodine induced thyrotoxicosis. J Clin Endocrinol Metab 1977;45:25

83. Amino N, Yabu Y, Miki Y, et al. Serum ratio of triiodothyronine to thyroxine, and thyroxine-binding globulin and calcitonin concentrations in Graves' disease and destruction-induced thyrotoxicosis. J Clin Endocrinol Metab 1981;53:113

84. Surks MI, Schadlow AR, Oppenheimer JH. A new radioimmunoassay for plasma L-triiodothyronine: measurements in thyroid disease and in patients maintained on hormonal replacement. J Clin Invest 1972;51:3104

85. Larsson M, Pettersson T, Carlström A. Thyroid hormone binding in serum of 15 vertebrate species: isolation of thyroxine-binding globulin and prealbumin analogs. Gen Comp Endocrinol 1985; 58:360

86. Refetoff S, Robin NI, Fang VS. Parameters of thyroid function in serum of 16 selected vertebrate species: a study of PBI, serum T$_4$, free T$_4$, and the pattern of T$_4$ and T$_3$ binding to serum proteins. Endocrinology 1970;86:793

87. Smallridge RC, Mehlman I, Pamplin CL III, et al. Pituitary and thyroid function in male cynomolgus monkeys. Lab Anim Sci 1981;31:693

88. Williams DA, Scott-Moncrieff JC, Bruner J, et al. Canine serum thyroid stimulating hormone following induction of hypothyroidism (abstract). J Vet Intern Med 1995;9:in press

89. Mendel CM, Frost PH, Kunitake ST, Cavalieri RR. Mechanism of the heparin-induced increase in the concentration of free thyroxine in plasma. J Clin Endocrinol Metab 1987;65:1259

90. Refetoff S. Inherited thyroxine-binding globulin abnormalities in man: update 1994. In: Braverman LE, Refetoff S, eds. Endocrine Reviews Monographs. 3. Clinical and molecular aspects of diseases of the thyroid. The Endocrine Society 1994:162

91. Refetoff S. Inherited thyroxine-binding globulin abnormalities in man. Endocr Rev 1989;10:275

92. Murata Y, Refetoff S, Sarne DH, et al. Variant thyroxine-binding globulin in serum of Australian aborigines: its physical, chemical and biological properties. J Endocrinol Invest 1985;8:225

93. Petersen CE, Scottolini AG, Cody LR, et al. A point mutation in the human serum albumin gene results in familial dysalbuminaemic hyperthyroxinaemia. J Med Genet 1994;31:355

94. Bartalena L. Thyroid hormone-binding proteins: update 1994. Endocr Rev Monographs. 1994;3:140

95. Lalloz MRA, Byfield PGH, Himsworth RL. A prealbumin variant with an increased affinity for T$_4$ and reverse T$_3$. Clin Endocrinol 1984;21:331

96. Blackett PR, Fry H, Garnica A, Blick K. Thyroxine and triiodothyronine autoantibodies in Hashimoto's thyroiditis with severe hormone-resistant hypothyroidism. J Pediatr Endocrinol 1994;7:65

97. Chopra IJ, Solomon DH, Huang T-S. Serum thyrotropin in hospitalized psychiatric patients: evidence for hyperthyrotropinemia as measured by an ultrasensitive thyrotropin assay. Metabolism 1990;39:538

98. Wortsman J, Premachandra BN, Williams K, et al. Familial resistance to thyroid hormone associated with decreased transport across the plasma membrane. Ann Intern Med 1983;98:904

99. Kleinhaus N, Faber J, Kahana L, et al. Euthyroid hyperthyroxinemia due to a generalized 5'-deiodinase defect. J Clin Endocrinol Metab 1988;66:684

100. Stockigt JR. Free thyroid hormone puzzle in critical illness. Eur J Endocrinol 1994;131:7

101. Wilcox RB, Nelson JC, Tomei RT. Heterogeneity in affinities of serum proteins for thyroxine among patients with nonthyroidal illness as indicated by serum free thyroxine response to serum dilution. Eur J Endocrinol 1994;131:9

102. Chopra IJ, Hershman JM, Hornabrook RW. Serum thyroid hormone and thyrotropin levels in subjects from endemic goiter regions of New Guinea. J Clin Endocrinol Metab 1975;40:326

103. Inada M, Nishikawa M, Kawai I. Hypothyroidism associated with positive results of the perchlorate discharge test in elderly patients. Am J Med 1983;74:1010

104. Stockigt JR, Dyer SA, Mohr VS, et al. Specific methods to identify plasma binding abnormalities in euthyroid hyperthyroxinemia. J Clin Endocrinol Metab 1986;62:230

105. Newnham HH, Hamblin PS, Long F, et al. Effect of oral furosemide on diagnostic indices of thyroid function. Clin Endocrinol 1987;26:423

106. Van den Berghe G, de Zegher F, Lauwers P. Dopamine and the sick euthyroid syndrome in critical illness. Clin Endocrinol 1994;41:731

107. Re RN, Kourides IA, Ridgeway EC, et al. The effect of glucocorticoid administration on human pituitary secretion of thyrotropin and prolactin. J Clin Endocrinol Metab 1976;43:338

108. Smith PJ, Surks MI. Multiple effects of diphenylhydantoin on the thyroid hormone system. Endocr Rev 1984;5:514

109. Topliss DJ, White EL, Stockigt JR. Significance of TSH excess in untreated primary adrenal insufficiency. J Clin Endocrinol Metab 1980;50:52

110. Miyai K, Onishi T, Hosokawa M, et al. Inhibition of thyrotropin and prolactin secretions in primary hypothyroidism by 2-Br-α-ergocryptine. J Clin Endocrinol Metab 1974;39:391

111. Bakker O, van Beeren HC, Wiersinga WM. Desethylamiodarone is a noncompetitive inhibitor of the binding of thyroid hormone to the thyroid hormone β_1-receptor protein. Endocrinology 1994;134:1665

112. Melmed S, Nademanee K, Reed AW, et al. Hyperthyroxinemia with bradycardia and normal thyrotropin secretion after chronic amiodarone administration. J Clin Endocrinol Metab 1981;53:997

113. Stockigt JR. Hyperthyroxinemia secondary to drugs and acute illness. The Endocrinologist 1993;3:67

114. Lambert M, Burger AG, De Nayer, Beckers C. Decreased TSH response to TRH induced by amiodarone. Acta Endocrinol 1988;118:449

115. Stockigt JR, Lim CF, Barlow JW, et al. High concentrations of furosemide inhibit plasma binding of thyroxine. J Clin Endocrinol Metab 1984;59:62

116. Spaulding SW, Burrow GN, Bermudez F, Himmelhoch JM. The inhibitory effect of lithium on thyroid hormone release in both euthyroid and thyrotoxic patients. J Clin Endocrinol Metab 1972;35:905

117. Berson SA, Yalow RS. The effect of cortisone on the iodine accumulating function of the thyroid gland in euthyroid subjects. Metabolism 1952;12:407

118. Williams DE, Chopra IJ, Orgiazzi J, Solomon DH. Acute effects of corticosteroids on thyroid activity in Graves' disease. J Clin Endocrinol Metab 1975;41:354

119. Ain KB, Refetoff S. Relationship of oligosaccharide modification to the cause of serum thyroxine-binding globulin excess. J Clin Endocrinol Metab 1988;66:1037

120. Chetkowski RJ, Meldrum DR, Steingold KA et al. Biologic effects of transdermal estradiol. N Engl J Med 1986;314:1615

121. English TN, Ruxton D, Eastman CJ. Abnormalities in thyroid function associated with chronic therapy with methadone. Clin Chem 1988;34:2202

122. Braverman LE, Ingbar SH. Effects of norethandrolone on the transport in serum and peripheral turnover of thyroxine. J Clin Endocrinol Metab 1967;27:389

123. Oppenheimer JH, Werner SC. Effect of prednisolone on thyroxine-binding proteins. J Clin Endocrinol Metab 1966;26:715

124. Kurtz AB, Capper SJ, Clifford J, et al. The effect of fenclofenac on thyroid function. Clin Endocrinol 1981;15:117

125. Lim C-F, Curtis AJ, Barlow JW, et al. Interactions between oleic acid and drug competitors influence specific binding of thyroxine in serum. J Clin Endocrinol Metab 1991;73:1106

126. Larsen PR. Salicylate-induced increases in free triiodothyronine in human serum. J Clin Invest 1972;51:1125

127. Lim C-F, Bai Y, Topliss DJ, et al. Drug and fatty acid effects on serum thyroid hormone binding. J Clin Endocrinol Metab 1988;67:682

128. Bishnoi A, Carlson HE, Gruber BL, et al. Effects of commonly prescribed nonsteroidal anti-inflammatory drugs on thyroid hormone measurements. Am J Med 1994;96:235

129. Stockigt JR, Lim C-F, Barlow JW, Topliss DJ. Drug-induced disturbances of in vitro thyroid testing: effects of circulating competitors for protein binding. Exp Clin Endocrinol 1994;102(suppl 2):110

130. Mendel CM, Frost PH, Cavalieri RR. Effect of free fatty acids on the concentration of free thyroxine in human serum: the role of albumin. J Clin Endocrinol Metab 1986;63:1394

131. Schatz DL, Sheppard RH, Steiner G, et al. Influence of heparin on serum free thyroxine. J Clin Endocrinol Metab 1969;29:1015

132. Mendel CM, Jaume JC, Frost PH, et al. Extremely low doses of heparin can cause artifactual elevations in the serum free thyroxine concentration as measured by equilibrium dialysis. Thyroid 1994;4(suppl 1):S63

133. Felicetta JV, Green WL, Nelp WB. Inhibition of hepatic binding of thyroxine by cholecystographic agents. J Clin Invest 1980;65:1032

134. Larkin JG, Macphee GJA, Beastall GH, Brodie MJ. Thyroid hormone concentrations in epileptic patients. Eur J Clin Pharmacol 1989;36:213

135. Northcutt RC, Stiel JN, Hollifield JW, Stant EG Jr. The influence of cholestyramine on thyroxine absorption. JAMA 1969;208:1857

136. Pinchera A, MacGillivray MH, Crawford JD, Freeman AG. Thyroid refractoriness in an athyreotic cretin fed soybean formula. N Engl J Med 1965;273:83

137. Sherman SI, Tielens ET, Ladenson PW. Sucralfate causes malabsorption of L-thyroxine. Am J Med 1994;96:531

138. Campbell NRC, Hasinoff BB, Stalts H, et al. Ferrous sulfate reduces thyroxine efficacy in patients with hypothyroidism. Ann Intern Med 1992;117:1010

139. Sperber AD, Liel Y. Evidence for interference with the intestinal absorption of levothyroxine sodium by aluminum hydroxide. Arch Intern Med 1992;152:183

140. Arafah BM. Decreased levothyroxine requirement in women with hypothyroidism during androgen therapy for breast cancer. Ann Intern Med 1994;121:247

141. Brabant G, Bergmann P, Kirsch CM, et al. Early adaptation of thyrotropin and thyroglobulin secretion to experimentally decreased iodine supply in man. Metabolism 1992;41:1093

142. Oppert J-M, Dussault JH, Tremblay A, et al. Thyroid hormones and thyrotropin variations during long term overfeeding in identical twins. J Clin Endocrinol Metab 1994;79:547

143. Hugues J, Burger AG, Pekary AE, Hershman JM. Rapid adaptations of serum thyrotropin, triiodothyronine and reverse triiodothyronine levels to short term starvation and refeeding. Act Endocrinol 1984;105:194

144. Kopp P, Van Sande J, Parma J, et al. Congenital hyperthyroidism caused by a mutation in the thyrotropin-receptor gene. N Engl J Med 1995;332:150

145. Kew MC. Thyroxine binding globulin, hyperthyroxinemia and hepatocellular carcinoma. Hepatology 1991;13:808

146. Maye P, Bisetti A, Burger A, et al. Hyperprealbuminemia, euthyroid hyperthyroxinemia, Zollinger-Ellison-like syndrome and hypercorticism in a pancreatic endocrine tumour. Acta Endocrinol 1989;120:87

147. Cooper DS, Daniels GH, Ladenson PW, Ridgway EC. Hyperthyroxinemia in patients treated with high-dose propranolol. Am J Med 1982;73:867

148. Goodwin TM, Montoro M, Mestman JM, Pekary AE, Hershman JM. The role of chorionic gonadotropin in transient hyperthyroidism of hyperemesis gravidarum. J Clin Endocrinol Metab 1992;75:1333

149. Morley JE, Shafer RB, Elson MK, et al. Amphetamine-induced hyperthyroxinemia. Ann Intern Med 1980;93:707

150. Mordes JP, Blume FD, Boyer S, et al. High-altitude pituitary-thyroid dysfunction on Mount Everest. N Engl J Med 1983;30:1135

151. Cogan E, Abramow M. Transient hyperthyroxinemia in symptomatic hyponatremic patients. Arch Intern Med 1986;146:545

Werner and Ingbar's The Thyroid, Seventh Edition,
edited by Lewis E. Braverman and Robert D. Utiger.
Lippincott–Raven Publishers, Philadelphia, © 1996

Section B
Miscellaneous Tests

19

Metabolic, Physiologic, and Clinical Indexes of Thyroid Function

Robert C. Smallridge

Laboratory confirmation of thyroid dysfunction appeared approximately 70 years ago, with early tests relying on physiologic measurements such as tendon reflexes[1] and the basal metabolic rate.[2] Not until the latter half of the twentieth century did biochemical tests of thyroid function emerge. Beginning with the protein-bound iodine test, specificity rapidly improved with radioimmunoassay and other methods to measure serum T_4, T_3, and TSH concentrations. Further technology has recently led to tests to directly measure serum free T_4 and T_3 and second- and third-generation TSH assays.

Given the available sophisticated methods for determining levels of thyroid hormones, is there now a need for less specific tests of thyroid function? The answer is decidedly yes, for just as the detection of circulating thyroid hormone concentrations has become more precise, so too has the clinician's appreciation of the diversity of thyroid diseases. The syndrome of thyroid hormone resistance, the "euthyroid sick" syndrome, the variety of thyroid hormone protein-binding abnormalities, the recognition of "subclinical" hyper- and hypothyroidism, and the numerous effects of drugs on thyroid hormone measurements are all instances in which circulating hormone concentrations are at variance with the patient's clinical state. Thus, a resurgence in the need for

"peripheral markers" of thyroid hormone effects has emerged. Although no such single marker exists, numerous nonspecific indices of thyroid hormone action in various tissues have been proposed.

The purpose of this chapter is to provide a resource for identifying potentially useful techniques to assess thyroid hormone action. The organ system manifestations of thyrotoxicosis and hypothyroidism are discussed in greater detail in Part IV, Section C, and Part V, Section C, respectively. Alterations in serum (and occasionally urine) concentrations of substances produced by selected organs have been reported in thyroid diseases. In most instances the proximate cause of the abnormality is unclear, although the usual postulated mechanisms include enhanced or delayed production or clearance of a chemical marker (i.e., protein or enzyme); enhanced release from injured tissues is proposed on occasion. Physiologic examination of certain organs has been helpful, as have tests of cognitive function and symptom-related questionnaires.

Some tests are reasonably specific, with good separation of values among hyperthyroid, euthyroid, and hypothyroid patients; others, while demonstrating statistical differences across patient groups, overlap too much to be of diagnostic use. However, when used longitudinally on the same patient,

TABLE 19-1.
Biochemical and Metabolic Measurements in Thyroid Disorders

Tissue	Test	Hyperthyroid	Hypothyroid	References
Blood cells				
Erythrocytes	Na/K-ATPase	↓	↑	3–5
	[Na+]$_i$	↑	↓	3–6
	Li-Na countertransport	↓	↑	6
	Ca-ATPase	↑	↓	7
	Carbonic anhydrase	↓	N, ↑	8, 9
	Glucose-6-phosphate dehydrogenase	↑	↓	10, 11
	Transketolase	↓	ND	10
Leukocytes	Na/K-ATPase activity	↑	↓	4
	[³H]-ouabain–binding capacity	ND	↓	4
	Alkaline phosphatase	ND	↑	12
	Interleukin-2 receptor	↑	↓	13
Platelets	Adhesion	ND	↓	14
	Volume	↑	↑	15
	Epidermal growth factor	↑	N	16
Bone	Osteocalcin	↑	N, ↓	17–19
	Alkaline phosphatase	↑	ND	19
	Hydroxyproline (urine)	↑	ND	19
	Pyridinoline cross-links (urine)	↑	ND	19
Endothelium	Factor VIII–related antigen (von Willebrand factor)	↑	↓	23–25
	Angiotensin-converting enzyme	↑	↓	24, 28
	Ristocetin cofactor activity	↑	↓	23
	Fibronectin	↑	N, ↓	24, 25, 29
	Thrombomodulin	↑	↓	30
	Tissue plasminogen activator	↑	ND	24
Hormones	Atrial natriuretic hormone	↑	↑, N, ↓	39
	Arginine vasopressin	↑	↓	25
	17-OHCS (urine)	↑	↓	40
	Aldosterone	N	↓	41
	Norepinephrine	N	↑	41, 42
Lipids	Cholesterol (total, low-density lipoprotein)	↓	↑	46–49
	Lp(a); apolipoprotein B	↓	↑	47
	Lipases (hepatic/lipoprotein)	↑/N	↓/↓	46
Liver	Ferritin	↑	N, ↓	50
	Factor VIII coagulant activity	↑	↓	23
	Sex hormone–binding globulin	↑	N, ↓	51–54
Metabolic	Tyrosine (plasma/urine)	↑/↑	↓/N	63
	Glutamic acid (plasma/urine)	↑/↑	N/N	63
	Nitrogen excretion (urine)	↑	ND	64
	Heat production rate (blood cells)	↑	N	65
	Procollagen III peptide	ND	↓	66
Muscle	Myoglobin	N	↑	69
	Creatine phosphokinase	↓	↑	69
	3-Methylhistidine (urine)	↑	ND	70
Thymus	Thymulin activity	↑	↓	87
Miscellaneous	Cyclic nucleotides (serum/urine)	↑	N	88

N; normal
NO; not done

TABLE 19-2.
Physiologic Measurements in Thyroid Disorders

Tissue	Test	Hyperthyroid	Hypothyroid	References
Bone	Bone mineral density	N, ↓	↑, N	20–22
Heart	Holter or electrocardiogram (heart rate)	↑	↓	31, 32
	Contractility			
	$\quad$ QK$_d$ (msec)	↓	↑	33, 34
	$\quad$ Systolic time intervals	↓	↑	35, 36
	$\quad$ Fiber-shortening velocity	↑	ND	31, 32
	$\quad$ Diastolic function	↑	↓	37
Intestine	Breath H$_2$ excretion (transit time)	↓	↑	43–45
Lungs	Respiratory muscle strength	↓	ND	55, 56
	Ventilatory drive (hypoxic/hypercapnic)	↑	↓	57–59
Metabolic	Basal metabolic rate	↑	↓	2, 60–62
Muscle	Achilles reflex time (msec)	↓	↑	1, 68
	Dynamometry (isokinetic)	↓	↓	71
Nerves	Evoked potentials (amplitude/latency)			
	$\quad$ Visual	↑/N	↓/↑	83–85
	$\quad$ Somatosensory	↑/N	ND	83
	Conduction time (median/ulnar)	N	↑	84
Skin	Flowmetry (laser Doppler)			
	$\quad$ Capillary flow (amplitude/velocity)	↑/↑	↓/↓	86

N; normal
ND; not done

even these tests offer some utility to the clinician. In considering the availability of these "peripheral markers," an alphabetic organ- or tissue-based classification has been adopted wherever possible and summaries of the biochemical, metabolic, and physiologic markers of thyroid dysfunction are listed in Tables 19-1 and 19-2.

TEST BY SPECIFIC ORGAN OR TISSUE

Blood Cells

ERYTHROCYTES

Circulating blood cells have been investigated for many years because of their availability. The erythrocyte has received the most attention, with alterations in Na$^+$ transport often reported. Red blood cell (RBC) Na/K-ATPase activity is reduced in hyperthyroidism, owing to fewer Na$^+$ pumps per cell; RBC intracellular Na$^+$ content is concomitantly increased.[3-5] A reduced sodium pump V$_{max}$ has also been reported. In hypothyroidism and nonthyroidal illness, mean enzyme activity is increased[3]; a small, significant decrease in Na$^+$ content has been noted.[3,6] Lithium-sodium (Li-Na) countertransport increases in hypothyroidism, and decreases by 40% in hyperthyroid patients.[6]

In contrast to the disturbances described in Na$^+$ transport, Ca^{2+}-ATPase activity is increased in hyperthyroidism and decreased in hypothyroidism.[7] Although the mechanisms responsible for changes in membrane transporters are unclear, alterations in membrane phospholipids in thyroid disorders have been proposed.

Erythrocyte carbonic anhydrase is affected variably in hypothyroidism but is consistently reduced in hyperthyroidism,[8,9] with as many as 88% of Graves' disease patients having values below the normal range.[9] Short-duration thyrotoxicosis, as seen in subacute thyroiditis, is not sufficient to alter carbonic anhydrase levels.[9]

Several RBC enzymes examined in the 1960s have not received recent attention. Glucose-6-phosphate dehydrogenase activity is increased above the normal range in about 50% of patients with thyrotoxicosis.[10,11] Hypothyroidism produces only a small decrease in activity[11] and provides no discrimination from normal levels. Transketolase was reduced in thyrotoxic patients in one study.[10]

LEUKOCYTES

White blood cells (WBCs) have been studied much less frequently than RBCs in thyroid disorders. Na/K-ATPase activity is affected in the opposite direction to that reported in RBCs, with small, significant increases in hyperthyroidism and decreases in hypothyroidism[4]; the [^{3}H]-ouabain binding capacity in hypothyroid WBCs was also below the normal range in six of eight subjects in one study,[4] and leukocyte alkaline phosphatase activity was elevated in seven of nine hypothyroid patients in another.[12] The latter two measurements warrant further study as potentially useful markers of thyroid hormone action. Serum interleukin-2 receptor varies directly with thyroid status in both immune and non-autoimmune dis-

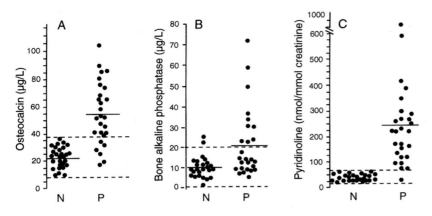

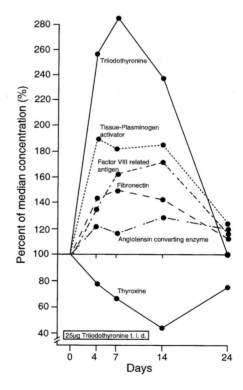

FIGURE 19-1. Serum osteocalcin *(A)*, bone alkaline phosphatase *(B)*, and urinary pyridinoline *(C)* are measured in patients with hyperthyroidism. Values in age-matched normal (N) subjects (left column) are compared to patient (P) values (right column). Dotted lines represent the lower and upper limits of the normal ranges (mean ± 2 SD). (From Garnero P, Vassy V, Bertholin A, et al. Markers of bone turnover in hyperthyroidism and the effects of treatment. J Clin Endocrinol Metab 1994;78:955, The Endocrine Society, Bethesda, MD)

eases;[13] serum interleukin 6 is increased in hyperthyroidism and returns to normal with therapy.[13a]

PLATELETS

Platelet adhesiveness is low in 75% of hypothyroid patients,[14] and the increased platelet volume in both hyper- and hypothyroid patients is too small to be of diagnostic utility.[15] Serum epidermal growth factor, derived from platelets, is increased twofold in hyperthyroid patients but reduced only marginally in hypothyroidism.[16]

Bone

Considerable attention has focused on the effects of thyroid hormone on skeletal metabolism. Hyperthyroidism increases serum osteocalcin[17–19] and bone specific alkaline phosphatase[19]—markers of bone formation—approximately twofold; osteocalcin levels are variably reduced in hypothyroidism.[17,18] Measures of bone resorption—urine hydroxyproline and pyridinoline cross-link excretion (Fig. 19-1)—are increased more than sixfold in hyperthyroid patients.[19] Bone density measurements are also reduced in hyperthyroid patients, but substantial overlap exists with euthyroid subjects.[20–22]

Endothelium

The endothelium is particularly sensitive to alterations in thyroid hormone levels. Factor VIII related antigen (F VIII R-Ag; von Willebrand's factor) is elevated in more than two thirds of hyperthyroid patients[23–25]; it is reduced much less often in hypothyroidism but, on occasion, has resulted in clinically significant acquired von Willebrand's disease.[26,27] Angiotensin converting enzyme activity (ACE),[24,28] ristocetin cofactor activity,[23] fibronectin,[24,25,29] and thrombomodulin[30] also vary directly with thyroid status, with the latter three being elevated in the majority of hyperthyroid patients. Tissue plasminogen activator (t-PA) responds to exogenous T_3 administration to a greater degree than do most other endothelial markers[24] (Fig. 19-2).

Heart

Increased heart rate is a cardinal physiologic manifestation of hyperthyroidism. Holter monitoring revealed a higher mean heart rate throughout a 24-hour period, and more frequent atrial premature beats in patients taking TSH suppressive doses of thyroid hormone.[31] These effects were inhibited by β-adrenergic blockade.[32]

An early measure of cardiac performance was the pulse wave arrival time, or QK_d interval. This test determines the time (in msec) from the Q wave onset to the Korotkoff sound in diastole at the brachial artery.[33,34] Although a very sensitive test for distinguishing and monitoring longitudinally hyper- and hypothyroidism, lack of availability of appropriate recording devices has limited its utility.

FIGURE 19-2. Mean concentrations of fibronectin, ACE, F VIII R-Ag, and t-PA before, during, and after oral T_3 administration (25 μg, three times daily) in seven normal women. (From Graninger W, Pirich KR, Speiser W, et al. Effect of thyroid hormones on plasma protein concentrations in man. J Clin Endocrinol Metab 1986;63:407, The Endocrine Society, Bethesda, MD)

Systolic time intervals have been employed for more than two decades but require simultaneous recording of an ECG, a phonocardiogram, and a carotid pulse tracing[35] (Fig. 19-3*A*). A recent modification uses a simultaneous ECG and M-mode echo of the aortic and mitral valves[36] (Fig. 19-3*B*). The echo can detect increased fractional and velocity of fiber shortening, and enhanced left ventricular (LV) mass index, even in mild exogenous thyrotoxicosis.[31,32] LV diastolic function, measured by Doppler echo, is also enhanced in hyperthyroidism and delayed in hypothyroidism.[37] Left ventricular ejection fraction is normal in younger adults with thyroid dysfunction.[37,38]

Hormones

Atrial natriuretic hormone is consistently elevated in hyperthyroidism, while levels in hypothyroid patients are more variable.[39] The finding of an elevated level of arginine vasopressin in all hyperthyroid subjects in one study suggests this hormone may be a useful diagnostic marker and should be further evaluated.[25] Cortisol metabolism, assessed by cortisol production rates and urinary 17-hydroxycorticosteroid (17-OHCS) excretion, varies directly with thyroid status,[40] whereas plasma aldosterone is reduced[41] and norepinephrine increased[41,42] in hypothyroidism.

Intestine

Gastrointestinal motility problems are frequent, with hyperdefecation (due to reduced intestinal transit time) occurring in hyperthyroidism and constipation (due to delayed transit) in hypothyroid patients. Documentation of these disturbances has been accomplished by measuring intestinal transit time, detecting breath H_2 excretion after lactulose ingestion.[43–45]

Lipids

The association of hypothyroidism with lipid abnormalities has been investigated for many years. Consistent findings of clinical significance include an increase in atherogenic total and low density lipoprotein (LDL) cholesterol, lipoprotein(a) (Lp[a]), and apolipoprotein B (Apo B),[46–49] as well as a reduction in hepatic and lipoprotein lipases.[46] In general, the opposite findings are seen in hyperthyroid patients.

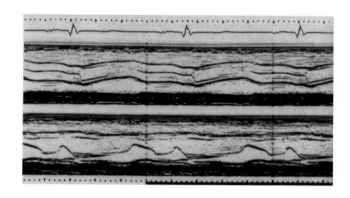

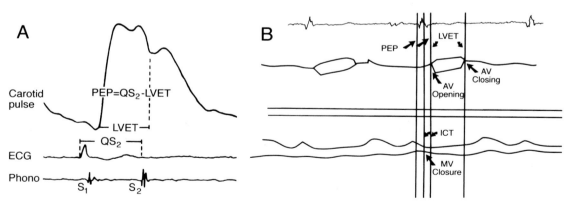

FIGURE 19-3. *(A)* Determination of systolic time intervals. The left ventricular ejection time (LVET) and the total electromechanical systole (QS_2) are measured directly from the carotid pulse curve, electrocardiogram, and phonocardiogram, whereas the pre-ejection period (PEP) is calculated by subtraction. (From Nuutila P, Irjala K, Saraste M, et al. Cardiac systolic time intervals and thyroid hormone levels during treatment of hypothyroidism. Scand J Clin Lab Invest 1992;52:467). *(B)* Simultaneous electrocardiographic and M mode echocardiographic aortic valve (AV) and mitral valve (MV) tracings. The lower panel is a graphic representation of the upper tracings. (Tseng KH, Walfish PG, Persaud JA, et al. Concurrent aortic and mitral valve echocardiography permits measurement of systolic time intervals as an index of peripheral tissue thyroid functional status. J Clin Endocrinol Metab 1989;69:633, The Endocrine Society, Bethesda, MD)

Liver

Many hepatic-derived proteins are unaffected or altered only modestly.[24] Serum ferritin levels provide little diagnostic utility in thyroid disorders; however, the response to exogenous T_3 is blunted in patients with thyroid hormone resistance (THR).[50] Factor VIII coagulant activity is affected more in hyper- than hypothyroidism.[23] The most sensitive test is serum sex hormone binding globulin (SHBG). Although affected little by hypothyroidism, almost all hyperthyroid patients have elevated values; it has been particularly useful in evaluating patients with THR.[51–54]

Lungs

Dyspnea on exertion is a common complaint in hyperthyroidism. Several authors have measured maximal static inspiratory and expiratory mouth pressures and determined that global respiratory muscle strength is reduced.[55,56] The ventilatory drive responses to hypercapnia and hypoxia vary directly with thyroid status,[57–59] and they may contribute to the hypoventilation that occurs occasionally in hypothyroidism.

Metabolism

The basal metabolic rate (BMR) has been used for many decades to assess thyroid status,[2] but many other conditions affect the test (Table 19-3) and it is now rarely utilized. Johansen and colleagues have shown that the BMR correlates with clinical index scores in hyper- and hypothyroidism,[60] and that the BMR correlates better with FT_3I than with FT_4I.[61] Also, newer equipment and methodology for measuring basal oxygen uptake (VO_2) has improved the sensitivity of this test to alterations in thyroid status.[62]

Plasma and urine levels of several amino acids (tyrosine and glutamic acid) were known to be elevated in hyperthyroidism more than 30 years ago; in particular, the tenfold increase in urinary glutamic acid could be a useful test.[63] Other indicators of metabolic function include urinary nitrogen excretion[64] and lymphocyte heat production rate,[65] which are both increased in hyperthyroidism.

TABLE 19-3.
Clinical States That Alter the Basal Metabolic Rate

INCREASE	DECREASE
Fever	Obesity
Pregnancy	Starvation or anorexia
Adrenergic agonist drugs	Hypogonadism
Pheochromocytoma	Adrenal insufficiency
Cancer	Cushing's syndrome
Congestive heart failure	Immobilization
Acromegaly	Sedative drugs
Polycythemia	
Paget's disease of bone	

Data from Becker DV. Metabolic indices. In: Ingbar SH, Braverman LE, eds. Werner's The Thyroid. 5th ed. Philadelphia: JB Lippincott, 1986:524.

Serum levels of procollagen-III-peptide (pIIIp) are low in subclinical hypothyroidism.[66] Recently, pIIIp was found to correlate positively with the BMR and was proposed as a possible marker of peripheral energy expenditure.[67]

Muscle

Perhaps the earliest physiologic measurement of muscle function in thyroid disease was the deep tendon reflex, an indicator of rate of muscle contractility. Attempts to quantify this response began more than 70 years ago, and measuring the half-relaxation time of the Achilles reflex was a popular thyroid function test. Although a delay in relaxation was observed in the majority of hypothyroid subjects in early studies,[1] a more recent paper found substantial overlap with euthyroid subjects.[68] Additionally, numerous other conditions can alter the test result.

Muscle weakness and myopathies develop commonly. In hypothyroidism, serum myoglobin and creatine kinase (CK) may be elevated, only occasionally to very high levels.[69] The CK band is almost totally MM, indicating a skeletal muscle source. Increased urinary excretion of 3-methylhistidine in hyperthyroid patients provides further evidence of muscle protein breakdown.[70] Thigh muscle efficiency has been assessed with an isokinetic dynamometer.[71] Peak torque and total work output improved after therapy in both hyper- and hypothyroid patients, and are useful parameters to follow longitudinally.

Nervous System

Thyroid dysfunction can dramatically alter central nervous system functions, and a variety of tests have been employed to assess the effects of hyper- and hypothyroidism on general and neurobehavioral symptoms (Table 19-4). Klein and coworkers[72] designed a 10-item hyperthyroid symptom scale (HSS) which has been used effectively in several reports.[32,37,73] Trzepacz and colleagues[73] administered a variety of self- and clinician-rated scales to ten patients with hyperthyroid Graves' disease, and found elevations of several of these including depression, anxiety, and hypomania. Symptoms often were improved with β-blockers, although not as effectively as with antithyroid drugs.[32,37,72,73] Neuropsychologic parameters (IQ, memory, and attention span) also improved when the patients became euthyroid.[73]

Hypothyroid symptoms have been quantified using[35,74–76] a diagnostic index described by Billewicz and coworkers[74] or several other questionnaires.[76,77] IQ, as well as neurologic and behavioral abnormalities, may be affected by congenital hypothyroidism.[78,79] In hypothyroid adults, memory-related abnormalities[80,81] as well as psychiatric features (anxiety, depression, obsessiveness, panic disorder)[81,82] have been reported. Brain metabolism measured by ^{31}P magnetic resonance imagery, is reduced in hypothyroidism.[82a]

Nerve conduction is also altered. Thyroid status affects evoked potentials, both visual and somatosensory; the amplitude of both measurements is increased in hyperthyroidism,[83] while the latency is normal.[83,84] In contrast, hypothyroidism prolongs latency and reduces the amplitude.[83–85] In addition, thyroid hormone deficiency delays both median and ulnar nerve conduction times.[84]

TABLE 19-4.
Tests Used in Assessment of Symptoms and Neurobehavioral Changes in Thyroid Disorders

Clinical Index	Instrument	References
HYPERTHYROID		
Symptoms	Hyperthyroid Symptom Scale	32, 37, 72, 73
Psychiatric	Schedule for Affective Disorders and Schizophrenia	73
	Beck Depression Inventory	73
	Spielberger State-Trait Anxiety Inventory	73
	Hopkins Symptom Checklist (SCL 90-R)	73
	Hamilton Depression Scale	73
	Mania Rating Scale	73
	Global Assessment Scale	73
Neuropsychologic	Wechsler Adult Intelligence Scale (WAIS-R)	73
	Wechsler Memory Scale	73
	Halstead-Reitan Battery	73
HYPOTHYROID		
Symptoms	Billewicz questionnaire	35, 74–76
	Profile of Mood States	76
	Symptom checklist	77
Psychiatric	Crown and Crisp Experiential Index	81
Neuropsychologic	Wechsler Memory Scale	80, 81
	Wechsler Intelligence Scale for Children (WISC-R)	78
	Schedule for Affective Disorders and Schizophrenia	82

Skin

Laser Doppler flowmetry has been used to examine skin perfusion.[86] Capillary flow velocity and pulse wave amplitude are both increased in hyperthyroid patients and reduced in hypothyroidism.

Thymus

The thymus produces factors that affect T-cell function. Thyroid status correlates strongly in a positive direction with serum thymulin activity and this activity is normalized when patients become euthyroid.[87]

Miscellaneous

Cyclic nucleotides (cAMP and cGMP) are elevated in the serum and urine of hyperthyroid patients, but remain normal in hypothyroidism.[88]

SUMMARY

Thyroid hormone affects biochemical and physiologic responses in many tissues, and a variety of tests have been used to characterize these responses. In the diagnosis of thyroid hormone resistance, several tests[54] have been particularly favored, as has a patient's response to exogenous T_3. Other tests (in Tables 19-1, 19-2, and 19-4) should also be clinically useful peripheral markers, thus improving the clinician's ability to di-

agnose and monitor therapy of patients with more difficult thyroid disorders.

References

1. Rives KL, Furth ED, Becker DV. Limitations of the ankle jerk test: Intercomparison with other tests of thyroid function. Ann Intern Med 1965;62:1139
2. Becker DV. Metabolic indices. In: Ingbar SH, Braverman LE, eds. Werner's the thyroid. 5th ed. Philadelphia: JB Lippincott, 1986;524
3. Dasmahapatra A, Cohen MP, Grossman SD, et al. Erythrocyte sodium/potassium adenosine triphosphatase in thyroid disease and nonthyroidal illness. J Clin Endocrinol Metab 1985;61:110
4. Khan FA, Baron DN. Ion flux and Na$^+$,K$^+$-ATPase activity of erythrocytes and leucocytes in thyroid disease. Clin Sci 1987;72:171
5. Arumanayagam M, Macdonald D, Cockram CS, et al. The effect of hyperthyroidism on in vivo aging of erythrocyte ouabain-binding sites and intracellular sodium and potassium. J Clin Endocrinol Metab 1990;71:260
6. Brent GA, Canessa M, Dluhy RG. Reversible alteration of red cell lithium-sodium countertransport in patients with thyroid disease. J Clin Endocrinol Metab 1989;68:322
7. Dube MP, Davis FB, Davis PJ, et al. Effects of hyperthyroidism and hypothyroidism on human red blood cell Ca^{2+}-ATPase activity. J Clin Endocrinol Metab 1986;62:253
8. Weatherall DJ, McIntyre PA. Developmental and acquired variations in erythrocyte carbonic anhydrase isozymes. Br J Haematol 1967;13:106
9. Kiso Y, Yoshida K, Kaise K, et al. Erythrocyte carbonic anhydrase-I concentrations in patients with Graves' disease and suba-

cute thyroiditis reflect integrated thyroid hormone levels over the previous few months. J Clin Endocrinol Metab 1991;72:515

10. Konttinen A, Viherkoski M. Blood transketolase and erythrocyte glucose-6-phosphate dehydrogenase activities in thyrotoxicosis. Clin Chim Acta 1968;22:145

11. Viherkoski M, Lamberg B-A. The glucose-6-phosphate dehydrogenase activity (G-6-PD) of the red blood cells in hyperthyroidism and hypothyroidism. Scand J Clin Lab Invest 1970;25:137

12. Barsano CP, Angulo M, Burke SF, et al. Leukocyte alkaline phosphatase in hypothyroidism and hyperthyroidism: response to initiation of thyroxine replacement therapy. Metabolism 1989;38:311

13. Mariotti S, Caturegli P, Barbesino G, et al. Thyroid function and thyroid autoimmunity independently modulate serum concentration of soluble interleukin 2 (IL-2) receptor (sIL-2R) in thyroid diseases. Clin Endocrinol 1992;37:415

13a. Celik I, Akalin S, Erbas T. Serum levels of interleukin 6 and tumor necrosis factor-α in hyperthyroid patients before and after propylthiouracil treatment. Eur J Endocrinol 1995;132:668

14. Edson JR, Fecher DR, Doe RP. Low platelet adhesiveness and other hemostatic abnormalities in hypothyroidism. Ann Intern Med 1975;82:342

15. Marongiu F, Conti M, Murtas ML, et al. What causes the increase in platelet mean volume in thyroid pathological conditions? Thromb Haemost 1990;63:323

16. Kung AWC, Hui WM, Ng ESK. Serum and plasma epidermal growth factor in thyroid disorders. Acta Endocrinol 1992;127:52

17. Martinez ME, Herranz L, de Pedro C, et al. Osteocalcin levels in patients with hyper- and hypothyroidism. Horm Metabol Res 1986;18:212

18. Kojima N, Sakata S, Nakamura S, et al. Serum concentrations of osteocalcin in patients with hyperthyroidism, hypothyroidism and subacute thyroiditis. J Endocrinol Invest 1992;15:491

19. Garnero P, Vassy V, Bertholin A, et al. Markers of bone turnover in hyperthyroidism and the effects of treatment. J Clin Endocrinol Metab 1994;78:955

20. Franklyn J, Betteridge J, Holder R, et al. Bone mineral density in thyroxine treated females with or without a previous history of thyrotoxicosis. Clin Endocrinol 1994;41:425

21. Ross DS. Hyperthyroidism, thyroid hormone therapy, and bone. Thyroid 1994;4:319

22. Faber J, Galloe AM. Changes in bone mass during prolonged subclinical hyperthyroidism due to L-thyroxine treatment: a meta-analysis. Europ J Endocrinol 1994;130:350

23. Rogers JS II, Shane SR, Jencks FS. Factor VIII activity and thyroid function. Ann Intern Med 1982;97:713

24. Graninger W, Pirich KR, Speiser W, et al. Effect of thyroid hormones on plasma protein concentrations in man. J Clin Endocrinol Metab 1986;63:407

25. Arnaout MA, Awidi AS, El-Najdawi AM, et al. Arginine-vasopressin and endothelium-associated proteins in thyroid disease. Acta Endocrinol 1992;126:399

26. Coccia MR, Barnes HV. Hypothyroidism and acquired von Willebrand disease. J Adolesc Health 1991;12:152

27. Aylesworth CA, Smallridge RC, Rick ME, Alving BM. Acquired von Willebrand disease: a rare manifestation of postpartum thyroiditis. Am J hematol 1995;50:217

28. Smallridge RC, Rogers J, Verma PS. Serum angiotensin-converting enzyme: Alterations in hyperthyroidism, hypothyroidism, and subacute thyroiditis. JAMA 1983;250:2489

29. Shirakami A, Hirai Y, Takeichi T, et al. Changes in plasma fibronectin levels in thyroid diseases. Horm Metabol Res 1986;18:345

30. Morikawa Y, Morikawa A, Makino I. Relationship of thyroid states and serum thrombomodulin (TM) levels in patients with Graves' disease: TM, a possible new marker of the peripheral activity of thyroid hormones. J Clin Endocrinol Metab 1993:76:609

31. Biondi B, Fazio S, Carella C, et al. Cardiac effects of long term thyrotropin-suppressive therapy with levothyroxine. J Clin Endocrinol Metab 1993;77:334

32. Biondi B, Fazio S, Carella C, et al. Control of adrenergic overactivity by β-blockade improves the quality of life in patients receiving long term suppressive therapy with levothyroxine. J Clin Endocrinol Metab 1994;78:1028

33. Young RT, Van Herle AJ, Rodbard D. Improved diagnosis and management of hyper- and hypothyroidism by timing the arterial sounds. J Clin Endocrinol Metab 1976;42:330

34. Osburne RC, Myers EA, Rodbard D, et al. Adaptation to hypocaloric feeding: physiologic significance of the fall in serum T_3 as measured by the pulse wave arrival time (QK_d). Metabolism 1983;32:9

35. Nuutila P, Irjala K, Saraste M, et al. Cardiac systolic time intervals and thyroid hormone levels during treatment of hypothyroidism. Scand J Clin Lab Invest 1992;52:467

36. Tseng KH, Walfish PG, Persaud JA, et al. Concurrent aortic and mitral valve echocardiography permits measurement of systolic time intervals as an index of peripheral tissue thyroid functional status. J Clin Endocrinol Metab 1989;69:633

37. Mintz G, Pizzarello R, Klein I. Enhanced left ventricular diastolic function in hyperthyroidism: noninvasive assessment and response to treatment. J Clin Endocrinol Metab 1991;73:146

38. Smallridge RC, Goldman MH, Raines K, et al. Rest and exercise left ventricular ejection fraction before and after therapy in young adults with hyperthyroidism and hypothyroidism. Am J Cardiol 1987;60:929

39. Rolandi E, Santaniello B, Bagnasco M, et al. Thyroid hormones and atrial natriuretic hormone secretion: study in hyper- and hypothyroid patients. Acta Endocrinol 1992;127:23

40. Kenny FM, Iturzaeta N, Preeyasombat C, et al. Cortisol production rate. VII. Hypothyroidism and hyperthyroidism in infants and children. J Clin Endocrinol Metab 1967;27:1616

41. Fraser R, Davies DL, Connell JM. Hormones and hypertension. Clin Endocrinol 1989;31:701

42. Del Rio G, Zizzo G, Marrama P, et al. α₂-Adrenergic activity is normal in patients with thyroid disease. Clin Endocrinol 1994; 40:235

43. Shafer RB, Prentiss RA, Bond JH. Gastrointestinal transit in thyroid disease. Gastroenterology 1984;86:852

44. Rahman Q, Haboubi NY, Hudson PR, et al. The effect of thyroxine on small intestinal motility in the elderly. Clin Endocrinol 1991;35:443

45. Wegener M, Wedmann B, Langhoff T, et al. Effect of hyperthyroidism on the transit of a caloric solid-liquid meal through the stomach, the small intestine, and the colon in man. J Clin Endocrinol Metab 1992;75:745

46. Valdemarsson S, Hansson P, Hedner P, et al. Relations between thyroid function, hepatic and lipoprotein lipase activities, and plasma lipoprotein concentrations. Acta Endocrinol 1983;104:50

47. de Bruin TWA, van Barlingen H, van Linde-Sibenius Trip M, et al. Lipoprotein(a) and apolipoprotein B plasma concentrations in hypothyroid, euthyroid, and hyperthyroid subjects. J Clin Endocrinol Metab 1993;76:121

48. Spandrio S, Sleiman I, Scalvini T, et al. Lipoprotein(a) in thyroid dysfunction before and after treatment. Horm Metab Res 1993; 25:586

49. Yamamoto K, Ozaki I, Fukushima N, et al. Serum lipoprotein(a) levels before and after subtotal thyroidectomy in subjects with hyperthyroidism. Metabolism 1995;44:4

50. Takamatsu J, Majima M, Miki K, et al. Serum ferritin as a marker of thyroid hormone action on peripheral tissues. J Clin Endocrinol Metab 1985;61:672

51. de Nayer Ph, Lambot MP, Desmons MC, et al. Sex hormone-binding protein in hyperthyroxinemic patients: a discriminator

for thyroid status in thyroid hormone resistance and familial dysalbuminemic hyperthyroxinemia. J Clin Endocrinol Metab 1986;62:1309

52. Smallridge RC, Parker RA, Wiggs EA, et al. Thyroid hormone resistance in a large kindred: physiologic, biochemical, pharmacologic, and neuropsychologic studies. Am J Med 1989;86:289

53. Beck-Peccoz P, Roncoroni R, Mariotti S, et al. Sex hormone-binding globulin measurement in patients with inappropriate secretion of thyrotropin (IST): evidence against selective pituitary thyroid hormone resistance in nonneoplastic IST. J Clin Endocrinol Metab 1990;71:19

54. Refetoff S, Weiss RE, Usala SJ. The syndromes of resistance to thyroid hormone. Endocr Rev 1993;14:348

55. Kendrick AH, O'Reilly JF, Laszlo G. Lung function and exercise performance in hyperthyroidism before and after treatment. Q J Med 1988;68:615

56. Siafakas NM, Milona I, Salesiotou V, et al. Respiratory muscle strength in hyperthyroidism before and after treatment. Am Rev Respir Dis 1992;146:1025

57. Zwillich CW, Matthay M, Potts DE, et al. Thyrotoxicosis: Comparison of effects of thyroid ablation and beta-adrenergic blockade on metabolic rate and ventilatory control. J Clin Endocrinol Metab 1978;46:491

58. Zwillich CW, Pierson DJ, Hofeldt FD, et al. Ventilatory control in myxedema and hypothyroidism. N Engl J Med 1975;292:662

59. Ladenson PW, Goldenheim PD, Ridgway EC. Prediction and reversal of blunted ventilatory responsiveness in patients with hypothyroidism. Am J Med 1988;84:877

60. Johansen K, Hansen JM, Skovsted L. Myxoedema and thyrotoxicosis: relations between clinical state and concentrations of thyroxine and triiodothyronine in blood. Acta Med Scand 1978;204:361

61. Johansen K, Hansen JM, Skovsted L. The preferential role of triiodothyronine in the regulation of basal metabolic rate in hyper- and hypothyroidism. Acta Med Scand 1978;204:357

62. Lim VS, Zavala DC, Flanigan MJ, et al. Basal oxygen uptake: A new technique for an old test. J Clin Endocrinol Metab 1986;62:863

63. Bélanger R, Chandramohan N, Misbin R, et al. Tyrosine and glutamic acid in plasma and urine of patients with altered thyroid function. Metabolism 1972;21:855

64. Georges LP, Santangelo RP, Mackin JF, et al. Metabolic effects of propranolol in thyrotoxicosis. I. Nitrogen, calcium, and hydroxyproline. Metabolism 1975;24:11

65. Valdemarsson S, Monti M. Increased ratio between anaerobic and aerobic metabolism in lymphocytes from hyperthyroid patients. Eur J Endocrinol 1994;130:276

66. Nyström E, Caidahl K, Fager G, et al. A double-blind cross-over 12-month study of L-thyroxine treatment of women with "subclinical" hypothyroidism. Clin Endocrinol 1988;29:63

67. Stenlöf K, Sjöström L, Fagerberg B, et al. Thyroid hormones, procollagen III peptide, body composition and basal metabolic rate in euthyroid individuals. Scand J Clin Lab Invest 1993;53:793

68. Ballantyne GH, Croxson MS. The effect of exercise, thyroid status and insulin-induced hypoglycaemia on the Achilles tendon reflex time in man. Eur J Appl Physiol 1981;46:77

69. Docherty I, Harrop JS, Hine KR, et al. Myoglobin concentration, creatine kinase activity, and creatine kinase B subunit concentrations in serum during thyroid disease. Clin Chem 1984;30:42

70. Adlerberth A, Angerås U, Jagenburg R, et al. Urinary excretion of 3-methylhistidine and creatinine and plasma concentrations of amino acids in hyperthyroid patients following preoperative treatment with antithyroid drug or β-blocking agent: results from a prospective, randomized study. Metabolism 1987;36:637

71. Zürcher RM, Horber FF, Grünig BE, et al. Effect of thyroid dysfunction on thigh muscle efficiency. J Clin Endocrinol Metab 1989;69:1082

72. Klein I, Trzepacz PT, Roberts M, et al. Symptom rating scale for assessing hyperthyroidism. Arch Intern Med 1988;148:387

73. Trzepacz PT, McCue M, Klein I, et al. Psychiatric and neuropsychological response to propranolol in Graves' disease. Biol Psychiatry 1988;23:678

74. Billewicz WZ, Chapman RS, Crooks J, et al. Statistical methods applied to the diagnosis of hypothyroidism. Q J Med 1969;38:255

75. Cooper DS, Halpern R, Wood LC, et al. L-Thyroxine therapy in subclinical hypothyroidism: a double-blind, placebo-controlled trial. Ann Intern Med 1984;101:18

76. Meier CA, Braverman LE, Ebner SA, et al. Diagnostic use of recombinant human thyrotropin in patients with thyroid carcinoma (phase I/II study). J Clin Endocrinol Metab 1994;78:188

77. Hayslip CC, Fein HG, O'Donnell VM, et al. The value of serum antimicrosomal antibody testing in screening for symptomatic postpartum thyroid dysfunction. Am J Obstet Gynecol 1988;159:203

78. Glorieux J, Desjardins M, Letarte J, et al. Useful parameters to predict the eventual mental outcome of hypothyroid children. Pediatr Res 1988;24:6

79. Porterfield SP, Hendrich CE. The role of thyroid hormones in prenatal and neonatal neurological development—Current perspectives. Endocr Rev 1993;14:94

80. Haggerty JJ Jr., Garbutt JC, Evans DL, et al. Subclinical hypothyroidism: a review of neuropsychiatric aspects. Int J Psychiatry Med 1990;20:193

81. Monzani F, Del Guerra P, Caraccio N, et al. Subclinical hypothyroidism: neurobehavioral features and beneficial effect of L-thyroxine treatment. Investig 1993;71:367

82. Joffe RT, Levitt AJ. Major depression and subclinical (grade 2) hypothyroidism. Psychoneuroendocrinology 1992;17:215

83. Takahashi K, Fujitani Y. Somatosensory and visual evoked potentials in hyperthyroidism. Electroenceph Clin Neurophysiol 1970;29:551

83a. Smith CD, Ain KB. Brain metabolism in hypothyroidism studied with ^{31}P magnetic-resonance spectroscopy. Lancet 1995;345:619

84. Abbott RJ, O'Malley BP, Barnett DB, et al. Central and peripheral nerve conduction in thyroid dysfunction: the influence of L-thyroxine therapy compared with warming upon the conduction abnormalities of primary hypothyroidism. Clin Sci 1983;64:617

85. Ladenson PW, Stakes JW, Ridgway EC. Reversible alteration of the visual evoked potential in hypothyroidism. Am J Med 1984;77:1010

86. Weiss M, Milman B, Rosen B, et al. Quantitation of thyroid hormone effect on skin perfusion by laser Doppler flowmetry. J Clin Endocrinol Metab 1993;76:680

87. Fabris N, Mocchegiani E, Mariotti S, et al. Thyroid function modulates thymic endocrine activity. J Clin Endocrinol Metab 1986;62:474

88. Peracchi M, Bamonti-Catena F, Lombardi L, et al. Plasma and urine cyclic nucleotide levels in patients with hyperthyroidism and hypothyroidism. J Endocrinol Invest 1983;6:173

Werner and Ingbar's The Thyroid, Seventh Edition,
edited by Lewis E. Braverman and Robert D. Utiger.
Lippincott–Raven Publishers, Philadelphia, © 1996

20

Thyroglobulin

Carole A. Spencer

Thyroglobulin (Tg) plays a central role in thyroid pathophysiology. It is involved in thyroid autoimmunity; genetic defects in Tg biosynthesis can result in inborn errors of thyroid hormone metabolism, and the tissue-specific origin of Tg has led to its use as a marker for differentiated thyroid cancer.[1–3] Despite three decades of serum Tg measurement, unsolved methodologic problems limit the clinical value of this biochemical test. These problems include limited assay sensitivity, lack of standardization, and thyroglobulin autoantibody (TgAb) interference.[4–7] Current immunoassay methods now detect Tg in the serum of all TgAb-negative euthyroid subjects.[6] Abnormal serum Tg concentrations result from abnormalities in thyroid mass, excess thyroidal stimulation, or physical thyroid damage.[8–11] This chapter will focus on the physiology of Tg and the methodology and clinical utility of serum Tg measurements.

THYROGLOBULIN BIOSYNTHESIS, SECRETION, AND METABOLIC CLEARANCE

Thyroglobulin is a large (660 kd[12]) homodimeric glycoprotein molecule, encoded by a gene on chromosome 8 that is secreted uniquely by thyroid follicular cells.[13–15] The factors controlling Tg gene expression include thyrotropin (TSH), insulin and insulin-like growth factor-1 (IGF-1), which act synergistically to stimulate transcription of the 8.5 kilobase (kb) Tg mRNA, whereas epidermal growth factor (EGF), interferon-γ, tumor necrosis factor (TNF-α), and retinoic acid are inhibitors of transcription (see chap 5).[10,16–21] The formation of mature Tg requires complex processing that involves dimerization and folding, glycosylation and modification in the Golgi apparatus, followed by incorporation into exocytotic vesicles for export into the lumen of thyroid follicles, after which thyroid peroxidase catalyses iodination of tyrosyl residues and coupling of some of them within the Tg polypeptide to form thyroxine (T_4) and triiodothyronine (T_3).[22–25]

Thyroglobulin in thyroid tissue and serum is heterogeneous.[26] All the steps involved in post-translational processing can affect the ultimate conformation and immunoreactivity of Tg. Antibodies used in Tg immunoassays are conformational, that is, directed against discontinuous regions of the protein.[27] Conformational differences in Tg arising from differences in its composition of carbohydrate[28,29] or iodine[30,31] can expose or mask epitopes[32] and cause antibody-dependent differences in immunoactivity.[33,34] Some monoclonal antibodies detect differences between the Tg isoforms present in the glandular extracts used for assay standardization as compared with Tg isoforms in the circulation.[33] This can have clinical consequences when using serum Tg as a marker for thyroid carcinomas that secrete conformationally abnormal Tg molecules.[32,33,35]

The processes involved in the release of Tg into and clearance from the circulation are poorly understood. Tg in the follicular lumen is internalized by micropinocytosis and undergoes proteolytic cleavage in lysosomes, a process that liberates T_4 and T_3 while degrading 90% or more of the Tg molecules.[36–38] Undigested Tg enters the circulation via the thyrolymphatic system by a poorly understood mechanism, either because lysosomal hydrolysis is incomplete or as a result of short-loop secretion that does not involve luminal storage.[39–41] The latter may represent the major route of secretion by thyroid carcinomas in which both glandular and circulating forms of Tg are poorly iodinated.[42]

During steady-state conditions, the serum Tg concentration is determined by the balance between its secretion and metabolism. The mechanisms for clearing Tg from the circulation are poorly understood, but they are thought to be influenced by the sialic acid content of the molecule; its presence appears to facilitate clearance.[43] Hepatocytes are thought to mediate most extrathyroidal Tg metabolism[44]; Tg binds to B-lymphocytes and other cells,[45] but the metabolic importance of this binding is unclear. In normal subjects the secretion rate and plasma half-life of Tg are 100 mg/60 kg/day and 29.6+/– 2.8 (± SD) hours, respectively.[46] The half-life after thyroidectomy is shorter in patients with Graves' disease or differentiated thyroid carcinoma and longer in patients with nodular goiter.[46–48] The different Tg half-life estimates, ranging from 2.3 hours to 6 days, may be due to variations in clearance resulting from release of Tg molecules of different size or sialic acid content.[29,48,49] In addition, there may be differences in immunoreactivity between the exogenously administered Tg preparations used for some clearance studies as compared with endogenous Tg measured in the post-thyroidectomy studies.[46,48] In the case of Graves' disease, formation of Tg-TgAb complexes might increase Tg clearance.[50,51]

LIMITATIONS OF SERUM THYROGLOBULIN MEASUREMENTS

Reliable serum Tg measurement is still technically challenging, especially in patients with serum TgAb. Isotopic[5] and non-isotopic[52] immunometric assay (IMA) methods utilizing monoclonal antibodies are now replacing double antibody radioimmunoassay (RIA) methods.[53] The newer assays are more sensitive and more rapid, but their utility is limited by problems of standardization, TgAb interference and sensitivity.

There is still no universal standardization of methods[4] and intermethod variability approaches 65%.[4,6] This precludes comparisons of both normal ranges and empiric cut-off values chosen to define patient status.[54–57] A recent collaborative effort, sponsored by the Community Bureau of Reference (CBR) of the Commission of the European Communities (CEC), produced a Tg standard for widespread distribution.[7] Although the use of this standard should reduce intermethod variability, differences in the anti-Tg antibodies used in different assays will continue to make comparisons of results difficult.

TgAb interference affects all Tg methods to some degree by causing over- or underestimation of serum Tg concentrations[4–6,58] (Fig 20-1). With RIA methods the direction of interference depends on the method used to separate antibody-bound and free Tg, the volume of serum used, and the concentration and affinity of the serum TgAb, because these factors affect the partitioning of Tg tracer between the antibody constituents.[59] Underestimation is the characteristic pattern of interference in immunometric assays because Tg complexed with TgAb appears to be blocked from participating in the two-site reaction.[60]

Some normal subjects have low serum TgAb concentrations,[61,62] whereas high serum TgAb concentrations are characteristic of autoimmune thyroid disorders.[61,63] It is unclear whether very low concentrations of naturally occurring TgAb are the cause of the interference found with some seemingly TgAb-negative serum samples.[64] Epitope mapping of Tg reveals six different antigenic domains (regions I–VI) with different specificity for naturally occurring TgAb.[65,66] Most laboratories still use insensitive hemagglutination techniques to detect TgAb in serum despite reports that TgAb concentrations too low to be detected by hemagglutination can interfere with serum Tg measurements.[58,67,68] Sensitive TgAb immunoassay methods are recommended for screening serum for interfering TgAb before Tg measurement is undertaken.[4,61] Using immunoassays, TgAb can be detected in 4% to 27% of normal subjects,[69] 20% to 45% of patients with thyroid carcinoma,[70–72] and 50% to 97% of patients with autoimmune thyroid disease.[73] It is difficult to predict which serum samples with TgAb will interfere with serum Tg measurements because the TgAb concentration does not correlate with the degree of interference assessed by recovery or dilution studies.[5,64] Attempts to overcome TgAb interference in immunometric assays by using monoclonal antibodies restricted to epitopes not involved in autoantibody formation has not overcome the interference problem,[5,74] either because the in vitro recovery approach is invalid, or because the TgAb in patients with thyroid carcinoma reacts with more epitopes than TgAb in patients with autoimmune thyroid disease.[6,75] Thus, any serum Tg value reported in patients with TgAb must be interpreted cautiously. In fact, it is probably better not to report serum Tg values at all in patients with TgAb in their serum, unless the Tg assay method can be shown to give serum Tg values concordant with clinical status.

Sensitive Tg methods are needed for monitoring patients with thyroid carcinoma receiving T_4 therapy to identify those with small amounts of thyroid tissue. This is especially important in patients who have recurrent thyroid carcinoma and may benefit from radioiodine therapy, particularly when recombinant human TSH (rhTSH) becomes available.[72]

SERUM THYROGLOBULIN CONCENTRATIONS IN NORMAL ADULTS

Thyroglobulin can be detected in the serum of all normal subjects when sensitive methods are used.[6] There is no diurnal or seasonal variability in serum Tg concentrations, but the concentration does appear to be under the control of a dominant gene.[76–78] The long-term intraperson biologic variation is relatively small (14% coefficient of variation), whereas interperson variability is high (35% coefficient of variation).[79]

Three factors determine serum Tg concentrations in most clinical situations: thyroid cell mass[80,81]; physical damage to the thyroid caused by biopsy,[82] surgery,[8,83,84] hemorrhage,[85] radioiodine administration,[86] external irradiation,[87] or inflammation[88]; and activation of TSH-receptors by either TSH,[10] chorionic gonadotropin (hCG),[89] or thyroid-stimulating antibodies (TSAb).[90] At steady state, thyroid size is the dominant factor modulating serum Tg concentrations.[80,81] Serum TSH and Tg concentrations are correlated only in patients with endemic goiter who have elevated serum TSH concentrations.[91] However, serum Tg changes in parallel with serum TSH when thyroid size remains constant; for example, serum Tg declines with serum TSH during fasting and rises in response to iodine-induced or hypothyroidism-induced increases in serum TSH.[92,92] Smokers have a higher frequency of goiter and higher serum Tg concentrations than nonsmokers, but their serum Tg and TSH concentrations are not correlated.[94] The changes in smokers may reflect the goitrogenic effects of thiocyanate exacerbated by iodine deficiency.[95,96]

Serum Tg concentrations tend to be higher in women than men, but the difference is small and the normal reference range is the same.[78,97] The intermethod variability in normal reference values is multifactorial (Table 20-1). Explanations for the variability include variations in standardization, variation in use of log-transformed values and use of varying criteria for

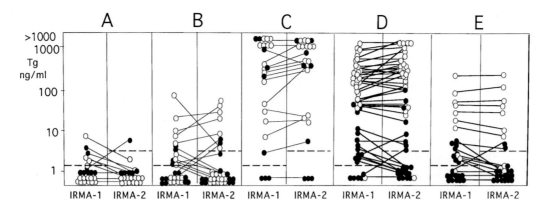

FIGURE 20-1. Serum Tg concentrations determined by two different immunoradiometric assays (IRMA). The Tg monoclonal antibodies used in IRMA-1 did not cross-react with Tg epitopes recognized by TgAB in serum from patients with thyroid disorders. The Tg antibodies used in IRMA-2 were polyclonal rabbit antibodies. Serum samples from TgAB-negative (*open symbols*) and TgAB-positive (*closed symbols*) patients with either thyroid carcinoma (A–C) or autoimmune thyroid disease (D–E) were assayed in each IRMA. Group A: patients with differentiated thyroid carcinoma with no clinical and scintigraphic evidence of residual thyroid tissue or metastases; group B: patients with residual thyroid tissue; group C: patients with lymph node or distant metastases; group D: patients with Graves' disease; and group E: patients with chronic autoimmune thyroiditis. (From Mariotti S, Barbesino G, Caturegli P, et al. Assay of thyroglobulin in serum with thyroglobulin autoantibodies: An unobtainable goal? J Clin Endocrinol Metab 1995; 80:468)

excluding subjects with TgAb, mild thyromegaly, thyroid nodules, or a smoking history.[5,7,80,94,98,99] Additionally, the various antibodies used may detect differences in immunoreactivity in circulating Tg isoforms.[33]

The role of estrogen in modulating serum Tg concentrations is unclear. Serum Tg concentrations change in parallel with the small changes in thyroid size that occur during the menstrual cycle and are higher in pregnant women than in nonpregnant women, especially during the third trimester.[80,81] At delivery serum Tg is correlated with both thyroid size as assessed by ultrasonography and serum TSH.[81] Factors responsible for the rise in serum Tg concentrations during pregnancy include hCG

TABLE 20-1.
Serum Thyroglobulin Concentrations in Normal Subjects and Patients With Various Thyroid Diseases

Clinical Status	Condition	Method	Reference	Sensitivity Limit (ng/mL)	Normal Values, mean (range) (ng/mL)	Mean ±SD (range) (ng/mL)
Euthyroid	Normal subjects	IRMA	53	0.4	10.0 (1.2–34.7)	
		IRMA	120	1.5	(3.0–35)	
		RIA	55	1.0	(<60)	
		RIA	72	1.0	5–50	
		RIA	3	3.0	2–30	
		RIA	57	1.0	11.7 (1–20)	
		IRMA	140	1.0	(<45)	
		IRMA	5	1.5	(3–35)	
	Pregnancy: 1st trimester	IRMA	81	0.4	10.0 (1.2–34.7)	31 ± 2 (SE)
	2nd trimester					31 ± 2 (SE)
	3rd trimester					38 ± 2 (SE)
	Benign nodules	RIA	129			86 ± 16 (SE)
		RIA	83			395 ± 168 (SE)
	Thyroid carcinoma	RIA	131			464 ± 248 (SE)
Thyrotoxicosis	Graves' disease	RIA	118	10.0		300 ± 247
		IRMA	5	1.5	(3–35)	<1.5 – 1000
Graves' disease	Thyroid adenoma	RIA	152		22 (5–74)	198 (144–337)
	Thyroiditis	RIA	88	1.5		268 ± 1684 (SD)
	Multinodular goiter	RIA	9		22 (6–81)	161 (<5–8250)

IRMA, immunoradiometric assay; RIA, radioimmunoassay.

(early in pregnancy) and TSH (later).[89] Serum Tg concentrations then decline during the first month postpartum.[81]

SERUM THYROGLOBULIN CONCENTRATIONS IN INFANTS AND CHILDREN

The thyroid gland differentiates and Tg gene expression is initiated in the absence of TSH, before thyrotrophs are detected.[13,100,101] TSH and thyroid hormone synthesis begins near mid-gestation in humans; thereafter, the pituitary-thyroid axis matures with the development of thyroid hormone feedback inhibition of TSH during the third trimester[102,103] (see chap 84). At birth the serum concentrations of T_4, free T_4, and T_3 are correlated positively, whereas serum Tg and TSH concentrations are correlated negatively with gestational age and birth weight.[103] Cord serum Tg and TSH concentrations are correlated positively[104] and are higher than maternal concentrations.[103,105] Although the fetal and maternal thyroid axes are controlled independently, maternal iodine intake influences fetal thyroid function such that cord serum Tg concentrations are correlated negatively with maternal urinary iodine excretion at the time of delivery.[104] The high cord serum Tg values typical of iodide-deficient areas presumably reflect either higher serum TSH concentrations,[104] enhanced secretion of poorly iodinated Tg,[106] or decreased clearance of Tg by the immature newborn liver.[107] Thyroid size and cord serum Tg concentrations are increased in infants born to smoking mothers.[108] This is thought to be secondary to a goitrogenic effect of thiocyanate, the concentrations of which are correlated positively in cord and maternal serum.[96]

Although infants with congenital hypothyroidism usually have abnormally low or high serum Tg concentrations depending on the underlying pathology, the serum Tg concentration is not diagnostic.[109] The Tg value together with the results of ultrasonography and radionuclide imaging of the thyroid can be used to determine the etiology of congenital hypothyroidism[2] (see also chap 56). Low but detectable serum Tg concentrations are characteristic of both thyroid agenesis and thyroid ectopy.[2,110] Serum Tg concentrations are high, sometimes very high (above 1000 ng/mL), in infants with thyroid hormone resistance, iodide transport or deiodinase defects, and other inborn errors of T_4 biosynthesis.[2,111,112] In normal full-term infants serum Tg increases in the first days after birth, presumably in response to the postnatal surge in TSH secretion[107]; this increase is attenuated in sick or preterm neonates.[113] Serum Tg concentrations fall approximately 50% during the first few months of life, after which they decline very gradually to reach adult levels after puberty.[114,115]

SERUM THYROGLOBULIN CONCENTRATIONS IN THYROID DISEASE

A low serum Tg concentration is rarely encountered except in patients who have very little or no thyroid tissue, as in thyroid agenesis, after total or near-total thyroidectomy or destruction by radioiodine, or when TSH secretion is suppressed.[116] Patients with other thyroid disorders have normal or high serum

Tg concentrations, the latter occurring as a result of autonomous thyroid function, thyroid injury, or activation of TSH receptors (see Table 20-1).

Thyrotoxicosis

Serum Tg concentrations are high in nearly all patients with hyperthyroidism caused by Graves' disease as a result of the stimulatory action of TSAb.[90] The few patients with normal or even low serum Tg values probably had TgAb that was undetected, because an insensitive TgAb assay was used to screen the serum samples for TgAb interference. When sensitive TgAb immunoassays are used, the majority of patients with Graves' hyperthyroidism have TgAb.[61,73]

Serum Tg concentrations decline during antithyroid drug treatment and may become normal if a remission of the Graves' disease occurs.[117] In contrast, although declining somewhat after therapy is initiated, the concentrations tend to remain elevated in those patients destined to have persistent hyperthyroidism, even though their serum T_4 and T_3 concentrations fall to normal as a result of the antithyroid drug therapy.[118] Although serum Tg concentrations and goiter size are positively correlated before and during antithyroid drug therapy, the correlation among serum Tg, TSAb, and subsequent remission is not strong.[119,120]

Both surgical and radioiodine treatment of patients with hyperthyroidism caused by Graves' disease result in an initial increase in serum Tg concentrations secondary to surgical trauma or radiation-induced thyroid destruction.[8,117] Serum Tg concentrations peak within one day after surgery and then decline over the subsequent month.[117] In contrast, serum Tg rises more slowly to peak between 1 to 3 months after radioiodine treatment.[117] After both surgery and radioiodine therapy, serum Tg concentrations later decline in parallel with the restoration of euthyroidism.

Serum Tg concentrations are also high in patients with thyroid hyperfunction caused by an autonomously functioning thyroid adenoma, multinodular goiter, or excess TSH secretion.[9,121,122] In contrast, serum Tg concentrations are normal or low in patients who are thyrotoxic as a result of exogenous thyroid hormone administration.[123] The concentration may be either high or low in patients with iodine-induced thyrotoxicosis, and high in patients with thyrotoxicosis caused by subacute thyroiditis, silent thyroiditis, or any other thyroid inflammatory process.[88,124,125]

Hypothyroidism

Serum Tg measurements have little clinical utility in the diagnosis or management of hypothyroidism. The reason is that hypothyroidism is most commonly caused by chronic autoimmune thyroiditis, in which the very high incidence of TgAb precludes serum Tg measurement.[5] In infants with congenital hypothyroidism the serum Tg value may be helpful in determining the cause, as noted earlier.[2]

Congenital goiter can result from synthesis of abnormal Tg molecules, defective Tg glycosylation, abnormal intracellular Tg trafficking, or a defect in thyroid peroxidase[126–129] (see chap 56). These patients typically have some degree of hypothyroidism and almost all have elevated serum TSH concentrations as the cause of the goiter.[129] The types of congenital goiters can be classified and distinguished from other causes of goiter by basal as well as TSH-stimulated serum Tg responses.[129] Typically patients with goiters resulting from quantitative defects in Tg synthesis have low basal serum Tg concentrations and no serum Tg response to exogenous TSH, whereas patients with qualitative defects usually have measurable or even elevated basal serum Tg concentrations and TSH-stimulated serum Tg responses comparable with those in patients with goiters resulting from organification defects.[130]

Serum Tg concentrations are high in patients with endemic goiter. This is especially true among patients with severe iodine deficiency in whom serum Tg and TSH concentrations are positively correlated.[91]

Thyroid Nodular Disease

Serum Tg concentrations are normal or high in euthyroid patients with benign thyroid nodules.[131] An increasing serum Tg concentration is indicative of the development of a nodule in patients with a history of head or neck irradiation.[132] Among patients with thyroid nodules who are treated with T_4, a decrease in serum Tg correlates with a reduction in nodule size as assessed by ultrasonography.[99]

Similarly, serum Tg concentrations are normal or elevated in euthyroid patients with multinodular goiter. The concentrations increase as goiter size increases (and serum TSH concentrations fall).[9] The genesis of elevated serum Tg concentrations in these patients is multifactorial and includes thyroid autonomy, thyroid follicular damage, and perhaps stimulation by thyroid growth factors other than TSH.[133] The Tg synthesized by some goiters may have increased carbohydrate or decreased iodine content.[134] The serum Tg elevations in patients with multinodular goiters are correlated with low intrathyroidal iodine stores as well as increased serum T_3/T_4 ratios and the degree of Tg iodination.[135,136] Poorly iodinated Tg produced by multinodular goiters may be released more rapidly after its resorption from the follicular lumen into thyroid follicular cells, thus explaining at least some part of the elevations in serum Tg. In these patients, serum Tg concentrations fall when iodine is administered, perhaps reflecting the production of more stable Tg molecules.[137]

Thyroiditis

Serum Tg concentrations are a sensitive marker of both acute and chronic thyroid inflammation. As noted previously, patients with thyrotoxicosis caused by subacute and silent (painless) thyroiditis (including postpartum thyroiditis) have high serum Tg concentrations.[138-141] The elevations in serum Tg can be used to distinguish thyrotoxic patients with silent thyroiditis from those with exogenous thyrotoxicosis, in whom serum Tg concentrations are low.[123,140] Although both subacute thyroiditis and silent thyroiditis subside in several weeks, serum Tg concentrations may remain elevated and thyroid iodine stores may remain depleted for 1 to 2 years.[142,143] The clinical utility of serum Tg measurements in patients with thyroiditis is limited by the interfering effects of the TgAb that are often present in these patients, especially those with postpartum thyroiditis.[5,141]

Patients with chronic autoimmune thyroiditis would be expected to have high serum Tg concentrations because of the chronic thyroid inflammation characteristic of this condition.[125] However, virtually all these patients have TgAb, so their serum Tg concentrations are not known. The undetectable serum Tg values recently found in some patients with chronic autoimmune thyroiditis who had no detectable TgAb may reflect underestimates of serum Tg caused by interference in the serum Tg assay by TgAb that were not detected by the TgAb method used[5] (Fig 20-1, panel E).

Thyroid Carcinoma

Tg is present in most differentiated thyroid carcinomas and some anaplastic thyroid carcinomas.[144,145] Immunostaining of tissue for Tg is a useful histologic probe for identifying metastases of thyroid carcinoma and for identifying neck masses as being of thyroid origin.[146,147] The Tg content of thyroid tumor tissue correlates poorly with serum Tg concentrations in patients with thyroid carcinoma.[144,146] Preoperatively, the diagnostic or prognostic value of serum Tg measurement is limited because the concentration may be increased in patients with either benign or malignant thyroid disease (see Table 20-1). Furthermore, a normal serum Tg value does not exclude carcinoma in any patient with thyroid nodular disease.

Among patients with thyroid carcinoma, serum Tg concentrations are usually higher in those with follicular carcinoma than in those with papillary carcinoma, probably because follicular carcinomas are more advanced at the time of diagnosis rather than because of any intrinsic differences between the two tumor types. Among patients with proven differentiated thyroid carcinoma, preoperative serum Tg concentrations are correlated positively with tumor mass.[11,144] A low preoperative serum Tg value in a patient with a large tumor burden suggests less tumor differentiation and predicts a poorer correlation between serum Tg values and tumor mass later on. Furthermore, the difference between pre- and postoperative serum Tg values is an indicator of the completeness of surgery.

Postoperatively, serum Tg measurements are most useful for detecting persistent or recurrent thyroid carcinoma in patients who have no remaining normal thyroid tissue.[57] In this setting, both serum Tg measurements and radioiodine imaging (see chap 17) are used for staging and long-term monitoring[148] (see chap 80, section on radioiodine and other traetments and outcomes). Periodic radioiodine imaging is inconvenient and costly, and serum Tg measurements have replaced or at least greatly reduced the need for imaging.[149] The combined use of serum Tg measurements and radioiodine imaging increases overall diagnostic sensitivity and specificity over either procedure alone, but the advantage of combined testing is very small.[54,55] With respect to testing protocol, exogenous thyroid therapy must be discontinued before radioiodine imaging. With respect to serum Tg measurements, the sensitivity for detecting thyroid tissue, particularly tumor, is increased to only a small degree after thyroid hormone therapy is discontinued.[53,54,57]

The relationship between basal and TSH-stimulated serum Tg concentrations may become a useful test for detecting the absence of any thyroid tissue and also providing information on the TSH sensitivity of any thyroid carcinoma

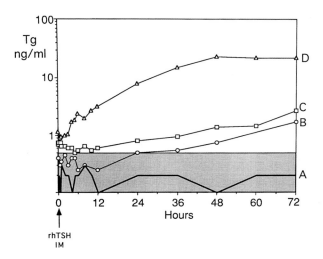

FIGURE 20-2. Patterns of changes in serum Tg concentrations in response to intramuscular administration of recombinant human TSH (rhTSH) in patients with thyroid carcinoma. Patient A: no response, suggesting the patient has no thyroid tissue; patient B: undetectable basal serum Tg concentration and minimal response to rhTSH, suggesting the presence of a small amount of thyroid tissue too small to be detected by radioiodine imaging; patient C: detectable basal serum Tg with minimal response to rhTSH, suggesting the presence of a poorly differentiated tumor with lower clinical efficacy for TSH suppression therapy; and patient D: detectable basal serum Tg with substantial response to rhTSH, suggesting the presence of TSH-responsive thyroid tissue.

tissue.[72] Patients who are athyreotic, as judged by no serum Tg response to TSH (Patient A, Fig 20-2), will likely need only T_4 replacement and not suppression therapy. Those with a low basal serum Tg concentration and a minimal response to TSH (Patient B) would probably have only a small amount of thyroid tissue unlikely to be detected by radioiodine imaging. A detectable basal serum Tg concentration but a poor response to TSH (Patient C) would suggest the presence of a poorly differentiated tumor with lower clinical efficacy for TSH suppression therapy. In contrast, a detectable basal serum Tg concentration associated with a substantial response to TSH (Patient D) would suggest the presence of a remnant of normal thyroid tissue or of some well-differentiated carcinoma tissue that will respond to TSH suppression.

Studies comparing the sensitivity of measurements of serum Tg and radioiodine imaging for detecting persistent or recurrent thyroid carcinoma are complicated by differences in TSH secretory status, imaging technique, and disparities between serum Tg assay methods.[4] Serum Tg values, ranging from 5 to 30 ng/mL have been chosen to classify patients as not having or having thyroid carcinoma after initial treatment.[54–57] Serum Tg should be undetectable, even during TSH stimulation, if successful treatment has rendered a patient athyreotic. The number of false-negative serum Tg values is increased by selecting a higher serum Tg cut-off value, because patients with some remaining thyroid tissue who may be at risk for late recurrence may be classified as being disease-free.[150] The combination of a detectable serum Tg value with a negative whole-body radioiodine scan is the most common discordance encountered in follow-up of patients with thyroid carcinoma.[56] This set of results usually occurs because the radioiodine scan is falsely negative rather than the serum

Tg value being falsely positive.[150] Discordance characterized by an undetectable serum Tg value and a positive radioiodine scan is infrequent[151]; this discordance may reflect a false-negative serum Tg value due to assay insensitivity, the selection of a high cut-off value, or an underestimation of serum Tg as a result of TgAb interference.[5] A false-negative serum Tg value also can occur if a tumor secretes a conformationally abnormal Tg molecule that is not detected in the Tg assay used.[33]

References

1. Mariotti S, Chiovato L, Vitti P, et al. Recent advances in the understanding of humoral and cellular mechanisms implicated in thyroid autoimmune disorders. Immunopathol 1989;50:S73
2. Heinze HJ, Shulman DI, Diamond FB, Bercu BB. Spectrum of serum thyroglobulin elevation in congenital thyroid disorders. Thyroid 1993;3:37
3. Baskin HJ. Effect of postoperative ^{131}I treatment on thyroglobulin measurements in the follow-up of patients with thyroid cancer. Thyroid 1994;4:239
4. Feldt-Rasmussen U, Schlumberger M. European interlaboratory comparison of serum thyroglobulin measurement. J Endocrinol Invest 1988;11:175
5. Mariotti S, Barbesino G, Caturegli P, et al. Assay of thyroglobulin in serum with thyroglobulin autoantibodies: an unobtainable goal? J Clin Endocrinol Metab 1995;80:468
6. Spencer CA, Takeuchi M, Kazarosyan M. Current status and performance goals for thyroglobulin (Tg) assays. Clin Chem, 1996. In press
7. Feldt-Rasmussen U, Profilis C, Colinet E, Schlumberger M, Black E. Purification and assessment of stability and homogeneity of human thyroglobulin reference material (CRM 457). Exp Clin Endocrinol 1994;102:87
8. Date J, Blichert-Toft M, Feldt-Rasmussen U, Haas V. Lacking evidence for release of thyroid hormones from circulating thyroglobulin during subtotal thyroidectomy. Acta Endocrinol 1988; 117:219
9. Berghout A, Wiersinga WM, Smits NJ, Touber JL. Interrelationships between age, thyroid volume, thyroid nodularity, and thyroid function in patients with sporadic nontoxic goiter. Am J Med 1990;89:602
10. Vassart G, Dumont J. The thyrotropin receptor and the regulation of thyrocyte function and growth. Endocr Rev 1992;13:596
11. Schlumberger M. Follow-up of patients with differentiated thyroid cancer. In: Johnson JT, Didolkar MS, eds. Head and Neck Cancer. Amsterdam: Elsevier Science Publishers BV, 1993:903
12. Edelhoch H. The structure of thyroglobulin and its role in iodination. Recent Prog Horm Res 1965;21:1
13. Van Herle AJ, Vassart G, Dumont JE. Control of thyroglobulin synthesis and secretion. (Second of two parts). N Engl J Med 1979;301:307
14. Baas F, Bikker H, Van Geurts KA, et al. The human thyroglobulin gene: A polymorphic marker localized distal to c-myc on chromosome 8 band q 24. Hum Genet 1985;69:138
15. Malthiery Y, Marriq C, Berge-Lefranc J, et al. Thyroglobulin structure and function. Biochimie 1989;71:195
16. Kung AW, Lau KS. Interleukin-1 beta modulates thyrotropin-induced thyroglobulin mRNA transcription through 3',5'-cyclic adenosine monophosphate. Endocrinology 1990;127:1369
17. Kung AW, Lau KS. Interferon-gamma inhibits thyrotropin-induced thyroglobulin gene transcription in cultured thyroid thyrocytes. J Clin Endocrinol Metab 1990;70:1512
18. Santisteban P, Acebron A, Schwarz MP, Di Lauro R. Insulin and insulin-like growth factor 1 regulate a thyroid-specific nuclear protein that binds to the thyroglobulin promoter. Mol Endocrinol 1992;6:1310

19. Namba H, Yamashita S, Morita S, et al. Retinoic acid inhibits human thyroid peroxidase and thyroglobulin gene expression. J Endocrinol Invest 1993;16:87

20. Farid NR, Shi YH, Zou M. Molecular basis of thyroid cancer. Endocr Rev 1994;15:202

21. Tang KT, Braverman LE, DeVito WJ. Tumor necrosis factor-alpha and interferon-gamma modulate gene expression of type I 5′-deiodinase, thyroid peroxidase, and thyroglobulin in FRTL-5 rat thyroid cells. Endocrinology 1995;136:881

22. Ring P, Bjorkmann U, Ekholm R. Localization of the incorporation of 3H-sialic acid into thyroglobulin in relation to the block of intracellular transport induced by monensin. Studies with isolated procine thyroid follicles. Cell Tissue Res 1987;250:149

23. Kim PS, Arvan P. Folding and assembly of newly synthesized thyroglobulin occurs in a pre-Golgi compartment. J Biol Chem 1991;266:12412

24. Zimmer KP, Hengst K, Carayon P, Bramswig J, Harms E. Different concentrations of thyroid peroxidase and thyroglobulin in the nuclear envelope and the endoplasmic reticulum throughout the cytoplasm. Eur J Cell Biol 1992;57:12

25. Takamatsu J, Hosoya T, Tsuji M, et al. Peroxidase and coupling activities of thyroid peroxidase in benign and malignant thyroid tumor tissues. Thyroid 1992;2:193

26. Bertaux F, Noel M, Malthiery Y, Fragu P. Demonstration of a heterogeneous transcription pattern of thyroglobulin mRNA in human thyroid tissues. Biochem Biophys Res Commun 1991; 178:586

27. Kiso Y, Furmaniak J, Morteo C, Smith BR. Analysis of carbohydrate residues on human thyroid peroxidase (TPO) and thyroglobulin (Tg) and effects of deglycosylation, reduction and unfolding on autoantibody binding. Autoimmunity 1992;12:259

28. Kumar A, Shah DH, Thakare UR. Biochemical characterization of serum thyroglobulin from patients with bone metastases from follicular carcinoma of the thyroid. Indian J Biochem Biophys 1991;28:198

29. Sinadinovic J, Cvejic D, Savin S, Jancic-Zuguricas M, Micic JV. Altered terminal glycosylation of thyroglobulin in papillary thyroid carcinoma. Exp Clin Endocrinol 1992;100:124

30. Gardas A, Domek H. Iodine induced alteration in immunological and biochemical properties of thyroglobulin. Am J Physiol 1993; 265:237

31. Saboori AM, Rose NR, Kuppers RC, Butscher WG, Bresler HS Burek CL. Immunoreactivity of multiple molecular forms of human thyroglobulin. Clin Immunol Immunopathol 1994;72:121

32. Sugawa H, Smith E, Imura H, Mori T. A thyroid cancer specific monoclonal antibody which recognizes cryptic epitope(s) of human thyroglobulin. Mol Cell Endocrinol 1993;93:207

33. Schulz R, Bethauser H, Stempka L, Heilig B, Moll A, Hufner M. Evidence for immunological differences between circulating and tissue-derived thyroglobulin in men. Eur J Clin Invest 1989; 19:459

34. Hufner M, Kiehne B, Stempka L, Bethauser H, Schulz R. Description of a variably expressed and labile epitope of thyroglobulin and its occurrence in different thyroid diseases using a monoclonal antibody. Clin Physiol Biochem 1992;9:35

35. Narkar AA, Shah DH, Yadav J, Swaroop D, Mulherkar R. Monoclonal antibodies to human thyroglobulin: evaluation of immunoreactivity. Hybridoma 1992;11:803

36. Bernier-Valentin F, Kostrouch Z, Rabilloud R, Rousset B. Analysis of the thyroglobulin internalization process using in vitro reconstituted thyroid follicles: evidence for a coated vesicle-dependent endocytic pathway. Endocrinology 1991;129:2194

37. Kostrouch Z, Munari-Silem Y, Rajas F, Bernier-Valentin F, Rousset B. Thyroglobulin internalized by thyrocytes passes through early and late endosomes. Endocrinology 1991;129:2202

38. Dunn AD, Crutchfield HE, Dunn JT. Proteolytic processing of thyroglobulin by extracts of thyroid lysosomes. Endocrinol 1991;128:3073

39. Daniel PM, Pratt OE, Roitt IM, Torrigiani G. The release of thyroglobulin from the thyroid gland into thyroid lymphatics; the identification of thyroglobulin in the thyroid lymph and in the blood of monkeys by physical and immunological methods and its estimation by radioimmunoassay. Immunology 1967;12:489

40. Gebel F, Studer H. Malignant follicles of a differentiated thyroid carcinoma releasing iodinated thyroglobulin into the lymphatic vessels. Clin Endocrinol 1984;20:457

41. Monaco F, Napolitano G, Lio S, Roche J. Existe-t-il une double voie de secretion de la thyroglobuline: un ″circuit court″ faiblement glycosylo-iode et un ″circuit long″ fortement glycoysloiode. CR Seances Soc Biol Fil 1989;183:108

42. Schneider A, Ikekubo K, Kuma K. Iodine content of serum thyroglobulin in normal individuals and patients with thyroid cancer. J Clin Endocrinol Metab 1983;57:1251

43. Ikekubo K, Pervos R, Schneider AB. Clearance of normal and tumor-related thyroglobulin from the circulation of rats: Role of the terminal sialic acid residues. Metabolism 1980;29:673

44. Ashwell G, Morell AG. The role of surface carbohydrates in the hepatic recognition and transport of circulating glycoproteins. Adv Enzymol 1974;41:99

45. Ludwig H, Schernthaner G, Richter E, Zambelis N, Wick G. Thyroglobulin binding cells: a diagnostic marker of Hashimoto's thyroiditis. Acta Endocrinol [Suppl] 1978;215:78

46. Izumi M, Kubo I, Taura M, et al. Kinetic study of immunoreactive human thyroglobulin. J Clin Endocrinol Metab 1986;62:410

47. Lo Gerfo P, Colacchio T, Colacchio D, Feind C. Serum clearance rates of immunologically reactive thyroglobulin. Cancer 1978; 42:164

48. Feldt-Rasmussen U, Petersen PH, Date J, Madsen CM. Serum thyroglobulin in patients undergoing subtotal thyroidectomy for toxic and nontoxic goiter. J Endocrinol Invest 1982;5:161

49. Feldt-Rasmussen U, Petersen PH, Nielsen H, Date J. Thyroglobulin of varying molecular sizes with different disappearance rates in plasma following subtotal thyroidectomy. Clin Endocrinol 1978;9:205

50. Weigle WO High GJ. The behaviour of autologous thyroglobulin in the circulation of rabbits immunized with either heterologous or altered homologous thyroglobulin. J Immunol 1967; 98:1105

51. Feldt-Rasmussen U, Petersen PH, Date J, Madsen CM. Sequential changes in serum thyroglobulin (Tg) and its autoantibodies (TgAb) following subtotal thyroidectomy of patients with preoperatively detectable TgAb. Clin Endocrinol 1980;12:29

52. Preissner CM, Klee GG, Krco CJ. Nonisotopic "sandwich" immunoassay of thyroglobulin in serum by the biotin-streptavidin technique: evaluation and comparison with an immunoradiometric assay. Clin Chem 1988;34:1784

53. Schlumberger M, Fragu P, Gardet P, Lumbroso J, Violot D, Parmentier C. A new immunoradiometric assay (IRMA) system for thyroglobulin measurement in the follow-up of thyroid cancer patients. Eur J Nucl Med 1991;18:153

54. Ronga G, Fiorentino A, Paserio E, et al. Can iodine-131 whole-body scan be replaced by thyroglobulin measurement in the post-surgical follow-up of differentiated thyroid carcinoma? J Nucl Med 1990;31:1766

55. Dadparvar S, Krishna L, Brady LW, et al. The role of iodine-131 and thallium-201 imaging and serum thyroglobulin in the management of differentiated thyroid cancer. Cancer 1993;71:3767

56. Lubin E, Mechlis-Frish S, Zatz S, et al. Serum thyroglobulin and iodine-131 whole-body scan in the diagnosis and assessment of treatment for metastatic differentiated thyroid carcinoma. J Nucl Med 1994;35:257

57. Ozata M, Suzuki S, Miyamoto T, Liu RT, Fierro-Renoy F, DeGroot LJ. Serum thyroglobulin in the follow-up of patients with treated differentiated thyroid cancer. J Clin Endocrinol Metab 1994;79:98

58. Feldt-Rasmussen U, Rasmussen AK. Serum thyroglobulin (Tg) in presence of thyroglobulin autoantibodies (TgAb). Clinical and methodological relevance of the interaction between Tg and TgAb in vitro and in vivo. J Endocrinol Invest 1985;8:571

59. Schneider AB, Pervos R. Radioimmunoassay of human thyroglobulin: Effect of antithyroglobulin autoantibodies. J Clin Endocrinol Metab 1978;47:126

60. Bayer M, Kriss JP. A solid phase, sandwich-type radioimmunoassay for antithyroglobulin: Elimination of false positive results and semiquantitative measurement of antithyroglobulin in the presence of elevated thyroglobulin. J Clin Endocrinol Metab 1979;49:565

61. Tamaki H, Katsumaru H, Amino N, Nakamoto H, Ishikawa E, Miyai K. Usefulness of thyroglobulin antibody detected by ultrasensitive enzyme immunoassay: a good parameter for immune surveillance in healthy subjects and for prediction of post-partum thyroid dysfunction. Clin Endocrinol 1992;37:266

62. Bouanani M, Dietrich G, Hurez V, et al. Age-related changes in specificity of human natural autoantibodies to thyroglobulin. J Autoimmunity 1993;6:639

63. Tamaki H, Amino N, Iwatani Y, Matsuzuka F, Kuma K, Miyai K. Detection of thyroid microsomal and thyroglobulin antibodies by new sensitive radioimmunoassay in Hashimoto's disease: Comparison with conventional hemagglutination. Endocrinol Jpn 1991;38:97

64. Ligabue A, Poggioli MC, Zacchini A. Interference of specific autoantibodies in the assessment of serum thyroglobulin. J Nucl Biol Med 1993;37:273

65. Piechaczyk M, Bouanani M, Salhi SL, et al. Antigenic domains on the human thyroglobulin molecule recognized by autoantibodies in patient's sera and by natural autoantibodies isolated from the sera of healthy subjects. Clin Immunol Immunopathol 1987;45:114

66. Bouanani M, Piechaczyk M, Pau B, Bastide M. Significance of the recognition of certain antigenic regions on the human thyroglobulin molecule by natural autoantibodies from healthy subjects. J Immunol 1989;143:1129

67. Fulthorpe AN, Roitt IM, Doniach D, Couchman K. A stable sheep cell preparation for detecting thyroglobulin autoantibodies and its clinical application. J Clin Pathol 1961;16:654

68. College of American Pathologists. 1990 CAP Surveys. Diagnostic Immunology Series 2, Survey, Set S-A. College of American Pathologists, 1990

69. Ericsson UB, Christensen SB, Thorell JI. A high prevalence of thyroglobulin autoantibodies in adults with and without thyroid disease as measured with a sensitive solid-phase immunosorbent radioassay. Clin Immunol Immunopathol 1985;37:154

70. Black EG, Hoffenberg R. Should one measure serum thyroglobulin in the presence of anti-thyroglobulin antibodies? Clin Endocrinol 1983;19:597

71. Aiello DP, Manni A. Thyroglobulin measurement vs iodine 131 total-body scan for follow-up of well-differentiated thyroid cancer. Arch Intern Med 1990;150:437

72. Meier C, Braverman L, Ebner S, et al. Diagnostic use of recombinant human thyrotropin in patients with thyroid carcinoma (phase I/II study). J Clin Endocrinol Metab 1994;78:188

73. Prentice LM, Phillips DIW, Sarsero D, Beever K, McLachlan S, Rees-Smith B. Geographical distribution of subclinical autoimmune thyroid disease in Britain: a study using highly sensitive direct assays for autoantibodies to thyroglobulin and thyroid peroxidase. Acta Endocrinol 1990;123:493

74. Piechaczyk M, Baldet L, Pau B, Bastide JM. Novel immunoradiometric assay of thyroglobulin in serum with use of monoclonal antibodies selected for lack of cross-reactivity with autoantibodies. Clin Chem 1989;35:422

75. Ruf J, Carayon P Lissitzky S. Various expressions of a unique anti-human thyroglobulin antibody repertoire in normal state and autoimmune disease. Eur J Immunol 1985;15:268

76. Van Herle AJ, Klandorf H, Uller RP. A radioimmunoassay for serum rat thyroglobulin. Physiologic and pharmacologic studies. J Clin Invest 1975;56:1073

77. Feldt-Rasmussen U, Hegedus L, Perrild H, Rasmussen N, Hansen JM. Relationship between serum thyroglobulin, thyroid volume and serum TSH in healthy non-goitrous subjects and the relationship to seasonal variations in iodine intake. Thyroidology 1989;3:115

78. Premawardhana LDKE, Phillips dIW, Prentice LM, Smith BR. Variability of serum thyroglobulin levels is determined by a major gene. Clin Endocrinol 1994;41:725

79. Feldt-Rasmussen U, Petersen PH, Blaabjerg O, Horder M. Long-term variability in serum thyroglobulin and thyroid related hormones in healthy subjects. Acta Endocrinol 1980;95:328

80. Rasmussen NG, Hornnes PJ, Hegedus L, Feldt-Rasmussen U. Serum thyroglobulin during the menstrual cycle, during pregnancy, and post partum. Acta Endocrinol 1989;121:168

81. Glinoer D, De Nayer P, Bourdoux P, et al. Regulation of maternal thyroid during pregnancy. J Clin Endocrinol Metab 1990;71:276

82. Bayraktar M, Ergin M, Boyacioglu A, Demir S. A preliminary report of thyroglobulin release after fine needle aspiration biopsy of thyroid nodules. J Int Med Res 1990;18:253

83. Djurica S, Djordjevic DJ, Sinadinovic J. Long-term follow up of serum thyroglobulin levels and its clinical implications in subjects after surgical removal of "cold" thyroid nodule. Exp Clin Endocrinol 1992;99:137

84. Tegler L, Ericsson UB, Gillquist J, Lindvall R. Basal and thyrotropin-stimulated secretion rates of thyroglobulin from the human thyroid gland during surgery. Thyroid 1993;3:213

85. Kawamura S, Kishino B, Tajima K, Mashita K, Tarui S. Elevated serum thyroglobulin as a manifestation of acute haemorrhage into the thyroid gland. Clin Endocrinol 1984;20:213

86. Van Herle AJ, Demeester-Mirkine N, Van Heuverswyn B, Dumont J. The effect of 131-I for diagnostic purposes on serum thyroglobulin (hTg) levels in subjects with thyroid disorders. J Endocrinol Invest 1981;4:107

87. Schlumberger M, Sebagh M, De Vathaire F, Bayle C, Fragu P, Parmentier C. Thyroid iodine content and serum thyroglobulin level following external irradiation to the neck for Hodgkin's disease. J Endocrinol Invest 1990;13:197

88. Madeddu G, Casu AR, Costanza C, et al. Serum thyroglobulin levels in the diagnosis and follow-up of subacute 'painful' thyroiditis. Arch Intern Med 1985;145:243

89. Kraiem Z, Sadeh O, Blithe DL, Nisula BC. Human chorionic gonadotropin stimulates thyroid hormone secretion, iodide uptake, organification, and adenosine $3',5'$-monophosphate formation in cultured human thyrocytes. J Clin Endocrinol Metab 1994;79:595

90. Filetti S, Belfiore A, Amir SM, et al. The role of thyroid stimulating antibodies of Graves' disease in differentiated thyroid cancer. N Engl J Med 1988;318:753

91. Hershman JM, Due DT, Sharp B, et al. Endemic goiter in Vietnam. J Clin Endocrinol Metab 1983;57:243

92. Unger J. Fasting induces a decrease in serum thyroglobulin in normal subjects. J Clin Endocrinol Metab 1988;67:1309

93. Namba H, Yamashita S, Kimura H, et al. Evidence of thyroid volume increase in normal subjects receiving excess iodide. J Clin Endocrinol Metab 1993;76:605

94. Bertelsen JB, Hegedus L. Cigarette smoking and the thyroid. Thyroid 1994;4:327

95. Hegedus L, Karstrup S, Veirang D, Jacobsen B, Skovsted L, Feldt-Rasmussen U. High frequency of goitre in cigarette smokers. Clin Endocrinol 1985;22:287

96. Fukayama H, Nasu M, Murakami S, Sugawara M. Examination of antithyroid effects of smoking products in cultured thyroid follicles: only thiocyanate is a potent antithyroid agent. Acta Endocrinol 1992;127:520

97. Feldt-Rasmussen U, Petersen PH, Date J. Sex and age-correlated reference values of serum thyroglobulin measured by a modified radioimmunoassay. Acta Endocrinol 1979;90:440

98. Feldt-Rasmussen U, Bech K, Date J. Serum thyroglobulin in patients with toxic and non-toxic goitres compared to sex- and age-matched control subjects. Acta Endocrinol 1979;91:264

99. Kuo SW, Hu CA, Pei D, Ni KB, Shian LR. Efficacy of thyroxine-suppressive therapy and its relation to serum thyroglobulin levels in solitary nontoxic thyroid nodules. J Formos Med Assoc 1993;92:55

100. Begeot M, Dupouy JP, Dubois MP, Dubois PM. Immunocytological determination of gonadotropic and thyreotropic cells in fetal rat anterior pituitary during normal development and under experimental conditions. Neuroendocrinology 1981;32:285

101. Rodriguez M, Santisteban P, Acebron A, Hernandez LC, Del Valle M, Jolin T. Expression of thyroglobulin gene in maternal and fetal thyroid in rats. Endocrinology 1992;131:415

102. Fisher DA. Maternal-fetal function in pregnancy. Clin Perinatol 1983;10:615

103. Hashimoto H, Sato T, Horita S, Kubo M, Ohki T. Maturation of the pituitary-thyroid axis during the perinatal period. Endocrinol Jpn 1991;38:151

104. Glinoer D, Delange F, Laboureur I, et al. Maternal and neonatal thyroid function at birth in an area of marginally low iodine intake. J Clin Endocrinol Metab 1992;75:800

105. Sava L, Tomaselli L, Runello F, Belfiore A, Vigneri R. Serum thyroglobulin levels are elevated in newborns from iodine-deficient areas. J Clin Endocrinol Metab 1986;62:429

106. Lamas L, Ingbar SH. The effect of varying iodine content on the susceptability of thyroglobulin to hydrolysis by thyroid acid protease. Endocrinology 1978;102:199

107. Pezzino V, Filetti S, Belfiore A, Proto S, Donzelli G, Vigneri R. Serum thyroglobulin levels in the newborn. J Clin Endocrinol Metab 1981;52:364

108. Chanoine JP, Toppet V, Bourdoux P, Spehl M, Delange F. Smoking during pregnancy: a significant cause of neonatal thyroid enlargement. Br J Obstet Gynaecol 1991;98:65

109. Fisher DA. Management of congenital hypothyroidism. J Clin Endocrinol Metab 1991;72:523

110. Ilicki A, Ericsson UB, Larsson A, Mortensson W, Thorell J. The value of neonatal serum thyroglobulin determinations in the follow-up of patients with congenital hypothyroidism. Acta Paediatr Scand 1990;79:769

111. Vulsma T, Rammeloo JA, Gons MH, de Vijlder JJM. The role of serum thyroglobulin concentration and thyroid ultrasound imaging in the detection of iodide transport defects in infants. Acta Endocrinol 1991;124:405

112. Refetoff S, Weiss RE, Usala SJ. The syndromes of resistance to thyroid hormone. Endocr Rev 1993;14:348

113. Black EG, Bodden SJ, Hulse JA, Hoffenberg R. Serum thyroglobulin in normal and hypothyroid neonates. Clin Endocrinol 1982;16:267

114. Ket JL, De Vijlder JJM, Bikker H, Gons MH, Tegelaers WHH. Serum thyroglobulin levels: The physiological decrease in infancy and the absence in athyroidism. J Clin Endocrinol Metab 1981;53:1301

115. Penny R, Spencer CA, Frasier SD, Nicoloff JT. Thyroid-stimulating hormone and thyroglobulin levels decrease with chronological age in children and adolescents. J Clin Endocrinol Metab 1983;56:177

116. Gardner DF, Rothman J, Utiger RD. Serum thyroglobulin in normal subjects and patients with hyperthyroidism due to Graves' disease: effects of T_3, iodide, ^{131}I and antithyroid drugs. Clin Endocrinol 1979;11:585

117. Uller RP, Van Herle AJ. Effect of therapy on serum thyroglobulin levels in patients with Graves' disease. J Clin Endocrinol Metab 1978;46:747

118. Aizawa T, Ishihara M, Koizumi Y, et al. Serum thyroglobulin concentration as an indicator for assessing thyroid stimulation in patients with Graves' disease during antithyroid drug therapy. Am J Med 1990;89:175

119. Talbot JN, Duron F, Feron R, Aubert P, Mihaud G. Thyroglobulin, thyrotropin and thyrotropin binding inhibiting immunoglobulins assayed at the withdrawal of antithyroid drug therapy as predictors of relapse of Graves' disease within one year. J Endocrinol Invest 1989;12:589

120. Werner RS, Romaldini JH, Farah CS, Werner MC, Bromberg N. Serum thyroid-stimulating antibody, thyroglobulin levels, and thyroid suppressibility measurement as predictors of the outcome of combined methimazole and triiodothyronine therapy in Graves' disease. Thyroid 1991;1:293

121. Madeddu G, Casu AR, Marrosu A, Marras G, Langer M. Serum thyroglobulin in patients with autonomous thyroid nodules. Clin Endocrinol 1984;21:377

122. Dorey F, Strauch G, Gayno JP. Thyrotoxicosis due to pituitary resistance to thyroid hormones, successful control with D-thyroxine: a study in three patients. Clin Endocrinol 1990;32:221

123. Cohen JH, Ingbar SH, Braverman LE. Thyrotoxicosis due to ingestion of excess thyroid hormone. Endocr Rev 1989;10:113

124. Martino E, Aghini-Lombardi F, Mariotti S, Bartalena L, Braverman L, Pinchera A. Amiodarone: a common source of iodine-induced thyrotoxicosis. Horm Res 1987;26:158

125. Singer PA. Thyroiditis, acute, subacute and chronic. Med Clin North Am 1991;75:61

126. Targovnik HM, Varela V, Juvenai GJ, et al. Differential levels of thyroid peroxidase and thyroglobulin messenger ribonucleic acids in congenital goiter with defective thyroglobulin synthesis. J Endocrinol Invest 1990;13:797

127. Grollman EF, Doi SQ, Weiss P, Ashwell G, Wajchenberg BL, Medeiros-Neto G. Hyposialated thyroglobulin in a patient with congenital goiter and hypothyroidism. J Clin Endocrinol Metab 1992;74:43

128. Ohyama Y, Hosoya T, Kameya T, et al. Congenital euthyroid goitre with impaired thyroglobulin transport. Clin Endocrinol 1994;41:129

129. Medeiros-Neto G, Targovnik HM, Vassart G. Defective thyroglobulin synthesis and secretion causing goiter and hypothyroidism. Endocr Rev 1993;14:165

130. Medeiros-Neto GA, Marcondes JA, Cavaliere H, Wajchenberg BL, Knobel M. Serum thyroglobulin (Tg) stimulation with bovine TSH: a useful test for diagnosis of congenital goitrous hypothyroidism due to defective Tg synthesis. Acta Endocrinol 1985; 110:61

131. Ongphiphadhanakul B, Rajatanavin R, Chiemchanya S, Chailurkit L, Kongsuksai A, Ayuthya WIN. Systematic inclusion of clinical and laboratory data improves diagnostic accuracy of fine-needle aspiration biopsy in solitary nodules. Acta Endocrinol 1992;126:233

132. Schneider AB, Shore-Freedman E, Ryo UY, Bekerman C, Pinsky SM. Prospective serum thyroglobulin measurements in assessing the risk of developing thyroid nodules in patients exposed to childhood neck irradiation. J Clin Endocrinol Metab 1985;61:547

133. Gebel F, Ramelli G, Burgi U, Ingold U, Studer H, Winand R. The site of leakage of intra follicular thyroglobulin into the blood stream in simple human goiter. J Clin Endocrinol Metab 1983;57:915

134. Mories T, Miralles JM, Reglero A, Felipe S, Corrales JJ, Garcia LC. A study of thyroglobulin and peroxidase activity in the thyroid tissue of patients with non-endemic non-toxic nodular goitre. Clin Sci 1991;80:301

135. Pezzino V, Vigneri R, Squatrito S, Filetti S, Camus M, Polosa P. Increased serum thyroglobulin levels in patients with nontoxic goiter. J Clin Endocrinol Metab 1978;46:653

136. Unger J, De Maertelaer V, Golstein J, Decoster C, Jonckheer MH. Relationship between serum thyroglobulin and intrathyroidal stable iodine in human simple goiter. Clin Endocrinol 1985;23:1

137. Djurica SN, Cirovic M, Tasovac-Ponomarev D. Serum thyroglobulin level in patients with diffuse and nodular goiter after therapeutic application of stable iodine. Exp Clin Endocrinol 1992; 99:21

138. Woolf PD. Transient painless thyroiditis with hyperthyroidism: a variant of lymphocytic thyroiditis? Endocr Rev 1980;1:411

139. Yamamoto M, Saito S, Sakurda T, et al. Effect of prednisolone and salicylate on serum thyroglobulin level in patients with subacute thyroiditis. Clin Endocrinol 1987;27:339

140. Hidaka Y, Nishi I, Tamaki T, et al. Differentiation of postpartum thyrotoxicosis by serum thyroglobulin: usefulness of a new multisite immunoradiometric assay. Thyroid 1994;4:275

141. Parkes AB, Black EG, Adams H, et al. Serum thyroglobulin: an early indicator of autoimmune post-partum thyroiditis. Clin Endocrinol 1994;41:9

142. Fragu P, Rougier P, Schlumberger M, Tubiana M. Evolution of thyroid 127-I stores measured by x-ray fluorescence in subacute thyroiditis. J Clin Endocrinol Metab 1982;54:162

143. Smallridge RC, De Keyser FM, Van Herle AJ, Butkus NE, Wartofsky L. Thyroid iodine content and serum thyroglobulin: clues to the natural history of destruction-induced thyroiditis. J Clin Endocrinol Metab 1986;62:1213

144. Dralle H, Schwarzrock R, Lang W, et al. Comparison of histology and immunohistochemistry with thyroglobulin serum levels and radioiodine uptake in recurrences and metastases of differentiated thyroid carcinomas. Acta Endocrinol 1985; 108:504

145. Heldin NE, Westermark B. The molecular biology of the human anaplastic thyroid carcinoma cell. Thyroidology 1991;3:127

146. Harach HR, Franssila KO. Thyroglobulin immunostaining in follicular thyroid carcinoma: relationship to the degree of differentiation and cell type. Histopathology 1988;13:43

147. Pacini F, Fugazzola L, Lippi F, et al. Detection of thyroglobulin in fine needle aspirates of nonthyroidal neck masses: A clue to the diagnosis of metastatic differentiated thyroid cancer. J Clin Endocrinol Metab 1992;74:1401

148. Dulgeroff AJ, Hershman JM. Medical therapy for differentiated thyroid carcinoma. Endocr Rev 1994;15:500

149. Black EG, Sheppard MC, Hoffenberg R. Serial serum thyroglobulin measurements in the management of differentiated thyroid carcinoma. Clin Endocrinol 1987;27:115

150. Black EG, Sheppard MC. Serum thyroglobulin measurements in thyroid cancer: evaluation of 'false' positive results. Clin Endocrinol 1991;35:519

151. Grant S, Luttrell B, Reeve T, et al. Thyroglobulin may be undetectable in the serum of patients with metastatic disease secondary to differentiated thyroid carcinoma. Follow-up of differentiated thyroid cancer. Cancer 1984;54:1625

152. Labouvie ST, Schmidt KG, Reiser HH, Rothenbuchner G, Schmidt KJ. Serum thyroglobulin (hTg) in patients of an endemic goiter area. In: Labouvie ST, Schmidt KG, Reiser HH, Rothenbuchner G, Schmidt KJ, eds. Thyroglobulin and thyroglobulin antibodies in the follow-up of thyroid cancer and endemic goiter. Stuttgart-New York: Georg Thieme Verlag, 1987:85

Werner and Ingbar's The Thyroid, Seventh Edition,
edited by Lewis E. Braverman and Robert D. Utiger
Lippincott–Raven Publishers, Philadelphia, © 1996

21

Antibodies in Autoimmune Thyroid Disease

J. Maxwell McKenzie
Margita Zakarija

The spontaneous development of antibodies to antigenic components of the thyroid gland is a well-established feature of autoimmune thyroid disease (AITD) (Table 21-1). This phenomenon was first described in 1956[1] in a report showing the presence of antibody to thyroglobulin in the serum of some patients who had chronic autoimmune (Hashimoto's) thyroiditis (in this chapter the term Hashimoto's thyroiditis refers to both the atrophic and goitrous forms of chronic autoimmune thyroiditis). Since then many other thyroid-reactive antibodies have been identified and methods for their assay have proliferated.

This review will focus primarily on autoantibodies to thyroglobulin (Tg), thyroid peroxidase (TPO), and the thyrotropin (TSH) receptor (TSH-R). These proteins have been cloned and studied in great detail in recent years, leading to a large body of data relating to the mode of action and significance of their respective antibodies (TgAb, TPOAb, TRAb). Therefore, we shall cite only work of historic significance and only the most recent publications and reviews that contain pertinent references to the rest of the field. The complex mechanisms regulating the immune response to antigens and production of antibodies[2–6] are also beyond the scope of this presentation, except for some statements to aid in the understanding of data regarding antibodies in patients with AITD (see also the section on pathogenesis of Graves' disease in chaps 30 and 55).

Antibodies, in general, recognize protein antigens in their native conformation; that is, an antigenic determinant or epitope of the antigen encompasses 15 to 22 amino acid residues discontinuous in sequence but forming a contiguous surface on a folded protein.[7,8] A protein molecule may have several discontinuous epitopes and may therefore elicit several epitope-specific antibodies. If the antigen is an enzyme, binding of antibody to an epitope that includes a catalytic site would affect its biologic activity. Antibodies may also recognize short linear sequences on antigens, but these linear epitopes are usually not accessible to antibodies unless the protein is unfolded, that is, denatured. In this instance antigen binding to antibody will occur, such as on Western blots, but not with the native antigen in solution. Antibodies of this type can arise in vivo owing to antigen degradation and the exposure of otherwise cryptic peptide sequences.

Although studies of antigen-antibody interactions can provide insight into the structure-function relationships of the antigen and its immunogenic regions, the only precise method for defining a binding epitope is by x-ray diffraction analysis of crystals of complexes of antigen and Fab or Fv fragments of an antibody containing the antigen-combining region.[7,8] This has not yet been accomplished with antigens and their respective antibodies in AITD. Autoantibodies are usually polyclonal, that is, they are derived from many distinct B-cell clones. Only with single clone-derived antibodies can their individual binding characteristics[8] and molecular genetic origin[3] be defined. The hybridoma technique, used to generate monoclonal antibodies (mAb) from a polyclonal response in immunized mice,[9] was not very successful when applied to production of human mAb of IgG class.[10] A combinatorial library approach,[11,12] a new technique for production of recombinant monoclonal Fab fragments of antibodies, has been more successful.

Whereas the variable regions of antibodies determine their antigen specificity, the constant regions confer effector function.[13] For example, antibodies of IgG class, which includes the autoantibodies in AITD, and of specific subclass, can fix complement or participate in antibody-dependent cell-mediated cytotoxic reactions.[14] In addition, IgG is the most abundant immunoglobulin class in the serum; it freely diffuses

TABLE 21-1.
Autoantibodies Found in Patients With Autoimmune Thyroid Disease

Antibody	Method of Assay
Antithyroglobulin (TgAb)	Hemagglutination, agglutination, ELISA, RIA
Antithyroid peroxidase (TPOAb)	Hemagglutination, agglutination, ELISA, RIA
Anti-TSH receptor (TRAb)	
Thyroid-stimulating (TSAb) (mimics TSH action)	Human thyroid, FRTL-5 and CHO-TSH-R cells, in culture Receptor assay
Thyroid-blocking (TBAb) (blocks TSH binding and action)	Inhibition of TSH or TSAb effects in cultured cells Receptor assay
Anti-T$_4$ or -T$_3$	Binding of ^{125}I-T$_4$ or ^{125}I-T$_3$ to IgG in patient's serum
Anti-TSH	Binding of ^{125}I-TSH to IgG in patient's serum

ELISA, enzyme-linked immunoassay; RIA, radioimmunoassay; TRAb, TSH receptor antibodies; FRTL-5, a rat thyroid cell line; CHO-TSH-R, Chinese hamster ovary cells stably transfected with cloned human TSH receptor (TSH-R); IgG, immunoglobulin G. For other antibodies, see text.

to extravascular sites and is the only class transported across the placenta, but it does not cross the epithelial barrier.

This short preamble disregards the fact that a prerequisite for B-cell activation and antibody production is the contact with activated antigen-specific T helper (T$_H$) lymphocytes.[2] It is at the T-cell level that the break of self-tolerance leads to autoimmunity.[4,5]

ANTIBODIES TO THYROGLOBULIN

As noted above, antithyroglobulin antibodies (TgAb) were the first autoantibodies to be recognized in patients with AITD.[1] A hemagglutination technique was the most common procedure for their identification[15,16] until other, more sensitive methods, such as enzyme-linked immunoassay (ELISA)[17] and radioimmunoassay (RIA)[18] were developed. By whichever technique used for assessment of TgAb and TPOAb, the latter are found more often than the former (Fig 21-1); when both antibodies are present, the titer of TPOAb tends to be higher.[15,18] Consequently, in practical (cost-effective) terms, measurement of TPOAb alone is usually sufficient to confirm a diagnosis of AITD. An exception applies to patients with differentiated thyroid cancer, who may have TgAb.[19] These antibodies interfere with assays for Tg, thus limiting the value of measurements of serum Tg as a marker of tumor persistence or recurrence in these patients[20] (see chap 20) and therefore should be sought before serum Tg is measured.

TgAb are primarily of IgG class, without restriction to any particular subclass or light chain, and are poor activators of the complement cascade.[6,21–25] The inability of TgAb to fix complement cannot be explained by the skewness of their subclass distribution (i.e., over-representation of IgG4 and low representation of IgG3),[25] which is also found in complement-fixing TPOAb.[6] The difference may be due to the low density of the relevant epitopes on the large Tg molecule, which does not allow the binding of the first component of complement to widely spaced TgAb. Thus, without a defined biologic action, TgAb appear to have no pathogenetic importance.

Unlike TgAb in animals immunized with Tg,[26] spontaneously occurring TgAb recognize a restricted number of epitopes on conformationally intact Tg molecules.[27–29] The exact number of identified epitopes and qualitative differences in epitope recognition by TgAb from different groups of patients varies (summarized in references 6 and 28). Five human monoclonal TgAb, produced by a hybridoma technique, had even more restricted epitope reactivity[29]; they recognized only two slightly overlapping epitopes, with two of the antibodies binding to one epitope (type I) and three to the other (type II). Mixtures of type I and type II mAb were effective in inhibiting binding of Tg to TgAb in serum from patients with AITD and normal subjects; type II TgAb predominated in the patients with AITD and type I in the normal subjects.

A small proportion of TgAb also binds to TPO.[30] This is puzzling, because there are no sequence similarities between the two antigens.[31] Similar antibodies can be induced in mice by immunization with Tg but not TPO, thus leading to the assumption that the Tg-combining site is responsible for the dual specificity. However, recent data suggest that TPO may bind to a region (idiotope) on the surface of these TgAb and not to the combining site for Tg; similar data were obtained with mouse mAb with comparable epitope-specifity for human Tg.[32] The importance of these highly unusual TgAb is not known.

ANTIBODIES TO THYROID PEROXIDASE

Thyroid microsomal antigen, the original term for TPO,[33,34] is a component of the exocytotic vesicles in which newly synthesized Tg is transferred to the follicular lumen.[35] In this process, TPO fuses with the thyroid follicular cell membrane,[36] thus explaining the restriction of the antigen, as identified by immunofluorescence, to the apical (luminal) portion of the membrane in intact follicles.[37] The expression of TPO is under positive control by TSH,[38] an action that can be modified by some cytokines.[39]

Anti-TPO antibodies (TPOAb) were first recognized by complement fixation[40] and indirect immunofluorescence staining of unfixed sections of thyroid tissue.[41] Most clinical data, however, have been obtained using a hemagglutination assay technique[15,16] that is still in use,[42] despite being superseded by more sensitive and specific tests.[18,43–46] Continued use of the hemaglutination-agglutination procedures may be due to their lower cost and the fact that the results are closely correlated with those of other assays.[18,44,47] A comparison of TPOAb titers measured by an agglutination method and a RIA method is shown in Figure 21-1. Regardless of the technique used, TPOAb are present in the serum of almost all patients with Hashimoto's thyroiditis, in more than 70% of those with Graves' disease, and, to a variable degree, in patients with nonthyroid autoimmune diseases and some normal subjects. Although the highest titers of TPOAb are found in hypothyroid patients with Hashimoto's thyroiditis, they can also be present in euthyroid patients with Hashimoto's thyroiditis or Graves' disease,[15] that is, the titers do not correlate with thyroid functional status. Individual patients with either disorder may have decreases in TPOAb titers during therapy, but others have no change.[47] There are conflicting results as to the relationship between the outcome of patients with Graves' hyperthyroidism treated with an antithyroid drug and TPOAb; in one study, the relapse rate was lower in those patients who had TPOAb (and TgAb) when therapy was discontinued,[48] but it was higher in another study.[49] On the other hand, there is a good correlation between the degree of lymphocytic infiltration of the thyroid gland and the presence or titer of TPOAb.[50–52] These studies clearly establish TPOAb as a marker of AITD but do not define their role as a pathogenetic agent.

The recognition that the microsomal antigen is TPO[33,34] led to testing the effect of TPOAb on the catalytic activity of the enzyme, with conflicting results. The findings varied from no inhibition of TPO activity at all with TPOAb-positive serum samples[53–55] and with 45 human monoclonal TPOAb,[55,56] to an inhibitory effect that did[57,58] or did not[59,60] correlate with TPOAb titers. The IgG subclass distribution of TPOAb, important for the effector function of antibodies,[13] was a subject of numerous studies (summarized in reference 61). The differences in the results—restriction or predominance of TPOAb in IgG1 and IgG4 or no subclass restriction but over-representation of IgG4 in relation to its concentration in serum—have been blamed on the peculiarities of the reagents used in the different studies and in assaying whole serum vs. affinity-purified subclass fractions.[61] There was also no restriction of light chains in any of the subclasses, with 79% of overall TPOAb activity associated with κ light chain, a value close to the normal $\kappa{:}\lambda$ ratio of approximately 70:30. The relative functional affinity was the highest in the IgG2 and lowest in the IgG4 fractions.[61] These findings confirm early results on the polyclonal nature of TPOAb, but the quantitative and qualitative prominence of the IgG2 antibodies makes them less important participants in cytotoxic reactions.

The search for binding epitopes on TPO and qualitative differences in TPOAb that might have pathogenetic or prognostic significance in AITD has led to a large body of literature and some controversies (summarized in references 38, 56, and 62). Even before recombinant TPO was available, it was found that TPOAb can bind not only to the native but also to dena-

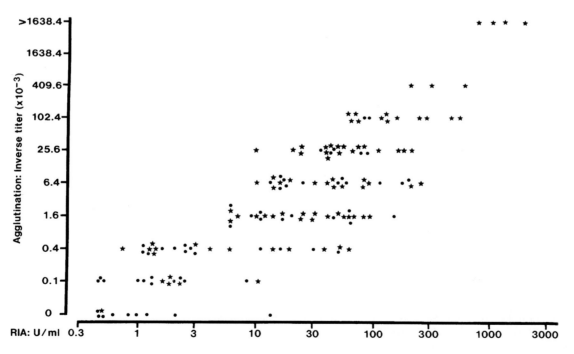

FIGURE 21-1. Comparison of two techniques, agglutination and radioimmunoassay (RIA), for the assay of TPOAb in serum. The 154 serum samples were identified by RIA as TPOAb-positive. Ten samples were negative by agglutination, but otherwise there was good correlation between the two methods. All samples were also tested for TgAb by RIA, and 89 (58%) were positive (*noted as stars*). The agglutination kits were obtained from Miles Inc., Elkhart, IN, and RIA kits were provided by KRONUS, San Clemente, CA.

tured and reduced TPO,[63] suggesting involvement of multiple, conformational, and linear epitopes and heterogeneity of TPOAb. For example, in one study all TPOAb-positive serum samples bound to TPO under denaturing and reducing conditions, and there was a highly significant correlation between the binding and the titers of TPOAb.[58] In another study, the results varied; 20% of TPOAb-positive serum samples did not react with denatured TPO, and of the 80% that were reactive only 20% recognized the reduced form of TPO.[60] These results, combined with the pattern of inhibition of enzyme activity, suggest there are at least six distinct binding epitopes on the TPO molecule.[60] There was no uniformity of results even with the use of recombinant TPO and its fragments (summarized in references 38 and 62), except for the identification of an immunogenic region containing two linear epitopes for the binding of TPOAb.[62] In the most representative study with whole serum, in which four slightly overlapping recombinant fragments, constituting almost the whole length of TPO, and the Western blot technique to analyze TPOAb binding were used, only 7% of 75 TPOAb-positive serum samples did not react with any of the fragments and 86% recognized the fragment spanning the immunogenic region containing the two linear epitopes, with other fragments being recognized less frequently.[62] The pattern of binding was similar with all TPOAb-positive serum samples, regardless of the antibody titer and its source (normal subjects or patients with AITD), indicating a lack of disease-specific epitopes. Almost all samples containing antigastric parietal cell antibodies, some positive and some negative for TPOAb, reacted with TPO peptides, confirming previous findings of an epitope shared by TPO and gastric parietal cells.[30] The fact that a majority of serum samples recognizing native TPO in a RIA also reacted with TPO fragments led to speculation that some linear sequences of the fragments may be part of a discontinuous conformational epitope,[62] but this is unlikely in view of what is known about antigen-antibody interactions.[7,8]

The single TPOAb generated by the hybridoma method was an IgG1κ with a high affinity for human TPO that had no effect on TPO enzyme activity.[55] It did not react with reduced human TPO, native porcine TPO, related peroxidases, or human Tg.[55] By a combinatorial library approach,[11,12] 44 recombinant TPOAb-Fab, with a high affinity for TPO, were obtained and characterized.[56,64] They all belonged to the IgG1 or IgG4 subclasses and all but one were associated with κ light chains. They only recognized native intact TPO[56,64] but did not inhibit its enzymatic activity and did not react with related peroxidases or Tg.[65] Four representative Fab were used to define the immunodominant region on TPO (Fig 21-2), which is recognized by all TPOAb-positive serum samples, with approximately 85% of TPOAb in individual samples directed at this region.[64] Use of the four individual Fab to compete with patients' TPOAb for binding to TPO identified TPOAb epitopic profiles ("fingerprints") in individual samples. The question of disease-specific epitopes, raised by some earlier studies, and possible spreading of epitopes, that is, emergence of antibodies with new specificities during the course of disease, was addressed recently.[66,67] TPOAb epitopic profiles, while distinct in individual serum samples,[66,67] were not different in hypothyroid and euthyroid elderly women[66] and did not change for up to 12 months postpartum in women who developed postpartum thyroid dysfunction or those who remained euthyroid.[67] Concerns about recombinant Fab being representative of TPOAb in serum, the contribution of heavy and light chains in determining epitope recognition, and the somewhat restricted usage of germ-line genes encoding these Fab have been discussed elsewhere.[56]

In summary, TPOAb in most serum samples react with both linear and conformational epitopes on TPO,[62] while mAb recognize only the latter.[55,56,64] Screening of combinatorial libraries with native TPO could have missed Fab reacting with cryptic linear epitopes.[38] Thus, it seems likely that TPOAb in serum are a mixture of antibodies to both types of epitopes, but only those to the intact TPO may have biologic importance.[7]

Postpartum thyroiditis, usually a transient disorder, occurs with high frequency in women who have TPOAb (see chap 89).[68,69] Clinically, these women develop hypothyroidism 3 to 6 months after delivery; in some it is preceded by an evanescent episode of thyrotoxicosis. Postpartum thyroiditis coincides with heightened immune function, a rebound phenomenon after the immunosuppression of pregnancy.[70,71] This is also reflected in TPOAb titers: they fall as pregnancy progresses and rise in the postpartum period.[72] The possible pathogenetic importance of this rise was tested by determining the contribution of individual IgG subclasses to the overall TPOAb titers, but differences in results led to contradictory conclusions.[72–74] Nevertheless, if TPOAb are to be used as a prognostic index for the development of postpartum thyroiditis, they should be measured in the first trimester.[71,72] The cost-effectiveness of such screening can be challenged on the grounds that only about 5% of women develop postpartum thyroiditis, and many of them have few symptoms. In contrast, the 25% incidence of postpartum thyroid dysfunction in

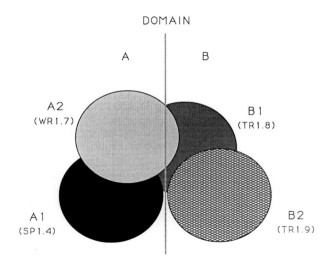

FIGURE 21-2. Schematic representation of the immunodominant regions on TPO. Recombinant TPOAb-FAbs SP1.4 and WR1.7 define the A1 and A2 components of the A domain, and TR1.8 and TR1.9 define the B1 and B2 components of the B domain. (Jaume JC, Costante G, Nishikawa T, Phillips IW, Rapoport B, McLachlan SM. Thyroid peroxidase autoantibody fingerprints in hypothyroid and euthyroid individuals. I. Cross-sectional study in elderly women. J Clin Endocrinol Metab 1995; 80:994, The Endocrine Society, Bethesda, MD)

women with insulin-dependent diabetes mellitus warrants screening and careful follow-up of these women.[75,76]

Unlike autoantibodies to Tg, TPOAb are rare in animal models of spontaneous and experimentally induced autoimmune thyroiditis.[6] Only recently was thyroiditis successfully induced in mice by immunization with porcine TPO, but antibodies to murine TPO were undetectable.[77] These findings are in keeping with the known primary pathogenetic role of T-cells in such animal models (reviewed in reference 6).

From what is known about TPOAb and the known sequestration of TPO,[37] it seems likely that TPOAb arise as a consequence of thyroid damage, and their biologic importance is limited. Still, they are excellent markers of an underlying autoimmune process in the thyroid.

CYTOTOXIC MECHANISMS

There are three cytotoxic mechanisms that may cause thyroid cell injury. Although thyroid cell destruction is the hallmark of Hashimoto's thyroiditis, there is evidence that all three mechanisms may be relevant to a certain degree to both Hashimoto's thyroiditis and Graves' disease.

Cytotoxic T-Lymphocytes

Cytotoxic T-lymphocytes are usually associated with CD8[+] phenotype; they recognize the antigen presented on MHC class I molecules and for activation are dependent on T_H lymphocytes.[78] The various mechanisms and requirements involved in the binding to and lysis of target cells by cytotoxic T-lymphocytes were reviewed recently.[79]

There is no good evidence for the presence of thyroid-specific cytotoxic T-cells in Hashimoto's thyroiditis,[6] and most of the data implicating such cells have come from in vitro cloning of human lymphocytes or animal models of autoimmune thyroiditis. However, T-cells containing perforin are found in thyroid infiltrates,[80] the expression of perforin being a marker for activated cytotoxic T-cells in situ.[81] Although the percentage of perforin-positive cells in the thyroid in five patients with Graves' disease and two patients with Hashimoto's thyroiditis was similar and varied from 0.5% to 8% and 1.5% to 5%, respectively, there was a major difference in the phenotype of these T-cells in the two diseases. CD4[+] perforin-expressing cells (9%–12%) were found only in Hashimoto's thyroiditis, suggesting a MHC class II–restricted component of cytotoxicity. In the infiltrates of thyroid tissue from patients with Graves' disease the predominant perforin-containing cells were CD3αβ[+]CD4[-]CD8[-], that is, double-negative, while in Hashimoto's thyroiditis 41% were CD8[+] (14% in Graves' disease). The number of CD3αβ[+] double-negative cells is increased in thyroid tissue of patients with AITD,[82] but the origin, site of selection or education, and the restricting element of these T-cells are not known.[80] The data suggest that cytotoxic T-cells participate in the pathogenesis of AITD, and that there are differences in cytotoxic autoimmune mechanisms between Graves' disease and Hashimoto's thyroiditis, with more activation of classic cytotoxic T-cells in the latter.

Antibody-Dependent Cell-Mediated Cytotoxicity

Cell effectors in antibody-dependent cell-mediated cytotoxicity (ADCC) are natural killer (NK) cells, defined as large granular lymphocytes bearing specific surface markers (e.g., CD56, CD16) and constitutively expressing perforin.[83] They can bind to, in a non-MHC-restricted fashion, and lyse target cells, whether virus-infected or malignant, directly or through binding of their CD16 receptor (FcγR III) to IgG (subclasses 1 and 3) antibody-coated cells.[83] Although normal cells,[83] including thyroid cells,[84,85] are relatively resistant to lysis by NK cells, assays exploring the role of ADCC in AITD have been performed using human thyroid cells exposed to serum from patients with AITD and NK cells isolated from the peripheral blood of normal subjects. With this assay system the results have varied substantially.

In one study,[86] the specific lysis of thyroid cells exposed to serum from patients with Hashimoto's thyroiditis was higher (27.3% lysis) than that of cells exposed to serum from normal subjects (10.6%) or patients with Graves' disease (13.3%). There was a positive correlation between percent specific lysis and the titers of TPOAb and TgAb. In another report,[87] the results of ADCC with serum from patients with Hashimoto's thyroiditis (80% positive) were confirmed, but there was no attempt to correlate percent specific lysis with TPOAb titers. In contrast, a high proportion of serum samples from patients with Graves' disease were positive without a correlation of ADCC with TPOAb. This was the first indication that antibodies distinct from TPOAb might also participate in ADCC. A subsequent report[88] corroborated the findings with serum from patients with Hashimoto's thyroiditis (63% positive), but a correlation with TPOAb titers was not confirmed. In addition, the degree of lysis was not influenced by preincubation of positive serum samples with TPO. The results suggested the presence of antibodies to an unidentified antigen on thyroid cells. Recently the same group reported a significant difference between patients with atrophic thyroiditis (80% positive) and goitrous thyroiditis (only 39% positive).[89] Again, there was no correlation of ADCC with either TPOAb or TgAb titers.

Other studies had different results. In one, specific lysis elicited by serum samples from patients with thyroid-associated ophthalmopathy was significantly greater than with serum from normal subjects, patients with Hashimoto's disease, and patients with Graves' disease but no ophthalmopathy, all of which gave similar degrees of lysis.[90] There was a significant positive correlation of ADCC activity against thyroid cells in prolonged culture (which lose the expression of surface TPO[39]) with the activity against eye muscle cells, but no correlation with TPOAb titers. ADCC activity against thyroid cells was abolished by preincubation of serum with either thyroid or eye muscle cells, but not vascular endothelium or chondrocytes. These results were interpreted as being due to antibodies against an antigen shared by thyroid and eye muscle cells. The second set of results[91] was obtained using thyroid cells cultured for only 2 days and still expressing surface TPO.[38] ADCC activity against thyroid cells, but not eye muscle cells, correlated with TPOAb titers; activity against both target cells did not correlate with either TRAb or TgAb titers. Lysis of eye muscle cells correlated with some measures of ophthalmopathy but not with the degree of proptosis. Orbital fibroblasts appeared to be a minor target of ADCC with the serum samples tested.[91]

Heterologous targets, namely porcine thyroid cells, have also been used in studies of ADCC.[92] Culture of porcine thyroid cells with TSH increased their susceptibility to ADCC; in the absence of TSH they were resistant to lysis after 7 days in culture. Serum samples from 75% of patients with autoimmune thyroiditis were effective; there was no difference in the mean percent specific lysis elicited by serum from goitrous or agoitrous patients, and only in the latter did ADCC correlate with TPOAb titers. Serum samples from 43% of patients with Graves' disease and ophthalmopathy were positive, with similar ADCC elicited by serum from hyperthyroid patients and euthyroid patients with ophthalmopathy. Although ADCC was positive with seven TPOAb-negative serum samples, there was a significant positive correlation with TPOAb titers but not with the severity of ophthalmopathy. ADCC was also assayed with serum from 39 mothers who gave birth to children with permanent congenital hypothyroidism and their children. The samples were obtained from 4 days to 17 years (6 ± 5 years, mean ± SD) after delivery. All mothers were positive for TPOAb, but none had hypothyroidism, while all children were receiving thyroxine (T_4) therapy at the time of sampling. Congenital hypothyroidism was due to thyroid agenesis in 11, ectopy in 19, and dyshormonogenesis in 3; the cause was not determined in 6 children. Positive ADCC was found with the serum from 36 mothers and 38 children, giving a concordance rate of 87% and reaching 100% in 9 mother-child pairs from whom serum was obtained 4 days to 9 months after birth. There was a positive correlation between ADCC and TPOAb titer in the mothers' serum. However, because of discrepancies between TPOAb titers and ADCC with some samples, the overall conclusion (in agreement with that reached by others[87,88,90]) was that antibodies to an antigen distinct from TPO may also participate in ADCC.[92]

Troubling aspects of the ADCC story in AITD are not only the intra- and interlaboratory inconsistencies of results but also the finding of ADCC in serum from patients with congenital hypothyroidism due to thyroid ectopy.[92,93] By the time the maternal IgG first appears in the fetal circulation, the thyroid is in place and fully differentiated,[94] which argues against the possibility of a maternal antibody, directly or through ADCC, affecting fetal thyroid development. Similar considerations apply to thyroid agenesis, but it is conceivable that high titer antibodies participating in cytotoxic reactions can damage the fetal thyroid in later stages of gestation, leading to thyroid atrophy and the diagnosis of agenesis at birth. Precedents for such a scenario exist,[95,96] but all mothers of corresponding hypothyroid children were clinically affected, unlike the mothers found positive in ADCC assays.[92,93]

A discussion about ADCC would be incomplete without including the status of NK cells, but there is no consensus on either their number or their activity in patients with AITD. The percentage (or absolute number) of NK cells in peripheral blood of patients with Graves' disease was reported to be decreased[97] or normal,[98–102] and in Hashimoto's thyroiditis, increased[97] or normal.[98,100–102] When comparing peripheral blood and thyroid-infiltrating lymphocytes, NK cells were found to be increased among the latter in patients with Graves' disease or Hashimoto's thyroiditis,[82] or decreased in Graves' disease.[103] The percentage of NK cells in peripheral blood was increased in subacute thyroiditis.[97,99] NK cell activity in peripheral blood of patients with Hashimoto's thyroiditis was reported to be normal[90,101,102,104] or increased,[87,98] normal in patients with Graves' hyperthyroidism after treatment,[87,103,105] and decreased,[100,102,105] normal[101] or increased[98] in patients with Graves' hyperthyroidism. NK cell activity against autologous thyroid cells[85,103] or K562 cells[103] was low in thyroid-infiltrating lymphocytes (TIL) from patients with Graves' hyperthyroidism after treatment and patients with Hashimoto's thyroiditis[85,103]; preincubation of TIL with interleukin-2 augmented the activity[103] or failed to do so.[85]

Even in postpartum thyroiditis there are discordant results.[98,106] One group[106] reported comparable NK cell activity in women with postpartum thyroiditis and normal postpartum women 4, 6, and 9 months after delivery; the activity in all postpartum women was lower than in the nonpregnant women. Another group[98] found no difference between nonpregnant and postpartum women or between normal postpartum women and women with postpartum thyroiditis. The activity in individual women with postpartum thyroiditis was increased during the thyrotoxic phase, as compared with the preceding euthyroid phase, as it was in women who developed Graves' hyperthyroidism postpartum. Only in this latter group was there an increase in NK cell number and activity as compared with all appropriate groups.[98]

To summarize, if, as is likely, ADCC occurs in patients with AITD, TPOAb are not the only offending antibodies. First, unlike with thyroid cells in culture, TPO is expressed only on the apical surface of follicular cells in vivo,[37] and as such is not accessible to circulating antibodies unless the follicular structure is already damaged. Secondly, the frequency of TPOAb in pregnant women is much greater than the finding of abnormal thyroid function in the newborn and, conversely, there is no correlation between the presence of maternal TPOAb and congenital hypothyroidism.[107] Rather, it is probable that ADCC also involves distinct antibodies directed at an uncharacterized antigen(s) that would have to be expressed on the basement membrane to be the target in the fetal thyroid. In addition, since among perforin-containing thyroid-infiltrating lymphocytes, NK cells are a minor population[80] with low lytic activity,[85,103] it can be inferred that ADCC is not an important cytotoxic mechanism in AITD. On the other hand, the ability of NK cells to lyse virus-infected cells, without the involvement of antibodies, might be responsible for thyroid damage in the initial phase of subacute thyroiditis,[97,99] which is believed to have a viral etiology (see chap 34).

Complement-Fixing Antibodies

The complement system, encompassing numerous proteins, plays an important role in inflammation and phagocytosis.[108] Its activation leads to various biologic effects, including complement-mediated cell lysis. The classic pathway of activation of the complement cascade is well defined.[108] It starts with binding of C1q, a part of the first component of complement, to antigen-antibody complexes on cell surfaces. (In such complexes, C1q has high avidity for single IgM molecules and aggregated IgG of certain subclasses; i.e., IgG3 > IgG1 > IgG2.) The subsequent steps of the cascade proceed until terminal complement components are available for the formation of a membrane attack complex, resulting in cell injury. Certain steps of the cascade are kept in check by inhibitors or regulators found in the fluid phase and on the target cells.[108] The complexity of the process is reflected in the various techniques used to assess the relevance of complement to AITD.[69,109–112]

From the first description of complement-fixing antibodies in Hashimoto's thyroiditis,[40] numerous reports[69,109–112] have implicated complement in the pathogenesis of AITD. The concentration of the terminal component of complement, C9, was increased in the serum of patients with Graves' disease; immunohistochemical staining identified C9 bound to the basement membrane of thyroid cells in Graves' disease but not normal thyroid cells.[109] The serum concentrations of terminal complement components were increased in both Graves' disease and Hashimoto's thyroiditis and the complexes were deposited around the thyroid follicles in the glands from such patients.[110] Membrane-bound and fluid phase regulators of complement activation were found in AITD glands.[111] The control of expression of these regulators and their modulation of the action of membrane attack complexes on thyroid cells have been discussed in detail.[6,111] It is clear that complement activation does occur in many patients with AITD.

The antibodies responsible for fixing complement leading to thyroid cell lysis were studied using cultured human thyroid cells incubated with IgG that was purified from the serum of patients with Hashimoto's thyroiditis or normal subjects and rabbit complement.[112] All the former samples were positive for TPOAb and 67% of them also contained TgAb. The main findings were that cytotoxic activity, expressed as percent specific lysis, was significantly higher with Hashimoto's thyroiditis IgG than with normal IgG; samples from 30% of patients with atrophic thyroiditis, 59% of patients with subclinical hypothyroidism, and 55% of overtly hypothyroid patients were positive. Preincubation of Hashimoto's thyroiditis IgG with purified TPO completely abolished the activity of some samples and partially abolished that of others; purified Tg had no effect. The lysis did not occur when the TPOAb titer was low, but some high-titer samples were also ineffective. Overall, there was no significant correlation between cytotoxicity and either TPOAb or TgAb titers. These data implicated TPOAb–TPO complexes as the main initiators of complement activation, but also suggested the involvement of an unknown antigen(s) on thyroid cells, reminiscent of the findings in ADCC.[87,88,92,93]

Activation of complement by TPOAb has also been implicated in the pathogenesis of postpartum thyroiditis.[69] Comparisons were made between two groups of postpartum women. All had TPOAb, but one group had developed postpartum thyroiditis. In all the women there was an increase in TPOAb titer, complement fixation, complement component C3 activation (expressed as an index), and TPOAb bioactivity (TPOAb levels × C3 index); at 2 to 8 months the increases were significantly greater in the postpartum thyroiditis group. None of the women negative for TPOAb, who served as controls, developed postpartum thyroiditis, whereas 50% of those with TPOAb did.[69]

In summary, compelling evidence has been provided for complement activation in AITD and the possible involvement of an unidentified antigen.[112] Could this be the main mechanism for thyroid cell damage in vivo? All nucleated cells, including thyroid cells,[111] have defense mechanisms that protect them from lysis by homologous complement. Despite this resistance, nonlethal membrane attack complexes inhibit thyroid cell function and induce release of proinflammatory substances (summarized in reference 6) so that the process could cause injury even in the absence of direct cell lysis. For this to occur, it is likely that the follicular structure has to be already damaged, as is the case for ADCC. This view is also supported by the findings in postpartum thyroiditis, in which signs of thyroid dysfunction precede the rise of TPOAb (discussed in reference 69), suggesting that there is a disruptive process already in place.

An integrated view of cytotoxic mechanisms in AITD is not possible at present because of often discrepant findings in vitro and the known complexities of interactions in vivo. Still, cytotoxic T-lymphocytes are the best candidates as initiators of thyroid cell damage, which can be exaggerated and perpetuated in the presence of activated complement. Circumstantial evidence for the participation of ADCC is the most controversial and is weak. Rare instances of permanent thyroid damage in children born to mothers with AITD do favor antibody-mediated mechanisms. Involvement of antibodies, distinct from TPOAb, in cytotoxic reactions has been suggested and their identification, as well as of the corresponding antigen(s) on thyroid cells, should help to clarify the present dilemma.

ANTIBODIES TO THE TSH RECEPTOR

Autoantibodies to the TSH receptor, termed TRAb, have a well-defined direct pathogenetic role in AITD.[113,114] Two major categories of TRAb have been identified. Thyroid-stimulating antibody (TSAb), with action analogous to TSH, is accepted as the cause of hyperthyroidism in Graves' disease. Thyroid-blocking antibody (TBAb), which inhibits the binding of TSH and the biologic actions of both TSH and TSAb, is the cause of hypothyroidism in some patients with Hashimoto's thyroiditis. The final proof that TRAb interact with the TSH-R came from work with the cloned receptor.[115–117]

Recognition of what has been known by a variety of names and acronyms, here termed TSAb, dates from 1956. In that year, thyroid-stimulating activity was detected in serum from patients with Graves' disease that was qualitatively different from TSH in that it was more slow-acting.[118] The initial bioassay in guinea pigs[118] was superseded by a similar assay using mice,[119] and the agreed terminology for the bioactivity was long-acting thyroid stimulator (LATS).[120] LATS was clearly identified as an IgG,[121] but was found in only a minority of patients with Graves' disease. Marked improvement in sensitivity of assays for TSAb occurred with the development of in vitro procedures.[113,114]

The finding of only inhibitory activity in the serum of a patient with atrophic thyroiditis[122] was the first clue to the existence of TBAb, and this type of antibody was subsequently found to be the cause of transient neonatal hypothyroidism in two children of a hypothyroid woman.[123] Further studies confirmed the primary pathogenetic role of TBAb in this syndrome.[124–126]

Assays for TRAb

Much of our current knowledge of TSAb comes from studies of the effect of TSAb on adenylyl cyclase activity or cAMP production in human thyroid homogenates or slices,[127–131] and more recently in cultured human thyroid cells,[132] the latter procedure made more sensitive by use of a hypotonic medium.[133,134] The nonhuman thyroid preparation that is most successful for the assay of TSAb is FRTL-5 cells.[135–137] More recently, cloning of the human TSH-R[115,116] led to, in place of thyroid cells, the use of Chinese hamster ovary (CHO) cells transfected with the recombinant receptor (CHO-TSH-R).[138,139] With most of these assays TSAb can be detected in almost 100% of patients with Graves' hyperthyroidism.

TSAb may also be assayed by its ability to inhibit binding of ^{125}I-TSH to the TSH-R.[114] This technique (TSH binding inhibition [TBI]) was developed[140] after recognition that TSAb, having the same effect on the thyroid as TSH, might compete with TSH for binding to TSH receptors (summarized in reference 140). Refinement of this assay has led to its widespread use,[114,141] and commercial TBI kits with solubilized porcine thyroid cell membranes as a source of the receptor are now available. A receptor preparation from CHO-TSH-R can also be used and compares favorably with a commercial kit.[142] TBI assays using thyroid[143,144] and CHO-TSH-R cells,[145] both having a single high-affinity binding site for TSH and comparable K_d values,[146] are confined to research laboratories. Not all serum samples from patients with Graves' hyperthyroidism are posi-

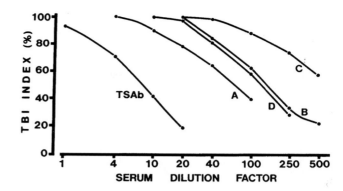

FIGURE 21-4. TBI assay of serum of mothers with AITD whose infants had transient neonatal hypothyroidism. TBI activity was measured using a commercial kit (KRONUS, San Clemente, CA) with minor modifications of the method recommended by the manufacturer. The maternal serum samples were diluted with pooled normal serum. A through D refer to individual mothers who had children with transient neonatal hypothyroidism. TSAb indicates the laboratory standard serum, which was from a woman who had a child with neonatal hyperthyroidism. Note the greater potency of serum samples A through D compared with TSAb. (Zakarija M, McKenzie JM, Eidson MS. Transient neonatal hypothyroidism: Characterization of maternal antibodies to the thyrotropin receptor. J Clin Endocrinol Metab 1990;70:1239, The Endocrine Society)

tive in TBI assays; negative results usually coincide with low stimulating activity.[147]

TBAb can be measured in both types of assays. In the stimulation assay it blocks the effect of TSH[113,124,148–150] and TSAb (Fig 21-3),[113,125,143,151] and the activity is often designated thyroid stimulation blocking Ab (TSBAb). TBAb are equally potent in blocking the binding of TSH in the TBI assay (an activity termed TSH binding inhibiting Ab [TBIAb]), with the highest titers found in mothers of infants with transient neonatal hypothyroidism (Fig 21-4).[125]

Recognition that there is no absolute distinction among AITD based on the type of TRAb came from the finding that TSAb and TBAb may coexist in individual patients with either Graves' disease or Hashimoto's thyroiditis.[113,125,143,152,153] This is reflected in a biphasic dose response in the stimulation-type assays (Fig 21-5)[113,125,152] and more inhibition of TSH binding than expected from the TSAb activity alone. Such a biphasic response was identified with purified IgG from the serum of 33% of patients with Graves' disease[154] and of some patients with Hashimoto's thyroiditis.[125] The relevance of such a mixture of antibodies to the clinical presentation was recognized 12 years ago.[155]

Clinical Application of Assays of TRAb

The assay of TSAb may be of clinical value in establishing the diagnosis of Graves' disease, estimating its prognosis, and forecasting neonatal hyperthyroidism. The first of these areas—the diagnostic usefulness—is clearly limited. Although a positive assay would be expected in all patients with Graves' hyperthyroidism, clinical criteria and the commonly used tests of thyroid status make the assay of TSAb unnecessary for diagnostic evaluation. Even in euthyroid patients with ophthalmopathy, in whom one is seeking evidence of a thyroid

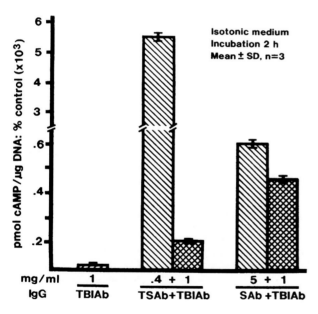

FIGURE 21-3. Comparison of the effect of TBIAb on the stimulation of CHO-TSH-R cells (JP-26 cell line) by TSAb and a novel stimulator (SAb) from a woman who initially had Graves' hyperthyroidism but became hypothyroid and gave birth to five infants with transient neonatal hypothyroidism (patient C in Fig. 21-4). cAMP was measured in the extracts of cells after incubation with the preparations and concentrations of IgG indicated. Note the large inhibitory effect of TBIAb on the activity of TSAb and the weak effect on the SAb activity. (Zakarija M, De Forteza R, McKenzie JM, Ghandur-Mnaymneh L. Characteristics and clinical correlates of a novel thyroid-stimulating autoantibody. Autoimmunity 1994; 19:31, Harwood Academic Publishers GmbH)

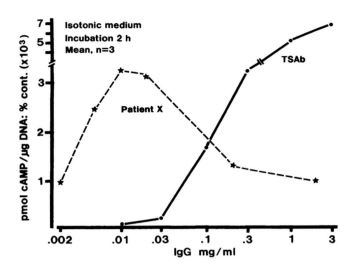

FIGURE 21-5. Stimulation of CHO-TSH-R cells (JP-26 cell line) by IgG from a patient (X) known to have multiple TRAb and by our laboratory standard TSAb. The biphasic effect of the patient's IgG is evident, as is the straight-line effect of the TSAb.

disorder, orbital imaging procedures and thyroid tests provide more information than the TSAb assay.

TSAb assays have some prognostic usefulness. In patients with Graves' hyperthyroidism who have been treated with antithyroid drug therapy, the presence of TSAb is a strong predictor of relapse after drug withdrawal. The strength of this association is probably greater when TSAb is measured as such, rather than in a TBI assay.[131,134,156–159] While the test could be a substantial contribution to patient management, of even greater value are the implications of results obtained in a predominantly retrospective study of patients who had been treated for hyperthyroidism with either antithyroid drug or destructive therapy. Those patients who had a high level of TSAb at the time of initial diagnosis were likely to have persistently detectable TSAb, regardless of the type of therapy.[131] Such results suggest that patients with high initial titers of TSAb might as well receive thyroid destructive therapy immediately.

Transplacental passage of TSAb as the likely cause of neonatal Graves' disease was recognized over 30 years ago.[160] This relation has been confirmed using many different TSAb assays. It appears clear that a high maternal titer of TSAb in the third trimester of pregnancy accurately forecasts neonatal Graves' disease (see chaps 86 and 90).[94,161,162] The emphasis on the third trimester reflects the fact that the titer of TSAb may be high early in pregnancy and fall during gestation, and the infants of such mothers are likely to be euthyroid. A low titer of TSAb in the mother at the time of parturition may be followed by an increase a few weeks postpartum.[163] These observations no doubt reflect the immunosuppressive effect of pregnancy that has been documented in other autoimmune diseases.[70,71]

Regarding the relevance of a history of AITD in the mother, some clinical features deserve emphasis. A current state of treated hypothyroidism that may be due to prior destructive therapy (i.e., by ^{131}I or surgery) for Graves' hyperthyroidism has little direct bearing on the persistence of TSAb;

such patients may still have high levels of TSAb and thus give birth to a hyperthyroid child.[161] Indeed, the mother may never have had hyperthyroidism but is euthyroid, taking T_4 for hypothyroidism caused by Hashimoto's thyroiditis, and yet have a very high level of TSAb, persisting for years, leading to successive children being born with neonatal hyperthyroidism.[155,164]

The clinical importance of TBAb lies in two areas: transient hypothyroidism in neonates and thyroid failure in adults. The former was first identified in 1980, but the syndrome is rare.[123,125,126] TBAb may also cause hypothyroidism in adults. The prevalence of TBAb usually is higher in hypothyroid patients with atrophic thyroiditis than in those with goitrous thyroiditis.[148] Among a group of patients with hypothyroidism who earlier had Graves' hyperthyroidism and were treated with an antithyroid drug, one third were thought to be hypothyroid because of the presence of TBAb and the remainder because of cell-mediated thyroid destruction.[165] TBAb may appear in a patient after there is clinical evidence of hypothyroidism,[125] so that identifying TBAb in a hypothyroid patient is not proof that the antibody is the cause of the hypothyroidism.

In some patients, TSAb or TBAb may persist for years, with little change in titer.[151,164] The presence of a circulating autoantibody and its effect, however, need not be permanent, not only during pregnancy but also in other settings. For instance, a patient who has hypothyroidism for a time and then develops typical Graves' hyperthyroidism might have produced a potent TSAb that overcame or replaced the effects of a TBAb.[166,167] The coexistence of stimulating and blocking antibodies in an individual patient is not unusual and the clinical consequence reflects the action of the predominant TRAb.[125,152]

TBAb-induced hypothyroidism in adults may be spontaneously reversible.[168] Among a group of 15 hypothyroid patients with TBAb in their serum in whom the antibodies disappeared during T_4 therapy, six remained euthyroid and nine became hypothyroid again after the T_4 was discontinued. All six patients studied who remained TBAb-positive during T_4 therapy became hypothyroid after it was discontinued. These results indicate that the occurrence of TBAb in a patient with Hashimoto's thyroiditis is not necessarily the cause of their hypothyroidism.

Characteristics of TRAb

The term *restricted heterogeneity* is used to imply that an antibody is not polyclonal, but has characteristics indicating that the B-lymphocytes that synthesize and secrete the antibody originate from only a few clones (oligoclonality) or conceivably only one clone (monoclonality). The biologic activity of a monoclonal IgG should be limited to molecules that have a single heavy-chain subclass and light chains that are of only one type (i.e., either κ or λ) and have a single isoelectric point (pH), as identified by isoelectric focusing. Polyclonal antibodies, such as TgAb and TPOAb, are widely spread by this technique.

Regarding TRAb, preparative isoelectric focusing of IgG revealed peak TSAb activity coincident with a pI of 8.5 to 9.0,[168a] compatible with an oligoclonal origin. Other studies supported polyclonality, since the TRAb had both κ and λ light chains.[169,170] In a recent study of 31 patients, the TSAb bioactivity in 27 patients was in IgG molecules with a single type of light chain (λ light chains, 23 patients; κ light chains, 4 patients);[171–173] in 15 samples tested in two studies all thyroid-stimulating activity was restricted to IgG1.[171,174] In contrast to TSAb, TBAb activity in serum of 11 patients was not subclass-restricted, although IgG1 was predominant in most samples and almost exclusive in two.[175] Light chain association has not been tested systematically, but in one patient TBAb was exclusively IgGκ[125] and in another mostly IgGλ.[125,176] Isoelectric focusing of TBAb showed progressive inhibitory activity from pI 8-10,[114,176] with the peak at more than 9.5.[176]

Restriction as high as that of TSAb has not been reported for any other autoantibodies. An unorthodox explanation would be that this is due to specific V region germ-line genes giving rise to TSAb (also not found with other antibodies, including TgAb[29] and TPOAb[56]) or to an unspecified primary B-cell abnormality.[6] Further characterization of TRAb, especially at a molecular level, has not been feasible, since all available techniques failed to produce monoclonal TRAb.[9,11,12]

The presence of other stimulating antibodies, directed at the TSH-R, has been documented in some patients with AITD. A woman considered to have hypothyroidism caused by Hashimoto's thyroiditis had three children with delayed onset of neonatal hyperthyroidism.[143,155,164] This woman's IgG, at low concentrations, enhanced TSH binding to human thyroid membranes (by as much as 250%) and at high concentrations completely inhibited TSH binding.[143] The enhancement was found only when particulate human thyroid membranes were used as the TSH-R; with solubilized membranes or FRTL-5 cells the IgG was only inhibitory.[143] A similar biphasic pattern, in terms of stimulation of cAMP accumulation, was found using human thyroid slices and cells and CHO-TSH-R cells[143,155] (Fig 21-5). The finding of intrauterine and delayed onset of hyperthyroidism in fetuses and neonates,[164] respectively, when maternal IgG concentrations in the fetus and neonate were low[94] confirmed the in vitro data. Unlike classic TSAb activity that is retained by the Fab fragment of IgG,[114,143] both the enhancement of TSH binding and the stimulation of thyroid preparations required a divalent molecule (i.e., the whole IgG or F[ab']$_2$ fragment).[143] In summary, this patient's IgG contained not only a potent TBAb, but also an antibody, distinct from TSAb, that enhanced TSH binding; whether this antibody stimulated the human thyroid directly or indirectly by enhancing the binding and action of TSAb is not known.

The serum of another patient, who initially had Graves' disease, contained not only TSAb and TBAb but also an additional stimulator. Its action was not inhibited by either its own or a TRAb from another patient (see Fig 21-3),[125,151,176] in keeping with the finding that its peak activity (pI > 9.5) coincided with that of TBAb in the same sample.[176] Of the three antibodies in this serum, the most potent was TBAb, which caused transient hypothyroidism in five consecutive neonates, but the stimulator was a probable cause of an enlarging goiter in the mother.[151] The incidence of these unusual stimulating antibodies, distinct from TSAb, is unknown, since different bioactivities cannot be detected by regular screening methods.

There is some confusion as to the heterogeneity of TBAb, based on occasional findings that some TBI-positive serum samples also affect post-receptor processes and some block

TSH-induced stimulation without altering TSH binding.[177] A suggestion was put forward that some species of TBAb with high TBI activity may exert a blocking effect by interacting with a component of thyroid cell membranes and not the TSH-R.[178] Many of these data were obtained with different thyroid cell types and assays, and mostly with crude IgG preparations, sometimes in large quantities. Still, some experimental evidence exists to support the notion that not all TBAb activity is associated with the TBI effect. Antibodies raised in rabbits to the recombinant TSH-R and short peptides, related to unique sequences of the TSH-R, have been tested for their ability to interact with the TSH-R.[179] Anti-TSH-R antibodies inhibited both TSH-induced stimulation and TSH binding, whereas the most potent blocking anti-peptide antibody was TBI-negative, despite its ability to bind the receptor, as shown by immunoprecipitation. The anti-peptide antibody data were interpreted as due to induction of a conformational change in the receptor, still allowing binding of TSH but influencing post-ligand-binding steps.[179]

A definite advancement in understanding of the interactions between TSH, TSAb, and TBAb came with the cloning of TSH-R.[115] Since then, an enormous amount of literature related to characterization of the structure-function relationships of the receptor and of binding sites of TRAb has accumulated.[115–117,180–183] Although the results are not absolutely concordant, certain generalizations can be made. TRAb bind to highly-conformational epitopes on the extracellular domain of TSH-R[115,116] and do not recognize linear epitopes.[184] TSAb, TBAb, and TSH interact with different sites on the receptor,[116,181–183] but there appears to be some overlap of epitopes in the carboxyl terminal region.[116] Based on studies of TSH-LH receptor chimeras, the serum of patients with Graves' disease contained at least two populations of stimulating antibodies.[180] The coexistence of TSAb and TBAb in hypothyroid patients[125,153] was confirmed using TSH-R mutants.[183] Further progress in this field is expected when monoclonal TRAb become available. The lack of animal models is another impediment to better understanding of Graves' disease.[6,185]

Site(s) of Synthesis of TRAb

The thyroid gland has been implicated as a major site of TgAb and TPOAb production,[6,114] but some of these antibodies are produced in regional lymph nodes and bone marrow.[186] (Antibody-secreting cells home to the bone marrow, a major site of all antibody production.[187,188]) A single report documented spontaneous secretion of TSAb, as measured in the TBI assay, by thyroid but not lymph node lymphocytes.[189] Although it is indisputable that antibody production occurs at the site of inflammation, some facts have been overlooked. For example, TSAb is present in the serum of patients with Graves' hyperthyroidism whose thyroids contain few or no lymphocytes,[147,190] and titers of TRAb may remain high despite subtotal thyroidectomy.[151] These data imply that the thyroid is a site, but not the major one, of TSAb production only when there is substantial lymphocytic infiltration of the gland. Even in infiltrated thyroid glands, T_H lymphocytes and elaborated cytokines are of a pro-inflammatory type,[191,192] known to inhibit thyroid function and expression of thyroid autoantigens,[6,39] and not conducive for antibody production.[6] We suggested that the size of the thyroid in patients with Graves' disease might be inversely correlated with the degree of lymphocytic infiltration,[190] and another group confirmed such a relationship for patients whose disease was of short duration.[147]

Regardless of the initial site of TRAb synthesis, the events that initiate it are not at all clear.[6] A satisfactory overall model of AITD, based on the diverse mechanisms known to lead to autoimmunity,[4,5] has yet to be developed.

ANTIBODIES TO THYROID HORMONES AND THYROTROPIN

Antibodies to Thyroid Hormones

Autoantibodies to T_4 or triiodothyronine (T_3) occur predominantly in patients who have AITD.[193] In most, if not all, patients this is a reflection of thyroid hormone in Tg acting as a hapten, and being recognized by the resulting antibody. Among different patients, the antibodies bind T_4, T_3, or both. As a consequence, such autoantibodies may interfere in immunoassays for serum T_4 and T_3; depending on the method used, the value may be falsely elevated or decreased (see also chap 18). However, such interference appears to be rare, perhaps due to low affinity of most antibodies for the hormones. The overall effect is similar to an increase in thyroxine-binding globulin (TBG). The total hormone concentration increases, but the free hormone concentration does not, so there is usually no identifiable clinical effect or alteration in TSH secretion. The importance of these anti-T_4 and anti-T_3 antibodies is their ability to cause serum T_4 and T_3 values that are inappropriate for a given clinical presentation.

Antibodies to Thyrotropin

Spontaneously occurring autoantibodies to TSH, causing error in immunoassays for TSH, have been recognized for more than a decade. Unless specifically sought, such antibodies are likely to be identified by the astute interpretation of clinically unexpected serum TSH values in patients with AITD.[194] Alternatively, these antibodies may be uncovered by their interference in assays for TRAb that use solubilized thyroid membranes as the receptor.[194-196] The result is an absurdly negative value (e.g., −74% to −170%) for the index of inhibition, due to precipitation by polyethylene glycol of not only [^{125}I]TSH-receptor but also [^{125}I]TSH-TSH antibody complexes.[194]

The other source of falsely abnormal results in TSH assays is the presence of heterophilic antibodies that interact with the reagent antibodies used to measure the hormone, usually in patients who have worked with animals[197,198] (see chap 18). Constant vigilance is required, by both assayists and clinicians who depend on assay results, to detect erroneous results arising from the presence of heterophilic antibodies to mouse immunoglobulins.

ANTIBODIES TO ORBITAL ANTIGENS

Theories of pathogenetic mechanisms that underlie the ophthalmopathy (or orbitopathy) of Graves' disease are more distinguished by their quantity than by their clarity and acceptance (see the section on opthalmopathy in chap 30). Nonetheless, an autoimmune basis for the disorder and an ill-defined relation to the thyroid component of Graves' disease are generally accepted. An autoimmune pathogenesis may be inferred from the histologic changes in the affected extraocular muscles; lymphoid follicles and less structured lymphoid infiltration were recognized long before it was realized that they were hallmarks of autoimmunity.[199] A relation to hyperthyroidism is unassailable, but precisely what that relation may be remains conjectural. Certainly the temporal relation to hyperthyroidism is variable,[200] and ophthalmopathy may occur without overt concomitant thyroid functional abnormality.[131]

Investigations into the pathogenesis of Graves' ophthalmopathy have focused on retroorbital antigens that may be involved in a primary autoimmune reaction. Two recent reviews consider the importance of eye muscle membrane protein vs. retroorbital fibroblasts as targets.[201,202] There are two possible pathogenetic scenarios, neither of which is supported unequivocally by available data nor touches on the truly primary pathogenic event(s). One is an immune attack on eye muscle membrane proteins, particularly one characterized by a molecular weight of 64 kd.[201] The other focuses on retroorbital fibroblasts as the primary antigenic target, with resultant release of cytokines that influence adversely the extraocular muscles.[202]

Some have supported a role for thyroglobulin, or related peptides, as being a common antigen linking the thyroid gland and retroorbital tissues.[203,204] There has recently been a suggestion that the link may be the TSH-R being expressed in retroorbital tissue.[205,206] TSH-R variant transcripts have been found in thyroid tissue from normal subjects and patients with Graves' disease, and also in extraocular muscle, peripheral blood mononuclear cells, and, to a lesser extent, in fat and fibroblasts.[207] This receptor, lacking the transmembrane segment, would not be functional, but could be relevant to the pathogenesis of ophthalmopathy.

The continuing controversy regarding the relation of autoantibodies to retroorbital antigens[201,208] may be solved by cloning mAb from retroorbital tissues.[209,210]

OTHER AUTOIMMUNE PHENOMENA

Localized myxedema (dermopathy) is a component of the Graves' disease syndrome that is pathogenetically unrelated to hyperthyroidism. It occurs in approximately 2% of patients with Graves' disease[211] and is characterized by accumulation of glycosaminoglycans in the extracellular matrix and fragmentation of collagen fibers. Consequently skin fibroblasts have been studied for their possible role in dermopathy both as a source of glycosaminoglycans and collagen and as targets for circulating autoantibodies[212] (see the section on localized myxedema in chap 30).

Serum and IgG from 20 patients with localized myxedema stimulated glycosaminoglycan synthesis in FRTL-5 cells[213] (known to respond to TRAb[214]) but had no effect on glycosaminoglycan synthesis by skin fibroblasts. Serum and IgG from normal subjects was inactive in both systems. Another approach to the understanding of localized myxedema has been to assess the importance of a 23-kd protein in fibroblasts that binds in vitro to antibodies in serum from patients with Graves' disease.[215] However, there was no specificity for the site of origin of the fibroblasts (i.e., skin affected by localized myxedema or not), so the pathogenesis of localized myxedema remains unknown.

The existence of thyroid growth-stimulating and blocking antibodies distinct from TRAb[216–218] has not been independently confirmed[219] and will not be reviewed here.

Serum antibodies to nuclear (tissue-nonspecific) antigens have been found in patients with Graves' disease.[220–222] One group described finding antibodies to double-stranded (ds) DNA,[220] an antibody normally considered to be specific for systemic lupus erythematosus, but others found no anti-ds-DNA antibodies in their patients.[221,222] The conflicting results may relate to the ready in vitro breakdown of dsDNA to single-stranded (ss) DNA (i.e., antibodies in the dsDNA assay were actually directed against ssDNA). Whatever type, if any, of antinuclear antibodies may be present in Graves' disease, their role in the pathogenesis of the disorder is not known.

References

1. Roitt IM, Doniach D, Campbell PN, Hudson RV. Autoantibodies in Hashimoto's disease (lymphadenoid goiter). Lancet 1956;2:820
2. Parker DC. T cell-dependent B cell activation. Annu Rev Immunol 1993;11:331
3. Tonegawa S. Somatic generation of antibody diversity. Nature 1983;302:575
4. Sercarz EE, Datta SK. Mechanisms of autoimmunization: perspective from the mid-90s. Curr Opin Immunol 1994;6:875
5. Mamula MJ, Craft J. The expression of self-antigenic determinants: implications for tolerance and autoimmunity. Curr Opin Immunol 1994;6:882
6. Weetman AP, McGregor AM. Autoimmune thyroid disease: further developments in our understanding. Endocr Rev 1994; 15:788
7. Laver WG, Air GM, Webster RG, Smith-Gill SJ. Epitopes on protein antigens: Misconceptions and realities. Cell 1990;61:553
8. Poljak RJ, Braden BC. Structural features of the reactions between antibodies and protein antigens. FASEB J 1995;9:9
9. Kohler G, Milstein C. Continuous cultures of fused cells secreting antibody of predefined specificity. Nature 1975;256:495
10. Kalsi JK, Isenberg DA. Immortalization of human antibody producing cells. Autoimmunity 1992;13:249
11. Huse WD, Sastry L, Iverson SA, et al. Generation of a large combinatorial library of the immunoglobulin repertoire in phage lambda. Science 1989;246:1275
12. Winter G, Griffiths AD, Hawkins RE, Hoogenboom HR. Making antibodies by phage display technology. Annu Rev Immunol 1994;12:433
13. Spiegelberg HL. Biological activities of immunoglobulins of different classes and subclasses. Adv Immunol 1974;19:259
14. Burton DR. Immunoglobulin G: functional sites. Molec Immunol 1985;22:161
15. Amino N, Hagan SR, Yamada N, Refetoff HS. Measurement of circulating thyroid microsomal antibodies by the tanned red cell haemagglutination technique: its usefulness in the diagnosis of autoimmune thyroid disease. Clin Endocrinol 1976;5:115
16. Cayzer I, Chalmers SR, Doniach D, Swana G. An evaluation of two new haemagglutination tests for the rapid diagnosis of autoimmune thyroid disease. J Clin Pathol 1978;31:1147
17. Goodburn R, Williams DL, Marks V. A simple micro-ELISA method for the assay of anti-thyroglobulin autoantibodies in human serum. J Clin Pathol 1981;34:1026

18. Beever K, Bradbury J, Phillips D, et al. Highly sensitive assay of autoantibodies to thyroglobulin and to thyroid peroxidase. Clin Chem 1989;35:1949
19. Pacini F, Mariotti S, Formica N, et al. Thyroid autoantibodies in thyroid cancer: incidence and relationship with tumour outcome. Acta Endocrinol 1988;119:373
20. Dulgeroff AJ, Hershman JM. Medical therapy for differentiated thyroid carcinoma. Endocr Rev 1994;15:500
21. Torrigiani G, Roitt IM, Doniach D. Quantitative distribution of human thyroglobulin autoantibodies in different immunoglobulin classes. Clin Exp Immunol 1968;3:621
22. Hay FC, Torrigiani G. The distribution of anti-thyroglobulin antibodies in the immunoglobulin G subclasses. Clin Exp Immunol 1973;15:517
23. Nye L, Decarvalho LP, Roitt IM. An investigation of the clonality of human autoimmune thyroglobulin antibodies and their light chains. Clin Exp Immunol 1981;46:161
24. Belyavin G, Trotter WR. Investigations of thyroid antigens reacting with Hashimoto sera. Evidence for an antigen other than thyroglobulin. Lancet 1959;1:648
25. Caturegli P, Kuppers RC, Mariotti S, et al. IgG subclass distribution of thyroglobulin antibodies in patients with thyroid disease. Clin Exp Immunol 1994;98:464
26. Heidelberger M. The molecular composition of immune precipitates from rabbit sera. J Am Chem Soc 1938;60:242
27. Nye L, Decarvalho LP, Roitt IM. Restrictions in the response to autologous thyroglobulin in the human. Clin Exp Immunol 1980;41:252
28. Caturegli P, Mariotti S, Kuppers RC, Burek CL, Pinchera A, Rose NL. Epitopes on thyroglobulin: A study of patients with thyroid disease. Autoimmunity 1994;18:41
29. Prentice L, Kiso Y, Fukuma N, et al. Monoclonal thyroglobulin autoantibodies: Variable region analysis and epitope recognition. J Clin Endocrinol Metab 1995;80:977
30. Ruf J, Ferrand M, Durand-Gorde JM, Carayon P. Significance of thyroglobulin antibodies cross-reactive with thyroperoxidase (TGPO antibodies) in individual patients and immunized mice. Clin Exp Immunol 1993;92:65
31. Ludgate M, Vassart G. The molecular genetics of three thyroid autoantigens: Thyroglobulin, thyroid peroxidase and the thyrotropin receptor. Autoimmunity 1990;7:201
32. Ruf J, Ferrand M, Durand-Gorde J-M, Carayon P. Autoantibodies and monoclonal antibodies directed to an immunodominant antigenic region of thyroglobulin interact with thyroperoxidase through an interspecies idiotype. Autoimmunity 1994;19:55
33. Czarnocka B, Ruf J, Ferrand M, Carayon P, Lissitzky S. Purification of the human thyroid peroxidase and its identification as the microsomal antigen involved in autoimmune thyroid disease. FEBS Lett 1985;190:147
34. Libert F, Ruf J, Ludgate M, et al. Complete nucleotide sequence of the human thyroid peroxidase-microsomal antigen cDNA. Nucl Acids Res 1987;15:6735
35. Roitt IM, Ling NR, Doniach D, Couchman KG. The cytoplasmic autoantigen of the human thyroid. I. Immunological and biochemical characteristics. Immunology 1964;7:375
36. Ekholm R. Biosynthesis of thyroid hormones. Int Rev Cytol 1990;120:243
37. Khoury EL, Bottazzo GF, Roitt IM. The thyroid "microsomal" antibody revisited: Its paradoxical binding in vivo to the apical surface of the follicular epithelium. J Exp Med 1984;159:577
38. McLachlan SM, Rapoport B. The molecular biology of thyroid peroxidase: Cloning, expression and role as autoantigen in autoimmune thyroid disease. Endocr Rev 1992;13:192
39. Chiovato L, Pinchera A. The microsomal/peroxidase antigen: modulation of its expression in thyroid cells. Autoimmunity 1991;10:319

40. Trotter WR, Belyavin G, Waddams A. Precipitating and complement fixing antibodies in Hashimoto's disease. Proc R Soc Med 1957;50:961

41. Holborow EJ, Brown PC, Roitt IM, Doniach D. Cytoplasmic localization of complement fixing autoantigen in human thyroid epithelium. Br J Exp Pathol 1959;40:583

42. Chiovato L, Bassi P, Santini F, et al. Antibodies producing complement-mediated thyroid cytotoxicity in patients with atrophic or goitrous autoimmune thyroiditis. J Clin Endocrinol Metab 1993;77:1700

43. Schardt CW, McLachlan SM, Matheson J, Rees Smith B. An enzyme-linked immunoassay for thyroid microsomal antibodies. J Immunol Methods 1982;55:155

44. Ludgate M, Mariotti S, Libert F, et al. Antibodies to human thyroid peroxidase in autoimmune thyroid disease: Studies with a cloned recombinant complementary deoxyribonucleic acid epitope. J Clin Endocrinol Metab 1989;68:1091

45. Kaufman KD, Filetti S, Seto P, Rapoport B. Recombinant human thyroid peroxidase generated in eukaryotic cells: a source of specific antigen for immunological assay of antimicrosomal antibodies in the sera of patients with autoimmune thyroid disease. J Clin Endocrinol Metab 1990;70:724

46. Ruf J, Czarnocka B, Ferrand M, Doullais F, Carayon P. Novel routine assay of thyroperoxidase autoantibodies. Clin Chem 1988;34:2231

47. Mariotti S, Caturegh P, Piccolo P, Barbesino G, Pinchera A. Antithyroid peroxidase autoantibodies in thyroid diseases. J Clin Endocrinol Metab 1990;71:661

48. Takaichi Y, Tamai H, Honda K, Nagai K, Kuma K, Nakagawa T. The significance of antithyroglobulin and antithyroidal microsomal antibodies in patients with hyperthyroidism due to Graves' disease treated with antithyroidal drugs. J Clin Endocrinol Metab 1989;68:1097

49. Romaldini JH, Bromberg N, Werner RS, et al. Comparison of effects of high and low dosage regimens of antithyroid drugs in the management of Graves' hyperthyroidism. J Clin Endocrinol Metab 1983;57:563

50. Schade ROK, Owen SG, Smart GA, Hall R. The relation of thyroid autoimmunity to round-celled infiltration of the thyroid gland. J Clin Pathol 1960;13:499

51. Yoshida H, Amino N, Yagawa K, et al. Association of serum antithyroid antibodies with lymphocytic infiltration of the thyroid gland: study of 70 autopsied cases. J Clin Endocrinol Metab 1978;46:859

52. Paschke R, Vogg M, Swillens S, Usadel KH. Correlation of microsomal antibodies with the intensity of the intrathyroidal autoimmune process in Graves' disease. J Clin Endocrinol Metab 1993;77:939

53. Portman L, Hamada N, Heinrich G, DeGroot LJ. Anti-thyroid peroxidase antibody in patients with autoimmune thyroid disease: Possible identity with antimicrosomal antibody. J Clin Endocrinol Metab 1985;61:1001

54. Saller B, Hörmann R, Mann K. Heterogeneity of autoantibodies against thyroid peroxidase in autoimmune thyroid disease: evidence against antibodies directly inhibiting peroxidase activity as regulatory factors in thyroid hormone metabolism. J Clin Endocrinol Metab 1991;72:188

55. Horimoto M, Petersen VS, Pegg CAS, et al. Production and characterisation of a human monoclonal peroxidase autoantibody. Autoimmunity 1992;14:1

56. Rapoport B, McLachlan SM. Thyroid peroxidase as an autoantigen in autoimmune thyroid disease: update 1994. Endocr Rev Monographs 1994;3:96

57. Okamoto Y, Hamada N, Saito H, et al. Thyroid peroxidase activity-inhibiting immunoglobulins in patients with autoimmune thyroid disease. J Clin Endocrinol Metab 1989;68:730

58. Yokoyama N, Taurog A, Dorris ML, Klee GG. Studies with purified human thyroid peroxidase and thyroid microsomal autoantibodies. J Clin Endocrinol Metab 1990;70:758

59. Kohno Y, Hiyama Y, Shimojo N, Niimi H, Nakajima H, Hosoya T. Autoantibodies to thyroid peroxidase in patients with chronic thyroiditis: Effect of antibody binding on enzyme activities. Clin Exp Immunol 1986;65:534

60. Doble ND, Banga JP, Pope R, Lalor E, Kilduff P, McGregor AM. Antibodies to the thyroid microsomal/thyroid peroxidase antigen are polyclonal and directed to several distinct antigenic sites. Immunology 1988;64:23

61. Weetman AP, Black CM, Cohen SB, Tomlinson R, Banga JP, Breimer CB. Affinity purification of IgG subclasses and the distribution of thyroid autoantibody reactivity in Hashimoto's thyroiditis. Scand J Immunol 1989;30:73

62. Tonacchera M, Cetani F, Costagliola S, et al. Mapping thyroid peroxidase epitopes using recombinant protein fragments. Eur J Endocrinol 1995;132:53

63. Hamada N, Jaeduck N, Portman L, Ito K, DeGroot LJ. Antibodies against denatured and reduced thyroid microsomal antigen in autoimmune thyroid disease. J Clin Endocrinol Metab 1987;64:230

64. Hexham JM, Partridge LJ, Furmaniak J, et al. Cloning and characterisation of TPO autoantibodies using combinatorial phage display libraries. Autoimmunity 1994;17:167

65. Nishikawa T, Jaume JC, McLachlan SM, Rapoport B. Human monoclonal autoantibodies against the immunodominant region on thyroid peroxidase: lack of cross-reactivity with related peroxidases or thyroglobulin and inability to inhibit thyroid peroxidase enzymatic activity. J Clin Endocrinol Metab 1995;80:1461

66. Jaume JC, Costante G, Nishikawa T, Phillips IW, Rapoport B, McLachlan SM. Thyroid peroxidase autoantibody fingerprints in hypothyroid and euthyroid individuals. I. Cross-sectional study in elderly women. J Clin Endocrinol Metab 1995;80:994

67. Jaume JC, Parkes AB, Lazarus JH, et al. Thyroid peroxidase autoantibody fingerprints. II. A longitudinal study in postpartum thyroiditis. J Clin Endocrinol Metab 1995;80:1000

68. Amino N, Mori H, Iwatani Y, et al. High prevalence of transient postpartum thyrotoxicosis and hypothyroidism. N Engl J Med 1982;306:849

69. Parkes AB, Othman S, Hall R, John R, Richards CJ, Lazarus JH. The role of complement in the pathogenesis of postpartum thyroiditis. J Clin Endocrinol Metab 1994;79:395

70. Jansson R, Karlsson FA, Linde A, Sjoberg O. Post-partum activation of autoimmunity: transient increase of total IgG levels in normal women and in women with autoimmune thyroiditis. Clin Exp Immunol 1987;70:68

71. Stagnaro-Green A, Roman SH, Cobin RH, El-Harazy E, Wallenstein S, Davies TF. A prospective study of lymphocyte-initiated immunosuppression in normal pregnancy: evidence of a T-cell etiology for postpartum thyroid dysfunction. J Clin Endocrinol Metab 1992;74:645

72. Jansson R, Thompson PM, Clark F, McLachlan SM. Association between thyroid microsomal antibodies of subclass IgG-1 and hypothyroidism in autoimmune postpartum thyroiditis. Clin Exp Immunol 1986;63:80

73. Briones-Urbina R, Parkes AB, Bogner U, Mariotti S, Walfish PG. Increase in antimicrosomal antibody-related IgG1 and IgG4, and titers of antithyroid peroxidase antibodies, but not antibody dependent cell-mediated cytotoxicity in post-partum thyroiditis with transient hyperthyroidism. J Endocrinol Invest 1990;13:879

74. Weetman AP, Fung HYM, Richards CJ, McGregor AM. IgG subclass distribution and relative functional affinity of thyroid mi-

crosomal antibodies in postpartum thyroiditis. Eur J Clin Invest 1990;20:133

75. Gerstein HC. Incidence of postpartum thyroid dysfunction in patients with type I diabetes mellitus. Ann Intern Med 1993;118:419

76. Alvarez-Marfany M, Roman SH, Drexler AJ, Robertson C, Stagnaro-Green A. Long-term prospective study of postpartum thyroid dysfunction in women with insulin dependent diabetes mellitus. J Clin Endocrinol Metab 1994;79:10

77. Kotani T, Umeki K, Yagihashi S, Hirai K, Ohtaki S. Identification of thyroiditogenic epitope on porcine thyroid peroxidase for C57BL/6 mice. J Immunol 1992;148:2084

78. Bass HZ, Yamashita N, Clement LT. Heterogenous mechanisms of human cytotoxic T lymphocyte generation. I. Differential helper cell requirement for the generation of cytotoxic effector cells from CD8+ precursor subpopulations. J Immunol 1992; 149:2489

79. Berke G. The binding and lysis of target cells by cytotoxic lymphocytes: molecular and cellular aspects. Ann Rev Immunol 1994;12:735

80. Wu Z, Podack ER, McKenzie JM, Olsen KJ, Zakarija M. Perforin expression by thyroid-infiltrating T cells in autoimmune thyroid disease. Clin Exp Immunol 1994;98:470

81. Podack ER. T-cell effector functions: mechanisms for delivery of cytotoxicity and help. Annu Rev Cell Biol 1991;7:479

82. Iwatani Y, Hidaka Y, Matsuzuka F, Kuma K, Amino N. Intrathyroidal lymphocyte subsets, including unusual CD4+CD8+ cells and CD3^{lo}TCRαβ$^{lo/-}$CD4$^-$CD8$^-$ cells, in autoimmune thyroid disease. Clin Exp Immunol 1993;93:430

83. Robertson MJ, Ritz J. Biology and clinical relevance of human natural killer cells. Blood 1990;76:2421

84. Kitagawa Y, Greiner DL, Keynolds CW, et al. Islet cells but not thyrocytes are susceptible to lysis by NK cells. J Autoimmun 1991;4:703

85. Matsubayashi S, Akasu F, Kosuga Y, Jamieson C, Volpé R. Interleukin 2-activated killer cells do not mediate autologous lysis in autoimmune thyroid disease in vitro. Thyroid 1991;1:151

86. Bogner U, Schleusener H, Wall JR. Antibody-dependent cell mediated cytotoxicity against human thyroid cells in Hashimoto's thyroiditis but not Graves' disease. J Clin Endocrinol Metab 1984;59:734

87. Bogner U, Wall J, Schleusener H. Cellular and antibody mediated cytotoxicity in autoimmune thyroid disease. Acta Endocrinol 1987;281(Suppl):133

88. Bogner U, Kotulla P, Peters H, Schleusener H. Thyroid peroxidase/microsomal antibodies are not identical with thyroid cytotoxic antibodies in autoimmune thyroiditis. Acta Endocrinol 1990;123:431

89. Bogner U, Hegedüs L, Hansen JM, Finke R, Schleusener H. Thyroid cytotoxic antibodies in atrophic and goitrous autoimmune thyroiditis. Eur J Endocrinol 1995;132:69

90. Hiromatsu Y, Fukazawa H, Guinard F, Salvi M, How J, Wall JR. A thyroid cytotoxic antibody that cross-reacts with an eye-muscle cell surface antigen may be the cause of thyroid-associated ophthalmopathy. J Clin Endocrinol Metab 1988;67:565

91. Hiromatsu Y, Cadarso L, Salvi M, Wall JR. Significance of cytotoxic eye muscle antibodies in patients with thyroid-associated ophthalmopathy. Autoimmunity 1990;5:205

92. Rodien P, Madec AM, Morel Y, Stefanutti A, Bornet H, Orgiazzi J. Assessment of antibody dependent cell cytotoxicity in autoimmune thyroid disease using porcine thyroid cells. Autoimmunity 1992;13:177

93. Bogner U, Grüters A, Sigle B, Helge H, Schleusener H. Cytotoxic antibodies in congenital hypothyroidism. J Clin Endocrinol Metab 1989;68:671

94. McKenzie JM, Zakarija M. Fetal and neonatal hyperthyroidism and hypothyroidism due to maternal TSH receptor antibodies. Thyroid 1992;2:155

95. Blizzard RM, Chandler RW, Landing BH, Pettit MD, West CD. Maternal autoimmunization to thyroid as a probable cause of athyrotic cretinism. N Engl J Med 1960;263:327

96. Sutherland JM, Esselborn VM, Burket RL, Skillman TB, Benson JT. Familial nongoitrous cretinism apparently due to maternal antithyroid antibody. Report of a family. N Engl J Med 1960;263:336

97. Amino N, Aozasa M, Tamaki H, et al. Peripheral natural killer (NK) lymphocytes in autoimmune thyroid disease. In: Medeiros-Neto G, Gaitan E, eds. Frontiers in thyroidology. New York:Plenum Medical, 1985:1381

98. Hidaka Y, Amino N, Iwatani Y, et al. Increase in peripheral natural killer cell activity in patients with autoimmune thyroid disease. Autoimmunity 1992;11:239

99. Wall JR, Baur R, Schleusener H, Bandy-Dafoe P. Peripheral blood and intrathyroidal mononuclear cell populations in patients with autoimmune thyroid disorders enumerated using monoclonal antibodies. J Clin Endocrinol Metab 1983;56:164

100. Papic M, Stein-Streilein J, Zakarija M, McKenzie JM, Guffee J, Fletcher MA. Suppression of peripheral blood natural killer cell activity by excess thyroid hormone. J Clin Invest 1987;79:404

101. Pedersen BK, Feldt-Rasmussen U, Bech K, Perrild H, Klarlund K, Hoier-Madsen M. Characterization of natural killer activity in Hashimoto's and Graves' diseases. Allergy 1989;44:477

102. Wang P, Luo S, Huang B, Lin J, Huang M. Depressed natural killer activity in Graves' disease and during antithyroid medication. Clin Endocrinol 1988;28:205

103. Tezuka H, Eguchi K, Fukuda T, et al. Natural killer and natural killer-like cell activity of peripheral blood and intrathyroidal mononuclear cells from patients with Graves' disease. J Clin Endocrinol Metab 1988;66:702

104. Sack J, Baker JR Jr, Weetman AP, Wartofsky L, Burman KD. Killer cell activity and antibody-dependent cell-mediated cytotoxicity are normal in Hashimoto's disease. J Clin Endocrinol Metab 1986;62:1059

105. Marazuela M, Vargas JA, Alvarez-Mon M, Albarrán F, Lucas T, Durántez A. Impaired natural killer cytotoxicity in peripheral blood mononuclear cells in Graves' disease. Eur J Endocrinol 1995;132:175

106. Hayslip CC, Baker JR Jr, Wartofsky L, Klein TA, Opsahl MS, Burman KD. Natural killer cell activity and serum autoantibodies in women with postpartum thyroiditis. J Clin Endocrinol Metab 1988;66:1089

107. Dussault JH, Letarte J, Guyda H, Laberge C. Lack of influence of thyroid antibodies on thyroid function in the newborn infant and on a mass screening program for congenital hypothyroidism. J Pediatr 1980;96:385

108. Janeway CA Jr, Travers P. Immunobiology—The immune system in health and disease. New York:Garland, 1994

109. Oleesky DA, Ratanachaiyavong S, Ludgate M, Morgan BP, Campbell AK, McGregor AM. Complement component C9 in Graves' disease. Clin Endocrinol 1986;25:623

110. Weetman AP, Cohen SB, Oleesky DA, Morgan BP. Terminal complement complexes and C1/C1 inhibitor complexes in autoimmune thyroid disease. Clin Exp Immunol 1989;77:25

111. Tandon N, Yan SL, Morgan BP, Weetman AP. Expression and function of multiple regulators of complement activation in autoimmune thyroid disease. Immunology 1994;81:643

112. Chiovato L, Bassi P, Santini F, et al. Antibodies producing complement-mediated thyroid cytotoxicity in patients with atrophic or goitrous autoimmune thyroiditis. J Clin Endocrinol Metab 1993;77:1700

113. Zakarija M, McKenzie JM. The spectrum and significance of autoantibodies reacting with the thyrotropin receptor. Endocrinol Metab Clin North Am 1987;16:343

114. Smith BR, McLachlan SM, Furmaniak J. Autoantibodies to the thyrotropin receptor. Endocr Rev 1988;9:106

115. Vassart G, Dumont JE. The thyrotropin receptor and the regulation of thyrocyte function and growth. Endocr Rev 1992;13:61

116. Rapoport B, Nagayama Y. The thyrotropin receptor 25 years after its discovery: new insight after its molecular cloning. Mol Endocrinol 1992;6:145

117. Vassart G, Parma J, Van Sande J, Dumont JE. The thyrotropin receptor and the regulation of thyrocyte function and growth: update 1994. Endocr Rev Monographs 1994;3:77

118. Adams DD, Purves HD. Abnormal responses in the assay of thyrotrophin. Proc Univ Otago Med Sch 1956;34:11

119. McKenzie JM. Delayed thyroid response to serum from thyrotoxic patients. Endocrinology 1958;62:865

120. McKenzie JM. Humoral factors in the pathogenesis of Graves' disease. Physiol Rev 1968;34:252

121. Kriss JP, Pleshakov V, Chien JR. Isolation and identification of the long acting thyroid stimulator and its relation to hyperthyroidism and circumscribed pretibial myxedema. J Clin Endocrinol Metab 1964;24:1005

122. Endo K, Kasagi K, Konishi J, et al. Detection and properties of TSH-binding inhibitor immunoglobulins in patients with Graves' disease and Hashimoto's thyroiditis. J Clin Endocrinol Metab 1978;46:734

123. Matsuura N, Yamada Y, Nohara Y, et al. Familial neonatal transient hypothyroidism due to maternal TSH-binding inhibitor immunoglobulins. N Engl J Med 1980;303:738

124. Konishi J, Iida Y, Kasagi K, et al. Primary myxedema with thyrotrophin-binding inhibitor immunoglobulins. Ann Intern Med 1985;103:26

125. Zakarija M, McKenzie JM, Eidson MS. Transient neonatal hypothyroidism: Characterization of maternal antibodies to the thyrotropin receptor. J Clin Endocrinol Metab 1990;70:1239

126. Brown RS, Keating P, Mitchell E. Maternal thyroid-blocking immunoglobulins in congenital hypothyroidism. J Clin Endocrinol Metab 1990;70:1341

127. Orgiazzi J, Williams DE, Chopra IJ, Solomon DH. Human thyroid adenyl cyclase stimulating activity in immunoglobulin G of patients with Graves' disease. J Clin Endocrinol Metab 1976; 42:341

128. Holmes SD, Dirmikis SM, Martin TJ, Munro DS. Effects of human thyroid-stimulating hormone and immunoglobulins on adenylate cyclase activity and the accumulation of cyclic AMP in human thyroid membranes and slices. J Endocrinol 1978;79:121

129. Bech K, Madsen SN. Thyroid adenylate cyclase stimulating immunoglobulins in thyroid disease. Clin Endocrinol 1979;11:47

130. McKenzie JM, Zakarija M. A reconsideration of a thyroid-stimulating-immunoglobulin as the cause of hyperthyroidism in Graves' disease. J Clin Endocrinol Metab 1976;42:778

131. Zakarija M, McKenzie JM, Banovac K. Clinical significance of assay of thyroid-stimulating antibody in Graves' disease. Ann Intern Med 1980;93:28

132. Rapoport B, Filetti S, Takai N, Seto P, Halverson G. Studies on the cyclic AMP response to thyroid stimulating immunoglobulin (TSI) and thyrotropin (TSH) in human thyroid cell monolayers. Metabolism 1982;31:1159

133. Kasagi K, Konishi J, Iida Y, et al. A new in vitro assay for human thyroid stimulator using cultured thyroid cells: effect of sodium chloride on adenosine 3'5'-monophosphate increase. J Clin Endocrinol Metab 1982;54:108

134. Rapoport B, Greenspan FS, Filetti S, Pepitone M. Clinical experience with a human thyroid cell bioassay for thyroid-stimulating immunoglobulin. J Clin Endocrinol Metab 1984;58:332

135. Ambesi-Impiombato FS, Parks LAM, Coon HF. Culture of hormone-dependent epithelial cells from rat thyroids. Proc Natl Acad Sci U S A 1980;77:3455

136. Vitti P, Rotella CM, Valente WA, et al. Characterization of the optimal stimulatory effects of Graves' monoclonal and serum IgGs on cyclic AMP production in FRTL-5 cells: a potential clinical assay. J Clin Endocrinol Metab 1983;57:782

137. Kasagi K, Konishi J, Iida Y, et al. A sensitive and practical assay for thyroid-stimulating antibodies using FRTL-5 thyroid cells. Acta Endocrinol 1987;115:30

138. Ludgate M, Perret J, Parmentier M, et al. Use of a recombinant human receptor (TSH-R) expressed in mammalian cell lines to assay TSH-R autoantibodies. Mol Cell Endocrinol 1990;73:R13

139. Vitti P, Elisei R, Tonacchera M, et al. Detection of thyroid-stimulating antibody using Chinese hamster ovary cells transfected with cloned human thyrotropin receptor. J Clin Endocrinol Metab 1993;76:499

140. Mehdi SQ, Nussey SS. A radio-ligand receptor assay for the long-acting thyroid stimulator. Biochem J 1975;145:105

141. Southgate K, Creagh F, Teece M, Kingswood C, Smith BR. A receptor assay for the measurement of TSH receptor antibodies in unextracted serum. Clin Endocrinol 1984;20:539

142. Costagliola S, Swillens S, Niccoli P, Dumont JE, Vassart G. Binding assay for thyrotropin receptor autoantibodies using the recombinant receptor protein. J Clin Endocrinol Metab 1992; 75:1540

143. Zakarija M, Garcia A, McKenzie JM. Studies on multiple thyroid cell membrane-directed antibodies in Graves' disease. J Clin Invest 1985;76:1885

144. Lu C, Kasagi K, Hidaka A, Hatabu H, Iida Y, Konishi J. Simultaneous measurement of TSH-binding inhibitor immunoglobulin and thyroid stimulating autoantibody activities using cultured FRTL-5 cells in patients with untreated Graves' disease. Acta Endocrinol (Copenh) 1990;123:282

145. Filetti S, Foti D, Costante G, Rapoport B. Recombinant human thyrotropin (TSH) receptor in a radioreceptor assay for the measurement of TSH receptor antibodies. J Clin Endocrinol Metab 1991;72:1096

146. De Forteza R, Smith CU, Amin J, McKenzie JM, Zakarija M. Visualization of the thyrotropin receptor on the cell surface by potent autoantibodies. J Clin Endocrinol Metab 1994;78:1271

147. Kawai K, Tamai H, Mori T, et al. Thyroid histology of hyperthyroid Graves' disease with undetectable thyrotropin receptor antibodies. J Clin Endocrinol Metab 1993;77:716

148. Chiovato L, Vitti P, Santini F, et al. Incidence of antibodies blocking thyrotropin effect in vitro in patients with euthyroid or hypothyroid autoimmune thyroiditis. J Clin Endocrinol Metab 1990; 71:40

149. Cho BY, Shong YK, Lee HK, Koh C-S, Min HK. Inhibition of thyrotrophin-stimulated adenylate cyclase activation and growth of rat thyroid cells, FRTL-5, by immunoglobulin G from patients with primary myxedema: comparison with activities of thyrotrophin-binding inhibitor immunoglobulins. Acta Endocrinol 1989;120:99

150. Chiovato L, Vitti P, Bendinelli G, et al. Detection of antibodies blocking thyrotropin effect using Chinese hamster ovary cells transfected with the cloned human TSH receptor. J Endocrinol Invest 1994;17:809

151. Zakarija M, De Forteza R, McKenzie JM, Ghandur-Mnaymneh L. Characteristics and clinical correlates of a novel thyroid-stimulating autoantibody. Autoimmunity 1994;19:31

152. Macchia E, Concetti R, Carone G, Borgoni F, Fenzi GF, Pinchera A. Demonstration of blocking immunoglobulins G, having a heterogenous behaviour, in sera of patients with Graves' disease: possible coexistence of different autoantibodies directed at the TSH receptor. Clin Endocrinol 1988;28:147

153. Kasagi K, Takeda K, Goshi K, et al. Presence of both stimulating and blocking types of TSH-receptor antibodies in sera from three patients with primary hypothyroidism. Clin Endocrinol 1990;32:253

154. McKenzie JM, Zakarija M. The clinical use of thyrotropin receptor antibody measurements. J Clin Endocrinol Metab 1989;69:1093

155. Zakarija M, McKenzie JM, Munro DS. Evidence of an IgG inhibitor of thyroid-stimulating antibody (TSAb) as a cause of delay in the onset of neonatal Graves' disease. J Clin Invest 1983;72:1352

156. Edan G, Massart C, Hody B, et al. Optimum duration of antithyroid drug treatment determined by assay of thyroid antibody in patients with Graves' disease. BMJ 1989;298:359

157. Schleusener H, Schwander J, Fischer C, et al. Prospective multicentre study on the prediction of relapse after antithyroid drug treatment in patients with Graves' disease. Acta Endocrinol 1980;120:689

158. Wilson R, McKillop JH, Thomson JA. The prognostic value of thyrotropin receptor antibody (TRAb) levels in Graves' disease. Ann Clin Biochem 1990;27:601

159. Ikenoue H, Okamura K, Sato K, et al. Prediction of relapse in drug-treated Graves' disease using thyroid stimulation indices. Acta Endocrinol 1991;125:643

160. McKenzie JM. Neonatal Graves' disease. J Clin Endocrinol Metab 1964;24:660

161. Zakarija M, McKenzie JM. Pregnancy-associated changes in the thyroid-stimulating antibody of Graves' disease and the relationship to neonatal hyperthyroidism. J Clin Endocrinol Metab 1983;57:1036

162. Dirmikis SM, Munro DS. Placental transmission of thyroid-stimulating immunoglobulin. BMJ 1975;2:665

163. Tamaki H, Amino N, Aozasa M, Mori M, Tanizawa O, Miyai K. Serial changes in thyroid-stimulating antibody and thyrotropin binding inhibitor immunoglobulin at the time of postpartum occurrence of thyrotoxicosis in Graves' disease. J Clin Endocrinol Metab 1987;65:324

164. Zakarija M, McKenzie JM, Hoffman WH. Prediction and therapy of intrauterine and late-onset neonatal hyperthyroidism. J Clin Endocrinol Metab 1986;62:368

165. Tamai H, Kasagi K, Takaichi Y, et al. Development of spontaneous hypothyroidism in patients with Graves' disease treated with antithyroidal drugs: clinical, immunological, and histological findings in 26 patients. J Clin Endocrinol Metab 1989;69:49

166. Fatourechi V, Gharib H. Hyperthyroidism following hypothyroidism: data on six cases. Arch Intern Med 1988;148:976

167. Takasu N, Yamada T, Sato A, et al. Graves' disease following hypothyroidism due to Hashimoto's disease: studies of eight cases. Clin Endocrinol 1990;6:687

168. Takasu N, Yamada T, Takasu M, et al. Disappearance of thyrotropin-blocking antibodies and spontaneous recovery from hypothyroidism in autoimmune thyroiditis. N Engl J Med 1992;326:513

168a. Zakarija M, McKenzie JM. Isoelectric focusing of thyroid-stimulating antibody of Graves' disease. Endocrinology 1978;103:1469

169. Kriss JP. Inactivation of long-acting thyroid stimulator (LATS) by anti-kappa and anti-lambda antisera. J Clin Endocrinol Metab 1968;24:1440

170. Maisey MN. The Ig class and light chain type of the long-acting thyroid stimulator. Clin Endocrinol 1972;1:189

171. Zakarija M. Immunochemical characterization of the thyroid-stimulating antibody (TSAb) of Graves' disease: evidence for restricted heterogeneity. J Clin Lab Immunol 1983;10:77

172. Knight J, Laing P, Knight A, Adams D, Ling N. Thyroid-stimulating autoantibodies usually contain only λ-light chains: evidence for the "forbidden clone" theory. J Clin Endocrinol Metab 1986;62:342

173. Williams RC, Marshall NJ, Kilpatrick K, et al. Kappa/lambda immunoglobulin distribution in Graves' thyroid-stimulating antibodies. J Clin Invest 1988;82:1306

174. Weetman AP, Yateman ME, Ealey PA, et al. Thyroid-stimulating antibody activity between different immunoglobulin G subclasses. J Clin Invest 1990;86:723

175. Kraiem Z, Cho BY, Sadeh O, Shong MH, Pickerill P, Weetman AP. The IgG subclass distribution of TSH receptor blocking antibodies in primary hypothyroidism. Clin Endocrinol 1992;37:135

176. Zakarija M, McKenzie JM. A novel thyroid-stimulating antibody that is distinct from TSAb. In: Gordon A, Gross J, Hennemann G, eds. Progress in thyroid research. Rotterdam: AA Balkema, 1991:461

177. Tokuda Y, Kasagi K, Iida Y, et al. Inhibition of thyrotropin-stimulated iodide uptake in FRTL-5 thyroid cells by crude immunoglobulin fractions from patients with goitrous and atrophic autoimmune thyroiditis. J Clin Endocrinol Metab 1988;67:251

178. Chen W, Inui T, Ochi Y, Kajita Y. Studies on the action of thyroid stimulation blocking antibody (TSBAb) on thyroid cell membrane. Thyroid 1994;4:479

179. Desai RK, Dallas JS, Gupta MK, et al. Dual mechanism of perturbation of thyrotropin-mediated activation of thyroid cells by antibodies to the thyrotropin receptor (TSHR) and TSH-derived peptides. J Clin Endocrinol Metab 1993;77:658

180. Nagayama Y, Rapoport B. Thyroid stimulatory autoantibodies in different patients with autoimmune thyroid disease do not all recognize the same components of the human thyrotropin receptor: selective role of receptor amino acids Ser 25-Glu 30. J Clin Endocrinol Metab 1992;75:1425

181. Kosugi S, Ban T, Akamizu T, Kohn LD. Identification of separate determinants on the thyrotropin receptor reactive with Graves' thyroid-stimulating antibodies with thyroid-stimulating blocking antibodies in idiopathic myxedema: these determinants have no homologous sequence on gonadotropin receptors. Mol Endocrinol 1992;6:168

182. Kosugi S, Ban T, Kohn LD. Identification of thyroid-stimulating antibody-specific interaction sites in the N-terminal region of the thyrotropin receptor. Mol Endocrinol 1993;7:114

183. Kosugi S, Ban T, Akamizu T, Valente W, Kohn LD. Use of thyrotropin receptor (TSHR) mutants to detect stimulating TSHR antibodies in hypothyroid patients with idiopathic myxedema, who have blocking TSHR antibodies. J Clin Endocrinol Metab 1993;77:19

184. Libert F, Ludgate M, Dinsart C, Vassart G. Thyroperoxidase, but not the thyrotropin receptor, contains sequential epitopes recognized by autoantibodies in recombinant peptides expressed in the pUEX vector. J Clin Endocrinol Metab 191;73:857

185. Carayanniotis G, Huang GC, Nicholson LB, et al. Unaltered thyroid function in mice responding to a highly immunogenic thyrotropin receptor: implications for the establishment of a mouse model for Graves' disease. Clin Exp Immunol 1995;99:294

186. Weetman AP, McGregor AM, Wheeler MH, Hall R. Extrathyroidal sites of autoantibody synthesis in Graves' disease. Clin Exp Immunol 1984;56:330

187. Tew JG, DiLosa RM, Burton GF, et al. Germinal center and antibody production in bone marrow. Immunol Rev 1992;126:99

188. Bachmann MF, Kündig TM, Odermatt B, Hengartner H, Zinkernagel RM. Free recirculation of memory B cells versus antigen-dependent differentiation to antibody-forming cells. J Immunol 1994;153:3386

189. McLachlan SM, Pegg CAS, Atherton MC, Middleton SL, Clark F, Smith BR. TSH receptor antibody synthesis by thyroid lymphocytes. Clin Endocrinol 1986;24:223

190. Levis S, Ghandur-Mnaymneh L, McKenzie JM, Zakarija M. Evaluation of the biological significance of leukocyte infiltration of the thyroid in Graves' disease. Int Arch Allergy Immunol 1992; 99:37

191. Grubeck-Loebenstein B, Turner M, Pirich K, et al. CD4⁺ T-cell clones from autoimmune thyroid tissue cannot be classified according to their lymphokine production. Scand J Immunol 1990;32:433

192. Watson PF, Pickerill AP, Davies R, Weetman AP. Analysis of cytokine gene expression in Graves' disease and multinodular goiter. J Clin Endocrinol Metab 1994;79:355

193. Sakata S. Autoimmunity against thyroid hormones. Crit Rev Immunol 1994;14:157

194. Akamizu T, Mori T, Kasagi K, et al. Anti-TSH antibody with high specificity to human TSH in sera from a patient with Graves' disease: Its isolation from, and interaction with, TSH receptor antibodies. Clin Endocrinol 1987;26:311

195. Noh J, Hamada N, Saito H, et al. Evidence against the importance in the disease process of antibodies to bovine thyroid-stimulating hormone found in some patients with Graves' disease. J Clin Endocrinol Metab 1989;68:107

196. Ochi Y, Nagamune T, Nakajima Y, et al. Anti-TSH antibodies in Graves' disease and their failure to interact with TSH receptor antibodies. Acta Endocrinol 1989;120:773

197. Boscato LM, Stuart MC. Heterophilic antibodies: a problem for all immunoassays. Clin Chem 1988;34:27

198. Kahn BB, Weintraub BD, Csako G, Zweig MH. Factitious elevation of thyrotropin in a new ultrasensitive assay: implications for the use of monoclonal antibodies in "sandwich" immunoassay. J Clin Endocrinol Metab 1988;66:526

199. Naffziger HC. Pathologic changes in the orbit in progressive exophthalmos, with special reference to alterations in the extraocular muscles and the optic disks. Arch Ophthalmol 1933;9:1

200. Gorman CA. Temporal relationship between onset of Graves' ophthalmopathy and diagnosis of thyrotoxicosis. Mayo Clin Proc 1983;58:515

201. Kiljanski JI, Nebes V, Wall JR. The ocular muscle cell is a target of the immune system in endocrine ophthalmopathy. Int Arch Allergy Immunol 1995;106:204

202. Bahn RS. The fibroblast is the target cell in the connective tissue manifestations of Graves' disease. Int Arch Allergy Immunol 1995;106:213

203. Mullin BR, Levinson RE, Friedman A, Henson DE, Winand RJ, Kohn LD. Delayed hypersensitivity in Graves' disease and exophthalmos: identification of thyroglobulin in normal human eye muscle. Endocrinology 1977;100:351

204. Tao TW, Chang PJ, Phan PH, Leu SL, Kriss JP. Monoclonal antithyroglobulin antibodies derived from immunizations of mice with human eye muscle and thyroid membranes. J Clin Endocrinol Metab 1986;63:577

205. Feliciello A, Porcellini A, Ciullo I, Bonavolonta G, Avvedimento EV, Fenzi G. Expression of thyrotropin-receptor mRNA in healthy and Graves' disease retro-orbital tissue. Lancet 1993; 342:337

206. Heufelder AE, Dutton CM, Sarkar G, Donovan KA, Bahn RS. Detection of TSH receptor RNA in cultured fibroblasts from patients with Graves' ophthalmopathy and pretibial dermopathy. Thyroid 1993;3:297

207. Paschke R, Metcalfe A, Alcalde L, Vassart G, Weetman A, Ludgate M. Presence of nonfunctional thyrotropin receptor variant transcripts in retroocular and other tissues. J Clin Endocrinol Metab 1994;79:1234

208. Tandon N, Yan SL, Arnold K, Metcalfe RA, Weetman AP. Immunoglobulin class and subclass distribution of eye muscle and fibroblast antibodies in patients with thyroid-associated ophthalmopathy. Clin Endocrinol 1994;40:629

209. McLachlan SM, Prummel MF, Dallow RL, Wiersinga WM, Rapoport B. Amplification by polymerase chain reaction of immunoglobulin heavy and light chain genes from orbital tissue of patients with Graves' ophthalmopathy. Autoimmunity 1993; 16:149

210. Prummel MF, Chazenbalk G, Jaume JC, Rapoport B, McLachlan SM. Profile of lambda light chain variable region genes in Graves' orbital tissue. Mol Immunol 1994;31:793

211. Fatourechi V, Pajouhi M, Fransway A. Dermopathy of Graves' disease (pretibial myxedema). Review of 150 cases. Medicine 1994;73:1

212. Smith TJ, Bahn RS, Gorman CA. Connective tissue, glycosaminoglycans, and diseases of the thyroid. Endocr Rev 1989;10:366

213. Tao TW, Leu SL, Kriss JP. Biological activity of autoantibodies associated with Graves' dermopathy. J Clin Endocrinol Metab 1989;69:90

214. Kohn LD, Alvarez F, Marcocci C, et al. Monoclonal antibody studies defining the origin and properties of autoantibodies in Graves' disease. Ann NY Acad Sci 1986;475:157

215. Bahn RS, Gorman CA, Johnson CM, Smith TJ. Presence of antibodies in the sera of patients with Graves' disease recognizing a 23 kilodalton fibroblast protein. J Clin Endocrinol Metab 1989; 69:622

216. Drexhage HA, Bottazzo GF, Doniach D. Thyroid growth stimulating and blocking immunoglobulins. In: Chayen J, Bitensky L, eds. Cytochemical bioassays. New York: Marcell Dekker, 1983:153

217. Wilders-Truschnig MM, Drexhage HA, Leb G, et al. Chromatographically purified immunoglobulin G of endemic and sporadic goiter patients stimulates FRTL-5 cell growth in a mitotic arrest assay. J Clin Endocrinol Metab 1990;70:444

218. Boyages SC, Halpern JP, Maberly GF, et al. Endemic cretinism: possible role for thyroid autoimmunity. Lancet 1989;2:529

219. Zakarija M, McKenzie JM. Do thyroid growth-promoting immunoglobulins exist? J Clin Endocrinol Metab 1990;70:308

220. Katakura M, Yamada T, Aizawa T, et al. Presence of antideoxyribonucleic acid antibody in patients with hyperthyroidism of Graves' disease. J Clin Endocrinol Metab 1987;64:405

221. Baethge BA, Levine SN, Wolf RE. Antibodies to nuclear antigens in Graves' disease. J Clin Endocrinol Metab 1988;66:485

222. McDermott MT, West SG, Emlen JW, Kidd GS. Antideoxyribonucleic acid antibodies in Graves' disease. J Clin Endocrinol Metab 1990;71:509

Werner and Ingbar's The Thyroid, Seventh Edition,
edited by Lewis E. Braverman and Robert D. Utiger.
Lippincott–Raven Publishers, Philadelphia, © 1996

22

Non-isotopic Techniques for Imaging the Thyroid

Anthony S. Jennings

During the past 25 years, our ability to image organs for clinical diagnosis and research has expanded rapidly. With the use of high resolution real-time ultrasonography, computed tomography, and magnetic resonance imaging, we can now visualize anatomic detail within the thyroid gland and the relationships between the thyroid gland and other structures within the neck and mediastinum as never before. The techniques require varying degrees of sophistication, expense, and patient cooperation, and each has inherent advantages and disadvantages. However, technical advances in thyroid imaging have not been accompanied by increased specificity for tissue diagnosis. Furthermore, these techniques are not cost-effective or necessary in most clinical situations. This chapter reviews the non-isotopic thyroid imaging techniques, and provides a framework for using them in clinical practice.

ULTRASONOGRAPHY

The superficial location of the thyroid gland makes it an ideal structure to study with ultrasound. After its introduction in the 1960s, ultrasound proved valuable in determining the volume, size, and dimensions of the thyroid.[1] In the 1970s, it was found to distinguish cystic from solid lesions of the thyroid.[2] The introduction of the small-parts transducer and high-resolution real-time sonography made thyroid ultrasonography easier to perform and greatly increased its use. The present-generation equipment allows high-resolution, real-time imaging of the thyroid, including visualization of vascular flow to and from the gland.[3–7] Ultrasound is highly sensitive in detecting thyroid lesions and distinguishing solid lesions from simple and complex cysts.[8] However, it cannot distinguish between benign and malignant lesions, and its clinical value is now limited.[2,5,7,9–11]

Principles

Ultrasonography is based on the interaction with and reflection of high frequency sound waves by tissues. This reflection depends on the ultrasound frequency and a property of tissues called *acoustic impedance*. Sound waves entering tissue can be either transmitted through it or reflected (echoed). Transmitted sound waves undergo progressive loss of intensity (attenuation), which is greater for high-frequency waves. The depth of tissue penetration is inversely related to wave attenuation and therefore is the least for high-frequency waves. Conversely, structural resolution is best attained with sound waves of high frequency. The frequency used to visualize the thyroid (7.5 to 10.0 million cycles/sec [mHz]) is a compromise between the need for depth of penetration and that for resolution.

The ease and clarity with which tissues can be distinguished depends on differences in their accoustic impedance. Small punctate calcifications have a much higher accoustic impedance than other tissues, so that calcifications of 1 mm or less in size can be seen. In contrast, large thyroid nodules with accoustic characteristics similar to normal thyroid tissue may be impossible to distinguish by ultrasound.

Ultrasound systems consist of a transducer that alternately transmits pulses of ultrasound and then receives the echoes and converts them to electrical signals that are processed and presented on a video screen as an image. Present ultrasound equipment produces images on a gray-scale monitor and has real-time capabilities, that is, 20 to 30 images per second are created. The real-time capabilities allow tissues that move or pulsate (arteries, veins, or the esophagus) to be distinguished from static structures such as the thyroid or lymph nodes and permits more rapid and thorough visualization of the thyroid. Newer transducers equipped with color-flow Doppler capabilities allow detection of blood vessels and determination of the velocity of blood flowing in them. Calibration of the equipment permits accurate determinations of the dimensions and volume of the thyroid and surrounding structures that correlate highly with pathologic determinations.[2,11–13]

Imaging Technique

Ultrasonography of the thyroid is best performed using real-time equipment with a small-parts high-resolution transducer. The transducer is coupled to the skin with oil or gel since ultrasound does not pass through air. With the patient supine and the neck hyperextended, the thyroid is palpated and its location in the neck noted. Images are obtained in the transverse (axial), longitudinal (sagittal), and oblique planes to visualize the lobes, isthmus, and surrounding structures. The lower poles of the thyroid occasionally extend into the thorax, in which case visualization is enhanced by having the patient swallow. Images can be recorded on film or videotape. The image quality and its clinical value are proportional to the diligence, skill, and knowledge of the person performing the procedure.

The Normal Thyroid Gland

The normal thyroid is characterized by its high-intensity, homogeneous echo pattern (Fig 22-1), and it can be distinguished from the anterior neck muscles because of their low echogenecity. The thyroid lobes are bordered posterolaterally by the sonolucent carotid artery and internal jugular vein and medially by the trachea. The internal jugular vein can be collapsed or expanded by having the patient perform a Valsalva maneuver. The tracheal rings are seen as cylinders of high echogenicity. The air in the trachea does not transmit ultrasound waves, making visualization of the posterior wall of the trachea difficult. The long muscle of the neck and neurovascular bundle containing the inferior thyroid artery and recurrent laryngeal nerve lie posteriorly to the lobes; the neurovascular bundle may be seen at the lower pole as a distinctive zone. The esophagus with its echogenic mucosa can be visualized behind the trachea on a lateral projection; seeing peristaltic activity with swallowing helps to identify it. The vertebrae behind the esophagus reflect ultrasound waves completely and may distort the scan.

Using a 10 mHz transducer, 1- to 3-mm cystic areas can be seen in 20% of persons with a normal thyroid gland; these areas may represent dilated thyroid follicles. Inspissated colloid within cystic follicles is seen as echogenic areas. Small nodules or areas of abnormal echogenicity are seen in the thyroid in 14% to 72% of normal subjects, the frequency being higher in women, increasing with each decade, and varying between countries.[14–20] In a recent study of healthy North American adults, 45% had multiple nodules and 22% had single nodules.[21] The importance of these abnormalities is unclear, but since incidental sonographic nodules are common, a conservative clinical approach is warranted.

The prevalence of goiter determined by ultrasonography is 3% to 10% and is higher in iodine-deficient countries.[20,22] Ultrasonography is the most sensitive technique for screening populations for goiter.

The parathyroid glands are not usually seen on routine thyroid ultrasound, but they can be identified with special effort if present in their usual locations.[23] They appear as flat or oval structures that are more sonolucent than the thyroid. Ultrasonography has a high sensitivity and specificity for localizing normally situated parathyroid adenomas, but it often fails to find adenomas in ectopic locations.[23–28] Adenomas appear as discrete solid nodules that are more hypoechoic than thyroid tissue. However, they vary from solid to predominantly cystic in appearance and may be indistinguishable from the thyroid.

The Abnormal Thyroid Gland

THYROID CYSTS

Thyroid cysts appear as circumscribed areas of greatly reduced or absent echogenicity,[2,11] because they reflect no echoes and minimally absorb the echo energy. As a result, the tissue behind a cyst has enhanced echogenicity. Varying degrees of echogenicity are seen when the cyst fluid contains debris or necrotic tissue.

True simple cysts are generally round, have a smooth discrete wall, and are anechoic (Fig 22-2). They represent less than 1% of all nodules; in one series of 550 patients with nodules, only one had a simple cyst.[7] Simple cysts are lined with squamous or columnar epithelium and are virtually always benign. Complex cysts have no epithelial lining (Fig 22-2) and are as likely to be a carcinoma as is a solid nodule. High-resolution ultrasonography has greatly improved visualization of septi and solid components within cysts, which has resulted in reclassification of many cysts previously thought to be simple into the complex cyst category. Cystic degeneration is present in 19% to 32% of thyroid carcinomas and up to 33% of all solid nodules.[29,30,31]

Acute hemorrhagic cysts of the thyroid appear as well-defined masses containing sonolucent areas with irregular borders and multiple internal septations. Hemorrhagic cysts occur most commonly in follicular adenomas, but occasionally they occur after trauma or needle aspiration biopsy. With time, the cyst develops a more sharply defined inner wall and may have a fluid-fluid level reflecting the presence of blood breakdown products and debris.

DIFFUSE THYROID DISEASE

The thyroid in goitrous autoimmune thyroiditis (Hashimoto's thyroiditis) is always abnormal on ultrasound studies, with decreased and inhomogeneous echogenicity.[5,7,32] The gland may be normal or increased in size and may have an irregular surface.[33] Small punctate calcifications appearing as hyperechoic areas with acoustic shadowing are occasionally present. Small discrete nodules are often seen, but sizable nodules are unusual and should raise the possibility of lymphoma or carcinoma.[33] Hashimoto's thyroiditis and multinodular goiter may appear similar on ultrasonography, and distinguishing between them may be difficult. The presence of areas of normal-appearing thyroid favors the diagnosis of multinodular goiter. In Graves' disease, the thyroid is usually enlarged and its echogenicity is inhomogeneous and normal to low in intensity, whereas normal-sized glands have a more uniform echo texture. Studies performed using color-flow Doppler equipment easily demonstrate the intense vascularity of the thyroid in Graves' disease.

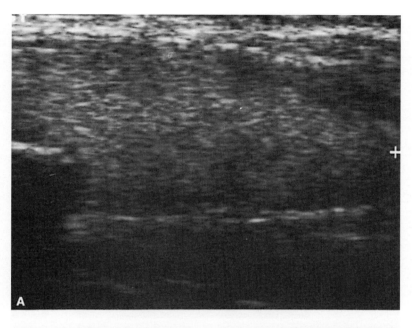

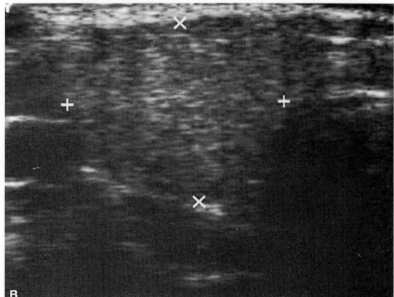

FIGURE 22-1. Ultrasound image of the normal thyroid gland showing longitudinal (A) and transverse (B) sections.

Simple goiters appear as diffusely enlarged glands with a uniform or irregular low-intensity echo pattern. Subacute thyroiditis appears as a normal to slightly enlarged gland with multiple areas of low echogenicity but no enhanced shadowing behind these areas.

MULTINODULAR GOITER

Multinodular goiters appear as large symmetric or asymmetric glands with an echographic texture that may be diffusely heterogenous or may have multiple discrete nodules interspersed throughout an otherwise normal-appearing gland.[7] Punctate calcifications are seen in 60% to 80% of patients. Many patients evaluated for single nodules are found to have additional small thyroid nodules; for example, in two studies of patients with single palpable nodules, 20% and 40% had additional nodules or a diffuse glandular abnormality.[5,34] Multiple nodules may be present in patients with a normal thyroid on physical examination.[4,21,35] It is often stated that demonstration of multiple nodules on ultrasonography (or another imaging study) in a patient with a single palpable nodule makes carcinoma unlikely, but several recent studies refute this notion; the malignant potential of any individual nodule should be based on clinical, cytologic, or histologic criteria.[34–36] In this regard, ultrasonography may be useful in guiding needle biopsy.[37–40]

Ultrasonography is rarely helpful in assessing the substernal extent of a goiter or mediastinal thyroid tissue. The transducer cannot usually be positioned to echo into the mediastinum and the bony thorax prevents penetration of sound waves.

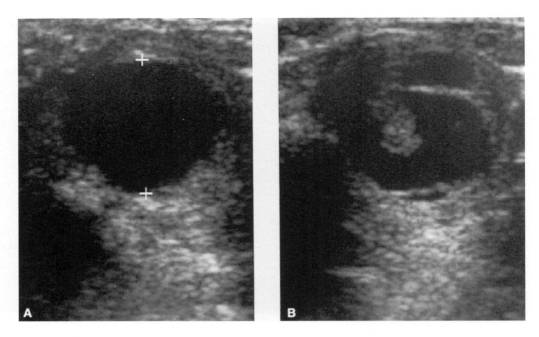

FIGURE 22-2. Ultrasound image of a simple thyroid cyst (A) and a complex thyroid cyst (B).

THYROID ADENOMAS

Both macrofollicular adenomas and cellular adenomas (microfollicular, fetal, embryonal, and Hürthle) appear on ultrasonography as discrete lesions of variable size and echogenicity (Fig 22-3). In a study of 79 patients with single follicular adenomas, 64 of the nodules showed decreased echogenicity, 10 had increased echogenicity, and 5 had the same echogenicity as normal thyroid tissue.[7] A sonolucent rim or halo demarcated the adenoma from the normal thyroid in 43 lesions, but was also seen in 2 patients with papillary carci-

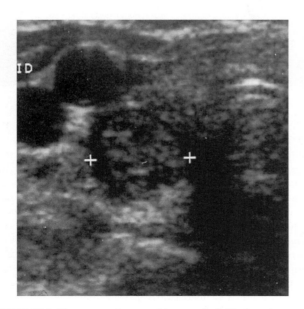

FIGURE 22-3. Transverse ultrasound image of a follicular adenoma of the thyroid (*seen between + symbols*).

noma. An echographic halo has also been seen in patients with follicular carcinoma. These observations render the finding of a sonographic halo nonspecific.[7,41,42]

Cysts of varying size and sonographic homogeneity are reported in 16% to 73% of follicular adenomas.[7,42] Adenomas greater than 2.5 to 3 cm in diameter commonly display the echographic characteristics of complex cysts; the cysts are irregularly shaped and have thick walls and irregular borders.

Small solid adenomas with uniformly low echogenicity can be mistaken for cysts but are distinguishable from cysts by the absence of enhanced echogenicity behind the area of low echogenicity. Increasing the gain setting may also increase the nodule's echogenicity.

THYROID CARCINOMA

The ultrasound appearance of thyroid carcinoma is highly variable. The carcinoma can be of any size and appear as a solid, partially cystic, or largely cystic mass, or even as a frond protruding into a large cyst. It is usually hypoechoic relative to normal thyroid, but can have the same echo texture as normal thyroid.[7,28,42] Calcifications are present in 50% to 80% of thyroid carcinomas.

Thyroid lymphomas appear as extremely hypoechoic masses, usually within a gland of decreased echogenicity because of coexisting Hashimoto's thyroiditis.[43] In approximately 50% of patients ultrasound studies show that the lymphoma involves both lobes, and it may extend into the soft tissues or lymph nodes of the neck.

In patients with medullary thyroid carcinoma, the tumors are solid masses containing punctate bright echogenic foci that correspond pathologically to deposits of calcium surrounded by amyloid.[44] Ultrasound is highly sensitive in detecting cervical lymph node metastases in these patients.[44,45]

Because of its sensitivity for detecting nodules as small as 1.5 to 2 mm, ultrasonography may be helpful in localizing and determining the extent of thyroid carcinoma in patients with lymphadenopathy or other evidence of metastatic disease in the neck. However, its specificity for carcinoma is quite low. No sonographic finding is characteristic of any type of thyroid carcinoma, and ultrasonography cannot differentiate benign from malignant nodules. Extension of tumor out of the thyroid into adjacent tissues or lymphadenopathy may suggest the diagnosis of thyroid carcinoma, but does not prove it. The presence of a prominent or discrete hypoechoic lesion in a patient with Hashimoto's thyroiditis should raise suspicion of lymphoma or carcinoma, but again is nonspecific. Because of the nonspecificity of ultrasonography, the need for biopsy or excision can be determined in most patients with clinically detected nodules without performing thyroid ultrasonography.[46,47]

In patients with known thyroid carcinoma, ultrasonography can detect local recurrence at a very early stage.[48] Recurrent cancer appears as sonolucent masses in the thyroid bed and adjacent tissues. In one series ultrasound was highly sensitive (96%) in detecting recurrent disease before clinically palpable abnormalities were detected.[49] However, the specificity of these findings was lower (83%), and abnormal findings on ultrasonography did not always indicate recurrent disease. Thus, ultrasonography is a sensitive technique for detecting recurrent thyroid carcinoma, especially in patients with carcinomas that do not concentrate radioactive iodine or in whom thyroidectomy was not completed.

ECTOPIC THYROID TISSUE

Ultrasound can identify neck masses as thyroidal in origin when there is clinical uncertainty.[50,51] Midline neck masses can be identified as ectopic thyroid tissue or a thyroglossal duct cyst, and occasionally thyroid carcinoma can be suspected in patients with midline cysts containing solid areas. In one study of 22 children with neck masses, ultrasonography localized the lesion to the thyroid in 12.[51]

COMPUTED TOMOGRAPHY

Computed tomography (CT) increases anatomic resolution by greatly increasing the distinction of differences in density between soft tissues. CT detects density differences as small as 0.5%, whereas conventional x-ray techniques detect density differences of 5% to 10%. CT also allows accurate measurement of the absorption of x-rays by tissues (the attenuation measurement), enabling individual tissues to be studied. This provides the basis for discriminating normal from abnormal tissues and allows exact localization of tumors. The noninvasive nature of CT further enhances its appeal.

The thyroid is visualized on CT because of its high endogenous iodine content, and serial sections through the gland provide a three-dimensional image. The resolution of CT is excellent and approximates the slice thickness (2–4 mm). The relationship of the thyroid to the trachea, esophagus, and surrounding structures is clearly evident and any extension of thyroid tissue into the mediastinum can be seen. The radiation dose to the thyroid is small (1–4 rads; 0.01–0.04 Gy) and collimation of the x-rays minimizes radiation exposure to the rest of the body. Short scanning times (1–3 sec/section) minimize the need for prolonged cooperation of the patient. The associated computer capabilities permit accurate, precise measurement of the dimensions, volume, and density of the normal thyroid and

of focal abnormalities. With proper calibration the iodine content of the thyroid can be quantified.[52,53]

Although most of the useful information regarding the thyroid can be obtained with unenhanced CT, intravenous administration of a radiographic contrast agent may be necessary to diagnose thyroid cysts and to visualize vascular relationships.[54] This poses the risk of an allergic reaction to the contrast agent, which is the most important complication of CT. Patients with large goiters occasionally cannot lie supine long enough to complete the study. Rarely, claustrophobic patients cannot tolerate being placed in the gantry, but this is much less common than with magnetic resonance imaging.

Principles of CT Imaging

CT depends on the attenuation of an x-ray beam as it passes through tissues. The extent of attenuation depends on the tissue constituents and density and the photon energy of the x-ray beam. The resolution is high because of the cumulative attenuation of x-ray beams passing through sections of the body from hundreds of angles and all directions within the plane of investigation. The x-rays are recorded by multiple detectors that generate and amplify an electrical signal. The data are digitized and stored in a computer, which reconstructs the thousands of data bits into an image. The brightness of each portion (pixel) of the final image is proportional to the degree that it attenuates the x-rays passing through it. The image is conventionally depicted in shades of gray, but it can also be shown in different colors.

Computer software programs allow the dimensions, volume, and density of the thyroid and abnormalities of it to be determined. The volume is determined by summing the volumes of the thyroid in each section; calculated CT volumes are usually within 10% of directly measured volumes.[54,55] The accuracy of the calculated volume may be affected by a low CT density at the periphery of the thyroid, observer error, or movement during the scanning. Density values are expressed in CT numbers (Hounsfield units, HU), which are related to the attenuation value of water. Using this scale, water has a value of 0 HU; air, −1000 HU; and bone, +1000 HU. In a typical section of the neck, muscle has a density of 40 to 70 HU; thyroid, 80 to 130 HU; and fat, −70 to −50 HU.[52-54] The CT density of the thyroid is closely correlated with its iodine content, and density can be used to estimate the iodine content.[52,53] There are considerable differences in the absolute CT numbers between most scanners and in the same tissue in different portions of the scan.[56] Finally, there is considerable overlap of CT density numbers in various thyroid abnormalities.[52] Thus, the absolute CT number is best used for making comparisons between tissues, such as the thyroid-to-muscle ratio.

Imaging Technique

CT of the thyroid is performed with the patient supine with the neck hyperextended.[54,57,58] This position maximally elevates the thyroid in the neck and minimizes streak artifacts caused by the shoulders. A frontal scan locates the landmarks of the neck, after which scanning is begun at the level of the vocal cords. During each scan (1–3 sec), the patient is asked to lie quietly without swallowing. Serial transverse sections of

2 to 5 mm thickness are taken from top to bottom through the entire gland. Thinner sections (1.5–2 mm) are used when searching for small lesions. The thyroid is usually visible 6 to 8 mm below the vocal cords and ends above the thoracic outlet. In patients with substernal extension of the thyroid, scanning is continued into the thorax to the lowest extent of the gland.

Injection of a radiographic contrast agent followed by a dynamic scanning sequence through areas of interest provides additional information.[54] The density of normal thyroid tissue and vascularized lesions increases as the contrast agent distributes within the vascular space. The density change of normal and abnormal areas is calculated and compared. The normal thyroid increases in density by 30 to 40 HU after contrast injection.

The Normal Thyroid Gland

The normal thyroid is sharply outlined on CT (Fig 22-4). Its density (80–130 HU) is always higher than surrounding tissues, and is usually 1½- to twofold greater than that of muscle. Administration of iodine for 3 to 7 days before the scan does not further enhance the density in subjects in the United States,[54] but modestly increases density in persons in areas of mild iodine deficiency.[58] The slight differences in density reported from country to country likely reflect differences in dietary iodine intake. The density decreases slightly with advancing age, and is similar in men and women. In older persons, the thyroid may not be as sharply demarcated from surrounding tissues as in younger persons without contrast injection.[59] Treatment with thyroid hormone decreases the CT density of the thyroid.[53,60]

The volume of the thyroid is greatest in young adults (range, 10–25 mL) and progressively declines with age, reaching mean volumes of 6 to 7 mL in persons older than 50 years.[54] The right lobe is on average about 20% larger than the left in all age groups. The inferior thyroid veins may be visible on two to three sections of the upper mediastinum, in which they appear as round areas of low signal intensity that enhance after contrast injection.[61]

The Abnormal Thyroid Gland

When the thyroid is diseased, its ability to concentrate iodine is usually decreased. Thus, most thyroid abnormalities have reduced density on CT and can be seen against a background of normal thyroid or when compared with the contralateral lobe. The exact density measurements have not been useful in distinguishing various disorders. The most useful information is obtained by comparing the density of a lesion to that of normal thyroid or the adjacent muscle.

THYROID CYSTS

Simple cysts appear as discrete smooth-walled homogeneous hypodense lesions surrounded by a rim of compressed normal thyroid tissue (Fig 22-5).[54] The rim thickness varies with the size and position of the cyst within the gland. The density of cyst fluid is always less than muscle, and there is little or no enhancement after contrast injection. Solid components and tissue fronds protruding into a cyst are easily seen and distinguish complex from simple cysts (Fig 22-5). Thick-walled cysts with an irregular inner surface suggest hemorrhage into an adenoma or carcinoma.

DIFFUSE THYROID DISEASE

Graves' disease causes thyroid enlargement with homogeneous or slightly inhomogeneous density on CT.[57] The total iodine content is increased, but the iodine concentration is decreased and accordingly so is the CT density[52,53,62,63]; the density is usually 50% to 70% of the normal value.[53,63]

Patients with Hashimoto's thyroiditis have a large thyroid gland with an irregular surface and inhomogeneous distribution of iodine. The CT density is decreased by 50% and is slightly lower in hypothyroid than in euthyroid patients.[53,64] As the CT number decreases, the thyroid volume typically increases.[64] Discrete asymmetric hypodense areas are uncommon in Hashimoto's thyroiditis and should raise the suspicion of lymphoma or carcinoma.

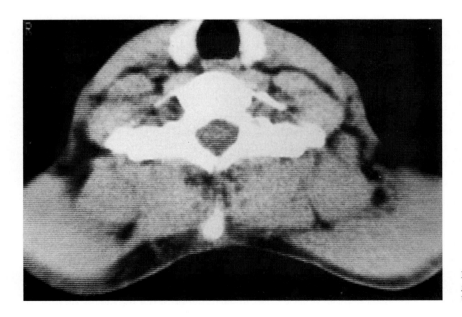

FIGURE 22-4. CT image of the normal thyroid gland. Each lobe can be seen lying alongside the trachea at the top of the picture.

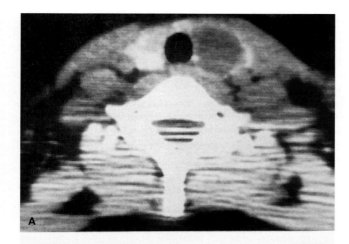

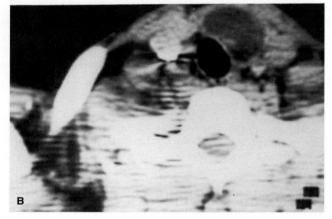

FIGURE 22-5. CT image of a simple thyroid cyst (A) and a complex thyroid cyst (B).

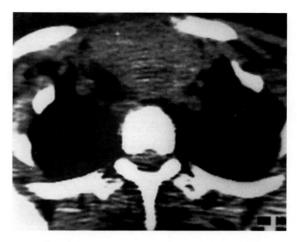

FIGURE 22-6. CT image of a multinodular goiter with substernal extension.

In subacute thyroiditis the gland is normal or increased in size and has decreased attenuation, which can be diffuse or focal depending on the extent of the disease.[65] Patients with acute suppurative thyroiditis have inhomogeneous enlargement of the affected lobe. As the infection progresses, loculated abscesses with decreased density may appear within the lobe, and the tissue overlying the thyroid may be thickened, suggestive of cellulitis.

Amyloid goiter can be recognized on CT as an enlarged thyroid gland with diffusely decreased density similar to fat.[66]

MULTINODULAR GOITER

Multinodular goiters appear as enlarged symmetric or asymmetric glands containing multiple low-density areas of varying degrees of discreteness[54,57] (Fig 22-6). The CT density is decreased but is highly variable from section to section. After contrast injection, the goiter may enhance uniformly; the areas that do not enhance contain hemorrhage, necrosis, or cysts. Areas of calcification are present in 50% to 60% of multinodular goiters. Compression of the trachea, esophagus, and great vessels is easily ascertained. Normal values for the area of the trachea have been established and permit estimation of tracheal compression.[67]

Multinodular goiters extend into the thorax in 20% of patients.[68-70] The extension is usually into the anterior mediastinum, but may be posterior as well. Several characteristics identify mediastinal masses as thyroidal in origin.[60,69,71] Intrathoracic thyroid tissue almost always arises from the thyroid, and demonstration of anatomic continuity with the cervical thyroid on serial sections or coronal images provides compelling evidence that the intrathoracic tissue is thyroidal. A CT density greater than muscle also suggests a thyroidal origin; mediastinal lymphoma, lymphadenopathy, and thymus rarely have CT densities exceeding that of muscle. An increase in the CT density and prolonged enhancement after contrast injection (2 min or more) excludes an aneurysm and favors substernal goiter. All of these features are not present in every patient, but the presence of several should suggest that an intrathoracic mass is composed of thyroid tissue.

THYROID ADENOMAS

Thyroid adenomas appear as circumscribed round or oval lesions of low density (Fig 22-7). After contrast injection, the density increases variably. Poorly enhancing central areas correspond to areas of hemorrhage, necrosis, or cyst formation. Focal calcifications are seen in approximately 10% of adenomas. Adenomas are usually single, but multiple small adenomas may be seen; they were present in 18% of patients in one study.[54] No CT characteristics distinguish follicular adenomas from carcinomas.

THYROID CARCINOMA

Papillary carcinomas are usually irregular lesions of low density, but occasionally are discrete.[54,58] Calcification is present in approximately 60% and may be dense. Enhancement after contrast injection is minimal to moderate. Some carcinomas contain a thick-walled cyst with an irregular inner surface that enhances little. No CT feature is highly predictive of carcinoma when the lesion is confined to the thyroid, but extrathyroidal extension or lymphadenopathy is suggestive of carcinoma.

Medullary thyroid carcinoma appears as single or multiple areas of decreased density and variable size in one or both

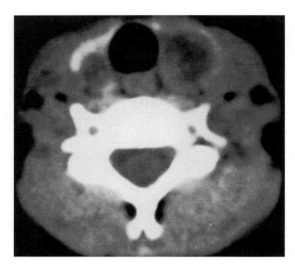

FIGURE 22-7. CT image of bilateral follicular adenomas of the thyroid.

lobes. In one series multiple or bilateral lesions were present in 10 of 13 patients.[58] CT scanning may reveal discrete loci not evident on scintigraphic scanning in some patients and infiltration of surrounding tissues and lymph node metastases in others. Lesions 1 to 2 mm in size can be detected. Small calcifications are scattered throughout the gland in 30% to 40% of patients. Hepatic metastases also are associated with multiple small round calcifications.[72] In patients with borderline calcitonin stimulation tests, discrete abnormalities on CT strongly suggest medullary carcinoma. Patients with C-cell hyperplasia have normal CT scans.[73]

Thyroid lymphomas usually appear as large masses of low to intermediate density that enhance poorly after contrast injection.[43] Both lobes are involved in approximately 50% of patients. Because most patients with thyroid lymphoma have coexistent Hashimoto's thyroiditis, which also decreases the thyroid's density, this distinction can be difficult and largely depends on the degree and extent of thyroidal involvement. Other CT characteristics of thyroid lymphoma include displacement or compression of the trachea or esophagus, lymphadenopathy, and invasion of the carotid artery. Calcification occurs in only 10% of patients, and areas of necrosis are unusual.

Anaplastic carcinomas appear as a large irregular mass of low attenuation with central cystic or necrotic areas. Calcification is present in 60% to 80% of these tumors. They may invade the trachea, cricoid cartilage, or thyroid cartilage, and may compress the trachea or grow into its lumen. However, a normal CT does not exclude minor degrees of tracheal destruction.

Recurrent thyroid carcinoma is evident on CT as discrete masses within or outside the thyroid bed. Lymph node metastases are suggested by the presence of lymph nodes 10 mm in size or greater; normal nodes are typically 3 to 5 mm in size. The presence of three or more contiguous ill-defined nodes 8 to 10 mm in diameter strongly suggests metastatic disease. Lymph nodes containing carcinoma typically have a regular rim and an area of central lucency that does not enhance after contrast injection. Calcifications or cystic degeneration may

also be present.[74] Obliteration or distortion of fascial planes may be seen with metastatic involvement but can also be seen in inflammatory disease, after surgical trauma, or after radiation therapy.

CT scanning is a sensitive technique for detection of pulmonary metastases. Lung nodules can be detected in patients with negative chest x-rays and strongly correlates with tumor mass and serum thyroglobulin concentrations.[75] CT scanning is therefore complementary to whole-body scanning with radioactive iodine and is useful in detecting nonfunctioning pulmonary metastatic disease.

ECTOPIC THYROID TISSUE

Ectopic thyroid tissue usually lies in the midline between the base of the tongue and thyroid isthmus.[76] Ectopic thyroid may appear in unusual locations such as the hyoid bone, where it can expand to destroy part of the cartilaginous structure.[77] Thyroglossal duct cysts appear as midline, round or elongated cystic lesions. These cysts rarely contain foci of papillary carcinoma; the presence of nodular excrescences in a midline cystic neck mass should raise this possibility.[78] True ectopic thyroid tissue in the chest is rare.[79]

OTHER NECK MASSES

Lipomas in the lower neck may simulate thyroid nodules. They are identified as fat on CT by their very low density.[80] Rarely thyroid masses rotate the laryngotracheal system, creating the illusion of a mass of the vocal apparatus.[81] CT can identify the primary tumor in patients presenting with lymphadenopathy or suggest the correct diagnosis when causes of lymphadenopathy other than carcinoma are present.[82] Distinction of thyroid abnormalities from cervical parenchymal cysts and normal salivary glands can usually be made with CT.[81,83]

MAGNETIC RESONANCE IMAGING

The multiple capabilities of magnetic resonance (MR) imaging make it an excellent choice for evaluating normal and diseased organs, including the thyroid. MR is noninvasive and images tissues based on their magnetic properties. The absence both of ionizing radiation and of the need for iodinated radiographic contrast agents make it an attractive alternative for pediatric patients and for adults requiring repetitive examinations. Its improved soft tissue contrast permits superior definition of many anatomic structures in the neck, and its ability to generate images in multiple planes further enhances visualization of anatomic relationships. High-field-strength MR units (1.5 Tesla) permit thinner sections, higher resolution, and shorter scanning times, and specially shaped surface coils for the neck have greatly enhanced the image quality.[84,85,86] In contrast to ultrasonography, MR can visualize the retrotracheal area, thoracic inlet, and mediastinum and is less operator-dependent.[87] Tumor vascularity can be assessed by using the paramagnetic contrast agent, gadolinium.[88]

MR imaging also has limitations. The image quality is sensitive to patient and physiologic tissue movement, and is highly dependent on the use of properly designed surface coils and other technical factors. MR does not identify calcification as readily as does CT.[89,90,91]

Absolute contraindications to MR imaging include the presence of a cardiac pacemaker, implantable defibrillators, central nervous system aneurysmal clips, auditory implants, and ferromagnetic ocular fragments. Small metal objects or shrapnel may likewise delay or prevent imaging. Stainless steel surgical clips and orthopedic devices cause local field inhomogeneity and loss of resolution but do not absolutely preclude MR imaging. Most dental amalgams are nonferromagnetic, and ferromagnetic dental substances generally cause only image distortion.

The safety of MR imaging has been questioned. There are no long-term studies of its safety, but there is little in vivo or in vitro evidence to suggest adverse effects with the field strengths used clinically. The only adverse effect reported is claustrophobia, which occurs in 5% of patients and may preclude MR examination.[92]

Principles of MR Imaging

The technology for producing MR images depends on the magnetic properties of certain atomic nuclei.[93] This is usually associated with nuclei containing an odd number of protons such as H^+, ^{31}P, ^{13}C, and ^{19}F. Hydrogen is the most prevalent in biologic tissues, in the form of water and lipids. Protons have a positive electrical charge and generate a magnetic field as they spin. When in the magnetic field of the scanner, protons align their axes parallel to the direction of the field. The protons spin about this axis at a frequency that is dependent on the magnetic field strength. If the aligned protons are exposed to an alternating magnetic field of the same radiofrequency, some of the nuclei absorb energy and are forced to a higher energy state with their axes perpendicular to the magnetic field. Immediately after being tipped 90 degrees, the protons are spinning in synchrony but quickly lose their phase coherence. The rate of decay of this synchronous spinning after a single excitation is related to spin–spin interactions of adjacent protons. When the radiofrequency is turned off, the protons recover and realign themselves in the magnetic field through a process known as relaxation. As realignment occurs, protons return to a lower energy state and release energy as a small voltage. This voltage is detected by a surface coil receiver, relayed to a computer, and used to reconstruct an image.

The reconstructed images show the density and energy loss of protons in tissues. The MR signal contains several variable components. *P* reflects the density, concentration, and biologic environment of the hydrogen protons. The *T1 relaxation time* (longitudinal or spin–lattice relaxation time) reflects the time for protons deflected perpendicular to the field to give up their energy to the surrounding environment (lattice) and return to their original alignment parallel to the magnetic field. The *T2 relaxation time* (transverse or spin–spin relaxation time) is the time needed for synchronous transverse spinning to decay after excitation. Although synchronized initially, some nuclei move more rapidly or slowly because of magnetic interactions with their neighbors. The T2 relaxation time indicates the realignment response of large numbers of nuclei. The superior images of MR result because the relatively independent magnetic properties of tissue, including the proton density, T1, and T2, are simultaneously incorporated into the final image. Adjustment of the radiofrequency pulse sequence can favor one or the other of these magnetic properties (proton, T1-weighted, or T2-weighted images).

MR Scanning Technique

The varied anatomy and pathologic abnormalities of the thyroid preclude a single approach with reference to the type of coil or imaging sequence used, and each study should be tailored to address the clinical question at hand. Proper patient positioning assures superior symmetric imaging and patient comfort. A typical examination requires 30 to 60 minutes, and patient motion must be minimized for optimal images. Children frequently require sedation to complete the examination. When the examination is confined to the thyroid, the surface coil provides the highest quality images. If the field of examination needs to be extended, the use of another surface coil or the head or body coil may be required.

MR scanning is performed with the patient supine and the neck extended. A surface coil is centered and taped in place over the thyroid.[92,94] Images are obtained while the patient breathes quietly without swallowing. Imaging usually begins with T1-weighted transverse images being obtained from the hyoid bone to the apex of the lungs. Coronal scans are useful for correlation with radionuclide scanning techniques or for evaluating substernal goiters.[95] The T1-weighted images are then followed by the T2-weighted images. T2-weighted images require longer scan times, are more sensitive to patient motion, and should be performed before the patient becomes restless. T2-weighted images have reduced signal-to-noise ratio and anatomic image clarity, but their contrast resolution provides additional insights regarding areas of tumor or inflammation.

The Normal Thyroid Gland

On T1-weighted images, fat appears hyperintense, muscle intermediate in intensity, and cortical bone hypointense. The normal thyroid shows a nearly homogeneous signal with an intensity similar to or slightly greater than that of the adjacent neck muscles[92–98] (Fig 22-8). The carotid arteries, jugular veins, neck muscles, and trachea are well visualized. Flowing blood, which gives a weak signal when moving rapidly, and vessels appear black in most imaging sequences. Blood moving slowly paradoxically gives rise to an increased signal. The esophagus appears as a thin line of intermediate signal intensity and is poorly distinguished from surrounding muscles.

On T2-weighted images, the normal thyroid has a much greater signal intensity than adjacent muscles (Fig 22-8). Its intensity is usually less than that of surrounding fat but occasionally is equal to it. The thyroid is homogeneous in most persons but can be inhomogeneous. Blood vessels and lymph nodes are easily identified and distinguished from the thyroid. The esophagus is clearly seen because its mucosa generates a high signal intensity on T2-weighted images. Cortical bone is hypointense. Focal abnormalities of the thyroid are evident in 21% to 46% of normal subjects[92,99]; most are solitary, 3- to 5-mm nodules, but occasionally multiple nodules are seen.

Air in the hypopharynx, larynx, and trachea produces no MR signal and provides a clear definition of the inner margin of these structures. The thyroid and cricoid cartilages and trachea have an intermediate intensity on T1- and T2-weighted images in younger

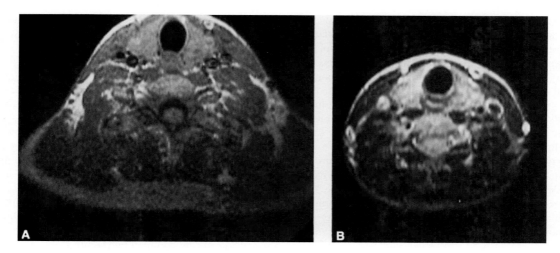

FIGURE 22-8. T1-weighted (A) and T2-weighted (B) MR images of a normal thyroid gland.

persons.[100] These structures calcify with age, and asymmetric medullary cavities filled with fat may form within them. Eventually, they appear as ossified structures with hypointense margins and central hyperintensity on T1-weighted scans. The posterior lamina of the cricoid cartilage contains marrow, resulting in an area of increased signal on T1-weighted images.

Normal parathyroid glands are not seen on MR images, but enlarged parathyroid glands can be seen.[85,90,94,96,101,102] Resolution is best on T1-weighted images; parathyroid adenomas are usually isointense with muscle and hypointense or isointense with thyroid, but distinct from surrounding hyperintense fat. Contrast resolution is markedly improved on T2-weighted images, on which adenomas are hyperintense relative to surrounding structures.[103] MR imaging detects parathyroid adenomas with a sensitivity of 60% to 80%.

The Abnormal Thyroid Gland

THYROID CYSTS

Thyroid cysts are characterized by homogenous high-intensity signals on both T1- and T2-weighted imaging.[92] As a group, hemorrhagic cysts have the highest thyroid-to-muscle signal ratio,[97] and the intense signal of hemorrhagic cysts is consistent with the signal intensity of methemoglobin. When hemorrhage has been present for 3 weeks or longer, T2-weighted images may reveal a low-intensity peripheral rim resulting from hemosiderin-laden macrophages.[104]

Colloid cysts also appear hyperintense on T2-weighted images. However, on T1-weighted images, they may be either hypointense or hyperintense relative to normal thyroid tissue,[91,92,105] and occasionally can be mistaken for carotid aneurysms.[106,107] Noncolloid cysts have low intensity on T1-weighted images and high intensity on T2-weighted images.[95,108] Thyroglossal duct cysts have a signal of heterogeneous increased intensity on both T1- and T2-weighted images, probably as a result of their high protein content.[92]

DIFFUSE THYROID DISEASE

The thyroid in Graves' disease is enlarged, sometimes lobulated, and has a slightly heterogeneous, diffusely increased signal on both T1- and T2-weighted images.[97,109] The intensity frequently exceeds that of fat on T2-weighted images. Numerous coarse bandlike structures and dilated vascular channels may traverse the parenchyma.[108] The thyroid-to-muscle signal ratio is linearly related to both the serum thyroxine (T_4) concentration and the 24-hour radioiodine uptake.[109] After treatment with radioiodine, the signal ratio falls in proportion to changes in the serum T_4 and radioactive iodine uptake. These changes may reflect a change in tissue water content, thyroglobulin content, blood flow, or vascularity of the thyroid. No similar correlation exists in patients with other thyroid abnormalities.

Hashimoto's thyroiditis causes a heterogeneous signal intensity on T1-weighted images. The signal on T2-weighted images is diffusely increased as compared with fat. Linear bands of increased intensity on both T1- and T2-weighted images are apparent in many glands and probably correspond to areas of fibrosis.[108]

The presence of hypointense lesions on T1- and T2-weighted images when associated with infiltration of adjacent neck structures suggests Riedel's thyroiditis.[110]

Magnetic resonance imaging can detect tissue deposition of iron because it markedly shortens the T2 relaxation time. Hemachromotosis of the thyroid is characterized by a marked reduction of the signal intensity on T1- and especially T2-weighted images.[111]

MULTINODULAR GOITER

Multinodular goiters have minimal to moderate heterogeneity and areas of low, normal, or increased signal intensity on T1-weighted images[95,97,109] (Fig 22-9). Areas of very high signal intensity are consistent with focal hemorrhage or cystic degeneration.[92,95,108] The extent of the goiter and its relationship to the trachea and esophagus are clearly delineated. T2-weighted images show more marked heterogeneity with multiple areas of increased intensity. MR can detect nodules as small as 3 to 5 mm. Nodules are better visualized on T2-weighted images because their signal intensity may exceed that of normal thyroid and surrounding fat,[97] and some nodules can only be seen on T2-weighted images.[108] Hyperfunc-

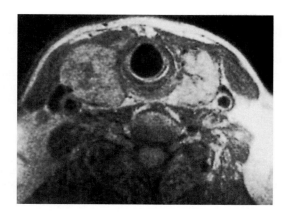

FIGURE 22-9. T1-weighted MR image of a multinodular goiter.

tioning and hypofunctioning nodules have similar MR characteristics. Calcifications are seen as low intensity areas that do not continue in several contiguous sections.

THYROID ADENOMAS

Follicular adenomas appear on T1-weighted images as round or oval circumscribed lesions with a heterogeneous signal that is equal to or slightly greater than that of normal thyroid tissue.[95,98,108] On T2-weighted images, the nodules have increased signal intensity. Hemorrhage is evidenced by central areas of high signal intensity. In one study, there were varying degrees of hemorrhagic degeneration in all adenomas, but only in 5 of 12 carcinomas. Functioning adenomas are isointense with surrounding thyroid tissue on both T1- and T2-weighted images.[92,109]

Most adenomas have a smooth capsule that is thicker and more uniform than is seen in carcinomas. The exact thickness of the capsule is often difficult to measure, but it is easily recognized when it is 1 mm or greater in thickness.[98] Most carcinomas have capsules that are partially destroyed or uneven in thickness; in some, however, the capsule is intact but its outer or inner surface is irregular.

THYROID CARCINOMA

Thyroid carcinomas appear as focal or nonfocal lesions with smooth or irregular borders and are variable in size. They are isointense or slightly hyperintense on T1-weighted images and are hyperintense on T2-weighted images, both in the thyroid and in lymph nodes. The imaging characteristics of all types of thyroid carcinomas, including medullary thyroid carcinomas and lymphomas, are similar.[92,95,97,98,108,112,113]

The MR characteristics of benign and malignant thyroid nodules differ in some respects both in vitro and in vivo.[91,95,97,114-116] Normal thyroid has the fastest T1 relaxation time, followed by thyroid adenomas and then thyroid carcinomas. The T2 values have more tissue specificity than T1 values.[115] However, the MR values overlap substantially, preventing discrimination of benign from malignant nodules in individual patients.

The extent of thyroid carcinoma can be determined preoperatively using MR, which may occasionally be useful in planning surgery. Extension into adjacent structures, including the larynx, trachea, and surrounding muscles, is usually evi-

dent. The contrast between muscle and tumor is greater on MR than CT.[91] Normal lymph nodes are hypointense relative to fat on T1-weighted images, and nodes as small as 3 mm can be identified on both T1- and T2-weighted images; metastatic nodes are most conspicuous on T2-weighted images because of their hyperintense signal relative to adjacent muscles and fat.[74,96] MR cannot distinguish metastatic from inflammatory adenopathy because both appear hyperintense on T2-weighted images.

Gadolinium may prove useful in distinguishing malignant from benign lymph nodes.[88] Gadolinium shortens the T1 and T2 relaxation times of tissues accumulating it and increases signal intensity on T1-weighted images. Metastases to nodes are enhanced centrally after gadolinium injection. Gadolinium may also help to distinguish recurrent carcinoma from postoperative fibrosis; carcinoma enhances with gadolinium, whereas scarring does not.

After surgery, MR may be useful for detecting residual or recurrent carcinoma and identifying tumor tissue in the neck when other techniques fail.[117] The thyroid remnant is usually seen as a small peritracheal rim of tissue that has low signal intensity on T1- and T2-weighted images. In contrast, recurrent carcinoma and lymph node metastases have low-to-medium signal intensity on T1-weighted images and medium-to-high signal intensity on T2-weighted images.[95,118] Early fibrosis and edema both have a high intensity signal on T2-weighted images and can mimic recurrent carcinoma. Recurrent carcinoma is best distinguished from fat using T1-weighted images and from muscle using T2-weighted images.[119] Muscle invaded by carcinoma has a higher intensity than that of the contralateral normal muscle, but so also does inflammation caused by carcinoma as compared with actual invasion. Other features suggesting recurrent carcinoma include assymetry or an increased signal intensity in the thyroid bed, invasion or displacement of adjacent tissues, and enlarged lymph nodes with an increased signal intensity. Using these criteria, MR imaging had a positive predictive value of 82%, a negative predictive value of 86%, and an overall diagnostic accuracy of 83% in predicting recurrence in one study of 32 patients.[120] When a quantitative assessment of tissue intensity was made, the best predictive results were obtained when abnormal tissue was compared with muscle as opposed to fat. MR imaging may find its major use in detecting recurrent carcinoma, because recurrent tumor can be distinguished from fibrous tissue, and lymph node metastases can be seen.

ROLE OF IMAGING TECHNIQUES

The role of ultrasonography, CT imaging, and MR imaging in clinical practice is to amplify and clarify the clinical, laboratory, nuclear medicine, and cytopathologic observations routinely obtained in patients with thyroid problems. There is no absolute clinical indication for performing any of these imaging procedures, and they are presently used far more often than is justified by the information they impart. Given their considerable expense and inability to distinguish benign and malignant thyroid lesions, they should be reserved for patients in whom clinically useful information can be obtained.

Of these techniques, thyroid ultrasonography is by far the most commonly performed. It is often but inappropriately ordered as part of the evaluation of patients with a thyroid nodule.[121] It is the definitive technique for demonstrating cystic thyroid lesions and is able to do this accurately. However, simple thyroid cysts are rare, and the information obtained does not usually provide insight into the nature of the problem. Many physicians order thyroid ultrasonography to confirm the presence of a thyroid nodule after a thyroid radionuclide scan reveals a hypofunctioning nodule. This is difficult to justify, since defects on a thyroid radionuclide scan are virtually always within the gland. Other physicians order ultrasonography to confirm their findings on palpation, and yet it would be less expensive to have another examiner palpate the neck. Thyroid ultrasound studies are occasionally ordered to look for other nodules, on the premise that the presence of a multinodular goiter makes the initially detected nodule less likely to be a carcinoma. There is no basis for this premise, particularly given the high prevalence of small thyroid nodules in normal persons. Ultrasonography may be used to monitor changes in the size of nodules during T_4 therapy, but palpation is nearly always adequate for this purpose. Thus, ultrasonography should not be routinely used in the evaluation or management of patients with nodular thyroid disease.

Thyroid ultrasonography is useful in patients in whom there is real uncertainty about the origin of a neck mass, such as in children in whom adenopathy and other neck masses are common. Patients with metastatic thyroid carcinoma may present with cervical adenopathy and no palpable thyroid nodule; ultrasonography is the simplest and most sensitive imaging technique for identifying small thyroid abnormalities. Thyroid ultrasound studies also can be used to guide needle biopsy of poorly localized nodules that are of clinical concern. Ultrasound guidance for injection of alcohol into thyroid cysts and adenomas may improve the efficacy of this treatment.

Ultrasonography is highly sensitive in identifying recurrent thyroid carcinoma, either in the thyroid bed or in cervical lymph nodes, and can be used to guide needle biopsy of these lesions.[48] It is not as sensitive as radionuclide scanning to identify carcinomas, if they concentrate iodine, but it may be useful for detecting and localizing nonfunctioning thyroid carcinomas. Thyroid ultrasound studies may be useful in evaluating thyroid nodules in pregnant women in whom radionuclide scanning is contraindicated. Thus, ultrasonography should be reserved for situations in which clinical uncertainty is present or when guided needle placement is indicated. As it is the least expensive of the newer imaging techniques, it should generally be the first to be used.

The clinical value of CT and MR imaging is much more limited. CT and MR imaging cannot distinguish benign from malignant nodules and, therefore, have no role in the routine evaluation of patients with thyroid nodules. CT can provide much of the information that can be obtained with ultrasound, but its greater expense, slight radiation exposure, and risk of reaction to contrast agent argue against its use most of the time. The primary indication for CT is to determine the substernal extent of a goiter or to diagnose a substernal goiter in a patient with a mediastinal mass. CT is occasionally useful in the evaluation of thyroid carcinomas, especially when the trachea, larynx, or bone are involved.

MR imaging may also be useful in assessing substernal goiters. MR outlines the relationship of the substernal thyroid to the intrathoracic vessels as well as CT does but without the need for contrast injection. The ease with which coronal sections can be obtained further facilitates understanding the anatomic relationships, including the degree of compression or displacement of the trachea and esophagus. MR imaging is especially useful in identifying recurrent thyroid carcinoma in the thyroid bed and in regional lymph nodes, and its greatest clinical utility unquestionably is for this purpose.

References

1. Fujimoto Y, Oka A, Omotto R, Hirose M. Ultrasound scanning of the thyroid gland as a new diagnostic approach. Ultrasonics 1967;5:177
2. Blum M, Goldman AB, Herskovic A, Hernberg J. Clinical aplications of thyroid echography. N Engl J Med 1972;287:11
3. Huang HK, Aberle DR, Lufkin R, Grant EG, Hanafee WN, Kangarloo H. Advances in medical imaging. Ann Intern Med 1990; 112:203
4. Radecki PD, Arger PH, Arenson RL, et al. Thyroid imaging: comparison of high-resolution real-time ultrasound and computed tomography. Head Neck Radiology 1984;153:145
5. Scheible W, Leopold GR, Woo VL, Gosink BB. High-resolution real-time ultrasonography of thyroid nodules. Radiology 1979; 133:413
6. Sigel B, Machi J, Beitler JC, Justin JR, Coelho JCU. Variable ultrasound echogenicity in flowing blood. Science 1982;218:1321
7. Simeone JF. High-resolution realtime sonography of the thyroid. Radiology 1982;145:431
8. Ikekubo K, Niga T, Hirasa M, Ishihara T, Waseda N, Mori T. Evaluation of radionuclide imaging and echography in the diagnosis of thyroid nodules. Clin Nucl Med 1985;145
9. Sackler JP, Passalaqua M, Blum M, Amorocho L. A spectrum of diseases of the thyroid gland as imaged by gray scale water bath sonography. Radiology 1977;125:467
10. Taylor KJW, Carpenter DA, Barrett JJ. Gray scale ultrasonography in the diagnosis of thyroid swellings. J Clin Ultrasound 1974;2:327
11. Thijs LG, Wiener JD. Ultrasonic examinations of the thyroid gland: possibilities and limitations. Am J Med 1976;60:96
12. Hansen JM, Kampmann J, Madsen SN, et al. Determination of thyroid volume by ultrasonic scanning. Endocrinol Exp 1974;8:223
13. Rasmussen SN, Hjorth L. Determination of thyroid volume by ultrasonic scanning. J Clin Ultrasound 1974;2:143
14. Berghout A, Wiersinga WM, Smits NJ, Touber JL. Determinants of thyroid volume as measured by ultrasonography in healthy adults in a non-iodine deficient area. Clin Endocrinol 1987; 26:273
15. Brander A, Viikinkoski P, Nickels J, Kivisaari L. Thyroid gland: US screening in middle-aged women with no previous thyroid disease. Radiology 1989;173:507
16. Carroll BA. Asymptomatic thyroid nodules: incidental sonographic detection. Am J Roentgenol 1982;138:499
17. Mazzaferri EL. Management of a solitary thyroid nodule. N Engl J Med 1993;328:553
18. Hsiao YL, Chang TC. Ultrasound evaluation of thyroid abnormalities and volume in Chinese adults without palpable thyroid glands. J Formosan Med Assoc 1994;93:140
19. Miki H, Oshimo K, Inoue H, et al. Incidence of ultrasonographically-detected thyroid nodules in healthy adults. Tokushima J Exp Med 1993;40:43
20. Gonczi J, Szabolcs I, Kovacs Z, Kakosy T, Goth M, Szilagyi G. Ultrasonography of the thyroid gland in hospitalized, chronically ill geriatric patients: thyroid volume, its relationship to age and disease, and the prevalence of diffuse and nodular goiter. J Clin Ultrasound 1994;22:257

21. Ezzat S, Sarti DA, Cain DR, Braunstein GD. Thyroid incidentalomas. Prevalence by palpation and ultrasonography. Arch Intern Med 1994;154:1838
22. Vitti P, Martino E, Aghini-Lombardi F, et al. Thyroid volume measurement by ultrasound in children as a tool for the assessment of mild iodine deficiency. J Clin Endocrinol Metab 1994;79:600
23. Mallette LE, Malini S. The role of parathyroid ultrasonography in the management of primary hyperparathyroidism. Am J Med Sci 1989;298:51
24. Edis AJ, Evans TC. High-resolution, real-time ultrasonography in the preoperative location of parathyroid tumors. Pilot study. N Eng J Med 1979;301:532
25. Krudy AG, Doppman JL, Brennan MF, et al. The detection of mediastinal parathyroid glands by computed tomography, selective arteriography, and venous sampling: an analysis of 17 cases. Radiology 1981;140:739
26. Randel SB, Gooding GAW, Clark OH, Stein RM, Winkler B. Parathyroid variants: US evaluation. Radiology 1987;165:191
27. Roses DF, Sudarsky LA, Sanger J, Raghavendra BN, Reede DL, Blum M. The use of preoperative localization of adenomas of the parathyroid glands by thallium-technetium substraction scintigraphy, high-resolution ultrasonography and computed tomography. Surg Gynecol Obstet 1989;168:99
28. Simeone JF, Mueller PR, Ferrucci JT, et al. High-resolution real-time sonography of the parathyroid. Radiology 1981;141:745
29. Evans DM. Diagnostic discriminants of thyroid cancer. Am J Surg 1987;153:569
30. Hammer M, Wortsman J, Folse R. Cancer in cystic lesions of the thyroid. Arch Surg 1982;117:1020
31. Rosen IB, Provias JP, Walfish PG. Pathologic nature of cystic thyroid nodules selected for surgery by needle aspiration biopsy. Surgery 1986;100:606
32. Ivarsson SA, Ericsson U-B, Fredriksson B, Persson PH. Ultrasonic imaging in the differential diagnosis of diffuse thyroid disorders in children. Am J Dis Child 1989;143:1369
33. Gutekunst R, Hafermann W, Mansky T, Scriba PC. Ultrasonography related to clinical and laboratory findings in lymphocytic thyroiditis. Acta Endocrinol 1989;121:129
34. Witterick IJ, Abel SM, Hartwick W, Mullen B, Salem S. Incidence and types of non-palpable thyroid nodules in thyroids removed for palpable disease. J Otolaryngol 1993;22:294
35. Kumar A, Ahuja MM, Chattopadhyay TK, et al. Fine needle aspiration cytology, sonography and radionuclide scanning in solitary thyroid nodule. J Assoc Physicians India 1992;40:302
36. Price R, Horvath K, Moore GD Jr. Surgery for solitary thyroid nodules: assessment of methods to select patients at low risk for unsuspected malignancy in the unaffected lobe and the possible utility of preoperative thyroid ultrasound. Thyroid 1993;3:87
37. Boland GW, Lee MJ, Mueller PR, May-Smith W, Dawson SL, Simeone JF. Efficacy of sonographically guided biopsy of thyroid masses and cervical lymph nodes. Am J Roentgenol 1993;161:1053
38. Sanchez RB, vanSonnenberg E, D'Agostino HB, et al. Ultrasound guided biopsy of nonpalpable and difficult to palpate thyroid masses. J Am Coll Surg 1994;178:33
39. McIvor NP, Freeman JL, Salem S, Elden L, Noyek AM, Bedard YC. Ultrasonography and ultrasound-guided fine-needle aspiration biopsy of head and neck lesions: a surgical perspective. Laryngoscope 1994;104:669
40. Cochand-Priollet B, Guillausseau PJ, Chagnon S, et al. The diagnostic value of fine-needle aspiration biopsy under ultrasonography in nonfunctional thyroid nodules: a prospective study comparing cytologic and histologic findings. Am J Med 1994;97:152
41. Propper RA, Skolnick ML, Weinstein BJ, Deker A. The nonspecificity of the thyroid "halo" sign. J Clin Ultrasound 1980;8:129
42. Hayashi N, Tamaki N, Yamamoto K, et al. Real-time ultrasonography of thyroid nodules. Acta Radiologica 1986;27:403
43. Takashima S, Ikezoe J, Morimoto S, et al. Primary thyroid lymphoma: evaluation with CT. Radiology 1988;168:765
44. Gorman B, Charboneau JW, James EM, et al. Medullary thyroid carcinoma: role of high-resolution ultrasound. Radiology 1987;162:147
45. Sutton RT, Reading CC, Charboneau JW, James EM, Grant CS, Hay ID. US-guided biopsy of neck masses in postoperative management of patients with thyroid cancer. Radiology 1988;168:769
46. Aggarwal SK, Jayaram G, Kakar A, Goel GD, Prakash R, Pant CS. Fine needle aspiration cytologic diagnosis of the solitary cold thyroid nodule: comparison with ultrasonography, radionuclide perfusion study and xeroradiography. Acta Cytol 1989;33:41
47. McLaughlin SJ, Gray JG, Marshall T. Aspiration cytology and ultrasonography of cold thyroid nodules. Aust NZ J Surg 1986;56:331
48. Reading CC, Gorman CA. Thyroid imaging techniques. Clin Lab Med 1993;13:711
49. Simeone JF, Daniels GH, Hall DA, et al. Sonography in the follow-up of 100 patients with thyroid carcinoma. Am J Radiol 1987;148:45
50. Bachrach LK, Daneman D, Daneman A Martin, David J. Use of ultrasound in childhood thyroid disorders. J Pediatr 1983;547
51. Sherman NH, Rosenberg HK, Heyman S, Templeton J. Ultrasound evaluation of neck masses in children. J Ultrasound Med 1985;4:127
52. Iida Y, Konishi J, Harioka T, Misaki T, Endo K, Torizuka K. Thyroid CT number and its relationship to iodine concentration. Radiology 1983;147:793
53. Kaneko T, Matsumoto M, Fukui K, Hori T, Katayama K. Clinical evaluation of thyroid CT values in various thyroid conditions. J Comput Tomogr 1979;3:1
54. Arger PH, Jennings AS, Gordon LF, et al. Computed tomography findings in clinically normal and abnormal thyroid patients. J Comput Tomogr 1985;9:111
55. Brenner DE, Whitley NO, Houk TL, Aisner J, Wiernik P, Whitley J. Volume determinations in computed tomography. JAMA 1982;247:1299
56. Levi C, Gray JE, McCullough EC, Hattery RR. The unreliability of CT numbers as absolute values. Am J Radiol 1982;139:443
57. Silverman PM, Newman GE, Korobkin M, Workman JB, Moore AV, Coleman RE. Computed tomography in the evaluation of thyroid diseases. Am J Radiol 1983;141:897
58. Vette JK. Computed tomography of the thyroid gland. Acta Endocrinol 1985;Suppl. 268:1
59. Reede DL, Whelan MA, Bergeron RT. Computed tomography of the infrahyoid neck. I. Normal anatomy. Radiology 1982;145:389
60. Reede DL, Bergeron RT, McCauley DA. CT of the thyroid and other thoracic inlet disorders. J Otolaryngol 1982;11:349
61. Belli A-M, Ingram CE, Heron CW, Husband JE. The appearance of the inferior thyroid veins on computed tomography. Br J Radiol 1988;61:125
62. Sekiya T, Tada S, Kawakami K, Kino M, Fukuda K, Watanabe H. Clinical application of computed tomography to thyroid disease. J Comput Tomogr 1979;3:185
63. Kamijo K. Clinical studies on thyroid CT number in Graves' disease and destructive thyrotoxicosis. Endocr J 1994;41:25
64. Kamijo K. Clinical studies on thyroid CT number in chronic thyroiditis. Endocr J 1994;41:19
65. Bernard PJ, Som PM, Urken ML, Lawson W, Biller HF. The CT findings of acute thyroiditis and acute suppurative thyroiditis. Otolaryngol Head Neck Surg 1988;99:489
66. Miyake H, Maeda H, Isomoto I, Nagatomo H, Nakashima A, Ashizawa A. Computed tomography in amyloid goiter. J Comput Assist Tomogr 1988;12:621
67. Breatnach E, Abbott GC, Fraser RG. Dimensions of the normal human trachea. Am J Radiol 1984;141:903
68. Michel LA, Bradpiece HA. Surgical management of substernal goitre. Br J Surg 1988;75:565

69. Morris UL, Colletti PM, Ralls PW, et al. CT demonstration of intrathoracic thyroid tissue. J Comput Assist Tomogr 1982;6:821

70. Sanders LE, Rossi RL, Shahian DM, Williamson WA. Mediastinal goiters. The need for an aggressive approach. Arch Surg 1992; 127:609

71. Glazer GM, Axel L, Moss AA. CT diagnosis of mediastinal thyroid. Am J Radiol 1982;138:495

72. McDonnell CH, Fishman EK, Zerhouni EA. CT demonstration of calcified liver metastases in medullary thyroid carcinoma. J Comput Assist Tomogr 1986;6:976

73. Wells SA, Donis-Keller H. Current perspectives on the diagnosis and management of patients with multiple endocrine neoplasia type 2 syndromes. Endocrinol Metab Clin North Am 1994;23:215

74. Som PM, Brandwein M, Lidov M, Lawson W, Biller HF. The varied presentations of papillary thyroid carcinoma cervical nodal disease: CT and MR findings. Am J Neuroradiol 1994;15:1123

75. Piekarski J-D, Schlumberger M, Leclere J, Couanet D, Masselot J, Parmentier C. Chest computed tomography (CT) in patients with micronodular lung metastases of differentiated thyroid carcinoma. Int J Radiol Oncol Biol Phys 1985;11:1023

76. Willinsky RA, Kassel EE, Cooper PW, Chin-Sang HB, Haight J. Computed tomography of lingual thyroid. J Comput Assist Tomogr 1987;11:182

77. Bourjat P, Cartier J, Woerther J-P. Thyroglossal duct cyst in hyoid bone: CT confirmation. J Comput Assist Tomogr 1988;12:871

78. Silverman PM, Degesys GE, Ferguson BJ, Bierre AR. Papillary carcinoma in a thyroglossal duct cyst: CT findings. J Comput Assist Tomogr 1985;9:806

79. Ladenson PW, Vineyard GC, Pinkus GS, Ridgway EC. Sequestered substernal goiter. Arch Intern Med 1983;143:1015

80. Leonidas J-R, Goldman JM, Wheeler MF. Cervical lipomas masquerading as thyroid nodules. JAMA 1985;253:1436

81. Som P, Sacher M, Lanzieri CF, et al. Parenchymal cysts of the lower neck. Radiology 1985;157:399

82. Muraki AS, Mancuso AA, Harnsberger HR. Metastatic cervical adenopathy from tumors of unknown origin: the role of CT. Radiology 1984;152:749

83. Bryan RN, Miller RH, Ferreyro RI, Sessions RB. Computed tomography of the major salivary glands. Am J Radiol 1981; 139:547

84. Axel L. Surface coil magnetic resonance imaging. J Comput Assist Tomogr 1984;8:381

85. Kier R, Herfkens RJ, Blinder RA, Leight GS, Utz JA, Silverman PM. MRI with surface coils for parathyroid tumors. Am J Roent 1986;147:497

86. Eisenberg B, Velchick MG, Spritzer C, Kressel H, Alavi A. Magnetic resonance imaging and scintingraphic correlation in thyroid disorders. Am J Physiol Imaging 1990;5:8

87. Mancuso AA, Dillon WP. The neck. Radiol Clin North Am 1989;27:407

88. Crawford SC, Harnsberger HR, Lufkin RB, Hanafee WN. The role of gadolinium-DTPA in the evaluation of extracranial head and neck mass lesions. Radiol Clin North Am 1989;27:219

89. Baker HL, Berquist TH, Kispert DB, et al. Magnetic resonance imaging in a routine clinical setting. Mayo Clin Proc 1985;60:75

90. Stark DD, Clark OH, Moss AA. Magnetic resonance imaging of the thyroid, thymus, and parathyroid glands. Surgery 1984; 96:1083

91. Stark DD, Moss AA, Gamsu G, Clark OH, Gooding GAW, Webb WR. Magnetic resonance imaging of the neck. II. Pathologic findings. Radiology 1984;150:455

92. Gefter WB, Spritzer CE, Eisenberg B, et al. Thyroid imaging with high-field strength surface-coil MR. Radiology 1987;164:483

93. Makow LS. Magnetic resonance imaging: a brief review of image contrast. Radiol Clin North Am 1989;27:195

94. Rafto SE, Gefter WB. MRI of the upper aerodigestive tract and neck. Radiol Clin North Am 1988;26:547

95. Higgins CB, McNamara MT, Fisher MR, Clark OH. MR imaging of the thyroid. Radiology 1986;147:1255

96. Higgins CB, Auffermann W. MR imaging of the thyroid and parathyroid glands: a review of current status. Am J Roentgenol 1988; 151:1095

97. Mountz JM, Glazer GM, Dmuchowski C, Sisson JC. MR imaging of the thyroid: Comparison with scintigraphy in the normal and diseased gland. J Comput Assist Tomogr 1987;11:612

98. Noma S, Kanaoka M, Minami S, et al. Thyroid masses: MR imaging and pathologic correlation. Radiology 1988;168:759

99. Funari M, Campos Z, Gooding GA, Higgins CB. MRI and ultrasound detection of asymptomatic thyroid nodules in hyperparathyroidism. J Comput Assist Tomogr 1992;16:615

100. Castelijns JA, Doornbos J, Verbeeten B, Vielvoye GJ, Bloem JL. MR imaging of the normal larynx. J Comput Assist Tomogr 1985;9:919

101. Kier R, Blinder RA, Herfkens RJ, Leight GS, Spitzer CE, Carroll BA. MR imaging with surface coils in primary hyperparathyroidism. J Comput Assist Tomogr 1987;11:863

102. Sandler MP, Patton JA. Multimodality imaging of the thyroid and parathyroid glands. J Nucl Med 1987;28:122

103. Seelos KC, DeMarco R, Clark OH, Higgins CB. Persistent and recurrent hyperparathyroidism: assessment with gadopentetate dimeglumine-enhanced MR imaging. Radiology 1990; 177:373

104. Rubin JI, Gomori JM, Grossman RI, Gefter WB, Kressel HY. High-field MR imaging of extracranial hematomas. Am J Roentgenol 1987;148:813

105. Stark DD, Moss AA, Gamsu G, Clark OH, Gooding GAW, Webb WR. Magnetic resonance imaging of the neck. I. Normal anatomy. Radiology 1984;150:447

106. Anderson CM, Gooding GA, Lee RE. Thyroid cyst mistaken for carotid pseudoaneurysm by MR angiography. Case report. Clin Imaging 1992;16:198

107. Fujimoto H, Yasuda S, Kashimada A, et al. Diagnosis of aneurysm of superior thyroid artery by CT and MR imaging. Acta Radiol 1992;33:420

108. Noma S, Nishimura K, Togashi K, et al. Thyroid gland: MR imaging. Radiology 1987;164:495

109. Charkes ND, Mauer AH, Siegel JA, Rakecki PD, Malmud LS. MR imaging in thyroid disorders: correlation of signal intensity with Graves' disease activity. Radiology 1987;164:491

110. Perez Fontan FJ, Cordido Carballido F, Pombo Felipe F, Mosquera Oses J, Villalba Martin C. Riedel thyroiditis: US, CT, and MR evaluation. J Comput Assist Tomogr 1993; 17:324

111. Noma S, Konishi J, Morikawa M, Yoshida Y. MR imaging of thyroid hemochromatosis. J Comput Assist Tomogr 1988;12:623

112. Takashima S, Ikezoe J, Morimoto S, Harada K, Kozuka T, Matsuzuka F. MR imaging of primary thyroid lymphoma. J Comput Assist Tomogr 1989;13:517

113. Shibata T, Moma S, Nakano Y, Konishi J. Primary thyroid lymphoma: MR appearance. J Comput Assist Tomogr 1991; 15:629

114. Johnson M, Selinsky B, Davis M, et al. In vitro NMR evaluation of human thyroid lesions. Invest Radiol 1989;24:666

115. Tennvall J, Biorklund A, Moller T, Olsson M, Persson B, Akerman M. Studies of NMR-relaxation-times in malignant tumours and normal tissues of the human thyroid gland. Prog Nucl Med 1984;8:142

116. Tennvall J, Olsson M, Moller T, et al. Thyroid tissue characterization by proton magnetic resonance relaxation time determination. Acta Oncol 1987;26:27

Werner and Ingbar's The Thyroid, Seventh Edition,
edited by Lewis E. Braverman and Robert D. Utiger.
Lippincott–Raven Publishers, Philadelphia, © 1996

23

Evaluation of Thyroid Nodules by Needle Biopsy

Joel I. Hamburger
Michael M. Kaplan

DEVELOPMENT AND ACCEPTANCE OF THYROID NEEDLE BIOPSY

Thyroid nodules are common but thyroid cancer is uncommon. Most thyroid cancers are not aggressive, but the uncommon anaplastic carcinomas are almost never curable. These considerations lead most physicians to conclude that excision of all thyroid nodules to preserve life is not only inappropriate but might produce more morbidity and mortality than it could prevent. Instead, these physicians select for surgery nodules that seem probably malignant, while advising observation for the rest. In the past, selection was based on imprecise clinical methods. Clinical findings that most conclusively suggest malignancy, such as rapid growth, vocal cord paralysis, local invasion, or distant metastases, are present in few thyroid cancer patients, most of whom have incurable disease. Other features, such as sex and age, nodule firmness, normality to palpation of extranodular thyroid tissue, prior radiation therapy to the upper body, or nodular response to exogenous thyroid hormone, are nonspecific and insensitive. Therefore, reliance on clinical evaluation results in many false-positive diagnoses, with a substantial risk of false-negative diagnosis.

The use of needle biopsy in the evaluation of thyroid nodules began with the 1930 report of Hayes Martin.[1] He used a large-needle aspiration technique to secure tissue fragments for conventional histologic evaluation. Subsequently, Silverman or Tru-Cut needles were used to obtain larger tissue cores.[2–5] Currently, nearly all centers rely primarily on fine-needle biopsy (FNB). It produces small tissue aspirates that are evaluated on the basis of cytologic criteria. Credit for the introduction of the FNB method is due especially to European cytopathologists who reported their experience in the years between 1952 and 1977.[6–12]

Through the mid-1980s in North America, opinion about the value of thyroid FNB was divided. In 1981 Ashcraft and van Herle exhaustively reviewed preoperative diagnostic techniques for thyroid nodules and concluded that needle biopsy was the best of those available.[13] Nevertheless, skepticism was expressed as late as 1984.[14–16] In the decade since then, FNB has gained progressively wider acceptance and use, because its advantages have been confirmed by numerous investigators.[17–31] They include the following:

- FNB is easy to learn for any physician who can palpate thyroid nodules well.
- One can sample nodules as small as 1 cm and even smaller if the nodule is easily accessible.
- FNB is essentially risk-free.
- FNB is cost-effective.
- Skill in the interpretation of FNB specimens is readily acquired by qualified cytopathologists after study of reference material and the acquisition of reasonable experience.[18,32–34]

The fears that led to hesitation about thyroid FNB have not been borne out. They included doubt that the number of thyroid operations would be reduced, concern that there would be a significant number of thyroid cancers missed because of false-negative FNB results, and worry that tumor could be seeded along a needle track. Seeding has been described only in 1973 and 1976 reports involving large-needle biopsies.[5,35]

This chapter deals in depth with FNB method, pitfalls and how to avoid them, and the integration of FNB data into the evaluation and treatment planning for thyroid nodule patients. Although not widely employed, large-needle biopsy procedures are described, mainly to compare them with FNB. The uses of thyroid FNB are listed in Table 23-1.

TABLE 23-1.
Uses of Thyroid Fine Needle Biopsy

COMMON

Selection of therapy for a thyroid nodule
   Surgery versus observation ± thyroxine
   Extent of surgery
Diagnosis of a thyroid nodule

LESS COMMON

Diagnosis of the cause of thyroid enlargement
Elimination of a thyroid nodule
   Removal of cyst fluid or blood from a cystic nodule
   Injection of a sclerosing agent, for a recurrent cyst
   Ablation of an autonomous nodule by ethanol injection
Postoperative evaluation of cervical lymph nodes
Diagnosis of infective thyroiditis
Obtaining thyroid DNA or RNA for amplification and analysis

FINE-NEEDLE BIOPSY TECHNIQUE

FNB provides specimens for cytologic evaluation. Different FNB techniques are used in various centers. We shall describe our method, one that has been refined during more than 15 years' experience with about 9000 patients.

Selecting the Needle

We use 25-gauge, 1½-inch needles. They produce excellent specimens and are less likely than larger needles to cause the bleeding that dilutes specimens and thereby greatly reduces their usefulness. The ease with which bleeding is induced depends not only on needle size but also on the structure of the nodule. Some nodules are dense and relatively avascular. Others are more loosely organized and bloody. It is difficult to judge prospectively the internal consistency of a nodule. Occasionally, a 22- or 23-gauge needle may be best for particularly hard papillary carcinomas and other fibrotic nodules.

Obtaining the Specimen

The skin is cleaned with alcohol and infiltrated with 1 to 2 ml of 1% lidocaine. The nodule is fixed by the fingers of the opposite hand, and the needle (attached to a 10-mL syringe) is inserted in a direction perpendicular to the anterior surface of the neck. Withdrawing the plunger about two thirds of the way produces negative pressure, and one looks for bloody fluid in the hub of the needle. At the first appearance of fluid, negative pressure is released and the needle withdrawn. No fluid should enter the syringe. If this happens, the specimen will be too dilute and may be lost in the syringe.

Material may appear in the syringe if too large a needle is used, if negative pressure is too vigorous, if the nodule is extensively degenerated or unusually vascular, or if the nodule is a fluid-filled cyst. For the first two possibilities, adjustments can be made to improve the chances for success with subse-

quent punctures. The last two situations are beyond the control of the operator, although it may help to insert the needle at the nodule periphery, where degeneration is less likely. The initial aspiration may produce no specimen if the needle is not in the nodule, if the needle is too fine, if negative pressure is not vigorous enough, or if the nodule is fibrotic.

If negative pressure fails to produce fluid in the hub of the needle and one is confident that the needle is in the nodule, some maneuver is necessary to disrupt the tissue integrity to permit aspiration of a specimen. The simplest method is to move the needle in and out within the nodule through a vertical distance of 1 to 2 mm.[36] This nearly always yields a specimen. If this maneuver fails, one can combine the in-and-out movement with a rotation of the needle through 360 degrees within the nodule. The rotating sharp bevel of the needle severs small tissue fragments for aspiration. This technique is seldom necessary and, for most nodules, produces a worthless and excessively voluminous bloody specimen. Some workers find that satisfactory specimens can often be obtained using only a needle, with no syringe and no suction. The needle is moved in and out over 1 to 2 mm and is then kept still for about 10 seconds, to allow the freed cells to flow into the needle by capillary action. This technique minimizes dilution of the thyroid cells by blood. The comparative yield of satisfactory specimens using syringe suction vs. no suction for thyroid nodule FNBs has not been studied systematically, to our knowledge.

If the nodule is a cyst, it will collapse with aspiration unless there is a solid component. FNB should be tried on any residual mass. We rarely obtain useful information from examining the sediment from cyst fluid.

After withdrawal, the needle is detached, and 3 to 4 mL of air is forced through the needle to evacuate the specimen onto a slide. After FNB, the area is dressed with an adhesive pad, and the patient may depart after a few minutes of observation to rule out local swelling. We obtain diagnostically useful FNB specimens about 80% of the time. This figure may be less than that claimed by some, but this relates to our relatively strict criteria for adequacy of cytologic material to exclude malignancy, as discussed later.

Some physicians place the syringe in a pistol grip designed to facilitate a one-handed biopsy.[37] We do not recommend this technique because it removes the operating hand further from the nodule, with an apparent loss of the tactile sense that we find helpful in assuring proper needle placement.

A grossly satisfactory FNB specimen consists of one drop of red-orange fluid (Fig 23-1A). Although gross inspection does not guarantee adequate numbers of epithelial cells, one can be sure that more voluminous and bloody specimens or specimens that consist of watery, greenish-brown degeneration fluid, crystal-clear jelly-like fluid, thick oily fluid, or cheesy white material contain insufficient epithelial cells. In some clinics, specimens can be stained and examined while the patient waits, so that an unsatisfactory procedure can be repeated immediately.

We have done nearly all of our FNBs guided by palpation alone. Some groups advocate real-time ultrasound imaging to direct placement of the biopsy needle.[38–40] This method will increase the expense of the biopsy procedure and requires ad-

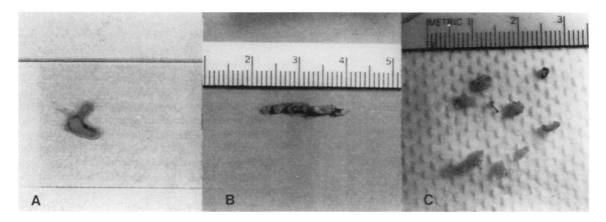

FIGURE 23-1. Needle biopsy specimens. *(A)* A satisfactory FNB specimen, consisting of a single drop of red-orange fluid. *(B)* A large-needle cutting biopsy specimen. *(C)* A large-needle aspiration biopsy specimen consisting of multiple tissue fragments. (Hamburger JI, Miller JM, Kini SR. Clinical pathological evaluation of thyroid nodules: Handbook and atlas. Southfield, MI: private publication, 1979)

vance scheduling unless ultrasound equipment is present in the office. It is unnecessary for easily palpable nodules but may be helpful for small, flat, or deep nodules, especially if an initial FNB attempt was made using just palpation produces unsatisfactory specimens.

Preparing the Smear

After expelling the specimen onto a glass slide, it should be smeared and fixed immediately to prevent air drying. A common technique is that used for a blood smear, in which a second slide is held at a 45- to 60-degree angle to the specimen on an underlying slide. The specimen is allowed to spread out along the edge of the upper slide, which is then advanced along the long axis of the underlying slide, drawing out the specimen into a smear. We find that this method too often produces thick, uneven smears. Instead, we recommend the following method of smearing the specimen. A top slide is placed flat on top of the specimen. With the index finger, the top slide is pressed down onto the specimen and drawn over the bottom slide. This simple maneuver produces flat, uniformly dispersed smears.

Although the Scandinavians have used air-dried smears stained with May-Giemsa-Grünwald stain, a stain that enhances cytoplasmic details, American cytopathologists prefer the crisp nuclear detail that Papanicolaou's stain provides. For Papanicolaou's stain, the specimens must be fixed immediately, before air drying has taken place. Even Löwhagen et al use the Papanicolaou method as a supplement to their usual technique in some cases.[36]

Some cytopathology laboratories prefer FNB specimens to be expelled from the needle into a preservative/fixative solution so that the slides can be prepared in the laboratory. This permits the use of methods that concentrate the thyroid cells and eliminate the red blood cells. The choice of direct smears fixed immediately with spray fixative or another technique needs to be made cooperatively between the FNB operator and the cytopathologist.

LARGE-NEEDLE BIOPSY TECHNIQUE

Large-needle biopsy procedures provide tissue cylinders or fragments for conventional histologic evaluation. Two methods of large-needle biopsy may be employed: large-needle cutting biopsy and large-needle aspiration biopsy.

Large-Needle Cutting Biopsy

Large-needle cutting biopsy (LNCB) provides a tissue cylinder for histologic evaluation. Hamlin and Vickery,[3] Wang and coworkers,[5] and more recently, LoGerfo,[4] have used LNCB for the diagnosis of thyroid nodules. LoGerfo reports an accuracy of 90%, provided that adequate specimens are obtained and studied by an experienced thyroid pathologist. Large-needle biopsy procedures are safely performed on outpatients and are not likely to disseminate malignant disease.

TECHNIQUES

Either the 14-gauge, 2 3/8-inch or 3 1/8-inch Silverman needle or the 14-gauge, 3-inch Tru-Cut disposable needle may be used. The techniques are different and are described individually.

Silverman Needle Procedure. The area down to the nodule capsule is infiltrated with 2 mL of 0.5% lidocaine. Because the needle is withdrawn through the skin and reinserted several times, the skin is prepared with iodine and alcohol, the biopsy site is draped with a disposable plastic drape, and the operator maintains sterile technique. The surgical pack contains the needle, gauze sponges, filter paper strips to receive the specimens, and a number-11 scalpel blade. The latter is used to make a skin nick because the needle is too large to insert through the intact skin. To avoid incising underlying structures, the nick is made in a skin fold pinched between thumb and forefinger.

The Silverman needle, obturator in place, is inserted at an angle of 60 degrees with the anterior neck surface, just proximal to the superior pole of the nodule, directed away from the trachea. After the needle penetrates the nodule, the angle is reduced to 30 degrees, and the needle is aligned parallel to the trachea to avoid the major neck vessels. The obturator is replaced by the cutting insert, which projects beyond the tip of the outer sheath. The outer sheath is advanced by rotation over the cutting insert to its tip, severing the specimen within the blades of the cutting insert. The needle is withdrawn, and the severed tissue (see Fig 23-1B) can be found on one of the blades. The specimen is placed on filter paper and immersed in Bouin's solution, a fixative that preserves cytologic details.[22] Bouin's fixation is especially helpful for follicular neoplasms. After the needle is withdrawn, pressure is maintained on the biopsy site. Control of bleeding is important per se, and also because excessive bleeding within the nodule may make it impossible to obtain further specimens. When possible, we secure three specimens, each from a different portion of the nodule. A cutting insert with retention tabs is helpful for firm nodules.

The Silverman needle may fail if extensive degeneration and unusual vascularity are present, or if the nodule is particularly soft.

Tru-Cut Needle Procedure. Preparation of the patient is the same as for the Silverman needle biopsy. Because the Tru-Cut needle has a relatively blunt tip, and the overlying sheath may not fit flush with the inner shaft bearing the biopsy notch, this needle is more difficult to insert into a nodule than the Silverman needle. If used as the manufacturer recommends, the outer sheath may catch on the subcutaneous tissues or the capsule so that the inner shaft retracts, and no specimen or a poor specimen is obtained. This problem and its solution are illustrated in Figure 23-2. Again, when feasible, we secure three specimens, each from a different part of the nodule. Specimens are fixed in Bouin's solution.

After completion of the biopsy with either the Silverman or Tru-Cut needle, the wound is dressed with an adhesive pad and the patient is asked to apply pressure for 20 to 30 minutes. The neck is inspected for swelling before the patient departs.

Large-Needle Aspiration Biopsy

Large-needle aspiration biopsy (LNAB) was first reported in 1930 by Martin and Ellis,[1] and later modified by Rudowski.[41]

Crile and Hawk[35] concluded that the routine use of LNAB for nodules that were not obviously malignant on clinical grounds would reduce the need for thyroidectomy by "a factor of 10 to 1."

TECHNIQUE

The LNAB technique is similar to that used for FNB; however, considerably larger needles are used. We employ 16- or 18-gauge needles, the smaller ones for smaller nodules, although success is rather low for nodules smaller than 2 cm. The skin is prepared and anesthetized as for FNB. The needle is attached to a 20-mL syringe containing heparin or 1 mL of sodium citrate solution to prevent specimen coagulation. Fixation and penetration of the nodules are accomplished as for FNB. As the needle enters the nodule, vigorous continuous negative pressure is applied. The syringe is rotated through 360 degrees, and the sharp bevel of the needle severs tissue fragments, which are aspirated along with blood into the syringe. Maintaining negative pressure, the needle is withdrawn to the capsule, redirected, and reinserted. The rotational biopsy maneuver is repeated four to six times at different sites, depending on the nodule size. The needle is then withdrawn, releasing negative pressure before the tip leaves the capsule. The biopsy site is dressed with an adhesive pad, and the patient maintains firm pressure for 20 minutes. The neck is examined for swelling before the patient leaves.

PREPARING THE SPECIMEN

After the biopsy, 5 to 10 mL of saline is aspirated into the syringe, washing any tissue in the needle into the syringe barrel. The syringe is up-ended over a paper filter, and the plunger is withdrawn, pouring the specimen onto the filter. This avoids the further fragmentation of the specimen that might occur if evacuation were through the needle. After the fluid drains off, the tissue fragments (see Fig 23-1C) are placed in Bouin's fixative.

Tissue may not be obtained if the nodule is composed entirely of degenerated material or if there is densely packed tissue with a considerable fibrotic component.

Table 23-2 compares the technical aspects of FNB, LNAB, and LNCB. Currently, we employ one of the larger needle procedures on less than 1% of our patients. The principal use of large-needle biopsy is for large nodules that have under-

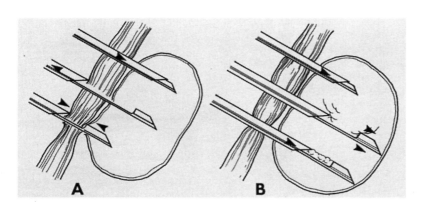

FIGURE 23-2. Tru-Cut needle biopsy technique. *(A)* Technique as recommended for thyroid by manufacturer. Needle is inserted into nodule. Outer sheath is withdrawn, opening biopsy notch. Outer sheath is then advanced but, as illustrated, catches on extranodular tissue because it offers more resistance than nodular tissue; the needle retracts rather than the sheath advancing as desired. *(B)* Preferred technique. Needle is inserted into nodule just through the capsule. Inner shaft is then advanced into nodule, opening biopsy notch to permit nodular tissue to prolapse into notch. Outer sheath is advanced, severing specimen. (Hamburger JI, Miller JM, Kini SR. Clinical pathological evaluation of thyroid nodules: Handbook and atlas. Southfield, MI: private publication, 1979)

TABLE 23-2.
Comparison of Technical Aspects of Fine-Needle, Large-Needle Aspiration, and Large-Needle Cutting Biopsies

	Fine-Needle Biopsy	Large-Needle Aspiration Biopsy	Large-Needle Cutting Biopsy
Relative difficulty	+	++	+++
Needle size (gauge)	22–25	16–18	14
Skin incision	No	No	Yes
Suitable for nodules with least diameter size (cm)			
Usual	1	2	2.5
Favorably located	0.5	1	1.5
Patient discomfort	0 to +	+	++
Relative potential for damage to adjacent structures	0	+	++
Success rate in obtaining specimens adequate for diagnostic purposes	80%	60%	90%

gone extensive degeneration so that FNB specimens produce only degeneration fluid. LNAB may aspirate useful small tissue fragments.

FNB is not only simpler than the larger needle procedures but may also be more sensitive when multiple aspirations are taken. This is especially so in larger pleomorphic follicular neoplasms. We have had experiences in which LNCB specimens by chance were taken from the more normal-appearing portion of a follicular carcinoma. The more complete sampling provided by multiple FNB samples produced suspicious cells that correctly indicated the need for operation.

POTENTIAL COMPLICATIONS OF NEEDLE BIOPSY

It is virtually impossible to do any serious damage with FNB. FNB is safe even in patients taking anticoagulants. Nevertheless, patients should be advised that trauma to adjacent structures is possible. Occasionally, there is a local hematoma after FNB. An ice pack is adequate treatment. Rarely, the entire thyroid gland swells acutely; this spontaneously resolves within 24 to 48 hours or less.

We have observed a transient recurrent nerve palsy after a large-needle biopsy and mild pain radiating to the ear that persisted for several months after one FNB. Although seeding a malignancy in the needle track has been reported after large-needle biopsies,[5,35] we are aware of no such occurrences after FNB. The reported seedings were easily excised and had no unfavorable impact on prognosis. Infection has not been associated with thyroid FNB.

The legal consequences of false-positive or false-negative diagnoses are of concern to some physicians. These risks are inherent in selecting thyroid nodules for operation. Needle biopsy improves diagnostic precision and reduces the potential for error. However, biopsies are neither successful nor reliable 100% of the time, and patients must be told this in advance. This ensures informed consent and defuses the potential for future litigation.

FINE-NEEDLE BIOPSY RESULTS AND DIAGNOSTIC ACCURACY

Figures 23-3 and 23-4 depict composites of FNB specimens and illustrate the important cytologic features of the principal thyroid nodular lesions. Table 23-3 shows the correlation between FNB diagnoses and the surgical diagnoses for our patients operated on between 1985 and 1989.

Avoiding False-Negative Diagnoses

To minimize sampling errors and to increase chances of adequate cellular material, we routinely perform enough aspirations to provide at least six separate specimens that appear grossly satisfactory. For each aspiration, the needle is inserted at a different location at the periphery of the nodule (if size permits). A single smear with just one cluster of obviously malignant cells may be enough to diagnose malignancy; because most thyroid nodules are benign, however, the principal objective of needle biopsy is to exclude malignancy and thus minimize unnecessary surgery. Although one does not obtain benign cells from a malignant nodule, malignant nodules have adjacent benign tissue. Therefore, if the needle is misplaced, benign cells can be aspirated even though the nodule is malignant. Also, in some areas of a malignancy, the cells may be more obviously malignant than in others, especially in follicular tumors. For these reasons, we have established a more stringent criterion to exclude than to establish a diagnosis of malignancy.[42–44] To exclude malignancy, we require at least six clusters of benign cells on at least two smears, and no malignant or suspicious cells. Because one cannot be absolutely certain by gross inspection whether any given FNB specimen has epithelial cells, we advise multiple aspirations.

Most reports indicate that one to four aspirates are adequate.[17,23,25,45–48] These reports include varying numbers of false-negative diagnoses (Table 23-4). The avoidable false-negative diagnoses we made in our first 1000 cases, however, proved to us the danger of making a diagnosis of benign disease on the basis of a few clusters of benign-appearing cells

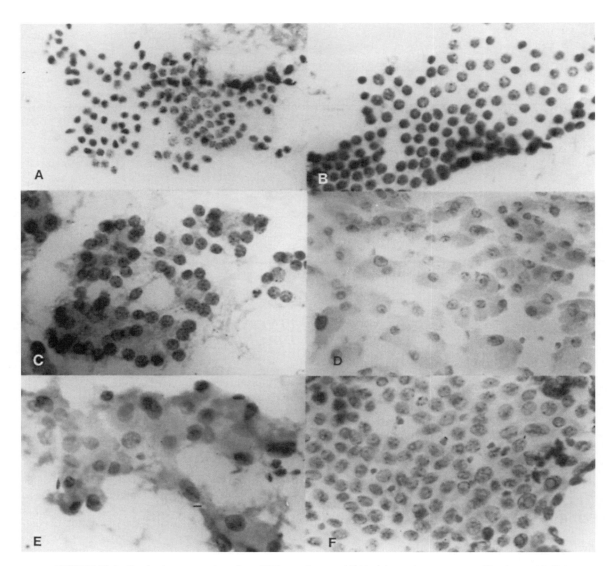

FIGURE 23-3. Cytologic preparations from FNB specimens. *(A)* Nodular goiter: a group of benign epithelial cells forming sheets and follicles. *(B)* Nodular goiter: a large, monolayered sheet of follicular cells containing uniform nuclei with finely granular chromatin. *(C)* Cellular adenoma: a tissue fragment with uniform, slightly enlarged nuclei with compact chromatin. There is marked crowding and overlapping of the nuclei. *(D)* Hürthle cell tumor: large polygonal cells, isolated and forming sheets with distinct cell borders and abundant, dense granular cytoplasm. Nuclei are mostly eccentric with prominent macronucleoli. *(E)* A tissue fragment of Hürthle cells showing ill-defined cell borders and large pleomorphic hyperchromatic nuclei with irregular nucleoli. *(F)* Papillary carcinoma: a monolayered sheet of cancer cells with large pleomorphic nuclei, exhibiting loss of polarity and numerous nuclear "holes". (Hamburger JI, Miller JM, Kini SR. Clinical pathological evaluation of thyroid nodules: Handbook and atlas. Southfield, MI: private publication, 1979)

on a single slide. The validity of this concept was shown in a later report of nine thyroid cancer patients, seven of whom had FNB specimens with only a few clusters of benign-appearing cells.[43] Sensitized by our previous experience, we did not make diagnoses of benign lesions. Instead, we reported that the specimens contained too few cells to exclude malignancy. Cancers were confirmed by repeat FNB and at operation. To determine whether the problem might have been a lack of expertise on the part of our cytopathologist, slides from six of these patients were reviewed at four major medical centers, intermingled with 14 others. The review pathologists were not forewarned of the objective of the study. Of 24 possible false-negative diagnoses (six cases, each studied at four institutions), 6 false-negative diagnoses were made.[44] The participating pathologists were then asked whether they used any quantitative criteria for adequacy of FNB sampling, or just evaluated the specimens qualitatively. None of them had quantitative guidelines for adequacy.

In the large Mayo Clinic study (6346 FNBs), one to four aspirations were performed, and five or six clusters of cells on

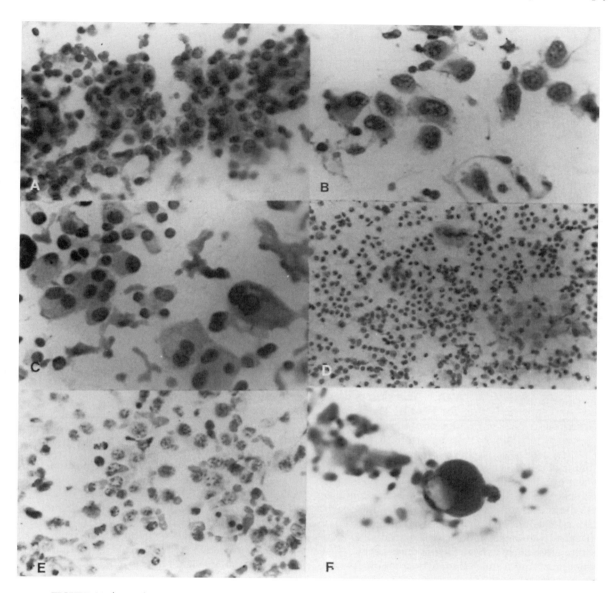

FIGURE 23-4. Cytologic preparations from FNB specimens. *(A)* Follicular carcinoma: a tissue fragment composed of cells with large hyperchromatic nuclei, extremely crowded, with overlapping and a tendency toward a follicular orientation. *(B)* Anaplastic carcinoma: large, noncoherent irregular cells with large, bizarre plemorphic nuclei containing multiple nucleoli and clumped chromatin. *(C)* Medullary carcinoma: a cellular specimen with cells of varying size that strongly resemble plasma cells. Nuclei are eccentric, with coarse chromatin and prominent nucleoli. *(D)* Hashimoto's thyroiditis: a profuse mixture of lymphocytes and plasma cells with large thyroid epithelial cells containing polymorphic nuclei with a fine chromatin pattern. *(E)* Malignant lymphoma of the thyroid: large discrete cells with scanty cytoplasm, large nuclei, and multiple nucleoli. *(F)* Colon carcinoma metastatic to the thyroid: a single large carcinoma cell with a large secretory vacuole. (Hamburger JI, Miller JM, Kini SR. Clinical pathological evaluation of thyroid nodules: Handbook and atlas. Southfield, MI: private publication, 1979)

a single slide were considered adequate to exclude malignancy. Inadequate sampling was blamed for eight false-negative diagnoses, five of them on papillary carcinomas.[48] False-negative diagnoses were also attributed to inadequate sampling in a report from the University of California, Los Angeles.[49]

In our hands, the criterion of at least six clusters of benign-appearing cells on at least two separate aspirates has virtually eliminated false-negative diagnoses. Of 86 patients in our recent series (see Table 23-3), operated on despite FNB diagnoses of benign disease, only one had a cancer, a well-differentiated follicular carcinoma. One should not conclude that as many as one of 86 of our benign diagnoses was false-negative, since the patients who had operations despite the benign FNB findings were not representative of the FNB benign nodule population as a whole. For example, in the same time pe-

TABLE 23-3.
Correlation of Fine-Needle Biopsy Diagnoses and Surgical Diagnoses, 1985–1989

Fine-Needle Biopsy Diagnoses	NUMBER	BENIGN	FOLLICULAR ADENOMA	HÜRTHLE CELL TUMOR	HÜRTHLE CELL CARCINOMA	ATYPICAL ADENOMA	PAPILLARY CARCINOMA	FOLLICULAR CARCINOMA	THYROGLOSSAL DUCT CYST	MISCELLA-NEOUS*
							Surgical Diagnoses			
Unsatisfactory	50	34	6	—	—	—	9	1	—	—
Hashimoto's thyroiditis	8	6	1	1	—	—	—	—	—	—
Nodular goiter	78	63	13	1	—	—	—	1	—	—
Follicular adenoma	83	25	45	2	1	3	3	4	—	—
Hürthle cell tumor	34	8	7	11	7	—	—	1	—	—
Hürthle cell carcinoma	2	—	—	—	1	—	1	—	—	—
Suspected papillary carcinoma	25	6	4	—	1	—	10	2	1	1
Suspected follicular carcinoma	4	1	1	—	—	—	—	2	—	—
Papillary carcinoma	91	—	1	—	—	—	87	3	—	—
Follicular carcinoma	3	—	—	—	—	—	—	3	—	—
Miscellaneous	7	—	—	—	—	—	—	—	—	7
TOTALS	385	143	78	15	10	3	113	14	1	8

*Miscellaneous diagnoses include 2 lymphomas, 2 medullary carcinomas, 1 undifferentiated carcinoma, 1 metastatic carcinoma to the thyroid, 1 lipoma, and 1 neurilemmoma.

riod, two thirds of our patients with benign FNB findings were subsequently treated with thyroxine. Contrary to the findings of Gharib and colleagues,[50] 19% of our thyroxine-treated nodules regressed to the size of 0.5 cm or smaller and an additional 9% regressed by at least 50%. These patients were not operated on. Younger patients with larger nodules that did not respond to thyroxine were more likely to have their nodules excised.

Assuming that our semiquantitative criterion for adequacy of sampling to exclude malignancy is effective, an-

other question is, how many aspirations are required to maximize the percentage of specimens that meet this criterion? To settle this issue, we numbered our aspirates sequentially for each patient, and they were evaluated individually by our cytopathologist until 100 consecutive FNB studies were completed for which the cellularity of the aspirates fulfilled our criterion for adequacy. All patients had at least six aspirations; 59 patients had eight aspirations. More than six aspirations were performed when some of the first six were of

TABLE 23-4.
False-Negative Diagnoses in Fine-Needle Biopsy and the Number of Aspirations Performed in a Fine-Needle Biopsy Procedure

References	No. of Excised Nodules with FNB Diagnoses of Benign	False-Negative Diagnoses		No. of Aspirations
		NO.	%	
Schwartz et al, 1982[45]	84	6	7	1
Ramacciotti et al, 1984[46]	64	6	10	2
Boey et al, 1984[47]	112	6	5	3–4
Anderson and Webb, 1987[17]	312	4	1	1
Hawkins et al, 1987[22]	336	10	3	≥2
Goellner et al, 1987[48]	130	8	6	1–4
Hamming et al, 1990[24]	92	3	3	1*

*Not stated in the report; information supplied in response to a query directed to the authors.

dubious quality grossly, being either scanty or bloody. For 77% of these cases, two to four aspirations would have been adequate; for the remaining 23%, however, five to eight aspirations were needed.[44] We advise at least six aspirations as the initial minimal evaluation, both to ensure adequate sampling at the first FNB and to minimize the need for repeating the FNB. When it is possible to study the aspirates cytologically at the time the FNB is performed, it may be suitable to make only two to four aspirations initially, and then to perform further aspirations until adequate sampling has been accomplished.

The use of local anesthesia facilitates patient comfort and cooperation throughout the procedure. Many physicians assert that local anesthesia is unnecessary, probably because they take fewer aspirates. We are very concerned about avoiding the false-negative diagnoses that result from inadequate sampling, and prefer to be able to take multiple samples with minimal pain.

False-Positive Diagnoses and the Problem of Follicular Tumors

False-positive diagnoses are made because aspirates from benign nodules have cytologic features that resemble those of malignant lesions. However, cytologic diagnoses of definite malignancy made by experienced cytopathologists are nearly always confirmed at operation.[25,28–30,42,48] The principal cause of false-positive FNB diagnoses is detection of the less decisive cytologic features that neither confirm nor exclude diagnoses of malignancy. FNB diagnoses of "suspected" papillary or follicular carcinoma should then be made, diagnoses that in our experience predicted the presence of a malignancy 50% or more of the time (see Table 23-3). Diagnoses of Hürthle cell tumor were indicative of underlying malignancy about 25% of the time, whereas diagnoses of follicular adenoma were indicative of an underlying malignancy only 13% of the time (including atypical adenomas). It is essential for each institution to establish its own statistics relative to the probabilities of malignancy for specific FNB diagnoses, if FNB data are to be used effectively in management planning.

In contrast to our approach, Gharib and Goellner[30] suggest that all lesions with FNB findings of "suspicious" require operation, because they find a 30% incidence of malignancy. They do not segregate those lesions with highly suspicious FNB findings (those we diagnose as "suspected papillary or follicular carcinoma") from those for which there is a much lower level of suspicion (those we diagnose as "follicular adenomas"). Hence, the management implications of FNB diagnoses depend on the cytologic criteria for the specific diagnoses. We too initially employed nonspecific terminology of *benign, suspicious,* and *malignant* for FNB. We believe it is more helpful to use the tissue diagnoses listed in Table 23-3; others use similar classifications.[28]

It can be argued that FNB diagnoses of follicular adenoma, Hürthle cell tumor, or suspected follicular carcinoma that lead to the excision of a benign nodule are not false-positive diagnoses. They are just diagnoses that neither exclude nor establish the presence of a malignancy. LiVolsi[51] comments that FNB cytology alone is not an adequate *diagnostic* technique for follicular tumors, for reasons intrinsic to the nature of these lesions. Rather, FNB cytology is a *screening* technique to help select nodules that should be surgically excised.

IMPACT OF NEEDLE BIOPSY DATA ON THYROID NODULE MANAGEMENT

Deciding When to Operate

With experience, needle biopsy diagnoses of benign or definite malignancy approximate the accuracy of diagnoses based on study of permanent sections from surgical specimens. Our study of needle biopsy has been ongoing since October 1976. Before needle biopsy, all patients with thyroid nodules were evaluated by conventional clinical methods. By those methods, about half of the patients were referred for operation, while only about one quarter of the patients operated on had thyroid cancer. Nevertheless, some cancers were overlooked. The use of needle biopsy has reduced to less than 20% the proportion of patients for whom surgery is advised, and increased to about 50% the proportion of those operated on who have malignancies (data from Table 23-3, excluding patients who had surgery for nodule size or who requested operation in spite of benign biopsy diagnoses). Reported yields of malignancy in other series vary between about 30% and 50%.[27–30]

The primary objective of needle biopsy is to reduce the number of unnecessary operations for thyroid nodules, that is, to identify nodules that are safely left in situ. By "safely," we mean that the risk of cancer is so small that the risks of operation would be greater. Even this statement needs amplification. Needle biopsy can achieve about 98% to 99% reliability for the exclusion of cancer when adequate specimens are obtained. For an occasional low-grade follicular carcinoma, FNB may produce cells that are indistinguishable from those of benign nodules. Nevertheless, the risk to the patient of such biopsy errors is not the same as their 1% to 2% frequency. Missing the diagnosis of such a cancer is not equivalent to a sentence of death. If the patient returns for periodic reevaluations, any subsequent growth indicates that a repeat FNB is prudent.[52] Indeed, repeat FNB may be desirable even in the absence of growth if the nodule is unchanged after 1 to 2 years, especially despite treatment with thyroxine.[52] A repeat FNB occasionally produces suspicious cells, which indicate the need for operation. Fortunately, the types of thyroid cancers for which an initial FNB may provide false-negative findings are most likely low-grade tumors that are usually still curable even if the diagnosis is delayed for a few years.

In contrast, the principal risk of operation (i.e., operative mortality) is faced entirely at the time of the procedure. Hence, an operative mortality of 0.1% may be a greater immediate risk to the patient than a 1% risk of a false-negative FNB diagnosis. Obviously, to assess these relative risks, each institution must develop its own statistics relative to both FNB accuracy and surgical morbidity and mortality.

With these reservations in mind, we can say that FNB diagnoses of definite papillary or follicular carcinoma, lymphoma of the thyroid, medullary carcinoma, undifferentiated carcinoma, and metastatic carcinoma to the thyroid are nearly always confirmed at operation. Surgery is advised for the potentially resectable lesions, and other appropriate management can be instituted for lymphoma, anaplastic, and metastatic lesions. In some instances, FNB diagnoses of follicular carcinoma are made when the lesion is the follicular variant of papillary carcinoma.

For FNB diagnoses of suspected papillary or follicular carcinoma or Hürthle cell tumor, the chances of malignancy are 25% to 50%, high enough that operation would be prudent unless there is a major contraindication to surgery. For FNB diagnoses of follicular adenoma with a microfollicular component, the chances of malignancy are only 10% to 15%. This risk is usually considered great enough to advise operation for young healthy patients; an 85% to 90% probability that the nodule is benign, however, might make observation an acceptable choice if the patient is elderly or infirm. At the Mayo Clinic, where the cytologic categories are benign, suspicious, and malignant, repeat biopsy of 41 nodules with an initial suspicious cytology resulted in benign cytology findings about half of the time.[53] However, since only two of the latter patients had surgery, the diagnostic implications of this sequence of results is uncertain. Observation is advised if the FNB diagnosis is Hashimoto's thyroiditis, nodular goiter, or macrofollicular adenoma without atypia.

About 20% of the time, one is not able to obtain enough material by needle biopsy to exclude malignancy reliably. In the series shown in Table 23-3, about 20% of the nodules were malignant. This is somewhat more than the overall 10% frequency of malignancy in solid hypofunctional thyroid nodules in our practice. The 20% rate of malignancy observed relates in part to clinical selectivity in our recommendation for operation. In another series, 9% of patients operated on with FNB specimens inadequate for diagnosis had thyroid cancers.[54] In the absence of reliable FNB data, we consider other clinical features that might affect the probabilities of malignancy before advising observation or operation,[25,29,55] recognizing the limited preoperative diagnostic accuracy of this approach.

Deciding Which Operation to Perform

The conventional surgical approach to thyroid nodules has been lobectomy (usually including the isthmus) with a frozen section, after which the operation is terminated or extended depending on the frozen section findings. This strategy is flawed, since frozen section diagnoses on thyroid lesions may be erroneous, and the diagnosis is frequently deferred pending review of the permanent sections.[51,56,57] Then, the surgeon sometimes performs an unnecessarily aggressive operation, with the attendant increased risks, or an inadequate cancer operation, having to take the patient back for a second procedure when the permanent sections reveal a malignancy. Patients dislike complications that might have been avoided by a more conservative procedure; however, they may like even less the prospect of a second operation when the necessary excision could have been done initially.

Could needle biopsy data improve the accuracy of surgical planning? After all, because needle biopsies are performed almost routinely in the initial evaluation of thyroid nodules, the data are available for use in surgical planning. Impressed by the frequency with which frozen section diagnoses were inaccurate or deferred in hospitals in the metropolitan Detroit area, we undertook a comparison of the relative accuracy of FNB findings with those of frozen section.[56]

Because FNB diagnoses of definite thyroid cancer were about 99% reliable, it seemed unlikely that frozen section could provide more reliable data. Indeed, frozen section, although accurate, was less reliable than FNB. Similarly, FNB diagnoses of benign disease were about 99% reliable, and frozen section was less reliable for those patients.

FNB was less specific in the diagnosis of malignancy for follicular and Hürthle cell tumors; however, frozen section was also unreliable for those lesions because multiple sections are usually necessary to search for evidence of vascular or capsular invasion before cancer can be confirmed or excluded. Hence, when decisive frozen section diagnoses would be most useful, they are least likely to be forthcoming.

From this analysis, we arrived at the following conclusions:

- If surgery is elected for a patient despite an FNB diagnosis of a benign nodule, the operation should be a lobectomy, without frozen section.
- If surgery is elected for a patient with an FNB diagnosis of follicular adenoma, an initial lobectomy will be the correct procedure more than 85% of the time. Even if the nodule is malignant, if it is a small, low-grade follicular carcinoma, some but not all thyroidologists would consider a lobectomy an adequate operation. Frozen section will not be needed.
- For FNB diagnoses of Hürthle cell tumor or suspected carcinoma (papillary or follicular), the chances of cancer are increased. In these circumstances, we advise a full disclosure of the possibilities to the patient in advance of the operation, rather than relying on frozen section for guidance. This reduces the potential for postoperation recriminations. In our experience, when faced with a substantial risk of a second operation, if the first procedure is limited to a lobectomy, most patients prefer to have a cancer operation as the initial procedure. They are willing to accept the additional operative risks to avoid the risks and unpleasantness of a second operation.
- For FNB diagnoses of definite malignancy, the chances of a false-positive diagnosis are so small that it is best to proceed with an appropriate cancer operation as the initial procedure, without bothering with frozen section.
- When FNB fails to provide diagnostic data, or in the occasional patient for whom an additional unexpected nodule is first discovered at the operation, frozen section may be helpful. In our experience, frozen section diagnoses of malignancy are only infrequently reversed by the findings on permanent sections.
- For FNB diagnoses of definite malignancy, the exact surgical procedure may be guided by frozen section evaluation of lymph nodes, parathyroid glands, and tumor invasion into fat and muscle.

Kopald and coworkers[57] also found FNB more reliable than frozen section. Keller and colleagues[24] and LiVolsi[51] found that FNB is reliable for surgical planning whenever diagnoses of benign or definite malignancy are made.

QUESTIONS COMMONLY ASKED ABOUT NEEDLE BIOPSY

Should All Thyroid Nodules Undergo Biopsy?

We do not perform biopsies on autonomously functioning thyroid nodules, functional hyperplastic nodules, or, of course, purely cystic nodules that disappear after aspiration. FNB findings on autonomous nodules may be confusingly suspicious.[58] In our opinion, the very small number of reported cancers in nodules that are hyperfunctioning by radioactive iodine imaging[59] does not mandate FNB of all such nodules, although we do perform FNB evaluation of hypofunctioning areas within functioning nodules. We also biopsy hypofunctioning nodules in multinodular goiters, a new hypofunctioning nodule in a thyroid that has other nodules, and any solid remnant after fluid has been removed from a cystic nodule, because the prevalence rates of cancers in multinodular goiters and in nodules with cystic components are not sufficiently lower than the rates in solitary nodules to allow reliance on these variables in deciding on management.[55,60,62]

We also advise prompt FNB evaluation of thyroid nodules discovered during pregnancy for two reasons. First, the detection of the nodule raises concern about malignancy that can usually be alleviated simply and quickly. Second, FNB offers maximum scheduling flexibility for those nodules that should be excised, including the options of surgery in the second trimester, as soon as possible after delivery, or at a time most consistent with breastfeeding plans.

We perform biopsies on nodules we think are benign, because we may be wrong. We perform biopsies on those we think are malignant, not only because we are often wrong but also because confirmatory biopsy information is helpful, for the following reasons:

- Patients with a biopsy diagnosis of malignancy will comply with a recommendation for surgery more readily than if cancer is suspected only from nonspecific clinical findings.
- When a biopsy diagnosis of unequivocal malignancy is made by an experienced pathologist, the surgeon can plan a proper cancer operation in advance.
- Biopsy findings may eliminate unnecessary surgery for certain malignancies such as lymphoma of the thyroid, anaplastic carcinoma, and metastatic carcinoma to the thyroid.
- Biopsy may identify patients with medullary carcinoma, who should have preoperative calcitonin and carcinoembryonic antigen measurements and preoperative evaluation for pheochromocytoma.

What Are the Limitations of Needle Biopsy?

The principal limitation is inexperience, both in obtaining adequate specimens and in interpreting the specimens once they have been secured. Illustrative material is available that permits one to use FNB without recapitulating the more elementary errors,[22,51,63,64] but there is no substitute for actual experience. It would be best to concentrate this work in a limited number of institutions to ensure a high volume.

FNB is not applicable to all nodules. Some are too small and too inaccessible for accurate needle placement, or too far down in the chest to be aspirated safely. Others are so degenerated that useful material cannot be obtained.

Finally, FNB diagnosis of benign for one nodule says nothing about other nodules, whether palpable or impalpable. Occult carcinomas may exist elsewhere within a gland with a benign nodule. There is no proof, however, that excising occult cancers before they are clinically detectable is important, and to do so would require the removal of an absurdly large number of thyroid glands. Therefore, the possibility of an occult lesion is not a practical limitation of needle biopsy.

Does Needle Biopsy Make Scanning or Diagnostic Ultrasound Obsolete?

Scintiscanning is useful to identify autonomously functioning thyroid nodules and hyperplastic functional nodules for which biopsy is unnecessary, and to locate most suspicious lesions in multinodular goiters and individual nodules that have both functioning and nonfunctioning areas. On the other hand, ultrasound is unnecessary, since palpable cystic nodules should be evaluated by FNB, and the enormous number of impalpable "nodules" visualized by ultrasound[31] have too low a risk of containing a clinically significant cancer to require FNB.

Does Radiation Therapy to the Upper Body Increase the Risk of Malignancy So Much That Surgery Is Indicated Regardless of Needle Biopsy Findings?

Therapeutic radiation to the upper body increases chances of developing thyroid cancer, especially 10 to 20 years later.[65] However, it also increases the frequency of benign nodules. Hence, it is appropriate to ask whether the prevalence of malignancy in a thyroid nodule increases if there is a history of prior radiation.

Table 23-5 provides our data for two periods: 1976 to 1980, when we were introducing FNB; and 1981 to 1987, after the usefulness of FNB had been established. During 1976 to 1980, we were more aggressive in advising operation in irradiated patients because we were not sure we could rely on FNB. Consequently, nearly 40% of irradiated patients were operated on, compared with 25% of nonirradiated patients. The prevalence of malignancy in the specimens from the irradiated patients was correspondingly lower at 27%, compared with 37% in the nonirradiated patients. In the 1981 to 1987 period, we operated on almost the same proportion of irradiated (24%) and nonirradiated (23%) patients, and the prevalence of malignancy was similar in the two groups, 40% and 47%, respectively. The prevalence of identified malignancies in all nodules studied by FNB in the two groups in both periods was virtually constant at about 10%.

These findings are nearly identical to those reported by Crile and colleagues in a smaller series.[66] Because the prognosis for thyroid cancer seems to be no different whether there is

TABLE 23-5.
Prevalence of Malignancy in Irradiated and Nonirradiated Patients

	Irradiated		Nonirradiated	
	1976–1980	1981–1987	1976–1980	1981–1987
Number of nodules	176	248	1549	2569
Number excised	70 (40%)	60 (24%)	390 (25%)	596 (23%)
Number malignant	19	24	146	281
Percentage of malignancy in nodules excised	27%	40%	37%	47%
Percentage of malignancy in nodules studied	11%	10%	9%	11%
Percentage of malignancy in all nodules studied	10%		10.4%	

a history of radiation therapy to the upper body or not, we evaluate nodules in irradiated patients in the same way as those in nonirradiated patients. A word of caution is in order: physicians in different localities should generate their own data, because in patient populations exposed to different average radiation doses, thyroid nodule findings could be different. Our conclusions are consistent with those of thyroidologists in several other locations[25,65,67,78] and may be representative of the usual situation.

OTHER USES OF THYROID FNB

We use FNB to evaluate diffuse enlargement of the entire thyroid gland or selective enlargement of one lobe, if blood tests and scintiscanning leave the etiology of the abnormality uncertain, or if the scan shows a discrete area of hypofunction. The area of concern is surveyed by aspirating six to eight sites, using the same technique as for nodules. Such survey FNBs can help distinguish antibody-negative Hashimoto's thyroiditis, lymphoma, or diffuse multifocal carcinoma from a colloid or adenomatous goiter.

There are several types of thyroid nodules that can be eliminated by fine-needle techniques. The most straightforward is aspiration of cyst fluid or blood from a purely cystic or hemorrhagic nodule, which disappears and does not recur. About half of cystic thyroid nodules do recur each time that fluid is removed.[69] The usual recommendation is that continued reaccumulation of fluid after three aspirations calls for surgical intervention. However, some cystic thyroid nodules will ultimately disappear after repeating the aspiration more than three times.[69] Sclerosing agents, such as tetracyclines, have been used to prevent recurrences of cystic nodules.[69] We have not used this method in recent years, because of the possible complication of extravasation of the sclerosing agent, including anecdotal reports of recurrent laryngeal nerve damage. Several groups have begun to ablate solid, autonomously functioning thyroid nodules by repeated injections of ethanol into them under ultrasound guidance.[70,71] The long-term efficacy and safety of this procedure remain to be established.

FNB can be used in patients who have had surgery for thyroid carcinoma and who have cervical lymphadenopathy. If the nodes are palpable, they can be sampled by FNB in the usual fashion. Some high-risk patients are evaluated by ultra-

sound or other imaging techniques and are found to have deep nodes that are impalpable. FNB of such nodes can be accomplished under ultrasound guidance. In clinics with extensive ultrasound experience, the yield of diagnostically useful material in this setting is high and the results are reported to be complementary to tumor marker testing.[72,73]

If the rare entity of acute suppurative thyroiditis is suspected, FNB can provide material for Gram stain and culture, and special stains have identified *Pneumocystis carinii* as the cause of both painful and painless thyroid enlargement in patients with the acquired immune deficiency syndrome.[74]

A recent report[75] described a mutation in the TSH receptor gene in autonomously functioning thyroid adenomas, using RNA obtained by FNB as a template for complementary DNA synthesis, followed by polymerase chain reaction amplification.

References

1. Martin HE, Ellis EB. Biopsy made by needle puncture and aspiration. Ann Surg 1930;92:169
2. Broughan TA, Esselstyn CB Jr. Large-needle thyroid biopsy: still necessary. Surgery 1986;100:1138
3. Hamlin E Jr, Vickery AL Jr. Needle biopsy of the thyroid gland. N Engl J Med 195;254:742
4. LoGerfo P. Coarse-needle biopsy of the thyroid. In: Hamburger JI, ed. Diagnostic methods in clinical thyroidology. New York: Springer-Verlag, 1989:205
5. Wang C, Vickery AL Jr, Maloof F. Needle biopsy of the thyroid. Surg Gynecol Obstet 1976;143:365
6. Einhorn J, Franzen S. Thin-needle biopsy in the diagnosis of thyroid disease. Acta Radiol 1962;58:321
7. Galvan G. Thin needle aspiration biopsy cytological examination of hypofunctional "cold" thyroid nodules in routine clinical work. Clin Nucl Med 1977;2:413
8. Ljunberg O. Cytologic diagnosis of medullary carcinoma of the thyroid gland with special regard to the demonstration of amyloid in smears of fine needle aspirates. Acta Cytol 1972;16:253
9. Löwhagen T, Sprenger E. Cytologic presentation of thyroid tumors in aspiration biopsy smear. Acta Cytol 1974;18:192
10. Nilsson LR, Persson PS. Cytological aspiration biopsy in adolescent goiter. Acta Paediatr 1964;53:333
11. Persson PS. Cytodiagnosis of thyroiditis. A comparative study of cytological, histological, immunological and clinical findings in thyroiditis, particularly in diffuse lymphoid thyroiditis. Acta Med Scand (Suppl) 1967;483:7

12. Soderstrom N. Puncture of goiters for aspiration biopsy. A preliminary report. Acta Med Scand 1952;144:235
13. Ashcraft MW, Van Herle AJ. Management of thyroid nodules. II. Scanning techniques, thyroid suppressive therapy, and fine needle aspiration. Head Neck Surgery 1981;3:297
14. Blum M. The diagnosis of the thyroid nodule using aspiration biopsy and cytology. Arch Intern Med 1984;144:1140
15. Hajdu SI, Melamed MR. Limitations of aspiration cytology in the diagnosis of primary neoplasms. Acta Cytol 1984;28:337
16. Molitch ME, Beck JR, Dresiman M, Gottlieb JE, Pauker SG. The cold thyroid nodule: an analysis of diagnostic and therapeutic options. Endocr Rev 1984;5:185
17. Anderson JB, Webb AJ. Fine-needle aspiration biopsy and the diagnosis of thyroid cancer. Br J Surg 1987;83:489
18. Asp AA, Georgitis W, Waldton EJ, Sims JE, Kidd SG II. Fine needle aspiration of the thyroid. Am J Med 1987;83:489
19. Esselstyn CB, Crile G Jr. Needle aspiration and needle biopsy of the thyroid. World J Surg 1978;2:45
20. Gershengorn MC, McClung MR, Chu EW, Hanson TAS, Weintraub BD, Robbins J. Fine-needle aspiration cytology in the preoperative diagnosis of thyroid nodules. Ann Intern Med 1977;87:265
21. Walfish PG, Hazani E, Strawbridge HTG, Miskin M, Rosen IB. Combined ultrasound and needle aspiration cytology in the assessment and management of the hypofunctioning thyroid nodule. Ann Intern Med 1977;87:270
22. Hamburger JI, Miller JM, Kini SR. Clinical pathological evaluation of thyroid nodules: Handbook and atlas. Southfield, MI: Authors, 1979
23. Hawkins F, Bellido D, Bernal C, et al. Fine needle aspiration biopsy in the diagnosis of thyroid cancer and thyroid disease. Cancer 1987;59:1206
24. Keller MP, Crabbe MM, Norwood SH. Accuracy and significance of fine-needle aspiration and frozen section in determining the extent of thyroid resection. Surgery 1987;101:632
25. Hamming JF, Goslings BM, van Steenis GH, Claasen HR, Hermans SJ, van deVelde, JH. The value of fine-needle aspiration biopsy in patients with nodular thyroid disease divided into groups of suspicion of malignant neoplasms on clinical grounds. Arch Intern Med 1990;150:113
26. Jones AJ, Aitman TJ, Edmonds CJ, Burke M, Hudson E, Tellez M. Comparison of fine needle aspiration cytology, radioisotopic and ultrasound scanning in the management of thyroid nodules. Postgrad Med J 1990;66:914
27. Zappi ME, Moussouris HF, Gillooley JF, Young I, Eberle R. Fine-needle aspiration of the thyroid. JAMA 1991;266:218
28. La Rosa GL, Belfiore A, Giuffrida D, et al. Evaluation of the fine needle aspiration biopsy in the preoperative selection of cold thyroid nodules. Cancer 1991;67:2137
29. Ridgway EC. Clinician's evaluation of a solitary thyroid nodule. J Clin Endocrinol Metab 1991;74:231
30. Gharib H, Goellner JR. Fine-needle aspiration biopsy of the thyroid: An appraisal. Ann Intern Med 1993;118:282
31. Mazzaferri EL. Management of a solitary thyroid nodule. N Engl J Med 1993;328:553
32. Silverman JF, West RL, Larkin EW, et al. The role of fine-needle aspiration biopsy in the rapid diagnosis and management of thyroid neoplasm. Cancer 1986;57:1164
33. Pepper GM, Zwickler D, Rosen Y. Fine-needle aspiration biopsy of the thyroid nodule. Results of a start-up project in a general teaching hospital setting. Arch Intern Med 1989;149:594
34. Dwarakanathan AA, Ryan WG, Staren ED, Martirano M, Economou SG. Fine-needle aspiration biopsy of the thyroid. Diagnostic accuracy when performing a moderate number of such procedures. Arch Intern Med 1989;149:2007
35. Crile G Jr, Hawk WA Jr. Aspiration biopsy of thyroid nodules. Surg Gynecol Obstet 1973;136:241
36. Lowhagen T, Willems JS, Lundel, Sundblad R, Granberg PO. Aspiration biopsy cytology in diagnosis of thyroid cancer. World J Surg 1981;18:192
37. Hamaker RC, Singer MI, DeRossi RV, Shockley WW. Role of needle biopsy in thyroid nodules. Arch Otolaryngol Head Neck Surg 1983;109:225
38. Sanchez RB, vanSonnenberg E, D'Agostino HB, et al. Ultrasound guided biopsy of nonpalpable and difficult to palpate thyroid mass. J Am Coll Surg 1994;178:33
39. Cochand-Priollet B, Guillausseau PJ, Chagnon S, et al. The diagnostic value of fine-needle aspiration biopsy under ultrasonography in nonfunctional thyroid nodules: a prospective study comparing cytologic and histologic findings. Am J Med 1994;97:152
40. Nobrega J, Reading C, Gharib H, Goellner J. Fine needle aspiration of thyroid nodules under real-time ultrasound guidance: A review of 100 cases. Thyroid 1993;3(Suppl):T6
41. Rudowski W. Critical evaluation of aspiration biopsy in the diagnosis of tumors of the thyroid. Am J Surg 1958;95:40
42. Hamburger JI, Hamburger SW. Fine needle biopsy of thyroid nodules: Avoiding the pitfalls. NY State J Med 1986;86:241
43. Hamburger JI, Husain M. Semiquantitative criteria for fine-needle biopsy diagnosis: reduced false-negative diagnoses. Diagn Cytopathol 1988;4:14
44. Hamburger JI, Husain M, Nishiyama R, Nunez C, Solomon D. Increasing the accuracy of fine-needle biopsy for thyroid nodules. Arch Pathol Lab Med 1989;113:1035
45. Schwartz AE, Nieburgs HE, Davies TF, Gilbert PL, Friedman EW. The place of fine needle biopsy in the diagnosis of nodules of the thyroid. Surg Gynecol Obstet 1982;155:54
46. Ramacciotti CE, Pretourius HT, Chu EW, Barsky SH, Brennan MF, Robbins J. Diagnostic accuracy and use of aspiration biopsy in the management of thyroid nodules. Arch Intern Med 1984;144:1169
47. Boey J, Hsu C, Collins RJ, Wong J. A prospective controlled study of fine-needle aspiration and Tru-Cut biopsy of dominant thyroid nodules. World J Surg 1984;8:458
48. Goellner JR, Gharib H, Grant CS, Johnson DA. Fine needle aspiration cytology of the thyroid, 1980 to 1986. Acta Cytol 1987;31:587
49. Hall TL, Layfield LJ, Philippe A, Rosenthal DL. Sources of diagnostic error in fine needle aspiration of the thyroid. Cancer 1989;63:718
50. Gharib H, James EM, Charboneau JW, et al. Suppressive therapy with levothyroxine for solitary thyroid nodules: a double-blind controlled clinical study. N Engl J Med 1987;317:70
51. LiVolsi VA. Cytology and needle biopsy. In: LiVolsi VA. Surgical pathology of the thyroid. Philadelphia: W.B. Saunders. 1990:367
52. Hamburger JI. Consistency of sequential needle biopsy findings for thyroid nodules. Arch Intern Med 1987;147:97
53. Cersosimo E, Gharib H, Suman VJ, Goellner JR. "Suspicious" thyroid cytologic findings: outcome in patients without immediate surgical treatment. Mayo Clin Proc 1993;68:343
54. McHenry CR, Walfish PG, Rosen IB. Non-diagnostic fine needle aspiration biopsy: a dilemma in management of nodular thyroid disease. Am Surg 1993;59:415
55. Belfiore A, LaRosa GL, LaPorta GA, et al. Cancer risk in patients with cold thyroid nodules: relevance of iodine intake, sex, age, and multinodularity. Am J Med 1992;93:363
56. Hamburger JI, Husain M. Contribution of intraoperative pathology evaluation to surgical management of thyroid nodules. Endocrinol Metab Clin North Am 1990;19:509.
57. Kopald KH, Layfield LJ, Mohrmann R, Foshag LJ, Giuliano AE. Clarifying the role of fine-needle aspiration cytologic evaluation and frozen section examination in the operative management of thyroid cancer. Arch Surg 1989;124:1201

58. Walfish PG, Strawbridge HTG, Rosen IB. Management implications from routine needle biopsy of hyper-functioning thyroid nodules. Surgery 1985;98:1179

59. Rubenfeld S, Wheeler TM. Thyroid cancer presenting as a hot thyroid nodule: Report of a case and review of the literature. Thyroidology 1988;1:63

60. de los Santos ET, Keyhani-Rofagha S, Cunningham JJ, Mazzaferri EL. Cystic thyroid nodules. The dilemma of malignant lesions. Arch Intern Med 1990;150:1422

61. Hammer M, Wortsman J, Folse R. Cancer in cystic lesions of the thyroid. Arch Surg 1982;117:1020

62. McCall A, Jaross H, Lawrence AM, Paloyan E. The incidence of thyroid carcinoma in solitary cold nodules and in multinodular goiters. Surgery 1986;100:1128

63. Kini SR. Guides to clinical aspiration biopsy. Thyroid. New York: Igaku-Shoin, 1987

64. Abele JS, Miller TR. Fine-needle aspiration of the thyroid nodule. In: Clark OH, ed. Endocrine surgery of the thyroid and parathyroid glands. St Louis: CV Mosby, 1985:293

65. Schneider AB, Recant W, Pinsky SM, Ryo UY, Bekerman C, Shore-Freedman E. Radiation-induced thyroid carcinoma. Ann Intern Med 1986;105:405

66. Crile G Jr, Esselstyn CB Jr, Hawk WA. Needle biopsy in the diagnosis of thyroid nodules appearing after radiation. N Engl J Med 1979;301:997

67. DeGroot LJ. Diagnostic approach and management of patients exposed to irradiation to the thyroid. J Clin Endocrinol Metab 1989;69:925

68. Utiger RD. Is external irradiation a risk factor for thyroid disease and thyroid carcinoma? JAMA 1979;242:2702

69. Lee J-K, Tai F-T, Lin H-D, Chou Y-H, Kaplan MM, Ching K-N. Treatment of recurrent thyroid cysts by injection of tetracycline or minocycline. Arch Intern Med 1989;149:599

70. Monzani F, Goletti O, Caraccio N, et al. Percutaneous ethanol injection treatment of autonomous thyroid adenoma: hormonal and clinical evaluation. Clin Endocrinol 1992; 36:491

71. Papini E, Panunzi C, Pacella CM, et al. Percutaneous ultrasound-guided ethanol injection: a new treatment of toxic autonomously functioning thyroid nodules. J Clin Endocrinol Metab 1993; 76:411

72. Sutton RT, Reeding CC, Charboneau JW, James EM, Grant CS, Hay ID. US-guided biopsy of neck masses in postoperative management of patients with thyroid cancer. Radiology 1988; 168:769

73. Lee MJ, Ross DS, Mueller PR, et al. Fine-needle biopsy of cervical lymph nodes in patients with thyroid cancer: a prospective comparison of cytopathologic and tissue marker analysis. Radiology 1993;187:851

74. Guttler R, Singer PA. *Pneumocystis carinii* thyroiditis report of three cases and review of the literature. Arch Intern Med 1993; 153:393

75. Porcellini A, Ciullo I, Laviola L, Amabile G, Fenzi G, Avvedimento V. Novel mutations of thyrotropin receptor gene in thyroid hyperfunctioning adenomas. J Clin Endocrinol Metab 1994; 79:335

THREE

Introduction to Thyroid Diseases

Werner and Ingbar's The Thyroid, Seventh Edition,
edited by Lewis E. Braverman and Robert D. Utiger.
Lippincott–Raven Publishers, Philadelphia, © 1996

24

Surgical Anatomy

Orlo H. Clark

The thyroid gland has historically been thought to round out and beautify the neck; thus, women were given larger thyroid glands than men. The gland was also thought to lubricate the larynx, to serve as a vascular shunt to maintain an adequate blood flow to the brain despite changes in position, and to be a blood-forming organ. Today, the thyroid gland is accepted as two endocrine organs in one. The follicular cells secrete the thyroid hormones, and the parafollicular cells secrete calcitonin.

Understanding the embryology and anatomy of the thyroid gland and the relation of the thyroid to the parathyroid glands, thymus, and other vital structures in the neck helps the physician not only to perform a proper physical examination but also to evaluate various images (radionuclide, ultrasonographic, computed tomographic, and magnetic resonance) and to perform thyroid operations. The purpose of this chapter is to describe the clinically relevant thyroid anatomy and the technique of thyroidectomy and modified radical neck and mediastinal dissection.

CLINICAL FEATURES AND SURGICALLY RELEVANT ANATOMY

Enlargement of the thyroid can cause dysphagia, pain that radiates to the ears, hoarseness due to invasion or stretching of the recurrent laryngeal nerve or distortion of the larynx, and superior vena cava obstruction with a positive Pemberton sign (distention of the external and anterior jugular veins with elevation of the arms above the head due to partial obstruction of the superior vena cava; Fig 24-1).

The normal thyroid gland weighs 15 to 20 g in adults who live in iodine-sufficient areas. It is shieldlike in shape, with two lobes and an isthmus (Fig 24-2). The right lobe of the thyroid gland is usually larger than the left, and some people have a pyramidal lobe that extends from the upper midportion of the thyroid gland to, or cephalad to, the hyoid bone. The isthmus of the thyroid gland is situated immediately caudal to the cricoid cartilage, although rarely there may be no isthmus

or the thyroid gland may be positioned in an ectopic position. When palpating the thyroid gland, one should first palpate the cricoid cartilage, which will indicate where the isthmus should be situated and thus where the thyroid lobes can be palpated. Posterior extension of the neck elevates the thyroid gland and also moves it anteriorly, but it causes the strap muscles to tighten so that palpation of the thyroid gland is more difficult. In kyphotic and older patients with short necks, the cricoid cartilage may be positioned at the suprasternal notch. In these patients, the thyroid gland is situated in a substernal position in the thoracic inlet rather than in its usual cervical position, making thyroid palpation and operation more difficult. Patients with substernal thyroid glands require a longer surgical incision because the thyroid gland is less accessible.

For all thyroid operations, the patient should be positioned with the neck extended. The head needs to be supported, or the patient will awaken with posterior neck pain. Also, the elbows should be padded so that injury to the ulnar and radial nerves is avoided.

THE INCISION

A transverse incision is made 1 cm caudal to the cricoid cartilage. This places the incision directly over the thyroid gland. It is most important that the incision be symmetric and that it conform to the normal skin lines. I mark the site of the incision using a 2-0 silk thread (Fig 24-3*A*). This incision should be neither a straight line nor too curved (Fig 24-3*B*). When necessary, the incision can be extended laterally to perform a neck dissection and remove clinically involved lymph nodes (Fig 24-4). Vertical cross-marks can be made with a marking pen for proper skin realignment after completion of the thyroidectomy, but this should never be done with a scalpel. The length of the incision should correspond with the amount of thyroid tissue to be removed, the degree to which the neck can be extended, and the position of the thyroid. Patients with

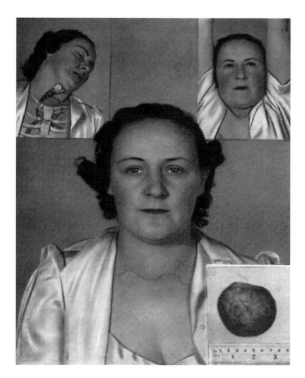

FIGURE 24-1. Retrosternal goiters can cause superior vena cava obstruction with nocturnal dyspnea and orthopnea when supine, and congestion of the face and dilation of the cervical veins when the arms are elevated (positive Pemberton sign). Some patients feel weak or faint when their arms are elevated and develop tachycardia and hypotension. (Bailey H. Demonstrations of physical science in clinical surgery. Baltimore: Williams & Wilkins, 1960:239)

long, thin necks with marked mobility and a small thyroid nodule require a short incision, whereas patients with large goiters or tumors, patients with short necks or with limited motion, and patients with low-lying thyroid glands require larger incisions. The skin incision is carried through the subcutaneous fat and platysma muscle. The anterior jugular veins are then identified in the midline and just lateral to the median raphe deep to the platysma muscle.

The dissection is continued on the midline raphe superiorly between the sternohyoid muscles from the suprasternal notch inferiorly to the thyroid cartilage superiorly. The midline is best identified just above the suprasternal notch because the strap muscles—the more superficial sternohyoid muscle and the deeper sternothyroid muscle—are further apart at this site. Usually, few vessels cross the midline, but the anterior jugular veins can have a large connecting vessel that crosses the midline just inferior to the thyroid cartilage.

The sternohyoid muscles arise from the clavicle and posterior sternum and run superiorly to insert on the hyoid bone. They function to depress the hyoid bone. The sternothyroid muscles are situated immediately beneath the sternohyoid muscles. They also run from the posterior aspect of the sternum anterior to the thyroid gland and insert on the thyroid cartilage. In most patients, the sternothyroid muscles do not meet in the midline. These muscles help to depress the larynx with deglutition. Dissecting between the sternohyoid and sternothyroid muscles provides better exposure of the thyroid and

deeper structures in the neck. Situated at the lateral aspect of these muscles is the ansa hypoglossal or ansa cervicalis nerve, which is just medial to the internal jugular vein and anterior to the common carotid artery.

The omohyoid muscles run obliquely in the neck deep to the sternocleidomastoid muscle. The inferior belly arises from the lateral border of the scapula and subscapular ligament. Its midportion is often tendinous, and it then joins the superior belly, crosses the carotid sheath, and inserts on the lateral aspect of the hyoid bone. It stabilizes the hyoid bone in deglutition.

The thyrohyoid muscle arises on the superior surface of the thyroid cartilage and inserts on the hyoid bone. It elevates the larynx, depresses the hyoid, or both, depending on the extent of fixation of the suprahyoid muscles. The function of these muscles is clinically minor since they may all be denervated, divided, or removed without appreciable changes in deglutition. If the sternohyoid or sternothyroid muscles are divided for better exposure of the vessels, this should be done at their superior end to minimize the degree of denervation, because these muscles are innervated from below by the ansa hypoglossi nerves. It is rarely necessary, however, to transect these muscles, because separating them from one another usually provides excellent exposure. Transection of the upper midportion of the sternothyroid muscle does provide better exposure of the superior pole vessels in patients with large goiters. When a thyroid nodule is adherent to the muscle, this portion of the muscle should be removed with the thyroid lobe because it may be invaded by tumor.

THE THYROID GLAND

The thyroid gland is situated immediately below the second layer of deep cervical fascia or prethyroidal fascia. As mentioned, the isthmus of the thyroid gland is just caudal to the cricoid cartilage. The normal thyroid gland is reddish brown in color, has a rich venous plexus on its surface, and has two lobes and a pyramidal lobe (see Fig 24-2). The structures immediately adjacent to the thyroid gland can usually be separated from the thyroid gland by blunt dissection. The middle thyroid veins should be seen laterally and the superior pole vessels superiorly. The middle thyroid vein or veins should be ligated and divided. Traction of the thyroid gland in a caudal and lateral direction helps identify the plane of dissection medial to the superior pole vessels. It is important during this part of the dissection to skeletonize the superior pole vessels and to dissect laterally to the cricothyroid muscle to avoid injury to the external laryngeal nerve (Fig 24-5). In about 80% of patients the external laryngeal nerve runs on the cricothyroid muscle, but in some patients it runs beneath the surface of the muscle. This nerve is the motor nerve to the cricothyroid muscle and provides tension to the vocal cord, which is what enables singers to reach high notes. In 15% of patients, this nerve loops down with the superior thyroid vessels onto the thyroid gland so that, to avoid injury and vocal difficulties, the surgeon should ligate and divide the superior pole vessels individually on the thyroid gland (Fig 24-5).

As the external laryngeal nerve runs superiorly, it joins the internal laryngeal nerve to form the superior laryngeal nerve. The internal laryngeal nerve provides sensation to the larynx. By applying traction on the thyroid in an inferior and

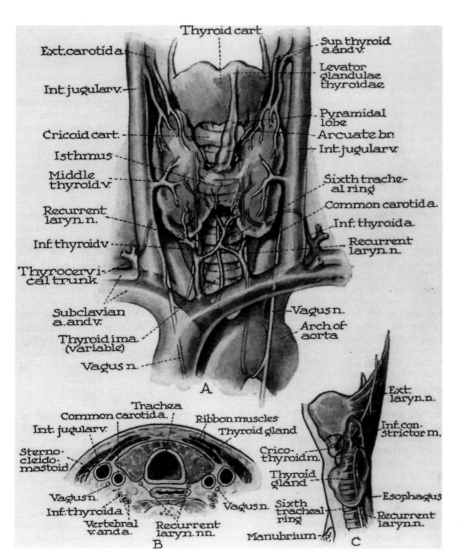

FIGURE 24-2. (*A*) The thyroid gland with vascular supply and recurrent laryngeal nerves Cross section (*B*) and lateral view (*C*) of the thyroid gland with relationships of recurrent laryngeal and external laryngeal nerves to thyroid gland. The parathyroid glands are not shown. (Thorek P. Anatomy in surgery. Philadelphia: JB Lippincott, 1951:205)

lateral direction, the superior pole vessels are usually easily identified. The fascia is then divided between the superior pole vessels and the upper portion of the thyroid and the cricothyroid muscle. The superior pole thyroid vessels are ligated and individually divided close to the thyroid gland to avoid injury to the external laryngeal nerve. Because the recurrent laryngeal nerve on each side consistently enters the larynx at the posterior medial aspect of the cricothyroid muscle inferior to the cricoid cartilage, dissection superior to the cricoid cartilage can be accomplished quickly. Once the superior thyroid vessels and middle thyroid veins have been ligated, the thyroid gland can be mobilized medially and the parathyroid glands and recurrent laryngeal nerve on each side identified.

The recurrent laryngeal nerves innervate the trachea and subglottic areas of the larynx and all the muscles of the larynx except the cricothyroid muscle. In some patients, a sensory branch from the recurrent laryngeal nerve joins the internal branch of the superior laryngeal nerve to form Galen's loop. The main motor function of the recurrent laryngeal nerve is to allow abduction and adduction of the vocal cords. Injury to

one recurrent laryngeal nerve usually results in the ipsilateral cord assuming a paramedian position, so that the patient usually becomes hoarse. Patients who have bilateral vocal cord paralysis have both vocal cords situated in a paramedian position. Unless there is a broad anterior glottic space between the vocal cords, these patients require immediate intubation to avoid suffocation and, if the injury is permanent, a subsequent tracheotomy. Injury to a recurrent laryngeal nerve, however, should be a rare occurrence when thyroidectomy is performed by an experienced surgeon.[1]

The right recurrent laryngeal nerve is a branch of the vagus nerve (see Fig 24-2*A*). It runs in a more oblique course than the left recurrent nerve, because the right recurrent laryngeal nerve passes behind the right subclavian artery, whereas the left recurrent laryngeal nerve originates from the vagus at the aortic arch and loops around the ligamentum arteriosum. The left recurrent laryngeal nerve then ascends superiorly in the tracheoesophageal groove. In some patients, the recurrent laryngeal nerves branch in the lower neck; this is more common on the left side. In other patients (about 1%), there may be a nonrecurrent nerve. In these patients, the laryngeal nerve

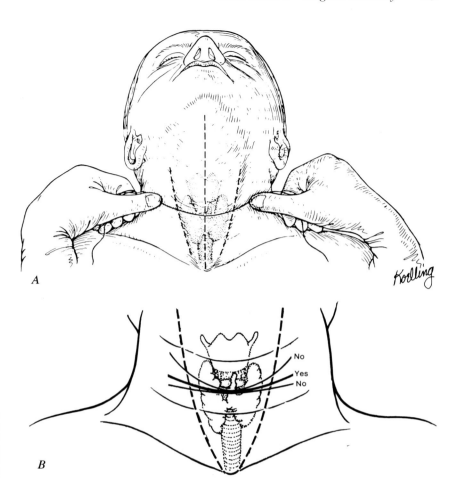

A

B

FIGURE 24-3. (*A*) Technique of marking the neck for skin incision. (*B*) The center of the incision should be 1 cm caudal to the cricord cartilage, and the incision should conform to the normal skin lines. (Clark OH. Endocrine surgery of the thyroid and parathyroid glands. St Louis: CV Mosby, 1995)

comes directly from the vagus to the larynx without descending first into the mediastinum. This occurs almost exclusively on the right side unless there is a right-sided aortic arch. The recurrent nerve is best identified by applying medial traction to the thyroid and lateral traction to the carotid sheath. This nerve can be differentiated from an artery because of its white color and its anatomic course in the neck and because a vaso nervorum runs in the same direction as the nerve (Fig 24-6).

It may be difficult to identify the recurrent laryngeal nerve during thyroid reoperations because of scar tissue. In these patients, one should either identify the recurrent laryngeal nerve low in the neck, if this area was not previously dissected, or at the site where the recurrent nerve enters the posterior medial aspect of the cricothyroid muscle. To identify the recurrent laryngeal nerve at this site, the superior pole vessels are divided as described previously, the isthmus of the thyroid gland is divided, and the thyroid gland is pulled inferiorly and laterally. Once the recurrent laryngeal nerve has been identified, it can usually be dissected from the scar or neoplastic tissue. In general, it is not necessary to sacrifice a recurrent laryngeal nerve if the vocal cords are functioning preoperatively. Rarely, however, the nerve may still function despite infiltration of tumor within it. When a recurrent laryngeal nerve is injured either purposely or unintentionally, it should be repaired in order to minimize atrophy of the larynx. If the injury occurs near the cricothyroid muscle, the recurrent nerve should be mobilized and the cut end placed in the cricothyroid muscle.

The four parathyroid glands are usually situated on the posterior surface of the thyroid gland immediately adjacent to the recurrent laryngeal nerves. A normal parathyroid gland measures about 6 mm × 3 mm × 3 mm, weighs less than 65 mg, is usually spherical, and is light beige or tan in color. The upper pair of parathyroid glands are most consistent in position; they are situated near where the recurrent laryngeal nerves enter the cricothyroid muscle and are usually cephalad to where the inferior thyroid artery crosses the recurrent laryngeal nerve. The inferior parathyroid glands are almost always situated anterior to the recurrent laryngeal nerves on the inferior lateral surface of the thyroid. When not there, they are often in the thymus or perithymic fat. To avoid injury to the parathyroid glands, they should be carefully dissected from the thyroid gland on a broad pedicle with as little manipulation as possible. The inferior thyroid artery should be divided at its terminal branches on the thyroid gland rather than the main trunk. In some patients, a tongue of thyroid tissue (Zuckerkandl's peduncle) extends over the recurrent laryngeal nerve just before the nerve penetrates Berry's ligament to enter the cricothyroid muscle. Within Berry's ligament is always a branch of the inferior thyroid artery and a vein (Fig 24-6). When bleeding occurs in this area, the recurrent nerve must be precisely identified before the vessels are ligated or the nerve may be injured. In some patients, a small amount of thyroid tissue extends behind the recurrent laryngeal nerve. If there is no tumor in

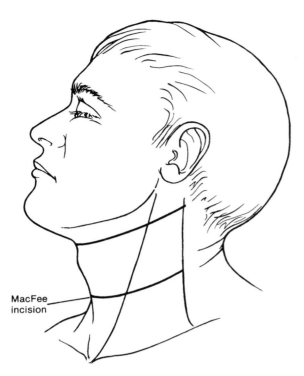

FIGURE 24-4. MacFee extension of transverse thyroidectomy incision for access to lateral neck for neck dissections. It occasionally is necessary to make a higher parallel incision to remove all involved nodes. (Clark OH. Endocrine surgery of the thyroid and parathyroid glands. St Louis: CV Mosby, 1985)

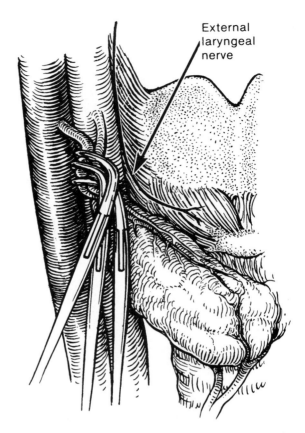

FIGURE 24-5. The external laryngeal nerve runs on (80%) or in (20%) the cricothyroid muscle. In about 15% of patients, it runs with the vessels that enter the superior pole of the thyroid. These vessels should therefore be skeletonized and ligated on the thyroid gland to avoid injury to this nerve. (Clark OH. Endocrine surgery of the thyroid and parathyroid glands. St Louis: CV Mosby, 1985)

this area, it is perhaps preferable to leave a few cells in this area to avoid injury to the nerve. When there is a little oozing from this area, some thrombin-soaked Gelfoam can be applied to stop the bleeding.

Once the parathyroid glands and recurrent nerve have been identified, the entire lobe is mobilized in a lateral to medial fashion. A total lobectomy and isthmectomy is performed and the specimen is sent for frozen section examination. If a pyramidal lobe is present, it should be removed. This is done by retracting the thyroid inferiorly and dissecting immediately adjacent to the pyramidal lobe to avoid injury to the external laryngeal nerve. The pyramidal lobe usually ends just cephalad to the thyroid cartilage.

When a total or near-total thyroidectomy is planned, a similar approach is used on the contralateral side. Briefly, the middle thyroid veins are individually ligated and divided, as are the superior thyroid vessels. After the parathyroid glands and recurrent laryngeal nerve are identified, the contralateral lobe is removed in total. When one or more parathyroid glands are attached to the thyroid, a small remnant of thyroid tissue may be left to avoid injury to the parathyroid glands. The thyroid gland should also be examined after removal to be sure that no parathyroid glands are removed with it. If a parathyroid gland is situated on the removed thyroid, a biopsy specimen should be taken to confirm its identity, and it should be transplanted in 1-mm pieces into individual sites within the sternocleidomastoid muscle.

All lymph nodes immediately adjacent to the thyroid gland and medial to the carotid sheath should be removed. If a patient has palpable nodes in the lateral neck, a modified neck dissection should be done. A prophylactic modified radical neck dissection is not recommended, except for patients with medullary thyroid cancer.

MODIFIED RADICAL NECK DISSECTION

Controversy exists about when to perform a neck dissection and how extensive this operation should be. In the United States, prophylactic neck dissections are generally not done because differentiated thyroid carcinomas do not seem to metastasize from lymph nodes to the rest of the body.

Part of the controversy about neck dissection concerns the fact that about 80% of patients with papillary thyroid carcinoma have microscopic lymph node metastases even when no nodes are clinically palpable. Despite the presence of microscopic carcinoma in the nodes, only about 8% of patients ever develop clinical evidence of recurrence even if the involved nodes are not removed. Treatment with radioactive iodine after total thyroidectomy appears to be beneficial in destroying micrometastases and returning serum thyroglobulin concentrations to normal, but radioactive iodine is relatively ineffective for ablating palpable metastatic carcinoma.[2–4] External

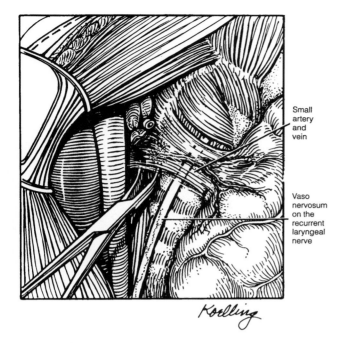

Koelling

FIGURE 24-6. The recurrent laryngeal nerve traverses through the posterior superior suspensory ligament of the thyroid (ligament of Berry) before entering cricothyroid muscle. An artery and a vein are always present in this area. (Clark OH. Endocrine surgery of the thyroid and parathyroid glands. St Louis: CV Mosby, 1995)

radiation is also generally ineffective for treating cervical node metastases.[4] Some surgeons recommend excision of only the palpable nodes. The studies of Noguchi and coworkers,[5,6] however, document that whenever thyroid carcinoma in a node is larger than 3 mm, there is always carcinoma in the smaller lymphatics. Therefore, I perform modified radical neck dissections for patients with thyroid carcinoma and clinically palpable cervical nodal metastases. This is an en bloc dissection that removes all the fibrofatty tissue in the lateral neck but does not cause a cosmetic or functional abnormality. I preserve the sternocleidomastoid muscle and the spinal accessory nerve unless they are directly invaded. This operation is performed by extending the thyroid incision laterally (MacFee extension; see Fig 24-4). The results are cosmetically preferable to vertical incisions in the neck, even when a second incision is required superiorly that parallels the initial incision. A modified radical neck dissection is preferable to a radical neck dissection because the clinical results are equivalent and the functional and cosmetic results are more desirable.[4]

It is important that surgeons understand the surgical anatomy in the lateral neck. Numerous sensory and motor nerves traverse this area, including the vagus nerve, the phrenic nerve, the sympathetic chain, the spinal accessory nerve, the hypoglossal nerve, and the brachial plexus.

Because the lateral neck is usually explored after the thyroidectomy and central neck dissection have been completed, the carotid sheath containing the carotid artery, vagus nerve, and internal jugular veins are already identified. The cervical sympathetic chain lies deep to the carotid sheath just anterior to the prevertebral fascia. The retropharyngeal lymphatics connect with the anterior cervical and jugular lymphatics across the sympathetic chain and may be involved in patients with

metastatic thyroid carcinoma. Injury to the sympathetic chain results in Horner's syndrome, with enophthalmos, ptosis, miosis, anhidrosis, and warm skin on the involved side of the face.

When performing a neck dissection, one dissects deep to the sternocleidomastoid muscle and anterior to the carotid sheath just above the clavicle. The carotid sheath thus remains deep to the plane of dissection. As one dissects more deeply, the phrenic nerve in the prevertebral fascia on the anterior scalene muscle (scalenus anticus) should be identified (Fig 24-7). It crosses from a lateral to a medial position on this muscle during its descent. On the left side, the phrenic nerve is close to the thoracic duct, where the internal jugular vein joins the subclavian vein. The phrenic nerve originates from C-3 and C-4. Large sensory nerves join the phrenic nerve and may be sacrificed (Fig 24-7).

During a modified radical neck dissection, all tissues between the superficial and prevertebral fascia should be removed except for the carotid artery, jugular vein, vagus, phrenic and spinal accessory nerves, sympathetic chain, and sternocleidomastoid muscle. The dissection begins just above the clavicle. The phrenic nerve is identified on the anterior scalene muscle and the brachial plexus between the anterior scalene and middle scalene. As the dissection continues in a cephalad direction, the spinal accessory nerve is identified at the deep and lateral surface of the sternocleidomastoid muscle (Fig 24-7). This nerve runs inferiorly at the lateral aspect of the posterior triangle of the neck. As one traces this nerve superiorly, it gives a branch to the sternocleidomastoid muscle, then passes deep to the posterior aspect of the digastric muscle and occipital artery across the internal jugular vein to the jugular foramen.

The hypoglossal nerve crosses anterior to the internal carotid artery and internal jugular vein and deep to the anterior facial vein. It follows the stylohyoid muscle into the submandibular triangle to innervate the tongue muscles. When ligating the internal jugular vein, care must be taken not to injure the hypoglossal nerve as it crosses the internal and external carotid arteries.

In general, it is not necessary to dissect in the suprahyoid area for thyroid carcinoma unless there is extensive lymph node involvement, because these nodes are involved in only about 1% of patients. The cervical lymph nodes contralateral to the carcinoma are only involved in about 10% of patients, and it is usually the lower cervical nodes immediately adjacent to the thyroid that are involved. In patients who have invasive tumors that involve nerves, the nerve when functioning should be dissected from the tumor and preserved, unless this is the only site in which tumor remains and all other tumor has been removed.

ANTERIOR MEDIAN STERNOTOMY

Nearly all benign and malignant thyroid tumors can be removed by means of a cervical incision. A median sternotomy may be required for patients who need reoperation, for patients with large invasive tumors, and for patients with low-lying thyroid glands who have virtually no thyroid tissue in the neck. When performing a median sternotomy, a midline incision is made from the midportion of the cervical wound. I usually split the sternum through the 3rd and 4th in-

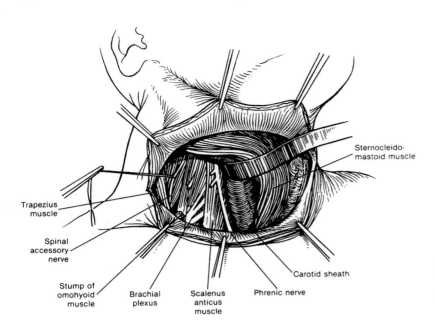

FIGURE 24-7. The phrenic nerve is situated on the scalenus anticus muscle. Also illustrated are the brachial plexus and spinal accessory nerve. (Clark OH. Endocrine surgery on the thyroid and parathyroid glands. St Louis: CV Mosby, 1985)

terspace bilaterally (Fig 24-8). Before dividing the sternum, the tissues deep to the sternum are swept bluntly from beneath the sternum with the index finger. When dividing the sternum laterally, it is important to avoid injuring the internal mammary arteries that run vertically about 1 to 2 cm lateral to the sternum.

The edges of the sternum are coagulated, and the tissues beneath the sternum again swept laterally by blunt dissection to avoid injuring the parietal pleura and causing a pneumothorax. A Finochietto retractor is used to obtain good exposure of the mediastinum. The anterior mediastinal fat and thymus are swept in a cephalad direction from the pericardium superiorly. Laterally, one must dissect carefully to avoid entering the parietal pleura or injuring the phrenic nerves. The innominate vein is identified just deep to the thymus. All fibrofatty tissue is swept from the innominate vein, and several vertical veins from the innominate vein to

the thymus are divided and ligated. Excellent exposure of the trachea, aortic arch, innominate vein, and central neck is obtained by a median sternotomy.

The sternum is closed with wire. A chest tube catheter may or may not be used, depending on whether the parietal pleura has been entered. A postoperative chest radiograph is essential.

CONCLUSION

Understanding the surgical anatomy of the neck makes the physical examination more accurate and thyroid operations safer. Despite the intricate nature of thyroid operations and neck dissections, complications such as hypoparathyroidism, injury to the recurrent laryngeal nerve, bleeding, or infection are unusual. Blood transfusions are almost never required. Most patients can be discharged from the hospital after a thyroidectomy within 1 or 2 days and within 2 or 3 days after a modified radical neck dissection or a median sternotomy.

References

1. Clark OH, Levin KE, Zeng GH, et al. Thyroid cancer: the case for total thyroidectomy. Eur J Cancer Clin Oncol 1988;24:305
2. DeGroot LJ, Kaplan EL, McCormick M, Straus FH. Natural history, treatment, and course of papillary thyroid carcinoma. J Clin Endocrinol Metab 1990;71:414
3. Schlumberger J, Tibiana M, DeVathaire F, et al. Long term results of treatment of 283 patients with lung and bone metastases from differentiated thyroid carcinomas. J Clin Endocrinol Metab 1986;663:960
4. Wilson SM, Block GE. Carcinoma of the thyroid metastatic to lymph nodes. Arch Surg 1971;102:285
5. Noguchi S, Murakami N. The value of lymph-node dissection in patients with differentiated thyroid cancer. Surg Clin North Am 1987;67:251
6. Noguchi S, Noguchi A, Murakami N. Papillary carcinoma of the thyroid: Developing pattern of metastases. Cancer 1970;26:1053

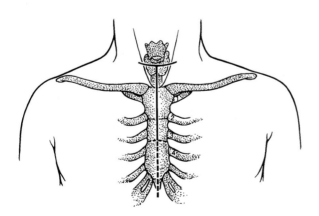

FIGURE 24-8. Incision for median sternotomy through second and third, as in illustration, or third and fourth interspaces. A median sternotomy provides excellent visualization of the innominate vein, thyroid, and carotid arteries. (Clark OH. Endocrine surgery of the thyroid and parathyroid glands. St. Louis: CV Mosby, 1985:62)

Werner and Ingbar's The Thyroid, Seventh Edition,
edited by Lewis E. Braverman and Robert D. Utiger.
Lippincott–Raven Publishers, Philadelphia, © 1996

25

Physical Examination of the Thyroid Gland

Gilbert H. Daniels

Palpation of the thyroid gland is a lost or unlearned art for too many physicians. Yet a careful, systematic examination of the thyroid should be part of every physical examination for two important reasons: palpation is the only way to detect certain diseases of the thyroid, and determination of the size, consistency, nodularity, and tenderness of the thyroid often is necessary to interpret the historical and other physical findings and laboratory test results.

The following examples illustrate how important a thorough thyroid examination can be in making the correct diagnosis.

A patient complains of fatigue, apathy, constipation, and depression. Although these complaints are nonspecific, if the patient's thyroid is slightly enlarged and firm, and has an irregular surface, the likely diagnosis is hypothyroidism secondary to the goitrous form of chronic autoimmune thyroiditis (Hashimoto's thyroiditis).[1] These findings on examination of the thyroid are helpful clues to the diagnosis of hypothyroidism. Palpation of the thyroid will not yield early clues to the diagnosis of hypothyroidism if the patient has had radioactive iodine therapy for hyperthyroidism or the atrophic form of chronic autoimmune thyroiditis.

A patient has a fever and sore throat. Palpation of the neck reveals exquisite tenderness over the thyroid gland, thus suggesting subacute thyroiditis as the likely cause of the symptoms.[2] If this physical finding had been ignored or missed, an inappropriate conclusion might have been reached.

A patient with unexplained weight loss has warm, moist hands. Physical examination reveals sinus tachycardia, systolic hypertension, hand tremor, a hyperdynamic precordium, and muscle weakness. On the basis of these findings, a diagnosis of thyrotoxicosis can be made. The presence of exophthalmos would indicate Graves' hyperthyroidism. In the absence of exophthalmos, the thyroid examination provides important clues about the cause of thyrotoxicosis.

A patient has hoarseness and a thyroid nodule. If ipsilateral vocal cord palsy also is present, the likely diagnosis is thyroid carcinoma.

A patient complains of shortness of breath, thought to be due to either asthma or emphysema. The discovery of a large goiter clearly suggests upper airway obstruction secondary to the thyroid mass.[3]

A patient taking suppressive doses of thyroid hormone is found to have a normal-sized or slightly enlarged thyroid gland. This physical finding suggests not only that the patient's thyroid gland is abnormal in structure, but also that its function may be autonomous. A normal thyroid gland ceases to be palpable in a patient who is receiving exogenous thyroid hormone.

EXAMINATION OF THE NECK

The thyroid can be seen most easily by tilting the patient's head backward (Fig 25-1). This position raises the thyroid up from the supraclavicular region and throws it into relief against the superficial structures of the neck. Because the thyroid is fixed to the pretracheal fascia, it rises with the trachea when the patient swallows. Many goiters and nodules are, therefore, clearly visible when the patient swallows in this position. Cervical adiposity does not rise with swallowing. This distinction is particularly important in differentiating between a goiter and a transverse band of cervical fat in young women.

The lymph nodes of the neck should be carefully palpated, particularly those of the anterior and posterior cervical chains and the submental, supraclavicular, and pretracheal regions.

The trachea also should be palpated, since lateral deviation of the trachea suggests a large thyroid lobe, a substernal goiter, or some other intrathoracic abnormality. Place the thumb and index finger on either side of the trachea, and fol-

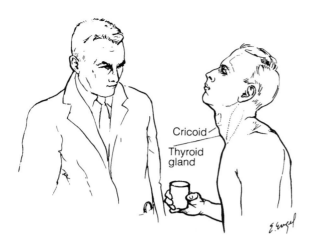

FIGURE 25-1. Inspection of the thyroid gland. The thyroid is inspected as the patient extends his neck and swallows, which causes the gland to rise. The thyroid isthmus crosses the trachea below the cricoid cartilage. (Morgan WL Jr, Engel GL. The clinical approach to the patient. Philadelphia: WB Saunders, 1969:105)

low the path of the trachea to the suprasternal notch. With a normally placed midline trachea, the fingers will descend to the middle of the suprasternal notch. If the fingers trace a path either to the right or to the left of the midline, the trachea is laterally deviated in that direction. A deviated trachea may itself be misinterpreted as a thyroid or other neck mass.

Although most physicians are taught to stand behind the patient when examining the thyroid, I believe that it is easier to learn thyroid palpation when facing the patient, who should be seated (it is very difficult to examine the thyroid when the patient is supine) (Fig 25-2). The patient's neck should be slightly flexed, since palpation is more difficult when the sternomastoid muscles are stretched. With care and practice, the thyroid gland can be palpated in many normal people.

The first step in thyroid palpation is to locate the cricoid cartilage, since the isthmus of the thyroid gland lies horizon-

tally just below this cartilage. Many young women with thin necks have a superiorly located cricoid cartilage and thyroid gland (Fig 25-3). In many older men, particularly those with kyphosis or emphysema, the cricoid cartilage and thyroid gland lie below the suprasternal notch, and therefore the thyroid gland may be hidden by the sternum. Thyroid palpation is extremely difficult in such people.

The thyroid isthmus can be examined by placing the thumb in a horizontal position with its upper edge along the lower margin of the cricoid cartilage. The thumb should then pass over the isthmus when the patient swallows. Even physicians who have had difficulty palpating normal thyroid lobes find that they can palpate the isthmus quite easily by following this procedure. The normal isthmus has the consistency of felt and is several millimeters in width (the anatomic isthmus often measures 1 cm). An enlarged, firm, or nodular isthmus often is an indication of a thyroid abnormality.

The thumb also should be used to locate the pyramidal lobe, if one is present. This roughly triangular structure has a vertical orientation and most often arises from the isthmic border of the left lobe. If a pyramidal lobe is present, it may extend to the thyroid cartilage or higher. The pyramidal lobe is most easily palpated by rubbing the thumb back and forth in the horizontal plane above the isthmus. An easily palpable pyramidal lobe may be an indication of a general abnormality of the thyroid gland (e.g., Hashimoto's thyroiditis or Graves' disease), but it occasionally can be found in a patient whose thyroid is otherwise normal.

There are two equally satisfactory ways of examining the thyroid lobes from the front.

Method 1. The examiner steps to the patient's right and places two fingers of the right hand along the lateral aspect of the trachea (see Fig 25-2). The fingers usually meet the trachea at a 45-degree angle and point in a lateral direction, while the heel of the hand is kept in a medial position. Starting high in the neck and working down, the fingers "massage" the trachea with a circular, rubbing motion, applying gentle pressure as they

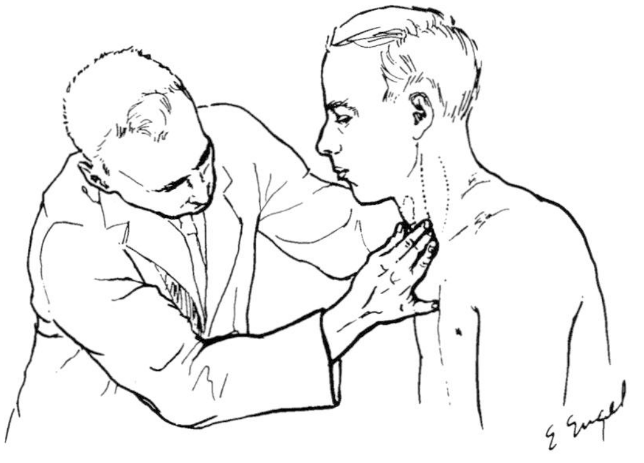

FIGURE 25-2. Palpation of the thyroid gland. The left lobe of the thyroid is palpated from the anterior position with the patient's neck sufficiently flexed to relax the sternocleidomastoid muscle. As the patient swallows, the gland is felt to ride up under the examiner's fingers. (Morgan WL Jr., Engel GL. The clinical approach to the patient. Philadelphia: WB Saunders, 1969:106)

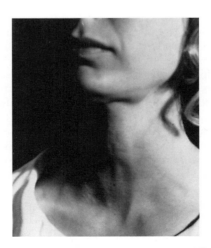

FIGURE 25-3. A normal thyroid gland simulating a diffuse goiter because of its anterior position. The thyroid is clearly visible. The neck is long and the gland lies high above the suprasternal notch. (Gwinup G, Morton ME. The high lying thyroid: a cause of pseudogoiter. J Clin Endocrinol Metab 1975;40:38)

reach the left thyroid lobe. Sometimes a large thyroid lobe is missed because palpation is begun too low in the neck, with the fingers already on the surface of the lobe. It is important that the fingers be medial to the sternomastoid muscle. Some examiners use their left thumb to stabilize the right side of the trachea.

The examiner proceeds down the trachea, paying particular attention to the region of the cricoid cartilage. It is helpful for the patient to swallow small sips of water during this part of the examination, since swallowing causes the thyroid to rise, so that the ends of the lobe or the boundaries of a nodule are more noticeable. The size, texture, and consistency of the thyroid lobe can then be estimated. If nodules are present, they also should be examined "on the way up" as the patient swallows, and then trapped between the fingers. The examiner must be careful to apply increased pressure to the trachea as the patient swallows or else the thyroid will slide between the fingers and the trachea without being palpated. The right lobe is similarly palpated with the left hand while standing to the patient's left.

Method 2. Standing on the right, as in Method 1, the examiner's left thumb is used to palpate the left lobe of the thyroid gland. When palpating the right thyroid lobe, two fingers of the left hand or the right thumb can be used.

Auscultation of the thyroid gland should be performed in any patient with thyrotoxicosis or goiter. Either of two types of vascular sounds may be heard in patients with diffuse goiters in which thyroid blood flow is greatly increased: a continuous, low-pitched sound (venous hum), or a systolic or diastolic murmur (bruit). The cause of such vascular sounds is nearly always Graves' disease.

THYROID NODULES

Thyroid nodules are more frequently detected by ultrasonography or autopsy examination than they are by physical examination (Table 25-1). The ease with which a nodule can be palpated depends both on its location and size and the anatomy of the patient's neck. In young, thin patients, most nodules of 1 cm or larger can be palpated; if anteriorly located, some nodules of 0.5 cm or less can be palpated. In older patients and in those of any age with muscular necks, nodules usually must be larger to be palpated.

It is essential to measure the vertical and horizontal dimensions of all nodules. Two methods are commonly used. (1) A ruler, tape measure, or caliper is placed on the patient's neck and the measurements are recorded. (2) Several pieces of paper tape are placed on the patient's neck, and an outline of the nodule is traced directly onto the tape; the tape is then placed in the patient's record. Both of these methods are reasonably accurate and permit serial observation.

A single, palpable thyroid nodule with no contralateral palpable thyroid tissue suggests an autonomously functioning thyroid adenoma, although laboratory tests are needed to confirm this diagnosis. Contralateral hypertrophy owing to agenesis of one lobe (usually the left) can mimic a nodule.[4] Although an autonomously functioning thyroid adenoma and lobe hypertrophy may appear similar on thyroid radionuclide imaging, the serum thyrotropin (TSH) concentrations in these two conditions are different: they are low in the patient with a thyroid adenoma and normal in thyroid agenesis.

Most benign thyroid nodules are freely movable, have a smooth surface, and are rubbery. The mobility of a nodule should not be confused with its texture. Texture is best appreci-

TABLE 25-1.
Summary of Findings on Physical Examination of the Thyroid Gland

Physical Finding	Differential Diagnosis	Special Features
Single nodule	Autonomously functioning adenoma	Opposite lobe not palpable
	Adenoma or adenomatous nodule	Rubbery, firm; tenderness suggests recent hemorrhage or infarction
	Carcinoma	Firm or hard; may have associated lymph node enlargement or vocal cord palsy
	Hyperplasia secondary to unilobar agenesis	Opposite lobe not palpable
Multiple nodules	Multinodular goiter	
	Goitrous autoimmune thyroiditis	Firm lobes or irregular surface misinterpreted as multiple nodules
Diffuse goiter	Graves' disease	Bruit or thrill; pyramidal lobe
	Goitrous autoimmune thyroiditis	Irregular surface; pyramidal lobe; rubbery or firm; occasionally tender; fibrous variant may be hard
	Subacute thyroiditis	Unilateral or bilateral tenderness; often hard
	Painless (silent) thyroiditis	Small to medium size; no bruit
	Thyroid lymphoma	Rapidly growing goiter, particularly in setting of preexisting goitrous autoimmune thyroiditis
	Multinodular goiter	Nodules may be hidden within gland
Tenderness	Subacute thyroiditis	Unilateral or bilateral; tenderness often severe
	Hemorrhagic or infarcted adenoma	Discrete nodule with tenderness
	Goitrous autoimmune thyroiditis	See above; mild tenderness
	Carcinoma	Irregular, firm thyroid nodule with chronic tenderness

ated by squeezing the nodule between the fingers; mobility refers to the ease of movement of the nodule as a whole within the neck. Benign thyroid nodules may be hard, especially those that are calcified or tensely distended with fluid. A painful, tender nodule probably indicates hemorrhage or infarction within a benign nodule, but some malignant thyroid nodules also are tender.

A nodule that does not rise with swallowing requires special attention; it may not be of thyroid origin. Alternatively, it may represent a thyroid carcinoma that is fixed to neck structures, or a nodule that is part of a large substernal goiter. When thyroglossal duct cysts are near the thyroid isthmus, they may mimic midline thyroid nodules. Thyroglossal duct cysts usually are found in the midline, anywhere from the base of the tongue to the thyroid isthmus, but a few of these cysts are more laterally placed. They rise with swallowing, just like thyroid nodules, but their attachment to the base of the tongue also causes them to rise when the tongue is protruded.

Malignant thyroid nodules may be firm or hard and irregular, but most are indistinguishable from benign nodules. Fixation of a nodule to the surrounding neck structures suggests that it is malignant. Because a history of head and neck irradiation increases the prevalence of both benign and malignant thyroid nodules, the examiner should be alert to signs of radiation skin damage (e.g., scarring, atrophy, and telangiectasis of the face and neck skin), although the doses used to treat lymphoid and thymic hyperplasia in children in the past that are associated with thyroid tumors were not sufficient to damage the skin. Ipsilateral lymphadenopathy suggests thyroid carcinoma. The Delphian, or upper pretracheal, node often is involved in thyroid cancer, but it also can become enlarged in patients with goitrous autoimmune thyroiditis.[5] A firm pyramidal lobe can mimic an enlargement of the Delphian node. A thyroid nodule in a patient with hoarseness secondary to an ipsilateral vocal cord palsy is likely to be a thyroid carcinoma, but on rare occasions, benign thyroid nodules or goiters cause hoarseness by compressing the recurrent laryngeal nerve.[6]

The examiner should be aware of the following clinical situations:

1. A thyroid nodule in a patient with marked diastolic hypertension might suggest medullary carcinoma of the thyroid in association with pheochromocytoma (multiple endocrine neoplasia type II).
2. The sudden appearance of a mass or growth of a goiter in a patient with known goitrous autoimmune thyroiditis should raise concern about a thyroid lymphoma.[7]
3. Rapid enlargement of a previously stable nodule, with or without local pain or pain radiating to the ear, suggests hemorrhage into an adenoma or the development of an anaplastic carcinoma of the thyroid.[8]
4. The appearance of a rapidly growing thyroid mass in a patient with previous extrathyroidal cancer (e.g., breast or renal cell carcinoma) may be due to a metastasis to the thyroid gland.

GOITER

A goiter is an enlarged thyroid gland, whatever the cause (see Table 25-1). An anteriorly placed normal thyroid gland

may simulate a goiter (pseudogoiter; see Fig 25-3).[9] A goiter may be symmetric, asymmetric, or nodular. A good estimate of the size of the goiter can be obtained by direct measurement of the thyroid lobes using a ruler, a tape measure, or calipers. It is helpful to draw a picture of the goiter and to record the length and width of each lobe on this picture. It is difficult to estimate the depth of the lobes with accuracy. Serial measurement and recording of the maximum neck circumference facilitate the follow-up of patients with large goiters.

Some examiners describe goiters as 1×, 2×, 3×, and so on, to indicate that a goiter is one, two, three, or more times the size of the normal thyroid. Others assign an estimated maximum weight to their approximations of size (e.g., 20, 40, or 60 g).[10] These numbers provide an individual "bookkeeping" system but should not be taken literally. An initial approximation would add together the volume of each lobe (length × width × depth) to estimate the weight of the gland (e.g., right lobe [5 cm × 3 cm × 2 cm] + left lobe [5 cm × 3 cm × 2 cm] = 60 g). The more accurate measurements provided by ultrasonography or computed tomography usually are unnecessary.

Diffuse enlargement of the thyroid gland in a clinically euthyroid or hypothyroid patient residing in an area of iodine sufficiency usually is caused by goitrous autoimmune thyroiditis. The thyroid gland in these patients has several important characteristics: (1) it normally is symmetric; (2) it is rubbery or firm and, occasionally, hard (fibrous variant)[11]; (3) its surface usually is irregular; (4) thyroid tenderness is uncommon; and (5) true nodules seldom are present. However, it may be very difficult to distinguish goitrous autoimmune thyroiditis from multinodular goiter by physical examination.

The goiter associated with Graves' hyperthyroidism is firm or rubbery and sometimes has a bruit. The presence of exophthalmos or other signs of infiltrative ophthalmopathy helps to confirm the diagnosis of Graves' disease. The texture of the thyroid becomes firmer if the condition has been present or treated with antithyroid drugs for many years.

A diffuse goiter in a thyrotoxic patient suggests Graves' disease, painless (silent) thyroiditis, or, more rarely, TSH-induced hyperthyroidism. The goiter of a patient with thyrotoxicosis caused by subacute thyroiditis often is firm and invariably exquisitely tender. Most uninodular (autonomously functioning thyroid adenoma) and multinodular goiters that cause thyrotoxicosis can be distinguished from the other causes by careful palpation. The thyroid gland of some thyrotoxic patients cannot be palpated. Although these patients may be thyrotoxic as a result of a struma ovarii or exogenous thyroid hormone administration, the cause is more likely to be painless thyroiditis or Graves' disease, especially in elderly patients.

Multinodular goiter is the probable diagnosis when multiple thyroid nodules are palpable, although thyroid cancer can present in this manner. In some patients, thyroxine therapy of what was thought to be a diffuse goiter unmasks the presence of nodules by decreasing the size of the paranodular tissue. The size of multinodular goiters can range from slight to massive. These goiters normally rise with swallowing. When a nodular goiter does not rise, several possibilities should be considered: a large substernal component; tissue fixation secondary to cancer, prior thyroid surgery; or a nonthyroidal nodular neck mass.

Multinodular goiters may cause tracheal obstruction, leading to dyspnea. Inspiratory stridor often is evident on auscultation over the trachea or anterior chest. Flow-volume loop study[3] and a computed tomography scan may be necessary to confirm the diagnosis of airway obstruction. Massive benign goiters may block venous outflow and result in distended neck veins.

Goiters may cause pressure symptoms and signs when they are trapped in a retroclavicular location. Extending the arms over the head (Pemberton's maneuver) raises the goiter into the thoracic inlet ("thyroid cork"),[12] resulting in shortness of breath, stridor, distention of neck veins, or facial plethora. Medium-sized goiters caused by Hashimoto's thyroiditis or Graves' disease also can create this clinical picture when they are strategically located.

Most goiters remain stable or increase slowly in size. However, thyroid enlargement may develop and subside in days or weeks in patients with painless (silent) thyroiditis or subacute thyroiditis; it may be even more transient in patients with pheochromocytomas.[13] Sudden enlargement, pain, and tenderness of a preexisting goiter may be the result of either a hemorrhage into a thyroid nodule or a rapidly growing carcinoma. Previously benign or low-grade malignant nodules may develop into anaplastic carcinomas.[8] Sudden symmetric or asymmetric growth of the thyroid gland in a patient with goitrous autoimmune thyroiditis suggests the development of a thyroid lymphoma.[7]

References

1. Fisher DA, Oddie TH, Johnson DE, Nelson JC. The diagnosis of Hashimoto's thyroiditis. J Clin Endocrinol Metab 1975;40:795

2. Simon H, Daniels GH. Hormonal hyperthermia: endocrinological causes of fever. Am J Med 1979;66:257

3. Kryger M, Bode F, Antic R, Anthonisen N. Diagnosis of obstruction of the upper and central airways. Am J Med 1976;61:85

4. Melnick JC, Stemkowski PE. Thyroid hemiagenesis (hockey stick sign): a review of the world literature and a report of four cases. J Clin Endocrinol Metab 1981;52:247

5. Cope O, Dobyns BM, Hamlin E Jr, Hopkirk J. What thyroid nodules are to be feared? J Clin Endocrinol Metab 1949;9:1012

6. Cerise EJ, Randall S, Ochsner A. Carcinoma of the thyroid and nontoxic nodular goiter. Surgery 1952;31:552

7. Hamburger JI, Miller JM, Kini SR. Lymphoma of the thyroid. Ann Intern Med 1983;99:685

8. Nel CJC, Van Heerden JA, Goellner JR, et al. Anaplastic carcinoma of the thyroid: a clinicopathologic study of 82 cases. Mayo Clin Proc 1985;60:51

9. Gwinup G, Morton ME. The high lying thyroid: a cause of pseudogoiter. J Clin Endocrinol Metab 1975;40:37

10. Berghout A, Wiersinga WM, Smits NJ, Touber JL. Determinants of thyroid volume as measured by ultrasonography in healthy adults in a non-iodine deficient area. Clin Endocrinol 1987; 26:273

11. Katz SM, Vickery AL. The fibrous variant of Hashimoto's thyroiditis. Hum Pathol 1974;5:161

12. Blum M, Biller BJ, Bergman DA. The thyroid cork. Obstruction of the thoracic inlet due to retroclavicular goiter. JAMA 1974; 227:189

13. Buckels JAC, Webb AMC, Rhodes A. Is paroxysmal thyroid swelling due to phaeochromocytoma a forgotten physical sign? BMJ 1983;287:1206

Werner and Ingbar's The Thyroid, Seventh Edition,
edited by Lewis E. Braverman and Robert D. Utiger.
Lippincott–Raven Publishers, Philadelphia, © 1996

26

The Epidemiology of Thyroid Diseases

Mark P.J. Vanderpump

W. Michael G. Tunbridge

The most common cause of thyroid disorders worldwide is iodine deficiency. In iodine-replete areas, most persons with thyroid disorders have autoimmune disease, ranging from hyperthyroidism to hypothyroidism. The problems encountered in epidemiologic studies of thyroid disorders are those of definition, including overt hypothyroidism vs. subclinical hypothyroidism; the selection criteria used; the influence of age, sex, and environmental factors; and the different techniques used for the measurement of thyroid function. The most commonly used initial tests in epidemiologic surveys are measurements of serum total thyroxine (T_4), a derived free thyroxine index (FT_4I) to correct for protein binding, and thyrotropin (TSH).

There have been cross-sectional studies on the prevalence of goiter, hypothyroidism, and thyrotoxicosis and the frequency and distribution of thyroid autoantibodies in different communities. Most studies have concentrated on middle-aged women and elderly people in the community, healthy persons undergoing routine medical examinations, or hospital inpatients, and only a few have documented the prevalence of thyroid disorders in a cross-section of the adult population in the community. Longitudinal studies are necessary to determine incidence rates, etiologic risk factors, and the natural history of the disease process. The logistic and administrative difficulties of such studies explain their relative paucity. The limitations of epidemiologic studies of thyroid disorders should therefore be borne in mind when considering the purported frequency of thyroid diseases in different communities. This chapter is concerned primarily with benign thyroid disorders in iodine-replete white communities. Postpartum thyroiditis, endemic goiter, and thyroid carcinoma are considered in other chapters.

THYROTOXICOSIS

In epidemiologic studies, the clinical diagnosis of thyrotoxicosis should be supported by measurements of serum T_4 (or triiodothyronine [T_3]) and TSH concentrations. A rise in serum T_3 and fall in serum TSH are the earliest measures of thyroid overactivity, followed by a rise in serum T_4. The most common causes of thyrotoxicosis are Graves' disease, followed by toxic multinodular goiter, an autonomously functioning thyroid adenoma, and thyroiditis. In epidemiologic studies, however, the etiology of thyrotoxicosis is rarely ascertained.

Prevalence of Thyrotoxicosis

A cross-sectional study of the community in Whickham, a mixed urban and rural area in northeast England, documented the prevalence of thyroid disorders.[1] The 2779 subjects examined in the survey represented a 1 in 6 sample of the adult population, and closely resembled the British population as a whole in terms of age, sex, and social class. The prevalence of undiagnosed thyrotoxicosis, based on clinical features and elevated serum T_4 and FT_4I values, was 4.7 per 1000 women. Thyrotoxicosis had been previously diagnosed and treated in 20 per 1000 women, rising to 27 per 1000 women when possible but unproven cases were included, as compared with 1.6 to 2.3 per 1000 men, in whom no cases were found at the time of the survey. The mean age at diagnosis was 48 years.

In the few other cross-sectional studies of the adult population the results were comparable to the Whickham data[2–5] (Table 26-1). The prevalence data in elderly persons are conflicting. In a survey of 1210 persons over 60 years of age in a single general practice in Birmingham, England, only one sub-

TABLE 26-1.
Prevalence of Previously Undiagnosed Overt Thyrotoxicosis and Incidence of Overt Thyrotoxicosis
in Epidemiologic Surveys of Thyroid Dysfunction

Study Names and References	No. of Subjects	Sex	Age	Test	Prevalence/1000		Incidence/1000/y		
					MEN	WOMEN	FOLLOW-UP (y)	MEN	WOMEN
Whickham, UK[1,13]	2779	M, F	18+	T_4, FT_4I	0	4.7	20	<0.1	0.8
Mölnlycke, Sweden[2]	2000	M, F	18+	TSH	0	2.5	—	—	—
Hisayama, Japan[3]	2421	M, F	40+	TSH	0	2.0	—	—	—
Kisa, Sweden[4]	3885	F	39–60	TSH, FT_4I	—	5.1	—	—	—
Göteborg, Sweden[5,23]	1283	F	44–66	TSH	—	6.0	6	—	1.3
Oakland, USA[22]	2704	M, F	18+	TSH, T_4, T_3	0	5.4	1	0.2	0.8
Birmingham, UK[6]	1210	M, F	60+	TSH	0.9		1	0.9	
Kisa, Sweden[7]	1442	F	60+	TSH, FT_4I	—	19.4	—	—	—
Gothenburg, Sweden[24]	1148	F	70+	TSH	—	—	10	—	1.0
Olmstead County, USA[16]	?	M, F	0+	BMR, PBI	—	—	32	0.1	0.3
Funen, Denmark[17]	450,000	M, F	0+	PBI, T_4, T_3	—	—	3	0.1	0.5
Iceland[18]	230,000	M, F	0+	T_4, T_3	—	—	3	0.1	0.4
Malmö, Sweden[19]	257,764	M, F	0+	PBI	—	—	5	0.1	0.4
112 Towns in UK[20]	1,641,949	M, F	0+	T_4	—	—	1	0.1	0.4

BMR, basal metabolic rate; PBI, protein-bound iodine (serum).

ject (sex not identified) was found to be thyrotoxic.[6] Among 1442 women over 60 years of age in Sweden, 28 (2%) were found to be thyrotoxic on the basis of biochemical screening.[7] In studies of patients in hospital, the point prevalence rates for previously undiagnosed thyrotoxicosis are consistent with the rate in the Whickham survey.[8–12]

Subclinical Thyrotoxicosis

Subclinical thyrotoxicosis is defined as a low serum TSH concentration in the presence of normal serum T_4 and T_3 concentrations, and the absence of hypothalamic or pituitary disease, nonthyroidal illness, or ingestion of drugs that inhibit TSH secretion. The available studies differ in the definition of a low serum TSH concentration and whether the subjects included were receiving thyroid hormone therapy. In a study of 2000 consecutive adults attending a primary care center in Sweden, 65 (3%) who were not receiving T_4 and were not new cases of overt thyrotoxicosis had a serum TSH concentration of 0.2 mU/L or less (normal range, 0.2–4.0 mU/L).[2] Among the 53 subjects in this group who were reexamined 2 to 3 weeks later, the value was normal in 51%, indicating that, whatever the cause, low serum TSH values often do not persist. At the 20-year follow-up of the 2779 subjects in the Whickham survey cohort, at which time 1704 of the 1877 known survivors of the cohort (over 38 years of age) were reexamined, 4% had a serum TSH concentration less than 0.5 mU/L (normal range, 0.5–5.2 mU/L), decreasing to 3% if those subjects taking T_4 and those with newly diagnosed overt thyrotoxicosis were excluded.[13] Use of a more sensitive TSH assay provided no additional diagnostic information.

The prevalence of subclinical thyrotoxicosis has been investigated in older populations. In 2575 survivors of the Framingham Heart Study over 60 years of age, 4% had a low serum TSH concentration (<0.1 mU/L), of whom half were taking T_4.[14] In the community survey in Birmingham, 6% had low serum TSH concentrations, and 2% of women and 1% of men had undetectable values (<0.05 mU/L).[6] Only 5% of these subjects with low or undetectable serum TSH concentrations were taking T_4. In a follow-up investigation of 15 elderly inpatients and outpatients with a low serum TSH and normal free T_4 and T_3 concentrations, two required antithyroid treatment and almost 50% had normal serum TSH concentrations when restudied during a mean follow-up of 8 months.[15]

Incidence of Thyrotoxicosis

The incidence data available for overt thyrotoxicosis for men and women from large population studies are comparable (Table 26-1). The age-specific incidence varies considerably. The peak age-specific incidence of Graves' disease was between 20 and 49 years in two studies,[16,17] but increased with age in Iceland[18] and peaked at 60 to 69 years in Malmö, Sweden.[19] The peak age-specific incidence of thyrotoxicosis caused by toxic nodular goiter and autonomously functioning thyroid adenomas in the Malmö study was over 80 years. In a prospective study of 12 towns in England and Wales, the annual incidence of thyrotoxicosis was strongly correlated with the prevalence of endemic goiter among schoolchildren 60 years earlier.[20] Subsequent to this survey, serum samples from 216 of the 290 cases identified were assayed for TSH-receptor antibodies. The incidence of antibody-negative thyrotoxicosis correlated closely with the previous prevalence of endemic goiter, indicating a high current incidence of toxic nodular goiter in towns in which the incidence of goiter had been high many years ago. The frequency of antibody-positive thyrotoxicosis, an indicator of Graves' disease, did not correlate with goiter in the past.[21]

In the 20-year follow-up of the Whickham cohort, 825 subjects had died.[13] In addition to death certificates, two thirds had information from medical records or postmortem reports to document morbidity before death. Of the 1877 known survivors, 91% were examined for clinical, biochemical, and immunologic evidence of thyroid dysfunction. Among the survivors, 11 women had been diagnosed and treated for thyrotoxicosis after the first survey and five women were diagnosed as having thyrotoxicosis at the second survey. The etiology in these 16 new cases was Graves' disease in 10 subjects, multinodular goiter in 3 subjects, an autonomously functioning thyroid adenoma in 1, chronic autoimmune thyroiditis in 1, and unknown in 1. The mean incidence of thyrotoxicosis in women was 0.8/1000 survivors per year (95% confidence interval, 0.5–1.4). The incidence rate was similar in the women who had died. No new cases were detected in men. An estimate of the probability of the development of thyrotoxicosis in women at a particular time (i.e., the hazard rate), averaged 1.4 per 1000 between the ages of 35 and 60 years (Fig 26-1). Neither thyroid antibody status nor the presence of a goiter during the first survey was associated with the development of thyrotoxicosis at follow-up. Other cohort studies provide comparable incidence data, which suggests that many cases of thyrotoxicosis remain undiagnosed in the community unless routine testing is undertaken.[22–24]

At the 1-year follow-up of the subjects over 60 years of age in Birmingham who initially had serum TSH values below normal, only one (sex not identified) developed thyrotoxicosis; 88% with undetectable serum TSH values (<0.05 mU/L) continued to have a subnormal value, and 76% with a value of between 0.05 and 0.5 mU/L had normal values at follow-up.[6]

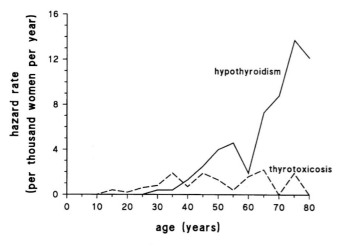

FIGURE 26-1. The age-specific hazard rates for the development of overt hypothyroidism and thyrotoxicosis in women at 20-year follow-up of the community survey in Whickham, United Kingdom. (Adapted from Vanderpump MPJ, Tunbridge WMG, French JM, et al. The incidence of thyroid disorders in the community: a twenty-year follow-up of the Whickham Survey. Clin Endocrinol 1995;43:55).

CHRONIC AUTOIMMUNE THYROIDITIS

A substantial proportion of the population, particularly elderly women who live in iodine-replete areas, have circulating thyroid antibodies (antithyroid peroxidase [microsomal] and antithyroglobulin antibodies) and normal thyroid function. The presence of these antibodies correlates with the presence of focal thyroiditis in biopsy and in postmortem material of patients with no evidence of hypothyroidism during life.[25,26] In an analysis of thyroid tissue from several hundred necropsies, histologic evidence of chronic autoimmune thyroiditis was found in 27% of adult women and 7% of adult men, and it was diffuse in 5% of women and 1% of men.[27]

Patients with hypothyroidism caused by either atrophic or goitrous autoimmune thyroiditis usually have high serum titers of these same antibodies (see chap 21), and they also are often detected in the serum of patients with Graves' disease and other thyroid diseases, but the titers are usually lower. There is considerable variation in the frequency and distribution of thyroid antibodies because of variations in techniques of detection, definition of abnormal titers, and inherent differences in the populations tested. Most of the available data are based on studies using hemagglutination and complement fixation tests for thyroglobulin and thyroid microsomal antibodies, respectively, and not the newer radioimmunoassays for antibodies against either thyroglobulin or thyroid peroxidase.

In all the early studies, regardless of the methodology, the prevalence of thyroid antibodies increased progressively with age in women, as compared with a uniformly low prevalence with no age trend in men.[28–30] Those trends were confirmed in the Whickham survey, but the frequency of positive tests was lower.[1] Specifically, 2% of the subjects surveyed had positive tests for antithyroglobulin antibodies, and only 0.7% had these antibodies and no antithyroid microsomal antibodies. The latter, measured by an immunofluorescent technique with serum diluted 1:10, were found in 7% (women, 10%; men, 3%). The mean serum TSH concentrations were significantly higher in both men and women with positive antibody tests, and 3% of the sample (5% of women, 1% of men) had both positive antibody tests and a serum TSH value greater than 6 mU/L.

In a random sample of 507 adults in southern Finland, the prevalence of asymptomatic chronic autoimmune thyroiditis was between 2% and 5%, based on elevated serum TSH values and high titers of either antithyroglobulin or antithyroid microsomal antibodies.[31] The prevalence of antithyroid microsomal antibodies was 7% (women, 10%; men, 3%) in an Australian survey,[32] and the prevalence of chronic autoimmune thyroiditis as defined by an elevated serum TSH and a positive antibody test was 5% if the serum TSH was even minimally elevated, and 3% if it was greater than 10 mU/L. The prevalence in women in the sixth decade was 15%, with a subsequent fall that suggests selective mortality in more elderly women. A lower prevalence of thyroid antibodies in the very elderly was also found in an Italian study.[33] In the Framingham cohort of subjects over 60 years of age, two thirds of those with serum TSH concentrations greater than 10 mU/L had positive tests for antithyroid microsomal antibodies,[34] and among 414 asymptomatic elderly people over 70 years of age in the United Kingdom, 15% and 13% had elevated titers of antithyroid microsomal and antithyroglobulin antibodies, respectively; 9% had elevated titers of both antibodies.[35] In summary, a significant proportion of subjects in the community have asymptomatic chronic autoimmune thyroiditis, of whom a substantial proportion have subclinical hypothyroidism.

In recent studies, in which antithyroid peroxidase antibodies were measured by radioimmunoassay, the results were similar. For example, positive tests were found in 18% of 698 female blood donors from seven towns in England and Wales,[36] with a rise in prevalence from 15% at age 18 to 24 years to 24% at age 55 to 64 years. In contrast to many of the earlier studies, the prevalence of antithyroid peroxidase antibodies and antithyroglobulin antibodies was similar. Geographic differences in the prevalence of thyroid antibodies were not significant and did not correlate with either the prevalence of goiter or with current differences in iodine intake. In another study of 342 elderly subjects in Italy (mean age, 80 years), 10% of the women and 2% of the men had antithyroid peroxidase antibodies measured by radioimmunoassay.[37]

At the 20-year follow-up of the Whickham survey, 1704 survivors had tests for antithyroid peroxidase or antithyroglobulin antibodies;[13] 19% had positive tests for the former and 5% had positive tests for the latter. Seventeen percent of women and 7% of men who initially had negative tests now had positive tests, 9% of women and 2% of men had positive tests on both occasions, and 2% of women and 0.5% of men no longer had positive tests. The thyroid antibodies were most often detected in women 55 to 65 years of age at follow-up (and who were therefore 35 to 45 years of age at the time of the first survey). There was no evidence that a positive antithyroid antibody test at the original survey was a risk factor for premature death in this cohort. Over 50% of the women in whom the tests changed from positive to negative were receiving T_4 treatment for hypothyroidism, a change noted previously by others.[38,39] In other, shorter longitudinal studies, one third of 160 subjects who were initially antibody-positive in a population survey no longer had detectable antibodies 6 years later,[32] whereas in another study of 51 elderly subjects all remained thyroid-antibody positive at a 5-year follow-up.[35]

HYPOTHYROIDISM

The earliest biochemical abnormality in hypothyroidism is a rise in serum TSH concentration associated with normal serum T_4 and T_3 concentrations (subclinical hypothyroidism) (see chap 87). Subsequently, serum T_4 falls, at which stage most patients have symptoms and benefit from treatment (overt hypothyroidism). In persons living in iodine-replete areas, the cause is most likely either chronic autoimmune disease (atrophic autoimmune thyroiditis or goitrous autoimmune thyroiditis [Hashimoto's thyroiditis]) or destructive treatment for thyrotoxicosis, but this is rarely discussed in the available studies.

Prevalence of Hypothyroidism

In the Whickham survey, the prevalence of newly diagnosed overt hypothyroidism was 3 per 1000 women. The prevalence of previously diagnosed and treated hypothyroidism was 14 per 1000 women, rising to 19 per 1000 women when possible but unproven cases were included. The overall prevalence in men was less than 1 case per 1000. The mean age at diagnosis was 57 years. One third had been previously treated by surgery or radioiodine for thyrotoxicosis. Excluding iatrogenic causes, the prevalence of hypothyroidism was 10 per 1000 women, rising to 15 per 1000 when possible but unproven cases were included. The diagnosis was based on clinical features and high serum TSH and low FT_4I values in the new cases, and from the original records in the previously diagnosed and treated cases.[1]

The figure of 3 new cases per 1000 women in the Whickham survey is comparable to the 2 per 1000 in a Finnish community study[40] and other studies (Table 26-2). The prevalence was higher in surveys of the elderly in the community. The overall prevalence of hypothyroidism, including those already taking T_4, in Birmingham was 4% of women and 0.8% of men over 60 years of age.[6] In people 60 years of age or more in Framingham, 4% had serum TSH concentration greater than 10 mU/L, of whom one third had low serum T_4 concentrations.[41]

The testing of hospital inpatients, predominantly elderly women, might be expected to reveal a higher proportion of unsuspected hypothyroidism,[42] but this is not supported by recent studies. Overt hypothyroidism, very rarely suspected clinically, was found in approximately 2% of a total of 1027 patients admitted for treatment of an acute illness in three studies.[8,10,11] In another similar study, however, 6% of 364 patients admitted consecutively to an acute care teaching hospital had unrecognized or untreated thyroid failure (low serum FT_4I and elevated TSH values).[12]

Subclinical Hypothyroidism

Serum TSH concentrations do not change as a function of age among adult men, but in women over 40 years the concentrations increase. If, however, women with antibodies are excluded, there is no age-related increase.[1] Nearly all older women with elevated serum TSH values have subclinical hypothyroidism. With respect to epidemiologic studies, the definition of subclinical hypothyroidism varies from any increase in serum TSH to values greater than 10 mU/L to, most stringently, a serum TSH value greater than 10 mU/L and a positive test for thyroid antibodies in serum. The most common etiology in the community is chronic autoimmune thyroiditis.

In the Whickham survey 8% of women (10% of women over 55 years of age) and 3% of men had subclinical hypothyroidism.[1] The results were similar in a study of a Japanese population 40 years of age and over; the prevalence of subclinical hypothyroidism was 6% in women and 3% in men.[3] Community studies of elderly persons have confirmed the high prevalence in this age group; approximately 10% of subjects over 60 years having serum TSH values above the normal range.[6,7,34] In surveys of hospital inpatients the point prevalence rates were similar, being between 3% and 6%.[10-12]

Incidence of Hypothyroidism

After destructive treatment of thyrotoxicosis, the incidence of overt hypothyroidism is greatest in the first year after either radioiodine therapy or surgery. If the serum TSH remains raised,

TABLE 26-2.
Prevalence of Previously Undiagnosed Overt Hypothyroidism and Incidence of Overt
Hypothyroidism in Epidemiologic Surveys of Thyroid Dysfunction

Study Names and References	No. of Subjects	Sex	Age	Test	Prevalence/1000		Incidence/1000/y		
					MEN	WOMEN	FOLLOW-UP (y)	MEN	WOMEN
Whickham, UK[1,13]	2779	M, F	18+	T_4, FT_4I	0	3.3	20	0.6	3.5
South Finland[40]	3000	M, F	18+	TSH	2.0		—	—	—
Mölnlycke, Sweden[2]	2000	M, F	18+	TSH	1.3	12.0	—	—	—
Hisayama, Japan[3]	2421	M, F	40+	TSH	4.0	7.0	—	—	—
Kisa, Sweden[4]	3885	F	39–60	TSH, FT_4I	—	0	—	—	—
Göteborg, Sweden[5,23]	1283	F	44–66	TSH	—	6.4	4	—	1–2
Oakland, USA[22]	2704	M, F	18+	TSH, T_4, T_3	3.5	6.1	1	8.0	
Birmingham, UK[6]	1210	M, F	60+	TSH	7.8	20.5	1	11.1	
Kisa, Sweden[7]	1442	F	60+	TSH, FT_4I	—	5.5	—	—	—
Gothenburg, Sweden[24]	1148	F	70+	TSH	—	—	10	—	2
Western Australia[32]	1587	M, F	18+	TMA	—	—	6	3	
Barry, Wales[35]	414	M, F	70+	TMA, TGA	4.8		5	4	

TMA, antithyroid microsomal antibodies; TGA, antithyroglobulin antibodies.

then the rate of progression to overt hypothyroidism is between 2% to 6% per year after either treatment.[43,44] In a long-term follow-up study conducted in a Birmingham, England, clinic, 1918 patients with thyrotoxicosis were treated with either radioiodine at a dose calculated from thyroid size and radioiodine uptake or an empirical dose of radioiodine (3, 5, or 10 mC [110, 185, or 370 MBq]), or partial thyroidectomy.[45] All three treatments resulted in control of hyperthyroidism in more than 90% of patients. After the calculated dose of radioiodine, 18% were hypothyroid at 5 years and 42% at 20 years, equivalent to a constant annual incidence of 2%. The results in the patients treated with an empirical dose of radioiodine were only available for 5 years, at which time just less than 40% were hypothyroid (8% per year). After partial thyroidectomy only 2% were hypothyroid at 5 years, but 28% were hypothyroid at 20 years; the annual incidence was 0.4% for the first decade and almost 3% for the second decade. The incidence of hypothyroidism after surgery, external radiation therapy, or both, for head and neck cancer is as high as 50% within the first year after treatment, particularly in patients who undergo both treatments.[46–48]

The 20-year follow-up of the Whickham cohort has provided incidence data and allowed the determination of risk factors for hypothyroidism in this period.[13] The mean incidence of spontaneous hypothyroidism in the surviving women over the 20-year follow-up period was 3.5/1000 per year (95% confidence interval, 2.8–4.5), rising to 4.1/1000 per year (95% confidence interval, 3.3–5.0) if all cases including those who had received destructive treatment for thyrotoxicosis are included. Only 9% of cases of spontaneous hypothyroidism in surviving women were diagnosed when they were less than 45 years old, and 51% were diagnosed between the ages of 45 to 64 years. The hazard rate (the estimate of the probability of a woman developing hypothyroidism at a particular time) increased with

age to 13.7 per 1000 in women between 75 and 80 years of age (Fig 26-1). The mean incidence during the 20-year follow-up period in men (all spontaneous except for one case of lithium-induced hypothyroidism) was 0.6/1000 per year (95% confidence interval, 0.3–1.2). The incidence rates for the deceased women and men were similar.

The risk of having developed hypothyroidism was examined with respect to risk factors identified in the first survey. In female survivors the annual risk of developing spontaneous hypothyroidism was 4% per year in those who had both raised TSH values and positive thyroid-antibody tests, 3% per year if only serum TSH was raised, and 2% per year if only thyroid antibodies were positive; at the time of follow-up the respective rates of hypothyroidism in these groups were 55%, 33%, and 27%. The probability of developing hypothyroidism was higher in those women who had serum TSH concentrations above 2 mU/L and higher titers of antithyroid microsomal antibodies at the first survey. Neither a positive family history of any form of thyroid disease, nor the presence of a goiter at either the first or the follow-up survey, nor parity at the first survey was associated with an increased risk of hypothyroidism. These results confirm those from a 4-year follow-up of a subgroup of women in the Whickham cohort in whom overt hypothyroidism had developed at a rate of 5% per year in those who initially had a raised serum TSH and a positive test for thyroid antibodies.[49] Either finding alone, however, was not associated with an increased risk of hypothyroidism at 4 years.

The other incidence data for hypothyroidism are from short (and often small) follow-up studies (Table 26-2). Among 22 women with asymptomatic chronic autoimmune thyroiditis, overt hypothyroidism developed at a rate of 7% per year, increasing to 10% per year in those who initially had serum TSH values greater than 19 mU/L.[50,51] In a recent follow-up study of 437 healthy women 40 to 60 years old in the Netherlands, 24% of those who initially had a positive test for antithyroid microsomal antibodies and normal serum TSH concentrations had an elevated serum TSH concentration (>4.2 mU/L) 10 years later, as compared with 3% in the antibody-negative group.[52] As in the 20-year follow-up of the Whickham cohort, serum TSH concentrations in the upper part of the normal range in this study also appeared to have a predictive value. These studies therefore indicate that the higher the serum TSH level, the greater is the risk of development of overt hypothyroidism in subjects with chronic autoimmune thyroiditis. The prognostic importance of positive thyroid antibody tests and raised serum TSH values in elderly subjects has also been confirmed.[6,34,53]

SPORADIC GOITER

The single most common thyroid disease in the community is simple (diffuse) goiter, notwithstanding that the clinical grading of thyroid size is subjective and imprecise. The widely used World Health Organization (WHO) grading system recognizes that an enlarged thyroid gland may be palpably but not visibly enlarged.[54] Examiner variation is greatest in deciding whether a thyroid that is palpable but not visible is normal (WHO grade O-A) or enlarged (WHO grade O-B).[55] Interexaminer variation may also lead to differences in classification of the type of thyroid disease, for example, diffuse goiter vs. multinodular goiter.[56] There is also considerable overlap between the five WHO grades as compared with thyroid volume estimated by ultrasonography.[57] More recently, ultrasonography has been used in epidemiologic studies to assess thyroid size,[58–60] leading to much higher estimates of goiter prevalence than in studies in which goiter size was assessed by physical examination.

Most studies define a thyroid that is visible as well as palpable as a goiter (WHO grade 1 or above). Considerable regional variations exist even in nonendemic goiter areas. In cross-sectional surveys, the prevalence of goiter declines with age, the greatest prevalence is in premenopausal women, and the ratio of women to men is at least 4:1.[28,61] In the Whickham survey, 16% of the cohort had small but easily palpable diffuse or multinodular goiters. In men, the prevalence of goiter declined with age from 7% in those less than 25 years of age to 4% in those 65 to 74 years of age. No goiters were detected in men over 75 years of age. Among the women 26% had a goiter; the frequency ranged from 31% in those less than 45 years of age to 12% in those over 75 years of age.[1] This decline in frequency of goiters with age is in contrast to the increase in frequency of thyroid nodules and thyroid antibodies with age. Fewer than 1% of the men but 5% of the women had thyroid nodules detected clinically, and this frequency was 9% in women over 75.

In 5234 subjects over 60 years of age studied over a 5-year period in Framingham, the prevalence of single thyroid nodules was 3% and multinodular goiter nodules was 1%.[41] In a survey of 101 women between 49 to 58 years of age, thyroid nodules were detected by ultrasonography in 36% of subjects, of whom less than a third were detected by palpation.[62]

Longitudinal studies confirm the decreasing frequency of goiter with age. In the 20-year follow-up of the Whickham cohort, 10% of women and 2% of men had a goiter, as compared to 23% and 5%, respectively, in the same subjects at the first survey.[18] In a 20-year follow-up study of a sample of a southwestern United States population 11 to 18 years of age, spontaneous regression by the age of 30 years occurred in 60% of the subjects who initially had diffuse goiters.[63] Among 108 patients with diffuse goiter followed for an average of 8 years in a thyroid clinic in Japan, the goiter disappeared in only 5% and another 7% developed thyroid dysfunction.[64] In contrast, in the 20-year follow-up of the Whickham cohort, the presence of a diffuse goiter was not predictive of any clinical or biochemical evidence of thyroid dysfunction. In women, an association was found between the development of a goiter and thyroid-antibody status at follow-up, but not initially. Although the order in which these events occurred is unknown, it would suggest an autoimmune etiology. Relative iodine deficiency may account for some cases of sporadic goiter. Serum TSH concentrations are elevated only in severe iodine deficiency, and in the non-iodine-deficient population of Whickham, thyroid function was similar in the goitrous and nongoitrous subjects at the first survey.

TESTING FOR THYROID DYSFUNCTION

It is desirable to detect any disease in its early stage, particularly when treatment is available that will benefit the affected person and forestall or improve the natural history of the condition. Thyroid disorders are amongst the most prevalent of medical conditions. Their symptoms and signs may be subtle and nonspecific and they can be mistakenly attributed to other illnesses, particularly in the elderly. On the basis of the epidemiologic studies of benign thyroid disorders in iodine-replete communities reviewed in this chapter, who should be tested for thyroid dysfunction, when, and by what method?

The evidence from the community studies is that general testing of the population will detect only a few cases of overt thyroid disease and is unjustified. Among postmenopausal women, however, up to 10% have subclinical hypothyroidism. Does this condition warrant detection? It may not have any ill effects and treatment is not without risk (see chaps 87 and 88). However, hypothyroidism is an insidious condition and can be readily overlooked, and questionnaires that aim to identify at-risk subjects in the community do not differentiate between those with and those without elevated serum TSH values.[65] Also, there is some evidence that nonspecific symptoms can be improved by T_4 with a retrospective awareness of disability,[66] and T_4 may have beneficial effects on cardiovascular function and lipoprotein metabolism in subjects with subclinical hypothyroidism.[67–69] Most clinicians treat those subjects who have both raised serum TSH concentrations and positive thyroid-antibody tests, even if symptoms are absent, provided that no contraindication is present, in view of the annual risk of developing hypothyroidism of approximately 5%. If serum TSH alone is raised the annual risk of developing hypothyroidism is approximately 3% per year. The risks of lifelong T_4 can be balanced against the need for regular long-term follow-up in the expectation that one third of these women will become hypothyroid within 20 years. If thyroid antibodies alone are found, serum TSH should be measured approximately every 3 to 5 years.

The case for detection of subclinical thyrotoxicosis, which will be an inevitable consequence of screening with serum TSH determinations, is even less clear (see chap 88). In addition to the risk of subsequent development of overt thyrotoxicosis, atrial fibrillation[70,71] and osteoporosis[72] are other possible long-term complications. The annual incidence of overt thyrotoxicosis, which is usually more clinically obvious than hypothyroidism, is as little as 1 per 1000 per year in women and negligible in men.[13]

Certain groups (see below) do have a high risk of developing thyroid disease and require at least annual surveillance of thyroid function. This can be part of a computerized testing program of serum TSH measurements in primary care, with a recall system and follow-up serum free T_4 measurements if the TSH is found to be abnormal. Those who would benefit most from this surveillance are patients who have been treated for thyrotoxicosis and who are therefore at risk for either recurrent thyrotoxicosis or hypothyroidism, and patients treated with external beam radiotherapy for head and neck cancer or lymphoma who have an increased risk of hypothyroidism as well as thyroid cancer. Other patients who should have a one-time assessment of thyroid function include those with atrial fibrillation or hyperlipidemia,[73,74] whereas periodic assessment is indicated in those receiving amiodarone and lithium[75] (see section on effect of excess iodide in chap 14 and chap 58). The evidence from the studies of patients hospitalized for acute illness is that the occurrence of thyroid disease is no more common than in the general population. Therefore, testing should be limited but with a high index of clinical suspicion, particularly in elderly women, and with an awareness of the difficulties in interpreting thyroid function tests in the presence of acute illness (see section on nonthyroidal illness in chap 14). For most purposes a determination of serum TSH, done by a sensitive immunoradiometric assay, is the single most useful test for screening thyroid function in any subject at risk.[76]

References

1. Tunbridge WMG, Evered DC, Hall R, et al. The spectrum of thyroid disease in the community: The Whickham Survey. Clin Endocrinol 1977;7:481
2. Eggertsen R, Petersen K, Lundberg P-A, Nyström E, Lindstedt G. Screening for thyroid disease in a primary care unit with a thyroid stimulating hormone assay with a low detection limit. BMJ 1988;297:1586
3. Okamura K, Ueda K, Sone H, et al. A sensitive thyroid stimulating hormone assay for screening of thyroid functional disorder in elderly Japanese. J Am Geriatr Soc 1989;37:317
4. Kågedal B, Månson JC, Norr A, Sörbo B, Tegler L. Screening for thyroid disorders in middle-aged women by computer-assisted evaluation of a thyroid hormone panel. Scand J Clin Lab Invest 1981;41:403
5. Nyström E, Bengtsson C, Lindquist O, Lindberg S, Lindstedt G, Lundberg P-A. Serum triiodothyronine and hyperthyroidism in a population sample of women. Clin Endocrinol 1984;20:31
6. Parle JV, Franklyn JA, Cross, KW, Jones SC, Sheppard MC. Prevalence and follow-up of abnormal thyrotrophin (TSH) concentrations in the elderly in the United Kingdom. Clin Endocrinol 1991;34:77

7. Falkenberg M, Kågedal B, Norr A. Screening of an elderly female population for hypo- and hyperthyroidism by use of a thyroid hormone panel. Acta Med Scand 1983;214:361
8. Kaplan MM, Reed Larsen P, Cranzt FR, Dzau VJ, Rossing TH. Prevalence of abnormal thyroid function test results in patients with acute medical illnesses. Am J Med 1982;72:9
9. Simons RJ, Simon JM, Demers LM, Santen RJ. Thyroid dysfunction in elderly hospitalized patients. Effect of age and severity of illness. Arch Intern Med 1990;150:1249
10. Gow SM, Elder A, Caldwell G, et al. An improved approach to thyroid function testing in patients with non-thyroidal illness. Clin Chim Acta 1986;158:49
11. Small M, Buchanan L, Evans R. Value of screening thyroid function in acute medical admissions to hospital. Clin Endocrinol 1990;32:185
12. DeGroot LJ, Mayor G. Admission screening by thyroid function tests in an acute general care teaching hospital. Am J Med 1992; 93:558
13. Vanderpump MPJ, Tunbridge WMG, French JM, et al. The incidence of thyroid disorders in the community: a twenty-year follow-up of the Whickham Survey. Clin Endocrinol 1995; 43:55
14. Sawin CT, Geller A, Kaplan MM, Bacharach P, Wilson PWF, Hershman JM. Low serum thyrotropin (thyroid-stimulating hormone) in older persons without hyperthyroidism. Arch Intern Med 1991;151:165
15. Stott DJ, McLellan AR, Finlayson J, Chu P, Alexander WD. Elderly patients with suppressed serum TSH but normal free thyroid levels usually have mild thyroid overactivity and are at increased risk of developing overt hyperthyroidism. Q J Med 1991;78:77
16. Furszyfer J, Kurland LT, McConahey WM, Elveback LR. Graves' disease in Olmsted County, Minnesota, 1935 through 1967. Mayo Clin Proc 1970;45:636
17. Mogensen EF, Green A. The epidemiology of thyrotoxicosis in Denmark. Incidence and geographical variation in the Funen region 1972–1974. Acta Med Scand 1980;208:183
18. Haraldsson A, Gudmundsson ST, Larusson G, Sigurdsson G. Thyrotoxicosis in Iceland 1980–1982. An epidemiological survey. Acta Med Scand 1985;217:253
19. Berglund J, Christensen SB, Hallengren B. Total and age-specific incidence of Graves' thyrotoxicosis, toxic nodular goitre and solitary toxic adenoma in Malmö 1970–1974. J Intern Med 1990;227:137
20. Barker DJB, Phillips DIW. Current incidence of thyrotoxicosis and past prevalence of goitre in 12 British towns. Lancet 1984; 2:567
21. Phillips DIW, Barker DJ, Rees Smith B, Didcote S, Morgan D. The geographical distribution of thyrotoxicosis in England according to the presence or absence of TSH-receptor antibodies. Clin Endocrinol 1985;23:283
22. dos Remedios LV, Weber PM, Feldman R, Schurr DA, Tsoi TG. Detecting unsuspected thyroid dysfunction by the free thyroxine index. Arch Intern Med 1980;140:1045
23. Nyström E, Bengtsson C, Lindquist O, Noppa H, Lindstedt G, Lundberg P-A. Thyroid disease and high concentration of serum thyrotrophin in a population sample of women. Acta Med Scand 1981;210:39
24. Sundbeck G, Lundberg P-A, Lindstedt G, Jagenburg R, Edén S. Incidence and prevalence of thyroid disease in elderly women: results from the longitudinal population study of elderly people in Gothenburg, Sweden. Age Ageing 1991;20:291
25. Goudie RB, Anderson JR, Gray KG. Complement fixing thyroid antibodies in hospital patients with asymptomatic thyroid lesions. J Pathol Bacteriol 1959;90:389

26. Basterie PA, Neve P, Bonnyns M, Vanhaelst L, Chailly M. Clinical and pathological significance of asymptomatic atrophic thyroiditis. Lancet 1967;1:915

27. Williams ED, Doniach I. The post mortem incidence of focal thyroiditis. J Pathol Bacteriol 1962;83:255

28. Dingle PR, Ferguson A, Horn DB, Tubmen J, Hall R. The incidence of thyroglobulin antibodies and thyroid enlargement in a general practice in north-east England. Clin Exp Immunol 1966;1:277

29. Couchman KG, Wigley RD, Prior IA. Autoantibodies in the Carterton population survey. J Chronic Dis 1970;23:45

30. Hooper B, Whittingham S, Mathews JD, Mackay IR, Curnow DH. Autoimmunity in a rural community. Clin Exp Immunol 1972;12:79

31. Gordin A, Maatela J, Miettinen A, Helenius T, Lamberg B-A. Serum thyrotrophin and circulating thyroglobulin and thyroid microsomal antibodies in a Finnish population. Acta Endocrinol 1979;90:33

32. Hawkins BR, Cheah PS, Dawkins RL, et al. Diagnostic significance of thyroid microsomal antibodies in randomly selected population. Lancet 1980;2:1057

33. Mariotti S, Sansoni P, Barbesino G, et al. Thyroid and other organ-specific autoantibodies in healthy centenarians. Lancet 1992;339:1506

34. Sawin CT, Castelli WP, Hershman JM, McNamara P, Bacharach P. The aging thyroid. Thyroid deficiency in the Framingham Study. Arch Intern Med 1985;145:1386

35. Lazarus JH, Burr ML, McGregor, AM, et al. The prevalence and progression of autoimmune thyroid disease in the elderly. Acta Endocrinol 1984;106:199

36. Prentice LM, Phillips DIW, Sarsero D, Beever K, McLachlan SM, Rees Smith B. Geographical distribution of subclinical autoimmune thyroid disease in Britain: a study using highly sensitive direct assays for autoantibodies to thyroglobulin and thyroid peroxidase. Acta Endocrinol 1990;123:493

37. Roti E, Gardini E, Minelli R, Bianconi L, Braverman LE. Prevalence of anti-thyroid peroxidase antibodies in serum in the elderly: comparison with other tests for anti-thyroid antibodies. Clin Chem 1992;38:88

38. Jansson R, Karlsson A, Dahlberg PA. Thyroxine, methimazole, and thyroid microsomal autoantibody titres in hypothyroid Hashimoto's thyroiditis. BMJ 1985;290:11

39. Takusu N, Yamada T, Takusu M, et al. Disappearance of thyrotropin-blocking antibodies and spontaneous recovery from hypothyroidism in autoimmune thyroiditis. N Engl J Med 1992;326:513

40. Gordin A, Heinonen OP, Saarinen P, Lamberg B-A. Serum-thyrotrophin in symptomless autoimmune thyroiditis. Lancet 1972;1:551

41. Sawin CT, Bigos ST, Land S. Bacharach P. The aging thyroid. Relationship between elevated serum thyrotropin level and thyroid antibodies in elderly patients. Am J Med 1985;79:591

42. Bahemuka M, Hodkinson HM. Screening for hypothyroidism in elderly inpatients. Br Med J 1975;2:601

43. Toft AD, Irvine WJ, Seth J, Hunter WM, Cameron EHD. Thyroid function in the long-term follow-up of patients treated with iodine-131 for thyrotoxicosis. Lancet 1975;2:576

44. Lundström B, Gillquist J. The importance of elevated TSH in serum after subtotal thyroidectomy for hyperthyroidism. Acta Chir Scand 1981;147:645

45. Franklyn JA, Daykin J, Droic Z, Farmer M, Sheppard MC. Long term follow-up of treatment of thyrotoxicosis by three different methods. Clin Endocrinol 1991;34:71

46. Buisset E, Leclerc L, Lefebvre JL, et al. Hypothyroidism following combined treatment for hypopharyngeal and laryngeal carcinoma. Am J Surg 1991;162:345

47. Grande C. Hypothyroidism following radiotherapy for head and neck cancer: multivariate analysis of risk factors. Radiother Oncol 1992;25:31

48. Tami TA, Gomez P, Parker GS, Gupta MB, Frassica DA. Thyroid dysfunction after radiation therapy in head and neck cancer patients. Am J Otolaryngol 1992;13:357

49. Tunbridge WMG, Brewis M, French JM, et al. Natural history of autoimmune thyroiditis. BMJ 1981;282:258

50. Gordin A, Lamberg B-A. Natural course of symptomless autoimmune thyroiditis. Lancet 1975;2:1234

51. Gordin A, Lamberg B-A. Spontaneous hypothyroidism in symptomless autoimmune thyroiditis. A long-term follow-up study. Clin Endocrinol 1981;15:537

52. Geul KW, van Sluisveld ILL, Grobbee DE, et al. The importance of thyroid microsomal antibodies in the development of elevated serum TSH in middle-aged women: associations with serum lipids. Clin Endocrinol 1993;39:275

53. Rosenthal KJ, Hunt WC, Garry PJ, Goodwin JS. Thyroid failure in the elderly. Microsomal antibodies as discriminant for therapy. JAMA 1987;258:209

54. Querido A, Delange F, Dunn JT, et al. Definitions of endemic goitre and cretinism, classification of goitre size and severity of endemias, and survey techniques. Pan American Health Organisation Scientific Publication 1974;292:267

55. MacLennan R, Gaitán E, Clinton Miller M. Observer variation in grading and measuring the thyroid in epidemiological surveys. Pan American Health Organisation Scientific Publication 1969;193:67

56. Jarlov AE, Hegedüs L, Gjorup T. Hansen MJ. Observer variation in the clinical assessment of the thyroid gland. J Intern Med 1991;229:159

57. Jarlov EA, Hegedüs L, Gjorup T, Hansen MJ. Inadequacy of the WHO classification of the thyroid gland. Thyroidology 1992;4:107

58. Brander A, Viikinkoski P, Nickels J, Kivisaari L. Thyroid gland: US screening in random adult population. Radiology 1991;181:683

59. Hintze G, Windeler J, Baumert J, Stein H, Kobberling J. Thyroid volume and goitre prevalence in the elderly as determined by ultrasound and their relationships to laboratory indices. Acta Endocrinol 1991;124:12

60. Nygaard B, Gideon P, Dige-Petersen H, Jespersen N, Solling K, Veje A. Thyroid volume and morphology and urinary iodine excretion in a Danish municipality. Acta Endocrinol 1993;129:505

61. Kilpatrick R, Milne JS, Rushbrooke M, Wilson ESB, Wilson GM. A survey of thyroid enlargement in two general practices in Great Britain. BMJ 1963;i:29

62. Brander A, Viikinkoski P, Nickels J, Kivisaari L. Thyroid gland: US screening in middle-aged women with no previous thyroid disease. Radiology 1989;173:507

63. Rallison ML, Dobyns BM, Meikle AW, Bishop M, Lyon JL, Stevens W. Natural history of thyroid abnormalities: prevalence, incidence, and regression of thyroid diseases in adolescents and young adults. Am J Med 1991;91:363

64. Hara T, Tamai H, Mukuta T, Fukata S, Kuma K, Nakagawa T. A long-term follow-up study of patients with non-toxic diffuse goitre in Japan. Clin Endocrinol 1993;39:541

65. Parle JV, Franklyn JA, Cross KW, Jones SC, Sheppard MC. Assessment of a screening process to detect patients aged 60 years and over at high risk of hypothyroidism. Br J Gen Pract 1991;41:414

66. Cooper DS, Halpern R, Wood LC, Levin AA, Ridgeway ED. L-thyroxine therapy in subclinical hypothyroidism: a double-blind, placebo-controlled trial. Ann Intern Med 1984;101:18

67. Bell GM, Todd WTA, Forfar JC, et al. End-organ responses to thyroxine therapy in subclinical hypothyroidism. Clin Endocrinol 1985;22:83

68. Nyström E, Caidahl K, Fager G, Wikkelsö C, Lundberg P-A, Lindstedt G. A double-blind cross-over 12-month study of L-thyroxine treatment of women with subclinical hypothyroidism. Clin Endocrinol 1988;29:63

69. Franklyn JA, Daykin J, Betteridge J, et al. Thyroxine replacement therapy and circulating lipid concentrations. Clin Endocrinol 1993;38:453

70. Tenerz A, Forberg R, Jansson R. Is a more active attitude warranted in patients with subclinical thyrotoxicosis? J Intern Med 1990;228:229

71. Sawin CT, Geller A, Wolf PA, et al. Low serum thyrotropin concentrations as a risk factor for atrial fibrillation in older persons. N Engl J Med 1994;331:1249

72. Földes J, Tarján G, Szathmari M, Varga F, Krasznai I, Horvath C. Bone mineral density in patients with endogenous subclinical hyperthyroidism: is this thyroid status a risk factor for osteoporosis? Clin Endocrinol 1993;39:521

73. Glueck CJ, Lang J, Tracy T, Speirs J. The common finding of covert hypothyroidism at initial clinical evaluation for hyperlipoproteinaemia. Clin Chim Acta 1991;201:113

74. O'Kane MJ, Neely RDG, Trimble ER, Nicholls DP. The incidence of asymptomatic hypothyroidism in new referrals to a hospital lipid clinic. Ann Clin Biochem 1991;28:509

75. Vanderpump MPJ, Tunbridge WMG. The effects of drugs on endocrine function. Clin Endocrinol 1993;39:389

76. Caldwell G, Kellett HA, Gow SM, et al. A new strategy for thyroid function testing. Lancet 1985;1:1117

Werner and Ingbar's The Thyroid, Seventh Edition,
edited by Lewis E. Braverman and Robert D. Utiger.
Lippincott–Raven Publishers, Philadelphia, © 1996

27

Genetic Factors in Thyroid Disease

Sandra M. McLachlan

Basil Rapoport

Many thyroid diseases have a genetic basis. Like other genetically determined conditions,[1] these diseases can be subdivided into two main categories. The genetic changes involved in the first category, whether mutations, polymorphisms, or abnormalities, are in the germ line. The second category involves somatic mutations, such as occur commonly in thyroid tumors. The focus of this chapter will be on the first category, which comprises three groups. In one group are those disorders transmitted by classic mendelian recessive or dominant inheritance that can be attributed to differences at a single genetic locus, for example, the enzymatic defects of thyroid hormone synthesis. A second group is characterized by diseases with complex inheritance patterns in which multiple genes appear to be involved, for example, autoimmune thyroid disease. In the third group are disorders caused by chromosomal abnormalities. Some of these abnormalities, for example, Down's syndrome, are associated with thyroid disorders, but none directly causes them.

CLASSIC MENDELIAN INHERITANCE OF THYROID DISEASES

Non-autoimmune hyperthyroidism is an example of a thyroid disorder which is inherited as an autosomal dominant trait (Fig 27-1). This form of hyperthyroidism is caused by germ line mutations of the TSH receptor (TSH-R) gene.[2] Mutations in the nucleotide sequence encoding the membrane-spanning region give rise to receptors that constitutively activate adenylyl cyclase in thyroid follicular cells, thereby causing autonomous thyroid hypersecretion. In contrast to these germ line mutations, a number of somatic mutations in the TSH-R gene are responsible for autonomously functioning thyroid adenomas.[3]

Other thyroid disorders with simple patterns of mendelian inheritance include defects in enzymes involved in thyroid hormone synthesis, the syndromes of thyroid hormone resistance, abnormalities of thyroid-binding proteins, conditions that predispose to some thyroid tumors, and miscellaneous syndromes (Table 27-1). On the one hand, the same phenotype, for example, goitrous hypothyroidism, can result from different defects of thyroid hormonogenesis. Most of these defects are inherited in an autosomal recessive manner (see chap 56). On the other hand, mutations in the same gene (such as the thyroxine-binding globulin gene) can give rise to different phenotypes. In addition, indistinguishable phenotypes may have different modes of inheritance.

GENETIC VERSUS ENVIRONMENTAL FACTORS

Diseases determined by a single gene may be influenced by other genes. Further, the interaction between environmental factors and genetic factors, particularly iodine, influences expression of many thyroid diseases. Endemic goiter, for example, appears to have a familial basis. Thus, within the same village, the proportion of children with goiter is higher in families with goitrous than with nongoitrous mothers,[4] and the concordance rate is higher between monozygotic than dizygotic twins.[5] Similar observations have been made in twin studies of simple goiter.[6]

The basis for genetic differences in endemic or simple goiter is unknown, but multiple genes likely are involved.[7] However, the balance between "nature and nurture" in endemic goiter is obviously tipped toward an environmental fac-

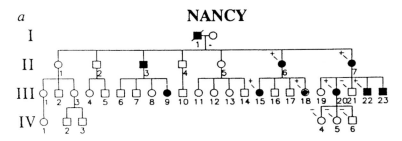

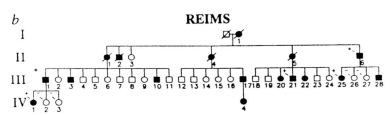

FIGURE 27-1. Two pedigrees, (*a*) Nancy and (*b*) Reims, illustrating autosomal dominant inheritance of non-autoimmune hyperthyroidism caused by a mutation in the thyrotropin (TSH) receptor gene. *Closed symbols*, persons with goiter identified as clinically and biochemically thyrotoxic; *oblique bars*, persons whose DNA was analyzed; (+) or (-), presence or absence of the mutation, which was different in each family. (From Duprez L, Parma J, Van Sande J, et al. Germline mutations in the thyrotropin receptor gene cause non-autoimmune autosomal dominant hyperthyroidism, Nature Genet 1994;7:396)

tor, iodine deficiency. The opposite seems to be the case for autoimmune thyroid disease. Although environmental factors such as iodine,[8] and possibly infectious organisms,[9] play a role in the development of autoimmune thyroid disease, genetic factors appear to predominate.

GENETIC MARKERS

A key requirement for detailed dissection of the genetic basis for thyroid diseases with simple mendelian inheritance, such as non-autoimmune hyperthyroidism, is knowing the protein molecule likely to be responsible for the defect. In contrast, there may be little or no information regarding the proteins (or processes) responsible for complex traits. However, it is possible to discover the genes responsible for a particular disease without prior knowledge of their function.[10] This method, called positional cloning, involves comparison of the inheritance pattern of a particular trait, in this case disease, with the inheritance pattern of defined chromosomal regions.

Positional cloning requires a chromosomal map of highly polymorphic markers. The markers initially available for human studies, blood group antigens and serum proteins, had limited polymorphisms. Recombinant DNA technology has expanded the number and types of suitable markers. For example, genomic DNA can be digested with restriction enzymes and the fragments then probed with radiolabeled sequences. Mutations, insertions, or deletions in different persons yield fragments of different lengths called restriction fragment polymorphisms (RFLPs).

More recently, there has been an explosion in the number of genetic markers based on the presence in the genome of short, repetitive DNA sequences, called satellite DNAs. These repeats, arranged in tandem fashion, vary extensively between unrelated persons. Variable numbers of tandem repeat (VNTR) minisatellites may be analyzed in restriction digests of genomic DNA by hybridization with probes unique to sequences outside the VNTRs. A recent development in this type of analysis involves amplification of genomic DNA by the polymerase chain reaction (PCR) for the detection of di-, tri-, or tetranucleotide minisatellite repeats.

By 1987, using classic markers and RFLPs, a map of 403 loci, at a resolution of 16 centimorgans (cM), had been constructed. Seven years later, a comprehensive human genetic map containing 5840 markers at an average density of 0.7 cM was produced, based on RFLP and PCR-based markers.[11] This map has opened the door to positional cloning of complex (multigenic) disease traits in humans.

GENETIC DISSECTION OF MULTIGENIC TRAITS

Four different approaches may be used to determine the inherited basis of multigenic traits.[10] First, experimental crosses of mice or rats (Fig 27-2*A*) provide the opportunity, impossible in humans, of investigating multiple offspring from a single set of parents. Suitable animal models may provide insight into key genes responsible for similar disorders in humans. For example, analysis of autoimmune type I diabetes in nonobese diabetic (NOD) mice[12] has demonstrated that susceptibility is determined by genes in the major histocompatibility (MHC) region. However, disease onset is influenced by two other genes on different chromosomes.

The second approach, association studies (Fig 27-2*B*), involves comparison of the frequency of a genetic marker in a group of patients with the frequency in a group of unaffected persons. The strength of an association is often measured by the relative risk, which is calculated as follows[13]:

$$\text{Relative risk} = \frac{a/c}{b/d} \left(= \frac{ad}{bc} \right)$$

in which *a* equals the number of patients with the marker, *b* equals the number of control subjects with the marker, *c* equals the number of patients without the marker, and *d* equals the number of control subjects without the marker.

Association studies are most meaningful using polymorphic markers of potential candidate genes. A positive association can occur if the genetic marker (the allele) of the gene

TABLE 27-1.
Thyroid Diseases Inherited According to Simple Mendelian Patterns

Disease	Thyroid Abnormality	MIM No.*
AUTOSOMAL RECESSIVE INHERITANCE		
DISORDERS OF THYROID HORMONOGENESIS		
Iodide transport defect	Goitrous hypothyroidism	274400
Organification (peroxidase) defect	Goitrous hypothyroidism	274500
Pendred's syndrome (goiter and deafness)	Goitrous hypothyroidism	274600
Iodotyrosine coupling defect	Goitrous hypothyroidism	274700
Iodotyrosine dehalogenase defect	Goitrous hypothyroidism	274800
Thyroglobulin synthesis defect	Goitrous hypothyroidism	274900
PITUITARY DEFECTS		
Isolated thyrotropin (TSH) deficiency	No goiter; hypothyroidism	275100
Pituitary dwarfism:		
Type III	No goiter; hypothyroidism	262600
Type IV	No goiter; hypothyroidism	262500
Small sella turcica	No goiter; hypothyroidism	262700
Large sella turcica	No goiter; hypothyroidism	262710
Thyrotropin-releasing hormone (TRH) deficiency	No goiter; hypothyroidism	275120
MISCELLANEOUS SYNDROMES AND DEFECTS		
Impaired thyroid response to TSH	Hypothyroidism without goiter, no response to TSH	275200
Ectopic thyroid with hypothyroidism	Hypothyroidism	225250
Athyreotic cretinism	Congenital hypothyroidism	218700
X-LINKED RECESSIVE INHERITANCE		
ABNORMALITIES OF SERUM THYROID HORMONE-BINDING PROTEINS		
Thyroxine-binding globulin deficiency	Decreased serum total T_4; normal free T_4	314200
Thyroxine-binding globulin increase	Increased serum total T_4; normal free T_4	314200
AUTOSOMAL DOMINANT INHERITANCE		
DISORDERS OF THYROID HORMONOGENESIS		
Thyroglobulin defect	Goitrous hypothyroidism	188450
ABNORMALITIES OF SERUM THYROID HORMONE–BINDING PROTEINS		
Thyroxine-binding globulin deficiency	Decreased serum total T_4; normal free T_4	188600
Familial dysalbuminemic hyperthyroxinemia	Increased serum total T_4 (and free T_4 index); normal free T_4	103600
Familial prealbuminemic hyperthyroxinemia	Increased serum total T_4 (and free T_4 index); normal free T_4	176300
THYROID HORMONE RESISTANCE		
Generalized	Clinical hypothyroidism or euthyroidism; increased serum total and free T_4	188570
MISCELLANEOUS SYNDROMES AND DEFECTS		
Thyrotoxic periodic paralysis	Hyperthyroidism	188580
Nonautoimmune hyperthyroidism	Hyperthyroidism	
Familial thyroglossal duct cyst	Associated hypothyroidism	188455
CONDITIONS THAT PREDISPOSE TO THYROID TUMORS		
Multiple endocrine neoplasia		
Type IIA	Medullary thyroid carcinoma	171400
Type IIB	Medullary thyroid carcinoma	162300
Cowden's (multiple hamartoma) syndrome	Thyroid hamartomas	158350

*MIM, Mendelian Inheritance in Man.[1]

causes the disease. Alternatively, the association can be positive if the allele itself is in linkage disequilibrium, that is, it occurs on the same chromosome near to the gene responsible for the disease. The major problem of association studies is the choice of the control group. For example, if one of the groups is drawn from a mixed population in which the marker is present at a higher frequency in one ethnic group, an artefactual positive association may be observed. Nevertheless, association studies have shed light, for example, on the role of the genes encoding the MHC in some autoimmune diseases.

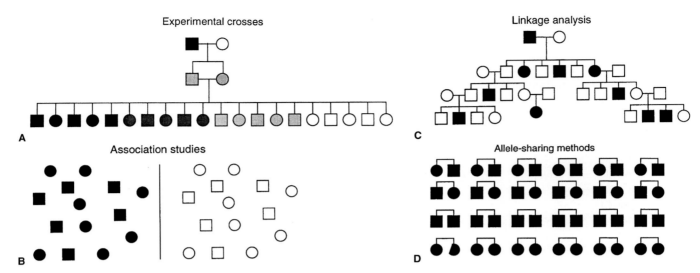

FIGURE 27-2. Approaches to genetic dissection of multigenic disorders (*A*) Experimental crosses between genetically homogeneous parental animal strains. Animals homozygous for two different genes are shown by solid and open symbols, and heterozygotes are shown with gray symbols. (*B*) Association studies in human populations. Two different populations are shown; persons with disease (*solid symbols*) and persons without disease (open symbols). (*C*) Linkage analysis of a pedigree. Affected persons are represented by closed symbols. (*D*) Allele sharing between affected relatives. All persons in this analysis have the disease. (From Lander ES, Schork NJ. Genetic dissection of complex traits. Science 1994;265:2037.)

In the third approach, linkage analysis (Fig 27-2*C*), a model is proposed to explain the pattern of inheritance of the disease and another genetic marker from one generation to another in a family pedigree. This analysis is based on the fact that, after meiosis, alleles at two genetic loci will be inherited together if the two genes are close to one another on the same chromosome but not if the genes are far apart (or on different chromosomes). As the distance between the two genes increases, the frequency of recombination (the recombination fraction) between two alleles increases. The model is tested by determining a likelihood ratio, the ratio of the probability of observing the pattern of the disease and the genetic marker under the hypothesis of linkage, to the probability under the hypothesis of no linkage (the null hypothesis). The data are usually reported as the $\log_{10}$ of the likelihood ratio, the LOD score. Traditionally, the threshold for the likelihood of linkage existing between an observed polymorphic locus and the putative second (pathogenic locus) is a LOD value of 3.

Linkage analysis is most readily applied to the inheritance of simple Mendelian traits such as non-autoimmune hyperthyroidism, for which one pedigree is illustrated in Fig 27-1. It is possible, although more difficult, to find suitable models for diseases with complex inheritance patterns. One problem in defining a model is that the expression of a disease trait, the penetrance, may vary. However, methods are available for performing linkage analysis when penetrance is unknown. Further, the analysis can be used to investigate situations in which two or more genes are involved in disease inheritance.

Allele-sharing methods (Fig 27-2*D*), the fourth approach, involve testing whether affected relatives inherit identical copies of a chromosomal region more often than expected under random Mendelian segregation. This method differs from linkage in that a model is rejected rather than constructed. The

simplest form of this approach is affected sib pair analysis. Under random segregation, the expected distribution for the sharing of zero, one or two copies of a locus that is identical by descent in two sibs is 25%-50%-25%. A chi-square test can then be used to evaluate whether or not there is significant excess allele sharing among a group of sibs. This analysis, which does not require prior knowledge of the mode of inheritance, demonstrated the importance of MHC genes in insulin-dependent diabetes mellitus.[10] More recently, sib pair analysis, in combination with dense genetic maps of highly polymorphic microsatellite markers, was used to confirm the major susceptibility locus for insulin-dependent diabetes mellitus, namely the MHC locus on chromosome 6, as well as to localize another susceptibility locus on chromosome 11.[14,15]

SPECTRUM OF AUTOIMMUNE THYROID DISEASE

One approach to reduce some of the problems associated with genetic dissection of complex diseases is to restrict the analysis to a clearly defined subset of patients. However, this is more easily said than done for autoimmune thyroid disease, which ranges from hyperthyroidism to hypothyroidism. Multiple mechanisms are responsible for this clinical spectrum. Thus, autoantibodies to the TSH-R, which mimic the stimulatory effects of TSH, are responsible for Graves' hyperthyroidism.[16] The processes leading to thyroid cell destruction or hypofunction in chronic autoimmune thyroiditis are poorly understood. Cytotoxic T-cells,[17] autoantibodies to thyroid peroxidase (TPO),[18] TSH-R blocking antibodies,[16] and possibly autoantibodies to thyroglobulin (Tg) may play a role. Finally, it is well known that many persons without thyroid dysfunction have autoantibodies to TPO or Tg.[19]

In addition to the multiple mechanisms outlined above, the influence of modulatory factors must be considered. Like many autoimmune diseases, Graves' disease and chronic autoimmune thyroiditis occur predominantly in women. It seems likely that sex hormones play a role but the precise mechanisms involved are not known. Further (as already mentioned), environmental factors, in particular iodine, influence expression of autoimmune thyroid disease.

MAJOR CANDIDATE IMMUNE RESPONSE GENES

The use of association studies for investigating the genetic basis of complex traits requires information about potentially relevant genetic loci. The single characteristic that links all forms of autoimmune thyroid disease is the presence of IgG class autoantibodies to thyroid autoantigens. In order to appreciate the range of candidate genes that may be involved in this process, some background is needed on the cellular and molecular interactions leading to antibody production.

Briefly, antigen is cleaved by proteolytic enzymes to form polypeptide fragments (10–20 amino acids in length) that bind to MHC molecules on the surface of an antigen-presenting cell, such as a macrophage. The recognition of this MHC-peptide complex by a T-lymphocyte leads to T-cell activation. Finally, the activated T-cell provides help for a B-lymphocyte, which then differentiates into a plasma cell secreting antibody against the same antigen. Therefore, the genes encoding three different cell surface glycoprotein receptors are candidate genes of potential importance in the inheritance of thyroid autoimmunity: the MHC molecule on the antigen-presenting cell, the T-cell antigen receptor, and the B-cell receptor, which is the membrane-bound immunoglobulin molecule that binds the same antigen as the antibody ultimately secreted by the plasma cell. All three types of molecule exhibit polymorphism.

The major cell surface receptors involved in the immune response are constructed from combinations of two different chains. MHC molecules are of two types. MHC class I molecules consist of a heavy chain (the α-chain) with three subunits and a much smaller nonpolymorphic β_2-microglobulin chain (Fig 27-3A). MHC class II molecules consist of an α-chain and a β-chain (Fig 27-3B). The polymorphic regions of both MHC molecules are located on the outer domains, namely α_1 for class I and α_1 and β_1 for class II. Elucidation of the three-dimensional structures of MHC molecules has shown that the α_1 domains form a binding pocket in which a peptide resides.[20] Amino acid polymorphisms at different locations within this region determine which peptides will (or will not) bind.

The polymorphic regions of T-cell receptors and immunoglobulin receptors are also located on the outer domains of the molecules. T-cell antigen receptors are composed of an α-chain and a β-chain, each of which contains an outer variable (V) and an inner constant (C) region (Fig 27-3C). Immunoglobulin receptors consist of a pair of identical heavy (H) and light (L) chains, each of which is subdivided into an outer VH (or VL) domain and an inner C domain, one for the L chain and three for the H chain of IgG (Fig 27-3D). The structures of the V regions of immunoglobulins and T-cell antigen receptors are similar. For example, the V region of an individual immunoglobulin heavy chain is produced by the selection of one of about 80 VH genes, one of about 40 diversity genes, and one of 6 JH genes. Diversity in the V region is generated by the combination of these three units, as well as by the random addition or deletion of nucleotides at the V-D and D-J junctions (N region diversification). In the immunoglobulin receptor, this diversity is later increased by somatic mutations.

It is important to realize that some of the approximately 80 VH genes present in the genome are polymorphic. For example, the 51pl group of VH genes is highly polymorphic. Some variants of 51pl are found in nearly 58% of persons. In contrast, other variants, like the gene hv1263 are found in a much smaller proportion (4%–8%) of persons.[21] Similarly, diversity exists in the germ line components of T-cell antigen receptors.[22]

OTHER CANDIDATE IMMUNE RESPONSE GENES

Interactions between the MHC-peptide complex and T-cell antigen receptors provide the first signal in T-cell activation. Binding between other proteins on the antigen-presenting cell and the T-cell (and later between the T-cell and B-cell), provides the second signal. In addition to adhesion molecules, the CD28 molecules (on T-cells) and B-7 molecules (on B-cells or macrophages) are crucial for costimulation.[23] Another ligand for B7 is CTLA-4, which is expressed on activated T-cells and may play a role in amplifying, or perhaps downregulating, T- or B-cell function. Additional factors involved in the series of events leading to autoantibody production include antigen processing, intracellular binding of peptide to MHC, transport of the peptide-MHC complex to the surface of the antigen-presenting cell, the characteristics of the antigen-presenting cell, as well as the cytokines secreted by antigen-presenting cells and T-cells. Polymorphisms in genes encoding any of these non-antigen-specific regulatory proteins may be important in the genetic basis for thyroid autoimmunity.

APPROACHES TO DETERMINING THE GENETIC BASIS OF AUTOIMMUNE THYROID DISEASE

It should be stated at the outset that the genetic basis for autoimmune thyroid disease has still to be defined. Nevertheless, some progress has been made in determining which genetic factors are likely to play key roles.

Genetic Insight from Animal Models of Thyroiditis

In mice immunized with Tg or TPO, the development of thyroiditis is controlled by genes within the MHC complex.[24,25] More appropriate animal models for human disease are those in which disease develops spontaneously, but there is no spontaneous animal model of Graves' disease. However, thyroiditis in obese-strain (OS) chickens shares many features with chronic autoimmune thyroiditis, including lymphocytic infiltration of the gland, a role for thyroid autoantibodies in thyroid destruction, and hypothyroidism.[26] As described for experimentally induced

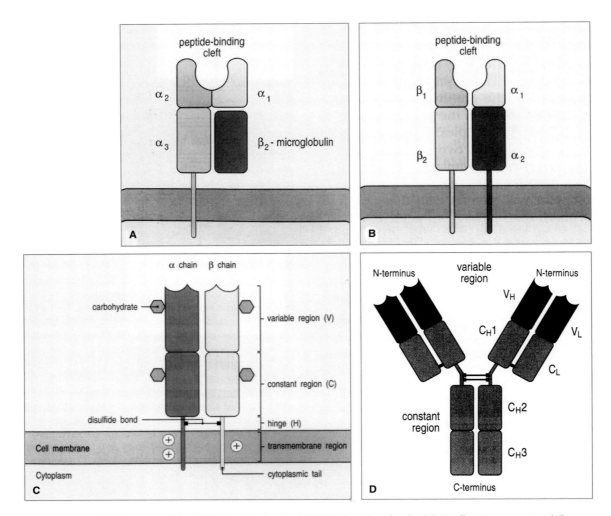

FIGURE 27-3. Structure if the MHC class I molecule (*A*) MHC class II molecule. (*B*) T-cell antigen receptor. (*C*) and an immunoglobulin molecule (*D*). The membrane form of the immunoglobulin molecule is the B-cell receptor. (From Janeway CA Jr, Travers P. Immunobiology: the immune system in health and disease, New York: Garland, 1994;4:4[A], 4:5[B], 4:31[C], 3:2[D]).

thyroiditis in mice, MHC genes play a role in spontaneous thyroiditis in OS chickens. However, development of thyroiditis is critically dependent on two other sets of genes. One genetic component determines abnormal immune responses, including the production of thyroid autoantibodies. The other component determines the susceptibility of the target organ to damage from cellular or humoral effector mechanisms.[27]

From this spontaneous model of thyroiditis, the following conclusions can be drawn. In addition to MHC genes, development of human autoimmune thyroid disease is likely to depend on non-MHC genes controlling the immune response, and genes controlling the susceptibility of the thyroid to the autoimmune thyroid response.

Nomenclature of the MHC Locus

Because of the crucial role of MHC molecules in antigen presentation, many studies directed at dissecting the genetic basis for autoimmune thyroid disease have focused on associations between disease and MHC (termed HLA in humans). To facilitate a review of these observations, the nomenclature of the MHC locus needs to be outlined.[28,29]

The MHC region, on the short arm of chromosome 6, encodes proteins in three different groups (Fig 27-4): (1) the class I region containing the genes that encode HLA antigens A, C, and B; (2) the class III region containing the genes for complement components (e.g., C4A, C4B), heat shock protein 70, the cytokines tumor necrosis factor and lymphotoxin β; and (3) the class II region including the HLA-D genes, of which there are three subgroups, DP, DR, and DQ. Each D subregion contains one α- and one or more β-chain genes. The class II region also includes the transporter (TAP) genes that encode proteins responsible for transporting peptides into class I molecules.

Class II molecules are among the most polymorphic proteins known. Initially, their polymorphism was defined serologically using antibodies and by the mixed lymphocyte reaction (the proliferation of T-cells in response to cells from

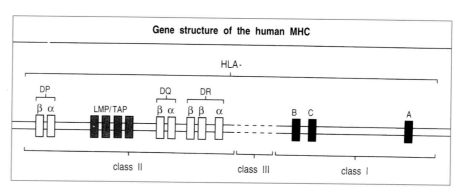

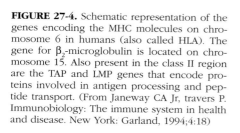

FIGURE 27-4. Schematic representation of the genes encoding the MHC molecules on chromosome 6 in humans (also called HLA). The gene for β$_2$-microglobulin is located on chromosome 15. Also present in the class II region are the TAP and LMP genes that encode proteins involved in antigen processing and peptide transport. (From Janeway CA Jr, travers P. Immunobiology: The immune system in health and disease. New York: Garland, 1994;4:18)

other persons expressing different class II molecules). More recently, class II polymorphisms have been defined by RFLPs. Now that the the alleles have been defined by direct sequencing, class II polymorphisms are determined on PCR-amplified DNA products using allele-specific oligonucleotide probes. Further, it is now clear that the polymorphism is much greater than was detected serologically or by mixed lymphocyte reactions. Consequently, a new nomenclature has been introduced for the HLA system, which provides a way of describing the alleles for individual α- and β- (now renamed A and B) chains.[29]

The relationship between this new nomenclature and the older terminology is illustrated for genes in the DR and DP regions in Figure 27-5.[30] For example, the serologic determinants of HLA-DR and HLA-DQ reflected polymorphisms in the

DRB1 and DQB1 chains. In contrast, the alleles of DRA (which displays little polymorphism) and DQA1 (which is polymorphic) were not detected serologically. The combination of DRA and polymorphisms of DRB3, indicated by DR52, were defined using mixed lymphocyte reactions.

ASSOCIATION STUDIES IN AUTOIMMUNE THYROID DISEASE

HLA Class I and Class II Markers and Disease

The association between Graves' disease and HLA-B8 and HLA-DR3, which has been observed in many studies of

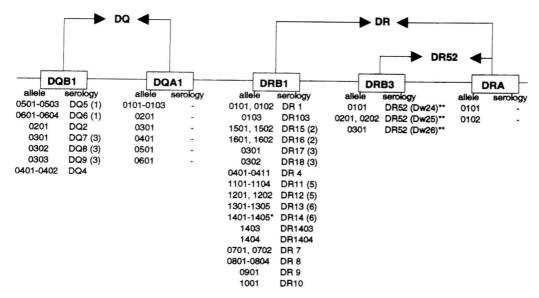

FIGURE 27-5. Alleles of HLA class II DQ and DR polymorphisms defined by serology, mixed lymphocyte reactions (Dw alleles), or by allele identification using oligonucleotide probes of PCR-amplified DNA. Each class II molecule is encoded by an A chain gene and a B chain gene. In the case of DQ, a DQA1 chain pairs with a DQB1 chain. With respect to DR, the DRA chain, which is relatively conserved (only two alleles) combines with one of the DRB1 alleles or one or the DRB3 alleles. The alleles listed under DQA1, DRB1, and DRB3 refer to polymorphisms in the outer domains of the molecules (seen as α$_1$ and β$_1$ in Fig. 27-3). Although called DRB3, the polymorphisms in this molecule are still within the β$_1$ (outer) domain. The DRB1 alleles defined serologically have been renamed. The old nomenclature is shown in parentheses (for example, DR3 is now DR17). (From Yanagawa T, Mangklabruks A, Chang Y-B, et al. Human histocompatibility leukocyte antigen-DQA1* 0501 allele associated with genetic susceptibility to Graves disease in a Caucasian population. J Clin Endocrinol Metab 1993;76:1569)

whites,[31–36] has also been observed in South African blacks (Table 27-2).[37] However, Graves' disease is associated with different class I and II HLA antigens in other ethnic groups, as well as in subdivisions of a major ethnic group (Chinese).[38,39]

The relevance of disease associations with MHC class I, rather than MHC class II (or vice versa), becomes clear when it is appreciated that antigen presentation and T-cell activation by class I or class II molecules is different. Class I molecules are expressed on virtually all nucleated cells and present endogenously processed peptides, such as viral proteins, to T-cells of the CD8 subset. Class II molecules, usually restricted to antigen-presenting cells, present exogenous antigen to T-cells of the CD4 subset. Antibody production by B-cells requires help from CD4 T-cells. In contrast, the CD8 subset includes the precursors of cytotoxic cells. Consequently, cytotoxic immune responses are likely to be associated with polymorphisms of class I molecules. A good example is the association between a class I allele and protection from cytotoxic damage in malaria.[40]

Subacute thyroiditis involves thyroid damage, possibly from the cytotoxic effects of a thyrotropic virus.[9] For this reason, an association between subacute thyroiditis and a class I marker (B35) was expected.[41,42] On the other hand, the major characteristic of autoimmune thyroid disease is thyroid autoantibody production. Thus, associations between Graves' disease and MHC are potentially more meaningful for class II molecules (like HLA-DR3) than for class I molecules (such as HLA-B). In this light, the recent focus on the class II region is understandable.

Although there are still insufficient data for a consensus, present evidence suggests that associations are stronger when subsets of patients are considered. For example, the prevalence of HLA-BW46 is increased in Chinese men (but not women) with Graves' disease, and the relative risk for this allele is higher in men with early-onset disease (10–19 years old) than in the group of men as a whole (relative risk 17.5 vs. 4.2).[39] Similarly, the association between Graves' disease and

TABLE 27-2.
Associations Between Genetic Markers in the MHC Locus and Graves' Disease

Serologic Markers	Class II HLA-DR	Class I HLA-B	References
SUSCEPTIBILITY			
Whites	DR3	B8	31–33, 34–36, 55
Blacks (South Africa)	DR3		37
Japanese	DR5		74
		B46	87
Chinese			
Northern		B5	38
Southern	DR9	B46	39
Koreans	DR5, DR8	B13	88
RESISTANCE			
Whites	DR5		76

Molecular and/or Serologic Markers	Class II				Class I	References
	DPB1	DQB1	DQA1	DR	B	
SUSCEPTIBILITY						
Whites (M + F)		None	0501			30
Whites (M + F)				DRB1*0301[a]		36
Whites (M + F)	0402				B8	36
Whites				DRB3*0101[b]		89
Whites (M)		0301	0501	DR11		43
Whites (F)			0501	DR3		43
Chinese (M)		0303		DR9	B46	90
Japanese (early onset)		0501				87
RESISTANCE						
Whites			0201	DR7		43
Japanese		0501				91
Chinese		0301	0401	DR12		90

Previous nomenclature: (a) DR17 (b) Dw24.

the allele DQA1*0501 is much higher in men than in women (relative risk 9.1 vs. 2.7, respectively).[43]

In chronic autoimmune thyroiditis and postpartum thyroiditis, associations have been observed for both disorders between HLA-DR3, HLA-DR4, or HLA-DR5 in whites (Table 27-3). As in Graves' disease, there is some evidence for preferential associations in subsets of patients. For example, atrophic autoimmune thyroiditis is associated with HLA-DR3[44] whereas goitrous autoimmune thyroiditis is associated with HLA-DR5.[45] Based on HLA analysis using PCR-amplified DNA and oligonucleotide probes, susceptibility or resistance between chronic autoimmune disease appears to be associated with HLA-DQ (but not HLA-DP) antigens.

Associations between autoimmune thyroid disease and polymorphisms of the peptide transporters TAP1 and TAP2 have not yet been studied. However, it is likely that associations of this kind may result from linkage disequilibrium with HLA-DR and HLA-DQ alleles, as was previously reported for insulin-dependent diabetes mellitus.[46]

HLA Class II Markers and Thyroid Autoantibody Production

Instead of focusing on disease as the phenotype, the relationship between thyroid autoantibody production and HLA has been examined. Thus, there is an association between TPO autoantibodies and HLA-DR5 in men,[47] and HLA-DQ alleles influence the ability to produce thyroid autoantibodies in Japanese subjects.[48] Further support for this possibility comes from genetic analyses of patients with and without TSH-R antibodies. Thus, the frequency of HLA-DPw2 is decreased in Japanese patients with Graves' disease who have TSH-R blocking antibodies and, conversely, increased in patients with chronic autoimmune thyroiditis.[49] In Koreans, increased frequencies of HLA-DR8 and HLA-DQB1*0302 are found only in TSH-R blocking antibody-positive patients and in Graves' patients with TSH binding-inhibiting immunoglobulins.[50] Despite these differences in ethnic groups and disease phenotypes, the conclusions from both groups are the

TABLE 27-3.
Associations Between Genetic Markers for MHC and Hashimoto's Thyroiditis or Postpartum Thyroiditis

	Hashimoto's Thyroiditis			Postpartum Thyroiditis		
	Class II HLA-D	Class I HLA-B	References	Class II HLA-D	Class I HLA-B	References
SEROLOGIC MARKERS						
SUSCEPTIBILITY						
Chinese	DR9	B46	92			
	DR9		93			
Japanese	DRw53		48			
Whites	DR4		94	Whites	DR5		95
Whites	DR3		96, 97	Whites	DR3	B8	98
Whites	DR5		95	Whites	DR4		94
Whites	DR3, DR4		99	Whites	DR4		100

	Class II				References
	DPA1/B1	DQB1	DQA1	DR	
MOLECULAR AND/OR SEROLOGIC MARKERS					
SUSCEPTIBILITY					
Whites	None	0201[a]		DR3	101
Whites		0201		DR3	102
Whites			0301	DR3	102
Whites*		0201			103
Whites	None	0301	0301/2		104
Whites	None	0301[b]	0201/0301		52
RESISTANCE					
Japanese		0602	0102		91
Whites		0602			102, 104
Whites		0501–03[c]			95
Whites		0302			103

Graves' disease and chronic autoimmune thyroiditis.
Previous nomenclature: (a) DQw2; (b) DQw7; (c) DQw1.

same: Patients with an autoimmune response to the TSH-R (either stimulating or blocking antibodies) are genetically different in terms of HLA from patients whose thyroid autoimmune response does not involve TSH-R antibodies. This shifts the emphasis from HLA associations with disease to associations with thyroid autoantibodies.

Many studies of the role of MHC in immune responses involve the use of simple antigens such as peptides that are 10 to 20 amino acids in length. In contrast, the TSH-R is a very large glycoprotein (764 amino acids).[16] An antigen of this type is potentially capable of activating a wide range of T-lymphocytes that can, in turn, activate B-lymphocytes to secrete antibodies that recognize multiple epitopes on the same antigen. However, there is evidence that the human autoimmune response to thyroid autoantigens is relatively restricted. In particular, there is partial overlap between the B-cell epitopes recognized by stimulatory and blocking TSH-R antibodies.[16] This suggests that T-lymphocytes may recognize only a limited number of TSH-R peptides. A restricted T-cell response is likely to involve a restricted number of HLA molecules.

Building on these observations, the association of HLA markers with the presence of TSH-R antibodies[49,50] would result from the ability of particular MHC molecules to bind the relevant TSH-R peptides. If correct, this opens the way to a more fundamental understanding of the immune response to thyroid antigens. However, it is disappointing to find that the relative risk between a particular HLA and TSH-R autoantibodies (about 4.4) is not much higher than the relative risk between HLA and disease. The complexity of the interactions leading to an autoantibody response (reviewed earlier) is likely to explain why HLA markers alone are not more closely associated with the autoimmune response to TSH-R.

Class III Polymorphisms

The locus for the cytokine tumor necrosis factor-β (TNF-β) lies in the class II region (see Fig 27-4). Because of its role in inflammation, as well as tentative associations with some autoimmune diseases, polymorphisms of the TNF-β gene[51] may be involved in autoimmune thyroid disease. Indeed, an association was found in whites between TNF-β polymorphisms and Graves' disease[34] but not chronic autoimmune thyroiditis.[52] However, this particular TNF polymorphism is linked to HLA-DR3, which was increased in the Graves' patients. A similar analysis of Chinese patients with Graves' disease, in whom there is no association with HLA-DR3 (Table 27-3), suggests that the TNF-β gene is not a susceptibility gene.[53] Associations between autoimmune thyroid disease and other genes in the MHC class III locus, such as heat shock protein 70,[54] probably also reflect linkage disequilibrium with class III antigens.

Associations with Non-MHC Markers

Potential associations have been sought between autoimmune thyroid disease, MHC markers, and non-MHC markers. Non-MHC markers include polymorphisms of immunoglobulin and T-cell receptor genes, as detected serologically or by RFLP. For example, immunoglobulin polymorphism has been studied with respect to serologic differences in heavy- and light-chain

constant regions (Gm and Km allotypes), as well as by RFLP analysis of the immunoglobulin switch regions. A combination of HLA and immunoglobulin polymorphisms was found to predispose to Graves' ophthalmopathy in one study,[55] but another study found no association between HLA and immunoglobulin gene switch regions.[56] In fact, no consensus has been reached on genetic factors in whites with Graves' opthalmopathy using polymorphisms of HLA, immunoglobulin markers, T-cell receptors, or blood group antigens (Table 27-4). However, in Japanese patients with Graves' disease, combinations of class I and II polymorphisms appeared to correlate with four different subpopulations classified according to the presence of ophthalmopathy, family history, early or late onset of disease, and goiter size.[57]

Turning to T-cell receptor polymorphisms and HLA, association studies have yielded inconsistent results. One investigation found an association between Graves' disease and HLA but not T-cell receptor polymorphisms.[58] In contrast, other studies have observed associations between HLA and T-cell receptor β-chain polymorphisms in different forms of autoimmune thyroid disease: for example, in chronic autoimmune thyroiditis but not in Graves' disease[59]; in Graves' disease[60]; and in both Graves' disease and chronic autoimmune thyroiditis.[61] Intriguingly, T-cell receptor β-chain polymorphisms in combination with HLA-DR were associated with the presence of Tg autoantibodies but not with disease.[62] This observation is reminiscent of the HLA polymorphisms described earlier, which appeared to influence the immune response rather than disease.

A novel approach has explored the possibility of a contribution to thyroid autoimmunity by the CTLA4 molecule, which plays a role in the second signal required for T-cell activation. Using highly polymorphic microsatellite markers, associations were found between one CTLA4 allele and Graves' disease.[63] Further, the frequency of this allele was higher in women with protective HLA specificities (DQA1*0201 positive/DQA1*0501 negative) than in those with susceptible specificities (DQA1*0201 negative/DQA1*0501 positive). These data, like those already mentioned for T-cell receptor polymorphisms, emphasize the potential importance of the interaction between polymorphisms of MHC and non-MHC genes.

FAMILY STUDIES OF AUTOIMMUNE THYROID DISEASE

Inheritance of the Ability to Produce Thyroid Autoantibodies

Turning from genetic associations in a population to genetic studies in families, early studies demonstrated that autoantibodies to thyroid peroxidase or thyroglobulin aggregate in families.[64] This could have arisen because ascertainment of probands from specialized hospital clinics led to over-representation in the sample of families with more than one affected member. However, clustering of thyroid autoantibodies was still found in families in which the proband was the only affected member.[65]

Using classic segregation analysis, autosomal dominant[64,66,67] or multifactorial models[65,68–70] of inheritance were proposed. Based on the dominant model with reduced penetrance in males, linkage was excluded between genes in the

TABLE 27-4.
Associations Between Genetic Markers in Graves' Ophthalmopathy (GO) and Graves' Disease
Without Ophthalmopathy (GD) or Normal Subjects (N)

Ethnic Group	Marker	Comparison	Observations	References
Whites	HLA-A, B, C, DR Gm allotypes	GO vs GD	B8 + DR7 increased B8 + Gm fb B35 + DR4 decreased	55
Whites	HLA, red-cell enzymes, serum proteins	GO vs N	Blood group P increased	33
Whites	Blood group P	GO vs GD	No difference	105
Whites	HLA-DR, DQ T-cell receptor RFLPs, immunoglobulin switch RFLPs	GO vs GD and GO vs N	No difference	56
Whites	Light-chain RFLP	GO vs GD	No difference	106
Whites	HLA-DQ, DP	GO vs GD and GO vs N	DPB 2.1/8 decreased DQw3.1 decreased	107
Japanese	HLA-A, B, C, DR, DQ	GO, FH+ve, LO GO, FH+ve, EO GO, FH-ve, EO GD, goiter	A31+ DQw4+ B5+ Dw12+ A11+ Dw2− DRw8+	57

FH, family history (+ve or −ve); LO, late onset; EO, early onset; RFLP, restriction fragment length polymorphism.
+ and − refer to people with, and without, the MHC marker.

HLA region and the ability to produce thyroid autoantibodies.[66,67] Further analysis of this model, using RFLPs for genes encoding the T-cell receptor and the immunoglobulin H-chain, as well as a number of highly polymorphic mini- and microsatellite markers on a variety of chromosomes, provided no evidence for linkage although a number of loci could be excluded.[71]

The prevalence of thyroid autoantibodies in the general population is high. Using sensitive assays, about 25% of women and about 10% of men have autoantibodies to TPO or Tg.[19] Further, pedigree analysis cannot distinguish between genetic and environmental factors shared in a family. Consequently, classic segregation analyses that suggest autosomal dominant inheritance could also be explained by recessive or multifactorial models. Complex segregation analysis is required for the examination of a wide range of genetic models. For example, the data may be tested against the following hypotheses: no transmission; transmission due to a major genetic locus with polygenic background (the mixed-model); a single locus with no polygenic background; and polygenic inheritance (no single locus).[72] Using this approach to analyze inheritance of the ability to produce autoantibodies to TPO or Tg, vertical transmission was confirmed in families unselected for autoimmune thyroid disease. One study could not distinguish between a single-gene and a multifactorial model.[73] In contrast, the data from large extended kindreds of the Old Order Amish population were consistent with a mixed model, in which the major gene is transmitted in a dominant fashion.[72]

Genetic Markers Associated with Inheritance of Disease

Although a number of investigators have addressed the mode of inheritance or the part played by candidate genes, there has been no consensus. Studies of Japanese families provided evidence for a major contribution by genes encoding HLA and Gm.[74,75] Sib pair analysis of Chinese families supported dominant inheritance in association with HLA.[76] However, in whites, HLA studies of sib pairs provided models compatible with dominant[77] or recessive[76,78] inheritance. Alternatively, no simple pattern could be determined.[79] Using a different approach, and assuming either dominant or recessive inheritance patterns, HLA genes were excluded from linkage with autoimmune thyroid disease.[80,81] It must be emphasized that the data that exclude HLA from linkage do not negate a role for HLA in Graves' disease and chronic autoimmune thyroiditis. Indeed, associations with HLA were confirmed within these families.[80] However, these observations indicate that a stronger genetic susceptibility must lie elsewhere in the genome and not in the HLA region.

TARGET ORGAN DEFECTS IN AUTOIMMUNE THYROID DISEASE

Thyroid functional abnormalities, unrelated to HLA, have been found frequently in relatives of patients with Graves' disease and chronic autoimmune thyroiditis.[82] However, there are no data suggesting that the autoimmune thyroid response arises because of gross defects in TPO or Tg. In this connection, a polymorphism in the portion of the TSH-R gene coding for the extracellular region of the receptor has been described which, in the heterozygous condition, does not influence thyroid function.[83] In contrast, other investigators have suggested that this polymorphism is associated with the autoimmune response.[84,85] It is of interest that another autoantibody-mediated disease, myasthenia gravis, is associated with a polymorphism in the target of the immune response, the acetylcholine receptor α-subunit.[86]

FUTURE GENETIC STUDIES OF AUTOIMMUNE THYROID DISEASE

Strategies for determining the genetic basis of autoimmune thyroid disease are likely to be based on those succesfully used for insulin-dependent diabetes.[14,15] This approach involves the analysis of a panel of highly polymorphic mini- or microsatellite markers[11] on PCR-amplified DNA from sib pairs with rigorously defined phenotypes of autoimmune disease. The initial objective is the identification of chromosomal loci showing linkage with the phenotypic disease marker. Once a chromosomal region has been located, the gene which is responsible has to be identified. In the absence of potential candidate genes, this is likely to be a formidable task. Indeed, it is likely that such investigations will require multicenter collaborations and substantial resources. However, ultimately this approach should provide the answer to the questions of which genetic loci in humans determine the autoimmune response to thyroid antigens, and which determine the development of the spectrum of autoimmune thyroid disease?

References

1. McKusick VA. Mendelian inheritance in man. Baltimore and London: The Johns Hopkins University Press, 1994
2. Duprez L, Parma J, Van Sande J, et al. Germline mutations in the thyrotropin receptor gene cause non-autoimmune autosomal dominant hyperthyroidism. Nature Genet 1994;7:396
3. Parma J, Duprez L, Van Sande J, et al. Somatic mutations in the thyrotropin receptor gene cause hyperfunctioning thyroid adenomas. Nature 1993;365:649
4. Hadjidakis SG, Koutras DA, Daikos GK. Endemic goitre in Greece: family studies. J Med Genet 1994;1:82
5. Malamos B, Koutras DA, Kostamis P, Rigopoulos GA, Zerefos NS, Yataganas XA. Endemic goitre in Greece: a study of 379 twin pairs. J Med Genet 1967;4:16
6. Greig WR, Boyle JA, Duncan A, et al. Genetic and non-genetic factors in simple goitre formation: evidence from a twin study. Q J Med 1994;36:175
7. Malamos B, Miras K, Koutras DA, et al. Endemic goiter in Greece: metabolic studies. J Clin Endocrinol 1966;26:696
8. Tajiri J, Higashi K, Morita M, Umeda T, Sato T. Studies of hypothyroidism in patients with high iodine intake. J Clin Endocrinol Metab 1986;63:412
9. Tomer Y, Davies TF. Infection, thyroid disease, and autoimmunity. Endocr Rev 1993;14:107
10. Lander ES, Schork NJ. Genetic dissection of complex traits. Science 1994;265:2037
11. Murray JC, Buetow KH, Weber JL, et al. A comprehensive human linkage map with centimorgan density. Science 1994;265:2049
12. Todd JA, Aitman TJ, Cornall RJ, et al. Genetic analysis of autoimmune type 1 diabetes mellitus in mice. Nature 1994;351:542
13. Woolf B. On estimating the relation between blood group and disease. Am J Hum Genetics 1955;19:251
14. Davies JL, Kawaguchi Y, Bennett ST, et al. A genome-wide search for human type 1 diabetes susceptibility genes. Nature 1994;371:130
15. Hashimoto L, Habita C, Beressl JP, et al. Genetic mapping of a susceptibility locus for insulin-dependent diabetes mellitus on chromosome 11q. Nature 1994;371:161
16. Nagayama Y, Rapoport B. The thyrotropin receptor twenty five years after its discovery: new insights following its molecular cloning. Mol Endocrinol 1992;6:145
17. Mackenzie WA, Davies TF. An intrathyroidal T-cell clone specifically cytotoxic for human thyroid cells. Immunology 1987; 61:101
18. McLachlan SM, Rapoport B. The molecular biology of thyroid peroxidase: cloning, expression and role as autoantigen in autoimmune thyroid disease. Endocr Rev 1992;13:192
19. Prentice LM, Phillips DIW, Sarsero D, Beever K, McLachlan SM, Rees Smith B. Geographical distribution of subclinical autoimmune thyroid disease in Britain: a study using highly sensitive direct assays for autoantibodies to thyroglobulin and thyroid peroxidase. Acta Endocrinol 1990;123:493
20. Bjorkman PJ, Saper MA, Samraoui B, Bennett WS, Strominger JL, Wiley DC. Structure of the human class I histocompatibility antigen, HLA-A2. Nature 1987;329:506
21. Sasso EH, van Dijk KW, Bull AP, Milner ECB. A fetally expressed immunoglobulin VH1 gene belongs to a complex set of alleles. J Clin Invest 1993;91:2358
22. Cornelis F, Pile K, Loveridge J, et al. Systematic study of human alpha beta T cell receptor V segments shows allelic variations resulting in a large number of distinct T cell receptor haplotypes. Eur J Immunol 1993;23:1277
23. Clark EA, Ledbetter JA. How B and T cells talk to each other. Nature 1994;367:425
24. Kong YM. The mouse model of autoimmune thyroid disease. In: McGregor AM, ed. Immunology and medicine. Lancaster: MTP Press Limited, 1986:1–24
25. Kotani T, Umeki K, Hirai K, Ohtaki S. Experimental murine thyroiditis induced by porcine thyroid peroxidase and its transfer by the antigen-specific T cell line. Clin Exp Immunol 1990; 80:11
26. Wick G, Most J, Schauenstein K, et al. Spontaneous autoimmune thyroiditis—a bird's eye view. Immunol Today 1985;6:359
27. Maczek C, Neu N, Wick G, Hala K. Target organ susceptibility and autoantibody production in an animal model of spontaneous autoimmune thyroiditis. Autoimmunity 1992;12:277
28. Campbell RD, Trowsdale J. Map of the human MHC. Immunol Today 1993;14:349
29. Bodmer JG, Marsh SGE, Albert ED, et al. Nomenclature for factors of the HLA system, 1991. Tissue Antigens 1992;39:161
30. Yanagawa T, Mangklabruks A, Chang YB, et al. Human histocompatibility leukocyte antigen-DQA1*0501 allele associated with genetic susceptibility to Graves' disease in a Caucasian population. J Clin Endocrinol Metab 1993;76:1569
31. Farid NR, Stone E, Johnson G. Graves' disease and HLA: clinical and epidemiologic associations. Clin Endocrinol 1980; 15:535
32. Frecker M, Mercer G, Skanes VM, Farid NR. Major histocompatibility complex (MHC) factors predisposing to and protecting against Graves' eye disease. Autoimmunity 1988;1:307
33. Kendall-Taylor P, Stephenson A, Stratton A, Papiha SS, Perros P, Roberts DF. Differentiation of autoimmune opthalmopathy from Graves' hyperthyroidism by analysis of genetic markers. Clin Endocrinol 1988;28:601
34. Badenhoop K, Schwarz G, Schleusener H, et al. Tumor necrosis factor β gene polymorphisms in Graves' disease. J Clin Endocrinol Metab 1992;74:287
35. Ratanachaiyavong S, Gunn CA, Bidwell EA, Darke C, Hall R, McGregor AM. DQA2 U Allele: a genetic marker for relapse of Graves' disease. Clin Endocrinol 1990;32:241
36. Ratanachaiyavong S, Fleming D, Janer M, et al. HLA-DPB1 polymorphisms in patients with hyperthyroid Graves' disease and early onset myasthenia gravis. Autoimmunity 1994;17:99
37. Omar MⁱK, Hammond MG, Desai RK, Motala AA, Aboo N, Seedat MA. HLA class I and II antigens in South African blacks with Graves' disease. Clin Immunol Immunopathol 1990;54:98
38. Hawkins BR, Ma JTC, Lam KSL, Wang CCL, Yeung RTT. Association of HLA antigens with thyrotoxic Graves' disease and peri-

odic paralysis in Hong Kong Chinese. Clin Endocrinol 1985; 23:245

39. Yeo PPB, Chan SH, Thai AC, et al. HLA Bw46 and DR9 associations in Graves' disease of Chinese patients are age- and sex-related. Tissue Antigens 1989;34:179

40. Hill AVS, Allsopp CEM, Kwiatkowski D, et al. Common West African HLA antigens are associated with protection from severe malaria. Nature 1991;252:595

41. Nyulassy S, Hnilica P, Stefanovic J. The HL-A system and subacute thyroiditis. A preliminary report. Tissue Antigens 1975; 6:105

42. Goto H, Uno H, Tamai H, et al. Genetic analysis of subacute (de Quervain's) thyroiditis. Tissue Antigens 1985;26:110

43. Yanagawa T, Mangklabruks A, DeGroot LJ. Strong association between HLA-DQA1*0501 and Graves' disease in a male Caucasian population. J Clin Endocrinol Metab 1994;79:227

44. Moens H, Barnard JM, Bear J, Farid NR. The association of HLA-B8 with atrophic thyroiditis. Tissue Antigens 1979;13:342

45. Farid NR, Sampson L, Moens H, Barnard LM. The association of goitrous autoimmune thyroiditis with HLA-DR5. Tissue Antigens 1981;17:265

46. Ronningen KS, Undlien DE, Ploski R, et al. Linkage disequilibrium between TAP2 variants and HLA class II alleles; no primary association between TAP2 variants and insulin-dependent diabetes mellitus. Eur J Immunol 1993;23:1050

47. Roman SH, Davies TF, Witt ME, Ginsberg-Fellner F, Rubinstein P. Thyroid autoantibodies in HLA-genotyped type 1 diabetic families: Sex-limited DR5 association with thyroid microsomal antibody. Clin Endocrinol 1986;25:23

48. Honda K, Tamai H, Morita T, Kuma K, Nishimura Y, Sasazuki T. Hashimoto's thyroiditis and HLA in Japanese. J Clin Endocrinol Metab 1989;69:1268

49. Inoue D, Sato K, Sugawa H, et al. Apparent genetic difference between hypothyroid patients with blocking-type thyrotropin receptor antibody and those without, as shown by restriction fragment length polymorphism analyses of HLA-DP loci. J Clin Endocrinol Metab 1993;77:606

50. Cho BY, Chung JH, Shong YK, et al. A strong association between thyrotropin receptor-blocking antibody-positive atrophic autoimmune thyroiditis and HLA-DR8 and HLA-DQB1*0302 in Koreans. J Clin Endocrinol Metab 1993;77:611

51. Jongeneel CV, Briant L, Udalova IA, Sevin A, Nedospasov SA, Cambon-Thomsen A. Extensive genetic polymorphism in the human tumor necrosis factor region and relation to extended HLA haplotypes. Proc Natl Acad Sci USA 1991;88:9717

52. Badenhoop K, Schwarz G, Walfish PG, Drummond V, Usadel KH, Bottazzo GF. Susceptibility to thyroid autoimmune disease: molecular analysis of HLA-D region genes identifies new markers for goitrous Hashimoto's thyroiditis. J Clin Endocrinol Metab 1990;71:1131

53. Cavan DA, Penny MA, Jacobs KH, et al. Analysis of a Chinese population suggests that the TNFB gene is not a susceptibility gene for Graves' disease. Hum Immunol 1994;40:135

54. Ratanachaiyavong S, Demaine AG, Campbell RD, McGregor AM. Heat shock protein 70 (HSP70) and complement C4 genotypes in patients with hyperthyroid Graves' disease. Clin Exp Immunol 1991;84:48

55. Frecker M, Stenszky V, Balazs C, Kozma L, Kraszits E, Farid NR. Genetic factors in Graves' ophthalmopathy. Clin Endocrinol 1986;25:479

56. Weetman AP, So AK, Warner CA, Foroni L, Fells P, Shine B. Immunogenetics of Graves' ophthalmopathy. Clin Endocrinol 1988;28:619

57. Inoue D, Sato K, Enomoto T, et al. Correlation of HLA types and clinical findings in Japanese patients with hyperthyroid Graves' disease: Evidence indicating the existence of four subpopulations. Clin Endocrinol 1992;36:75

58. Mangklabruks A, Cox N, DeGroot LJ. Genetic factors in autoimmune thyroid disease analyzed by restriction fragment length polymorphisms of candidate genes. J Clin Endocrinol Metab 1991; 73:236

59. Weetman AP, So AK, Roe C, Walport MJ, Foroni L. T-cell receptor alpha chain V region polymorphism linked to primary autoimmune hypothyroidism but not Graves' disease. Hum Immunol 1987;20:167

60. Demaine A, Welsh KI, Hawe BS, Farid NR. Polymorphism of the T cell receptor β-chain in Graves' disease. J Clin Endocrinol Metab 1987;65:643

61. Ito M, Tanimoto M, Kamura H, et al. Association of HLA antigen and restriction fragment length polymorphism of T cell receptor β-chain gene with Graves' disease and Hashimoto's thyroiditis. J Clin Endocrinol Metab 1989;69:100

62. Demaine AG, Ratanachaiyavong S, Pope R, Ewins D, Millward BA, McGregor AM. Thyroglobulin antibodies in Graves' disease are associated with T-cell receptor beta chain and major histocompatibility complex loci. Clin Exp Immunol 1989;77:21

63. Yanagawa T, Hidaka Y, Guimaraes V, Soliman M, DeGroot LJ. CTLA-4 gene polymorphism associated with Graves' disease in a Caucasian population. J Clin Endocrinol Metab 1995;80:41

64. Hall R, Owen SG, Smart GA. Evidence for genetic predisposition to formation of thyroid autoantibodies. Lancet 1960;2:187

65. Roitt IM, Doniach D. A reassessment of studies on the aggregation of thyroid autoimmunity in families of thyroiditis patients. Clin Exp Immunol 1967;2:727

66. Phillips D, McLachlan S, Stephenson A, et al. Autosomal dominant transmission of autoantibodies to thyroglobulin and thyroid peroxidase. J Clin Endocrinol Metab 1990;70:742

67. Phillips D, Prentice L, Upadhyaya M, et al. Autosomal dominant inheritance of autoantibodies to thyroid peroxidase and thyroglobulin—Studies in families not selected for autoimmune thyroid disease. J Clin Endocrinol Metab 1991;72:973

68. Evans AWH, Woodrow JC, McDougall CDM, Chew AR, Evans RW. Antibodies in the families of thyrotoxic patients. Lancet 1967;1:636

69. Hall R, Dingle PR, Roberts DF. Thyroid antibodies: a study of first degree relatives. Clin Genet 1972;3:319

70. Burek CL, Hoffman WH, Rose NR. The presence of thyroid autoantibodies in children and adolescents with autoimmune thyroid disease and in their siblings and parents. Clin Immunol Immunopathol 1982;25:395

71. Prentice L, Phillips DIW, Premawardhana LDKE, Rees Smith B. Genetic linkage analysis of thyroid autoantibodies. Autoimmunity 1993;15:225

72. Pauls DL, Zakarija M, McKenzie JM, Egeland JA. Complex segregation analysis of antibodies to thyroid peroxidase in old order Amish families. Am J Med Genet 1993;47:375

73. Phillips DIW, Shields DC, Dugoujon JH, Prentice L, McGuffin P, Rees Smith B. Complex segregation analysis of thyroid autoantibodies: are they inherited as an autosomal dominant trait? Hum Hered 1993;43:141

74. Uno H, Sasasuk T, Tamai H, Matsumoto H. Two major genes, linked to HLA and Gm, control susceptibility to Graves' disease. Nature 1981;292:768

75. Tamai H, Uno H, Hirota Y, et al. Immunogenetics of Hashimoto's and Graves' diseases. J Clin Endocrinol Metab 1985;60:62

76. Payami H, Joe S, Farid NR, et al. Relative predispositional effects (RPEs) of marker alleles with disease: HLA-DR alleles and Graves' disease. Am J Hum Genet 1989;45:541

77. Torfs CP, King M-C, Huey B, Malmgren J, Grumet FC. Genetic interrelationship between insulin-dependent diabetes mellitus, the autoimmune thyroid diseases, and rheumatoid arthritis. Am J Hum Genet 1986;38:170

78. Stenszky V, Kozna L, Balazs C, Rochlitz S, Bear JC, Farid NR. The genetics of Graves' disease: HLA and disease susceptibility. J Clin Endocrinol Metab 1985;61:735

79. Ratanachaiyavong S, Lloyd L, Darke C, McGregor AM. MHC-extended haplotypes in families of patients with Graves' disease. Hum Immunol 1993;36:99

80. Roman SH, Greenberg D, Rubinstein P, Wallenstein S, Davies TF. Genetics of autoimmune thyroid disease: Lack of evidence for linkage to HLA within families. J Clin Endocrinol Metab 1992;74:496

81. O'Connor G, Neufeld DS, Greenberg DA, Concepcion ES, Roman SH, Davies TF. Lack of disease associated HLA-DQ restriction fragment length polymorphisms in families with autoimmune thyroid disease. Autoimmunity 1993;14:237

82. Chopra IJ, Solomon DH, Chopra U, Yoshihara E, Terasaki PI, Smith F. Abnormalities in thyroid function in relatives of patients with Graves' disease and Hashimoto's thyroiditis: lack of correlation with inheritance of HLA-B8. J Clin Endocrinol Metab 1977;45:45

83. Sunthornthepvarakul T, Hayashi Y, Refetoff S. Polymorphism of a variant human thyrotropin receptor (hTSHR) gene. Thyroid 1994;4:147

84. Bohr URM, Behr M, Loos U. A heritable point mutation in an extracellular domain of the TSH receptor involved in the interaction with Graves' immunoglobulins. Biochim Biophys Acta 1993; 1216:504

85. Bahn RS, Dutton CM, Heufelder AE, Sarkar G. A genomic point mutation in the extracellular domain of the thyrotropin receptor in patients with Graves' ophthalmopathy. J Clin Endocrinol Metab 1994;78:256

86. Garchon H-J, Djabiri F, Viard J-P, Gajdos P, Bach J-F. Involvement of human muscle acetylcholine receptor alpha-subunit gene (CHRNA) in susceptibility to myasthenia gravis. Proc Natl Acad Sci U S A 1994;91:4668

87. Onuma H, Ota M, Sugenoya A, Inoko H. Association of HLA-DPB1*0501 with early-onset Graves' disease in Japanese. Hum Immunol 1994;39:195

88. Cho BY, Rhee BD, Lee DS, et al. HLA and Graves' disease in Koreans. Tissue Antigens 1987;31:119

89. Semana G, Allanic H, Quillivic F, et al. Implication of the HLA-DRB3 gene in Graves' disease: predominance of allele Dw24. Hum Immunol 1990;29:143

90. Cavan DA, Penny MA, Jacobs KH, et al. The HLA association with Graves' disease is sex-specific in Hong Kong Chinese subjects. Clin Endocrinol 1994;40:63

91. Tamai H, Kimura A, Dong R-P, et al. Resistance to autoimmune thyroid disease is associated with HLA-DQ. J Clin Endocrinol Metab 1994;78:94

92. Hawkins BR, Lam KSL, Ma JTC, Wang C, Yeung RTT. Strong association between HLA DRw9 and Hashimoto's thyroiditis in Southern Chinese. Acta Endocrinol 1987 114:543

93. Wang FW, Yu ZQ, Xy JJ, Wang XL, Zhang DQ, Chen JL. HLA and hypertrophic Hashimoto's thyroiditis in Shanghai Chinese. Tissue Antigens 1988;32:235

94. Thompson C, Farid NR. Post-partum thyroiditis and goitrous (Hashimoto's) thyroiditis are associated with HLA-DR4. Immunol Lett 1985;11:301

95. Vargas MT, Briones-Urbina R, Gladman D, Papsin FR, Walfish PG. Antithyroid microsomal autoantibodies and HLA-DR5 are associated with postpartum thyroid dysfunction: evidence supporting an autoimmune pathogenesis. J Clin Endocrinol Metab 1988;67:327

96. Thomsen M, Ryder LP, Bech K, et al. HLA-D in Hashimoto's thyroiditis. Tissue Antigens 1983;21:173

97. Stenszky V, Balazs C, Kraszits E, et al. Association of goitrous autoimmune thyroiditis with HLA-DR3 in Eastern Hungary. J Immunogenet 1987;14:143

98. Kologlu M, Fung H, Darke C, Richards CJ, Hall R, McGregor AH. Postpartum thyroid dysfunction and HLA status. Eur J Clin Invest 1990;20:56

99. Jenkins D, Penny MA, Fletcher JA, et al. HLA class II gene polymorphism contributes little to Hashimoto's thyroiditis. Clin Endocrinol 1992;37:141

100. Jansson R, Safwenberg J, Dahlberg PA. Influence of HLA-DR4 antigen and iodine status on the development of autoimmune post-partum thyroiditis. J Clin Endocrinol Metab 1985;60:168

101. Tandon N, Zhang L, Weetman AP. HLA associations with Hashimoto's thyroiditis. Clin Endocrinol 1991;34:383

102. Shi Y, Zou M, Robb D, Farid NR. Typing for major histocompatibility complex class II antigens in thyroid tissue blocks: association of Hashimoto's thyroiditis with HLA-DQA0301 and DQB0201 alleles. J Clin Endocrinol Metab 1992;75:943

103. Santamaria P, Barbosa JJ, Lindstrom AL, Lemke TA, Goetz FC, Rich SS. HLA-DQB1-associated susceptibility that distinguishes Hashimoto's thyroiditis from Graves' disease in type I diabetic patients. J Clin Endocrinol Metab 1994;78:878

104. Wu Z, Stephens HAF, Sachs JA, et al. Molecular analysis of HLA-DQ and -DP genes in Caucasoid patients with Hashimoto's thyroiditis. Tissue Antigens 1994;43:116

105. Westman AP, Poole J. Failure to find an association of blood group P1 with thyroid-associated ophthalmopathy. Clin Endocrinol 1992;37:423

106. Williams RC Jr, Marshall NJ, Kilpatrick K, et al. Kappa/lambda immunoglobulin distribution in Graves' thyroid-stimulating antibodies. J Clin Invest 1988;82:1306

107. Weetman AP, Zhang L, Webb S, Shine B. Analysis of HLA-DQB and HLA-DPB alleles in Graves' disease by oligonucleotide probing of enzymatically amplified DNA. Clin Endocrinol 1990; 33:65

108. Janeway Jr CA, Travers P. Immunobiology: the immune system in health and disease. New York: Garland, 1994

Werner and Ingbar's The Thyroid, Seventh Edition,
edited by Lewis E. Braverman and Robert D. Utiger.
Lippincott–Raven Publishers, Philadelphia, © 1996

28

Pathology

Virginia A. LiVolsi

PHYSIOLOGY OF THE THYROID GLAND

Normal Thyroid

The normal thyroid gland is a bilobed structure, connected by an isthmus. The thyroid capsule is thin, does not strip easily, and contains sizable venous channels that become strikingly prominent when vascularity is increased. The normal gland is soft and yellowish red; the colloid gives the cut surfaces a glistening, translucent appearance. Normal thyroid glands in the United States weigh from 10 to 20 g.

The functional unit of the thyroid is the follicle, which averages about 20 μm in diameter.[1] A thyroid lobule consists of 20 to 40 follicles bound together by a thin sheath of connective tissue and supplied with blood by a lobular artery.[2] The thyroid follicles are formed by a single layer of low-cuboidal epithelium. The nucleus of the follicular cell is round to ovoid, sometimes irregular in shape, centrally placed, and uniform in size. The nucleolus is inconspicuous. A basal lamina envelops the entire follicle. Numerous capillaries and lymphatics surround the follicle. Considerable interstitial connective tissue and fat cells may be present.[3] The follicular lumen is occupied by colloid, partly composed of thyroglobulin, which is evenly applied to the luminal cell borders. Calcium oxalate crystals are common in the colloid of adults.[4,5] Electron microscopy demonstrates that the normal flat to low-cuboidal follicular cells interdigitate and overlap one another, and that they are intimately related to the capillaries that surround the follicle; microvilli on the apical surface are numerous near the cellular margins.[6–8]

C-cells are intrafollicular and lie next to the follicular cells and within the basal lamina that surrounds each follicle of the normal gland. C-cells are most numerous in the central portions of the middle and upper thirds of the thyroid lobes.[9–12] They are believed to originate from the last branchial pouches (ultimobranchial bodies). C-cells are typically more numerous in infant thyroids than in adult glands.[9,13]

Sizable C-cell aggregates have been observed in some adults without any known endocrinologic abnormality.[10,11,14] The C-cells are polygonal to spindle-shaped, have "light" (low-density) cytoplasm, and contain numerous membrane-limited cytoplasmic granules, which contain calcitonin. A small number of C-cells (or cells similar to them) contain somatostatin and have been said to increase in number in some patients.[15,16] Guyetant and coworkers[17] define C-cell hyperplasia as consisting of more than 40 C-cells/cm² and the presence of at least three low-power microscopic fields containing more than 50 C-cells.

The tiny solid cell nests of ovoid to spindle-shaped epidermoid cells are also considered to be of ultimobranchial origin.[18–21] Typically, the nests have about the same distribution in the thyroid lobes as the C-cells. Tiny cysts that contain fluid and a few mucous cells may lie within or accompany the solid cell nests. So-called mixed follicles[19] are lined by follicular cells and epidermoid cells (and sometimes C-cells) and contain both colloid and mucoid material. The ultimobranchial structures probably also contribute a small proportion of normal thyroid follicles.[21–25]

Oxyphil cells (oncocytes, Askanazy cells, Hürthle cells) are altered follicular cells; they are enlarged, have granular eosinophilic cytoplasm, and have large, hyperchromatic, or bizarre nuclei.[26,27] The cytoplasm is filled with swollen mitochondria. They are commonly found in long-standing Graves' disease, autoimmune thyroiditis, thyroids damaged by radiation, neoplasms, and some adenomatous nodules.[28]

Small clusters of lymphoid cells in the thyroid stroma are so common that they are essentially a normal finding.[29] Also present in the interstitial tissue are antigen-presenting dendritic cells; these are sparse in the normal gland but increased in autoimmune thyroid disease.[30]

Developmental Variations

The thyroglossal tract extends in the midline from the foramen cecum at the base of the tongue to the isthmus of the normal gland (see also chap 2).[31] The tract consists of connective tissue, the thyroglossal duct, lymphoid tissue, and thyroid follicles; it is attached to and may extend through the center of the hyoid bone and is intimately related to the surrounding skeletal muscle. Thyroid tissue may persist at the base of the tongue and in some patients may represent the only thyroid present.[32] The thyroglossal duct typically is a tube lined by ciliated pseudostratified epithelium. If the duct is traumatized or infected, the epithelium may be transitional or squamous, or it may be partially or completely lost and replaced by fibrous tissue. Foreign-body reaction and chronic inflammation may be conspicuous. If fluid accumulates in part of the thyroglossal duct, a thyroglossal cyst may develop.[31,33] Any type of diffuse thyroid disease can involve lingual thyroid[34] and thyroid tissue along the tract.

Occasionally, segments of thyroglossal duct are included within the thyroid gland proper and, rarely, may serve as the origin of an intrathyroidal cyst.[35] Parathyroid glands, thymic tissue, tiny masses of cartilage, and tiny glands lined by ciliated cells may be seen in normal thyroid glands and are presumably related to anomalies in the development of the branchial pouches.[36–38]

Because of the intimate relationship that exists in the embryo between the immature thyroid tissue and the adjacent developing skeletal muscle, strips of striated muscle are occasionally included within the thyroid.[2,39,40] Conversely, thyroid tissue may be found in perithyroidal skeletal muscle. Such nodules of thyroid tissue are particularly prominent when the gland is hyperplastic, and they should not be confused with carcinoma.

Groups of thyroid follicles in lymph nodes nearly always represent metastatic carcinoma (papillary carcinoma). According to some experienced pathologists, normal thyroid follicles rarely occur in cervical lymph nodes.[41–43] Hence, normal thyroid tissue lying only within the capsule of a node, especially if the node is located in the midline, may represent an embryologic remnant and not metastatic cancer.

GOITER

Goiter is a diffuse or nodular enlargement of the gland usually resulting from a benign process or a process of unknown origin (see also chap 78).

When there is a deficiency of circulating thyroid hormone because of inborn errors of metabolism, iodine deficiency, or goitrogenic agents, and if the hypothalamic-pituitary axis is intact, production of thyroid-stimulating hormone (TSH; thyrotropin) is increased; consequently, cellular activity and increased glandular activity and glandular mass result in an attempt to attain the euthyroid state.

Worldwide, the most common cause for a deficient output of thyroid hormone is an inadequate amount of iodine in the diet, leading to iodine-deficiency goiter.[44] Other causes of such hyperplasia include inborn errors of thyroidal metabolism (dyshormonogenetic goiter),[45,46] dietary goitrogens, and goitrogenic drugs and chemicals.

The pathologic changes of simple nontoxic goiter include one or more of the following: hyperplasia, colloid accumulation, and nodularity.[44,47,48] Hyperplasia represents the response of the thyroid to TSH, other growth factors, or to circulating stimulatory antibodies.[49] The hyperplasia may compensate for thyroid hormonal deficiency, but in some patients, even severe hyperplasia does not produce sufficient hormonal output to avoid development of hypothyroidism.

If the deficiency of thyroid hormone occurs at birth or early in life, cretinism or juvenile myxedema may result, even though the gland is enlarged and hyperplastic; this is especially likely when an inborn error of thyroidal metabolism is present. A hyperplastic gland is hyperemic, diffusely enlarged, and not nodular. The epithelium is tall and columnar; the follicles are collapsed and contain only scanty colloid. When the hyperplastic stage is extreme and prolonged, there may be confusion with carcinoma because of the degree of cellularity and the presence of enlarged cells. The nuclei are enlarged, hyperchromatic, and even bizarre. Because of follicular collapse and epithelial hyperplasia and hypertrophy, papillary changes can be seen.[50] This pattern occurs most often in untreated dyshormonogenetic goiter.[45,46] Recognition of the benign nature of the process is possible because all the glandular tissue is abnormal, unlike carcinoma, in which the neoplastic masses constitute one or more localized groups of abnormal cells with a background of non-neoplastic parenchyma.

Thyroid follicles may not remain in a state of continuous hyperplasia but instead undergo a process called *involution,* in which the hyperplastic follicles reaccumulate colloid. The epithelium becomes low-cuboidal or flattened and resembles that of the normal gland. Some follicles become much larger than normal, contain excessive colloid, and are lined with flat epithelium (overinvolution; exhaustion atrophy). The gland is diffusely enlarged, soft, and has a glistening cut surface because of the excess of stored colloid. In addition to large follicles filled with colloid, there are foci in the gland where hyperplasia is still evident. This phase of nontoxic goiter is often termed *colloid goiter.*

Patients with long-standing thyroid disorders associated with deficiency of circulating thyroid hormone typically develop nodular goiters that result from overdistention of some involuted follicles, and persistence of regions of epithelial hyperplasia. The new follicles form nodules and may be heterogeneous in their appearance, in their capacity for growth and function, and in their responsiveness to TSH. The vascular network is altered through the elongation and distortion of vessels, which leads to hemorrhage, necrosis, inflammation, and fibrosis. These localized degenerative and reparative changes produce some nodules that are poorly circumscribed and others that are well demarcated and resemble true adenomas (adenomatous goiter).[47,50,51] Because the nodules distort vascular supply to some areas of the gland, some zones will contain larger than normal amounts of TSH and/or iodide and others will have relative TSH and/or iodide deficiency. Growth of goiters, therefore, may be related to focally excessive stimulation by TSH, stimulation by growth factors, focally abnormal iodide concentration, growth-promoting thyroid antibodies, and poorly understood intrathyroidal factors.

Nodular goiter is essentially a process involving the entire gland, but the nodularity may be asymmetric, and individual nodules within the same gland may vary greatly in size. If one nodule is much larger or more prominent than the others, distinguishing it from a true neoplasm may not be possible. Several studies have shown that about 70% of dominant nodules in nodular goiter are indeed clonal proliferations.[52-55] The formation of cysts, hemorrhage, fibrosis, and calcification further complicates the assessment of the gland.

The heterogeneity of the generations of replicating follicular cells in response to outside stimuli, functional capacity, and rate of growth causes groups of cells to appear that are hyperfunctional or autonomous, or both. These form "hot" nodules that may cause hyperthyroidism (Plummer's disease).[56] However, studies with radioactive iodine administered before operation have not always demonstrated correlations between the morphology of a nodule and its iodine metabolism.[57]

GRAVES' HYPERPLASIA

In this disorder, also termed diffuse toxic goiter, the thyroid is diffusely enlarged up to several times normal size. The capsule is smooth and the gland is hyperemic. The cut surfaces are fleshy and lack normal translucence because of loss of colloid. If the patient is untreated, treated briefly, or receives only propranolol, the microscopic appearance shows cellular hypertrophy and hyperplasia (Fig 28-1).[6,9] There is almost no colloid. The cells are tall columnar cells and are thrown into

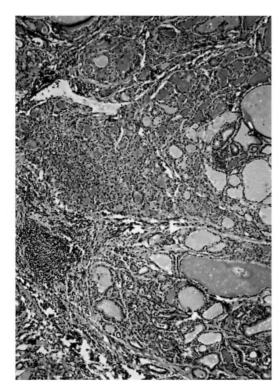

FIGURE 28-1. Diffuse hyperplasia of Graves' disease. Some colloid has accumulated (*right side*) because of the preoperative antithyroid drug therapy.

papillary folds that extend into the lumina of the follicles. Blood vessels are congested. At the ultrastructural level, microvilli are increased in number and elongated, the Golgi apparatus and endoplasmic reticulum are large, and mitochondria are numerous.[6] Infiltrates of lymphocytes that lie between the follicles range from minimal to extensive. T-cells predominate among the epithelial cells (cytotoxic-suppressor cells) and in the interstitial tissue (helper-inducer cells), where there are no lymphoid follicles.[58-60] B-cells are numerous in the lymphoid follicles. Class II major histocompatibility complex antigens are expressed on the epithelial cells, and these epithelial cells induce the proliferation of T-cells, helping to perpetuate the process.[58,61] Lymphoid hyperplasia may occur elsewhere in the body: in the thymus, lymph nodes, or spleen.

Because nearly all patients now receive antithyroid medication and then iodide before surgery, the glands have undergone varying degrees of involution.[63] Some appear almost normal except for numerous large follicles filled with colloid; a few papillae may remain. The hyperemia is notably decreased, especially if there has been preoperative administration of iodide.[63] If hyperplasia continues for many months or several years, oxyphilic metaplasia of the cells begins to occur, the amount of stroma increases in an irregular fashion, and nodularity develops, just as in diffuse euthyroid goiter. If the process subsides spontaneously or because of maintenance on antithyroid medication, the involution may be remarkably complete, it may be irregular (with some foci of hyperplasia evident), or the gland may be altered by chronic lymphocytic thyroiditis.[64]

DYSHORMONOGENETIC GOITER

When an inborn error of thyroid metabolism exists, and sufficient amount of circulating thyroid hormone is not available, the normal physiologic response of the pituitary to increase TSH causes a larger, more active thyroid, which may or may not be able to produce enough hormone to reach a normal equilibrium. If TSH stimulation is marked and prolonged, the thyroid becomes large and nodular; microscopically, enlargement of follicular cells, virtual absence of colloid, and increased stroma are seen.[45,46]

Large follicular cells with bizarre, hyperchromatic nuclei may be numerous. The enlarged gland, the bizarre cells, and the cellular nodules have at times been mistaken for carcinoma. Cancer can occur in a dyshormonogenetic goiter, but it is very rare.[65] (See also chap 56.)

IATROGENIC AND RELATED HYPERPLASIAS

Chronic ingestion of excess iodide, for whatever reason, occasionally leads to diffuse hyperplasia. Papillary formations and small nodules may be numerous. Infiltration of lymphocytes may occur.

About 3% of patients given lithium salts for a prolonged period develop goiter or hypothyroidism, or both. Patients so treated have been reported to have diffuse hyperplasia with considerable cellular and nuclear pleomorphism.[66]

Bromide ingestion may lead to hypothyroidism because of loss of iodide from the gland. There are hyperplastic cells, foci of papillary proliferation, and loss of colloid.[67]

AUTOIMMUNE THYROIDITIS

Common synonyms for autoimmune thyroiditis include Hashimoto's thyroiditis, lymphocytic thyroiditis, and struma lymphomatosa.

The disorder, most common in women, encompasses a spectrum of clinical and pathologic changes,[44] ranging from an absence of symptoms of thyroid dysfunction to hypothyroidism and rarely, hyperthyroidism, from a large goiter to an atrophic gland, and from scattered clusters of infiltrating lymphocytes to extensive chronic inflammation and scarring with almost complete loss of follicular epithelium.

Various circulating antithyroid antibodies and other immune phenomena occur, including in situ immune complex deposition and basement membrane changes in the gland and expression of major histocompatibility complex antigens on the thyroid cells.[58,59,68] The thyroiditis may be found in the same families in which idiopathic hypothyroidism and Graves' disease are common. It may follow typical Graves' disease.[64]

The hyperthyroid variant of autoimmune thyroiditis is closely related to Graves' disease and may be almost identical in its gross and microscopic appearance to the latter condition,[69] suggesting that this variant may indeed be Graves' disease. The presence of thyroid-stimulating TSH receptor antibodies in such patients would confirm the diagnosis of Graves' disease.

If the thyroiditis is slight and focal, then the thyroid is normal in size and contains scattered infiltrates of lymphocytes, predominantly T-cells. Some of the infiltrates contain lymphoid follicular centers, mostly B-cells. The thyroid follicles involved by the infiltrates appear atrophic; they have lost part or all of their colloid.

A small number of plasma cells (mostly IgG-positive) are mixed with lymphocytes.[68] Glands involved by this focal thyroiditis typically are asymptomatic; therefore, the thyroiditis is discovered when thyroid tissue is surgically removed for other reasons, or the process is found at autopsy. Focal lymphocytic thyroiditis probably represents the mild or early form of autoimmune thyroiditis.[29] When focal lymphocytic thyroiditis is more than minimal and the foci of involvement are larger and more numerous, occasional follicular cells undergo metaplasia toward oxyphilic cells. Part of a lobe sometimes may be extensively involved by lymphocytic thyroiditis, with minor changes occurring elsewhere in the gland; hence, nodularity may result (nodular Hashimoto's thyroiditis).

In more advanced cases of autoimmune thyroiditis, little or no normal parenchyma is visible. The gland on gross examination is enlarged, and its cut surfaces are fleshy and pale.

Microscopic examination shows that many follicles are small, the amount of colloid is decreased, and infiltrates of lymphocytes, plasma cells, and macrophages are extensive (Fig 28-2).[70,71] Lymphoid follicular centers are numerous, and their antibody-producing B-cells are polyclonal; those containing immunoglobulin G are the most numerous.[59–61,68,72] T-

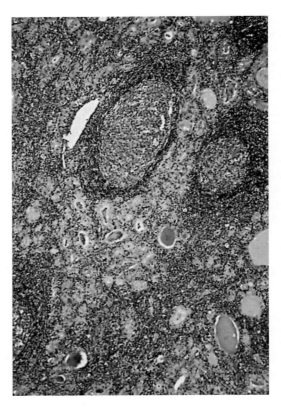

FIGURE 28-2. Autoimmune thyroiditis. Lymphoid follicles are conspicuous. Only a few colloid-filled thyroid follicles remain; most of these follicles are small and formed by hyperplastic and metaplastic cells.

cells are most frequent among the epithelial cells and in the interstitial tissue away from lymphoid follicles. Inflammatory giant cells may be scattered through the damaged follicles; their presence should not lead the pathologist to mistake autoimmune thyroiditis for de Quervain's thyroiditis.[71] The amount of connective tissue in the gland often increases. Some follicular cells appear atrophic or damaged; many are hyperplastic or metaplastic (oncocytic or Hürthle cells; squamous metaplasia).[73,74] The solid cell nests have been suggested as the origin of the latter.[21,74] Possibly related rare cystic lesions have also been noted.[38,40,75,76]

Most cases of adult hypothyroidism (idiopathic myxedema) not related to pituitary failure, radiation, or surgical removal probably represent a form of autoimmune thyroiditis. These glands are fibrotic and usually small, with a few nests of abnormal epithelial cells; scattered small groups of lymphocytes and plasma cells are present.

SILENT THYROIDITIS

Some patients with autoimmune thyroiditis have one or more episodes of painless enlargement of the gland accompanied by transient thyrotoxicosis and reduced radioiodine uptake followed by transient and less commonly permanent hypothyroidism.[77–79] The episodes often occur postpartum.[79] Biopsies have demonstrated that the thyroid may have diffuse or focal lymphocytic thyroiditis. The entities of "silent thyroiditis" or postpartum thyroiditis have been shown to fall into the spectrum of autoimmune thyroid disease.[77,79]

SPECIFIC INFECTIOUS THYROIDITIS

Acute suppurative thyroiditis results from infection by pyogenic organisms. Tuberculosis, syphilis, parasitic infestation, and fungal infections may occur.[80,81] In children, suppurative thyroiditis may occur by direct extension of infection from the pyriform sinus.[82] *Pneumocystis carinii* thyroiditis and cytomegalovirus infection have been identified in patients with acquired immunodeficiency syndrome.[83,84] Thyroidal infection usually is associated with the presence of the organism elsewhere in the body and takes place in a patient who lacks a normal immune system (e.g., transplant recipients, patients with acquired immune deficiency syndrome) or who is debilitated by a chronic disease.

GRANULOMATOUS THYROIDITIS

Synonyms for granulomatous thyroiditis are subacute thyroiditis, and de Quervain's thyroiditis. This disorder, probably of viral origin, is characteristically self-limiting, lasting 1 to 3 months. Grossly, the gland is slightly enlarged. The pathologic changes may be bilateral or asymmetric or focal. The involved regions are firm, poorly defined, and resemble carcinoma grossly.[85] Microscopic changes in the regions involved consist of follicles disrupted, with fragmentation of the colloid and many macrophages present (Fig 28-3).[85]

Microabscesses form as some follicles are filled with polymorphonuclear leukocytes. Both follicular cells and colloid are destroyed focally. Giant cells of the foreign-body type arise from the fusion of macrophages, and they lie adjacent to or surround the disrupted colloid. Fibrous tissue proliferates around the damaged follicles, and lymphocytes infiltrate the connective tissue. Because the damaged foci contain necrotic cells, macrophages, and giant cells, and because they are surrounded by proliferating connective tissue that contains lymphocytes, there is a distinct resemblance to pathologic processes characterized by the formation of granulomas.

The thyroid tissue between the damaged regions appears normal. Healing occurs by fibrosis and by proliferation of remaining follicular cells; new follicles appear.

PALPATION THYROIDITIS

In many thyroid specimens, particularly surgically resected ones, an occasional follicle is disorganized, which entails breakdown of colloid, macrophages, and foreign-body giant cell reaction. This incidental microscopic finding is believed to be the result of clinical palpation of the gland and, hence, is a post-traumatic thyroiditis.[86]

AMIODARONE INJURY WITH THYROTOXICOSIS

Administration of amiodarone may cause thyrotoxicosis, primarily because of the large quantity of iodine in the drug. Tissue changes are usually focal. Groups of follicles contain degenerated follicular cells (with granular or vacuolated cytoplasm); some follicles have lost follicular cells; and there is partial or complete loss of colloid. Zones of fibrosis are evident. The intervening thyroid tissue is normal.[87,88]

FIBROSCLEROSIS

Fibrosclerosis (invasive fibrous thyroiditis and Riedel's struma)[89,90] is a very rare condition that represents one manifestation of a systemic collagenosis. It may include sclerosing mediastinitis, retroperitoneal fibrosis, pseudotumor of the orbit, and sclerosis of the biliary tract.[90] The involvement of the thyroid seems to be incidental. Typically, a lobe of the thyroid and the adjacent skeletal muscle, nerves, blood vessels, and trachea are extensively replaced by dense, inflamed fibrous tissue. The mass formed is firm to hard, pale gray, and easily mistaken for cancer on clinical examination or by the surgeon at operation. Inflammatory cells, especially lymphocytes and plasma cells, are present in the dense connective tissue; angiitis usually involving veins may be conspicuous. There is no atypia of the fibroblasts or of the inflammatory cells; no oxyphilic metaplasia is found.

Carcinomas with extensive fibrosis and sclerosing lymphomas should be considered in the differential diagnosis; absence of cytologic atypia is helpful in this distinction.

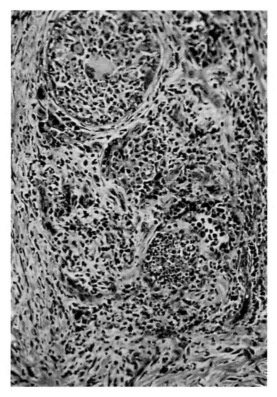

FIGURE 28-3. de Quervain's thyroiditis. The five follicles shown are distended by inflammatory cells.

There does not appear to be any relation to other types of thyroiditis. Riedel's struma may be unilateral, with the portion of the gland not involved by the process remaining normal. In some cases, remnants of a nodule or adenoma are found.

MISCELLANEOUS DISORDERS

Effects of Radiation

Ionizing radiation delivered in small doses to the thyroid glands of infants, children, and adolescents causes a marked increase in the later incidence of benign and malignant neoplasms.[91–95] The neoplasms begin to appear about 5 to 10 years later, but many occur decades after the radiation. Larger doses produce more numerous nodules; many of these nodules are particularly cellular, and some are atypical in their structure and cytologic features, suggesting premalignant characteristics.[91] The cancers that develop after small doses of radiation are mostly papillary carcinomas, are often multicentric or bilateral, and are frequently small.[94] In addition to the nodules and neoplasms that occur, other changes are believed to be more common, including focal epithelial hyperplasia (possibly incipient nodules), chronic lymphocytic thyroiditis, oxyphilic metaplasia of follicular cells, and slight fibrosis.[95]

Large doses of ionizing radiation (e.g., therapeutic radiation for head and neck cancer; or radioiodine therapy) initially cause injury to vessels, irregular necrosis and sloughing of the follicular epithelium, and breakdown of some follicles. Hemorrhages, edema, and small numbers of the usual inflammatory cells appear. As the damage heals, sclerosis and dilatation of vessels occur, the fibrous stroma of the gland increases, and a mixture of atrophic, hyperplastic, and metaplastic changes take place in the follicular epithelium.[96,97] Some follicles are lined by oxyphilic cells that have bizarre nuclei. (See also chaps 16 and 80.)

Amyloidosis

The thyroid may be involved by primary or secondary amyloidosis.[98,99] The amyloid deposition may be sufficiently uneven to produce an amyloid tumor or mass. Such an accumulation must be differentiated from that occurring in some instances of medullary carcinoma.

Black Thyroid

Prolonged therapy with tetracycline antibiotics, especially minocycline, may cause the accumulation of sufficient pigment in the follicular cells to produce a dark brown to black gland.[100,101] Much of the pigment is lipofuscin, but part may be a metabolite of the drug. Rarely, there may be interference with thyroid function.[100]

NEOPLASMS

Thyroid neoplasms demonstrate a variety of morphologic patterns which complicate their pathologic interpretation. All neoplasms that arise from thyroid epithelial cells may have some functional capacities. They may respond to TSH and may even produce ex-

cessive amounts of thyroid hormones[56,102–104] or, if medullary carcinoma, may release abnormal quantities of calcitonin or other hormones. Immunohistochemical evaluation has been of diagnostic value. Localization of thyroglobulin or calcitonin aids in the classification of unusual thyroidal tumors and in providing definite identification of metastatic thyroid carcinomas.[105]

In general, evaluation of nuclear ploidy[27,106–109] has been of little use in assessing malignancy in thyroid tumors. Some apparently diploid tumors are malignant; some aneuploid tumors are benign.[107,109–112] Measurements of steroid receptors,[113] oncogenes,[114] proliferation indices,[115,116] particular antigens,[117] and studies of the nucleolar organizing regions[118] have provided some limited diagnostic or prognostic data (see chap 80).

Changes that occur with moderate frequency in thyroid epithelial tumors are the appearance of clear cells[119] and oxyphilic cells (oncocytes, Hürthle cells, Askanazy cells).[120,121]

Benign Neoplasms: Adenomas and Adenomatous Nodules

Nearly all adenomas have follicular patterns. Those follicular adenomas with papillary hyperplasia (some of which are functional) should not be classified as papillary adenomas,[56] but as papillary hyperplastic nodules. An adenoma is defined as a solitary, encapsulated lesion having a uniform internal architecture that is substantially different from the surrounding thyroidal parenchyma and is compressing the adjacent gland.[46,122]

On gross examination, adenomas and nodules are well circumscribed and are often sharply demarcated from the adjacent tissue. They vary in size from about 1 mm in diameter to several centimeters (Fig 28-4). The typical nodule contains so much colloid that it appears translucent, whereas the classic adenoma is cellular, fleshy, and pale. Hemorrhage, fibrosis, and cystic change may be evident in both nodules and adenomas.

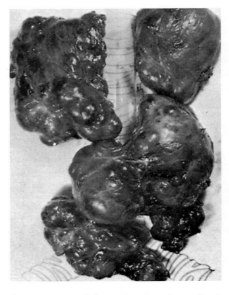

FIGURE 28-4. Nontoxic nodular goiter, largely mediastinal. The trachea and main-stem bronchi are represented diagrammatically.

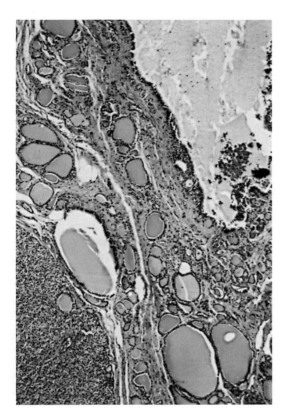

FIGURE 28-5. Adenomatous nodules. The left inferior one is solid; the superior one has undergone cystic degeneration.

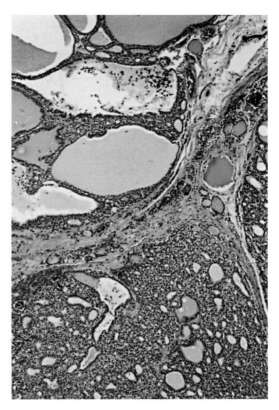

FIGURE 28-6. Adenomatous nodules. The superior one contains large colloid-filled follicles.

Microscopically, a typical adenomatous nodule has a varied pattern consisting of large and small follicles, usually with a large amount of colloid present (Figs 28-5 and 28-6). Giant follicles (colloid cysts), often irregular in shape, are common. The cells range from flat to cuboidal or columnar, and their nuclei are small, round, uniform, and compact. The stroma often appears loose and edematous. Chronic inflammation, groups of macrophages, hemosiderin, fibrosis, and even calcification can be found.

The characteristic adenoma is encapsulated, cellular in comparison with the usual nodule, and relatively uniform in pattern (Figs 28-7 and 28-8). It may present as a solid mass of cells with only a hint of follicular pattern, but more often adenomas are composed of relatively uniform follicles (Fig 28-9). Adenomas sometimes have unusual patterns and cellular features (Fig 28-10). Some, described as atypical adenomas, are hypercellular and may contain mitotic figures,[44,122–125] therefore resembling well-encapsulated follicular carcinoma. Such a tumor requires careful study to avoid missing a carcinoma. Another group of atypical adenomas is also cellular but contains spindle cells or polygonal cells with large and bizarre nuclei.[125]

The hyalinizing trabecular adenoma is a small, well-circumscribed tumor characterized by a trabecular and nesting pattern with the nested, usually elongated, cells surrounding hyaline connective tissue.[126–128] Nuclei may contain cytoplasmic inclusions.[126–128] Small psammoma bodies may occur. Gradations between typical follicular adenomas, trabecular adenomas, and the hyalinizing trabecular adenomas are seen.[126–129] The differential diagnosis for these neoplasms is encapsulated medullary carcinoma; the adenomas contain thyroglobulin and no calcitonin.

A rare variant of follicular adenoma is composed of vacuolated, signet-ring-type cells (sometimes called *mucinous*), in which droplets of thyroglobulin and mucin-like material (possibly a carbohydrate or breakdown product of colloid) are

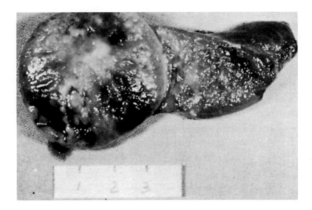

FIGURE 28-7. Follicular adenoma and normal thyroid tissue (gross). A capsule is visible, and the tumor contains central fibrosis and foci of hemorrhage.

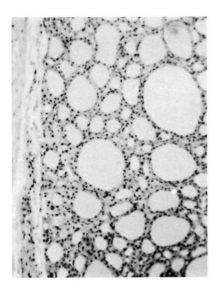

FIGURE 28-8. Follicular adenoma. The capsule is at left.

present.[130] An even more uncommon adenoma is the lipid-rich cell adenomas.[131]

Cystic change is common, especially in adenomatous nodules, and almost all the typical architecture may disappear except for tiny remnants of the periphery. Cystic changes in nodules are frequently accompanied by the formation of papillae (Fig 28-11).

Critical examination of adenomatous nodules shows that many of these lesions are not solitary, that encapsulation and compression are inconstant phenomena, and that their internal architecture is quite variable. Studies of clonality[52–55] suggest that they are true neoplasms. Most adenomas or nodules take up little or no radioiodine and are thus "cold" on scan.

A few of these benign lesions are hyperfunctional, or "hot"; usually this occurs with nodules of nodular goiter rather than with a classic adenoma.[56] In adolescents and young women, many of the hot, or toxic, nodules contain numerous papillae, often sufficient in number to cause a pathologist to suggest a diagnosis of papillary carcinoma.

Teratomas of the thyroid and of the tissues adjacent to the thyroid occur predominantly in infants and are usually diagnosed at the time of birth.[132] They may become large, sufficiently so to cause dystocia by hyperextension of the neck. They are often associated with polyhydramnios. These tumors are almost always benign. Teratomas of the thyroid and the perithyroidal region are rare in adults and may be malignant.[133] Microscopically, the teratoma is composed of multiple elements, often with a preponderance of neural components.

MALIGNANT NEOPLASMS

The most common malignant neoplasms that originate in the thyroid are the well-differentiated carcinomas of follicular epithelial origin; most are papillary carcinomas. They constitute about 80% of the thyroid neoplasms.

In arriving at a prognosis for thyroid cancer, one must consider the patient's age and sex, the size of the primary tumor, the presence or absence of direct extension into the juxtathyroidal

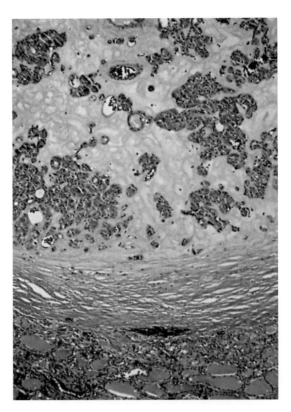

FIGURE 28-9. Follicular adenoma with a thick capsule. Extensive fibrous stroma is evident. Normal thyroid is at bottom.

tissues, and the presence or absence of metastatic foci. In some neoplasms, features such as DNA content and the presence of certain cells and antigens must be considered.[27,107,134–137]

Most non-neoplastic diseases of the thyroid do not seem to be precursors of malignant diseases, with the exception of autoimmune thyroiditis, which may predispose to malignant

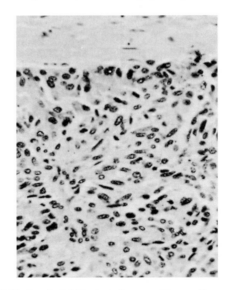

FIGURE 28-10. Atypical follicular adenoma. Many cells are elongated; some have large and irregular nuclei; and there is only a suggestion of follicle formation.

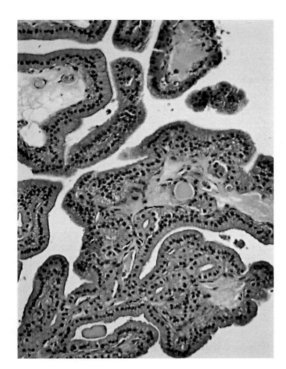

FIGURE 28-11. Adenoma or adenomatous nodule with papillae. The patient was 10 years old, and the nodule was hyperfunctional. The nuclei appear compact and regular.

lymphoma. An occasional adenoma or adenomatous nodule appears to contain a focus of papillary carcinoma when removed at operation, but this is a rare occurrence.

Anaplastic carcinomas often have arisen in goitrous thyroids, and careful examination of the resected tissues has frequently demonstrated benign tumors or well-differentiated carcinomas in close association with the anaplastic neoplasm. Such findings have led to suggestions that the benign tumor or low-grade carcinoma has become "transformed" into the anaplastic carcinoma.[125,138,139]

The characteristics of well-differentiated carcinoma can be appreciated only by careful microscopic examination of multiple, well-prepared sections. Frozen sections at times may be misleading,[140] and the surgeon must accept this limitation.

Papillary Carcinoma

About 80% of thyroid carcinomas are papillary carcinomas. More common in women than in men and rarely familial,[141] papillary carcinoma occurs most frequently in those parts of the world where ample iodine is present in the diet and the environment.[142,143] The association of radiation, especially low-dose external radiation in childhood with the development of adult papillary thyroid cancer is well documented.[144,145] Recent studies from the areas of the former Soviet Union near the Chernobyl nuclear plant indicate an "epidemic" of thyroid carcinoma in children and teenagers following the nuclear accident and release of radioactive iodine. Virtually all of these tumors are papillary carcinomas.[146]

Grossly, papillary cancers are predominantly solid, although small cystic foci may be present. A distinctly cystic

character is evident in some cases, with one or more cystic spaces occupying most of the neoplasm.[125,147] Bits of calcified material and crystals may be present in the cyst fluid. Papillae may protrude into the cysts and at times are so numerous that portions of the cut surfaces appear granular.

Papillary carcinomas usually are infiltrative, and their margins often are poorly defined; however, about 10% to 20% of papillary cancers appear grossly encapsulated.

Fibrosis is common in and around papillary carcinomas[147–149] and it may be distributed in an extremely irregular fashion, grossly and microscopically.[147–151] Occasionally, fibrosis is so extensive that almost no neoplastic cells can be found. Rarely, the stroma of the carcinomas is myxoid or similar to that of nodular fasciitis.[152,153] Nonlamellated calcification is also common; small papillary carcinomas ("occult" carcinomas), are defined as 1 cm in diameter or less and may be called minimal, tiny, or minute carcinomas.[125,154–158] The prevalence of these lesions ranges from 6% to 36%.[125] When visible on gross examination, they present as small, irregular, firm scars, as soft foci of discoloration, or as tiny calcific lesions. Occasionally, such a tumor presents as a metastatic focus, usually as an enlarged cervical lymph node, and rarely in a distant site.[159–163] Microscopically, they contain neoplastic follicles or papillae, with the smallest ones showing a predominance of follicular pattern.[159,162] They may be encapsulated or infiltrative.

Microscopic examination shows that most clinically evident papillary cancers contain papillae (Fig 28-12); however, papillae may constitute only a tiny part of the neoplasm. Papillary cancer may be solid, may be composed of follicles (Fig 28-13), or may be almost entirely papillary.[125,148–151,164] Trabecular,[150,164] cribriform,[150] and diffuse[125,151,166–171] patterns also occur (Fig 28-14).

The most diagnostic single feature in papillary carcinoma is the epithelial cell, which is usually cuboidal to low columnar, and contains a distinctive nucleus (see Fig 28-13).[125,147–151,172–174]

The nucleus is relatively large and irregular in shape, with folds, indentations, and cytoplasmic inclusions.[147–151,172–174] The nucleolus is often inconspicuous because it lies near the nuclear membrane. The nuclear heterochromatin tends to be concentrated near the nuclear membrane, causing the central portion of the nucleus to appear relatively pale, empty, or like ground glass. When the cells form papillae or follicles, often most of the cytoplasm is concentrated in the apical or basal portions of the cells, thereby causing neighboring nuclei to appear to touch or overlap one another.

The papillae are distinctive, typically gnarled, with well-developed fibrovascular cores, and covered with a single layer of the characteristic cells.[172] When papillae are crowded close together, the cancer may appear almost solid. Many papillary carcinomas have a substantial number of follicles (indeed, they may predominate).[125,147–151] An occasional papillary carcinoma, however, is composed almost entirely of distended, colloid-filled follicles of moderately uniform size and shape, thereby closely resembling a common pattern of an adenomatoid nodule.[151] Rare papillae, an occasional focus of infiltration at the periphery, and the characteristic nuclei confirm the diagnosis.

Papillary carcinoma may be largely or exclusively solid. In young people, it is not known if this pattern may affect the

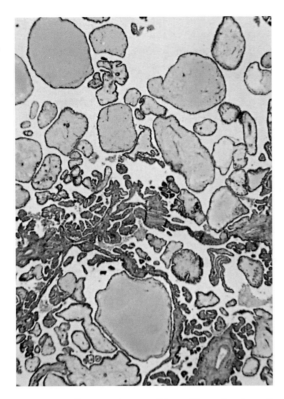

FIGURE 28-12. Papillary carcinoma with papillae of various sizes.

Rarely, a papillary carcinoma is composed of oxyphilic cells (oncocytes, Askanazy cells, Hürthle cells)[26,125,151,177] and arises in a thyroid altered by lymphocytic thyroiditis. These lesions may show central cystic change.[177] This variant appears to have the same spectrum of behavior as the common variety.

Encapsulation of the primary carcinoma is associated with a lower frequency of lymph node involvement.[125,147–151,178,179]

About one third to one half of papillary carcinomas form laminated calcific spherules, known as psammoma bodies (Fig 28-15).[125,147–151,164,180] They measure 5 to 100 μm in diameter and probably begin in damaged or dying cells of papillary carcinomas. Anytime a psammoma body is found in normal thyroid tissue, cervical lymph nodes, or juxtathyroidal soft tissue, a search of the resected tissues should be instituted for papillary thyroid carcinoma. Structures resembling psammoma bodies are occasionally found inside the follicles of adenomas or adenomatous nodules, especially those composed of oxyphilic cells, where they seem to arise from calcification of inspissated colloid.

Lymphocytic infiltration is often present within and around papillary carcinomas[148,149] (Fig 28-16).

Lymphatic invasion accounts for the frequency of multiple intrathyroidal foci of the tumor and commonly found metastasis to cervical lymph nodes (Fig 28-17). Occasionally, cervical nodal enlargement representing metastatic papillary carcinoma is the presenting complaint. If a nodal metastasis is cystic, it must be differentiated from a branchial cleft cyst.[125] If the node is enlarged by well-differentiated neoplastic follicles,

prognosis,[125,146,148] but in the middle-aged and elderly, it may be associated with a loss of differentiation that suggests an aggressive neoplasm. Follicles or papillae may be rare or nonexistent in the primary focus, although they are more likely to be present in the metastatic foci in the lymph nodes.

The characteristic nuclei, the frequent presence of psammoma bodies, the tendency for focal metaplasia suggestive of squamous metaplasia, and the infiltration by lymphocytes in and around the neoplasm help distinguish this variant from medullary carcinoma, solid follicular carcinoma, and insular carcinoma.[125] Immunoreactive thyroglobulin can be demonstrated focally in these variants; no calcitonin is present.

Rarely, papillary thyroid carcinoma appears as a diffuse involvement of all the lymphatic channels of one lobe or of the entire thyroid,[125,148,166–171] accompanied by severe lymphocytic thyroiditis or interstitial fibrosis. Psammoma bodies are numerous. A primary mass lesion (epicenter) may not be found in the gland. This variant occurs more often in young people, is usually accompanied by lymph node metastases, and often has pulmonary metastases.

The tall cell variant is an unusual type of papillary carcinoma that appears to be more aggressive than the usual variety.[125,147,150,175,176] Some of these tumors are composed of cells with oncocytic cytoplasm, but the cells are narrow and elongated (at least twice as long as they are wide). These tumors often show extrathyroidal soft tissue extension and vascular invasion (20%–25%). Most occur in older persons, on average 20 years older than persons with usual papillary cancer. A mortality rate of 25% is reported.[176]

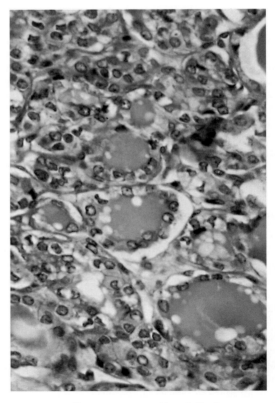

FIGURE 28-13. Papillary carcinoma with a follicular pattern. Nuclei vary in size and shape, and some have clear centers.

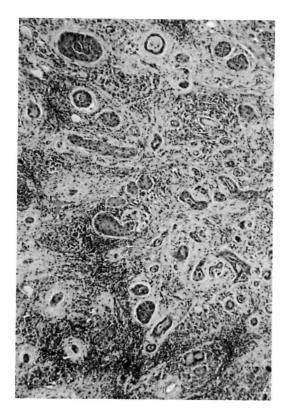

FIGURE 28-14. Papillary carcinoma with extensive fibrosis, chronic inflammation, and squamous metaplasia.

it must not be mistaken for a sequestered thyroid nodule.[40,181] The nuclear features of papillary carcinoma may not be present in these differentiated follicular-patterned metastases. Blood vessel invasion by papillary carcinoma is uncommon,[125,147–151] and metastatic foci in distant sites are unusual, with the lungs most frequently involved.[125,147–151,182,183]

The presence of easily found mitotic figures, enlarged or hyperchromatic nuclei, abnormal DNA content, deviation from the usual recognized histologic patterns, and regions of nondescript neoplastic cells not clearly recognizable as typical of papillary carcinoma (loss of differentiation) constitute characteristics believed to indicate that more aggressive behavior is likely.[137,150,183] These features occur most often in the cancers diagnosed in older people and in extensive cancers, that is, those tumors that are already extrathyroidal.

Follicular Carcinoma

Follicular carcinoma accounts for about 5% or less of all thyroid carcinomas in the United States. It is more common in women than in men and may occur at any age but is more frequent with increasing age (especially after 30 years). The incidence is higher in regions of the world where iodine deficiency occurs.[142,143]

Follicular carcinoma is an expansile neoplasm that nearly always is more or less encapsulated and has many similarities to follicular adenoma.[125,184–190] Grossly, it usually presents as a fleshy, solid, encapsulated mass, sometimes focally fibrotic and calcified. The capsule is usually well developed, but if the tumor is aggressive, extensions beyond the capsule may be readily apparent. Sometimes invasion of sinusoids or veins can be appreciated at the periphery of the neoplasm.[125,184]

On microscopic examination, follicular carcinomas most often have a microfollicular pattern and resemble a cellular follicular adenoma. Trabecular or solid patterns are fairly common. Medium-sized to large follicles filled with colloid typically are a minor component or are absent; only rarely do they comprise most of the cancer[184] (Fig 28-18). Thyroglobulin immunostaining may be used to detect colloid droplets, thereby demonstrating that some of the apparently solid neoplasms do contain microfollicles[191] and confirming the follicular derivation of the tumor.

The cells of follicular carcinoma are slightly to moderately larger than those present in most adenomas and adenomatous nodules, but otherwise they are similar. Mitotic figures range from rare to easily identified.

Follicular carcinomas are divided into (1) localized, minimally invasive cancers and (2) more widely invasive cancers.[125,184–190] Because follicular carcinomas are nearly always encapsulated, the distinction between adenoma and minimally invasive carcinoma may be difficult to make. Carcinoma is recognized by its extension into vessels at its periphery, by its penetration into and through the capsule that surrounds it, and (occasionally) by the presence of distant metastasis.[184,189] Even a minimally invasive carcinoma can present as a metastatic lesion.[185,189] Multiple sections of the periphery of the neoplasm

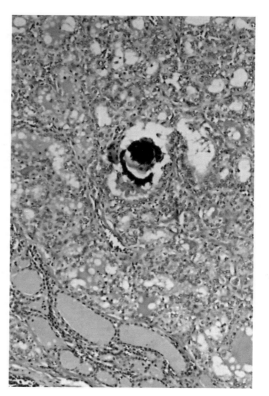

FIGURE 28-15. Papillary carcinoma containing a psammoma body. Normal thyroid is at lower left.

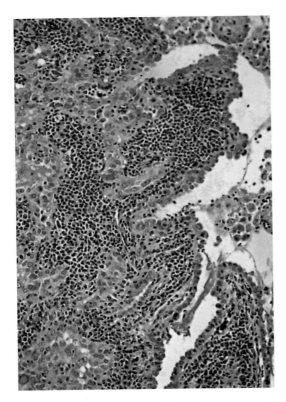

FIGURE 28-16. Papillary carcinoma with extensive infiltration by lymphocytes and plasma cells.

than Hürthle cell (or oncocytic) neoplasms. Clinicians and pathologists alike have disagreed, since such tumors do not "follow the rules" for histopathologic diagnosis of malignancy.[26,27,195–199]

Over the past decade, studies from numerous institutions throughout the world have shown that oncocytic or Hürthle cell tumors can be divided into benign and malignant categories by careful adherence to strict pathologic criteria. More importantly, these pathologic distinctions predict clinical behavior.[26,27,120,121,195,198,199]

Most oncocytic neoplasms behave as follicular carcinomas; that is, pathologically the capsule or vessels should be assessed for invasion.[26,27,199] However, some papillary carcinomas show oncocytic cytology; these behave as usual papillary cancers and often arise in glands with chronic thyroiditis.[177]

Hürthle cell carcinomas should be separated into a category of thyroid neoplasms different from true follicular cancers. First, Hürthle cell cancers can metastasize to regional lymph nodes as well as spread hematogenously[30]; in addition, histologic evidence of invasive characteristics is found more commonly in oncocytic cancers.[192]

Since approximately one third of oncocytic thyroid tumors show invasion (i.e., are cancers) as compared with 2% to 5% of non-oncocytic follicular tumors, the finding of Hürthle cell cytology in a fine-needle aspiration sample of a thyroid nodule should lead to surgical resection of the lesion to assess malignancy.[26,199]

may be necessary to find the evidence of invasion, although most follicular cancers will be diagnosed on examination of 10 different sections of the capsule-tumor interface.[184,185,189]

A follicular carcinoma that invades only two or three small vessels may be called *encapsulated.* A lesion which penetrates or invades its capsule to a limited extent but does not show vascular invasion is termed *minimally invasive* (Figs 28-19 and 28-20). The term invasive adenoma should be avoided; these are cancers.

The minimally invasive neoplasms rarely recur or spread to distant sites, so the outlook for most patients is good. However, since the literature contains numerous studies in which distributions between the follicular variant of papillary carcinoma and true follicular carcinoma were not made,[192,193] accurate data on long-term prognosis for *minimally invasive* follicular carcinoma are not available. Follicular carcinoma has little tendency to invade lymphatic vessels and to spread to lymph nodes.[184–190,192,194] Metastatic spread to the skeleton, lungs, brain, liver, and other tissues through the bloodstream may occur.

The follicular carcinomas that are not localized or minimally invasive have been grouped as *widely invasive*; these include examples in which multiple fingers of neoplastic cells extend into the surrounding thyroid or in which there is extensive replacement of the thyroid gland and soft tissue of the neck.

Oncocytic (Hürthle Cell) Tumors

Perhaps no thyroid neoplasm has elicited more confusion or debate

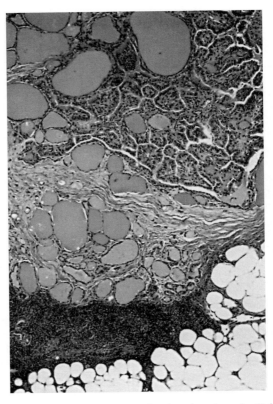

FIGURE 28-17. Papillary carcinoma lies in a lymph node. Half of it has a follicular pattern; half is composed of papillae.

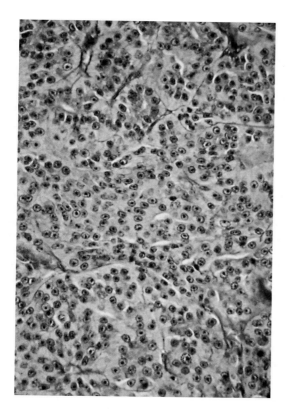

FIGURE 28-18. Follicular carcinoma with a mostly solid pattern. A few closed follicles are evident. Nucleoli are conspicuous.

Clear Cell Tumors

Clear cell change can be identified focally in many follicular-derived lesions in the thyroid—in thyroiditis, nodules, and neoplasms.[119] Most clear cell metaplasia is associated with oncocytic or Hürthle cell change. Hence, distinction of proliferative from neoplastic nodules relies on adherence to accepted criteria for usual follicular lesions. Of greatest import is the differentiation of clear cell change in follicular thyroid lesions from clear cell renal cell carcinomas metastatic to the thyroid.[119,125] Immunostains for thyroglobulin may be helpful in sorting out this diagnostic problem.

Poorly Differentiated Carcinoma

Reviews of large numbers of thyroid carcinomas[200-202] have often included examples of carcinomas that are recognizable as originating from follicular epithelium (often with evidence of coexistent papillary or follicular carcinoma), but with some notable differences: moderate to high rates of mitotic activity, composed of solid masses or trabeculae of relatively uniform epithelial cells, tiny follicles present in varying numbers, regions of acute necrosis, and more aggressive than the usual well-differentiated carcinomas. Included among these lesions are insular carcinoma; columnar cell, tall cell, and trabecular types of papillary cancer[147,176,203-207]; and "poorly differentiated" carcinoma of Sakamoto.[202] These tumors generally lack the usual histologic features and exceptional aggressiveness of anaplastic carcinomas, but they are neither typical follicular nor papillary carcinomas.

The role of oncogenes in thyroid carcinogenesis is not discussed in detail in this chapter. However, several investigators have reported results of immunostaining for p 53, bcl-2, Ras oncogenes, and nM23 gene.[125,208-215] Well-differentiated thyroid cancers are rarely positive with immunostaining for p 53, whereas many anaplastic carcinomas show positivity (40%–60%).[212,213] Correspondingly, bcl-2 (related to the mechanism of apoptosis) oncogene is often expressed in well-differentiated cancers and rarely in undifferentiated lesions. Tumors in the poorly differentiated group (tall cell or columnar cell papillary cancer, and insular carcinoma) show intermediate patterns of expression of p 532 (about 25% of cases) and of bcl-2.[212,213] Immunoreactions for oncogene nM23 have not proved useful in evaluating thyroid tumors.[125]

Evaluation for proliferative indices in thyroid neoplasms (immunostaining for PCNA or Ki67 antigen) have shown, as expected, low proliferation rates for well-differentiated tumors and high rates in poorly differentiated or undifferentiated lesions. The value of these tests is not evident in the clinical evaluation of affected patients.[115,116]

Anaplastic Carcinoma

Fewer than 10% of thyroid carcinomas may be classified as anaplastic or undifferentiated. They are most common in regions of the world where iodine is deficient.[142,143] Traditionally,

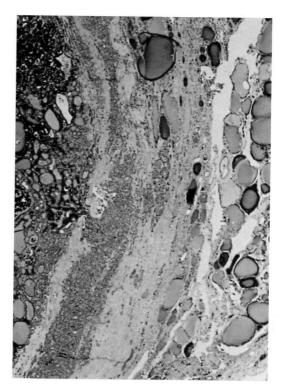

FIGURE 28-19. Follicular carcinoma that is small, hemorrhagic, and associated with skeletal metastases. Irregular infiltrates of neoplastic cells are visible in its capsule.

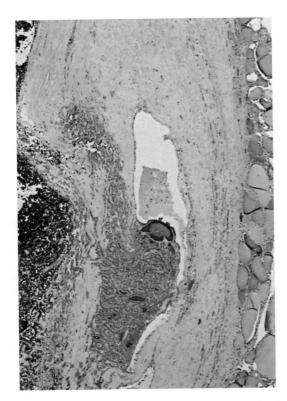

FIGURE 28-20. Follicular carcinoma (same as in Fig. 28-19). The cells protrude into a vessel in its capsule.

these tumors include the rare small-cell carcinomas and the more common spindle- cell and giant-cell types. However, most lesions originally classified as small-cell anaplastic carcinomas represent either medullary carcinoma, insular carcinoma, or small-cell malignant lymphoma.[216] An oat cell thyroid carcinoma, apparently separate from small-cell variant medullary carcinoma, has been described and could be another small-cell thyroid cancer.[217] The possibility of a metastatic carcinoma from another organ always has to be considered.

The following discussion will focus on spindle-cell and giant-cell tumors. Both are aggressive neoplasms that usually occur in elderly people, more often women. The patient may relate a history of a thyroid nodule that, after many years of stability, suddenly begins to grow rapidly. Some patients are known to have had low-grade thyroid carcinoma; some have low-grade thyroid carcinoma discovered at the time of diagnosis of the anaplastic tumor; and some have no history of thyroid disease.

Careful pathologic examination of thyroids that contain anaplastic carcinomas has demonstrated a high (50%–70%) incidence of remnants of well-differentiated follicular or papillary carcinoma[138,139,200,218,219] or sometimes an adenoma or adenomatoid nodules,[219] confirming the clinical impression that anaplastic carcinomas arise out of tumors of low-grade neoplasm.

Gross examination demonstrates a hard, pale, infiltrative mass that may contain soft foci of necrosis and hemorrhage. These tumors invade the cervical soft tissues and involve the regional lymph nodes, often by direct extension. Microscopic examination reveals varied histologic patterns, many mitotic figures, and regions of acute necrosis.

Anaplastic carcinomas are usually pleomorphic (Fig 28-21) and are composed of medium-sized to large cells with a vaguely epithelial appearance.[138,139,218,219] There may be squamous cell differentiation[138,139] (or a tendency toward this pattern). Others appear sarcomatous (Fig 28-22), especially resembling malignant fibrous histiocytoma, fibrosarcoma, and angiosarcoma.[138,139,218,219] Spindle cells may dominate. The giant-cell carcinomas often have malignant spindle cells. The most common type has bizarre giant cells, frequently multinucleated, and containing abnormal mitotic figures. Less commonly, some giant cells resemble osteoclasts.[139,219,220]

Ultrastructural studies have demonstrated the presence of structures resembling tiny follicles and junctions between the cells, supporting an epithelial phenotype.[138,139,218,219] Immunohistochemical evidence of thyroglobulin has been found in a few anaplastic carcinomas; it is likely that in most of these cases, the thyroglobulin staining represents diffusion of thyroglobulin cells from destroyed thyroid follicles[138,218]; 50% to 100% of these tumors contain keratin.[138,139,218,219] Carcinosarcoma of the thyroid[221] has been described.

Squamous Cell Carcinoma, Mucoepidermoid Carcinoma, and Intrathyroidal Thymoma-like Neoplasms

Chronic inflammation and scarring in the thyroid may cause the affected epithelium to undergo benign squamous metapla-

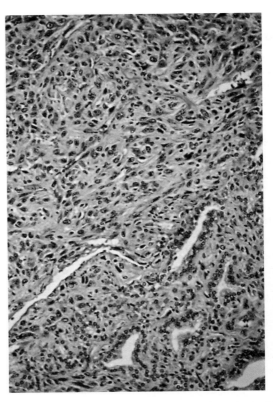

FIGURE 28-21. Anaplastic carcinoma. Remnants of neoplastic follicles are present in the lower portion.

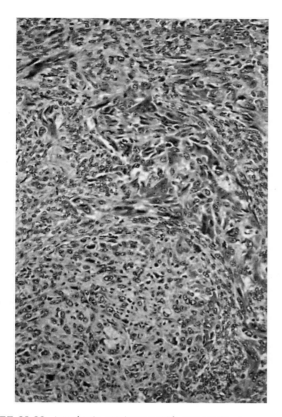

FIGURE 28-22. Anaplastic carcinoma with sarcomatous appearance.

sia.[122,222] Squamous metaplasia may occur in papillary carcinoma[125,148] and in anaplastic carcinoma.[138,139,218,219] Sometimes, typical squamous cell carcinoma occurs in association with papillary or anaplastic carcinoma.[202,222–224] Occasionally, squamous cell carcinoma appears as an entity independent of any other form of thyroid cancer.[224] Variants associated with leukocytosis and hypercalcemia have been described.[225] The major differential diagnosis is metastatic squamous carcinoma, especially from a head and neck, lungs, or esophagus. Primary squamous carcinoma of the thyroid is usually aggressive with a poor prognosis.[224]

Mucoepidermoid carcinoma in thyroid is rare[226–230] and may originate from ultimobranchial remnants,[227] from included salivary gland tissue,[230] or from thyroglossal tract remnants.

The tumor presents as a firm mass with conspicuous fibrosis. The epidermoid elements consist of irregular nests of squamous cells. Irregular ductlike or glandlike elements contain mucin. Some of these tumors that have a clinical behavior of low-grade malignancy have arisen in glands with chronic thyroiditis; this subgroup is associated with extensive eosinophilic leukocyte infiltration of the tumor without peripheral eosinophilia.[226]

Rare thyroid tumors have been reported, which are composed of spindled epithelial cells arranged in nests, sometimes associated with mucous microcysts, and resembling thymomas (SETTLE tumors—spindled and epithelial tumor with thymus-like differentiation).[231] A few examples of neoplasms resembling thymic carcinomas have been described, (CASTLE

tumor—carcinoma with thymus-like differentiation).[233] These lesions may originate from branchial pouch remnants within and adjacent to the thyroid.[231,232]

Medullary Carcinoma

C-cell proliferation has been reported in adults as a possible change with advancing age,[12,15] as a familial disorder associated with medullary carcinoma with or without multiple endocrine neoplasia,[233–235] as an association with hypercalcemia,[13] in areas of thyroid abutting follicular tumors,[236] in chronic thyroiditis,[237] and as an isolated event of unknown significance.[11,18,236] Medullary carcinoma[238–240] constitutes about 5% of thyroid carcinomas, originates from C-cells,[240] may be sporadic or familial, and may be associated with disorders of other endocrine glands.

On gross examination, most medullary carcinomas are found to be firm, white or yellow, and infiltrative. Some are well defined and even encapsulated; the latter have a better prognosis.[106,241]

On light microscopic examination, the cells are rounded or polygonal or may be spindled (Figs 28-23 and 28-24).[238–240] They appear as a diffuse solid mass, as islands separated by fibrous tissue (usually dense or hyalinized), as trabeculae or ribbons of cells, and (uncommonly) as glandular structures (Figs 28-25 and 28-26).[238–242] Small vessels in the tumor may be conspicuous, with the cells oriented around them. Pseudopapillary formations[243] and even true papillary pat-

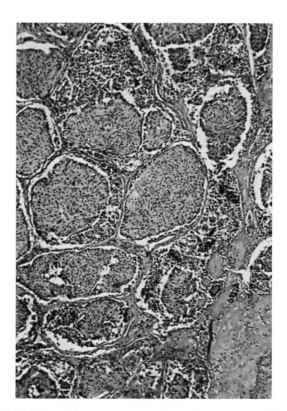

FIGURE 28-23. Medullary carcinoma with insular pattern. Amyloid is present at lower right.

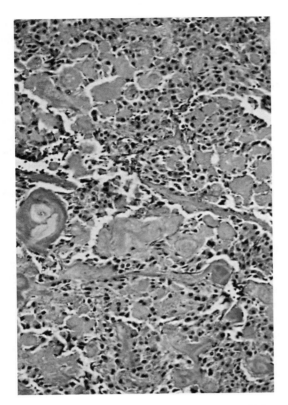

FIGURE 28-24. Medullary carcinoma with numerous small deposits of amyloid.

terns[242–244] have been reported. The carcinomas may be composed of small cells (in the past confused with small-cell anaplastic carcinoma),[242,244] may contain numerous giant cells,[244,245] and like some anaplastic carcinomas, may have large cells with eosinophilic cytoplasm, resembling oncocytic follicular cells[247]; these carcinomas can also contain glands.[248] Clear cell medullary carcinomas have been reported.[249] Cells producing mucus may be present in varying numbers.[250,251] Rarely, these carcinomas produce melanin.[252,253]

The nuclei are rounded or elongated; occasional nuclei are large and irregular. Cytoplasmic inclusions in nuclei may occur. Aneuploid DNA patterns indicate a less favorable outlook.[106,254]

Multiple small foci of necrosis sometimes are present, especially in the medullary carcinomas composed of small cells. Anaplastic variants of medullary carcinoma have been described, but these are extremely rare.[138,218,242,245]

Amyloid deposits formed by the secretory products of the neoplastic cells are frequently present, both in the primary neoplasms and in the metastatic foci. About 20% of medullary cancers lack amyloid.[106,242] The presence of amyloid indicates a better outlook.[106] Tumor stroma and the amyloid may undergo calcification.

Medullary carcinomas nearly always produce calcitonin, although a few may lack this peptide.[217,242] Other substances detected include chromogranins, calcitonin gene-related peptide, carcinoembryonic antigen, somatostatin, β-endorphin, adrenocorticotropic hormone, serotonin, bombesin, chorionic gonadotropin, histaminase, and prostaglandins.[255–258] The

demonstration of small amounts of calcitonin by immunostaining has been associated with a worse prognosis.[259,260]

Invasion of lymphatic and blood vessels and metastasis in cervical nodes are common. A few patients develop widespread disease and die in 2 or 3 years. A few have extraordinary indolent tumors (initially misdiagnosed as adenoma) that persist for as long as 30 years. Some reports indicate familial medullary carcinomas (especially patients with Sipple's syndrome) have a better prognosis.[259–261] Several authors indicate that patients with MEN-II B have tumors that are particularly aggressive.[260]

Most cases of medullary carcinoma are sporadic, particularly in patients over 40 years old, may involve only one lobe, and may not be associated with other endocrine lesions. A considerable number of cases are familial, however, especially in younger patients.[233–235] Such cancers may be associated with bilateral pheochromocytomas or adrenal medullary hyperplasia and with parathyroid hyperplasia (Sipple's syndrome, multiple endocrine neoplasia MEN-II A).

Some patients have a variant syndrome, with mucosal and cutaneous neuromas and skeletal abnormalities (MEN-II B).[234] The familial medullary carcinomas are usually bilateral and multicentric. Other family members may have C-cell hyperplasia and medullary carcinomas of microscopic size, some of which may have already spread to lymph nodes. In this situation, the C-cell hyperplasia must be regarded as premalignant.

Recent evidence suggests that immunostaining for neural adhesion molecule component can distinguish familial C-cell

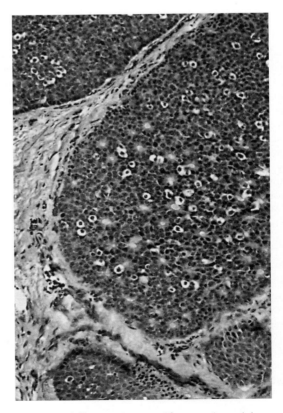

FIGURE 28-25. Medullary carcinoma with many tiny acini present in the islands of cells.

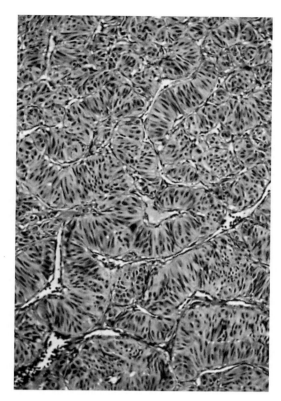

FIGURE 28-26. Medullary carcinoma with a trabecular pattern.

Malignant lymphoma presenting as a primary neoplasm in the thyroid is uncommon but not rare.[274–277] Its apparent rarity in the older literature reflects diagnosis of lymphoma as anaplastic carcinoma. Most patients may have a history of diffuse goiter (probably the result of autoimmune thyroiditis) that has suddenly increased in size.

Gross examination reveals firm, fleshy tissue that is usually pale. Evidence of previous lymphocytic thyroiditis is present in most cases in which some thyroid parenchyma still persists.[274,276]

Most thyroid lymphomas are of diffuse type (Fig 28-27). Virtually all examples are B-cell types[274,275,278–280]; many may be extranodal lymphomas that arise in mucosa-associated lymphoid tissue (MALT).[274,278] Some patients have typical plasmacytomas[281,282]; these have a good prognosis. Hodgkin's disease is extremely rare.

Invasion of lymphoma into and through the thyroid capsule, extension into the adjacent soft tissues, and involvement of regional lymph nodes occur fairly often and represent unfavorable prognostic factors. Some reports in the literature have suggested that gastrointestinal involvement is fairly common in patients having thyroid lymphoma, but experience varies in this regard.[274]

Distinguishing lymphoma from small-cell carcinoma, either primary or metastatic, may be difficult; appropriate special procedures usually allow this to be done.[283] Malignant lymphoma also has to be differentiated from advanced autoimmune thyroiditis; this distinction may require assessment

hyperplasia from secondary reactive states.[262] However, with the advent of genetic testing for familial medullary carcinoma, the pathologist can be relieved of the burden of defining C-cell hyperplasia in glands removed for medullary carcinoma.[263–265] C-cell adenoma ("medullary adenoma") has not been identified, pathologically; even though lesions diagnosed as C-cell adenoma are small and circumscribed, they are cancers.

A few medullary carcinomas are discovered incidental to thyroid operations for other conditions,[266] at autopsy,[267,268] or because of an elevated serum calcitonin.[269] The nontumoral parenchyma should be examined for evidence of C-cell hyperplasia in a thyroid removed for a medullary carcinoma. Occasionally, the gland contains moderate to severe autoimmune thyroiditis,[237,266] adenomatoid nodules, or another follicular-derived thyroid cancer.[236]

Some medullary carcinomas grow sufficiently slowly to allow them to trap thyroid follicles. A few neoplasms have been reported that appear to represent joint C-cell and follicular cell proliferations,[270–273] but these are rare. A putative example must be evaluated critically because of the possibility of collision tumors.[273] (See also chap 81.)

Lymphoma

Secondary involvement of the thyroid by malignant lymphoma that first appeared elsewhere in the body has been reported in 20% of patients dying from generalized lymphoma.[122]

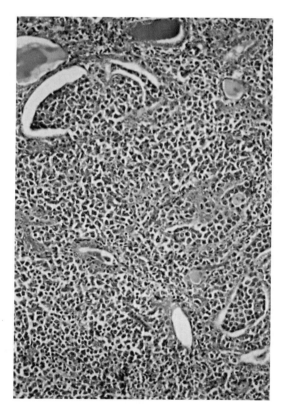

FIGURE 28-27. Malignant lymphoma. Several thyroid follicles are distended by the infiltrate.

of lymphocyte clonality by special studies (e.g., flow cytometry, gene rearrangement).

Sarcoma

Sarcomas of the thyroid are rare and compose fewer than 1% of all thyroid malignancies. There is a tendency to overdiagnose sarcoma of the thyroid.[284] On complete, critical examination most proposed sarcomas prove to be anaplastic carcinomas. Reports of acceptable angiosarcoma[285–287] and leiomyosarcoma[288] have been published.

Carcinoma in Ectopic Thyroid Tissue

The neoplasms that arise in the thyroglossal tract have been mostly papillary carcinomas.[289–291] In contrast with the thyroglossal carcinomas, neoplasms of sublingual and lingual ectopic thyroid tissue constitute the various types encountered in the main gland.

Carcinomas, usually the papillary subtype,[292] and lesions that resemble carcinoid tumors[293] have been reported in struma ovarii.

Metastatic Neoplasms

The most common metastatic tumors in the thyroid are malignant melanoma and carcinomas of the lung, breast, and kidney.[294]

Metastatic neoplasms in the thyroid that masquerade as primary tumors are rare. They have been reported to be most often carcinomas from breast, lung, and kidney.[294] Metastatic renal cell carcinoma probably is the secondary neoplasm that not only may appear clinically as a primary thyroidal neoplasm but also may be mistaken as a thyroid tumor by the pathologist.[119,295] Immunostaining for thyroglobulin may be helpful in making the distinction. Sometimes the thyroid mass represents the initial manifestation of the renal neoplasm; on other occasions, it appears so long after the nephrectomy that the possibility of a metastasis has been forgotten by the patient and the physician.

References

1. Toda S, Yonemitsu N, Hikichi Y, Sugihara H, Koike N. Differentiation of human thyroid follicle cells from normal subjects and Basedow's disease in three dimensional collagen gel culture. Pathol Res Pract 1992;188:874
2. Klinck GH. Structure of the thyroid. In: Hazard JB, Smith DE, eds. The thyroid. Baltimore: Williams & Wilkins, 1964:1
3. Gnepp DR, Ogorzalek JM, Heffess CS. Fat-containing lesions of the thyroid gland. Am J Surg Pathol 1989;13:605
4. MacMahon HE, Lee HY, Rivelis CF. Birefringent crystals in human thyroid. Acta Endocrinol 1968;58:172
5. Reid JD, Choi CH, Oldroyd NO. Calcium oxalate crystals in the thyroid: their identification, prevalence origin and possible significance. Am J Clin Pathol 1987;87:443
6. Heimann P. Ultrastructure of human thyroid: a study of normal thyroid, untreated and treated diffuse toxic goiter. Acta Endocrinol 1966;53(Suppl 110):1
7. Klinck GH, Oertel JE, Winship T. Ultrastructure of normal human thyroid. Lab Invest 1970;22:2
8. Sobrinho-Simoes M, Johannessen JV. Scanning electron microscopy of the normal human thyroid. J Submicrosc Cytol 1981;13:209
9. Gibson W, Croker B, Cox C. C cell populations in normal children and young adults. Lab Invest 19890;42:119
10. Gibson WGH, Peng TC, Croker BP. C cell nodules in adult human thyroid. A common autopsy finding. Am J Clin Pathol 1981;75:347
11. Gibson WGH, Peng TC, Croker BP. Age associated C cell hyperplasia in human thyroid. Am J Pathol 1982;106:388
12. Wolfe HJ, Voelkel EF, Tashjian AH. Distribution of calcitonin-containing cells in the nromal adult human thyroid gland: a correlation of morphology with peptide content. J Clin Endocrinol Metab 1974;38:688
13. Wolfe HJ, DeLellis RA, Voelkel EF, Tashjian AH. Distribution of calcitonin-containing cells in neonatal human thyroid gland: a correlation of morphology with peptide content. J Clin Endocrinol Metab 1975;41:1076
14. O'Toole K, Fenoglio-Preiser C, Pushparaj N. Endocrine changes associated with the human aging process III. Effect of age on the number of calcitonin immunoreactive cells in the thyroid gland. Hum Pathol 1985:16:991
15. Baschieri L, Castagna M, Fierabracci A, Antonelli A, Del Guerra P, Squartini F. Distribution of calcitonin- and somatostatin-containing cells in thyroid lymphoma and in Hashimoto's thyroiditis. Appl Pathol 1989;7:99
16. Kameda Y, Oyama H, Endoh M, Horino M. Somatostatin immunoreactive C-cells in thyroid glands from various mammaliam species. Anat Rec 1982;204:161
17. Guyetant S, Wion-Barbot N, Rousselet MC, Franc B, Bigorgne JC, Saint-Andre JP. C-cell hyperplasia associated with chronic lymphocytic thyroiditis. Hum Pathol 1994;25:514
18. Harach JR. Solid cell nests of the thyroid: an anatomical survey and immunohistochemical study for the presence of thyroglobulin. Acta Anat 1985;122:249
19. Harach JR. Mixed follicles of the human thyroid gland. Acta Anat 1987;129:27
20. Harach JR. Solid cell nests of the thyroid. J Pathol 1988;155:191
21. Harach HR, Viyanic GM, Jasani B. Ultimobranchial body nest in human fetal thyroid: an autopsy histological and immunohistochemical study in relation to solid cell nests and mucoepidermoid carcinoma of the thyroid. J Pathol 1993;169:465
22. Cameselle-Teijeero J, Valera-Duran J, Sambade C, Villanueva JP, Valera-Nunez R, Sobrinho-Simoes M. Solid cell nests of the thyroid. Hum Pathol 1994;25:684
23. Mizukami Y, Nonomura A, Mishigishi T, et al. Solid cell nests of the thyroid. Am J Clin Pathol 1994;101:186
24. Parham DM. Laterally situated neck cysts derived from the embryological remnants of thyroid development. Histopathology 1988;12:95
25. Williams ED, Toyn CE, Harach HR. The ultimobranchial gland and congenital thyroid abnormalities in man. J Pathol 1989;159:135
26. Bronner MP, LiVolsi VA. Oxyphilic (Askanazy/Hürthle cell) tumors of the thyroid: Microscopic features predict biologic behavior. Surg Pathol 1988;1:137
27. Flint A, Davenport RD, Lloyd RV, Beckwith AL, Thompson NW. Cytomorphometric measurements of Hurthle cell tumors of the thyroid gland: correlation with pathologic features and clinical behavior. Cancer 1988;61:110
28. Friedman NB. Cellular involution in the thyroid gland. Significance of Hürthle cells in myxedema, exhaustion atrophy, Hashimoto's disease and the reactions to irradiation, thiouracil therapy and subtotal resection. J Clin Endocrinol Metab 1949;9:874

29. Mitchell JD, Kirkham N, Machin D. Focal lymphocytic thyroiditis in Southampton. J Pathol 1984;144:269
30. Kabel PJ, Voorbij HAM, DeHaan M, van der Gaag RD, Drexhage HA. Intrathyroidal dendritic-cells. J Clin Endocrinol Metab 1988; 66:199
31. Allard RHB. The thyroglossal cyst. Head Neck Surg 1982;5:134
32. Neinas FW, Goman CA, Devine KD, Woolner LB. Lingual thyroid: Clinical characteristics of 15 cases. Ann Intern Med 1973; 79:205
33. Pollock WF, Stevenson EO. Cysts and sinuses of the thyroglossal duct. Am J Surg 1966;112:225
34. Sauk JJ. Ectopic lingual thyroid. J Pathol 1970;102:239
35. Shareef DS, Salm R. Ectopic vestigial lesions of neck and shoulders. J Clin Pathol 1981;34:1155
36. Apel RL, Asa SL, Chalvardjian A, LiVolsi VA. Intrathyroidal lymphoepithelial cysts of probable branchial origin. Hum Pathol 1994;25:1238
37. Carpenter GR, Emery JL. Inclusions in the human thyroid. J Anat 1976;122:77
38. LiVolsi VA. Branchial and thymic remnants in the thyroid and cervical region. An explanation for unusual tumors and microscopic curiosities. Endocr Pathol 1993;4:115
39. Gardiner WR. Unusual relationships between thyroid gland and skeletal muscle in infants: a review of the literature and four case reports. Cancer 1956;9:681
40. Hathaway BM. Innocuous accessory thyroid nodules. Arch Surg 1965;90:222
41. Gerard-Merchant R, Caillou B. Thyroid inclusions in cervical lymph nodes. Clin Endocrinol Metab 1981:10:337
42. Meyer JS, Steinberg LS. Microscopically benign thyroid follicles in cervical lymph nodes: serial section study of lymph node inclusions and entire thyroid gland in 5 cases. Cancer 1969;24:302
43. Roth LM. Inclusions of nonneoplastic thyroid tissue within cervical lymph nodes. Cancer 1965;18:105
44. Doniach I. The thyroid gland. In: Symmers W StC, ed. Systemic Pathology. 2nd ed. Edinburgh: Churchill Livingstone, 1978:1976
45. Kennedy JS. The pathology of dyshormonogenetic goitre. J Pathol 1969;99:251
46. Moore GH. The thyroid in sporadic goitrous cretinism: a report of three new cases, description of the pathologic anatomy of the thyroid glands and a review of the literature. Arch Pathol 1962; 74:35
47. Studer H, Ramelli F. Simple goiter and its variants; euthyroid and hyperthyroid multinodular goiters. Endocr Rev 1982;3:40
48. Taylor S. The evolution of nodular goiter. J Clin Endocrinol Metab 1953;13:1232
49. van der Gaag RD, Drexhage HA, Wiersinga WM, et al. Further studies on thyroid growth-stimulating immunoglobulins in euthyroid nonendemic goiter. J Clin Endocrinol Metab 1974;9:719
50. Ramelli F, Studer H, Bruggisser D. Patholgenesis of thyroid nodules in multinodular goiter. Am J Pathol 1982;109:215
51. Studer H, Gerber H, Zbaeren J, Peter HJ. Histomorphological and immunohistochemical evidence that nodular goiters grow by episodic replication of multiple clusters of thyroid follicular cells. J Clin Endocrinol Metab 1992;75:1151
52. Aeschemann S, Kopp PA, Kemura ET, et al. Morphological and functional polymorphism within clonal thyroid nodules. J Clin Invest 1993;77:846
53. Apel RL, Ezzat S, Bapat BV, Pan N, LiVolsi VA, Asa SL. Clonality of thyroid nodules in sporadic goiter. Diagn Molec Pathol 1995;4:113
54. Hicks DG, LiVolsi VA, Neidich JA, Puck J, Kant J. Clonal analysis of solitary follicular nodules in the thyroid. Am J Pathol 1990; 137:553
55. Namba H, Matsuo K, Fagin JA. Clonal composition of benign and malignant thyroid tumors. J Clin Invest 1990;86:120
56. Mizukami Y, Michigishi T, Nonomura A, et al. Autonomously functioning (hot) nodule of the thyroid gland. A clinical and histopathologic study of 17 cases. Am J Clin Pathol 1994;101:29
57. Campbell WL, Santiago HE, Perzin KH, Johnson PM. The autonomous thyroid nodule: correlation of scan appearance and histopathology. Radiology 1973;107:133
58. DeGroot LJ, Quintans J. The causes of autoimmune thyroid disease. Endocr Rev 1989;10:537
59. Wick MR, Sawyer MD. Antigenic alterations in autoimmune thyroid diseases: observations and hypotheses. Arch Pathol Lab Med 1989;113:77
60. Derwahl M, Huber G, Studer H. Slow growth but intense hypertrophy of thyrocytes in longstanding Graves' goitre. Acta Endocrinol 1989;121:389
61. Margolick JB, Hsu SM, Volkman DJ, Burman KD, Fauci AS. Immunohistochemical characterization of intrathyroid lymphocytes in Graves' disease: interstitial and intraepithelial populations. Am J Med 1984;76:815
62. Matsunaga M, Eguchi K, Fukuda T, et al. Class II major histocompatibility complex antigen expression and cellular interactions in thyroid glands of Graves' disease. J Clin Endocrinol Metab 1986; 62:723
63. Eggen PC, Seljelid R. The histological appearance of hyperfunctioning thyroids following various preoperative treatments. Acta Pathol Microbiol Immunol Scand (A) 1973;71:1663
64. Hirota Y, Tamai H, Hayashi Y, et al. Thyroid function and histology in forty-five patients with hyperthyroid Graves' disease in clinical remission more than ten years after thionamide drug treatment. J Clin Endocrinol Metab 1986;62:165
65. Vickery AL. The diagnosis of malignancy in dyshormonogenetic goiter. Clin Endocrinol Metab 1985;2:90
66. Fauerholdt L, Vendsborg P. Thyroid gland morphology after lithium treatment. Acta Pathol Microbiol Immunol Scand (A) 1981;89:339
67. Mizukami Y, Funaki N, Hashimoto T, Kawato M, Michigishi T, Matsubara F. Histologic features of thyroid gland in a patient with bromide induced hypothyroidism. Am J Clin Pathol 1988; 89:802
68. Aichinger G, Fill H, Wick G. In situ immune complexes, lymphocyte subpopulations, and HLA-DR-positive epithelial cells in Hashimoto's thyroiditis. Lab Invest 1985;52:132
69. Fatourechi V, McConahey WM, Woolner LB. Hyperthyroidism associated with histologic Hashimoto's thyroiditis. Mayo Clin Proc 1971;46:682
70. LiVolsi VA. The pathology of autoimmune thyroid disease: A review. Thyroid 1994;4:333
71. Mizukami Y, Michigishi T, Kawato M, et al. Chronic thyroiditis: Thyroid function and histologic correlation in 601 cases. Hum Pathol 1992;23:980
72. Ben-Ezra J, Wu A, Sheibani K. Hashimoto's thyroiditis lacks detectable clonal immunoglobulin and T cell receptor gene rearrangements. Hum Pathol 1988;19:1444
73. LiVolsi VA, Merino MJ. Squamous cells in the human thyroid gland. Am J Surg Pathol 1978;2:133
74. Vollenweider I, Hedinger C. Solid cell nests (SCN) in Hashimoto's thyroiditis. Virchows Arch (A) 1988;412:357
75. Carney JA. Thyroid cysts. Am J Surg Pathol 1989;13:1072
76. Louis DN, Vickery AL, Rosai J, Wang CA. Multiple branchial cleft-like cysts in Hashimoto's thyroiditis. Am J Surg Pathol 1989;13:45
77. Mizukami Y, Michigishi F, Hashimoto T, et al. Silent thyroiditis: a histologic and immunohistochemical study. Hum Pathol 1988; 19:423
78. Woolf PD. Transient painless thyroiditis with hyperthyroidism: a variant of lymphocytic thyroiditis? Endocr Rev 1980;1:411
79. LiVolsi VA. Postpartum thyroiditis. The pathology slowly unravels. Am J Clin Pathol 1993;100:193

80. deMont SH, Smith RRL, Karp JE, Merz WG. Pulmonary, cardiac, and thyroid involvement in disseminated *Pseudoallescheria boydii*. Arch Pathol Lab Med 1984;108:859

81. Loeb JM, Livermore BM, Wofsy D. Coccidioidomycosis of the thyroid. Ann Intern Med 1979;91:409

82. Lucaya J, Bordon WE, Enriquez G, Regas J, Carreno JC. Congenital pyriform sinus fistula: a cause of acute left-sided suppurative thyroiditis and neck abscess in children. Pediatr Radiol 1990; 21:27

83. Drucker DJ, Bailey D, Rotstein L. Thyroiditis as the presenting manifestation of disseminated extrapulmonary *Pneumocystis carinii* infection. J Clin Endocrinol Metab 1990;71:1663

84. Frank TS, LiVolsi VA, Connor AM. Cytomegalovirus infection of the thyroid in immunocompromised adults. Yale J Biol Med 1987;60:1

85. Lindsay S, Dailey ME. Granulomatous or giant cell thyroiditis. Surg Gynecol Obstet 1954;98:197

86. Carney JA, Moore SB, Northcutt RC, Woolner LB, Stillwell GK. Palpation thyroiditis (multifocal granulomatous folliculitis). Am J Clin Pathol 1975;64:639

87. Leung WH, Lau CP, Wong CK, Wang C. Amiodarone induced thyroiditis. Am Heart J 1989;118:848

88. Smyrk TC, Goellner JR, Brennan MD, Carney JA. Pathology of the thyroid in amiodarone associated thyrotoxicosis. Am J Surg Pathol 1987;11:197

89. Schwaegerle SM, Bauer TW, Esselstyn CB. Riedel's thyroiditis. Am J Clin Pathol 1988;90:715

90. Comings DE, Skubi KB, Van Eyes J, Motulsky AG. Familial multifocal fibrosclerosis: findings suggesting that retroperitoneal fibrosis, mediastinal fibrosis, sclerosing cholangitis, Riedel's thyroiditis and pseudotumor of the orbit may be different manifestations of a single disease. Ann Intern Med 1967;66:884

91. Carr RF, LiVolsi VA. Morphologic changes in the thyroid after irradiation for Hodgkin's and non-Hodgkin's lymphoma. Cancer 1989;64:825

92. Conrad RA, Dobyns BM, Sutow WW. Thyroid neoplasia as late effect of exposure to radioactive iodine in fallout. JAMA 1970; 214:316

93. Komorowski RA, Hanson GA. Morphologic changes in the thyroid following low dose childhood radiation. Arch Pathol Lab Med 1977;101:36

94. Schneider AB, Pinsky S, Bekerman C, Ryo UY. Characteristics of 108 thyroid cancers detected by screening in a population with a history of head and neck irradiation. Cancer 1980;46:1218

95. Spitalnick PF, Strauss FH. Patterns of human thyroid parenchymal reaction following low dose childhood irradiation. Cancer 1978;41:1098

96. Curran RC, Eckert H, Wilson GM. The thyroid gland after treatment of hyperthyroidism by partial thyroidectomy or iodine 131. J Pathol 1958;76:541

97. Dobyns BM, Vickery AI, Maloof F, Chapman EM. Functional and histologic effects of therapeutic doses of radioactive iodine on the thyroid of man. J Clin Endocrinol Metab 1953;13:548

98. Kanoh T, Shimada H, Uchino H, Matsumara K. Amyloid goiter with hypothyroidism. Arch Pathol Lab Med 1989;113:542

99. Kennedy JS, Thomson JA, Buchanan WM. Amyloid in the thyroid. Q J Med 1974;43:127

100. Alexander CB, Herrera GA, Jaffe K, Yu H. Black thyroid: clinical manifestations, ultrastructural findings, and possible mechanisms. Hum Pathol 1985;16:72

101. Landas SK, Schelper RL, Tio FO, Turner JW, Moore KC, Bennett-Gray J. Black thyroid syndrome: exaggeration of a normal process? Am J Clin Pathol 1986;85:411

102. McConahey WM, Hay ID, Woolner LB, van Heerden JA, Taylor WF. Papillary thyroid cancer treated at the Mayo Clinic, 1946 through 1970: initial manifestations, pathological findings, therapy and outcome. Mayo Clin Proc 1986;61:978

103. McConnon JK, Von Westarp C, Mitchell RI. Follicular carcinoma of the thyroid with functioning metastases and clinical hyperthyroidism. Can Med Assoc J 1975;112:724

104. Panke TW, Croxson MS, Parker JW, Carriere DP, Rosoff L, Warner NE. Triiodothyronine secreting (toxic) adenoma of the thyroid gland: light and electron microscopic characteristics. Cancer 1978;12:95

105. Ryff-de Leche A, Staub JJ, Kohler-Faden R, Muller-Brand J, Heitz PU. Thyroglobulin production by malignant thyroid tumors: an immunocytochemical and radioimmunassay study. Cancer 1986; 57:1145

106. Bergholm U, Adami HO, Auer G, et al. Histopathologic characteristics and nuclear DNA content as prognostic factors in medullary thyroid carcinomas: a nationwide study in Sweden. Cancer 1989;64:135

107. Bronner MP, Clevenger CV, Edmonds PR, Lowell DM, McFarland MM, LiVolsi VA. Flow cytometric analysis of DNA content in Hurthle cell adenomas and carcinoma of the thyroid. Am J Clin Pathol 1988;89:764

108. Joensuu H, Klemi PJ. Comparison of nuclear DNA content in primary and metastatic differentiated thyroid carcinoma. Am J Clin Pathol 1988;89:35

109. Joensuu H, Klemi PJ, Eerola E. DNA aneuploidy in follicular adenomas of the thyroid gland. Am J Pathol 1986;124:373

110. Fukunga M, Shinozaki N, Endo Y, Ushigome S. Atypical adenoma of the thyroid. Acta Pathol Jpn 1992;42:432

111. Oyama T, Vickery AL, Preffer FI, Colvin RB. A comparative study of flow cytometric and histopathologic findings in thyroid follicular carcinomas and adenomas. Hum Pathol 1994;25:271

112. Zedenuis J, Auer G, Backdahl M, et al. Follicular tumors of the thyroid gland: Diagnosis, clinical aspects and nuclear DNA analysis. World J Surg 1992;16:589

113. van Hoeven KH, Menendez-Botel CJ, Strong EW, Huvos AG. Estrogen and progesterone receptor content in human thyroid disease. Am J Clin Pathol 1993;99:175

114. Farley DR, Eberhardt NL, Grant CS, et al. Expression of a potential metastasis suppressor gene (nm23) in thyroid neoplasms. World J Surg 1993;17:615

115. Shimizu T, Usuda N, Yamanda T, Sugenoya A, Iida F. Proliferative activity of human thyroid tumors evaluated by proliferating cell nuclear antigen/cyclin immunohistochemical studies. Cancer 1993;71:2807

116. Tateyama H, Yang YP, Ermoto T, et al. Proliferative cell nuclear antigen expression in follicular tumors of the thyroid with special reference to oxyphilic cell lesions. Virchows Arch 1994; 424:533

117. Loy TS, Darkow GV, Spollen LE, Diaz-Arias AA. Immunostaining for Leu-7 in the diagnosis of thyroid carcinoma. Arch Pathol Lab Med 1994;118:172

118. Nairn ER, Crocker J, McGovern J. Limited value of AgNOR enumeration in assessment of thyroid neoplasms. J Clin Pathol 1988;41:1136

119. Carcangiu ML, Sibley RK, Rosai J. Clear cell change in primary thyroid tumors: a study of 38 cases. Am J Surg Pathol 1989; 13:1041

120. Arganini M, Behar R, Wu T-C, et al. Hürthle cell tumors: a twenty-five year experience. Surgery 1986;100:1108

121. Bondeson L, Bondeson AG, Ljungberg O, Tibblin S. Oxyphil tumors of the thyroid: followup of 42 surgical cases. Ann Surg 1981;194:677

122. Meissner WA, Warren S. Tumors of the thyroid gland. In: Atlas of tumor pathology. 2nd series, fascicle 4. Washington, DC: Armed Forces Institute of Pathology, 1969

123. Hazard JB, Kenyon R. Atypical adenoma of the thyroid. Arch Pathol 1954;58:554

124. Lang W, Georgii A, Stauch G, Kienzle E. The differentiation of atypical adenomas and encapsulated follicular carcinomas in the thyroid gland. Virchows Arch (A) 1980;385:125

125. Rosai J, Carcangiu ML, DeLellis RA. Tumors of the thyroid gland. In: Atlas of tumor pathology. 3rd series, fascicle 5. Washington, DC: Armed Forces Institute of Pathology, 1992

126. Chan JKC, Tse CCH, Chiu HS. Hyalinizing trabecular adenoma-like lesions in multinodular goitre. Histopathology 1990;16:611

127. LiVolsi VA, Gupta PK. Thyroid fine needle aspiration-paraganglioma-like adenoma of the thyroid. Diagn Cytopathol 1992; 8:82

128. Sambade C, Franssila KO, Cameselle-Trejeiro J, Nesland J, Sobrinho-Simoes M. Hyalinizing trabecular adenoma: a misnomer for a peculiar tumor of the thyroid gland. Endocr Pathol 1991; 2:83

129. Bronner MP, LiVolsi VA, Jennings TA. PLAT: paraganglioma-like adenomas of the thyroid. Surg Pathol 1988;1:383

130. Gherardi G. Signet ring cell "mucinous" thyroid adenomas: a follicle cell tumour with abnormal accumulation of thyroglobulin and a peculiar histochemical profile. Histopathology 1987;11:317

131. Toth K, Peter I, Kremmer T, Sugar J. Lipid rich cell thyroid adenoma: histopathology and comparative lipid analysis. Virchows Arch (A) 1990;417:273

132. Bale GF. Teratoma of the neck in the region of the thyroid gland: a review of the literature and report of four cases. Am J Pathol 1950;26:565

133. Kimler SC, Muth WF. Primary malignant teratoma of the thyroid: case report and literature review of cervical teratomas in adults. Cancer 1978;42:311

134. Hrafnkelsson J, Stal O, Enestrom S, et al. Cellular DNA pattern, S-phase frequency and survival in papillary thyroid cancer. Acta Oncol 1988;27:329

135. Schroder S, Schwarz W, Rehpenning W, Loning T, Bocker W. Prognostic significance of Leu-M1 immunostaining in papillary carcinomas of the thyroid gland. Virchows Arch (A) 1987; 411:435

136. Schroder S, Schwarz W, Rehpenning W, Loning T, Bocker W. Dendritic/Langerhans cells and prognosis in patients with papillary thyroid carcinomas: Immunohistochemical study of 106 thyroid neoplasms correlated with followup data. Am J Clin Pathol 1988;89:295

137. Tennvall J, Biorklund A, Moller T, Ranstam J, Akerstrom M. Prognostic factors of papillary, follicular and medullary carcinomas of the thyroid gland: retrospective multivariate analysis of 216 patients with a median followup of 11 years. Acta Radiol Oncol 1985;24:17

138. LiVolsi VA, Brooks JJ, Arendash-Durand B. Anaplastic thyroid tumors: immunohistology. Am J Clin Pathol 1987;87:434

139. Carcangiu ML, Steeper T, Zampi G, Rosai J. Anaplastic thyroid carcinoma: a study of 70 cases. Am J Clin Pathol 1985;83:135

140. Bronner MP, Hamilton R, LiVolsi VA. Utility of frozen section analysis on follicular lesions of the thyroid. Endocr Pathol 1994;5:154

141. Lote K, Andersen K, Nordal E, Brennhovd IO. Familial occurrence of papillary thyroid carcinoma. Cancer 1980;46:1291

142. Cuello C, Correa P, Eisenberg H. Geographic pathology of thyroid carcinoma. Cancer 1969;23:230

143. Hofstadter F. Frequency and morphology of malignant tumours of the thyroid before and after the introduction of iodine prophylaxis. Virchows Arch (A) 1980;385:263

144. Samaan NA. Papillary carcinoma of the thyroid: Hereditary or radiation induced? Cancer Invest 1989;7:399

145. Kerber RA, Till JE, Simon SL, et al. A cohort study of thyroid disease in relation to fallout from nuclear weapons testing. JAMA 1993;270:2076

146. Nikiforov Y, Grepp DR. Pediatric thyroid cancer after the Chernobyl disaster. Cancer 1994;74:748

147. Hawk WA, Hazard JB. The many appearances of papillary carcinoma of the thyroid. Cleve Clin Q 1976;43:207

148. Carcangiu ML, Zampi G, Pupi A, Castognoli A, Rosai J. Papillary carcinoma of the thyroid: a clinicopathologic study of 241 cases treated at the University of Florence, Italy. Cancer 1985;55:805

149. Carcangiu ML, Zampi G, Rosai J. Papillary thyroid carcinoma: a study of its many morphologic expressions and clinical correlates. Pathol Annu 1985;20(Pt 1):1

150. Tscholl-Ducommun J, Hedinger CE. Papillary thyroid carcinomas: morphology and prognosis. Virchows Arch (A) 1982; 396:19

151. Vickery AI, Carcangiu ML, Johannessen JV, Sobrinho-Simoes M. Papillary carcinoma. Semin Diagn Pathol 1985;2:90

152. Chan JKC, Rosai J. Papillary carcinoma of thyroid with exuberant nodular fasciitis-like stroma: report of three cases. Am J Clin Pathol 1991;95:309

153. Ostrowski MA, Asa SL, Chamberlain D, Moffat FL, Rotstein LE. Myxomatous change in papillary carcinoma of the thyroid. Surg Pathol 1989;2:249

154. Salvadori B, DelBo R, Pilotti S, Grassi M, Cusumano F. Occult papillary carcinoma of the thyroid: a questional entity. Eur J Cancer 1993;13:1817

155. Franssila KO, Harach HR. Occult papillary carcinoma of the thyroid in children and young adults: a systematic autopsy study in Finland. Cancer 1986;58:715

156. Harach HR, Franssila KO, Wasenius VM. Occult papillary carcinoma of the thyroid: a "normal" finding in Finland. A systematic autopsy study. Cancer 1985;56:531

157. Kasai, N, Sakamoto A. New subgrouping of small thyroid carcinomas. Cancer 1987;60:1767

158. Komorowski RA, Hanson GA. Occult thyroid pathology in the young adult: an autopsy study of 138 patients without clinical thyroid disease. Hum Pathol 1988;19:689

159. Yamamoto Y, Maeda T, Izumi K, Otsuka H. Occult papillary carcinoma of the thyroid: a study of 408 autopsy cases. Cancer 1990;65:1173

160. Harach HR, Franssila KO. Occult papillary carcinoma of the thyroid appearing as lung metastasis. Arch Pathol Lab Med 1984; 108:529

161. Patchefsky AS, Keller IB, Mansfield CM. Solitary vertebral column metastasis from occult sclerosing carcinoma of the thyroid gland. Am J Clin Pathol 1970;53:596

162. Sampson RJ, Key CR, Buncher CR, Iijima S. Smallest forms of papillary carcinoma of the thyroid: a study of 141 microcarcinomas less than 0.1 cm in greatest dimension. Arch Pathol 1971; 91:334

163. Strate SM, Lee EL, Childers JH. Occult papillary carcinoma of the thyroid with distant metastases. Cancer 1984;54:1093

164. Hedinger CE, Williams ED, Sobin LH. Histological typing of thyroid tumours. 2nd ed. International Histological Classification of Tumours, no. 11. Berlin: Springer-Verlag, 1988

165. Lindsay S. Papillary thyroid carcinoma revisited. In: Hedinger CE, ed. Thyroid cancer. Berlin: Springer-Verlag, 1969

166. Carcangiu ML, Bianchi S. Diffuse sclerosing variant of papillary thyroid carcinoma: clinicopathologic study of 15 cases. Am J Surg Pathol 1989;13:1041

167. Fujimoto Y, Obara T, Ito Y, Kodama T, Aiba M, Yamaguchi K. Diffuse sclerosing variant of papillary carcinoma of the thyroid. Cancer 1990;66:2306

168. Chan JKC, Tsui MS, Tse CH. Diffuse sclerosing variant of papillary carcinoma of the thyroid: a histological and immunohistochemical study of three cases. Histopathology 1987;11:191

169. Schroder S, Bay V, Dumke K, et al. Diffuse sclerosing variant of papillary thyroid carcinoma: S-100 protein immunocytochemistry and prognosis. Virchows Arch (A) 1990;416:367

170. Soares J, Limbert E, Sobrinho-Simoes M. Diffuse sclerosing variant of papillary thyroid carcinoma: a clinicopathologic study of 10 cases. Pathol Res Pract 1989;185:200

171. Moreno-Egea A, Rodriguez-Gonzalez JM, Sola-Perez J, Sorea T, Parillo-Paricio P. Clinicopathological study of the diffuse sclerosing variety of papillary cancer of the thyroid. Europ J Surg Oncol 1994;20:7

172. Kini SR. Guides to clinical aspiration biopsy: Thyroid. New York: Igaku-Shoin, 1987

173. Gray A, Doniach I. Morphology of the nuclei of papillary carcinoma of the thyroid. Br J Cancer 1969;23:49

174. Johannessen JV, Gould VE, Jao W. The fine structure of human thyroid cancer. Hum Pathol 1978;9:385

175. Akslen LA, Varhaug JE. Thyroid carcinoma with mixed tall cell and columnar cell features. Am J Clin Pathol 1990;94:442

176. Johnson TL, Lloyd RV, Thompson NW, Beierwaltes WH, Sisson JC. Prognostic implications of the tall cell variant of papillary thyroid carcinoma. Am J Surg Pathol 1988;12:22

177. LiVolsi VA, Apel RL, Asa SL. Papillary Hürthle cell carcinoma with lymphocytic stroma: "Warthin-like tumor" of the thyroid. Am J Surg Pathol, 1995. In press

178. Evans HL. Encapsulated papillary neoplasms of the thyroid: a study of 14 cases followed for a minimum of 10 years. Am J Surg Pathol 1987;11:592

179. Schroder S, Bocker W, Dralle H, Kortmann KB, Stern C. The encapsulated papillary carcinoma of the thyroid: a morphologic subtype of the papillary thyroid carcinoma. Cancer 1984; 54:90

180. Johannessen JV, Sobrinho-Simoes M. The origin and significance of thyroid psammoma bodies. Lab Invest 1980;43:287

181. Sisson JC, Schmidt RW, Beierwaltes WH. Sequestered nodular goiter. N Engl J Med 1964;270:927

182. Russell WO, Ibanez ML, Clark RL, White EC. Thyroid carcinoma: classification, intraglandular dissemination and clinicopathological study based upon whole organ sections of 80 glands. Cancer 1963;16:1425

183. Smith SA, Hay ID, Goellner JR, Ryan JJ, Mc Conahey WM. Mortality from papillary thyroid carcinoma: a case control study of 56 lethal cases. Cancer 1988;62:1381

184. Franssila KO, Ackerman LV, Brown CL, Hedinger CE. Follicular carcinoma. Semin Diagn Pathol 1985;2:101

185. Yamashina M. Follicular neoplasms of the thyroid. Am J Surg Pathol 1992;16:392

186. Kahn NF, Perzin KH. Follicular carcinoma of the thyroid. An evaluation of the histologic criteria used for diagnosis. Pathol Annu 1983;18(Pt 1):221

187. Lang W, Choritz H, Hundeshagen H. Risk factors in follicular thyroid carcinoma: a retrospective followup study covering a 14 year period with emphasis on morphologic findings. Am J Surg Pathol 1986;10:246

188. Hazard JB, Kenyon R. Encapsulated angioinvasive carcinoma (angioinvasive adenoma) of thyroid gland. Arch Pathol 1954; 19:152

189. Evans HL. Follicular neoplasms of the thyroid: a study of 44 cases followed for a minimum of 10 years with emphasis on differential diagnosis. Cancer 1984;54:535

190. Schroder S, Pfannschmidt N, Dralle H, Arps H, Bocker W. The encapsulated follicular carcinoma of the thyroid: a clinicopathologic study of 35 cases. Virchows Arch (A) 1984;402:259

191. Harach HR, Franssila KO. Thyroglobulin immunostaining in follicular thyroid carcinoma: relationship to the degree of differentiation and cell type. Histopathology 1988;13:43

192. LiVolsi VA, Asa SL. The demise of follicular carcinoma of the thyroid gland. Thyroid 1994;4:233

193. van Heerden JA, Hay ID, Goellner JR, et al. Follicular thyroid carcinoma with capsular invasion alone. A nonthreatening malignancy. Surgery 1992;112:1130

194. Franssila KO. Is the differentiation between papillary and follicular thyroid carcinoma valid? Cancer 1973;32:853

195. Watson DG, Brennan MD, Goellner JR, van Heerden JA, McConahey WM, Taylor WF. Invasive Hürthle cell carcinoma of the thyroid: natural history and management. Mayo Clin Proc 1984; 59:851

196. Gundry SR, Burney RE, Thompson NW, Lloyd R. Total thyroidectomy for Hürthle cell neoplasm of the thyroid. Arch Surg 1983; 118:529

197. Thompson NW, Dunn EL, Batsakis JG, Nishiyama RH. Hürthle cell lesions of the thyroid gland. Surg Gynecol Obstet 1974; 139:555

198. Flint A, Lloyd RV. Hürthle cell neoplasms of the thyroid gland. Pathol Annu 1990;25 (Pt 1):37

199. Tallini G, Carcangiu ML, Rosai J. Oncocytic neoplasms of the thyroid gland. Acta Pathol Jpn 1992;42:305

200. Rosai J, Saxen EA, Woolner LB. Undifferentiated and poorly differentiated carcinoma. Semin Diagn Pathol 1985;2:123

201. Carcangiu ML, Zampi G, Rosai J. Poorly differentiated ("insular") thyroid carcinoma. Am J Surg Pathol 1984;8:655

202. Sakamoto A, Kasai N, Sugano H. Poorly differentiated carcinoma of the thyroid: a clinicopathologic entity for a high risk group of papillary and follicular carcinomas. Cancer 1983;52:1849

203. Evans HL. Columnar cell carcinoma of the thyroid: a report of two cases of an aggressive variant of thyroid carcinoma. Am J Clin Pathol 1986;85:77

204. Mizukami Y, Nonomura A, Michigishi T, Noguchi M, Nakamura S, Hashimoto T. Columnar cell carcinoma of the thyroid gland. Hum Pathol 1994;25:1098

205. Robbins J, Merino MJ, Boice JD, et al. Thyroid cancer: a lethal endocrine neoplasm. Ann Int Med 1991;115:133

206. Sobrinho-Simoes M, Nesland JM, Johannessen JV. Columnar cell carcinoma. Another variant of poorly differentiated carcinoma of the thyroid. Am J Clin Pathol 1988;89:264

207. Sobrinho-Simoes M, Sambade C, Nesland JM, Johannessen JV. Tall cell papillary carcinoma. Am J Surg Pathol 1989;13:79

208. Auguste LJ, Masood S, Westerband O, Belluco C, Valderamma E, Attie JO. Oncogene expression in follicular neoplasms of the thyroid. Am J Surg 1992;164:592

209. Dobashi Y, Sakamoto A, Sugimura H, et al. Overexpression of p53 as a possible prognostic factor in human thyroid carcinoma. Am J Surg Pathol 1993;17:375

210. Dobashi Y, Sugimura H, Sakamoto A, Mernyei M, Mori M, Oyama T, Machinami R. Stepwise participation of p 53 gene mutation during dedifferentiation of human thyroid carcinomas. Diagn Molec Pathol 1994;3:9–14

211. Matias-Guiu X, Cuatrecasas M, Musulen E, Prat J. P 53 expression in anaplastic carcinomas arising from papillary carcinomas. J Clin Pathol 1994;47:337

212. Pilotti S, Collini P, DelBo R, Cattoretti G, Pierotti MA, Rilke F. A novel panel of antibodies that segregates immunocytochemically poorly differentiated carcinoma from undifferentiated carcinoma of the thyroid gland. Am J Surg Pathol 1994;18:1054

213. Pilotti S, Collini P, Rilke F, Cattoretti G, DelBo R, Pierotti M. Bcl-2 protein expression in carcinomas originating from the follicular epithelium of the thyroid gland. J Pathol 1994;172:337

214. Soares P, Cameselle-Teijeiro J, Sobrinho-Simoes M. Immunohistochemical detection of p 53 in differentiated, poorly differentiated and undifferentiated carcinomas of the thyroid. Histopathology 1994;24:205

215. Fagin JA, Matsuo K, Karmakar A, Chen DL, Tang S-H, Koeffler HP. High prevalence of mutations of the p 53 gene in poorly differentiated human thyroid carcinomas. J Clin Invest 1993;91:179

216. Mambo NC, Irwin SM. Anaplastic small cell neoplasms of the thyroid: an immunoperoxidase study. Hum Pathol 1984:15:55

217. Eusebi V, Damiani S, Riva C, Lloyd RV, Capella C. Calcitonin free oat cell carcinoma of the thyroid gland. Virchows Arch (A) 1990; 14:737

218. Hurlimann J, Gardiol D, Scazziga B. Immunohistology of anaplastic thyroid carcinoma: a study of 43 cases. Histopathology 1987;11:567

219. Venkatesh YSS, Ordonez NG, Schultz PN, Hickey RS, Goepfert H, Samaan NA. Anaplastic carcinoma of the thyroid: a clinicopathologic study of 121 cases. Cancer 1990;66:321

220. Hashimoto H, Koga S, Watanabe H, Enjoji M. Undifferentiated carcinoma of the thyroid gland with osteoclast-like giant cells. Acta Pathol Jpn 1980;30:323

221. Donnell CA, Pollock WJ, Sybers WA. Thyroid carcinosarcoma. Arch Pathol Lab Med 1987;111:1169

222. Katoh R, Sakamoto A, Kasai N, Yagawa K. Squamous differentiation in thyroid carcinoma: with special reference to histogenesis of squamous cell carcinoma of the thyroid. Acta Pathol Jpn 1989;39:306

223. Mikukami Y, Matsubara F, Hashimoto T et al. Primary mucin producing adenosquamous carcinoma of the thyroid gland. Acta Pathol Jpn 1987;37:1157

224. Huang TY, Assor D. Primary squamous cell carcinoma of the thyroid gland: a report of four cases. Am J Clin Pathol 1971; 11:567

225. Riddle PE, Dinesoy HP. Primary squamous cell carcinoma of the thyroid associated with leukocytosis and hypercalcemia. Arch Pathol Lab Med 1987;111:373

226. Chan JKC, Albores-Saavedra J, Battifora H, Carcangiu ML, Rosai J. Sclerosing mucoepidermoid thyroid carcinoma with eosinophilia. Am J Surg Pathol 1991;15:438

227. Franssila KO, Harach HR, Wasenius VM. Mucoepidermoid carcinoma of the thyroid. Histopathology 1984;8:847

228. Katoh R, Sugai T, Ono S, et al. Mucoepidermoid carcinoma of the thyroid gland. Cancer 1990;65:2020

229. Mizukami Y, Matsubara F, Hashimoto T, et al. Primary mucoepidermoid carcinoma in the thyroid gland: a case report including an ultrastructural and biochemical study. Cancer 1984;53:1741

230. Rhatigan RM, Roque J, Bucker RL. Mucoepidermoid carcinoma of the thyroid gland. Cancer 1977;39:210

231. Chan JKC, Rosai J. Tumors of the neck showing thymic or related branchial pouch differentiation. Hum Pathol 1991;22:349

232. Miyauchi A, Kuma K, Matsuzuka F, et al. Intrathyroidal epithelial thymoma: an entity distinct from squamous cell carcinoma of the thyroid. World J Surg 1985;9:128

233. Bigner SH, Mendelsohn G, Wells SA, Cox EB, Baylin SB, Eggleston JO. Medullary carcinoma of the thyroid in the multiple endocrine neoplasia lIB syndrome. Am J Surg Pathol 1981;5:459

234. Carney JA, Sizemore GW, Hayles AB. C cell disease of the thyroid gland in multiple endocrine neoplasia type 2b. Cancer 1979;44:2173

235. Melvin KEW, Tashjian AH, Miller HH. Studies in familial medullary thyroid carcinoma. Rec Prog Horm Res 1972;28:399

236. Albores-Saavedra J, Montfonte H, Nadji M, Morales AR. C-cell hyperplasia in thyroid tissue adjacent to follicular cell tumors. Hum Pathol 1988;19:795

237. Libbey NP, Nowakowski KJ, Tucci JR. C cell hyperplasia of the thyroid in a patient with goitrous hypothyroidism and Hashimoto's thyroiditis. Am J Surg Pathol 1989;13:71

238. Hazard JB, Hawk WA, Crile G. Medullary (solid) carcinoma of the thyroid: a clinicopathologic entity. J Clin Endocrinol Metab 1959;19:152

239. Williams ED, Brown CL, Doniach I. Pathological and clinical findings in a series of 67 cases of medullary carcinoma of the thyroid. J Clin Pathol 1966;19:103

240. Hazard JB. The C (parafollicular) cells of the thyroid gland and medullary thyroid carcinoma: a review. Am J Pathol 1977;88:214

241. Huss LJ, Mendelsohn G. Medullary carcinoma of the thyroid gland: an encapsulated variant resembling the hyalinizing trabecular (paraganglioma-like) adenoma of thyroid. Mod Pathol 1990;3:581

242. Albores-Saavedra J, LiVolsi VA, Williams ED. Medullary carcinoma. Semin Diagn Pathol 1985;2:137

243. Kakudo K, Miyauchi A, Takai S, Katayama S, Kuma K, Kitamura H. C cell carcinoma of the thyroid: papillary type. Acta Pathol Jpn 1979;29:653

244. Sambade C, Baldaque-Faria A, Cardoso-Oliveira M, Sobrinho-Simoes M. Follicular and papillary variants of medullary carcinoma of the thyroid. Pathol Res Pract 1989;184:98

245. Nieuwenhuizjen-Kruseman AC, Bosman FT, van Bergen-Henegouw JC, Cramier-Knynburg G, Brutel de la Riviere G. Medullary differentiation of anaplastic thyroid carcinoma. Am J Clin Pathol 1992;77:541

246. Kakudo K, Miyauchi A, Ogihara T, et al. Medullary carcinoma of the thyroid: giant cell type. Arch Pathol Lab Med 1978;102:445

247. Harach HR, Bergholm U. Medullary (C cell) carcinoma of the thyroid with features of follicular oxyphilic cell tumours. Histopathology 1988;13:645

248. Harach HR, Williams ED. Glandular (tubular and follicular) variants of medullary carcinoma of the thyroid. Histopathology 1983;7:83

249. Landon G, Ordonez NG. Clear cell variant of medullary carcinoma of the thyroid. Hum Pathol 1985;16:844

250. Martin-Lacavel, Gonzalez-Campora R, Moreno-Fernandez, A, Sanchez-Gallego F, Montero C, Galera-Davidson, H. Mucosubstances in medullary carcinoma of the thyroid. Histopathology 1988;13:55

251. Zaatari GS, Saigo PE, Huvos AG. Mucin production in medullary carcinoma of the thyroid. Arch Pathol Lab Med 1983;107:70

252. Beerman H, Rigaud C, Bogomoletz WV, HollanderH, Veldhuizen RW. Melanin production in black medullary thyroid carcinoma (MTC). Histopathology 1990;16:227

253. Marcus JN, Dise CA, LiVolsi VA. Melanin production in a medullary thyroid carcinoma. Cancer 1982;49:2518

254. Schroder S, Bocker W, Baisch H, et al. Prognostic factors in medullary thyroid carcinoma: survival in relation to age, sex, stage, histology, immunocytochemistry and DNA content. Cancer 1988;61:806

255. Capella C, Bordi C, Monga G et al. Multiple endocrine cell types in thyroid medullary carcinoma: evidence for calcitonin, somatostatin, ACTH, 5HT and small granule cells. Virchows Arch (A) 1978;377:111

256. Dasovic-Knezevic M, Bormer O, Holm R, Hoie J, Sobrinho-Simoes M, Nesland JM. Carcinoembryonic antigen in medullary thyroid carcinoma: an immunohistochemical study applying six novel monoclonal antibodies. Mod Pathol 1989;2:610

257. Pacini F, Elisei R, Anelli S, Basolo F, Cola A, Pinchera A. Somatostatin in medullary thyroid cancer: in vitro and in vivo studies. Cancer 1989;63:1189

258. Lippman SM, Mendelsohn G, Trump DL, Wells SA, Baylin SB. The prognostic and biological significance of cellular heterogeneity in medullary thyroid carcinoma: a study of calcitonin, L-dopa decarboxylase, and histaminase. J Clin Endocrinol Metab 1982;54:233

259. Saad MF, Ordonez NG, Rashid RK, et al. Medullary carcinoma of the thyroid: a study of the clinical features and prognostic factors in 161 patients. Medicine 1984;63:319

260. Samaan NA, Schultz PN, Hickey RC. Medullary thyroid carcinoma: Prognosis of familial versus sporadic disease and the role of radiotherapy. J Clin Endocrinol Metab 1988;67:801

261. Charib H, McConahey WM, Tregs RD, et al. Medullary thyroid carcinoma: Clinicopathologic features and longterm followup of 65 patients treated during 1946 through 1970. Mayo Clin Proc 1992;67:934

262. Komminoth P, Roth J, Saramaslani P, Matias Guiu X, Wolfe HJ, Heitz P. Polysialic acid of the neural adhesion molecule in the human thyroid: a marker for medullary thyroid carcinoma and primary C-cell hyperplasia. Am J Surg Pathol 1994;18:399

263. Feldman GL, Kambouris M, Talpos GB, Mulligan LM, Ponder BAJ, Jackson CE. Clinical value of direct DNA analysis of the RET protooncogene in families with multiple endocrine neoplasia type 2A. Surgery 1994;116:1042

264. O'Riordain DS, O'Brien T, Weaver A, et al. Medullary thyroid carcinoma in multiple endocrine neoplasia types 2A and 2B. Surgery 1994;116:1017

265. Utiger RD. Medullary thyroid carcinoma, genes and the prevention of cancer. N Engl J Med 1994;331:870

266. Weiss LM, Weinberg DS, Warhol MJ. Medullary carcinoma arising in a thyroid with Hashimoto's thyroiditis. Am J Clin Pathol 1983; 80:534

267. Bondeson L, Ljungberg O. Occult thyroid carcinoma at autopsy in Malmo, Sweden. Cancer 1981;47:319

268. Lang W, Borrusch H, Bauer L. Occult carcinoma of the thyroid: evaluation of 1020 consecutive autopsies. Am J Clin Pathol 1988; 90:72

269. White IL, Vimadalal SD, Catz B, Van de Velde R, LaGanga T. Occult medullary carcinoma of thyroid: an unusual clinical and pathological presentation. Cancer 1981;47:1364

270. Apel RL, Alpert LC, Rizzo A, LiVolsi VA, Asa SL. A metastasizing composite carcinoma of the thyroid with distinct medullary and papillary components. Arch Pathol Lab Med 1994;118:1143

271. Holm R, Sobrinho-Simoes M, Nesland JM, Sambade C, Johannessen JV. Medullary thyroid carcinoma with thyroglobulin immunoreactivity: a special entity? Lab Invest 1987;57:258

272. Kovacs CS, Mase RM, Kovacs K, Nguyen GK, Chik CL. Thyroid medullary carcinoma with thyroglobulin immunoreactivity in sporadic multiple endocrine neoplasia type 2B. Cancer 1994; 74:928

273. Lax SF, Beham A, Kronberger-Schonecker D, Langsteger W, Denk H. Coexistence of papillary and medullary carcinoma of the thyroid gland-mixed or collision tumor? Virchows Arch (A) 1994;424:441

274. Anscombe AM, Wright DH. Primary malignant lymphoma of the thyroid-a tumor of mucosa-associated lymphoid tissue: review of seventy-six cases. Histopathology 1985;9:81

275. Aozasa K, Inoue A, Tajima K, Miyauchi A, Matsuzuka F, Kuma K. Malignant lymphomas of the thyroid gland. Analysis of 79 patients with emphasis on histologic prognostic factors. Cancer 1986;58:100

276. Compagno J, Oertel JE. Malignant lymphoma and other lymphoproliferative disorders of the thyroid gland: a clinicopathologic study of 245 cases. Am J Clin Pathol 1980;74:1

277. Oertel JE, Heffess CS. Lymphoma of the thyroid and related disorders. Semin Oncol 1987;14:333

278. Hyjek E, Isaacson PG. Primary B-cell lymphoma of the thyroid and its relationship to Hashimoto's thyroiditis. Hum Pathol 1988; 19:1315

279. Aozasa K, Inoue A, Yoshimura H, et al. Intermediate lymphocytic lymphoma of the thyroid. An immunologic and immunohistologic study. Cancer 1986;57:1762

280. Faure P, Chittal S, Woodman-Memeteau F, et al. Diagnostic features of primary malignant lymphomas of the thyroid with monoclonal antibodies. Cancer 1988;61:1852

281. Aozasa K, Inoue A, Yoshimura H, Miyauchi A, Matsuzuka F, Kuma K. Plasmacytoma of the thyroid gland. Cancer 1986; 58:105

282. Kovacs CA, Mant MJ, Nguyen GK, Ginsberg J. Plasma cell lesions of the thyroid. Thyroid 1994;4:65

283. Burke JS. Histologic criteria for distinguishing between benign and malignant extranodal lymphoid infiltrates. Semin Diagn Pathol 1985;2:152

284. Hedinger CE. Sarcomas of the thyroid gland. In: Hedinger CE, ed. Thyroid cancer. Berlin: Springer-Verlag, 1969:47

285. Eusebi V, Carcangiu ML, Dina R, Rosai J. Keratin positive epithelioid angiosarcoma of thyroid: a report of four cases. Am J Surg Pathol 1990;14:737

286. Pfaltz M, Hedinger CE, Saremaslani P, Egloff B. Malignant hemangioendothelioma of the thyroid and factor VIII-related antigen. Virchows Arch (A) 1983;401:177

287. Ruchti C, Gerber HA, Schaffner T. Factor VIII-related antigen in malignant hemangioendothelioma of the thyroid: additional evidence for the endothelial origin of this tumor. Am J Clin Pathol 1984;82:474

288. Kawahara E, Nakanishi T, Terahata S, Ikegaki S. Leiomyosarcoma of the thyroid gland: a case report with a comparative study of five cases of anaplastic carcinoma. Cancer 1988; 62:2558

289. Bhagavan BS, Govinda Rao DR, Weinberg T. Carcinoma of thyroglossal duct cyst: Case reports and review of the literature. Surgery 1970;67:281

290. Boswell WC, Zoller M, Williams JS, Lord SA, Check W. Thyroglossal duct carcinoma. Am Surg 1994;60:650

291. LiVolsi VA, Perzin KH, Savetsky L. Carcinoma arising in median ectopic thyroid (including thyroglossal duct tissue). Cancer 1974;34:577

292. Devaney K, Snyder R, Norris HJ, Tavassoli FA. Proliferative struma ovarii and histologically malignant struma ovarii—a clinicopathologic study of 54 cases. Int J Gynecol Pathol 1993; 12:333

293. Snyder RR, Tavassoli FA. Ovarian strumal carcinoid: immunohistochemical, ultrastructural and clinicopathologic observations. Int J Gynecol Pathol 1986;5:187

294. Czech JM, Lichtor TR, Carneu JA, van Heeredn JA. Neoplasms metastatic to the thyroid gland. Surg Gynecol Obstet 1982; 155:503

295. Green LK, Ro JY, Mackay B, Ayala AG, Luna MA. Renal cell carcinoma metastatic to the thyroid. Cancer 1989;63:1810

FOUR

Thyroid Diseases: Thyrotoxicosis

Werner and Ingbar's The Thyroid, Seventh Edition,
edited by Lewis E. Braverman and Robert D. Utiger.
Lippincott–Raven Publishers, Philadelphia, © 1996

Section A
Introduction

29

Introduction to Thyrotoxicosis

Lewis E. Braverman
Robert D. Utiger

This chapter introduces the section on thyrotoxicosis, a common and important thyroid disorder. It has multiple causes, and its recognition and management are important components of endocrine practice.

We use the term thyrotoxicosis to mean the clinical syndrome of hypermetabolism that results when the serum concentrations of free thyroxine (T_4), free triiodothyronine (T_3), or both are increased. The term hyperthyroidism is used to mean sustained increases in thyroid hormone biosynthesis and secretion by the thyroid gland. Thus, the terms thyrotoxicosis and hyperthyroidism are not synonymous. Although many patients with thyrotoxicosis have hyperthyroidism, others—for example, those in whom thyrotoxicosis is caused by thyroiditis or exogenous thyroid hormone administration—do not.

The clinical manifestations of thyrotoxicosis are, for the most part, independent of its cause. However, certain features of the illness often provide clues about the cause of thyrotoxicosis in an individual patient. These features include the duration of thyrotoxicosis, the size and shape of the thyroid gland, and the presence or absence of the extrathyroidal manifestations of Graves' disease. An attempt should be made to determine the cause of thyrotoxicosis in all patients, whether it is done by clinical examination or laboratory studies, because knowledge of the cause determines prognosis and guides therapy.

The causes of thyrotoxicosis can be subdivided into the disorders that are associated with hyperthyroidism and those that are not (Table 29-1). All of these disorders are discussed in detail in the following chapters. Among the causes of spontaneously occurring thyrotoxicosis, Graves' disease is the most common; its frequency as the cause of thyrotoxicosis ranges from approximately 60% to 90% in different regions of the world. Most of the remaining cases are caused by toxic nodular goiter, autonomously functioning thyroid adenomas (toxic adenomas), or the several types of thyroiditis.[1-3] Except for exogenous thyrotoxicosis, the other causes of thyrotoxicosis are rare.[4-6]

Although many patients with thyrotoxicosis have overt clinical and biochemical disease, thyrotoxicosis may be subclinical. Subclinical thyrotoxicosis is defined as normal serum free T_4 and T_3 concentrations and low serum thyrotropin (TSH) concentrations; the patients may or may not have symptoms of thyrotoxicosis, but if present, the symptoms are mild and nonspecific (see chap 88). The causes of overt and subclinical thyrotoxicosis are similar, but the most common cause of subclinical thyrotoxicosis is exogenous thyroid hormone administration rather than Graves' disease. Whether and how patients with subclinical thyrotoxicosis should be treated, excluding those who can be treated by decreasing the dosage of thyroid hormone, are controversial issues.

TABLE 29-1.
Causes of Thyrotoxicosis

Type of Thyrotoxicosis	Pathogenic Mechanism
COMMON CAUSES	
THYROTOXICOSIS ASSOCIATED WITH HYPERTHYROIDISM*	
Production of abnormal thyroid stimulator (Graves' disease)	TSH receptor antibodies
Intrinsic thyroid autonomy	
Toxic adenoma	Benign tumor
Toxic multinodular goiter	Foci of functional autonomy
THYROTOXICOSIS NOT ASSOCIATED WITH HYPERTHYROIDISM†	
Inflammatory disease	
Silent thyroiditis‡	Release of stored hormones
Subacute thyroiditis	Release of stored hormones
Extrathyroidal source of thyroid hormone	
Exogenous hormone	Hormone in medication or food
UNCOMMON CAUSES	
THYROTOXICOSIS ASSOCIATED WITH HYPERTHYROIDISM*	
Production of thyroid stimulators	
TSH hypersecretion	Thyrotroph adenoma
	Thyrotroph resistance to T_4
Trophoblastic tumor	Chorionic gonadotropin
Hyperemesis gravidarum	Chorionic gonadotropin
Intrinsic thyroid autonomy	
Thyroid carcinoma	Foci of functional autonomy
Nonautoimmune autosomal dominant hyperthyroidism	Constitutive activation of TSH receptors
Struma ovarii†	Toxic adenoma in a dermoid tumor of ovary
Drug-induced hyperthyroidism	
Iodine and iodine-containing drugs and radiographic contrast agents†	Iodine excess plus thyroid autonomy
Lithium	? Thyroid autonomy
THYROTOXICOSIS NOT ASSOCIATED WITH HYPERTHYROIDISM†	
Inflammatory disease	
Drug-induced thyroiditis (amiodarone, interferon-α)	Release of stored hormone
Infarction of thyroid adenoma	Release of stored hormone
Radiation thyroiditis	Release of stored hormone

Thyroid radioiodine uptake high.
†*Thyroid radioiodine uptake low.*
‡*Including postpartum thyroiditis.*

The more common clinical manifestations of thyrotoxicosis are listed in Table 29-2, and they are discussed in detail in the following chapters. None of the clinical manifestations is specific; it is usually the combination of several of them that brings to mind the possibility of the disorder in a particular patient. The frequency and severity of these symptoms and signs vary considerably among patients; some patients have only a few symptoms or signs and others many, and their severity varies widely. The clinical findings that point to a particular disorder as a cause of thyrotoxicosis are shown in Table 29-3.

Among the factors that determine the manifestations of thyrotoxicosis are the age of the patient[7] and the presence of concomitant disturbances in the function of one or another organ system, so that the impact of thyrotoxicosis is either enhanced or diminished. For example, as compared with younger patients, older patients have fewer symptoms and signs of sympathetic activation, such as anxiety, hyperactivity, and tremor, and more symptoms and signs of cardiovascular dysfunction, such as dyspnea and atrial fibrillation. The extent and severity of the clinical manifestations of thyrotoxicosis are not strongly correlated with its biochemical severity.[8]

TABLE 29-2.
Common Clinical Manifestations of Thyrotoxicosis

SYMPTOMS

Nervousness

Fatigue

Weakness

Increased perspiration

Heat intolerance

Tremor

Hyperactivity

Palpitation

Appetite change (usually increase)

Weight change (usually loss)

Menstrual disturbances

GENERAL SIGNS

Hyperactivity

Tachycardia or atrial arrhythmia

Systolic hypertension

Warm, moist, smooth skin

Stare and eyelid retraction

Tremor

Hyperreflexia

Muscle weakness

TABLE 29-3.
Clinical Manifestations of the Common Causes of Thyrotoxicosis

Symptom and Sign	Cause
Diffuse goiter	Graves' disease, silent thyroiditis
Uninodular goiter	Thyroid autonomy
Multinodular goiter	Thyroid autonomy
Thyroid pain and tenderness	Subacute thyroiditis
Ophthalmopathy	Graves' disease
Localized myxedema	Graves' disease

It is now easy to obtain biochemical confirmation of thyrotoxicosis by measurements of serum TSH and direct or indirect measurements of the serum concentrations of free T_4, free T_3, or both. In contrast, use of biochemical tests to determine the cause of thyrotoxicosis is much less convenient and reliable, and fortunately it is not routinely necessary. Finally, while the various antithyroid treatments available effectively ameliorate hyperthyroidism and therefore thyrotoxicosis, preferences for them vary widely,[9] and none are ideal because they do not address the fundamental abnormality that causes thyrotoxicosis in most patients.

References

1. Brownlie BEW, Wells JE. The epidemiology of thyrotoxicosis in New Zealand: incidence and geographical distribution in North Canterbury, 1983–1985. Clin Endocrinol 1990;33:249

2. Reinwein D, Benker G, Konig MP, Pinchera A, Schatz H, Schleusner A. The different types of hyperthyroidism in Europe. Results of a prospective study of 924 patients. J Endocrinol Invest 1988;11:193

3. Williams I, Ankrett VO, Lazarus JH, Volpe R. Aetiology of hyperthyroidism in Canada and Wales. J Epidemiol Comm Health 1983;37:245

4. Kasagi K, Takeuchi R, Miyamoto S, et al. Metastatic thyroid cancer presenting as thyrotoxicosis. Clin Endocrinol 1994;40:429

5. Barclay ML, Brownlie BEW, Turner JG, Wells JE. Lithium associated thyrotoxicosis: a report of 14 cases, with statistical analysis of incidence. Clin Endocrinol 1994;40:759

6. Duprez L, Parma J, Van Sande J, et al. Germline mutations in the thyrotropin receptor gene cause non-autoimmune autosomal dominant hyperthyroidism. Nature Genetics 1994;7:396

7. Nordyke RA, Gilbert FI Jr, Harada ASM. Graves' disease: influence of age on clinical findings. Arch Intern Med 1988;148:626

8. Trzepacz PT, Klein I, Robert M, Greenhouse J, Levey GS. Graves' disease: an analysis of thyroid hormone levels and hyperthyroid signs and symptoms. Am J Med 1989;87:558

9. Solomon B, Glinoer D, Lagasse R, Wartofsky L. Current trends in the management of Graves' disease. J Clin Endocrinol Metab 1990;70:1518

Werner and Ingbar's The Thyroid, Seventh Edition,
edited by Lewis E. Braverman and Robert D. Utiger.
Lippincott–Raven Publishers, Philadelphia, © 1996

Section B
Causes of Thyrotoxicosis

30

Graves' Disease

THE PATHOGENESIS OF GRAVES' DISEASE

Terry F. Davies

INTRODUCTION

Graves' disease is an autoimmune disease, and in recent years much has occurred to further our understanding of autoimmune mechanisms.[1-3] The importance of thyroid autoantibodies, especially thyrotropin (TSH) receptor autoantibodies, and the concept of genetic susceptibility are discussed in chapters 21 and 27, respectively. This chapter will concentrate on the pathogenesis of Graves' disease as we currently understand it. In Graves' disease, both B- and T-lymphocytes are known to be directed at the three well known thyroid autoantigens, thyroglobulin (Tg), thyroid peroxidase (TPO), and the TSH receptor (TSHR). However, evidence suggests that it is the TSHR itself which is the primary autoantigen of Graves' disease.

Definition of an Autoantigen

There are a number of simple rules concerning the self-molecules with which T cells and autoantibodies interact. Autoantigens are not unique structures and there is no example of an antigen of abnormal structure being the cause of the abnormal immune response. In fact, autoantigens are often highly conserved structural proteins coded for by genes with low muta-

tion rates. Autoantigens are also present from birth and do not appear later during development. Their molecular recognition sites, the epitopes, for autoantibodies and T cells usually differ, and immunization of animals with the antigen induces a specific T-cell and B-cell response.

Antibody and T-Cell Interactions with Antigen

Immunoglobulins, whether in the free state or when expressed on the surface of B cells, are able to bind to antigenic molecules directly. The strength of this binding, or the affinity of the antibody, is dependent to a large degree on the number of antigen binding sites on the antibody (Fig. 30-1). Hence, the binding energy is greater for nonlinear antigens than for the binding to a small linear antigen.[4] Pathogenic antibodies of high affinity are, therefore, most likely to interact with nonlinear antigens. The T-cell antigen receptor is also a member of the immunoglobulin family, except that it has a transmembrane domain that anchors it within the cell surface.[5] In contrast to immunoglobulins, T cells interact with a complex of antigen and HLA molecule (Fig. 30-2). The CD8+ T cells recognize antigens complexed with HLA class I molecules (A,C,B) and CD4+ T cells recognize antigen with HLA class II molecules (DR,DP,DQ). T cells are able to recognize small linear peptides as long as they are complexed with an HLA molecule and, therefore, are termed "HLA restricted" and will only interact with the appropriate HLA molecule.[6] Hence, thyroid antigens are engulfed by antigen-presenting cells (APCs) such as macrophages and then digested within these cells. Antigen breakdown products (peptides) are then bound

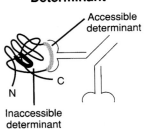

Conformational Determinant

Linear Determinant

Accessible determinant

Inaccessible determinant

FIGURE 30-1. Antigen–antibody interactions. (*Left*) An IgG antibody interacts with a conformational (nonlinear) determinant involving noncontiguous parts of the antigen. (*Right*) An IgG antibody reacts with a linear (accessible) determinant; an inaccessible determinant is buried within the antigen. (Adapted from Abbas AK, Lichtman AH, Pober JS. Anonymous cellular and molecular immunology. Philadelphia, WB Saunders, 1991)

to HLA molecules and the complexes are transported onto the cell surface.

Second Signals

Both B cells and T cells rely on secondary signals once antigen has been identified in order to enter a proliferative and secretory state.[7] A variety of cytokines serve as second B-cell signals, whereas the most important T-cell second signals appear to be a family of cell-surface molecules (the B7 family) found on APCs such as macrophages and dendritic cells. B cells and T cells that interact with specific antigen in the absence of a second signal become desensitized; a state referred to as *anergy*. Hence, anergy is one of the mechanisms used for controlling and suppressing the immune response.

Criteria for an Autoimmune Disease

The original criteria for an autoimmune disease were the need for an antibody or cell-mediated response, an identified corresponding antigen, and the induction of an analogous autoimmune response in experimental animals.[8] However, a secondary immune response may also meet these criteria.[9] Three types of evidence need to be marshalled to establish that a human disease is autoimmune in origin:

1. Direct evidence from transfer of pathogenic antibody or pathogenic T cells
2. Indirect evidence based on studies in experimental animals
3. Circumstantial evidence from clinical studies

In Graves' disease the antibody and cell-mediated thyroid antigen-specific immune responses are well defined, but there are no animal models of Graves' disease. Nevertheless, the induction of thyroid hyperfunction by TSHR antibodies in normal subjects by the transfer of serum from patients with Graves' disease[10] and the passive transfer of TSHR antibodies to the fetus in pregnant women[11] serve as major examples of the type of direct proof needed to illustrate immune mechanisms in human autoimmune disease.

Restriction vs. Polyclonality

Much effort has been expended in recent years to learn whether autoimmune reactions are multireactive and representative of a secondary polyclonal immune response, or whether the immune response is much more focused, involving a restricted number of B cells and T cells.[1] In an autoimmune disease, the immune system is where the abnormality is to be found and, therefore, the primary autoimmune response at the onset of the disease should be restricted. This has, indeed, proven to be the case for most of the human autoimmune diseases. We discuss below some of the evidence for this as it relates to Graves' disease.

THE INTRATHYROIDAL LYMPHOCYTIC INFILTRATE

Much of the early evidence that Graves' disease is an autoimmune disease was based on the discovery of TSHR antibodies. However, supporting evidence could have been found much earlier in the thyroid gland itself. The thyroid in Graves' disease is characterized by a nonhomogeneous lymphocytic infiltration in addition to thyroid follicular hyperplasia[12] (Fig. 30-3). Antithyroid drug treatment may markedly reduce the degree of lymphocytic infiltration, which should be kept in mind when examining individual patient samples.[13]

Immunohistochemistry

Although the intrathyroidal lymphocyte population is mixed, immunohistologic staining has shown that the majority of cells

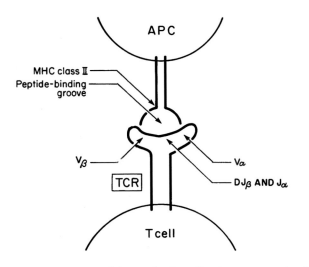

FIGURE 30-2. Diagram of the mechanism of antigen presentation by an antigen-presenting cell (APC) to the T-cell antigen receptor (TCR) of a T-cell.

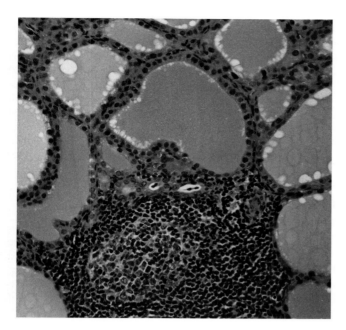

FIGURE 30-3. Histologic section from a patient with Graves' disease shows the patchy lymphocytic infiltrate that is characteristic of the disease.

TABLE 30-1.
Phenotypic Characteristics of Intrathyroidal T Cells*

T-Cell Subset	Thyroid (%)	PBMC (%)
CD2+	47 ± 11	
CD4+	18 ± 4	
CD8+	25 ± 6	
CD4:CD8	**0.7 ± 0.1**	**2.9 ± 10**
% CD4+ CD29+	85 ± 3	
% CD4+ CD45RA+	41 ± 5	
CD29:CD45RA+	**2.6 ± 1.0**	**8.2 ± 2.0**
Activated (DR+)	19 ± 5	

Note that the number of CD8+ T cells within the thyroid glands was high and that the CD29+ cells (helper-inducer, memory-type T cells) make up the majority of CD4+ T cells. Double-positive CD4+ cells caused the total of stained cells to be >100%.
The results (mean ± SE) were derived from the analysis of thyroid tissue from five patients with Graves' disease glands.
PBMC, peripheral blood mononuclear cells.
(Martin A, Goldsmith NK, Friedman EW, Schwartz AE, Davies TF, Roman SH. Intrathyroidal accumulation of T-cell phenotypes in autoimmune thyroid disease. Autoimmunity 1990;6:269–281)

are T cells and that B-cell germinal centers are much less common than in chronic autoimmune thyroiditis.[14] Intra-epithelial T cells and plasma cells can be seen both adjacent to and within the thyroid follicles.[14–16] Follicular epithelial cell size has been correlated with the intensity of the local infiltrate, which suggests local thyroid cell stimulation by TSHR antibodies.[17] Within the T-cell population, there is sometimes a preponderance of memory T cells, but this can be quite variable from patient to patient. However, activated B-cells and T cells are more frequent in intrathyroidal lymphocyte cultures than peripheral blood cultures (Table 30-1).

B CELLS AND TSH RECEPTOR ANTIBODIES

B-Cell Function

The B cells that accumulate within the thyroid gland of patients with Graves' disease have reduced proliferative responses to B-cell mitogens and greater basal immunoglobulin secretion than peripheral blood B cells.[18] B cells from Graves' thyroid tissue may also secrete thyroid autoantibodies spontaneously in vitro, implying pre-activation. Hence, the thyroid gland is a primary site of thyroid autoantibody secretion in autoimmune thyroid disease, perhaps best described by studies in mice with severe combined immunodeficiency (SCID) (Fig. 30-4). Transplantation of Graves' thyroid tissue into T-cell and B-cell deficient SCID mice results in the detection of human thyroid autoantibodies in the serum of the recipient mice.[19] Additional evidence comes from direct animal models of thyroiditis and, indirectly, from the decline in thyroid autoantibodies after antithyroid drug treatment,[20,21] thyroidectomy, and radioiodine therapy.[22] However, in long-

term studies of post-thyroidectomy patients and patients who received radioiodine treatment, some patients had no decline in serum antithyroid antibody concentrations, implying there must be additional important extrathyroidal sources of production.

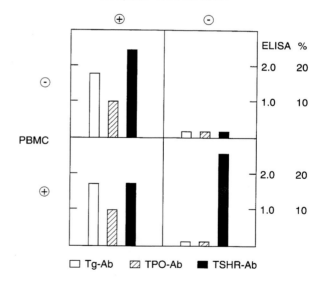

FIGURE 30-4. Production of antibodies in mice with subacute combined immunodeficiency disease (SCID) after thyroid tissue engraftment or intraperitoneal injection of peripheral blood mononuclear cells (PBMC) from a patient undergoing surgery for the treatment of Graves' disease. Thyroid antibodies were measured in mouse serum 4 to 6 weeks after transplantation. In the absence of thyroid tissue and PBMC, no thyroid antibodies were detectable *(upper right)*. In contrast, transplantation of thyroid tissue resulted in the production of Tg, TPO, and TSH receptor (TSH-R) antibodies (Ab) by the mice.

Autoantibodies to the Human TSH Receptor

Long-acting thyroid stimulator (LATS) was discovered by Adams and Purves[23] almost 40 years ago during a search for thyroid-stimulating activity in the serum of patients with Graves' disease using a bioassay for pituitary TSH (see chap 21). The patient's serum stimulated radioiodine release from the prelabeled thyroid glands of guinea pigs for a much longer time period than did a pituitary TSH preparation. This prolonged stimulating activity was then found to reside in the IgG fraction of serum. With the advent of biologically active radiolabeled TSH, it became possible to detect TSH receptors on thyroid membranes, and subsequently this IgG activity was found to compete with TSH for receptor occupancy[24] and was indeed a TSHR antibody acting as a TSH agonist. Hence, in patients with Graves' disease, the thyroid gland is no longer under the control of pituitary TSH but is continuously stimulated by circulating antibodies with TSH-like activity.

Bioactivity of TSHR Antibodies

Antibodies that bind to the TSH receptor may or may not initiate an intracellular signal transduction process (Fig. 30-5) and may, therefore, be either TSHR-stimulating or TSHR-blocking antibodies.[25] Further complicating this issue has been the observation of the simultaneous presence of TSHR-stimulating and TSHR-blocking antibodies in the same serum samples with the effective degree of thyroid stimulation dependent on the relative concentration and bioactivities of the different antibodies.[26] The original self-infusion of serum from patients with Graves' disease by Adams and colleagues and the resulting thyroid stimulation[10] was the first evidence for the role of TSHR antibodies in the induction of hyperthyroidism in humans. Another early demonstration of the in vivo effects of TSHR antibodies came from studies demonstrating stimulation of the thyroid in neonates by transplacental passage of TSHR antibodies from their mothers.[11]

Prevalence of TSHR Antibodies in Graves' Disease

TSHR antibodies are detectable only in patients with autoimmune thyroid disease. Such antibodies are, therefore, disease-specific, in great contrast to the high prevalence of Tg and TPO antibodies in normal subjects. Furthermore, TSHR antibodies are unique human antibodies; there are no animal models of TSHR antibodies or of Graves' disease. Eighty percent to 100% of untreated patients with thyrotoxicosis caused by Graves' disease have detectable TSHR antibodies that are biologically active in their serum. The titers of TSHR antibodies are altered by treatment of thyrotoxicosis[13] (see chap 53) and when present in higher concentrations may predict the response to antithyroid drug treatment.[27,28] TSHR-blocking antibodies may in time become the more prevalent antibody after treatment of thyrotoxic patients with Graves' disease.

Immunologic Characteristics of TSHR Antibodies

TSHR antibodies in many patients with Graves' disease demonstrate light chain restriction,[29] and the TSH agonist bioactivity is found mostly in the IgG_1 subclass, again suggesting oligoclonality.[30] This evidence of a pauciclonal B-cell response is in contrast to the variable biologic nature of the antibodies when examined in vitro. However, TSHR antibody V genes have not yet been analyzed, and it remains unclear how restricted the B-cell immune response is in Graves' disease.

TSHR Antibody Epitopes

The cloning of the TSHR has permitted the initiation of detailed studies of its epitopes and structure—function relationships.[31–33] The extracellular domain of the TSHR is the major immunogenic region, and TSHR antibodies bind to this domain of the receptor (see Fig. 30-5). The difference in functional activity of different TSHR antibodies may relate to molecular binding characteristics dependent on conformational changes and affinity. The extracellular domain of prokaryotic TSHR has been used to identify immunogenic regions in the extracellular domain of the human TSHR in both immunized mice and patients with Graves' disease.[34] The results suggest that some TSHR antibodies also recognize linear epitopes and, therefore, lack a conformational requirement (see Fig. 30-1).

TSH Receptor Regulation in Graves' Disease

Like TSH, TSH stimulating antibodies cause cAMP-mediated release of thyroid hormone and Tg; and they stimulate iodine uptake, protein synthesis, and thyroid growth. Although desensitization of the thyroidal cAMP response by prolonged exposure to TSHR antibodies occurs in vitro, this cannot occur in vivo or patients would not remain hyperthyroid.[35,36] In fact, hyperthyroid patients clearly have little desensitization of their thyroid glands. This dichotomy is most likely explained as a dose effect, with very high concentrations of TSH or TSHR antibodies being necessary for desensitization. At lower levels of stimulation, there is good evidence for positive regulation of the TSH receptor by TSH both in vivo and in vitro[37,38]; resistance to desensitization by lower concentrations of TSH antibodies will allow the hyperthyroid state to persist.

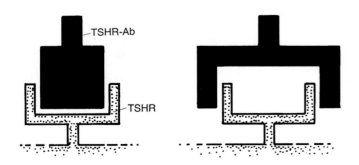

FIGURE 30-5. TSH-R antibodies may act as TSH agonists *(left)* or antagonists *(right)*, depending on their interaction with the TSH receptor.

Other Thyroid Antibodies in Graves' Disease

The majority of patients with Graves' disease have circulating antibodies to other autoantigens, particularly Tg and TPO. Since these antibodies are polyclonal in nature,[39] and the role of TSHR antibodies is so important in the disease, the anti-Tg and anti-TPO antibodies appear to have little role in disease etiology. However, they are likely to be markers for susceptibility to clinical thyroid disease. Indeed, Graves' disease may develop on a background of autoimmune thyroiditis and many patients will become hypothyroid in time, even if they do not receive thyrodestructive therapy.

THE PRIMARY ROLE OF T CELLS

The Nature of T Cells

The T cells that survive intrathymic deletion and appear in the peripheral circulation are a complex mixture of cells of different phenotype. Both CD4+ and CD8+ cells consist of many subsets and a full discussion of them is not possible here. To complicate matters further, many T cells are in transition between immature and mature forms, and this may occur within an autoimmune infiltrate.[14] However, biologic function is probably more important than phenotype. On the whole, the CD4+ cells tend to be regulatory cells and the CD8+ cells tend to be cytotoxic cells capable of lysing target cells. Many T cells exert their function by the secretion of cytokines. In general, CD4+ cells, when stimulated by bacterial antigens, secrete interleukin-2 (IL-2), γ-interferon, and tumor necrosis factor-β, a so-called Th1 helper-type response.[40] In contrast, stimulation with allergens results in the development of CD4+ cells that secrete IL-4 and IL-5 but not γ-interferon; this is the Th2 regulatory response.

Analysis of Intrathyroidal T Cells

T cells in patients with autoimmune thyroid disease are reactive to processed thyroid antigens (as peptides)[41–45] (see Fig. 30-2). Such activated T cells enhance antibody (anti-Tg, anti-TPO, and TSHR antibody) secretion and have helper, regulatory, and cytotoxic T-cell activity. About 10% of activated T cells infiltrating the thyroid gland in patients with autoimmune thyroid disease proliferate in response to thyroid cell antigens.[46] In Graves' disease the intrathyroidal T-cell clones are more than 75% CD45RO+ (memory T cells), with considerable T-cell helper activity[47] (Table 30-2).In support of the concept that the functional role of T cells in Graves' disease is primarily a helper role rather than a suppressor or cytotoxic cell role is the failure to characterize a T-cell clone as specifically cytolytic to autologous thyroid cells in patients with Graves' disease, whereas this has been accomplished in patients with chronic autoimmune thyroiditis.[48] Although characterization of intrathyroidal T cells from patients with Graves' disease as Th1 or Th2 helper T-cell subsets has been difficult,[49] they are known to secrete considerable amounts of δ-interferon, suggesting that most of the CD4+ T cells may be Th1.[50,51]

The T-Cell Receptor V Gene Repertoire

Most T-cell antigen receptors on the surface of T cells consist of two noncovalently linked chains (α and β), each with variable (V), diversity (D) (mainly β), and junctional (J) regions with common constant (Cα and Cβ) regions (see Figs. 30-2 and 30-6). Other T cells of uncertain function have γ/δ receptors. The V, D, and J genes code for the antigen-HLA recognition site on the T-cell antigen receptor, affording antigen specificity. In addition to the many V (>100) and J (>50) genes present in the genome, random nucleotide (N) additions and deletions to the D region add immense complexity to the T-cell antigen receptor repertoire[5,52] causing this region, referred to as the *third complementarity determining region* (CDR3), to be of prime importance in antigen recognition.

The Intrathyroidal T-Cell Repertoire

As discussed earlier, restricted heterogeneity of T-cell antigen receptor V-gene families in an autoimmune disease would implicate the T cells as etiologic. In order to examine the T-cell antigen receptor V gene use for T-cell antigen receptors among intrathyroidal T cells, the polymerase chain reaction (PCR) has been used with multiple oligonucleotide amplimers to test for the Vα and Vβ families used by intrathyroidal T cells from patients with Graves' disease[53,54] (Fig. 30-7). The results demonstrated bias in V gene utilization by T cells from within the thyroid as compared with peripheral blood from the same patient. Evidence was also sought for clonally expanded T-cell populations within the thyroid gland of patients by direct sequencing of the CDR3 regions of the T-cell antigen receptors of intrathyroidal T cells generated by PCR. The most prominent V-gene families were indeed representative of clonally expanded T cells, based on the evidence of multiple identical sequences within the generated fragments.[55,56] Such information supports the concept of restricted T-cell heterogeneity in Graves' disease and points to the primacy of T-cells in disease etiology. A similar situation has been observed in rheumatoid arthritis, multiple sclerosis, and a variety of other autoimmune diseases.[57,58] We and others, therefore, have suggested that highly restricted T-cell responses occur early in autoimmune disease, but that as the pathologic process progresses the response is less restricted, secondary to "determinant spreading."[54,59,60]

Suppressor Effects of T Cells

The reduced numbers of circulating CD8+ T cells in patients with Graves' hyperthyroidism support the possibility that lack of suppressor/cytotoxic T cells might be responsible for the breakdown of tolerance in Graves' disease.[61] Earlier studies had led to the suggestion that the production of thyroid antibodies was due to a defect in thyroid-antigen specific suppressor T cells.[62] Whether true antigen-specific human suppressor T cells commonly exist is uncertain,[63] but there is no doubt that the immune system exerts some of its overall control via "suppression." This suppression can occur in a variety of ways, including via cytokines and "anergized" T cells. Although antigen-specific suppressor T-cell factors have been hypothesized, there is no evidence for such a factor in Graves' disease. Indeed, sufficient other mechanisms exist to

Table 30-2
Characteristics of Intrathyroidal T-Cell Clones*

Source	No.	CD4+ (%)	CD8+ (%)	MLR (%)	Thyroid (%)	Cytotoxic (%)
PBMC	21	100	0	55	0	ND
Graves'	21	75	25	50	33	0
Hashimoto's	36	41	58	55	11	14

*Data are expressed as percentage of cells exhibiting autologous mixed lymphocyte reactions (MLR), proliferation in response to crude thyroid antigen (thyroid), or lysis of autologous thyroid cells (cytotoxic).
PBMC, peripheral blood mononuclear cells.
(Data from Mackenzie WA, Schwartz AE, Friedman EW, Davies TF. Intrathyroidal T-cell clones from patients with autoimmune thyroid disease. J Clin Endocrinol Metab 1987;64:818–824)*

explain antigen-specific tolerance. Positive and negative selection of immature T cells and B cells occurs in the thymus, and deletion of immature immune cells also occurs in the peripheral immune system.[64,65] Deletion probably occurs when immature T cells and B cells bind antigen in the absence of second signals, as discussed earlier. In contrast, when mature immune cells bind antigen in the absence of second signals, they may be desensitized rather than deleted (the phenomenon of anergy). Together, deletion and anergy may be sufficient to account for immune suppression. Anergized T cells have potent suppressive actions and may act as regulatory cells.[66] It is also important to note that certain HLA-DR haplotypes confer a reduced nonspecific suppressor T-cell function. For example, normal subjects with HLA-DR3[67,68] have reduced suppressor T-cell activity as compared with non-DR3 subjects. Since many patients with Graves' disease are HLA-DR3, data regarding suppressor T-cell activity obtained without HLA typing of patients and normal subjects cannot be fairly interpreted.

IMMUNE MECHANISMS IN THE PATHOGENESIS OF GRAVES' DISEASE

A number of possible explanations for the onset of Graves' disease can be hypothesized on the basis of how the immune system works (Table 30-3). Here we review some of these possibilities and the evidence for or against involvement with Graves' disease.

Self-Antigen Expression

Viral infection may lead to the virus becoming a persistent endogenous antigen or to exposure of previously unexposed antigens. For example, transgenic mice expressing LCM virus antigens in pancreatic beta cells, when challenged with LCM virus, developed lymphocytic infiltrates in their beta cells and then diabetes mellitus.[69] Expression of retroviral protein has been detected in thyroid tissue from patients with autoimmune thyroid disease but confirmation has not been forthcoming (see the section on infection below).

Specificity Crossover

Structural similarity between antigens encoded by different genes can lead to crossover of specificity (molecular mimicry). Antigenic similarity between infectious agents and host cell proteins is common, and in one analysis of 600 monoclonal antibodies raised against a large variety of viruses, 4% of the monoclonal antibodies cross-reacted with host determinants expressed in uninfected tissues.[70] Mice infected with reovirus type 1 develop an autoimmune polyendocrinopathy and generate antibodies directed against normal pancreas, pituitary,

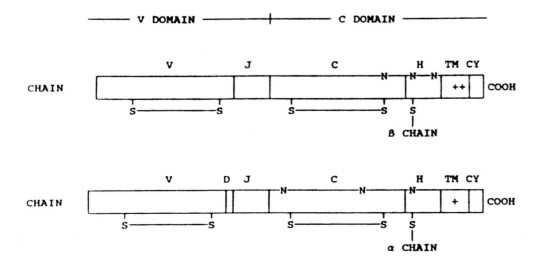

FIGURE 30-6. The structure of the α and β polypeptide chains of the T-cell antigen receptor. V is the variable region, D the diversity segment, J the joining segment, C the constant region, H the hinge region, TM the transmembrane region, and CY the cytoplasmic domain. (Adapted from Bona CA, Siminovitch KA, Zanetti M, Theofilopoulos AN. The molecular pathology of autoimmune diseases. Chur, Switzerland: Harwood Acedemic, 1993)

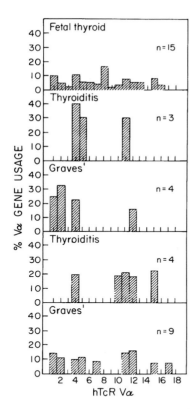

FIGURE 30-7. Results of Southern blot analyses of thyroid tissue from a normal fetus, two patients with Graves' disease, and two patients with autoimmune thyroiditis. Results are shown as densitometric measurements of Vα gene fragments. Note the reduced V gene use in the tissue from the four patients as compared with the widespread use in very vascular fetal thyroid. n, number of V gene families detected.

thyroid, and gastric mucosa, which suggests antigenic similarity between a retroviral antigen and a tissue antigen expressed in multiple endocrine tissues.[71] Molecular mimicry has also been reported between *Yersinia enterocolitica* and TSHR, based on the cross-reaction between *Yersinia* and serum from patients with Graves' disease as well as between retroviral sequences and the TSH receptor.[72]

Superantigens

Superantigens are potent T-cell stimulatory molecules that bind to major histocompatibility complex (MHC) class II molecules. The complex of MHC molecules and superantigen is recognized by particular T cells, that are then activated and may be deleted. Individual superantigens activate a restricted proportion of T cells, which is determined by the T-cell antigen receptor V gene used.[73] Superantigens stimulate T cells exclusively via the V-β chain of the T-cell antigen receptor by binding to the MHC molecules at the external surface of their β-pleated sheets. This reaction activates T-cell clones expressing only that specific V-β chain.[74] Superantigenic stimulation of a V-β specific T-cell clone can lead to stimulation, anergy, or deletion of that particular clone, depending on the developmental state of the T cell.[73] Superantigens may be extrinsic or intrinsic. Extrinsic superantigens currently constitute a group

of bacterial toxins (e.g., staphylococcal, streptococcal, and mycoplasmal toxins). Intrinsic superantigens have so far been reported only in mice, in which they comprise the minor lymphocyte-stimulating antigens encoded by several endogenous murine retroviruses.[73] In persons in whom the T-cell repertoire includes low concentrations of autoreactive T cells, stimulation by a superantigen may obliterate any tolerance mechanisms and may activate these autoreactive T cells to proliferate and cause tissue injury.[74] However, no common preferential use of particular V genes of the T-cell antigen receptor has yet been found in thyroid tissue from patients with Graves' disease.

The Idiotypic Network

Auto-anti-idiotypic antibodies and T-suppressor cells are generated in the course of the normal immune response to a foreign invading pathogen, and serve to regulate the normal immune response.[75] Anti-idiotypic antibodies produced in response to an exogenous pathogen during the primary immune response carry the internal image of the epitopes on the pathogen that binds to its receptor in the host. Consequently, the development of receptor-binding anti-idiotypes can be harmful to the host and initiate autoimmunity (reviewed in reference 76). Alterations in the idiotypic network have been implicated in the pathogenesis of Graves' disease, based on the findings that immunization of animals with TSH led to the development of anti-idiotypic antibodies that recognized and were able to activate TSH receptors.[77] Furthermore, formation of monoclonal antibodies to the TSHR with TSH agonist activity have been reported after TSH immunization. However, there is no evidence that the majority of TSHR antibodies in patients with Graves' disease are anti-idiotypic in their derivation.

TABLE 30-3.
Potential Pathogenic Mechanisms in Graves' Disease

IMMUNE MECHANISMS

Self-antigen expression of a viral antigen or a previously hidden antigen

Specificity crossover between different self antigens or with an infectious agent

Superantigenic alteration of the T-cell repertoire

Idiotypic antibodies becoming pathogenic autoantibodies

Heat shock proteins as the autoantigen

New expression of HLA class II antigens on thyroid epithelial cells

PRECIPITATING FACTORS

Infection

Stress

Sex steroids

GENETIC SUSCEPTIBILITY

HLA genes

Non-HLA genes (eg, sex, polymorphisms of T-cell antigen receptors)

Heat Shock Proteins

Heat shock protein synthesis can be induced not only by heat shock but also by other stressful stimuli, including exposure to oxidative radicals, alcohol, heavy metals, anoxia, or infection, and are produced in small quantities under normal conditions. Heat shock proteins are immunogenic, and bacterial infection can induce an antibody and T-cell response to microbial heat shock proteins.[78] These antibodies and T cells may then cross-react with self-cellular heat shock proteins containing conserved epitopes. Heat shock protein 72 has recently been demonstrated to be expressed in thyroid tissue from patients with Graves' disease but not in that from normal subjects,[79] which implies that Graves' disease is associated with an autoimmune response to certain heat shock proteins,[80] although indirect factors may also be responsible.

Nonimmune Cell Expression of MHC Molecules

HLA-DR molecules are expressed on thyroid cells from patients with autoimmune thyroid disease but not in the cells from normal subjects[81,82] (Fig. 30-8). A local viral infection could stimulate production of γ-interferon or other cytokines by thyroid follicular cells that, in turn, induce expression of HLA class II molecules on these cells, leading to presentation of autoantigens and activation of autoreactive T cells. Indeed, in vivo induction of MHC class II molecules on thyroid follicular cells by γ-interferon can induce autoimmune thyroiditis in susceptible mice.[83] Viruses are also known to be able to induce the expression of class II MHC molecules directly and independently of cytokine secretion.[84] Cultured rat thyroid cells infected with reovirus types 1 and 3 express MHC class II antigens in a dose-dependent manner in the absence of T cells.[85] Cytomegalovirus (CMV) infection of primary cultures of human thyroid cells also result in induction of HLA-DR expression on the cells.[86]

Thyroid Cells as Antigen-Presenting Cells

Cells that express HLA molecules have the potential of presenting antigen directly to T cells (see Fig. 30-2; Table 30-4). Thyroid follicular cells bearing such determinants can present preprocessed viral peptide antigens to cloned human T cells.[87] In addition, thyroid antigen-specific T-cell clones react specifically with cloned autologous thyroid cells in the absence of conventional antigen presenting cells.[88] These findings support the view that infection may induce the expression of MHC class II molecules on thyroid cells and that these cells may act as antigen presenting cells and may be involved in the induction of thyroid autoimmune disease. T-cell accumulation and cytokine secretion would then perpetuate the disease process. In addition, local intrathyroidal dendritic cells[89] and B cells themselves[90] may serve as antigen-presenting cells. However, as discussed earlier, HLA antigen expression in the absence of second signal would have the opposite effect, exerting a suppressive influence on the local immune response.

KNOWN PRECIPITATING FACTORS

Infection

For infection to be defined as the cause of Graves' disease, an identifiable agent should be present in the majority of patients and transfer of the agent should transfer the disease. As discussed earlier, some data have directly and indirectly implicated infectious agents in the possible immune mechanisms involved in the pathogenesis of Graves' disease; the disease has been associated with a variety of infectious agents (e.g., *Y. enterocolitica*[91,92]), but there is no evidence that such infections lead directly to autoimmune thyroid disease.[93] Possible infections of the thyroid gland itself (e.g., subacute thyroiditis, congenital rubella) are associated with thyroid autoimmune phenomena (for review, see reference 94). However, the causative role of infectious agents in Graves' disease is unproven, although autoimmune thyroid disease can be induced

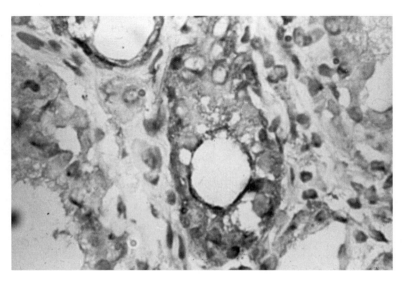

FIGURE 30-8. HLA-DR antigen expression (the dark immunoperoxidase-stained areas) in thyroid tissue from a patient with Graves' disease. (x 200.)

TABLE 30-4.
Summary of Evidence That Thyroid Cells May Act as
Antigen-Presenting Cells

HLA-DR–positive thyroid cells will stimulate an autologous mixed lymphocyte reaction with proliferation of helper T cells.[88,112]

Co-culture of thyroid cells and peripheral blood mononuclear cells from patients with Graves' disease leads to γ-interferon production and thyroid cell HLA-DR expression.[113]

Human thyroid epithelial cells were able to present an influenza-specific peptide to a peptide-specific human T-cell clone a reaction that was blocked by HLA-class II antibody. However, the thyroid cells were unable to process complex antigen (intact influenza virus) for presentation.[87]

Thyroid epithelial cells were capable of phagocytosis but at a slower rate than macrophages. This function was inhibited by interleukin-1, methimazole, and dexamethasone but enhanced by interleukin-2 and interferon-β.[114]

A cloned line of thyroid cells from Wistar rats was able to interact directly with cloned antigen-specific T cells in the absence of other antigen-presenting cells.[115]

in experimental animals by certain viral infections.[94,95] Reports of retroviral sequences in the thyroid glands of patients with Graves' disease have not been substantiated.[96–100]

Stress

The second case of thyrotoxicosis originally described by Parry in 1825[101] was a 21-year-old woman who became symptomatic after she had fallen accidentally down the stairs in a wheelchair. Since that time, a major stress has often been associated with the onset of Graves' disease, including data on the high incidence of thyrotoxicosis among refugees from German concentration camps.[102] Both acute and chronic stress induces an overall state of immune suppression by non–antigen-specific mechanisms,[103] perhaps secondary to the effects of cortisol and corticotropin-releasing hormone action at the level of the immune cell. In several recent studies, more patients with Graves' disease had a history of major stresses than control subjects.[104–106] Acute stress-induced immune suppression may be followed by immune system hyperactivity, which could precipitate autoimmune thyroid disease, as in the postpartum period in which Graves' disease may occur 3 to 9 months after delivery.[107,108]

Sex Steroids

Far more women than men have Graves' disease. Some evidence suggests that sex steroids are responsible for this difference rather than undefined genes on the X or Y chromosome. Graves' disease is uncommon before puberty, and estrogen may influence the immune system, particularly the B-cell repertoire.[109] During pregnancy, both T-cell and B-cell function is diminished, and the rebound from this immunosuppression is thought to contribute to the development of the postpartum thyroid syndromes.[43,110] Furthermore, androgen protects against and estrogen enhances thyroiditis after thyroglobulin immunization. These results provide evidence for a major influence of sex steroids on the development of Graves' disease.

CONCLUSIONS

The intrathyroidal lymphocytic infiltrate is the initial abnormality in autoimmune thyroid disease and can be correlated with the titer of thyroid antibodies.[111] With this background in susceptible persons, mostly women, thyroid-specific T cells in patients developing Graves' disease must be further activated either extra-thyroidally, perhaps via stress-related mechanisms, or as a result of a direct infectious assault on the thyroid cells which changes their antigen presenting status. Extrathyroidal activation may also imply crossover specificity between a thyroid antigen and an infectious agent. Once activated, the thyroid-specific T cells induce B-cell proliferation and secretion of TSHR antibodies, and hyperthyroidism ensues.

References

1. Martin A, Davies TF. T-cells and human autoimmune thyroid disease: Emerging data show lack of need to invoke suppressor T-cell problems. Thyroid 1992;2:247

2. Weetman AP. Autoimmune endocrine disease. Cambridge: Cambridge University Press, 1991

3. Mariotti S, Chiovato L, Vitti P, Marcocci C, Fenzi GF, Del Prete GF, et al. Recent advances in the understanding of humoral and cellular mechanisms implicated in thyroid autoimmune disorders. Clin Immunol Immunopathol 1989;50:S73

4. Tainer JA, Deal CD, Geysen HM, Roberts VA, Getzoff ED. Defining antibody-antigen recognition: towards engineered antibodies and epitopes. Int Rev Immunol 1991;7:165

5. Weiss A. Structure and function of the T cell antigen receptor. J Clin Invest 1990;86:1015

6. Brown JH, Jardetzky S, Gorga JC, Stern LJ, Urban RG, Strominger JL, et al. Three-dimensional structure of the human class II histocompatibility antigen HLA-DR1. Nature 1993;364:33

7. Schwartz RH. T cell anergy. Sci Am 1993;269:66

8. Witebsky E, Rose NR, Terplan K, Paine JR, Egan RW. JAMA 1957;164:1439

9. Rose NR, Bona C. Defining criteria for autoimmune diseases (Witebsky's postulates revisited). Immunol Today 1993;14:426

10. Adams DD, Fastier FN, Howie JB, Kennedy TH, Kilpatrick JA, Stewart RDH. Stimulation of the human thyroid by infusions of plasma containing LATS protector. J Clin Endocrinol Metab 1974;39:826

11. Zakarija M, McKenzie JM. Pregnancy-associated changes in thyroid-stimulating antibody of Graves' disease and the relationship to neonatal hyperthyroidism. J Clin Endocrinol Metab 1983;57:1036

12. Livolsi VA. Surgical pathology of the thyroid. Philadelphia: WB Saunders, 1990

13. Weetman AP, McGregor AM, Hall R. Evidence for an effect of antithyroid drugs on the natural history of Graves' disease. Clin Endocrinol 1984;21:163

14. Martin A, Goldsmith NK, Friedman EW, Schwartz AE, Davies TF, Roman SH. Intrathyroidal accumulation of T cell phenotypes in autoimmune thyroid disease. Autoimmunity 1990;6:269

15. Paschke R, Bruckner N, Schmeidl R, Pfiester P, Usadel KH. Predominant intraepithelial localization of primed T-cells and immunoglobulin-producing lymphocytes in Graves' disease. Acta Endocrinol 1991;124:630

16. Roman SH, Goldsmith NK, Leiderman IZ, Davies TF. Induction of microsomal antigen and comparison with histologic localization of HLA-DR in Graves thyroid tissue. Autoimmunity 1989;2:253

17. Paschke R, Bruckner N, Eck T, Schaaf L, Back W, Usadel KH. Regional stimulation of thyroid epithelial cells in Graves' disease by lymphocytic aggregates and plasma cells. Acta Endocrinol 1991;125:459

18. Ueki Y, Eguchi K, Otsubo T, Kawabe Y, Shimomura C, Tezuka H, et al. Abnormal B lymphocyte function in thyroid glands from patients with Graves' disease. J Clin Endocrinol Metab 1989; 69:939

19. Martin A, Valentine M, Unger P, Yeung SW, Shultz LD, Davies TF. Engraftment of human lymphocytes and thyroid tissue into Scid and Rag2-deficient mice: absent progression of lymphocytic infiltration. J Clin Endocrinol Metab 1994;79:716

20. McGregor AM, Petersen MM, McLachlan SM, Rooke P, Smith BR, Hall R. Carbimazole and the autoimmune response in Graves' disease. N Engl J Med 1980;303:302

21. Weetman AP. The immunomodulatory effects of antithyroid drugs. Thyroid 1994;4:145

22. McGregor AM, Petersen MM, Capiferri R, Evered DC, Rees Smith B, Hall R. Effects of radioiodine on thyrotrophin binding inhibiting immunoglobulins in Graves' disease. Clin Endocrinol 1979; 11:437

23. Adams DD, Purves HD. Abnormal responses in the assay of thyrotropin. Proc Univ Otago Medical School 1956;34:11

24. Rees Smith B, McLachlan SM, Furmaniak J. Autoantibodies to the thyrotropin receptor. Endocr Rev 1988;9:106

25. Kraiem Z, Lahat N, Glaser B, Baron E, Sadeh O, Sheinfeld M. Thyrotropin receptor blocking antibodies: incidence, characterization and in-vitro synthesis. Clin Endocrinol 1987;27:409

26. Zakarija M, McKenzie JM, Eidson MS. Transient neonatal hypothyroidism: characterization of maternal antibodies to the thyrotropin receptor. J Clin Endocrinol Metab 1990;70:1239

27. Davies TF, Yeo PP, Evered DC, Clark F, Smith BR, Hall R. Value of thyroid-stimulating-antibody determinations in predicting short-term thyrotoxic relapse in Graves' disease. Lancet 1977; 1:1181

28. Wilson R, McKillop JH, Henderson N, Pearson DW, Thomson JA. The ability of the serum TSH receptor antibody index and HLA status to predict long-term remission of thyrotoxicosis following medical therapy for Graves' disease. Clin Endocrinol 1986; 25:151

29. Zakarija MJ. Immunochemical characterization of the thyroid-stimulating antibody (TSab) of Graves' disease: evidence for restricted heterogeneity. J Clin Lab Immunol 1983;10:77

30. Weetman AP, Yateman ME, Ealey PA, Black CM, Reimer CB, Williams RC, et al. Thyroid-stimulating antibody activity between different immunoglobulin G subclasses. J Clin Invest 1990;86:723

31. Lechler RI, Lombardi G, Batchelor JR, Reinsmoen N, Bach FH. The molecular basis of alloreactivity. Immunol Today 1990;11:83

32. Loosfelt H, Misrahi M, Atger M, Salesse R, Vu H, Thi MT, et al. Science 1989;245:525

33. Nagayama Y, Kaufman KD, Seto P, Rapoport B. Molecular cloning, sequence and functional expression of the cDNA for the human thyrotropin receptor. Biochem Biophys Res Commun 1989;165:1184

34. Vlase H, Graves PN, Magnusson R, Davies TF. Human autoantibodies to the TSH receptor: recognition of linear, folded and glycosylated recombinant extracellular domain. J Clin Endocrinol Metab 1995;80:46

35. Damante G, Foti D, Catalfamo R, Filetti S. Desensitization of thyroid cyclic AMP response to thyroid stimulating immunoglobulin: comparison with TSH. Metabolism 1987;36:768

36. Kraiem Z, Alkobi R, Sadeh O. Sensitization and desensitization of human thyroid cells in culture: effects of thyrotropin and thyroid-stimulating immunoglobulin. J Endocrinol 1988;119:341

37. Davies TF. Positive regulation of the guinea pig thyrotropin receptor. Endocrinology 1985;117:201

38. Huber G, Concepcion LE, Graves P, Davies TF. Positive regulation of the human TSH receptor mRNA by recombinant human TSH is at the nuclear level. Endocrinology 1992;130:2858

39. Parks VA, McLachlan SM, Bird P, Rees Smith B. Distribution of microsomal antibody and thyroglobulin antibody activity amongst IgG subclasses. Isr J Med Sci 1984;57:239

40. Romagnani S, Del Prete GF, Maggi F, Parronchi P, De Carli M, Macchia D, et al. Human Th1 nad Th2 subsets. Int Arch Allergy Immunol 1992;99:242

41. Male DK, Champion BR, Pryce G, Matthews H, Shepherd P. Antigenic determinants of human thyroglobulin differentiated using antigen fragments. Immunology 1985;54:419

42. Dayan CM, Londei M, Corcoran AE, Grubeck-Loebenstein B, James RF, Rapoport B, et al. Autoantigen recognition by thyroid-infiltrating T-cells in Graves disease. Proc Natl Acad Sci USA 1991;88:7415

43. Acuto O, Reinhertz EL. The human T cell receptor—Structure and function. N Engl J Med 1985;312:1100

44. Benacerraf B. Role of MHC gene products in immune regulation. Science 1981;212:1229

45. Tandon N, Freeman MA, Weetman AP. T cell response to synthetic TSH receptor peptides in Graves' disease. Clin Exp Immunol 1992;89:468

46. Mackenzie WA, Schwartz AE, Friedman EW, Davies TF. Intrathyroidal T cell clones from patients with autoimmune thyroid disease. J Clin Endocrinol Metab 1987;64:818

47. Martin A, Schwartz AE, Friedman EW, Davies TF. Successful production of intrathyroidal human T cell hybridomas: evidence for intact helper T cell function in Graves' disease. J Clin Endocrinol Metab 1989;69:1104

48. Mackenzie WA, Davies TF. An intrathyroidal T-cell clone specifically cytotoxic for human thyroid cells. Immunology 1987; 61:101

49. Grubeck-Loebenstein B, Turner M, Pirich K, Kassal H, Londei M, Waldhausl W, et al. CD4+ T-cell clones from autoimmune thyroid tissue cannot be classified according to their lymphokine production. Scand J Immunol 1990;32:433

50. Del Prete GF, Tiri A, Mariotti S, Pinchera A, Ricci M, Romagnani S. Enhanced production of gamma-interferon by thyroid-derived T cell clones from patients with Hashimoto's thyroiditis. Clin Exp Immunol 1987;69:323

51. Watson PF, Pickerill AP, Davies R, Weetman AP. Analysis of cytokine gene expression in Graves' disease and multinodular goiter. J Clin Endocinol Metab 1994;79:355

52. Davis MM, Bjorkman PJ. T-cell antigen receptor genes and T-cell recognition. Nature 1988;334:395

53. Davies TF, Martin A, Concepcion ES, Graves P, Cohen L, Ben-Nun A. Evidence of limited variability of antigen receptors on intrathyroidal T-cells in autoimmune thyroid disease. N Engl J Med 1991;325:238

54. Davies T, Concepcion E, Ben-Nun A, Graves P, Tarjan G. T-cell receptor V gene usage in autoimmune thyroid disease: direct assessment by thyroid aspiration. J Clin Endocrinol Metab 1993;76:660

55. Matsuoka N, Martin A, Concepcion ES, Unger P, Shultz LD, Davies TF. Preservation of functioning human thyroid organoids in the *scid* mouse: II. Biased use of intrathyroidal T cell receptor V genes. J Clin Endocrinol Metab 1993;77:311

56. De Riu A, Martin A, Valentine M, Concepcion ES, Shultz LD, Davies TF. Graves' disease thyroid transplants in Scid mice: persistent selectivity in hTcR V alpha gene family use. Autoimmunity 1995;19:271

57. Oksenberg JR, Stuart S, Begovich AB, Bell RB, Erlich HA, Steinman L, et al. Limited heterogeneity of rearranged T cell receptor V alpha transcripts in brains of multiple sclerosis patients. Nature 1990;345:344

58. Ben-Nun A, Liblau RS, Cohen L, Lehmann D, Tournier-Lasseru E, Rosenzwig A, et al. Restricted T cell receptor V beta usage by myelin basic protein-specific T cell clones in multiple sclerosis: predominant genes vary in individuals. Proc Natl Acad Sci USA 1991;88:2466

59. Davies TF. Preferential use of T-cell receptor V genes in human autoimmune thyroid disease. Autoimmunity 1992;13:11

60. Lehmann PV, Sercarz EE, Forsthuber T, Dayan CM, Gammon G. Determinant spreading and the dynamics of the autoimmune repertoire. Immunol Today 1993;14:203

61. Sridama V, Pacini V, DeGroot LJ. Decreased suppressor T lymphocytes in autoimmune thyroid diseases detected by monoclonal antibodies. J Clin Endocrinol Metab 1982;54:316

62. Volpe R. The immunoregulatory disturbance in autoimmune thyroid disease. Autoimmunity 1988;2:55

63. Moller G. Do suppressor T-cells exist ? Scand J Immunol 1988; 27:247

64. Jenkins M. The role of cell division in the induction of clonal anergy. Immunol Today 1992;13:69

65. Morahan G, Hoffmann M, Miller J. A nondeletional mechanism of peripheral tolerance in T-cell receptor transgenic mice. Proc Natl Acad Sci U S A 1992;88:11421

66. Lombardi G, Sidhu S, Batchelor R, Lechler R. Anergic T-cells as suppressor cells in vitro. Science 1994;264:1587

67. Ambinder JM, Chiorazzi N, Gibofsky A, Fotino M, Kunkel HG. Special characteristics of cellular immune function in normal individuals of the HLA-DR3 type. Clin Immunol Immunopathol 1982;23:269

68. Kallenberg CGM, Klaassen RJL, BeelenM, The TH. HLA-B8/DR3 phenotype and the primary immune response. Clin Immunol Immunopathol 1985;34:135

69. Oldstone MBA, Nerenberg M, Southern P, Price J, Lewicki H. Virus infection triggers insulin-dependent diabetes mellitus in a transgenic model: role of anti-self (virus) immune response. Cell 1991;65:319

70. Srinivasappa J, Saegusa J, Prabhakar BS, Gentry MK, Buchmeier MJ, Wiktor TJ, et al. Molecular mimicry: frequency of reactivity of monoclonal antiviral antibodies with normal tissues. J Virol 1986;57:397

71. Haspel MV, Onodera T, Prabhakar BS, Horita M, Suzuki H, Notkins AL. Virus-induced autoimmunity: monoclonal antibodies that react with endocrine tissues. Science 1983;220:304

72. Burch HB, Nagy EV, Lukes YG, Cai WY, Wartofsky L, Burman KD. Nucleotide and amino acid homology between the human thyrotropin receptor and HIV-1 nef protein: identification and functional analysis. Biochem Biophys Res Commun 1991; 181:498

73. Acha-Orbea H, Palmer E. Mls-a retrovirus exploits the immune system. Immunol Today 1991;12:356

74. Marrack P, Kappler J. The staphylococcal enterotoxins and their relatives. Science 1990;248:705

75. Jerne NK. Towards a network theory of the immune system. Ann Immunol (Paris) 1974;125c:373

76. Tomer Y, Shoenfeld Y. Idiotypes, anti-idiotypic antibodies and autoimmunity. In: Khamashta MA, Font J, Hughes GRV, eds. Autoimmune connective tissue diseases. Barcelona: Ediciones Doyma, 1993:27

77. Islam MN, Pepper BM, Briones-Urbina R, Farid NR. Biological activity of anti-thyrotropin and anti-idiotypic antibody. Eur J Immunol 1983;13:57

78. Lamb JR, Young DB. T cell recognition of stress proteins. A link between infectious and autoimmune disease. Mol Biol Med 1994;7:311

79. Bahn RS, Heufelder AE, Gorman CA, Goellner JR. Immunohistochemical detection and localization of a 72 kDa heat shock protein (HSP) in Graves' and Hashimoto's thyroid glands. Thyroid 1991;1(Suppl 1):S-62

80. Trieb K, Sztankay A, Hermann M, Gratzl R, Szabo J, Jindal S, et al. Do heat shock proteins play a role in Graves' disease? J Clin Endocrinol Metab 1993;77:528

81. Hanafusa T, Pujol Borrell R, Chiovato L, Russell RC, Doniach D, Bottazzo GF. Aberrant expression of HLA-DR antigen on thyrocytes in Graves' disease: relevance for autoimmunity. Lancet 1983;2:1111

82. Bottazzo GF, Pujol Borrell R, Hanafusa T, Feldmann M. Role of aberrant HLA-DR expression and antigen presentation in induction of endocrine autoimmunity. Lancet 1983;2:1115

83. Kawakami Y, Kuzuya N, Watanabe T, Uchiyama Y, Yamashita K. Induction of experimental thyroiditis in mice by recombinant interferon gamma administration. Acta Endocrinol (Copenh) 1990;122:41

84. Massa PT, Dorries R, Meulen V. Viral particles induce Ia antigen expression on astrocytes. Nature 1986;320:543

85. Neufeld DS, Platzer M, Davies TF. Reovirus induction of MHC class II antigen in rat thyroid cells. Endocrinology 1989;124:543

86. Khoury EL, Pereira L, Greenspan FS. Induction of HLA-DR expression on thyroid follicular cells by cytomegalovirus infection in vitro. Evidence for a dual mechanism of induction. Am J Pathol 1991;138:1209

87. Londei M, Lamb JR, Bottazzo GF, Feldmann M. Epithelial cells expressing aberrant MHC class II determinants can present antigen to cloned human T-cells. Nature 1984;312:639

88. Davies TF. Co-culture of human thyroid monolayer cells and autologous T-cells: Impact of HLA class II antigen expression. J Clin Endocrinol Metab 1985;61:418

89. Kabel PJ, Voorbij HA, De Haan M, van der Gaag RD, Drexhage HA. Intrathyroidal dendritic cells. J Clin Endocrinol Metab 1988;66:199

90. Hutchings P, Rayner DC, Champion BR, Marshall Clarke S, Macatonia S, Roitt I, et al. High efficiency antigen presentation by thyroglobulin-primed murine splenic B cells. Eur J Immunol 1987;17:393

91. Lidman K, Eriksson U, Norberg R, Fagraeus A. Indirect immunofluorescence staining of human thyroid by antibodies occurring in *Yersinia enterocolitica* infections. Clin Exp Immunol 1976;23:429

92. Wenzel BE, Heeseman J, Wenzel KW, Scriba PC. Antibodies to plasmid-encoded proteins of enteropathogenic *Yersinia* in patients with autoimmune thyroid disease. Lancet 1988;1:56

93. Toivanen P, Toivanen A. Does *Yersinia* induce autoimmunity? Int Arch Allergy Immunol 1994;104:107

94. Tomer Y, Davies TF. Infection, thyroid disease and autoimmunity. Endocr Rev 1993;14:107

95. Carter JK, Smith RE. Rapid induction of hypothyroidism by an avian leukosis virus. Infect Immun 1983;40:795

96. Ciampolillo A, Mirakian R, Schulz T, Vittoria M, Buscema M, Pujol Borrell R, et al. Retrovirus-like sequences in Graves' disease: Implications for human autoimmunity. Lancet 1989;1:1096

97. Wick G, Trieb K, Aguzzi A, Recheis H, Anderl H, Grubeck-Loebenstein B. Possible role of human foamy virus in Graves' disease. Intervirol 1993;35:101

98. Lagaye S, Vexiau P, Morozov V, Guenebaut-Claudet V, Tobaly-Tapiero J, Canivet M, et al. Human spumaretrovirus-related sequences in the DNA of leukocytes from patients with Graves' disease. Proc Natl Acad Sci USA 1992;89:10070

99. Humphrey M, Baker JR Jr, Carr FE, Wartofsky L, Mosca J, Drabick JJ, et al. Absence of retroviral sequences in Graves' disease. Lancet 1991;337:17

100. Neumann-Haefelin D, Fleps U, Renne R, Schweizer M. Foamy viruses. Intervirol 1993;35:196

101. Parry CH. Disease of the heart. In: Anonymous collections from the unpublished writings. Vol 2. London: Underwoods, 1825:111

102. Weisman SA. Incidence of thyrotoxicosis among refugees from Nazi prison camps. J Clin Endocrinol Metabol 1958;48:747

103. Locke S, Ader R, Besedovsky H, Hall N, Solomon G, Strom T. Foundations of psychoneuroimmunology. New York: Aldine, 1985

104. Leclere J, Germain M, Weryha G, Duquenne M, Hartemann P. Role of stressful life-events in the onset of Graves' disease. 10th Int Thyroid Conf, The Hague, 1991. Abstract 100

105. Winsa B, Adami H, Bergstrom R, Gamstedt A, Dahlberg PA, Adamson U, et al. Stressful life events and Graves' disease. Lancet 1991;338:1475

106. Sonino N, Girelli M, Boscaro M, Fallo F, Busnardo B, Fava GA. Life events in the pathogenesis of Graves' disease. A controlled study. Acta Endocrinologica 1993;128:293

107. Amino N, Miyai K. Postpartum autoimmune endocrine syndromes. In: Davies TF, ed. Autoimmune endocrine disease. New York: Wiley, 1983:247

108. Stagnaro-Green A, Roman SH, Cobin RH, El-Harazy E, Wallenstein S, Davies TF. A prospective study of lymphocyte-initiated immunosuppression in normal pregnancy: evidence of a T-cell etiology for postpartum thyroid dysfunction. J Clin Endocrinol Metab 1992;74:645

109. Kincade PW, Medina KL, Smithson G, Scott DC. Pregnancy: a clue to normal regulation of B lymphopoiesis. Immunol Today 1994;15:539

110. Hall R, Smith BR, Mukhtar ED. Thyroid stimulators in health and disease. Clin Endocrinol 1975;4:213

111. Doniach D. Hashimoto's thyroiditis and primary myxedema viewed as separate entities. Eur J Clin Invest 1981;11:245

112. Eguchi K, Otsubo T, Kawabe K, Ueki Y, Fukuda T, Mayumi M, et al. The remarkable proliferation of helper T cell subset in response to autologous thyrocytes and intrathyroidal T-cells from patients with Graves' disease. Isr J Med Sci 1987;70:403

113. Iwatani Y, Gerstein HC, Iitaka M, Row VV, Volpe R. Thyrocyte HLA-DR expression and gamma interferon production in autoimmune thyroid disease. J Clin Endocrinol Metab 1986;63:695

114. Matsunaga M. The effects of cytokines, antithyroidal drugs, and glucocorticoids on phagocytosis by thyroid cells. Acta Endocrinol 1988;119:413

115. Kimura H, Davies TF. Thyroid-specific T-cells in the normal Wistar rat. II. T cell clones interact with cloned Wistar rat thyroid cells and provide direct evidence for autoantigen presentation by thyroid epithelial cells. Clin Immunol Immunopathol 1991;58:195

Ophthalmopathy

Henry B. Burch
Colum A. Gorman
Rebecca S. Bahn
James A. Garrity

Hyperthyroidism in Graves' disease is a consequence of the action of thyrotropin (TSH) receptor-stimulating antibodies (TSAb) on TSH receptors. In contrast, the cause of the extrathyroidal manifestations of Graves' disease, such as ophthalmopathy, localized myxedema, and thyroid acropachy, is not known. In this chapter we review current concepts in the pathogenesis and management of Graves' ophthalmopathy.

EPIDEMIOLOGY

Estimates of the prevalence of ophthalmopathy in patients with Graves' disease are influenced by several variables, including the sensitivity of the detection method, the inclusion of thyrotoxic patients with eyelid changes alone, and selection bias in the study group.[1] Clinically evident ophthalmopathy occurs in 10% to 25% of unselected patients with Graves' disease if eyelid signs are excluded, 30% to 45% if eyelid changes are included, and in most patients if a sensitive technique such as computed tomography (CT) is used to detect eye involvement.[2,3] When patients with Graves' hyperthyroidism who did not have clinically evident ophthalmopathy were examined by CT, 70% had increases in the volume of extraocular muscles, retrobulbar connective tissue, or both.[3] Fortunately, fewer than 5% of patients with Graves' disease have severe ophthalmopathy.[4,5] The incidence of Graves' ophthalmopathy was recently determined in the population of Olmsted County, Minnesota, for the years 1976 to 1990.[6] A total of 120 cases were found, yielding an age-adjusted incidence rate of 16 cases per year for women and 2.9 for men per 100,000 population. The distribution was bimodal, with peak incidence in the age groups 40 to 44 and 60 to 64 years in women and 45 to 49 and 65 to 69 years in men. There was no seasonal variation in the diagnosis of new cases.

A sex-related difference in the severity of Graves' ophthalmopathy has been noted, with men comprising a relatively greater proportion of cases of severe ophthalmopathy.[7] The prevalence of cigarette smokers is higher in patients with Graves' ophthalmopathy as compared with patients with Graves' disease without ophthalmopathy or patients with other thyroid disorders.[8–11] The mechanisms underlying this finding are unclear, although smokers are more likely to have goiter[12] and higher serum thyroglobulin concentrations[13] than nonsmokers, suggesting that thyroid damage may contribute to the association.

ANATOMY OF THE ORBIT

An understanding of orbital anatomy is important in illuminating differential diagnosis, the mechanical components of pathogenesis, and the opportunities and difficulties presented by several forms of therapy of Graves' ophthalmopathy. Of special importance are the proximity of the bony orbit to the paranasal sinuses, the location of the cribriform plate of the ethmoid bone, which can easily be injured during ethmoidal decompression,[14] and the passage of the infraorbital nerve through its canal on the orbital floor until it exits at the infraorbital foramen. Retraction of the nerve during transantral orbital decompression accounts for numbness of the upper lip postoperatively (Fig. 30-9).[15]

The extraocular muscles originate at Zinn's annulus (Fig. 30-10), which is the fibrous periosteal extension located at the apex of the orbit that forms the posterior attachment site of the muscles. Anteriorly, the muscles insert onto the sclera.[16] The visual axis and the axis of the orbit are not precisely parallel. As a result, the superior rectus muscles elevate and rotate the eyes inwardly and the inferior rectus muscles lower and outwardly rotate the eyes. Both oblique muscles run posteriorly to their

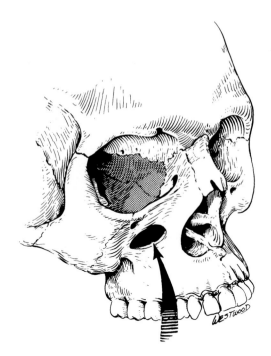

FIGURE 30-9. Surgical approach to transantral orbital decompression for Graves' ophthalmopathy. Through an anterior antrostomy, bone is removed to the inferior orbital fissure and superiorly to the cribriform plate of the ethmoid bone. The infraorbital nerve traverses the orbital floor and emerges through the infraorbital foramen, which is visible just above the antrostomy. (Gorman CA, DeSanto LW, MacCarty CS, Riley FC. Optic neuropathy of Graves' disease: Treatment by transantral or transfrontal orbital decompression. N Engl J Med 1974;290:70. Reproduced with permission)

attachment on the eye (see Fig. 30-10*A*). The superior oblique muscles depress, abduct, and rotate the eyes inwardly. The inferior oblique muscles elevate, abduct, and rotate the eyes outwardly. In contrast, the medial and lateral rectus muscles are straightforward abductors and adductors, respectively.

The extraocular muscles are invested by a fibrous connective tissue sheath that envelops the muscle (Fig. 30-10) and coalesces between muscles to create a velamentous boundary between the intraconal compartment and the extraconal space.[16] Anteriorly, the periosteal connective tissue reflects from the orbital rim to form the orbital septum that inserts in the eyelids and that, together with the limited extensibility of the extraocular muscles, restricts anterior motion of the eyes when retrobulbar pressure increases. Recession of the rectus muscles while correcting diplopia may increase proptosis.[14]

The major radiographic finding in Graves' ophthalmopathy is the swollen extraocular muscles (but not their tendons).[17] In contrast, in orbital myositis, the muscle bellies and tendons are both swollen (Fig. 30-11).[18]

PATHOLOGY

The average volume of each orbital cavity in humans is 26 mL.[19] Normally this cavity is occupied anteriorly by the globe and posteriorly by the extraocular muscles, connective tissue, vessels, and nerves (Table 30-5). The extent of orbital protru-

sion (proptosis, exophthalmos) is determined by the extent to which the orbital soft tissues fill the orbital cavity. Assuming an orbital volume of 25 mL and specific gravity of 0.96, an increase in orbital volume of only 4 mL should result in 6 mm of proptosis.[19] Computed tomographic imaging studies have shown that the volume of extraocular muscle normally ranges from 3.0 to 6.8 mL and that of the retrobulbar fat and connective tissue ranges from 8.2 to 14.0 mL.[2]

In patients with ophthalmopathy, muscle volume as high as 21.6 mL and fat and connective tissue volume as high as 22.6 mL have been recorded.[2]

Extraocular Muscles and Retrobulbar Connective Tissue

Few detailed studies of orbital histology have been made (Fig. 30-12).[20–23] In one young man with severe Graves' ophthalmopathy, the extraocular muscles showed edema, mononuclear cell infiltration, glycosaminoglycan deposition, and fibrosis.[20] Although the extraocular muscles are generally enlarged, the extraocular muscle fibers themselves are usually normal.[20,23–25] The muscle enlargement is due to muscle fiber separation by edematous ground substance,[26] fibrosis, and sometimes aggregates of lymphocytes. Immunoglobulin E deposition has been noted.[21] As seen on orbital CT scans, extraocular muscles are affected with varying frequency. Among 71 patients with Graves' ophthalmopathy, 63% had superior rectus enlargement, 61% had medial rectus enlargement, and 57% had inferior rectus enlargement.[27] Solitary muscle enlargement most frequently involved the superior rectus (6%), and isolated involvement of the lateral rectus was rare.

Extraocular muscle tissue from patients with Graves' ophthalmopathy contains B- and T-lymphocytes, monocytes, and macrophages, and abnormal human leukocyte antigen (HLA)-DR expression on the perimysial fibroblasts.[22] In three carefully studied patients, most lymphocytes were T cells that were members of a group of cells that may include memory cells.[28] Few lymphocytes were seen in the orbital fat and connective tissue, and extraocular muscle cells did not express HLA-DR molecules. Interstitial cells, probably including fibroblasts and vascular endothelial cells, were HLA-DR-molecule positive. The connective tissue septa between fat lobules were thickened in varying degrees. These results suggest that the T cells and to a lesser extent B cells may be directed against interstitial cells. Suppressor-cytotoxic T cells predominate among interleukin-2-responsive retroocular lymphocytes in patients with Graves' ophthalmopathy; these cells proliferate in response to autologous retroocular fibroblasts but not crude eye muscle extract, suggesting that the former represent the major target in these patients.[29] Focal accumulation of lymphocytes, plasma cells, and occasional polymorphonuclear leukocytes also have been seen.[25] In some patients, fat may be completely replaced by fibrous tissue. Clusters of newly formed collagen may be interspersed with glycolipid deposits that contain material with the staining characteristics of hyaluronic acid,[20,30] which is produced by fibroblasts, including retroocular fibroblasts[31,32] (see chap 37).

The osmotic characteristics of hyaluronic acid lead to orbital edema and the expansion of orbital tissues. Urinary excretion of acid mucopolysaccharide may be increased in

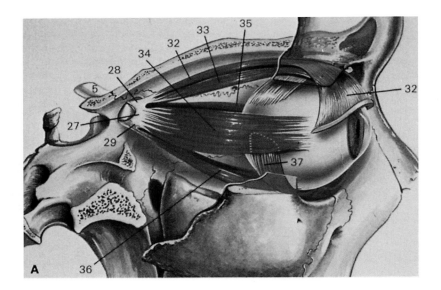

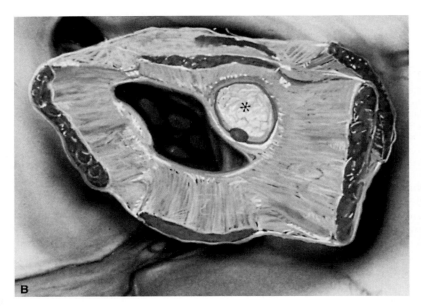

FIGURE 30-10. Anatomy of the orbit. *(A)* Cutaway lateral view of the right orbit showing the optic nerve (35) as it passes through the annulus of Zinn (27–29). The levator palpebrae muscle (32) lies above the superior rectus muscle (33). With high-resolution coronal computed tomography or magnetic resonance imaging, these two structures can often be distinguished. The inferior oblique muscle (37) passes under the inferior rectus muscle (36). Note the insertion of the superior oblique muscle under the superior rectus muscle (33). (Rootman J, Stewart B. Atlas of orbital anatomy. In: Rootman J, ed. Diseases of the orbit. Philadelphia: JB Lippincott, 1988:19). *(B)* View of apex of right orbit. The optic nerve *(asterisk)* and ophthalmic artery *(below asterisk)* pass through the medial half of the annulus of Zinn. The origins of the lateral rectus, inferior rectus, medial rectus, superior oblique, superior rectus, and levator palpebrae muscles are illustrated. (Zibe BM, Jelks GW. Surgical anatomy of the orbit. New York: Raven Press, 1985)

patients with active ophthalmopathy.[33] Tissue accumulation of glycosaminoglycans is suggested by histochemical stains of orbital biopsies,[34] but the glycosaminoglycan content in orbital tissues from patients with Graves' ophthalmopathy has not been measured.

Optic Nerve

Histologic studies of the optic nerve in Graves' ophthalmopathy are rare. Damage to the nerve is believed to be the consequence of mechanical compression at the apex of the muscle cone (Fig. 30-13). This may result in fibrous and fatty areolar connective tissue replacement[35] and segmental degeneration in the nerve, with loss of myelin and destruction of axis cylinders.

PATHOGENESIS

In a mechanical sense, the proximate causes of Graves' ophthalmopathy are enlargement of extraocular muscles and retroocular connective tissue behind the globe. As a result, the globe is displaced anteriorly so that proptosis occurs. The efficacy of proptosis as an adaptation to increased retroorbital pressure is limited by the restraining effect of the extraocular muscles and the orbital septum. The enlarged and fibrotic extraocular and eyelid muscles are restricted in their motion, resulting in diplopia and lid retraction. Combined with proptosis, eyelid retraction may allow exposure keratitis to develop. Enlargement of the muscles at the posterior apex of the muscle cone may compress the optic nerve and cause optic neuropathy. Chemosis and periorbital edema result from local inflam-

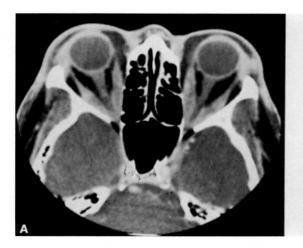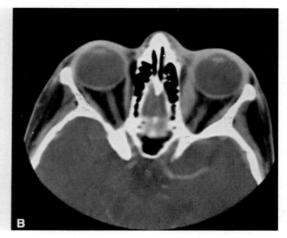

FIGURE 30-11. Computed tomographic images of Graves' ophthalmopathy and orbital myositis. *(A)* Graves' ophthalmopathy (axial view). Note the enlarged medial and lateral rectus muscles, which taper toward slender tendons, and the orbital septum bulging anteriorly. *(B)* Orbital myositis (axial view). The left medial rectus muscle and tendon are both swollen. The orbital septum does not bulge anteriorly.

mation and impaired orbital venous drainage.[36,37] The enlargement of the extraocular muscles and retroocular connective tissue is mainly a consequence of edema within the perimysial connective tissues,[25] an effect that is compounded by the resulting impairment of orbital venous drainage.

Glycosaminoglycan synthesis and glucose utilization are increased in retroocular fibroblasts from patients with Graves' ophthalmopathy (co-cultured with human lymphocytes).[38] This stimulation occurs with lymphocytes from both normal subjects and patients with Graves' ophthalmopathy. Activated T cells and macrophages present within the orbit in Graves' ophthalmopathy produce various cytokines, including interferon-γ, tumor necrosis factor-β, and interleukin-1α.[39] These cytokines are capable of stimulating the proliferation of orbital fibroblasts[40] as well as production of glycosaminoglycans by these cells.[41,42] In addition, these cytokines stimulate the expression of HLA-DR and various immunomodulatory proteins (intercellular adhesion molecules, 72-kDa heat-shock protein) in orbital fibroblasts, and these latter substances may play a

role in the local propagation of the autoimmune inflammatory response.[43,44,45] These changes ultimately lead to the characteristic histologic, anatomic, and clinical findings of Graves' ophthalmopathy.

The serum of patients with Graves' ophthalmopathy contains antibodies that are directed against various retroorbital tissue components, including fibroblasts[46] and extraocular muscle.[47] The importance of these antibodies is unclear; they may be produced as a consequence of tissue damage rather than being the cause of it.[48,49]

One explanation for the involvement of the eyes in Graves' disease is the existence of a target antigen common to the thyroid and the retroocular tissues and against which the autoimmune response is directed. Because the TSH receptor is the autoantigen involved in Graves' hyperthyroidism, it is attractive to postulate that this protein serves as the link between the thyroid and the ocular manifestations of Graves' disease. Indeed, TSH receptor protein[50] or RNA encoding the entire[51] or a variant fragment[52] of the extracellular domain of the receptor has been demonstrated in orbital fibroblasts. In addition, this receptor (or a variant) may be present in orbital muscle[52] or fat cells.[53] However, whether the protein is present in the orbit in sufficient quantity to serve as an autoantigen is unknown.

In summary, the following scheme has been proposed to explain the development of Graves' ophthalmopathy[36] (Fig. 30-14). Circulating T cells in patients with Graves' disease, directed against an antigen in thyroid follicular cells, recognize this same or a similar antigen in orbital tissue. As a consequence, activated T cells infiltrate the orbit and release cytokines (including interferon-γ, interleukin-1α, and tumor necrosis factor-β) into the surrounding tissue. These or other cytokines then stimulate the expression of immunomodulatory proteins and the production of glycosaminoglycans by orbital fibroblasts. The subsequent local accumulation of glycosaminoglycans and edema leads to the mechanical changes within the orbit that are recognized clinically as Graves' ophthalmopathy.

TABLE 30-5.
Composition and Weight of Retrobulbar and Peribulbar Tissues in Normal Subjects

Tissues	Weight (g)
Extraocular muscles	3.3
Lacrimal gland	0.6
Fat	12.0
Nerves and vessels	0.6
Fibrofatty residue	2.4
TOTAL	18.9

(Rundle FF, Pochin EE. The orbital tissues in thyrotoxicosis: a quantitative analysis relating to exophthalmos. Clin Sci 1944;5:51)

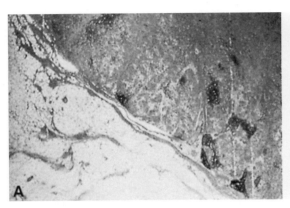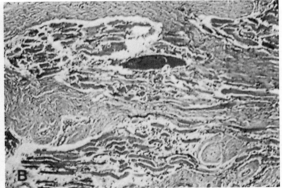

FIGURE 30-12. Photomicrographs of extraocular muscle from patients with Graves' ophthalmopathy. *(A)* Lymphocytic infiltration in extraocular muscle. Fat is not inflamed. *(B)* Perimysial fibrosis in extraocular muscle. (Trokel SL, Jakobiec FA. Correlation of CT scanning and pathologic features of ophthalmic Graves' disease. Ophthalmology 1981; 88:553)

CLINICAL PRESENTATION

Patients with Graves' ophthalmopathy may complain of a gritty, sandy sensation in the eyes or of retroocular pressure. Lacrimation, photophobia, blurring of vision, and diplopia are other frequent symptoms. The sensation of retroocular pressure presumably is caused by expansion of the retrobulbar structures within the confined orbital space. Visual blurring due to an alteration of the tear film on the surface of the cornea (either an excess of fluid associated with tearing, or a deficiency associated with a dry eye) may be cleared or modified by blinking. Another form of visual blurring is caused by minor degrees of extraocular muscle imbalance not yet perceived as diplopia. This type of blurring clears when either eye is closed. The visual blurring that is of greatest concern, however, continues for days or weeks, and persists when one eye is closed. It is commonly associated with a perceived reduction in color brightness or as an alteration in visual quality

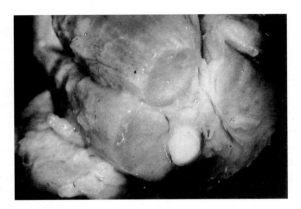

FIGURE 30-13. Compression of the optic nerve at the orbital apex by swollen extraocular muscles in a patient with Graves' ophthalmopathy. (Hufnagel TJ, Hickey WF, Cobbs WH, Jakobiec FA, Iwamoto T, Eagle RC. Immunohistochemical and ultrastructural studies of the exenterated orbital tissues of a patient with Graves' disease. Ophthalmology 1984;91:1411)

in one portion of the visual field. This type of blurring usually indicates optic neuropathy.

Diplopia in Graves' ophthalmopathy is caused by restriction of antagonist muscles rather than weakness of agonist muscles.[24,54] Initially it may be intermittent, being present early in the morning, when the patient is tired, or at the extremes of gaze. As the condition progresses, images separate further, and diplopia becomes persistent.

The most common presentation of Graves' ophthalmopathy is awareness of proptosis or a staring appearance. For example, these were the initial complaints in 32 of 50 consecutive patients referred to us for severe ophthalmopathy. Fifteen patients first noted inflammatory changes, and only three described diplopia as their first symptom. When the patient is thyrotoxic, the stare is worsened because of sympathetic overactivity resulting in contraction of the levator muscle and can be reversed by β-adrenergic blockade.[55] In euthyroid patients, stare may result from severe proptosis or from fibrosis and scarring of the eyelid levator muscles.

Whether due to proptosis or to eyelid retraction, the exposed cornea tends to become dry and inflamed. Protection of the cornea by avoidance of smoke, air currents, and other irritants is of great importance in management of patients with opthalmopathy. The varied clinical presentations of ophthalmopathy are illustrated in Figure 30-15.[56]

In most patients the ophthalmopathy appears coincident with or soon after the appearance of thyrotoxicosis (Fig. 30-16). The term *euthyroid ophthalmopathy* or *euthyroid Graves' disease* is applied to those patients who do not have thyrotoxicosis before the emergence of ophthalmopathy and are euthyroid when they seek care.[57] These patients are seldom without some stigmata of thyroid disease,[58] and may become thyrotoxic months or years later.

DIAGNOSIS

In patients who are thyrotoxic and at the same time have most or all of the characteristic findings of Graves' ophthalmopathy, or were thyrotoxic in the recent past, the diagnosis

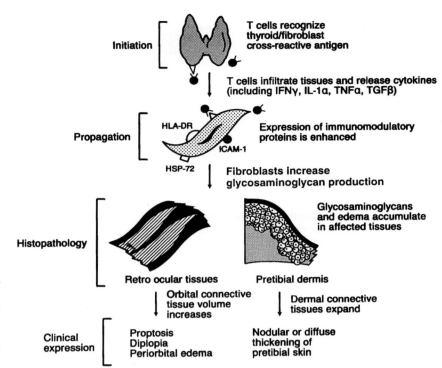

FIGURE 30-14. Proposed sequence of events leading to the development of Graves' ophthalmopathy. IFN-γ, interferon-γ; TNFα, tumor necrosis factor α; TGF β, transforming growth factor B; ICAM-1, intercellular adhesion molecule-1; HSP-72, 72-kDa heat-shock protein. (Bahn RS, Heufelder AE. Pathogenesis of Graves' ophthalmopathy. N Engl J Med 1993;329:1468. Reproduced with permission)

is straightforward, and specialized diagnostic tests are not necessary (Fig. 30-17). When a history of thyrotoxicosis is absent and the eye findings are few, subtle in expression, or monocular, the diagnosis is more difficult. In these circumstances, one may seek evidence of abnormal thyroid regulation. If such evidence is found, it is presumed to link the diagnostically nonspecific eye findings to Graves' disease. Some patients with abnormal thyroid regulation, however, may have unrelated eye disorders,[59] and conversely, some patients with Graves' ophthalmopathy have no thyroid abnormality whatsoever.[58,60] In most patients, however, as noted previously, the onset of thyroid dysfunction and ophthalmopathy are temporally related. In considering a diagnosis of Graves' ophthalmopathy, one seeks to establish that the eye findings are at least consistent with that diagnosis, that thy-

roid function or regulation is somehow disordered, or that conditions such as orbital tumors, that may mimic it, have been adequately excluded.

Specificity of Eye Findings

Ocular findings are most specific for Graves' ophthalmopathy when they occur bilaterally and in certain combinations (Fig. 30-17). The concurrence of bilateral lid retraction with proptosis and restrictive ophthalmoplegia is virtually diagnostic, whereas markedly asymmetric or unilateral occurrence of most of the manifestations of ophthalmopathy should raise the suspicion of other ocular disease. Even in patients in whom the ophthalmopathy is obviously due to Graves' disease, measurements of proptosis, which can be done using a

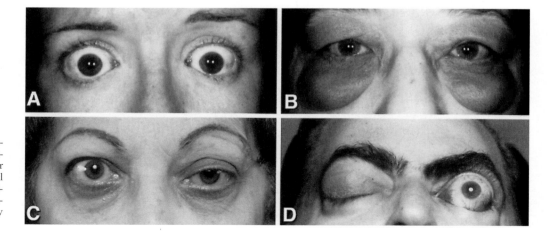

FIGURE 30-15. Clinical presentations of Graves' ophthalmopathy. *(A)* Retraction of both upper eyelids. *(B)* Severe periorbital edema. *(C)* Predominantly unilateral involvement. *(D)* Spontaneous subluxation of a severely proptotic left eye.

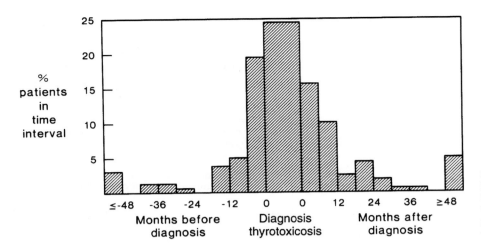

FIGURE 30-16. Onset of eye symptoms in relation to time of diagnosis of thyrotoxicosis (zero on horizontal axis). The number of patients who first noticed eye symptoms within a given 6-month period is expressed as the percentage of the entire group.

variety of exophthalmometers, frequently vary by 1 or 2 mm even between experienced examiners.[61] Ethnic differences exist for normal proptosis measurements; Asians have an upper limit of 18 mm of protrusion as measured from the lateral orbital rim, as compared with 20 mm for whites and 22 mm for blacks.[62,63]

Conversely, bilateral proptosis alone is not diagnostic of Graves' ophthalmopathy. It may be a consequence of shallow orbits as in Crouzon's disease or to large globes, as are characteristic of severe myopia, or to retroocular fat accumulation, as occurs in exogenous steroid administration,[64] spontaneously occurring Cushing's syndrome, or obesity.[65] Bilateral proptosis also has been reported with lithium therapy,[66] cirrhosis,[67] orbital pseudotumor,[59] Wegener's granulomatosis,[68] lymphoma, arteriovenous malformations, and metastatic tumors.[59,69,70] Unilateral proptosis is, of course, even less specific; nevertheless, Graves' ophthalmopathy is the single most common cause of unilateral proptosis, representing from 15% to 28% of cases, followed by a variety of primary and metastatic tumors in about 25% of cases.[59,69]

Evaluation of the Eyes

A subjective assessment of the patient's eye status helps to define the stage of the patient in the natural history of the disease.[71] How long ago did the first eye symptom develop? Are eye pain, lacrimation, photophobia, visual blurring, or diplopia present? Are the symptoms stable or progressive? Are they tolerable or does the patient demand relief? If diplopia is present, is it intermittent or constant? What is the status of the cornea, optic nerve, and extraocular muscles? Are the patient and physician in agreement as to the most severe eye problem? Physicians may be most concerned about subtle optic neuropathy that the patient perceives as slight blurring of color vision or a barely detectable field defect,[72] whereas patients may be most concerned about diplopia that physicians recognize as likely to subside or readily correctable with prisms or extraocular muscle surgery. Effective communication between the patient and physician to reconcile their priorities helps to avoid later misunderstandings.

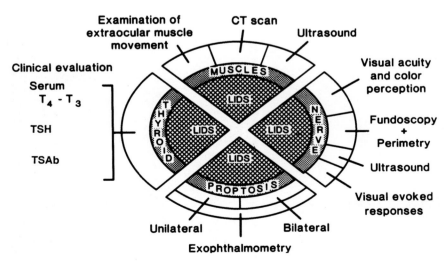

FIGURE 30-17. Diagnostic eye findings in patients with Graves' ophthalmopathy. The diagnosis is likely if all features from one quadrant are present. Eyelid changes *(inner ring)*, particularly lid reaction and lid lag, are among the most consistent and specific findings in Graves' ophthalmopathy. In patients with severe ophthalmopathy, all four quadrants of the figure may apply, but in less severe cases, the concurrence of lid changes with alterations in extraocular muscles, optic nerve, proptosis, or thyroid function is sufficient for diagnosis. Listed in the outer ring are the means by which these abnormalities are recognized. TSAB, TSH receptor-stimulating antibodies.

The objective eye examination begins with a determination of visual acuity in each eye separately. The pupillary responses are then carefully evaluated for the presence or absence of an afferent pupillary defect. When both a reduction in visual acuity and an afferent pupillary defect are present, optic neuropathy is likely and formal field testing is mandatory. Color vision, tested in each eye separately, can provide additional evidence of optic nerve dysfunction, except in the 8% of men who have congenital impairment of color perception. The eyes are then inspected for periorbital edema, lid edema, and lid lag. Lid fissure width and position of the lids relative to the limbus are measured with a ruler (Fig. 30-18). The patient is asked to close the lids lightly to check for incomplete lid closure (lagophthalmos). Lid lag is demonstrated by having the patient follow the finger of the examiner as it is moved slowly from the up gaze to the down gaze position. Conjunctival injection and chemosis, while frequently present, are nonspecific findings. Injection in Graves' disease is typically first seen over the insertions of the medial and lateral rectus muscles. A perilimbal pattern of injection is seen with ocular inflammation and may accompany exposure keratitis. Superior limbic keratoconjunctivitis may cause localized injection evident on down gaze and when the upper eyelid is retracted. With severe ophthalmopathy both types of conjunctivitis may coexist. Detection of exposure keratitis can be enhanced with the use of fluorescein. Motility disturbances can be recognized by asking the patient to move the eyes upward, downward, and from side to side. Diplopia field testing and use of the Lancaster or Hess screens allow quantitation of the degree of extraocular muscle impairment. Rigidity of the inferior rectus muscle pulling against the globe with up gaze can elevate the intraocular pressure reading and lead to an incorrect diagnosis of glaucoma. Measurement of the degree of proptosis with an exophthalmometer is followed by fundus examination to search for papilledema or choroidal folds which, when present in Graves' ophthalmopathy, tend to be associated with optic neuropathy or marked orbital inflammation.

Orbital Imaging

The advent of high resolution orbital imaging, first by ultrasonography and then by CT and magnetic resonance imaging (MRI), has greatly simplified the differential diagnosis of proptosis. CT imaging may be used to estimate the volume of extraocular muscle and retroocular fat tissue.[2,3,17,73] The primary indications for radiographic evaluation include confirming the diagnosis in patients in whom uncertainty exists and before orbital decompression. Both CT and MRI allow measurements of extraocular muscle thickness and the degree of proptosis and provide good visualization in the critical area at the orbital apex, where ultrasonography is least applicable. MRI after gadolinium-DTPA administration can distinguish between muscles that are swollen due to fatty degeneration, fibrosis, and edema, and T2-weighted MRI images may provide evidence of active inflammation.[74,75,76] Another advantage of MRI is the absence of radiation exposure to the lens; it is 0.017 to 0.032 Gy (1.7 to 3.2 rad) with CT scanning.[17] MRI, however, currently requires up to 60 minutes per examination and is more expensive.

CT imaging, with axial and coronal views, is the preferred study because of its ability to provide bony detail and lower cost. The earlier confusion on CT images between Graves' ophthalmopathy causing extraocular muscle enlargement near the apex and apical orbital tumors has been relieved by higher resolution images and multiplanar imaging.[23,77] Iodinated contrast material is usually not given to patients with thyrotoxicosis because it delays radioiodine treatment.

NATURAL HISTORY

Understanding the natural history of Graves' ophthalmopathy is very important in formulating a rational treatment plan. Ophthalmopathy in Graves' disease characteristically worsens over an initial period of 3 to 6 months. A lengthy plateau ensues, followed eventually in many patients by gradual spontaneous improvement. During the phase of progression, vision-threatening complications such as optic neuropathy or corneal ulceration may develop that demand urgent therapy. Measures taken to reduce orbital inflammation may have greatest efficacy during this stage. During the plateau phase, the patient's tolerance of the ophthalmopathy may wane before improvement is apparent. During the resolution phase, the extraocular muscles may heal by progressive fibrosis, resulting in fibrotic contractures and diplopia.

The Effect of Therapy for Thyrotoxicosis

Thyrotoxicosis may precede or follow Graves' ophthalmopathy. When it comes first, it has been suggested that antithyroid treatment rather than the natural course of the illness is responsible for subsequent onset or exacerbation of ophthalmopathy. This notion is based on the theory that thyroid damage accompanying treatment of thyrotoxicosis activates the autoimmune response against antigens co-expressed in the thyroid and retroocular tissues.[78] Because radioiodine therapy evokes at least transient increases in serum concentrations of TSH recep-

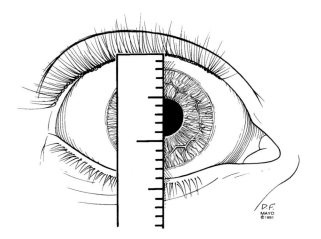

FIGURE 30-18. Eyelid position and fissure width measurement can be easily and reproducibly measured with the ruler centered on the pupil while the facial muscles are relaxed and gaze is directed straight ahead. The lid fissure measures 14 mm; the upper lid is retracted 2 mm from the limbus, while the lower lid is retracted 1 mm from the limbus. (Garrity JA. Graves' ophthalmopathy: An ophthalmologist's perspective. Thyroid Today 1992;15:1-9. Reproduced with permission)

tor antibodies,[79,80] which may cross-react with orbital tissues, it has received special attention as a potential causative agent for ophthalmopathy.[81] Here, we use the term post-radioiodine ophthalmopathy to refer only to a temporal and not an etiologic sequence. The evidence that radioiodine therapy causes or exacerbates ophthalmopathy is unconvincing.[82] Two recent controlled trials have examined this issue. In one trial,[83] the rate of development or worsening of ophthalmopathy was studied in patients with thyrotoxicosis caused by Graves' disease who were randomly assigned to receive an antithyroid drug alone, thyroidectomy, or radioiodine. Ophthalmopathy occurred or worsened during a 24-month follow-up period in 33% of the radioiodine-treated patients, as compared with 10% and 16% of patients treated medically or surgically, respectively. However, the radioiodine treatment group had a greater percentage of smokers, many were transiently hypothyroid, and many appeared to have refractory Graves' disease, with nearly one half requiring repeated doses of ^{131}I to control thyrotoxicosis. Further, only 6 of the patients had sufficiently severe ophthalmopathy to warrant specific treatment. In a second randomized trial,[84] the efficacy of concomitant treatment with corticosteroids in patients receiving ^{131}I to prevent treatment-associated worsening of ocular status was evaluated. During an 18-month follow-up period, worsening of pre-existing ophthalmopathy occurred in 56% of patients who were treated with radioiodine alone, as compared with no worsening in similar patients who received radioiodine and concurrent corticosteroid therapy. The finding that early corticosteroid therapy attenuates the subsequent course of Graves' ophthalmopathy does not prove that radioiodine aggravates eye disease. The benefit may have been independent of the method chosen to treat thyrotoxicosis. In a retrospective analysis of 426 patients with thyrotoxicosis caused by Graves' disease treated with an antithyroid drug, radioiodine, or thyroidectomy, there was no association between the type of therapy and the progression of ophthalmopathy.[85]

Other recent trials have examined the effects of thyroid hormone therapy on the course of Graves' ophthalmopathy. In one study[86] eye disease deteriorated in 11% of patients receiving thyroxine (T_4) therapy starting 2 weeks after administration of radioiodine, as compared with 18% of patients who became hypothyroid before T_4 therapy was begun. In a second study,[87] patients receiving a combined regimen of triiodothyronine (T_3) and antithyroid drug therapy before radioiodine had a slightly lower incidence of progression of eye disease than patients pretreated with an antithyroid drug alone, but the T_3-treated patients also received higher drug doses. A third study[88] found that pretreatment with an antithyroid drug plus T_4 had no effect on the incidence of worsening of ophthalmopathy, but serum TSH concentrations were elevated after radioiodine therapy more frequently in patients having new or worsened eye disease. These studies suggest that thyroid hormone therapy may provide modest benefit in reducing the development or progression of ophthalmopathy after thyroid ablation, and that this effect may be due to prevention of a post-therapy rise in serum TSH concentrations.

TREATMENT

The vast majority of patients with Graves' ophthalmopathy are successfully treated with reassurance and local protective measures alone. Patients with more severe ophthalmopathy, such as those with advanced soft tissue inflammation, ophthalmoplegia, moderate to severe proptosis, or optic neuropathy, are considered for more aggressive management. These patients have an illness that may last for months or years and may involve thyrotoxicosis, hypothyroidism, severe corticosteroid side effects, and disconcerting changes in their appearance. They may also encounter an array of specialists, each of whom tends to focus on a small component of their condition, so that all too frequently management is not comprehensive. It is the role of the internist or endocrinologist to provide perspective, continuity, and structure in the management of patients with Graves' eye disease.

The Eye Condition In Context

In a comprehensive evaluation, the examiner should determine what other medical conditions are present and the degree of threat they pose to the patient's life and well-being. Specifically, are there contraindications to corticosteroid therapy or to surgery? If the patient had received systemic corticosteroids in the past, what side effects resulted? Skin bruising, weight gain, and abnormal fat distribution are reversible in time, but bone loss may be irreversible, and compression fractures should be considered a contraindication to further corticosteroid therapy. It is important to define the patient's thyroid status since thyrotoxicosis may induce lid retraction and lid lag, which disappear when it is corrected. Conversely, periorbital edema may be a consequence of hypothyroidism that disappears when T_4 is given. The physician should define what treatment has been directed against the thyroid gland in the past, the degree to which it was successful, and the probability that it will be needed again. Aberrant thyroid function should be corrected with T_4, an antithyroid drug or radioiodine; the authors do not hesitate to treat a patient with thyrotoxicosis with radioiodine regardless of the stage of the ophthalmopathy.[82] It is important to establish the stage in evolution of the ophthalmopathy. Typically treatment is called for in the ascendant phase because of concern about symptoms or protecting vision. In the plateau phase the patient's weariness with the persistent manifestations of the illness is a motivating factor to seek treatment. In the late phase the treatments are often rehabilitative and intended to relieve pain, provide better coverage of the globe, correct diplopia, and improve appearance. Some of the treatments and the criteria used to select them are summarized in Table 30-6 and in Figure 30-19.

Local Protective Measures

For all patients with ophthalmopathy, measures to protect the cornea are appropriate. Use of tinted spectacle lenses worn out of doors should protect against wind and wind-borne particles. Artificial tears instilled as eye drops often diminish the foreign-body sensation that is sometimes troublesome. A protective eye patch, taping the eyelids shut at night, or the use of an artificial tear ointment at bedtime may further reduce the tendency of the cornea to dry as a result of exposure. Topical application of guanethidine to combat lid retraction is best avoided because it causes local irritation with variable effectiveness.[55,89]

TABLE 30-6.
Available Treatment Options for Graves' Ophthalmopathy

Objectives	Modes	Mechanism of Effect
Protection of cornea	Lubricants	Prevent corneal drying and exposure keratopathy
	Taping eyelids shut	
	Protective eye patches	
	Dark spectacle lenses	
	Eyelid surgery	
Reduction of intraorbital soft tissue volume	Diuretics	Decrease fluid content
	Radiotherapy	? Eliminates pathogenetic retroocular lymphocytes
	Plasmapheresis	? Removes pathogenetic antibodies
	Corticosteroids and other immunomodulatory drugs	Nonspecific immune suppression, antiinflammatory effects
Expansion of orbital space	Decompression surgery	Relieves intraorbital pressure by allowing expansion of orbital tissues into adjacent areas
Correction of diplopia	Prisms	Corrects minor degrees of diplopia
	Monocular occlusion	Eliminates diplopia not correctable by prisms or extraocular muscle surgery
	Extraocular muscle surgery	Modifies tension to allow realignment of eyes deviated by extraocular muscle fibrosis
Improvement of appearance	Müller's muscle recession or levator tarsorraphy	Corrects eyelid malposition and exposure keratitis

Treatments Intended to Modify the Immune Response

The treatments in this category are directed against effectors of the retroocular immune response believed responsible for the pathogenesis of Graves' ophthalmopathy. As opposed to surgical methods for expanding orbital volume, these therapies attempt to decrease the mass of tissue occupying this space while reducing damage to the components of the orbit such as the extraocular muscles. Hence, corticosteroids and orbital radiation therapy are believed to eliminate established clones of activated retroocular lymphocytes, while drugs such as cyclosporine A may act to prevent re-emergence of these clones. Plasmapheresis removes circulating antibodies or other noxious substances presumably involved in the retroocular immune response. Determining the efficacy of any therapy for Graves' ophthalmopathy requires circumspection if one is to avoid confusing natural disease regression with therapeutic benefit.[90] Therefore, when available, adequately controlled, prospective trials will be emphasized in this section. Unfortunately, such trials are few or nonexistent for several commonly used treatments for this disorder.

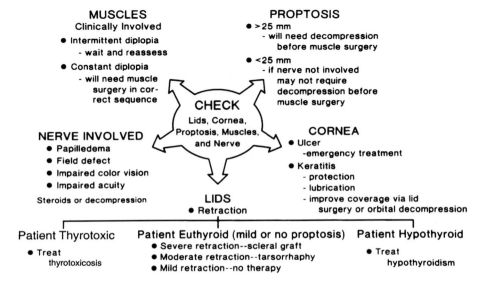

FIGURE 30-19. Flow chart of eye examination for comprehensive care decision-making in patients with Graves' ophthalmopathy.

SYSTEMIC CORTICOSTEROID THERAPY

Corticosteroids have been used in the treatment of Graves' ophthalmopathy for over 40 years.[1] In addition to their anti-inflammatory and immunomodulatory effects, they may directly inhibit glycosaminoglycan synthesis and release from fibroblasts.[26] Corticosteroid therapy provides rapid amelioration of the pain, injection, and conjunctival edema associated with the inflammatory soft tissue changes in Graves' ophthalmopathy, and may also provide substantial relief from compressive optic neuropathy while awaiting disease regression or more definitive therapy.[91] Improvement in proptosis and ophthalmoplegia may also occur, but to a lesser degree and with a higher likelihood of exacerbation after discontinuation of treatment.[1,92]

Therapy is usually initiated with a relatively high dose of corticosteroid such as 60 to 80 mg of prednisone per day for 2 to 4 weeks, after which the daily dose is tapered by 2.5 to 10.0 mg every 2 to 4 weeks, as permitted by the patient's response.[93,94,95] Regression of chemosis and attendant symptoms occurs within 48 hours, while improvement in extraocular muscle function, if it occurs at all, may require several weeks of therapy. Optic nerve dysfunction may improve after as little as 2 weeks, and may continue to improve for several months. Adverse effects associated with high-dose corticosteroid therapy include weight gain, psychosis, osteoporosis, and glucose intolerance.[1] Depot subconjunctival or retrobulbar corticosteroid injections[96] have been used as a means of limiting the systemic effects of corticosteroids, but the associated risk[97] and patient discomfort limit the usefulness of this approach. Recently, intravenous pulse therapy with large doses of methylprednisolone has been advocated as a means of delivering immunosuppressive doses of corticosteroid while reducing the side effects associated with chronic high-dose oral prednisone therapy.[98–100] Corticosteroid preparations appear to act synergistically with other anti-inflammatory treatments such as radiation therapy[101,102] and cyclosporine A.[103,104]

Corticosteroid therapy is most efficacious in patients with a shorter duration of disease.[1] Other predictors of response to anti-inflammatory therapy include the presence of classic signs of inflammation, as assessed by activity score[105] and the degree of signal intensity on MRI.[74,106] In summary, corticosteroid therapy provides rapid relief from the inflammatory changes occurring in Graves' ophthalmopathy, but the benefit is associated with important side effects, and tapering or discontinuation frequently results in disease exacerbation.

OTHER IMMUNOSUPPRESSIVE AGENTS

Cyclosporine A inhibits the proliferation of helper T cells and the production of cytokines, prevents activation of cytotoxic T cells, and suppresses immunoglobulin production by B cells.[107] After initial anecdotal reports and several uncontrolled trials, two prospective randomized studies examined the efficacy of cyclosporine A in Graves' ophthalmopathy.[103,104] In one study,[103] patients receiving prednisone alone were compared with those given both prednisone and cyclosporine A. Patients receiving combined therapy had a more rapid fall in eye activity score, a greater decrease in extraocular muscle thickness by CT, and a lower frequency of exacerbation after prednisone was withdrawn. In the second trial,[104] cyclosporine A and prednisone initially were compared as single drug therapies, and combination therapy with both was then given to patients failing either alone. Prednisone was superior to cyclosporine A as single drug therapy, but nearly 60% of patients not responding to either alone subsequently improved with combined therapy. Early high-dose corticosteroid therapy may result in lysis of clones of activated helper T cells, while maintenance cyclosporine A therapy prevents re-emergence of effector T cells, thereby allowing expansion of suppressor T cells.[108] Despite this apparent efficacy, the high cost of cyclosporine A and the requirement for frequent drug monitoring, coupled with a side effect profile that includes hypertension, renal insufficiency, hepatic dysfunction, gum hypertrophy, hypertrichosis, and paresthesia,[107,109] limit the utility of this drug.

Patients with active Graves' ophthalmopathy have also been treated with azathioprine,[110,111] cyclophosphamide,[112,113] ciamexone,[114] and intravenous immunoglobulin.[115] Only azathioprine[111] and ciamexone[114] have been studied in adequately controlled trials, and neither proved efficacious. Total thyroid ablation, using meticulous thyroid bed dissection or high doses of radioactive iodine in an effort to eradicate all thyroidal antigens, has not proven useful and may expose the patient to unnecessary risk.

PLASMAPHERESIS

The efficacy of removal of circulating immunoglobulins with plasmapheresis in ophthalmopathy patients has been examined in several small trials.[1] In a study[116] in which 18 patients underwent plasma exchange for several weeks, there was no significant improvement in proptosis, extraocular muscle dysfunction, visual acuity, visual fields, intraocular pressure, or appearance of extraocular muscles on ultrasonography or CT. Conversely, in another study involving 11 patients with severe ophthalmopathy,[117] plasma exchange followed by immunosuppressive therapy resulted in significant improvement in soft tissue inflammation, proptosis, intraocular pressure, and extraocular muscle function. Other studies of plasma exchange also yielded conflicting results.[1] The concurrent use of immunosuppressive therapy in most of these studies and the absence of suitable control groups prevent any conclusions regarding the efficacy of plasmapheresis in Graves' ophthalmopathy.

ORBITAL RADIATION THERAPY

The rationale for the use of supervoltage orbital radiation therapy in Graves' ophthalmopathy depends on the exquisite radiosensitivity of lymphocytes, thought to be a primary effector in this disorder. Radiation to the orbits is generally administered using 20 Gy (2000 rads) delivered in 10 fractions over 2 weeks, although several European centers have used a lower total dosage effectively.[118] The largest experience reported to date involved more than 300 patients treated with megavoltage radiation,[119,120] of whom approximately one third received concurrent corticosteroid therapy. After orbital radiation, 80% of patients had improvement in soft tissue inflammation, 51% had recession of proptosis, 56% had improvement in eye muscle function, and 67% had improvement in vision. Despite this improvement, 29% of patients required one or more eye operations after the radiation therapy, most of which were performed to correct strabismus. In a recent randomized double-blind trial comparing orbital radiation with prednisone in patients with Graves' ophthalmopathy, the efficacy of the two therapies was similar, but orbital radiation had fewer side effects.[121] In a review of 14 uncontrolled studies of orbital radiotherapy in Graves' ophthalmopathy,[1] the authors concluded that orbital radiation is well tolerated and generally effective. The benefit occurs within 1 to 4 weeks after the initiation of therapy,[122,123] and may continue for as long as 12 months after its completion. Soft tissue inflammatory changes are often reduced, and in many patients muscle function, proptosis, and optic neuropathy improve. The effects on proptosis and ophthalmoplegia are generally insufficient to avoid orbital decompression and strabismus surgery in patients with indications for these procedures, but radiation may shorten the interval before surgical intervention may be attempted.[92] In general, the duration of eye disease correlates inversely with the likelihood of response to radiotherapy.[1]

Combined orbital radiation and corticosteroid therapy is more effective than either alone.[101] Lastly, although orbital radiation has few adverse effects, it can cause retinopathy and cataracts, emphasizing the importance of patient referral to a center having expertise with this technique.[124,125,126]

Nonimmunomodulatory Treatments

Several novel therapies have been examined for efficacy in the management of Graves' ophthalmopathy.[1,107] The presence of receptors for insulin-like growth factor-I on retroocular connective tissue and extraocular muscle[127] provided the rationale for a trial of the somatostatin analogue octreotide in patients with ophthalmopathy.[128] Each of six patients treated with octreotide for 3 months had improvement in extraocular muscle function. Amelioration of soft tissue changes occurred in two patients, and localized myxedema, present in three patients, also resolved. Other agents with less apparent rationale for use, including bromocriptine[129] and metronidazole,[130] were effective in a few patients; however, it is not possible to distinguish therapeutic benefit from spontaneous disease regression. Acupuncture was useful in an uncontrolled trial in some patients with ophthalmopathy,[131] but it had no benefit in a more recent trial.[132]

Surgical Therapy

In general, the surgical approaches produce results much more quickly than the nonsurgical approaches[133] (Fig. 30-20). If surgical treatment is chosen, it is important that the different approaches be considered in proper sequence. Orbital decompression, if required, should be performed first. Extraocular muscle surgery, if required, should follow orbital decompression. Any eyelid surgery should follow extraocular muscle surgery.

Orbital decompression can be considered at any point in the course of the disease. It is not necessary that it be stable, and surgery can be performed while the process is worsening. There are many indications for orbital decompression, but the central theme is any circumstance in which expansion of the bony orbital volume is desired (Table 30-7). Another type of

decompression removes only orbital fat without removing any bone[134-137]; this procedure is typically considered only after the ophthalmopathy has been quiescent for at least 6 months, and as such its utility for congestive ophthalmopathy is limited. Patients with large extraocular muscles but little fat evident on CT scanning would be poor candidates for this type of procedure.

The optic neuropathy of Graves' ophthalmopathy is most likely due to apical compression of the optic nerve by enlarged extraocular muscles,[138,139] although stretching of this nerve due to excessive proptosis may present similarly in exceptional cases.[140] The key to successful surgery for compressive optic neuropathy is apical orbital decompression. The apex can be adequately decompressed only by removing the roof or medial wall. Therefore, effective therapy of optic neuropathy requires inclusion of one of these walls in the decompression. The medial wall is the one most frequently chosen, in which case it is essential to decompress the posterior ethmoid air cells adequately.[141]

Patients with severe orbital inflammation that worsens when the dosage of corticosteroid is reduced beyond a certain threshold level or is associated with deep orbital pain generally respond well to decompression. Much of their soft tissue swelling is due to venous congestion that rapidly improves after decompression.[37]

Corneal exposure related to excessive proptosis is best managed by orbital decompression. The amount of globe recession obtained is roughly proportional to the number of orbital walls decompressed[142] (Table 30-8). The relative merits of four types of decompression are shown in Table 30-9. In our practice, the transantral route is most frequently used. We believe this procedure offers an acceptable balance between ease of operation, safety, and effectiveness with an acceptable range of side effects (Table 30-10).

Patients with moderate proptosis and an obvious requirement for extraocular muscle surgery should be considered for orbital decompression before muscle surgery. As the swollen retroocular tissues push the globe forward, the extraocular muscles resist this trend. A recession of the muscle would theoretically allow the globe to come forward, exacerbating the proptosis. There is no specific measurement of proptosis that defines the need for orbital decompression, although a reading of more than 25 mm should lead to consideration for operation. An important further consideration is that recession of the inferior rectus muscle will result in lower lid retraction, thereby compounding any exposure keratitis.

We approach orbital decompression for cosmetic reasons cautiously. While the procedure is effective for an appropriately motivated patient, some patients have unrealistic expectations of the benefit of the operation.

The surgical treatment of diplopia after decompression should be delayed for at least 6 weeks or until any orbital inflammation has subsided and any motility disturbance has remained stable for 6 to 9 months. The most frequently performed procedure is a recession (a weakening procedure) of the medial or inferior rectus muscles. Eye muscle surgery will not restore the eyes to their normal premorbid state, but rather its goal is to restore single binocular vision in primary gaze and in the reading position. Multiple operative procedures may be required.

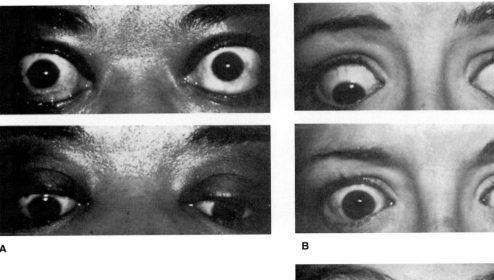

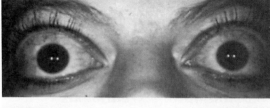

FIGURE 30-20. Results of orbital surgery in patients with Graves' ophthalmopathy. *(A)* Transantral orbital decompression before *(top)* and after *(bottom)*. *(B)* Extraocular muscle surgery before *(top)* and after *(bottom)*. *(C)* Scleral graft insertion to correct eyelid malposition before *(top)* and after *(bottom)*. (Courtesy of Drs. LW DeSanto, J Dyer, and R Waller. Photographs *A* and *C* are from Gorman CA. The presentation and management of endocrine ophthalmopathy. Clin Endocrinol Metab 1978;7:67)

Non-urgent eyelid surgery represents the final phase of surgical rehabilitation for patients with severe ophthalmopathy. We reevaluate patients approximately 6 weeks after completion of extraocular muscle surgery, especially vertical muscle surgery, for consideration of lid procedures. Inferior rectus restriction indirectly affects upper lid position and lid retraction may resolve following recession of this muscle, while superior rectus recession will cause more upper lid retraction. If no decompression or eye muscle surgery was required, stable lid findings for at least 6 months and normal thyroid function are essential before determining the need for lid surgery.

Upper lid retraction, up to 2 mm, can be treated with a recession of Müller's muscle. Recession of the levator, especially along its temporal aspect, is included if the degree of retraction is greater. Lower lid retraction can be more challenging since it is antigravity. Simple lateral tarsorrhaphies will sometimes improve lower lid retraction, but ultimately some type of

TABLE 30-7.
Indications for Orbital Decompression

Optic neuropathy
Severe orbital inflammation
Excessive proptosis
   Before extraocular muscle surgery
   Exposure keratitis
   Cosmesis
Pain relief
Corticosteroid dependence

TABLE 30-8.
Proptosis Reduction as a Function of Number of Walls Decompressed

Walls Decompressed	Globe Recession
1 (medial wall)	0–4 mm
2 (lateral wall + floor, or floor + medial wall)	3–6 mm
3 (medial + lateral walls + floor)	6–10 mm
4 (all 4 walls)	10–17 mm

(Kennerdell JS, Maroon JC, Buerger GF. Comprehensive surgical management of proptosis in dysthyroid orbitopathy. Orbit 1987;6:153)

TABLE 30-9.
Advantages and Disadvantages of Four Types of Orbital Decompression

Advantages	Disadvantages
TRANSANTRAL DECOMPRESSION (FLOOR AND MEDIAL WALL)	
No external scar	Anatomy unfamiliar to most ophthalmologists
Good operative visualization and control of intraoperative sinus bleeding	More postoperative facial swelling
Decompresses posterior ethmoid sinuses (important for relief of optic nerve compression)	More postoperative diplopia
Short operative period (2 h for bilateral procedure) and brief hospitalization (1–2 days)	Numb upper lip
ANTERIOR DECOMPRESSIONS (1, 2, 3, OR ALL 4 WALLS)	
Easy to individualize therapy	External scar
Anatomy familiar	Visualization of medial wall can be difficult
Less postoperative diplopia	Difficulty treating intraoperative sinus bleeding
Nasal endoscope may be used for medial wall and medial floor	More postoperative diplopia
Shorter hospital stay (1 inpatient day)	Numb upper lip
	Longer surgery (4–5h for bilateral 3-wall operation)
TRANSFRONTAL DECOMPRESSION (ROOF + LATERAL WALL)	
Less postoperative diplopia	Haircut
Upper lip not numb	External scar with burr holes
Effective for optic neuropathy	Possible frontalis paresis
Effective for failed prior decompression	Postoperative pulsating globe
	Longer surgery (4–5 h for both eyes)
	Longer hospital stay (4–5 days)
ORBITAL FAT DECOMPRESSION	
Upper lip not numb	Not useful with active disease
No postoperative sinus complications	Not useful if minimal fat apparent on imaging studies
Can perform blepharoplasty at same time	Temporary diplopia possible due to trauma to inferior oblique muscle
Short hospital stay (usually 1 day)	Minimal proptosis reduction (usually)

spacer might have to be inserted. A hard palate graft suits this purpose as well or better than scleral grafts.

In summary, the elements of successful care of the patient with Graves' ophthalmopathy include careful medical and endocrine assessment to establish the setting in which ophthalmopathy occurs. A careful examination of the eyes and orbit including establishment of priorities for physician and patient is followed by coordinated management. This sometimes involves the endocrinologist, otolaryngologist, and ophthalmologist.

TABLE 30-10.
Side Effects of Transantral Orbital Decompression

Diplopia
Sinusitis
Cerebrospinal fluid leak, meningitis
Lip numbness
Entropion (inversion of eyelid)
Nasolacrimal duct obstruction

References

1. Burch HB, Wartofsky L. Graves' ophthalmopathy: current concepts regarding pathogenesis and management. Endocr Rev 1993;14:747
2. Forbes G, Gorman CA, Brennan MD, Gehring DG, Ilstrup DM, Earnest F. Ophthalmopathy of Graves' disease: computerized volume measurements of the orbital fat and muscle. Am J Neuroradiol 1986;7:651
3. Forbes G, Gorman CA, Gehring DG, Baker HL. Computer analysis of orbital fat and muscle volumes in Graves' ophthalmopathy. Am J Neuroradiol 1983;4:737
4. Hamilton RD, Mayberry WE, McConahey WM, Hanson KC. Ophthalmopathy of Graves' disease: a comparison between patients treated surgically and patients treated with radioiodine. Mayo Clin Proc 1967;42:812
5. Kriss JP. Pathogenesis and treatment of Graves' ophthalmopathy. Thyroid Today 1984;7:1
6. Bartley GB, Fatourechi V, Kadrmas EF, et al. The incidence of Graves' ophthalmopathy in Olmsted County. Am J Ophthalmol 1995;120:511
7. Perros P, Kendall-Taylor P. Pathogenetic mechanisms in thyroid-associated ophthalmopathy. J Intern Med 1992;231:205

8. Bartalena L, Martino E, Marcocci C, et al. More on smoking habits and Graves' ophthalmopathy. J Endocrinol Invest 1989; 12:733

9. Hägg E, Asplund K. Is endocrine ophthalmopathy related to smoking? BMJ 1987;295:634

10. Prummel MF, Wiersinga WM. Smoking and risk of Graves' disease. JAMA 1993;269:518

11. Shine B, Fells P, Edwards OM, Weetman AP. Association between Graves' ophthalmopathy and smoking. Lancet 1990; 335:1261

12. Hegedüs L, Karstrup S, Veiergang D, Jacobsen B, Skovsted L, Feldt-Rasmussen U. High frequency of goiter in cigarette smokers. Clin Endocrinol 1985;22:287

13. Christensen SB, Ericsson UB, Janzon L, Tibblin S, Melander A. Influence of cigarette smoking on goiter formation, thyroglobulin, and thyroid hormone levels in women. J Clin Endocrinol Metab 1984;58:615

14. Garrity JA, Gorman CA. Pitfalls associated with orbital decompression for thyroid associated orbitopathy. Exp Clin Endocrinol 1991;97:338

15. DeSanto LW, Gorman CA. Selection of patients and choice of operation for orbital decompression in Graves' ophthalmopathy. Laryngoscope 1973;83:945

16. Koornneef L. Orbital bony and soft tissue anatomy. In: Gorman CA, Campbell RJ, Dyer JA, eds. The eye and orbit in thyroid disease. New York: Raven Press, 1984:5

17. Markl AF, Hilbertz T, Mann K. Graves' ophthalmopathy: Standardized evaluation of computed tomography examinations and magnetic resonance imaging. Dev Ophthalmol 1989;20:38

18. Forbes G. Computerized imaging evaluation: CT and NMR scanning and computed volume measurement. In: Gorman CA, Campbell RJ, Dyer JA, eds. The eye and orbit in thyroid disease. New York: Raven Press, 1984:173

19. Rundle FF, Pochin EE. The orbital tissues in thyrotoxicosis: a quantitative analysis relating to exophthalmos. Clin Sci 1944;5:51

20. Hufnagel TJ, Hickey WF, Cobbs WH, Jakobiec FA, Iwamoto T, Eagle RC. Immunohistochemical and ultrastructural studies of the exenterated orbital tissues of a patient with Graves' disease. Ophthalmology 1984;91:1411

21. Raikow RB, Dalbow MH, Kennerdell JS, et al. Immunohistochemical evidence for IgE involvement in Graves' orbitopathy. Ophthalmology 1990;97:629

22. Tallstedt L, Norberg R. Immunohistochemical staining of normal and Graves' extraocular muscle. Invest Ophthal Vis Sci 1988; 29:175

23. Trokel SL, Jakobiec FA. Correlation of CT scanning and pathologic features of ophthalmic Graves' disease. Ophthalmology 1981;88:553

24. Kroll AJ, Kuwabara T. Dysthyroid ocular myopathy: anatomy, histology, and electron microscopy. Arch Ophthalmol 1966; 76:244

25. Riley FC. Orbital pathology in Graves' disease. Mayo Clin Proc 1972;47:975

26. Smith TJ, Bahn RS, Gorman CA. Connective tissue, glycosaminoglycans, and diseases of the thyroid. Endocr Rev 1989;10:366

27. Nugent RA, Belkin RI, Neigel JM, Rootman J, Robertson WD, Spinelli J, Graeb DA. Graves' orbitopathy: correlation of CT and clinical findings. Radiology 1990;177:675

28. Weetman AP, Cohen S, Gatter KC, Fells P, Shine B. Immunohistochemical analysis of the retrobulbar tissues in Graves' ophthalmopathy. Clin Exp Immunol 1989;75:222

29. Grubeck-Loebenstein B, Trieb K, Sztankay A, Holter W, Anderl H, Wick G. Retrobulbar T cells from patients with Graves' ophthalmopathy are CD8+ and specifically recognize autologous fibroblasts. J Clin Invest 1994;93:2738

30. Bahn RS, Smith TJ, Gorman CA. The central role of the fibroblast in the pathogenesis of extrathyroidal manifestations of Graves' ophthalmopathy. Acta Endocrinol 1989;121(Suppl 2):75

31. Smith TJ, Bahn RS, Gorman CA. Hormonal regulation of hyaluronate synthesis in cultured fibroblasts: evidence for differences between retroocular and dermal fibroblasts. J Clin Endocrinol Metab 1989;69:1019

32. Stanley RJ, McCaffrey TV, Offord KP, DeSanto LW. Superior and transantral orbital decompression procedures. Effects on increased intraorbital pressure and orbital dynamics. Arch Otolaryngol Head Neck Surg 1989;115:369

33. Kahaly G, Schuler M, Sewell AC, Bernhard G, Beyer G, Krause U. Urinary glycosaminoglycans in Graves' ophthalmopathy. Clin Endocrinol 1990;33:35

34. McGregor AM. Immunoendocrine interactions in autoimmunity. N Engl J Med 1990;332:1739

35. Merrill HG, Oaks LW. Extreme bilateral exophthalmos: report of two cases with autopsy findings in one. Am J Ophthalmol 1933;16:231

36. Bahn RS, Heufelder AE. Pathogenesis of Graves' ophthalmopathy. N Engl J Med 1993;329:1468

37. Hudson HL, Levin L, Feldon SE. Graves' exophthalmos unrelated to extraocular muscle enlargement. Superior rectus muscle inflammation may induce venous obstruction. Ophthalmology 1991;98:1495

38. Sisson JC. Stimulation of glucose utilization and glycosaminoglycan production by fibroblasts derived from retrobulbar tissue. Exp Eye Res 1971;12:285

39. Heufelder AE, Bahn RS. Detection and localization of cytokine immunoreactivity in retroocular connective tissue in Graves' ophthalmopathy. Eur J Clin Invest 1993;23:10

40. Heufelder AE, Bahn RS. Modulation of orbital fibroblast proliferation by cytokines and glucocorticoid receptor antagonists. Invest Ophthalmol Vis Sci 1994;35:120

41. Korducki JM, Loftus SJ, Bahn RS. Stimulation of glycosaminoglycan production in cultured human retroocular fibroblasts. Invest Ophthalmol Vis Sci 1992;33:2037

42. Smith TJ, Bahn RS, Gorman CA, Cheavens M. Stimulation of glycosaminoglycan accumulation by interferon gamma in human cultured retroocular fibroblasts. J Clin Endocrinol Metab 1991;72:1169

43. Heufelder AE, Bahn RS. Graves' immunoglobulins and cytokines stimulate the expression of intercellular adhesion molecule-1 (ICAM-1) in cultured Graves' orbital fibroblasts. Eur J Clin Invest 1992;22:529

44. Heufelder AE, Smith TJ, Gorman CA, Bahn RS. Increased induction of HLA-DR by interferon gamma in cultured fibroblasts derived from patients with Graves' ophthalmopathy and pretibial dermopathy. J Clin Endocrinol Metab 1991;73:307

45. Heufelder AE, Wenzel BE, Gorman CA, Bahn RS. Detection, cellular localization and modulation of heat shock proteins in cultured fibroblasts from patients with extrathyroidal manifestations of Graves' disease. J Clin Endocrinol Metab 1991;73:739

46. Bahn RS, Gorman CA, Johnson CM, Smith TJ. Presence of antibodies in the sera of patients of patients with Graves' disease recognizing a 23 kilodalton fibroblast protein. J Clin Endocrinol Metab 1989;69:622

47. Salvi M, Miller A, Wall JR. Human orbital tissue and thyroid membranes express a 64 kDa protein which is recognized by autoantibodies in the serum of patients with thyroid-associated ophthalmopathy. FEBS Lett 1988;232:135

48. Weetman AP. Thyroid-associated ophthalmopathy. Autoimmunity 1992;12:215

49. Kendler DL, Rootman J, Huber GK, Davies TF. A 64 kDa membrane antigen is a recurrent epitope for natural autoantibodies in patients with Graves' thyroid and ophthalmic disease. Clin Endocrinol 1991;35:539

50. Burch HB, Selletti D, Barnes SG, Nagy EV, Bahn RS, Burman KD. Thyrotropin receptor antisera for the detection in immunoreactive protein species in retroocular fibroblasts obtained from pa-

tients with Graves' ophthalmopathy. J Clin Endocrinol Metab 1994;78:1384

51. Heufelder AE, Dutton CM, Sarkar G, Donovan KA, Bahn RS. Detection of TSH receptor RNA in cultured fibroblasts from patients with Graves' ophthalmopathy and pretibial dermopathy. Thyroid 1993;3:297

52. Paschke R, Metcalfe A, Alcalde G, Vassart G, Weetman A, Ludgate M. Presence of nonfunctional thyrotropin receptor variant transcripts in retroocular and other tissues. J Clin Endocrinol Metab 1994;79:1234

53. Feliciello A, Porcellini A, Ciullo I, Bonavolonta G, Avvedimento EV, Fenzi GF. Expression of thyrotropin-receptor in RNA in healthy and Graves' disease retro-orbital tissues. Lancet 1993;342:337

54. Dyer JA. The oculorotary muscles in Graves' disease. Trans Am Ophthalmol Soc 1976;74:425

55. Crombie AL, Lawson AAH. Long-term trial of guanethidine in treatment of eye signs of thyroid dysfunction and idiopathic lid retraction. BMJ 1967;4:592

56. Hay ID. Clinical presentations of Graves' ophthalmopathy. In: Gorman CA, Campbell RJ, Dyer JA, eds. The eye and orbit in thyroid disease. New York: Raven Press, 1984:129

57. Gorman CA. Temporal relationship between onset of Graves' ophthalmopathy and diagnosis of thyrotoxicosis. Mayo Clin Proc 1983;58:515

58. Tamai H, Nakagawa T, Ohsako N, Fukino O, Takahashi H, Matsuzuka F, Kuma K, Nagataki S. Changes in thyroid functions in patients with euthyroid Graves' disease. J Clin Endocrinol Metab 1980;50:108

59. Henderson JW. Orbital tumors. Philadelphia: WB Saunders, 1973:705

60. Solomon DH, Chopra IJ, Chopra U, Smith FJ. Identification of subgroups of euthyroid Graves' ophthalmopathy. N Engl J Med 1977;296:181

61. Musch DC, Freuh BR, Landis JR. The reliability of Hertel exophthalmometry. Observer variation between physician and lay readers. Ophthalmology 1985;92:1177

62. Migliori ME, Gladstone GJ. Determination of the normal range of exophthalmometric values for black and white adults. Am J Ophthalmol 1984;98:438

63. Amino N, Yuasa T, Yabu Y, Miyai K, Kumahara Y. Exophthalmos in autoimmune thyroid disease. J Clin Endocrinol Metab 1980;51:1232

64. Cohen BA, Som PA, Haffner PH, Friedman AH. Steroid exophthalmos. J Comput Assist Tomogr 1981;5:907

65. Peyster RG, Ginsberg F, Silber JH, Adler LP. Exophthalmos caused by excessive fat: CT volumetric analysis and differential diagnosis. Am J Neuroradiol 1986;7:35

66. Segal RL, Rosenblatt S, Eliasoph I. Endocrine exophthalmos during lithium therapy of manic-depressive disease. N Engl J Med 1973;289:136

67. Summerskill WHJ, Molnar GD. Eye signs in hepatic cirrhosis. N Engl J Med 1962;266:1244

68. Cassan SH, Divertie MB, Hollenhorst TW, Harrison EG. Pseudotumor of the orbit and limited Wegener's granulomatosis. Ann Intern Med 1970;72:687

69. Dallow RL. Evaluation of unilateral exophthalmos with ultrasonography: Analysis of 258 consecutive cases. Laryngoscope 1975;85:1905

70. Grove AS Jr. Evaluation of exophthalmos. N Engl J Med 1975;292:1005

71. Gorman CA. Comprehensive care. In: Gorman CA, Campbell RJ, Dyer JA, eds. The eye and orbit in thyroid disease. New York: Raven Press, 1984:325

72. Feldon SE, Maramatsu S, Weiner JM. Clinical classification of Graves' ophthalmopathy: identification of risk factors for optic neuropathy. Arch Ophthalmol 1984;102:1469

73. Feldon SE, Weiner JM. Clinical significance of extraocular muscle volumes in Graves' ophthalmopathy. A quantitative computed tomography study. Arch Ophthalmol 1982;100:1266

74. Hiromatsu Y, Kojima K, Ishisaka N, Tanaka K, Sato M, Nonaka K, Nishimura H, Nishida H. Role of magnetic resonance imaging in thyroid-associated ophthalmopathy: its predictive value for therapeutic outcome of immunosuppressive therapy. Thyroid 1992;2:299

75. Just M, Kahaly G, Higer HP, Rösler HP, Kutzner J, Beyer J, Thelen M. Graves' ophthalmopathy: role of MR imaging in radiation therapy. Radiology 1991;179:187

76. Sato M, Hiromatsu Y, Tanaka K, Nonaka K. Role of magnetic resonance imaging in thyroid-associated ophthalmopathy: prediction of therapeutic outcome of active eye disease. Abstract. Thyroid 1992;2 (Suppl 1):S34

77. Trokel SL, Hilal SK. Submillimeter resolution CT scanning of orbital diseases. Ophthalmology 1981;87:412

78. Kriss JP, Pleshakov V, Rosenblum AL, Holderness M, Sharp G, Utiger R. Studies on the pathogenesis of the ophthalmopathy of Graves' disease. J Clin Endocrinol 1967;27:582

79. Bech K, Feldt-Rasmussen U, Bliddal H, Date J, Blichert-Toft M. The acute changes in thyroid stimulating immunoglobulins, thyroglobulin, and thyroglobulin antibodies following subtotal thyroidectomy. Clin Endocrinol 1982;16:235

80. Bech K, Madsen N. Influence of treatment with radioiodine and propylthiouracil on thyroid stimulating immunoglobulins in Graves' disease. Clin Endocrinol 1980;13:417

81. Barth A, Probst P, Bürgi H. Identification of a subgroup of Graves' disease patients at higher risk for severe ophthalmopathy after radioiodine. J Endocrinol Invest 1991;14:209

82. Gorman CA. Radioiodine therapy does not aggravate Graves' ophthalmopathy. J Clin Endocrinol Metab 1995;80:340

83. Tallstedt L, Lundell G, Tørring O, Wallin G, Ljunggren J-G, Blomgren H, Taube A, and the Thyroid Study Group. Occurrence of ophthalmopathy after treatment for Graves' hyperthyroidism. N Engl J Med 1992;326:1733

84. Bartalena L, Marcocci C, Bogazzi F, Panicucci M, Lepri A, Pinchera A. Use of corticosteroids to prevent progression of Graves' ophthalmopathy after radioiodine therapy for hyperthyroidism. N Engl J Med 1989;321:1349

85. Sridama V, DeGroot LJ. Treatment of Graves' disease and the course of ophthalmopathy. Am J Med 1989;87:70

86. Tallstedt L, Lundell G, Blomgren H, Bring J. Does early administration of thyroxine reduce the development of Graves' ophthalmopathy after radioiodine treatment? Eur J Endocrinol 1994;130:494

87. Bromberg N, Romaldini JH, Werner RS, Sgarbi JA, Werner MC. The evolution of Graves' ophthalmopathy during treatment with antithyroid drag alone and combined with triiodothyronine. J Endocrinol Invest 1992;15:191

88. Kung AW, Yau CC, Cheng A. The incidence of ophthalmopathy after radioiodine therapy for Graves' disease: prognostic factors and the role of methimazole. J Clin Endocrinol Metab 1994;79:542

89. Dorian W, Schirmer KE. Guanethidine and pupillary reaction. Can Med Assoc J 1964;90:932

90. Bahn RS, Gorman CA. Choice of therapy and criteria for assessing treatment outcome in thyroid-associated ophthalmopathy. Endocrinol Metab Clin North Am 1987; 16:391

91. Day RM, Carroll FD. Corticosteroids in the treatment of optic nerve involvement associated with thyroid dysfunction. Arch Ophthalmol 1968;79:279

92. Wiersinga WM. Immunosuppressive treatment of Graves' ophthalmopathy. Thyroid 1992;2:229

93. Burman KD. Treatment of autoimmune ophthalmopathy. The Endocrinologist 1991;1:102

94. McConahey WM. Medical therapy. In: Gorman CA, Campbell RJ, Dyer JA, eds. The eye and orbit in thyroid disease. New York: Raven Press, 1984:317

95. Wiersinga WM. Immunosuppressive treatment of Graves' ophthalmopathy. Trends Endocrinol Metab 1990;1:377

96. Marcocci C, Bartalena L, Panicucci M, Marconcini C, Cartei F, Cavallacci G, Laddaga M, Campobasso G, Baschieri L, Pinchera A. Orbital cobalt irradiation combined with retrobulbar or systemic corticosteroids for Graves' ophthalmopathy: a comparative study. Clin Endocrinol 1987;27:33

97. Kahaly G, Beyer J. Immunosuppressant therapy of thyroid eye disease. Klin Wochenschr 1988;66:1049

98. Guy JR, Fagien S, Donovan JP, Rubin ML. Methylprednisolone pulse therapy in severe dysthyroid optic neuropathy. Ophthalmology 1989;96:1048

99. Kendall-Taylor P, Crombie AL, Stephenson AM, Hardwick M, Hall K. Intravenous methylprednisolone in the treatment of Graves' ophthalmopathy. BMJ 1988;297:1574

100. Nagayama Y, Izumi M, Kiriyama T, Yokoyama N, Morita S, Kakezono F, Ohtakara S. Treatment of Graves' ophthalmopathy with high-dose intravenous methylprednisolone pulse therapy. Acta Endocrinol 1987;116:513

101. Bartalena L, Marcocci C, Chiovato L, Lepri A, Andreani D, Cavallacci G, Baschieri L Pinchera A. Orbital cobalt irradiation combined with systemic corticosteroids for Graves' ophthalmopathy: comparison with systemic corticosteroids alone. J Clin Endocrinol Metab 1983;56:1139

102. Marcocci C, Bartalena L, Bogazzi F, Bruno-Bossio G, Lepri A, Pinchera A. Orbital radiotherapy combined with high dose systemic glucocorticoids for Graves' ophthalmopathy is more effective than radiotherapy alone: results of a prospective-randomized study. J Endocrinol Invest 1991; 14:853

103. Kahaly G, Schrezenmeir J, Krause U, Schweikert B, Meuer S, Muller W, Dennebaum R, Beyer J. Ciclosporin and prednisone v. prednisone in treatment of Graves' ophthalmopathy: a controlled, randomized and prospective study. Eur J Clin Invest 1986;16:415

104. Prummel MF, Mourits MP, Berghout A, Krenning EP, van der Gaag R, Kornneef L, Wiersinga WM. Prednisone and cyclosporine in the treatment of severe Graves' ophthalmopathy. N Engl J Med 1989;321:1353

105. Mourits MP. Koornneef L, Wiersinga WM, Prummel MF, Berghout A, van der Gaag R. Clinical criteria for the assessment of disease activity in Graves' ophthalmopathy: a novel approach. Br J Ophthalmol 1989;73:639

106. Laitt RD, Hoh B, Wakeley C, Kabala J, Harrad R, Potts M, Goddard P. The value of short tau inversion recovery sequence in magnetic resonance imaging of thyroid eye disease. Br J Radiol 1994;67:244

107. Wiersinga WM. Novel drugs for the therapy of Graves' ophthalmopathy. In: Wall JR, How J, Eds. Graves' ophthalmopathy. Cambridge: Blackwell Press, 1990:111

108. Cyclosporin in autoimmune disease. Lancet 1985;1:909

109. Gayno JP, Strauch G. Ciclosporine and Graves' ophthalmopathy. Horm Res 1987;26:190

110. Burrow GN, Mitchell MS, Howard RO, Morrow LB. Immunosuppressive therapy for the eye changes of Graves' disease. J Clin Endocrinol 1970;31:307

111. Perros P, Weightman DR, Crombie AL, Kendall-Taylor P. Azathioprine in the treatment of thyroid-associated ophthalmopathy. Acta Endocrinol 1990;122:8

112. Bigos ST, Nisula BC, Daniels GH, Eastman RC, Johnston HH, Kohler PO. Cyclophosphamide in the management of advanced Graves' ophthalmopathy. A preliminary report. Ann Intern Med 1979;90:921

113. Wall JR, Strakosch CR, Fang SL, Ingbar SH, Braverman LE. Thyroid binding antibodies and other immunological abnormalities in patients with Graves' ophthalmopathy: effect of treatment with cyclophosphamide. Clin Endocrinol 1979;10:79

114. Kahaly G, Lieb W, Müller-Forell W, Mainberger M, Beyer J, Vollmar J, Staiger C. Ciamexone in endocrine orbitopathy. A randomized double-blind, placebo-controlled study. Acta Endocrinol (Copenh) 1990;122:13

115. Antonelli A, Saracino A, Alberti B, Canapicchi R, Cartei F, Lepri A, Laddaga M, Baschieri L. High-dose intravenous immunoglobulin treatment in Graves' ophthalmopathy. Acta Endocrinol 1992;126:13

116. Kelly W, Longson D, Smithard D, Fawcitt R, Wensley R, Noble J, Keeley J. An evaluation of plasma exchange for Graves' ophthalmopathy. Clin Endocrinol 1983;18:485

117. Glinoer D, Schrooyen M. Plasma exchange therapy for severe Graves' ophthalmopathy. Horm Res 1987;26:184

118. Sautter-Bihl M-L, Heinze HG. Radiotherapy of Graves' ophthalmopathy. Dev Ophthalmol 1989;20:139

119. Kriss JP, Peterson IA, Donaldson SS, McDougall IR. Supervoltage orbital radiotherapy for progressive Graves' ophthalmopathy: Results of a twenty year experience. Acta Endocrinol 1989; 121(Suppl 2):154

120. Peterson IA, Kriss JP, McDougall IR, Donaldson SS. Prognostic factors in the radiotherapy of Graves' ophthalmopathy. Int J Radiat Oncol Biol Phys 1990;19:259

121. Prummel MF, Mourits MP, Blank L, Berghout A, Koornneef L, Wiersinga WM. Randomized double-blind trial of prednisone versus radiotherapy in Graves' ophthalmopathy. Lancet 1993;342:949

122. Palmer D, Greenberg P, Cornwell P, Parker RG. Radiation therapy for Graves' ophthalmopathy: a retrospective analysis. Int J Radiat Oncol Biol Phys 1987;13:1815

123. Pigeon P, Orgiazzi J, Berthezene F, Gerard JP, Haguenauer JP, Mornex R. High voltage orbital radiotherapy and surgical orbital decompression in the management of Graves' ophthalmopathy. Horm Res 1987;26:172

124. Kinyoun JL, Kalina RE, Brower SA, Mills RP, Johnson RH. Radiation retinopathy following orbital irradiation for Graves' ophthalmopathy. Arch Ophthalmol 1984;102:1473

125. Parsons JT, Fitzgerald CR, Hood CI, Ellingwood KE, Bova FJ, Million RR. The effects of irradiation on the eye and optic nerve. Int J Radiation Oncol Biol Phys 1983;9:609

126. Pinchera A, Bartalena L, Chiovata L, Marcocci C. Radiotherapy of Graves' ophthalmopathy. In: Gorman CA, Campbell RJ, Dyer JA, eds. The eye and orbit inthyroid disease. New York: Raven Press, 1984:301

127. Postema PTE, Krenning EP, Wijngaarde R, et al. [I-131-In-DTPA-D-Phe¹] octreotide scintigraphy in thyroidal and orbital Graves' disease:a parameter for disease activity? J Clin Endocrinol Metab 1994;79:1845

128. Chang TC, Kao SCS, Huang KM. Octreotide and Graves' ophthalmopathy and pretibial myxoedema. BMJ 1992; 304:158

129. Lopatynsky MO, Krohel GB. Bromocriptine therapy for thyroid ophthalmopathy. Am J Ophthalmol 1989;107:680

130. Harden RM, Chisholm CJS, Cant JS. The effect of metronidazole on thyroid function and exophthalmos in man. Metabolism 1967;16:890

131. Zesen W, Shubai J, Zutong Z. The effect of acupuncture in 40 cases of endocrinic ophthalmopathy. J Tradit Chin Med 1985;5:19

132. Rogvi-Hansen B, Perrild H, Christensen T, Detmar SE, Siersbaek-Nielsen K, Hansen JEM. Acupuncture in the treatment of Graves' ophthalmopathy. A blinded randomized study. Acta Endocrinol 1991;124:143

133. Garrity JA, Fatourechi V, Bergstralh EJ, et al. Results of transantral orbital decompression in 428 patients with severe Graves' ophthalmopathy. Am J Ophthalmol 1993; 116:533

134. Olivari N. Transpalpebral decompression of endocrine ophthalmopathy (Graves' disease) by removal of intraorbital fat: Experience with 147 operations over 5 years. Plast Reconstr Surg 1991;87:627

135. Roncevic R, Jackson IT. Surgical treatment of thyrotoxic exophthalmos. Plast Reconstr Surg 1989;84:754

136. Stark B, Olivari N. Treatment of exophthalmos by orbital fat removal. Clin Plast Surg 1993;20:285

137. Trokel S, Kazim M, Moore S. Orbital fat removal. Decompression for Graves orbitopathy. Ophthalmology 1993;100:674

138. Kennerdell JS, Rosenbaum AE, El-Hoshy MH. Apical optic nerve compression of dysthyroid optic neuropathy on computed tomography. Arch Ophthalmol 1981;99:807

139. Trobe JD. Optic nerve involvement in dysthyroidism. Ophthalmology 1981;88:488

140. Anderson RL, Tweeten JP, Patrinely JR, Garland PE, Thiese SM. Dysthyroid optic neuropathy without extraocular muscle involvement. Ophthalmic Surg 1989;20:568

141. DeSanto LW. The total rehabilitation of Graves' ophthalmopathy. Laryngoscope 1980;90:1652

142. Kennerdell JS, Maroon JC, Buerger GF. Comprehensive surgical management of proptosis in dysthyroid orbitopathy. Orbit 1987;6:153

LOCALIZED MYXEDEMA AND THYROID ACROPACHY

Vahab Fatourechi

LOCALIZED MYXEDEMA

Localized myxedema, an uncommon manifestation of autoimmune thyroid disease, is almost always associated with Graves' ophthalmopathy.[1–3] Although most of the patients have a history of thyrotoxicosis, the condition can occur in its absence and also in patients with chronic autoimmune thyroiditis.[3,4] The characteristic abnormality—skin thickening—is usually limited to the pretibial area. Thus, the disorder has been called pretibial myxedema, but because it occurs occasionally in other areas, localized myxedema, thyroid dermopathy, and dermopathy of Graves' disease are more appropriate terms. Community-based epidemiologic studies have shown that 4% of patients with clinically evident ophthalmopathy have localized myxedema,[5] and it occurs in from 12% to 15% of patients with severe Graves' ophthalmopathy.[2,4] A subclinical form of the disorder identified by forearm and pretibial skin biopsies in patients without clinically obvious changes may be more common.[6,7] Because most affected patients have relatively severe ophthalmopathy[3] and virtually all have high serum concentrations of thyrotropin (TSH) receptor antibodies,[8,9] dermopathy most likely indicates more severe Graves' disease.

The lesions are characterized by accumulation of glycosaminoglycan (GAG) in the dermis and subcutaneous tissues.[10–13] Although localized myxedema is uncommon, histologic similarities between fibroblast activation and GAG production in retroorbital tissue of Graves' ophthalmopathy and dermal tissue of localized myxedema suggest that insights into the pathogenesis of the latter would be helpful in the understanding and treatment of the more common and clinically important condition of ophthalmopathy.[14]

Clinical Manifestations

The lesions of localized myxedema of Graves' disease usually occur in the pretibial area. The feet and toes are also often involved.[2,3] Clinical involvement of the upper extremity occurred in only 1 of 150 consecutive patients[3] (Fig. 30-21). Isolated cases of involvement of the upper extremity, shoulders, upper back, pinnae, nose, and scar tissues have been reported.[15–19] The lesions occur most frequently in the sixth decade of life in both sexes, and the female-to-male ratio is 3.5:1.[3] Of the patients, over 90% have a history of thyrotoxicosis, but, as noted above, some may never have been clinically thyrotoxic and a few have or have had hypothyroidism caused by chronic autoimmune thyroiditis.[3,4]

Although more diffuse subclinical forms of the condition may exist,[6,7] localized myxedema commonly begins with raised waxy lesions in the pretibial area. They are usually light-colored but may be flesh-colored or yellowish brown.[2,3,20,21] Hyperpigmentation and hyperkeratosis may be present,[2,3] as may hyperhidrosis.[22] The lesions may be indurated and the hair follicles prominent, so that the lesions have an orange peel (peau d'orange) appearance and texture. The lesions are usually asymptomatic and of only cosmetic importance but occasionally cause impairment of function, such as difficulty wearing shoes, or rarely may be painful or pruritic. Nerve entrapment and reversible foot drop were reported in one patient.[23] The lesions are usually aggravated by trauma, and exuberant recurrence may ensue if they are surgically excised.[24]

Localized myxedema may appear in several distinct clinical forms (Fig. 30-22): diffuse, nonpitting edema, the most common form[3]; raised plaque lesions on a background of nonpitting edema; sharply circumscribed tubular or nodular le-

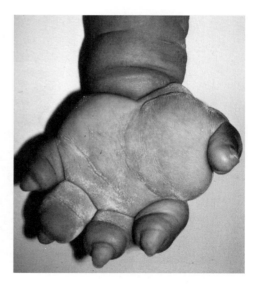

FIGURE 30-21. Extensive elephantiasic localized myxedema of the hands and forearm in a patient with Graves' disease. (From Smith TJ, Bahn RS, Gorman CA. Connective tissue, glycosaminoglycans, and diseases of the thyroid. Endocr Rev 1989;10:366. By permission of The Endocrine Society)

sions; and the relatively rare elephantiasic form, consisting of nodular lesions mixed with lymphedema. Very rarely, the lesions are polypoid or fungating. They usually do not ulcerate.

In a recent review of 150 consecutive patients with localized myxedema, only one did not have ophthalmopathy. The most common time of onset of ophthalmopathy was 0 to 12 months after diagnosis of thyrotoxicosis, and for localized myxedema the onset was 12 to 24 months after the diagnosis of thyrotoxicosis[3] (Fig. 30-23). Most patients with localized myxedema had relatively severe ophthalmopathy, and 88% had proptosis, with exophthalmometer readings greater than 20 mm.[3] Many of these patients required systemic corticosteroid therapy or decompressive surgery for their ophthalmopathy. The presence of localized myxedema does not alter the beneficial effect of orbital decompression in the treatment of ophthalmopathy.[4]

Biochemical Nature and Histopathology

Light microscopy of biopsy specimens of lesions of localized myxedema shows large amounts of GAG diffusely dispersed in the reticular part of the dermis. GAG does not usually accumulate in the papillary dermis. There is some infiltration of T-lymphocytes in the perivascular spaces, and mast cells are moderately increased in number. Collagen fiber fragmentation and fraying are seen when the tissue is stained with hematoxylin and eosin (Fig. 30-24). Mucinous material with and without connective tissue separation is seen when the tissue is stained with alcian blue and the periodic acid-Schiff stain. Collagen fibers are relatively reduced, and there is marked edema. Hyperkeratosis, acanthosis, and papillomatosis are occasionally seen.[25] Ultrastructural studies show dilated endoplasmic reticulum in fibroblasts, which indicates secretory activity and formation of GAG. The epidermis is usually normal

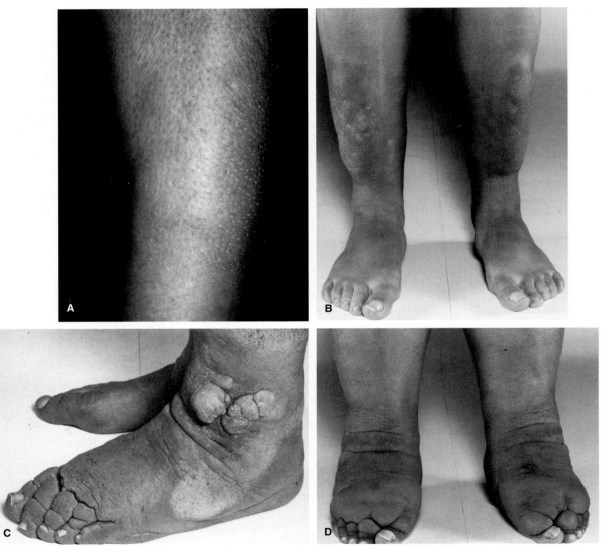

FIGURE 30-22. Photographs of localized myxedema in four patients. *(A)* Nonpitting edema form in the pretibial area. *(B)* Plaque form in the pretibial area. *(C)* Mixed nodular and elephantiasic forms on the ankles and feet. *(D)* Elephantiasic form. (From Fatourechi V, Pajouhi M, Fransway AF. Dermopathy of Graves' disease [pretibial myxedema]: Review of 150 cases. Medicine 1994;73:1. By permission of Williams & Wilkins)

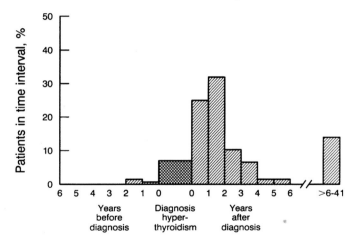

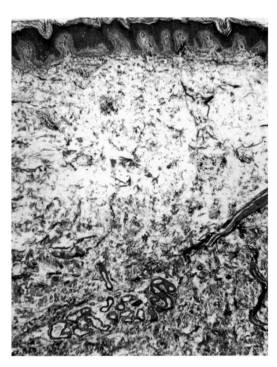

FIGURE 30-23. Onset of localized myxedema in relation to time of diagnosis of thyrotoxicosis in 136 patients. The cross-hatched bar represents onset of localized myxedema within 3 months of diagnosis of thyrotoxicosis. (From Fatourechi V, Pajouhi M, Fransway AF. Dermopathy of Graves' disease [pretibial myxedema]: Review of 150 cases. Medicine 1994;73:1. By permission of Williams & Wilkins)

FIGURE 30-24. Photomicrograph of a skin biopsy specimen from the pretibial area of a patient with localized myxedema showing separation and fraying of connective tissue fibers and edema. The epidermis *(top)* is normal. (Hematoxylin and eosin, original magnification x 40). (From Fatourechi V, Pajouhi M, Fransway AF. Dermopathy of Graves' disease [pretibial myxedema]: Review of 150 cases. Medicine 1994;73:1. By permission of Williams & Wilkins)

except for widened intercellular spaces. Amorphous electron-dense material is seen close to the surface of the fibroblasts. There are structural similarities with hypothyroid myxedema. However, hyperkeratosis, greater abundance of mucin, and mononuclear cell infiltration are more typical for localized myxedema.[25–27] The characteristics that distinguish localized myxedema from mucinosis associated with stasis dermatitis include preservation of a zone of normal-appearing collagen in the superficial papillary dermis, mucin deposition in the reticular dermis, lack of angioplasia, and relative absence of hemosiderin.[28] Quantitative lymphoscintigraphy and fluorescence microlymphography have shown that the deposited mucin promotes dermal edema by retention of fluid, which, in turn, causes compression or occlusion of small peripheral lymphatics and lymphedema.[29] Characteristically, immuno-staining does not show immunoglobulin G (IgG) deposition, but in one report, IgM deposits in the basement membrane zone were observed by direct immunofluorescence.[25]

Pathogenesis

Graves' hyperthyroidism results from direct stimulation of thyroid follicular cells by TSH receptor antibodies (see subchapter on pathogenesis of Graves' hyperthyroidism in chap 30). The reason for the increased GAG production by dermal fibroblasts in localized myxedema is unclear despite evidence for a common antigen between thyroid and dermal fibroblasts.[30,31] All patients with localized myxedema have high serum concentrations of TSH receptor antibodies, as determined by a variety of different methods.[2,8,9,32–34] By using the polymerase chain reaction, RNA encoding of the extracellular domain of the TSH receptor has been demonstrated in cultured orbital, abdominal skin, and peripheral skin fibroblasts from patients with ophthalmopathy or localized myxedema and from normal subjects.[30] The serum of patients with localized myxedema may stimulate fibroblast GAG production in vitro.[35,36] Other studies do not support a

role for circulating IgG in mediating localized myxedema. In these latter studies, patient IgGs enhanced GAG, protein, and DNA synthesis by cultured FRTL-5 thyroid cells but their effect on dermal fibroblasts did not differ from that of IgG from normal subjects.[31] The fibroblast activation could be indirect, through sensitized T cells. One can postulate that if T cells recognize an antigen shared by thyroid follicular cells and fibroblasts, one likely candidate being a portion of the TSH receptor, sensitized T cells could infiltrate tissues and release cytokines, including interleukin-1α and transforming growth factor β. These cytokines are capable of stimulating GAG synthesis and activating immunomodulatory proteins in dermal fibroblasts.[14,37] These proteins, which include the 72-kDa heat shock protein,[38] may aid in propagation of the autoimmune response in dermal connective tissues.[39] Local GAG accumulation leads to accumulation of fluid, expansion of dermal connective tissue, and characteristic nodular or diffuse thickening of the pretibial skin.[14] Secondarily, obstruction of lymphatic microcirculation may aggravate the lesions.[29]

More puzzling is the predominance of the lower extremities as sites for the lesions. Traditionally, roles for dependency and trauma have been proposed,[2] but evidence for differences in the regulation of GAG synthesis by fibroblasts from various anatomic sites has been presented.[40] Also, the profile of GAGs may differ according to the anatomic region. The principal proteoglycan synthesized by orbital fibroblasts is chondroitin sulfate, whereas skin fibroblasts produce mostly dermatan sulfate or heparan sulfate.[12,41] Also, retroorbital and pretibial fibroblasts may be more sensitive than normal skin fibroblasts to induction of HLA-DR, which could aid in perpetuating the lesions, after exposure to interferon-γ.[42]

In summary, despite demonstration of RNA-encoding portions of TSH receptor in orbital and pretibial fibroblasts, recognition of the role of various cytokines in fibroblast simulation and GAG production, and demonstration of high concentrations of TSH receptor antibodies in the serum of patients with localized myxedema (suggesting a common antigenic site in the skin and the thyroid as a putative target for TSH receptor antibodies or sensitized lymphocytes), the pathogenesis of localized myedema and the reason for site-specific involvement of the pretibial skin remain unexplained.

Differential Diagnosis

Localized myxedema should be differentiated from simple edema of fluid retention or venous insufficiency, generalized myxedema, chronic or lichenified dermatitis, hypertrophic lichen planus, and urticarial phases of certain blistering eruptions, such as bullous pemphigoid. Cutaneous mucinoses, such as lichen myxedematosus (papular mucinosis), reticular erythematous mucinosis, and follicular mucinosis, are relatively rare dermatologic conditions in which accumulation of mucin in the dermis is a prominent feature.[2,43] However, most of these conditions involve the upper extremities, and stigmata of Graves' disease, such as thyroid dysfunction and ophthalmopathy, are absent. Usually, the diagnosis of localized myxedema is obvious because of classic features of ophthalmopathy and typical pretibial lesions. However, biopsy may be necessary in some cases.[3,28] The diagnosis should be considered doubtful if Graves' ophthalmopathy is not present.

Treatment

Information about the natural course of untreated localized myxedema is scant.[3] In most patients, no therapy is required because the lesions are asymptomatic and not particularly unsightly, or they can be covered by clothing to the patient's satisfaction. Also, the lesions progress little and may partially or completely regress with time.[3]

When treatment becomes necessary because of cosmetic concerns, functional impairment, or local discomfort, topical application of a corticosteroid is the treatment of choice.[44,45] Kriss and colleagues noted regression of dermopathy in all 11 patients treated by nighttime application of 0.2% fluocinolone acetonide cream under occlusive plastic film dressings.[44] The dressings were removed in the morning. Initially, the cream was applied nightly or every other night, but the frequency could ultimately be reduced to two to four times a month. Nightly application of 0.05% to 0.1% triamcinolone acetonide in a cream base under occlusive dressing with plastic film (Saran Wrap) for 3 to 10 weeks, followed by intermittent maintenance therapy, also results in satisfactory partial remission, although patient compliance may modify results.[3] Because of fluid accumulation associated with the abundant amounts of GAG and some degree of superficial lymphatic obstruction, compressive bandages result in additional benefit. Jobst stockings and compressive bandages may be particularly useful in the elephantiasic form of localized myxedema. These patients

may require many months of therapy, the goal of which is to limit the degree of disfigurement, improve function, and avoid tissue breakdown and compressive complications. Intradermal injections of corticosteroids[46] and hyaluronidase have been used, but they are not recommended because the benefits are doubtful. Surgical excision of nodules and skin grafting should be avoided because of the possibility of recurrence of dermopathy at the site of surgical scars.[24]

When ophthalmopathy overshadows the localized myxedema, as is usually the case, systemic corticosteroid therapy for the former may cause regression of the skin lesions.[3,47] Corticosteroids are rarely, if ever, indicated for localized myxedema alone. Experimental treatments that have been beneficial in a few patients include plasmapheresis, the somatostatin analogue octreotide, and intravenous administration of high doses of immunoglobulin.[48–52]

THYROID ACROPACHY

Thyroid acropachy is the least common manifestation of autoimmune thyroid disease. Only 7% of patients with localized myxedema have thyroid acropachy.[3] Unlike other manifestations of Graves' disease, the female:male ratio is 1:1.[53] Acropachy almost always occurs in association with ophthalmopathy and localized myedema, although an isolated case without them has been reported.[54]

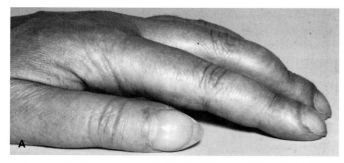

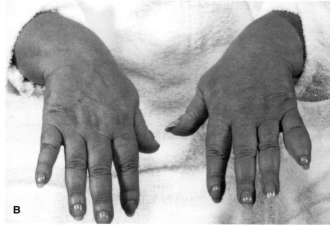

FIGURE 30-25. *(A and B)* Photographs of the hands in two patients with thyroid acropachy, showing clubbing of fingertips and soft tissue swelling. In *B*, note asymmetric involvement of the fingers.

Typically, the process involves soft tissue swelling of the hands and feet, usually in association with clubbing of the fingers and toes (Fig. 30-25). The skin is commonly pigmented and hyperkeratotic. Joints are not involved in thyroid acropachy, and the local warmth and increased blood flow characteristic of pulmonary osteoarthropathy are usually absent. The upper and lower extremities are equally involved.[53,55] The process may be asymmetrical, and the involvement of a single digit has been reported.[56] Acropachy is often painless, but some patients have lymphatic obstruction, extreme swelling, loss of function, and pain.[57] Like localized myxedema, the condition usually occurs in patients with a history of thyrotoxicosis but can occur in euthyroid or hypothyroid patients with chronic autoimmune thyroiditis.[53] It is unusual for acropachy to occur before thyroid dysfunction, and in general the developmental chronology is thyroid dysfunction, ophthalmopathy, dermopathy, and, lastly, acropachy.[53,55] Although it can occur as late as 40 years after the onset of thyroid dysfunction, the median interval between diagnosis of thyroid dysfunction and acropachy is 2 to 3 years.[53]

Radiologic findings show fusiform soft tissue swelling of the digits and subperiosteal bone formation, which usually involves the metacarpals, the proximal and middle phalanges of the fingers, and the metatarsal and proximal phalanges of the toes. The subperiosteal reaction does not occur in the long bones of the forearms or the legs, in contrast to pulmonary osteoarthropathy. The new bone formation is most marked in the midportion of the diaphysis. Radiographs show a characteristic subperiosteal spiculated, frothy, or lacy appearance (Fig. 30-26),[53,55] quite different from laminal periosteal proliferation of classic pulmonary osteoarthropathy. In the earlier stages of acropachy, when bone x-ray results are normal, ^{99m}Tc pyrophosphate bone scans show focal accumulation of the radionuclide in the affected areas.[58] Skin pathologic features are similar to those of localized myxedema, including fibroblast activation and GAG deposition.[53,59]

Little is known about the pathologic characteristics and pathogenesis of thyroid acropachy. One study of bone histology revealed nodular fibrosis of the periosteal area, subperiosteal bone formation, and fibrosis of the marrow space.[60] One can speculate that the process involves autoimmune activation of periosteal fibroblasts.

The natural history of the condition is not known. Although local corticosteroid therapy under occlusive compression dressings has been of benefit in patients with symptoms,[59] no therapy proved to be effective is available.

References

1. Beierwaltes WH. Clinical correlation of pretibial myxedema with malignant exophthalmos. Ann Intern Med 1954;40:968
2. Kriss JP. Pathogenesis and treatment of pretibial myxedema. Endocrinol Metab Clin North Am 1987;16:409
3. Fatourechi V, Pajouhi M, Fransway AF. Dermopathy of Graves disease (pretibial myxedema): Review of 150 cases. Medicine 1994;73:1
4. Fatourechi V, Garrity JA, Bartley GB, Bergstralh EJ, Gorman CA. Orbital decompression in Graves' ophthalmopathy associated with pretibial myxedema. J Endocrinol Invest 1993;16:433
5. Bartley GB, Fatourrechi V, Kadrinas EF, et al. Clinical features of Graves' ophthalmopathy in an incidence cohort. Am J Ophthalmol. 1996;121:in press
6. Wortsman J, Dietrich J, Traycoff RB, Stone S. Preradial myxedema in thyroid disease. Arch Dermatol 1981;117:635
7. Salvi M, De Chiara F, Gardini E, et al. Echographic diagnosis of pretibial myxedema in patients with autoimmune thyroid disease. Eur J Endocrinol 1994;131:113
8. Morris JC III, Hay ID, Nelson RE, Jiang NS. Clinical utility of thyrotropin-receptor antibody assays: Comparison of radioreceptor and bioassay methods. Mayo Clin Proc 1988;63:707
9. Schermer DR, Roenigk HH Jr, Schumacher OP, McKenzie JM. Relationship of long-acting thyroid stimulator to pretibial myxedema. Arch Dermatol 1970;102:62
10. Watson EM, Pearce RH. The mucopolysaccharide content of the skin in localized (pretibial) myxedema. Am J Clin Pathol 1947;17:507
11. Sisson JC. Hyaluronic acid in localized myxedema. J Clin Endocrinol Metab 1968;28:433
12. Smith TJ, Bahn RS, Gorman CA. Connective tissue, glycosaminoglycans, and diseases of the thyroid. Endocr Rev 1989;10:366
13. Hanke CW, Bergfeld WF, Guirguis MN, Lewis LJ. Hyaluronic acid synthesis in fibroblasts of pretibial myxedema. Cleve Clin Q 1983;50:129
14. Bahn RS, Heufelder AE. Pathogenesis of Graves' ophthalmopathy. N Engl J Med 1993;329:1468
15. Cohen BD, Benua RS, Rawson RW. Localized myxedema involving the upper extremities. Arch Intern Med 1963;111:641
16. Noppakun N, Bancheun K, Chandraprasert S. Unusual locations of localized myxedema in Graves' disease. Report of three cases. Arch Dermatol 1986;122:85
17. Akasu F, Takazawa K, Akasu R, Onaya T. Localized myxedema on the nasal dorsum in a patient with Graves' disease: report of a case. J Endocrinol Invest 1989;12:717
18. Slater DN. Cervical nodular localized myxoedema in a thyroidectomy scar: light and electron microscopy and histochemical findings. Clin Exp Dermatol 1987;12:216
19. Wright AL, Buxton PK, Menzies D. Pretibial myxedema localized to scar tissue. Int J Dermatol 1990;29:54
20. Frisch DR, Roth I. Pretibial myxedema: a review of the literature and case report. J Am Podiatr Med Assoc 1985;75:147
21. Truhan AP. Pretibial myxedema. Am Fam Physician 1985;31:135

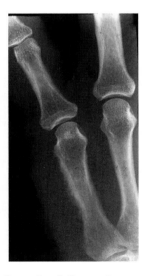

FIGURE 30-26. Radiograph of fingers in a patient with thyroid acropachy. Note the asymmetric frothy appearance of subperiosteal bone formation in the midportion of the proximal phalanx on the left.

22. Gitter DG, Sato K. Localized hyperhidrosis in pretibial myxedema. J Am Acad Dermatol 1990;23:250

23. Siegler M, Refetoff S. Pretibial myxedema—a reversible cause of foot drop due to entrapment of the peroneal nerve. N Engl J Med 1976;294:1383

24. Chremos PN. Relentless localized myxedema, with exophthalmos, clubbing of the fingers and hypertrophic osteoarthropathy: observations on an unusual case. Am J Med 1965;38:954

25. Konrad K, Brenner W, Pehamberger H. Ultrastructural and immunological findings in Graves' disease with pretibial myxedema. J Cutan Pathol 1980;7:99

26. Kobayasi T, Danielsen L, Asboe-Hansen G. Ultrastructure of localized myxedema. Acta Dermatovener 1976;56:173

27. Ishii M, Nakagawa K, Hamada T. An ultrastructural study of pretibial myxedema utilizing improved ruthenium red stain. J Cutan Pathol 1984;11:125

28. Somach SC, Helm TN, Lawlor KB, Bergfeld WF, Bass J. Pretibial mucin. Histologic patterns and clinical correlation. Arch Dermatol 1993;129:1152

29. Bull RH, Coburn PR, Mortimer PS. Pretibial myxoedema: a manifestation of lymphoedema? Lancet 1993;341:403

30. Heufelder AE, Dutton CM, Sarkar G, Donovan KA, Bahn RS. Detection of TSH receptor RNA in cultured fibroblasts from patients with Graves' ophthalmopathy and pretibial dermopathy. Thyroid 1993;3:297

31. Metcalfe RA, Davies R, Weetman AP. Analysis of fibroblast-stimulating activity in IgG from patients with Graves' dermopathy. Thyroid 1993;3:207

32. Kriss JP, Pleshakov V, Chien JR. Isolation and identification of the long-acting thyroid stimulator and its relation to hyperthyroidism and circumscribed pretibial myxedema. J Clin Endocrinol Metab 1964;24:1005

33. Chang T-C, Wu S-L, Hsiao Y-L, et al. TSH and TSH receptor antibody-binding sites in fibroblasts of pretibial myxedema are related to the extracellular domain of entire TSH receptor. Clin Immunol Immunopathol 1994;71:113

34. Tao T-W, Leu S-L, Kriss JP. Biological activity of autoantibodies associated with Graves' dermopathy. J Clin Endocrinol Metab 1989;69:90

35. Cheung HS, Nicoloff JT, Kamiel MB, Spolter L, Nimni ME. Stimulation of fibroblast biosynthetic activity by serum of patients with pretibial myxedema. J Invest Dermatol 1978;71:12

36. Shishiba Y, Imai Y, Odajima R, Ozawa Y, Shimizu T. Immunoglobulin G of patients with circumscribed pretibial myxedema of Graves' disease stimulates proteoglycan synthesis in human skin fibroblasts in culture. Acta Endocrinol 1992;127:44

37. Umetsu DT, Katzen D, Jabara HH, Geha RS. Antigen presentation by human dermal fibroblasts: activation of resting T lymphocytes. J Immunol 1986;136:440

38. Heufelder AE, Wenzel BE, Gorman CA, Bahn RS. Detection, cellular localization, and modulation of heat shock proteins in cultured fibroblasts from patients with extrathyroidal manifestations of Graves' disease. J Clin Endocrinol Metab 1991;73:739

39. Korducki JM, Loftus SJ, Bahn RS. Stimulation of glycosaminoglycan production in cultured human retroocular fibroblasts. Invest Ophthalmol Vis Sci 1992;33:2037

40. Smith TJ, Bahn RS, Gorman CA. Hormonal regulation of hyaluronate synthesis in cultured human fibroblasts: evidence for differences between retroocular and dermal fibroblasts. J Clin Endocrinol Metab 1989;69:1019

41. Shishiba Y, Tanaka T, Ozawa Y, Shimizu T, Kadowaki N. Chemical characterization of high buoyant density proteoglycan accumulated in the affected skin of pretibial myxedema of Graves' disease. Endocrinol Jpn 1986;33:395

42. Heufelder AE, Smith TJ, Gorman CA, Bahn RS. Increased induction of HLA-DR by interferon-γ in cultured fibroblasts derived from patients with Graves' ophthalmopathy and pretibial dermopathy. J Clin Endocrinol Metab 1991;73:307

43. Truhan AP, Roenigk HH Jr. The cutaneous mucinoses. J Am Acad Dermatol 1986;14:1

44. Kriss JP, Pleshakov V, Rosenblum A, Sharp G. Therapy with occlusive dressings of pretibial myxedema with fluocinolone acetonide. J Clin Endocrinol 1967;27:595

45. Benoit FL, Greenspan FS. Corticoid therapy for pretibial myxedema: observations on the long-acting thyroid stimulator. Ann Intern Med 1967;66:711

46. Lang PG Jr, Sisson JC, Lynch PJ. Intralesional triamcinolone therapy for pretibial myxedema. Arch Dermatol 1975; 111:197

47. Koshiyama H, Mori S, Fujiwara K, Hayakawa K, Koh T. Successful treatment of hypothyroid Graves' disease with a combination of levothyroxine replacement, intravenous high-dose steroid and irradiation to the orbit. Intern Med 1993; 32:421

48. Kuzuya N, DeGroot LJ. Effect of plasmapheresis and steroid treatment on thyrotropin binding inhibitory immunoglobulins in a patient with exophthalmos and a patient with pretibial myxedema. J Endocrinol Invest 1982;5:373

49. Noppen M, Velkeniers B, Steenssens L, Vanhaelst L. Beneficial effects of plasmapheresis followed by immunosuppressive therapy in pretibial myxedema. Acta Clin Belg 1988; 43:381

50. Chang TC, Kao SCS, Huang KM. Octreotide and Graves' ophthalmopathy and pretibial myxoedema. BMJ 1992;304:158

51. Priestley GC, Aldridge RD, Sime PJ, Wilson D. Skin fibroblast activity in pretibial myxoedema and the effect of octreotide (Sandostatin) in vitro. Br J Dermatol 1994;131:52

52. Antonelli A, Navarranne A, Palla R, et al. Pretibial myxedema and high-dose intravenous immunoglobulin treatment. Thyroid 1994;4:399

53. Winkler A, Wilson D. Thyroid acropachy: case report and literature review. Mo Med 1985;82:756

54. Goette DK. Thyroid acropachy. Arch Dermatol 1980;116:205

55. Kinsella RA Jr, Back DK. Thyroid acropachy. Med Clin North Am 1968;52:393

56. Chapman ME, Beggs I, Wu PS-C. Thyroid acropachy in a single digit. Clin Radiol 1993;47:58

57. Rothschild BM, Yoon BH. Thyroid acropachy complicated by lymphatic obstruction. Arthritis Rheum 1982;25:588

58. Seigel RS, Thrall JH, Sisson JC. ^{99m}Tc-Pyrophosphate scan and radiographic correlation in thyroid acropachy: case report. J Nucl Med 1976;17:791

59. Parker LN, Wu S-Y, Lai MK, Ramadan MB, Rajan RK, Yusi AM. The early diagnosis of atypical thyroid acropachy. Arch Intern Med 1982;142:1749

60. King LR, Braunstein H, Chambers D, Goldsmith R. A case study of peculiar soft-tissue and bony changes in association with thyroid disease. J Clin Endocrinol Metab 1959;19:1323

Werner and Ingbar's The Thyroid, Seventh Edition,
edited by Lewis E. Braverman and Robert D. Utiger.
Lippincott–Raven Publishers, Philadelphia, © 1996

31

Thyrotropin-Induced Hyperthyroidism

Neil Gesundheit

Hyperthyroidism results much more commonly from immune stimulation or a primary disease of the thyroid gland than from excessive secretion of thyroid-stimulating hormone (TSH; thyrotropin) from the pituitary. With the advent of sensitive TSH immunoassays,[1,2] however, an increasing number of patients are now recognized who demonstrate normal or elevated immunoreactive TSH in the presence of increased total and free serum thyroid hormone levels. Because TSH is normally suppressed by high free thyroid hormone levels, this entity has been termed *inappropriate TSH secretion*.[3,4] In these conditions there is no intrinsic derangement of the thyroid gland or of the immune system; instead, TSH itself is responsible for thyroid hyperstimulation.

Hyperthyroidism induced by TSH results from either a TSH-secreting pituitary adenoma or from nontumorous TSH hypersecretion due to thyroid hormone resistance. In this latter condition (discussed in chap 90), thyrotoxicosis results only if the pituitary gland is more resistant to thyroid hormone feedback than the periphery is to thyroid hormone action (thus called *selective pituitary* or *central* thyroid hormone resistance). More common reasons for referral to the endocrinologist are various clinical conditions that can be confused with inappropriate TSH hypersecretion; these are listed in Table 31-2 and are discussed in a later section of this chapter. Finally, a particular diagnostic challenge is provided by patients with apparent inappropriate TSH secretion who have undergone prior thyroid gland ablation. The clinical approach to these patients also will be discussed.

TSH-SECRETING PITUITARY ADENOMAS

These tumors of the pituitary gland are unusual but recognized with increasing frequency. The first patient with indisputable hyperthyroidism secondary to a TSH-secreting pituitary adenoma diagnosed by modern radioimmunoassay techniques was reported in 1970.[5] Since then more than 100 patients have been described (reviewed in references 6–10). Whereas earlier reports describe these tumors as large, locally invasive, and causing high morbidity,[11] several patients have now been cured owing to earlier diagnosis. Because the measurement of TSH has recently assumed a pivotal role in thyroid diagnostics, it is expected that more of these patients will be diagnosed at the microadenoma stage, permitting an improved clinical outcome.

Diagnosis

The patient with a TSH-secreting pituitary adenoma presents with clinical features consistent with a hormonally active pituitary tumor. Goiter and clinical thyrotoxicosis are the most common presenting symptoms. Headache, visual disturbance, and other symptoms of pituitary mass are common if the tumor has not been recognized and, instead, antithyroid therapy has been administered. Partial hypopituitarism is common—in particular, loss of gonadal function. The co-secretion of other pituitary hormones, such as growth hormone,[12] prolactin,[13] or follicle-stimulating hormone,[14] is present in approximately one third of patients.[10]

The associated stigmata of Graves' disease, such as infiltrative ophthalmopathy, dermopathy, and acropachy, are absent. One unusual patient was reported who had unilateral exophthalmos, suggesting Graves' disease, due to a TSH-secreting pituitary tumor invading the orbit.[15] Most patients are between the ages of 30 and 60 when they first come to clinical attention. In contrast to autoimmune thyroid disease, which shows about a 5:1 to 10:1 female to male ratio, there is no sex predilection for TSH-secreting pituitary tumors.

Patients with TSH-secreting pituitary tumors are frequently treated inappropriately with thyroid-lowering therapy owing to a failure to recognize the underlying cause of the hyperthyroidism. An interesting feature in this regard is that the thyroid gland, which is intrinsically normal in this disorder, may be difficult to ablate and may regrow even after near-total resection. Thus, patients with TSH-secreting pituitary tumors may present to the specialist with hyperthyroidism that has been refractory to prior attempts at ablation.

Laboratory and Biochemical Features

Laboratory investigations demonstrate elevated total and free thyroid hormone levels, increased thyroidal radioiodine uptake, and evidence of peripheral hypermetabolism (as measured, for instance, by basal metabolic rate, Achilles reflexometry, or the pulse-wave arrival time). Antithyroid peroxidase and antithyroglobulin antibodies are absent unless there is coexistent autoimmune thyroid disease. Importantly, TSH levels are within the normal range or frankly elevated rather than suppressed as they are in more common causes of hyperthyroidism, such as Graves' diseases, toxic multinodular goiter, a hyperfunctioning thyroid nodule, or the hyperthyroid phase of thyroiditis. Because measurement of TSH was not performed routinely in hyperthyroid patients prior to the 1990s, the majority of patients with TSH-secreting pituitary adenomas reported to date received prior thyroid ablation. In one such series, the average time from the onset of hyperthyroidism to the recognition of a TSH-secreting pituitary adenoma was 6.2 years.[9]

Several distinctive biochemical features are present in the patient with a TSH-secreting pituitary tumor. Patients with these tumors usually have a blunted or absent TSH response to thyrotropin-releasing hormone (TRH) and fail to suppress fully with exogenous administration of triiodothyronine (T_3). In addition, measurement of the free α-subunit has proven to be a useful biochemical marker for the presence of a TSH-secreting adenoma. TSH is a heterodimeric glycoprotein composed of an α-subunit and a hormone-specific β-subunit; under normal physiologic conditions, the production of these subunits is coordinately regulated (reviewed in reference 16). As was shown by Kourides and coworkers,[17] TSH-secreting pituitary tumors are characterized by excessive production and secretion of α-subunit, which can be measured by radioimmunoassay at specialized laboratories. The molar ratio in serum of α-subunit to TSH in patients with TSH-secreting tumors is nearly always greater than 1.[17]

Several other pharmacologic tests have been described that attempt to discriminate between tumorous and nontumorous TSH hypersecretion,[8] based on potential mediators of TSH secretion.[18] No single test has proven diagnostic, however, and each patient needs to be assessed individually. One can be confident of the diagnosis of a TSH-secreting pituitary tumor in the patient with the constellation of (1) inappropriate serum TSH; (2) clinical hyperthyroidism without stigmata of Graves' disease; and (3) a pituitary mass. Assuming that a patient is evaluated after steady-state thyroid hormone levels have been achieved and that no laboratory artifacts are present (discussed later), the only clinical setting that can fulfill these three features would be the patient with selective pituitary thyroid hormone resistance (next section) and a coincident pituitary mass. Such an unlikely patient would be expected to have a normal serum α-subunit level (Table 31-1).

A greater diagnostic challenge is provided by the patient with a TSH-secreting microadenoma. Several such patients have now been described,[9,19–21] and the prognosis appears to be excellent when a diagnosis is made at this early stage. In these patients, in addition to elevation of the α-subunit tumor marker, high-resolution nuclear magnetic resonance scanning with gadolinium may disclose the pituitary abnormality,[22] or inferior venous petrosal sampling may disclose a gradient and lateralization consistent with tumor.[23]

Only one patient with a TSH-secreting pituitary tumor in the context of multiple endocrine neoplasia syndrome type I has been described.[24] Ectopic production of TSH has not been reported.

Anatomic and Histologic Features

The cell type of origin for these tumors is the thyrotroph of the anterior pituitary. TSH-secreting tumors are nearly always benign and exert their central nervous system effects by local suprasellar extension or invasion into neighboring sinuses. On immunohistochemical analysis these tumors typically stain positively for both α- and TSH-β-subunits, and they can co-secrete other pituitary hormones, most commonly prolactin and growth hormone.[13,25,26] The clinical confirmation of the multihormonal potential of these tumors has been provided by numerous reports of patients with coexistent TSH hypersecretion and acromegaly.[9,11,12,27–29] As with other pituitary tumors, fibrosis can be a prominent feature, even in the absence of prior surgery or radiotherapy.

The pathogenesis of these tumors has not been clearly elucidated. A hypothalamic basis with excessive TRH production has been suggested,[6,30] although the data supporting this view are not compelling. One possible explanation is that these patients have an acquired or hereditary loss of normal negative regulatory feedback by thyroid hormone(s). Pituitary growth in such a setting is supported by the example of dramatic thyrotroph hyperplasia that can occur with prolonged primary hypothyroidism[31,32] and by the one patient reported to have had thyroid hormone resistance prior to the development of a TSH-secreting pituitary tumor.[9] An alternative explanation is that pituitary-specific growth and differentiation factors/protooncogenes may be activated by unknown environmental factors in a patient with a susceptible genetic background. Both of these explanations provide intriguing hypotheses for the pathogenesis of these and other pituitary tumors and are the subject of current investigation.

In vitro studies performed on tissue explants or dispersed tumor cells have demonstrated variable responses to regulatory agents such as dopamine, somatostatin, and TRH.[13,33–35] These have generally supported the notion that these tumors respond in a blunted but expected manner (i.e., TRH functions as a positive secretagogue; somatostatin, dopamine, T_3, and glucocorticoids function as negative secretagogues[18]). Biochemical characterization of tumor-derived TSH has suggested interesting properties such as heterogeneity of molecular weight associated with enhanced biologic activity[27] and heterogeneous glycosylation shown by altered binding to various lectins.[36]

Although TSH-secreting pituitary tumors are almost always benign and present clinical symptoms either due to TSH-induced hyperthyroidism or to a mass effect, an unusual patient was reported with a pituitary carcinoma metastatic to distant parts of the central nervous system, liver, and lung. This patient underwent two resections for a pituitary adenoma, and after several years of observation, during which α-subunit relative to TSH rose dramatically, she ultimately developed fatal metastatic disease.[37]

Treatment

Pituitary surgery is the cornerstone of treatment. Short-term administration of thionamides or potassium iodide in preparation for surgery may be necessary in thyrotoxic patients whose symptoms cannot be controlled by beta-blockers alone; however, long-term antithyroid therapy should be avoided because of the possibility that thyroid-lowering therapy may promote tumor growth.[9] In addition, permanent thyroid ablation by either surgery or radioiodine is unnecessary and may complicate the postoperative management of these patients; for example, in the patient who has undergone thyroid ablation, the recurrence of functioning pituitary tumor can no longer be easily gauged by the return of hyperthyroidism. As mentioned previously, early diagnosis and prompt surgery, preferably by a transsphenoidal route, provide the best opportunity for cure. Several patients have been reported who were diagnosed and treated at the stage of a pituitary microadenoma (diameter < 10 mm), and these patients have had favorable outcomes.[9,19–21] In patients with macroadenomas, surgical therapy is recommended to debulk tumor and permit management by radio- and pharmacotherapy. Radiation therapy in the form of 3000 to 4500 rad (30–45 Gy) fractionated over 4 to 6 weeks has been employed to control further tumor growth, but the efficacy of this treatment has not been specifically documented with TSH-secreting pituitary tumors. Octreotide acetate, a long-acting somatostatin analogue, has been shown to decrease TSH secretion in these patients[38–40] and has been shown in some patients to improve visual fields, suggesting a possible tumoricidal effect.[40] A common complication of octreotide therapy, however, is the development of cholestasis and cholelithiasis. Nevertheless, this agent appears useful as an adjunct to the therapy of these tumors, and its use can be considered in either the preoperative or postoperative period.

THYROID HORMONE RESISTANCE

Hyperthyroidism can occasionally occur as a result of nontumorous hypersecretion of TSH. This syndrome of thyroid hormone resistance[41] has several variants, as described in chapter 90. The most common form of thyroid hormone resistance is one in which all tissues, including the pituitary, are resistant to thyroid hormone action. If the pituitary and peripheral tissues are equally resistant, the patient is eumetabolic, although goiter and elevated levels of free thyroid hormones are present in order to overcome the generalized resistance. These patients are usually discovered incidentally, and they are frequently subjected to inappropriate lowering of thyroid hormone levels (by either thyroidectomy, radioiodine ablation, or thionamide

therapy) in attempts to treat biochemical hyperthyroidism. As shown in Table 31-1, TSH levels are usually within the normal range but inappropriately detectable for the high levels of circulating free thyroid hormones.

Linkage of generalized thyroid hormone resistance to the β thyroid hormone receptor gene (c-*erb*Aβ) has been demonstrated,[42] and the exact molecular defect has been elucidated now in numerous kindreds (reviewed in references 41, 43, and 43a), permitting a more complete understanding of this syndrome. A defect in the ligand binding domain of the beta form of the thyroid hormone receptor (c-*erb*Aβ), encoded by a gene on the short arm of chromosome 3, is the most common molecular basis for the syndrome. Decreased affinity of T_3 for the ligand-binding domain of a defective thyroid hormone receptor may result in a dominant negative effect on thyroid hormone-responsive genes. The dominant negative effect occurs because a putative dimerization motif within the T_3 receptor is preserved in the autosomal dominant form of this syndrome; the function of the wild-type T_3 receptor is impaired after dimerization with the defective receptor. If the level of resistance at the pituitary is equivalent to that in the periphery, the patient is eumetabolic, although thyroid hormone levels will be elevated. Within kindreds with generalized thyroid hormone resistance, however, there appears to be discernible tissue-to-tissue variability in the degree of thyroid hormone sensitivity.[44] For example, the pituitary—functioning as the central regulator—may sense "normal" thyroid hormone levels, whereas the heart may be more sensitive to thyroid hormone and manifest symptomatic tachyarrhythmias. Thus, even within the category of generalized thyroid hormone resistance, there exist patients with different spectra of clinical manifestations; at one end are patients who are clinically euthyroid in every endorgan; and at the other end are patients who demonstrate increased sensitivity to thyroid hormone in some organ systems and decreased sensitivity in others.

Selective Pituitary Thyroid Hormone Resistance

At one extreme of the syndrome of thyroid hormone resistance are the patients who have profound pituitary resistance but nearly normal responsiveness to thyroid hormones in other tissues. This variant of thyroid hormone resistance produces clinical hyperthyroidism that is TSH-mediated and is referred to as *selective pituitary* or *central resistance* to thyroid hormones.

DIAGNOSIS AND CLINICAL FEATURES

The dominant clinical features are goiter and clinical thyrotoxicosis without stigmata of Graves' disease. In contrast to patients with TSH-secreting pituitary tumors, however, the pituitary gland is morphologically normal in these patients. Indeed, imaging studies of the pituitary disclose a normal gland unless the patient has been rendered hypothyroid inappropriately, in which case the pituitary may enlarge, as can occur with prolonged primary hypothyroidism. Thyroid-stimulating immunoglobulins and antithyroid antibodies are absent unless the patient has coexisting autoimmune thyroid disease. Thyroid hormone values demonstrate elevated total and free thyroid hormones and TSH that is either in the normal or elevated range.

TABLE 31-1.
Conditions That Demonstrate Elevated Serum Thyroid Hormone and Nonsuppressed TSH Levels

Condition	Clinical States	TSH	TSH Response to TRH	T_4	Free T_4	T_3	Free T_3	α Subunit	TSH Suppression by T_3	Sellar Radiograph
TSH-secreting pituitary tumor	Hyperthyroid	nl or ↑	Blunted or nl	↑	↑	↑	↑	↑	None or partial	Microadenoma or macroadenoma
Generalized thyroid hormone resistance	Euthyroid	nl or ↑	nl or ↑	↑	↑	↑	↑	nl	partial or complete	nl
Selective pituitary thyroid hormone resistance	Hyperthyroid	nl or ↑	nl or ↑	↑	↑	↑	↑	nl	Partial or complete	nl
Increased TBG	Euthyroid	nl	nl	↑	nl	↑	nl	nl	Complete	nl
Increased albumin or TBPA binding	Euthyroid	nl	nl	↑	nl	nl or slight ↑	nl	nl	Complete	nl
Iopanoic acid, ipodate, amiodarone	Euthyroid or hypothyroid*	nl or ↑ or ↓	nl or ↑ or ↓	nl or ↑	nl or ↑	nl or ↓	nl or ↓	nl	Complete	nl

nl, normal.
Amiodarone can also cause hyperthyroidism; see text and references 54 and 55.

In patients with selective pituitary resistance to thyroid hormones as well as in those with TSH-secreting microadenomas, imaging studies of the sella are usually normal. An important and distinguishing feature, therefore, is that the serum level of α-subunit is elevated in the patient with a TSH-secreting pituitary adenoma but is normal in the patient with thyroid hormone resistance.

TREATMENT

In contrast to patients with generalized thyroid hormone resistance who usually require no treatment, patients with selective pituitary resistance have symptomatic hyperthyroidism. If symptoms are mild, beta-blocker therapy can be administered, although these patients may still be susceptible to possible deleterious effects of chronic excessive thyroid hormones, such as osteopenia. Alternatively, radioiodine or chronic thionamide therapy can be instituted; however, if these antithyroid treatments are employed, the serum TSH level typically rises dramatically and imaging studies of the pituitary should be performed at appropriate intervals to rule out untoward pituitary enlargement.

Several pharmacologic therapies have been utilized in these patients. Rosler and coworkers[45] reported that a moderate daily dose (25 to 50 μg) of triiodothyronine administered over several months was effective in decreasing TSH secretion, thyroid hormone levels, and clinical thyrotoxicosis in several members of a kindred with selective pituitary resistance. This paradoxical result implies that TSH is better suppressed in some of these patients by a single daily high serum level of T_3 than it is by a continuous moderately high level of

T_3. Beneficial effects of D-thyroxine administration have also been reported.[46] Several investigators have shown the possible utility of triiodothyroacetic acid (TRIAC) in these patients.[47,48] Although TRIAC is not widely available, it appears capable of suppressing TSH while exerting minimal peripheral thyromimetic actions. TRIAC must be used cautiously, however, because its long-term efficacy and safety are unknown. There is limited experience with octreotide acetate or bromocriptine in this syndrome, but these agents deserve mention because they can suppress TSH secretion by acting as somatostatin and dopamine analogues, respectively.[38,49]

The most sensible approach to these patients, given that thyroid hormone resistance is a life-long condition, is to cautiously experiment with conservative therapy, such as the use of additional small doses of T_3 and beta-blockers, and to reserve antithyroid therapy for those patients with significant, symptomatic hyperthyroidism refractory to conservative measures. Because selective ablation of thyrotrophs is not feasible, neither pituitary surgery nor radiotherapy is recommended.

CONDITIONS COMMONLY CONFUSED WITH TSH-INDUCED HYPERTHYROIDISM

Table 31-2 lists various abnormalities in pituitary and thyroid physiology that are confused with inappropriate TSH secretion. These conditions are more common than is inappropriate TSH secretion and should be excluded *before* performing an extensive evaluation of the pituitary-thyroid axis. The hallmark

TABLE 31-2.
Conditions Commonly Confused with TSH-Induced Hyperthyroidism

LABORATORY ARTIFACTS

Antibodies to TSH,[51] T$_3$, or T$_4$[50]

Human antimouse antibodies[52]

INHIBITION OF T$_4$ TO T$_3$ CONVERSION

Drugs (amiodarone, iopanoic acid, sodium ipodate)[54]

5'-Deiodinase deficiency[56]

Nonthyroidal illness (see Chap. 14)

ABNORMAL THYROID HORMONE TRANSPORT BY SERUM PROTEINS

Increased T$_4$ binding to variant albumins or TTR[57]

Increased thyroxine-binding globulin levels

Congenital

Acquired (ie, drugs, estrogens, liver disease, porphyria)[59]

NONEQUILIBRIUM CONDITIONS

T$_4$ replacement of hypothyroid patients

Neonatal period (see Chap. 84)

OTHERS

Acute psychiatric illness (usually with agitation)[59]

Amphetamine use[59]

---

of these conditions is that total thyroid hormone levels and TSH appear inappropriate due to either a laboratory artifact, inhibition of T$_4$ to T$_3$ conversion, abnormal thyroid hormone binding by serum protein(s), or disequilibrium (nonsteady state) of thyroid hormone(s) and TSH. Examples of each of these conditions are presented here:

Laboratory Artifact

Circulating antibodies to thyroid hormones, present in some patients with autoimmune thyroid disease, can artifactually elevate thyroid hormone levels measured by radioimmunoassay. These antibodies can bind labeled ligand, and because they are of human origin, they will not be precipitated by second antibody (usually an anti-mouse or anti-rabbit antisera, depending on origin of the first antibody in the assay). Thus, the second antibody precipitate contains decreased amounts of labeled ligand, consistent with high endogenous (displacing) thyroid hormones. Numerous methods have been described to test and counteract the effects of such antithyroid hormone antibodies,[50] but the simplest solution is to determine free thyroid hormone levels by equilibrium dialysis. In the patient with inappropriate TSH secretion, both total and free thyroid hormone levels are elevated, whereas in the patient with antithyroid hormone antibodies, total thyroid hormone levels are elevated while free levels are normal because the confounding immunoglobulin is excluded by the dialysis membrane. Similarly, factitiously high TSH levels have been reported in patients with anti-TSH antibodies (such as in patients previously treated with bovine TSH[51]) or with anti-mouse IgG anti-

bodies (in assays that use mouse monoclonal antibodies[52]). Various improvements in commercial TSH assays have made these artifacts uncommon; nevertheless, they should be suspected in patients who are clinically euthyroid and have inappropriate elevated TSH values.

Inhibition of T$_4$ to T$_3$ Conversion

Certain drugs can produce a biochemical profile that can be confused with inappropriate TSH secretion, in particular, the iodine-containing radiocontrast agents sodium ipodate and iopanoic acid, and the iodine-containing antiarrhythmic, amiodarone. These agents can produce hyperthyroxinemia and nonsuppressed TSH. The mechanism of this effect is presumed to be inhibition of 5'-deiodinase activity in both pituitary and periphery and thus decreased T$_4$ to T$_3$ as well as reverse T$_3$ (rT$_3$) to T$_2$ conversion. Because intrapituitary T$_3$ is felt to be the major regulator of TSH biosynthesis and release, the decrease in intrapituitary T$_3$ results in a compensatory increase in TSH secretion. With amiodarone, this effect is most significant in the first 3 months of therapy.[53] Although these patients appear to have inappropriate TSH secretion, their levels of T$_3$ are normal or low-normal, and their levels of reverse T$_3$ are elevated. In the patient who develops amiodarone-associated thyrotoxicosis, there is usually a background of iodine deficiency[54] and TSH levels are actually suppressed.[55]

Unusual inherited defects in T$_4$ to T$_3$ conversion may also exist.[56] These patients are clinically euthyroid, and their TSH is appropriate for the level of circulating T$_3$.

Abnormal Thyroid Hormone Binding by Serum Proteins

Increases in thyroxine-binding globulin (TBG) or in variants of albumin or transthyretin (TTR) that bind excess thyroid hormones can lead to increases in total serum thyroid hormone(s) levels and thus produce a biochemical profile that can be confused with inappropriate TSH secretion.[57] In these conditions, the levels of free thyroid hormones by equilibrium dialysis are normal. In addition, patients with albumin and TTR variants typically have much greater elevation of total T$_4$ than total T$_3$ (total T$_3$ is usually in the high normal range). Because these conditions are familial (TBG excess is an x-linked codominant trait; familial dysalbuminemic hyperthyroxinemia an autosomal dominant trait), the proper diagnosis of a single case can lead to the identification of multiple affected members within a kindred. It is of particular importance to identify other affected family members to preclude iatrogenic complications, such as thyroid ablation or thionamide treatment in these euthyroid patients. An unusual patient with a TSH-secreting pituitary adenoma and increased thyroxine binding to TTR has been described.[58]

Thyroid Hormone–TSH Disequilibrium (Nonsteady State)

Nonsteady state is a common condition in which patients may transiently demonstrate measurable TSH levels despite elevated levels of free thyroid hormone(s). An extreme example is the patient with thyroid cancer after ablation who is withdrawn from thyroid hormone. In such a patient, TSH becomes elevated, and if the patient is given aggressive thyroid replacement therapy, a period may occur in which the biochemical definition of inappropriate TSH is met (i.e., TSH is not fully suppressed by elevated total and free thyroid hormones). Thus, the diagnosis of inappropriate TSH may be very difficult to establish in any patient who has had a dramatic change in thyroid hormone replacement therapy either due to physician instruction or to poor compliance. Typically, thyroid hormone replacement for 6 to 8 weeks at a constant dose is necessary to achieve steady-state conditions; this should be a prerequisite to applying the definition of inappropriate TSH secretion.

Table 31-1 illustrates thyroid and pituitary test results in patients with clinical entities that produced elevated thyroid hormone levels and nonsuppressed TSH. The first three entities have been discussed under the rubric of inappropriate TSH secretion because in these conditions, total and free thyroid hormones are elevated at a time that TSH is (inappropriately) measurable or elevated. The last three clinical entities, as mentioned previously, can be confused with inappropriate TSH secretion but are altogether different. In these conditions, free thyroid hormone levels are normal, and TSH is therefore appropriate for the level of (free) thyroid hormone; thus, these abnormalities are more appropriately termed conditions of *euthyroid hyperthyroxinemia* (reviewed in reference 59). No therapy is necessary for patients with the majority of the clinical conditions listed in Table 31-1, except for patients with TSH-secreting pituitary tumors and those with symptomatic thyroid hormone resistance. In addition, in those conditions with an inheritable pattern, affected family members should be identified and advised of their condition to prevent iatrogenic intervention.

THE APPROACH TO THE PATIENT WITH SUSPECTED INAPPROPRIATE TSH SECRETION AND PRIOR THYROID ABLATION

It is imperative before testing patients suspected of having inappropriate TSH secretion that thyroid hormone levels be allowed to reach equilibrium. Thus, in a hypothyroid patient, thyroid hormone replacement should ideally be at a constant level for 6 to 8 weeks to reflect steady-state kinetics before thyroid testing. In addition, pituitary imaging studies should be interpreted cautiously in patients with prior hypothyroidism, because pituitary size may not return to normal for several months. If there are no medical contraindications, thyroid hormone replacement should be somewhat aggressive (i.e., 2.0–2.5 μg/kg of T_4) in the patient with prior thyroid ablation who is suspected of having inappropriate TSH secretion so as to provide sufficient free thyroid hormones to suppress TSH. It is only in the context of *elevated levels* of *free* thyroid hormones that TSH, if measurable, is inappropriate.

CONCLUSION

Excessive secretion of TSH can cause hyperthyroidism, and with increasing use of sensitive TSH assays for the evaluation of patients with suspected thyrotoxicosis, more patients will be recognized with elevated free thyroid hormone levels and nonsuppressed (inappropriate) TSH. Common conditions that can be confused with inappropriate TSH should be considered (see Table 31-2); these conditions should be suspected, particularly in the patient who is clinically euthyroid. In the hyperthyroid patient in whom these conditions have been ruled out, evaluation and treatment for a possible TSH-secreting pituitary tumor or selective pituitary thyroid hormone resistance should be undertaken.

References

1. Nicoloff JT, Spencer CA. Clinical review 12: the use and misuse of the sensitive thyrotropin assays. J Clin Endocrinol Metab 1990;71(3):553
2. Ridgway EC. Thyrotropin radioimmunoassays: birth, life, and demise. Mayo Clin Proc 1988;63(10):1028
3. Gershengorn MC, Weintraub BD. Thyrotropin-induced hyperthyroidism caused by selective pituitary resistance to thyroid hormone: a new syndrome of "inappropriate secretion of TSH." J Clin Invest 1975;56:633
4. Weintraub BD, Gershengorn MC, Kourides IA, Fein H. Inappropriate secretion of thyroid-stimulating hormone. Ann Intern Med 1981;95:339
5. Hamilton CR Jr, Adams LC, Maloof F. Hyperthyroidism due to thyrotropin-producing pituitary chromophobe adenoma. N Engl J Med 1970;283:1077
6. Emerson CH, Utiger RD. Hyperthyroidism and excessive thyrotropin secretion. N Engl J Med 1972;287:328
7. Brenner-Gati L, Gershengorn MC. Thyroid-stimulating hormone-induced hyperthyroidism. In: Imura H, ed. The pituitary gland. New York: Raven Press, 1985:467
8. Faglia G, Beck-Peccoz P, Piscitelli G, Medri G. Inappropriate secretion of thyrotropin by the pituitary. Horm Res 1987;26(1-4):79
9. Gesundheit N, Petrick PA, Nissim M, et al. Thyrotropin-secreting pituitary adenomas: clinical and biochemical heterogeneity. Ann Intern Med 1989;111:827
10. Smallridge RC. Thyrotropin-secreting pituitary tumors. Endocrinol Metab Clin North Am 1987;16(3):765
11. Hill SA, Falko JM, Wilson CB, Hunt WE. Thyrotrophin-producing pituitary adenomas. J Neurosurg 1982;57:515
12. Kovacs K, Horvath E, Ezrin C, Weiss MH. Adenoma of the human pituitary producing growth hormone and thyrotropin. Virchows Arch Pathol Anat 1982;395:59
13. Jaquet P, Hassoun J, Delori P, Gunz G, Grisoli F, Weintraub BD. A human pituitary adenoma secreting thyrotropin and prolactin: immunohistochemical, biochemical, and cell culture studies. J Clin Endocrinol Metab 1984;59:817
14. Koide Y, Kugai N, Kimura S, et al. A case of pituitary adenoma with possible simultaneous secretion of thyrotropin and follicle-stimulating hormone. J Clin Endocrinol Metab 1982;54:397
15. Yovos JG, Falko JM, O'Dorisio TM, Malarkey WB, Cataland S, Capen CC. Thyrotoxicosis and a thyrotropin-secreting pituitary tumor causing unilateral exophthalmos. J Clin Endocrinol Metab 1981;53:338
16. Magner JA. Thyroid-stimulating hormone: biosynthesis, cell biology, and bioactivity. Endocr Rev 1990;11:354
17. Kourides IA, Ridgway EC, Weintraub BD, Bigos ST, Gershengorn MC, Maloof F. Thyrotropin-induced hyperthyroidism: use of α and β subunit levels to identify patients with pituitary tumors. J Clin Endocrinol Metab 1977;45:534
18. Morley JE. Neuroendocrine control of thyrotropin secretion. Endocr Rev 1981;2:396
19. Kellett HA, Wyllie AH, Dale BAB, Best JJK, Toft AD. Hyperthyroidism due to a thyrotrophin-secreting microadenoma. Clin Endocrinol 1983;10:57
20. Mashiter K, Van Noorden S, Fahlbusch R, Fill H, Skrabal K. Hyperthyroidism due to a TSH secreting pituitary adenoma: case

report, treatment and evidence for adenoma TSH by morphological and cell culture studies. Clin Endocrinol 1983;18:473

21. Jackson JA, Smigiel M, Greene JF. Hyperthyroidism due to a thyrotropin-secreting pituitary microadenoma. Henry Ford Hosp Med J 1987;4:198

22. Newton DR, Dillon WP, Norman D, Newton TH, Wilson CB. Gd-DTPA-enhanced MR imaging of pituitary adenomas. Am J Neuroradiol 1989;10:949

23. Frank SJ, Gesundheit N, Doppman JL, et al. Preoperative lateralization of pituitary microadenomas by petrosal sinus sampling: utility in two patients with non-ACTH-secreting tumors. Am J Med 1989;87:679

24. Wynne AG, Gharib H, Scheithauer BW, et al. Hyperthyroidism due to inappropriate secretion of thyrotropin in 10 patients. Am J Med 1992;92;15

25. Saeger W, Ludecke DK. Pituitary adenomas with hyperfunction of TSH. Frequency, histological classification, immunocytochemistry and ultrastructure. Virchows Arch Pathol Anat 1982;394:255

26. Grisoli F, Leclercq T, Winteler P, et al. Thyroid-stimulating hormone pituitary adenomas and hyperthyroidism. Surg Neurol 1986;25:361

27. Beck-Peccoz P, Piscitelli G, Amr S, et al. Endocrine, biochemical and morphological studies of a pituitary adenoma secreting growth hormone, thyrotropin (TSH) and α-subunit: evidence for secretion of TSH with increased bioactivity. J Clin Endocrinol Metab 1986;62:704

28. Carlson HE, Linfoot JA, Braunstein GD, Kovacs K, Young RT. Hyperthyroidism and acromegaly due to a thyrotropin- and growth hormone-secreting pituitary tumor. Lack of hormonal response to bromocriptine. Am J Med 1983;74:915

29. Lamberg BA, Pekonen R, Gordin A, et al. Hyperthyroidism and acromegaly caused by a pituitary TSH- and GH-secreting tumour. Acta Endocrinol (Copenh) 1983;103:7

30. Kamoi K, Mitsuma T, Sato H, et al. Hyperthyroidism caused by a pituitary thyrotrophin-secreting tumour with excessive secretion of thyrotrophin-releasing hormone and subsequently followed by Graves' disease in a middle-aged woman. Acta Endocrinol (Copenh) 1985;110(3):373

31. Vagenakis AG, Dole K, Braverman LE. Pituitary enlargement, pituitary failure, and primary hypothyroidism. Ann Intern Med 1976;85:195

32. Samaan NA, Osborne BM, Mackay B, Leavens ME, Duello TM, Halmi NS. Endocrine and morphologic studies of pituitary adenomas secondary to primary hypothyroidism. J Clin Endocrinol Metab 1977;45:903

33. Filetti S, Rapoport B, Aron DC, Greenspan FC, Wilson CB, Fraser W. TSH and TSH-subunit production by human thyrotropic tumor cells in monolayer culture. Acta Endocrinol 1982;99:224

34. Simard M, Mirell CJ, Pekary AE, Drexler J, Kovacs K, Hershman JM. Hormonal control of thyrotropin and growth hormone secretion in a human thyrotrope pituitary adenoma studied in vitro. Acta Endocrinol (Copenh) 1988;119:283

35. Samuels MH, Wood WM, Gordon DF, Kleinschmidt-DeMasters BK, Lillehei K, Ridgway EC. Clinical and molecular studies of a thyrotropin-secreting pituitary adenoma. J Clin Endocrinol Metab 1989;68:1211

36. Magner J, Klibanski A, Fein H, Smallridge R, Blackard W, Young W Jr, Ferriss JB, Murphy D, Kane J, Rubin D. Ricin and lentil lectin-affinity chromatography reveals oligosaccharide heterogeneity of thyrotropin secreted by 12 human pituitary tumors. Metabolism 1992;41:1009

37. Mixson AJ, Friedman TC, Katz DA, Feuerstein IM, Taubenberger JK, Colandrea JM, Doppman JL, Oldfield EH, Weintraub BD. Thyrotropin-secreting pituitary carcinoma. J Clin Endocrinol Metab 1993;76:529

38. Comi RJ, Gesundheit N, Murray L, Gorden P, Weintraub BD. Response of thyrotropin-secreting pituitary adenomas to a long-acting somatostatin analogue. N Engl J Med 1987;317(1):12

39. Wemeau JL, Dewailly D, Leroy R, et al. Long term treatment with the somatostatin analog SMS 201-995 in a patient with a thyrotropin- and growth hormone secreting pituitary adenoma. J Clin Endocrinol Metab 1988;66:636

40. Chanson P, Weintraub BD, Harris AG. Octreotide therapy for thyroid-stimulating hormone-secreting pituitary adenomas. A follow-up of 52 patients. Ann Intern Med 1993;119(3):236

41. Refetoff S, Weiss RE, Usala SJ. The syndromes of resistance to thyroid hormone. Endocr Rev 1993;14(3):348

42. Usala SJ, Bale AE, Gesundheit N, et al. Tight linkage between the syndrome of generalized thyroid hormone resistance and the human c-erbAβ gene. Mol Endocrinol 1988;2:1217

43. Adams M, Matthews C, Collingwood TN, Tone Y, Beck-Peccoz P, Chatterjee KK, Genetic analysis of 29 kindreds with generalized and pituitary resistance to thyroid hormone. Identification of thirteen novel mutations in the thyroid hormone receptor beta gene. J Clin Invest 1994;94:506

43a. Brucker-Davis F, Skarulis MC, Crace MB, et al. Genetic and clinical features of 42 kindreds with resistance to thyroid hormone. Ann Intern Med 1995;123:572

44. Beck-Peccoz P, Chatterjee VK. The variable clinical phenotype in thyroid hormone resistance syndrome. Thyroid 1994;4(2):225

45. Rosler A, Litvin Y, Hage C, Gross J, Cerasi E. Familial hyperthyroidism due to inappropriate thyrotropin secretion successfully treated with triiodothyronine. J Clin Endocrinol Metab 1982;54:76

46. Hamon P, Bovier-Lapierre M, Robert M, Peynaud D, Pugeat M, Orgiazzi J. Hyperthyroidism due to selective pituitary resistance to thyroid hormones in a 15-month-old boy: efficacy of D-thyroxine therapy. J Clin Endocrinol Metab 1988;67:1089

47. Beck-Peccoz P, Piscitelli G, Cattaneo MG, Faglia G. Successful treatment of hyperthyroidism due to non-neoplastic pituitary TSH hypersecretion with 3,5,3′-triiodothyroacetic acid (TRIAC). J Endocrinol Invest 1983;6:217

48. Salmela PI, Wide L, Juustila H, Ruokonen A. Effects of thyroid hormones (T4, T3), bromocriptine and TRIAC on inappropriate TSH hypersecretion. Clin Endocrinol (Oxf) 1988;28:497

49. Connell JMC, Mc Cruden DC, Davies DL, Alexander WD. Bromocriptine for inappropriate thyrotropin secretion. Ann Intern Med 1982;96:251

50. Sakata S, Nakamura S, Miura K. Autoantibodies against thyroid hormones or iodothyronine. Ann Intern Med 1985;103:579

51. Frohman LA, Baron MA, Schneider AB. Plasma immunoreactive TSH: spurious elevation due to antibodies to bovine TSH which cross-react with human TSH. Metabolism 1982;31:834

52. Kahn BB, Weintraub BW, Csako G, Zweig MH. Factitious elevation of thyrotropin in a new ultrasensitive assay: implications for the use of monoclonal antibodies in "sandwich" immunoassay. J Clin Endocrinol Metab 1988;66:526

53. Melmed S, Nademanee K, Reed AW, Hendrickson JA, Singh BN, Hershman JM. Hyperthyroxinemia with bradycardia and normal thyrotropin secretion after chronic amiodarone administration. J Clin Endocrinol Metab 1981;53:997

54. Martino E, Safran M, Aghini-Lombardi F, et al. Environmental iodine intake and thyroid dysfunction during chronic amiodarone therapy. Ann Intern Med 1984;101:28

55. Brennan MD, van Heerden JA, Carney JA. Amiodarone-associated thyrotoxicosis (AAT): experience with surgical management. Surgery 1987;102,6:1062

56. Kleinhaus N, Faber J, Kahana L, Schneer J, Scheinfeld M. Euthyroid hyperthyroxinemia due to a generalized 5′-deiodinase defect. J Clin Endocrinol Metab 1988;66:684

57. Ruiz M, Rajatanavin R, Young RA, et al. Familial dysalbuminemic hyperthyroxinemia. N Engl J Med 1982;306:635

58. Lind P, Langsteger W, Koltringer P, et al. Transient prealbumin-associated hyperthyroxinemia in TSH-producing pituitary adenoma. Nuklearmedizin 1990;29:40

59. Borst GC, Eil C, Burman KD. Euthyroid hyperthyroxinemia. Ann Intern Med 1983;98:366

Werner and Ingbar's The Thyroid, Seventh Edition,
edited by Lewis E. Braverman and Robert D. Utiger.
Lippincott–Raven Publishers, Philadelphia, © 1996

32

Toxic Adenoma and Toxic Multinodular Goiter

Ian D. Hay
John C. Morris

AUTONOMOUSLY FUNCTIONING THYROID NODULES

Autonomously functioning thyroid nodules (AFTNs) are discrete thyroid nodules that function independently of the normal pituitary-thyroid negative feedback control mechanism.[1] Their ability to synthesize and secrete thyroid hormones autonomously suppresses thyrotropin (TSH) secretion, so that the extranodular tissue becomes functionally and anatomically quiescent.[2] On radionuclide imaging, these nodules appear hyperfunctioning (hot), because they concentrate radioiodide or ^{99m}Tc-pertechnetate to a greater extent than the atrophic paranodular and contralateral tissue deprived of its normal tonic stimulation by TSH.[3] Administration of thyroxine (T_4) or triiodothyronine (T_3) does not decrease radionuclide uptake in the nodules (Fig. 32-1), and TSH administration restores uptake in the quiescent extranodular tissue (Fig. 32-2).

AFTNs may be solitary in otherwise normal glands or they may appear as single or multiple nodules in preexisting multinodular goiters,[4] although traditionally the term is applied to nodules that are solitary. Rather than being distinct entities, these lesions probably constitute a spectrum of autonomously functioning thyroid tissues.[3,5] AFTNs are by definition always hyperactive.[6,7] Depending on the available iodine supply,[8,9] the age of the patient,[4,10,11] and the mass of hyperfunctioning tissue,[4,12] the patient clinically may be either euthyroid or thyrotoxic. In a large series of patients with AFTNs studied over two decades 76% were euthyroid, 19% were thyrotoxic, and 5% were borderline thyrotoxic.[11]

Pathology

AFTNs are most commonly classified by pathologists as either adenomas or adenomatous nodules. The term *adenoma* has been defined by the World Health Organization as a "benign encapsulated tumor showing evidence of follicular cell differentiation."[13] Such a hypercellular tumor is usually solitary and has a well-defined fibrous capsule. The tumor's uniform but abnormal architectural pattern differs from that of the surrounding gland, the adjacent glandular tissue may be compressed, and degenerative changes such as hemorrhage, edema, fibrosis, calcification, and cyst formation may be present in the tumor.[13,14] The term *adenomatous nodule* has been used to describe lesions that are circumscribed but not encapsulated, typically with areas of normal follicular architecture and cellularity and with a prominent stromal component[14] (see also chap 28). AFTNs that are differentiated carcinomas, principally papillary carcinomas, are rare, but carcinoma has been found in as many as 2% to 6% of AFTNs in adults[4,15] and 11% of AFTNs in children.[10]

It has been said that "a true hot adenoma is an exquisite rarity in thyroid pathology."[16] The scintigraphic term *toxic adenoma* more often refers to a polyclonal and heterogeneous cohort of follicles with relatively high iodine metabolism.[17] Studies of the variations in function between different follicles within an individual nodule have led to the suggestion that individual follicles are derived from single cells with differing heritable function[18] or growth properties.[19] Recent histochemical studies performed in female mice heterozygous for an X-linked polymorphism revealed that true thyroid adenomas are monoclonal and that adenomatous nodules are polyclonal.[14]

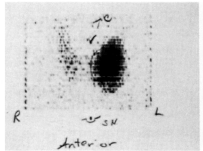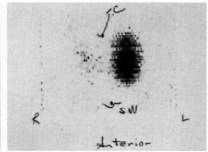

FIGURE 32-1. ^{99m}Tc-pertechnetate scans in a 34-year-old woman with an autonomously functioning nodule of the left lobe of the thyroid before (baseline) (*left*) and after (*right*) the administration of 100 μg/day of T$_3$ for 5 days. The baseline scan shows the nodule and a small amount of uptake in the right lobe; the latter is decreased in the scan performed after T$_3$ administration. TC, thyroid cartilage

In a series of 30 consecutive patients with an AFTN operated on in the United States, adenomas, as opposed to adenomatous nodules, accounted for 94%.[15] In a report from an iodine-deficient area in Europe, however, 10% of AFTNs were histologically diagnosed as "epithelial hyperfunction in multinodular goiters."[4]

Pathogenesis

AFTNs consist of hyperfunctioning thyroid cells whose function is uncoupled from normal physiologic control. Thus, they fit the definition of "minimal deviation benign tumors."[1] In vitro biochemical studies suggest that AFTNs are caused by an inherent defect and not by a circulating factor. This suggestion is supported by the coexistence in the same organ of an autonomous lesion and of quiescent tissue, the persistence of hyperactivity in AFTNs grafted into nude mice[20] and in cell culture,[21] and the persistence in vitro of the characteristics of iodine metabolism resulting from an increased capacity of the iodide-trapping system.[1]

Recent evidence suggests some AFTNs have a mutation of the gene for the TSH receptor (TSHR) that results in constitutive activation of the receptor. Somatic mutations resulting in single amino acid substitutions (Asp 619-Gly and Ala 623-Ile) within the third intracellular loop of the TSHR were detected in 3 of 11 AFTNs but not in the surrounding thyroid tissue in one study.[22] Expression of these mutant receptors in vitro resulted in constitutive activation of the cAMP cascade as well as an enhanced response to TSH. In other studies additional acti-

vating mutations were found within other regions of the transmembrane domain of TSHR, particularly the sixth transmembrane spanning segment; these other mutations include Ala 623-Ser, Phe 631-Cys, Thr 632-Ile, and Asp 633-Glu.[23,24] By activating cAMP generation in the absence of TSH, the mutant receptors offer a growth and functional advantage to these cells. This advantage eventually produces a tumor mass and, when sufficient autonomously functioning tissue is present, TSH secretion is inhibited and thereby the function of the remainder of the gland is decreased.

Another mutational event is responsible for other AFTNs, namely mutations of the gene for the α-subunit (G$_s$α) of the stimulatory guanine nucleotide-binding (G) protein.[24,25] Mutations affecting this protein (involving codons 201 and 227) also result in constitutive activation of the cAMP cascade and produce a similar phenotype to activating mutations of the TSHR gene. The overall frequency of mutations in either the G$_s$α gene or the TSHR gene is not known. In one study of 37 AFTNs, nine tumors had G$_s$α gene mutations and three tumors had TSHR gene mutations (only mutations of the third intracellular loop of the TSHR gene were sought in this study),[24] whereas in another study of 11 AFTNs (in which all of exon 10 of the TSHR gene was examined) mutations were found in 9 tumors.[25a]

Occurrence and Natural History

The annual incidence rates for thyrotoxicosis from all causes in three European studies were between 24 and 26 per 100,000 inhabitants[26–28] (see also chap 26). In Iceland, an area of high iodine intake, multinodular and uninodular goiter accounted for 6% and 7% of the cases, respectively,[27] while in Malmö, Sweden, an area with relatively low iodine intake, the respective rates were 21% and 11%.[26] In a study of seven English towns the incidence of toxic nodular goiter correlated closely with the previous prevalence of endemic goiter,[28] whereas in a retrospective study in Sicily, AFTNs were almost twice as common in an iodine-deficient area as in an iodine-sufficient area.[8] In a prospective multicenter study performed in six European countries 9% of thyrotoxic patients had AFTNs, and in the United Kingdom the rate was higher (10%) in iodine-deficient areas as compared with iodine-sufficient areas (3%).[16] In retrospective studies of referred thyrotoxic patients in three clinics in the United Kingdom and Canada, 8% to 25% of patients had toxic nodular goiter, and more patients had a toxic multinodular goiter (5% to 15%) than a toxic uninodular goiter (3% to 10%).[29,30]

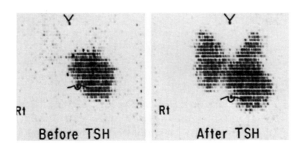

FIGURE 32-2. ^{99m}Tc-pertechnetate scans in a 67-year-old woman with an autonomously functioning nodule of the left lobe of the thyroid before (baseline) (*left*) and after (*right*) TSH administration. The baseline scan shows uptake only in the nodule, whereas the scan performed after TSH administration shows uptake not only in the nodule but also in the right lobe and above the nodule in the left lobe.

The AFTN is an unusual thyroid lesion in the United States, being present in only about 1% of patients referred for thyroid evaluation, and accounting for only about 5% of patients with solitary or dominant nodules.[12] In a study of 349 patients, the AFTNs were toxic in 56% of patients over 60 years of age but only in 12% of younger patients.[12] An increase in nodule size of at least 1 cm in diameter occurred in only 9% of patients followed for up to 15 years. Of 142 patients with nontoxic AFTNs followed for at least 6 years, 14 (10%) became thyrotoxic. During the 15-year period, no patient with an AFTN smaller than 2 cm became thyrotoxic, whereas one patient in five with an AFTN 3 cm or larger did become thyrotoxic. Based on these results, euthyroid patients with AFTNs are most likely to become thyrotoxic within 6 years if their nodule is 2.5 cm or larger, the patient is younger than 20 or older than 60 years of age, and the patient's serum T_3 concentration is near the upper limit of normal at the time of initial evaluation (sensitive serum TSH assays were not available when these patients were initially evaluated).[2,11,12] Some of the nodules degenerated during follow-up, precluding the development of or eliminating already-present thyrotoxicosis; a few patients had transient thyrotoxicosis as a result of necrosis of their AFTN.[2]

The results of other long-term follow-up studies were similar. For example, among 74 euthyroid patients, 46 (62%) with solitary or predominant AFTNs and 28 (38%) with multifocal autonomy on scintican, who were followed for 5 to 22 years (mean 9 years), 24 (32%) had major increases in nodule size or became thyrotoxic.[31] Most of the patients with solitary AFTNs had either major changes or no change in size or function; minor biochemical or scintigraphic changes prevailed in those patients with multifocal autonomy. Major changes occurred in 9 of the 12 patients who were younger than 40 years initially, and were less common in older patients. In a study of 375 euthyroid patients with AFTN followed for 3 to 204 months (mean 53 months), 34% received treatment; the reasons for treatment were thyrotoxicosis in 44%, patient request in 14%, mechanical symptoms in 13%, the presence of hypofunctioning nodules in 6%, and unstated in 23%.[32] There was no correlation between age (or sex) or nodule size and the occurrence of thyrotoxicosis during follow-up in this study. The results of all these studies suggest that progressive increases in function or size of AFTNs are uncommon.

Diagnosis

Because the development of thyrotoxicosis in patients with AFTN is often delayed and the thyrotoxicosis is usually mild,[12] the patients most frequently present for evaluation of a nodule. Recognition that a nodule is an AFTN has changed with the emergence of two relatively new methods of thyroid diagnosis. In the past, most AFTNs were detected by thyroid scintiscanning, whether the patient was euthyroid or thyrotoxic. Fine-needle aspiration biopsy of thyroid nodules has reduced the need for thyroid scintiscanning in patients with solitary nodules. Therefore, AFTNs are now less likely to be discovered by detection of a hyperfunctioning nodule. Second, use of newer serum TSH assays has meant that the finding of a low basal serum TSH concentration is often the first indication that a patient with a thyroid nodule who has no symptoms of thyrotoxicosis has an AFTN. Accordingly, the finding of a low serum TSH concentration in a patient with a thyroid nodule, whether the patient has symptomatic thyrotoxicosis or high serum thyroid hormone concentrations or not, should suggest that the nodule is an AFTN.

Diagnostic confirmation of an AFTN is obtained by the scintigraphic demonstration that the nodule concentrates a radionuclide in excess of, or to the exclusion of, the extranodular tissue. The term *warm nodule* refers to those nodules in which the uptake of radionuclide by adjacent tissue is incompletely suppressed. The imaging can be performed with ^{123}I, ^{131}I, or ^{99m}Tc-pertechnetate (see also chap 17).

In the past, patients sometimes were given bovine TSH to demonstrate that the inactive extranodular tissue retained the ability to become functional in the presence of TSH, therefore confirming the autonomy of the hyperfunctioning nodule (Fig. 32-2). In addition, T_3 was given to determine that the activity of the AFTN did not diminish when TSH secretion was (further) suppressed (see Fig. 32-1). These are cumbersome, expensive, and impractical tests, and most of the information they provide can be obtained by a basal serum TSH measurement.[33,34]

Serum total and free T_4 measurements have relatively limited utility in the evaluation of patients with AFTNs because many of the nodules preferentially secrete T_3. Therefore, serum T_3 concentrations are more likely to be high than are serum T_4 concentrations.[12] In addition, a borderline or high serum T_3 concentration can serve as a marker of impending thyrotoxicosis in an asymptomatic patient. As noted above, however, the earliest indication that a thyroid nodule is an AFTN is a low serum TSH value (subclinical thyrotoxicosis).[33]

The results of fine-needle aspiration biopsy of the nodule in patients with an AFTN are not generally different from those in patients whose nodule is hypofunctioning (see chap 23). No specific cytologic finding is characteristic of an AFTN.[35] Furthermore, up to 40% of AFTNs show cytologic evidence of lymphocytic thyroiditis, and some may show features suggestive of thyroid carcinoma, such as marked hypercellularity and cellular atypia.[35] Thus, fine-needle aspiration biopsy may be used to exclude cancer in the evaluation of patients with a nodule but should not be expected to contribute otherwise to the diagnosis. Likewise, ultrasonographic examination of an AFTN is rarely of value because the nodules are solid, like most poorly functioning and nonfunctioning nodules. A report on the use of color-coded duplex ultrasonography in the evaluation of thyroid diseases suggests, however, that AFTNs are more likely to show increased vascularity than nonfunctioning nodules, nontoxic multinodular goiters, and lymphocytic thyroiditis.[36]

Treatment

In a patient who has an AFTN and is thyrotoxic, or has local symptoms, ablation of the AFTN is indicated. An asymptomatic patient with an AFTN should be followed until symptoms appear, especially if the patient is otherwise young and healthy.[37] In older patients and those whose nodule is more than 3 cm in diameter, in whom the risk of developing thyrotoxicosis is greater,[12] ablation of the AFTN may be indicated. Three options exist for ablative therapy: surgery, ^{131}I therapy, or percutaneous ethanol injection.

SURGERY

Surgery for AFTN is simple and effective. Excision of the nodule itself with sparing of the remaining tissue is the procedure of choice. Because the resection is much less extensive, the operative risk is substantially lower than that of the operative treatment of toxic diffuse goiter (Graves' disease) or multinodular goiter. Because the thyrotoxicosis is generally mild, little preparation other than administration of a beta-adrenergic antagonist drug and inorganic iodide for 7 to 10 days preoperatively is needed. Surgery offers the advantage of avoiding radiation exposure of the remaining thyroid tissue. Recurrence of thyrotoxicosis after successful surgery for AFTN has not been reported. Postoperative hypothyroidism is infrequent, although it may be more common than previously recognized; in one study, a 42% cumulative incidence at 9 years was reported in 24 patients treated surgically for AFTN.[38]

RADIOIODINE THERAPY

Therapy with ^{131}I is as effective as surgery for the treatment of AFTNs. Because the nodules are relatively radioresistant, larger doses are generally required for treatment of AFTN than for Graves' disease. Thirty thousand rads (300 Gy) delivered to the center of the nodule cured 83% of AFTN patients in one study.[39] For a 3.5-cm diameter nodule in which the ^{131}I uptake is 30% of the administered dose, 28.6 mCi (1058 MBq) [131]I is required.[40] Patients with larger nodules require larger doses of ^{131}I to achieve the same dosage within the nodule, so that a patient who had a 6-cm nodule with equivalent ^{131}I uptake would require a dose of 135 mCi (4995 MBq). A concern relative to these doses is the radiation exposure of the surrounding tissue. As shown in Figure 32-3, the opposite lobe of a 4-cm thyroid nodule that receives 30,000 rad (300 Gy) to its center is itself exposed to considerable radiation. The risk of thyroid carcinoma in children exposed to x-ray irradiation increases linearly between 20 and 1125 rads (0.2 and 11.25 Gy),[41] doses that are routinely achieved in the tissue surrounding an AFTN treated with [131]I (see also section on pathogenesis in chap 80). Nevertheless, reports of thyroid carcinoma after ^{131}I therapy for an AFTN are rare.

Patients with AFTNs can be treated with smaller doses of ^{131}I, but the cure rates are usually lower (<75%) than those reported with doses of 20 mCi (740 MBq) or greater.[39,42–44] An exception was a study in which treatment was successful in 29 of 30 patients (97%) given a standard dose of 15 mCi (555 MBq) [131]I,[45] although the period of follow-up was relatively short (6 months to 3 years). Even if thyrotoxicosis is adequately treated, the AFTN may persist (see following). Overall, we agree with Hamburger's statement about the choice of ^{131}I dose for patients with AFTNs: "Those who prefer to avoid, rather than relive, the disasters that can result from inadequate ^{131}I therapy for toxic AFTNs should heed the advice of the older workers who advise larger ablative doses."[2]

The cumulative rates of hypothyroidism after ^{131}I therapy for AFTN have varied from as low at 0% to as high as 44%.[43,44,46–48] Its occurrence appears to be related inversely to the degree of TSH suppression and the resultant reduction in ^{131}I uptake by the extranodular tissue.[46,47] Because of this concern, some authors have advocated the administration of T_3 to AFTN patients with incomplete TSH suppression before ^{131}I is

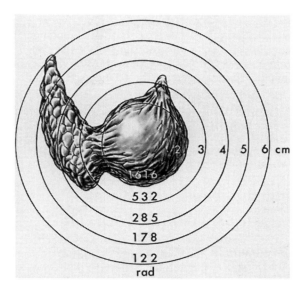

FIGURE 32-3. Diagram of the spatial relation between an autonomously functioning nodule and the remainder of the thyroid gland. The size of the thyroid and the location of the nodule are assumed to be such that the center of the nodule is 6 cm from the tip of the opposite lobe. Concentric circles are used to indicate the dose (in rads) at various distances from the center of a nodule 4 cm in diameter receiving 30,000 rads (300 Gy) from [131]I. (From Gorman CA, Robertson JS. Radiation dose in the selection of ^{131}I or surgical treatment for toxic thyroid adenoma. Ann Intern Med 1978;89:85, with permission of the American College of Physicians)

given in order to protect the paranodular tissue. The presence of Hashimoto's thyroiditis in the paranodular tissue may increase the risk of hypothyroidism; in one study patients with an AFTN treated with ^{131}I who had antithyroid antibodies in their serum were more likely to develop hypothyroidism than similar patients without these antibodies.[49] These results contrast with an earlier report of 97 patients in whom the incidence of posttreatment hypothyroidism was similar in those treated with ^{131}I and those treated surgically (5% vs 7%, respectively); Hashimoto's disease was not specifically identified in the glands of the surgically treated patients.[42]

Repeat thyroid scintigraphy after treatment of a patient with AFTN with ^{131}I may reveal persistent autonomy, even in those who remain euthyroid. In a recent study of 66 patients (55 with thyrotoxicosis) treated 1 to 16 years (median 8 years) earlier, 50% had autonomous nodules with suppression of the extranodular tissue.[50] Many of the patients had normal serum TSH concentrations for several years before the follow-up scan. Therefore, therapy need not destroy the nodule to be effective.

PERCUTANEOUS ETHANOL INJECTION

Percutaneous injection of an AFTN with ethanol is an alternative to ^{131}I therapy and surgery.[51–53] The procedure involves the instillation of ethanol (1 to 9 mL) directly into the nodule, generally using ultrasound guidance. Multiple injections are required to destroy a nodule successfully (3 to 8 treatments over 2 to 4 weeks).[51,54,55] Although the number of patients treated in this way is still small, it appears to be safe and effective. Complications include transient vocal cord dysfunction in 3% and mild to moderate local pain in the thyroid region.[56,57] From 80% to 100% of nodules become impalpable, although scintiscans reveal persistence of autonomous tissue in many patients, and long-term data are not yet available.

In treating thyrotoxic patients with AFTNs, we generally recommend surgical therapy for young patients and those with relatively large nodules (>3 cm). [131]I treatment is best suited for older patients and those with smaller nodules in whom radiation exposure of the extranodular tissue is not an important consideration. The role of percutaneous ethanol injection remains to be defined. Currently, inconvenience and unknown long-term outcome limit our enthusiasm for its use.

TOXIC MULTINODULAR GOITER

Pathogenesis

Thyrotoxicosis occurs in patients with a multinodular goiter whenever the number of newly generated follicles with at least some degree of autonomous capability to synthesize T_4 and T_3 becomes large enough so that overall hormone production exceeds the need of the organism (Fig. 32-4). Because the generation of new follicles is a slow process (see also chap 78), this type of thyrotoxicosis (Plummer's disease) develops insidiously over a period of years,[58,59] usually in older people with long-standing goiters,[60] in sharp contrast with Graves' hyperthyroidism. Subclinical thyrotoxicosis is a common finding in patients with a multinodular goiter, and invariably precedes the appearance of overt thyrotoxicosis.[60,61] It disappears after surgical removal of the diseased parts of the thyroid gland.[62]

Because multinodular goiters contain new follicles with widely varying degrees of autonomous function, iodine-induced thyrotoxicosis readily occurs when the iodine supply increases.[63,64] In normal subjects, an acute increase in iodine supply may result in a small increase in thyroid secretion.[65,66] Consequently, TSH secretion decreases, and then thyroid secretion declines. This mechanism is no longer operative in patients with nodular goiters. On the one hand, TSH secretion may already be inhibited, or nearly so, by the nodules that produce T_4 and T_3 autonomously. On the other hand, the transient iodine-induced overproduction of T_4 and T_3 characteristic of normal follicles may be more marked in autonomous goiter follicles with greater capacity to synthesize T_4 and T_3 but more limited ability to trap iodide when iodide intake is normal.[65] Therefore, even a small increase of iodide supply may induce a clinically important increase in T_4 and T_3 production.[58] The true incidence of iodine-induced thyrotoxicosis is not known. In some reports,[64,67] thyrotoxicosis was considered to occur in up to half of goitrous patients exposed to excess iodine; however, in other studies,[68] the prevalence was near 20%. In Switzerland, with its postendemic goiter pattern, few toxic nodular goiter patients have been exposed to iodine overload.[69,70]

Treatment

Because toxic multinodular goiter results from gradual multiplication of autonomous follicles, removal of the excessive number of follicles by partial thyroidectomy or their destruction by administration of ^{131}I is the treatment of choice (see also chap 53). The younger the patient, the better the patient's general health, and the larger the goiter, the more easily it is to recommend thyroidectomy. [131]I therapy is the best choice for

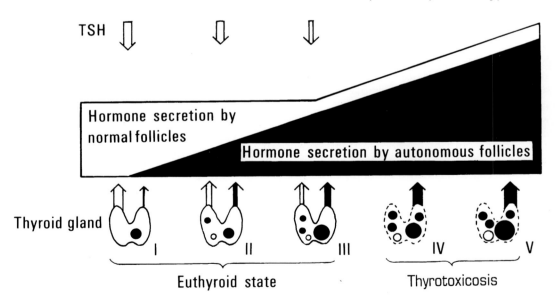

FIGURE 32-4. Evolution of thyrotoxicosis in multinodular goiter. As the goiter progresses over many years or decades from stage I to V, an increasing number of follicles with high rates of autonomous iodine turnover are generated. Some functioning follicles form large clusters, mimicking hyperfunctioning adenomas (black areas), while others are scattered throughout the gland. Overall T_4 and T_3 production rises insidiously and eventually (stage III) becomes supranormal. At this point, endogenous TSH secretion is inhibited and T_4 and T_3 production by normal follicles declines ultimately to its lowest possible level (which is always somewhat above zero). Simultaneously, nodules that consist of hypofunctioning follicles (white areas) may also develop but do not contribute to hormone synthesis.

elderly patients with multiple health problems. It may be desirable to treat the patient with an antithyroid drug before either surgery or ^{131}I therapy is undertaken, because the patient becomes euthyroid more quickly and the risk of treatment-induced exacerbation of thyrotoxicosis is lower.

The aim of surgical treatment of multinodular toxic goiter is the removal of all diseased micro- or macronodular tissue.[71,72] Even so, goiter recurrence, although rare, is not entirely eliminated. T_4 therapy probably does not prevent recurrences outside endemic goiter areas. It is, therefore, indicated only for patients with postoperative hypothyroidism. Serum TSH concentrations should be measured at yearly intervals to detect impending hypothyroidism. Although, theoretically, hypothyroidism is not an anticipated complication of ^{131}I therapy of toxic multinodular goiter, since ^{131}I is preferentially accumulated in the hyperfunctioning nodules, it can occur.[46]

Thyrotoxicosis is reversible by treatment with an antithyroid drug. This therapy is not advisable, however, because it must be life-long.

References

1. Van Sande J, Lamy F, Lecocq R, et al. Pathogenesis of autonomous thyroid nodules: in vitro study of iodine and adenosine 3′,5′-monophosphate metabolism. J Clin Endocrinol Metab 1988;66:570

2. Hamburger JI. The autonomously functioning thyroid nodule: Goetsch's disease. Endocr Rev 1987;8:439

3. Thomas CG, Croom RD. Current management of the patient with autonomously functioning nodular goiter. Surg Clin North Am 1987;67:315

4. Goretski P, Wahl RA, Branscheid D, et al. Indication for operation of patients with autonomously functioning thyroid tissue in endemic goiter areas. World J Surg 1985;9:149

5. Wiener JD, van der Gaag RD. Autoimmunity and the pathogenesis of localized thyroid autonomy (Plummer's disease). Clin Endocrinol 1985;23:635

6. Gheri RG, Borrelli D, Cicchi P, et al. Thyroxine and triiodothyronine levels in thyroid vein blood and in thyroid tissue of patients with autonomous adenomas. Clin Endocrinol 1981;15:485

7. Solter M, Tislaric D, Banovac K, et al. Thyroidal thyroxine and triiodothyronine in autonomously functioning thyroid nodule and paranodular tissue. Exp Clin Endocrinol 1985;85:369

8. Belfiore A, Sava L, Runello F, et al. Solitary autonomously functioning thyroid nodules and iodine deficiency. J Clin Endocrinol Metab 1983;56:283

9. Safa AM, Nakhjavani MK. Autonomously functioning thyroid nodule: a study of 67 patients from an iodine deficient area. Cleve Clin J Med 1988;55:227

10. Croom RD, Thomas CG Jr, Reddick RL, et al. Autonomously functioning thyroid nodules in childhood and adolescence. Surgery 1987;102:1101

11. Hamburger JI. Should all autonomously functioning thyroid nodules be ablated to prevent the subsequent development of thyrotoxicosis? In: Hamburger JI, Miller JM, eds. Controversies in clinical thyroidology. New York: Springer-Verlag, 1981:69

12. Hamburger JI. Evolution of toxicity in solitary nontoxic autonomously functioning thyroid nodules. J Clin Endocrinol Metab 1980;50:1089

13. Hedinger C, Williams ED, Sobin LH. Histological typing of thyroid tumors. 2nd ed. Berlin: Springer-Verlag, 1988:5

14. Thomas GA, Williams D, Williams ED. The clonal origin of thyroid nodules and adenomas. Am J Pathol 1989;134:141

15. Smith M, McHenry C, Jarosz H, Lawrence, AM, Paloyan E. Carcinoma of the thyroid in patients with autonomous nodules. Am Surg 1988;54:448

16. Reinwein D, Benker G, Konig MP, et al. The different types of hyperthyroidism in Europe. Results of a prospective survey of 924 patients. J Endocrinol Invest 1988;11:193

17. Studer H. A fresh look at an old thyroid disease: euthyroid and hyperthyroid nodular goiter. J Endocrinol Invest 1982;5:57

18. Peter HJ, Studer H, Forster R, et al. The pathogenesis of "hot" and "cold" follicles in multinodular goiters. J Clin Endocrinol Metab 1982;55:941

19. Peter HJ, Gerber H, Studer H, et al. Pathogenesis and heterogeneity in human multinodular goiter: a study on growth and function of thyroid tissue transplanted onto nude mice. J Clin Invest 1985;76:1992

20. Vignaud J, Duprez A, Bene M, et al. Transplantation of human hyperthyroid tissue to the nude mouse: an experimental model. Am J Pathol 1984;117:355

21. Sugenoya A, Yamada Y, Kaneko G, et al. In vitro study on release of thyroid hormone in solitary autonomously functioning thyroid nodules using cell culture. Endocrinol Jpn 1984;31:749

22. Parma J, Duprez L, Van Sande J, et al. Somatic mutations in the thyrotropin receptor gene cause hyperfunctioning thyroid adenomas. Nature 1993;365:649

23. Porcellini A, Ciullo I, Laviola L, Amabile G, Fenzi G, Avvedimento VE. Novel mutations of thyrotropin receptor gene in thyroid hyperfunctioning adenomas. J Clin Endocrinol Metab 1994;79:657

24. Russo D, Arturi F. Wicker R, et al. Genetic alterations in thyroid hyperfunctioning adenomas. J Clin Endocrinol Metab 1995;80:1347

25. Lyons J, Landis CA, Harsh G, et al. Two G protein oncogenes in human endocrine tumors. Science 1990;249:655

25a. Van Sande J, Parma J, Tonacchera M, Swillens S, Dumont J, Vassart G. Somatic and germline mutations of the TSH receptor in thyroid diseases. J Clin Endocrinol Metab 1995;80:2577

26. Berglund J, Borup Christensen S, Hallengren B. Total and age-specific incidence of Graves' thyrotoxicosis, toxic nodular goiter and solitary toxic adenoma in Malmö 1970–74. J Intern Med 1990;227:137

27. Haroldsson A, Godmundsson ST, Larusson G, et al. Thyrotoxicosis in Iceland 1980–1882: an epidemiologic survey. Acta Med Scand 1985;217:253

28. Phillips DIW, Parker DJP, Rees Smith B, et al. The geographical distribution of thyrotoxicosis in England according to the presence or absence of TSH-receptor antibodies. Clin Endocrinol 1985;23:283

29. Fogelman I, Cooks SG, Maisey MN. The role of thyroid scanning in hyperthyroidism. Eur J Nucl Med 1986;11:397

30. Williams I, Ankrett VO, Lazarus JH, et al. Aetiology of hyperthyroidism in Canada and Wales. J Epidemiol Community Health 1983;37:245

31. Wiener JD. Long term follow-up in untreated Plummer's disease (autonomous goiter). Clin Nucl Med 1987;12:198

32. Sandrock D, Olbricht T, Emrich D, Benker G, Reinwein D. Long-term follow-up in patients with autonomous thyroid adenoma. Acta Endocrinol 1993;128:51

33. Foldes J, Banos CS, Csillag J, et al. Examination of serum thyrotropic hormone level by "supersensitive" immunoradiometric assay in functioning thyroid adenoma. Acta Med Hung 1987;44:329

34. Klee GG, Hay ID. Assessment of sensitive thyrotropin assays for an expanded role in thyroid function testing: proposed criteria for analytic performance and clinical utility. J Clin Endocrinol Metab 1987;64:461

35. Walfish PG, Strawbridge HTG, Rosen IB. Management implications from routine needle biopsy of hyperfunctioning thyroid nodules. Surgery 1985;98:1179

36. Fobbe F, Finke R, Reichenstein E, et al. Appearance of thyroid diseases using color-coded duplex sonography. Eur J Radiol 1989;9:29

37. Burman KD, Earll JM, Johnson MC, et al. Clinical observations on the solitary autonomous thyroid nodule. Arch Intern Med 1974;134:915

38. Kinser JA, Roesler H, Furrer T, et al. Nonimmunogenic hyperthyroidism: cumulative hypothyroidism incidence after radioiodine and surgical treatment. J Nucl Med 1989;30:1960

39. Horst W, Rosler H, Schneider C, et al. 306 cases of toxic adenoma: clinical aspects, findings in radioiodine diagnostics, radiochromatography and histology—results of ^{131}I and surgical treatment. J Nucl Med 1967;8:515

40. Gorman CA, Robertson JS. Radiation dose in the selection of ^{131}I or surgical treatment for toxic thyroid adenoma. Ann Intern Med 1978;89:85

41. Hempelmann LH. Risk of thyroid neoplasms after irradiation in childhood. Science 1968;160:159

42. Eyre-Brooks IA, Talbot CH. The treatment of autonomous functioning thyroid nodules. Br J Surg 1982;69:577

43. Goldstein R, Hart IR. Follow-up of solitary autonomous thyroid nodules treated with [131]I. N Engl J Med 1983;309:1473

44. Clerc J, Dagousset F, Izembart M, et al. Radioiodine therapy of the autonomous thyroid nodule in patients with and without visible extranodular activity. J Nucl Med 1995;36:217

45. Ng Tang Fui SC, Maisey MN. Standard dose ^{131}I therapy for hyperthyroidism caused by autonomously functioning thyroid nodules. Clin Endocrinol 1979;10:69

46. Fontana B, Curti G, Biggi A, et al. The incidence of hypothyroidism after radioactive iodine (^{131}I) therapy for autonomous hyperfunctioning thyroid nodules evaluated by means of life-table method. J Nucl Med Allied Sci 1980;24:85

47. Hegedus L, Veiergang D, Karstrup S, et al. Compensated ^{131}I-therapy of solitary autonomous thyroid nodules: effect on thyroid size and early hypothyroidism. Acta Endocrinol 1986;113:226

48. Ross DS, Ridgway EC, Daniels GH. Successful treatment of solitary toxic thyroid nodules with relatively low-dose iodine-131, with low prevalence of hypothyroidism. Ann Intern Med 1984;101:488

49. Mariotti S, Martino E, Francesconi M, et al. Serum thyroid autoantibodies as a risk factor for development of hypothyroidism after radioactive iodine therapy for single thyroid "hot" nodule. Acta Endocrinol 1986;113:500

50. Nygaard B, Jarlov AE, Hegedus L, Schaadt B, Kristensen LO, Hansen JM. Long-term follow-up of thyroid scintigraphies after ^{131}I therapy of solitary autonomous thyroid nodules. Thyroid 1994;4:167

51. Monzani F, Goletti O, Caraccio N, et al. Percutaneous ethanol injection treatment of autonomous thyroid adenoma: hormonal and clinical evaluation. Clin Endocrinol 1992;36:491

52. Martino E, Murtas ML, Loviselli A, et al. Percutaneous intranodular ethanol injection for treatment of autonomously functioning thyroid nodules. Surgery 1992;112:1161

53. Goletti O, Monzani F, Caraccio N, et al. Percutaneous ethanol injection treatment of autonomously functioning single thyroid nodules: optimization of treatment and short term outcome. World J Surg 1992;16:784

54. Papini E, Panunzi C, Pacella CM, et al. Percutaneous ultrasound-guided ethanol injection: a new treatment of toxic autonomously functioning thyroid nodules. J Clin Endocrinol Metab 1993;76:411

55. De Lelio A, Rivolta M, Casati M, Capra M. Treatment of autonomous thyroid nodules: value of percutaneous ethanol injection. Am J Roentg 1994;164:207

56. Ozdemir H, Ilgit ET, Yucel C, et al. Treatment of autonomous thyroid nodules: safety and efficacy of sonographically guided percutaneous injection of ethanol. Am J Roentg 1994; 163:929

57. Livraghi T, Paracchi A, Ferrari C, Reschini E, Macchi RM, Bonifacino A. Treatment of autonomous thyroid nodules with percutaneous ethanol injection: 4-year experience. Radiology 1994; 190:529

58. Studer H, Peter HJ, Gerber H. Toxic nodular goitre. Clin Endocrinol Metab 1985;14:351

59. Plummer HS. The clinical and pathological relationship of simple and exophthalmic goiter. Am J Med Sci 1913;146:790

60. Berghout A, Wiersinga WM, Smits NJ, Touber JL. Interrelationships between age, thyroid volume, thyroid nodularity, and thyroid function in patients with sporadic nodular goiter. Am J Med 1990;89:602.

61. Rieu M, Bekka S, Sambor B, Berrod J-L, Fombeur J-P. Prevalence of subclinical hyperthyroidism and relationship between thyroid hormonal status and thyroid ultrasonographic parameteres in patients with non-toxic nodular goitre. Clin Endocrinol 1993; 39:67

62. Gemsenjager E, Staub JJ, Girard J. Pituitary thyroid recovery following surgery in TRH-unresponsive patients with uni- and multinodular goiter. Horm Res 1977;8:139

63. Fradkin JE, Wolff J. Iodide-induced thyrotoxicosis. Medicine 1983;62:1

64. Vagenakis AG, Wang C, Burger A, Maloof F, Braverman LE, Ingbar SH. Iodide-induced thyrotoxicosis in Boston. N. Engl J Med 1972;287:523

65. Emrich D, Karkavitsas N, Facorro U, et al. Influence of increasing iodine uptake on thyroid function in euthyroid and hyperthyroid states. J Clin Endocrinol Metab 1982;54:1236

66. Studer H, Burgi H, Kohler H, Garcia MC, Moreal de Escobar G. A transient rise of hormone secretion: a response of the stimulated rat thyroid gland to small increments of iodide supply. Acta Endocrinol 1976;81:507

67. Mahlstedt J, Joseph K. Dekompensation autonomer Adenome der Schilddruse nach prolongierter Jodzufuhr. Dtsch Med Wochenschr 1973;98:1748

68. Haberman J, Leisner B. Witte A, Pickardt CR, Scriba PC. Iodine contamination as a cause of hyperthyroidism or lack of TSH response to TRH stimulation (results based on a screening investigation). J Endocrinol Invest 1982;5:153

69. Burgi H, Supersaxo Z, Selz B. Iodine deficiency diseases in Switzerland one hundred years after Theodor Kocher's survey: a historical review with some new goiter prevalence data. Acta Endocrinol 1990;127:577

70. Mordasini C, Abetel G, Lauterburg H, et al. Untersuchungen zum Kochsalzkonsum und zur Jodversorgung der schweizerischen Bevolkerung. Schweiz Med Wochenschr 1984;114:1924

71. Gemsenjager E, Heitz PU, Staub JJ, Girard J, Barthe P, Benz UF. Surgical aspects of thyroid autonomy in multinodular goiter. World J Surg 1983;7:363

72. Teuscher J, Peter HJ, Gerber H, Berchtold R, Studer H. Pathogenesis of nodular goiter and its implications for surgical management. Surgery 1988;103:87

Werner and Ingbar's The Thyroid, Seventh Edition,
edited by Lewis E. Braverman and Robert D. Utiger.
Lippincott–Raven Publishers, Philadelphia, © 1996

33

Trophoblastic Tumors

Jerome M. Hershman

Thyrotoxicosis occurs in patients with trophoblastic tumors, which are either hydatidiform moles or choriocarcinomas. Since the first report of thyrotoxicosis in women with hydatidiform mole in 1955,[1] many additional cases have been reported.[2–6] These reports revealed that the thyrotoxicosis disappeared rapidly after removal of the tumor, thus suggesting that the tumor produced a substance responsible for the thyrotoxicosis. It is now clear that human chorionic gonadotropin is the thyroid stimulator that causes the thyrotoxicosis in patients with throphoblastic tumors.

Hydatidiform mole occurs in about 1 in 1500 pregnancies in the United States and is 10 times more common in Asian and Latin American countries. Choriocarcinoma occurs in 1 in 40,000 pregnancies; about one-half of the cases occur in women with previously diagnosed hydatidiform moles. Although thyrotoxicosis has been reported more frequently in women with hydatidiform mole than in those with choriocarcinoma, there have been many case reports of thyrotoxicosis in women with choriocarcinoma[7–12] as well as some in men with testicular tumors[13,14] and in one man with a colon choriocarcinoma.[15] The precise prevalence of thyrotoxicosis in patients with trophoblastic tumors is unknown. It was found in 5 of 20 patients with trophoblastic disease evaluated at a referral center in one year;[16] three of the five thyrotoxic patients had choriocarcinoma and two had hydatidiform moles. In another study, 30 of 52 patients with gestational trophoblastic tumors were found to be thyrotoxic.[2]

GRADATIONS OF SEVERITY

In trophoblastic disease, the spectrum of alterations of thyroid function ranges from a minimal increase in serum thyroxine (T_4) and triiodothyronine (T_3) concentrations, as evidenced by a subnormal serum thyrotropin (TSH) response to thyrotropin-releasing hormone (TRH),[17] to moderate increases in serum T_4

and T_3 concentrations without symptoms of hypermetabolism, to marked increases in thyroid secretion with severe clinical thyrotoxicosis, to thyroid storm. The lack of clear clinical features of thyrotoxicosis in many patients with elevated serum T_4 and T_3 concentrations may be attributable to the relatively brief duration of the increased thyroid function, so that there is insufficient time to develop overt clinical thyrotoxicosis.[3,18] Also, the clinical manifestations of thyrotoxicosis may be overlooked because attention is focused on the toxemia that frequently accompanies the chorionic tumor. In addition, the toxemia may lower serum T_3 concentrations, as occurs in patients with nonthyroidal illness. Thyrotoxic patients with trophoblastic tumors have lower serum T_3/T_4 ratios than patients with Graves' hyperthyroidism.[2]

CLINICAL FEATURES

Whereas many women with trophoblastic tumors lack clinical evidence of thyrotoxicosis despite having elevated serum T_4 and T_3 concentrations, others have typical clinical findings that include weight loss, muscle weakness, fatigue, excessive sweating, heat intolerance, tachycardia, nervousness, and tremor. The thyroid gland is either not enlarged or only minimally enlarged, rarely to more than twice normal size. Ophthalmopathy is absent, in contrast with the usual presentation of Graves' disease in young women. In addition there are characteristic features of the trophoblastic tumor. Hydatidiform mole may present as a pregnancy in which the size of the uterus is large for the duration of the gestation. There is uterine bleeding between the sixth and sixteenth week of pregnancy in more than 95% of patients with trophoblastic tumors. Nausea, vomiting, and toxemia of pregnancy occur commonly in molar pregnancy and may obscure the features of thyrotoxicosis.

Although choriocarcinoma in women may be confined to the uterus, the tumor is usually widely metastatic and may involve the pelvis, liver, lungs, and even the brain. The diagnosis of metastatic cancer is usually obvious and dominates the clinical picture. As in patients with hydatidiform mole, there may be laboratory evidence of increased thyroid function without clinically evident thyrotoxicosis.[19] In men, choriocarcinoma nearly always arises in the testis and in those men with thyrotoxicosis is usually widely metastatic.[13,14] Gynecomastia is a common complaint in men with choriocarcinoma, but because gynecomastia can occur in any man with thyrotoxicosis, this finding does not indicate that a trophoblastic tumor is the cause of the thyrotoxicosis.

DIAGNOSIS

Chorionic gonadotropin (hCG) is secreted by the trophoblastic tissue—both hydatidiform moles and choriocarcinomas. Therefore, hCG serves as a marker for the tumor. It can be measured by a specific radioimmunoassay using an antibody directed against the β-subunit of hCG. Patients with trophoblastic tumors have very high serum hCG concentrations and urinary hCG excretion, with values that greatly exceed the threshold for diagnosis of pregnancy. In patients with thyrotoxicosis caused by trophoblastic tumors, serum hCG concentrations usually exceed 300 U/mL and always exceed 100 U/mL,[5,10,11,20] the peak concentration that occurs in pregnant women at 10 to 12 weeks' gestation. However, not all patients with trophoblastic tumors with very high serum hCG concentrations have thyrotoxicosis.

The diagnosis of thyrotoxicosis, or increased thyroid function, is established by finding elevated serum T_4, free T_4 and T_3 concentrations. Trophoblastic tumors secrete less estrogen than normal placental tissue, so that the increase of serum thyroxine-binding globulin (TBG) concentration is less in molar pregnancy than in normal pregnancy.[2] Thyroid radioiodine uptake is greatly increased.[3] Even when serum T_4 and T_3 concentrations are only slightly elevated, both serum TSH concentrations and serum TSH responses to TRH are low.[17] In severely thyrotoxic patients with trophoblastic tumors who have very high serum hCG concentrations, serum TSH was often inappropriately detectable in the normal range in older TSH radioimmunoassays due to the weak cross-reaction of hCG in these assays. With the improved specificity of current sensitive TSH assays, this cross-reaction does not occur.[2,16] TSH-receptor antibodies are not detectable, excluding Graves' disease as the cause of thyrotoxicosis in patients with trophoblastic tumors.

Ultrasonography of the uterus shows a characteristic snowstorm pattern in patients with hydatidiform mole. The definitive diagnosis of hydatidiform mole or choriocarcinoma is based on the histopathology of the tissue removed by curettage or surgery.

HYPEREMESIS GRAVIDARUM

Elevated serum T_4 and T_3 concentrations are a common finding in women with hyperemesis gravidarum.[21–23] Women with hyperemesis and elevated serum T_4 and T_3 values have higher serum hCG concentrations than normal pregnant women.[22]

Their serum hCG concentrations correlate with the degree of elevation of serum T_4 and T_3 concentrations and with serum thyrotropic activity. Vomiting is also more severe in those women with higher serum hCG concentrations, suggesting that another factor induced by hCG, perhaps estradiol, may be responsible for the vomiting.[22] Although clinical features of thyrotoxicosis are usually absent, or overlooked, in women with hyperemesis gravidarum, some have had a few signs and symptoms of thyrotoxicosis; but thyroid enlargement is lacking.[24,25] The thyrotoxicosis resolves spontaneously within several weeks as the vomiting disappears.[22,25]

HUMAN CHORIONIC GONADOTROPIN

Human chorionic gonadotropin is composed of α- and β-subunits. The α-subunit is identical to the α-subunit of TSH, luteinizing hormone, and follicle-stimulating hormone. The β-subunit of hCG has considerable structural homology with the β-subunit of TSH, but it is larger because it contains a 33-amino-acid carboxy-terminal tail.

The material with thyrotropic activity that can be extracted from hydatidiform moles and choriocarcinoma copurifies with hCG.[8,26] The thyrotropic activity of hCG has been demonstrated in mice, rats, chicks, and humans.[26–28] Injection of large amounts of hCG (100,000–150,000 U) into normal men stimulates thyroid iodine release.[27] In normal pregnant women, serum TSH concentrations decrease at 9 to 12 weeks of gestation when serum hCG concentrations are highest;[29–31] the high hCG concentrations correlate with increased thyroid-stimulating activity in a mouse bioassay. Serum thyrotropic activity measured by a thyroid cell culture assay also is increased during the first trimester in normal pregnant women, and this activity correlates with serum hCG and free T_4 concentrations.[32] The thyrotropic activity of purified hCG is equivalent to about 0.2 μU bovine TSH/U hCG in a mouse bioassay,[30] and 0.04 μU bovine TSH/U hCG in a rat thyroid cell culture bioassay (Fig. 33-1), but equivalent to only 0.0013 μU human TSH/U hCG in a human thyroid cell culture bioassay.[33] Nevertheless, this thyrotropic activity may be substantial in patients with trophoblastic tumors whose serum hCG concentrations may reach 300 to 2000 U/mL. Serum hCG and T_3 concentrations were correlated in patients with hydatidiform moles.[5] In five women with trophoblastic thyrotoxicosis, serum hCG concentrations correlated with serum T_4, free T_4, and T_3 concentrations.[16]

Early work on the thyrotropic activity of hCG assayed with human thyroid membrane TSH receptors gave equivocal results, and the role of hCG as a thyroid-stimulating hormone in humans was controversial.[34] However, recent data using recombinant human TSH receptors and cell culture systems have clarified this issue. hCG inhibits the binding of labeled TSH to its plasma membrane receptors on thyroid follicular cells[35,36]; hCG activates adenylyl cyclase in rat thyroid cells and in cells transfected with human TSH receptors[36,37]; and hCG with greatly increased thyrotropic potency against human and rodent TSH receptors that was extracted from hydatidiform moles[6,38] was enriched in the more basic isoelectric forms of the molecule that contained less sialic acid as compared with normal hCG. Asialo-hCG purified from a patient with choriocarcinoma had very potent thyrotropic activity in a

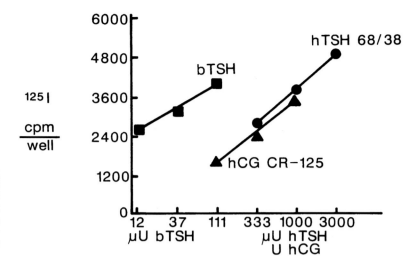

FIGURE 33-1. Comparison of the effects of bovine TSH and purified hCG on iodide uptake in cultured rat thyroid (FRTL-5) cells. Relative potencies are 1 U hCG = 0.72 μU hTSH = 0.042 μU bTSH. (Hershman JM, Lee H-Y, Sugawara M, et al. Human chorionic gonadotropin stimulates iodide uptake, adenylate cyclase, and deoxyribonucleic acid synthesis in cultured rat thyroid cells. J Clin Endocrinol Metab 1988;67:74)

bioassay that used human thyroid follicles.[33] Although asialo-hCG has much greater thyrotropic activity in vitro than sialated hCG, the lack of sialic acid greatly accelerates its clearance from plasma and thus reduces its physiologic action.[39] Removal of several amino residues from the β-subunit of hCG increases its thyrotropic activity several-fold.[40] Recombinant mutant hCG lacking the 31-amino-acid carboxy-terminal tail of the β-subunit stimulates the human TSH receptor about tenfold more potently than does intact hCG.[36] Presumably the long C-terminal tail and the high sialic acid content restrict the interaction of hCG with the TSH receptor.

The basis for the thyrotropic effect of hCG is, therefore, the molecular similarity of hCG to TSH. Although hCG is a very weak thyrotropin in comparison with TSH, it is likely that molecular variants of hCG that are secreted by trophoblastic tumors have considerably greater thyrotropic activity than hCG secreted in normal pregnancy.

THERAPY

Surgical removal of the hydatidiform mole in a thyrotoxic patient rapidly cures the thyrotoxicosis, as shown in Figure 33-2, and should be carried out as soon as possible. Other treatment of the thyrotoxicosis should be based on anticipation of the benefit of surgery. Propylthiouracil and methimazole will not control the thyrotoxicosis within only a few days. Therapy with potassium iodide given orally or sodium iodide given intravenously will rapidly lower serum T_4 and T_3 concentrations.[5] Propranolol and other beta-adrenergic antagonist drugs are useful in controlling tachycardia and other symptoms of sympathetic activation, and other supportive measures such as fluid and electrolyte replacement should be administered as needed.

Treatment of choriocarcinoma requires appropriate chemotherapy, which is best given in a referral center that specializes in this disorder. Cure of gestational choriocarcinoma cures the thyrotoxicosis.[9,10,16,20] Unfortunately, patients with choriocarcinomas who have thyrotoxicosis usually have a large tumor mass, as indicated by very high serum hCG concentrations, so that cure of the tumor with chemotherapy is

less likely to be achieved than in the usual woman with choriocarcinoma, in whom the cure rate is over 90%. Nevertheless, several women with metastatic choriocarcinoma and thyrotoxicosis have achieved complete remission with chemotherapy. The prognosis of men with testicular choriocarcinoma and related hCG-secreting testicular tumors, however, is poor.[13] In thyrotoxic patients with choriocarcinoma, the thyrotoxicosis should be treated by any of the usual medical therapies (see chap 53), but surgical thyroidectomy is ill advised.

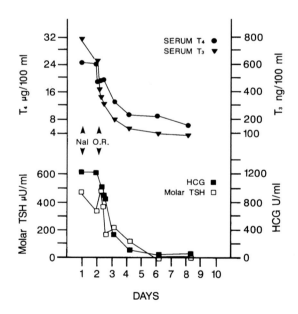

FIGURE 33-2. Serum T_4, T_3, TSH, and hCG concentrations in a 40-year-old woman who was moderately thyrotoxic at 16 weeks of gestation with a hydatidiform mole. She was given 1 g sodium iodide intravenously (NaI) and the mole was removed operatively (O.R.). There was a parallel fall in the serum hCG concentration, measured by radioimmunoassay, and in the serum molar TSH concentration, which was measured by a mouse bioassay. The patient's serum T_4 and T_3 concentrations also fell rapidly after removal of the mole (Higgins HP, Hershman JM, Kenimer JG, Patillo RA, Bayley TA, Walfish P. The thyrotoxicosis of hydatidiform mole. Ann Intern Med 1975;83:307)

References

1. Tisne L, Barzelatto J, Stevenson C. Study of thyroid function during pregnancy and the post-partum period with radioactive iodine. (Span). Bol Soc Chil Obstet Ginecol 1955;20:246

2. Desai RK, Norman RJ, Jialal I, Joubert SM. Spectrum of thyroid function abnormalities in gestational trophoblastic neoplasia. Clin Endocrinol 1988;29:583

3. Galton VA, Ingbar SH, Jimenez-Fonseca J, Hershman JM. Alterations in thyroid hormone economy in patients with hydatidiform mole. J Clin Invest 1971;50:1345

4. Hershman JM, Higgins HP. Hydatidiform mole—a cause of clinical hyperthyroidism. N Engl J Med 1971;284:573

5. Higgins HP, Hershman JM, Kenimer JG, Patillo RA, Bayley TA, Walfish P. The thyrotoxicosis of hydatidiform mole. Ann Intern Med 1975;83:307

6. Pekary AE, Jackson IMD, Goodwin TM, Pang X-P, Hein MD, Hershman JM. Increased in vitro thyrotropic activity of partially sialated human chorionic gonadotropin extracted from hydatidiform moles of patients with hyperthyroidism. J Clin Endocrinol Metab 1993;76:70

7. Anderson NR, Lokich JJ, McDermott WV, Jr, Trey C, Falchuk KR. Gestational choriocarcinoma and thyrotoxicosis. Cancer 1979;44:304

8. Cave WT Jr, Dunn JT. Choriocarcinoma with hyperthyroidism: probable identity of the thyrotropin with human chorionic gonadotropin. Ann Intern Med 1976;85:60

9. Cohen JD, Utiger RD. Metastatic choriocarcinoma associated with hyperthyroidism. J Clin Endocrinol Metab 1970;30:423

10. Morley JE, Jacobson RJ, Melamed J, Hershman JM. Choriocarcinoma as a cause of thyrotoxicosis. Am J Med 1976;60:1036

11. Nisula BC, Taliadouros GS. Thyroid function in gestational trophoblastic neoplasia: Evidence that the thyrotropic activity of chorionic gonadotropin mediates the thyrotoxicosis of choriocarcinoma. Am J Obstet Gynecol 1980;138:77

12. Soutter WP, Green-Thompson RW. The management of choriocarcinoma causing severe thyrotoxicosis. Br J Obstet Gynaecol 1981;88:938

13. Giralt SA, Dexeus F, Amato R, Sella A, Logothetis C. Hyperthyroidism in men with germ cell tumors and high levels of beta-human chorionic gonadotropin. Cancer 1992;69:1286

14. Karp PJ, Hershman JM, Richmond S, Goldstein DP, Selenkow HA. Thyrotoxicosis from molar thyrotropin. Arch Intern Med 1973;132:432

15. Orgiazzi J, Rousset B, Cosentino C, Tournaire J, Dutrieux N. Plasma thyrotropic activity in a man with choriocarcinoma. J Clin Endocrinol Metab 1974;39:653

16. Rajatanavin R, Chailurkit LO, Srisupandit S, Tungtrakul S, Bunyaratvej S. Trophoblastic hyperthyroidism: clinical and biochemical features of five cases. Am J Med 1988;85:237

17. Miyai K, Tanizawa O, Yamamoto T, et al. Pituitary-thyroid function in trophoblastic disease. J Clin Endocrinol Metab 1976;42:254

18. Nagataki S, Mizuno M, Sakamoto S, Irie M, Shizume K. Thyroid function in molar pregnancy. J Clin Endocrinol Metab 1977;44:254

19. Odell WD, Bates RW, Rivlin RS, Lipsett MB, Hertz R. Increased thyroid function without clinical hyperthyroidism in patients with choriocarcinoma. J Clin Endocrinol Metab 1963;29:658

20. Norman RJ, Green-Thompson W, Jialal I, Soutter WP, Pillay NL, Jourbert SM. Hyperthyroidism in gestational trophoblastic neoplasia. Clin Endocrinol 1981;15:395

21. Goodwin TM, Montoro M, Mestman JH. Transient hyperthyroidism and hyperemesis gravidarum: Clinical aspects. Am J Obstet Gynecol 1992;167:648

22. Goodwin TM, Montoro M, Mestman JH, Pekary AE, Hershman JM. The role of chorionic gonadotropin in transient hyperthyroidism of hyperemesis gravidarum. J Clin Endocrinol Metab 1992;75:1333

23. Swaminathan R, Chin RK, Lao TTH, Mak YT, Panesar NS, Cockram CS. Thyroid function in hyperemesis gravidarum. Acta Endocrinol 1989;120:155

24. Chin RKH, Lao TTH, Cockram CS, Swaminathan R. Transient hyperthyroidism in pregnancy. Case report. Br J Obstet Gynecol 1987;94:483

25. Kimura M, Amino N, Tamaki H, et al. Gestational thyrotoxicosis and hyperemesis gravidarum: possible role of hCG with higher stimulating activity. Clin Endocrinol 1993;38:345

26. Kenimer JG, Hershman JM, Higgins HP. The thyrotropin in hydatidiform moles is human chorionic gonadotropin. J Clin Endocrinol Metab 1975;40:482

27. Sowers JR, Hershman JM, Carlson HE, Pekary AE. Effect of human chorionic gonadotropin on thyroid function in euthyroid men. J Clin Endocrinol Metab 1978;47:898

28. Pekary AE, Azukizawa M, Hershman JM. Thyroidal responses to human chorionic gonadotropin in the chick and rat. Horm Res 1983;7:36

29. Braunstein GD, Hershman JM. Comparison of serum pituitary thyrotropin and chorionic gonadotropin concentrations throughout pregnancy. J Clin Endocrinol Metab 1976;42:1123

30. Harada A, Hershman JM, Reed AW, et al. Comparisons of thyroid stimulators and thyroid hormone concentrations in the sera of pregnant women. J Clin Endocrinol Metab 1979;48:793

31. Pekonen F, Alfthan H, Stenman U-H, Ylikorkala O. Human chorionic gonadotropin (hCG) and thyroid function in early human pregnancy: circadian variation and evidence for intrinsic thyrotropic activity of hCG. J Clin Endocrinol Metab 1988;66:853

32. Yoshikawa N, Nishikawa M, Horimoto M, et al. Thyroid-stimulating activity in sera of normal pregnant women. J Clin Endocrinol Metab 1989;69:891

33. Yamazaki K, Sato K, Shizume K, et al. Potent thyrotropic activity of human chorionic gonadotropin variants in terms of ^{125}I incorporation and de novo-synthesized thyroid hormone release in human thyroid follicles. J Clin Endocrinol Metab 1995;80:473

34. Amir SM. Human chorionic gonadotropin: a neglible human thyroid stimulator. In: Ingbar SH, Braverman LE, eds. The thyroid. A fundamental and clinical text. 5th ed. Philadelphia: JB Lippincott, 1986:1088

35. Azukizawa M, Kurtzman G, Pekary AE, Hershman JM. Comparison of the binding characteristics of bovine thyrotropin and human chorionic gonadotropin to thyroid plasma membranes. Endocrinology 1977;202:1880

36. Yoshimura M, Hershman JM, Pang X-P, Berg L, Pekary AE. Activation of the thyrotropin (TSH) receptor by human chorionic gonadotropin and luteinizing hormone in Chinese hamster ovary cells expressing functional human TSH receptors. J Clin Endocrinol Metab 1993;77:1009

37. Hershman JM, Lee H-Y, Sugawara M, et al. Human chorionic gonadotropin stimulates iodide uptake, adenylate cyclase, and deoxyribonucleic acid synthesis in cultured rat thyroid cells. J Clin Endocrinol Metab 1988;67:74

38. Yoshimura M, Pekary AE, Pang X-P, Berg L, Goodwin TM, Hershman JM. Thyrotropic activity of basic isoelectric forms of human chorionic gonadotropin extracted from hydatidiform mole tissues. J Clin Endocrinol Metab 1994;78:862

39. Hoermann R, Kubota K, Amir SM. Role of subunit sialic acid in hepatic binding, plasma survival rate, and in vivo thyrotropic activity of human chorionic gonadotropin. Thyroid 1993;3:41

40. Carayon P, AMR S, Nisula B, Lissitzky S. Effects of carboxypeptidase digestion of the human choriogonadotropin molecule on its thyrotropic activity. Endocrinology 1981;108:1891

Werner and Ingbar's The Thyroid, Seventh Edition,
edited by Lewis E. Braverman and Robert D. Utiger.
Lippincott–Raven Publishers, Philadelphia, © 1996

34

Silent Thyroiditis and Subacute Thyroiditis

John H. Lazarus

For the purpose of this chapter, silent thyroiditis and subacute thyroiditis refer to the clinical syndromes that occur in conjunction with certain histopathologic changes in the thyroid gland. *Silent thyroiditis* is used to describe lymphocytic thyroiditis with transient thyrotoxicosis and transient hypothyroidism. Silent thyroiditis and postpartum thyroiditis are similar in many respects, although postpartum thyroiditis has a wider clinical spectrum in that it also includes transient thyrotoxicosis, transient hypothyroidism, persistent hypothyroidism, and euthyroid goiter (see chap 89). *Subacute thyroiditis* is used to describe only granulomatous or nonsuppurative thyroiditis. In most studies of these two disorders, the cases were classified according to clinical characteristics without histologic confirmation. The features of the two conditions are shown in Table 34-1.

SILENT THYROIDITIS

Silent (painless) thyroiditis associated with transient thyrotoxicosis was identified with increasing frequency during the late 1970s and early 1980s, but its frequency now seems to be waning. Although the terms silent thyroiditis and painless thyroiditis[1–5] are most often used to describe this syndrome, other descriptive nomenclature includes thyrotoxicosis with painless thyroiditis[6]; painless, atypical, or occult subacute thyroiditis[7–10]; lymphocytic thyroiditis with spontaneously resolving thyrotoxicosis[11]; and transient thyrotoxicosis with lymphocytic thyroiditis.[12] Silent thyroiditis was initially described as a painless form of subacute thyroiditis (a disorder dominated by thyroid pain and tenderness) because of its similar clinical course[5,6,9]; histologic studies, however, showed it to be a form of lymphocytic thyroiditis,[11–13] similar to, although usually less extensive than, that found in chronic autoimmune thyroiditis.

The same disorder occurs in the postpartum period.[14,15] When thyrotoxicosis is present, silent thyroiditis, postpartum thyroiditis, and subacute thyroiditis all have a similar clinical course,[16] but the last differs from the former two both clinically and pathologically. Histopathologically, silent thyroiditis and postpartum thyroiditis are indistinguishable forms of lymphocytic thyroiditis, whereas subacute thyroiditis is characterized by granulomatous and giant-cell inflammation. The several disorders may be overlapping forms of thyroid inflammation induced by different infectious, autoimmune, or other processes. Silent thyroiditis is usually recognized because the duration of symptoms of thyrotoxicosis before presentation is short, and is confirmed by the finding of a low thyroid radioactive iodine uptake. It follows a self-limited course of a few weeks to several months, and transient hypothyroidism often occurs during recovery. An unknown factor apparently causes a rather sudden onset of inflammation, damaging thyroid follicles, and activating thyroglobulin proteolysis, so that sufficient thyroxine (T_4) and triiodothyronine (T_3) are released into the circulation to cause the thyrotoxicosis. Some thyroglobulin is released as well. Multiple episodes may occur in the same person.[11]

Incidence

Silent thyroiditis has been reported in North and South America, Europe, India, and Japan. Its recognition increased in the 1970s such that in some areas (e.g., Wisconsin) it accounted for as many as 23% of all cases of thyrotoxicosis.[11] However, this high relative frequency of silent thyroiditis as a cause of thyrotoxicosis has not been reported in other parts of the United States or in Europe. In a retrospective survey of 100 consecutive thyrotoxic patients in Toronto and 100 in Cardiff, silent thyroiditis accounted for 6% in the former city but no

TABLE 34-1.
Comparative Features of Silent Thyroiditis and Subacute Thyroiditis

	Silent Thyroiditis	Subacute Thyroiditis
Age of onset (ys)	5–93	20–60
Sex ratio (F/M)	2:1	5:1
Incidence (cf Graves' disease)*	≤5%–10%	≤20%
Etiology	Autoimmune	Viral
Pathology	Lymphocytic infiltration	Follicular cell destruction and inflammation
Painful goiter	No	Yes
Fever and malaise	No	Yes
Permanent hypothyroidism	Occasionally	Very rare
Reduced thyroid ^{131}I uptake	Yes	Yes
Ultrasonography	Hypoechogenicity	Hypoechogenicity
Thyroid peroxidase and thyroglobulin antibodies	Yes	Occasionally
TSH receptor antibodies	Usually not	Up to 40%
Treatment	None or β-adrenergic antagonist drugs	Prednisone, analgesic drugs
HLA haplotype	DR3, low risk	B35, high risk

Incidence (compared with that of Graves' disease) varies with geography, ethnic background, and method of ascertainment.

cases in the latter.[17] In the United States the condition was found to account for less than 5% of all cases of thyrotoxicosis in Philadelphia,[18] Brooklyn,[19] and coastal Virginia,[6] but 15% in Texas.[1] In a random poll of endocrinologists in 1983, silent thyroiditis was a rare finding on the East and West coasts of the United States and in Europe and Argentina but common around the Great Lakes in the United States and Canada.[20] One factor that may explain some of the variation in incidence is that the transient and painless nature of the illness and its symptoms may be attributed to a "flulike" illness by those unfamiliar with the disease. Some asymptomatic patients are also found to have silent thyroiditis by routine testing. Although differences in ascertainment are probably the main reason for the differences in the frequency of the condition, there are probably true geographic variations in frequency as well. Two minor epidemics of thyrotoxicosis first believed to be silent thyroiditis have occurred in the midwestern United States, but both outbreaks proved to be due to the contamination of ground beef with thyroid tissue.[21,22]

The affected patients are usually white or Asian. Women predominate in a ratio of 1.5 to 2:1, which is a much lower ratio than reported for almost all other types of thyroid disease, for which the ratios range from 3 to 10:1. Most patients are in the third through sixth decade of life, but patients as young as 5 years and as old as 93 years have been reported.[11]

Etiology

The initial suggestion that silent thyroiditis might represent a silent form of subacute or granulomatous thyroiditis has been disproved by multiple reports describing only lymphocytic thyroiditis in biopsy specimens.[11–13,23] A search for antibodies to influenza viruses A and B; parainfluenza viruses types 1, 2,

and 3; adenovirus; respiratory syncytial virus; mumps virus; measles virus; and coxsackieviruses types 1 through 6 in 18 patients with silent thyroiditis revealed only 1 patient with a substantial rise in antibody titer during the course of the disease.[11] In contrast, over 40% of patients with subacute thyroiditis have illness-related changes in viral antibody titers.[24] No positive cultures for viruses or bacteria or electron microscopic evidence of viral inclusion bodies have been reported. A history of an illness such as an upper respiratory infection, which often occurs before the onset of subacute thyroiditis, is unusual in silent thyroiditis. However, infection with rubella virus was implicated in one case[25] and an unidentified antecedent infection or exposure to antigen causing a transient increase in serum IgM concentration was reported in another.[26] A seasonal cluster in summer and late autumn, the simultaneous occurrence of subacute thyroiditis and silent thyroiditis in a wife and husband,[10] and the occurrence, in a short period of time, in five nursery school coworkers,[27] suggest an infectious agent. However, viral serologic studies of acute and convalescent serum in the last group were negative.

Strong evidence suggests that silent thyroiditis is a variant or a new form of lymphocytic thyroiditis (see chap 55), because of the uniform finding of lymphocytic thyroiditis on biopsy.[11–13,23] Although most patients have a partial or complete remission, follow-up study for 1 to 10 years has shown the persistence of or later development of thyroid autoantibodies, thyroid enlargement, or permanent hypothyroidism in about half of patients, whereas those having subacute thyroiditis rarely develop permanent thyroid disease.[28] A substantial percentage of patients who have silent thyroiditis have personal or family histories of autoimmune thyroid disease. HLA haplotype studies show an increased frequency of HLA-DR3 in patients with silent thyroiditis, and HLA-DR3 and HLA-

DR5 in those with postpartum thyroiditis,[29] whereas the frequency of HLA-B35 is increased in patients with subacute thyroiditis.[30] Intrathyroidal T-cell phenotypes are similar in silent thyroiditis and chronic lymphocytic thyroiditis.[31] Taken together, these results suggest that silent thyroiditis is an early and unusual presentation of chronic lymphocytic thyroiditis, with an unknown factor causing the onset or exacerbation of the destructive process. Variant or atypical forms characterized by thyroid pain or tenderness similar to subacute thyroiditis are recognized only when biopsies are done.[32,33]

Several factors have been suggested to be the initiating event in silent thyroiditis, but these factors are absent in the majority of cases. Excess iodide intake, especially from the antiarrhythmic drug amiodarone, leads the list.[34] An increase in serum interleukin-6, an inflammatory mediator, has been found in patients with amiodarone-induced destructive thyroiditis with thyrotoxicosis.[35] (Although thyroid iodine content and iodine intake may have an effect on the severity of the thyrotoxic and hypothyroid phases of postpartum thyroiditis, no evidence of an etiologic role for iodine in the postpartum period has been found.[36,37]) Thyroid iodine content has been found to be normal or slightly decreased during the thyrotoxic phase of silent thyroiditis,[38] and urinary iodide excretion is increased during this phase but is decreased during recovery.[11] This increase in urinary iodide reflects release of iodide and iodinated compounds from the damaged thyroid. Iodine-induced thyrotoxicosis and silent thyroiditis are sometimes indistinguishable, but the few patients with the former who have had thyroid biopsies have not had lymphocytic thyroiditis. Excessive iodine intake has been proposed as an aggravating or inciting factor because of its effects on lymphocytic thyroiditis in animals and on human thyroid disease (see section on the effects of excess iodide in chap 14). In the case of painless thyroiditis in the postpartum period, the initiating event may be related to the decline in immunologic tolerance that occurs at this time (see chap 89).

Other possible initiating factors include drugs such as lithium,[39] which has thyroid immunomodulatory effects,[40] and interleukin-2.[41,42] Alpha interferon therapy, given for hepatitis B and C[43–45] and metastatic cancer,[46] has caused episodes of silent thyroiditis both in patients who had evidence of chronic autoimmune thyroiditis before treatment and in those who did not. Reversible thyroid dysfunction has been reported after administration of granulocyte colony-stimulating factor.[47] Interestingly, no patients with hepatitis B treated with interferon gamma have developed thyroid dysfunction or thyroid autoimmunity.[48] Silent thyroiditis has also been reported in association with other immune disorders such as rheumatoid arthritis,[49] systemic lupus erythematosus,[50] Graves' disease,[51] and systemic sclerosis.[52] The importance of these associations is not clear, but these disorders may trigger a silent transient destructive thyroiditis. Simple palpation has been reported to cause thyroiditis (palpation thyroiditis) without any serum thyroid hormone concentration abnormalities.[53] Similarly, transient thyrotoxicosis can occur in patients recovering from parathyroid surgery for parathyroid adenoma; thyroiditis was confirmed by a low thyroid radioactive iodine uptake during these episodes.[54]

Although thyrotropin (TSH) is necessary for normal thyroid secretion, reduction of TSH secretion with T_4 therapy in postpartum women with thyroid antibodies did not prevent the occurrence of postpartum thyroiditis,[55] indicating that TSH need not be present in normal amounts for the disorder to occur. There are reports of the presence of TSH-receptor stimulating antibodies[56] and even TSH-receptor blocking antibodies in patients with silent thyroiditis.[57] Furthermore, there is evidence that antithyroid peroxidase antibodies are associated with the development of the hypothyroid phase[58] and that both types of TSH-receptor antibodies are associated with transient hypothyroidism in this disorder[59]; the presence of these antibodies may be related to more severe immunologic damage in the thyroid. The previously mentioned seasonal clustering of cases and near simultaneous occurrence in family members and coworkers suggest an infectious agent, but no such factor has been identified.

Pathology

Thyroid tissue (Fig. 34-1) obtained by needle biopsy or surgery during the thyrotoxic phase of silent thyroiditis shows prominent focal or diffuse lymphocytic infiltration.[11,12,31] Some thyroid follicles are disrupted or collapsed and contain intrafollicular macrophages, whereas adjacent follicles may be normal. Fibrosis is usually minimal but may be extensive. Lymphoid follicles are found in about half of patients, whereas Hürthle cells are sparse or absent (see chap 28). The pathologic changes of silent thyroiditis cannot be distinguished readily from those of chronic lymphocytic thyroiditis when unidentified biopsy specimens are compared.[11] The extent of the lymphocytic infiltration and fibrosis and the numbers of Hürthle cells and of lymphoid follicles are usually more extensive in the latter, whereas follicular disruption is more extensive in the former. A few multinucleated giant cells within and around disrupted thyroid follicles—characteristic of subacute thyroiditis—may be seen in the biopsy specimens of some patients with painless thyroiditis. The results of fine-needle aspiration biopsies are similar: the specimens contain lymphoid cells, thyroid follicular cells with Hürthle cell changes, and a few multinucleated giant cells.[31]

Thyroid tissue obtained during the hypothyroid or early recovery phase usually shows mild lymphocytic thyroiditis and regenerating thyroid follicles that contain little colloid. Thyroid biopsies done 6 months to 3 years later showed persistent mild lymphocytic thyroiditis in some patients and were normal in others.[28,31]

Clinical Features

The onset and severity of silent thyroiditis are variable. In one series, about 8% of patients were asymptomatic; the thyroiditis was detected by routine thyroid function testing.[11] Thyrotoxicosis is usually mild, resulting in little if any disability. The symptoms and signs are those of thyrotoxicosis in general (Table 34-2), and may include the rather unusual ones of atrial fibrillation, diffuse myalgia, and periodic paralysis.[8,13,60–63] Exophthalmos, localized myxedema, and thyroid acropachy do not occur, although lid lag and lid retraction are frequently present.

The thyroid is enlarged in 50% to 60% of patients.[63] The enlargement is usually symmetrical and is rarely more than

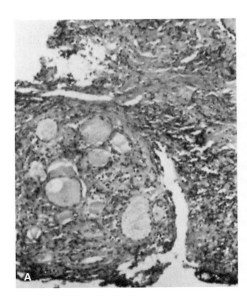 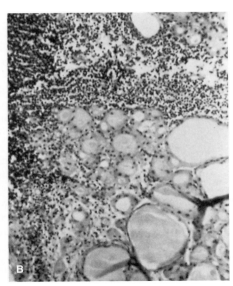

FIGURE 34-1. Histopathologic findings in silent thyroiditis. (*A*) Focal lymphocytic infiltration with partially or completely collapsed thyroid follicles. The thyroid follicular cells appear normal. (*B*) Extensive lymphocytic infiltration with collapsed thyroid follicles and follicles containing mononuclear cells. (Hematoxylin and eosin, × 100.)

two to three times normal. The thyroid is usually described as being firmer than normal, and the surface may be slightly irregular. The disease has been found in single nodules and in ectopic thyroid tissue.[11,64,65] Thyroid pain or tenderness is rare, and when present is mild. Preexisting goiter is unusual.

TABLE 34-2.
Presenting Symptoms and Signs in 89 Patients (112 Episodes) With Silent Thyroiditis

Symptoms and Signs	Percentage of Patients
SYMPTOMS	
None	8
Weight loss (5–40 lb)	67
Nervousness	84
Fatigue and weakness	83
Heat intolerance	75
Increased sweating	70
SIGNS	
Goiter	54
Diffuse	52
Multinodular	2
Uninodular	1
Tachycardia	88
Hyperactive reflexes	71
Resting tremor	67
Lid lag and lid retraction	53
Purposeless movements	32
Muscle weakness	8

(Modified to include data from 1978 through 1983 from Nikolai TF. Lymphocytic thyroiditis with spontaneously resolving hyperthyroidism [silent thyroiditis]. Thyroid Today 1979;2:1)

Painless thyroiditis characterized only by hypothyroidism, in which no thyrotoxic phase is recognized, has most often been reported in the postpartum period.[14,15,60,66–68] Sometimes, a goiter is the first abnormality in the woman, followed by transient thyrotoxicosis and hypothyroidism during the subsequent 12 to 20 weeks. Pain in the thyroid has also been reported in postpartum thyroiditis.[69] Other postpartum women develop a goiter that disappears within a few weeks but have no thyrotoxicosis or hypothyroidism.

Course

A schematic representation of the course of silent thyroiditis is shown in Figure 34-2. Most patients present in the thyrotoxic phase, but a few present in the eithyroid or hypothyroid phase. Most patients have had symptoms of thyrotoxicosis for 1 to 4 weeks when the disease is discovered, and these symptoms persist for about 1 to 5 weeks after discovery. About 40% then have a hypothyroid phase, which usually lasts between 4 to 16 weeks but occasionally persists indefinitely.

Laboratory Findings

The results of thyroid function tests vary substantially depending on the stage of the disease,[11,58,63] and relate directly to the pathologic state of the thyroid gland. The laboratory findings during the thyrotoxic phase are shown in Table 34-3. Initially, as noted above, when the thyroid gland becomes inflamed and the thyroid follicles are damaged, thyroglobulin proteolysis is activated and its products leak into the circulation, resulting in increased serum total and free T_4 and T_3 concentrations. The T_4 to T_3 ratio is higher than in Graves' hyperthyroidism. Serum TSH concentrations are low, and do not increase in response to thyrotropin-releasing hormone (TRH).[28] Other iodinated materials, such as thyroglobulin and iodinated albumin, are found in the serum in increased quantities; the concentration of the former may be as high as 400 ng/mL.

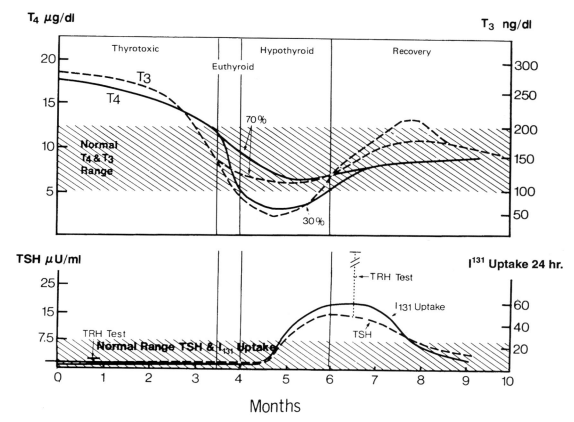

FIGURE 34-2. Schematic representation of the changes in serum T_4, T_3, and TSH concentrations and 24-hour thyroid ^{131}I uptake during the course of silent thyroiditis and of subacute thyroiditis. The hatched areas represent the normal stages. The serum T_4 and T_3 lines separate during the early part of the euthyroid phase to show that only about 30% of patients subsequently develop hypothyroidism. In the recovery phase, the serum T_3 line separates to show that about 15% of patients have transient elevations of the serum T_3 concentrations during this phase. To convert serum T_4 values to nmol/L; multiply by 12.87; to convert serum T_3 values to nmol/L, multiply by 0.015. (Modified from Woolf PD. Transient painless thyroiditis with hyperthyroidism: a variant of lymphocytic thyroiditis? Endocr Rev 1980;1:411, by permission of The Endocrine Society)

As a result of both thyroid follicular cell damage and decreased TSH secretion, the thyroid follicular cells are unable to transport iodine normally, so that the thyroid radioiodine (^{131}I) uptake falls to low values. The damaged thyroid gland does not respond to exogenous TSH stimulation. Serum inorganic iodide concentrations are slightly increased and urinary iodide excretion is increased two- to fivefold because of the leakage of iodide from the damaged thyroid.[6] The increase in serum inorganic iodide concentration may contribute to the decrease in fractional thyroid ^{131}I uptake.

About 25% of patients have serum antithyroglobulin antibodies, whereas antithyroid peroxidase antibodies are found in about 60%.[11,63] The erythrocyte sedimentation rate is elevated in about half of patients, but only rarely to values above 50 mm/hour.[11] Leukocyte counts and serum protein concentrations also are increased in about half of the patients.

Hypothyroid and Recovery Phases

As the thyrotoxic phase abates, the serum T_4 and T_3 concentrations fall into the normal range and either remain there, or, after 1 to 6 weeks in about 40% of patients, fall to subnormal concentrations (see Fig. 34-2). In the interval when the serum T_4 and T_3 concentrations are normal, serum TSH concentrations and the thyroid ^{131}I uptake values remain low. After 2 to 4 weeks, if the patient remains euthyroid, or toward the end of the hypothyroid phase, these latter two tests become normal or elevated. Within another 1 to 3 weeks, serum T_4 and T_3 concentrations return to normal if hypothyroidism has occurred earlier. The hypothyroid interval lasts 4 to 10 weeks, occasionally longer. Permanent hypothyroidism occurs in less than 5% of patients. Antithyroid antibody titers usually reach their highest levels during the hypothyroid phase, especially in women during the postpartum period,[66] after which the titers decrease. The antibodies disappear in about half of patients and persist indefinitely in low titer in the remainder.[11]

The intrathyroidal iodine content is decreased by 50% to 70% 1 to 3 months after the onset of thyroiditis and is still decreased by 20% to 30% at 10 to 12 months.[38] Serum thyroglobulin concentrations gradually fall during the recovery phase but are often still slightly elevated 1 to 2 years later, indicating persistent thyroid inflammation.[38] Urinary iodide excretion decreases during the recovery phase because the thyroid is relatively depleted of its iodine and thyroid hormone stores.[11]

TABLE 34-3.
Laboratory Test Results During the Thyrotoxic Phase of Silent Thyroiditis in 89 Patients (112 Episodes)

	Range	Mean	Normal Range
Serum T$_4$ (μg/dL)*	11.5–35.0	16.7	5–12
Serum T$_3$ (ng/dL)*	194–584	308	100–200
Erythrocyte sedimentation rate (mm/h)	2–65	28	0–30
Antithyroid antibody titers			
Microsomal	0–1:1,250,000	1:25,000	0–1:100
Thyroglobulin	0–1:600,000	1:800	0–1:100
Thyroid-^{131}I uptake (4–24 h)	0%–3%	<3	5–25
Serum TSH (μU/mL)	0–1	<1	0–7.5
Peak serum TSH after TRH (μU/mL)	0–2	<1	5–30

*To convert serum T$_4$ values to nmol/L, multiply by 12.87; to convert serum T$_3$ values to nmol/L, multiply by 0.015.

Diagnosis

The principal diagnostic features of silent thyroiditis are a mild to moderate degree of thyrotoxicosis with corresponding elevation in serum T$_4$ and T$_3$ concentrations, a low thyroid ^{131}I uptake, slight thyroid enlargement (in 50%–60% of patients), no thyroid tenderness, and no history of therapy with iodine-containing drugs or thyroid hormone. A fine-needle or core-needle biopsy of the thyroid gland showing lymphocytic thyroiditis confirms the diagnosis but is rarely needed.

Many patients with silent thyroiditis are thought to have Graves' thyrotoxicosis. The presence of TSH-receptor antibodies favors the latter diagnosis, but a few patients with silent thyroiditis have these antibodies; moreover, not all patients with Graves' thyrotoxicosis have them. Although a low thyroid ^{131}I uptake value is most useful in identifying silent thyroiditis, it is important to remember that the value may be low because of increased dietary iodine intake, therapy with an iodine-containing drug, or recent radiographic studies with contrast agents in any patient with thyrotoxicosis of any cause, and in patients receiving exogenous thyroid hormone therapy. Silent thyroiditis is, however, the predominant cause of low ^{131}I uptake among patients with thyrotoxicosis. In patients in whom increased iodine intake is not obvious, a urinary excretion of greater than 1000 to 1500 μg of inorganic iodide in a 24-hour urine specimen, or a serum inorganic iodide concentration of greater than 1.5 μg/dL indicates prior excess iodine intake. In Europe about 10% of thyrotoxic patients who would normally be expected to have an elevated ^{131}I uptake have normal or low values because of exposure to excess iodine in some form.[70]

Iodine-induced thyrotoxicosis can easily be confused with silent thyroiditis. It has been recognized in patients with numerous preexisting thyroid diseases, such as a solitary nodule or nontoxic diffuse or multinodular goiter, as well as in patients without any history of thyroid disease. The thyroid ^{131}I uptake in these patients is usually low (see section on the effect of excess iodide in chap 14). Once excess iodine intake ceases thyroid hypersecretion may disappear, but if it persists, ^{131}I uptake will become elevated in most patients.

Rare diseases that cause thyrotoxicosis with low thyroid ^{131}I uptake values are struma ovarii (if the struma is a thyroid adenoma), differentiated carcinoma of the thyroid, and thyrotoxicosis factitia. Struma ovarii is characterized by a pelvic mass and ^{131}I uptake over the tumor in the lower abdomen. Carcinoma of the thyroid is usually clinically obvious, since most patients have had previous thyroid surgery and have extensive metastatic disease. The most difficult entity to recognize is thyrotoxicosis factitia. Surreptitious intake of thyroid hormone should always be suspected in a patient with thyrotoxicosis with low ^{131}I uptake and no goiter (see chap 35). It may be differentiated from silent thyroiditis by history, if of long duration; patient behavior, often histrionic or denial; and the absence of thyroid antibodies and low serum thyroglobulin concentrations.

Ultrasonography usually reveals a slight increase in thyroid volume with decreased echogenicity. This examination may be useful in diagnosis and further monitoring of these patients.[4]

Treatment

Patients with silent thyroiditis may receive inappropriate treatment, such as an antithyroid drug, because of the failure to recognize the disorder. Most often, the thyrotoxicosis is mild and not particularly bothersome, so patients need only be counseled about the disorder and reassured that their symptoms will subside in a few weeks. They should be reminded that a short period of hypothyroidism may occur during recovery and that about 10% of patients have recurrent episodes of thyroiditis.

When symptoms of thyrotoxicosis are bothersome, the patient may be given beta-adrenergic antagonist, drug therapy. Therapy with propylthiouracil or methimazole is inappropriate because increased thyroid hormone biosynthesis is not the cause of thyrotoxicosis in painless thyroiditis. Indeed, propylthiouracil administration does not change the course or severity of thyrotoxicosis in patients with silent thyroiditis.[62]

The few patients in whom thyrotoxicosis is more disabling may benefit from anti-inflammatory therapy. Prednisone reduces the inflammatory process, causing decreases in both thyroid size and serum T_4 and T_3 concentrations, which may decline to the normal range within 7 to 10 days[62] (Fig. 34-3). The optimal starting dose of prednisone or duration of therapy has not been established, but therapy similar to that used successfully for many years in subacute thyroiditis (see later) works well. Initial therapy with 40 to 60 mg/d in single or divided doses and gradual reduction of the daily dose by 7.5 to 15 mg/wk for a 4-week course is usually adequate. In rare patients who have been disabled from recurring episodes of silent thyroiditis, subtotal thyroidectomy has been beneficial.[12,62] Ablation of the thyroid with ^{131}I could also be used in these instances, but one must wait until the thyroid ^{131}I uptake has recovered before this therapy can be given.

When hypothyroidism develops in silent thyroiditis, it is usually mild, and the patient can be advised that it will disappear within 4 to 10 weeks. If the symptoms of hypothyroidism are bothersome, sufficient T_4 should be given to relieve the hypothyroid symptoms but not so much as to decrease serum TSH to normal, since continued TSH secretion may hasten recovery. The therapy can then be slowly withdrawn. In the occasional patient who develops permanent hypothyroidism, the serum T_4 concentration falls and the serum TSH concentration rises when T_4 therapy is withdrawn. If hypothyroidism lasts for longer than 6 months, it is proba-

bly permanent, and no further attempts or withdrawal need be undertaken.

All patients who recover should be followed at 1- to 2-year intervals for evidence of goiter or hypothyroidism, because about half of patients who have an episode of silent thyroiditis eventually develop permanent thyroid disease.[28] Women who have a goiter and are not receiving treatment or who have had previous episodes of silent thyroiditis should be followed closely in the postpartum period for a recurrence and for postpartum depression.

SUBACUTE THYROIDITIS

Subacute thyroiditis has a multiplicity of synonyms that in part describe the historical evolution of information on the disorder. These include granulomatous thyroiditis, giant-cell thyroiditis, noninfectious thyroiditis, acute or subacute non-suppurative thyroiditis, pseudotuberculous thyroiditis, and de Quervain's thyroiditis.[71] De Quervain's name has been associated with the disorder because of his descriptions of the pathology of this condition in 1904 and 1936.[72,73] The credit for the first description of subacute thyroiditis, however, goes to Mygind, who described 18 cases of "thyroiditis acute simplex" in 1895.[74]

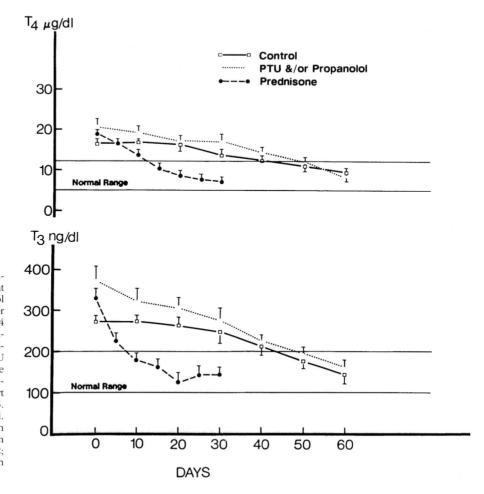

FIGURE 34-3. Serum T_4 and T_3 concentrations (mean ± SE) during the course of silent thyroiditis in three groups of patients: control (no treatment), 11 patients; propranolol or propylthiouracil (PTU) treatment, or both, 14 patients; and prednisone treatment, 14 patients. Note the dramatic response to prednisone and the lack of response in the PTU and propranolol group, compared with the no treatment group. To convert serum T_4 values to nmol/L, multiply by 12.87; to convert serum T_3 values to nmol/L, multiply by 0.015. (Nikolai TF, Coombs GJ, McKenzie AK, et al. Treatment of lymphocytic thyroiditis with spontaneously resolving hyperthyroidism [silent thyroiditis]. Arch Intern Med 1982; 142:2281, by permission of the American Medical Association)

Incidence

Subacute thyroiditis is much less common than Graves' disease, occurring at the rate of about one case in five of Graves' disease.[75] It is more common than silent thyroiditis, but accurate data on relative frequency are not available. It occurs widely in North America, Europe, Scandinavia, and Japan but is rarely reported in many other parts of the world, especially the tropical and subtropical areas. There is no difference in incidence rates among Japanese and whites, at least in Hawaii.[76] Whether the geographic variation reflects differences in actual frequency or merely in ascertainment is unknown. Subacute thyroiditis is most common between the third and sixth decades of life, and it is rare in children and the elderly. The female/male ratio is in the range of 3 to 6:1,[71] and the disorder tends to be recognized more often during the summer months.[77,78]

Etiology

The evidence is strong, though mostly indirect, that viral infections are the cause of subacute thyroiditis, as first proposed in 1952.[79] Subacute thyroiditis is often preceded by an upper respiratory infection, and sometimes there is an immediate prodromal phase characterized by muscular aches and pains, malaise, and fatigue. Its highest seasonal occurrence coincides with those of summer enterovirus infections. Circulating antibodies to mumps virus have been found in patients with subacute thyroiditis who did not develop clinical evidence of mumps[80]; and mumps virus was grown from thyroid tissue obtained by biopsy from two of these patients. Other reports associate subacute thyroiditis with mumps,[81,82] measles,[83] influenza,[84] and the common cold,[85] as well as adenovirus,[86] Epstein-Barr virus,[85] and coxsackievirus[87] infections and cat-scratch disease.[88] A cytopathic virus was isolated from 5 of 28 patients with subacute thyroiditis.[89] Viral inclusion bodies, however, have not been seen in thyroid tissue.[90]

Antibody studies of acute and convalescent phase serum also have implicated a variety of viruses, including coxsackievirus, adenovirus, influenza virus, and echovirus, as causes of subacute thyroiditis[24] (Fig. 34-4). In that study, which was from Canada, however, only 44% of the patients had changes in viral antibody titers, so either other viruses or other etiologic agents must be involved in many patients with subacute thyroiditis. Antibodies to a similar spectrum of viruses were not found in 10 patients with subacute thyroiditis in Singapore.[91] Subacute thyroiditis has rarely been reported in association with Q fever[92] and malaria,[93] but never with retrovirus infections.[94] Epidemics of subacute thyroiditis have also been described.[95,96]

Autoimmunity may play a role in the etiology of subacute thyroiditis.[24,97–100] Thyroid autoantibodies are found in some patients, but their presence is generally transitory, and they disappear within several months after recovery. TSH receptor antibodies may be present during the thyrotoxic phase of the illness or later,[56,101,102] but the correlation between the presence of these antibodies and thyroid status is poor.[99] Circulating immune complexes have been found to persist in patients with subacute thyroiditis for as long as 3 years after onset, suggesting that resolution of the immune response is very slow.[103] More recently, about 20% of 31 patients who had a prolonged hypothyroid phase had TSH-receptor blocking antibodies, whereas these antibodies were found in only 3% of patients who had only transient hypothyroidism.[100] It is probable that tissue damage in the thyroid leads to variable expression of TSH-receptor stimulating or blocking antibodies which may, in turn, influence the clinical expression of the disease. Thus, the role of autoantibodies in subacute thyroiditis may be secondary, and their importance is probably minimal.[71]

Patients with subacute thyroiditis have circulating T-lymphocytes sensitized to thyroid antigens,[97,98,104,105] and their thyroid tissue contains large numbers of antigen-reactive T-lymphocytes.[106] The overall percentage of T-lymphocytes in the peripheral blood is low.[105] The number of Fc receptor-bearing mononuclear cells may be either increased or decreased.[97] Peripheral blood killer cells from patients with subacute thyroiditis may cause antibody-dependent cytotoxicity.[107] Furthermore, analysis of lymphocyte subsets in peripheral blood has suggested that T-cell receptor negative T cells (as defined by specific monoclonal antibodies), as well as CD8 and CD4 cells, are important in thyroid destruction in subacute thyroiditis.[108] Also, thyroid follicular cells may express HLA-DR molecules and the percentage of intrathyroidal T cells that are CD8 (cytotoxic-suppressor) cells may be increased. All these findings are transitory and probably represent nonspecific responses to the inflammatory process and the release of thyroid antigens.

A strong association between subacute thyroiditis and HLA-B35 has been found in all ethnic groups.[30,109–113] Unlike the rather low relative risk for the association of some HLA haplotypes and Graves' disease or chronic autoimmune thyroiditis, the relative risk of HLA-B35 in subacute thyroiditis is high, ranging from 8.0 to 56.6. The HLA-B35 molecule presumably greatly augments the immune response to the infectious agent in subacute thyroiditis, thus permitting the expression of the disease. A report of the simultaneous development of subacute thyroiditis in identical twins who were both heterozygous for HLA-B35 provides additional evidence that this haplotype confers genetic susceptibility for the disease.[114] HLA-B35 is in linkage disequilibrium with HLA-Cw4[109–111] and HLA-Dw1,[110,111,115] both of which are found in increasing frequency in white patients with subacute thyroiditis. In Japanese patients there is a weak association of subacute thyroiditis with HLA-DRw8.[116]

Pathology

The thyroid gland is enlarged, somewhat edematous, and may be adherent to adjacent structures. Microscopically, the thyroid tissue shows a diffuse or irregular pattern of involvement, with various stages of the disease sometimes present within the same specimen (Fig. 34-5). Initially, there is extensive follicular cell destruction, extravasation of colloid, and infiltration with lymphocytes and histiocytes. The latter tend to congregate around masses of colloid and coalesce into giant cells. With time, there is a variable degree of fibrosis, and areas of follicular regeneration are seen. Caseation, hemorrhage, and calcification do not occur. After recovery, the thyroid appears normal except for minimal residual fibrosis. Thyroid tissue obtained by fine-needle aspiration biopsy shows a mixed

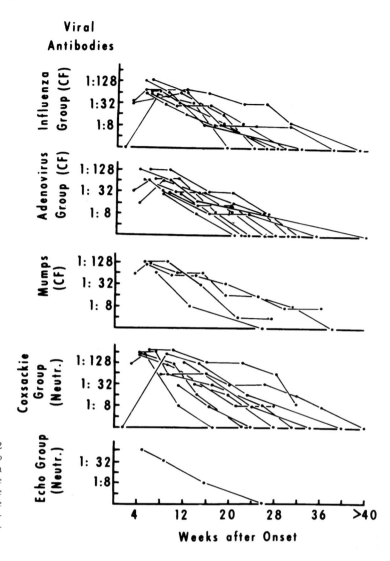

FIGURE 34-4. Viral antibody titers in subacute thyroiditis. Of 72 patients with this disorder, 32 were found to have antibodies to common viruses during their illness that changed sufficiently in titer to suggest that one or another of the viruses might have caused the thyroiditis. The antibodies detected most often were anti-coxsackievirus antibodies, although other antibodies were also commonly found. (Volpe R, Row VV, Ezrin C. Circulating viral and thyroid antibodies in subacute thyroiditis. J Clin Endocrinol Metab 1967;27:1275)

and polymorphous inflammatory infiltrate of neutrophils, lymphocytes, and histiocytes, single or clusters of follicular cells, and multinucleated giant cells, all in close relationship to masses of colloid material.[117–119] Further analysis of the giant cells has shown the occasional presence of carcinoma antigen 19–9 and carcinoembryonic antigen consistent with a histiocytic or follicular cell origin of these cells.[120] Some features characteristic of silent thyroiditis or chronic lymphocytic thyroiditis have been seen in a few cases,[58,102] but whether these findings are an aberration of the cytologic procedure or subacute thyroiditis occurring in a patient with lymphocytic thyroiditis is not known. Electron microscopy has not demonstrated viral inclusion bodies[90] but does show marked thickening of basement membranes.

Clinical Manifestations

Patients with subacute thyroiditis usually have neck pain, thyroid tenderness, and systemic symptoms of inflammatory illness with or without symptoms of thyrotoxicosis. Up to half of patients have a history of an antecedent upper respiratory in-

fection, followed in days or weeks by the clinical manifestations of subacute thyroiditis itself (Tables 34-4 and 34-5). The illness begins with the acute onset of malaise, feverishness, and pain of varying degree in the region of the thyroid gland. This pain usually involves the entire thyroid, is usually constant, and may be severe. It typically radiates from the thyroid to the angle of the jaw and to the ears. In occasional patients, the pain is initially unilateral and then spreads to the centralateral lobe of the thyroid within days or weeks, or the pain is most prominent in the throat, the ears, or the upper anterior chest. Whatever its location, the pain is often aggravated by coughing, swallowing, or turning the head. Some patients have neck pain only with swallowing or head movement or when wearing tight garments or their neck is palpated.

Although the symptoms may be limited to the head and neck, most patients have systemic symptoms as well. These include malaise, myalgia, fever, and anorexia (see Table 34-4). If thyrotoxicosis is present, the usual symptoms of nervousness, tremulousness, heat intolerance, and palpitations predominate.

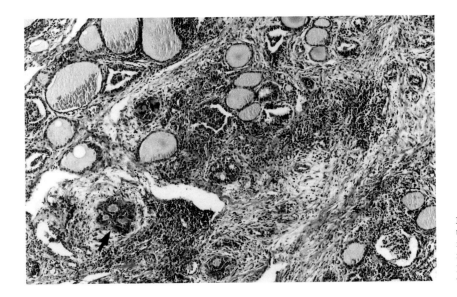

FIGURE 34-5. Histopathologic findings in subacute thyroiditis. Thyroid follicles are destroyed and there is a mixed inflammatory infiltrate, desquamated thyroid epithelial cells, edema, and colloid undergoing phagocytosis by histiocytes (foreign-body type giant cells, *arrow*). (Hematoxylin and eosin, × 40.)

On physical examination, the patient often appears acutely ill and uncomfortable. The thyroid is tender, often exquisitely so, and is mildly to moderately enlarged. Typically, like the pain, the enlargement is diffuse, but it may be unilateral. The consistency of the thyroid is usually firm or hard to the touch, if the patient will allow much palpation. With time or treatment, the thyroid tenderness subsides, and the goiter generally disappears within several weeks or months. Cervical lymphadenopathy is rarely present, but if enlarged the lymph nodes may be tender. Most patients have fever (temperature up to 40°C), and about half have clinical manifestations of thyrotoxicosis. If there are symptoms of thyrotoxicosis, they are mild as well as transient. A history of preexisting goiter is unusual[28,96,121] but has been found in 8% to 16% of patients.[122]

More rarely, subacute thyroiditis may present with painless nontender diffuse thyroid enlargement, a multinodular goiter, or even a solitary nodule. These variant forms of subacute thyroiditis have occasioned considerable discussion, and because of the absence of pain some consider them a form of silent (lymphocytic) thyroiditis. In two reviews of subacute thyroiditis a small number (about 5%) of patients had painless nontender goiter, low thyroid ^{131}I uptake, and granulomatous thyroiditis on biopsy.[123] As noted earlier, there are some histologic and cytologic similarities between subacute thyroiditis and silent thyroiditis,[117] and it is conceivable they are variant forms of the same process. More likely, in some patients subacute thyroiditis is superimposed on chronic lymphocytic thyroiditis. Other atypical features of subacute thyroiditis include the presence of HLA-B15,[95] confusion with papillary carcinoma,[124] and increased thyroid uptake after administration of radiogallium.[125]

Course

In most patients, subacute thyroiditis lasts from 8 to 16 weeks, although it may last up to a year. When the course is prolonged, the major manifestation is persistent, painful, tender thyroid enlargement, the thyrotoxicosis almost always having subsided earlier. In the 50% of patients who have clinical manifestations of thyrotoxicosis, its signs and symptoms usually last 4 to 10 weeks. The course of the disease is shortened by corticosteroid therapy (see later). As the acute phase of the disease progresses, the colloid stores are depleted and the patient becomes euthyroid even though symptomatic thyroid inflammation persists. In more severe cases, there is then transient hypothyroidism, which usually lasts 4 to 8 weeks. As recovery continues, the thyroid follicles regenerate, the colloid is repleted, and normal thyroid function is restored. In about 90% of patients thyroid morphology as evaluated by ultrasonography is normal after 2 years.[126,127] The occurrence of long-lasting subclinical hypothyroidism in Japanese patients who had subacute thyroiditis may have been related to high serum inorganic iodide concentrations.[128] Persistent or progressive thyroid disease is unusual, in contrast to silent thyroiditis,[28,128,129] but an occasional patient may develop permanent hypothyroidism.[24,90]

Laboratory Findings

With the onset of thyroid inflammation, there is unregulated release of T_4, T_3, thyroglobulin, other iodinated proteins, and iodide from the thyroid gland, as in painless thyroiditis.[130,131] Hence, serum T_4, T_3, and thyroglobulin concentrations increase, as do serum and urinary iodide, and serum TSH concentrations fall.[132–135] As the colloid is depleted and thyroiditis subsides, the serum T_4 and T_3 concentrations fall to normal and then, in 20% to 30% of patients, to subnormal before returning to normal. The serum T_3 concentrations are less elevated than in Graves' thyrotoxicosis.[135] Similar to the situation in silent thyroiditis, serum thyroglobulin concentrations may remain elevated for up to 1 year, long after other evidence of the thyroiditis has resolved.[136] Serum interleukin-6 concentrations, a major mediator of the acute phase response, are increased in the early stages of the illness, and fall to normal after 3 to 4 months.[137] This pattern of changes in thyroid function tests during the thyrotoxic, euthyroid, hypothyroid, and recovery phases of subacute thyroiditis is similar to that in silent thyroiditis (see Fig. 34-2).

TABLE 34-4.
Predominant Symptoms of Subacute Thyroiditis in 56 Patients

Symptoms	Percentage of Patients
LOCAL	
Pain in neck	91
Pain in region of thyroid	89
Anterior aspect of neck	25
Unilateral pain	27
Pain migrated from one side to the other	38
Radiation of pain to ears	64
Sore throat	36
Pain on swallowing	52
Pain on moving head	38
Constant, dull aching pain in neck	70
Sudden, sharp pain in neck	18
Constricting sensation in neck	21
Hoarseness	7
Noticeable swelling in neck	14
SYSTEMIC	
GENERAL	
Malaise, fatigue	84
Feverishness	46
Weight loss	38
Anorexia	18
Previous upper-respiratory infection	18
Chills	7
Muscle aches and pains	12
SUGGESTIVE OF THYROTOXICOSIS	
Nervousness	46
Perspiration	46
Heat intolerance	30
Tachycardia	18
Increased appetite (with weight loss)	11
Tremulousness	9

(Modified from Volpé R, Johnston MW. Subacute thyroiditis: a disease commonly mistaken for pharyngitis. Can Med Assoc J 1957;77:297)

TABLE 34-5.
Predominant Signs of Subacute Thyroiditis in 56 Patients

Signs	Percentage of Patients
LOCAL	
Both lobes of thyroid enlarged when first seen	45
One lobe enlarged, then the other	38
Only one lobe enlarged	18
Thyroid firm or hard in consistency	100
Tenderness in thyroid region	9
Tenderness present or more marked on one side	43
No tenderness	7
SYSTEMIC	
GENERAL	
Acutely ill	50
Chronically ill	9
Appeared well	41
Fever	57
No fever	43
SUGGESTIVE OF THYROTOXICOSIS	
Tense, restless appearance	46
Warm, moist skin	46
Wild pulse pressure	18
Tremor	16
Lid lag, stare	11

(Modified from Volpé R, Johnston MW. Subacute thyroiditis: a disease commonly mistaken for pharyngitis. Can Med Assoc J 1957;77:297)

The damage to the thyroid follicular cells results in impaired iodine transport, so that the thyroid ^{131}I uptake is characteristically low. It is low even if only part of the thyroid gland is involved, presumably owing to the suppression of TSH secretion and increased serum inorganic iodide concentration.[138] Thyroid radioisotope scans in the early stages reveal patchy and irregular uptake of the tracer or no uptake at all.[138,139] Ultrasonography of the thyroid reveals hypoechogenicity of the involved areas similar to that in silent thyroiditis and chronic lymphocytic thyroiditis.[127,140,141]

After the acute phase, the serum T_3 and T_4 concentrations fall to normal or sometimes subnormal levels. Serum TSH concentrations and thyroid ^{131}I uptake values begin to rise and may be elevated for 2 to 4 weeks (see Fig. 34-2). The serum T_4 and T_3 concentrations then return to normal 1 to 2 weeks after a rise in serum TSH. In most patients, the hypothyroid phase lasts only 4 to 8 weeks, although it may be longer.

Tests for thyroid antibodies are positive in 10% to 20% of patients during the thyrotoxic phase, antithyroglobulin antibodies being present more often than antithyroid peroxidase antibodies. These changes reflect a secondary immune response to antigens released from the damaged thyroid. The antibody titers tend to be highest during the hypothyroid phase and then decline to low levels or become negative within 1 to 6 months after recovery, and in most patients they remain undetectable.[28]

The erythrocyte sedimentation rate is characteristically elevated, often to above 100 mm/hour, in subacute thyroiditis.[90,96,121] If the test is normal or only slightly elevated and the thyroid is only slightly tender, the diagnosis of subacute thyroiditis should be reconsidered because these patients may well have silent thyroiditis.[6] The leukocyte count is usually normal, but it can be as high as 18,000/uL. Transient liver dysfunction may occur during the early phase of the illness.[142]

Diagnosis

The diagnosis of subacute thyroiditis is usually obvious when the patient is first seen because of the neck pain radiating to the jaw and ears and the exquisitely tender thyroid gland. In those patients who have only a sore throat or ear pain, however, the diagnosis is less obvious, although physical examination should reveal an enlarged, tender thyroid. Therefore, it is important that the thyroid be palpated in all patients presenting with upper respiratory infections and complaints of sore throat or earache. Occasional patients with chronic autoimmune thyroiditis and a few with silent thyroiditis may present with painful tender thyroid enlargement.[96]

Acute suppurative thyroiditis initially may mimic subacute thyroiditis, but with time, the findings of fever, localized tenderness, and swelling and erythema over the involved area of the thyroid should become obvious. Patients with globus hystericus complain of pressure or feeling of a ball or lump in the throat. They often have mild tenderness in the anterior neck, but it is not localized to the thyroid and they do not have thyroid enlargement. A rapidly growing anaplastic carcinoma of the thyroid or hemorrhage into a thyroid nodule can cause thyroid pain and tenderness, but these disorders usually can be recognized by differences in the history and physical examination.

Among the disorders that cause painful, tender thyroid enlargement, the most important laboratory tests indicating subacute thyroiditis are an increased erythrocyte sedimentation rate, increased serum T_4 and T_3 concentrations, and a low thyroid ^{131}I uptake. In addition, fine-needle aspiration biopsy provides the correct diagnosis in at least 90% of cases. Occasionally, however, a large-needle biopsy or a small, open surgical biopsy of the thyroid may be necessary to establish the diagnosis.

During the recovery or hypothyroid phase, thyroid test results may be confusing. For example, if the patient is first seen during the hypothyroid phase, a diagnosis of permanent hypothyroidism may erroneously be made unless the history of the earlier stages of the disease is obtained.[121] In this setting, needle biopsy of the thyroid can be helpful, but time alone usually suffices to distinguish between transient and permanent hypothyroidism.

Treatment

Salicylates and other nonsteroidal anti-inflammatory drugs have frequently been used successfully.[143,144] These drugs, however, are less effective than corticosteroids and result in relief of neck pain and tenderness only in patients with mild to moderate symptoms. In a study[145] comparing salicylate and prednisolone therapy, the latter, although it was used in the more severe cases, resulted in more rapid reduction in the sedimentation rate and elevated serum thyroid hormone concentrations. Information on the relative effectiveness of these two agents in providing symptomatic relief in this study was not reported.

The most effective therapy for subacute thyroiditis is a corticosteroid, because of its ability to provide prompt resolution of symptoms in most patients.[71,96] Specifically, this therapy results in partial or near complete relief in pain and neck tenderness within 24 to 48 hours. If the neck pain and tenderness do not improve within 72 hours, the diagnosis of subacute thyroiditis should be questioned. Corticosteroids act by suppressing the thyroid inflammation, but whether they alter the course of the disease is not known. Although a beta-adrenergic antagonist drug may be useful in controlling symptoms of thyrotoxicosis, such therapy is rarely necessary because corticosteroids or nonsteroidal anti-inflammatory drugs usually suffice to ameliorate thyrotoxicosis as well as thyroid pain and tenderness.

Prednisone or any other synthetic corticosteroid can be used.[144] The most effective regimen is prednisone in an initial dose of 40 to 60 mg/day for about a week, followed by rapid dose reduction and withdrawal in 4 weeks. Once-a-day dosage is adequate and most convenient. An exacerbation of the disease occurs in about 10% of patients when the dose of prednisone is reduced to the 10 to 20 mg/day range or soon after prednisone is discontinued. Later recurrences are unusual.[28] In those patients who have exacerbations, increasing or continuing the prednisone therapy for another month usually results in ultimate recovery. There are no historical, physical, or laboratory findings that help the clinician predict those patients likely to have an exacerbation of the disease when prednisone therapy is decreased or discontinued.

Although T_3 therapy has been reported to relieve symptoms in the acute phase of subacute thyroiditis,[81,135] it has not been tested adequately, and the improvement that occurred was probably coincidental. In those few patients who have repeated exacerbations of subacute thyroiditis, T_4 or T_3 therapy may be helpful in preventing further exacerbations,[96,144] suggesting that endogenous TSH may contribute to their occurrence. Also, in a few patients exogenous TSH either aggravated or precipitated thyroiditis.[96] In the rare patient with a prolonged course with persistent neck pain and tenderness and malaise, near total thyroidectomy or ablation of the thyroid with ^{131}I may be justified.[144]

References

1. Dorfman SG, Cooperman MT, Nelson RS, et al. Painless thyroiditis and transient hyperthyroidism without goiter. Ann Intern Med 1977;86:24
2. Gordon M. "Silent" thyroiditis with symptomatic hyperthyroidism in an elderly patient. J Am Geriatr Soc 1978;26:375
3. Hofeldt FD, Weled BJ, Brown JE, Adler RA, Ghaed N, Hirata RM. "Silent thyroiditis" versus thyrotoxicosis factitia. Minn Med 1976;59:380
4. Miyakawa M, Tsushima T, Onoda N, et al. Thyroid ultrasonography related to clinical and laboratory findings in patients with silent thyroiditis. J Endocrinol Invest 1992;15:289
5. Papapetrou PD, Jackson IMD. Thyrotoxicosis due to "silent" thyroiditis. Lancet 1975;1:36
6. Woolf PD, Daly R. Thyrotoxicosis with painless thyroiditis. Am J Med 1976;60:73
7. Blonde L, Witkin M, Harris R. Painless subacute thyroiditis simulating Graves' disease. West J Med 1976;125:75
8. Gegick CG, Herring WB. Painless subacute thyroiditis: a report of two cases. NC Med J 1977;38:387
9. Hamburger JI. Occult subacute thyroiditis—Diagnostic challenge. Mich Med 1971;70:1125
10. Morrison J, Caplan RH. Typical and atypical ("silent") subacute thyroiditis in a wife and husband. Arch Intern Med 1978;138:45
11. Nikolai TF, Brosseau J, Kettrick MA, et al. Lymphocytic thyroiditis with spontaneously resolving hyperthyroidism (silent thyroiditis). Arch Intern Med 1980;140:478
12. Gorman CA, Duick DS, Woolner LB, et al. Transient hyperthyroidism in patients with lymphocytic thyroiditis. Mayo Clin Proc 1978;53:359

13. Gluck FB, Nusynowitz MD, Plymate S. Chronic lymphocytic thyroiditis, thyrotoxicosis, and low radioactive iodine uptake. Report of four cases. N Engl J Med 1975;293:624

14. Jansson R, Dahlberg PA, Karlsson FA. Postpartum thyroiditis. Bailliere's Clin Endocrinol and Metabol. 1988;2:619

15. Nikolai TF, Turney S, Roberts R. Postpartum lymphocytic thyroiditis. Arch Intern Med 1987;147:221

16. Amino N, Yabu Y, Miyai K, et al. Differentiation of thyrotoxicosis induced by thyroid destruction from Graves' disease. Lancet 1978;2:344

17. Williams I, Ankrett VO, Lazarus JH, Volpe R. Aetiology of hyperthyroidism in Canada and Wales. J Epidemiol Commun Health 1982;37:245

18. Schorr AB, Miller JL, Shtasel P, Rose LI. Low incidence of painless thyroiditis in the Philadelphia area. Clin Nucl Med 1986; 11:379

19. Vitug AC, Goldman JM. Thyrotoxic silent thyroiditis: a geographic puzzle. Arch Intern Med 1985;145:2263

20. Schneeberg NG. Silent thyroiditis. Arch Intern Med 1983; 143:2214

21. Hedberg CW, Fishbein DB, Janssen RS, et al. An outbreak of thyrotoxicosis caused by the consumption of bovine thyroid gland in ground beef. N Engl J Med 1987;316:993

22. Kinney JS, Hurwitz ES, Fishbein DB, et al. Community outbreak of thyrotoxicosis: epidemiology, immunogenetic characteristics, and long-term outcome. Am J Med 1988;84:10

23. Ginsberg J, Walfish PG. Post-partum transient thyrotoxicosis with painless thyroiditis. Lancet 1977;1:1125

24. Volpe R, Row VV, Ezrin C. Circulating viral and thyroid antibodies in subacute thyroiditis. J Clin Endocrinol Metab 1967;27:1275

25. Nakamura S, Kosaka J, Sugimoto M, Watanabe H, Shima H, Takuno H. Silent thyroiditis following rubella. Endocrinol Jpn 1990;37(1):79

26. Masuno M, Kosaka J, Nakamura S. Silent thyroiditis in an eleven-year-old girl, associated with transient increase in serum IgM and thyroid hormone. Endocrinol Jpn 1991;38:219

27. Ogura T, Hirakawa S, Suzuki S, et al. Five patients with painless thyroiditis simultaneously developed in a nursery school. Endocrinol Jpn 1980;35:225

28. Nikolai TF, Coombs GJ, McKenzie AK. Lymphocytic thyroiditis with spontaneously resolving hyperthyroidism (silent thyroiditis) and subacute thyroiditis: long-term follow-up. Arch Intern Med 1981;141:145

29. Farid NR, Hawe BS, Walfish PG. Increased frequency of HLA-DR3 and 5 in the syndromes of painless thyroiditis with transient thyrotoxocisis: evidence for an autoimmune aetiology. Clin Endocrinol 1983;19:699

30. Fein HG, Metz S, Nikolai TF, Johnson AH, Smallridge RC. HLA antigens in thyroiditis: differences between silent and postpartum lymphocytic forms, and comparison with subacute and goitrous autoimmune thyroiditis. In: Walfish PG, Wall J, Volpe R, eds. Autoimmunity and the thyroid. Orlando, FL: Academic Press, 1985:373

31. Mizukami Y, Michigishi T, Hashimoto T, et al. Silent thyroiditis: a histologic and immunohistochemical study. Hum Pathol 1988; 19:423

32. Ishihara T, Mori T, Waseda N, et al. Histological, clinical and laboratory findings of acute exacerbation of Hashimoto's thyroiditis-comparison with those of subacute granulomatous thyroiditis. Endocrinol Jpn 1987;34:831

33. Shigemasa C, Ueta Y, Mitani Y, et al. Chronic thyroiditis with painful tender thyroid enlargement and transient thyrotoxicosis. J Clin Endocrinol Metab 1990;70:385

34. Gudbjornsson B, Kristinsson A, Geirsson G, et al. Painless autoimmune thyroiditis occurring on amiodarone therapy. Acta Med Scand 1987;221:219

35. Bartalena L, Grasso L, Brogioni S, Aghini-Lombardi F, Braverman LE, Martino E. Serum interleukin-6 in amiodarone-induced thyrotoxicosis. J Clin Endocrinol Metab 1994;78:423

36. Jansson R, Safwenberg J, Dahlberg PA. Influence of the HLA-DR4 antigen and iodine status on the development of autoimmune postpartum thyroiditis. J Clin Endocrinol Metab 1985;60:168

37. Othman S, Phillips DIW, Lazarus JH, Parkes AB, Richards C, Hall R. Iodine metabolism in postpartum thyroiditis. Thyroid 1992;2:107

38. Smallridge RC, De Keyser FM, Van Herle AJ, et al. Thyroid iodine content and serum thyroglobulin: clues to the natural history of destruction-induced thyroiditis. J Clin Endocrinol Metab 1986; 62:1213

39. Chow CC, Lee S, Shek CC, Wing YK, Ahuja A, Cockram CS. Lithium-associated transient thyrotoxicosis in 4 Chinese women with autoimmune thyroiditis. Aust NZ J Psychiatry 1993;27:246

40. Lazarus JH. Effect of lithium on the thyroid gland. In: Lazarus JH. Endocrine and metabolic effects of lithium. New York: Plenum Press, 1986:99

41. Vassilopoulou-Sellin R, Sella A, Dexeus FH, Theriault RL, Pololoff DA. Acute thyroid dysfunction (thyroiditis) after therapy with interleukin-2. Horm Metab Res 1992;24(9):434

42. Reid I, Sharpe I, McDevitt J, et al. Thyroid dysfunction can predict response to immunotherapy with interleukin-2 and interferon-2a. Br J Cancer 1991;64:915

43. Lisker-Melman M, Di Biscelglie AM, Usala SJ, Weintraub B, Murray LM, Hoofnagle JH. Development of thyroid disease during therapy of chronic viral hepatitis with interferon alfa. Gastroenterology 1992;102:2155

44. Kamikubo K, Takami R, Suwa T, et al. Silent thyroiditis developed during alpha-interferon therapy. Am J Med Sci 1993;306:174

45. Kodama T, Katabami S, Kamijo K, et al. Development of transient thyroid disease and reaction during treatment of chronic hepatitis-C with interferon. J Gastroenterology 1994;29:289

46. Sauter NP, Atkins MB, Mier JW, Lechan RM. Transient thyrotoxicosis and persistent hypothyroidism during acute autoimmune-thyroiditis after interleukin-2 and interferon-alpha therapy for metastatic carcinoma—a case report. Am J Med 1992;92:441

47. Hoekman K, von blomberg-van der Flier BM, Wagstaff J, Drexhage HA, Pinedo HM. Reversible thyroid dysfunction during treatment with GM-CSF. Lancet 1991;338:541

48. Kung AWC, Jones BM, Lai CL. Effects of interferon-γ therapy on thyroid function, T-lymphocyte subpopulations and induction of autoantibodies. J Clin Endocrinol Metab 1990;71:1230

49. Sakata S, Nagai K, Shibata T, et al. A case of rheumatoid arthritis associated with silent thyroiditis. J Endocrinol Invest 1992;15:377

50. Magaro M, Zoli A, Altomonte L, et al. The association of silent thyroiditis with active systemic lupus erythematosus. Clin Exp Rheumatol 1992;10:67

51. Iitaka M, Ishii J, Ishikawa N, et al. A case of Graves' disease with false hyperthyrotropinemia who developed silent thyroiditis. Endocrinol Jpn 1991;38:667

52. Yamamoto M, Fuwa Y, Chimori K, Yamakita N, Sakata S. A case of progressive systemic sclerosis (PSS) with silent thyroiditis and anti-bovine thyrotropin antibodies. Endocrinol Jpn 1991;38:265

53. Carney AG, Moore SB, Northcutt RC, Woolner LB, Stillwell GK. Palpation thyroiditis (multifocal granulomatous folliculitis). Am J Clin Pathol 1975;64:639

54. Walfish PG, Caplan D, Rosen IB. Postparathyroidectomy transient thyrotoxicosis. J Clin Endocrinol Metab 1992;75:224

55. Kampe O, Jansson R, Karlsson FA. Effects of L-thyroxine and iodide on the development of autoimmune postpartum thyroiditis. J Clin Endocrinol Metab 1990;70:1014

56. Mitani Y, Shigesmasa C, Kouchi T, et al. Detection of thyroid stimulating antibody in patients with inflammatory thyrotoxicosis. Horm Res 1992;37:196

57. Nakamura S, Sugimoto M, Kosaka J, Watanabe H, Shima H, Kawahira S. Silent thyroiditis with thyroid-stimulation-blocking antibodies (TSBAb). Japan J Med 1990;29:623

58. Yamamoto M, Sakurada T, Yoshida K, et al. Thyroid function and antimicrosomal antibody during the course of silent thyroiditis. Endocrinol Jpn 1987;34:357

59. Morita T, Tamai H, Oshima A, et al. The occurrence of thyrotropin binding-inhibiting immunoglobulins and thyroid-stimulating antibodies in patients with silent thyroiditis. J Clin Endocrinol Metab 1990;71:1051

60. Amino N, Mori H, Iwatani Y, et al. High prevalence of transient postpartum thyrotoxicosis and hypothyroidism. N Engl J Med 1982;306:849

61. Kreider KR. Hyperthyroidism without goiter. Ann Intern Med 1977;87:120

62. Nikolai TF, Coombs GJ, McKenzie AK, et al. Treatment of lymphocytic thyroiditis with spontaneously resolving hyperthyroidism (silent thyroiditis). Arch Intern Med 1982;142:2281

63. Woolf PD. Transient painless thyroiditis with hyperthyroidism: A variant of lymphocytic thyroiditis? Endocr Rev 1980;4:411

64. Hamburger JI. Subacute thyroiditis: diagnostic difficulties and simple treatment. J Nucl Med 1974;15:81

65. Radfar N, Kenny FM, Larsen PR. Subacute thyroiditis in a lateral thyroid gland: Evaluation of the pituitary-thyroid axis during the acute destructive and the recovery phases. J Pediatr 1975;87:34

66. Amino N, Miyai K, Kuro R, et al. Transient postpartum hypothyroidism: fourteen cases with autoimmune thyroiditis. Ann Intern Med 1977;87:155

67. Amino N, Miyai K, Onishi T, et al. Transient hypothyroidism after delivery in autoimmune thyroiditis. J Clin Endocrinol Metab 1976;42:296

68. Nikolai TF. Recovery of thyroid function in primary hypothyroidism. Am J Med Sci 1989;297:18

69. Othman S, Parkes AB, Richards CJ, Hall R, Lazarus JH. Postpartum thyroiditis can be painful. Postgrad Med J 1990;66:130

70. Reinwein D, Benker G, Konig MP, Pinchera A, Schatz H, Schleusener H. The different types of hyperthyroidism in Europe. Results of a prospective survey of 924 patients. J Endocrinol Invest 1988;11:193

71. Volpe R. Subacute thyroiditis. In: Burrow GN, Oppenheimer JH, Volpe R, eds. Thyroid function and disease. Philadelphia: WB Saunders, 1989:179

72. de Quervain F. Die akute nicht Eiterige Thyreoiditis und die Beteiligung der Schilddruse an akuten intoxikationen und infektionen Uberhaupt. Mitt Grenz Med Chir(Suppl) 1904;2:1

73. de Quervain F, Giodanengo D. Die akute und subakute nicht Eiterige Thyreoiditis. Mitt Grenz Med Chir 1936;44:538

74. Mygind H. Thyroiditis akuta simplex. J Laryngol 1895;9:181

75. Nikolai TF. Lymphocytic thyroiditis with spontaneously resolving hyperthyroidism. Thyroid Today 1989;2:1

76. Nordyke RA, Gilbert FI Jr, Lew C. Painful subacute thyroiditis in Hawaii. West J Med 1991;155(1):61

77. Martino E, Buratti L, Bartalena L, et al. High prevalence of subacute thyroiditis during summer season in Italy. J Endocrinol Invest 1987;10:321

78. Saito S, Sakurada T, Yamamoto M, et al. Subacute thyroiditis: observations on 98 cases for the last 14 years. Tohoku J Exp Med 1974;113:141

79. Fraser R, Harrison RJ. Subacute thyroiditis. Lancet 1952;1:382

80. Eylan E, Zmucky R, Sheba C. Mumps virus and subacute thyroiditis. Evidence of a causal association. Lancet 1957;1:1062

81. Hung W. Mumps, thyroiditis and hypothyroidism. J Pediatr 1969;74:611

82. McArthur AM. Subacute giant cell thyroiditis associated with mumps. Med J Aust 1964;1:116

83. Robertson WS. Acute inflammation of the thyroid gland. Lancet 1911;1:930

84. Saito S. Clinical studies of subacute thyroiditis. Gunma J Med Sci 1959;8:(Suppl 17):1

85. Hintze G, Fortelius P, Railo J. Epidemic thyroidits. Acta Endocrinol 1964;45:381

86. Swann NH. Acute thyroiditis: five cases associated with adenovirus infection. Metabolism 1964;13:908

87. Liberman U, Djaldetti M, Devries A. A case of herpangina, pleurodynia and subacute thyroiditis. Harefuah 1964;67:342

88. Shumway M, Davis PL. Catscratch thyroiditis treated with thyrotrophin hormone. J Clin Endocrinol Metab 1954;14:742

89. Stancek D, Stancekova-Gressnerova M, Janotka M, et al. Isolation and some serological and epidemiological data on the viruses recovered from patients with subacute thyroiditis de Quervain. Med Microbiol Immunol 1975;161:133

90. Bastenie PA, Ermans AM. Thyroiditis and thyroid function. Clinical, morphological and physiological studies. International series of monographs in pure and applied biology: Modern trends in physiological sciences. Vol 36. Oxford: Pergamon Press, 1972

91. Yeo PPB, Rauff A, Chan SH, et al. Subacute (de Quervain's) thyroiditis in the tropics. In: Stockigt JR, Nagataki S, eds. Thyroid Research. Vol VIII. Canberra: Australian Academy of Science 1980:570

92. Somlo FM, Kovalik M. Acute thyroiditis in a patient with Q fever. Can Med Assoc J 1966;95:1091

93. Sein M. Acute non-suppurative thyroiditis. Lancet 1938;2:673

94. Debons-Guillemin MC, Valla J, Gazeau J, et al. No evidence of spumaretrovirus infection markers in 19 cases of de Quervain's thyroiditis. AIDS Res Human Retroviruses 1992;8:1547

95. deBruin TWA, Riekhoff FPM, deBoer JJ. An outbreak of thyrotoxicosis due to atypical subacute thyroiditis. J Clin Endocrinol Metab 1990;70:396

96. Greene JN. Subacute thyroiditis. Am J Med 1971;51:97

97. Chartier B, Bandy P, Wall JR. Fc receptor-bearing blood mononuclear cells in thyroid disorders: increased levels in patients with subacute thyroiditis. J Clin Endocrinol Metab 1980;51:1014

98. Galluzzo A, Giordano C, Andronica F, et al. Leukocyte migration tests in subacute thyroiditis: hypothetical role of cell-mediated immunity. J Clin Endocrinol Metab 1980;59:1034

99. Strakosch CR, Joyner D, Wall JR. Thyroid stimulating antibodies in patients with subacute thyroiditis. J Clin Endocrinol Metab 1978;46:345

100. Tamai H, Nozaki T, Mukuta T, et al. The incidence of thyroid stimulating blocking antibodies during the hypothyroid phase in patients with subacute thyroiditis. J Clin Endocrinol Metab 1991;73:245

101. Fenzi G, Hashizume K, Roudebush CP, et al. Changes in thyroid-stimulating immunoglobulins during antithyroid therapy. J Clin Endocrinol Metab 1979;48:572

102. Karlsson FA, Dahlberg A, Ritzen EM. Thyroid blocking antibodies in thyroiditis. Acta Med Scand 1984;215:461

103. Bech K, Feldt-Rasmussen U, Bliddal H, Hoier-Madsen M, Thomsen B, Nielsen H. Persistence of autoimmune reactions during recovery of subacute thyroiditis. In: Pinchera A, Ingbar SH, McKenzie JM, Fenzi GF, eds. Thyroid autoimmunity. New York: Plenum Press, 1987:623

104. Volpe R. Acute and subacute thyroiditis. Pharmacol Ther 1976;1:171

105. Wall JR, Gravy B, Greenwood DM. Total and "activated" peripheral blood T lymphocytes in patients with thyroid disorders. Acta Endocrinol 1977;85:753

106. Totterman TH. Distribution of T, B and thyroglobulin binding lymphocytes infiltrating the thyroid gland in Graves' disease.

Hashimoto's thyroiditis and de Quervain's thyroiditis. Clin Immunol Immunopathol 1978;10:270

107. Fukazawa H, Sakurada T, Tamura K, et al. The influence of immunosuppressive acidic protein on the activity of peripheral K-lymphocytes in subacute thyroiditis. J Clin Endocrinol Metab 1990;71(1):193

108. Iwatani Y, Amino N, Hidaka Y, et al. Decreases in alpha beta T cell receptor negative T cells and CD8 cells, and an increase in CD4+ CD8+ cells in active Hashimoto's disease and subacute thryoiditis. Clin Exper Immunol 1992;87(3):444

109. Aiginger P, Weissel M, Fritzsche H, Kroiss A, Hoffer R, Mayr WR. HLA antigens and de Quervain's thyroiditis. Tissue Antigens 1978;11:59

110. Bech K, Nerup J, Thomsen M, et al. Subacute thyroiditis de Quervain: a disease associated with HLA-B antigen. Acta Endocrinol 1977;86:504

111. Nyulassy S. Hnilica P, Buc M, et al. Subacute (de Quervain's) thyroiditis: association with HLA-Bw35 antigen and abnormalities of the complement system, immunoglobulins and other serum proteins. J Clin Endocrinol Metab 1977;45:270

112. Tamai H, Goto H, Uno H, et al. HLA in Japanese patients with subacute (de Quervain's) thyroiditis. Tissue Antigens 1984;24:58

113. Yeo PPB, Chan SH, Aw TC, et al. HLA and Chinese patients with subacute (de Quervain's) thyroiditis. Tissue Antigens 1981; 17:249

114. Rubin RA, Guay AT. Susceptibility to subacute thyroiditis is genetically influenced: Familial occurrence in identical twins. Thyroid 1991;1:157

115. Buc M, Nyulassy S, Hnilica P, Busova B, Stefanovic J. The frequency of HLA-Dw1 determinants in subacute (de Quervain's) thyroiditis. Tissue Antigens 1979;14:63

116. Goto H, Uno H, Tamai H, et al. Genetic analysis of subacute (de Quervain's) thyroiditis. Tissue Antigens 1985;26:110

117. Jayaram G, Marwaha RK, Gupta RK, Sharma, SK. Cytomorphologic aspects of thyroiditis, a study of 51 cases with functional, immunologic and ultrasonographic data. Acta Cytol 1987;31:687

118. Mizukami Y, Michigishi T, Kawato M, et al. Immunohistochemcial and ultrastructural study of subacute thyroiditis with special references to multinucleated giant cells. Hum Pathol 1987;18:929

119. Sanders LR, Moreno A, Pittman DL, et al. Painless giant cell thyroiditis diagnosed by fine needle aspiration and associated with intense thyroidal uptake of gallium. Am J Med 1986;80:971

120. Schmid KW, Ofner C, Ramsauer T, et al. CA 19-9 expression in subacute (de Quervain's) thyroiditis: an immunohistochemical study. Mod Pathol 1992;5:268

121. Volpe R, Johnston MN. Subacute thyroiditis: a disease commonly mistaken for pharyngitis. Can Med Assoc J 1957;77:297

122. Woolner LB, McConahey WM, Beahrs OH. Granulomatous thyroiditis (de Quervain's thyroiditis). J Clin Endocrinol Metab 1957;17:1202

123. Skillern PG, Nelson HE, Crile G Jr. Some new observations on subacute thyroiditis. J Clin Endocrinol Metab 1956;16:1422

124. Yamashita T, Okamoto T, Kawada J, et al. Characteristics and clinical course of patients with subacute thyroiditis without typical signs and symptoms. Folia Endocrinol Jpn 1993; 69:1057

125. Miyake H, Tanaka R, Takeoka H, et al. Unsuspected painless subacute thyroiditis detected by radiogallium scintigraphy. Jap J Nucl Med 1992;29:1475

126. Brander A. Ultrasound appearances in de Quervain's subacute thyroiditis with long-term follow-up. J Intern Med 1992;232:321

127. Tokuda Y, Kasagi K, Iida Y, et al. Sonography of subacute thyroiditis: changes in the findings during the course of the disease. J Clin Ultrasound 1990;18:21

128. Ishizuki Y, Hirroka Y, Murata Y, Togashi K. The functional outcome of patients with subacute thyroiditis. Folia Endocrinol Jpn 1992;68:154

129. Steinberg FU. Subacute granulomatous thyroiditis: a review. Ann Intern Med 1960;52:1014

130. Dorta T, Beraud T. New investigations on subacute thyroiditis. Helv Med Acta 1961;28:19

131. Ingbar SH, Frienkel N. Thyroid function and metabolism of iodine in patients with subacute thyroiditis. Arch Intern Med 1958;101:339

132. Gordin A, Lamberg BA. Serum thyrotrophin response to thyrotrophin releasing hormone and the concentration of free thyroxine in subacute thyroiditis. Acta Endocrinol 1973;74:111

133. Larsen PR. Serum triiodothyronine and thyrotropin during hyperthyroid, hypothyroid and recovery phases of subacute nonsuppurative thyroiditis. Metabolism 1974;23:467

134. Staub JJ. TRH test in subacute thyroiditis. Lancet 1975;1:868

135. Weihl AC, Daniels GH, Ridgeway EC, et al. Thyroid function tests during the early phase of subacute thyroiditis. J Clin Endocrinol Metab 1977;44:1107

136. Izumi M, Larsen PR. Correlation of sequential changes in serum thyroglobulin, triiodothyronine and thyroxine in patients with Graves' disease and subacute thyroiditis. Metabolism 1978; 27:449

137. Bartalena L, Brogioni S, Grasso L, Martino E. Increased serum interleukin-6 concentration in patients with subacute thyroiditis: relationship with concomitant changes in serum T4-binding globulin concentration. J Endocrinol Invest 1993;16:213

138. Lewitus Z, Rechnic J, Lubin E. Sequential scanning of the thyroid as an aid in diagnosis of subacute thyroiditis. Isr J Med Sci 1967;3:847

139. Hamburger JI, Kadian G, Rossin HW. Subacute thyroiditis: evaluation depicted by serial ^{131}I scintigram. J Nucl Med 1965;6:560

140. Benker G, Olbricht TH, Windeck R, et al. The sonographical and function sequelae of de Quervain's subacute thyroiditis. Acta Endocrinol 1988;117:435

141. Birchall IW, Chow CC, Metreweli C. Ultrasound appearances of de Quervain's thyroiditis. Clin Radiol 1990;41:57

142. Babb RR. Association between diseases of the thyroid and the liver. Am J Gastroenterol 1984;79:421

143. Van Herle AJ, Vassart G, Dumont JE. Control of thyroglobulin synthesis and secretion. N Engl J Med 1979;301:239

144. Volpe R. The management of subacute (de Quervain's) thyroiditis. Thyroid 1993;3:253

145. Yamamoto M, Saito S, Sakurada T, et al. Effect of prednisolone and salicylate on serum thyroglobulin level in patients with subacute thyroiditis. Clin Endocrinol 1987;27:339

Werner and Ingbar's The Thyroid, Seventh Edition,
edited by Lewis E. Braverman and Robert D. Utiger.
Lippincott–Raven Publishers, Philadelphia, © 1996

35

Thyrotoxicosis of Extrathyroid Origin

Monte A. Greer

Extrathyroidal causes of thyrotoxicosis, although unusual, can present confusing diagnostic problems. Fortunately, once the disease is diagnosed, therapy is usually simple and effective. The three most frequent causes are thyrotoxicosis factitia,[1] metastatic thyroid cancer, and struma ovarii. The latter two are extremely rare causes of thyrotoxicosis.

THYROTOXICOSIS FACTITIA

The term *thyrotoxicosis factitia* is used to describe thyrotoxicosis produced by administration of exogenous thyroid hormone. Thyrotoxicosis factitia is also known by a variety of other names, including thyrotoxicosis medicamentosa, and is often hard to identify because patients may be secretive about their use of thyroid hormone.

The underlying background of thyrotoxicosis factitia is diverse. Thyroid hormone has been employed for diseases other than hypothyroidism since soon after Murray discovered its efficacy in treating myxedema in 1891. Obesity is the most common nonthyroid disorder for which thyroid hormone is used, but it has been used for almost every conceivable problem from menstrual irregularities and infertility to baldness. Since essentially no patient with these nonthyroid disorders is actually benefitted by treatment with thyroid hormone, either the physician or the patient may gradually, but inexorably, increase the dose of hormone in an attempt to gain the desired effect. At some point in this ascending scale of futility, thyrotoxicosis usually becomes manifest; however, it may not be recognized as such by either the patient or the physician.

Another common cause of thyrotoxicosis factitia is the purposeful and usually secretive ingestion of thyroid hormone by psychiatrically disturbed patients (most often with a medical or paramedical background) who wish to obtain attention, lose weight, or receive insurance compensation from an excessive use of thyroid hormone but who will not admit to using it. The accidental ingestion of a large number of thyroid pills by children is occasionally seen in emergency rooms.[2]

Thyrotoxicosis factitia can also occur when too large a dose of thyroid hormone is employed for conditions in which it is definitely beneficial, such as hypothyroidism or nontoxic goiter.

The clinical manifestations of thyrotoxicosis factitia are identical to those of hyperthyroidism of thyroid origin, except that thyroid enlargement, infiltrative ophthalmopathy, and dermopathy do not occur. Lid lag may be present, however, because catecholamine effects are enhanced. Although treatment with thyroid hormone does not induce goiter formation, a goiter present when exogenous hormone ingestion was instituted may confuse the diagnosis.

Any substance with thyromimetic activity can produce clinical thyrotoxicosis if taken in adequate amounts. It can even be absorbed through the skin.[3] It is not possible to distinguish which thyroactive agent is being used from the clinical effects. As with thyrotoxicosis of endogenous origin, the manifestations of thyrotoxicosis factitia vary considerably among patients. In some, weight loss and agitation may be most apparent. In others, atrial fibrillation or angina pectoris may be the primary finding.[4]

Exogenous thyroid hormone suppresses thyroid-stimulating hormone secretion by negative feedback on the pituitary thyrotrophs, maintaining a constant level of circulating thyroid hormone through normal homeostatic mechanisms. When the amount of thyroid hormone ingested is slightly less than or equal to that normally produced by the patient's own thyroid gland, a eumetabolic state is preserved. When the amount ingested produces a metabolic effect greater than that maintained by the patient's own thyroid hormone secretion, however, thyrotoxicosis results. Whether the negative feedback is partial or complete, the patient's endogenous thyroid gland function is always suppressed unless some preexisting autonomy of either the pituitary or thyroid exists. The thyroid gland is small, and the thyroid radioiodine or pertechnetate uptake is depressed to low levels. These findings are strong clues that thyrotoxicosis factitia might exist, because endogenous hyperthyroidism rarely occurs without significant thyroid enlargement.

Results of laboratory tests in patients with thyrotoxicosis factitia vary according to which preparation is responsible for the disease. If there is a large component of thyroxine (T_4) in the form of desiccated thyroid, purified thyroglobulin, or T_4 itself, both total and free serum T_4 levels will be elevated. If the responsible agent is triiodothyronine (T_3) or a material with a high T_3/T_4 ratio, the serum T_4 level may be low or normal and only the serum T_3 level will be elevated. When T_4 is the drug taken to produce thyrotoxicosis, the serum T_4/T_3 ratio is often elevated to a higher level than usually seen with endogenous thyrotoxicosis. This is because both T_4 and T_3 are normally secreted from the thyroid gland, and with a highly active thyroid the T_4/T_3 ratio of secreted hormone decreases, probably primarily due to the increased rate of turnover and thus decreased degree of iodination of intrafollicular thyroglobulin. The only source of serum T_3 when excess T_4 suppresses endogenous thyroid function is from extrathyroidal 5'-deiodination of T_4. The serum T_4/T_3 ratio can thus provide another clue of excessive T_4 ingestion.

Measurement of serum thyroglobulin (Tg) concentration is an extremely valuable laboratory aid in diagnosing thyrotoxicosis factitia.[1] Tg is normally secreted in small amounts by the thyroid gland and can be detected in serum by radioimmunoassay. When thyroid hormone is taken orally, however, no Tg or a very low amount of Tg is detectable in the serum. Neither T_4 nor T_3 contains Tg. When desiccated thyroid or purified Tg is taken orally, the Tg is degraded by proteolysis in the gastrointestinal tract before absorption; no significant amounts appear in the circulation. Very low or undetectable amounts of Tg in the serum thus allow differentiation of thyrotoxicosis factitia from other potentially confusing entities, such as silent thyroiditis, metastatic thyroid cancer, and struma ovarii, all of which result in normal or elevated levels of serum Tg. In occasional patients, the test may not be reliable because of circulating anti-Tg antibodies. Measurement of fecal thyroid hormones may also be useful.[5]

If a history of ingestion of thyroid material is elicited, diagnosis is not particularly difficult. Treatment with exogenous thyroid hormone is stopped, and clinical and laboratory evaluation is made 2 to 4 weeks later. If all evidence of thyrotoxicosis has disappeared, thyrotoxicosis factitia is firmly established. Often, however, there is surreptitious use of thyroid hormone, and elucidation of the underlying cause of the thyrotoxicosis may be difficult. Silent thyroiditis is the most difficult alternative diagnosis to exclude, but the serum Tg is helpful in the differentiation, providing Tg antibodies are absent. Once the physician is convinced that the patient is indeed ingesting sufficient exogenous thyroid hormone to cause thyrotoxicosis, delicate maneuvering is required to confront the patient, explain the basis of the condition, and urge the patient to stop ingesting thyroid hormone.

Although not usually necessary, further therapeutic measures may be required to treat children (or rarely adults) who ingest a large amount of thyroid hormone. Such measures include beta-blocking drugs and agents that block the peripheral conversion of T_4 to T_3, such as sodium ipodate or iopanoic acid, when T_4 is the primary medication ingested, or bile acid sequestrants.[6]

On rare occasions, thyrotoxicosis factitia is produced by ingestion of food contaminated with thyroid tissue due to the poor anatomic training or carelessness of the workers at the abattoir.[7,8]

METASTATIC THYROID CARCINOMA

Differentiated thyroid carcinomas are usually hypofunctional compared with normal thyroid tissue. They do produce Tg, however, which can become iodinated and form thyroid hormone that is secreted as T_4 and T_3. In metastatic carcinomas with relatively well-preserved function, and even in rather poorly functional carcinomas with metastases that form a large mass, sufficient thyroid hormone can be synthesized and secreted to cause thyrotoxicosis. In most instances, a previous diagnosis of thyroid malignancy has been made, so that some clue to the cause of the thyrotoxicosis exists. Since the treatment of patients with thyroid cancer is usually a total surgical thyroidectomy and iodine-131 (^{131}I) ablation of the thyroid remnant, followed by treatment with exogenous thyroid hormone, the correct diagnosis may not be made initially if the clinician suspects that the thyrotoxicosis is due to overtreatment with suppressive thyroid replacement. It is essential to stop thyroid hormone treatment to see if the signs and symptoms are alleviated and if the levels of T_4 and T_3 in the serum fall. If not, the hyperthyroidism may be due to functional thyroid metastases. This can be confirmed by whole-body radioiodine scanning.

In some patients, thyroid cancer coexists with Graves' disease or nonmalignant toxic nodular goiter. When thyrotoxicosis recurs or persists after thyroidectomy in these patients, it may be difficult to ascertain whether cervical masses that concentrate radioiodine are truly metastases or are merely ectopic thyroid remnants.

Laboratory studies (other than radioiodine or pertechnetate scans and tumor histologic findings) are usually not specific. Because the Tg in the tumors is usually poorly iodinated, a high T_3/T_4 ratio is found in the colloid, and a high proportion of patients have T_3-toxicosis.[9,10]

Treatment may be more easily achieved with ^{131}I than with surgery, especially in patients with widespread metastases. If a large and relatively accessible isolated metastasis is producing the thyrotoxicosis, however, surgery is preferable.

STRUMA OVARII

Struma ovarii, an extremely rare cause of thyrotoxicosis, is due to the presence of an ovarian teratoma that contains hyperfunctional autonomous thyroid tissue. Such teratomas can also be found in locations other than the ovary. Suspicion that this condition may exist in a thyrotoxic patient is the clinician's necessary first step in diagnosis. Suggestive clues are an absence of thyroid enlargement, a normal or elevated serum Tg level, and a very low thyroid radioiodine uptake. The diagnosis is then theoretically established by localization of functional heterotopic thyroid tissue by body scanning after radioiodine administration. Such cases, however, are extremely rare.[11,12]

Struma ovarii without associated thyrotoxicosis is much more common and is usually diagnosed only during surgery for an ovarian tumor. Only 9 of 233 patients mentioned in an extensive review had signs of thyrotoxicosis (usually without specific confirmatory laboratory data), which were relieved solely by tumor resection.[13] A more recent review[11] found only 10 patients in whom symptoms and basal metabolic rate (rarely were other thyroid function tests described) returned to normal after the ovarian struma was removed. The eutopic thyroid may have been at least in part responsible for the hyperthyroidism is some patients, since 42% of these patients also had a cervical goiter.[11]

Although a cure can theoretically be affected by treatment with ^{131}I, because the tissue is neoplastic and potentially malignant and often contains nonthyroid tissue,[13,14] surgical resection is more appropriate.

References

1. Cohen JH, Ingbar SH, Braverman LE. Thyrotoxicosis due to ingestion of excess thyroid hormone. Endocr Rev 1989;10:113

2. Gorman RL, Chamberlain JM, Rose SR, Oderda GM. Massive levothyroxine overdose: high anxiety—low toxicity. Pediatrics 1988;82:666

3. DelGuerra P, Caraccio N, Simoncini M, Monzani F. Occupational thyroid disease. Int Arch Occup Environ Health 1992;63:373

4. Shammas NW, Richeson JF, Pomerantz R. Myocardial dysfunction and necrosis after ingestion of thyroid hormone. Am Heart J 1994;127:232

5. Bouillon R, Verresen L, Staels F, Bex M, De Vos P, De Roo M. The measurement of fecal thyroxine in the diagnosis of thyrotoxicosis factitia. Thyroid 1993;3:101

6. Solomon BL, Wartofsky L, Burman KD. Adjunctive cholestyramine therapy for thyrotoxicosis. Clin Endocrinol (Oxf) 1993;38:39

7. Hedberg CW, Fishbein DB, Janssen RS, et al. An outbreak of thyrotoxicosis caused by the consumption of bovine thyroid gland in ground beef. N Engl J Med 1987;316:993

8. Kinney JS, Hurwitz ES, Fishbein DB, et al. Community outbreak of thyrotoxicosis: epidemiology, immunogenetic characteristics, and long-term outcome. Am J Med 1988;84:10

9. Baumann K, Weitzel M, Burgi H. Hormonproduzierendes Schilddruesenkarzinom mit Hyperthyreose. Schweiz Med Wschr 1979;109:309

10. Nakashima T, Inoue K, Shiro-ozu A, Yoshinari M, Okamura K, Itoh M. Predominant T3 synthesis in the metastatic thyroid carcinoma in a patient with T3-toxicosis. Metabolism 1981 30:327

11. Brown WW, Shetty KR, Rosenfeld PS. Hyperthyroidism due to struma ovarii: demonstration by radioiodine scan. Acta Endocrinol (Copenh) 1973;73:266

12. March DE, Desai AG, Park CH, Hendricks PJ, Davis PS. Struma ovarii: hyperthyroidism in a postmenopausal woman. J Nucl Med 1988;29:263

13. Brocq P, Rouvillois C, Gauchez G. A propos des varietes, de l'avenir, du diagnostic des tumeur thyroidiennes de l'ovaire. Presse Med 1959;67:165

14. Rosenblum NG, LiVolsi VA, Edmonds PR, Mikuta JJ. Malignant struma ovarii. Gynecol Oncol 1989;32:224

Werner and Ingbar's The Thyroid, Seventh Edition,
edited by Lewis E. Braverman and Robert D. Utiger.
Lippincott–Raven Publishers, Philadelphia, © 1996

Section C
Organ System Manifestations

36

The Skin in Thyrotoxicosis

Jeffrey D. Bernhard

Irwin M. Freedberg

Louis N. Vogel

Thyrotoxicosis is accompanied by cutaneous alterations that reflect the basic pathophysiologic process and by a number of changes that may have practical diagnostic significance. Because the skin plays a fundamental role in thermoregulation in all homeothermic species, changes in cutaneous function occur whenever there is an increase in metabolic rate and heat production. In addition, the epidermal and dermal tissues that form the skin and its appendages are target organs for the action of the thyroid hormones. The metabolism of these tissues changes with increases in the level of circulating thyroid hormones, and these changes are reflected in visible clinical abnormalities (Table 36-1).

The skin of thyrotoxic patients is usually warm, erythematous, and moist, with a smooth, silky texture.[1,2,3] Temperature elevation and erythema are consequences of increased dermal blood flow. Episodic flushing may occur over the face and the throat; telangiectatic vessels may develop in these same areas. The face may stay flushed. Palmar erythema and redness of the elbows may be observed. Increased capillary fragility has also been noted.[4] As a consequence of excessive perspiration found in about half of thyrotoxic patients, miliaria, caused by poral occlusion and subsequent intracutaneous sweat retention, may be present.[5]

The receptors for thyroid hormone in human skin are specific for triiodothyronine (T_3). The epidermis changes in structure and activation in thyroid disease. Epidermal cell division and anabolic activity are increased in thyrotoxicosis.[6] The changes are rapidly reversible.

THE SKIN'S APPENDAGES

Hair

Laboratory studies have proven that thyroid hormones affect hair growth. In rats, thyroxine (T_4) enhances initiation of the growth cycle in each hair follicle, stimulates the rate of hair growth, and potentiates the action of agents such as x-rays on the follicle.[7,8] Thyroxine also greatly accelerates passage of the molt.[9]

The mechanism and control of hair growth vary significantly among species, so that animal studies cannot be directly extrapolated to humans to explain the quantitative and qualitative hair abnormalities that occur in thyrotoxicosis. Diffuse loss of scalp hair occurs in 20% to 40% of thyrotoxic patients, although the severity of the loss is not directly related to

TABLE 36-1.
Cutaneous Changes in Thyrotoxicosis

FREQUENT

Warm skin

Erythema

Telangiectasia

Hyperhidrosis

Alopecia, localized or generalized

Hyperpigmentation

Abnormalities in nail growth

Eczematous dermatitis

INFREQUENT

Localized myxedema*

Thyroid acropachy*

Vitiligo*

Pruritus

Urticaria and dermographism

Xanthelasma

Features of Graves' disease rather than of thyrotoxicosis per se.

the severity of the endocrine abnormality.[10] Axillary hair may also decrease.[11] Alopecia areata and loss of axillary, pubic, body, and eyebrow hair have been noted since the initial description by Basedow. The hair itself is most commonly fine and soft, and holds a permanent wave poorly. The latter changes may be ascribable to a fundamental, although as yet undefined, alteration in the proteins synthesized by the hair follicle. When patients who present with alopecia areata are evaluated prospectively, as many as 24% may have evidence of thyroid hormone abnormalities and/or elevation of microsomal or TPO antibody levels,[12] although this is not a universal experience.[13] This suggests that autoimmune thyroid disease rather than thyrotoxicosis or hypothyroidism is the associated abnormality.

Nails

The nails in thyrotoxicosis become shiny and may be soft and friable. These abnormalities are caused by alterations in the keratinizing nail matrix and in its supporting dermal structures. The rate of nail growth is increased, and longitudinal striations associated with a flattening of the surface contour result in a scoop-shovel appearance.[14] Many patients develop onycholysis, that is, distal separation of the nail plate from its underlying bed, so-called Plummer's nails.[15,16] Onycholysis is not specific to thyrotoxicosis, but when it occurs in this setting it usually begins under the distal central portion of the fourth fingernail. It may eventually involve any of the finger and toe nails. The hyponychium of thyrotoxic patients is ragged and often dirty. Such nail changes are less common in thyrotoxic patients over 60 years of age.[17]

PIGMENTARY ALTERATIONS

Abnormalities of cutaneous pigment production are present in a significant number of patients. Hyperpigmentation has been reported in from 2% to as high as 40% of large series.[2,18] The hyperpigmentation is often diffuse, although a spectrum of abnormalities may be seen, ranging from localized hyperpigmented areas on the face to typical Addisonian hyperpigmentation with involvement of the oral mucous membranes, genitalia, body creases, and scars. Vitiligo of variable extent occurs in a substantial proportion of patients, and is seen especially in Graves' disease and in Hashimoto's thyroiditis as a marker of the autoimmune disease.[19]

The reason for these alterations in pigmentation has not been defined, although there are two major interrelationships between the thyroid and the melanocytic system. Tyrosine is a precursor of both T_4 and melanin, so that the abnormalities could be related to some alteration in the conversion of the precursor to its products.[20] The other, less direct relation, depends on the secondary elevation in adrenocorticotropic hormone level that may occur in thyrotoxicosis.[21] Because the melanocyte-stimulating hormone and adrenocorticotropic hormone (ACTH) have common areas of primary structure, hyperpigmentation may be expected in thyrotoxicosis as well as in other clinical conditions associated with elevated ACTH levels.

MISCELLANEOUS CUTANEOUS CHANGES

Among the less frequently reported cutaneous changes in thyrotoxicosis are dermographism, urticaria,[22,22a] purpura, and ill-defined, generalized erythematous eruptions.[23] Pruritus may be the chief complaint.[24,25] Xanthelasma has been reported.[26] Eczematous dermatitis has been described in one-third of a larger series of thyrotoxic patients, a higher incidence than in either a control group or in patients with nontoxic goiter. The significance of this association is not evident.[27]

Other disorders reported in association with thyrotoxicosis include systemic lupus erythematosus,[28] pustular variants of chronic recurrent hand dermatitis,[29,30] and subcorneal pustular dermatosis.[31] Rare or anecdotal associations are reviewed in greater detail in reference 3. Reports of patients with more than one autoimmune disease, including thyroid disease, are not uncommon.[32] The hypothesis that such associations are all due to autoimmunity has not been proven. Other autoimmune skin diseases, such as pemphigus vulgaris, may also be associated with an increased prevalence of autoimmune thyroid disease in family members.[33]

LOCALIZED MYXEDEMA AND THYROID ACROPACHY

These autoimmune manifestations of Graves' disease are discussed in detail in chapter 30 and elsewhere.[2,3,34]

References

1. Youmans JB. Changes in the skin in thyrotoxicosis. J Med Sci 1931;181:681

2. Rosen T, Kleman GA. Thyroid and the skin. In: Callen JP, Jorizzo JL, Greer KE, et al., eds. Dermatologic signs of internal disease. 2nd ed. Philadelphia: WB Saunders, 1995:189

3. Heymann WR. Cutaneous manifestations of thyroid disease. J Am Acad Dermatol 1992;26:885

4. Thomson JA. Alterations in capillary fragility in thyroid disease. Clin Sci 1964;25:55

5. Hyde JN, McEwen EL. The dermatoses occurring in exophthalmic goiter. Am J Med Sci 1903;125:1000

6. Holt PJA, Marks MB. The epidermal response to change in thyroid status. J Invest Dermatol 1977;68:299

7. Ebling FJ, Johnson E. The action of hormones on spontaneous growth cycles in the rat. J Endocrinol 1964;29:193

8. Griem ML, Malkinson FD. Some studies on the effects of radiation and radiation modifiers on growing hair. Radiat Res 1967; 30:431

9. Ebling FJ. Hair. J Invest Dermatol 1976;67:98

10. Rook A. Endocrine influences on hair growth. Br Med J 1965; 1:609

11. Rook A, Dawber R. Diseases of the hair and scalp. 2nd ed. Oxford: Blackwell Scientific Publications, 1991:147

12. Milgraum SS, Mitchell AJ, Bacon GE, et al. Alopecia areata, endocrine function, and autoantibodies in patients 16 years of age or younger. J Am Acad Dermatol 1987;17:57

13. Puavilai S, Puabilai G, Charuwichitratana S, et al. Prevalence of thyroid diseases in patients with alopecia areata. Int J Dermatol 1994;33:632

14. Luria MN, Asper SP Jr. Onycholysis in hyperthyroidism. Ann Intern Med 1958;49:102

15. Tosti A, Baran R, Dawber RPR. The nail in systemic diseases and drug-induced changes. In: Baran R, Dawber RPR, eds. Diseases of the nails and their management. Oxford: Blackwell, 1994:175

16. Locke W. Unusual manifestations of Graves' disease. Med Clin North Am 1967;51:915

17. Davis PJ, Davis FB. Hyperthyroidism in patients over the age of 60 years. Medicine 1974;53:161

18. Dore SE. Cutaneous affections occurring in the course of Graves' disease. Br J Dermatol 1900;12:353

19. Ortonne J-P, Mosher DB, Fitzpatrick TB. Vitiligo and other hypomelanoses of hair and skin. New York: Plenum, 1983:182

20. Lerner AB, Fitzpatrick TB. Biochemistry of melanin formation. Physiol Rev 1950;30:91

21. Kirkeby K, Hangaard G, Lingjærde P. The pigmentation of thyrotoxic patients. Acta Med Scand 1963;174:257

22. Leznoff A, Sussman GL. Syndrome of idiopathic chronic urticaria and angioedema with thyroid autoimmunity: a study of 90 patients. J Allergy Clin Immunol 1989;84:66

22a. Collet E, Petit J-M, LaCroix M, Bensa AF, Morvan C, Lambert D. Chronic urticaria and thyroid auto-immunity. Ann Dermatol Venereol 1995;122:413

23. Pegum JS, Grice K. Unusual skin eruption with eosinophilia associated with hyperthyroidism. Br J Dermatol 1973;88:295

24. Barrow MV, Bird ED. Pruritus in hyperthyroidism. Arch Dermatol 1966;93:237

25. Bernhard JD. Endocrine itches. In: Bernhard JD, ed. Itch: Mechanisms and management of pruritus. New York: McGraw-Hill, 1994:251

26. Thomson JA. Xanthelasma associated with thyrotoxicosis. J Clin Endocrinol Metab 1965;25:758

27. Readett MD. Constitutional eczema and thyroid disease. Br J Dermatol 1964;76:126

28. Rodrique S, LaBorde H, Cataggio PM. Systemic lupus erythematosus and thyrotoxicosis: a hitherto little recognized association. Am Rheum Disease 1989;48:424

29. Rosen K. Pustulosis palmoplantaris and chronic eczematous hand dermatitis. Treatment, epidermal Langerhans cells and association with thyroid disease. Acta Derm Venereol (Suppl) 1988;137:1

30. Rosen K, Lindstedt G, Mobacken H, Nystrom E. Thyroid function in patients with pustulosis palmoplantaris. J Am Acad Dermatol 1988;19:1009

31. Taniguchi S, Tsuruta D, Kutsuna H, Hamada T. Subcorneal pustular dermatosis in a patient with hyperthyroidism. Dermatology 1995;190:64

32. Ueki R, Ryusuke I, Takamori K, et al. Three patients with concurrent alopecia areata, vitiligo and chronic thyroiditis. Eur J Dermatol 1993;3:454

33. Firooz A, Mazhar A, Ahmed AR. Prevalence of autoimmune diseases in the family members of patients with pemphigus vulgaris. J Am Acad Dermatol 1994;31:434

34. Freinkel RK. Cutaneous manifestations of endocrine diseases. In: Fitzpatrick TB, Eisen AZ, Wolff K, et al., eds. Dermatology in general medicine, 4th ed. New York: McGraw-Hill, 1993: 2113

Werner and Ingbar's The Thyroid, Seventh Edition,
edited by Lewis E. Braverman and Robert D. Utiger.
Lippincott–Raven Publishers, Philadelphia, © 1996

37

Connective Tissue in Thyrotoxicosis

Terry J. Smith

COMPOSITION OF CONNECTIVE TISSUE

The shape and coherence of all mammalian tissues derive from the unique physicochemical properties of connective tissue. This tissue has both cellular and noncellular components. The cellular elements include fibroblasts and their more specialized derivatives (chondrocytes, osteocytes, adipocytes). These cells have largely secretory functions and are the source of many extracellular macromolecules. Fibroblasts synthesize and secrete fibrous proteins (collagen), attachment molecules (fibronectin and laminin), and ground substance (glycosaminoglycans and proteoglycans) in amounts that vary in different tissues.

Fibroblasts

Fibroblasts vary with respect to their anatomic sites of origin, both in terms of their morphology and the factors that influence their proliferation and metabolism. For instance, gingival fibroblasts respond to phenytoin, whereas fibroblasts derived from other regions do not. Testosterone metabolism in genital fibroblasts differs from that in nongenital fibroblasts. Skin fibroblasts are considerably more responsive to thyroid hormone than those derived from the orbital connective tissue.[1]

Fibroblasts have extensive Golgi apparatus and endoplasmic reticulum, and they synthesize and release numerous matrix molecules. Fibroblast cell morphology in vitro varies from fusiform (spindle shaped with two to three dendritic processes) to angular (stellate shaped with three or more dendritic processes). The cytoplasm can be either very granular or homogeneous. Fibroblasts are relatively inactive metabolically compared with some other cell types, such as renal epithelium, hepatocytes, and neural cells. Because they proliferate easily in cell culture, fibroblasts are extremely useful for the study of connective tissue and the diseases that affect connective tissue.

Fibroblast proliferation is stimulated by various molecular factors. Fibroblast growth factor, platelet-derived growth factor, cytokines, and corticosteroids all can influence proliferation. Some insulin-like peptides stimulate fibroblast metabolism but not proliferation. Thyroid hormone also may stimulate fibroblast proliferation.[2] Heparin sulfate can inhibit fibroblast proliferation, a property not shared by other abundant glycosaminoglycans. Human fibroblasts have multiple hormone receptors, including high-affinity, limited-capacity binding sites for triiodothyronine (T_3),[3,4] corticosteroids,[5] insulin,[6] androgens,[7] growth hormone,[8] bradykinin,[9] 1,25-dihydroxycholecalciferol,[10] epidermal growth factor,[11] endothelin-1,[12] and retinoic acid–binding protein.[13]

Fibroblasts respond to numerous factors that are potentially important in the regulation of connective tissue. Thyroid hormone stimulates glucose utilization and lactate production,[14] regulates the degradation of low-density lipoproteins,[15] and inhibits the synthesis of hyaluronic acid (or hyaluronan as it is now termed),[16] fibronectin,[17] and collagen[18] in cultured fibroblasts. T_3 and corticosteroids modulate the abundance of several fibroblast proteins.[19] In addition to their role as targets for the action of thyroid hormone, fibroblasts may be able to deiodinate thyroxine (T_4) and T_3.[20,21]

In some instances, skin fibroblasts from patients with peripheral resistance to thyroid hormone (see chap 90) and cultures from patients who are resistant to the actions of other hormones share the defects present in vivo. Abnormalities in hormone binding or action have been demonstrated in fibroblasts from patients who are resistant to T_3, cortisol, androgens, and 1,25-dihydroxyvitamin D.[22] These findings suggest the physiologic relevance of the respective hormone receptors present in fibroblasts.

FIBROBLAST DIVERSITY

The term fibroblast is used to describe a population of cells that share common morphologic features. In general, these cells are cast in a passive role; they synthesize and release extracellular molecules that form cohesive networks in which parenchymal cells function. Despite similar appearances, fibroblasts are a diverse cell type capable of producing numerous cytokines, growth factors, and other regulatory molecules. Fibroblasts may therefore affect the growth and differentiation of their cellular neighbors. For example, two discrete subsets of fibroblasts are present in the lung; those expressing Thy-1 and those in which detectable Thy-1 is absent.[23] In murine fibroblasts, Thy-1-negative fibroblasts respond to interferon-γ in regard to expression of class II MHC antigens, whereas those expressing Thy-1 do not.[23] In human lung fibroblasts, Thy-1 expression correlates positively with class II MHC induction by interferon-γ.[24]

The anatomic region from which fibroblasts emanate determines much about their protein synthetic capacity and response repertoire. Among dermal fibroblasts, there are substantial differences in the responses to lymphokines in cells from different anatomic sites. For instance, in pretibial skin fibroblasts the expression of plasminogen-activator inhibitor type-1 (PAI-1), a serine protease inhibitor, is increased in response to interferon-γ[25,26] and leukoregulin,[27] whereas PAI-1 expression is decreased by both lymphokines in fibroblasts from the skin of the abdominal wall.[25–28] These findings suggest the potential for functional specialization among fibroblasts. Moreover, the phenotypic attributes of fibroblasts in a particular region of the body may account for the site-specific vulnerability of the area to the localized manifestations of systemic disease. Such is the case in localized myxedema in which the pretibial skin is most often affected.

ORBITAL FIBROBLASTS AND THEIR POTENTIAL ROLE IN GRAVES' OPHTHALMOPATHY

A prominent feature of Graves' disease is ophthalmopathy, a condition characterized by the accumulation of hyaluronan in the soft tissues of the orbit.[22] Hyaluronan is an abundant, nonsulfated glycosaminoglycan that also accumulates in interstitial tissue in severe hypothyroidism (see chap 61). The extreme hydrophilicity of hyaluronan leads to the retention of water and volume expansion in tissues in which it accumulates, including the perimysium of the extraoccular musculature and orbital fatty connective tissue.

Fibroblasts are a major source of glycosaminoglycans. A number of studies have focused on potential differences in orbital fibroblasts that might set them apart from other fibroblasts. The major proteoglycan synthesized by orbital fibroblasts is chondroitin sulfate, in contrast to dermal fibroblasts, in which dermatan sulfate and heparan sulfate predominate.[29] Platelet-derived growth factor (PDGF) and insulin-like growth factor-1 (IGF-1) stimulate the production of hyaluronan and chondroitin sulfate in orbital fibroblasts.[30] Moreover, the increases are factor-dependent, in that PDGF stimulates the production of large chondroitin sulfate while IGF-1 stimulates that of small chondroitin sulfate proteoglycan. Orbital fibroblasts synthesize less hyaluronan than do dermal fibroblasts under basal culture conditions. When exposed to interferon-γ[30] or leukoregulin,[31] the rate of hyaluronan synthesis in orbital fi-

broblasts increases. The stimulatory effect of leukoregulin is dramatic, up to 15-fold, and site-selective in that hyaluronan synthesis in cultures of dermal fibroblasts is enhanced to a much lesser degree. Corticosteroids block the effects of leukoregulin on hyaluronan synthesis, an action that requires de novo protein synthesis.

In orbital fibroblasts, the constitutive expression of PAI-1 is very low as compared with that in dermal fibroblasts.[25,32] When cultures of orbital fibroblasts are treated with interferon-γ[25] or leukoregulin,[27] PAI-1 synthesis is increased and it is deposited in the undersurface of the fibroblasts where it complexes with the extracellular matrix. The induction of PAI-1 by leukoregulin is mediated through an increase in PAI-1 gene expression. The low levels of constitutive PAI-1 expression suggest that the pericellular proteolytic activity of orbital connective tissue is ordinarily governed by factors other than PAI-1, unlike dermal connective tissue. PAI-1, by virtue of massive increases during inflammatory processes, could be an important regulatory factor of extracellular matrix stability in orbital connective tissue. The net consequence of induction of PAI-1 should be a decreased rate of macromolecular degradation.

Orbital fibroblasts undergo striking morphologic changes when exposed to prostaglandin E_2.[33] Their typical fibroblastoid appearance is lost and they develop prominent cytoplasmic processes and become stellate in shape. A similar phenomenon has been reported in synovial cells derived from joints of patients with rheumatoid arthritis.[34] Particular patterns of cytokine production may be associated with cells undergoing changes in shape. The shape change in orbital fibroblasts may be the consequence of loss of actin stress-fibers. The functional importance of this cellular response is not known, but it does not occur in dermal fibroblasts, suggesting that the cytoskeleton of orbital fibroblasts is relatively less stable than that of other types of fibroblasts. In addition, orbital fibroblasts from patients with Graves' disease express immunoreactive heat shock proteins in a cellular-localization pattern that differs from that of normal orbital or dermal fibroblasts.[35]

A major search has been made for an antigenic determinant in fibroblasts displaying restricted anatomic-site expression. Such a determinant, acting as an autoantigen, could link the orbit and the thyroid. Messenger RNA encoding the thyrotropin (TSH) receptor has been detected in orbital tissues.[36] This mRNA was also found in orbital fibroblasts as well as in dermal fibroblasts from all anatomic regions tested.[37] Subsequently, expression of another transcript, a 1.3-kilobase variant, encoding the extracellular domain of the TSH receptor but lacking the membrane-spanning region, was found in orbital tissue.[38] The encoded protein could not couple to G-proteins and should not be functional in a manner analogous to the receptor. This variant could serve as an autoantigen, but its widespread tissue distribution makes it a less likely cause for the site-specific involvement of the orbit in Graves' disease.

Glycosaminoglycans and Proteoglycans

Proteoglycans are very-high-molecular-weight polyanionic molecules that consist of repeating disaccharide units covalently linked to core proteins. They differ from glycoproteins in that the greatest portion of their mass derives from the carbohydrate moieties rather than vice versa. Unlike glycoproteins, the physicochemical properties of proteoglycans resemble those of carbohydrates. Proteoglycans bind cations avidly, have large molecular volumes when fully hydrated, and can bind to fibrous protein molecules to form extracellular matrix.

The carbohydrate portion of proteoglycans, glycosaminoglycans, consist of alternating amino sugar and uronic acid residues (Fig. 37-1). Hyaluronan differs from the other major types of glycosaminoglycans in that it does not contain a core protein and is not sulfated. It is the most abundant glycosaminoglycan in mammals and it is the principal species altered in thyroid diseases. In Graves' disease hyaluronan accumulates in the lesions of localized myxedema and in the soft tissues of the orbit. Because these abnormalities in glycosaminoglycan accumulation do not occur in other forms of thyrotoxicosis, they are not a direct consequence of excess thyroid hormone but instead are related to the autoimmune features of Graves' disease.

Hyaluronan is synthesized at the plasma membrane through a process that is independent of ongoing protein synthesis.[39] The alternating residues of *N*-acetylglucosamine and glucuronic acid are transferred sequentially from their respective uridine diphosphate donors in reactions catalyzed by hyaluronan synthase. A bacterial hyaluronan synthase was recently cloned,[40] but the mammalian enzyme remains poorly characterized. Hyaluronan, like the other glycosaminoglycans, has large numbers of negative charges and is always associated with cations such as sodium. Its polyanionic character yields a metachromatic staining (violet-red) pattern after reaction with toluidine blue or alcian blue.[41]

The highly diffuse hyaluronan molecule (molecular weight about 1000 kilodaltons [kd]) occupies a volume of 3.3×10^{-14} mL and has a spherical diameter of 4000 A°.[42] In contrast, a molecule of collagen with a molecular weight of 345 kd has a volume of 4.3×10^{-19} mL. Thus, an equivalent mass of hyaluronan occupies 75,000 times the volume of collagen. The highly viscous nature of hyaluronan solutions probably relates to the molecular weight of those molecules. The other glycosaminoglycans have similar rheologic properties, which are altered by proteolytic digestion. The absence of a trypsin effect on the viscosity of a hyaluronan solution suggests that a protein backbone does not contribute to the rheologic properties of that glycosaminoglycan.

The interaction of hyaluronan with cells may be mediated by specific receptors. CD44, a surface glycoprotein, is a hyaluronan receptor associated with lymphocyte homing and tumor cell migration.[43] RHAMM is another hyaluronan receptor that may mediate the ability of hyaluronan to increase cell motility.[44] The interaction of this glycosaminoglycan with its receptors may activate a complex set of signal transduction mechanisms leading to locomotion.[45]

Human skin fibroblasts synthesize large amounts of glycosaminoglycans in vitro. Hyaluronan is by far the most abundant species,[46] there being considerably less chondroitin sulfate, dermatan sulfate, and heparan sulfate. The rate of hyaluronan synthesis is highly dependent on the culture density and is greatly enhanced by simian virus 40 transformation.

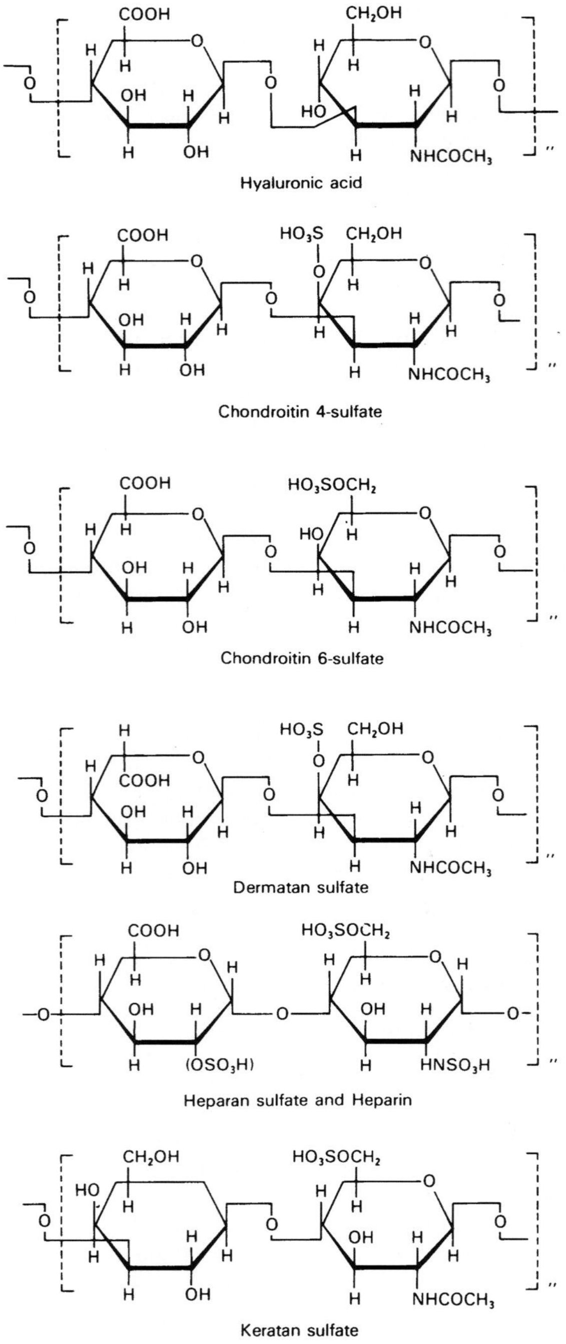

FIGURE 37-1. Molecular structures of the most abundant glycosaminoglycans.

Chondroitin sulfates are comprised of shorter chains than those in hyaluronan. They are abundant in skeletal and soft tissues and are the predominant glycosaminoglycan in cartilage. Each repeating unit in the chains consists of *N*-acetyl-D-galactosamine alternating with D-glucuronic acid in a $1 \rightarrow 3$ glycosidic linkage. The two forms, chondroitin 4-sulfate and chondroitin 6-sulfate, differ only in the position at which the sulfate occurs on the galactosamine residue. Dermatan sulfate (formerly designated chondroitin sulfate B) is composed of disaccharide units of iduronic acid residues alternating with N-acetyl-D-galactosamine. Chondroitin sulfates and dermatan sulfate are bound to core proteins by O-glycosidic linkages to serine residues.

Heparan sulfate is an important surface component of virtually all eukaryotic cells. This proteoglycan has a highly variable molecular weight, depending on the cell type. Heparan chains consist of alternating residues of glucosamine and either L-iduronic acid or D-glucuronic acid. Unlike other glycosaminoglycans, heparan sulfate contains $1\rightarrow4$ uronosyl linkages. It is abundant in blood vessel walls and in the lung.

Keratan sulfate consists of repeating disaccharides with alternating residues of N-acetylglucosamine $1\rightarrow3$ linked to galactose in a β-configuration.

GLYCOSAMINOGLYCAN DEGRADATION

Hyaluronan degradation occurs enzymatically through the actions of tissue- and species-specific hyaluronidases whose substrate specificities vary.[47] Hyaluronoglucosaminidase (testicular-type hyaluronidase, EC 3.2.1.35) acting as endo-N-acetyl-D-hexosaminidase, hydrolyzes the β $1\rightarrow4$ linkages of hyaluronan. It diminishes dramatically the viscosity of a hyaluronan solution. Other types of hyaluronidases have been useful probes in the investigation of glycosaminoglycan structure. They include leech hyaluronidase (EC 3.2.1.36), which acts as an endoglucuronidase on the β $1\rightarrow3$-glycosidic linkage, and microbial hyaluronidases (EC 4.2.99.1), which yield Δ-4,5-unsaturated disaccharides (by β elimination).

Testicular hyaluronidase is a cell-membrane glycoprotein composed of two forms with molecular weights of 61 and 67 kd. Unlike *Streptomyces* hyaluronidase, which has an absolute specificity for hyaluronan, testicular hyaluronidase also degrades chondroitin 4-sulfate, chondroitin 6-sulfate, and dermatan sulfate. The K_ms for these substrates varies widely. The products of hyaluronate degradation are even-numbered oligosaccharides, with tetrasaccharides predominating. The substrate specificity of lysosomal hyaluronoglucosaminidase from liver and other tissues is similar to that of testicular hyaluronidase. The lysosomal enzyme is apparently distinct from testicular hyaluronidase and may be necessary for the intralysosomal degradation of hyaluronan and other glycosaminoglycans. Endoglycosidases that are capable of acting on the iduronic acid residues of heparan and dermatan sulfates as well as those that degrade keratan sulfate have yet to be isolated from human tissue. The breakdown products of sulfated glycosaminoglycans are similar in size to those resulting from hyaluronan degradation.

The complete degradation of oligosaccharides to monosaccharides results from the actions of exoglycosidases such as the N-acetylhexosaminidases and glucuronidase. Desulfation of glycosaminoglycans occurs through the action of lysosomal-derived sulfatases. They are thought to act at the nonreducing end of short, sulfated chains. It would appear that the degradation of the glycosaminoglycan and protein portions of proteoglycans is well coordinated.[48]

Although hyaluronan and the sulfated glycosaminoglycans function in the extracellular compartment, both probably need to be internalized and transported into lysosomes for complete degradation to occur. Unlike hepatocytes and synovial cells, human skin fibroblasts cannot internalize hyaluronan and are therefore unable to degrade it to its monomeric components.[49] The absence of hyaluronidase activity in cultured human fibroblasts[50] and its presence in certain animal fibroblasts may reflect fundamental interspecies differences in hyaluronan metabolism. Alternatively, human cells may lose this particular phenotypic trait in culture, but may have the capacity to degrade hyaluronan in vivo. Caution must therefore be applied when extrapolating experimental results regarding the metabolism of hyaluronan obtained from animal models to human disease. The results of studies in which exogenous hyaluronan was administered to animals indicate that liver, spleen, and the lymphatics are important sites of hyaluronan degradation.[51,52] Cellular uptake of hyaluronan apparently involves receptor-mediated endocytosis,[53] and hyaluronan and chondroitin sulfate compete for the same surface receptors.[54]

Little is known about the molecular characteristics of mammalian hyaluronidases. Hemopexin, a heme-binding β-glycoprotein, may be the predominant hyaluronidase in the liver.[55] It has a conserved domain common to collagenases, stromelysin, and other enzymes involved in the degradation of the extracellular matrix. The expression of hemopexin is thought to be liver-specific, is constitutive, and is increased in the hepatic acute-phase response. It is probably one of several hyaluronidases present in serum.

THYROID HORMONE AS A REGULATOR OF GLYCOSAMINOGLYCAN SYNTHESIS

Thyroid hormone regulates the rate of synthesis of hyaluronan in human skin fibroblasts in vitro. When confluent cultures are shifted to a medium depleted of T_4 and T_3, hyaluronan synthesis increases, but the synthesis of sulfated glycosaminoglycans (chondroitin sulfate, heparan sulfate, and dermatan sulfate) is unaffected.[16,56] The addition of physiologic concentrations of T_3 (1 nmol/L [65 ng/dL] total T_3, 10 pmol/L [0.65 ng/dL] free T_3) to the culture medium inhibits the rate of synthesis of hyaluronan to levels that occur in cultures incubated in normal serum. The addition of supraphysiologic concentrations of T_3 does not further inhibit hyaluronan synthesis. Most studies of glycosaminoglycan synthesis have used metabolic labeling techniques.[16,56,57] The effects of T_3 on hyaluronan synthesis are probably not a consequence of changes in precursor pool sizes. The most convincing evidence for a direct T_3 effect derives from the finding that hyaluronan synthetase activity in cell sonicates changes in parallel with inhibition of metabolic incorporation of radiolabeled precursor.[16] The synthetase assay measures the incorporation of ^{14}C-UDP glucuronic acid into *Streptomyces* hyaluronidase– digestible material.

Besides its regulation of hyaluronan synthesis, thyroid hormone affects the synthesis of other macromolecular constituents of the extracellular matrix in fibroblast cultures. Whether the actions of T_3 in these isolated cell systems accurately reflect a physiologic role of the hormone in different tissues or in the intact organism is not known. In primary cultures of chick chondrocytes, T_3 stimulates the synthesis of hyaluronan (Kundu P, Schwartz NB, Smith TJ, unpublished observation), in contrast to its inhibitory action in fibroblast cultures.[16] These findings suggest the possibility that thyroid hormone may regulate hyaluronan synthesis in a tissue-specific manner.

T_3 directly stimulates the sulfation of glycosaminoglycans in chick embryo sternums in vitro.[58] When added alone, its effect is modest, but concomitant treatment of the explants with physiologic concentrations of T_3 and serum from hypophysectomized animals greatly (1.3- to 3-fold) enhances the sulfation. T_4 was 10-fold less potent than T_3. These effects were rapid, occurring within 1 to 4 hours after hormone addition.

The turnover of glycosaminoglycans is greatly accelerated in thyrotoxicosis. This acceleration probably reflects increases in both synthesis and degradation of several types of glycosaminoglycans. Their urinary excretion also is increased several-fold and is normalized with adequate therapy. That thyroid hormone alters hyaluronidase activity in vivo is suggested by studies in rats,[59] which disclose more rapid clearance of hyaluronan from the serum of hypothyroid rats treated with T_3 as compared with untreated rats.

OTHER REGULATORS OF GLYCOSAMINOGLYCAN SYNTHESIS

Two other compounds whose nuclear receptors, like those for T_3, are encoded by members of the c-*erb*A family of protooncogenes (see chap 9) appear to be regulators of hyaluronan synthesis in human skin fibroblasts. Corticosteroids[60,61] and retinoic acid,[62] like T_3, inhibit hyaluronan synthesis. The effects of all three compounds are additive at concentrations of each that are maximally inhibitory; thus, separate pathways mediate the actions of each. Cytokines such as interleukin-1 can stimulate glycosaminoglycan accumulation in fibroblast cultures[63] and in various other cell types. Several polypeptides derived from human tissues can stimulate macromolecular synthesis in fibroblasts.[64,65] These tissue-specific proteins, termed connective tissue-activating peptides, are secreted by leukocytes, lymphocytes, platelets, and tumors. They are capable of stimulating DNA synthesis, glucose uptake, lactate production, and glycosaminoglycan synthesis in cultured fibroblasts. The short-chain aliphatic carboxylic acid, *n*-butyrate, can both inhibit and stimulate hyaluronan synthesis in human skin and colonic fibroblasts, depending on the concentration of the compound.[66] Thus, thyroid hormone should be viewed as one of several factors that influence connective tissue metabolism in vitro. These other compounds may play a role in the connective tissue abnormalities associated with thyroid dysfunction.

Collagens

More than 14 types of collagen have been identified, and these molecules constitute the most abundant class of proteins in the body.[67] Collagens have key roles in cellular differentiation and morphogenesis as well as the maintenance of structural integrity. Collagen has a complex, multiexon gene structure. The proximate products are prepro-α peptides that are extensively processed posttranslationally. Each type of collagen is encoded by a distinct genetic locus. Three α-chains are arranged in a left-handed triple helix comprising either identical or nonidentical peptides, depending on the type of collagen. The relative abundance of the different collagens varies with respect to tissue type. Type I collagen has a wide tissue distribution and is especially abundant in skin, tendon, and bone. Type II collagen is found mainly in cartilage. Type III collagen is predominant in fetal skin and the cardiovascular system, and type IV collagen is found in the basement membrane in many tissues.

The basic structural unit of collagen is termed tropocollagen, which has a molecular weight of 285 kd. Nearly one-third of the amino acid residues are glycine and there are many proline residues as well. The hydroxylation of proline is catalyzed by prolyl hydroxylase; it also requires the presence of a reducing agent such as ascorbate. Proline becomes hydroxylated only when it is part of a large peptide chain. Collagen is glycosylated at hydroxylysine residues. The structure of collagen is stabilized greatly by intramolecular cross-linking, which occurs in nonhelical regions adjacent to the amino terminus. These cross-links involve aldehyde derivatives of two lysine residues, which undergo an aldol condensation, a reaction catalyzed by lysyl oxidase, a copper-containing enzyme that functions in the extracellular compartment.

Collagens interact with cells through specific surface receptors. These receptors have yet to be fully characterized, although a number of putative binding sites have been identified. Type I collagen binds to a single class of sites with a high affinity (K_d about 10^{-11} mol/L).

The effects of thyroid hormone on collagen synthesis may be tissue specific. In cultured human skin fibroblasts, T_3 inhibits collagen synthesis.[18] In contrast, collagen synthesis appears to be accelerated in thyrotoxic rats, and supraphysiologic concentrations of T_3 may stimulate collagen production in cultured sternal explants.

Collagenases initiate the degradation of collagen. Human skin fibroblasts synthesize and release two procollagenases, each of which is activated by trypsin. The structural gene for collagenase has been assigned to human chromosome 11, and its translational product can represent up to 1% of newly synthesized human skin fibroblast proteins.[68] The recent cloning of a full-length 2.1-kb collagenase cDNA from human synovial cells[69] and human skin fibroblasts[70] suggests that a single gene encodes the enzymes expressed in most tissues.

Thyroid hormone may influence collagen degradation through its effects on collagenase expression. T_4 increases collagenase activity in the tail of the tadpole, accounting for the resorption of that structure.[71] Thyrotoxic patients excrete greater quantities of hydroxyproline than do normal subjects, suggesting accelerated turnover of collagen in bone and soft tissues.

Fibronectin

Fibronectin exists in two forms: as a soluble plasma protein and as a cell surface protein. The cellular species has a subunit molecular weight of about 250 kd and secures cells to substratum and to adjacent cells. Two subunits form the mature protein. Cellular fibronectin forms complexes with the collagen, elastin, and hyaluronan that compose the extracellular matrix. The abundance of fibronectin on the cell surface appears to be regulated by numerous hormonal factors and is dependent on the state of cellular differentiation. In general, as cells become neoplastically transformed, they express less surface fibronectin. Moreover, as cells undergo mitosis, surface fibronectin expression diminishes substantially.

Fibronectin interacts with a recently characterized cell-surface receptor with moderate affinity; the K_d is 8×10^{-7} mol/L. There are as many as 500,000 fibronectin receptors per cell. The fibronectin receptor belongs to a family of glycoproteins called integrins. Other members of the β-integrin family function as receptors for collagen, vitronectin, intracellular adhesion molecule (ICAM), and laminin.[72] Fibronectin-binding activity derives from a 75-kd middle portion of the fibronectin molecule, although smaller fragments retain at least partial ligand binding activity.

Thyroid hormone inhibits the synthesis of fibronectin in human skin fibroblasts.[17] When confluent cultures are incubated in a medium depleted of T_3, the addition of T_3 reduces synthetic rates by 30% to 40%. The inhibitory effect is the consequence of a reduction by T_3 of steady-state fibronectin messenger RNA levels.

Other Important Components of Connective Tissue

Vitronectin is an adhesive glycoprotein involved in cell attachment and spread. The actions of this protein are independent of those ascribed to fibronectin, yet they have considerable functional similarity. Like fibronectin, vitronectin contains binding sites for heparin, collagen, and target cells. Vitronectin apparently binds to a specific cellular receptor, although the determinants of receptor specificity are still controversial. A unique vitronectin receptor, which also can function as a fibronectin receptor, has been described on neoplastic and non-neoplastic epithelial cells.

Elastin is a connective tissue protein strongly resembling collagen, and is found in skin, lung, blood vessel walls, and ligaments. This protein is the major component of the elastic fibers that are essential to the function of the organs in which it predominates. Like collagen, it contains one-third glycine residues and is enriched in proline. Its amino acid composition differs from that of collagen in that it contains few polar residues, no hydroxylysine, and little hydroxyproline.

Laminin is an adhesion glycoprotein of 900 kd that invests basement membranes. It comprises three polypeptide chains (α-chain, $β_1$-chain, and $β_2$-chain). There are discrete domains for binding collagen and heparin and for cellular attachment. Like fibronectin, laminin contains proteinase-resistant domains. Although laminin initially was thought to be an epithelial cell-attachment protein, other cell types, such as fibroblasts and sarcoma cells, can also adhere to it. Laminin interacts with the cell surface through members of the integrin family. The fibronectin receptor can also bind laminin, but with low affinity. Laminin binding to its cellular receptors is of high affinity (K_d about 2×10^{-9} mol/L) and target cells contain between 10^4 and 10^5 sites. The major binding site is a 67-kd glycoprotein that has been identified in human breast carcinoma, rat myoblasts, placenta, melanoma, and macrophages.[73,74]

MOLECULAR ACTIONS OF THYROID HORMONE ON FIBROBLASTS

The mechanisms of thyroid hormone action are discussed in detail in chapter 9. T_3 regulates the rate at which specific genes are transcribed and the abundance of various messenger RNAs. Nuclear-mediated T_3 effects are transduced through binding of T_3 to protein receptors encoded by the c-*erb*A superfamily of protooncogenes.[75] T_3 receptors, encoded by two separate genes, are expressed and regulated differentially. T_3 may also regulate cellular metabolism through its interaction with binding sites on the plasma membrane and the inner mitochondrial membrane.

Information concerning the mechanisms of action of T_3 in fibroblasts is limited. However, a priori there is no reason to suspect that the fundamental mechanisms operating in other tissues are not also involved in the hormone's action in connective tissue.

THYROID HORMONE EFFECTS ON ADIPOCYTES AND FAT METABOLISM

Thyroid hormone stimulates fatty acid biosynthesis, lipolysis, and oxidation in the liver.[76,77] Its effects on lipogenesis are mediated through the induction of lipogenic enzymes by increasing steady-state messenger RNA levels.[78] Hepatic glycerol and triglyceride synthesis is inhibited by thyrotoxicosis, which coincides with a decrease in the content of fatty acid synthetase.[79] The rate of fatty acid synthesis in the livers of euthyroid rats is threefold to fivefold higher than in hypothyroid rats and threefold to fourfold lower than in thyrotoxic rats.[80] T_3 also exerts direct effects on adipocytes.[76,81,82] In adipocytes from young rats, T_3 enhances lipogenesis by increasing the accumulation of glucose-6-phosphate and NADPH (the reduced form of nicotinamide-adenine dinucleotide phosphate)[82] and by increasing the activities of fatty acid synthetase and adenosine triphosphate citrate lyase, enzymes that partition the acetyl CoA destined for long-chain fatty acid synthesis. Thyroid status also conditions the response of fat cells to lipolytic hormones.[82] T_3 stimulates fatty acid synthesis in epididymal fat and in the remainder of the carcass. From 6% to 10% of the net differences in energy expenditure between hypothyroid and thyrotoxic rats could be attributed to lipogenesis.[80]

T_3 enhances the high affinity binding of low-density lipoprotein (LDL) to its receptors on human skin fibroblasts and, in so doing, accelerates cholesterol degradation.[15] Hypothyroid patients have an LDL receptor defect similar to that in patients with homozygous familial hypercholesterolemia.[83] T_4 administration reduces the elevated plasma LDL-cholesterol concentrations and normalizes LDL receptor-mediated catabolism as assessed by in vivo turnover studies.

ONYCHOLYSIS

Onycholysis is the process whereby a fingernail or toenail becomes detached from the underlying nail bed (Fig. 37-2). First described by Plummer, it is associated with thyro-

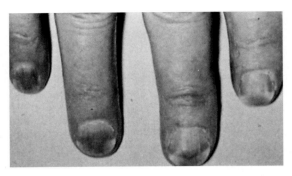

FIGURE 37-2. Photograph of the fingernails of a patient with thyrotoxicosis showing onycholysis. Note the separation of the nails from the nail beds.

toxicosis of any cause and is reversible after antithyroid therapy.

WOUND HEALING

The healing of wounds involves a complex set of events, including recruitment of circulating cells and fibroblasts and the deposition of macromolecules. Glycosaminoglycans and collagen play important roles in wound healing, a process that is influenced by several factors including thyroid hormone. In laboratory animals, large doses of T_4 reduce the tensile strength of wounds,[84] an effect that may be dependent on the action of ascorbic acid.[85] On the other hand, more modest doses of thyroid hormone may enhance wound healing and hasten wound closure.[86] Hypothyroidism results in increased ^{35}S incorporation into wounds.[87]

References

1. Smith TJ, Bahn RS, Gorman CA. Hormonal regulation of hyaluronate synthesis in cultured human fibroblasts: evidence for differences between retroocular and dermal fibroblasts. J Clin Endocrinol Metab 1989;69:1019
2. Vogelaar JPM, Erlichman E. The growth of human fibroblasts in media containing various amounts of thyroxin. Am J Cancer 1936;26:358
3. Bernal J, Refetoff S, DeGroot LJ. Abnormalities of triiodothyronine binding to lymphocyte and fibroblast nuclei from a patient with peripheral tissue-resistance to thyroid hormone action. J Clin Endocrinol Metab 1978;47:1266
4. Eil C, Fein HB, Smith TJ, et al. Nuclear binding of [^{125}I] triiodothyronine in dispersed, cultured skin fibroblasts from patients with resistance to thyroid hormone. J Clin Endocrinol Metab 1982;55:502
5. Bruning PF, Meyer WJ III, Migeon CJ. Glucocorticoid receptor in cultured human skin fibroblasts. J Steroid Biochem 1979;10:587
6. Gavin JR III, Roth J, Jen P, Freychet P. Insulin receptors in human circulating cells and fibroblasts. Proc Natl Acad Sci USA 1979;69:747
7. Griffin JE, Punyashthiti K, Wilson JD. Dehydrotestosterone binding by cultured human fibroblasts: comparison of cells from control subjects and from patients with hereditary male pseudohermaphrodism due to androgen resistance. J Clin Invest 1976;57:1342
8. Murphy LJ, Vrhovsek E, Lazarus L. Identification and characterization of specific growth hormone receptors in cultured human fibroblasts. J Clin Endocrinol Metab 1983;57:1117
9. Roscher AA, Manganiello VC, Jelsema CL, Moss J. Receptors for bradykinin in intact cultured human fibroblasts. J Clin Invest 1983;72:626
10. Liberman UA, Eil C, Marx SJ. Resistance to 1,25-dihydroxyvitamin D. Association with heterogeneous defects in cultured skin fibroblasts. J Clin Invest 1983;71:192
11. Philips PD, Kuhnle E, Cristofalo VJ. [^{125}I] EGF binding ability is stable throughout the replicative life-span of WI-38 cells. J Cell Physiol 1983;114:311
12. Smith TJ, Kottke RJ, Lum H, Andersen TT. Human orbital fibroblasts in culture bind and respond to endothelin. Am J Physiol 1993;265:C138
13. Lacroix A, Anderson GD, Lippman MC. Binding of retinoids to human fibroblast cell lines and their effects on growth. Proc NY Acad Sci 1981;359:405
14. Yoshizato K, Kikuyama S, Shioya N. Stimulation of glucose utilization and lactate production in cultured human fibroblasts by thyroid hormone. Biochim Biophys Acta 1980;627:23
15. Chait A, Bierman EL, Albers JJ. Regulatory role of triiodothyronine in the degradation of low density lipoprotein by cultured human skin fibroblasts. J Clin Endocrinol Metab 1979;48:887
16. Smith TJ, Murata Y, Horwitz AL, Philipson L, Refetoff S. Regulation of glycosaminoglycan synthesis by thyroid hormone in vitro. J Clin Invest 1982;70:1066
17. Murata Y, Ceccarelli P, Refetoff S, Horwitz AL, Matsui N. Thyroid hormone inhibits fibronectin synthesis by cultured human skin fibroblasts. J Clin Endocrinol Metab 1987;64:334
18. de Rycker C, Vandalem J-L, Hennen G. Effect of 3,5,3'-triiodothyronine on collagen synthesis by cultured human skin fibroblasts. FEBS Lett 1984;174:34
19. Davis R, Smith TJ. Triiodothyronine and dexamethasone regulate the abundance of specific cellular proteins in human skin fibroblasts in vitro. Endocr Res 1987;13:61
20. Refetoff S, Matalon R, Bigazzi M. Metabolism of L-thyroxine (T_4) and L-triiodothyronine (T_3) by human fibroblasts in tissue culture: evidence for cellular binding proteins and conversion of T_4 to T_3. Endocrinology 1972;91:934
21. Kaplan MM, Pan C, Gordon PR, Lee J-K, Gilchrest BA. Human epidermal keratinocytes in culture convert thyroxine to 3,5,3'-triiodothyronine by type II iodothyronine deiodination: a novel endocrine function of the skin. J Clin Endocrinol Metab 1988;66:815
22. Smith TJ, Bahn RS, Gorman CA. Connective tissue, glycosaminoglycans, and diseases of the thyroid. Endocr Rev 1989;10:366
23. Phipps RP, Penny DP, Keng P, et al. Characterization of two major populations of lung fibroblasts: distinguishing morphology and discordant display of Thy-1 and class II MHC. Am J Respir Cell Mol Biol 1989;1:65
24. Fries KM, Blieden T, Looney RJ, et al. Evidence of fibroblast heterogeneity and the role of fibroblast subpopulations in fibrosis. Clin Immunol Immunopath 1994;72:283
25. Smith TJ, Ahmed A, Hogg MG, Higgins PJ. Interferon gamma is an inducer of plasminogen activator inhibitor type-1 in human orbital fibroblasts. Am J Physiol 1992;263:C24
26. Smith TJ, Higgins PJ. Interferon gamma regulation of de novo protein synthesis in human dermal fibroblasts in culture is anatomic site-dependent. J Invest Dermatol 1993;100:288
27. Hogg MG, Evans CH, Smith TJ. Leukoregulin induces plasminogen activator inhibitor type-1 in human orbital fibroblasts. Am J Physiol 1995;269:359
28. Smith TJ, Higgins PJ. Bidimensional gel electrophoretic analysis of protein synthesis and response to interferon-r in cultured human dermal fibroblasts. Biochim Biophys Acta 1993;1181:300

29. Imai Y, Odajima R, Inoue Y, Shishiba Y. Effect of growth factors on hyaluronan and proteoglycan synthesis by retroocular tissue fibroblasts of Graves' ophthalmopathy in culture. Acta Endocrinol 1992;126:541

30. Smith TJ, Bahn RS, Gorman CA, Cheavens M. Stimulation of glycosaminoglycan accumulation by interferon gamma in cultured human retroocular fibroblasts. J Clin Endocrinol Metab 1991; 72:1169

31. Smith TJ, Wang H-S, Evans CH. Leukoregulin is a potent inducer of hyaluronan synthesis in cultured orbital fibroblasts. Am J Physiol 1995;268:C382

32. Higgins PJ, Smith TJ. Pleiotropic action of interferon gamma in human orbital fibroblasts. Biochim Biophys Acta 1993;1181:23

33. Smith TJ, Wang H-S, Hogg MG, Henrikson RC, Keese CR, Giaever I. Prostaglandin E_2 elicits a morphological change in cultured orbital fibroblasts from patients with Graves' ophthalmopathy. Proc Natl Acad Sci U S A 1994;91:5094

34. Goto M, Sasano M, Yamanaka H, et al. Spontaneous production of an interleukin 1-like factor by cloned rheumatoid synovial cells in long-term culture. J Clin Invest 1987;80:786

35. Heufelder AE, Wenzel BE, Bahn RS. Cell surface localization of a 72 kilodalton heat shock protein in retroocular fibroblasts from patients with Graves' ophthalmopathy. J Clin Endocrinol Metab 1992;74:732

36. Feliciello A, Porcellini A, Ciullo I, Bonavolonta G, Avvedimento EV, Fenzi G. Expression of thyrotropin-receptor mRNA in healthy and Graves' disease retro-orbital tissue. Lancet 1993;342:337

37. Heufelder AE, Dutton CM, Sarkar G, Donovan KA, Bahn RS. Detection of TSH receptor RNA in cultured fibroblasts from patients with Graves' ophthalmopathy and pretibial dermopathy. Thyroid 1993;3:297

38. Paschke R, Metcalfe A, Alcalde L, Vassart G, Weetman A, Ludgate M. Presence of nonfunctional thyrotropin receptor variant transcripts in retroocular and other tissues. J Clin Endocrinol Metab 1994;79:1234

39. Philipson LH, Schwartz NB. Subcellular localization of hyaluronate synthetase in oligodendroglioma cells. J Biol Chem 1984;259:5017

40. DeAngelis PL, Papaconstantinou J, Weigel PH. Molecular cloning, identification, and sequence of the hyaluronan synthase gene from group A *Streptococcus pyogenes*. J Biol Chem 1993;268:19181

41. Schubert M, Hamerman D. Metachromasia: chemical theory and histochemical use. J Histochem Cytochem 1956;4:159

42. Schubert M. Intercellular macromolecules containing polysaccharides. Biophys J 1964;4(Suppl):119

43. Stamenkovic I, Amiot M, Pesando JM, Seed B. A lymphocyte molecule implicated in lymph node homing is a member of the cartilage link protein family. Cell 1989;56:1057

44. Yang B, Zhang L, Turley EA. Identification of two hyaluronan-binding domains in the hyaluronan receptor RHAMM. J Biol Chem 1993;268:8617

45. Hall CL, Wang C, Lange LA, Turley EA. Hyaluronan and hyaluronan receptor RHAMM promote focal adhesion turnover and transient tyrosine kinase activity. J Cell Biol 1994;126:575

46. Hopwood JJ, Dorfman A. Glycosaminoglycan synthesis by cultured human skin fibroblasts after transformation with simian virus 40. J Biol Chem 1977;252:4777

47. Kresse H, Glössl J. Glycosaminoglycan degradation. Adv Enzymol Relat Areas Mol Biol 1987;60:217

48. Gross JI, Mathews MB, Dorfman A. Sodium chondroitin sulfate-protein complexes of cartilage. J Biol Chem 1960;235:2889

49. Truppe W, Basner R, von Figura K, Kresse H. Uptake of hyaluronate by cultured cells. Biochem Biophys Res Commun 1977;78:713

50. Arbogast B, Hopwood JJ, Dorfman A. Absence of hyaluronidase in cultured human skin fibroblasts. Biochem Biophys Res Commun 1975;67:376

51. Eriksson S, Fraser JRE, Laurent TC, Pertoft H, Smedsrod B. Endothelial cells are a site of uptake and degradation of hyaluronic acid in the liver. Exp Cell Res 1983;144:223

52. Fraser JRE, Laurent TC, Pertoft H, Baxter E. Plasma clearance, tissue distribution and metabolism of hyaluronic acid injected intravenously in the rabbit. Biochem J 1981;200:415

53. Smedsrod B, Pertoft H, Eriksson S, Fraser JR, Laurent TC. Studies *in vitro* on the uptake and degradation of sodium hyaluronate in rat liver endothelial cells. Biochem J 1984;223:617

54. Smedsrod B, Kjellen L, Pertoft H. Endocytosis and degradation of chondroitin sulphate by liver endothelial cells. Biochem J 1985;229:63

55. Zhu L, Hope TJ, Hall J, et al. Molecular cloning of a mammalian hyaluronidase reveals identity with hemopexin, a serum heme-binding protein. J Biol Chem 1994;269:32092

56. Smith TJ, Horwitz AL, Refetoff S. The effect of thyroid hormone on glycosaminoglycan accumulation in human skin fibroblasts. Endocrinology 1981;108:2397

57. Shishiba Y, Yanagishita M, Hascoll VC. Effect of thyroid hormone deficiency on proteoglycan synthesis by human skin fibroblast cultures. Connect Tissue Res 1988;17:119

58. Audhya TK, Gibson KD. Enhancement of somatomedin titres of normal and hypopituitary sera by addition of L-triiodothyronine *in vitro* at physiological concentrations. Proc Natl Acad Sci U S A 1975;72:604

59. Schiller S, Slover GA, Dorfman A. Effect of the thyroid gland on metabolism of acid mucopolysaccharides in skin. Biochim Biophys Acta 1962;58:27

60. Smith TJ. Dexamethasone regulation of glycosaminoglycan synthesis in human skin fibroblasts: similar effects of glucocorticoid and thyroid hormones. J Clin Invest 1984;74:2157

61. Smith TJ. Glucocorticoid regulation of glycosaminoglycan synthesis in cultured human skin fibroblasts: evidence for a receptor-mediated mechanism involving effects on specific de novo protein synthesis. Metabolism 1988;37:179

62. Smith TJ. Retinoic acid inhibition of hyaluronate synthesis in human skin fibroblasts in culture. J Clin Endocrinol Metab 1990;70:655

63. Postlethwaite AE, Smith Jr GN, Lachman LD, et al. Stimulation of glycosaminoglycan synthesis in cultured human dermal fibroblasts by interleukin I. J Clin Invest 1989;83:629

64. Castor CW, Furlong AM, Carter-Su C. Connective tissue activation: stimulation of glucose transport by connective tissue activating peptide III. Biochemistry 1985;24:1762

65. Myers SL, Castor CW. Connective tissue activation. XV. Stimulation of glycosaminoglycan and DNA synthesis by a polymorphonuclear leukocyte factor. Arthritis Rheum 1980;23:556

66. Smith TJ. n-Butyrate inhibition of hyaluronate synthesis in human cultured fibroblasts. J Clin Invest 1987;79:1493

67. Ramirez F, Di Liberto M. Complex and diversified regulatory programs control the expression of vertebrate collagen genes. FASEB J 1990;4:1616

68. Valle K-J, Dauer EA. Biosynthesis of collagenase by human skin fibroblasts in monolayer culture. J Biol Chem 1979; 254:10115

69. Brinckerhoff CE, Ruby PL, Austin SD, Fini ME, White HD. Molecular cloning of human synovial cell collagenase and selection of a single gene from genomic DNA. J Clin Invest 1987; 79:542

70. Goldberg GI, Wilhelm SM, Kronberger A, Bauer EA, Grant GA, Eisen AZ. Human fibroblast collagenase: complete primary structure and homology to an oncogene transformation induced rat protein. J Biol Chem 1986;261:6600

71. Davis BP, Jeffrey JJ, Eisen AZ, Derby A. The induction of collagenase by thyroxine in resorbing tadpole tailfin in vitro. Dev Biol 1975;44:217

72. Akiyama SK, Nagata K, Yamada KM. Cell surface receptors for extracellular matrix components. Biochim Biophys Acta 1990;1031:91

73. Douville PJ, Harvey WJ, Carbonetto S. Isolation and partial characterization of high affinity laminin receptors in neural cells. J Biol Chem 1988;263:14964

74. Wewer UM, Liotta LA, Jaye M, et al. Altered levels of laminin receptor mRNA in various human carcinoma cells that have different abilities to bind laminin. Proc Natl Acad Sci U S A 1986;83:7137

75. Evans RM. The steroid and thyroid hormone receptor superfamily. Science 1988;240:889

76. Diamant S, Gorin E, Shafrir E. Enzyme activities related to fatty acid synthesis in liver and adipose tissue of rats treated with triiodothyronine. Eur J Biochem 1972;26:553

77. Muller MJ, Seitz HJ. Thyroid hormone action on intermediary metabolism II. Lipid metabolism in hypo- and hyperthyroidism. Klin Wochenschr 1984;62:49

78. Goodridge AG, Black DW, Wilson SB, Goldman MJ. Regulation of genes for enzymes involved in fatty acid synthesis. Ann NY Acad Sci 1986;478:46

79. Roncari DAK, Murthy VK. Effects of thyroid hormones on enzymes involved in fatty acid and glycerolipid synthesis. J Biol Chem 1975;250:4134

80. Freake HC, Schwartz HL, Oppenheimer JH. The regulation of lipogenesis by thyroid hormone and its contribution to thermogenesis. Endocrinology 1989;125:2868

81. Gnoni GV, Landriscina C, Quagliariello E. Fatty acid biosynthesis in adipose tissue and lung subcellular fractions of thyrotoxic rats. FEBS Lett 1980;122:37

82. Correze C, Berriche S, Tamayo L, Nunez J. Effect of thyroid hormones and cAMP on some lipogenic enzymes of the fat cell. Eur J Biochem 1982;122:387

83. Thompson GR, Soutar AK, Spengel FA, Jadhav A, Gauigan SJ, Myant NB. Defects of receptor-mediated low density lipoprotein catabolism in homozygous familial hypercholesterolemia and hypothyroidism in vivo. Proc Natl Acad Sci U S A 1981;78 2591

84. Moltke E. Wound healing influenced by thyroxine and thyrotrophic hormone: a tensiometric study. Proc Soc Exp Biol Med 1955;88:596

85. Moltke E. Role of ascorbic acid in wound healing influenced by D, L-thyroxine. Acta Endocrinol 1956;23:105

86. Barclay THC, Cuthbertson DP, Isaacs A. The influence of metabolic stimulants on wound healing: the influence of thyroid and 2,4-f dinitrophenol. Q J Exp Physiol 1944;32:309

87. Moltke E, Lorenzen I. Effect of thyroidectomy and thyroxine on the mucopolysaccharides of wounds and skin. Acta Endocrinol 1960;34:407

Werner and Ingbar's The Thyroid, Seventh Edition,
edited by Lewis E. Braverman and Robert D. Utiger.
Lippincott–Raven Publishers, Philadelphia, © 1996

38

The Cardiovascular System in Thyrotoxicosis

Irwin Klein

Gerald S. Levey

The cardiovascular manifestations of thyrotoxicosis have been recognized for almost two centuries[1] and are some of the most profound and characteristic symptoms and signs of the disorder.[2,3] Understanding the cardiac physiology of thyrotoxicosis can further our insight into the actions of thyroid hormone and provide a rational basis for the management of thyrotoxic patients.[4,5] In this chapter we will review the molecular, cellular, and organ system responses to excessive thyroid hormone as it affects the cardiovascular system.

CARDIOVASCULAR HEMODYNAMICS

The changes in cardiovascular hemodynamics that accompany both naturally occurring and experimentally induced thyrotoxicosis in humans and animals are summarized in Table 38-1.[6,7] There are predictable decreases in systemic vascular resistance and increases in cardiac output, systolic blood pressure, heart rate, left ventricular ejection fraction, cardiac contractility and mass, and blood volume.[7]

One of the earliest cardiovascular responses to thyroid hormone administration in both humans and animals is a decrease in systemic vascular resistance.[8] It may decrease by as much as 50% to 70%, resulting in increased blood flow to the skin, muscles, kidneys, and heart.[6] The effects of thyroid hormone on systemic vascular resistance may be direct[9] or mediated by adrenergic receptors, because beta-adrenergic blockade blunts the thyroid hormone-mediated decrease in systemic vascular resistance and the accompanying increase in cardiac output.[10,11] Because the increase in forearm blood flow, which includes both skin and muscle, can be partially abolished by atropine, an acetylcholine-mediated vasomotor

response is also implicated.[12] The importance of the decrease in systemic vascular resistance in increasing cardiac output is further suggested by the observation that vasoconstrictor drugs, when administered to thyrotoxic patients, reverse the decrease in systemic vascular resistance and simultaneously decrease cardiac output.[13]

Thyroid hormone itself is a vasodilator that acts directly on vascular smooth muscle cells to cause relaxation.[8,9,11] This response to thyroid hormone may result from a direct effect on vascular smooth muscle cells or may be the result of thyroid hormone action on vascular endothelial cells to release other vasoactive substances such as nitric oxide.[14]

Increased cardiac contractility accompanies both spontaneously occurring and experimentally induced thyrotoxicosis.[2,15–18] Measures of systolic contractility, such as the rate of ventricular pressure development or velocity of contraction, are uniformly increased.[15] In addition, noninvasive measures of diastolic performance, including the rate of diastolic relaxation and compliance, are supranormal in thyrotoxic patients.[18]

The process of cardiac contraction, which is mediated by the interdigitation of the two major contractile proteins, actin and myosin, requires myosin-catalyzed ATP-hydrolysis and has an absolute requirement for calcium.[5,19] One determinant of systolic contractility is the maximum velocity of muscle fiber shortening, which correlates with the inherent ATPase activity of the myosin molecule.[16] There are two cardiac myosin isoforms, each characterized by the level of ATPase enzymatic activity located in the globular head structure of the myosin heavy chain molecule. The alpha-myosin heavy chain isoform is associated with a higher level of ATPase activity than the myosin composed of heavy chains of beta-myosin.

TABLE 38-1.
Cardiovascular Hemodynamics in Thyrotoxicosis

Parameter	Change	Comments
Systemic vascular resistance	↓	50%–70% lower, similar to exercise
Cardiac output	↑	200%–300% increase
Blood pressure		
Systolic	↑	Especially in elderly
Diastolic	↓	
Heart rate	↑	Most often sinus tachycardia; 10%–15% of patients have atrial fibrillation
Cardiac contractility	↑	Systolic and diastolic function both enhanced
Cardiac mass	↑	Hypertrophy from increased cardiac work
Blood volume	↑	Increased serum erythropoietin and sodium reabsorption

Each myosin heavy chain isomer is encoded by a different gene that is under separate transcriptional control.[20,21] The distribution of these two isomers of myosin in rats is under the control of various epigenetic and humoral factors including thyroid hormone.[2,5,21–23] Thyroid hormone acts to maintain or enhance the expression of the alpha-myosin heavy chain gene through changes at the level of gene transcription and by posttranscriptional mechanisms.[24] Hypothyroidism in rats results in a decrease in alpha-myosin and a predominance of beta-myosin in the heart.[20–23] Thus, thyroid hormone acting at the cellular level increases the rate of muscle fiber shortening as a consequence of the higher myosin ATPase activity inherent in the alpha-myosin heavy chain protein.

The ability to measure changes in expression of the genes for heavy-chain myosin in cardiac myocytes has led to major advances in our understanding in the cellular actions of triiodothyronine (T_3).[5,21,23,25] However, significant species differences in myosin heavy chain gene expression exist, such that samples of heart muscle obtained from euthyroid patients at the time of autopsy were found to contain mostly heavy chains of beta-myosin with low ATPase activity.[4,26] In a thyrotoxic patient who died suddenly, the ventricular myosin consisted predominantly of the beta-myosin heavy chain isoform.[27] Thus, in contrast to animals, it appears unlikely that thyroid hormone is the major determinant of myosin isoform expression or that significant alterations in myosin gene expression occur in humans with thyroid disease.[4]

Calcium release from and re-uptake into the sarcoplasmic reticulum of cardiac muscle regulates the rate of ventricular contraction and relaxation.[28] The gene for the cardiac-specific sarcoplasmic reticulum calcium ATPase that regulates the sequestration of calcium in the sarcoplasmic reticulum during diastole is activated by thyroid hormone.[5,29] In addition, the expression of the protein phospholamban, which is a negative regulator of calcium uptake by the sarcoplasmic reticulum, is inhibited by thyroxine (T_4) and T_3.[30] Taken together, these ob-

servations could account for the increase in calcium intake in the sarcoplasmic reticulum and explain the increased rate of development of systolic tension and diastolic relaxation in the heart of thyrotoxic patients.[15,16,31]

Increases in resting heart rate are characteristic of thyrotoxicosis; over 90% of patients have resting tachycardia and many have heart rates greater than 120 beats per minute.[32–34] The increases in heart rate and in left ventricular ejection fraction account for the increased cardiac work and cardiac output characteristic of thyrotoxicosis (Table 38-1).[6,35] Since these changes occur in the setting of reduced systemic vascular resistance, they are in many ways analogous to the hemodynamic responses to exercise and other high cardiac output states.[7,19]

Thyrotoxicosis is associated with an increase in blood volume.[35] There is a correlation between both blood volume and basal metabolic rate.[36] Serum erythropoietin concentrations also vary directly with changes in serum T_4 concentrations. These changes, coupled with increased renal sodium reabsorption, may explain the 25% increase in total blood volume, plasma volume, and erythrocyte mass reported for patients with thyrotoxicosis.[35,36]

CARDIOVASCULAR PATHOPHYSIOLOGY

Understanding the pathophysiology of the changes in cardiovascular function in thyrotoxicosis requires that two independent but interrelated hypotheses be addressed. The first proposes that thyroid hormone has direct cellular effects on the heart,[5] and the second that thyroid hormone exerts predominantly indirect effects on the heart. The latter would result from effects on the peripheral circulation, either a direct vasodilatory action or an indirect vasodilatory action (caused by thyroid hormone-stimulation of oxygen consumption of skeletal muscle, liver, and other organ systems), or both[2] (Fig. 38-1). Recognition of a hyperadrenergic component must be acknowledged to understand fully the cardiovascular manifestations of thyrotoxicosis, because many of the physiologic responses are ameliorated by beta-adrenergic blockade.[37,38]

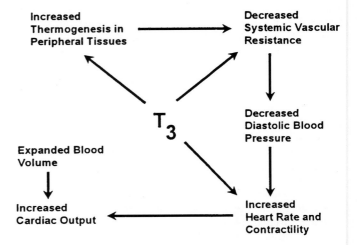

FIGURE 38-1. Thyroid hormone effects upon the heart and peripheral vascular system.

Cardiac Effects

The cellular actions of T_4 and T_3 on cardiac myocytes are mediated both at the level of the cell nucleus and at extranuclear sites.[5,14,21,39] T_3 exerts its genomic effects by binding to specific nuclear receptors that bind to specific DNA sequences (thyroid hormone response elements) located on target genes[40–42] (see chap 9). Thyroid hormone response elements have been identified on the promoter sequences for alpha-myosin heavy chain, sarcoplasmic reticulum calcium-ATPase, alpha-cardiac actin, and Na$^+$,K$^+$-ATPase, all of which are important regulatory proteins in the heart[2,5,21,23] (Table 38-2). Two T_3-binding isoforms of the thyroid hormone receptor (thyroid receptor-α_1 and thyroid receptor-β_1) and the non-T_3 binding isoform (α_2) have been identified in left ventricular muscle and in isolated cultured cardiac myocytes.[22,41] T_3 has direct effects on the rate of gene transcription in isolated cardiac myocytes.[21] These effects are associated with a 6- to 24-hour latent period and occur in association with changes in myocyte RNA content and protein synthesis.[5] T_3 also modulates the stability of mRNA and the rate of protein translation.[24] In the intact heart the myocytes are a minority of the total cells, but it is primarily these cells that respond to changes in cardiac work load and hormonal stimulation. Since thyroid receptors and thyroid-response elements are present in mammalian myocytes it is not surprising that T_3 has direct, nuclear-mediated effects on the heart.[5,29,41,42]

Both thyroid receptor-α and -β are expressed in cardiac myocytes, but the precise role of the different receptor isoforms in the heart has not been defined.[41] Mutations in the thyroid hormone receptor have been identified in the syndrome of thyroid hormone resistance.[43] The identification of a child with a homozygous mutation in thyroid receptor-β who had some cardiac manifestations (tachycardia) of thyrotoxicosis suggests a diminished role for this receptor isoform in the heart.[44] In addition, T_3 itself regulates the expression of thyroid receptor isoforms in myocytes, suggesting a feedback-type regulatory mechanism of T_3 on cellular hormone responsiveness.[22,41]

Plasma membrane Na$^+$,K$^+$-ATPase is responsive to thyroid hormone in heart and liver.[45,46] Similar to myosin, this enzyme is composed of multiple subunits and exists in several isoenzymic forms. Experimentally, thyroid hormone increases the expression of specific isoforms and the overall activity of Na$^+$,K$^+$-ATPase primarily in thyroid hormone-deficient states.[45] Other cardiac proteins that are directly thyroid hormone-responsive, and may in part mediate some of the changes in cardiovascular hemodynamics in thyrotoxicosis, include atrial naturetic hormone, alpha-actin, and the malic enzyme.[5]

In contrast to the genomic effects of thyroid hormone on the heart, a constellation of effects suggest a non-nuclear site of action. These responses, because of their rapid time course and lack of associated changes in mRNA or protein synthesis, imply action of thyroid hormone at the plasma membrane, sarcoplasmic reticulum, and mitochondria.[39] Effects at the plasma membrane include enhanced sinoatrial node pacemaker activity and calcium, sodium, and glucose transport.[11] Increased sarcoplasmic reticulum calcium transport and various effects on the mitochondria, including increases in nucleotide translocase activity, magnesium flux, and oxidative phosphorylation, may occur through non-nuclear pathways.[39]

The importance of the non-nuclear effects derive primarily from their rapid onset of action, and they may explain the results of some recent studies of the effects of T_3 in patients undergoing cardiopulmonary bypass surgery.[8,11,47] In these studies parenteral T_3 administration resulted in increases in cardiac output within 120 minutes.[8,47] Studies in animals confirm that T_3 can rapidly increase cardiac contractility.[48] A non-nuclear effect also explains the rapid chronotropic response of atrial cells to T_3.[49]

Peripheral Circulatory Effects

In thyrotoxicosis systemic vascular resistance is reduced from normal values (1700 dynes/sec/cm^{-5}) to values as low as 500 to 700 dynes/sec/cm^{-5}.[6,35] In animals given T_3 the decrease is rapid and occurs before changes in heart rate or cardiac contractility.[10] The decrease in resistance occurs in many organs. The result is an increase in blood flow to these organs, which serves to meet the increased demands for oxygen and substrate delivery.[7] This decrease in vascular resistance may result from either a local response to increased tissue formation of lactic acid or from a direct vasodilatory effect of T_3 on vascular smooth muscle cells.[9] As systemic vascular resistance declines,

TABLE 38-2.
Effect of Thyroid Hormone on Cardiac Gene Expression

Gene	Effect	Comment
Myosin heavy chain		Effect mainly in small animals
α	↑	Fast myosin
β	↓	Slow myosin
Sarcoplasmic reticulum Ca^{++}-ATPase	↑	May determine ventricular diastolic function through calcium regulation
Phospholamban	↓	Acts in concert with sarcoplasmic reticulum Ca-ATPase
Na,K-ATPase	↑	Tissue and isoform specific, regulation of transmembrane ion flux
Atrial naturetic hormone	↑	Reduces renal salt and water reabsorption, lowers blood pressure
Malic enzyme	↑	A lipogenic enzyme
Glucose transporter	↑	Isoform specific to alter glucose uptake
β-Adrenergic receptor	↑	Tissue specific, may in part explain the change in adrenergic tone characteristic of thyrotoxicosis through changes in adenylyl cyclase activity
G$_s$-protein*	↑	
G$_i$-protein†	↓	

*The guanine nucleotide–binding protein that mediates stimulation of adenylyl cyclase activity.
†The guanine nucleotide–binding protein that mediates inhibition of adenylyl cyclase activity.

so does diastolic blood pressure, which in turn causes a reflex increase in heart rate, stroke volume, and cardiac output (see Fig. 38-1). The reflex nature of these changes is further supported by the observation that pharmacologic prevention of the fall in systemic vascular resistance with the α-adrenergic agonist phenylephrine or the β-adrenergic antagonist propranolol mitigates or prevents the inotropic and chronotropic responses to T_3.[10–13]

Additional evidence for indirect effects of thyroid hormone on the heart comes from evaluation of the cardiac hypertrophic (growth) response to thyrotoxicosis. In humans[31] and animals,[4] chronic thyrotoxicosis causes variable degrees of cardiac hypertrophy. If this hypertrophy was caused by a direct effect of thyroid hormone on cardiac protein synthesis, then it should not be affected by β-adrenergic blockade, but in fact both propranolol and bisoprolol either block or reverse thyroid hormone-induced cardiac hypertrophy in animals and humans.[50,51] These results support the postulate that increased cardiac work is the major mediator of the cardiac growth response of thyrotoxicosis. Further confirmation comes from experiments with heterotopically transplanted hearts, in which the myocytes are exposed to increased serum thyroid hormone concentrations without the accompanying increase in cardiac work.[52] Under these circumstances, cardiac hypertrophy does not occur but changes in cardiac gene expression and heart rate do.[24]

The changes in cardiovascular hemodynamics also induce substantial changes in renal physiology. With the fall in systemic vascular resistance there is a decline in renal perfusion pressure that stimulates the release of renin, leading to increases in the production of angiotensin.[53] The resultant transient increase in aldosterone production augments renal sodium reabsorption and expands total body sodium content and plasma and blood volume[35,36] (see chap 40).

Whereas the changes in systemic vascular resistance characteristically occur in association with chronic thyrotoxicosis, thyroid hormone has acute effects. Within hours after T_3 administration to normal animals, peripheral vascular resistance decreases, potentially reflecting a direct effect of T_3 on arterial vascular smooth muscle tone.[8,9] Similarly, T_3 can rapidly (within minutes) cause relaxation of vascular smooth muscle cells in culture.[9] Therefore, T_3 may have acute as well as chronic vasodilator actions.[13,14]

Thyroid Hormone–Catecholamine Interactions

Many of the cardiovascular symptoms and signs of thyrotoxicosis mimic those that occur in states of increased β-adrenergic activity, such as pheochromocytoma.[37] These symptoms and signs include palpitations, tachycardia, widened pulse pressure, exercise intolerance, and cardiac hypertrophy.[38] The overlap of symptoms and signs between thyrotoxicosis and hyperadrenergic states suggested long ago that catecholamine metabolism might be altered in thyrotoxicosis,[3,37,54] but in fact plasma norepinephrine and epinephrine concentrations are normal or low and urinary excretion of catecholamine metabolites (including metanephrine, vanillylmandelic acid, and normetanephrine) is normal[3,54] (see chap 46). Sensitivity to catecholamines, as judged by increases in heart rate and

systolic blood pressure in response to administration of catecholamines, may be increased but is more often normal.[37,55–57]

Alternative explanations for the hyperadrenergic state include increased β-adrenergic receptor density in cardiac muscle[58,59]; an increase in catecholamine turnover at neural synapses or in the affinity of adrenergic receptors for catecholamines; an increase in the quantity of guanine nucleotide-binding (G) proteins, both G_s (stimulatory) and G_i (inhibitory)(see Table 38-2), that couple adrenergic receptors to adenylyl cyclase[60]; or a separate neurotransmitter that mimics the effects of catecholamines.[61] Finally, thyroid hormone could exert its actions independently of catecholamines, but by a common signalling pathway.[37] This latter possibility is supported by the structural similarities between T_4 and T_3 and catecholamines and by evidence that T_3 is taken up and released at nerve synapses and so might function as a sympathomimetic neurotransmitter.[61] Regardless of the mechanism, the similarities of the manifestations of thyrotoxicosis and the hyperadrenergic state have important implications for treatment of thyrotoxicosis.[37,38]

CLINICAL MANIFESTATIONS

The cardiovascular manifestations of thyrotoxicosis constitute some of the most profound and characteristic symptoms and signs of the disorder (Table 38-3).[2,3,62] The majority of patients have palpitations, which refer to both a rapid heart rate as well as the sensation of forceful cardiac contraction.[32,34,38,62] Occasional atrial rhythm disturbances, including atrial fibrillation or flutter, may produce the sensation of either an irregular or a rapid heart rate, or both. Patients often note that their heart rate declines slowly after exercise, with it staying above 90 beats per minute at rest in over 90% of patients.[32] The sensation of exercising while at rest reflects the continuous maintenance of a high cardiac output.[2,6]

The heart rate also is elevated during sleep, and the diurnal variation in the heart rate is less than normal, suggesting autonomic dysfunction.[3,7] Alterations in parasympathetic tone

TABLE 38-3.
Cardiovascular Symptoms of Thyrotoxicosis

Symptoms	Prevalence (%)
Palpitations	85
Exercise intolerance	65
Dyspnea on exertion	45
Angina pectoris	3–5
Orthopnea	3
Tachycardia	95
Atrial fibrillation	10–15
Hyperdynamic precordium	75
Widened pulse pressure	75
Cardiac flow murmurs	50
Pedal edema	5
Third (S_3) heart sound	3

are further supported by the loss of normal heart rate variability as measured by changes in the R-R interval on the electrocardiogram.

Other common cardiovascular symptoms include exercise intolerance and dyspnea on exertion.[18,64] The latter is most pronounced with sustained activity, but may arise with activity as limited as climbing a flight of stairs. Although thought to reflect impaired cardiac performance,[64] these symptoms are probably caused by weakness of skeletal and respiratory muscles.[2,65] Treatment of thyrotoxic patients with β-adrenergic antagonist drugs results in improvement in both muscle function and exercise performance within 24 hours.[62,65] Whether β-adrenergic blockade also improves exercise performance through a salutory effect on cardiovascular hemodynamics in these patients is discussed later.

In older patients the initial cardiac manifestations of thyrotoxicosis may be limited to resting tachycardia.[31] In this group of patients other classic thyrotoxic symptoms may be absent, possibly due to the relative paucity of adrenergic activity.[37,62,66] With the onset of atrial fibrillation,[67–69] the extent of cardiovascular manifestations may be exaggerated, leading to heart failure, peripheral edema, or tachypnea.[4,68]

Thyrotoxic patients may have chest pain similar in almost all respects to angina pectoris,[3,70] probably caused by either relative myocardial ischemia due to a mismatch between cardiac oxygen supply and demand[71] or coronary artery spasm.[70] The anginal symptoms almost always disappear after treatment of the thyrotoxicosis. In older patients, however, the imposition of increased myocardial oxygen demand due to thyrotoxicosis may unmask coronary artery disease,[2,71] and pathologic examination may reveal varying degrees of hypertrophy of left ventricular myocytes. In some patients the heart may be dilated consistent with impaired function.[27] A decrease in connective tissue content and myocyte necrosis or myocarditis have been reported in pathologic studies,[3] but they do not account for the development of heart failure.

Physical Examination

The measured heart rate is fast, often with bounding pulses in the larger arteries due to widened pulse pressure with elevated systolic and lowered diastolic blood pressure[6,7] (see Table 38-3). The mean blood pressure is most often normal. A subset of older patients may have an exaggerated rise in systolic blood pressure due to loss of the elastic components of the larger (capacitance) arteries; their mean blood pressure may also be elevated.[7]

The enhanced cardiac contractility can be evident from a rapid rise in the carotid upstroke, a sharp and easily audible first heart sound, and a hyperdynamic precordium and apical impulse. Auscultation may reveal a systolic murmur caused by rapid flow of blood through the aortic outflow tract. Systolic murmurs due to regurgitant flow across the mitral valve may arise from valve prolapse, left ventricular dilatation, or dysfunction of the mitral valve apparatus.[72–74] A "scratch" can occasionally be heard in the pulmonic area (second left intercostal space), corresponding to contact between the pleural and pericardial surfaces during the contraction cycle.

The occurrence of pedal edema or pleural effusions signifies the presence of fluid overload and increased total body sodium content secondary to either congestive heart failure or renal mediated changes in fluid balance. Rarely, as noted below, symptoms and signs of true congestive heart failure, including impaired left ventricular contractility, the presence of a third heart sound (S_3), and paroxysmal nocturnal dyspnea, may be present.[2,20,27,68]

Cardiac Rhythm Disturbances

Routine electrocardiographic tracings demonstrate sinus tachycardia in the majority of patients.[31–34] A subset, estimated at 10% to 15%, have atrial fibrillation,[2,67,69] a complication more common in the elderly.[69] The ventricular rate in atrial fibrillation is often rapid due to the increased rate of conduction of the electrical impulse through the atrioventricular node.[37] Most patients with atrial fibrillation have the arrhythmia for less than 4 to 8 weeks before the diagnosis of thyrotoxicosis. In the absence of evidence for chronicity the likelihood of spontaneous reversion to normal sinus rhythm within 8 to 12 weeks after restoration of euthyroidism is high.[67] In elderly patients with chronic atrial fibrillation or patients who have underlying heart disease, the likelihood of spontaneous reversion to sinus rhythm after treatment of the thyrotoxicosis is less. The presence of anatomic abnormalities of the mitral valve or left atrium also suggest that atrial fibrillation will not respond solely to normalization of serum T_4 and T_3 concentrations.[75]

Patients with subclinical thyrotoxicosis may have resting sinus tachycardia and also clinically unrecognized episodes of atrial fibrillation that spontaneously terminate[31] (see chap 88). In older patients with subclinical thyrotoxicosis the risk of developing persistent atrial fibrillation is approximately three times that of normal subjects.[69] When viewed overall, however, both overt and subclinical thyrotoxicosis account for approximately 5% or less of all cases of atrial fibrillation.

The development of atrial fibrillation poses the potential for systemic embolization and stroke. Although the prevalence of embolism is not known, it appears to be more common in older patients with coexistent heart disease.[69,75] Atrial flutter and other supraventricular tachyarrhythmias (including paroxysmal atrial tachycardia) are uncommon rhythm disturbances in thyrotoxic patients. Ventricular fibrillation and ventricular premature contractions are rare.[34,38,76,77]

Nonspecific electrocardiographic (ECG) changes may occur in thyrotoxic patients. A shortening of the P-R interval is common, secondary to the increased rate of conduction through the atrioventricular node. In patients with angina-like complaints there may be ST-segment elevations, suggesting myocardial ischemia.[70]

Noninvasive Cardiac Evaluation

Noninvasive cardiac diagnostic studies of the effects of thyrotoxicosis on cardiac contractility, including radionuclide angiography to measure left ventricular ejection fraction and Doppler echocardiography to assess cardiac systolic and diastolic performance characteristics, have revealed that all aspects of left ventricular contractility are enhanced in patients with thyrotoxicosis as compared with age-matched normal subjects or the same patients after treatment.[16–18,71,78] These findings also apply to patients with subclinical thyrotoxicosis.[51] Thus, the effects of thyroid hormone on the heart are to increase contractile performance and augment cardiac output and work.[2,3,7,38] The long-term effect of this increase in cardiac work is cardiac hypertrophy.[4] Studies of cardiac hypertrophy in other clinical situations, including valvular heart disease and hypertension, suggest that it is a pathologic response, but this does not necessarily apply in the newly diagnosed thyrotoxic patient in whom both systolic and diastolic function are supranormal.[19] Longer duration disease may, however, lead to impaired cardiac contractile performance.[79]

HEART FAILURE

Thyrotoxicosis alone may cause heart failure in old and, much less often, in young patients.[6,68,74] In light of the changes in cardiovascular hemodynamics and cardiac contractility described above, this is an unexpected result, and raises the question of whether there is a distinct thyrotoxic cardiomyopathy[64] or whether other factors can explain the occurrence of heart failure in the absence of underlying heart disease.[4]

In large clinical studies of thyrotoxic patients with evidence of heart failure the patients were generally older and therefore at risk for underlying heart disease and had chronic thyrotoxicosis.[32,68] Hypertension, valvular heart disease, or coronary artery disease predisposes a patient to cardiac contractile dysfunction if the work load and oxygen consumption increase, as occurs in thyrotoxicosis.[71] Elderly patients with rhythm disturbances, including atrial fibrillation, have the greatest risk for heart failure; even so, in the absence of atrial fibrillation, heart failure is rare.[32,68] These patients may not have the more typical symptoms and signs of thyrotoxicosis. Weight loss or muscle weakness may be the only findings to alert the physician to the underlying diagnosis.[66]

A comparison of thyrotoxic patients with heart failure with those with no cardiac symptoms reveals two major hemodynamic changes that distinguish the heart failure group. They are higher levels of systemic vascular resistance[6] and a disproportionate increase in systemic vascular resistance with exercise.[7]

In younger patients, or in the absence of underlying heart disease, the heart failure is thought to be "high output."[27] That an increase in cardiac output per se could lead to cardiac failure is controversial. High-output heart failure may not be heart failure but rather a circulatory congestion caused by fluid retention.[7,20,53] Support for this possibility comes from the finding of expanded blood volume with increased venous filling pressures and peripheral edema, with a good clinical response to treatment with a diuretic drug.[17,35,75]

In thyrotoxic patients cardiac output is potentially near maximal at rest and cannot increase in response to exercise, stress (infection), surgery, or pregnancy with the expected further increments.[64,71] As a result, atrial filling pressures rise, leading to pulmonary and peripheral edema. This situation is worsened by atrial fibrillation, which impairs atrial and ventricular filling.[32,38,68] Patients with thyrotoxicosis have a less than expected increase in left ventricular contractility during exercise; these same patients have the expected response after antithyroid treatment, which suggests the presence of a reversible thyrotoxic cardiomyopathy.[64] An alternative explanation is that before treatment, resting systemic vascular resistance was already maximally lowered and therefore could not decline further with exercise.[6,20] In the absence of such a decline, left ventricular afterload and contractility may not change, and so cardiac output would not increase. These observations further reinforce the importance of changes in systemic vascular resistance, blood volume, and loading conditions as determinants of the cardiovascular response in thyrotoxicosis.[7,16]

Perhaps the most compelling explanation of impaired left ventricular function (decreased ejection fraction, abnormal diastolic compliance, and an S3 on physical examination) in thyrotoxic patients is the observation that persistent tachyarrhythmias alter left ventricular contractile function, otherwise known as rate-related heart failure.[80] Sustained tachycardia causes abnormal ventricular systolic and diastolic function that resolves when the arrhythmia is treated. That thyrotoxicosis may cause heart rates of 120 beats per minute or higher for prolonged periods sufficient to impair ventricular contractility is consistent with this explanation.[19,27,32] The development of atrial fibrillation with an even higher ventricular heart rate would be expected to further compromise cardiac function. The occurrence of rate-related heart failure in thyrotoxicosis is further supported by the finding of greater degrees of heart disease in patients with the most chronic and severe forms of thyrotoxicosis.[27] Beta-adrenergic receptor blockade-mediated slowing of the heart rate can rapidly reverse even severe degrees of left ventricular dysfunction in these patients.[38] The finding that cardiac function returns to normal with treatment of the thyrotoxicosis obscures the fact that it is the heart rate that is simultaneously controlled and may be the primary cause for the heart failure.[75]

TREATMENT

Therapy is directed at reversing the hemodynamic changes that accompany thyrotoxicosis without impairing the ability of the heart to meet the oxygen and substrate demands of peripheral tissues[7,71] (Table 38-4). Ultimately this requires the establishment of a euthyroid state.[75] However, since the half-life of T_4 in serum and its biologic effects are relatively long and antithyroid therapies are inherently slow in action, palliative treatment is often necessary in these patients.[38,65,75,81,83]

Acute Interventions

Because of the importance of reduction in heart rate, initial therapy of the thyrotoxic patient with or without underlying heart disease is best accomplished with β-adrenergic receptor blockade.[37,38,81–83] Propranolol, a nonselective β-adrenergic blocking drug, has been used most often in divided doses of 80 to 240 mg given daily[65] (see chap 53). Intravenous treatment (1 mg) can be used in more acutely ill patients, provided that they are treated in a closely monitored setting. The goals of therapy are to slow the heart rate, decrease symptoms, and signs of cardiac decompensation, maintain blood pressure, and improve some of the noncardiac manifestations of thyrotoxicosis.[65,82,83] If angina pectoris is present, the decrease in cardiac work can improve the symptoms. Beta-adrenergic receptor blockade is contraindicated in patients with asthma.[38] Although heart failure is

TABLE 38-4.
Treatment of Cardiac Manifestations of Thyrotoxicosis

ACUTE TREATMENT OF TACHYCARDIA OR EXERCISE-RELATED SYMPTOMS

β-Adrenergic antagonist drugs

Calcium-channel–blocking drugs (when β-blockade is contraindicated)

ACUTE TREATMENT OF HEART FAILURE

β-Adrenergic antagonist drugs: indicated for rate-related heart failure and control of ventricular response in atrial fibrillation

Diuretic drugs

Digoxin: greater than usual loading and maintenance dosage needed

Anticoagulation: consider for patient with chronic atrial fibrillation

CHRONIC TREATMENT OF HYPERTHYROIDISM

Radioiodine

Antithyroid drug therapy

---

usually considered a contraindication to the use of β-adrenergic receptor blocking drugs, the importance of heart rate control in reversing left ventricular dysfunction in thyrotoxic patients usually outweighs the risks.

Acute therapy of the thyrotoxic patient with signs of heart failure, including peripheral (or pulmonary) edema, should include moderate diuresis with furosemide. The initial goal is to control and improve symptoms of fluid overload. Volume contraction should be avoided because it impairs cardiac filling and therefore lowers cardiac output. In addition to diuresis, digoxin can be beneficial in both controlling the symptoms and signs of heart failure and also slowing the ventricular rate in patients with atrial fibrillation. Thyrotoxic patients have increased digoxin clearance and decreased cardiac sensitivity to digoxin,[84] so that it is important to adjust the dose to provide the desired therapeutic response.

Calcium channel blockers may slow the heart rate in thyrotoxic patients when administered chronically.[33] Acute therapy with these drugs may lower systemic vascular resistance, leading to hemodynamic instability or cardiovascular collapse, which may be reversed by volume expansion. When β-adrenergic receptor blocking drugs are contraindicated, a calcium channel blocker can be given to control atrial fibrillation or other supraventricular arrhythmias, but it should be given very cautiously to avoid untoward hypotension or negative inotropic effects.[75]

Chronic Therapy

Antithyroid therapy of thyrotoxicosis is discussed in chapter 53. The results of radioactive iodine treatment of a large number of thyrotoxic patients documents both the utility and safety of this treatment.[32] Among 356 patients with cardiac involvement, including atrial fibrillation, angina pectoris or heart failure, over 90% had improvement in their cardiovascular symptoms and signs after treatment with radioactive iodine alone. The opportunity to combine β-adrenergic receptor blockade with radioactive iodine treatment should provide effective acute as well as long-term therapy.

The role of anticoagulation in thyrotoxic patients with atrial fibrillation is an unresolved issue.[75] The results that support this treatment have been accumulated in small numbers of patients studied retrospectively,[85] but they were not confirmed by a larger retrospective study.[67] In young patients with a short duration of atrial fibrillation and no underlying heart disease, anticoagulation does not seem warranted because sinus rhythm is usually restored soon after initiation of antithyroid therapy. A similar approach can be justified in older patients in the absence of organic heart disease and a defined duration of atrial fibrillation. In contrast, older patients with evidence of underlying heart disease or chronic atrial fibrillation should receive anticoagulant therapy, as is recommended for patients with atrial fibrillation who do not have thyrotoxicosis.[69,75] The effectiveness of aspirin as compared with coumadin remains to be determined.

SELECTED CLINICAL SITUATIONS

Pregnancy

The hemodynamic changes of pregnancy, which are similar to those of thyrotoxicosis, result from the increased blood flow and oxygen requirements of the developing fetus, which is perfused through a low resistance vascular bed.[86] For pregnant women with thyrotoxicosis the effects of the two conditions are additive.

In pregnant women with thyrotoxicosis appropriate antithyroid treatment usually prevents any untoward hemodynamic burden on the heart[75,86] (see chap 89). The development of peripheral edema, exaggerated tachycardia, or symptoms of cardiac decompensation should be managed in the same way in pregnant women as in other patients, except that β-adrenergic blocking drugs should be used sparingly, because of their possible ability to cause fetal growth retardation and their ability to prolong labor and delivery.[38,86]

Mitral Valve Prolapse

Patients with Graves' disease may have a higher than expected prevalence of mitral valve prolapse as diagnosed by echocardiography.[72,73] Initial studies suggested that the hemodynamic changes of thyrotoxicosis could explain this association, but more recent reports implicate genetic factors, because the prevalence of mitral valve prolapse may also be increased in patients with chronic autoimmune thyroiditis.[87] Regardless of the underlying pathophysiology, the presence of mitral valve dysfunction may decrease left ventricular performance in patients with thyrotoxicosis. Thus, any patient with thyrotoxicosis who has a prominent cardiac murmur should undergo echocardiography, with particular attention to the mitral valve. Thyrotoxic patients with substantial prolapse should be managed in the same way as any patient with prolapse with respect to antibiotic prophylaxis for dental and surgical procedures.[88]

References

1. Parry CH. Collections from the unpublished papers of the late Caleb Hilliel Parry. Dis Heart 1825;2:111

2. Klein I. Thyroid hormone and the cardiovascular system. Am J Med 1990;88:631

3. Polikar R, Albert G, Urs S, Nicod P. The thyroid and the heart. Circulation 1993;87:1435

4. Klein I, Ojamaa K. Thyroid hormone and the cardiovascular system: from theory to practice. J Clin Endocrinol Metab 1994; 78:1026

5. Dillmann WH. Biochemical basis of thyroid hormone action in the heart. Am J Med 1990;88:626

6. Graettinger JS, Muenster JJ, Selverstone LA, Campbell JA. A correlation of clinical and hemodynamic studies in patients with hyperthyroidism with and without heart failure. J Clin Invest 1959; 19:1316

7. Klein I, Ojamaa K. Thyroid hormone and blood pressure regulation. In: Laragh J, Brenner B, eds. Hypertension. New York: Raven Press, 1995:2247

8. Klemperer JD, Klein I, Gomez M, et al. Thyroid hormone treatment after coronary artery bypass surgery. N Engl J Med 1995; 333:1522

9. Ojamaa K, Balkman C, Klein I. Acute effects of triiodothyronine on arterial smooth muscle cells. Ann Thorac Surg 1993; 56:S61

10. Kapitola J, Vilimovska D. Inhibition of the early circulatory effects of triiodothyronine in rats by propranolol. Physiol Bohemoslov 1981;30:347

11. Klein I, Ojamaa K, Powell S. Potential clinical applications for parenteral thyroid hormone therapy. Hosp Formulary 1993; 28:848

12. Kontos HA, Shapiro W, Mauch P Jr, et al. Mechanism of certain abnormalities of the circulation to the limbs in thyrotoxicosis. J Clin Invest 1965;44:947

13. Theilen EO, Wilson WR. Hemodynamic effects of peripheral vasoconstriction in normal and thyrotoxic subjects. J Appl Physiol 1967;22:207

14. Palmer R, Ferrice A, Moncada S. Nitric oxide release accounts for the biological activity of endothelium-derived relaxing factor. Nature 1987;329:524

15. Buccino RA, Spann JF, Pool PE, Sonnenblick EH, Braunwald E. Influence of the thyroid state on the intrinsic contractile properties and energy stores of the myocardium. J Clin Invest 1967;46:1669

16. Morkin E, Flink IL, Goldman S. Biochemical and physiologic effects of thyroid hormone on cardiac performance. Prog Cardiovasc Dis 1983;25:435

17. Merillon JP, Passa P, Chastre J, Wolf A, Gourgon R. Left ventricular function and hyperthyroidism. Br Heart J 1981;46:137

18. Mintz G, Pizzarello R, Klein I. Enhanced left ventricular diastolic function in hyperthyroidism: noninvasive assessment and response to treatment. J Clin Endocrinol Metab 1991;73:146

19. Klein I, Ojamaa K. Cardiovascular manifestations of endocrine disease. J Clin Endocrinol Metab 1992;75:339

20. Umeda PK, Darling DS, Kennedy JM, et al. Control of myosin heavy chain expression in cardiac hypertrophy. Am J Cardiol 1987;59:49A

21. Morkin E: Regulation of myosin heavy chain genes in the heart. Circulation 1993;87:1451

22. Balkman C, Ojamaa K, Klein I. Time course of the effects of thyroid hormone on cardiac gene expression. Endocrinology 1992; 130:2001

23. Ojamaa K, Klein I. In vivo regulation of recombinant cardiac myosin heavy chain gene expression by thyroid hormone. Endocrinology 1993;132:1002

24. Ojamaa K, Samarel A, Kupfer J, Hong C, Klein I. Thyroid hormone effects on cardiac gene expression independent of cardiac growth and protein synthesis. Am J Physiol 1992;263:E534

25. Subramanian A, Gulick A, Neumann J, et al. Transgenic analysis of the thyroid response elements in the alpha cardiac myosin heavy chain gene promoter. J Biol Chem 1993;268:4331

26. Mercadier J, Bouveret P, Gorza L, et al. Myosin isoenzymes in normal and hypertrophied human ventricular myocardium. Circulation Res 1983;53:52

27. Magner JA, Clark W, Allenby P. Congestive heart failure and sudden death in a young woman with thyrotoxicosis. West J Med 1990;8:553

28. Bonow RO, Udelson JE. Left ventricular diastolic dysfunction as a cause of congestive heart failure. Ann Int Med 1992;117:502

29. Rohrer D, Dillmann WH. Thyroid hormone markedly increases the mRNA coding for sarcoplasmic reticulum Ca^{2+}-ATPase in the rat heart. J Biol Chem 1988;263:6941

30. Arat M, Masui H, Periasamy M. Sarcoplasmic reticulum gene expression in cardiac hypertrophy and heart failure. Circulation Res 1994;74:555

31. Biondi B, Fazio S, Carella C, et al. Cardiac effects of long term thyrotropin-suppressive therapy with levothyroxine. J Clin Endocrinol Metab 1993;77:334

32. Delit C, Silver S, Yohalen SB, Segal RL. Thyrocardiac disease and its management with radioactive iodine [131]I. JAMA 1961;176:262

33. Roti E, Montermin M, Roti S, et al. The effect of diltiazem, a calcium channel-blocking drug, on cardiac rate and rhythm in hyperthyroid patients. Arch Intern Med 1988;148:1919

34. Olshausen KV, Bischoff S, Kahaly G, et al. Cardiac arrhythmias and heart rate in hyperthyroidism. Am J Cardiol 1989;63:930

35. Anthonisen P, Holst E, Thomsen AA. Determination of cardiac output and other hemodynamic data in patients with hyper- and hypothyroidism, using dye dilution technique. Scand J Clin Lab Invest 1960;12:472

36. Gibson JG, Harris AW. Clinical studies of the blood volume of hyperthyroidism and myxedema. J Clin Invest 1938;18:59

37. Levey GS, Klein I: Catecholamine-thyroid hormone interactions and the cardiovascular manifestations of hyperthyroidism. Am J Med 1990;88:642

38. Ventrella S, Klein I. Beta-adrenergic receptor blocking drugs in the management of hyperthyroidism. Endocrinologist 1994; 4:391

39. Davis PJ. Cellular actions of thyroid hormone. In: Braverman LE, Utiger R, eds. The thyroid. 6th ed. Philadelphia: JB Lippincott, 1991:190

40. Oppenheimer JH, Samuels HH. Molecular basis of thyroid hormone action. New York, Academic Press, 1983:1

41. Hodin RA, Lazar MA, Chin WW. Differential and tissue-specific regulation of the multiple rat c-erbA mRNA species by thyroid hormone. J Clin Invest 1990;85:101

42. Brent G. The molecular basis of thyroid hormone action. N Engl J Med 1994;331:847

43. Refetoff S. Resistance to thyroid hormone. Clin Lab Med 1993; 13:563

44. Schwartz ID, Bercu BB. Dextrothyroxine in the treatment of generalized thyroid hormone resistance in a boy homozygous for a defect in the T_3 receptor. Thyroid 1992;2:15

45. Kamitani T, Ikeda U, Muto S, et al. Regulation of Na,K-ATPase gene expression by thyroid hormone in rat cardiocytes. Circulation Res 1992;71:1457

46. Edelman I, Ismail-Beigi F. Thyroid thermogenesis and active sodium transport. Recent Prog Horm Reg 1974;30:235

47. Salter DR, Dyke CM, Wechsler AS. Triiodothyronine (T_3) and cardiovascular therapeutics: a review. J Cardiac Surg 1992;7:363

48. Klemperer JD, Ojamaa K, Klein I, Isom W, Kreiger K. Triiodothyronine improves left ventricular function without oxygen wast-

ing effects following global hypothermic ischemia. J Thoracic Cardiovasc Surg 1995;109:457

49. Dudley SC Jr, Baumgarten CH. Bursting of sodium channels after acute exposure to 3,5,3'-triiodo-L-thyronine. Circulation Res 1993;73:301

50. Klein I. Thyroxine-induced cardiac hypertrophy: time course of development and inhibition by propranolol. Endocrinology 1988;123:203

51. Biondi B, Fazio S, Carella C, et al. Control of adrenergic overactivity by beta-blockade improves quality of life in patients on long-term suppressive therapy with levothyroxine. J Clin Endocrinol Metab 1994;78:1132

52. Klein I, Hong C. Effects of thyroid hormone on the myosin content and myosin isoenzymes of the heterotopically transplanted heart. J Clin Invest 1986;77:1694

53. Resnick LM, Laragh JH. Plasma renin activity in syndromes of thyroid hormone excess and deficiency. Life Sci 1982;30:585

54. Coulombe P, Dussault JH, Letarte J, Simard SJ. Catecholamines metabolism in thyroid disease. I. Epinephrine secretion rate in hyperthyroidism and hypothyroidism. J Clin Endocrinol Metab 1976;42:125

55. Martin WH, Spina RJ, Korte E. Effect of hyperthyroidism of short duration on cardiac sensitivity to beta-adrenergic stimulation. J Am Coll Cardiol 1992;19:1185

56. Liggett SB, Shah SD, Cryer PE. Increased fat cell and skeletal muscle beta-adrenergic receptor densities but unattended lipolytic, glycemic and cardiac chronotropic in vivo in experimental human thyrotoxicosis. J Clin Invest 1989;83:803

57. Bilezikian JP, Loeb JN. The influence of hyperthyroidism and hypothyroidism on alpha- and beta-adrenergic receptor systems and adrenergic receptor systems and adrenergic responsiveness. Endocr Rev 1983;4:378

58. Williams LT, Lefkowitz RJ, Watanabe AM, et al. Thyroid hormone regulation of beta-adrenergic number. J Biol Chem 1977;252:2787

59. Ikram H. The nature and prognosis of thyrotoxic heart disease. Q J Med 1985;54:19-28

60. Levine MA, Feldman AM, Robishaw JD. Influence of thyroid hormone status on expression of genes encoding G protein subunits in the rat heart. J Biol Chem 1990;25:3553

61. Dratman MB, Goldman M, Crutchfield FL, Gordon JT. Nervous system role of iodocompounds in blood pressure regulation. Life Sci 1982;30:611

62. Klein I, Trzepacz P, Roberts M, Levey GS. Symptom rating scale for assessing hyperthyroidism. Arch Intern Med 1988;148:387

63. Falcone M, Mixamoto T, Fierro-Renoy F, Macchia E, DeGroot L. Antipeptide polyclonal antibodies specifically recognize each human thyroid hormone receptor isoform. Endocrinology 1992;131:2419

64. Forfar JC, Muir AL, Sawers SA, et al. Abnormal left ventricular function in hyperthyroidism. N Engl J Med 1982;307:1165

65. Olson B, Klein I, Brenner R, Burdett R, Trzepacz P, Levey GS. Hyperthyroid myopathy and the response to treatment. Thyroid 1991;1:137

66. Thomas FB, Mazzaferri EL, Skillman TG. Apathetic thyrotoxicosis: a distinctive clinical and laboratory entity. Ann Intern Med 1970;72:679

67. Nakazawa HK, Sakurai K, Hamada N, Momotani N, Ito K. Management of atrial fibrillation in the post-thyrotoxic state. Am J Med 1982;72:903

68. Sandler G, Wilson GM. The nature and prognosis of heart disease in thyrotoxicosis. Q J Med 1959;28:347

69. Sawin CT, Geller A, Wolf PA, et al. Low serum thyrotropin levels as a risk factor for atrial fibrillation in older persons. N Engl J Med 1994;33:1249

70. Featherstone HJ, Stewart DK. Angina in thyrotoxicosis: thyroid-related coronary artery spasm. Arch Intern Med 1983;143:554

71. Grossman W, Robin NL, Johnson LW. The enhanced myocardial contractility of thyrotoxicosis. Ann Intern Med 1971;74:869

72. Channick BJ, Aetlin EJ, Marks AD, et al. Hyperthyroidism and mitral valve prolapse. N Engl J Med 1981;305;497

73. Brauman A, Algon M, Gilboa Y, et al. Mitral valve prolapse in hyperthyroidism of two different origins. Br Heart J 1985;53:374

74. Forfar JC, Caldwell GC. Hyperthyroid heart disease. Clin Endocrinol Metab 1985;14:491

75. Klein I, Becker D, Levey GS. Treatment of hyperthyroid disease. Ann Intern Med 1994;121:281

76. Polikar R, Reld GK, Dittrich HC, Smith J, Nicod P. Effect of thyroid replacement therapy on the frequency of benign atrial and ventricular arrhythmias. J Am Coll Cardiol 1989;14:999

77. Venkatesh N, Kuhle WG, Feld GK, Singh BN. Hypothyroidism elevates ventricular fibrillation threshold in rabbits. J Am Coll Cardiol 1988;1(Suppl A):41A

78. Smallridge RC, Goldman MH, Raines K, et al. Rest and exercise left ventricular ejection fraction before and after therapy in young adults with hyperthyroidism and hypothyroidism. Am J Cardiol 1987;60:929

79. Fazio S, Biondi B, Carella C, et al. Diastolic dysfunction in patients on thyroid-stimulating hormone suppressive therapy with levothyroxine: beneficial effect of beta-blockade. J Clin Endocrinol Metab 1995;80:2222

80. Cruz FES, Cherieu EC, Smeets RM, et al. Reversibility of tachycardiac-induced cardiomyopathy after cure of incessant supraventricular tachycardia. J Am Col Cardiol 1990;16:739

81. Hellman R, Kelly KL, Mason WD. Propranolol for thyroid storm. N Engl J Med 1977;297:671

82. Eber O, Buchinger W, Lindner W, et al. The effect of D-versus L-propranolol in the treatment of hyperthyroidism. Clin Endocrinol 1990;32:363

83. Zonszein J, Santangelo RP, Mackin JF, et al. Propranolol and the surgical treatment of thyrotoxicosis. Am J Med 1979;66:411

84. Kim D, Smith T. Effects of thyroid hormone on sodium pump site, sodium content and contractile response to cardiac glycosis in cultured heart cells. J Clin Invest 1984;74:H81

85. Dunn M, Alexander J, de Silva R, Hildner F. Antithrombotic therapy in atrial fibrillation. Chest 1989;95(2 Suppl):118S

86. Burrow GN. Thyroid function and hyperfunction during gestation. Endocr Rev 1993;14:194

87. Marks AD, Channick BJ, Adlin EV, et al. Chronic thyroiditis and mitral valve prolapse. Ann Intern Med 1985;102:479

88. Nishimura RA, McGoon MD, Shub C, et al. Echocardiographically documented mitral valve prolapse. Long term follow up of 237 patients. N Engl J Med 1985;313:1305

Werner and Ingbar's The Thyroid, Seventh Edition,
edited by Lewis E. Braverman and Robert D. Utiger
Lippincott–Raven Publishers, Philadelphia, © 1996

39

The Respiratory System in Thyrotoxicosis

David H. Ingbar

The respiratory system and the thyroid gland are interrelated in several major ways. First, the thyroid is in proximity to the trachea. Second, the functions of both systems are coupled to cellular oxidative metabolism. In this way, they each contribute to the regulation of the steady-state levels of carbon dioxide and tissue oxygen. Third, thyroid hormones probably play an important role in the development of the lung. This chapter briefly summarizes current knowledge about the biochemical interactions of thyroid hormones with the lungs and considers the ways in which the lungs are affected in thyrotoxicosis. Other conditions in which abnormalities of both the thyroid gland and the respiratory system coexist are reviewed.

BIOCHEMISTRY OF THYROID HORMONES IN THE LUNG

The actions and the metabolism of the thyroid hormones vary from one organ to another, and within one organ the effects on different cell types may differ. In addition, the effects may not be the same in the developing and the adult organ. Where do thyroid hormones act on the lung, and what are their effects?

Thyroid hormones may act directly on the cell membrane, nucleus, or mitochondria, as discussed in chapter 9, but relatively little is known about the mechanisms of thyroid hormone action in the lung. Thyroxine (T_4) and triiodothyronine (T_3) are small molecules and should be accessible to the lung in proportion to their free serum concentrations. The intracellular compartment of the rat lung has a high concentration of T_3 relative to T_4 (lung/plasma ratios of 2.6 and 0.04, respectively).[1,2] Although a similar intracellular concentration of T_3 exists in the liver and the kidney, the latter organs contain relatively more T_4 (ratios of 0.5).

There are many possible explanations for the relatively high concentration of T_3 in the lung. There could be rapid conversion of T_4 to T_3 in the lung, but Chopra[3] did not find significant conversion in rat lung tissue in vitro. However, McCann and Shaw[4] found significant type I 5'-deiodination of iodothyronine in rat lung homogenates, although not as much as in liver or kidney. This activity increased postnatally and was not increased further by corticosterone. It was depressed in lungs from thyrotoxic animals. Alternatively, the lung could contain a large number of high-affinity binding sites for T_3. High-affinity nuclear receptors for T_3 are present in nuclei from mixtures of lung cells, similar to the nuclear receptors for T_3 present in many other organ systems.[5–7] These receptors were present in nuclei from rat lung cells and from cells of the L-2 and A-549 cell lines,[8] which supposedly derive from rat and human type II alveolar pneumocytes, respectively. Gonzales and Ballard[5,6] demonstrated similar receptors in the lungs of human fetuses and of fetal and adult rabbits, with their number increasing during gestation.

The localization of the lung's high-affinity T_3-binding sites among the 40 cell types in the lung is not certain. In monolayers of a cell line cloned from rat type II pneumocytes stained with anti-T_3 and anti-T_4 antibodies, T_3 localized to the nucleus, more than the perinuclear and lammellar body regions; little T_4 was present.[9] Using autoradiography with labeled T_4 and T_3 of living hypothyroid rats and of organ culture of lungs from hypothyroid rats, type II pneumocytes were the primary site of binding, and T_3 bound to a much greater degree than T_4.[10] This localization is in agreement with other evidence discussed in chapter 63, suggesting that thyroid hormones play a role in the development of type II cells and in surfactant synthesis in the fetus. Adult rats made thyrotoxic with exogenous T_4 show increased size of their type II cells as well as the diameter and number of lamellar bodies.[11] Increased amounts of surfactant are released into the alveoli, while the phospholipid composition is normal. Similar changes occur in the fetal rat within 2 days after the intra-amniotic injection of high doses of T_4 at day 18 of gestation. This effect is promoted by hydrocortisone and partially blocked by metyrapone.[12] Rats made hypothyroid from day 18 of gestation display decreased lung weight and lung content of DNA, protein, and β-adrenergic receptors.[13]

Thyroid hormone may be of general importance in lung development, as discussed in chapter 63. The interaction of thyroid hormones and catecholamines stimulated interest, because many of the clinical manifestations of thyrotoxicosis resemble the effects of adrenergic agents. The β-adrenergic system of the lung regulates airway resistance and counteracts bronchoconstriction of the muscarinic cholinergic system.[14] In rat lungs, the number of beta-receptors increases throughout gestation and into the postnatal period.[13] Administration of exogenous thyroid hormone or propylthiouracil (PTU) does not change the number or affinity of adult rat lung beta-receptors.[13,15] The cell type bearing the affected beta-receptors is uncertain. In summary, there is relatively little biochemical evidence for an effect of T_3 and T_4 on beta-receptors in the adult rat or human lung; however, during gestation, the development of β-adrenergic receptors seems to require thyroid hormone, in at least some species.

Some clinical case reports have suggested that thyrotoxicosis may aggravate airway hyperreactivity in asthmatics—the opposite effect from that suggested by the hypothesized thyroid-catecholamine interaction. If thyroid hormones do affect the number of beta-receptors in adult humans, the consequences for the regulation of airway tone in patients with asthma or chronic obstructive pulmonary disease (COPD) could be important.

Another recently discovered commonality between the lung and the thyroid gland is a common, organ-specific transcription factor during development. In both organs, thyroid transcription factor-1 (TTF-1) is selectively expressed during early development and activates expression of tissue-specific genes. In the thyroid, this nuclear transcription factor is a positive regulator of thyroglobulin and thyroperoxidase gene transcription.[16] In the developing rat lung, it is expressed early in the lung bud and airway epithelium but not in the laryngotracheal groove. TTF-1 increases transcription of several lung epithelium specific genes: surfactant apoproteins A, B, and C and Clara cell secretory protein.[17] Since different genes are upregulated in the two organs, other organ-specific transcription factors also must be important determinants of gene expression.

In summary, the major effects of thyroid hormone seem to be promotion of development of the lung and of the type II pneumocyte-surfactant system. The role of thyroid hormone in the function of adult lungs is unclear. There is no evidence for a specific role in the lungs of adults beyond that exerted on all cells of the body; however, many questions remain unexplored. There is no information as to whether lung structure is altered in thyrotoxicosis. In the presence of exogenous T_3, cultured human skin fibroblasts decrease secretion of glycosaminoglycans.[18] Thyroid hormones might influence the nature of the extracellular matrix in the lung through changes in glycosaminoglycans, proteoglycans, elastin, and collagen.

THE LUNGS IN THYROTOXICOSIS

Dyspnea on exertion is a common complaint in thyrotoxic patients, but the causes of this symptom remain unclear and probably vary from one patient to another. Proposed explanations include respiratory muscle weakness, high-output left heart failure causing an engorged pulmonary capillary bed, increased ventilatory drive to breathe, increased airway resistance, diminished lung compliance, and tracheal compression by an enlarged thyroid gland.

Analysis of the effects of thyrotoxicosis on the lung is difficult because there are no large, detailed studies of the subject, despite the high incidence of Graves' disease. The results of the small series available frequently conflict with one another and confuse the overall picture. Table 39-1 summarizes the spectrum of respiratory changes that occur in thyrotoxicosis.

The increased metabolic rate stresses the lungs, necessitating a more rapid net rate of gas exchange to accommodate the increased oxygen consumption and carbon dioxide production. Although the normal person can easily accomplish this, a patient who is thyrotoxic may not be able to meet the demand for increased gas exchange when this stress is superimposed on underlying lung disease.

Lung Volumes and Flow Rates

Interest in the causes of dyspnea in thyrotoxicosis dates back at least to the early part of this century, when Peabody and Wentworth[19] demonstrated a decreased vital capacity (VC) in two of seven patients with clinical thyrotoxicosis. Difficulty in determining whether the patients also had left ventricular failure confounded attempts to correlate the change in VC with an increase in the basal metabolic rate (BMR). Using only clinical signs and symptoms as markers of congestive heart failure (CHF), Lemon and Moersch[20] found that a decreased VC correlated only with "cardiac decompensation" and not with either the BMR or the severity of the thyrotoxic symptoms. Other early studies found an inverse correlation between the VC and the BMR.[21] Despite several studies of the lung volumes in the subsequent 70 years, little more is known.

TABLE 39-1.
Respiratory Changes in Thyrotoxicosis

Increased oxygen consumption
Increased carbon dioxide production
Increased minute ventilation
Tachypnea
Decreased vital capacity
Decreased diffusing capacity for carbon monoxide
Decreased lung compliance
Respiratory muscle weakness
Increased ventilatory response to hypercapnia
Increased ventilatory response to hypoxia
High-output congestive left ventricular failure
Pulmonary artery dilation and hypertension

As the sophistication of pulmonary-function testing has increased, more detailed analysis of the subdivisions of lung volume has become possible. One older study noted that one quarter of patients had decreased residual volume (RV), vital capacity (VC), and total lung capacity (TLC), with normal ABGs and diffusing capacity for carbon monoxide.[22] In the most recent study of 12 patients and 12 normal subjects, there were no significant differences in the mean baseline VC, TLC, RV, static compliance, or pressure-volume curves.[23] After treatment, the VC and TLC increased significantly in eight patients. Airway resistance and flow rates were normal in essentially all studies.

These studies of the subdivisions of lung volumes present a confusing picture.[23–26] The VC often is diminished in thyrotoxicosis and increases in response to treatment. The reported changes in the other lung volumes are not consistent; in some studies, the RV is increased and the TLC is decreased, suggesting muscle weakness. Other investigators report decreases of RV and elevations of TLC from "normal" levels with treatment. These heterogeneous findings may reflect the presence of other underlying lung diseases in some of the patients that were not mentioned in the reports. Alternatively, thyrotoxicosis may cause several types of changes in the lungs, and they may not all occur in the same patient. For example, respiratory muscle weakness due to chronic thyrotoxic myopathy probably occurs only in some patients.

Arterial blood gas partial pressures and the oxygen and carbon dioxide–hemoglobin dissociation curves usually are normal.[27] The mixed venous oxygen saturation typically increases because the rise in cardiac output is greater than what is necessitated by the increased oxygen consumption. Although the total amount of oxygen extracted by the peripheral tissues is increased, the fractional extraction of the transported oxygen is decreased. Diffusing capacity of the lung for carbon dioxide (DLCO) at rest may be normal[23,27,28] or low,[29] but in most patients it is lower than expected for the high cardiac output. With exercise, the DLCO usually rises less than normal or even falls. The reason for this increased efficiency of gas exchange with exercise is not clear, but there may be disturbances either in the alveolar capillary wall or in the recruitment of reserve capillaries.

Lung Compliance and Respiratory Muscle Weakness

The ability to inhale or exhale a given tidal volume of gas is determined by the airway resistance, the compliance of the lung, and respiratory muscle function. Airway resistance is normal in thyrotoxic patients. Because some patients presumably can have chronic thyrotoxic myopathy that involves the diaphragm, assessment of whether there are simultaneous changes in the intrinsic lung compliance poses difficulties. Lung compliance could be altered by changes in the elastic properties (connective tissue) or by vascular engorgement. It usually is determined from the static pressure-volume curve of the lung, with measurement of intrathoracic pressure using an esophageal balloon manometer. The maximal expiratory pressure ($P_i$max) at RV, maximal expiratory pressure ($P_e$max) at TLC, maximal transdiaphragmatic pressure, and maximal voluntary minute ventilation (MVV) yield information about max-

imal respiratory muscle power. Even with these techniques, it is difficult to separate patients with pure respiratory muscle weakness from patients who have only decreased lung compliance. As expected, diaphragmatic dysfunction decreases $P_i$max and $P_e$max pressures, but it also may alter the static pressure-volume curve in these patients, possibly because of atelectasis. Manifestations of respiratory muscle dysfunction include rapid shallow respirations, decreased $P_i$max and $P_e$max pressures, decreased transdiaphragmatic pressure, respiratory dyskinesis, hypoventilation with carbon dioxide retention and respiratory acidosis, and easy fatigability.

Stein and associates[22] found that almost all of 13 thyrotoxic patients had decreased lung compliance and loss of $P_i$max and $P_e$max. There was significant improvement in all these parameters after therapy. These findings have been confirmed in some studies,[27] but not others.[28] Most of the patients whose lung compliance improved with treatment also displayed increases in VC, but TLC did not increase, as would be expected if muscle function had improved.

Most thyrotoxic patients who complain of exertional dyspnea have diminished proximal muscle strength.[29] In half the patients with proximal muscle weakness, $P_i$max improved significantly after 6 weeks of therapy. The mean values of $P_i$max and $P_e$max decrease in many thyrotoxic patients.[23,24,26,28,30,32] Static lung compliance and elastic recoil were normal and did not improve with treatment. In the only study that directly measured transdiaphragmatic pressures of seven thyrotoxic patients with proximal muscle weakness and decreased $P_i$max and $P_e$max, transdiaphragmatic pressure was decreased in only one of the four patients in whom it was measured. All four patients had significant increases of transdiaphragmatic pressure after treatment that correlated with their improvements in $P_i$max, $P_e$max, VC, and proximal muscle strength.[30] In another additional study, the $P_i$max and $P_e$max were decreased in 5 and 8 of 14 patients, respectively.[25] Significant increases in both values after correction of the thyrotoxicosis were typical.

These results suggest that chronic thyrotoxic myopathy affects the diaphragm and other respiratory muscles in up to half of thyrotoxic patients, causing loss of maximal respiratory muscle power. Because there are no specific pathologic or electromyographic hallmarks of chronic thyrotoxic myopathy, involvement of the diaphragm must be inferred from physiologic tests. Whether chronic thyrotoxic myopathy of the diaphragm also causes easy fatigability is unknown. To detect early fatigue, a shift in the high-low power spectrum of the diaphragmatic electromyogram should be looked for in future studies. Thyrotoxic dogs showed decreased transdiaphragmatic pressures and twitch shortening, accompanied by vacuolization and loss of diaphragm muscle fibers.[31] These changes occurred in both the costal and crural parts of the diaphragm but not in skeletal muscles. Easy fatigue could be another cause of exertional dyspnea. Rarely, myasthenia gravis associated with thyrotoxicosis causes respiratory muscle weakness and easy fatigue.

The biochemical basis of these changes in respiratory muscle function is not understood. Thyrotoxic rat diaphragm has depressed glycolytic, tricarboxylic acid cycle, and fatty acid oxidative activity.[32] Apart from respiratory muscle dysfunction, changes in lung structure may alter lung compliance; such changes could be looked for morphologically. Vascular engorgement is an unlikely cause of the changes in compliance because the DLCO is not increased, as in other high cardiac output or capillary engorgement conditions, such as asthma or mild CHF.

Ventilatory Control

The increased oxygen consumption and carbon dioxide production of thyrotoxicosis lead to a homeostatic increase in minute ventilation. Thyrotoxicosis may affect the central regulatory response to a blood gas perturbation. The traditional method of assessing ventilatory drive or response is to measure the increase of ventilation while breathing either hyperoxic hypercapnic (HCVR) or hypoxic isocapnic (HVR) gas mixtures.[32] Ventilatory response is measured as minute ventilation, transdiaphragmatic pressure, or mouth occlusion pressure. The latter two measures more directly reflect neural output and are not as confounded by the presence of other lung disease.

In early studies,[33] thyrotoxic patients and normal subjects given exogenous T_3 increased their minute ventilation normally in response to hypercapnia up to a level of 6% inhaled carbon dioxide, without a change in $PaCO_2$, suggesting that the increased respiratory activity was set by the metabolic rate. This contrasts with the increased ventilation in hypermetabolism of fever, salicylates, or dinitrophenol, in which $PaCO_2$ normally decreases. Using a carbon dioxide rebreathing method of assessing HCVR in 14 patients, Engel and Ritchie[34] showed an increased response to carbon dioxide. Catecholamines released during the testing might be synergized by the thyrotoxic state and directly augment the hypercapnic stimulation of ventilation. The ventilatory response to hypercapnia was increased and unaffected by propanolol (Figs. 39-1 and 39-2).[35]

Until recently, little information has been available on the HVR in thyrotoxicosis. HVR increases with exercise and fever, usually in proportion to the elevation of the metabolic rate. Stein and colleagues[22] believed that hypoxic drive might be an important cause of exertional dyspnea because oxygen supplementation during exercise in thyrotoxic patients decreased both their dyspnea and their minute ventilation. Stockley and Bishop[36] found that most untreated patients had a normal HVR; however, the fall in resting minute ventilation when

these patients were given oxygen was greater before than after therapy. Propranolol had no significant effect on the HVR. In 13 patients, Zwillich and coworkers[35] found a significant increase of the HVR that correlated with the increase in BMR. In each study, propranolol had no effect on the HVR.

In summary, both the HCVR and the HVR are increased in most thyrotoxic patients. This effect is independent of the β-adrenergic effects of catecholamines, and its mechanism is not understood. It is not clear whether thyroid hormones are affecting the peripheral chemoreceptors or the medullary respiratory center. The increased ventilatory drive may be, but is not necessarily, a contributing factor in the dyspnea. Thyrotoxicosis, with its increased ventilatory drive superimposed on underlying lung disease, certainly can worsen dyspnea and might cause frank respiratory failure.

Exercise

Thyrotoxicosis typically increases the resting heart rate, cardiac output, respiratory rate, and minute ventilation. The normal increases during exercise are magnified in thyrotoxic patients.[22,24,26,28,37] The amount of oxygen consumed to perform any work load is increased. Although the rate of the increase in oxygen consumption with increasing work is normal (Fig. 39-3),[38] both the minute ventilation and the cardiac output for a given level of oxygen consumption are elevated at all levels of oxygen consumption (Fig. 39-4). The minute ventilation and the mouth occlusion pressure may be disproportionately elevated for the carbon dioxide production rate,[23] possibly because of a rapid, shallow breathing pattern with more wasted dead-space ventilation[39] and consistent with an increased ventilatory drive beyond the hypermetabolism. When ventilatory drive was expressed as the ratio of mouth occlusion pressure to carbon dioxide, the drive increased with positive correlation with the T_3 level. Beta blockade decreased the ventilatory drive in the individuals with the highest T_3 levels. In one study, the anaerobic threshold was lower than predicted, but it was not clear if this was due to poorer oxygen extraction by the peripheral tissues, greater lactate production, or both.

Thyrotoxic patients may be predominantly limited by their cardiac[40] or by their pulmonary system. None of 15 patients achieved 80% of their predicted maximal oxygen uptake

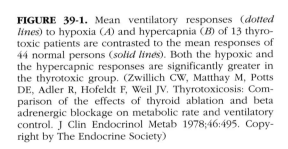

FIGURE 39-1. Mean ventilatory responses (*dotted lines*) to hypoxia (*A*) and hypercapnia (*B*) of 13 thyrotoxic patients are contrasted to the mean responses of 44 normal persons (*solid lines*). Both the hypoxic and the hypercapnic responses are significantly greater in the thyrotoxic group. (Zwillich CW, Matthay M, Potts DE, Adler R, Hofeldt F, Weil JV. Thyrotoxicosis: Comparison of the effects of thyroid ablation and beta adrenergic blockage on metabolic rate and ventilatory control. J Clin Endocrinol Metab 1978;46:495. Copyright by The Endocrine Society)

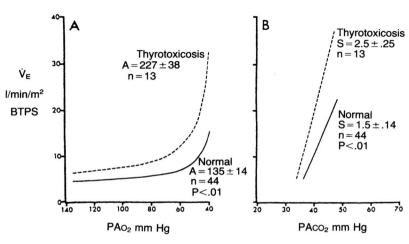

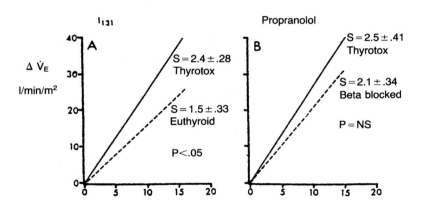

FIGURE 39-2. Effects of treatment with [131]I (*A*) and propranolol (*B*) on the mean ventilatory response to hypercapnia of 13 patients with thyrotoxicosis. The solid lines show the pretreatment responses, and the dotted lines indicate the post-treatment responses to hypercapnia. Radioactive iodine, but not propranolol, significantly diminished the hypercapnic ventilatory response. (Zwillich CW, Matthay M, Potts DE, Adler R, Hofeldt F, Weil JV. Thyrotoxicosis: Comparision of effects of thyroid ablation and beta adrenergic blockage on metabolic rate and ventilatory control. J Clin Endocrinol Metab 1978;46:496, Copyright by The Endocrine Society)

and only 7 exceeded 80% of their predicted maximal heart rates.[23] Because both organ systems are affected, and because normal people are cardiac-limited, cardiac limitation probably predominates in the absence of other lung disease or severe respiratory muscle weakness.

With treatment, the maximal work performed usually increases significantly. Surprisingly, the maximal oxygen uptake achieved during exercise testing did not increase in two studies,[23,28] even with improvements in maximal respiratory muscle pressures. The subjective sense of dyspnea also was not improved by therapy.

Pulmonary artery pressures of thyrotoxic patients may rise more than usual with exercise,[37] but this has not been carefully evaluated. Exercise normally decreases the mixed venous oxygen saturation and the dead space/tidal volume ratio[39]; the converse occurs in thyrotoxicosis.[21] The DLCO of some patients decreases with exercise,[29] especially at higher work loads. The elevated cardiac output may shorten capillary transit times and

prevent complete gas equilibration. Although exchange of oxygen should be affected more than that of carbon monoxide, oxygen desaturation with exercise has not been reported. The normal respiratory exchange ratio suggests that oxidative phosphorylation is not uncoupled.

Effects of Cardiac Changes on the Lungs

The lungs may be affected in two ways by the cardiac consequences of thyrotoxicosis (see chap 38). First, there may be high-output cardiac failure; second, there may be pulmonary artery dilatation, possibly accompanied by pulmonary hypertension, but the pulmonary capillary wedge pressure has been normal in most patients studied.

The pulmonary artery may appear dilated on the plain chest x-ray films. Physical findings of an accentuated pulmonic second heart sound and a right ventricular heave suggest pulmonary hypertension. Mild elevations of resting pulmonary

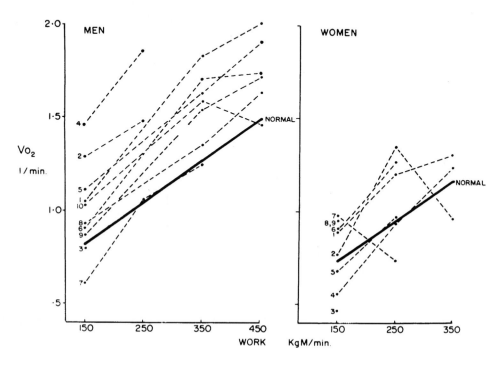

FIGURE 39-3. Oxygen consumption of 19 thyrotoxic patients at increasing work loads of bicycle exercise is shown. Most of the men (*left*) and women (*right*) have increased oxygen consumption at all work loads; the slope of the increase, however, is the same in the thyrotoxic patients as in the normal subjects. (Massey DG, Becklake MR, McKenzie JM, Bates DV. Circulatory and ventilatory response to exercise in thyrotoxicosis. N Engl J Med 1967;276:1107. Reprinted by permission of the New England Journal of Medicine).

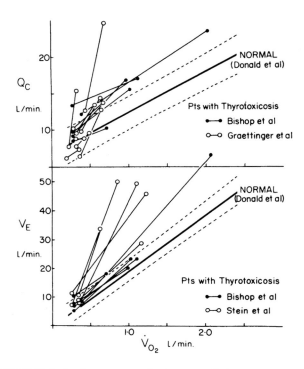

FIGURE 39-4. Cardiac output and minute ventilation responses to increasing oxygen consumption during exercise for patients with thyrotoxicosis. These are contrasted with the normal responses (*heavy lines*). The 95% confidence interval for the normal response is shown by the broken lines. (Data for cardiac output response are from Bishop[37] and Graettinger[30]; data for the minute ventilation response are from Bishop[37] and Stein and coworkers.[22]) Both the cardiac output and the minute ventilation are higher than normal at all levels of oxygen consumption. (Data synthesized and plotted by Massey DG, Becklake MR, McKenzie J, Bates DV. Circulatory and ventilatory response to exercise in thyrotoxicosis. N Engl J Med 1967;276:1106, reprinted by permission)

artery pressure were common with thyrotoxicosis, and the pressure frequently rose significantly during exercise.[37] Resting right ventricular stroke work often is elevated because an increased volume of blood is pumped against a somewhat increased pulmonary vascular resistance. The potential for severe pulmonary hypertension solely due to thyrotoxicosis is not clear. Another physical sign of thyrotoxicosis is the Means-Lerman sign, a scratchy, coarse systolic ejection rub or murmur that is heard best along the left sternal border at the base of the heart. It has been attributed either to rubbing of the dilated aorta or pulmonary artery against some other mediastinal structure or to turbulent pulmonary artery blood flow; the precise origin and physiologic significance of this sign are not known.

OTHER INTERACTIONS OF THE RESPIRATORY SYSTEM AND THYROID GLAND

There are several instances in which the thyroid gland and the respiratory system are both affected by a systemic process. Alternatively, abnormalities of one system may affect the actual or apparent function of the other. Table 39-2 outlines these situations.

Pulmonary Disorders That Influence the Thyroid

Pulmonary diseases can alter thyroid function tests. The sick euthyroid syndrome has become widely recognized over the past decade. In this syndrome, several patterns of change in the thyroid-function tests may occur and are discussed in chapter 14. A significantly higher percentage of patients with abnormal thyroid-function tests, especially a low serum T_4 value, do not survive. The presence of this syndrome may be a marker of severity of illness. Eighty-eight percent of 41 critically ill patients had suppressed TSH responses to TRH in a recent study and the degree of suppression correlated with outcome.[41] Similar suppression has been reported with severe COPD,[29] pulmonary tuberculosis,[42] and lung cancer. Rats with induced sepsis markedly decrease their T_3 levels over 20 to 30 hours.[43] Treatment with exogenous T_3 increased ventilatory drive and lung elastance, but did not affect mortality or gas exchange.

Elevated basal serum levels of calcitonin occur in medullary carcinoma of the thyroid, and they rise markedly after pentagastrin administration. Hypercalcitonemia also has been found in all pathologic types of bronchogenic carcinoma,[44] but it most commonly occurs in small cell carcinoma. Some patients with bronchogenic carcinoma and normal basal calcitonin levels may have a supranormal response to pentagastrin stimulation, but not to the degree seen in medullary carcinoma of the thyroid. The calcitonin can be produced ectopically by the tumor itself, or it may come from the thyroid gland owing to the presence of a factor secreted by the tumor.

Lung cancer can metastasize to the thyroid gland. A review of malignant thyroid disease over 25 years at the Mayo Clinic found that 5 of 30 cases of metastatic thyroid involvement were from a lung primary.[45] Typically, patients presented with a painful, tender thyroid mass. The lung lesion was found either concurrently or later than the thyroid mass. Both small cell and squamous cell carcinomas metastatic from the lung have been demonstrated by fine-needle aspiration of the thyroid.[46]

Thyroid Disorders That Influence the Respiratory System

THYROID CANCER METASTATIC TO THE LUNG

Thyroid diseases other than hyperthyroidism can affect the respiratory system. Thyroid cancer metastasizes to the lungs in 5% to 20% of cases,[47,48] most commonly with papillary carcinoma. The pulmonary metastases usually are asymptomatic, but they may cause dyspnea on exertion. Rarely these patients present with hemoptysis from airway involvement, Pancoast's syndrome, or polycythemia from hypoxemia that has been attributed to small arteriovenous shunts in the tumor. The chest radiograph may be normal or reveal diffuse miliary opacities that may have stippled calcification because of aggregation of psammoma bodies in the tumor. Less commonly, a smaller number of large nodules are present bilaterally on the chest radiograph.

Pulmonary metastases most commonly occur in younger patients and usually present within 1 to 2 years of diagnosis,

PULMONARY DISORDERS THAT INFLUENCE THE THYROID

Sick euthyroid syndrome

Hypercalcitonemia due to bronchogenic carcinoma

Lung cancer metastatic to the thyroid

**THYROID DISORDERS THAT INFLUENCE THE
RESPIRATORY SYSTEM**

Thyroid carcinoma with lung metastases

Compression syndrome due to enlarged thyroid

Tracheal obstruction

Superior vena cava syndrome

Mediastinal mass due to thyroid tissue

Cronic cough due to thyroiditis

? Increased airway reactivity in asthmatics

Increased serum angiotensin-converting enzyme in hyperthyroidism

Propylthiouracil-induced pleuritis or pneumonitis

? Increased risk of lung cancer in Hashimoto's thyroiditis

**SYSTEMIC CONDITIONS THAT AFFECT BOTH THE LUNG
AND THE THYROID GLAND**

Cystic fibrosis

Cigarette smoking

Acute respiratory distress after surgery or molar pregnancy

Associated autoimmune disorders: sytemic lupus erythematosus, Sjögren's syndrome, myasthenia gravis

Pneumocystis carinii infections

Histiocytosis X (eosinophilic granuloma)

rather than as a late complication. The metastases may or may not take up iodine and rarely may function as a site of thyroid hormone synthesis.[48] Functioning metastases have a better prognosis than nonfunctioning metastases, especially if the chest x-ray film is normal.[49] Radioiodine scans are most likely to reveal pulmonary involvement after surgical removal of the primary tumor and thyroid gland. In some series, half the patients with lung metastases had normal chest x-ray films and diffuse uptake on radioiodine scans.[48] Rarely, primary lung tumors, such as adenocarcinoma, concentrate iodine and are confused with metastatic thyroid cancer.

The presence of pulmonary metastases does not necessarily mean a poor clinical course. Even without treatment, densities in the chest radiograph may persist without progression for many years.[50] A sudden increase in pulmonary involvement after a long period of stability suggests that the tumor may have undergone an anaplastic change. Documentation by biopsy and more aggressive treatment may be necessary.

Thyroid cancer in the neck or mediastinum can obstruct the trachea by compression or displacement, or can erode into the trachea or esophagus, causing luminal obstruction. Rarely thyroid carcinomas originate in ectopic thyroid tissue located in the trachea.[51] Thyroid carcinoma involves the upper airway

in 1% to 6% of cases and causes hemoptysis and vocal cord paralysis more often than benign disease does.[52] Airway invasion may be more common in older men. A recently proposed staging system indicated that the 5-year prognosis for operated patients was significantly lower only if the tumor involved or expanded the tracheal mucosa as a nodule or ulcerated mass.[53] Lymphoma, in particular, infiltrates the tracheal wall, obstructing the lymphatics and causing laryngeal and subglottic edema. Compression or infiltration of the tracheal wall is more common than intraluminal tumor growth. Only 18 of 2000 cases of thyroid carcinoma seen at the Mayo Clinic had intraluminal growth of tumor.[54] Rarely, thyroid carcinoma can develop in substernal or intrathoracic goiters, causing rapid enlargement and compressive symptoms.

Surgical treatment of thyroid carcinoma with laryngotracheal involvement may be complex.[55–59] The tumor tends to grow along the trachea rather than causing early luminal obstruction. Resection often requires airway reconstruction, such as sleeve tracheal resection, tracheal and cricoid cartilage resection, or more complex procedures. Of the 34 patients at Massachusetts General Hospital undergoing resection, 3 died postoperatively, but only 2 patients had airway recurrence.[57,65] Patients who cannot be completely resected have a high mortality, whereas patients with total resection and external beam irradiation often do well.[58] Shave excision of thyroid carcinoma is dangerous because of the high likelihood of recurrence. Massive invasion prohibiting reconstruction, innominate artery invasion, or deep invasion into the mediastinum are considered major contraindications to resection.

NONMALIGNANT UPPER AIRWAY COMPRESSION

Enlargement of the thyroid due to a variety of nonmalignant conditions, most commonly multinodular goiter, can compress or displace the surrounding structures (Fig. 39-5) Intrathoracic goiters have an incidence of 1 in 5000 persons and up to 1 in 2000 in women over age 45.[60] The vast majority arise in the cervical thyroid and retain an anatomic connection to it and a similar blood supply. Of 144 patients with goiter, airway obstruction on flow volume loops occurred in 31% and was especially common in men.[61]

The consequences of thyroid enlargement depend on the location of the enlarged thyroid tissue. In the neck, it can obstruct the trachea or esophagus, or compress the superior vena cava or the recurrent laryngeal or cervical sympathetic nerves, resulting in exertional dyspnea, dysphagia, hoarseness, dysphonia, wheezing, stridor, or cough that may be positional.[62] Bilateral vocal cord paralysis also can cause respiratory distress and stridor that are mistaken for asthma.[63] About 15% to 20% of patients are asymptomatic. Sudden onset of stridor occurs in 2% to 3% of these patients, usually because of spontaneous or traumatic hemorrhage within a multinodular goiter. Stridor also may occur immediately after extubation. In some cases, it may be difficult to recognize that a thyroid abnormality is causing chronic cough, because of a lack of marked thyroid enlargement, as in subacute thyroiditis.[64] A markedly enlarged substernal or mediastinal thyroid is one of the rare benign causes of superior vena cava syndrome.[65] In toxic multinodular goiter, PTU may increase the size of the goiter and precipitate or worsen superior vena cava obstruc-

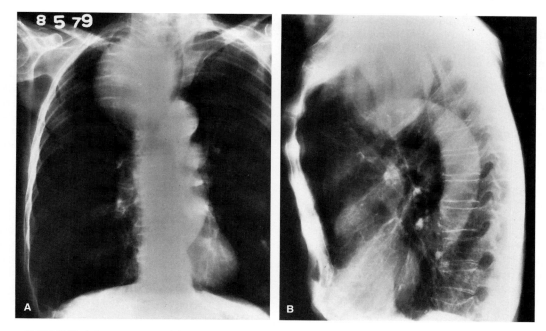

FIGURE 39-5. Posteroanterior (*A*) and lateral (*B*) chest radiographs show a large substernal goiter, which is causing compression and anterolateral displacement of the trachea towards the left chest.

tion.[66] Unilateral or bilateral Horner's sign also may occur with a large intrathoracic goiter that disrupts the cervical sympathetic nerves.

If the thyroid enlargement is at the level of the narrow thoracic inlet, compression of the trachea or esophagus is particularly likely, even with relatively small goiters. Elevating the arms or flexing the neck may raise the retroclavicular goiter into the inlet and aggravate the compression. Blum and colleagues[67] have termed this the "thyroid cork." Thoracic inlet compression results in decreased venous return, increased jugular venous pressure, facial plethora, dysphonia, hoarseness, dizziness, and shortness of breath. Precipitation of these findings by raising the arms has been termed Pemberton's sign. In contrast to superior vena cava syndrome, there is no venous dilation over the chest wall because the obstruction is not central.

The consequences of tracheal obstruction can be quite serious. The patient may be difficult to intubate or may develop airway obstruction after extubation. Seventy-five percent of the trachea's cross-sectional area needs to be lost before stridor and upper airway obstruction are clearly recognizable by the clinician. Bilateral vocal cord paralysis can occur from nerve compression, although it is far more common in malignant thyroid disease. Tracheomalacia may result from longstanding pressure on the trachea and may worsen after surgical tracheotomy. A sudden increase in the size of the thyroid mass, as may be caused by hemorrhage, can lead to acute tracheal obstruction and respiratory arrest.[68]

Forty-three of 269 patients (16%) with enlarged thyroid glands had some symptoms of obstruction to breathing or swallowing.[69] Of the 5% of patients with exertional dyspnea, most had tracheal deviation and hoarseness. Intraluminal involvement, vocal cord paralysis, or hemoptysis did not always indicate malignant disease. The degree of tracheal displacement was independent of the degree of compression.[70] Although the goiters frequently extended into the superior mediastinum and were visible on chest radiographs as a superior mediastinal mass, sternotomy usually was not required for surgical removal. In another series, 45 of 300 patients (15%) undergoing thyroidectomy had evidence of tracheal compression from benign thyroid disease.[71] Four patients presented with acute upper airway obstruction requiring intubation, and four patients developed life-threatening obstruction while hospitalized. About half of 20 consecutive nonsurgical patients with euthyroid benign goiters, on careful questioning, had exertional dyspnea and 80% had abnormalities of pulmonary-function tests or tracheal tomography.[72] Late recurrence has been reported in a patient with prior surgery who was maintained on chronic suppressive therapy with T_4.[73]

Pulmonary-function tests show decreased peak flow rates.[74] Extrathoracic obstruction primarily diminishes inspiratory airflow, whereas intrathoracic obstruction predominantly affects expiratory airflow. The peaks of the flow volume loop are cut off and flattened. Spirometric changes indicative of upper airway obstruction include a forced inspiratory flow measured at 50% of VC that is less than 100 L/min, a ratio of forced inspiratory to forced expiratory flow rates measured at 50% of VC that is greater than 1, and a ratio of forced expiratory volume in 1 second to peak expiratory flow that is greater than 10 L/min. Of these many tests, the inspiratory-expiratory flow volume loop is probably the most sensitive indicator, particularly if the test is performed with the patient in the supine position. One recent study found that although chest radiography and ultrasound predict retrosternal extension of goiter, they do not predict upper airway obstruction.[61]

Other tests also can help to define the presence of airway obstruction. Tracheal tomography or computed tomography (CT) delineates the extent of luminal narrowing and may help plan airway and surgical management. A barium swallow can determine whether the esophagus also is compressed or deviated, as is true in up to one-third of the patients. Fluoroscopy can identify a pulsatile mass, indicating the presence of an aortic aneurysm rather than thyroid tissue. A radioactive iodine scan can confirm that a mediastinal mass takes up iodine and is likely to be thyroid tissue, but a negative scan does not exclude the possibility that it is nonfunctioning thyroid tissue. This must be done before CT scanning with iodinated contrast. Bronchoscopy or esophagoscopy may be necessary to ensure that primary cancer of one of these organs is not coexisting with a goiter.

About 10% of anterior mediastinal masses are mediastinal thyroid tissue. Overall, 5% of mediastinal tumors prove to be intrathoracic goiters.[75] Suggestive CT features include anatomic continuity with the cervical thyroid, focal calcifications, high CT number (>70 HU), and a prolonged increase in CT numbers after iodinated intravenous contrast material (>100 HU).[75] Less commonly, mediastinal goiters occur in other parts of the mediastinum. Radionuclide scanning after administration of ^{123}I or ^{131}I may confirm this diagnosis.

Surgical management of a large substernal goiter with airway compression can be difficult.[52,76] Most intrathoracic goiters should be removed because of the risk of sudden enlargement, unless the patient is in a very high-risk group for surgical complications. Usually such goiters can be removed using a standard cervical collar incision, but sometimes a sternotomy or a thoracotomy is required. A combined surgical approach often is necessary for posterior mediastinal goiters. Tracheostomy should be avoided if possible, unless laryngeal edema is present. Intubation should be attempted only in life-threatening situations or at the time of definitive surgery, after the diagnostic work-up is otherwise complete. Peak and mid-inspiratory flow rates often double after removal of large goiters with significant tracheal obstruction. Two patients with hypercapnia preoperatively became normocapnic after removal of the goiter. Surgery usually is recommended for goiters that cause peak inspiratory flow rates of 1.5 L/sec or less. Substernal goiters can recur in as many as 20% of postoperative patients. Until recently, there was reluctance to treat patients with large multinodular goiters and compressive symptoms with ^{131}I, but a recent study of 21 patients demonstrated objective improvement in tracheal luminal size and tracheal deviation.[77]

THYROTOXICOSIS AND ASTHMA

Thyrotoxicosis has been said to worsen airway hyperreactivity in patients with asthma. Settipane and colleagues[78] reported 5 patients with severe intractable asthma who became responsive to therapy after several days of antithyroid treatment with PTU. Although this relation has been generally accepted,[79] there are only a few case reports to substantiate this effect.[80,81] Because asthma and thyrotoxicosis are both common illnesses, it is surprising that this deleterious effect of thyrotoxicosis is not better documented.

Exogenous T_3 given chronically to asthmatics can decrease their symptoms and increase their peak flow rates[82]; however, peak flow measurement is highly variable and significantly effort-dependent. Normal subjects who were made thyrotoxic with exogenous T_3 and challenged with methacholine inhalation did not increase their airway resistance.[83] Nonasthmatic thyrotoxic patients did not bronchoconstrict after histamine challenge or change responses after becoming euthyroid.[84] Mild asthmatics with T_3-induced thyrotoxicosis also did not have a change in methacholine-induced bronchospasm, pulmonary function tests, or exercise capacity.[85] To further confuse the subject, hyperthyroidism decreased bronchial reactivity to carbachol provocation in 8 of 11 patients studied before and after being treated for Graves' disease.[86] Acute hypothyroidism caused by thyroidectomy for cancer was associated with increased bronchial reactivity to carbachol in 11 patients without prior pulmonary disease.[87]

In summary, most data does not support a consistent relation between thyroid function and bronchial reactivity. It remains unclear whether or not hyperthyroidism and asthma are associated more frequently than expected based on their individual prevalence.

MISCELLANEOUS INTERACTIONS

Airway obstruction (asthma or COPD) and thyrotoxicosis interact in other ways. For example, beta-blockers may worsen airway obstruction. Theophylline metabolism can be accelerated[88] up to fourfold[89] because of increased hepatic metabolism by the cytochrome P450 system. Theophylline metabolism after intravenous dosing is accelerated, and there is no change in the volume of drug distribution. Theophylline can increase the serum T_4 level, at least transiently, in adults and children.[90]

Serum angiotensin-converting enzyme activity (SACE) usually is elevated in sarcoidosis, many other granulomatous diseases, and diabetes mellitus. It also is increased in thyrotoxicosis and decreased in hypothyroidism, independent of their cause.[91-93] In subacute thyroiditis, the SACE level changes in parallel with the level of thyroid function. In nonthyroidal illness, the SACE levels are variable, and may reflect the true functional status of the thyroid gland, particularly the T_3 level.[94] The tissue of origin of the elevated SACE in thyrotoxicosis is not known.

PTU can cause eosinophilic pleuritis or diffuse interstitial pneumonitis.[95,96] The latter has been documented by lung biopsies of two patients with dyspnea, a productive cough, and restrictive pulmonary-function tests within 1 to 3 months of beginning PTU therapy. The pulmonary findings resolved rapidly after discontinuation of PTU. Finally, Hashimoto's thyroiditis may be associated with a twofold increase in the frequency of bronchogenic carcinoma, especially adenocarcinoma.[97]

Systemic Conditions That Affect Both Lung and Thyroid

Several conditions can affect both the lung and the thyroid, such as cystic fibrosis. In the past, children with cystic fibrosis often were treated with potassium iodide as an expectorant. Their sensitivity to the goitrogenic effects of chronic iodide therapy was manifested by a very high incidence of goiter and hypothyroidism.[98] Children with cystic fibrosis not receiving iodides had normal serum T_4 and TSH levels and intrathyroidal iodine organification (perchlorate discharge test), but their serum T_3 levels were diminished, perhaps owing to decreased peripheral conversion of T_4 to T_3.[99] Other studies have found lower than normal serum T_4 levels and elevated T_3/T_4 ratios with an increased TSH response to TRH,[100] suggesting subclinical hypothyroidism. These studies did not control for the effects of malnutrition or exocrine pancreatic deficiency.

Iodinated glycerol (Organidin), used to increase mucus clearance and for symptomatic treatment of COPD, may cause thyrotoxicosis or hypothyroidism.[101,102] Very recently, iodine was removed from this medication. Chronic iodine intake also may cause pulmonary edema.[103]

Cigarette smoking can subtly alter thyroid function tests; however, the changes are not clinically significant in most people. Discontinuation of smoking led to a decrease in the serum T_4 and rT_3 levels, a small rise in the serum TSH level, and no change in the serum T_3 level.[104] In contrast, in another study, heavy smokers had lower T_4 and T_3 levels when compared with light smokers and control subjects.[105] Other measures of thyroid function did not differ among the three groups. The authors of the latter study suggest that the pyridine components of cigarette smoke may have a mild antithyroid effect. Alternatively, inhibition of thyroid function may reflect the higher serum thiocyanate concentrations in smokers. Smoking has also been associated with a higher prevalence of ophthalmopathy in patients with Graves' disease[106] and nontoxic goiter, and it has been recently reported to increase the serum TSH further in subclinical hypothyroidism and to impair the peripheral action of thyroid hormone.[106a].

Systemic autoimmune disorders may involve the lung and often are associated with thyroid disease. Examples include Sjögren's syndrome, systemic lupus erythematosus, and rheumatoid arthritis. Myasthenia gravis occurs in 0.1% of patients with Graves' disease, a 30-fold increase over the prevalence in the general population. Pulmonary manifestations can include thymoma, aspiration due to bulbar involvement, and respiratory muscle weakness leading to respiratory failure.

Other systemic diseases can involve both the lung and thyroid. *Pneumocystis carinii* (PCP) infection of the thyroid has been found in seven AIDS patients, six of whom were receiving aerosolized pentamidine prophylaxis against PCP pneumonia.[107] Their glands were enlarged. These goiters may or may not be tender and patients have been hyper- or hypothyroid. Radioactive iodine uptake usually is decreased in the region affected. The role of suppression of lung infection in promoting extrapulmonary PCP is not clear. Histiocytosis X (Eosinophilic granuloma, Langerhans' cell histiocytosis) has been found in the thyroid gland in patients with or without pulmonary involvement.[108,109]

References

1. Hitchcock KR, Reichlin S. Thyroid hormones in the adult rat lung. Am Rev Respir Dis 1978;117:807
2. Obregon MJ, Deescobar M, Escobar Del Rey, F. Concentrations of triiodo-L-thyronine in the plasma and tissue of normal rats, as determined by radioimmunoassay. Endocrinology 1979;103:2145
3. Chopra IJ. A study of extrathyroidal conversion of thyroxine to 3,5,3' triiodo-L-thyronine in the rat. J Clin Invest 1977;50:1124
4. McCann UD, Shaw EA. Iodothyronine deiodination reaction types in several rat tissues: effects of age, thyroid status, and glucocorticoid treatment. Endocrinology 1984;114:1513
5. Gonzales LW, Ballard PL. Identification and characterization of nuclear T_3-binding sites in fetal human lung. J Clin Endocrinol Metab 1981;53:21
6. Gonzales LW, Ballard PL. Nuclear 3',5'-tri-iodothyronine receptors in rabbit lung: characterization and developmental changes. Endocrinology 1982;111:542
7. Morishige WK, Geurnsey DL. Triiodothyronine receptors in rat lung. Endocrinology 1978;102:1628
8. Lindenberg JA, Brehier A, Ballard PL. Tri-iodothyronine nuclear binding in fetal an adult rabbit lung and cultured lung cells. Endocrinology 1979;103:1725
9. Wilson M, Hitchcock KR, Douglas WJ, et al. Hormones and the lung. III. Immunohistochemical localization of thyroid hormone binding in type II pulmonary epithelial cells clonally derived from adult rat lung. Anat Rec 1979;195:611
10. Smith DM, Hitchcock KR. Thyroid hormone binding to adult rat alveolar type II cells. Exp Lung Res 1983;5:141
11. Redding RA, Douglas WHJ, Stein M. Thyroid hormone influence on lung surfactant metabolism. Science 1972;175:994
12. Hitchcock KR. Hormones and the lung. I. Thyroid hormones and glucocorticoids in lung development. Anat Rec 1979;194:15
13. Whitsett JA, Darovec-Beckerman C, Adams K, et al. Thyroid dependent maturation of β-adrenergic receptors in the rat lung. Biochem Biophys Res Commun 1980;97;913
14. Baker SP. Effect of thyroid status on β-adrenoreceptors and muscarinic receptors in the rat lung. J Auton Pharmacol 1981;1:269
15. Scarpace PJ, Abrass IB. Thyroid hormone regulation of rat heart, lymphocyte, and lung β-adrenergic receptors. Endocrinology 1981;108:1007
16. Lazzaro D, Price M, De Felice M, et al. The transcription factor TTF-1 is expressed at the onset of thyroid and lung morphogenesis and in restricted regions of the foetal brain. Development 1991;113:1093.
17. Bohinski RJ, Di Lauro R, Whitsett JA. The lung-specific surfactant protein B gene promoter is a target for thyroid transcription factor 1 and hepatocyte nuclear factor 3, indicating common factors for organ-specific gene expression along the foregut axis. Molec Cell Biol 1994;14:5671.
18. Smith TJ, Murata Y, Horwitz AL, et al. Regulation of glycosaminoglycan synthesis by thyroid hormone in vitro. J Clin Invest 1982;70:1066
19. Peabody FW, Wentworth JA. Clinical studies of the respiration. IV. The vital capacity of the lungs and its relation to dyspnea. Arch Intern Med 1917;20:443
20. Lemon WS, Moersch JH. Basal metabolism and vital capacity. Arch Intern Med 1924;33:130
21. Rabinowitch IM. The vital capacity in hyperthyroidism with a study of the influence of posture. Arch Intern Med 1923;31:910
22. Stein M, Kimbel P, Johnson RL. Pulmonary function in hyperthyroidism. J Clin Invest 1961;40:348
23. McElvaney GN, Wilcox PG, Fairbarn MS, et al. Respiratory muscle weakness and dyspnea in thyrotoxic patients. Am Rev Respir Dis 1990;141:1221
24. Davies HW, Meakins J, Sands J. The influence of circulatory disturbances on the gaseous exchange of blood. V. Blood gases and circulation rate in hyperthyroidism. Heart 1924;11:299
25. Kendrick AH, O'Reilly JR, Laszlo G. Lung function and exercise performance in hyperthyroidism before and after treatment. Q U Med 1988;68:615
26. Bates DM, Macklem PT, Christie RV. Respiratory function in disease. Philadelphia: WB Saunders, 1971:430

27. Freedman S. Lung volumes and distensibility and maximum respiratory pressures in thyroid disease before and after treatment. Thorax 1978;33:785

28. Massey DG, Becklake MR, McKenzie JM, et al. Circulatory and ventilatory response to exercise in thyrotoxicosis. N Engl J Med 1967;276:1104

29. Ayres J, Clark TH, Maisey MN. Thyrotoxicosis and dyspnea. Clin Endocrinol (Oxf) 1982;164:645

30. Mier A, Brophy C, Wass JAH, et al. Reversible respiratory muscle weakness in hyperthyroidism. Am Rev Respir Dis 1989;139:529

31. Miyashita A, Suzuki S, Suzuki M, et al. Effect of thyroid hormone on in vivo contractility of the canine diaphragm. Am Rev Respir Dis 1992;145:1456

32. Ianuzzo CD, Chen V, O'Brien P, et al. Effect of experimental dysthyroidism on the enzymatic character of the diaphragm. J Appl Physiol 1984;56:117

33. Valtin H, Tenney SM. Respiratory adaptations to hyperthyroidism. J Appl Physiol 1960;15:1107

34. Engel LA, Ritchie B. Ventilatory response to inhaled carbon dioxide in hyperthyroidism. J Appl Physiol 1971;30:173

35. Zwillich CW, Matthay M, Potts DE, et al. Thyrotoxicosis: comparison of effects of thyroid ablation and beta-adrenergic blockade on metabolic rate and ventilatory control. J Clin Endocrinol Metab 1978;46:491

36. Stockley RA, Bishop JM. Effect of thyrotoxicosis on the reflex hypoxic respiratory drive. Clin Sci 1977;53:93

37. Bishop JM, Donald KW, Wade OL. Circulatory dynamics at rest and on exercise in the hyperkinetic states. Clin Sci 1956;14:329

38. McIlroy MD, Elridge FL, Stone RW. The mechanical properties of the lungs in anoxia, anaemia, and thyrotoxicosis. Clin Sci 1955;15:353

39. Small D, Gillons W, Levy RD, et al. Exertional dyspnea and ventilation in hyperthyroidism. Chest 1992;101:1268

40. Forfar JC, Muir AL, Sawers, et al. Abnormal left ventricular function in hyperthyroidism. N Engl J Med 1982;307:1165

41. Sumita S, Ujike Y, Namiki A, et al. Suppression of the thyrotropin response to thyrotropin-releasing hormone and its association with severity of critical illness. Crit Care Med 1994;22:1603

42. Post FA, Soule SG, Willcox PA, et al. The spectrum of endocrine dysfunction in active pulmonary tuberculosis. Clin Endocrinol 1994;40:367

43. Dulchavesky SA, Kennedy PR, Geller ER, et al. T$_3$ preserves respiratory function in sepsis. J Trauma 1991;31:753

44. Samaan NA, Castillo S, Schultz PN, et al. Serum calcitonin after pentagastrin stimulation in patients with bronchogenic carcinoma and breast cancer compared to that in patients with medullary thyroid carcinoma. J Clin Endocrinol Metab 1980;51:237

45. Ivey HK. Cancer metastatic to the thyroid: a diagnostic problem. Mayo Clin Proc 1984;59:856

46. Smith SA, Gharib H, Goellner JR. Fine-needle aspiration. Usefulness for diagnosis and management of metastatic carcinoma to the thyroid. Arch Intern Med 1987;147:311

47. Worm AM, Holten I, Teaning E. Nuclear imaging of pulmonary metastases in thyroid carcinoma. Acta Radiol Oncol Radiat Phys Biol 1960;19:410

48. Vassilopoulou-Sellin R, Klein MJ, Smith TH, et al. Pulmonary metastases in children and young adults with differentiated thyroid cancer. Cancer 1993;71:1348

49. Casara D, Rubello D, Saladini G, et al. Different features of pulmonary metastases in differentiated thyroid cancer: natural history and multivariate statistical analysis of prognostic variables. J Nucl Med 1993;34:809

50. Maruyama M, Sugenoya A, Kobayashi S, et al. A case of papillary carcinoma of the thyroid with more than 30 years long-term asymptomatic pulmonary metastases. Clin Endocrinol 1993;38:331

51. Rotenberg D, Lawson VG, Van Nostrand, AWP. Thyroid carcinoma presenting as a tracheal tumor: case report and literature review with reflections on pathogenesis. J Otolaryngol 1979;8:4601

52. Lawson V. The management of airway involvement in thyroid tumors. Arch Otolaryngol 1983;109:86

53. Shin DH, Mark EJ, Suen HC, et al. Pathologic staging of papillary carcinoma of the thyroid with airway invasion based on the anatomic manner of extension to the trachea. Hum Pathol 1993;24:866

54. Djalilian M, Bealirs OH, Devine KC, et al. Intraluminal involvement of the larynx and trachea by thyroid cancer. Am J Surg 1974;128:500

55. Friedman M. Surgical management of thyroid carcinoma with laryngotracheal invasion. Otolaryngol Clin North Am 1990;23:495

56. Melliere DJM, Yashia NEB, Becquemin JP, et al. Thyroid carcinoma with tracheal or esophageal involvement: limited or maximal surgery? Surgery 1993;113:166

57. Grillo HC, Suen HC, Mathisen DJ, Wain JC. Resectional management of thyroid carcinoma invading the airway. Ann Thorac Surg 1992;54:3

58. Lydiatt DD, Markin RS, Ogren FP. Tracheal invasion by thyroid carcinoma. Ear Nose Throat J 1990;69:145

59. Nomori H, Kobayashi K, Ishihara T, et al. Thyroid carcinoma infiltrating the trachea: clinical, histologic, and morphometric analyses. J Surg Oncol 1990;44:78

60. Katlic MR, Wang CA, Grillo HC. Substernal goiter. Ann Thorac Surg 1985;39:391

61. Miller MR, Pincock AC, Oates GD, Wilkinson R, Skene-Smith H. Upper airway obstruction due to goitre: detection, prevalence and results of surgical management. Q Med 1990;74:177

62. Shambaugh GE, Seed R, Korn A. Airway obstruction in substernal goiters: clinical and therapeutic implications. J Chronic Dis 1973;26:737

63. Godwin JE, Miller KS, Goang KG, Sahn SA. Benign thyroid hyperplasia presenting as bilateral vocal cord paralysis: complete remission following surgery. Chest 1991;99:1029

64. Irwin RS, Pratter MR, Hamolsky MW. Chronic persistent cough: an uncommon presenting complaint of thyroiditis. Chest 1982;81:386

65. Siderys H, Rowe GA. Superior vena caval syndrome caused by intrathoracic goiter. Am Surg 1970;36:446

66. Hershey CO, McVeigh RC, Miller RP. Transient superior vena cava syndrome due to porpylthiouracil therapy in intrathoracic goiter. Chest 1981;79:356

67. Blum M, Biller BJ, Bergman DA. The thyroid cork: obstruction of the thoracic inlet due to retroclavicular goiter. JAMA 1974;227:189

68. Torres A, Arroyo J, Kastanos N, et al. Acute respiratory failure and tracheal obstruction in patients with intrathoracic goiter. Crit Care Med 1983;11:265

69. Calcaterra TC, Macari DR. Aerodigestive dysfunction secondary to thyroid tumors. Laryngoscope 1981;91:701

70. Hassard AO, Holland JG. Benign thyroid disease and upper airway obstruction. J Otolaryngol 1982;11:77

71. Alfonso A, Christoudias G, Amarruin Q, et al. Tracheal or esophageal compression due to benign thyroid disease. Am J Surg 1981;142:350

72. Jaregui R, Liker ES, Bayley A. Upper airway obstruction in euthyroid goiter. JAMA 1977;238:2163

73. Canham EM, Sahn SA. Recurrent "suppressed" goiter causing upper airway obstruction. Am Rev Respir Dis 1982;125:757

74. Karbowitz SR, Edelman LB, Nath S, et al. Spectrum of advanced upper airway obstruction due to goiters. Chest 1985;87:18

75. Glazer GM, Axel L, Moss AA. CT diagnosis of mediastinal thyroid. AJR 1982;138:495

76. Shaha AR. Surgery for benign thyroid disease causing tracheoesophageal compression. Otolaryngol Clin North Am 1990;23:391

77. Huysmans DAKC, Hermus ARMM, Corstens FHM, Barentsz JO, Kloppenborg WC. Large, compressive goiters treated with radioiodine. Ann Intern Med 1994;121:757

78. Settipane GA, Schoenfeld E, Hamolsky MW. Asthma and hyperthyroidism. J Allergy Clin Immunol 1972;49:348

79. Bush RK, Ehrlich EN, Reed CE. Thyroid disease and asthma. J Allergy Clin Immunol 1977;59:398

80. Cockroft DW, Silverberg JDH, Dosman JA. Decrease in nonspecific bronchial reactivity in an asthmatic following treatment of hyperthyroidism. Ann Allergy 1978;41:163

81. White NW, Raine RI, Bateman ED. Asthma and hyperthyroidism. South African Med J 1990;78:750

82. Ismail AA, Shaleby E, Gadalla. Effect of tri-iodothyronine on bronchial asthma (part 2). J Asthma Res 1977;14:111

83. Irwin RS, Pratter MR, Stivers DH, et al. Airway reactivity and lung function in triiodothyronine-induced thyrotoxicosis. J Appl Physiol 1985;58:1485

84. Roberts JA, McLellan AR, Alexander WD. Effect of hyperthyroidism on bronchial reactivity in non-asthmatic patients. Thorax 1989;445:603

85. Hollingsworth HM, Pratter MR, Dubois JM, Braverman LE, Irwin RS. Effect of triiodothyronine-induced thyrotocixosis on airway hyperresponsiveness. J Appl Physiol 1991;71:438

86. Israel RH, Poe RH, Cave WT, et al. Hyperthyroidism protects against carbachol-induced bronchospasm. Chest 1987;91:243

87. Wieshammer S, Keck FS, Shauffelen AC, von Beauvais H, Seibold H, Homback V. Effects of hypothyroidism on bronchial reactivity in non-asthmatic subjects. Thorax 1990;45:947

88. Pokrajac M, Simic D, Varagic VM. Pharmacokinetics of theophylline in hyperthyroid and hypothyroid patients with chronic obstructive pulmonary disease. Eur J Clin Pharmacol 1987;33:483

89. Bauman JH, Teichman S, Wible DA. Increased theophylline clearance in a patient with hyperthyroidism. Ann Allergy 1984;52:94

90. Hiratani M, Muto K, Oshida Y, et al. Effect of sustained-release theophylline administration on pituitary-thyroid axis. J Allergy Clin Immunol 1982;70:481

91. Brent GA, Hershman JM, Reed AW, et al. Serum angiotensin converting enzyme in severe nonthyroidal illness associated with low serum thyroxine concentration. Ann Intern Med 1984;100:6840

92. Smallrige RC, Rogers J, Verma PS. Serum angiotensin converting enzyme alterations in hyperthyroidism, hypothyroidism, and subacute thyroiditis. JAMA 1983;250:489

93. Yotsumoto H, Imai Y, Kuzuya N. Increased levels of serum angiotensin-converting enzyme activity in hyperthyroidism. Ann Intern Med 1982;96:326

94. Smallridge RC, Chernow B, Snyder R, et al. Angiotensin-converting enzyme activity. Arch Intern Med 1985;145:1829

95. Miyazono K, Okazaki T, Uchida S, et al. Propylthiouracil-induced diffuse interstitial pneumonitis. Arch Intern Med 1984;144:1764

96. Middleton KL, Santella R, Couser JI. Eosinophilic pleuritis due to propylthiouracil. Chest 1993;103:955

97. Yamashita N, Maruchi N, Mori W. Hashimoto's thyroiditis: a possible risk factor for lung cancer among Japanese women. Cancer Lett 1979;7:9

98. Dolan TF, Gibson LE. Complications of iodide therapy in patients with cystic fibrosis. J Pediatr 1971;79:684

99. Segall-Blank M, Vagenakis AG, Schwachman H, et al. Thyroid gland function and pituitary TSH reserve in patients with cystic fibrosis. J Pediatr 1981;98:218

100. De Luca F, Trimarchi F, Sferlazzas C, et al. Thyroid function in children with cystic fibrosis. Eur J Pediatr 1982;138:327

101. Huseby JS, Benett SW, Hagensee ME. Hyperthyroidism induced by iodinated glycerol. Am Rev Respir Dis 1991;144:1403

102. Becker CB, Gordon JM. Iodinated glycerol and thyroid dysfunction; four cases and a review of the literature. Chest 1993;103:188

103. Geurian K, Branam C. Iodine poisoning secondary to long-term iodinated glycerol therapy. Arch Intern Med 1994;154:1153

104. Melander A, Nordenskjold E, Lundh B, et al. Influence of smoking on thyroid activity. Acta Med Scand 1981;2049:441

105. Sepkovic DW, Haley NJ, Wyner EL. Thyroid activity in cigarette smokers. Arch Intern Med 1984;144:501

106. Bertelsen JB, Heged s L. Cigarette smoking and the thyroid. Thyroid 1994;4:327

106a. Miller B, Zulewski H, Huber P, Ratcliffe JG, Staub JJ. Impaired action of thyroid hormone associated with smoking in women with hypothyroidism. N Engl J Med 1995; 333:964

107. Guttler R, Singer PA. Pneumocystis carinii thyroiditis. Arch Intern Med 1993;153:393

108. Tsang WYW, Lau MF, Chan JKC. Incidental Langerhans' cell histiocytosis of the thyroid. Histopathology 1994;24:397

109. Maurea S, Lastoria S, Klain M, et al. Diagnostic evaluation of thyroid involvement by histiocytosis X. J Nucl Med 1994;35:263

Werner and Ingbar's The Thyroid, Seventh Edition,
edited by Lewis E. Braverman and Robert D. Utiger.
Lippincott–Raven Publishers, Philadelphia, © 1996

40

The Kidneys and Electrolyte Metabolism in Thyrotoxicosis

Arnold M. Moses

Steven J. Scheinman

RENAL HEMODYNAMICS AND TUBULAR FUNCTION

Thyrotoxicosis causes changes in hemodynamics that closely resemble those associated with arteriovenous fistulae.[1] Cardiac output increases and peripheral vascular resistance decreases. Right-sided cardiac filling pressures tend to be moderately elevated and mean arterial pressure is somewhat diminished, reflecting redistribution of blood from the arterial to the venous side of the circulation, with increased venous volume and reduced effective arterial volume (see chap 38).

In both human thyrotoxicosis and in animals treated with excess thyroid hormone, renal plasma flow and glomerular filtration rate (GFR) are increased, probably because of the increase in cardiac output and decrease in peripheral resistance. Intrarenal vasodilatation also occurs.[2] The renal content of the endogenous vasoconstrictor substance endothelin is lower in thyrotoxic rats, and decreases in endothelin may play a role in the renal vasodilatation in thyrotoxicosis.[3]

The tendency of not only GFR but also extracellular fluid volume to be high in thyrotoxicosis suggests that serum creatinine concentrations should be low. Indeed, normal subjects given large doses of thyroid hormone have decreased serum creatinine concentrations before substantial muscle wasting occurs. The mean 24-hour urine creatinine excretion is significantly lower in thyrotoxic patients as compared with either the same patients after treatment or with normal subjects. This decrease has been ascribed to loss of muscle mass in thyrotoxic patients, and it occurs despite an increase in the renal tubular secretion of creatinine.[4–6] Presumably reflecting the protein catabolic state, blood urea nitrogen (BUN) concentrations are slightly elevated in thyrotoxicosis despite an increase in urea clearance,[7] and thus the BUN/creatinine ratio is elevated. In all

of these studies, these values were normalized by restoration of euthyroidism.[4,5,7] Urinary total protein excretion is mildly elevated, perhaps as a result of the increase in GFR.[6]

Thyroid hormones increase renal tubular mass by inducing both hypertrophy and hyperplasia of renal tubular epithelial cells. The increase in weight is proportional to the increase in GFR and renal plasma flow. Thyroid hormone also stimulates renal growth in young animals, an effect that is independent of protein intake and pituitary activity.[2]

The functional and morphologic changes that occur in renal tubules in thyrotoxicosis are accompanied by an increased renal tubular capacity for active transport. For example, transepithelial voltage is increased and Na^+,K^+-ATPase activity is increased, with consequent increases in sodium transport. Thyroid hormone also stimulates sodium-dependent phosphate transport in cultured renal tubular cells through an increase in transport capacity, rather than affinity of the transporter for phosphate,[8] without a change in Na^+-dependent transport of sulfate,[9] glucose, or proline.[10] In addition, proximal tubular sodium-proton exchange is increased in experimental thyrotoxicosis in rats.[10] These changes are not associated with clinically important increases in the reabsorption of phosphate or bicarbonate.

WATER AND ELECTROLYTE METABOLISM

Patients with thyrotoxicosis rarely have discernible abnormalities in water metabolism. Serum electrolyte concentrations are usually normal. Occasionally, however, these patients have polydipsia with 24-hour urine volumes as high as 3 or 4 liters,[11] associated at times with slightly hypotonic plasma. Thyrotoxicosis increases free water excretion in patients with diabetes insipidus. The polyuria is not due to increased solute excretion and is therefore not an osmotic diuresis. Some thyrotoxic patients have mild impairment in urinary concentrating ability,[12] but this is not clinically important.[13] The release of vasopressin in response to an osmotic stimulus is not impaired.[14] By exclusion, therefore, the polyuria in these patients is due to increased thirst, as in primary polydipsia. This explanation is supported by observations in thyrotoxic animals.[15,16] In patients with thyrotoxicosis, the sensation of thirst is initiated at a lower plasma osmolality than when they are euthyroid.[14] This polydipsia may be secondary to the dipsogenic effect of elevated plasma angiotensin-II concentrations.[17] The polydipsia and polyuria revert to normal after treatment of thyrotoxicosis.

Patients with thyrotoxicosis have increased plasma atrial natriuretic hormone concentrations and plasma renin activity.[18–20] In contrast, serum aldosterone concentrations are normal or low, particularly in relation to plasma renin activity.[20] These hormonal alterations seem to have no clinical consequences except for mild edema. The urinary excretion of sodium and potassium is normal when patients consume the usual amounts of those ions. However, there are no detailed studies on the effect of thyrotoxicosis on the ability of patients (or animals) to conserve sodium when sodium intake is low or to excrete sodium when sodium intake is high. Whereas total body exchangeable potassium is decreased in thyrotoxicosis due to a decrease in total muscle mass,[21] total exchangeable sodium is often increased.

EDEMA

Thyrotoxic patients may develop pitting edema involving the hands, ankles, legs, and sacrum. Some patients even develop periorbital edema, with apparent aging changes, leading them to seek blepharoplasty.[22] The edema in thyrotoxic patients results from renal salt and water retention in response to the reduction in effective arterial volume, and this retention contributes to an increase in blood volume and venous pressure. The edema that develops under these circumstances does not necessarily imply the presence of congestive heart failure. In support of this concept, exercise testing in thyrotoxic patients with edema may induce a substantial increase in cardiac output with little or no increase in right atrial or pulmonary artery pressure. If the additional circulatory load imposed by high cardiac output overwhelms myocardial reserve or if myocardial function is impaired by organic heart disease or by the thyrotoxic state itself, congestive failure ensues. Severe thyrotoxicosis may also be associated with protein-calorie malnutrition, with hypoalbuminemia, an additional cause of expansion of plasma volume.

HYPERCALCEMIA AND HYPERCALCIURIA

Thyrotoxicosis is associated with accelerated bone resorption, occasionally sufficiently intense to cause hypercalcemia (see chap 48). The thyrotoxicosis-induced bone resorption leads to increased urinary excretion of various markers of bone resorption such as hydroxyproline and the cross-linked N-telopep-

tide of type I collagen.[23] Parathyroid hormone release is inhibited as a consequence of the accelerated bone resorption, leading to decreased nephrogenous cAMP excretion and increased renal phosphate reabsorption. Decreased parathyroid hormone secretion also leads to a decrease in renal tubular production of 1,25-dihydroxyvitamin D from 25-hydroxyvitamin D, with a subsequent decrease in intestinal calcium absorption. The increase in bone resorption and decrease in parathyroid hormone secretion also lead to increases in urinary calcium excretion. This occasionally results in renal calculi, nephrocalcinosis, and reversible renal insufficiency.[24]

Serum magnesium concentrations may be decreased in as many as one-third of thyrotoxic patients. Although urinary magnesium excretion may be increased, magnesium balance is normal, and exchangeable magnesium is increased in thyrotoxic patients, suggesting enhanced cellular uptake of magnesium. The severity of hypomagnesemia has been reported to correlate with the clinical severity of the thyrotoxicosis. Abnormalities of magnesium metabolism are rarely of clinical importance, although it has been speculated that hypomagnesemia may explain some of the findings in apathetic thyrotoxicosis.[25]

THYROTOXIC PERIODIC PARALYSIS

Thyrotoxic periodic paralysis is characterized by localized or generalized attacks of muscular weakness or flaccid paralysis that last for a few hours to several days (for details of the muscular disease per se, see chap 43). Most thyrotoxic patients with the disorder have Graves' disease. However, thyrotoxic periodic paralysis has also been described in patients with toxic nodular goiter, toxic thyroid adenoma, thyroiditis, exogenous thyrotoxicosis, and TSH-producing pituitary tumors.[26,27] The episodes of muscle weakness are invariably associated with a decrease in serum potassium concentration, although the concentration is not always subnormal.[28] Total body potassium content is normal; the hypokalemia is the result of an intracellular shift of potassium. (This is in contrast to patients with idiopathic hypokalemic periodic paralysis, in whom total body potassium stores are reduced.[29]) The severity of the weakness appears to reflect the severity of the hypokalemia. As the potassium moves back out of the cells over a period of several hours to several days, the neuromuscular symptoms resolve. Episodes of paralysis can be precipitated in susceptible thyrotoxic patients by the ingestion of carbohydrate or ethanol, by strenuous physical exercise in hot humid weather, and by the administration of insulin and acetazolamide.[30] In spite of these precipitating factors the episodes occur erratically in most patients. Between attacks, serum potassium concentrations are within normal limits.

Asian patients seem to be particularly susceptible to thyrotoxic periodic paralysis, although its prevalence in this population may be decreasing. In three Japanese clinics in 1957, 8.6% of thyrotoxic men and 0.4% of thyrotoxic women had periodic paralysis; in the same clinics in 1991 the respective figures were 4.3% and 0.04%.[31] One possible cause of the decreased frequency of periodic paralysis was a change in food consumption; less carbohydrate and more potassium were eaten in 1991 than in 1957.[31] The prevalence of thyrotoxic periodic paralysis is much less in whites than in Asians, and it is very rare in Hispanic[32] and black[33] patients.

The cause of the susceptibility of some thyrotoxic patients to periodic paralysis is not known. The intracellular movement of potassium interferes with the contraction of actomyosin, which can cause paralysis. Thyroid hormone excess increases Na^+,K^+-ATPase activity in skeletal muscle, liver, and kidney and results in increased intracellular transport of potassium.[34] Platelet Na^+,K^+-ATPase activity in thyrotoxic patients with periodic paralysis was higher than in those without periodic paralysis,[35] but the activity of this enzyme was similar in treated thyrotoxic patients with and without a history of periodic paralysis. These results suggest that the activity of the sodium/potassium pump may be especially sensitive to thyroid hormone excess in those patients who have thyrotoxic periodic paralysis. Thyrotoxicosis also increases tissue responsiveness to beta-adrenergic stimulation, another activator of Na^+,K^+-ATPase activity,[36] and nonselective beta-adrenergic antagonist drugs decrease the frequency of paralytic attacks in these patients. The Na^+,K^+-ATPase is also activated by insulin,[36] which may explain the induction of paralytic attacks by carbohydrate meals and administration of insulin. In addition, potassium translocation independent of Na^+,K^+-ATPase may be an important feature of thyrotoxic periodic paralysis.[37] However, hypokalemia may not be the cause of the neuromuscular problems of thyrotoxic periodic paralysis,[27] because hypokalemia sufficient to provoke paralysis in a thyrotoxic patient has no effect when the same patient is euthyroid.

Restoration of the euthyroid state effectively prevents episodes of weakness or paralysis, but symptoms can return with recurrence of thyrotoxicosis. Potassium administration during acute attacks shortens the duration of the episodes, and treatment with potassium or spironolactone may prevent attacks in some patients, even if their thyrotoxicosis persists.[27]

RENAL TUBULAR ACIDOSIS

Renal tubular acidosis occasionally occurs in association with thyrotoxicosis. The renal tubular acidosis has been characterized as distal because there is failure to achieve maximal urinary acidification. Renal bicarbonate wasting (proximal renal tubular acidosis) has not been described. Hypokalemia, a common feature of renal tubular acidosis, may exacerbate a tendency to periodic paralysis. The renal tubular acidosis rarely results from hypercalcemia and hypercalciuria, which can cause nephrocalcinosis, tubular damage, and impairment of renal acidification.[38] Minimum urine pH, serum bicarbonate concentrations, and urine calcium excretion should be measured in the occasional thyrotoxic patient who has nephrolithiasis.

Renal tubular acidosis may also occur in association with thyrotoxicosis caused by Graves' disease in the absence of nephrocalcinosis and may persist despite resolution of the thyrotoxicosis.[39] The renal tubular acidosis in these patients may have an autoimmune basis; antibodies to renal tubular cells were demonstrated in the serum of a patient with Graves' hyperthyroidism and renal tubular acidosis.[40] Some patients with autoimmune thyroid disease and renal tubular acidosis also have Sjögren's syndrome, and this syndrome by itself may be associated with renal tubular acidosis.[41]

IMMUNE-COMPLEX GLOMERULONEPHRITIS AND THYROID DISEASE

Immune-complex glomerulonephritis has been documented in a number of thyrotoxic patients, and several reports have implicated circulating immune complexes, with thyroglobulin as the antigen, in these cases.[42–44] The histology is usually that of a proliferative glomerulonephritis. The same lesion has been reported in patients with chronic autoimmune thyroiditis and hypothyroidism.[45,46] The relative rarity of this clinical entity contrasts with the frequency of circulating immune complexes in thyroid disease, estimated to be as high as 17% in thyrotoxicosis and higher in other thyroid diseases.[47]

RENAL COMPLICATIONS OF ANTITHYROID DRUG TREATMENT

Renal complications of antithyroid therapy are very rare. The few cases of proteinuria that have been reported in patients taking propylthiouracil or methimazole during the past half century occurred mainly among patients having a drug-induced vasculitis[48–50] or a lupus-like reaction[51] to the drugs; the glomerular filtration rate in these patients was either normal or only mildly depressed. One case of nephrotic syndrome caused by minimal change nephropathy was reported in a patient taking methimazole, with rapid resolution after discontinuation of the drug.[52] Acute renal failure caused by acute allergic interstitial nephritis during therapy with propylthiouracil was reported in one patient[53]; that patient was unusual in having severe allergic reactions to several drugs.

Hypersensitivity reactions to iodide are not uncommon, and may rarely cause a periarteritis syndrome or thrombotic thrombocytopenic purpura. Lithium carbonate, which is rarely used in the treatment of thyrotoxicosis, can cause nephrogenic diabetes insipidus or chronic tubulointerstitial nephropathy.

References

1. Graettinger JS, Muenster JJ, Selverstone LA, Campbell JA. A correlation of clinical and hemodynamic studies in patients with hyperthyroidism with and without congestive heart failure. J Clin Invest 1959;38:1316
2. Bradley SE, Stephan F, Coelho JB, Reville P. The thyroid and the kidney. Kidney Int 1974;6:346
3. Singh G, Sharma AC, Thompson EB, Gulati A. Renal endothelin mechanism in altered thyroid states. Life Sci 1994;54:1901
4. Shirota T, Shinoda T, Yamada T, Aizawa T. Alteration of renal function in hyperthyroidism: increased tubular secretion of creatinine and decreased distal tubular delivery of chloride. Metabolism 1992;41:402
5. Adlerberth A, Angeras U, Jagenburg R, Lindstedt G, Stenstram G, Hasselgren PO. Urinary excretion of 3-methylhistidine and creatinine and plasma concentrations of amino acids in hyperthyroid patients following preoperative treatment with antithyroid drug or β-blocking agents: results from a prospective, randomized study. Metabolism 1987;36:637
6. Ford HC, Lim WC, Chisnall WN, Pearce JM. Renal function and electrolyte levels in hyperthyroidism: urinary protein excretion

and the plasma concentrations of urea, creatinine, urine acid, hydrogen ion and electrolytes. Clin Endocrinol 1989;30:293

7. Aizawa T, Hiramatsu K, Ohtsuka H, et al. An elevation of BUN/creatinine ratio in patients with hyperthyroidism. Horm Metab Res 1986;18:771

8. Noronha-Blob L, Lowe V, Sacktor B. Stimulation by thyroid hormone of phosphate transport in primary cultured renal cells. J Cell Physiol 1988;137:95

9. Beers KW, Dousa TP. Thyroid hormone stimulates the Na⁺-PO₄ symporter but not the Na⁺-SO₄ symporter in renal brush border. Am J Physiol 1993;265:F323

10. Kinsella J, Sacktor B. Thyroid hormones increase Na⁺/K⁺ exchange activity in renal brush border membranes. Proc Natl Acad Sci U S A 1985;82:3606

11. Evered DC, Hayter CJ, Surveyor I. Primary polydipsia in thyrotoxicosis. Metabolism 1972;21:393

12. Cutler RE, Glatte H, Dowling JT. Effect of hyperthyroidism on the renal concentrating mechanism in humans. J Clin Endocrinol 1967;27:453

13. Katz AI, Emmanouel DS, Lindheimer MD. Thyroid hormone and the kidney. Nephron 1975;15:223

14. Harvey JN, Nagi DK, Baylis PH, Wilkinson R, Belchetz PE. Disturbance of osmoregulated thirst and vasopressin secretion in thyrotoxicosis. Clin Endocrinol 1991;35:29

15. Thoday KL, Monney CT. Historial, clinical and laboratory features of 126 hyperthyroid cats. Vet Record 1992;131:257

16. Hoey A. Page A, Brown L, Atwell RB. Cardiac changes in experimental hyperthyroidism in dogs. Austral Vet J 1991;68:352

17. Phillips PA, Rolls BJ, Ledingham GG, Morton JJ, Forsling ML. Agiontensin II–induced thirst and vasopressin release in man. Clin Sci 1985;68:669

18. Rolandi E, Santaniello B, Bagnasco M, et al. Thyroid hormones and atrial natriuretic hormone secretion: study in hyper- and hypothyroid patients. Acta Endocrinol 1992;127:23

19. Tajiri J, Noguchi S, Naomi S, et al. Plasma atrial natriuretic peptide in patients with Graves' disease. Endocrinol Jpn 1990;37:665

20. Shigimatsu S, Iwasaki T, Aizawa T, et al. Plasma atrial natriuretic peptide, plasma renin activity and aldosterone during treatment of hyperthyroidism due to Graves' disease. Horm Metab Res 1989;21:514

21. Aikawa JK. Isotopic studies of the body potassium content in thyrotoxicosis. Proc Soc Exper Biol Med 1953;84:594

22. Klatsky SA, Manson PN. Thyroid disorders masquerading as aging changes. Ann Plastic Surg 1992;28:420

23. Rosen HN, Dresser-Pollak R, Moses AC, et al. Specificity of urinary excretion of cross-linked N-telopeptides of type I collagen as a marker of bone turnover. Calcif Tissue Int 1994;54:26

24. Epstein FH, Freedman LR, Levitan H. Hypercalcemia, nephrocalcinosis and reversible renal insufficiency associated with hyperthyroidism. N Engl J Med 1958;258:782

25. Marks P, Ashraf H. Apathetic hyperthyroidism with hypomagnesaemia and raised alkaline phosphatase concentration. BMJ 1978;1:821

26. Kiso Y, Yoshida K, Kaise K, et al. A case of thyrotropin (TSH)-secreting tumor complicated by periodic paralysis. Japan J Med 1990;29:399

27. Ober KP. Thyrotoxic periodic paralysis in the United States. Report of 7 cases and review of the literature. Medicine 1992;71:109

28. Yeo PP, O'Neill WC. Thyrotoxicosis and periodic paralysis. Med Grand Rounds 1984;3:10

29. Shizume K, Shishiba Y, Sakuma M, Yamauchi H, Nakao K, Okinaka S. Studies on electrolyte metabolism in idiopathic and thyrotoxic periodic paralysis. II. Total exchangeable sodium and potassium. Metabolism 1966;15:145

30. Shulkin D, Olson BR, Levey GS. Thyrotoxic periodic paralysis in a Latin-American taking acetazolamide. Am J Med Sci 1989;297:337

31. Shizume K, Shishiba Y, Kuma K, et al. Comparison of the incidence of association of periodic paralysis and hyperthyroidism in Japan in 1957 and 1991. Endocrinol Jpn 1992;39:315

32. Baumgartner FJ, Lee ET. Hyperthyroid hypokalemic periodic paralysis in a Hispanic male. J Nat Med Assoc 1990;82:133

33. Hackshaw KV, Coker E. Hypokalemic periodic paralysis in a hyperthyroid black woman. J Nat Med Assoc 1988;80:1343

34. Kubota K, Ingbar SH. Influences of thyroid states and sympathoadrenal system on extrarenal potassium disposal. Am J Physiol 1990;258:E428

35. Chan A, Shinde R, Chow CC, Cockram CS, Swaminathan R. In vivo and in vitro sodium pump activity in subjects with thyrotoxic periodic paralysis. BMJ 1991;303:1096

36. Sterns RH, Spital A. Disorders of internal potassium balance. Semin Nephrol 1987;7:399

37. Oh VMS, Taylor EA, Yeo SH, Lee KO. Cation transport across lymphocytic plasma membranes in euthyroid and thyrotoxic men with and without hypokalaemic periodic paralysis. Clin Sci 1990;78:199

38. Dash SC, Jain S, Khanna KN, Grewal K. Thyrotoxicosis, renal tubular acidosis and renal stone. J Assoc Physicians India 1980;28:323.

39. Jaeger P, Portmann L, Wauters JP, et al. Distal renal tubular acidosis and lymphocytic thyroiditis with spontaneously resolving hyperthyroidism. Report of 1 case without nephrocalcinosis. Am J Nephrol 1985;5:116

40. Konishi K, Hayashi M, Saruta T. Renal tubular acidosis with autoantibody directed to renal collecting-duct cells. N Engl J Med 1994;331:1593

41. Mason A, Golding PL. Renal tubular acidosis and autoimmune thyroid disease. Lancet 1970;2:1104

42. Jordan SC, Buckingham B, Sakai R, et al. Studies of immune complex glomerulonephritis mediated by human thyroglobulin. N Engl J Med 1981;304:121

43. O'Regan S, Fong JS, Kaplan BS, et al. Thyroid antigen-antibody nephritis. Clin Immunol Immunopathol 1976;6:341

44. Matsuura M, Kikkawa Y, Akashi K, et al. Thyroid antigen-antibody nephritis: possible involvement of fucosyl-GMI as the antigen. Endocrinol Jpn 1987;34:587

45. Horvath F, Teague P, Gaffney EF, et al. Thyroid antigen associated immune complex glomerulonephritis in Graves' disease. Am J Med 1979;67:901

46. Jordan SC, Johnston WH, Bergstein JM. Immune complex glomerulonephritis mediated by thyroid antigens. Arch Pathol Lab Med 1978;102:530

47. Calder EA, Penhale WJ, Barnes EW, Irvine WJ. Evidence for circulating immune complexes in thyroid disease. BMJ 1974;2:30

48. Griswold WR, Mendoza SA, Johnston W, Nichols S. Vasculitis associated with propylthiouracil. Evidence for immune complex pathogenesis and response to therapy. West J Med 1978;128:543

49. McCormick RV. Periarteritis occurring during propylthiouracil therapy. JAMA 1950;144:1453

50. Cassorla FG, Finegold DN, Parks JS, Tenore A, Thawerani H, Baker L. Vasculitis, pulmonary cavitation, and anemia during antithyroid drug therapy. Am J Dis Child 1983;137:118

51. Amrhein JA, Kenny FM, Ross D. Granulocytopenia, lupus-like syndrome, and other complications of propylthiouracil therapy. J Pediatr 1970;76:54

52. Reynolds LR, Bhathena D. Nephrotic syndrome associated with methimazole therapy. Arch Intern Med 1979;139:236

53. Reinhart SC, Moses AM, Cleary L, Scheinman SJ. Acute interstitial nephritis with renal failure associated with propylthiouracil therapy. Am J Kidney Dis 1994;24:575

Werner and Ingbar's The Thyroid, Seventh Edition,
edited by Lewis E. Braverman and Robert D. Utiger.
Lippincott–Raven Publishers, Philadelphia, © 1996

41

The Gastrointestinal Tract and Liver in Thyrotoxicosis

Rena Vassilopoulou-Sellin

Joseph H. Sellin

The classic gastrointestinal (GI) manifestations of thyrotoxicosis are rapid intestinal transit, increased frequency of semiformed stools, and weight loss from increased caloric requirement or malabsorption. This classic scenario is not necessarily common, and a caveat is in order. Although there are definite GI manifestations of thyrotoxicosis, their lack of specificity is such that they cannot serve as reliable diagnostic indices. One may find, instead, increased appetite, hyperphagia, and a paradoxical weight gain despite the hypermetabolic state. The absence of constipation in the elderly patient occasionally has pointed the astute clinician to the diagnosis of apathetic thyrotoxicosis. Thyrotoxicosis has been associated with a multiplicity of liver-function abnormalities; however, the interpretation of these derangements is clouded by the frequent coexistence of congestive heart failure, malnutrition, autoimmune liver disease, or propylthiouracil therapy. The clinical importance of a direct effect of thyrotoxicosis on the liver, through increased metabolic demand and a relative hypoxia, remains controversial.

Because the diagnosis of thyrotoxicosis is now made more accurately, easily, and earlier, and because effective treatment can promptly correct the symptoms and metabolic consequences of this disorder, prominent GI symptoms usually are confined to cases of noncompliance or diagnostic oversight.

The findings of GI dysfunction associated with thyrotoxicosis suggest that an excess of thyroid hormone disrupts the normal homeostatic mechanisms of the gut. Additionally, they point to a possible role for thyroid hormone in the physiology of the GI tract and liver and serve as a basis for further investigation into the peripheral effects of thyroid hormone.

HYPERTHYROIDISM AND GUT MOTILITY

Frequent bowel movements (more than two a day) are significantly more common in hyperthyroidism than in normal controls.[1] Most hyperthyroid patients, however, have one bowel movement daily. Although constipation is rare, 3% of hyperthyroid patients take laxatives, about the same as in the general population, thus limiting the value of stool frequency as a clue toward the clinical diagnosis of hyperthyroidism in the individual patient.

The physiologic basis for the increased stool frequency is attributed to hypermotility of the intestine, which is due to rapid transit[2-4] and changes in the migrating motor contractions through the small bowel.[5] In hyperthyroidism the mouth-to-cecum transit time is approximately 40% of normal.[6-7] These changes appear reversible after correction of the thyrotoxicosis.

Recent studies have emphasized several parameters of motility, including: (1) the electrical activity of the muscle, both the basal oscillations and the spike activity preceding a contraction; (2) the contractile activity of muscle, measured as the pressure generated within the esophageal or intestinal lumen and quantified as either the frequency or the duration of waves; and (3) the propulsive activity, estimated by the peristaltic propagation of waves over a length of gut or the movement of labeled markers through the GI tract. The interrelations among these measures of motility are complex, even in normals, and further clarification in disease states is needed.

A marked decrease in the force of propulsion of the pharyngeal muscles and in the closure of the upper esophageal sphincter has been observed in hyperthyroidism,[8] which may account for the swallowing difficulties occasionally encountered in thyrotoxic patients. The hyperthyroid esophagus has an increased rate of peristaltic propagation.[9]

Studies of gastric emptying have yielded variable results. In thyrotoxic rats, gastric emptying, as measured by intestinal recovery of carbon-14 triolein mixed in olive oil or by oral glucose tolerance, is more rapid. In clinical studies, gastric emptying time of a liquid meal containing glucose was mildly decreased,[10] whereas no difference in the gastric emptying of a technetium-labeled mixed protein-carbohydrate-fat meal was found when hyperthyroid patients were compared with normals.[11] Vomiting associated with thyrotoxicosis has been ascribed to either thyroid stimulation of a chemoreceptor trigger zone in the central nervous system[12] or to gastric stasis.[13]

Christensen and associates[14] demonstrated that the basic electrical rhythm or slow wave activity of the intestine was increased in hyperthyroidism, indicating that the hyperthyroid intestine is capable of more frequent contractions. In a more recent study, examining contractile rather than myoelectric activity, hyperthyroidism induced changes in both the fasted and fed states, including an increase in contraction frequency during phase 2 of the migrating motor complex and during the digestive state.[5] Occasional giant migrating complexes were observed in the hyperthyroid state but not in controls.

By using a noninvasive measure of orocecal transit time, the lactulose-hydrogen breath test, investigators have demonstrated a shortened transit time in hyperthyroid patients that normalizes with treatment.[7,15]

The clinical and experimental data on the effects of hyperthyroidism on gut motility provide some evidence that thyroid excess affects the orderly propulsion of ingested materials through the GI tract. Significant gaps exist, however, in our knowledge of the thyrotoxic effects on intestinal motility. Further investigation is required to clearly substantiate the clinical impression of intestinal hurry, specifically in the areas of gastric emptying, migrating motor complexes, and colonic motility.

GASTRIC FUNCTION IN THYROTOXICOSIS

The association between thyrotoxicosis and pernicious anemia was first described by Neuser[16] in 1899; there has since prevailed a strong clinical impression that spontaneous thyroid disease and autoimmune gastritis coincide more frequently than by statistical probability. Pernicious anemia has been reported in 2% to 5% of hyperthyroid patients.[3,17] The frequency of parietal cell or intrinsic factor antibodies, as well as low serum B_{12} or intrinsic factor levels, however, has been in the order of 20% to 30% of tested patients.[18,19] Atrophic gastritis, decreased acid secretion, and histamine-fast hypochlorhydria or achlorhydria have been found in thyrotoxic subjects, even without overt pernicious anemia.[20] Hypergastrinemia is occasionally found in association with hyperthyroidism. There is no increased incidence of ulcer disease; therefore, the hypergastrinemia may be secondary to decreased acid secretion.

It is likely that the frequently coexisting abnormalities of thyroid and gastric function reflect the association of autoimmune hyperthyroidism with other autoimmune diseases. The finding of decreased acid production in dogs rendered thyrotoxic, however, suggests a potential direct role for thyroid hormone in gastric acid production.[21]

ABSORPTION AND INTESTINAL FUNCTION

Steatorrhea has been observed in hyperthyroidism,[20,22] with daily fecal fat as high as 20g (normal, <7 g/d assuming daily intake of 100 g fat daily). This cannot be ascribed exclusively to fat hyperphagia; an element of malabsorption appears to exist, although the cause remains obscure. Pancreatic exocrine function, as measured by standard secretion tests, is normal.

Small bowel biopsies in hyperthyroid patients have not demonstrated any alteration in the normal villous architecture, although minor increases in lymphocytic infiltration and edema have been observed. Small bowel radiographs have noted occasional dilation and thickening of the circular folds.[23]

The absorptive function of the intestine in hyperthyroidism has been examined. Intestinal absorption of D-xylose is normal, although renal clearance may be increased. Studies of glucose metabolism in hyperthyroid laboratory animals have yielded conflicting results; whereas in vivo studies have suggested decreased or normal sugar absorption, in vitro gut sac studies have demonstrated increased glucose absorption.[9,24] It is unlikely that significant malabsorption of glucose occurs clinically because of the large glucose absorptive capacity of the intestine. Decreased calcium absorption has been demonstrated in clinical and animal studies,[25,26] perhaps due to deficient parathyroid-mediated synthesis of $1.25(OH)_2$ vitamin D.

Case reports have documented hyperthyroidism coincident with celiac sprue and inflammatory bowel disease[27–29] although no clear epidemiologic association has been established. Hyperthyroidism may exacerbate ulcerative colitis. Management of the intestinal disorder is simplified after therapy for hyperthyroidism. Secretory diarrhea may rarely occur with hyperthyroidism.[30]

Rapid intestinal transit, with resulting pancreaticocibal asynchronism, is the generally accepted explanation for the steatorrhea of hyperthyroidism. Analogous to the postgastrectomy states, inadequate mixing of food and pancreatic secretions occurs as the intestinal chyme precedes the digestive enzymes through the length of the small bowel; maldigestion results because dietary fat, protein, and carbohydrate are not adequately broken down into digestive components that a normal intestinal mucosa can absorb. Propranolol therapy may decrease both stool frequency and the amount of steatorrhea, suggesting that at least some of the intestinal findings can be mediated by β-agonists.[22]

THE LIVER IN THYROID DISEASE

The association between the liver and thyroid diseases has been a subject of investigation over the past 50 years, but the exact nature of the relation remains elusive. Possible thyroid-liver interactions include (1) liver damage secondary to the systemic effects of thyroid excess; (2) direct toxic effects of thyroid hormone on the liver; (3) association of intrinsic liver disease with intrinsic thyroid disease through autoimmune mechanisms; (4) alterations of thyroid hormone metabolism secondary to intrinsic liver disease; and (5) subclinical physiologic effects of thyroid hormone on liver function.

Early autopsy reports emphasized the severity of liver disease in patients dying with untreated thyrotoxicosis[31] and described marked hepatic inflammation, steatosis, necrosis, and cirrhosis. It is not clear whether these were a direct effect of thyrotoxicosis, or caused by associated conditions (congestive heart failure, infection, or malnutrition) that can in themselves lead to hepatic dysfunction. Hepatic changes seen on light microscopy include vacuolization of hepatocytes, balloon degeneration, nuclear glycogen, and mild portal infiltration of mononuclear cells; electron microscopy reveals subtle ultrastructural changes, including hyperplasia of the smooth endoplasmic reticulum, a paucity of glycogen, and mitochondrial abnormalities (increased size and number of mitochondria with increased crystal formation per mitochondrion).[32] These are all signs of mild, nonspecific liver injury. Abnormal liver-function tests occur in a significant minority of hyperthyroid patients,[33,34] with mild elevations of alkaline phosphatase or bilirubin; these abnormalities are reversible with correction of the hyperthyroidism. In patients undergoing medical therapy for hyperthyroidism, it is important to consider that liver function abnormalities may be drug-induced, because transient asymptomatic hepatotoxicity may occur with propylthiouracil therapy.[35]

Within the context of the generalized hypermetabolic state of thyrotoxicosis, resting metabolic rate and hepatic oxygen consumption increase,[36] probably secondary to increased $Na^+,-K^+$-ATPase activity. Increased hepatic oxygen uptake has been described in hyperthyroidism, despite normal fructose-6-phosphate and pentose cycling.[37] The metabolic impact of thyroid hormone on the liver appears multifactorial, mediated by alterations of insulin-like growth factor homeostasis[38], NADPH P450 regulation,[39] and changes of fatty acid synthesis and lipid secretion.[40] Although mitochondrial metabolism appears to be stimulated by thyroid hormone, it has been difficult to establish a clear-cut relationship between mitochondrial metabolism and thyroid function.[41,42] Because hepatic blood flow is not increased,[43] a combination of relative anoxia and increased metabolic demands develops that may lead to the centrizonal necrosis occasionally seen in severe hyperthyroidism. A similar hypermetabolic state has been described in alcohol-associated liver damage, and propylthiouracil has been used therapeutically in patients with alcoholic hepatitis[44,45] with conflicting short-term results. One study suggests that administration of propylthiouracil reduces mortality in alcoholic liver diseases over a 2-year period.[46]

There is still no firm evidence that thyroid hormone is directly toxic to the liver. Therefore, the hyperthyroid patient who presents with liver dysfunction requires a careful investigation for nonthyroidal illness; this frequently results in the detection of an autoimmune disorder, since multisystem autoimmune diseases may affect both the liver and the thyroid.[47] Perhaps the strongest association exists between lymphocytic thyroiditis and primary biliary cirrhosis.[48,49] In a survey of 95 patients with primary biliary cirrhosis, Crowe and colleagues[50] found that 26% had thyroid microsomal antibodies, 16% had thyroglobulin antibodies, and 16% had either clinical or biochemical evidence of hypothyroidism.

THYROID FUNCTION IN LIVER DISEASE

The interpretation of concomitant thyroid and liver-function abnormalities must take into account the fact that thyroid hormone metabolism is abnormal in severe liver disease. Both the thyroxine (T_4)-binding globulin and the peripheral conversion of T_4 to triiodothyronine (T_3) may be abnormal in patients with chronic disease or those with acute or chronic hepatitis. The increase in serum TBG in those patients with hepatitis is probably due to decreased clearance of TBG secondary to its increased sialic acid content.[51] Despite the increased energy expenditure found in cirrhosis,[52] most patients with cirrhosis are clinically euthyroid. In patients with chronic hepatitis C, therapeutic administration of interferon-α may precipitate clinical thyroid dysfunction, especially if anti-thyroid antibodies were present before treatment.[53]

Several investigators have systematically examined the thyroid hormone profiles associated with hepatitis and cirrhosis (usually alcohol-related). Despite considerable variability in serum total T_4 levels, the free T_4 index usually is normal or mildly increased; the serum T_3 level usually is decreased, whereas reverse-T_3 concentration is elevated.[54–56] In cirrhosis, basal thyroid-stimulating hormone (TSH) levels may be elevated, and the TSH response to thyrotropin-releasing hormone infusion is not different from that of normal subjects.[56,57] Overall, this picture is most consistent with the changes that occur in systemic nonthyroidal illness.

THYROID HORMONE EFFECTS ON PHYSIOLOGIC FUNCTION OF GUT AND LIVER

The liver handles thyroid hormone similarly to the way in which it handles several organic anions. T_4 and T_3 are glucuronidated and sulfated, secreted into the biliary canaliculus, and concentrated in bile. The daily biliary excretion of thyroid hormone (20 μmol) is miniscule compared with that of other organic anions (e.g., 600 mol bilirubin daily). Thyroid hormone has profound effects on hepatic organic anion transport and biliary excretion. Although bilirubin glucuronide formation is not changed in vitro, extrahepatic factors result in abnormal bilirubin metabolism in vivo.[58,59] In experimental models hyperthyroidism is associated with an increased bilirubin output in bile, which may result from increased degradation of hepatic heme.[60] Thyroid-induced alterations in hepatic metabolism of bilirubin, specifically a decrease in glucuronyltransferase, may be responsible for the clinical occurrence of unconjugated hyperbilirubinemia, possibly by unmasking a previously unrecognized case of Gilbert syndrome.[60]

Thyroid hormone influences bile acid production and total bile acid pool size. Studies of bile acid kinetics in humans suggest that hyperthyroidism is associated with a decrease in the synthesis of primary bile acids (principally cholic acid) and a decrease in the size of the bile acid pool. This may be related to T_4-induced inhibition of hepatic 12-hydroxylase.[61] Clinically, duodenal bile salt concentration in hyperthyroid humans appears to be normal.[11] The clinical import of thyroid-induced alterations in organic anion excretion, bile flow, and microsomal enzyme activity requires further investigation but points to the important effects of thyroid hormone in normal liver function.

SUMMARY

Thyroid hormones play an important role in the normal physiology of GI function; when present in excess, they may result most notably in hypermotility and malabsorption. Patients with hyperthyroidism may exhibit associated hepatic or gastric dysfunction because of underlying autoimmune disease. Overall, the early detection and effective treatments that are available have changed the clinical presentation of hyperthyroidism such that GI symptoms have become clinically subtle in most patients despite a significant subclinical role for thyroid hormone in the maintenance of normal gastric and hepatic function.

References

1. Baker JT, Harvey RF. Bowel habits in thyrotoxicosis and hyperthyroidism. Br Med J 1971;1:322
2. Nepotent MI, Spesivtseva VG. Motor function of gastrointestinal tract before and after I[131] therapy in patients with thyrotoxicosis. Fed Proc 1963;22:T1177
3. Schiller KRFR, Spray GH, Wangel AG, Wright R. Clinical and precursory forms of pernicious anaemia in hyperthyroidism. Q J Med 1968;174:451
4. Wegener M, Wedmann B, Langhoff T, Schaffstein J, Adamek R. Effect of hyperthyroidism on the transit of a caloric solid-liquid meal through the stomach, the small intestine, and the colon in man. J Clin Endocrinol Metab 1992;75:745
5. Karaus M, Wienbeck M, Grussendorf M, et al. Intestinal motor activity in experimental hyperthyroidism in conscious dogs. Gastroenterology 1989;97:911
6. Bozzani A, Camborsi AG, Tidone L. Gastrointestinal transit in hyperthyroid patients before and after propranolol. Am J Gastroentrol 1985;80:550
7. Shafer RB, Prentiss R, Bond JH. Gastrointestinal transit in thyroid disease. Gastroenterology 1984;86:852
8. Pope C. In: Schlessinger M, Fordtran J, eds. Gastrointestinal disease. Philadelphia: WB Saunders, 1978
9. Meshkinpour H, Afrasiabi MA, Valenta LJ. Esophageal motor function in Graves' disease. Dig Dis Sci 1979;24:159
10. Holdsworth DC, Besser GM. Influence of gastric emptying rates and of insulin response on oral glucose tolerance in thyroid disease. Lancet 1968;2:700
11. Wiley ZD, Lavigne ME, Liu KM, MacGregor IL. The effect of hyperthyroidism on gastric emptying rates and pancreatic exocrine and biliary secretion in man. Am J Dig Dis 1978;23:1003
12. Rosenthal DG, Jones C, Lewis SI. Thyrotoxic vomiting. Br Med J 1976;2:209
13. Parkin AJ, Bishop N, Nisbet AP. Vomiting due to gastric stasis as the presenting feature in thyrotoxicosis. Postgrad Med J 1982;57:405
14. Christensen J, Schedl HP, Clifton JA. The basic electrical rhythm of the duodenum in normal human subjects and in patients with thyroid disease. J Clin Invest 1964;43:1659
15. Tobin MV, Fisken RA, Diggory RT, Morris AI, Gilmore IT. Orocaecal transit time in health and in thyroid disease. Gut 1989;30:26
16. Neuser E. Anemia. Wein Klin Wschr 1899;122:288
17. Furszyfer J, McConahey WM, Kurland LT, Maldonado GE. On the increased association of Graves' disease with pernicious anemia. Mayo Clin Proc 1971;46:37
18. Doniach D, Roitt IM, Taylor KP. Autoimmune phenomena in pernicious anema: serological overlap with thyroiditis, thyrotoxicosis, and systemic lupus erythematosus. BMJ 1963;1:1374
19. Burman P, Kampe O, Kraaz W, et al. A study of autoimmune gastritis in the postpartum period and at a 5-year follow-up. Gastroenterology 1992;103:934
20. Siurala M, Julkunen H, Lamberg BA. Gastrointestinal tract in hyperthyroidism before and after treatment. Lancet 1966;1:79
21. Dotevall G, Rohrer V, Stefco P, Price W. Relationship between gastric and thyroid function. Am J Dig Dis 1967;12:1230
22. Thomas FB, Caldwell JH, Greenberger NJ. Steatorrhea thyrotoxicosis: relation to hypermotility and excessive dietary fat. Ann Intern Med 1973;78:669
23. Hellesen C, Friis Th, Larson S, Pock-Steen OCh. Small intestinal histology, radiology and absorption in hyperthyroidism. Scand J Gastroenterol 1968;4:169
24. Debiec H, Cross HS, Peterlik M. D-Glucose uptake is increased in jejunal brush-border membrane vesicles from hyperthyroid chicks. Acta Endocrinol (Copenh) 1989;120:435
25. Lin TH, Rubinstein R, Holmes WL. A study of the effect of D-and L-triiodothyronine on bile acid excretion of rats. J Lipid Res 1973;4:63
26. Noble HM, Matty AJ. The effect of thyroxine on the movement of calcium and inorganic phosphate through the small intestine of the rat. J Endocrinol 1967;37:111
27. Celle G, Dodero M, Fresco G. Hyperthyroidism and coaeliac sprue: simple association. Acta Hepatogastroenterol 1976;23:68
28. Clubb JS, Black PJ, Wallace DC. An association of thyroid disease, ulcerative colitis and diabetes mellitus. Aust Ann Med 1970;19:1519
29. Hammer B, Ashurst P, Haish J. Diseases associated with ulcerative colitis and Crohn's disease. Gut 1968;9:17
30. Culp KS, Piziak VK. Thyrotoxicosis presenting with secretory diarrhea. Ann Int Med 1986;105:216
31. Weller CV. Hepatic pathology in exophthalmic goiter. Ann Intern Med 1933;7:687
32. Klion FM, Segal R, Schaffner F. The effect of altered thyroid function on the ultrastructure of the human liver. Am J Med 1971;50:317
33. Ashkar FS, Miller R, Smoak WM, Gilson AJ. Liver disease in hyperthyroidism. South Med J 1971;64:462
34. Huang MJ, Li KL, Wei JS, Wu SS, Fan KD, Liaw YF. Sequential liver and bone biochemical changes in hyperthyroidism: prospective controlled follow-up study. Am J Gastroenterol 1994;89:1071
35. Liaw YF, Huang MJ, Fan KD, Li KL, Wu SS, Chen TJ. Hepatic injury during propylthiouracil therapy in patients with hyperthyroidism: a cohort study. Ann Int Med 1993;118:424
36. Iossa S, Liverini G, Barletta A. Relationship between the resting metabolic rate and hepatic metabolism in rats: effect of hyperthyroidism and fasting for 24 hours. J Endocrinol 1992;135:45
37. Magnusson I, Wennlund A, Chandramouli V, et al. Fructose-6-phosphate cycling and the pentose cycle in hyperthyroidism. J Clin Endocrinol Metab 1990;70:461
38. Angervo M, Tiihonen M, Leinonen P, Valimaaki M, Seppala M. Thyroxine treatment increases circulating levels of insulin-like growth factor binding protein-1: a placebo-controlled study. Clin Endocrinol 1993;38:547
39. Ram PA, Waxman DJ. Thyroid hormone stimulation of NADPH P450 reductase expression in liver and extrahepatic tissues. J Biol Chem 1992;267:3294
40. Castellani LW, Wilcox HC, Heimberg M. Relationships between fatty acid synthesis and lipid secretion in the isolated perfused rat liver: effects of hyperthyroidism, glucose and oleate. Biochim Biophys Acta 1991;1086:197
41. Lanni A, Moreno LM, Cioffi M, Goglia F. Effect of 3,3'-di-iodothyronine and 3,5-di-iodothyronine on liver mitochondria. J Endocrinol 1993;136:59

42. Soboll B, Horst C, Hummerich H, Schumacker JP, Seitz HJ. Mitochondrial metabolism in different thyroid states. Biochem J 1992;281:171

43. Myers JD, Brannon ES, Holland BC. A correlative study of the cardiac output and the hepatic circulation in hyperthyroidism. J Clin Invest 1950;29:1069

44. Halle P, Pare P, Kaptern E, et al. Double-blind controlled trial of propylthiouracil in patients with severe acute alcoholic hepatitis. Gastroenterology 1982;82:925

45. Kaplowitz N. Propylthiouracil treatment for alcoholic hepatitis: should it and does it work? Gastroenterology 1982;82:1468

46. Orrego H, Blake JE, Blendis LM, Compton KV, Israel Y. Long-term treatment of alcoholic liver disease with propylthiouracil. N Engl J Med 1987;317;1421

47. Doniach D, Roitt IM, Walker JG, Sherlock S. Tissue autoantibodies in primary biliary cirrhosis, active chronic hepatitis, cryptogenic cirrhosis. Clin Exp Immunol Immunopathol 1966; 237:262

48. Culp KS, Fleming CR, Duffy J, Baldus WP, Dickson ER. Autoimmune associations in primary biliary cirrhosis. Mayo Clin Proc 1983;57:365

49. Schussler GC, Schaffner F, Korn F. Increased serum thyroid hormone binding and decreased free hormone in chronic active liver disease. N Engl J Med 1978;299:510

50. Crowe JP, Christensen E, Butler J, et al. Primary biliary cirrhosis: prevalence of hypothyroidism and its relationship to thyroid antibodies. Gastroenterology 1980;78:1437

51. Ain KB, Refetoff S. Relationship of oligosaccharide modification to the cause of serum thyroxine-binding globulin excess. J Clin Endocrinol Metab 1988;66:1037

52. Schneeweiss B, Graninger W, Ferenci P, et al. Energy metabolism in patients with acute and chronic liver disease. Hepatology 1990;11:387

53. Watanabe U, Hashimoto E, Hisamitsu T, Obata H, Hayashi N. The risk factor for development of thyroid disease during interferon-α-therapy for chronic hepatitis C. Am J Gastroenterol 1994;89:399

54. Chopra IJ. An assessment of daily production and significance of thyroidal secretion of reverse T_3 in man. J Clin Invest 1976;58:32

55. Faber J, Thomsen JF, Lumholtz IB, et al. Kinetic studies of thyroxine, 3,5,3′-triiodothyronine, 3,3′,3′-triiodothyronine, 3′,5′-diiodothyronine, 3,3′-diiodothyronine, and 3′-monoiodothyronine in patients with liver cirrhosis. J Clin Endocrinol Metab 1981;53:1978

56. Nomura S, Pittman CS, Chambers JB Jr, et al. Reduced peripheral conversion of thyroxine to triiodothyronine in patients with hepatic cirrhosis. J Clin Invest 1975;56:643

57. Van Thiel DH, Smith WI, Wight B, Abuid J. Elevated basal and abnormal thyrotropin-releasing-hormone induced thyroid-stimulating hormone secretion in chronic alcoholic men with liver disease. Clin Exp Res 1979;3:301

58. Gartner LM, Arias IM. Hormonal control of hepatic bilirubin transport and conjugation. Am J Physiol 1972;222;1091

59. Reyes H, Levi J, Gatmaitan Z, Arias IM. Studies of Y and Z, two hepatic cytoplasmic organic anion-binding proteins: effect of drugs, chemicals, hormones, and cholestasis. J Clin Invest 1971; 50:2242

60. Van Steenbergen W, Fevery J, DeGroote J. Thyroid hormones and the hepatic handling of bilirubin: effects of hypothyroidism and hyperthyroidism on the apparent maximal biliary secretion of bilirubin in the Wistar rat. J Hepatol 1988;7:229

61. Pauletzki J, Stellare F, BPaumgartner G. Bile acid metabolism in human hyperthyroidism. Hepatology 1989;9:852

Werner and Ingbar's The Thyroid, Seventh Edition,
edited by Lewis E. Braverman and Robert D. Utiger.
Lippincott–Raven Publishers, Philadelphia, © 1996

42

The Blood in Thyrotoxicosis

Jack E. Ansell

Clinically recognizable hematologic abnormalities are not a prominent feature of thyrotoxic conditions, but well-characterized changes do occur in the formed elements of the blood, especially in red blood cells (RBCs) and, to a lesser extent, in leukocytes and platelets, as well as the coagulation proteins.

Erythropoietic tissue is particularly sensitive to the hormonal environment. Erythropoietin (EPO), synthesized mainly by the kidney, is the principal regulator of erythropoiesis.[1] It responds primarily to alterations in oxygen tension in the kidney and peripheral tissues (a complex balance between relative rates of supply and demand). Because thyroid hormone influences oxygen use in the peripheral tissues, it is not surprising that alterations of thyroid function affect erythropoiesis.

The following discussion focuses on the physiologic changes in hematopoietic tissue and the coagulation proteins in response to excessive thyroid hormone. These physiologic effects are then placed in a clinical context, as the clinically relevant hematologic disorders that occur in the setting of thyrotoxicosis are discussed.

PHYSIOLOGIC EFFECTS OF EXCESS THYROID HORMONE

Erythrocytes

The physiologic effects of thyroid hormone on erythropoiesis have been studied in thyrotoxic and hypothyroid patients, in animal models of thyroid disease, and in in vitro cell culture systems (Table 42-1). As early as 1938, Gibson and Harris[2] demonstrated in 25 patients with thyrotoxicosis an increase in blood volume that fell with treatment, coinciding with a reduction in basal metabolic rate. Conversely, patients with hypothyroidism were found to have a reduced blood volume. Muldowney and associates[3] and Das and colleagues[4] confirmed these changes in thyrotoxic patients by detecting an el-

evated RBC mass that correlated with the basal metabolic rate and oxygen consumption.[3] Donati and coworkers[5] also detected enhanced erythropoiesis on the basis of an elevated radiolabeled iron-59 incorporation and more rapid plasma iron turnover and clearance in thyrotoxic patients. These changes returned to normal after treatment.

It is well known that the major stimulus for erythropoiesis is the oxygen requirement of peripheral tissues.[1] Renal hypoxia stimulates the secretion of EPO from the kidney, and EPO, in turn, stimulates erythropoiesis. Because an elevated metabolic rate increases oxygen demand and consumption, it is thought that the thyroid's effect on erythropoiesis is mediated by EPO responding to relative degrees of hypoxia. This concept was supported by Das and associates,[4] who noted high EPO levels in patients with thyrotoxicosis and an elevated RBC mass, and by Peschle and colleagues,[6] who detected an erythropoietic response in thyroxine (T_4)-treated mice only after the appearance of EPO in the serum. Supportive but opposite findings were seen in rabbits after thyroidectomy, showing reduced erythropoiesis and EPO levels.[7] More recently, Fandrey and colleagues[8] and Brenner and coworkers[9] have further confirmed the stimulatory effect of thyroid hormone on EPO production in vitro and in vivo by use of a sensitive EPO assay. They found that EPO levels correlated inversely with the level of hemoglobin, as one would expect, in both thyrotoxic and hypothyroid individuals, but that there was a significantly higher level of EPO for a given level of hemoglobin in the thyrotoxic subjects. T_4 and triiodothyronine (T_3) stimulated EPO synthesis in vitro in the human liver cell line HepG2. This response developed acutely (within 3 hours), but its effect was sustained for up to 24 hours after T_4 and T_3 were removed. Thyroid hormone's suspected impact on EPO production is further supported by the presence of steroid/thyroid hormone–like DNA receptor response motifs flanking the EPO gene,[10] which may influence EPO promoter and enhancer DNA sequences. However, Brenner and colleagues[9] suggest that thyroid hormone is probably not respon-

TABLE 42-1.
Physiologic Effects of Thyroid Hormone on Hematopoetic Tissue in Thyrotoxicosis

Blood Cell	Physiologic Effect	Comment
Red blood cell (RBC)	Increase in erythropoiesis, RBC mass and plasma volume	Mediated by elevated erythropoietin responding to increased oxygen requirements
		Thyroid hormone also has a direct, non-erythropoietin–mediated stimulatory effect on erythropoiesis
	Bone marrow erythroid and myeloid hypercellularity	Response to the stimulation of erythropoiesis
	Possible increase in 2,3-diphosphoglycerate (2,3-DPG)	2,3-DPG facilitates oxygen release from hemoglobin; studies contradictory
	Increase in glucose-6-phosphate dehydrogenase	Associated with a decrease in RBC fragility
	Increase in hemoglobin A_2	Absolute increase in globin δ-chain synthesis
	Increase in serum ferritin	
	Shortened RBC survival	Decreased life-span may be due to reticuloendothelial hyperplasia and splenic hypertrophy
White blood cell	± Increase in lymphocytes	Reports in literature contradictory
	± Increase in T-lymphocytes	
	Occasional eosinophilia	
Platelets	Shortened platelet survival	A mild decrease in survival due to reticuloendothelial hyperplasia; more significant thrombocytopenia, usually immune mediated
	Thrombocytopenia	
	Increase in mean platelet volume	
Coagulation proteins	Increase in factor VIII activity	Probably not clinically significant
	Decrease in fibrinolytic activity	

sible for the diurnal swings in EPO levels because of the sustained effect. Rather, the hypophyseal system and thyroid-stimulating hormone (TSH) may be relevant given the parallel diurnal changes in TSH and EPO and the additional influence of hypophysectomy on EPO levels.

The morphologic appearance of bone marrow also supports the concept of a stimulatory effect of thyroid hormone on erythropoiesis, in that both generalized myeloid hyperplasia[11] and erythroid hyperplasia[4] are found when bone marrow samples are studied in thyrotoxic patients. Thus the major effect of thyroid hormone on erythropoiesis is to increase metabolism and oxygen use, which leads to variable and relative degrees of tissue hypoxia and stimulates EPO secretion and an erythropoietic response.

Evidence also suggests that thyroid hormone stimulates RBC growth by a noncalorigenic or non–EPO-related mechanism. Meineke and Crafts[12] found increased erythropoiesis in T_4-treated hypophysectomized polycythemic rats, animals that should have a muted EPO response because of the polycythemia. They also found that T_4, more than dinitrophenol, stimulated erythropoiesis, although the latter compound produced a greater increase in oxygen consumption. Donati and coworkers[13] and Shirakura and associates[14] added further support by showing an erythroproliferative response to both L-triiodothyronine (L-T_3) and D-triiodothyronine (D-T_3) when only the former hormone is metabolically active, producing an increase in oxygen consumption.

Studies using in vitro cell culture methodology provide additional evidence for a noncalorigenic effect of thyroid hormone. Golde and colleagues[15] found a potentiating effect of L-T_4, D-T_4, L-T_3, and reverse T_3 on erythroid colony growth primed with EPO. Dainiak and coworkers[16] showed that thyroid hormone affects not only the earliest (BFU-E) but also the more committed (CFU-E) erythroid precursors. Popovic and associates[17] and Boussios and colleagues[18] explored the mechanism of this effect by identifying T_4-sensitive β-adrenergic receptors on the cell membrane[17] or special receptors in the cell nucleus.[18] Lastly, Fandrey and colleagues[8] found that thyroid hormone stimulated hypoxia-induced EPO production in HepG2 cells that was not due to an increase in hypoxia as measured by oxygen consumption.

Thus, an elevated RBC mass is a well-documented response to excess thyroid hormone. This effect is mediated by EPO in response to relative tissue hypoxia secondary to increased oxygen requirements, as well as by a direct, probably receptor-mediated effect of thyroid hormone.

In addition to its ability to stimulate erythropoiesis, thyroid hormone can produce a number of other alterations in both RBCs and hemoglobin. Some investigators have detected an increase in erythrocyte 2,3-diphosphoglycerate (2,3-DPG) by in vitro and in vivo studies. Grosz and Farmer[19] first noted a rapid drop in the reduction-oxidation potential of blood from hypothyroid compared with thyrotoxic patients, which would correlate with a left-shifted oxyhemoglobin dissociation curve and a deficiency of an oxygen-releasing factor. Miller and associates[20] found increased 2,3-DPG levels in two patients with thyrotoxicosis, and Snyder and Reddy[21] detected an increase in 2,3-DPG when thyroid hormone was incubated with a crude, hemoglobin-free enzyme preparation from RBCs. Such a change in 2,3-DPG, which regulates hemoglobin's affinity for oxygen, would facilitate the release of oxygen from hemoglobin in thyrotoxic patients and increase the availability of oxygen in the setting of increased utilization. Zaroulis and coworkers, however,[22] were unable to show such changes in 2,3-DPG, or in adenosine triphosphate or the P_{50} of hemoglobin in vitro, from a large number of hypothyroid, thyrotoxic, and euthyroid subjects. Thus the situation remains unclear.

Erythrocytes in thyrotoxic patients also may be more resistant to osmotic lysis (i.e., decreased osmotic fragility). This was noted coincidentally when investigators were studying glucose-6-phosphate dehydrogenase (G-6-PD) activity in a thyrotoxic patient.[23] G-6-PD subsequently was found to be increased in six of eight thyrotoxic subjects,[23] possibly because of an increase in glucose metabolism along the hexose monophosphate shunt. Such changes return to normal after treatment.[24]

Erythrocyte life span, normally 100 to 120 days, occasionally is reduced in thyrotoxicosis.[4,25] This rarely causes anemia. Such RBCs survive normally when transfused into normal subjects, suggesting that a shortened survival is not an intrinsic defect,[25] and may be a function of a hypertrophic reticuloendothelial system, as reflected by the mild splenomegaly that commonly occurs.[26]

Finally, hemoglobin A_2 concentration may be elevated in thyrotoxicosis. This interesting finding is attributable to an absolute, rather than relative, increase in hemoglobin δ-chain synthesis.[27] The mechanism of this increase is unknown. In treated patients, hemoglobin A_2 levels return to normal.[28] This finding also is associated with the production of small RBCs (microcytosis), a well-described finding. At least in one case, this combination of an elevated hemoglobin A_2 and a microcytic anemia in a Jordanian individual with thyrotoxicosis, was mistaken for β-thalassemia trait, until the abnormalities returned to normal after treatment of the thyrotoxicosis.[29] Microcytosis may be due to an increased number of mitotic divisions (and loss of cytoplasm) as a result of accelerated erythropoiesis.[28] It also has been attributed to iron deficiency in these patients,[28] yet iron stores in the bone marrow usually are normal[4] and the level of serum ferritin, a major iron storage protein, typically is elevated[30,31] and returns to normal with treatment.[31,32] The cause for elevated serum ferritin levels is unknown. Iwasa and coworkers[33] found experimental evidence in cultured rat glioma C6 cells and other tissues that the addition of T_3 caused a time- and dose-dependent increase in the steady-state level of ferritin H mRNA due to an increase in the transcription rate of the ferritin H gene. The opposite was found in hypothyroid animals. Other explanations include ineffective iron use, cellular leakage of ferritin, decreased clearance, and increased synthesis.[32] Because of this elevation, some investigators caution against the use of ferritin levels in the diagnosis of iron deficiency in the setting of thyrotoxicosis.[30] In one case the diagnosis of hemochromatosis was even suspected because of a marked elevation of the ferritin and the concomitant finding of an elevated serum iron and high transferrin saturation attributable to ferritin's transport of iron into the plasma.[34]

Leukocytes

LYMPHOCYTES

There are relatively few known important effects on leukocytes in the presence of excess thyroid hormone. The changes that have been studied appear to affect lymphoid cells more than granulocytic elements, but the literature is contradictory regarding total lymphocyte populations or subpopulations of T and B lymphocytes.[35–39] Thyrotoxicosis may be associated with a mild lymphocytosis and increase in T cells,[36,40,41] but normal lymphocyte counts and subpopulations have also been reported,[38,39] as well as a reduction in T cells.[35] Activated lymphocytes, similar to the atypical lymphocytes seen in infectious mononucleosis, may be seen. Whether such changes in lymphocyte numbers are a reflection of an altered immune system, or, as some have suggested, attributable to a relative decrease in cortisol, an increase of which is known to suppress lymphoid tissue,[42] remains unknown. Based on a recent report of lymphoid subpopulations in toxic and nontoxic multinodular goiter, no abnormalities were found in the absolute or relative numbers of T, B, or NK cells, suggesting that hormone level was not influential.[43] However, these investigators did note a significant increase in absolute and relative numbers of activated T lymphocytes, cytotoxic T cells, and NK-related cells in patients with multinodular goiter versus controls regardless of whether the subjects were euthyroid or hyperthyroid.

GRANULOCYTES

Granulocytes are even less influenced by thyroid hormone, and only an occasional moderate eosinophilia may be noted in thyrotoxicosis. Once again, this finding has been attributed to a relative decrease in serum cortisol.[42] Recently, three thyrotoxic patients were reported with pancytopenia that disappeared when the patients became euthyroid.[43a] The mechanism remains obscure but might be more common than previously suspected.

Hemostasis

PLATELETS

Alterations in platelet count in the setting of thyrotoxicosis were first reported more than 50 years ago.[44] Since then, thrombocytopenia has been a documented phenomenon in thyrotoxic conditions. Herman and coworkers[45] summarized nearly 50 cases in 1978, and the impression at that time was that thrombocytopenia was immune mediated, presumably associated with other immunologic aberrations in thyrotoxicosis. Subsequent investigations suggest that thyroid hormone may have nonimmunologic effects on platelet kinetics. Kurata and associates[46] showed that a shortened platelet survival and platelet count could be induced in rats injected with T_3 and that platelets from these rats, when transfused into normal animals, survived normally. Similarly, platelets from a normal rat, when transfused to a T_3-treated rodent, demonstrated a shortened survival. These findings led the investigators to postulate splenic sequestration as the mechanism that shortened platelet survival in thyrotoxic states. More recent studies confirm these changes of an increased mean platelet volume and shortened survival that returns to normal with treatment.[47–49] This occurs whether or not the platelet-associated immunoglobulin (PAIgG) level is elevated. Changes in platelet function are less well characterized in thyroid disease, especially thyrotoxicosis. Evidence indicates that some patients may bruise more easily and that this finding is related to increased PAIgG and not to thrombocytopenia.[50]

COAGULATION

The coagulation proteins of the blood are altered to an even lesser extent than blood platelets, but some changes do occur. Findings include an elevation of factor VIII coagulant activity[51-53] and von Willebrand factor.[54] The elevation in von Willebrand factor was abrogated by the administration of propranolol, suggesting that β-adrenergic receptors are important mediators of this response. Effects on the fibrinolytic mechanism show both a prolonged euglobulin lysis time[52] implying a reduction in fibrinolytic activity, as well as evidence of enhanced fibrinolysis as determined by specific measurements of Bβ 15–42, a fibrin fragment produced by plasmin activity.[55] The latter has been studied both before and after treatment and found not to change, suggesting that the underlying autoimmunity accounting for some cases of thyrotoxicosis rather than excess hormone may be the cause of excess fibrinolytic activity. These same investigators also found an elevation in fibrinopeptide A, a thrombin-derived cleavage product of fibrinogen, indicative of coagulation activation. This could reflect an underlying hypercoagulable state and account for a potential increase in thromboembolism as has been reported in thyrotoxic states.[56,57]

Another interesting effect of thyroid hormone on coagulation is the recent finding of an elevation in circulating thrombomodulin, an endothelial-based receptor for thrombin that mediates the activation of protein C, an inhibitor of activated factor VIII and factor V. Morikawa and coworkers[58] showed that thrombomodulin levels are directly correlated with thyroid hormone concentrations. The latter may influence the synthesis or metabolism of thrombomodulin or the elevation may be a marker of endothelial damage. The relationship of this finding to changes in coagulation, however, is unknown.

Lastly, an increase in the presence of anticardiolipin antibodies has been noted in patients with thyrotoxicosis, first reported by Marongiu and colleagues.[59] Paggi and associates[60] subsequently detected high titers of IgG or IgM anticardiolipin antibodies in 17 of 31 patients with thyrotoxicosis, but none of these patients had manifestations of the antiphospholipid syndrome or clinical thrombosis.

CLINICAL CORRELATES AND ASSOCIATED HEMATOLOGIC ABNORMALITIES

Red Blood Cells

Anemia is not considered to be a common problem or clinical finding in patients with thyrotoxicosis although frequencies ranging from 8% to 20% are reported (Table 42-2).[41,61] Excess thyroid hormone produces an increase in RBC mass rather than a decrease, and it would be expected to cause polycythemia. The latter, however, is seldom found because thyrotoxicosis also produces an increase in plasma volume that keeps RBC parameters in the normal range because they are measured per unit volume of whole blood. The reticulocyte count also remains normal (about 1%) because about 1% of the RBC mass is renewed each day.

The most common RBC morphologic abnormality encountered is microcytosis, found in at least 37% of patients.[41,62] The cause for this change is unclear.[28] Iron deficiency often is cited as an occasional finding in thyrotoxic states, but a critical review of previous reports suggests that there is little, if any, documentation of this association.[41,61-64] Even though achlorhydria is common and may lead to decreased iron absorption, clinical iron deficiency is seldom encountered. Microcytosis usually resolves with treatment of the thyroid disease,[62] unless there is an underlying deficiency.

Some patients develop a normocytic anemia that possibly is attributable to severe excess of thyroid hormone.[63] Defective iron use has been shown to occur in thyrotoxicosis[64] and may be responsible for anemia in these cases.

Macrocytic anemias are the last major morphologic category of anemia seen in thyrotoxicosis. Macrocytic anemias are

---

TABLE 42-2.
Clinical Manifestations of Thyroid Hormone's Effects on Hematopoietic Tissue in Thyrotoxicosis

Blood Cell	Clinical Effect	Comment
Red blood cell (RBC)	(Polycythemia)	Physiologic increase in RBC mass virtually never clinically apparent because of concomitant increase in plasma volume
	Anemia	Occurs uncommonly
	Microcytic anemia	Most common change in RBC morphology, often in the absence of anemia; iron deficiency uncommon cause of microcytosis in this setting; often corrects with correction of thyrotoxicosis
	Normocytic anemia	Occasional finding; may be related to defective iron use
	Macrocytic anemia	Most often associated with vitamin B_{12} or folic acid deficiency; increased frequency of pernicious anemia as well as low levels of vitamin B_{12} or folic acid due to increased metabolism
White blood cell	Lymphocytosis	Occasionally found, but literature contradictory
	Leukopenia or agranulocytopenia	Can be seen with antithyroid medications
Platelets	Thrombocytopenia	Mild reduction in platelet count (usually still within normal range), possibly due to reticuloendothelial hyperplasia and usually not clinically significant; immune thrombocytopenia (idiopathic thrombocytopenic purpura) causes more serious thrombocytopenia and requires treatment

a common manifestation of hypothyroidism, even without vitamin B_{12} or folic acid deficiency, but in thyrotoxic conditions, macrocytosis usually is a result of megaloblastic erythroid maturation and a deficiency of vitamin B_{12} or folic acid. There is a well-described increase in folic acid and vitamin B_{12} metabolism and clearance[63,65,66] in thyrotoxicosis, with low serum and RBC folate levels, and low normal serum vitamin B_{12} levels, the latter rising with achievement of normal thyroid function. More recent studies question these earlier findings, and suggest that serum and RBC folate levels and serum vitamin B_{12} levels are no different from those found in a control group.[67,68]

The relationship between vitamin B_{12} homeostasis and thyroid disease is more complex. There is a higher incidence of pernicious anemia (PA) with all autoimmune thyroid disorders, especially hypothyroidism.[69,70] Gastric parietal tissue, important in the absorption of vitamin B_{12} by secretion of intrinsic factor, often is abnormal in the setting of thyroid disease,[71,72] and there is the frequent association of autoantibodies to one organ when the other is affected.[73–75] This is not surprising, given the fact that both organs have a common origin from the embryonic foregut, and that Graves' disease and PA are both autoimmune disorders. About one-third of patients with thyrotoxicosis have antibodies to gastric parietal cells,[76] and about one-half of patients with PA have antibodies to thyroid tissue.[74,76] As would be expected, there also is a higher incidence of hypochlorhydria and achlorhydria than in age-matched normal subjects.[71,72] PA is found in about 1% to 3% of patients with Graves' hyperthyroidism;[73,77] the latter is found in 2% of primarily European patients with PA[78] and up to 8% of American patients with PA.[79] Furthermore, the age of onset of PA is considerably lower in thyrotoxic patients than in age-matched controls, even occurring in childhood,[80] suggesting that the appropriate evaluation should be considered when confronted with a macrocytic anemia in a thyrotoxic patient.

A bone marrow evaluation traditionally is obtained when confronted with a possible megaloblastic anemia, but it may not be necessary, given the reliability of vitamin B_{12} and folate assays. If other hematologic problems are unlikely, assessment of the serum vitamin B_{12} level and the serum and RBC folate level are all that may be necessary after evaluating RBC indices and the peripheral blood smear. Vitamin B_{12} and folic acid levels must be evaluated simultaneously because of the enhanced metabolism and clearance of folic acid in thyrotoxicosis and the many indistinguishable characteristics of either deficiency. If vitamin B_{12} deficiency is found, then the appropriate diagnostic tests to elucidate its cause are in order.[81] These include intrinsic factor and parietal cell antibodies and radiolabeled B_{12} absorption tests (Schilling test) to determine the cause of vitamin B_{12} malabsorption. Folic acid deficiency should lead to a focus on dietary practices, which, even if borderline, might facilitate a clinical deficiency because of the greater turnover of folic acid in thyrotoxicosis.

White Blood Cells

Alterations in leukocyte number are relatively modest and apply principally to the lymphoid tissue. The mild relative or absolute lymphocytosis occasionally seen produces no known clinical sequelae. A generalized lymphadenopathy may be present, and the spleen, although not often palpable on physical examination, has been shown to be enlarged by imaging studies in 50% of the patients with thyrotoxicosis.[26] An interesting association recently described[82] identifies a threefold increase in thyroid disease, especially thyrotoxicosis, in patients with acute leukemia, primarily acute myeloid leukemia. Patients with Graves' and Hashimoto's disease tended to have a better outcome, and the authors raise the question of the influence of thyroid hormone on hematopoiesis and this improved outcome. The associated autoimmunity of these two thyroid disorders could also play a role.

One problem associated with the therapy for thyrotoxicosis is granulocytopenia, a direct effect of antithyroid medication.[83] About 0.5% to 1% of patients treated with methimazole, carbimazole, or propylthiouracil develop agranulocytosis from a few days to several months after initiating treatment. A slightly greater percentage may develop a mild to moderate leukopenia. One study found that people over age 40 may be more likely to develop this problem with methimazole and propylthiouracil, that the agranulocytosis is far less likely to develop after 4 months of therapy, and that higher doses (above 30 mg/d) are an important factor with methimazole.[84] This may not always be the case, because in an unpublished series of 10 patients with propylthiouracil-induced agranulocytosis, 8 were less than 40 years of age and 4 developed the disorder after more than 4 months of therapy (L. E. Braverman, unpublished observations). At least in some cases, peripheral destruction of granulocytes by leukoagglutinins is thought to be the mechanism involved.[85] Appropriate treatment calls for the prompt cessation of the suspected offending medication in the case of agranulocytosis, and recovery almost always occurs within 6 days, which can be shortened by giving rhG-CSF.[85a] With mild leukopenia, close observation and monitoring of counts may be adequate, rather than discontinuation of the drug. The diagnostic evaluation of agranulocytosis usually requires a bone marrow biopsy. If fever or documented infection is present, broad-spectrum antibiotics usually are required.

Platelets and Coagulation

The major alteration in the hemostatic system in thyrotoxicosis is thrombocytopenia. The shortened platelet survival and reduction in count that are presumed to be due to splenic sequestration appear to be mild and of little clinical importance.[46,47,49] Thrombocytopenia that appears to be immune mediated and indistinguishable from idiopathic thrombocytopenic purpura should be approached more vigorously. This thrombocytopenia resolves in some patients by treatment of the thyrotoxicosis, or it may resolve spontaneously, but in others, it may persist and require corticosteroids or other measures used in the therapy of idiopathic thrombocytopenic purpura.[86]

The minor changes in coagulation factors associated with thyrotoxicosis are of questionable clinical significance and require no specific evaluation or intervention. However, there is a possibility of a hypercoagulable state in thyrotoxicosis leading to a greater incidence of thromboembolism in thyrotoxic atrial fibrillation compared to other causes of atrial fibrillation.[57] Whether this phenomenon is due to activation of coagulation factors,[55] the presence of antiphospholipid antibodies,[59] endothelial injury,[58] or some other effect remains unknown.

SUMMARY

Thyrotoxicosis is not often associated with clinically significant alterations in the hematopoietic elements, but thyroid hormone does have recognized effects on hematopoiesis. By increasing the oxygen requirement of peripheral tissues and creating relative degrees of hypoxia, thyroid hormone stimulates the secretion of EPO, which, in turn, stimulates erythropoiesis, resulting in an increase in RBC mass. Thyroid hormone has a direct stimulatory effect on erythropoiesis as well.

Other effects of thyroid hormone include a potential increase in 2,3-DPG, providing for greater oxygen unloading from hemoglobin; an increase in G-6-PD, with decreased osmotic fragility; and an increase in hemoglobin A_2 production. Lastly, RBC survival is mildly reduced in thyrotoxicosis, probably the result of the reticuloendothelial hyperplasia that may occur.

Microcytic RBC morphology, reversible with treatment of the thyroid disease, often is seen in thyrotoxicosis. Anemia is a less common finding. A mild normocytic anemia occurs rarely, and a macrocytic anemia often is due to folic acid or vitamin B_{12} deficiency. Not only is the metabolism of these latter two vitamins increased in thyrotoxicosis, but PA also is more frequently encountered in autoimmune thyroid disease.

White blood cells are altered to a minor degree in thyrotoxicosis, with most reports describing a mild lymphocytosis. Antithyroid medication can induce a serious reduction in granulocyte counts, leading to an enhanced risk of infection.

Platelet survival is reduced in thyrotoxicosis, probably related to reticuloendothelial hyperplasia, and may lead to a mild thrombocytopenia. Immune thrombocytopenia also occurs and may require treatment with corticosteroids or other modalities as would be considered for any patient with immune thrombocytopenic purpura. Qualitative abnormalities of platelet function are unusual, and the changes in the coagulation mechanism are of uncertain significance.

References

1. Fisher JW. Control of erythropoietin production. Proc Soc Exp Biol Med 1983;173:289
2. Gibson JG, Harris AW. Clinical studies of the blood volume. V. Hyperthyroidism and myxedema. J Clin Invest 1939;18:59
3. Muldowney FP, Crooks J, Wayne EJ. The total red cell mass in thyrotoxicosis and myxedema. Clin Sci 1957;16:309
4. Das KC, Mukherjee M, Sarker TK, et al. Erythropoiesis and erythropoietin in hypo- and hyperthyroidism. J Clin Endocrinol Metab 1975;40:211
5. Donati RM, Warnecke MA, Gallagher NI. Ferrokinetics in hyperthyroidism. Ann Intern Med 1965;63:945
6. Peschle C, Zanjani ED, Gidari AS, et al. Mechanism of thyroxin action on erythropoiesis. Endocrinology 1971;89:609
7. Nakao K, Malkawa T, Shirakura T, Yaginuma M. Anemia due to hypothyroidism. Isr J Med Sci 1965;1:742
8. Fandrey J, Pagel H, Frede S, et al. Thyroid hormones enhance hypoxia-induced erythropoietin production in vitro. Exp Hematol 1994;22:272
9. Brenner B, Fandrey J, Jelkmann W. Serum immunoreactive erythropoietin in hyper- and hypothyroidism: clinical observations related to cell culture studies. Eur J Haematol 1994;53:6
10. Blanchard KL, Acquaviva AM, Galson DL, Bunn HF. Hypoxic induction of the human erythropoietin gene: cooperation between the promoter and enhancer, each of which contains steroid receptor response elements. Mol Cell Biol 1992;12:5373
11. Axelrod AR, Berman L. The bone marrow in hyperthyroidism and hypothyroidism. Blood 1951;6:436
12. Meineke HA, Crafts RC. Evidence for a non-calorigenic effect of thyroxin on erythropoiesis as judged by radioiron utilization. Proc Soc Exp Biol Med 1964;117:520
13. Donati RM, Warnecke MA, Gallagher NI. Effect of triiodothyronine administration on erythrocyte radioiron incorporation in rats. Proc Soc Exp Biol Med 1964;115:405
14. Shirakura T, Azuma M, Malkawa T. A study on the erythropoiesis stimulating effect of the thyroid hormone. Blut 1970;21:240
15. Golde DW, Bersch N, Chopra IJ, Cline MJ. Thyroid hormones stimulate erythropoiesis in vitro. Br J Haematol 1977;37:173
16. Dainiak N, Hoffman R, Maffei LA, Forget BG. Potentiation of human erythropoiesis in vitro by thyroid hormone. Nature 1978;272:260
17. Popovic WJ, Brown JE, Adamson JW. The influence of thyroid hormones on in vitro erythropoiesis. J Clin Invest 1977;60:907
18. Boussios T, McIntyre WR, Gordon AS, Bertles JF. Receptors specific for thyroid hormones in nuclei of mammalian erythroid cells: involvement in erythroid cell proliferation. Br J Haematol 1982;51:99
19. Grosz HJ, Farmer BB. Reduction-oxidation potential of blood determined by oxygen releasing factor in thyroid disorders. Nature 1969;222:875
20. Miller WW, Delivoria-Papadopoulos M, Miller L, Oski FA. Oxygen releasing factor in hyperthyroidism. JAMA 1970;211;1824
21. Snyder LM, Reddy WJ. Thyroid hormone control of erythrocyte 2,3-diphosphoglyceric acid concentrations. Science 1970;169:879
22. Zaroulis CG, Kourides IA, Valeri CR. Red cell 2,3-diphosphoglycerate and oxygen affinity of hemoglobin in patients with thyroid disorders. Blood 1978;52:181
23. Baikie AG, Lawson N. Glucose-6-phosphate dehydrogenase activity and an osmotic abnormality of erythrocytes in thyrotoxicosis. Lancet 1965;1:86
24. Vikerhoski M, Lamberg BA. The glucose-6-phosphate dehydrogenase activity of the red blood cells in hyperthyroidism and hypothyroidism. Scand J Clin Lab Invest 1970;25:137
25. McClellan JE, Donegan C, Thorup OA, Leavell BS. Survival time of the erythrocyte in myxedema and hyperthyroidism. J Lab Clin Med 1958;51:91
26. Metcalfe-Gibson C, Keddie N. Spleen size and previous tonsillectomy in autoimmune disease of the thyroid. Lancet 1978;1:944
27. Krishnamoorthy R, Elion J, Kuhn JM, et al. Hemoglobin A_2 is elevated in hyperthyroid patients. Nouv Rev Fr Hematol 1982;24:39
28. Kuhn JM, Riew M, Rochette J, et al. Influence of thyroid status on hemoglobin A_2 expression. J Clin Endocrinol Metab 1983;57:344
29. Akasheh MS. Graves' disease mimicking β-thalassemia trait. Postgrad Med J 1994;70:300
30. Macaron CI, Macaron ZG. Increase serum ferritin levels in hyperthyroidism. Ann Intern Med 1982;96:617
31. Van de Vyver FL, Blockx PP, Abs RE, Bekaert JL. Serum ferritin levels in hyperthyroidism. Ann Intern Med 1982;97:930
32. Takamatsu J, Majima M, Mikki K, et al. Serum ferritin as a marker of thyroid hormone action on peripheral tissues. J Clin Endocrinol Metab 1985;61:672
33. Iwasa Y, Aida K, Yokomori N, et al. Transcriptional regulation of ferritin heavy chain messenger RNA expression by thyroid hormone. Biochem Biophys Res Commun 1990;167:1279
34. Delfina M. Serum ferritin in hyperthyroidism. Ann Intern Med 1993;119:249

35. Aanderud S, Matre R, Varhaug JE. Immunological characterization of mononuclear cells in thyroid gland and blood in Graves' disease, multinodular goiter and papillary carcinoma. Int Arch Allergy Appl Immunol 1982;69:137

36. Farid NR, Munro RE, Row VV, Volpe R. Peripheral thymus dependent (T) lymphocytes in Graves' disease and Hashimoto's thyroiditis. N Engl J Med 1973;228:1313

37. Grinblat J, Shohat B, Lewitus Z, Joshua H. Quantitative and functional assessment of peripheral T-lymphocytes in thyroid diseases. Acta Endocrinol (Copenh) 1979;90:52

38. Lundell G, Wasserman J, Granberg PO, Blomgren H. Lymphocyte populations in peripheral blood in hyperthyroid and euthyroid subjects. Clin Exp Immunol 1976;23:33

39. Urbaniak SJ, Penhale WJ, Irvine WJ. Peripheral blood T and B lymphocytes in patients with thyrotoxicosis and Hashimoto's thyroiditis and in normal subjects. Clin Exp Immunol 1974;18:449

40. Aoki N, Wakisaka G, Nagata I. Increase of T cells in Graves' disease. Lancet 1973;2:49

41. Reddy J, Brownlie BEW, Heaton DC, et al. The peripheral blood picture in thyrotoxicosis. N Z Med J 1981;93:143

42. Herbert V. The blood. In: Ingbar SH, Braverman LE, eds. The thyroid. 5th ed. Philadelphia: JB Lippincott, 1986:878

43. Corrales JJ, Orfao A, Miralles JM, San Miguel J. The relationship between hyperthyroidism and the distribution of peripheral blood T, NK and B-lymphocytes in multinodular goiter. Horm Metab Res 1994;26:104

43a. Duquenne M, Lakonsky D, Humbert JC, et al. Pancytopénic résolutive par le traitement d'une hyperthyroïdie. Presse Méd 1995;24:807

44. Jackson AS. Acute hemorrhagic purpura associated with exophthalmic goiter. JAMA 1931;96:38

45. Herman J, Resnitzky P, Fink A. Association between thyrotoxicosis and thrombocytopenia. Isr J Med Sci 1978;14:469

46. Kurata Y, Nishioeda Y, Tadahiro T, Kitani T. Thrombocytopenia in Graves' disease: effect of T_3 on platelet kinetics. Acta Haematol (Basel) 1980;63:185

47. Ford HC, Toomath RJ, Carter JM, Delehunt JW, Fagerstrom JN. Mean platelet volume is increased in hyperthyroidism. Am J Hematol 1988;27:190

48. Marongiu F, Conti M, Murtas ML, et al. What causes the increase in platelet mean volume in thyroid pathological conditions. Thromb Haemost 1990;63:323

49. Panzer S, Haubenstock A, Minar E. Platelets in hyperthyroidism: studies on platelet counts, mean platelet volume, 111-indium-labeled platelet kinetics, and platelet associated immunoglobulins G and M. J Clin Endocrinol Metab 1990;70:491

50. Hymes K, Blum M, Lackner H, Karpatkin S. Easy bruising, thrombocytopenia and elevated platelet immunoglobulin G in Graves' disease and Hashimoto's thyroiditis. Ann Intern Med 1981;94:27

51. Egeberg O. Thyroid function and hemostasis. Scand J Clin Lab Invest 1964;16:511

52. Farid NR, Griffiths BL, Collins JR, et al. Blood coagulation and fibrinolysis in thyroid disease. Thromb Haemost 1976;35:415

53. Simone JV, Abildgaard CF, Schulman I. Blood coagulation in thyroid dysfunction. N Engl J Med 1965;273:1057

54. Liu L, Wang X, Lin Z, Wu H. Elevated plasma levels of VWF:Ag in hyperthyroidism are mediated through beta-adrenergic receptors. Endocr Res 1993;19:123

55. Marongiu F, Conti M, Murtas ML, et al. Activation of blood coagulation and fibrinolysis in Graves' disease. Horm Metab Res 1991;23:609

56. Haynes JH, Kageler WV. Thyrocardiotoxic embolic syndrome South Med J 1989;82:1292

57. Presti CF, Hart RG. Thyrotoxicosis, atrial fibrillation and embolism revisited. Am Heart J 1989;117:976

58. Morikawa Y, Morikawa A, Makino I. Relationship of thyroid states and serum thrombomodulin (TM) levels in patients with Graves' disease: TM, a possible new marker of the peripheral activity of thyroid hormones. J Clin Endocrinol Metab 1993;76:609

59. Marongiu F, Conti M, Murtas ML, et al. Anticardiolipin antibodies in Graves' disease: relationship with thrombin activity in vivo. Thromb Res 1991;64:745

60. Paggi A, Caccavo D, Ferri GM, et al. Anti-cardiolipin antibodies in autoimmune thyroid disease. Clin Endocrinol 1994;40:329

61. Nightingale S, Vitek PJ, Hemsworth RL. The haematology of hyperthyroidism. Q J Med 1978;47:35

62. How J, Davidson RJL, Bewsher PD. Red cell changes in hyperthyroidism. Scand J Haematol 1979;23:323

63. Fein HG, Rivlin RS. Anemia in thyroid disease. Med Clin North Am 1975;59:1133

64. Rivlin RS, Wagner HN. Anemia in hyperthyroidism. Ann Intern Med 1969;70:507

65. Alperin JB, Haggard ME, Haynie TP. A study of vitamin B_{12} requirements in a patient with pernicious anemia and thyrotoxicosis. Blood 1970;36:632

66. Lindenbaum J, Klipstein FA. Folic acid clearances and basal serum folate levels in patients with thyroid disease. J Clin Pathol 1964;17:666

67. Caplan RH, Davis K, Bengston B, Smith MJ. Serum folate and vitamin B_{12} levels in hypothyroid and hyperthyroid patients. Arch Intern Med 1975;135:701

68. Ford HC, Carter JM, Rendle MA. Serum and red cell folate and serum vitamin B_{12} levels in hyperthyroidism. Am J Hematol 1989;31:233

69. Erslev AJ. Anemia of endocrine disorders. In: Williams WJ, Beutler E, Erslev AJ, Lichtman MA, eds. Hematology. 4th ed. New York: McGraw-Hill, 1990:444

70. Green ST, Ng JP. Hypothyroidism and anemia. Biomed Pharmacother 1986;40:326

71. Bock OAA, Witts LJ. Gastric acidity and gastric biopsy in thyrotoxicosis. Br Med J 1963;2:20

72. Williams MJ, Blair DW. Gastric secretion in hyperthyroidism. Br Med J 1964;1:940

73. Ardeman S, Chanarin I, Krafchik B, Singer W. Addisonian pernicious anemia and intrinsic factor antibodies in thyroid disorders. Q J Med 1966;35:421

74. Doniach D, Roitt IM. An evaluation of gastric and thyroid autoimmunity in relation to hematologic disorders. Semin Hematol 1964;1:313

75. Doniach D, Roitt IM, Taylor KB. Autoimmunity in pernicious anemia and thyroiditis: a family study. Ann N Y Acad Sci 1965;124:605

76. Doniach D, Roitt IM, Taylor KB. Autoimmune phenomena in pernicious anemia. Br Med J 1963;1:1374

77. Schiller KFR, Spray GH, Wangel AG, Wright R. Clinical and precursory forms of pernicious anemia in hyperthyroidism. Q J Med 1968;37:451

78. Chanarin I. The megaloblastic anemias. 2nd ed. Oxford: Blackwell Scientific, 1979:

79. Carmel R, Spencer CA. Clinical and subclinical thyroid disorders associated with pernicious anemia. Arch Intern Med 1982;142:1465

80. Suzuki N, Mitamura R, Ohmi H, et al. Hashimoto's thyroiditis, distal renal tubular acidosis, pernicious anaemia and encephalopathy: a rare combination of autoimmune disorders in a 12 year old girl. Eur J Pediatr 1994;153:78

81. Babior BM. The megaloblastic anemias. In: Williams WJ, Beutler E, Erslev AJ, Lichtman MA, eds. Hematology. 4th ed. New York: McGraw-Hill, 1990:453

82. Moskowitz C, Dutcher JP, Wiernik PH. Association of thyroid disease with acute leukemia. Am J Hematol 1992;39:102

83. Wintrobe MM, Lee GR, Boggs DR, et al. Variations of leukocytes in disease. In: Wintrobe MM, Lee GR, Boggs DR, et al, eds. Clinical hematology. 8th ed. Philadelphia: Lea & Febiger, 1981:1308

84. Cooper DS, Goldminz D, Levin AA, et al. Agranulocytosis associated with antithyroid drugs. Ann Intern Med 1983;98:26

85. Wall JR, Fang SL, Kuroki T, et al. In vitro immunoreactivity to propylthiouracil, methimazole, and carbimazole in patients with Graves' disease: a possible cause of antithyroid drug-induced agranulocytosis. J Clin Endocrinol Metab 1984;58:868

85a. Tamai H, Mukuta H, Matsubayashi T, et al. Treatment of methimazole-induced agranulocytosis using recombinant human granulocyte colony-stimulating factor (rh G-CSF). J Clin Endocrinol Metab 1993;77:1356

86. Kelton JG, Gibbons S. Autoimmune platelet destruction: idiopathic thrombocytopenia purpura. Semin Thromb Hemost 1982;8:83

Werner and Ingbar's The Thyroid, Seventh Edition,
edited by Lewis E. Braverman and Robert D. Utiger.
Lippincott–Raven Publishers, Philadelphia, © 1996

43

The Neuromuscular System and Brain in Thyrotoxicosis

G. Robert DeLong

Excess activity of the thyroid gland produces well-recognized disorders of the neuromuscular system and of brain function. Neuromuscular disorders in thyrotoxic patients include generalized weakness and atrophy of muscles,[1] localized paralysis of ocular muscles,[2] periodic paralysis,[3] and myasthenia gravis.[4] These disorders are seen with greater frequency than would be expected if entirely unrelated diseases had appeared together by chance. Central nervous system (CNS) complications of thyrotoxicosis include disturbances of mental and emotional faculties,[5,6] chorea,[7] and, when severe, delirium, stupor, coma, and convulsions.[8]

MUSCULAR SYSTEM

One conclusion emerges from all studies of thyroid disease: excessive thyroid function induces changes in the skeletal musculature (Table 43-1). For the reader who seeks further information, several publications are recommended.[1,2,4,9]

Clinical Observations

Some reduction in the power of muscle contraction probably occurs in every patient with thyrotoxicosis. This myopathy usually is associated with easy fatigability and a varying degree of muscular atrophy. The symptoms may not be sufficiently prominent to attract notice and often are attributed to weight loss and general asthenia. To patients, the most obvious manifestation is a weakness of the legs on climbing stairs. Alternatively, they may describe rapid fatigue of shoulder muscles on elevation of the arms for a period of time. On clinical testing, this progressive weakness is more evident in the large proximal limb muscles than in the distal ones, despite the generalization of muscle involvement. In the quadriceps

test, sometimes used for its clinical demonstration, the patient with thyrotoxicosis can hold a leg out straight, in a horizontal position, when seated in a chair for only 20 to 25 seconds, whereas most normal people can do so for more than 60 seconds.[10]

The small, distal limb muscles also are affected, as shown in ergographic studies. These studies demonstrate a rapid diminution in the strength of repeated muscle contractions.[1] Facial, laryngeal, pharyngeal, and lingual muscles are seldom sufficiently involved to produce symptoms. Respiratory and bulbar musculature may be affected.[11,12] Respiratory muscle strength is consistently decreased in thyrotoxicosis, in an inverse linear relationship to triiodothyronine (T_3) and thyroxine (T_4) levels, at least partially explaining the dyspnea on exertion seen in thyrotoxic patients.[13] The muscle weakness varies from patient to patient and is roughly proportional to the severity and duration of the thyrotoxicosis. The weakness almost never progresses to total paralysis.

Muscular atrophy also occurs in thyrotoxicosis but is difficult to assess in the average patient. If weight loss has been extreme, the prominence of the ribs and scapulas gives the impression that the muscular atrophy is of a degree far in excess of actual weakness. In contrast, when the adipose tissue is abundant, even moderate atrophy may be obscured. The extent of atrophy can best be judged by inspection of the intrinsic muscles of the hands and the face. Concavity of the thenar and hypothenar muscle masses and deepening of the interosseous spaces appear, and there also are hollows above and below the cheekbones. The atrophy is never as extreme as it may be in progressive muscular atrophy or in other diseases that destroy lower motor neurons.

In contrast with other metabolic myopathies, in thyrotoxicosis the tendon reflexes are brisk and the relaxation phase is shortened[14]; these findings are variable, however, and the re-

TABLE 43-1.
Incidence of Neuromuscular Disorders Associated
With Thyrotoxicosis

Disorder	Incidence (%)
Myopathy	>50
Severe	4
Myasthenia gravis	<1
Periodic paralysis	2–8 (in male Asians mainly)

*(Kudrjavcev T. Neurologic complications of thyroid dysfunction.
Adv Neurol 1978;19:619)*

flexes may be difficult to elicit in some patients because of the normal individual variations of tendon reflex activity.

The presence of tremor may create the appearance of fascicular twitching. These twitchings of fascicles of muscles usually disappear when relaxation is complete. Benign fasciculation, sometimes incorrectly called myokymia, may coincide with any disease and often is present in normal people.

All the symptoms and signs of disturbed muscle function disappear when euthyroidism is reinstated.[15]

Pathophysiology

An outstanding recent clinical study of short-duration experimental thyrotoxicosis in 18 human subjects found that cardiac output increased at rest and after exercise, but muscle bulk and function decreased.[16] Activities of oxidative and glycolytic enzymes in skeletal muscle decreased 21% to 37%. The cross-sectional area of type IIA muscle decreased 15%, lean body mass was reduced, and rates of whole body protein breakdown were enhanced. During exercise, plasma lactic acid concentration was elevated 25%, and the arteriovenous oxygen difference was decreased, reflecting the imbalance between cardiac output and muscle function.

Findings in thyrotoxic myopathy include altered electrical responses, decreased muscle bulk, altered energy metabolism, and increased sensitivity to β-adrenergic stimuli.[17] Thyroid hormones have a profound effect on mitochondrial oxidative activity, synthesis and degradation of proteins, sensitivity of tissues to catecholamines, the differentiation of muscle fibers, capillary growth, and levels of antioxidant enzymes and compounds.[18] The contribution of these factors to thyrotoxic myopathy is reviewed here, but a clear understanding of the disorder remains to be discovered.

Myographic studies of patients with thyrotoxicosis, in which repeated contractions of a single group of muscles (eg, the flexors of the forearm and hand) are induced by electrical stimuli, show a weakness of contraction and a lack of the normal potentiation of contraction.[1]

The brevity of the Achilles tendon reflex in these patients has been studied physiologically. When the duration of the Achilles reflex responses was measured by the half-relaxation time alone, 66 of 70 thyrotoxic adults showed a reflex response of shortened duration.[19] The mean half-relaxation time for this group was 230 ms, significantly shorter than the mean

of 322 ms for an age-related group of 174 normal subjects. Because the measurement of Achilles reflex time usually correlates poorly with biochemical parameters of thyroid function, it has limited clinical applicability.[14]

Electromyographic (EMG) studies of skeletal muscle in thyrotoxic and hypothyroid patients have yielded limited information. Abnormal EMG results were found in the proximal muscles in 93% and in the distal muscles in 43% of 54 consecutive patients with thyrotoxicosis. The abnormalities included a reduced duration of mean action potentials and an increased mean percentage of polyphasic potentials.[20] Large action potentials frequently are seen in thyrotoxic myopathy but are not associated with neuropathic change histopathologically and probably do not indicate denervation.

Thigh muscle volume and muscle efficiency (total work output per square centimeter of muscle) are decreased in thyrotoxic patients and increase after therapy.[21] Urinary excretion of creatinine is low and increases after treatment, also suggesting reduced muscle mass.[22] The 3-methylhistidine/creatinine ratio is higher than after treatment, indicating accelerated protein breakdown in skeletal muscle during thyrotoxicosis. Muscle biopsies (vastus lateralis) of patients showed a significantly lower proportion of type I (red, mitochondria-rich, oxidative) fibers (30% versus 41%), a higher capillary density (23%), lower glycogen content (33%), and higher hexokinase activity (32%) compared with biopsies repeated after 10 months of treatment.[23] An electron microscopic study of quadriceps biopsy specimens of thyrotoxic patients revealed alterations in the normal structure of muscle fibers and changes in capillaries in muscle ranging from an increase in basement membrane thickness with reduplication to destruction of the capillaries.[24]

Thyrotoxicosis produces extensive changes in the metabolic character and protein composition of muscle. The nature and extent of these changes differ in different muscles; for example, heart muscle hypertrophies, whereas skeletal muscle shows a hypotrophic response. The changes in skeletal muscle occur particularly in extensor muscles, which contain a high proportion of type I fibers.[25] In skeletal muscle of thyrotoxic rats, basal oxygen consumption is increased 40%, and adenosine triphosphate (ATP) turnover in relation to the sum of force developed during stimulation is significantly increased compared with euthyroid animals.[26] Both oxidative capacity and stimulation of oxidative phosphorylation are increased in soleus muscle of thyrotoxic rats.[24,27] The concept that oxidative phosphorylation may be "uncoupled" in thyrotoxic muscle has not been corroborated.[28] Thyrotoxic animals show a greater capillarity in skeletal muscles than do normal animals.[24]

A striking increase in glucose metabolism occurs in muscle tissue in human thyrotoxicosis, as shown by a study of forearm muscle glucose uptake and oxidation in such patients.[29] These patients, compared with normal subjects, had a twofold increase in forearm glucose uptake (1286 versus 677 μmol/dL forearm·min with a threefold enhanced glucose oxidation (443 versus 147 μmol/dL forearm·min). Nonoxidative glucose metabolism also was greater in thyrotoxic patients (842 versus 529 μmol/dL forearm·min). Basal lipid oxidation rates in the forearm muscles of the thyrotoxic patients also were significantly higher than in normal subjects (0.290 versus 0.088 mg/dL forearm·min). Thyroid hormone increases the expression of the muscle/fat glucose transporter, which appears to be the major glucose transport protein in skeletal muscle.[30]

The effects of thyroid hormones on human and rat skeletal muscle energetics have been studied in vivo by phosphorus 31 magnetic resonance spectroscopy.[31] Five patients had a normal phosphocreatine/inorganic phosphate ratio (PCr/Pi) at rest, normal PCr depletion during exercise, and unusually rapid recovery of PCr/Pi after exercise.

Adrenergic activity contributes to the hypermetabolism and protein breakdown caused by thyroid excess.[17] β-Adrenergic blockade with intravenous propranolol abolished the calorigenic response to epinephrine, but it had no detectable effect on either the accelerated basal metabolic rate or the augmented body protein catabolism caused by thyroid hormone excess. Thus the increased basal metabolic rate and accelerated protein breakdown are presumably not adrenergically mediated. Under nonbasal conditions, enhanced responsiveness to adrenergic calorigenesis may exaggerate the hypermetabolic state and contribute to weight loss, including loss of muscle bulk.

Thyrotoxicosis causes important changes in protein composition of skeletal muscle. The number of sodium-potassium (Na-K) pumps, determined by ^{3}H-ouabain binding sites, was increased 68% in biopsy samples of muscle obtained from thyrotoxic patients.[27] Thyroid hormone, acting directly on fast muscle cells, orchestrates the transition from neonatal to adult myosin.[32] Long-term administration of sodium $3,3',5$-T_3 induces a transformation of the alkali-labile myofibrillar adenosine triphosphatase (M-ATPase) of the slow fibers of the rat soleus muscle to the alkali-stable M-ATPase more typical of fast fibers,[33] that is, thyrotoxicosis is capable of inducing a fiber-type change that is independent of innervation.[34] Experimental thyrotoxicosis produces an increase in the mitochondria of rat soleus muscle,[35] consistent with the increase in oxidative capacity already noted.

Triiodothyronine-induced thyrotoxicosis produces greater dystrophy in the mdx muscular dystrophy mouse. Cardiac hypertrophy and skeletal muscle atrophy were present after T_3 treatment. Both cardiac and type I skeletal muscle (but not fast-twitch muscle) had larger, more frequent dystrophic lesions in T_3-treated mdx mice.[36]

Clinical Thyrotoxic Myopathic Syndromes

CHRONIC THYROTOXIC MYOPATHY

Among patients with thyrotoxicosis, it is possible to distinguish a group with such pronounced muscular atrophy and weakness as to suggest the diagnosis of progressive muscular atrophy. In the literature, more than 300 such cases can be found.[1,15] It is the impression of some authors that a large number of the patients have been middle-aged and that men may be affected more often than women. It is rare, however, for the myopathy to be the presenting feature in thyrotoxicosis.[15]

The clinical picture in most patients is one of marked weakness and atrophy of muscles and weight loss. The onset is insidious and the course slowly progressive. The thyrotoxicosis often is of the masked type. Exophthalmos is not prominent. Nervousness, sweating, and intolerance to heat have appeared in several instances after the onset of the muscle disorder. For these reasons, the diagnosis may at first be difficult.

Muscle weakness predominantly involves the pelvic and shoulder girdles, although all muscles are affected to some extent. The shoulder and hand muscles undergo the most obvious atrophy, but the facial muscles also may be affected. Seldom does the weakness extend to bulbar and ocular muscles, and when it does, myasthenia gravis should be suspected.[15] The degree of weakness varies; most patients remain ambulatory. Tremors and coarse twitching of muscles during contraction may occur. Coarse fasciculations at rest, like those seen in motor system disease, have not been noted in thyrotoxic patients under personal observation. The tendon reflexes usually are normal or enhanced, and plantar reflexes are flexor. No sensory changes or other neurologic abnormalities have been described.

A few patients with chronic thyrotoxic myopathy presumably have died of the disease. Of the remainder, recovery has been complete, or nearly so, after successful treatment. Residual weakness has been noted in a few cases.

As for some laboratory findings, the basal metabolic rate has varied from +14% to +100%. Glucose tolerance has been normal or decreased. Serum levels of electrolytes, including potassium, have been normal. EMGs have disclosed abnormalities in most patients.[20] The results of prostigmine and curare tests have consistently been normal.

In 48 patients with thyrotoxicosis who had chronic myopathy, a search for EMG stigmata of latent myasthenia was done by performing repeated nerve stimulation. Eight patients had abnormal neuromuscular transmission, as in myasthenia gravis, of whom one patient later developed clinical ocular myasthenia. Three other cases showed abnormal facilitation, as in Eaton-Lambert syndrome.[37]

Relatively few detailed reports on muscle pathology in chronic thyrotoxic myopathy are available. We could find no definite pathologic changes in the biopsy specimens we examined. One can only conclude that the principal changes in thyrotoxicosis are mild atrophy and, in some patients, infiltration of fat cells, increase in sarcolemmal nuclei, and focal perivascular lymphorrhages.[38] The atrophy can be demonstrated by light microscopy only if micrometer measurements are made. Even electron microscopy has not shed much light on the subject. In two specimens, the only finding was an excessive number of abnormal mitochondria.[39]

The differential diagnosis of this myopathic disease usually is not difficult. Although chronic thyrotoxic myopathy is said to simulate progressive muscular atrophy, the weakness and atrophy are never as severe, and true fasciculations have not been demonstrated either clinically or electromyographically.

Chronic thyrotoxic myopathy can be differentiated from myasthenia gravis by the following features. In myasthenia gravis, there is (1) an involvement of bulbar and ocular muscles predominantly, (2) a lack of definite muscle atrophy, (3) rapid fatigue of muscle, (4) a beneficial effect of prostigmine, and (5) excessive weakening of muscle contraction by small doses of curare. Polymyositis, with or without skin changes, may lead to severe weakness or paralysis with atrophy, impairment of tendon reflexes, elevated basal metabolic rate, and creatinuria. This disorder occasionally has been confused with thyrotoxic myopathy. The EMGs of the involved muscles in polymyositis are abnormal, and biopsy discloses a characteristic pathologic picture consisting of infiltrations of inflammatory cells, together with severe degenerative and regenerative changes in muscle fibers. Hypothyroid myopathy is discussed in chapter 67.

EXOPHTHALMIC OPHTHALMOPLEGIA (GRAVES' OPHTHALMOPATHY)

Among the most frequent and troublesome of the peripheral complications in thyrotoxicosis are ocular abnormalities, including lid lag, lid retraction, and exophthalmos. A number of such cases progress to severe exophthalmos, ophthalmoplegia, chemosis, and panophthalmitis.[15] Definite pathologic changes, with degeneration and swelling of extraocular muscle fibers, infiltrations of inflammatory lymphocytes and mononuclear cells, and interstitial tissue inflammation and edema, have been observed.[38] Graves' ophthalmopathy is almost certainly an autoimmune disease and is the focus of intense research interest. The exact nature of the autoimmune ophthalmopathy remains to be elucidated and is discussed in chapter 30.

Severe extraocular muscle swelling in Graves' ophthalmopathy may produce optic nerve compression, endangering vision. Computed tomography or magnetic resonance imaging can evaluate the extent of disease and impingement on the optic nerve.[40] A more complete discussion of Graves' ophthalmopathy is presented in chapter 30.

THYROTOXICOSIS WITH MYASTHENIA GRAVIS

The coexistence of myasthenia gravis and thyrotoxicosis is relatively rare, in contrast to the myopathy of uncomplicated thyrotoxicosis and to the "ophthalmoplegic" syndrome. The subject has been reviewed extensively.[4,9] Less than 1% of patients have complicating myasthenia gravis,[41] whereas the incidence of thyrotoxicosis in myasthenia gravis has ranged from 3% to 6%.[9] In a recent study of 104 patients with myasthenia gravis, 5.7% had thyrotoxicosis, 10% had subclinical hyperthyroidism, 1.9% had hypothyroidism, and 3.4% had subclinical hypothyroidism. Twelve patients had antithyroid antibodies.[42] Graves' disease[43] and myasthenia gravis[44] both implicate autoimmune mechanisms in their pathogenesis; this may account in part for their coexistence. Antibodies to the nicotinic acetylcholine receptor, a specific test for the diagnosis of myasthenia gravis, were negative in the sera of patients with thyroid disease and ophthalmopathy or periodic paralysis, but were positive in patients with thyroid disease and concurrent myasthenia gravis.[45]

The myasthenia gravis syndrome does not differ from that in euthyroid patients. A variable weakness after the use of skeletal muscles, particularly those subserving ocular movement, mastication, facial expression, deglutition, and speech, is the principal feature of this disease. The muscles of the neck, trunk, and limbs frequently are involved, and when the disease is severe and generalized, failure of the respiratory muscles may lead to death. Cardiac and smooth muscles are not affected. In the early stages, weakness develops only after maintained contraction, but as the disease advances, the muscles first and most severely affected cease to contract normally even after prolonged rest.

The gross appearance of the involved muscles, although thin, is otherwise natural; microscopic sections have revealed no important changes except for collections of lymphocytes, termed lymphorrhages, and, in some instances, the degeneration of isolated muscle fibers.

The EMG of myasthenic muscle during exercise differs quantitatively from that of normal muscle; action currents of the former tend to be of lower amplitude, and gradually decrease in amplitude during sustained activity. This contrasts with normal muscle, in which the amplitude of action currents increases with fatigue. The EMG of patients with myasthenia gravis is the same, regardless of the presence or absence of thyrotoxicosis. Prostigmine improves the strength of contraction of myasthenic muscles; small doses of curare, insufficient to affect the normal patient, impair the strength of contraction of myasthenic muscles.

The largest reported series with myasthenia gravis and thyrotoxicosis consisted of 25 patients, of whom 20 were women.[9] Ophthalmoplegia was present in 16 patients, weakness of bulbar muscles in 12, and weakness of limb and trunk musculature in 8. This is almost identical with the distribution of muscle weakness in uncomplicated myasthenia gravis. No definite relation was found between the onset of the myasthenia gravis and the stage of thyrotoxicosis. In about one-third of patients, the thyrotoxicosis developed first; in another third, the myasthenia gravis preceded the thyrotoxicosis.

Hypothyroidism aggravates myasthenia gravis, increasing the requirement of prostigmine. The effects of the two diseases may be difficult to dissect, but the condition of the myasthenic patient worsens when any departure from the euthyroid state occurs.[4,46]

All patients have responded to prostigmine, although the improvement has almost invariably been less than complete. Prostigmine does not completely rectify the fundamental defect in myasthenia gravis, either in the uncomplicated disease or in the form accompanied by thyrotoxicosis. When thyrotoxicosis coexists with myasthenia, it adds the weakness of limbs resulting from thyrotoxic myopathy to the myasthenia, and so increases the patient's motor deficit. The requirements for prostigmine to control the myasthenia remain unchanged. In a recent report, a patient with concurrent myasthenia gravis, thyrotoxicosis, and polymyositis was successfully treated with prednisone alone.[47] Another report describes three patients presenting with both myasthenia gravis and thyrotoxicosis in whom control of the thyrotoxicosis with carbimazole was accompanied by deterioration of the myasthenic symptoms in two and persistence in one; thymectomy was performed with subsequent improvement in all three patients.[48] This suggests that attempts to bring concurrent autoimmune diseases under control should be directed at the autoimmune process.

Thyroidectomy has been attended by a high mortality rate in these patients, so that medical, rather than surgical, treatment is recommended. The myasthenia gravis persists after successful antithyroid treatment but may become less severe.[49]

THYROTOXICOSIS WITH PERIODIC PARALYSIS

Periodic paralysis is a rare and peculiar disorder. Its cardinal features are attacks of flaccid paralysis of the legs, arms, and trunk, with areflexia and abolition of electrical excitability.[50] The degree of paralysis varies from one attack to another. In severe episodes, there may be complete paralysis of all skeletal muscles, including those that control respiration. The muscles of facial expression, mastication, deglutition, and ocular movement usually are involved to a lesser degree. Smooth muscle is not affected, and cardiac function seldom is disturbed. The attacks may last from a few hours to several days, and their frequency is extremely variable. They may be precipitated by exercise followed by rest, by excessive ingestion of carbohydrate foods, and by the administration of insulin or epinephrine. A low serum potassium level has been noted during attacks in some cases, and the administration of potassium salts prevents or aborts an attack of paralysis. A vacuolar myopathy characterizes the pathology of muscle fibers seen in biopsy specimens from patients during and probably between attacks of primary hypokalemic periodic paralysis.[51] Electron microscopy has shown the fine vacuoles to be dilatations of endoplasmic reticulum.[52]

Data have been collected on hundreds of patients with periodic paralysis associated with thyrotoxicosis.[43,49] Many of the patients have been of Asian extraction with an overwhelming male predominance.[53] The following discussion is largely based on the summary of these cases.

Periodic paralysis in conjunction with thyrotoxicosis differs from the uncomplicated disease in only two respects. The patients have been older at the time of onset of paralytic attacks (20–39 years in 84%) and a family history of periodic paralysis has been absent in all but 2%.

Antithyroid treatment resulted in the cure of the thyrotoxicosis in 152 of 159 patients, with improvement in the remaining 7; the periodic paralysis was completely relieved in 141 patients and improved in 11 others. The last 11 may have been examples of coexistence of two separate diseases, a latent periodic paralysis becoming manifest after the development of thyrotoxicosis.

The favorable response of the paralytic attacks to the treatment of the thyrotoxicosis speaks in favor of therapeutically restoring all such patients to a euthyroid status. If the paralytic attacks continue, potassium salts should be used.

One report states that propranolol prevented the periodic paralysis in a Vietnamese man who suffered recurrent episodes of hypokalemic periodic paralysis during therapy for thyrotoxicosis.[54] Acetazolamide, which is useful in the prevention of attacks in familial–euthyroid periodic paralysis, was reported to worsen thyrotoxic periodic paralysis in a Latin American man.[55]

Abnormalities of Na^+-K^+ transport have been suggested in patients with thyrotoxic periodic paralysis,[56-58] but an explanation of the mechanism of thyrotoxic periodic paralysis has not been available.

NEUROLOGIC DISORDERS

Disorders of thyroid metabolism have profound effects on the normal functioning of the brain. As discussed in chapters 57 and 67 and the sections on congenital hypothyroidism and acquired juvenile hypothyroidism in chapter 85, thyroid deficiency of congenital type (ie, cretinism) or that which is acquired early in life hinders the growth and differentiation of the brain and the attainment of full intellectual potential. In the adult, thyroid deficiency results in a variety of neurologic disorders, which are discussed in detail in chapter 67.

Central Nervous System Syndromes in Thyrotoxicosis

Thyrotoxicosis induces a range of disorders of the CNS. These can be characterized as neuropsychiatric disorders, discrete neurologic syndromes (chorea), and severe acute systemic states with delirium, coma, and convulsions (thyroid storm or thyrotoxic crisis).

NEUROPSYCHIATRIC SYNDROMES

Nervousness, irritability, and tremulousness are common symptoms of thyrotoxicosis. Beyond this, major depression, anxiety disorder, hypomania or mania, and even schizophreniform disorder[59] are not uncommonly described. Such patients may be inappropriately referred to a psychiatrist before thyrotoxicosis is recognized. One study found that a history of psychiatric disease and a family history of psychiatric disease did not predict anxiety or depression in patients with thyrotoxicosis.[5] With treatment, psychiatric improvements parallel improvements in endocrine symptoms.[60] More provocative are reports of resolution of thyrotoxicosis after electroconvulsive therapy.[61]

Mild deficits in attention, memory, and complex problem solving have been documented in thyrotoxic patients. In one study,[62] propranolol treatment resulted in improvement in psychiatric symptoms, but improvements in accompanying neuropsychologic deficits of memory and attention were seen only after 6 months of antithyroid treatment. Another report describes marked to severe intellectual impairment on neuropsychological testing in 23% of a group of 26 patients studied 10 years after successful treatment of thyrotoxicosis.[6] This effect on cognitive function requires further study. The psychiatric manifestations of thyrotoxicosis are thoroughly reviewed in chapter 50.

NEUROLOGIC SYNDROMES

Chorea, indistinguishable in its features from Sydenham's chorea, seldom appears as a manifestation of thyrotoxicosis.[7] It may persist after the patient is rendered euthyroid.[63]

Chronic atrial fibrillation is associated with an increased risk of embolic stroke. In a recent study of 126 patients with atrial fibrillation, one-fourth of whom had an acute embolic stroke, 8 were found to have occult thyrotoxicosis. All 8 patients had reversion to sinus rhythm after antithyroid treatment, obviating the need for prolonged anticoagulation.[64]

Thyrotoxic crisis, a fulminant increase in all signs and symptoms of thyrotoxicosis, is a rare occurrence.[65] Its neurologic manifestations may rarely include coma and status epilepticus.[8,22]

These clinical facts emphasize the important role that thyroid hormone plays in the function of the mature nervous system, beyond its better-defined role in the development of the brain.

Pathologic Physiology of the Nervous System in Thyroid Disease

The electroencephalograms (EEGs) of most patients with thyrotoxicosis show an increase in frequency of the α rhythm that is greater than can be accounted for by elevation in temperature.[66–68] In hypothyroidism, the opposite change occurs, and as symptoms of cerebral disease become manifest, the EEG becomes grossly abnormal. The basal metabolic rate tends to correlate with the frequency of brain waves,[69] but in the extremes of thyroid abnormality, when nervous symptoms supervene, the correlation not uncommonly is poor. The rate of cerebral circulation, and hence oxygen utilization in hyperthyroidism, is now known to be significantly elevated.[70] By contrast, hypothyroidism causes a definite decrease in cerebral blood flow as well as in cerebral oxygen consumption and cerebral glucose consumption. After treatment with T_4, these parameters of cerebral function return to normal.[71] Such alterations in circulatory dynamics correlate reasonably well with EEG alterations and changes in mental functioning.

Biochemical Studies

The effects of thyroid hormone on brain tissue biochemistry are much more prominent during development than in adulthood. The effects of thyroid hormone and its deficiency on brain development are discussed in chapters 57 and 67 and the subchapter on congenital hypothyroidism in chapter 85. Here we are concerned with metabolic effects of thyrotoxicosis on the mature brain.

In brain and pituitary, iodothyronine 5′-deiodinases produce 50% or more of the T_3 found in these tissues, and show rapid threefold to fivefold changes in response to changes in the thyroid status.[72] Measurements in rat brain of the effects of chronic thyroid hormone deficiency or excess on brain iodothyronine economy demonstrate that despite extremes of T_4 availability, brain T_4 and T_3 concentrations and brain T_3 production and turnover rates are kept within narrow limits.[73,74] These responses suggest that brain iodothyronine homeostasis is strongly defended. Nevertheless, because signs of CNS dysfunction occur in thyrotoxic patients, it is possible that even small deviations of brain iodocompounds can produce significant changes in brain function.[73] Studies of brain mitochondria from rats made thyrotoxic show only marginal effects.[75] On the other hand, long-term hypothyroidism reduces mitochondrial respiratory enzymes[76] and oxidative metabolism, suggesting that the metabolic properties of brain mitochondria are sensitive to thyroid hormones. The brain may need less iodothyronines than other organs.[76] Different metabolic responses to thyroid hormones are seen in different areas of the brain.[77]

Activities of some brain enzymes are sensitive to thyroid hormones. Nuclear polymerase I activity in the brain declines promptly after thyroidectomy.[76] Thyrotoxicosis reduces the activity of glutamate dehydrogenase[77] and pyruvate dehydrogenase in the brain.[78] Several other enzymes have been found to be unchanged: transthyretin,[79] calcium channel binding sites,[80] and the erythroid glucose transporter (which is strongly expressed in cerebral cortex).[30]

In contrast, thyrotoxicosis has been shown to produce prominent and specific effects on neurotransmitter systems in brain. In the mature rat brain, thyroid status affects specific neurotransmitter receptors and levels. In adult rats, thyrotoxicosis resulted in an increase in β-adrenergic binding sites in cerebral cortex whereas γ-aminobutyric acid-binding sites were decreased.[81]

Thyrotoxicosis produced complex and regionally specific changes in brain nuclei levels of serotonin, 5-hydroxyindoleacetic acid, and substance P.[82] Thyrotoxicosis increased the number of opiate receptors and also increased native pain sensitivity.[83] In all these cases, affinity constants were never modified. These results, taken together, begin to clarify how thyrotoxicosis may affect psychological and emotional function in the human. We may ask whether the mechanism of action of psychopharmacologic drugs involves CNS thyroid hormone metabolism. Desmethylimipramine, a selective inhibitor of presynaptic uptake of norepinephrine, decreases the uptake into brain of T_3 and T_4.[84] The interaction of thyroid hormones, brain neurotransmitters, and psychopharmacologic agents continues to be a topic of increasing interest. It is becoming clear that thyroid hormones act directly on the adult nervous system in complex and important ways. The homeostasis of thyroid function of mature brain is strongly supported, and metabolic changes in the face of thyroid dysfunction are much more muted than in other organs.

References

1. Engel AG. Neuromuscular manifestations of Graves' disease. Mayo Clinic Proc 1972;47:919
2. Kroll AI, Kuwabara T. Dysthyroid ocular myopathy. Arch Ophthalmol 1966;76:244
3. Kelley DE. Thyrotoxic periodic paralysis. Arch Intern Med 1989: 149:2597
4. Gaelen LH, Levitan S. Myasthenia gravis and thyroid function. Arch Neurol 1968;18:107
5. Kathol RG, Delahunt JW. The relationship of anxiety and depression to symptoms of hyperthyroidism using operational criteria. Gen Hosp Psychiatry 1986;8:23
6. Perrild H, Hansen JM, Arnung K, et al. Intellectual impairment after hyperthyroidism. Acta Endocrinol (Copenh) 1986;112:185
7. Shahar E, Shapiro MS, Shenkman L. Hyperthyroid-induced chorea. Case report and review of the literature. Isr J Med Sci 1988;24:264
8. Safe AF, Griffiths KD, Maxwell RT. Thyrotoxic crisis presenting as status epilepticus. Postgrad Med 1990;66:150
9. Millikan CH, Haines SF. Thyroid gland in relation to neuromuscular disease. Arch Intern Med 1953;92:5
10. Lahey FH. The quadriceps test for the myasthenia of thyroidism. JAMA 1926;87:754
11. Gaan D. Chronic thyrotoxic myopathy with involvement of respiratory and bulbar muscles. Br Med J [Clin Res] 1967;3:415
12. McElvaney GN, Wilcox PG, Fairbarn MS, et al. Respiratory muscle weakness and dyspnea in thyrotoxic patients. Am Rev Respir Dis 1990;141:1221
13. Siafakas NM, Milona I, Salesiotou V, et al. Respiratory muscle strength in hyperthyroidism before and after treatment. Am Rev Respir Dis 1992;146:1025
14. Costin G, Kaplan SA, Ling SM. The Achilles reflex time in thyroid disorders. J Pediatr 1970;76:277
15. Bradley WG, Walton JN. Neurologic manifestations of thyroid disease. Postgrad Med 1971;50:118
16. Martin WH, Spina RJ, Korte E, et al. Mechanisms of impaired exercise capacity in short duration experimental hyperthyroidism. J Clin Invest 1991;88:2047
17. Gelfand RA, Hutchinson-Williams KA, Bonde AA, et al. Catabolic effects of thyroid hormone excess: the contribution of adrenergic activity to hypermetabolism and protein breakdown. Metabolism 1987;36:562

18. Asayama K, Kato K. Oxidative muscle injury and its relevance to hyperthyroidism. Free Radic Biol Med 1990;8:293

19. Reinfrank RF, Kaufman RP, Wetstone HJ, Glennon JA. Observations of the Achilles reflex test. JAMA 1967;199:1

20. Ramsay ID. Electromyography in thyrotoxicosis. Q J Med 1965;34:255

21. Zurcher RM, Horber FF, Grunig BE, et al. Effect of thyroid dysfunction on thigh muscle efficiency. J Clin Endocrinol Metab 1989;69:1082

22. Aiello DP, DuPlessis AJ, Pattishall EG, et al. Thyroid storm presenting with coma and seizures in a 3-year-old girl. Clin Pediatr (Phila) 1989;28:571

23. Celsing F, Blomstrand E, Melichna J, et al. Effect of hyperthyroidism on fibre-type composition, fibre area, glycogen content and enzyme activity in human skeletal muscle. Clin Physiol 1986;6:171

24. Capo LA, Sillau AH. The effect of hyperthyroidism on capillarity and oxidative capacity in rat soleus and gastrocnemius muscles. J Physiol (Lond) 1983;342:1

25. Brown JG, Millward DJ. Dose response of protein turnover in rat skeletal muscle to triiodothyronine treatment. Biochim Biophys Acta 1983;757:182

26. Everts ME, Vanhardeveld C, Ter-Keurs HE, et al. Force development and metabolism in perfused skeletal muscle of euthyroid and hyperthyroid rats. Horm Metab Res 1983;15:388

27. Leijendekker WJ, Vanhardeveld C, Kassenaar AA. The influence of the thyroid state on energy turnover during tetanic stimulation in the fast twitch (mixed type) muscle of rats. Metabolism 1983;32:615

28. Stocker WW, Samaha FJ, DeGroot LJ. Coupled oxidative phosphorylation in muscle of thyrotoxic patients. Am J Med 1968;44:900

29. Foss MC, Paccola GM, Saad MJ, et al. Peripheral glucose metabolism in human hyperthyroidism. J Clin Endocrinol Metab 1990;70:1167

30. Weinstein SP, Watts J, Haber RS. Thyroid hormone increases muscle/fat glucose transporter gene expression in rat skeletal muscle. Endocrinology 1991;129:455

31. Argov Z, Renshaw PF, Boden B, et al. Effects of thyroid hormones on skeletal muscle bioenergetics: in vivo phosphorus-31 magnetic resonance spectroscopy study of humans and rats. J Clin Invest 1988;81:1695

32. Gambke B, Lyons GE, Haselgrove J, et al. Thyroidal and neural control of myosin transitions during development of rat fast and slow muscles. FEBS Lett 1983;156:335

33. Ianuzzo D, Patel P, Chan V, et al. Thyroidal influence on skeletal muscle myosin. Nature 1977;270:74

34. Hall-Craggs EC, Wines MM, Max SR. Fiber type changes in denervated soleus muscles of the hyperthyroid rat. Exp Neurol 1983;80:252

35. Winder WW. Time course of the T_3- and T_4-induced increase in rat soleus muscle mitochondria. Am J Physiol 1979;236:C132

36. Anderson JE, Liu L, Kardami E. The effects of hyperthyroidism on muscular dystrophy in the mdx mouse: greater dystrophy in cardiac and soleus muscle. Muscle Nerve 1994;17:64

37. Puvanendran K, Cheah JS, Naganathan N, et al. Neuromuscular transmission in thyrotoxicosis. J Neurol Sci 1979;43:47

38. Kakulas B, Adams RD. Diseases of muscle: a study in pathology. 4th ed. New York: Blakiston, 1985:635

39. Engel AG. Electron microscopic observations in thyrotoxic and corticosteroid-induced myopathies. Mayo Clin Proc 1966;41:785

40. Shah KJ, Dasher BG, Brooks B. Computed tomography of Graves' ophthalmopathy. Diagnosis, management and posttherapeutic evaluation. Clin Imaging 1989;13:58

41. Ohno M, Hamada N, Yamakawa J, et al. Myasthenia gravis associated with Graves' disease in Japan. Jpn J Med 1987;26:2

42. Kiessling WR, Pflughaupt KW, Ricker K, et al. Thyroid function and circulating antithyroid antibodies in myasthenia gravis. Neurology 1981;31:771

43. Kidd A, Okita N, Row VV, Volpé R. Immunologic aspects of Graves' and Hashimoto's diseases. Metabolism 1980;29:80

44. Engel AG. Myasthenia gravis and myasthenic syndromes. Ann Neurol 1984;16:519

45. Ong BK, Chong PN, Tan SK, et al. Acetylcholine receptor antibody assay kit: establishment of controls in normals and nonmyasthenias and evaluation of sera from patients with thyroid disease. Ann Acad Med Singapore 1993;22:567

46. Drachman DB. Myasthenia gravis and the thyroid gland. N Engl J Med 1962;266:330

47. Haratis Y, Patten BM. Prednisone use in concurrent autoimmune diseases. Arch Neurol 1979;36:103

48. Teoh R, Chow CC, Kay R, et al. Response to control of hyperthyroidism in patients with myasthenia gravis and thyrotoxicosis. Br J Clin Pract 1990;44:742

49. Engel AG. Thyroid function and periodic paralysis. Am J Med 1961;30:327

50. Riggs JE. The periodic paralyses. Neurol Clin 1988;6:485

51. Engel AG, Lambert EH, Rosevers JW, Tauxe WN. Clinical and electromyographic studies in a patient with primary hypokalemic periodic paralysis. Am J Med 1965;38:626

52. Engel AG. Electron microscopic observations in primary hypokalemic and thyrotoxic periodic paralysis. Mayo Clin Proc 1966;41:797

53. Ferriero JE, Arguelles DJ, Rams H. Thyrotoxic periodic paralysis. Am J Med 1986;80:146

54. McHutchison JG, Melick RA, Wark JD. Hypokalemic periodic paralysis of thyrotoxic origin. Aust N Z J Med 1987;17:455

55. Shulkin D, Olson BR, Levey GS. Thyrotoxic periodic paralysis in a Latin-American taking acetazolamide. Am J Med Sci 1989;297:337

56. Lam KS, Yeung RT, Benson EA, et al. Erythrocyte sodium-potassium pump in thyrotoxic periodic paralysis. Aust N Z J Med 1989;19:6

57. Marx A, Ruppersberg JP, Pietrzyk C, et al. Thyrotoxic periodic paralysis and the sodium-potassium pump. Muscle Nerve 1989;12:810

58. Oh VM, Taylor EA, Yeo SH, et al. Cation transport across lymphocyte plasma membranes in euthyroid and thyrotoxic men with and without hypokalaemic periodic paralysis. Clin Sci 1990;78:199

59. Lazarus A, Jaffe R. Resolution of thyroid-induced schizophreniform disorder following subtotal thyroidectomy: case report. Gen Hosp Psychiatry 1986;8:29

60. Kudrjavcev T. Neurologic complications of thyroid dysfunction. Adv Neurol 1978;19:619

61. Diaz-Cabal R, Pearlman C, Kawecki A. Hyperthyroidism in a patient with agitated depression: resolution after electroconvulsive therapy. J Clin Psychiatry 1986;47:322

62. Trzepacz PT, McCue M, Klein I, et al. Psychiatric and neuropsychological response to propranolol in Graves' disease. Biol Psychiatry 1988;23:678

63. Javaid A, Hilton DD. Persistent chorea as a manifestation of thyrotoxicosis. Postgrad Med J 1988;64:789

64. Monreal M, Lafoz E, Foz M, et al. Occult thyrotoxicosis in patients with atrial fibrillation and an acute arterial embolism. Angiology 1988;39:981

65. Ingbar SH. Thyrotoxic storm. N Engl J Med 1966;274:1252

66. Jackson IMD, Renfrew S. The diagnostic value of the EEG in thyrotoxicosis. Acta Endocrinol (Copenh) 1966;52:399

67. Leubuscher HJ, Herrmann F, Hambsch K, et al. EEG changes in untreated hyperthyroidism and under the conditions of thyreostatic treatment. Exp Clin Endocrinol 1988;92:85

68. Ross DA, Schwab RS. The cortical alpha rhythm in thyroid disorders. Endocrinology 1939;25:75

69. Herrmann HTT, Quarton GC. Changes in alpha frequency with change in thyroid hormone level. Electroencephalogr Clin Neurophysiol 1964;16:515

70. Sokoloff L. Cerebral blood flow and oxygen consumption in hyperthyroidism before and after treatment. J Clin Invest 1953;32:202

71. Scheinberg P, Stead EA. Cerebral metabolism in hyperthyroidism and myxedema. Fed Proc 1950;9:112

72. Leonard JL, Silva JE, Kaplan MM, et al. Acute post-transcriptional regulation of cerebrocortical and pituitary iodothyronine 5'-deiodinases by thyroid hormone. Endocrinology 1984;114:998

73. Dratman MB, Crutchfield FL, Gordon JT, et al. Iodothyronine homeostasis in rat brain during hypo and hyperthyroidism. Am J Physiol 1983;245:E185

74. Vandoorn J, Vanderheide D, Roelfsema F. The contribution of local thyroxine monodeiodination to intracellular 3,5,3'-triiodothyronine in several tissues of hyperthyroid rats at isotopic equilibrium. Endocrinology 1984;115:174

75. Satav JG, Katyare SS. Effect of experimental thyrotoxicosis on oxidative phosphorylation in rat liver, kidney and brain mitochondria. Mol Cell Endocrinol 1982;28:173

76. Dembri A, Belkhiria M, Michel O, et al. Effects of short- and long-term thyroidectomy on mitochondrial and nuclear activity in adult rat brain. Mol Cell Endocrinol 1983;33:211

77. Fernandez-Pastor JM, Morell M, Menendez-Patterson A, et al. Effect of experimental changes in thyroid function on oxidative metabolism and glutamate dehydrogenase activity in the limbic system of the rat. Rev Esp Fisiol 1983;39:311

78. Murthy AS, Baquer NZ. Changes of pyruvate dehydrogenase in rat brain with thyroid hormones. Enzyme 1982;28:48

79. Blay P, Nilsson C, Owman C, et al. Transthyretin expression in the rat brain: effect of thyroid functional state and role in thyroxine transport. Brain Res 1993;632:114

80. Kosinski C, Gross G, Hanft G. Effect of hypo- and hyperthyroidism on binding of [3H]-nitrendipine to myocardial and brain membranes. Br J Clin Pharmacol 1990;30(Suppl 1):128S

81. Sandrini M, Marrama D, Vergoni AV, Bertolini A. Effects of thyroid status on the characteristics of alpha 1-, alpha 2-, beta, imipramine and GABA receptors in the rat brain. Life Sci 1991;48:659

82. Savard P, Merand Y, Dipaolo T, et al. Effects of thyroid state on serotonin, 5-hydroxyindoleacetic acid and substance P contents in discrete brain nuclei of adult rats. Neuroscience 1983;10:1399

83. Edmondson EA, Bonnet KA, Friedhoff AJ. The effect of hyperthyroidism on opiate receptor binding and pain sensitivity. Life Sci 1990;47:2283

84. Gordon JT, Martens DA, Tomlinson EE, et al. Desmethylimipramine, a potent inhibitor of synaptosomal norepinephrine uptake, has diverse effects on thyroid hormone processing in rat brain. I. Effects on in vivo uptake of ^{125}I-labeled thyroid hormones in rat brain. Brain Res 1993;626:175

Werner and Ingbar's The Thyroid, Seventh Edition,
edited by Lewis E. Braverman and Robert D. Utiger.
Lippincott–Raven Publishers, Philadelphia, © 1996

44

The Pituitary
in Thyrotoxicosis

Peter J. Snyder

Thyrotoxicosis affects the secretion of most pituitary hormones, but because the clinical consequences are not so great as are those in hypothyroidism, the abnormalities of pituitary hormone secretion have not been studied as well as those in hypothyroidism. The effects of thyrotoxicosis on the secretion of growth hormone (GH) and prolactin (PRL) are discussed in this chapter; the effects on the secretion of vasopressin, adrenocorticotropin, and follicle-stimulating hormone and luteinizing hormone are discussed elsewhere (see chaps 40, 45, and 47, respectively).

GROWTH HORMONE

Clinical Manifestations

Children with thyrotoxicosis grow more rapidly than normal children. In one study of five children studied before and during antithyroid treatment, the height ages were all more than 3 standard deviations (SD) above the mean for normal children.[1] The bone ages also were accelerated and to a similar degree, so that the relationship of bone age to height age remained normal. Consequently, when the patients were treated, it appeared that their final heights would be normal.

Hormonal Abnormalities

Growth acceleration in thyrotoxic children suggests that their GH secretion might be greater than normal. In one study of adults, both the production rate and metabolic clearance rate of GH were greater in thyrotoxic patients and less in hypothyroid patients than in normal subjects.[2] In 8 thyrotoxic patients, the mean (± SD) production rate was 529 ± 242

ng/min, as compared with 347 ± 173 ng/min in 22 normal subjects and 160 ± 69 ng/min in 6 hypothyroid patients. Serum GH concentrations, however, are lower in thyrotoxic patients than in normal subjects. This decrease is not due to a lower serum concentration of GH-binding protein because it was found to be similar in 15 thyrotoxic patients and 19 euthyroid subjects.[3] Serum GH concentrations increase in response to deep sleep less in thyrotoxic children and adolescents than in normal subjects and increase when the patients are treated with propylthiouracil (Fig 44-1).[4] Likewise, the increase in serum GH concentrations in response to insulin-induced hypoglycemia is less in thyrotoxic children and adults than in normal subjects,[5–7] especially in those with severe thyrotoxicosis.[6]

The decreased serum GH concentration, despite the increased production rate, is probably the result of the increased metabolic clearance rate.[2] In fact, studies of GH secretion in seven thyrotoxic patients, based on measurements of serum GH concentrations at 10-minute intervals for 24 hours and deconvolution analysis (which removes the effect of metabolic clearance mathematically) revealed more frequent GH secretory bursts, a larger mass of GH released per burst, and a fourfold higher GH production rate than in seven normal subjects.[8] Because GH secretion is greater than normal in thyrotoxicosis, the increase in linear growth in thyrotoxic children could be a GH effect. The finding of higher than normal serum insulin-like growth factor-1 concentrations in thyrotoxic patients (259 ± 34 μg/L) (± SD) and a fall to normal (189 ± 15 μg/L) during treatment[9] suggests that there is a greater than normal effect of GH in thyrotoxicosis. These results do not, however, exclude the possibility that increased linear growth in thyrotoxicosis could be at least partly due to the direct effect of thyroid hormone on bone.

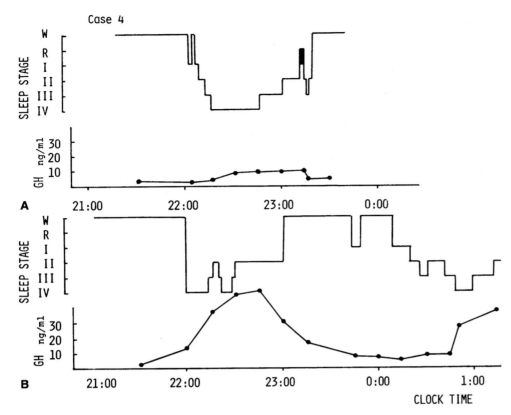

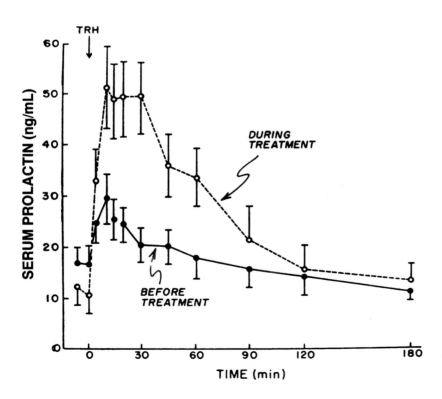

FIGURE 44-1. Serum GH concentrations during stages III and IV of sleep in a patient when thyrotoxic (*A*) and later after treatment when euthyroid (*B*). (Sasaki N, Tsuyusaki T, Nakamura H, et al. Sleep-related growth hormone release in thyrotoxic patients before and during propylthiouracil therapy. Endocrinol Jpn 1985;(32:39)

FIGURE 44-2. Serum PRL responses to TRH in 10 patients when they were thyrotoxic (*closed circles*) and when they were euthyroid (*open circles*). (Snyder PJ, Jacobs LS, Utiger RD, Daughaday WH. Thyroid hormone inhibition of the prolactin response to thyrotropin-releasing hormone. J Clin Invest 1973;52:2324)

PROLACTIN

Clinical Manifestations

Because galactorrhea is a manifestation of hypothyroidism, one might expect that difficulty in lactation would occur in postpartum women with thyrotoxicosis who attempt to nurse, but this difficulty has not yet been reported. Decreased lactation, if it does occur, might not be recognized because the ease of diagnosis of postpartum thyrotoxicosis would lead to its recognition before the decrease in lactation becomes clinically apparent. The physician then would probably advise the patient to discontinue nursing if she needed antithyroid treatment. Alternatively, PRL secretion and serum PRL concentrations in women with thyrotoxicosis may be sufficient for normal lactation.

Hormonal Abnormalities

Secretion of PRL in thyrotoxicosis is similar to that of GH, in that the production rate and metabolic clearance rate are somewhat greater than normal, but serum PRL concentrations, especially in response to stimulation, are less than normal. In one study, the mean (± SD) production rate of PRL in six thyrotoxic patients was 504 ± 91 μg/d and in six normal subjects was 367 ± 144 μg/d.[10] The serum PRL response to thyrotropin-releasing hormone (TRH), however, is distinctly subnormal in thyrotoxic patients, as compared with normal subjects, and returns to normal when the patients are treated (Fig 44-2).[11] The serum PRL response to arginine is also decreased in both women and men with thyrotoxicosis.[12] So far, no physiologic or clinical consequences of these abnormalities are known.

References

1. Schlesinger S, MacGillivray MH, Munschauer RW. Acceleration of growth and bone maturation in childhood thyrotoxicosis. Pediatrics 1973;83:233

2. Taylor AL, Finster JL, Mintz DH. Metabolic clearance and production rates of human growth hormone. J Clin Invest 1969;48:2349

3. Amit T, Hertz P, Ish-Shalom S, et al. Effects of hypo- or hyperthyroidism on growth hormone-binding protein. Clin Endocrinol 1991;35:159

4. Sasaki N, Tsuyusaki T, Nakamura H, et al. Sleep-related growth hormone release in thyrotoxic patients before and during propylthiouracil therapy. Endocrinol Jpn 1985;32:39

5. Burgess JA, Smith BR, Merimee TJ. Growth hormone in thyrotoxicosis: effect of insulin-induced hypoglycemia. J Clin Endocrinol 1966;26:1257

6. Giustina G, Reschini E, Valentini F, Cantalamessa L. Growth hormone and cortisol responses to insulin-induced hypoglycemia in thyrotoxicosis. J Clin Endocrinol 1971;32:571

7. Katz HP, Youlton R, Kaplan SL, Grumbach MM. Growth and growth hormone. III. Growth hormone release in children with primary hypothyroidism and thyrotoxicosis. J Clin Endocrinol 1969;29:346

8. Iranmanesh A, Lizarralde G, Johnson ML, Veldhuis JD. Nature of altered growth hormone secretion in hyperthyroidism. J Clin Endocrinol Metab 1991;72:108

9. Miell JP, Taylor AM, Zini M, et al. Effects of hypothyroidism and hyperthyroidism on insulin-like growth factors (IGFs) and growth hormone- and IGF-proteins. J Clin Endocrinol Metab 1993;76:950

10. Cooper DS, Ridgway EC, Kliman B, et al. Metabolic clearance and production rates of prolactin in man. J Clin Invest 1979;64:1669

11. Snyder PJ, Jacobs LS, Utiger RD, Daughaday WH. Thyroid hormone inhibition of the prolactin response to thyrotropin-releasing hormone. J Clin Invest 1973;52:2324

12. Ciccarelli D, Zini M, Grottoli S, et al. Impaired prolactin response to arginine in patients with hyperthyroidism. Clin Endocrinol 1994;41:371

Werner and Ingbar's The Thyroid, Seventh Edition,
edited by Lewis E. Braverman and Robert D. Utiger.
Lippincott–Raven Publishers, Philadelphia, © 1996

45

The Adrenal Cortex
in Thyrotoxicosis

Robert G. Dluhy

Thyrotoxicosis has several effects on adrenocortical function and the metabolism of adrenocortical hormones, serving especially to accelerate the latter. Because hypothalamic-pituitary feedback regulation is not altered, patients with thyrotoxicosis have increased cortisol secretion and therefore their serum cortisol concentrations are normal (Fig 45-1). However, if hypothalamic, pituitary, or adrenal function was impaired, the patient's serum cortisol concentrations would be low. Other possible effects of thyrotoxicosis on adrenocortical function include direct effects on adrenal steroidogenesis and alteration in serum corticosteroid-binding proteins.

Conversely, glucocorticoids could affect a variety of thyroid functions, such as thyrotropin (TSH) secretion, the production or clearance of thyroxine (T_4), peripheral conversion of T_4 to triiodothyronine (T_3), renal clearance of iodide, and the production or clearance of serum thyroid hormone-binding proteins.

Finally, thyroid and adrenal function may be altered by concurrent disease processes, such as autoimmunity, beyond the above-noted hormonal interactions. Additional potential interactions include those resulting from the alterations in both adrenal and thyroid function that occur during stress and acute and chronic illness.

THYROID-GLUCOCORTICOID INTERACTIONS IN PERIPHERAL TISSUES

In vitro, glucocorticoids act synergistically with T_3 to increase growth hormone production by pituitary tumor cells. The affinity of nuclear receptors for T_3 is reduced by 50% in the absence of cortisol.[1] Other interactions between thyroid hormones and glucocorticoids, for example, effects on the mRNAs for the receptors for the two hormones, in regulating

growth hormone gene expression have also been reported.[2–4] Thyroid hormone and glucocorticoid receptors are encoded by genes that are members of a single family, and the two types of receptors have some structural similarity. In one study of GH_3 cells (a pituitary tumor cell line), T_3 increased glucocorticoid action by increasing glucocorticoid receptor mRNA concentrations.[4] A reciprocal action of glucocorticoids on T_3 receptor mRNA was not found, even though T_3 action in GH_3 cells is augmented by glucocorticoids. In contrast to these interactions of glucocorticoids and thyroid hormone on growth hormone secretion, there are no data on such interactions in pituitary thyrotrophs or corticotrophs or in other tissues.

In addition, some negative findings have emerged. For example, patients with either primary cortisol resistance or the cortisol hyperreactive syndrome have normal serum TSH and thyroid hormone concentrations, and the responsiveness of their tissues to T_4 and T_3 is normal.[5,6]

THYROID-ADRENOCORTICAL INTERACTIONS IN THE CENTRAL NERVOUS SYSTEM AND ANTERIOR PITUITARY

Neither adrenocorticotropin (ACTH) nor cortisol is a major regulator of pituitary TSH secretion,[7] and the release of ACTH and TSH is governed by separate hypothalamic signals.[8,9] Thus, under physiologic conditions in humans, there is no functionally important feedback of cortisol on circadian rhythms of TSH, even though serum cortisol concentrations are lowest when serum TSH concentrations are highest at the same time in the late evening. On the other hand, chronic high-dose glucocorticoid administration inhibits thyrotropin-releasing hormone (TRH)-induced TSH secretion, a phenomenon that also occurs

NORMAL

$$SC = \frac{SR}{MCR}$$

THYROTOXICOSIS

$$SC = \frac{\uparrow SR}{*\uparrow MCR}$$

* initiating event

FIGURE 45-1. The relationship between the serum concentrations and the secretion and clearance rates of cortisol in normal subjects and in patients with thyrotoxicosis. In normal subjects the serum concentration (SC) of cortisol reflects its secretion at the time of measurement. The SC is dependent on two factors: the cortisol secretion rate (SR) and the rate at which cortisol is metabolized, ie, metabolic clearance rate (MCR). In patients with thyrotoxicosis, the hepatic clearance of cortisol is accelerated due to augmentation of Δ^4-reductase activity (see Fig. 45-2). If normal feedback relationships are preserved, the endogenous secretion rate should increase and normal serum cortisol concentrations should be maintained.

in patients with Cushing's syndrome. In addition, administration of glucocorticoids to normal subjects almost immediately reduces mean 24-hour serum TSH concentrations and the nocturnal surge in TSH secretion, and patients with Cushing's syndrome have similar changes in TSH secretion.[10] These changes are caused by a decrease in TSH pulse amplitude. TSH secretion returns to normal after the glucocorticoid is discontinued or Cushing's syndrome is treated. However, TSH secretion partially escapes from suppression during long-term glucocorticoid exposure, so that hypothyroidism does not occur.[11] The actions of glucocorticoids that affect TSH secretion occur at both the hypothalamic and pituitary levels.[11,12]

THYROTOXICOSIS AND ADRENOCORTICAL FUNCTION

In animals, thyrotoxicosis causes adrenocortical enlargement. However, it does not occur in hypophysectomized animals given thyroid hormone, indicating that the effect of thyroid hormone is indirect. In early studies of patients with thyrotoxicosis, urinary 17-ketosteroid excretion was usually low and 17-hydroxycorticosteroid excretion was slightly increased. Conversely, both were low in hypothyroid patients. Subsequent studies revealed that the metabolism of cortisol and other steroids is accelerated in thyrotoxicosis and delayed in hypothyroidism.[13] These metabolic abnormalities are discussed in the next section with respect to the C_{21}-corticosteroids cortisol and aldosterone.

Effects of Thyrotoxicosis on Cortisol Secretion and Metabolism

Infused cortisol is cleared from the circulation at an accelerated rate in thyrotoxicosis but not in other hypermetabolic states (Fig 45-2).[13] Kinetic studies have shown that in thyrotoxicosis the miscible pool of endogenous cortisol is normal, whereas the fractional turnover rate of the pool per unit time (metabolic clearance rate) and the secretion rate are increased, the latter occurring as a result of an increase in the number of cortisol secretory episodes.[14] The raised cortisol secretion rate

accounts for the increase in urinary 17-hydroxycorticoid excretion. These abnormalities are corrected after restoration of a euthyroid state by appropriate treatment.[13] In hypothyroidism, the opposite changes occur, again with a normal cortisol pool size (see Fig 45-2); the reduced cortisol secretion rate is concordant with low urinary 17-hydroxycorticoid excretion, and treatment with thyroid hormone restores cortisol metabolism to normal.[13]

In thyrotoxicosis, the normal pool of cortisol may be regarded as concordant with the normal serum cortisol concentrations. Serum corticosteroid-binding globulin concentrations are also normal, indicating that serum free cortisol concentrations should be normal. The latter is confirmed by the finding of normal urinary cortisol excretion in thyrotoxicosis. Therefore, it is not associated with abnormal adrenocortical function from the point of view of the peripheral tissues.[13]

Thyrotoxicosis accelerates the disposal rate of endogenous or exogenous cortisol by accelerating reduction of ring A of the corticosteroid molecule, chiefly by stimulating corticosteroid Δ^4-reductase activity in hepatic microsomes; this is the rate-limiting step in hepatic degradation of glucocorticoids (Fig 45-3). The clearance of one of these metabolites, tetrahydrocortisone, in thyrotoxic patients is normal. This finding indicates that the next step in the disposal of tetrahydro-

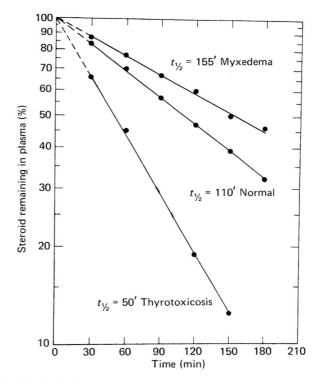

FIGURE 45-2. Disappearance of cortisol from plasma after its intravenous administration to a single normal subject, a patient with hypothyroidism (myxedema), and one with thyrotoxicosis. The slowing and acceleration, respectively, of the plasma half-life ($t^{1/2}$) are obvious. In this study, the results were similar after infusion of tracer doses of isotopic 4-14C-cortisol. (Peterson RE. The influence of the thyroid on adrenal cortical function. J Clin Invest 1958;37:736)

cortisone (and other ring A-reduced cortisol metabolites), which is conjugation with glucuronic acid, is normal.[13]

Thyrotoxicosis not only influences the rate of cortisol degradation but also affects its metabolism qualitatively (see Fig 45-3). It increases the fraction of cortisol metabolized to 11-keto as opposed to 11β-OH compounds; the quantities of tetrahydrocortisone and cortolones rise, whereas those of tetrahydrocortisol and cortols fall.[13] Thyrotoxicosis, by increasing hepatic 11β-hydroxysteroid dehydrogenase activity, leads to increased cortisol inactivation by enhancing conversion to the 11-keto product cortisone, which is biologically inactive.[13] As a result, the ratio of tetrahydrocortisone to tetrahydrocortisol is increased. Because these urinary cortisol metabolites provide an assessment of peripheral thyroid hormone action, a low ratio in the setting of high serum T_4 concentrations has been used as a marker of peripheral thyroid hormone resistance (see chap 90).[15] Cortisone, like cortisol, is also disposed of at an accelerated rate in thyrotoxicosis, as are corticosterone, deoxycorticosterone, aldosterone (see the next section), and most other steroids.

Effects of Thyrotoxicosis on the Pituitary-Adrenal Axis

Not only are basal serum cortisol concentrations normal in patients with thyrotoxicosis, but the responses to exogenous ACTH and insulin-induced hypoglycemia also are normal. The hormonal counterregulatory responses to insulin-induced hypoglycemia are variable, revealing heightened glucagon, blunted growth hormone and slightly heightened ACTH responses, all in the setting of a more rapid rise in serum glucose concentrations during the recovery phase, as compared with normal subjects.[16]

In thyrotoxicosis basal plasma epinephrine and norepinephrine concentrations are normal or slightly reduced, respectively (see chap 46).[17] However, the plasma epinephrine response to insulin-induced hypoglycemia is normal, whereas that of norepinephrine is reduced, consistent with a selective action of thyroid hormones on the sympathoadrenal system.[17]

Effects of Thyrotoxicosis on the Renin-Angiotensin-Aldosterone System

In patients with thyrotoxicosis, the metabolic clearance rate of aldosterone is slightly increased, resulting in a compensatory increase in aldosterone secretion; serum concentrations of aldosterone are usually normal (Table 45-1).[13,18,19] In hypothyroidism, the metabolic clearance rate and rate of secretion of aldosterone are slightly decreased, but the miscible pool and serum concentrations of aldosterone are also within normal limits. None of the changes in metabolism is of clinical importance, nor do the changes underlie the cardiovascular manifestations of thyrotoxicosis, which are dominated by heightened adrenergic activity (see chap 38).

In addition to increasing the hepatic degradation of aldosterone, thyrotoxicosis is associated with other alterations in the function of the renin-angiotensin-aldosterone system (see Table 45-1). Plasma renin activity basally and in response to upright posture is increased, probably caused by enhanced activity of the β-adrenergic nervous system.[19,20] Serum an-

TABLE 45-1.
Effects of Thyrotoxicosis on the Renin–Angiotensin–Aldosterone System

Hepatic clearance of aldosterone increased

Serum aldosterone concentrations normal*

Plasma renin activity increased

Serum angiotensin-converting enzyme concentrations increased

Serum angiotensinogen concentrations increased

Serum aldosterone concentrations were high in some studies and low in others, probably reflecting variable states of sodium and potassium balance as well as the severity of thyrotoxicosis at the time of study.

giotensin-converting enzyme concentrations are increased by thyroid hormone as well as by glucocorticoids. Finally, serum angiotensinogen concentrations are increased,[22] probably as a result of increased transcription of the angiotensinogen gene or increased stability of its mRNA.[23] As a result of the increase in serum angiotensinogen, the generation of angiotensin peptides is increased because the serum concentration of angiotensinogen is near the K_m of the proteolytic activity of renin. The actions of thyroid hormone on the production of angiotensinogen may in part explain the increased plasma renin activity in thyrotoxicosis.

Thus, the regulation of aldosterone secretion in patients with thyrotoxicosis reflects thyroid hormone-induced alterations in hepatic steroid metabolism as well as independent actions on the renin-angiotensin system. In addition, patients with thyrotoxicosis may have depleted total body potassium stores due to the kaliuretic effects of thyroid hormone; potassium depletion independently results in increased plasma renin activity and decreased production of aldosterone.[24,25] These variables, as well as overall sodium balance and the severity of thyrotoxicosis, mean that the results of studies of the renin-angiotensin-aldosterone system are variable in thyrotoxic patients. In general, plasma renin activity is increased[19,20] while basal serum aldosterone concentrations are normal, but may be high or low.[19,26,27] The serum aldosterone response to exogenous ACTH is normal,[19,26] but the response to exogenous angiotensin II is blunted.[26] The altered relationship between the renin-angiotensin system and aldosterone secretion may reflect potassium depletion, because in one study oral potassium loading corrected the abnormalities.[19] However, despite these alterations the overall function of the renin-angiotensin-aldosterone system is preserved in thyrotoxicosis, so that blood pressure regulation and sodium homeostasis are nearly always normal.

ANDROGENS AND ESTROGENS

Men with thyrotoxicosis have elevated serum estradiol concentrations, as a result of increased extraglandular conversion of androstenedione to estradiol, and some have gynecomastia (see chap 47). In addition, serum sex hormone-binding globulin concentrations are increased, leading to increases in serum total testosterone and estradiol and concomitant decreases in

11b-DEHYDROGENASE (11b-HSD)

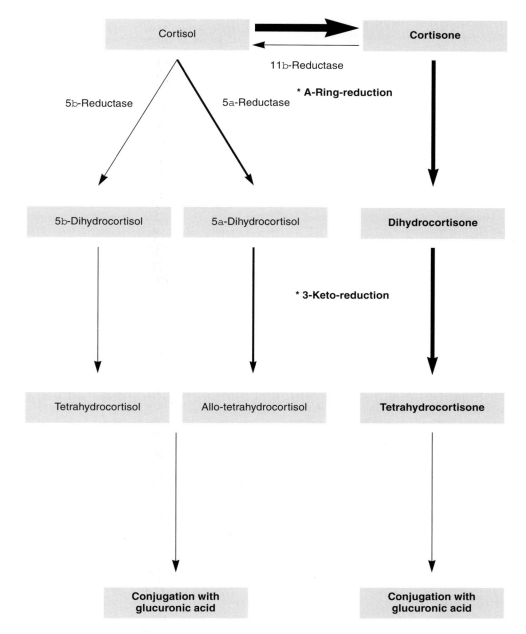

FIGURE 45-3. Alterations in cortisol metabolism in thyrotoxicosis. Cortisol is inactivated primarily by hepatic reduction of the α, β unsaturated ketone region in ring A, yielding as initial products the inactive dihydro, 3-oxo and subsequently the tetrahydro, 3-hydroxymetabolites. The enzymes that catalyze these reactions are the hepatic Δ^4-steroid reductases($*$); the Δ^4 reduction reactum is irreversible. Thyroid hormones stimulates the activity of the reductases, as well as 11β-hydroxysteroid dehydrogenase (11β-HSD), the enzyme that converts cortisol to the biologically inactive cortisone. Thyroid hormone does not change the hepatic conjugation of the metabolites of cortisol. As a result, in thyrotoxicosis there is an overall increase in the metabolic clearance of cortisol and is a qualitative alteration in the pattern of metabolites produced, with a small increase in the fraction of cortisol metabolized to tetrahydrocortisone, a small increase in the allo-tetrahydrocortisol fraction, and a decrease in the fraction of tetrahydrocortisol.

the clearance rate of both steroids.[28] In a human hepatoma cell line the mRNA for sex hormone-binding globulin is increased by T_3, suggesting that it increases expression of the gene for the binding protein.[29]

Thyroid hormones also preferentially stimulate hepatic 5α-steroid reductase activity (Fig 45-3). The result is a shift in the pattern of adrenal androgen metabolism, so that the formation and urinary excretion of androsterone are increased and those of etiocholanolone are decreased.[13]

References

1. DeNayer P, Dozin B, Vandeput Y, et al. Altered interaction between triiodothyronine and its nuclear receptors in absence of cortisol: a proposed mechanism for increased thyrotropin secretion in corticosteroid deficiency states. Eur J Clin Invest 1987; 17:106

2. Brent GA, Harney JW, Moore DD, Larsen PR. Multihormonal regulation of the human, rat, and bovine growth hormone promoters: differential effects of 3',5'-cyclic adenosine monophosphate, thyroid hormone, and glucocorticoids. Mol Endocrinol 1988;2:792

3. Brent GA. The molecular basis of thyroid hormone action. N Engl J Med 1994;331:847

4. Williams GR, Franklyn JA, Sheppard MC. Thyroid hormone and glucocorticoid regulation of receptor and target gene mRNAs in pituitary GH3 cells. Mol Cell Endocrinol 1991;80:127

5. Malchoff CD, Javier EC, Malchoff DM, et al. Primary cortisol resistance presenting as isosexual precocity. J Clin Endocrinol Metab 1990;70:503

6. Iida S, Nakamura Y, Fujii H, et al. A patient with hypocortisolism and Cushing's syndrome-like manifestations: cortisol hyperreactive syndrome. J Clin Endocrinol Metab 1990;70:729

7. Brabant A, Brabant G, Schuermeyer T, et al. The role of glucocorticoids in the regulation of thyrotropin. Acta Endocrinol 1989;121:95

8. Alford FP, Baker HWG, Burger HG, et al. Temporal patterns of integrated plasma hormone levels during sleep and wakefulness. I. Thyroid-stimulating hormone, growth hormone and cortisol. J Clin Endocrinol Metab 1973;37:841

9. Van Cauter E, Leclercq R, Vanhaelst L, Golstein J. Simultaneous study of cortisol and TSH daily variations in normal subjects and patients with hyperadrenalcorticism. J Clin Endocrinol Metab 1974;39:645

10. Adriaanse R, Brabant G, Endert E, Wiersinga WM. Pulsatile thyrotropin secretion in patients with Cushing's syndrome. Metabolism 1994;43:782

11. Nicoloff JT, Fisher DA, Appleman MD. The role of glucocorticoids in the regulation of thyroid function in man. J Clin Invest 1970;49:1922

12. Wilber JF, Utiger RD. The effect of glucocorticoids on thyrotropin secretion. J Clin Invest 1969;48:2096

13. Peterson RE. Metabolism of adrenal cortical steroids. In: Christy NP, ed. The human adrenal cortex. New York: Harper and Row, 1971:137

14. Gallagher TF, Hellman L, Finkelstein J, et al. Hyperthyroidism and cortisol secretion in man. J Clin Endocrinol Metab 1972; 34:919

15. Taniyama M, Honma K, Ban Y. Urinary cortisol metabolites in the assessment of peripheral thyroid hormone action: application of diagnosis of resistance to thyroid hormone. Thyroid 1993;3:229

16. Moghetti P, Castello R, Tosi F, et al. Glucose counterregulatory response to acute hypoglycemia in hyperthyroid human subjects. J Clin Endocrinol Metab 1994;78:169

17. Coulombe P, Dussault JH, Walker P. Catecholamine metabolism in thyroid diseases. II. Norepinephrine secretion rate in hyperthyroidism and hypothyroidism. J Clin Endocrinol Metab 1977;44:1185

18. Luetscher JA Jr, Camargo CA, Cohen AP, et al. Observations on metabolism of aldosterone in man. Ann Intern Med 1963;59:1

19. Cain JP, Dluhy RG, Williams GH, et al. Control of aldosterone secretion in hyperthyroidism. J Clin Endocrinol Metab 1973; 36:365

20. Resnick LM, Laragh JH. Plasma renin activity in syndromes of thyroid hormone excess and deficiency. Life Sci 1982;30:585

21. Brent GA, Hershman JM, Reed AW, et al. Serum angiotensin-converting enzyme in severe nonthyroidal illnesses associated with low serum thyroxine concentration. Ann Intern Med 1984; 100:680

22. Dzau VJ, Hermann HC. Hormonal regulation of angiotensinogen synthesis. Life Sci 1982;30:577

23. Deschepper CF, Hong-Brown LQ. Hormonal regulation of the angiotensinogen gene in liver and other tissues. In: Raizada MK, Phillips MI, Sumners C. eds. Cellular and molecular biology of renin-angiotensin system. Boca Raton, FL: CRC Press, 1993;152

24. Dluhy RG, Underwood RH, Williams GH. Influence of dietary potassium on plasma renin activity in normal man. J Appl Physiol 1970;28:299

25. Dluhy RG, Axelrod L, Underwood RH, Williams GH. Studies of the control of plasma aldosterone concentration in normal man. II. Effect of dietary potassium and acute potassium infusion. J Clin Invest 1972;51:1950

26. Kigoshi T, Kaneko M, Nakano S, et al. Aldosterone response to various stimuli in hyperthyroidism: in vivo and in vitro studies. Folia Endocrinol Jpn 1993;69:609

27. Shigematsu S, Iwasaki T, Aizawa T, et al. Plasma atrial natriuretic peptide, plasma renin activity and aldosterone during treatment of hyperthyroidism due to Graves' disease. Horm Metab Res 1989;21:514

28. Ridgway EC, Longcope C, Maloof F. Metabolic clearance and blood production rates of estradiol in hyperthyroidism. J Clin Endocrinol Metab 1975;41:491

29. Barlow JW, Crowe TC, Cowen NL, et al. Stimulation of sex hormone-binding globulin mRNA and attenuation of corticosteroid-binding globulin mRNA by triiodothyronine in human hepatoma cells. Eur J Endocrinol 1994;130:166

Werner and Ingbar's The Thyroid, Seventh Edition,
edited by Lewis E. Braverman and Robert D. Utiger.
Lippincott–Raven Publishers, Philadelphia, © 1996

46

Catecholamines and the Sympathoadrenal System in Thyrotoxicosis

J. Enrique Silva

The sympathetic nervous system and the adrenal medulla are often referred to as the sympathoadrenal system. Norepinephrine, the main sympathetic nervous system neurotransmitter, is synthesized and stored in peripheral sympathetic nerve endings and released in response to coordinated nerve impulses targeted to specific tissues or organs. Epinephrine, in contrast, is a hormone secreted by the adrenal medulla in response to impulses carried in the splanchnic nerves. As a hormone, epinephrine influences processes throughout the body. The activity of the sympathoadrenal system is centrally controlled at the level of the hypothalamus and brain stem. Both limbs of the system may be activated together, as in severe cold exposure and strenuous exertion, or independently, as for example in hypoglycemia, in which the adrenal medulla is stimulated and the activity of the sympathetic nervous system suppressed.

Catecholamines initiate their effects by interacting with specific cell surface receptors. Early pharmacologic and physiologic studies distinguished several types and subtypes of adrenergic receptors.[1] This functional variability reflects the existence of different genes for the receptors and variations in posttranscriptional processing.[2] The α-adrenergic receptors mediate effects such as vasoconstriction, inhibition of insulin secretion,[3] or the stimulation of brown adipose tissue type II thyroxine (T_4) 5'-deiodinase.[4] The β-adrenergic receptors mediate other processes, including cardiac stimulation, lipolysis, bronchodilation, vasodilation, and the production of metabolic heat. The α_2- and β-adrenergic receptors are coupled to adenylyl cyclase via guanosine phosphate-binding proteins (G-proteins). While β-adrenergic receptors stimulate the production of cyclic adenosine monophosphate (cAMP) by interacting with stimulatory G-proteins (Gs), α_2-receptors interact with inhibitory G-proteins (Gi) to inhibit adenylyl cyclase. cAMP activates protein kinases, generically called protein kinase A, that phosphorylate a wide variety of proteins ultimately leading to end effects. The α_1-adrenergic receptor second messengers are inositol triphosphate (IP_3) and diacylglycerol, both released from the hydrolysis of phosphatidylinositol. Diacylglycerol directly stimulates protein kinase C, which in turn phosphorylates several proteins mediating a variety of end effects, and IP_3 elevates cytosolic Ca^{++}, which influences cellular processes either directly or indirectly through the activation of Ca^{++}-calmodulin-dependent protein kinases.

EFFECTS OF THYROID HORMONES ON THE FUNCTIONAL STATE OF THE SYMPATHOADRENAL SYSTEM

The sympathoadrenal system and thyroid hormones normally interact in a coordinated manner. The sympathoadrenal system has a clear adaptive role providing the means for rapid adjustments to the environment, and thyroid hormones appear to introduce a positive gain in the capacity of many tissues to respond to the majority of the actions of catecholamines. This synergistic interaction plays an obvious adaptive role, for example, in the response to cold exposure, when both systems interact to increase heat production. In general, the need for a synergistic interaction is apparent in states when the delivery of substrate or release of energy by organs and systems is required. In the opposite situation, for example in starvation, both systems are turned down independently, at separate levels: sympathetic outflow decreases[5] and thyroidal secretion and conversion of T_4 to triiodothyronine (T_3) are reduced.

The pathophysiology of the sympathoadrenal system in thyrotoxicosis and hypothyroidism can be viewed as the result of the disruption of the interactions between the two systems in circumstances when one of them, the thyroid, is fixed at an abnormally high or low level. For example, in thyrotoxicosis, when obligatory thermogenesis is increased, there is less need for the calorigenic action of catecholamines. Moreover, because the responsiveness to catecholamines is increased by thyroid hormones, it would appear advantageous to reduce sympathetic outflow to thermogenic organs. Not surprisingly, norepinephrine turnover rate, a measure of sympathetic activity in the organs of experimental animals, is diminished in thyroid hormone-treated animals and is markedly increased by thyroid hormone deficiency.[6-9] In patients with thyrotoxicosis, plasma concentrations and urinary excretion of norepinephrine are normal or diminished,[10,11] whereas, in hypothyroidism, urinary norepinephrine excretion is increased and plasma norepinephrine concentrations are elevated,[11-13] reflecting proportional increases in production rate[14,15] (see chap 70). On the other hand, adrenal medullary activity is not altered by thyroid hormone excess or deficiency, as assessed by plasma concentrations and urinary excretion of epinephrine and kinetic studies in thyrotoxic and hypothyroid patients.[16] Therefore, the sympathomimetic features of thyrotoxicosis cannot be explained by enhanced sympathetic activity. Rather, the sympathomimetic symptoms and signs in thyrotoxicosis reflect the similarity of actions of thyroid hormones and catecholamines as well as synergistic interactions between them. An additional important source of variability of the sympathomimetic manifestations is the efficiency with which sympathetic outflow from the central nervous system is inhibited.

EFFECTS OF THYROID HORMONES ON PHYSIOLOGIC RESPONSES TO CATECHOLAMINES

In an attempt to explain the sympathomimetic features of thyrotoxicosis, as well as the widely recognized amelioration of some manifestations of thyrotoxicosis by β-adrenergic blockade, much attention has been devoted to the effects of thyroid hormone on numerous responses to catecholamines. Thyroid hormone enhances the β-adrenergic effects of catecholamines at the cellular level by a number of mechanisms. These mechanisms differ substantially, both qualitatively and quantitatively, in a tissue- and species-specific manner. They can be grouped into those in which T_3 increases the accumulation of cAMP in response to adrenergic stimulation and those in which T_3 potentiates or enhances the effects of cAMP. In addition, thyroid hormones play a role in the development of the sympathoadrenal system.[17,18] Regarding the other adrenergic signaling pathways, the effect of thyroid hormone is neither as

clear nor as physiologically important as on the β-adrenergic pathways.

Mechanisms Whereby Thyroid Hormone Enhances cAMP Responses to Adrenergic Receptor Stimulation

Thyroid hormone-induced increases in the number of β-adrenergic receptors as well as decreases in the number of α-adrenergic receptors have been documented in a number of tissues and cell systems from several species (see reference 19 for review). For example, in rats, thyroid hormones augment the density of β-adrenergic receptors in the heart,[19-24] in brown fat,[25] and in white fat.[19] In humans, T_3 administration increases the density of β-receptors on circulating monocytes[26] and thyrotoxicosis is associated with a doubling of the density of β-adrenergic receptors in white adipocytes.[27] In general, the gain in receptor number associated with thyroid hormone excess is modest, rarely more than twofold, and additional mechanisms have to be invoked to explain the much larger increase in cAMP and some responses to catecholamines in the transition from hypothyroidism to thyrotoxicosis.[27-29]

Thyroid hormones, indeed, have an important effect on cAMP production. Plasma concentrations of cAMP are reduced in hypothyroid patients and are increased in thyrotoxic patients.[30,31] In the latter, the increase was diminished by the β-receptor antagonist, propranolol, and the infusion of epinephrine markedly increased urinary cAMP excretion.[32] Thyroid hormones increase adenylyl cyclase activity in rat epididymal fat pads[33,34] and brown adipocytes,[28] and potentiate cAMP accumulation in response to catecholamines in isolated adipocytes from thyrotoxic patients or T_3-treated rats.[27,35,36] Probably the most important postreceptor mechanism whereby thyroid hormones enhance cAMP responses is by decreasing the cellular concentration of certain G-protein subunits; in several different systems, T_3 downregulates some species of $G_\alpha i$ and G_β subunits.[37-40] The former leads to less Gi-mediated inhibition of adenylyl cyclase, whereas the latter makes more $G_\alpha s$ subunits available to mediate stimulation of the cyclase. Thyroid hormone may also limit cAMP degradation in adipose tissue by downregulating some phosphodiesterases.[41] By other mechanisms less well characterized, such as an increase in cytosolic Ca^{++}, thyroid hormones can amplify cAMP accumulation in response to catecholamines.[42-44] Moreover, all these postreceptor mechanisms may enhance the cAMP responses to other hormones such as glucagon that act through adenylyl cyclase-coupled receptors.

Enhancement of cAMP Effects by Thyroid Hormone

In addition to increasing the availability of cAMP, thyroid hormone may enhance the effects of cAMP. Examples of this action of thyroid hormone are increases in the gluconeogenic enzyme phosphoenolpyruvate carboxykinase (PEPCK) and the uncoupling protein (UCP) in brown adipose tissue. Given the growing list of genes regulated by cAMP,[5] some of them also regulated by thyroid hormone, this novel mechanism may well turn out to be common.

In gluconeogenesis, PEPCK is a rate-limiting enzyme. PEPCK gene transcription is stimulated by cAMP produced in response to glucagon or epinephrine via cAMP response elements (CREs) in the PEPCK gene sequence.[46] Thyroid hormone stimulates gluconeogenesis and the activity of PEPCK,[47] interacting in a synergistic manner with cAMP.[48] Recent work has identified a thyroid hormone response element (TRE) in the PEPCK gene in close association with one of the CREs, and both CRE and TRE are necessary for T_3 stimulation and for the synergism between cAMP and T_3.[48]

The UCP is the key molecule in brown adipose tissue thermogenesis. Norepinephrine (via cAMP) and T_3 synergistically stimulate the expression of the UCP gene by a mechanism not requiring ongoing protein synthesis.[49] The stimulation of UCP gene transcription by norepinephrine or T_3 separately is two- to threefold, whereas together the stimulation is about 20-fold. As with PEPCK, a CRE has been identified within a critical enhancer sequence in the gene.[50] Two TREs, directly downstream of the CRE, within the same enhancer, have recently been identified and characterized.[51] Of the two, the downstream TRE and an adjacent downstream sequence seem essential for the synergism between cAMP and T_3.[51]

EFFECTS OF CATECHOLAMINES ON EXTRATHYROIDAL T_4 CONVERSION TO T_3

Catecholamines may stimulate T_4 5'-deiodination to T_3, and because T_3 is intrinsically at least 10 times more potent than T_4, this is a mechanism whereby catecholamines might enhance the potency of the thyroidal secretion. There are two types of 5'-deiodinating activity in various tissues[52,53] (see chap 8). Type I activity, a selenocysteine-containing protein,[54] is largely present in liver, kidney, and thyroid and is believed to be the main source of extrathyroidally generated plasma T_3; type II activity, clearly demonstrated in pituitary, central nervous system, placenta, and brown adipose tissue, but probably present in other tissues as well, is believed to provide, predominantly, a local source of T_3 that is subject to tissue-specific regulation.[55–58]

Catecholamines and Type I T_4-5'-Deiodinase

In humans, exogenous epinephrine has little effect on T_4 metabolism.[59] However, the possibility of an important effect of catecholamines on extrathyroidal conversion of T_4 to T_3 was suggested by studies demonstrating that β-adrenergic blockade, both in thyrotoxic and in hypothyroid patients maintained on a fixed dose of T_4, decreased the plasma concentration of T_3 (see reference 60 for review). Other nonselective β-blockers, such as alprenolol, and the $β_1$-selective antagonists metoprolol and atenolol have similar effects, leading to the hypothesis that these substances inhibited a $β_1$-adrenergic receptor-mediated effect of catecholamines.[60] Tracer kinetic studies[60,61] showing reduced fractional T_4 to T_3 conversion, along with increases in plasma 3,3,5'-triiodothyronine (reverse T_3, rT_3) concentrations after β-blocker administration,[62] pointed to type I T_4-5'-deiodinase as the site of action of propranolol. This effect of β-adrenergic antagonists

is the result of a direct inhibitory effect of these agents on the type I T_4-5'-deiodinase. These drugs block T_4 conversion to T_3 in crude homogenates of liver; furthermore, in these studies D- and L-propranolol are equally potent, and the potency of various compounds relates to their lipid solubility and not to their β-blocking potency.[63] In addition, catecholamines do not stimulate T_4 to T_3 conversion in isolated rat renal tubules, yet both D- and L-propranolol inhibit conversion by 35%, as does quinidine, while β-blockers like atenolol and sotalol that do not share the membrane-stabilizing properties of propranolol and quinidine have no effect.[64]

Catecholamines and Type II T_4-5'-Deiodinase

Type II T_4-5'-deiodinase is vigorously stimulated by catecholamines in brown adipose tissue of rats[4,55,56,65] and other species.[66,67] $α_1$-Adrenergic receptor agonists stimulate type II T_4-5'-deiodinase in vivo and the stimulation by norepinephrine, a nonselective agonist, can be obliterated by prazosin, a specific $α_1$-receptor antagonist.[4,65] However, in isolated brown adipocytes cAMP is needed for full stimulation,[68] suggesting that the stimulation of type II T_4-5'-deiodinase requires strong $α_1$-receptor stimulation in the presence of comparatively low concentrations of cAMP, which are provided in vivo by the sympathetic tone. The brain is another tissue in which type II T_4-5'-deiodinase is the major source of T_3.[58] The injection of epinephrine significantly increased the amount of tracer T_3 in the brain of mice after the injection of radiolabeled T_4, without detectable radiolabeled T_3 in the plasma,[69] suggesting that catecholamines could, directly or indirectly, stimulate the T_4-5'-deiodinase in some areas of the brain.

In rats, acute or sustained adrenergic stimulation of brown adipose tissue results in a striking increase in T_3 generation in this tissue,[65] such that the brown fat T_3 receptors become nearly saturated[70] and there is a substantial contribution to the plasma pool of T_3.[65] The increase in local T_3 production and the high level of nuclear T_3 occupancy have proven to be essential for a full response of UCP, α-glycerophosphate dehydrogenase, and other enzymes to adrenergic stimulation.[7,71] Without adrenergic activation of the deiodinase, this level of T_3 receptor occupancy would only be possible with more than 10-fold elevation of the plasma T_3 concentrations.[71,72] On the other hand, brown adipose tissue type II T_4-5'-deiodinase activity,[55,56] like that of brain and pituitary,[73] is increased in hypothyroidism and is rapidly and powerfully inhibited by T_4. Thus, type II T_4-5'-deiodinase plays a key role in coordinating the synergism between norepinephrine and T_3 in brown fat. In the euthyroid state, when stimulated by the sympathetic nervous system, the enzyme provides the large amount of T_3 required for a full thermogenic response to norepinephrine without causing systemic thyrotoxicosis, whereas in the thyrotoxic state, brown adipose tissue sympathetic stimulation is reduced and T_4 inhibits the deiodinase, limiting the thermogenic response.[74,75] The importance of these studies for humans, in whom brown adipose tissue becomes progressively less active with age, is not yet clear, but they indicate that the intracellular availability of T_3 and hence cell responses to catecholamines may depend on local mechanisms in tissues containing type II T_4-5'-deiodinase.

The contribution of the brown fat deiodinase to plasma T_3 in rats in hyperadrenergic states[65] raises the possibility that type II T_4-5'-deiodinase could contribute to the plasma T_3 pool in humans as well. It is conceivable that a significant fraction of plasma T_3 in humans derives from the activity of this enzyme,[76] and other tissues containing the type II enzyme (e.g., skin) could contribute to the plasma pool of T_3. However, because this enzyme is powerfully inhibited by T_4, this pathway of T_3 generation is not likely to operate in thyrotoxicosis.[55,56]

PHYSIOLOGIC AND CLINICAL CONSEQUENCES OF CATECHOLAMINE–THYROID HORMONE INTERACTIONS IN THYROTOXICOSIS

Cardiovascular Responses

The fact that the β-adrenergic receptor blockade ameliorates some of the cardiovascular manifestations of thyrotoxicosis suggests that catecholamines play a role in their genesis. Because the plasma concentrations of catecholamines are not elevated and there is a reduction in the sympathetic input to the heart,[9] the sympathetic component of the cardiovascular manifestations of thyrotoxicosis largely reflects enhanced cardiac sensitivity, responsiveness, or both, to catecholamines by virtue of the mechanisms discussed previously. In humans, most studies (with a few exceptions[77,78]) demonstrate exaggerated heart rate responses to catecholamines in thyrotoxicosis.[79] On the other hand, T_3 directly affects the myocardium leading to tachycardia and increased contractility[80] (see chaps 38 and 62), and it has not been possible to define the extent to which enhanced catecholamine responsiveness and sensitivity participate in the hemodynamic changes in thyrotoxicosis. Studies of the hemodynamic effects of β blockers in thyrotoxicosis (see references 79 and 81 for reviews) reveal that β-adrenergic blockade reduces, but does not normalize, heart rate and cardiac output, nor does it decrease the enhanced cardiac contractility in agreement with the observation that the reduction in cardiac output obtained with β blockers is proportional to the decrease in heart rate. It is likely that the participation of the sympathetic nervous system in the hyperdynamic cardiovascular state of thyrotoxicosis varies depending on the physiologic status and that the degree of reduction of sympathetic outflow in thyrotoxicosis is subject to individual variability.[9,82] Even if lower than normal, the adrenergic stimulation of the heart, such as in stressful situations or exercise, will result in exaggerated cardiovascular responses. Also, at high load rates the sympathetic nervous system may enhance myocardial performance, as suggested by the contractility curves of myocardium obtained from thyrotoxic cats with and without sympathetic blockade[83] and the negative effect of β-adrenergic blockade in the left ventricular ejection fraction during exercise in thyrotoxic patients.[84]

Metabolic Responses

Thyroid hormones accentuate the lipolytic effect of catecholamines in experimental animals and humans. T_3 not only enhances the strength of the norepinephrine signal by a variety of mechanisms, but it also may stimulate lipolysis by other, postcyclase mechanisms.[27,85,86] In thyrotoxicosis, the sensitivity, responsiveness, or both of adipose tissue or adipocytes to catecholamines is increased.[27,36,87,88] The mechanisms increasing the norepinephrine signal vary depending on the species. In rats, for example, thyroid hormone inhibits the expression of G_β subunit[39,40] and Gi subunits.[90,91] These proteins are underexpressed in adipocytes exposed to excess thyroid hormone as they are overexpressed in hypothyroidism. The increased lipolytic response to catecholamines in thyrotoxicosis in humans may be partly explained by an increase in β-adrenergic receptors,[27] but the increment in lipolytic response to norepinephrine in adipocytes from thyrotoxic patients is greater (eightfold) than the increment in β-adrenergic receptor number (less than twofold). This increment cannot be explained either by an increase in adenylyl cyclase activity or a reduction in phosphodiesterase activity, and is better explained by the changes in G-protein subunits mentioned above. As in the heart, it is likely that the increased lipolysis and lipolytic responses to catecholamines in thyrotoxicosis are multifactorial. The augmented basal rate of lipolysis[85] may represent predominantly direct effects of thyroid hormone on the adipose tissue, for example, on the expression of hormone-sensitive lipase. Thyroid hormone also directly stimulates lipogenesis and fatty acid oxidation,[92,93] contributing to accelerated fatty acid turnover. α_2-Adrenergic receptors, which inhibit adenylyl cyclase via Gi proteins, do not play a role in the increased lipolytic responses.[94]

The relationship between catecholamines and thyroid hormones in the regulation of metabolic heat production (or thermogenesis) in mammalian organisms is complex. Both thyroid hormones and the sympathetic nervous system participate in thermogenesis.[75,95–98] The sympathetic nervous system is concerned chiefly with rapid adjustments in heat production above basal rates in response to low environmental temperature or dietary intake,[96] whereas thyroid hormone has the double role of being the main controller of basal metabolic rate and a positive modulator for catecholamine-induced thermogenesis. The increase in resting energy expenditure induced by thyroid hormone is the direct consequence of the numerous biochemical reactions accelerated or stimulated by this hormone, and can be readily demonstrated ex vivo in tissues from T_3- or T_4-treated rats.[97] The participation of thyroid hormone in catecholamine-driven facultative thermogenesis is twofold. It augments the availability of fuel substrate to keep up with increased energy needs, and directly enhances the thermogenic effect of catecholamines at the cellular level.[95] In addition to amplifying the lipolytic responses, T_3 magnifies the response to glycogenolytic[44,99] and gluconeogenic[100–102] stimuli such as epinephrine and glucagon. Besides, T_3 stimulates heat-generating mechanisms such as Na^+, K^+-ATPase (see chaps 49 and 73), Ca^{++} turnover through the sarcoplasmic reticulum in muscle[103] and brown fat uncoupling protein,[71] all of which are directly or indirectly stimulated by catecholamines.

Brown adipose tissue, a unique heat-producing organ in mammals, is an important site of metabolic heat production regulated by catecholamines.[104,105] This tissue plays an important role in temperature regulation and diet-induced thermogenesis in small animals and during the newborn period in larger species, including humans.[104,105] It has been mentioned that brown adipose tissue is a site of reciprocal synergism between the sympathetic nervous system and thyroid hormone wherein T_3 amplifies the responses to norepinephrine and the sympathetic nervous system augments the local availability of T_3. While in the cold and overfeeding the sympathetic stimulation of the deiodinase in brown fat is of obvious adaptive value, in thyrotoxicosis the mechanisms regulating this deiodinase may prevent an unwanted thermogenic synergism between thyroid hormone and catecholamines because of the sensitivity of the enzyme to inhibition by elevated plasma T_4 concentrations.[6] Indeed, in rats with T_4-induced thyrotoxicosis, the response to cold in brown fat is blunted.[74,75] Skeletal muscle is likely an important site of facultative thermogenesis in adult humans[106] and may be directly or indirectly (e.g., via fatty acids) stimulated by catecholamines.[107] Regardless of the site of thermogenesis, it is conceivable that the rather sudden hyperthermia that occurs in patients with thyrotoxic storm represents the failure of the body to suppress central sympathetic outflow, in accord with the observations that thyrotoxic storm may be triggered by stressful situations or by sympathomimetic agents[108] and may benefit from sympathetic blockade.

Thyrotoxicosis also modifies the effect of catecholamines on insulin secretion in rats and in humans.[109–111] Depending on the circumstances, catecholamines may either inhibit or stimulate insulin secretion; suppression is mediated by an α-adrenergic mechanism,[3] whereas stimulation involves the β-adrenergic receptor.[112] In both experimental and clinical thyrotoxicosis, β-receptor-mediated stimulation of insulin secretion is enhanced.[109]

Catecholamines increase calcium mobilization from the skeleton,[113,114] which is believed to be mediated by β-adrenergic receptors recently described in osteoblasts from rats and humans.[115] The stimulation of calcium release from bone in thyrotoxicosis may be mediated at least in part by catecholamines because β blockers may reduce serum calcium in hypercalcemic, but not in normocalcemic, thyrotoxic patients.[116–118]

Thyrotoxicosis is usually associated with loss of muscle protein (see chap 43). This effect, however, is not likely to be mediated by catecholamines because muscle sympathetic activity is frequently reduced in thyrotoxicosis[2] and β-blocking drugs have no effects on protein degradation in thyrotoxicosis, in rats or humans, as judged by 3-methylhistidine excretion.[119,120] The improvement in nitrogen balance induced by β blockers is probably mediated by other mechanisms[121] (see below).

ADRENERGIC BLOCKADE IN HYPERTHYROIDISM

It follows from the foregoing discussion that the suppression of *residual* sympathetic activity, in view of the enhanced tissue responses to catecholamines, may be beneficial in thyrotoxicosis. Reserpine, guanethidine, and propranolol reverse some of the clinical manifestations of thyrotoxicosis.[81] Because most of the catecholamine effects enhanced by thyroid hormone are mediated by β-adrenergic receptors, β-adrenergic antagonists probably represent the most specific way to accomplish the sympathetic blockade. The efficacy of propranolol in the symptomatic management of thyrotoxicosis has

been demonstrated in a number of studies.[81] β-Adrenergic blockade does not reduce thyroidal secretion (see chap 53), and although several β-blockers cause a modest fall in plasma T_3 concentrations,[60] this action plays a minor role in the beneficial effects of sympathetic blockade. Although studies comparing D- and L-propranolol[122] indicate that some of the beneficial effects of this drug may be due to actions independent of β-adrenergic antagonism, studies on the level of cAMP[31] and comparisons with pure β_1-antagonists[23] suggest that most of the clinical benefit, particularly of lower doses, is due to β_1-receptor blockade.

Clinical and Physiologic Effects of Adrenergic Blockade

Adrenergic blockade reduces weight loss in thyrotoxic patients but does not restore weight to normal.[81,121] Nitrogen balance, however, is improved by propranolol and lean body mass is preserved better than body fat stores.[21] This improvement may result from a reduction in intestinal hypermotility and improved absorption.[24] Although the increased metabolic rate, heat intolerance, and sweating are ameliorated by β adrenergic-blockade,[81,125] it does not significantly reduce the hypermetabolism,[121] and when it does, the fall correlates with the reduction in plasma T_3 that may occur.[26,127] As noted above, β-adrenergic blockade has also been reported to reduce the hypercalcemia associated with thyrotoxicosis.[117,118,128] Lid lag, lid retraction, widened palpebral fissures, as well as tremor and hyperreflexia, all of which are expressions of increased adrenergic responses, are correspondingly reduced by sympathetic blockade.[129–131] Nervousness and irritability are also diminished.[32] Some of the more unusual and dramatic neurologic manifestations of thyrotoxicosis are also ameliorated by β-adrenergic blockade, for example, thyrotoxic periodic paralysis,[133] choreoathetosis,[134] and upper motor neuron weakness and spasticity.[135]

The hemodynamic effects of adrenergic blockade in experimental and spontaneous thyrotoxicosis have been particularly well studied. Heart rate, cardiac output, systolic blood pressure, and pulse pressure are decreased, and circulation time is prolonged.[79,81,136] As mentioned earlier, the reduction of cardiac output during sympathetic blockade in thyrotoxicosis closely correlates with the decrease in heart rate, and there is little or no effect on myocardial contractility,[78,137,138] supporting the idea that most of the enhanced contractility reflects a direct action of T_3 on cardiac muscle. However, it is important to recall here that in exercise and in conditions of overload or impending congestive failure, the sympathetic nervous system significantly contributes to maintain cardiac output and, in such conditions, the indiscriminate use of adrenergic-blocking agents is likely to be detrimental.[84,139–141]

Clinical Usefulness of Adrenergic Blockade in the Treatment of Thyrotoxicosis

β-Adrenergic antagonist drugs have significantly improved the management of symptomatic thyrotoxic patients. In mild-to-moderate thyrotoxicosis, subjective symptomatic improvement can often be achieved with 40 to 80 mg propranolol daily (see chap 53). Reversal of weight loss, however, tends to require higher doses.[142,143] Thyrotoxicosis may increase plasma clearance of propranolol, so that drug dosage should be adjusted in each patient depending on the clinical features and the clinical response.[142–144] Reduction in pulse rate, particularly after moderate exercise, often provides a useful guide.

Probably because of direct, unrestrained participation of the sympathetic nervous system, the effect of these drugs in patients with thyrotoxic storm is often dramatic.[81] In them, doses of propranolol in excess of 160 mg/d will often be necessary. Nevertheless, the clinical efficacy of these drugs in this situation depends on the extent of the sympathetic participation because β blockers do not significantly antagonize the catabolic effects of thyroid hormones excess or their direct thermogenic effects.[21,145–148] Indeed, there are reports of failure of propranolol to prevent thyrotoxic storm.[149,150]

β-Adrenergic blockade is also useful in thyrotoxic patients undergoing treatment with radioactive iodine, particularly in elderly patients who might worsen clinically if the radioactive iodine induces a substantial degree of radiation thyroiditis. Propranolol, with or without concomitant inorganic iodide therapy,[23,151–154] or even with dexamethasone[155] has been safely used in thyrotoxic patients allergic to thionamides requiring thyroid surgery or for nonthyroidal emergency surgery in thyrotoxic patients. Although it has been used alone, there is consensus that it is safer to include inorganic iodide to decrease thyroidal secretion.[153,156] The metabolic and endocrine responses to surgical stress appear to be diminished by propranolol.[156,157]

Propranolol has also been used in the treatment of thyrotoxicosis during pregnancy[158–160] and in the preoperative preparation of pregnant women for thyroidectomy.[161] Although it is effective for controlling the symptoms of thyrotoxicosis in the mother, it has potential adverse effects on the fetus and on the course of labor. Neonatal apnea, bradycardia, hypoglycemia, polycythemia, hyperbilirubinemia, and premature labor have been described,[158–160] and congestive heart failure in the newborn is a dreaded potential complication.[162] Propranolol also may be useful in the management of neonatal thyrotoxicosis,[163–165] but as in the case of the fetus receiving propranolol by the transplacental route, it may also cause severe side effects.[166]

β-Adrenergic blockade certainly has an important place in the management of thyrotoxicosis. However, it should be used judiciously, and it must be emphasized that in patients with severe thyrotoxicosis or thyrotoxic storm, β-adrenergic blockade is only a *palliative* treatment and must be used in conjunction with other measures (thionamides, iodides).

References

1. Insel PA. Adrenergic receptors. Evolving concepts on structure and function. Am J Hypertens 1989;2:112S

2. Emorine LJ, Feve B, Pairault J, et al. Structural basis for functional diversity of β$_1$-, β$_2$-, and β$_3$-adrenergic receptors. Biochem Pharmacol 1991;41:853

3. Chan SL. Role of alpha 2-adrenoceptors and imidazoline-binding sites in the control of insulin secretion. Clin Sci 1993;85:671

4. Silva JE, Larsen PR. Adrenergic activation of triiodothyronine production in brown adipose tissue. Nature 1983;305:712

5. Young JB, Saville E, Rothwell NJ, et al. Effect of diet and cold exposure on norepinephrine turnover in brown adipose tissue of the rat. J Clin Invest 1982;69:1061

6. Landsberg L, Axelrod J. Influence of pituitary, thyroid and adrenal hormones on norepinephrine turnover and metabolism in the rat heart. Circ Res 1968;22:559

7. Matsukawa T, Mano T, Gotoh E, et al. Altered muscle sympathetic nerve activity in hyperthyroidism and hypothyroidism. J Auton Nerv Syst 1993;42:171

8. Tu T, Nash CW. The influence of prolonged hyper- and hypothyroid states on the noradrenaline content of rat tissues and on the accumulation and efflux rates of tritiated noradrenaline. Can J Physiol Pharmacol 1975;53:74

9. Gross G, Lues I. Thyroid-dependent alterations of myocardial adrenoceptors and adrenoceptor-mediated responses in the rat. Naunyn Schmiedebergs Arch Pharmacol 1985;329:427

10. Bayliss RIS, Edwards OM. Urinary secretion of free catecholamines in Graves' disease. Endocrinology 1971;49:167

11. Coulombe P, Dussault JH, Walker P. Plasma catecholamine concentrations in hyperthyroidism and hypothyroidism. Metabolism 1976;25:973

12. Christensen NJ. Increased levels of plasma noradrenaline in hypothyroidism. J Clin Endocrinol Metab 1972;35:359

13. Manhem P, Bramnert M, Hallengren B, et al. Increased arterial and venous plasma noradrenaline levels in patients with primary hypothyroidism during hypothyroid as compared to euthyroid state. J Endocrinol Invest 1992;15:763

14. Polikar R, Kennedy B, Ziegler M, et al. Plasma norepinephrine kinetics, dopamine-beta-hydroxylase, and chromogranin-A, in hypothyroid patients before and following replacement therapy. J Clin Endocrinol Metab 1990;70:277

15. Coulombe P, Dussault JH. Catecholamine metabolism in thyroid disease. II. Norepinephrine secretion rate in hyperthyroidism and hypothyroidism. J Clin Endocrinol Metab 1977;44:1185

16. Coulombe P, Dussault JH, Letarte J, Simard SJ. Catecholamine metabolism in thyroid diseases. I. Epinephrine secretion rate in hyperthyroidism and hypothyroidism. J Clin Endocrinol Metab 1976;42:125

17. Pracyk JB, Slotkin TA. Thyroid hormone regulates ontogeny of beta adrenergic receptors and adenylate cyclase in rat heart and kidney: effects of propylthiouracil-induced perinatal hypothyroidism. J Pharmacol Exp Ther 1992;261:951

18. Gripois D, Valens M, Diarra A, Roffi J. Influence of neonatal hypothyroidism on the response of the adrenal medulla of young rats to a physiological stimulation. Pathol Biol (Paris) 1985;33:993

19. Bilezikian JP, Loeb JN. The influence of hyperthyroidism and hyperthyroidism on α- and β-adrenergic receptor systems and adrenergic responsiveness. Endocr Rev 1983;4:378

20. Allely MC, Ungar A. Interactions of beta-adrenoceptor antagonists and thyroid hormones in the control of heart rate in the dog. Br J Pharmacol 1985;86:393

21. Williams LT, Lefkowitz RJ, Watanabe AM, et al. Thyroid hormone regulation of beta-adrenergic receptor number. J Biol Chem 1977;252:2787

22. Crozatier B, Su JB, Corsin A, Bouanani N el-H. Species differences in myocardial beta-adrenergic receptor regulation in response to hyperthyroidism. Circ Res 1991;69:1234

23. Tsai JS, Chen A. Effect of L-triiodothyronine on (−)^{3}H-dihydroalprenolol binding and cyclic AMP response to (−)adrenaline in cultured heart cells. Nature 1978;275:138

24. Kupfer LE, Bilezikian JP, Robinson RB. Regulation of alpha and beta adrenergic receptors by triiodothyronine in cultured rat myocardial cells. Naunyn Schmiedebergs Arch Pharmacol 1986;334:275

25. Rothwell NJ, Stock MJ, Sudera DK. Changes in adrenoreceptor density in brown adipose tissue from hyperthyroid rats. Eur J Pharmacol 1985;114:227

26. Ginsberg AM, Clutter WE, Shah SD, Cryer PE. Triiodothyronine-induced thyrotoxicosis increases mononuclear leukocyte β-adrenergic receptor density in man. J Clin Invest 1981;67:1785

27. Wahrenberg H, Wennlund A, Arner P. Adrenergic regulation of lipolysis in fat cells from hyperthyroid and hypothyroid patients. J Clin Endocrinol Metab 1994;78:898

28. Sundin U, Mills I, Fain JN. Thyroid-catecholamine interactions in isolated brown adipocytes. Metabolism 1984;33:1028

29. Garcia-Sainz JA, Litosch L, Hoffman BB, et al. Effect of thyroid status on α- and β-catecholamine responsiveness of hamster adipocytes. Biochim Biophys Acta 1981;648:334

30. Karlberg BE, Henriksson KG, Andersson RG. Cyclic adenosine 3′,5′-monophosphate concentration in plasma, adipose tissue and skeletal muscle in normal subjects and in patients with hyper- and hypothyroidism. J Clin Endocrinol Metab 1974;39:96

31. Guttler RB, Croxson MS, DeQuattro VL, et al. Effects of thyroid hormone on plasma adenosine 3′,5′-monophosphate production in man. Metabolism 1977;26:1155

32. Guttler RG, Shaw JW, Otis CL, Nicoloff JT. Epinephrine-induced alterations in urinary cyclic AMP in hyper- and hypothyroidism. J Clin Endocrinol Metab 1975;41:707

33. Krishna G, Hynic S, Brodie BB. Effects of thyroid hormones on adenyl cyclase in adipose tissue and on free fatty acid mobilization. Proc Natl Acad Sci U S A 1968;59:884

34. Bumgarner JR, Ramkumar V, Stiles GL. Altered thyroid status regulates the adipocyte A_1 adenosine receptor-adenylate cyclase system. Life Sci 1989;44:1705

35. Mills I, Garcia-Sainz JA, Fain JN. Pertussis toxin effects on adenylate cyclase activity, cyclic AMP accumulation and lipolysis in adipocytes from hypothyroid, euthyroid and hyperthyroid rats. Biochim Biophys Acta 1986;876:619

36. Elks ML, Manganiello VC. Effects of thyroid hormone on regulation of lipolysis and adenosine 3′,5′-monophosphate metabolism in 3T3-L1 adipocytes. Endocrinology 1985;117:947

37. Michel-Reher MB, Gross G, Jasper JR, et al. Tissue- and subunit-specific regulation of G-protein expression by hypo- and hyperthyroidism. Biochem Pharmacol 1993;45:1417

38. Orford MR, Leung FCL, Milligan G, Saggerson ED. Treatment with triiodothyronine decreases the abundance of the α-subunits of G_i1 and G_i2 in the cerebral cortex. J Neurol Sci 1992;112:34

39. Levine MA, Feldman AM, Robishaw JD, et al. Influence of thyroid hormone status on expression of genes encoding G proteins subunits in rat heart. J Biol Chem 1990;265:3553

40. Rapiejko PJ, Watkins DC, Ros M, Malbon CC. Thyroid hormones regulate G-protein β-subunit mRNA expression in vivo. J Biol Chem 1989;264:16183

41. Goswami A, Rosenberg IN. Effects of thyroid status on membrane-bound low K_m cyclic nucleotide phosphodiesterase activities in rat adipocytes. J Biol Chem 1985;260:82

42. Goswami A, Rosenberg IN. Thyroid hormone modulation of epinephrine-induced lipolysis in rat adipocytes: a possible role of calcium. Endocrinology 1978;103:2223

43. Tse J, Wrenn RW, Kuo JF. Thyroxine-induced changes in characteristics and activities of beta-adrenergic receptors and adenosine 3′,5′-monophosphate and guanosine 3′,5′-monophosphate systems in the heart may be related to reputed catecholamine supersensitivity in hyperthyroidism. Endocrinology 1980;107:6

44. Storm H, van Hardeveld C. Effect of thyroid hormone on intracellular Ca2+ mobilization by noradrenaline and vasopressin in relation to glycogenolysis in rat liver. Biochim Biophys Acta 1985;846:275

45. Meyer TE, Habener JF. Cyclic adenosine 3′,5′-monophosphate response element binding protein (CREB) and related transcription-activating deoxyribonucleic acid-binding proteins. Endocr Rev 1993;14:269

46. Liu J, Park EA, Gurney AL, et al. Cyclic AMP induction of phosphoenolpyruvate carboxykinase (GTP) gene transcription is mediated by multiple promoter elements. J Biol Chem 1991;266:19095

47. Hoppner W, Sussmuth W, Seitz HJ. Effect of thyroid state on cyclic AMP-mediated induction of hepatic phosphoenolpyruvate carboxykinase. Biochem J 1985;226:67

48. Giralt M, Park EA, Gurney AL, et al. Identification of a thyroid hormone response element in the phosphoenolpyruvate carboxykinase (GTP) gene. Evidence for synergistic interaction between thyroid hormone and cAMP cis-regulatory elements. J Biol Chem 1991;266:21991

49. Bianco AC, Sheng X, Silva JE. Triiodothyronine amplifies norepinephrine stimulation of uncoupling protein gene transcription by a mechanism not requiring protein synthesis. J Biol Chem 1988;263:18168

50. Kozak UC, Kopecky J, Teisinger J, et al. An upstream enhancer regulating brown-fat specific expression of the mitochondrial uncoupling protein gene. Mol Cell Biol 1994;14:59

51. Rabelo R, Schifman A, Rubio A, et al. Delineation of thyroid hormone responsive sequences within a critical enhancer in the rat uncoupling protein gene. Endocrinology 1995;136:1003

52. Silva JE, Leonard JL, Crantz FR, Larsen PR. Evidence for two tissue-specific pathways for in vivo thyroxine 5′-deiodination in the rat. J Clin Invest 1982;69:1176

53. Visser TJ, Leonard JL, Kaplan MM, Larsen PR. Kinetic evidence suggesting two mechanisms for iodothyronine 5′-deiodination in rat cerebral cortex. Proc Natl Acad Sci U S A 1982;79:5080

54. Berry MJ, Banu L, Larsen PR. Type I iodothyronine deiodinase is a selenocysteine-containing enzyme. Nature 1991;349:438

55. Silva JE, Larsen PR. Hormonal regulation of iodothyronine 5′-deiodinase in rat brown adipose tissue. Am J Physiol 1986;251:E639

56. Silva JE, Larsen PR. Interrelationships among thyroxine, growth hormone, and the sympathetic nervous system in the regulation of 5′-iodothyronine deiodinase in rat brown adipose tissue. J Clin Invest 1986;77:1214

57. Bianco AC, Silva JE. Intracellular conversion of thyroxine to triiodothyronine is required for the optimal thermogenic function of brown adipose tissue. J Clin Invest 1987;79:295

58. Silva JE, Matthews PS. Production rates and turnover of triiodothyronine in rat-developing-cerebral cortex and cerebellum: responses to hypothyroidism. J Clin Invest 1984;74:1035

59. Hays MT, Solomon DH. Effect of epinephrine on the peripheral metabolism of thyroxine. J Clin Invest 1969;48:1114

60. Wiersinga WM. Propranolol and thyroid hormone metabolism. Thyroid 1991;1:273

61. Perrild H, Hansen JM, Skovsted L, Christensen LK. Different effects of propranolol, alprenolol, sotalol, atenolol and metoprolol on serum T$_3$ and serum rT$_3$ in hyperthyroidism. Clin Endocrinol 1983;18:139

62. Kallner G, Ljunggren J, Tryselius M. The effect of propranolol on serum levels of T$_4$, T$_3$, and reverse-T$_3$ in hyperthyroidism. Acta Med Scand 1978;204:35

63. Shulkin BL, Peele ME, Utiger RD. Beta-adrenergic antagonist inhibition of hepatic 3,5,3′-triiodothyronine production. Endocrinology 1984;115:858

64. Heyma P, Larkins RG, Campbell DG. Inhibition by propranolol of 3,5,3′-triiodothyronine formation from thyroxine in isolated rat renal tubules: an effect independent of β-adrenergic blockade. Endocrinology 1980;106:1437

65. Silva JE, Larsen PR. Potential of brown adipose tissue type II thyroxine 5′-deiodinase as a local and systemic source of triiodothyronine in rats. J Clin Invest 1985;76:2296

66. Kopecky J, Sigurdson L, Park IRA, Himms-Hagen J. Thyroxine 5′-deiodinase in hamster and rat brown adipose tissue: effect of cold and diet. Am J Physiol 1986;251:E1

67. Kates AL, Zaror-Behrens G, Himms-Hagen J. Adrenergic effects of thyroxine 5'-deiodinase in brown adipose tissue of lean and ob/ob mice. Am J Physiol 1990;258:R430

68. Raasmaja A, Larsen PR. α_1- And β-adrenergic agents cause synergistic stimulation of the iodothyronine deiodinase in rat brown adipocytes. Endocrinology 1989;125:2502

69. Grinberg R. Effect of epinephrine on metabolism of thyroxine by pituitary and brain. Proc Soc Exp Biol Med 1963;116:35

70. Bianco AC, Silva JE. Cold exposure rapidly produces virtual saturation of brown adipose tissue nuclear T_3 receptors. Am J Physiol 1988;255:E496

71. Bianco AC, Silva JE. Optimal response of key enzymes and uncoupling protein to cold in brown adipose tissue depends on local T_3 generation. Am J Physiol 1987;253:E255

72. Bianco AC, Silva JE. Nuclear 3,4,3'-triiodothyroxine (T_3) in brown adipose tissue: receptor occupancy and sources of T_3 as determined by in vivo techniques. Endocrinology 1987;120:55

73. Silva JE, Leonard JL. Regulation of rat cerebrocortical and adenohypohyseal type II 5'-deiodinase by thyroxine, triiodothyronine and reverse triiodothyronine. Endocrinology 1985;116:1627

74. Sundin U. GDP binding to rat brown fat mitochondria: effects of thyroxine at different ambient temperature. Am J Physiol 1981;241:C134

75. Triandafillou J, Gwilliam C, Himms-Hagen J. Role of thyroid hormone in cold-induced changes in rat brown adipose tissue mitochondria. Can J Biochem 1982;60:530

76. Lum SM, Nicoloff JT, Spencer CA, Kaptein EM. Peripheral tissue mechanism for maintenance of serum triiodothyronine values in a thyroxine-deficient state in man. J Clin Invest 1984;73:570

77. Aoki VS, Wilson WR, Thellen EO. Studies of the reputed augmentation of the cardiovascular effects of catecholamines in patients with spontaneous hyperthyroidism. J Pharmacol Exp Ther 1972;181:362

78. Forfar JC, Stewart J, Sawers A, Toft AD. Cardiovascular responses in hyperthyroidism before and during β-adrenoreceptor blockade: evidence against adrenergic hypersensitivity. Clin Endocrinol 1982;16:441

79. Levey GS, Klein I. Catecholamine-thyroid hormone interactions and the cardiovascular manifestations of hyperthyroidism. Am J Med 1990;88:642

80. Dillmann WH. Biochemical basis of thyroid hormone action in the heart. Am J Med 1990;88:626

81. Geffner DL, Hershman JM. Beta-adrenergic blockade for the treatment of hyperthyroidism. Am J Med 1992;93:61

82. Matsukawa T, Mano T, Gotoh E, et al. Altered muscle sympathetic nerve activity in hyperthyroidism and hypothyroidism. J Auton Nerv Syst 1993;42:171

83. Buccino RA, Spann JF Jr, Pool PE, et al. Influence of the thyroid state on the intrinsic contractile properties and energy stores of the myocardium. J Clin Invest 1967;46:1669

84. Forfar JC, Muir AL, Sawers SA, Toft AD. Abnormal left ventricular function in hyperthyroidism. Evidence for a possible reversible cardiomyopathy. N Engl J Med 1982;307:1165

85. Beylot M, Martin C, Laville M, et al. Lipolytic and ketogenic fluxes in human hyperthyroidism. J Clin Endocrinol Metab 1991;73:42

86. Saffari B, Ong JM, Kern PA. Regulation of adipose tissue lipoprotein lipase gene expression by thyroid hormone in rats. J Lipid Res 1992;33:241

87. Arner P, Wennlund A, Ostman J. Regulation of lipolysis by human adipose tissue in hyperthyroidism. J Clin Endocrinol Metab 1979;48:415

88. Rapiejko PJ, Malbon CC. Short-term hyperthyroidism modulates adenosine receptors and catalytic activity of adenylate cyclase in adipocytes. Biochem J 1987;241:765

89. Port JD, Hadcock JR, Malbon CC. Cross-regulation between G-protein-mediated pathways. Acute activation of the inhibitory pathway of adenylylcyclase reduces β_2-adrenergic receptor phosphorylation and increases β-adrenergic responsiveness. J Biol Chem 1992;267:8468

90. Milligan G, Spiegel AM, Unson CG, Saggerson ED. Chemically induced hypothyroidism produces elevated amounts of the α subunit of the inhibitory guanine nucleotide binding protein (G_i) and the β subunit common to all G-proteins. Biochem J 1987;247:223

91. Milligan G, Saggerson ED. Concurrent up-regulation of guanine-nucleotide-binding proteins Gi1 alpha, Gi2 alpha and Gi3 alpha in adipocytes of hypothyroid rats. Biochem J 1990;270:765

92. Freake HC, Schwartz HL, Oppenheimer JH. The regulation of lipogenesis by thyroid hormone and its contribution to thermogenesis. Endocrinology 1989;125:2868

93. Oppenheimer JH, Schwartz HL, Lane JT, Thompson MP. Functional relationship of thyroid hormone-induced lipogenesis, lipolysis and thermogenesis in the rat. J Clin Invest 1991;87:125

94. Del Rio G, Zizzo G, Marrama P, et al. Alpha 2-adrenergic activity is normal in patients with thyroid disease. Clin Endocrinol 1994;40:235

95. Silva JE. Hormonal control of thermogenesis and energy dissipation. Trends Endocrinol Metab 1993;4:25

96. Landsberg L, Saville ME, Young JB. The sympathoadrenal system and regulation of thermogenesis. Am J Physiol 1984;247:E181

97. Sestoft L. Metabolic aspects of the calorigenic effect of thyroid hormone in mammals. Clin Endocrinol 1980;13:489

98. Mory G, Ricquier D, Pesquies P, Hemon P. Effects of hypothyroidism on the brown adipose tissue of adult rats: comparison with the effects of adaptation to the cold. J Endocrinol 1981;91:515

99. Chu DT, Shikama H, Khatra BS, Exton JH. Effects of altered thyroid status on beta-adrenergic actions on skeletal muscle glycogen metabolism. J Biol Chem 1985;260:9994

100. McCulloch AJ, Steele NR, Kendall-Taylor P, et al. Enhanced gluconeogenic capacity from glycerol in hyperthyroid man: evidence in favour of a beta-adrenergic mechanism. Clin Endocrinol 1984;21:399

101. Betley S, Peak M, Agius L. Triiodo-L-thyronine stimulates glycogen synthesis in rat hepatocyte cultures. Mol Cell Biochem 1993;120:151

102. Comte B, Vidal H, Laville M, Riou JP. Influence of thyroid hormones on gluconeogenesis from glycerol in rat hepatocytes: a dose-response study. Metabolism 1990;39:259

103. Leijendeckker WJ, van Hardeveld C, Elzinga G. Heat production during contraction in skeletal muscle of hypothyroid mice. Am J Physiol Endocrinol Metab 1987;253:E124

104. Himms-Hagen J. Brown adipose tissue metabolism and thermogenesis. Annu Rev Nutr 1985;5:69

105. Cannon B, Nedergaard J. The biochemistry of an inefficient tissue: brown adipose tissue. Essays Biochem 1985;2:110

106. Astrup A, Bulow J, Madsen J, Christensen NJ. Contribution of BAT and skeletal muscle to thermogenesis induced by ephedrine in man. Am J Physiol 1985;248:E507

107. Block BA. Thermogenesis in muscle. Annu Rev Physiol 1994;56:535

108. Wilson BE, Hobbs WN. Pseudoephedrine-associated thyroid storm: thyroid hormone-catecholamine interactions. Am J Med Sci 1993;306:317

109. Wajchenberg BL, Cesar FP, Leme CE, et al. Effects of adrenergic stimulating and blocking agents on glucose-induced insulin responses in human thyrotoxicosis. Metabolism 1978;27:1715

110. Casla A, Arrieta F, Grant C, et al. Effect of short- and long-term experimental hyperthyroidism on plasma glucose level and insulin secretion during an intravenous glucose load and on insulin binding, insulin receptor kinase activity, and insulin action in adipose tissue. Metabolism 1993;42:814

111. O'Meara NM, Blackman JD, Sturis J, Polonsky KS. Alterations in the kinetics of C-peptide and insulin secretion in hyperthyroidism. J Clin Endocrinol Metab 1993;76:79

112. Young JB, Landsberg L. Catecholamines and the regulation of hormone secretion. Clin Endocrinol Metab 1977;6:657

113. Skrabanek P. Catecholamines cause the hypercalciuria and hypercalcaemia in phaeochromocytoma and in hyperthyroidism. Med Hypotheses 1977;3:59

114. McPherson ML, Prince SR, Atamer ER, et al. Theophylline-induced hypercalcemia. Ann Intern Med 1986;105:52

115. Moore RE, Smith CK 2d, Bailey CS, et al. Characterization of beta-adrenergic receptors on rat and human osteoblast-like cells and demonstration that beta-receptor agonists can stimulate bone resorption in organ culture. Bone Miner 1993;23:301

116. Hayes JR, Ritchie CM. Hypercalcaemia due to thyrotoxicosis. Irish J Med Sci 1983;152:422

117. Feely J. Propranolol and the hypercalcaemia of thyrotoxicosis. Acta Endocrinol 1981;98:528

118. Rude RK, Oldham SB, Singer FR, Nicoloff JT. Treatment of thyrotoxic hypercalcemia with propranolol. N Engl J Med 1976; 294:431

119. Angeras U, Jagenburg R, Lindstedt G, Hasselgren PO. Effects of beta-blocking agents on urinary excretion of 3-methylhistidine during experimental hyperthyroidism in rats. Eur Surg Res 1987; 19:23

120. Adlerberth A, Angeras U, Jagenburg R, et al. Urinary excretion of 3-methylhistidine and creatinine and plasma concentrations of amino acids in hyperthyroid patients following preoperative treatment with antithyroid drug or beta-blocking agent: results from a prospective, randomized study. Metabolism 1987;36:637

121. Georges LP, Santangelo RP, Mackin JF, Canary JJ. Metabolic effects of propranolol in thyrotoxicosis. I. Nitrogen, calcium, and hydroxyproline. Metabolism 1975;24:11

122. Eber O, Buchinger W, Lindner W, et al. The effect of D- versus L-propranolol in the treatment of hyperthyroidism. Clin Endocrinol 1990;32:363

123. Vickers P, Garg KM, Arya R, et al. The role of selective beta 1-blocker in the preoperative preparation of thyrotoxicosis: a comparative study with propranolol. Int Surg 1990;75:179

124. Bozzani A, Camboni MG, Tidone L, et al. Gastrointestinal transit in hyperthyroid patients before and after propranolol treatment. Am J Gastroenterol 1985;80:550

125. Allen JA, Lowe DC, Roddie IC, Wallace WF. Studies on sweating in clinical and experimental thyrotoxicosis. Clin Sci Mol Med 1973;45:765

126. Jung RT, Shetty PS, James WP. The effect of beta-adrenergic blockade on metabolic rate and peripheral thyroid metabolism in obesity. Eur J Clin Invest 1980;10:179

127. Saunders J, Hall SE, Crowther A, Sonksen PH. The effect of propranolol on thyroid hormones and oxygen consumption in thyrotoxicosis. Clin Endocrinol 1978;9:67

128. Shahshahani MN, Palmieri GM. Oral propranolol in hypercalcemia associated with apathetic thyrotoxicosis. Am J Med Sci 1978;275:199

129. Sneddon JM, Turner P. Adrenergic blockade and the eye signs of thyrotoxicosis. Lancet 1966;2:525

130. Marsden CD, Gimlette TM, McAllister RG, et al. Effect of beta-adrenergic blockade on finger tremor and Achilles reflex time in anxious and thyrotoxic patients. Acta Endocrinol 1968;57:353

131. Abila B, Lazarus JH, Kingswood JC, et al. Tremor: an alternative approach for investigating adrenergic mechanisms in thyrotoxicosis? Clin Sci 1985;69:459

132. Trzepacz PT, McCue M, Klein I, et al. Psychiatric and neuropsychological response to propranolol in Graves' disease. Biol Psychiatry 1988;23:678

133. Shayne P, Hart A. Thyrotoxic periodic paralysis terminated with intravenous propranolol. Ann Emer Med 1994;24:736

134. Shahar E, Shapiro MS, Shenkman L. Hyperthyroid-induced chorea. Case report and review of the literature. Isr J Med Sci 1988;24:264

135. Rothberg MP, Shebert RT, Levey GS, Daroff RB. Propranolol and hyperthyroidism. Reversal of upper motor neuron signs. JAMA 1974;230:1017

136. Grossman W, Robin NI, Johnson LW, et al. The enhanced myocardial contractility of thyrotoxicosis: role of the beta adrenergic receptor. Ann Intern Med 1971;74:869

137. Morkin E, Flink IL, Goldman S. Biochemical and physiological effects of thyroid hormone on cardiac performance. Metabolism 1983;25:435

138. Valensi P, Simon A, Pithois-Merli I, Levenson J. Non–beta-adrenergic-mediated peripheral circulatory hyperkinesia in hyperthyroidism. Angiology 1992;43:996

139. Tulea E, Schneider F, Lungu G, Stefaniga P. Functional response of the hyperthyroid patients with beta adrenoreceptor blockade to exercise. Physiologie 1985;22:263

140. Ikram H. Haemodynamic effects of beta-adrenergic blockade in hyperthyroid patients with and without heart failure. BMJ 1977;1:1505

141. Martin WH, 3d. Triiodothyronine, beta-adrenergic receptors, agonist responses, and exercise capacity. Ann Thorac Surg 1993;56:S24

142. Feely J, Forrest A, Gunn A, et al. Propranolol dosage in thyrotoxicosis. J Clin Endocrinol Metab 1980;51:658

143. Feely J, Stevenson IH, Crooks J. Propranolol dynamics in thyrotoxicosis. Clin Pharmacol Ther 1980;28:40

144. Wells PG, Feely J, Wilkinson GR, Wood AJ. Effect of thyrotoxicosis on liver blood flow and propranolol disposition after long-term dosing. Clin Pharmacol Ther 1983;33:603

145. Angeras U, Hasselgren PO. Protein degradation in skeletal muscle during experimental hyperthyroidism in rats and the effect of beta-blocking agents. Endocrinology 1987;120:1417

146. Morrison WL, Gibson JN, Jung RT, Rennie MJ. Skeletal muscle and whole body protein turnover in thyroid disease. Eur J Clin Invest 1988; 18:62

147. Martin WH 3d, Korte E, Tolley TK, Saffitz JE. Skeletal muscle beta-adrenoceptor distribution and responses to isoproterenol in hyperthyroidism. Am J Physiol 1992;262:E504

148. Hasselgren PO, Adlerberth A, Angeras U, Stenstrom G. Protein metabolism in skeletal muscle tissue from hyperthyroid patients after preoperative treatment with antithyroid drug or selective beta-blocking agent. Results from a prospective, randomized study. J Clin Endocrinol Metab 1984;59:835

149. Eriksson M, Rubenfeld S, Garber AJ, Kohler PO. Propranolol does not prevent thyroid storm. N Engl J Med 1977;296:263

150. Strube PJ. Thyroid storm during beta blockade. Anaesthesia 1984;39:343

151. Feely J, Crooks J, Forrest AL, et al. Propranolol in the surgical treatment of hyperthyroidism, including severely thyrotoxic patients. Br J Surg 1981;68:865

152. Lennquist S, Jortso E, Anderberg B, Smeds S. Beta blockers compared with antithyroid drugs as preoperative treatment in hyperthyroidism: drug tolerance, complications, and postoperative thyroid function. Surgery 1985;98:1141

153. Lee KS, Kim K, Hur KB, Kim CK. The role of propranolol in the preoperative preparation of patients with Graves' disease. Surg Gynecol Obstet 1986;162:365

154. Cook DR, Chodoff P. Anesthetic management of an incompletely controlled hyperthyroid patient for thyroidectomy. Anesthesiology 1970;33:562

155. Baeza A, Aguayo J, Barria M, Pineda G. Rapid preoperative preparation in hyperthyroidism. Clin Endocrinol 1991;35:439

156. Peden NR, Browning MC, Feely J, et al. The clinical and metabolic responses to early surgical treatment for hyperthyroid Graves' disease: a comparison of three pre-operative treatment regimens. Q J Med 1985;56:579

157. Feely J, Crooks J, Forrest AL, et al. Altered endocrine response to partial thyroidectomy in propranolol-prepared hyperthyroid patients. Clin Endocrinol 1981;14:597

158. Sherif IH, Oyan WT, Bosairi S, Carrascal SM. Treatment of hyperthyroidism in pregnancy. Acta Obstet Gynecol Scand 1991; 70:461

159. Bullock JL, Harris RE, Young R. Treatment of thyrotoxicosis during pregnancy with propranolol. Am J Obstet Gynecol 1975; 121:242

160. Pruyn SC, Phelan JP, Buchanan GC. Long-term propranolol therapy in pregnancy: maternal and fetal outcome. Am J Obstet Gynecol 1979;135:485

161. Levy CA, Waite JH, Dickey R. Thyrotoxicosis and pregnancy: use of preoperative propranolol for thyroidectomy. Am J Surg 1977; 133:319

162. Lightner ES, Allen HD, Loughlin G. Neonatal hyperthyroidism and heart failure. A differential approach. Am J Dis Child 1977;131:68

163. Smith CS, Howard NJ. Propranolol in treatment of neonatal thyrotoxicosis. J Pediatr 1973;83:1046

164. Pemberton PJ, McConnell B, Shanks RG. Neonatal thyrotoxicosis treated with propranolol. Arch Dis Child 1974;49:813

165. Orbeck H. Neonatal hyperthyroidism. Acta Paediatr Scand 1973; 62:313

166. Gardner LI. Is propranolol alone really beneficial in neonatal thyrotoxicosis? Bradycardia and hypoglycemia evoke the doctrine of primum non nocere. Am J Dis Child 1980;134:819

Werner and Ingbar's The Thyroid, Seventh Edition,
edited by Lewis E. Braverman and Robert D. Utiger.
Lippincott–Raven Publishers, Philadelphia, © 1996

47

The Male and Female Reproductive Systems in Thyrotoxicosis

Christopher Longcope

THYROTOXICOSIS IN THE FEMALE REPRODUCTIVE SYSTEM

The incidence of thyroid disease, including thyrotoxicosis, is far more common in women than in men.[1] Whether this is directly or indirectly related to the hormonal status of women remains uncertain. For a better understanding of the effect of thyrotoxicosis on the female reproductive system, a brief review of the normal development and physiology of the female reproductive system follows.

The emergence and differentiation of the female genital tract occurs at a later developmental period than in the male,[2] and the fetal ovary does not participate in the differentiation of the reproductive tract.[3] However, steroid secretion from ovarian tissue can be demonstrated by 6 to 8 weeks of fetal life,[4] and estradiol levels in the fetus do rise throughout gestation,[5] but the role of estrogen in the development of the female fetus is uncertain because its absence does not appear to be lethal.[6] The growth of the fetal ovary is under partial control of the fetal pituitary because anencephalic fetuses have hypoplastic ovaries and a decreased number of primordial follicles.[5] After delivery and in the first days after birth, there is a transient rise in serum estradiol and testosterone levels, but these levels then rapidly decrease and remain low throughout the prepubertal years.[5]

During the first year, the circulating levels of gonadotropins increase somewhat, with higher values for follicle-stimulating hormone (FSH) than for luteinizing hormone (LH), and then these levels decrease and remain relatively constant until the seventh to eighth year.[7] Before the onset of puberty, gonadotropin levels begin to increase, with the rise in LH greater than that of FSH.[8] The gonadotropins stimulate ovarian steroidogenesis and the levels of estrogens rise with consequent onset of breast development.[8,9] The adrenals,

stimulated by uncertain mechanisms,[9] secrete increasing amounts of the androgen precursors, dehydroepiandrosterone, dehydroepiandrosterone sulfate, and androstenedione,[9,10] which are associated with pubic hair growth.

These events are followed by the first episode of vaginal bleeding. Menstrual cycles are irregular and anovulatory in the first year after menarche, but ovulatory cycles increase in frequency thereafter and finally achieve the regularity that is seen in the adult female.[11] For normal ovulatory cycles to occur, it appears that the gonadotropin-releasing hormone (GnRH) must be released in secretory episodes occurring approximately every 1 to 2 hours.[12] These episodes, controlled in part by opioid peptides,[13] not only trigger a release of LH, but also FSH.

In the early days of the ovulatory cycle, there is an orderly pattern of follicle recruitment and selection leading to the growth of a dominant follicle.[14,15] The levels of estradiol increase markedly just before ovulation and result in a positive feedback effect causing the surge of LH and FSH,[16] which is necessary for ovulation and subsequent corpus luteum formation. There is also evidence that rising levels of circulating progesterone may act at the pituitary level to influence the midcycle gonadotropin surge.[17,18]

The endometrium, which has been proliferating under the influence of estradiol, now changes to a secretory pattern through the stimulation of progesterone secreted by the corpus luteum. If implantation does not occur, the corpus luteum function declines, estrogen and progesterone levels fall, and the endometrium is shed during the menses. This pattern of regular cycles is maintained in the majority of normal women through the reproductive years. When pregnancy occurs, the cycles are interrupted until they are re-established after delivery. Following delivery, the pituitary responsiveness to GnRH is decreased[19] and gradually returns to its prepregnant state

671

within 6 weeks.[20] In women who breast-feed, suckling will stimulate prolactin release,[21] and this periodic increase in prolactin may play a role in the amenorrhea seen in women who breast-feed. However, prolactin does not appear to play a major role in the control of normal cycles.

In the perimenopausal years, ovulatory cycles become more irregular,[22] frequently associated with an increase in FSH levels. With cessation of menses, LH and FSH rise to postmenopausal levels.[22] Ovarian function is then essentially nonexistent in many women although 50% or more women will continue to have some ovarian function in their postmenopausal years; at this point, the ovary is primarily secreting testosterone.[23]

Influence of Thyroid Hormone on the Female Reproductive Tract

ANIMAL STUDIES

There are few data on the effects of excess thyroid hormone on the fetal development of the female reproductive tract; however, it has been noted that small doses of thyroid hormone given to young female mice result in the early attainment of sexual maturity with an early opening of the vagina and onset of estrous cycles.[24] The ovaries of these mice revealed multiple corpora lutea and follicles. The administration of large doses of thyroxine (T_4) to the neonatal rat, however, resulted in a delay in vaginal opening and first estrous.[25] Because the period of administration was brief (5 days) and was followed by a period of hypothyroidism, whether the excess T_4 or the subsequent hypothyroidism caused the delay in sexual development is uncertain. In the adult female rat, administration of T_4 in high doses resulted in long periods of diestrus with few mature follicles or corpora lutea.[26] The administration of excess thyroid hormone has been reported to cause an increase or no change in pituitary LH[27,28] and a decrease in serum LH.[28] Thyroid hormone has been reported to synergize with FSH to stimulate differentiation of porcine granulosa cells.[29]

Because thyroid hormone receptors have been reported to be present in the uterus,[30] changes in the uterus could be expected after administration of thyroid hormone. Feeding thyroid hormone in excess to mice causes thickened endometria,[31] and Ruh and associates reported that T_4 decreased estradiol uptake and retention by the rat uterus.[32] Schultze and Noonan reported a reduced uterine response to estrogen in thyrotoxic rats.[33]

A marked excess of thyroid hormone would seem to be deleterious to pregnancy and has been reported to cause abortion and neonatal death,[34] perhaps through a direct effect on trophoblastic function.[35] However, a lesser degree of thyrotoxicosis was reported to help in the maintenance of implantation of delayed blastocysts and an increase in litter size.[33]

HUMAN STUDIES

Children born with neonatal Graves' disease have no defects in the reproductive system that can be related to this disease. Thyrotoxicosis occurring before puberty has been reported to delay sexual maturation and the onset of menses[36] although Saxena did note that, in thyrotoxic girls, the mean age of menarche was slightly advanced over that of their control population without endocrine disease.[37] Polyostotic fibrous dysplasia (McCune-Albright syndrome) is associated with thyrotoxicosis and sexual precocity, but the association of the two conditions in this syndrome may be coincidental.[38–40]

Although ovulatory menstrual cycles occur in women with thyrotoxicosis, oligo- or amenorrhea is common, and LH, FSH and estrogen levels are frequently increased.[36,41] The gonadotropin response to GnRH is increased[42] although the midcycle LH peak may be reduced or absent.[41] Colon and colleagues have reported that there is a significant increase, in both phases of the cycle, of serum LH, but not FSH, after the administration of thyrotropin-releasing hormone (TRH).[43]

Women with thyrotoxicosis have an elevated sex hormone-binding globulin (SHBG) concentration,[44] a decrease in the metabolic clearance rates of testosterone and of estradiol,[45–47] an increase in the $5\alpha/5\beta$-reduced metabolites in the urine, and an increase in catechol estrogens in the urine at the expense of estriol and other 16-hydroxylated estrogen metabolites.[48]

An increase in the peripheral aromatization of androgens to estrogens occurs in some thyrotoxic women.[47] This would appear due to an alteration in peripheral blood flow and not to the direct effect of T_4 on the aromatase complex.[49,50]

Sex Steroid Hormone Effects on Thyroid Function

Thyroid cells contain estrogen receptors, but whether these receptors play a role in the higher incidence of papillary carcinoma in women compared with men is uncertain.[51] Thyroid size, as measured by ultrasonography, varies during the menstrual cycle, being greatest at midcycle.[52] The administration of estrogen increases the circulating level of T_4-binding globulin (TBG), probably due to decreased clearance of TBG rather than increased production.[53] Nevertheless, except for transient alterations in free T_4, a new steady-state level will be achieved with stable, high T_4 and triiodothyronine (T_3) levels and T_4-TBG complexes, but normal levels of free T_4 and T_3. During the normal menstrual cycle, thyroid hormone levels fluctuate slightly due to the changes in circulating estrogen levels.[54] The administration of androgens, which lower the concentration of serum TBG, have no effect on free T_4.[55,56] However, in hypothyroid women on appropriate L-T_4 replacement therapy, androgen administration for breast cancer results in a rise in the serum free T_4 and a decrease in the serum thyroid-stimulating hormone (TSH) concentrations requiring a lower dose of L-T_4.[57] This is due to the absence of the thyroid to adapt to the decreased TBG induced by androgens. Certain progestins such as norethindrone, which have androgenic potency, will also result in a decrease in TBG and in serum T_4 concentrations.[55]

The responses of both TSH and prolactin to a given dose of TRH are greater in women than in men,[58] and both responses are greater in women in the preovulatory phase compared to the luteal phase of the cycle.[59] After the administration of oral contraceptives, both the prolactin and TSH responses to TRH are increased compared with the control period,[60] and the levels of reverse T_3 in the serum are increased, due to the increase in TBG.[60,61]

Both choriocarcinomas and hydatidiform moles can be associated with the signs and symptoms of thyrotoxicosis.[36] The thyrotoxicosis in such instances appears to be due to increased secretion of T_4 secondary to thyroid stimulation from the high levels of human chorionic gonadotropin (hCG), especially asialo-hCG.[62a]

Thyroid Function and Pregnancy

In early pregnancy, but not later, thyroid hormone is necessary for proper placental trophoblast function.[35] In a normal pregnancy, there are changes in maternal thyroid activity and an increase in thyroid size, especially in areas of low iodine intake.[63] In part, the changes are due to the effects of increased circulating estrogens and the associated increases in serum TBG levels and the thyroid-stimulating effects of the elevated levels of hCG, highest during the first trimester. The increase in thyroid size during pregnancy is associated with an increase in radioactive iodine uptake and an increase in histologic secretory activity and total production of thyroid hormone.[63–65] There is a transient decrease in TSH levels early in pregnancy, after which the levels increase within the normal range and then remain constant until parturition[63] or continue to increase through the latter stages of pregnancy.[66] Although it has been reported that the serum free hormone levels remain constant during pregnancy, the free T_4 may increase in early pregnancy and then decrease to slightly below levels seen in nonpregnant controls.[63] Total T_3 increases slightly, but not significantly, but free T_3 falls throughout pregnancy.[66] There is an increase in serum prolactin levels and the prolactin response to TRH,[67] but the TSH responses are variable. The normal nocturnal surge in TSH is preserved during pregnancy.[68]

Substances with TSH activity are produced by the placenta and trophoblastic tissue such as choriocarcinoma and hydatidiform mole.[62,69] The latter two diseases can be associated with thyrotoxicosis, probably due to the increased thyroid stimulation caused by the large amounts of hCG produced, particularly asialo-hCG.[62a]

Thyrotoxicosis during and after pregnancy and postpartum thyroiditis are discussed in detail in chapters 34 and 89.

Clinical Signs and Symptoms in the Reproductive System

One of the earliest reports of clinical changes in thyrotoxicosis was the occurrence of amenorrhea, which was reported in 1840.[70] Amenorrhea has been reported frequently since then, but a number of other changes in menstrual cycles have been noted, including anovulation, oligomenorrhea,[36] and menometrorrhagia, which is more common in hypothyroidism. Whether these changes are due to a direct action of T_4 on the ovary and uterus, on the pituitary and hypothalamus, or in combination is uncertain. The effect of T_4 on fertility is less well established although the disturbances in menstrual cycles will obviously disturb fertility. With therapy, the menstrual cycles return to their regular pattern for the individual.

In summary, thyrotoxicosis occurring in prepubertal girls may result in slightly delayed menarche. In adult women, the effects of thyrotoxicosis on the reproductive system are seen on the hypothalamic-pituitary axis with alterations in gonadotropin release and also in the circulating levels of SHBG, which alter steroid metabolism or biologic activity. These effects produce the variable clinical picture seen in women with thyrotoxicosis.

THYROTOXICOSIS IN THE MALE REPRODUCTIVE SYSTEM

The fetal gonad in the male begins to differentiate and secrete testosterone by the sixth to seventh week of gestation.[71] The secreted testosterone and müllerian duct–inhibiting substance are responsible for the differentiation of the internal reproductive tract in the male;[3,71] however, the development of the prostate and external genitalia require the presence of the enzyme 5α-reductase to convert testosterone to the more active 5α-dihydrotestosterone.[71] Testicular secretion of testosterone in the fetus reaches a peak late in the first trimester and then declines until parturition.[71]

In the first year of life, there is a transient rise in testosterone secretion,[4] after which the testis remains relatively quiescent until the onset of puberty. At that time, there is an increase in gonadotropin secretion from the pituitary and a gradual stimulation of the testis, not only Leydig cells but also seminiferous tubules and spermatogenesis, until full adult development occurs.

In the adult male, GnRH and the gonadotropins are secreted in discrete pulses.[12] LH stimulates the Leydig cells to secrete testosterone and, to a minor extent, estradiol;[72,73] testicular aromatization in the Leydig cells appears to be governed by LH.[74] The testosterone concentration in the testis is maintained at a high concentration relative to serum by androgen-binding protein secreted by the Sertoli cells under the influence of FSH.[75,76] The high intratesticular concentration of testosterone may be necessary for normal Sertoli cell function or may play a role in spermatogenesis or sperm transport.[76] There is a decline in testicular function due to age,[77,78] although the interplay of life-style and disease processes probably play a role.[79] In certain tissues, especially the prostate, circulating testosterone enters the cell and is metabolized to more active products, notably dihydrotestosterone (DHT), through the action of the enzyme 5α-reductase II.[80] In other tissues 5α-reductase I is the major isoenzyme.[51] Although DHT is the active androgen in some areas, testosterone itself is an active androgen, especially in muscle, which lacks the enzyme 5α-reductase.[81] In other tissues, notably the liver, there is metabolism to other relatively inactive products, primarily androsterone and etiocholanolone, which are reduced at the 5α and 5β positions.

In the male, although the testicular secretion of estradiol is important,[72,73] the other major source of circulating estradiol is from aromatization of testosterone in peripheral tissues, including adipose tissue, muscle, and skin;[49] however, little aromatization appears to occur in the liver.[82] The estrogens so formed are further metabolized, primarily in the liver, to estriol and the catechol estrogens.[83] The hypothalamus and pituitary can aromatize androgens so it is uncertain whether testosterone itself or the estrogens formed locally from testosterone are the main negative feedback mechanisms for LH release,[84] but there is good evidence that one of the major factors controlling LH release is testosterone itself.[85] Inhibin is a major factor in the control of FSH secretion.[86]

Therefore, masculinization in men depends on the actions of both testosterone and DHT. The exact role of estradiol is uncertain, but it appears to be of importance in modulating gonadotropin release.

In the normal adult male, testosterone, DHT, and, to some degree, estradiol circulate in the plasma bound in part to a β globulin, SHBG, which arises in the liver, and L-T_4 and D-T_4 can influence SHBG levels.[44,87] The testosterone, DHT, and estradiol bound to this SHBG are inactive and appear not to be readily metabolized.[44,56] The biologically active testosterone, DHT, and estradiol circulate in the blood unbound or bound to albumin. Because SHBG binds testosterone to a greater degree than it binds estradiol,[44] fluctuations in SHBG levels can influence testosterone activity to a greater degree than estradiol activity. Although bound with high affinity to SHBG, circulating DHT itself may not be as important in its effect on its target tissues as the DHT formed in the target tissues from precursors.

Animal Studies

Studies on the effects of alterations in thyroid hormone levels on the reproductive system have been carried out extensively in animals.[88] Changes from normal have generally resulted in a decrease in fertility and sexual activity. Unfortunately there is no clear-cut mechanism that is constant throughout all species studied and the results of all studies are not in total agreement as to the effect of excess thyroid hormone on the development and physiology of the male reproductive tract. In intact rats, the administration of T_4 resulted in decreases in both serum LH and FSH concentrations.[89,90] This decrease in concentration can also be produced, however, by thyroidectomy, in which case, the levels are returned to normal on administration of T_4.[89] Thyroid hormone receptors have been found in rat Sertoli cells and $T_3(10^{-7}M)$ stimulated glucose uptake in cultured Sertoli cells from immature, but not mature, rats.[91]

When administered to male mice in doses that are slightly greater than physiologic, T_4 appears to shorten the time of development and there is a tendency toward early maturation.[88] However, large doses of thyroid hormone result in a decrease in the weights of the testes and seminal vesicles in mice and rabbits.[88] In immature rats, excess T_3 results in a decrease in androgen-binding protein production by Sertoli cells.[92] In ram lambs, the induction of testosterone results in a decrease in testis volume and serum testosterone levels and in an impairment of sexual development, in part, due to alterations in LH pulse frequency.[93,94] In certain species of cockerels, excess thyroid hormone results in a decrease in semen volume and sperm density.[88] Studies on the effect of T_4 directly on the testes have indicated that there is minimal change in oxygen consumption when T_4 is present in testicular slice incubations.[95] This may be due, in part, to the fact that the number of nuclear binding sites for T_3 in the testis was fewer than those found in the liver.[96] The administration of excess T_4 to mature male rats has been reported to decrease total lipids, cholesterol, and phospholipids in the testes[97] and to increase testicu-

lar pyruvate kinase activity.[98] Testes from rats made thyrotoxic by T_4 administration synthesized increased amounts of testosterone.[90] Leydig cells from goat testis secrete increased amounts of testosterone when incubated with T_3 at concentrations deemed supraphysiologic (50 ng/mL).[99] The increase in testosterone secretion appeared to be mediated by a 100-k protein the synthesis of which was increased by T_3.[99] There are conflicting reports on the effect of T_4 on spermatogenesis; it would appear that T_4 does not exert a direct effect on spermatogenesis in mature rats[100] or rams.[101]

Levels of SHBG in humans and in female, but not male, rabbits are increased by the administration of L-thyroxine and D-thyroxine.[87,102,103] In male cynomolgus monkeys made thyrotoxic by the administration of excess T_4, the metabolic clearance rates of androgens and estrogens did not change significantly compared to control values, although the percent free testosterone fell, and the concentration of SHBG rose significantly. The peripheral aromatization of androstenedione to estrone fell but the aromatization of testosterone to estradiol was unchanged.[104]

Human Studies and Clinical Findings

Human studies related to the administration of excess T_4 on the reproductive system generally are acute in nature. The administration of excess T_3 for up to 3 weeks to men or women was associated with a marked increase in the SHBG levels and in the amount of testosterone bound to this protein with a decrease in free testosterone; there was also a resultant increase in LH concentration.[105,106] It was felt that the increase in SHBG was a result of the T_3 administration and the subsequent LH increase was secondary to a decrease in biologically active testosterone.[105] Those studies were carried out for a maximum of 3 weeks only and whether the changes would continue with continuation of the thyrotoxic state has not been elucidated.

An increase in SHBG is a prominent feature of thyrotoxicosis, occurring regularly in men,[44,107] and is responsible for many of the aberrations in steroid metabolism. Studies in thyrotoxic men have shown that the concentration of unbound or free testosterone was not different from that seen in normal men although the increase in SHBG resulted in an increase in total testosterone.[107] Plasma levels of LH in both induced and spontaneous thyrotoxicosis have been reported as normal or increased.[105,107]

Because of the increase in SHBG, the metabolic clearance rates of testosterone and, to some extent, of estradiol are decreased in thyrotoxicosis.[47] As noted, however, the change in SHBG affects testosterone more than estradiol because of the differences in binding affinity.[44]

The pathways of metabolism of androgens and estrogens are also affected in thyrotoxicosis. In thyrotoxicosis, there is an increase in the excretion of 5α-reduced metabolites and the α:β ratio increases[48] although the mechanism for this is uncertain.

The peripheral aromatization of androgens to estrogens may be increased in some men with thyrotoxicosis probably due to changes in peripheral blood flow[47,49] and not to a direct effect of T_4 on the aromatase complex. In thyrotoxic monkeys the aromatization either was unchanged or fell.[104] Nevertheless, circulating estradiol levels are increased in many men with thyrotoxicosis.[107] Some of this increase in estradiol is secondary to the increase in SHBG and more estradiol being bound to it.[107] Nevertheless, there is an increase in the production rates of estrogens in some men with thyrotoxicosis,[47] and whether this is due to an increased production of adrenal androgen precursors (specifically, androstenedione) or to other mechanisms remains uncertain.[47]

Thyrotoxicosis also affects estrogen metabolism, and there is a marked increase in the excretion of the 2-hydroxyestrogens and a correlated decrease in the excretion of 16α-hydroxyestrogens.[108] Whether this shift in the type of estrogen metabolite excreted plays a role in the disease presentation or is merely the result of the thyrotoxicosis remains uncertain.

Men with thyrotoxicosis often present with indications of increased estrogen biologic activity; gynecomastia, spider angiomas, and a decrease in libido are frequent complaints.[100,109] Gynecomastia is probably the most common finding and has been reported to be present in up to 83% of men with thyrotoxicosis.[109] This high incidence was based on breast biopsy in men with thyrotoxicosis, and palpable gynecomastia would appear to be less common. The gynecomastia appears to be secondary to the increase in estrogen production in these individuals. Circulating levels of testosterone will be increased due to the increase in SHBG,[107] and the levels of estrogen will be at the upper limit of normal and occasionally increased.[47] There are often increases in circulating LH concentration as well,[100,107] and these increases, along with impaired spermatogenesis, have been suggested as due, in part, to Leydig cell failure.[100] The decrease in libido may be a nonspecific finding and usually does not respond to testosterone, which may make the gynecomastia worse. With proper treatment—either drug, surgery, or radioactive [131]I—the findings can be reversed. The SHBG level falls and the reproductive system returns to its baseline state in that individual.

In summary, men with thyrotoxicosis display evidence of excess estrogen biologic activity. This excess activity appears to be brought about by the interplay of T_4 in several areas, notably the liver and probably the hypothalamic-pituitary axis. The changes induced appear to be reversible with proper therapy for the thyrotoxicosis.

References

1. Jackson IMD, Cobb WE. Disorders of the thyroid. In: Kohler PO, ed. Clinical endocrinology. New York: John Wiley & Sons, 1986:73

2. Dennefors BL, Janson PO, Knutson F, Hamberger L. Steroid production and responsiveness to gonadotropin in isolated stromal tissue of human postmenopausal ovaries. Am J Obstet Gynecol 1980;136:997

3. Byskov AG, Hoyer PE. Embryology of mammalian gonads and ducts. In: Knobil E, Neill JD, eds. The physiology of reproduction. New York: Raven Press, 1994:487

4. Imperato-McGinley J. Sexual differentiation: normal and abnormal. In: Martini L, James VHT, eds. Fetal endocrinology and metabolism. New York: Academic Press, 1983:231

5. Forest MG, De Peretti E, Bertrand J. Hypothalamic-pituitary-gonadal relationships in man from birth to puberty. Clin Endocrinol 1976;5:551

6. Smith EP, Boyd J, Frank GR, et al. Estrogen resistance caused by a mutation in the estrogen-receptor gene in a man. N Engl J Med 1994;331:1056

7. Mulchahey JJ, DiBlasio AM, Martin MC, et al. Hormone production and peptide regulation of the human fetal pituitary gland. Endocr Rev 1987;8:406

8. Ojeda SR, Andrews WW, Advis JP, White SS. Recent advances in the endocrinology of puberty. Endocr Rev 1980;1:228

9. Odell W, Parker L. Control of adrenal androgen secretion. In: Genazzani AR, ed. Adrenal androgens. New York: Raven Press, 1980:27

10. Pintor C, Genazzani AR, Carboni G, et al. Adrenal androgens and pubertal development in physiological and pathological conditions. In: Genazzani AR, ed. Adrenal androgens. New York: Raven Press, 1980:173

11. Plant TM. Puberty in primates. In: Knobil E, Neill JD, eds. The physiology of reproduction. New York: Raven Press, 1994:453

12. Crowley WF Jr, Filicori M, Spratt DI, Santoro NF. The physiology of gonadotropin-releasing hormone (GnRH) secretion in men and women. Recent Prog Horm Res 1985;41:473

13. Evans W, Weltman J, Johnson M, et al. Effects of opioid receptor blockade on luteinizing hormone (LH) pulses and interpulse LH concentrations in normal women during the early phase of the menstrual cycle. J Endocrinol Invest 1992;15:525

14. Gougeon A. Influence of cyclic variations in gonadotrophin and steroid hormones on follicular growth in the human ovary. In: de Brux J, Gautray J-P, eds. Clinical pathology of the endocrine ovary. Lancaster, England: MTP Press Limited, 1984:63

15. Glasier AF, Baird DT, Hillier SG. FSH and the control of follicular growth. J Steroid Biochem 1989;32:167

16. Ross GT, Cargille CM, Lipsett MB, et al. Pituitary and gonadal hormones in women during spontaneous and induced ovulatory cycles. Recent Prog Horm Res 1970;26:1

17. Batista M, Cartledge TP, Zellmer AW, et al. Evidence for a critical role of progesterone in the regulation of the midcycle gonadotropin surge and ovulation. J Clin Endocrinol Metab 1992;74:565

18. Batista M, Cartledge TP, Zellmer AW, et al. The antiprogestin RU486 delays the midcycle gonadotropin surge and ovulation in gonadotropin-releasing hormone-induced cycles. Fertil Steril 1994;62:28

19. Keye WR Jr, Jaffe RB. Changing patterns of FSH and LH response to gonadotropin-releasing hormone in the puerperium. J Clin Endocrinol Metab 1976;42:1133

20. Yen SSC. Physiology of human prolactin. In: Yen SC, Jaffe RB, eds. Physiology, pathophysiology and clinical management. Philadelphia: WB Saunders, 1978:152

21. Frantz AG, Kleinberg DL, Noel GL. Studies on prolactin in man. Recent Prog Horm Res 1972;28:527

22. Buckler HM, Anderson DC. The perimenopausal state and incipient ovarian failure. In: Lobo RA, ed. Treatment of the postmenopausal woman. New York: Raven Press, 1994:11

23. Longcope C, Hunter R, Franz C. Steroid secretion by the postmenopausal ovary. Am J Obstet Gynecol 1980;138:564

24. Atalla F, Reineke EP. Influence of environmental temperature and thyroid status on reproductive organs of young female mice. Fed Proc 1951;10:1

25. Gellert RJ, Bakke JL, Lawrence NL. Delayed vaginal opening in the rat following pharmacologic doses of T_4 administered during the neonatal period. J Lab Clin Med 1971;77:410

26. Leathem JH. Nutritional effects on endocrine secretions. In: Young WC, ed. Sex and internal secretions. Baltimore: Williams & Wilkins, 1961:666

27. Cohen RS. Effect of experimental hyperthyroidism upon the reproductive organs of the rat. Am J Anat 1935;56:143

28. Howland BE, Ibrahim EA. Hyperthyroidism and gonadotropin secretion in male and female rats. Experientia 1973;29:1398

29. Maruo T, Hiramatsu S, Otani T, et al. Increase in the expression of thyroid hormone receptors in porcine granulosa cells early in follicular maturation. Acta Endocrinol 1992;127:152

30. Evans RW, Farwell AP, Braverman LE. Nuclear thyroid hormone receptors in the rat uterus. Endocrinology 1983;113:1459

31. Reineke EP, Soliman FA. Role of thyroid hormone in reproductive physiology in the female. Iowa State Col J Sci 1953;28:67

32. Ruh MF, Ruh TS, Klitgaard HM. Uptake and retention of estrogens by uteri from rats in various thyroid states. Proc Soc Biol Med 1970;134:558

33. Schultze AB, Noonan J. Thyroxine administration and reproduction in rats. J Anim Sci 1970;30:774

34. Leathem JH. Role of the thyroid. In: Balin H, Glasser S, eds. Reproductive biology. Amsterdam: Excerpta Medica, 1972:23

35. Maruo T, Matsuo H, Mochizuki M. Thyroid hormone as a biological amplifier of differentiated trophoblast function in early pregnancy. Acta Endocrinol 1991;125:56

36. Thomas R, Reid RL. Thyroid disease and reproductive dysfunction: a review. Obstet Gynecol 1987;70:789

37. Saxena KM, Crawford JD, Talbot NB. Childhood thyrotoxicosis: a long-term prospective. Br Med J 1964;2:1153

38. Martin JB, Reichlin S. Clinical neuroendocrinology. 2nd ed. Philadelphia: FA Davis, 1987:332

39. Feuillan P, Shawker T, Rose S, et al. Thyroid abnormalities in the McCune-Albright syndrome: ultrasonography and hormonal studies. J Clin Endocrinol Metab 1990;71:1596

40. Cavanah SF, Dons RF. McCune-Albright syndrome: how many endocrinopathies can one patient have? South Med J 1993;86:364

41. Akande EO, Hockaday TR. Plasma concentration of gonadotrophins, oestrogen and progesterone in thyrotoxic women. Br J Obstet Gynaecol 1975;82:541

42. Erfurth EM, Hedner P. Increased plasma gonadotropin levels in spontaneous hyperthyroidism reproduced by thyroxine but not by triiodothyronine administration to normal subjects. J Clin Endocrinol Metab 1987;64:698

43. Colon JM, Lessing JB, Yavetz C, et al. The effect of thyrotropin-releasing hormone stimulation on serum levels of gonadotropins in women during the follicular and luteal phases of the menstrual cycle. Fertil Steril 1988;49:809

44. Rosner W. The functions of corticosteroid-binding globulin and sex hormone-binding globulin: recent advances. Endocr Rev 1990;11:80

45. Ridgway EC, Longcope C, Maloof F. Metabolic clearance and blood production rates of estradiol in hyperthyroidism. J Clin Endocrinol Metab 1975;41:491

46. Gordon GG, Southren AL. Thyroid-hormone effects on steroid-hormone metabolism. Bull N Y Acad Med 1977;53:241

47. Ridgway EC, Maloof F, Longcope C. Androgen and oestrogen dynamics in hyperthyroidism. J Endocrinol 1982;95:105

48. Gallagher TF, Fukushima DK, Noguchi S, et al. Recent studies in steroid hormone metabolism in man. Recent Prog Horm Res 1966;22:283

49. Longcope C. Methods and results of aromatization studies in vivo. Cancer Res 1982;42:3307s

50. Longcope C. Peripheral aromatization: studies on controlling factors. Steroids 1987;50:253

51. Jenkins EP, Andersson S, Imperato-McGinley J, et al. Genetic and pharmalogical evidence for more than one human steroid 5 alpha-reductase. J Clin Invest 1992;89:293

52. De Remigis P, Raggiunti B, Nepa A, et al. Thyroid volume variation during the menstrual cycle in healthy subjects. In: Hayes DK, Pauly JE, Reiter RJ. Chronobiology: its role in clinical medicine, general biology, and agriculture. New York: Wiley-Liss, 1990:169

53. Ain KB, Mori Y, Refetoff S. Reduced clearance rate of thyroxine-binding globulin (TBG) with increased sialylation: a mechanism for estrogen-induced elevation of serum TBG concentration. J Clin Endocrinol Metab 1987;65:689

54. Beck RP, Fawcett DM, Morcos F. Thyroid function studies in different phases of the menstrual cycle and in women receiving norethindrone with or without estrogen. Am J Obstet Gynecol 1972;112:369

55. Bartalena L. Recent achievements in studies on thyroid hormone-binding proteins. Endocr Rev 1990;11:47

56. Mendel CM. The free hormone hypothesis: a physiologically based mathematical model. Endocr Rev 1989;10:232

57. Arafah BM. Decreased levothyroxine requirement in women with hypothyroidism during androgen therapy for breast cancer. Ann Intern Med 1994;121:247

58. Noel GL, Dimond RC, Wartofsky L, et al. Studies of prolactin and TSH secretion by continuous infusion of small amounts of thyrotropin-releasing hormone. J Clin Endocrinol Metab 1974; 39:6

59. Sanchez-Franco F, Garcia MD, Cacicedo L, et al. Influence of sex phase of the menstrual cycle on thyrotropin (TSH) response to thyrotropin-releasing hormone (TRH). J Clin Endocrinol Metab 1973;37:736

60. Ramey JN, Burrow GN, Polackwich RJ, Donabedian RK. The effect of oral contraceptive steroids on the response of thyroid-stimulating hormone to thyrotropin-releasing hormone. J Clin Endocrinol Metab 1975;40:712

61. Pansini F, Bassi P, Cavallini AR, et al. Effect of the hormonal contraception on serum reverse triiodothyronine levels. Gynecol Obstet Invest 1987;23:133

62. Kenimer JG, Hershman JM, Higgins HP. The thyrotropin in hydatidiform moles is human chorionic gonadotropin. J Clin Endocrinol Metab 1975;40:482

62a. Yamazaki K, Sato K, Shizume K, et al. Potent thyrotropic activity of human chorionic gonadotropin variants in terms of ^{125}I incorporation and de novo synthesized thyroid hormone release in human thyroid follicles. J Clin Endocrinol Metab 1995;80:473

63. Burrow GN, Fisher DA, Larsen PR. Maternal and fetal thyroid function. N Engl J Med 1994;331:1072

64. Noble MD, Rowlands S. Utilization of radioiodine during pregnancy. J Obstet Gynaecol Br Commonw 1953;60:892

65. Hall R, Richards CJ, Lazarus JH. The thyroid and pregnancy. Br J Obstet Gynaecol 1993;100:512

66. Glinoer D, De Nayer P, Bourdoux P, et al. Regulation of maternal thyroid during pregnancy. J Clin Endocrinol Metab 1990; 71:276

67. Hershman JM, Kojima A, Friesen HG. Effect of thyrotropin-releasing hormone on human pituitary thyrotropin, prolactin, placental lactogen, and chorionic thyrotrophin. J Clin Endocrinol Metab 1973;36:497

68. Roti E, Bartalena L, Minelli R, et al. Circadian thyrotropin variations are preserved in normal pregnant women. Europ J Endocrinol 1995;133:71

69. Higgins HP, Hershman JM, Kenimer JG, et al. The thyrotoxicosis of hydatidiform mole. Ann Intern Med 1975;83:307

70. Von Basedow CA. Exophthalmos durch hypertrophie des Zellgewebes in der Augenhohl. Wochenschrift Heilk 1840;6:197

71. George F, Wilson JD. Sex determination and differentiation. In: Knobil E, Neill JD, eds. The physiology of reproduction. New York: Raven Press, 1994:3

72. Longcope C, Widrich W, Sawin CT. The secretion of estrone and estradiol-17B by human testis. Steroids 1972;20:439

73. Weinstein RL, Kelch RP, Jenner MR, et al. Secretion of unconjugated androgens and estrogens by the normal and abnormal human testis before and after human chorionic gonadotropin. J Clin Invest 1974;53:1

74. Valladares LE, Payne AH. Induction of testicular aromatization by luteinizing hormone in mature rats. Endocrinology 1979; 105:431

75. Bardin CW, Yan Cheng C, Mustow NA, Gunsalus GL. The Sertoli cell. In: Knobil E, Neill JD, eds. The physiology of reproduction. New York: Raven Press, 1994:1291

76. Sharpe RM. Regulation of spermatogenesis. In: Knobil E, Neill JD, eds. The physiology of reproduction. New York: Raven Press, 1994:1363

77. Morley JE, Kaiser FE. Testicular function in the aging male. In: Armbrecht HJ, Coe RM, Wongsurawat N, eds. Endocrine function and aging. New York: Springer-Verlag, 1990:99

78. vom Saal FS, Finch CE, Nelson JF. Natural history and mechanisms of reproductive aging in humans, laboratory rodents, and other selected vertebrates. In: Knobil E, Neill JD, eds. The physiology of reproduction. New York: Raven Press, 1994:1213

79. Gray A, Feldman HA, McKinlay JB, Longcope C. Age, disease, and changing sex hormone levels in middle-aged men: results of the Massachusetts male aging study. J Clin Endocrinol Metab 1991;73:1016

80. Luke M, Coffey DS. The male sex accessory tissues. In: Knobil E, Neill JD, eds. The physiology of reproduction. New York: Raven Press, 1994:1435

81. Wilson JD, Gloyna RE. The intranuclear metabolism of testosterone in the accessory organs of reproduction. Recent Prog Horm Res 1970;26:309

82. Longcope C, Sato K, McKay C, Horton R. Aromatization by splanchnic tissue in men. J Clin Endocrinol Metab 1984;58:1089

83. Bolt HM. Metabolism of estrogens: natural and synthetic. Pharmacol Ther 1979;4:155

84. Sheckter CB, Matsumoto AM, Bremner WJ. Testosterone administration inhibits gonadotropin secretion by an effect directly on the pituitary. J Clin Endocrinol Metab 1989;68:397

85. Santen RJ, Bardin CW. Episodic luteinizing hormone secretion in man. J Clin Invest 1973;52:2617

86. Vale W, Bilezikjian LM, Rivier C. Reproductive and other roles of inhibins and activins. In: Knobil E, Neill JD, eds. The physiology of reproduction. New York: Raven Press, 1994:1861

87. Yosha S, Fay M, Longcope C, Braverman LE. Effect of D-thyroxine on serum sex hormone binding globulin, testosterone and pituitary-thyroid function in euthyroid subjects. J Endocrinol Invest 1984;7:489

88. Gomes WR. Metabolic and regulatory hormones influencing testis function. In: Johnson AD, Gomes WR, Vandemark NL, eds. The testis. Vol. III. Influencing factors. New York: Academic Press, 1970:67

89. Bruni JF, Marshall S, Dibbett JA, Meites J. Effect of hyper- and hypothyroidism on serum LH and FSH levels in intact and gonadectomized male and female rats. Endocrinology 1975; 97:558

90. Schneider G, Kopach K, Ohanian H, et al. The hypothalamic-pituitary-gonadal axis during hyperthyroidism in the rat. Endocrinology 1979;105:674

91. Ulisse S, Jannini EA, Pepe M, et al. Thyroid hormone stimulates glucose transport and GLUT1 mRNA in rat Sertoli cells. Mol Cell Endocrinol 1992;87:131

92. Palmero S, de Marchis M, Gallo G, Fugassa E. Thyroid hormone affects the development of Sertoli cell function in the rat. J Endocrinol 1989;123:105

93. Chandrasekhar Y, D'Occhio MJ, Setchell BP. Delayed puberty caused by hyperthyroidism in ram lambs is not a result of suppression in body growth. J Reprod Fertil 1986;76:763

94. Chandrasekhar Y, D'Occhio MJ, Holland MK, Setchell BP. Activity of the hypothalamo-pituitary gonadal axis and testicular development in prepubertal ram lambs with induced hypothyroidism or hyperthyroidism. Endocrinology 1985;117:1645

95. Massie ED, Gomes WR, Vandemark NL. Effects of thyroidectomy or thyroxine on testicular tissue metabolism. J Reprod Fertil 1969;17:173

96. Oppenheimer JH, Schwartz HL, Surks MI. Tissue differences in the rat: liver, kidney, pituitary, heart, brain, spleen and testis. Endocrinology 1974;95:897

97. Aruldhas MM, Valivullah HM, Srinivasan N, Govindarajulu P. Role of thyroid on testicular lipids in prepubertal, pubertal, and adult rats. I. Hyperthyroidism. Biochim Biophys Acta 1986;881:462

98. Aruldhas MM, Valivullah HM, Govindarajulu P. Specific effect of thyroid hormone on testicular enzymes involved in carbohydrate metabolism. II. Hyperthyroidism. Biochim Biophys Acta 1982;715:121

99. Jana NR, Bhattacharya S. Binding of thyroid hormone to the goat testicular Leydig cell induces the generation of a proteinaceous factor which stimulates androgen release. J Endocrinol 1994; 143:549

100. Kidd GS, Glass AR, Vigersky RA. The hypothalamic-pituitary-testicular axis in thyrotoxicosis. J Clin Endocrinol Metab 1979;48:798

101. Chandrasekhar Y, Holland MK, D'Occhio MJ, Setchell BP. Spermatogenesis, seminal characteristics and reproductive hormone levels in mature rams with induced hypothyroidism and hyperthyroidism. J Endocrinol 1985;105:39

102. Tremblay RR, Braithwaite S, Ho-Kim MA, Dube JY. Effect of thyroid state on estradiol-17B metabolism in the rabbit. Steroids 1977;20:649

103. Yosha S, Longcope C, Braverman LE. The effect of D- and L-thyroxine on sex hormone-binding globulin in rabbits. Endocrinology 1984;115:1446

104. Bourget C, Femino A, Franz C, et al. The effects of l-thyroxine and dexamethasone on steroid dynamics in male cynomologous monkeys. J Steroid Biochem 1987;28:575

105. Ruder H, Corvol P, Mahoudeau JA, et al. Effects on induced hyperthyroidism on steroid metabolism in man. J Clin Endocrinol Metab 1971;33:382

106. Sarne DH, Refetoff S, Rosenfield RL, Farriaux JP. Sex hormone-binding globulin in the diagnosis of peripheral tissue resistance to thyroid hormone: the value of changes after short term triiodothyronine administration. J Clin Endocrinol Metab 1988; 66:740

107. Chopra IJ, Tulchinsky D. Status of estrogen-androgen balance in hyperthyroid men with Graves' disease. J Clin Endocrinol Metab 1974;38:269

108. Michnovicz JJ, Galbraith RA. Effects of exogenous thyroxine on C-2 and C-16a hydroxylations of estradiol in humans. Steroids 1990;55:22

109. Carlson HE. Current concepts—gynecomastia. N Engl J Med 1980;303:795

Werner and Ingbar's The Thyroid, Seventh Edition,
edited by Lewis E. Braverman and Robert D. Utiger.
Lippincott–Raven Publishers, Philadelphia, © 1996

48

The Skeletal System
in Thyrotoxicosis

Daniel T. Baran

Disorders of the skeleton and mineral metabolism are rarely the presenting symptoms of patients with thyrotoxicosis. However, thyroid disease can alter hormonal regulation of calcium metabolism and can contribute to bone loss and the development of osteoporosis. Calcium metabolism is controlled through the interactions of parathyroid hormone (PTH), $1\alpha,25$-dihydroxyvitamin D_3 ($1\alpha,25(OH)_2D_3$), and calcitonin. These hormones, along with growth factors produced by bone cells, regulate the activity of the bone cells, subsequent bone remodeling, and calcium metabolism.[1] Thyroid hormone can act directly on bone to increase resorption and alter normal metabolism.[2] To more clearly understand the mechanism by which thyroid hormone can alter mineral metabolism and skeletal remodeling, it is necessary to briefly review calcium physiology and bone structure.

CALCIUM PHYSIOLOGY

Less than 1% of total body calcium is located in extracellular fluids. The biologically active calcium fraction is the free ionized form. Sixty percent of the extracellular calcium is bound to albumin (50%) or anions such as citrate, lactate, or sulfate (10%); 40% is the free, ionized form. The free calcium level (normal range 4.5–5.5 mg/dL) can be estimated from the formula:

Total serum calcium (mg/dL) – 0.8 + serum albumin (mg/dL) = free calcium (mg/dL)

Because the formula does not consider the impact of changes in H^+ ion concentration, which may alter the binding of calcium to albumin, or of changes in the other anions that may bind calcium, it is best to measure the ionized calcium directly when there is suspicion of altered serum calcium levels.

HORMONAL REGULATION OF CALCIUM

Serum calcium levels depend on bone resorption and formation, gastrointestinal absorption, and renal excretion. These processes are in large part regulated by PTH, $1\alpha,25(OH)_2D_3$, and calcitonin.

Parathyroid Hormone

Parathyroid hormone is an 84 amino acid polypeptide secreted by the chief cells of the parathyroid gland. Decreasing levels of calcium in the cytoplasm of the chief cells stimulate the secretion of PTH. The target organs of PTH are bone, kidney, and intestine. PTH acts on the osteoblasts and osteoclasts to stimulate bone resorption and release calcium and phosphate from hydroxyapatite crystals in bone. $1\alpha,25(OH)_2D_3$ augments the skeletal effects of PTH. In the kidney, PTH decreases tubular reabsorption of phosphate (phosphate wasting), increases tubular reabsorption of calcium (calcium retention), increases renal mitochondrial production of $1\alpha,25(OH)_2D_3$, and augments cyclic adenosine monophosphate production. The effects of PTH on the intestine are indirect and mediated by its actions on renal vitamin D metabolism.

Radioimmunoassays for PTH measure the intact 84 amino acid polypeptide, the 34 amino acid amino terminal fragment, or various regions of the 50 amino acid carboxyl terminal fragment. As with the ultrasensitive thyroid-stimulating hormone (TSH) assay, the intact PTH measurement will play an increasingly important role in the investigation of disorders of mineral metabolism. The intact assay is able to separate those patients with elevated, normal, and suppressed PTH levels.[3]

In addition to regulating serum calcium and phosphorus levels, PTH exerts both anabolic and catabolic effects on the skeleton. Anabolic effects occur at physiologic levels of the hormone and probably result from PTH regulation of growth factor production by bone cells.[4] The catabolic effects are mediated by enhanced osteoclastic activity resulting in release of calcium and phosphate from the bone matrix. The enhanced osteoclastic activity is in part the result of increased recruitment of osteoclasts.[5]

The rapid release of PTH in response to decreased serum calcium is essential for normal calcium homeostasis. This is exemplified in those patients developing hypocalcemia after thyroid surgery. Hypocalcemia, usually transient, has been reported in up to 83% of patients undergoing total thyroidectomy.[6-8] Its cause has been attributed to inadvertent parathyroid resection or vascular compromise and a fall in serum albumin due to stress and hemodilution. Damage to the parathyroid glands impairs the normal increase of PTH in response to hypocalcemia in these patients.

Vitamin D

Vitamin D, a steroid, is also essential for normal calcium balance. The most potent form of the steroid, $1\alpha,25(OH)_2D_3$, is a hormone whose production in the kidney is regulated by PTH, calcium, and phosphorus. $1\alpha,25(OH)_2D_3$ exerts its effects through binding to nuclear receptors. Receptors are found in enterocytes, osteoblasts, renal tubular cells, parathyroid cells, and in tissues not associated with normal calcium balance, for example, islet cells of the pancreas.[9] The steroid also appears to act directly on cell membranes to cause immediate increments in cytosolic calcium mediated by alterations in membrane phospholipids.[10]

Calcitonin

Calcitonin is a 32 amino acid polypeptide produced by the C cells of the thyroid. Elevations in serum calcium and gastrin stimulate calcitonin secretion. Calcitonin is the most potent endogenous inhibitor of osteoclastic bone resorption.[11-13] It acts on the kidneys to enhance the excretion of calcium.

Calcitonin production has been demonstrated by extrathyroidal C cells in multiple organs, including brain, gastrointestinal tract, urinary bladder, thymus, and lungs. This extrathyroidal production of calcitonin contributes to circulating levels and may explain the presence of measurable levels of calcitonin in patients who have undergone total thyroidectomy.[14]

The physiologic role of calcitonin in man is unclear. Although calcitonin levels are increased in patients with medullary carcinoma of the thyroid, calcium, phosphate, and PTH levels in these patients are normal. In fact, abnormal calcium balance due to either excess or deficient calcitonin production has not been demonstrated in man. Therefore, there is no evidence that the decreased calcitonin levels after thyroidectomy are detrimental.

The role of calcitonin in the development of osteoporosis is unclear. Basal and stimulated calcitonin levels are variable in women with osteoporosis. Calcitonin deficiency, as occurs after thyroidectomy or radioactive iodine treatment, does not appear to affect the incidence of osteoporosis when thyroid replacement is such as to maintain the patient euthyroid.[15-17]

In contrast, the hormone has been shown to increase bone mass in some women with osteoporosis[18] and to prevent bone loss in the perimenopausal period.[19]

BONE STRUCTURE

Bone is composed of organic and inorganic components. The organic component consists of 95% type I collagen and 5% noncollagenous proteins (e.g., osteocalcin, osteonectin, bone morphogenic protein, proteoglycans, and sialoproteins). Collagen is produced by the osteoblasts. Approximately 10% of the amino acid residues in mammalian collagen are the unique amino acid hydroxyproline. The amino acid is formed by hydroxylation of proline residues that have been incorporated into the polypeptide chains.[20] The hydroxyproline that is released during the degradation of collagen cannot be reincorporated into new collagen molecules. It is either metabolized further or excreted in the urine and thus serves as a marker for collagen degradation.[21]

The functions of the noncollagenous proteins are not well understood. Osteocalcin (bone Gla protein) comprises 20% to 40% of the noncollagenous proteins. It is produced by the osteoblasts and is thought to be involved in the calcification of bone.[22,23] Its production is stimulated by $1\alpha,25(OH)_2D_3$[24,25] and thyroid hormone.[26] Osteonectin comprises 20% of the noncollagenous proteins.[27] The osteonectin-collagen complex potentiates the deposition of calcium phosphate salts onto the organic matrix.

The inorganic component makes up 70% of the bone mass and consists of hydroxyapatite, an insoluble crystal. The mineral is initially deposited on the organic matrix as calcium phosphate salts and later transformed into apatite crystals. Bone apatite is relatively impure, containing varying amounts of carbonate, magnesium, fluoride, sodium, and potassium.

There are two types of bone: trabecular (cancellous) and cortical (compact). The trabecular bone is found primarily in vertebrae and the ends of long bones. The cortical bone is found in the shafts of long bones. Although the majority of bone in the skeleton is cortical, alterations in bone turnover are usually noted in the trabecular component because of its higher metabolic activity.

BONE FORMATION AND REMODELING

Skeletal growth and development begin in utero. Peak trabecular and cortical bone mass is attained during the third decade. Bone is never at rest metabolically and continuously remodels. The factors controlling bone resorption and formation under normal remodeling situations are not known. However, under normal circumstances, bone resorption and formation are somewhat balanced, a situation often referred to as "coupling."

The remodeling sequence is an orderly one involving: (1) *initiation*, the generation of an impulse that alters the status of a resting bone surface, lowering its threshold for activation; (2) *activation*, the provocation of the earliest cellular responses to the initiating stimulus; (3) *resorption*, the removal of organic and inorganic components of bone; (4) *reversal*, the termination of resorption and initiation of formation; and (5) *formation*, osteoblastic repair of the resorption cavity.[28] In the long term, bone mass is not preserved. This long-term progressive loss in bone mass is the summation of short-term losses (failure of formation to equal resorption) at the individual remodeling loci. Bone loss can be accelerated by excessive resorption or diminished formation. The cells that mediate these processes are the osteoclast (resorption) and the osteoblast (formation). Their functions are controlled not only by hormones, but also by substances produced by the bone cells and adjacent tissues.

The Osteoclast

The osteoclast is a multinucleated cell that resorbs bone. The active osteoclast is characterized by a ruffled border at the site where the cell attaches to bone. Tartrate-resistant acid phosphatase is an enzyme produced by the osteoclast and reflects osteoclastic activity.[29–31] The ruffled border is the site where resorption occurs. Although the exact mechanism is unclear, H^+ secretion by the osteoclast promotes hydroxyapatite dissolution.[32] The osteoclast also causes the breakdown of the organic component of bone (collagen) by releasing proteases.[33,34] It is postulated that the protease produced by the osteoclasts is cathepsin B.[35] Inhibitors of this protease block PTH-induced bone resorption in vitro and indices of bone resorption in vivo.[36] The measurement of collagen cross-links in urine is a sensitive and specific biochemical marker of bone resorption.[37] These markers are increased in patients with thyrotoxicosis[38,39] and in patients on TSH-suppressive doses of thyroxine (T_4).[39]

The osteoclast is derived from a hematopoietic stem cell by fusion. A large body of evidence supports the hypothesis that cells of the monocyte-macrophage series are the pre-osteoclasts.

The Osteoblast

The osteoblast is a cuboidal cell that lines bone surfaces. The principal protein produced by osteoblasts is type I collagen, the predominant collagen of bone. In addition to collagen, the osteoblast synthesizes a variety of noncollagenous proteins, including osteocalcin[22,23] and osteonectin.[27]

Evidence now exists that the osteoblast plays a key role in the activation of bone remodeling. Osteoblasts, not osteoclasts, have receptors for PTH and $1\alpha,25(OH)_2D_3$.[5,40] PTH and $1\alpha,25(OH)_2D_3$ cause changes in osteoblast function but not that of osteoclasts.[41] Osteoblasts are required for the hormonal inducement of bone resorption by osteoclasts,[42] and isolated osteoclasts alone will not resorb bone.[43] Osteoblasts also mediate thyroid hormone stimulation of bone resorption, indicating that thyroid hormone can act on osteoblasts to indirectly stimulate osteoclastic bone resorption.[44]

Growth Factors Produced by Bone Cells

Recent studies indicate that factors produced by the bone cells themselves modulate the remodeling process. PTH regulates the production of insulin-like growth factor I (IGF-I) by osteoblasts.[4,45] IGF-I in turn increases bone formation.[45] This may explain the anabolic effects of PTH.[45,46] In addition, PTH induces the release of granulocyte-macrophage colony-stimulating factor and macrophage-stimulating factor from osteoblasts. Both substances appear to enhance the recruitment of osteoclasts from precursors.[47,48] Transforming growth factor β (TGF-β) appears to be released from the organic matrix of bone during osteoclastic resorption.[49] TGF-β itself stimulates osteoblastic activity and bone formation.[50,51]

Other Growth Factors

Factors produced by cells that are involved in the immune response may also contribute to bone remodeling. The interleukins are polypeptides produced by cells of the monocyte-macrophage lineage. Interleukin-1 (IL-1) contributes to the bone resorption of osteoclast activating factor.[52] At low doses IL-1 stimulates osteoblastic synthesis of collagen. Like PTH,[5] IL-1 stimulates osteoclasts only in the presence of osteoblasts.[53] PTH and IL-1 act synergistically to enhance bone resorption.[54] Low concentrations of PTH and IL-1, which alone have minimal effects on resorption, produce striking increments together. Interleukin-6 (IL-6) may also regulate bone resorption and IL-6 may effect thyroid hormone metabolism.[55]

Tumor necrosis factor α (TNF-α) is produced by activated macrophages and plays a role in events associated with the immune response. It stimulates bone resorption and inhibits bone formation in vitro.[56] TNF-α stimulates IL-1 production by macrophages and this may mediate some of the effects of TNF-α on bone remodeling.

ALTERATIONS IN MINERAL METABOLISM IN THYROTOXICOSIS

Thyrotoxicosis accelerates the rate of bone remodeling. The increased turnover of bone that develops in thyrotoxicosis is characterized by an increase in the number of osteoclasts, the number of resorption sites, and the ratio of resorptive to formative bone surfaces, with the net result of bone loss.[57–62] As a consequence of this acceleration in bone resorption, hypercalcemia may occur in thyrotoxicosis. Hypercalcemia, although mild, has been reported in approximately 20% of patients with thyrotoxicosis.[63–65] Studies examining ionized calcium levels have suggested that as many as 50% of patients with thyrotoxicosis have hypercalcemia.[66–68] However, the patient is rarely symptomatic due to the hypercalcemia. The calcium is felt to originate from the increase in bone resorption because immunoreactive PTH levels and PTH bioactivity are suppressed,[58,68] serum levels of $1\alpha,25(OH)_2D_3$ are decreased,[61,69] and intestinal calcium absorption is impaired[70,71] in patients with thyrotoxicosis.

Increased urinary calcium excretion is also common in thyrotoxicosis. The increased excretion is normalized after treatment of the thyrotoxicosis.[63] Administration of thyroid hormone to normal subjects promptly increases urinary calcium excretion.[72] Hypercalciuria frequently occurs in thyrotoxic patients who are not hypercalcemic. The thyroid hormone-induced decrease in PTH secretion and resultant decrease in renal tubular calcium reabsorption mediated by PTH is thought to be the mechanism to explain the increased urinary calcium excretion in these patients.[63,73]

Excretion of calcium in the feces is also increased in thyrotoxic patients.[65,67] Administration of excess thyroid hormone to normal subjects increases fecal calcium excretion within a week.[74] The secretions of the gastrointestinal tract are altered in thyrotoxicosis and the transit time of calcium in the intestine is decreased.[75,76] In addition, steatorrhea is common in patients with thyrotoxicosis[72] and thyroid hormone alters the enteric circulation of bile in the rat.[77,78] The combination of these effects of thyroid hormone on the intestine account for the increased fecal calcium excretion noted in thyrotoxicosis.

ALTERATIONS IN SKELETAL METABOLISM IN THYROTOXICOSIS

Thyrotoxicosis is one of the known risk factors for osteoporosis.[79] T_4 and triiodothyronine (T_3) can directly stimulate bone resorption in vitro over a 5-day period.[2] The minimum free concentrations of these hormones that cause detectable bone resorption are within a 100-fold concentration of the free circulating concentrations. The effect of thyroid hormone can be inhibited by propranolol. This may explain the normalization

of calcium levels in patients with thyrotoxicosis treated with propranolol.

In thyrotoxicosis there is an increase in osteoid, the unmineralized bone matrix.[80] The microscopic appearance of the bone is similar to osteomalacia, in which there is increased osteoid due to decreased mineralization. In contrast to osteomalacia, mineralization rates are even greater than in euthyroid normal subjects.[58,62,81–84]

Osteoblast-like cell lines possess receptors for T_3.[26,85–87] Bone cell-specific T_3 responses appear to be associated with differing patterns of receptor gene expression and stages of osteoblast phenotype expression[88] and respond to the hormone with an increase in the production of osteocalcin,[26] alkaline phosphatase,[85,87] and IGF-I.[89] This direct effect of thyroid hormone on the osteoblasts accounts for the increased circulating levels of alkaline phosphatase[90] and osteocalcin[91–93] frequently noted in patients with thyrotoxicosis. Despite the increased mineralization rate and osteoblastic activity, the enhanced bone formation cannot compensate for thyroid hormone-induced increments in bone resorption. The consequence of this osteoclastic activity is progressive bone demineralization (Fig 48-1).

Bone mass in thyrotoxic patients is decreased.[94–97] Recent studies have suggested that the detrimental effects of

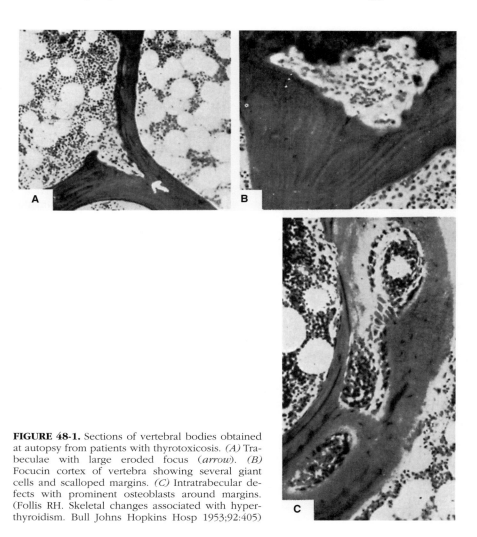

FIGURE 48-1. Sections of vertebral bodies obtained at autopsy from patients with thyrotoxicosis. *(A)* Trabeculae with large eroded focus *(arrow).* *(B)* Focucin cortex of vertebra showing several giant cells and scalloped margins. *(C)* Intratrabecular defects with prominent osteoblasts around margins. (Follis RH. Skeletal changes associated with hyperthyroidism. Bull Johns Hopkins Hosp 1953;92:405)

thyroid hormone on bone may be more likely to occur in female patients.[94]

Individuals with a history of thyrotoxicosis have a slightly increased risk of fracture[98] and sustain fractures at an earlier age than individuals who have never been thyrotoxic.[99] The decreased bone density associated with thyrotoxicosis is reversible after effective treatment[100-103] (Fig 48-2).

It is clear that thyrotoxicosis is detrimental to bone mass. However, the skeletal effects of thyroid hormone replacement therapy and TSH-suppressive doses of thyroid hormone are unclear.[104] Bone mineral density has been reported to be decreased by thyroid hormone replacement therapy of hypothyroid patients.[105-108] In contrast, other studies suggest that T_4 replacement therapy does not represent a significant risk factor for loss of bone mineral density.[109-111]

Administration of high doses of T_4 to suppress TSH secretion in patients with differentiated thyroid cancer and nontoxic goiter is considered appropriate therapy for those conditions. In patients prone to osteoporosis, this therapy may aggravate fracture risk.[112] There are disagreements whether TSH-suppressive doses of T_4 have a detrimental effect on bone mineral density. Initial studies demonstrated that supraphysiologic doses of thyroid hormone in premenopausal women were associated with decreased forearm[113] and femoral neck[114] bone mineral density. These studies were confounded by the inclusion of women who had previously been thyrotoxic. Subsequent cross-sectional and prospective studies of premenopausal women who had never been thyrotoxic confirmed that TSH-suppressive doses of thyroid hormone decreased axial and appendicular bone mass.[115-117] Other studies have not shown a decrease in bone mineral density in premenopausal women receiving supraphysiologic doses of T_4.[106,118-122] These reports have been confounded by the absence of TSH suppression[120] or failure to use the new sensitive TSH assays to assess suppression.[106]

Similarly, in postmenopausal women, TSH-suppressive doses of thyroid hormone have been reported to decrease[115,117-119,122-124] or have no effect[106,120,125] on bone mineral density. In general, supraphysiologic doses of T_4 do not appear to decrease bone mineral density in men.[118,120] A meta-analysis of the reports in which bone mineral density was as-

sessed in women receiving TSH-suppressive doses of T_4 concluded that treatment did not appear to significantly reduce bone mass in premenopausal women, but that it led to a 1% increase in annual bone loss in postmenopausal women.[126] Although this meta-analysis suggests that TSH-suppressive doses of T_4 are not detrimental to bone mass in premenopausal women, there is no reason that premenopausal women will not be at risk over a long period of time.

At present, it is prudent to assess bone mineral density in patients requiring TSH-suppressive doses of thyroid hormone. Measurements at 1- or 2-year intervals will detect those with accelerated bone loss. In experimental animal models, the bisphosphonates, but not calcitonin, inhibit the detrimental effects of thyroid hormone on the skeleton.[127-130] The bisphosphonates inhibit the short-term effects of thyroid hormone on the biochemical markers of bone turnover in man,[131] and estrogen appears to prevent thyroid hormone-induced bone loss in postmenopausal women.[132] These therapies should be considered for individuals at increased fracture risk who demonstrate increased rates of bone loss due to thyroid hormone.

ARTHROPATHIES ASSOCIATED WITH THYROTOXICOSIS

Thyroid acropachy is an uncommon manifestation of Graves' disease that is always associated with exophthalmos and pretibial myxedema. It seldom is present with active thyrotoxicosis but usually develops after the thyrotoxicosis is treated.[133] The bone changes usually occur in the peripheral skeleton and consist of clubbing, periostitis (typically in the metacarpals), and swelling. Pain is usually not a presenting symptom, whereas stiffness is a common complaint. The disorder occurs with equal frequency in men and women.

The incidence of collagen vascular diseases in patients with Graves' disease is probably not increased, despite the presence of high titers of rheumatoid factor.[134] Propylthiouracil treatment of Graves' disease has been associated with the development of the lupus syndrome.[135] Giant cell arteritis has been reported to occur more frequently in patients with

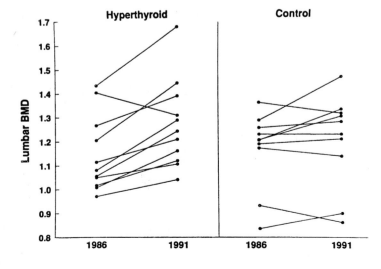

FIGURE 48-2. Lumbar BMD (gm^2) in 11 hyperthyroid patients and 10 controls in 1986 measured by DPA and in 1991 by DXA. All of the hyperthyroid patients were successfully treated and remained euthyroid for more than 3 years (mean TSH, 2.25 ± 0.80 mU/L at 5 years). The controls were euthyroid in both 1986 and 1991. Lumbar BMD increased by 11.02 ± 2.38% ($P < 0.001$) in previously thyrotoxic subjects, but only 2.67 ± 2.15% ($P = 0.10$) in controls over the time period. (Rosen CJ, Adler RA. Longitudinal changes in lumbar bone density among thyrotoxic patients after attainment of euthyroidism. J Clin Endocrinol Metab 1992;75:1531-1534. Copyright The Endocrine Society)

Graves' disease.[136] Likewise, patients with systemic vasculitis have a high frequency of hyperthyroidism.[137]

The incidence of restricted painful shoulders in patients with thyrotoxicosis varies between 1.7% and 27%.[138–140] Relief of shoulder pain appears to coincide with treatment of the thyroid disease.[138,139] There does not appear to be any relationship between periarthritis and alterations in calcium metabolism. The relationship between disturbances in mineral metabolism in thyrotoxicosis and adhesive capsulitis of the shoulder is unknown. Likewise, the significance of antibodies to thyroglobulin in the synovial fluid of patients with arthritides is unknown.[141]

References

1. Canalis E, McCarthy T, Centrella M. Growth factors and the regulation of bone remodeling. J Clin Invest 1988;81:277

2. Mundy GR, Shapiro JL, Bandelin JG, et al. Direct stimulation of bone resorption by thyroid hormones. J Clin Invest 1976;58:529

3. Woodhead JS, Silver AC, Aston JP, Brown RC. Measurement of circulating parathyroid hormone. Horm Res 1989;32:97

4. McCarthy TL, Centrella M, Canalis E. Parathyroid hormone enhances the transcript and polypeptide levels of insulin-like growth factor I in osteoblast-enriched cultures from fetal rat bone. Endocrinology 1989;124:1247

5. McSheeny PMJ, Chambers TJ. Osteoblast-like cells in the presence of parathyroid hormone release soluble factor that stimulates osteoclastic bone resorption. Endocrinology 1986;119:1654

6. Falk SA, Birken EA, Baran DT. Temporary postthyroidectomy hypocalcemia. Arch Otolaryngol Head Neck Surg 1988;114:168

7. Scanlon EF, Kellogg JE, Winchester DP, Larsen RH. The morbidity of total thyroidectomy. Arch Surg 1981;116:568

8. Wingert DJ, Friesen SR, Iliopoulos JI, et al. Post-thyroidectomy hypocalcemia. Am J Surg 1986;152:606

9. DeLuca HF. The vitamin D story: a collaborative effort of basic science and clinical medicine. FASEB J 1988;2:224

10. Baran DT, Sorensen AM, Honeyman TW, et al. 1α,25-dihydroxyvitamin D$_3$-induced increments in hepatocyte cytosolic calcium and lysophosphatidylinositol: inhibition by pertussis toxin and 1β,25-dihydroxyvitamin D$_3$. J Bone Miner Res 1990;5:517

11. Malgaroli A, Meldolesi J, Zallone AZ, Teti A. Control of cytosolic free calcium in rat and chicken osteoclasts. J Biol Chem 1989;264:14342

12. Murrills RJ, Shane E, Lindsay R, Dempster DW. Bone resorption by isolated human osteoclasts in vitro: effects of calcitonin. J Bone Miner Res 1989;4:259

13. Nicholson GC, Moseley JM, Yates AJP, Martin TJ. Control of cyclic adenosine 3′,5′-monophosphate production in osteoclasts: calcitonin-induced persistent activation and homologous desensitization of adenylate cyclase. Endocrinology 1987;120:1902

14. Becker KL, Snider RH, Moore CF, et al. Calcitonin in extrathyroidal tissues of man. Acta Endocrinol (Copenh) 1979;92:746

15. Hurley DL, Tiegs RD, Wahner HW, Heath H III. Axial and appendicular bone mineral density in patients with long-term deficiency or excess of calcitonin. N Engl J Med 1987;317:537

16. Lowery WD, Thomas CG, Awbrey BJ, et al. The late effect of subtotal thyroidectomy and radioactive iodine therapy on calcitonin secretion and bone mineral density in women treated for Graves' disease. Surgery 1986;100:1142

17. McDermott MT, Kidd GS. The role of calcitonin in the development and treatment of osteoporosis. Endocr Rev 1987;8:377

18. Civitelli R, Gonnelli S, Zacchei F, et al. Bone turnover in postmenopausal osteoporosis: effect of calcitonin treatment. J Clin Invest 1988;82:1268

19. Reginster JY, Albert A, Lecart MP, et al. 1-year controlled randomised trial of prevention of early postmenopausal bone loss by intranasal calcitonin. Lancet 1987;II:1481

20. Grant ME, Prockop DJ. The biosynthesis of collagen. N Engl J Med 1972;286:194

21. Kivirikko KI. Urinary excretion of hydroxyproline in health and disease. Int Rev Connect Tissue Res 1970;5:93

22. Price PA, Nishimoto SK. Radioimmunoassay for the vitamin K-dependent protein of bone and its discovery in plasma. Proc Natl Acad Sci U S A 1980;77:2234

23. Slovik DM, Gundberg CM, Neer RM, Lian JB. Clinical evaluation of bone turnover by serum osteocalcin measurements in a hospital setting. J Clin Endocrinol Metab 1984;59:228

24. Demay MB, Gerardi JM, DeLuca HF, Kronenberg HM. DNA sequences in the rat osteocalcin gene that bind the 1,25-dihydroxyvitamin D$_3$ receptor and confer responsiveness to 1,25-dihydroxyvitamin D$_3$. Proc Natl Acad Sci U S A 1990;87:369

25. Markose ER, Stein JL, Stein GS, Lian JB. Vitamin D-mediated modifications in protein-DNA interactions at two promoter elements of the osteocalcin gene. Proc Natl Acad Sci U S A 1990;87:1701

26. Rizzoli R, Poser J, Burgi U. Nuclear thyroid hormone receptors in cultured bone cells. Metabolism 1986;35:71

27. Gehron Robey P, Termine JD. Human bone cells in vitro. Calcif Tissue Int 1985;37:453

28. Peck WA, Woods WL. The cells of bone. In: Riggs BL, Melton LJ, eds. Osteoporosis: etiology, diagnosis and management. New York: Raven Press, 1988:1

29. Azria M. The value of biomarkers in detecting alterations in bone metabolism. Calcif Tissue Int 1989;45:7

30. de la Piedra C, Torres R, Rapado A, et al. Serum tartrate-resistant acid phosphatase and bone mineral content in postmenopausal osteoporosis. Calcif Tissue Int 1989;45:58

31. Stepan JJ, Pospichal J, Schreiber V, et al. The application of plasma tartrate-resistant acid phosphatase to assess changes in bone resorption in response to artificial menopause and its treatment with estrogen or norethisterone. Calcif Tissue Int 1989;45:273

32. Blair HC, Teitelbaum SL, Ghiselli R, Gluck S. Osteoclastic bone resorption by a polarized vacuolar proton pump. Science 1989;245:855

33. Baron R. Molecular mechanisms of bone resorption by the osteoclast. Anat Rec 1989;224:317

34. Blair HC, Kahn AJ, Crouch EC, et al. Isolated osteoclasts resorb the organic and inorganic components of bone. J Cell Biol 1986;102:1164

35. Delaisse J-M, Eeckhout Y, Vaes G. In vivo and in vitro evidence of the involvement of cysteine proteinases in bone resorption. Biochem Biophys Res Commun 1984;125:441

36. Delaisse J-M, Eeckhout Y, Vaes G. Inhibition of bone resorption in culture by inhibitors of thiol proteinases. Science 1980;192:1340

37. Webelhart D, Gineyts EC, Chapuy M-C, Delmas PD. Urinary excretion of pyridinium cross-links: a new marker of bone resorption in metabolic bone disease. Bone Miner 1990;8:87

38. Garnero P, Vassy V, Bertholin A, et al. Markers of bone turnover in hyperthyroidism and the effects of treatment. J Clin Endocrinol Metab 1994;78:955

39. Harvey RD, McHardy KC, Reid IW, et al. Measurement of bone collagen degradation in hyperthyroidism and during thyroxine replacement therapy using pyridinium cross-links as specific urinary markers. J Clin Endocrinol Metab 1991;72:1189

40. McSheeny PMJ, Chambers T. 1,25-Dihydroxyvitamin D$_3$ stimulates rat osteoblastic cells to release a soluble factor that increases osteoclastic bone resorption. J Clin Invest 1987;80:425

41. Sakamoto S, Sakomoto M. Osteoblast collagenase: collagenase synthesis by clonally derived mouse osteogenic (MC3T3-E1) cells. Biochem Int 1984;9:51

42. Burger EH, Van der Meer JWM, Nijweide PJ. Osteoclast formation from mononuclear phagocytes: role of bone-forming cells. J Cell Biol 1984;99:1901

43. Zambonin-Zallone A, Teti A, Primavera MV. Resorption of vital or devitalized bone by isolated osteoclasts in vitro. Cell Tissue Res 1984;235:561

44. Britto JM, Fenton AJ, Holloway WR, Nicholson GC. Osteoblasts mediate thyroid hormone stimulation of osteoclastic bone resorption. Endocrinology 1994;134:169

45. Canalis E, Centrella M, Burch W, McCarthy TL. Insulin-like growth factor I mediates selective anabolic effects of parathyroid hormone in bone cultures. J Clin Invest 1989;83:60

46. Hock JM, Gera I, Fonseca GJ, Raisz LG. Human parathyroid hormone-(1-34) increases bone mass in ovariectomized and orchidectomized rats. Endocrinology 1988;122:2899

47. Felix R, Fleisch H, Elford PR. Bone-resorbing cytokines enhance release of macrophage colony-stimulating activity by the osteoblastic cell MC3T3-E1. Calcif Tissue Int 1989;44:356

48. MacDonald BR, Mundy GR, Clark S, et al. Effects of human recombinant CSF-GM and highly purified CSF-1 on the formation of multinucleated cells with osteoclast characteristics in long-term bone marrow cultures. J Bone Miner Res 1986;1:227

49. Centrella M, McCarthy TL, Canalis E. Skeletal tissue and transforming growth factor β. FASEB J 1988;2:3066

50. Centrella M, McCarthy TL, Canalis E. Mitogenesis in fetal rat bone cells simultaneously exposed to type β transforming growth factor and other growth regulators. FASEB J 1987;1:312

51. Centrella M, McCarthy TL, Canalis E. Transforming growth factor β is a bifunctional regulator of replication and collagen synthesis in osteoblast-enriched cell cultures from fetal rat bone. J Biol Chem 1987;262:2869

52. Dewhirst FE, Stashenko PP, Mole JE, Tsurumachi T. Purification and partial sequence of human osteoclast-activating factor: identity with interleukin 1β. J Immunol 1985;135:2562

53. Thomson BM, Saklatvala J, Chambers TJ. Osteoblasts mediate interleukin 1 stimulation of bone resorption by rat osteoclasts. J Exp Med 1986;164:104

54. Dewhirst FE, Ago JM, Peros WJ, Stashenko P. Synergism between parathyroid hormone and interleukin 1 in stimulating bone resorption in organ culture. J Bone Miner Res 1987;2:127

55. Stouthard JML, vanderPoll T, Endert E, et al. Effects of acute and chronic interleukin-6 administration on thyroid hormone metabolism in humans. J Clin Endocrinol Metab 1994;79:1342

56. Bertolini DR, Nedwin GE, Bringman TS, et al. Stimulation of bone resorption and inhibition of bone formation in vitro by human tumor necrosis factors. Nature 1986;319:516

57. Eriksen EF, Mosekilde L, Melsen F. Trabecular bone remodeling and bone balance in hyperthyroidism. Bone 1985;6:421

58. Fallon MD, Perry HM III, Bergfeld M, et al. Exogenous hyperthyroidism with osteoporosis. Arch Intern Med 1983;143:442

59. Hasling C, Eriksen EF, Charles P, Mosekilde L. Exogenous triiodothyronine activates bone remodeling. Bone 1987;8:65

60. High WB, Capen CC, Black HE. Effects of thyroxine on cortical bone remodeling in adult dogs: a histomorphometric study. Am J Pathol 1981;102:438

61. Jastrup B, Mosekilde L, Melsen F, et al. Serum levels of vitamin D metabolites and bone remodeling in hyperthyroidism. Metabolism 1982;31:126

62. Mosekilde L, Melsen F. A tetracycline-based histomorphometric evaluation of bone resorption and bone turnover in hyperthyroidism and hyperparathyroidism. Acta Med Scand 1978;204:97

63. Baxter JD, Bondy PK. Hypercalcemia of thyrotoxicosis. Ann Intern Med 1966;65:429

64. Farnsworth AE, Dobyns BM. Hypercalcemia and thyrotoxicosis. Med J Aust 1974;2:782

65. Gordon DL, Suvanich S, Erviti V, et al. The serum calcium level and its significance in hyperparathyroidism: a prospective study. Am J Med Sci 1974;268:31

66. Burman KD, Monchik JM, Earll JM, Wartofsky L. Ionized and total serum calcium and parathyroid hormone in hyperthyroidism. Ann Intern Med 1976;84:668

67. Frizel D, Malleson A, Marks V. Plasma levels of ionized calcium and magnesium in thyroid disease. Lancet 1967;I:1360

68. Mosekilde L, Christensen MS. Decreased parathyroid function in hyperthyroidism: interrelationships between serum parathyroid hormone, calcium-phosphorus metabolism and thyroid function. Acta Endocrinol (Copenh) 1977;84:566

69. Bouillon R, Muls E, DeMoor P. Influence of thyroid function on the serum concentration of 1,25-dihydroxyvitamin D_3. J Clin Endocrinol Metab 1980;51:793

70. Haldimann B, Kaptein EM, Singer FR, et al. Intestinal calcium absorption in patients with hyperthyroidism. J Clin Endocrinol Metab 1980;51;995

71. Singhelakis P, Alevizaki CC, Ikkos DG. Intestinal calcium absorption in hyperthyroidism. Metabolism 1974;23:311

72. Thomas FB, Caldwell JH, Greenberger NJ. Steatorrhea in thyrotoxicosis: relation to hypermotility and excessive dietary fat. Ann Intern Med 1973;78:669

73. Mundy GR, Raisz LG. Thyrotoxicosis and calcium metabolism. Miner Electrolyte Metab 1979;2:285

74. Aub JC, Bauer W, Heath C, Ropes M. Studies of calcium and phosphorus metabolism III. The effects of thyroid hormone and thyroid disease. J Clin Invest 1929;7:97

75. Middleton WRJ. Thyroid hormones and the gut. Gut 1971;12:172

76. Siurala M, Julkunen H, Lamberg BA. Gastrointestinal tract in hyperthyroidism before and after treatment. Scand J Gastroenterol 1966;1:79

77. Eriksson S. Influence of thyroid activity on excretion of bile acids and cholesterol in the rat. Proc Soc Exp Biol Med 1957;94:582

78. Lin TH, Rubenstein R, Holmes WL. A study of the effect of D- and L-triiodothyronine on bile acid excretion of rats. J Lipid Res 1963;4:63

79. Riggs BL, Melton LJ III. Involutional osteoporosis. N Engl J Med 1986;314:1676

80. Adams PH, Jowsey J, Kelly PJ, et al. Effects of hyperthyroidism on bone and mineral metabolism in man. Q J Med 1967;36:1

81. Bordier Ph, Miravet L, Matrajt H, et al. Bone changes in adult patients with abnormal thyroid function (with specific reference to ^{45}Ca kinetics and quantitative histology). Proc R Soc Med 1967;60:1132

82. Melsen F, Mosekilde L. Morphometric and dynamic studies of bone changes in hyperthyroidism. Acta Pathol Microbiol Scand [A] 1977;85A:141

83. Meunier PJ, Bianchi GGS, Edouard CM, et al. Bony manifestations of thyrotoxicosis. Orthop Clin North Am 1972;3:745

84. Mosekilde L, Jastrup B, Melsen F, et al. Effect of propranolol treatment on bone mass, bone mineral content, bone remodeling, parathyroid function and vitamin D metabolism in hyperthyroidism. Eur J Clin Invest 1984;14:96

85. Kasono K, Sato K, Han DC, et al. Stimulation of alkaline phosphatase activity by thyroid hormone in mouse osteoblast-like cells (MC3T3-E1): a possible mechanism of hyperalkaline phosphatasia in hyperthyroidism. Bone Miner 1988;4:355

86. LeBron BA, Pekary AE, Mirell C, et al. Thyroid hormone 5'-deiodinase activity, nuclear binding, and effects on mitogenesis in UMR 106-osteoblastic osteosarcoma cells. J Bone Miner Res 1989;4:173

87. Sato K, Han DC, Fujii Y, et al. Thyroid hormone stimulates alkaline phosphatase activity in cultured rat osteoblastic cells (ROS

17/2.8) through 3,5,3′-triiodo-L-thyronine nuclear receptors. Endocrinology 1987;120:1873

88. Williams GR, Bland R, Sheppard ML. Characterization of thyroid hormone (T_3) receptors in three osteosarcoma cell lines of distinct osteoblast phenotype: interactions among T_3, vitamin D_3 and retinoid signalling. Endocrinology 1994;135:2375

89. Schmid C, Schlapter I, Futo E, et al. Triiodothyronine stimulates insulin-like growth factor 1 and IGF binding protein 2 production by rat osteoblast in vitro. Acta Endocrinol 1992;126:467

90. Cooper DS, Kaplan MM, Ridgway EC, et al. Alkaline phosphatase isoenzyme patterns in hyperthyroidism. Ann Intern Med 1979;90:164

91. Faber J, Perrild H, Johansen JS. Bone Gla protein and sex hormone-binding globulin in nontoxic goiter: parameters for metabolic status at the tissue level. J Clin Endocrinol Metab 1990;70:49

92. Garrel DR, Delmas PD, Malaval L, Tourniaire J. Serum bone Gla protein: a marker of bone turnover in hyperthyroidism. J Clin Endocrinol Metab 1986;62:1052

93. Lukert BP, Higgins JC, Stoskopf MM. Serum osteocalcin is increased in patients with hyperthyroidism and decreased in patients receiving glucocorticoids. J Clin Endocrinol Metab 1986; 62:1056

94. Lee MS, Kim SY, Lee MC, et al. Negative correlation between the change in bone mineral density and serum osteocalcin in patients with hyperthyroidism. J Clin Endocrinol Metab 1990;70:766

95. Linde J, Friis T. Osteoporosis in hyperthyroidism estimated by photon absorptiometry. Acta Endocrinol (Copenh) 1979;91:437

96. Toh SH, Claunch BC, Brown PH. Effect of hyperthyroidism and its treatment on bone mineral content. Arch Intern Med 1985; 145:883

97. Krolner B, Vesterdal Jorgensen J, Pors Nielsen S. Spinal bone mineral content in myxoedema and thyrotoxicosis: effects of thyroid hormone(s) and antithyroid treatment. Clin Endocrinol 1983;18:439

98. Bauer DC, Cummings SR, Tao JL, Browner WS. Hyperthyroidism increases the risk of hip fractures: a prospective study. J Bone Mineral Res 1992;7(suppl 1):121

99. Solomon BL, Wartofsky L, Burman KD. Prevalence of fractures in postmenopausal women with thyroid disease. Thyroid 1993;3:17

100. Diamond T, Vine J, Smart R, Butler P. Thyrotoxic bone disease in women: a potentially reversible disorder. Ann Intern Med 1994; 120:8

101. Rosen C, Adler RA. Longitudinal changes in lumbar bone density among thyrotoxic patients after attainment of euthyroidism. J Clin Endocrinol Metab 1992;75:1531

102. Wakasugi M, Wakao R, Tawata M, et al. Changes in bone mineral density in patients with hyperthyroidism after attainment of euthyroidism by dual energy x-ray absorptiometry. Thyroid 1994; 4:179

103. Mudde AH, Houben AJ, Nieuwenhuijzen HM, Kruseman AC. Bone metabolism during antithyroid drug treatment of endogenous subclinical hyperthyroidism. Clin Endocrinol 1994;41:421

104. Baran DT. Thyroid hormone and bone mass: the clinician's dilemma. Thyroid 1994;4:143

105. Krolner B, Jorgensen JV, Nielsen SP. Spinal bone mineral content in myxoedema and thyrotoxicosis. Effects of thyroid hormone(s) and antithyroid treatment. Clin Endocrinol (Oxf) 1983;18:439

106. Ribot C, Tremollieres F, Pouilles JM, Louvet JP. Bone mineral density and thyroid hormone therapy. Clin Endocrinol (Oxf) 1990; 33:143

107. Lakatos P, Tarjan G, Foldes J, et al. The effect of thyroid hormone treatment on bone mineral content in patients with hypothyroidism and euthyroid benign adenoma. In: Christiansen C, Johansen JS, Riis BJ, eds. Osteoporosis 1987. Viborg, Denmark: Norhaven A/S, 1987:452

108. Demeester-Mirkine N, Bergmann P, Body J-J, Corvilain J. Calcitonin and bone mass status in congenital hypothyroidism. Calcif Tissue Int 1990;46:222

109. Toh SH, Brown PH. Bone mineral content in hypothyroid male patients with hormone replacement: a 3-year study. J Bone Miner Res 1990;5:463

110. Duncan WE, Chung A, Solomon B, Wartofsky L. Influence of clinical characteristics and parameters associated with thyroid hormone therapy on the bone mineral density of women treated with thyroid hormone. Thyroid 1994;4:183

111. Franklyn J, Betteridge J, Holder R, et al. Bone mineral density in thyroxine treated females with or without a previous history of thyrotoxicosis. Clin Endocrinol 1994;4:425

112. Baran DT. Detrimental skeletal effects of thyrotropin suppressive doses of thyroxine: fact or fantasy? J Clin Endocrinol Metab 1994;78:816

113. Ross DS, Neer RM, Ridgway EC, Daniels GH. Subclinical hyperthyroidism and reduced bone density as a possible result of prolonged suppression of the pituitary-thyroid axis with L-thyroxine. Am J Med 1987;82:1167

114. Paul TL, Kerrigan J, Kelly AM, et al. Long-term L-thyroxine therapy is associated with decreased hip bone density in premenopausal women. JAMA 1988;259:3137

115. Diamond T, Nevy L, Hales I. A therapeutic dilemma: suppressive doses of thyroxine significantly reduce bone mineral measurements in both premenopausal and postmenopausal women with thyroid carcinoma. J Clin Endocrinol Metab 1991;72:1184

116. Pioli G, Pedrazzoni M, Palummeri E, et al. Longitudinal study of bone loss after thyroidectomy and suppressive therapy in premenopausal women. Acta Endocrinol 1992;126:238

117. Greenspan S, Resnick NM, Block JE, et al. Skeletal integrity in premenopausal and postmenopausal women receiving long-term L-thyroxine therapy. Am J Med 1991;91:5

118. Stepan JJ, Limanova Z. Biochemical assessment of bone loss in patients on long term thyroid hormone treatment. Bone Miner 1992;17:377

119. Taelman P, Kaufman JM, Jannssen X, et al. Reduced forearm bone mineral content and biochemical evidence of increased bone turnover in women with euthyroid goiter treated with thyroid hormone. Clin Endocrinol (Oxf) 1990;33:107

120. Franklyn JA, Betteridge J, Daykin J, et al. Long-term thyroxine treatment and bone mineral density. Lancet 1992;340:9

121. Marcocci C, Golia F, Bruno-Bossio G, et al. Carefully monitored levothyroxine suppressive therapy is not associated with bone loss in premenopausal women. J Clin Endocrinol Metab 1994; 78:817

122. Lehmke J, Bogner V, Felsenberg D, et al. Determination of bone mineral density by quantitative computed tomography and single photon absorptiometry in subclinical hyperthyroidism: a risk of early osteopenia in postmenopausal women. Clin Endocrinol 1992;36:511

123. Stall GM, Harris S, Sokoll LJ, Dawson-Hughes B. Accelerated bone loss in hypothyroid patients overtreated with L-thyroxine. Ann Intern Med 1990;113:265

124. Adlin EV, Maurer AH, Marks AD, Channick BJ. Bone mineral density in postmenopausal women treated with L-thyroxine. Am J Med 1991;90:360

125. Gam AN, Jensen GF, Hasselstrom K, et al. Effect of thyroxine therapy on bone metabolism in substituted hypothyroid patients with normal or suppressed levels of TSH. J Endocrinol Invest 1991;14:451

126. Faber J, Galloe AM. Changes in bone mass during prolonged subclinical hyperthyroidism due to L-thyroxine treatment: a meta-analysis. Eur J Endocrinol 1994;130:350

127. Ongphiphadhanakul B, Jenis LG, Braverman LE, et al. Etidronate inhibits the thyroid hormone-induced bone loss in rats assessed

by bone mineral density and messenger ribonuclei acid markers of osteoblast and osteoclast function. Endocrinology 1993; 133:2502

128. Rosen HN, Sullivan EK, Middlebrooks VL, et al. Parenteral pamidronate prevents thyroid hormone-induced bone loss in rats. J Bone Miner Res 1993;5:1255

129. Yamamoto M, Markatos A, Seedor JG, et al. The effects of the amino bisphosphonate alendronate on thyroid hormone-induced osteopenia in rats. Calcif Tissue Int 1993; 53:278

130. Rosen HN, Middlebrooks VL, Sullivan EK, et al. Subregion analysis of the rat femur: a sensitive indicator of changes in bone density following treatment with thyroid hormone or bisphosphonate. Calcif Tissue Int 1994;55:173

131. Rosen HN, Moses AC, Gundberg C, et al. Therapy with parenteral pamidronate prevents thyroid hormone-induced bone turnover in humans. J Clin Endocrinol Metab 1993;77:664

132. Schneider DL, Barrett-Connor EL, Morton DJ. Thyroid hormone use and bone mineral density in elderly women: effects of estrogen. JAMA 1994;271:1245

133. Gimlette TMD. Thyroid acropachy. Lancet 1960;I:22

134. Silverberg J, Volpe R. Rheumatoid factors in Graves' disease. Ann Intern Med 1978;88:216

135. Amrhein JA, Kenny FM, Ross D. Granulocytopenia, lupus-like syndrome, and other complications of propylthiouracil therapy. J Pediatr 1970;76:54

136. Thomas RD, Croft DN. Thyrotoxicosis and giant cell arteritis. Br Med J 1974;2:408

137. Arnaout MA, Nasrallah NS, El-Khateeb MS. Prevalence of abnormal thyroid function tests in connective tissue disease. Scand J Rheumatol 1994;23:128

138. Chapman EM, Maloof F. Bizarre clinical manifestations of hyperthyroidism. N Engl J Med 1956;254:1

139. Meulengracht E, Schwartz M. Course and prognosis of humeroscapular periarthrosis, especially in cases with general symptoms. Nord Med 1951;46:1629

140. Skillern PG. The association of periarthritis of the shoulder with hyperthyroidism. In: Transactions of the American Goiter Association. Springfield, IL: Charles C. Thomas, 1953:100

141. Blake DR, McGregor AM, Stansfield E, Rees-Smith B. Antithyroid-antibody activity in the synovial fluid of patients with various arthritides. Lancet 1979;II:224

Werner and Ingbar's The Thyroid, Seventh Edition,
edited by Lewis E. Braverman and Robert D. Utiger.
Lippincott–Raven Publishers, Philadelphia, © 1996

49

Metabolic Changes in Thyrotoxicosis

METABOLIC CHANGES IN THYROTOXICOSIS

John N. Loeb

BASAL METABOLIC RATE AND CALORIGENESIS

Extensive weight loss despite normal or increased caloric intake is one of the earliest metabolic derangements to occur in thyrotoxicosis. Loss of weight (which averaged about 15 pounds in one large series of men with thyrotoxicosis caused by Graves' disease[1]) reflects not only depletion of body adipose tissue stores but also loss of muscle mass.[2] The weight loss in thyrotoxicosis is caused by accelerated catabolism of foodstuffs and is accompanied by increased oxygen consumption.[3] In experimental thyrotoxicosis an enhanced rate of oxygen consumption is demonstrable in nearly all tissues with the exception of spleen, testis, and adult brain.[4]

All but a small fraction of the total oxygen consumption of the body occurs in mitochondria, where about 40% of the energy derived from the metabolism of primary foodstuffs is trapped in the form of adenosine triphosphate (ATP) for use in a wide variety of energy-requiring cellular functions. The increased energy utilization and production in the thyrotoxic state are ultimately reflected in increased heat production and heat elimination clinically manifested by a slightly elevated basal body temperature, heat intolerance, weight loss, and increased appetite.

Consistent with the increase in total oxygen consumption in vivo, various tissues in experimental thyrotoxicosis show increased mitochondrial size, number, and surface area.[5–8] These changes appear to be a secondary response to the increase in substrate utilization and oxygen consumption induced by excess thyroid hormone. Under certain conditions mitochondria from thyrotoxic animals consume oxygen more rapidly per unit mass than mitochondria from normal animals,[9] and increased tissue oxygen consumption can be induced considerably earlier than can be accounted for by increases in mitochondrial size and number.

High concentrations of thyroid hormones added to isolated mitochondria in vitro can result in a decreased yield of ATP per molecule of oxygen consumed.[9] This reduction in the efficiency of mitochondrial ATP generation is referred to as "uncoupling" of oxidative phosphorylation. The same phenomenon can be induced in mitochondria from laboratory animals under certain conditions of extreme thyrotoxicosis.[9] Under most conditions, however, oxidative phosphorylation in most tissues from thyrotoxic animals is not uncoupled despite a substantial increase in tissue oxygen consumption, and the earlier suggestion that uncoupling itself might account for the widespread calorigenic action of thyroid hormones is now recognized as incorrect.[10]

An important exception is brown adipose tissue, a tissue that responds through mechanisms triggered by the sympathetic nervous system with a large increase in oxygen consumption and heat production, and that, in several species, including rats, plays a major role in cold adaptation.[11] In brown adipose tissue, the thyroxine (T_4)-5'-deiodinase isoform (type 2) that catalyzes the deiodination to triiodothyronine (T_3) is markedly activated by sympathetic stimulation,[12,13] and local production of high concentrations of T_3 in turn stimulates the production of a mitochondrial protein that uncouples oxidative phosphorylation.[14,15] Cold exposure results in a large increase in the messenger RNA for this uncoupling protein[16] that is at least in part mediated by enhanced local production of T_3.[17,18] The effects of T_3 and catecholamines on brown adipose tissue in vivo can likewise be demonstrated in freshly dispersed brown adipocytes in vitro[19] as well as in cultured fetal rat brown adipocytes.[20]

Although ATP formation remains normally coupled to oxygen consumption in most tissues, the sites of increased ATP utilization in these tissues that account for the increased oxygen consumption in thyrotoxicosis are for the most part not known. Although as much as 20% of the resting metabolic rate in normal subjects may be due to energy requirements related to protein turnover,[21] inhibition of protein synthesis, whether in isolated mitochondria[22] or in liver slices from thyrotoxic or normal animals,[23] has a negligible effect on the rate of oxygen consumption.

A major component of the increase in oxygen consumption by a variety of thyrotoxic tissues in vitro can be blocked by the addition of ouabain,[24,25] a specific inhibitor of the sodium-potassium pump ($Na^+_1K^+$ pump; $Na^+_1K^+$-ATPase), whose primary function is to maintain normal intracellular-to-extracellular sodium and potassium ion gradients. This observation, in conjunction with an estimate that active extrusion of Na^+ from cells might account for 20% to 45% of the total energy requirement of resting cells,[26,27] led to the suggestion that, in the thyrotoxic state, a substantial proportion of the increase in oxygen consumption is attributable to increased activity of the $Na^+_1K^+$ pump, with a parallel enhancement of active Na^+ extrusion, active K^+ accumulation, and associated ATP utilization.[24,25,28] The increase in pump activity in the thyrotoxic state is accompanied by a rise in $Na^+_1K^+$-ATPase enzymatic activity[25] and number of $Na^+_1K^+$ pump units in plasma membrane preparations,[29] and the time course of the increase in enzymatic activity after administration of thyroid hormone parallels that of the increase in cellular oxygen consumption.[28,30] Addition of thyroid hormone also increases $Na^+_1K^+$-ATPase in primary cultures of rat hepatocytes[31] and chick ventricular cells[32] as well as in some continuously cultured rat liver cell lines.[33–35] In skeletal muscle[36] and heart[37] the increase in $Na^+_1K^+$-ATPase is selective for certain isoforms of the enzyme.

The magnitude of the contribution of active monovalent cation transport to overall cellular energy requirements, however, has been questioned, and earlier estimates of the energy cost of active Na^+ and K^+ transport may have been too high.[38–42] Moreover, the increase in $Na^+_1K^+$ pump units in response to thyroid hormone cannot be exclusively attributed to a direct effect of the hormone itself, but is at least in part a secondary, adaptive response to other cellular alterations induced by thyroid hormone (e.g., an enhancement of passive fluxes of monovalent cations in the directions opposite to those of their active transport[34,42–45]). Although thyroid hormone, both in vivo[37] and in vitro,[46] can lead to early increases in the messenger RNA that codes for $Na^+_1K^+$-ATPase, there is a substantial increase in passive K^+ efflux rate in liver slices from T_3-treated rats that appears to precede any detectable increase in $Na^+_1K^+$-ATPase activity.[42] Exposure to T_3 also facilitates passive Na^+ influx in a number of cell types.[34,47,48]

FAT METABOLISM

Thyroid hormones exert an enormous range of effects on lipid metabolism, and in the thyrotoxic state lipid synthesis, mobilization, and degradation are all accelerated. The turnover of plasma triglyceride is markedly enhanced, and both lipoprotein lipase activity and chylomicron triglyceride clearance are increased in skeletal muscle.[49] Although fatty acid synthesis is increased in both adipose tissue and liver,[50,51] degradation of most lipids appears to be stimulated out of proportion to synthesis; body lipid depots consequently become depleted and plasma concentrations of various lipid components fall. Although most of these effects have of necessity been studied in laboratory animals, such data as are available from humans with thyrotoxicosis are similar (see later discussion).

Rates of fatty acid oxidation and free fatty acid release from adipose tissue are increased in both human and experimental thyrotoxicosis. Adipose tissue from thyrotoxic animals releases fatty acids at an enhanced rate under basal conditions,[52] and in humans the normal mobilization of lipid stores and rise in plasma free fatty acid concentrations in response to both fasting[53–56] and catecholamines[55] are enhanced. Although norepinephrine significantly enhances lipolysis in adipose tissue from thyrotoxic humans,[57] the role of sympathomimetic amines in mediating a number of the metabolic abnormalities of adipose tissue in the thyrotoxic state remains unclear. Adipose tissue from thyrotoxic rats demonstrates both increased adenylyl cyclase activity[58] and an increased lipolytic response to catecholamines.[52] Increased lipolysis in humans with thyrotoxicosis is accompanied by increased triglyceride-fatty acid cycling, which may contribute to excessive energy expenditure.[59] High concentrations of thyroid hormones also have direct (in vitro) effects on a variety of functions of isolated fat cells. These include both an increase in oxygen consumption[60] and a potentiation of the lipolytic actions of supraphysiologic concentrations of epinephrine[61,62] and of adrenocorticotropin, thyrotropin, and glucagon.[61] Isolated white fat cells from thyrotoxic rats accumulate more cyclic adenosine monophosphate in response to epinephrine than do the same cells from normal rats, even though the number of β-adrenergic receptors per cell appears to be unaltered.[63] Increased hydrolysis of triglyceride results in release of glycerol, which, in turn, becomes available for increased hepatic gluconeogenesis.[64]

In rats, increased lipolysis is accompanied by an increased rate of fatty acid re-esterification,[59,65] but there is a net loss of triglyceride stores. It has been estimated that the increase in oxygen consumption of adipose tissue from thyrotoxic animals can be accounted for quantitatively by the energy requirement for accelerated re-esterification.[65] This is consistent with the finding that, in contrast to its effects on many other cells, ouabain (a selective inhibitor of $Na^+_1K^+$-ATPase) has no effect on the T_3-induced increment in oxygen consumption in isolated white fat cells in vitro.[66]

In addition to a more than 50% rise in the fasting plasma concentration of free fatty acids,[53–56] there is about a 50% increase in plasma triglyceride concentrations in patients with thyrotoxicosis.[56] The latter reflects augmented production of triglycerides by the liver without concomitant change in the fractional rate of peripheral removal. The increase in overall plasma triglyceride turnover is accompanied by a rise in plasma postheparin lipolytic activity, and in association with these changes there is as much as a doubling of both free fatty acid and glycerol concentrations in plasma.[56]

Plasma phospholipid and low-density lipoprotein cholesterol concentrations fall, and an enhanced rate of cholesterol synthesis is counterbalanced by a concomitant increase in the rate of cholesterol degradation and excretion. The rate of cholesterol excretion in the bile is strikingly enhanced in thyrotoxic rats.[67] Increased excretion, as well as a reduction in the concentration of low-density lipoprotein cholesterol- and phospholipid-binding apolipoproteins because of their accelerated catabolism, probably accounts for the corresponding reductions in plasma cholesterol and phospholipids in humans.[68]

CARBOHYDRATE METABOLISM

Utilization of carbohydrate by extrahepatic tissues is enhanced in thyrotoxicosis,[69] and glucose absorption, utilization, and production are increased. The increased rate of glucose utilization is accompanied by enhanced hepatic gluconeogenesis from both lactate (by way of the Cori cycle)[64,70] and glycerol.[64] The magnitude of the contribution of endogenous amino acids derived from muscle breakdown to gluconeogenesis in the thyrotoxic state remains unknown, but the rate of conversion of alanine to glucose is markedly increased in the livers of thyrotoxic rats.[71]

Hepatic glycogen stores are depleted in thyrotoxic animals[7,72,73] and liver biopsy samples from humans with thyrotoxicosis.[74] The mechanisms remain uncertain, but T_3 may increase the activity of both liver phosphorylase kinase and lysosomal α-glucosidase.[75] Hepatic α- and β-adrenergic receptor numbers are decreased in the thyrotoxic state,[76,77] cyclic adenosine monophosphate generation is reduced in response to β-adrenergic agonists, and maximal glycogen phosphorylase responses to both α- and β-agonists are blunted.[78]

Carbohydrate Tolerance

Although fasting plasma glucose concentrations are usually normal in patients with thyrotoxicosis,[79,80] the concentrations tend to increase supranormally after oral glucose administration. Perhaps the most common abnormality is an abnormally rapid rise in plasma glucose after glucose ingestion, but some patients have a delayed peak plasma glucose or a peak value that is higher than in normal subjects.[54,79,80] These abnormalities may reflect changes in glucose absorption rather than metabolism inasmuch as many of the patients who have abnormal oral glucose tolerance have normal responses to intravenous glucose administration.[81,82] Glucose intolerance, depending on the criteria used, has been reported in up to 57% of patients with thyrotoxicosis,[83] and the incidence of postprandial glycosuria has been reported to be as high as 38%.[84] The incidence of clinically important diabetes mellitus is considerably less, perhaps as low as 2% to 3%.[84] Preexisting diabetes is almost always aggravated during thyrotoxicosis; there is usually an increase in insulin requirement, and there may be an increased tendency for the development of ketoacidosis. Latent diabetes may become unmasked; sustained hyperglycemia sufficient to require insulin therapy is almost always a sign of underlying diabetes mellitus.[85]

Glucose Uptake

The rate of glucose uptake by many peripheral tissues is increased in thyrotoxicosis. Forearm muscle glucose uptake is markedly increased in patients with thyrotoxicosis, with increased fluxes of glucose through both the oxidative and nonoxidative pathways,[86] and treatment of rats with T_3 increases the expression of the muscle/fat cell glucose transporter-gene in skeletal muscle.[87] Administration of T_3 to humans results in a marked increase in muscle glucose uptake, muscle alanine and glutamine release, and hepatic gluconeogenesis, even in the absence of changes in plasma insulin concentrations.[88,89] Thyroid hormone also stimulates both glucose production and glucose disposal in humans even when pancreatic hormone secretion is blocked by the administration of somatostatin.[90] These effects reflect an influence of thyroid hormone on target tissues independent of any effect of the hormone on plasma insulin concentrations. Indeed, in humans thyroid hormone excess induces appreciable insulin resistance at a postbinding site in both the liver and peripheral tissues, and this resistance is accompanied by increased insulin clearance and a compensatory increase in insulin secretion,[91] consistent with earlier demonstrations of a decrease in plasma insulin half-life in thyrotoxic animals.[92] Although insulin secretion rates under basal conditions are similar to those in normal subjects, patients with spontaneous thyrotoxicosis have an enhanced insulin secretory response to meals.[93] Insulin receptor number is decreased in adipocytes from thyrotoxic patients[94] but unchanged in liver membranes from thyrotoxic rats.[95]

A direct stimulatory effect of thyroid hormone on glucose uptake is demonstrable in chick embryo heart cells,[96] human fibroblasts,[97] rat thymocytes,[98] and in several continuous cell lines derived from normal rat liver.[35,99] In some of these systems the increase in glucose uptake is accompanied by an increase in lactate production.[35,97] Although the time course of the stimulation of glucose uptake and the mechanism by which it is mediated appear to vary among different cell types, the enhancement of glucose uptake in at least some of these systems represents facilitation of glucose transport at the level of the plasma membrane.[96,99–101] The stimulation of glucose transport appears to be mediated by an increase in plasma membrane glucose transporter abundance as well as activation of glucose transporters pre-existing in the plasma membrane.[101]

PROTEIN METABOLISM

Thyrotoxicosis in laboratory animals results in stimulation of both synthesis and degradation of protein. Under most circumstances degradation predominates, and in both experimental and human thyrotoxicosis there is net protein catabolism, negative nitrogen balance, and loss of muscle mass. The administration of T_3 markedly increases the release of alanine and other gluconeogenic amino acids from muscle,[88] and a variable degree of muscle atrophy is common.[2] The rate of urea synthesis, reflecting enhanced amino-nitrogen metabolism, is increased substantially in patients with thyrotoxicosis.[89] Although an increase in protein degradation thus accompanies the increased catabolism of fat and carbohydrate, it can be minimized, and indeed in some instances reversed, if dietary protein and calorie intake are increased sufficiently,[102] and some thyrotoxic patients are able to gain weight. There may be loss of protein from body stores other than muscle, and decreased collagen synthesis and increased degradation may, for example, account in part for the typical thinning of the skin in thyrotoxicosis.[103] There may be mild hypoalbuminemia. Mitochondrial and microsomal protein synthesis are both enhanced by excess thyroid hormone, but the mechanisms remain unknown. Treatment of normal rats with T_4 increases in vitro amino acid incorporation by liver mitochondria,[104] and the addition of mitochondria from T_4-treated rats stimulates amino acid incorporation into protein by microsomes from normal rats in vitro.[105] High concentrations of T_4 added directly to mitochondria in vitro can stimulate mitochondrial amino acid incorporation,[106] and the administration of thyroid hormone to rats markedly stimulates both the synthesis and degradation of mitochondrial protein in liver and heart.[107] The mechanisms by which the thyroid hormones may stimulate protein synthesis are reviewed elsewhere (see chap 9). Despite widespread stimulation of both protein synthesis and protein degradation, it is unlikely that increased protein synthesis itself accounts for more than a small fraction of the increased energy demand in thyrotoxicosis.[22,23]

In addition to stimulating overall synthesis and degradation of protein in a variety of tissues, thyroid hormone excess influences the rates of synthesis or degradation, or both, of a large number of individual enzymes to result in either increases or decreases in enzyme activity.[108,109] The physiologic importance of most of these changes is obscure, but one of the changes that may have important physiologic consequences is the increase in $Na^+_1K^+$-ATPase[25] discussed earlier. Another widely studied enzyme is α-glycerophosphate dehydrogenase,[110,111] an enzyme important in carbohydrate catabolism, which under some circumstances increases as much as 90-fold under the influence of thyroid hormone. Thyroid hormones also are potent stimulators of hepatic malic enzyme synthesis.[110,111]

MINERAL METABOLISM

Thyrotoxicosis may result in marked abnormalities of calcium and phosphorus metabolism and can cause as much as a threefold increase in urinary and fecal calcium excretion.[112] Bone formation and resorption in bone are both enhanced,[113] although intestinal absorption of calcium is decreased.[114] In a large older series about 15% of patients with thyrotoxicosis had plasma calcium concentrations above 10.6 mg/dL (2.6 mmol/L)[115]; today the proportion with hypercalcemia would certainly be smaller. Derangements in the metabolism of calcium, phosphorus, other minerals, and bone are considered in greater detail elsewhere (see chap 48).

DRUG AND HORMONE METABOLISM

The metabolism and excretion of many drugs are accelerated in the thyrotoxic state, and the maintenance doses of a number of drugs must be increased in patients with thyrotoxicosis. As an example, the daily administration of 0.5 mg digoxin for a week in one study resulted in substantially lower plasma digoxin concentrations in thyrotoxic than in hypothyroid patients (mean plasma concentrations 0.7 and 1.5 ng/mL, respectively), and the plasma half-life of digoxin was shorter in the former group.[116] The reduced plasma half-life of digoxin in thyrotoxic patients was attributed to both an enhanced glomerular filtration rate and an increased rate of digoxin degradation.[116] Administration of thyroid hormone to rats re-

sults in the acceleration of the hepatic metabolism of a variety of other drugs.[117,118] The magnitude of the effect is variable, however, and the rate of metabolism of certain drugs is in fact reduced in the thyrotoxic state.[117]

Patients with thyrotoxicosis are particularly sensitive to the anticoagulant effects of warfarin, despite the fact that the plasma half-life of the drug in these patients is unchanged.[119] The heightened response may be caused by more rapid clearance of vitamin K-dependent coagulation factors rather than changes in the action or metabolism of warfarin.[119] Thyrotoxic rats similarly have increased sensitivity to warfarin.[120]

The effects of thyrotoxicosis on hormone metabolism have received considerable attention. In general, both synthetic and degradative rates are increased, so that plasma hormone concentrations remain normal. For example, the plasma half-life of insulin is decreased in rabbits[92] and humans[91] with experimental thyrotoxicosis, but the secretion rate is correspondingly increased so that plasma insulin concentrations do not change.[88,92] In contrast, growth hormone secretion is decreased without an appreciable change in the half-life of the hormone.[121] Changes in adrenal and gonadal steroid and catecholamine metabolism are discussed in chapters 45, 47, and 46, respectively.

The metabolism of the thyroid hormones themselves is markedly accelerated in thyrotoxicosis. The plasma half-lives of T_4[122] and T_3[110] may be reduced by as much as 40% to 50% in humans, and the turnover of both hormones is correspondingly increased.[123–125] In thyrotoxic rats the total T_4 clearance rate is more than doubled as a consequence of increases in both fecal and deiodinative clearances.[126,127] In humans, the metabolic clearance and production rates of 3,3',5'-triiodothyronine (reverse T_3)[128] and of 3',5'-diiodothyronine[129] are increased as well. The rate of conversion of T_4 to T_3 is increased in liver from thyrotoxic rats,[130] an increase that is largely attributable to an increase in type 1 T_4-5'-monodeiodinase activity.[131]

References

1. Blahd WH, Hays MT. Graves' disease in the male: a review of 241 cases treated with an individually calculated dose of sodium iodide I 131. Arch Intern Med 1972;129:33
2. Ramsay I. Thyroid disease and muscle dysfunction. Chicago: Heinemann, 1974:1
3. Magnus-Levy A. Über den respiratorischen Gaswechsel unter dem Einfluss der Thyroidea sowie unter verschiedenen pathologischen Zuständen. Klin Wochenschr 1895;32:650
4. Barker SB, Klitgaard HM. Metabolism of tissues excised from thyroxine-injected rats. Am J Physiol 1952;170:81
5. Schulz H, Low H, Ernster L, Sjöstrand FS. Electronenmikroscopische Studien an Leberschnitten von Thyroxin-behandelten Ratten. In: Sjöstrand FS, Rhodin J, eds. Electron microscopy: proceedings of the Stockholm conference. September 1956. New York: Academic Press, 1957:134
6. Paget GE, Thorp JM. An effect of thyroxin on the fine structure of the rat liver cell. Nature 1963;199:1307
7. Douglas JE. Thyroxine-induced alterations in the fine structure of rat liver cells. Johns Hopkins Med J 1964;114:253
8. Engel AG. Electron microscopic observations in thyrotoxic and corticosteroid-induced myopathies. Mayo Clin Proc 1966;41:785
9. Hoch FL, Lipmann F. The uncoupling of respiration and phosphorylation by thyroid hormones. Proc Natl Acad Sci U S A 1954;40:909

10. Hoch FL. Biochemical actions of thyroid hormones. Physiol Rev 1962;42:605

11. Himms-Hagen J. Brown adipose tissue metabolism and thermogenesis. Annu Rev Nutr 1985;5:69

12. Silva JE, Larsen PR. Adrenergic activation of triiodothyronine production in brown adipose tissue. Nature 1983;305:712

13. Silva JE, Larsen PR. Potential of brown adipose tissue type II thyroxine 5′-deiodinase as a systemic source of triiodothyronine in rats. J Clin Invest 1985;76:2296

14. Bianco AC, Silva JE. Intracellular conversion of thyroxine to triiodothyronine is required for the optimal thermogenic function of brown adipose tissue. J Clin Invest 1987;79:295

15. Bianco AC, Silva JE. Cold exposure rapidly induces virtual saturation of brown adipose tissue nuclear T_3 receptors. Am J Physiol 1988;255:E496

16. Rehnmark S, Bianco AC, Kieffer JD, Silva JE. Transcriptional and post-transcriptional mechanisms in uncoupling protein response to cold. Am J Physiol 1992;262:E58

17. Reiter RJ, Klaus S, Ebbinghaus C, et al. Inhibition of 5′-deiodination of thyroxine suppresses the cold-induced increase in brown adipose tissue messenger ribonucleic acid for mitochondrial uncoupling protein without influencing lipoprotein lipase activity. Endocrinology 1990;126:2550

18. Carvalho SD, Kimura ET, Bianco AC, Silva JE. Central role of brown adipose tissue thyroxine 5′-deiodinase on thyroid hormone-dependent thermogenic response to cold. Endocrinology 1991;128:2149

19. Bianco AC, Kieffer JD, Silva JE. Adenosine 3′,5′-monophosphate and thyroid hormone control by uncoupling protein in freshly dispersed brown adipocytes. Endocrinology 1992;130:2625

20. Guerra C, Porras A, Roncero C, et al. Triiodothyronine induces the expression of the uncoupling protein in long term fetal rat brown adipocyte primary cultures: role of nuclear thyroid hormone receptor expression. Endocrinology 1994;134:1067

21. Welle S, Nair KS. Relationship of resting metabolic rate to body composition and protein turnover. Am J Physiol 1990;258:E990

22. Buchanan JL, Primack MP, Tapley DF. Effect of inhibition of mitochondrial protein synthesis in vitro upon thyroxine stimulation of oxygen consumption. Endocrinology 1971;89:534

23. Ismail-Beigi F, Dietz T, Edelman IS. Thyroid thermogenesis: minimal contribution of energy requirement for protein synthesis. Mol Cell Endocrinol 1976;5:1

24. Ismail-Beigi F, Edelman IS. Mechanism of thyroid calorigenesis: role of active sodium transport. Proc Natl Acad Sci USA 1970;67:1071

25. Ismail-Beigi F, Edelman IS. The mechanism of the calorigenic action of thyroid hormone: stimulation of $Na^+ + K^+$-activated adenosine triphosphatase activity. J Gen Physiol 1971;57:710

26. Whittam R. The interdependence of metabolism and active transport. In: Hoffman JF, ed. The cellular functions of membrane transport. Englewood Cliffs, NJ: Prentice-Hall, 1964:139

27. Smith TJ, Edelman IS. The role of sodium transport in thyroid thermogenesis. Fed Proc 1979;38:2150

28. Guernsey DL, Edelman IS. Regulation of thermogenesis by thyroid hormones. In: Oppenheimer JH, Samuels HH, eds. Molecular basis of thyroid hormone action. New York: Academic Press, 1983:293

29. Lin MH, Akera T. Increased (Na^+, K^+)-ATPase concentrations in various tissues of rats caused by thyroid hormone treatment. J Biol Chem 1978;253:723

30. Edelman IS. Thyroid thermogenesis. N Engl J Med 1974;290:1303

31. Ismail-Beigi F, Bissell DM, Edelman IS. Thyroid thermogenesis in adult rat hepatocytes in primary monolayer culture: direct action of thyroid hormone in vitro. J Gen Physiol 1979;73:369

32. Kim D, Smith TW. Effects of thyroid hormone on sodium pump sites, sodium content, and contractile responses to cardiac glycosides in cultured chick ventricular cells. J Clin Invest 1984;74:1481

33. Gregg VA, Edelman IS. The response of an established line of rat liver cells to thyroid hormone. Biochim Biophys Acta 1986;887:319

34. Ismail-Beigi F, Haber RS, Loeb JN. Stimulation of active Na^+ and K^+ transport by thyroid hormone in a rat liver cell line: role of enhanced Na^+ entry. Endocrinology 1986;119:2527

35. Haber RS, Ismail-Beigi F, Loeb JN. Time course of Na,K transport and other metabolic responses to thyroid hormone in clone 9 cells. Endocrinology 1988;123:238

36. Haber RS, Loeb JN. Selective induction of high-ouabain-affinity isoform of Na^+-K^+-ATPase by thyroid hormone. Am J Physiol 1988;255:E912

37. Gick GG, Melikian J, Ismail-Beigi F. Thyroidal enhancement of rat myocardial Na,K-ATPase: preferential expression of α_2 activity and mRNA abundance. J Membrane Biol 1990;115:273

38. Chinet A, Clausen T, Girardier L. Microcalorimetric determination of energy expenditure due to active sodium-potassium transport in the soleus muscle and brown adipose tissue of the rat. J Physiol 1977;265:43

39. Folke M, Sestoft L. Thyroid calorigenesis in perfused rat liver: minor role of active sodium-potassium transport. J Physiol (Lond) 1977;269:407

40. Biron R, Burger A, Chinet A, et al. Thyroid hormones and the energetics of active sodium-potassium transport in mammalian skeletal muscle. J Physiol 1979;297:47

41. van Hardeveld C, Kassenaar AAH. Evidence that the thyroid state influences Ca^{++}-mediated processes in perfused skeletal muscle. Horm Metab Res 1981;13:33

42. Haber RS, Loeb JN. Early enhancement of passive potassium efflux from rat liver by thyroid hormone: relation to induction of Na,K-ATPase. Endocrinology 1984;115:291

43. Asano Y. Increased cell membrane permeability to Na^+ and K^+ induced by thyroid hormone in rat skeletal muscle. Experientia [Suppl] 1978;32:199

44. Haber RS, Loeb JN. Effect of T_3 treatment on potassium efflux from isolated rat diaphragm: role of increased permeability in the thermogenic response. Endocrinology 1982;111:1217

45. Loeb JN, Haber RS, Ismail-Beigi F. Thyroid hormone and Na,K transport. Trans Am Clin Clim Assoc 1986;98:176

46. Gick GG, Ismail-Beigi F. Thyroid hormone induction of Na,K-ATPase and its mRNAs in a rat liver cell line. Am J Physiol 1990;258:C544

47. Kinsella J, Sacktor B. Thyroid hormones increase Na^+-H^+ exchange activity in renal brush border membranes. Proc Natl Acad Sci U S A 1985;82:3606

48. Yonemura K, Cheng L, Sacktor B, Kinsella JL. Stimulation by thyroid hormone of Na^+-H^+ exchange activity in cultured opossum kidney cells. Am J Physiol 1990;258:F333

49. Kaciuba-Uscilko H, Dudley GA, Terjung RL. Influence of thyroid status on skeletal muscle LPL activity and TG uptake. Am J Physiol 1980;238:E518

50. Freake HC, Schwartz HL, Oppenheimer JH. The regulation of lipogenesis by thyroid hormone and its contribution to thermogenesis. Endocrinology 1989;125:2868

51. Blennemann B, Moon YK, Freake HC. Tissue-specific regulation of fatty acid synthesis by thyroid hormone. Endocrinology 1992;130:637

52. Debons AF, Schwartz IL. Dependence of the lipolytic action of epinephrine in vitro upon thyroid hormone. J Lipid Res 1961;2:86

53. Rich C, Bierman EL, Schwartz IL. Plasma nonesterified fatty acids in hyperthyroid states. J Clin Invest 1959;38:275

54. Marks BH, Kiem I, Hills AG. Endocrine influences on fat and carbohydrate metabolism in man. I. Effect of hyperthyroidism on

fasting serum nonesterified fatty acid concentration and on its response to glucose ingestion. Metabolism 1960;9:1133

55. Harlan WR, Lazlo J, Bogdonoff MD, Estes EH. Alterations in free fatty acid metabolism in endocrine disorders. I. Effect of thyroid hormone. J Clin Endocrinol Metab 1963;23:33

56. Nikkila EA, Kekki M. Plasma triglyceride metabolism in thyroid disease. J Clin Invest 1972;51:2103

57. Wahrenberg H, Wennlund A, Arner P. Adrenergic regulation of lipolysis in fat cells from hyperthyroid and hypothyroid patients. J Clin Endocrinol Metab 1994;78:898

58. Brodie BB, Davies JI, Hynie S, et al. Interrelationships of catecholamines with other endocrine systems. Pharmacol Rev 1966;18:273

59. Beylot M, Martin C, Laville M, et al. Lipolytic and ketogenic fluxes in human hyperthyroidism. J Clin Endocrinol Metab 1991;73:42

60. Challoner DR. A direct effect of triiodothyronine on the oxygen consumption of rat fat cells. Am J Physiol 1969;216:905

61. Vaughan M. An in vitro effect of triiodothyronine on rat adipose tissue. J Clin Invest 1967;46:1482

62. Challoner DR, Allen DO. An in vitro effect of triiodothyronine on lipolysis, cyclic AMP-C^{14} accumulation and oxygen consumption in isolated fat cells. Metabolism 1970;19:480

63. Malbon CC, Moreno FJ, Cabelli RJ, Fain JN. Fat cell adenylate cyclase and β-adrenergic receptors in altered thyroid states. J Biol Chem 1978;253:671

64. Freedland RA, Krebs HA. The effect of thyroxine treatment on the rate of gluconeogenesis in the perfused rat liver. Biochem J 1967;104:45P

65. Fisher JN, Ball EG. Studies on the metabolism of adipose tissue. XX. The effect of thyroid status upon oxygen consumption and lipolysis. Biochemistry 1967;6:637

66. Fain JN, Rosenthal JW. Calorigenic action of triiodothyronine on white fat cells: effects of ouabain, oligomycin, and catecholamines. Endocrinology 1971;89:1205

67. Friedman M, Byers SO, Rosenman RH. Changes in excretion of intestinal cholesterol and sterol digitonides in hyper- and hypothyroidism. Circulation 1952;5:657

68. Walton KW, Scott PJ, Dykes PW, Davies JWL. The significance of alterations in serum lipids in thyroid dysfunction. II. Alterations of the metabolism and turnover of ^{131}I-low-density lipoproteins in hypothyroidism and thyrotoxicosis. Clin Sci 1965;29:217

69. Mirsky IA, Broh-Kahn RH. The effect of experimental hyperthyroidism on carbohydrate metabolism. Am J Physiol 1936;117:6

70. Svedmyr N. Studies on the relationships between some metabolic effects of thyroid hormones and catecholamines in animals and man. Acta Physiol Scand [Suppl] 1966;68:274

71. Singh S, Snyder AK. Effect of thyrotoxicosis on gluconeogenesis from alanine in the perfused rat liver. Endocrinology 1978;102:182

72. Kuriyama S. The influence of thyroid feeding upon carbohydrate metabolism. I. The storage and mobilization of the liver glycogen in thyroid-fed animals. J Biol Chem 1918;33:193

73. Coggeshall HC, Greene JA. The influence of desiccated thyroid gland, thyroxin and inorganic iodine upon the storage of glycogen in the liver of the albino rat under controlled conditions. Am J Physiol 1933;105:103

74. Pipher J, Poulsen E. Liver biopsy in thyrotoxicosis. Acta Med Scand 1947;127:439

75. Nebioglu S, Wathanaronchai P, Nebioglu D, et al. Mechanisms underlying enhanced glycogenolysis in livers of 3,5,3'-triiodothyronine-treated rats. Am J Physiol 1990;258:E109

76. Malbon CC, LoPresti JJ. Hyperthyroidism impairs the activation of glycogen phosphorylase by epinephrine in rat hepatocytes. J Biol Chem 1981;256:12199

77. Malbon CC, Greenberg ML. 3,3',5-Triiodothyronine administration in vivo modulates the hormone-sensitive adenylate cyclase system of rat hepatocytes. J Clin Invest 1982;69:414

78. Bilezikian JP, Loeb JN. The influence of hyperthyroidism and hypothyroidism on α- and β-adrenergic receptor systems and adrenergic responsiveness. Endocr Rev 1983;4:378

79. Hales CN, Hyams DE. Plasma concentrations of glucose, nonesterified fatty acid, and insulin during oral glucose-tolerance tests in thyrotoxicosis. Lancet 1964;2:69

80. Woeber KA, Arky R, Braverman LE. Reversal by guanethidine of abnormal oral glucose tolerance in thyrotoxicosis. Lancet 1966;1:895

81. Althausen TL, Stockholm M. Influence of thyroid gland on absorption in the digestive tract. Am J Physiol 1938;123:577

82. Amatuzio DS, Schultz AL, Vanderbilt MJ, et al. The effect of epinephrine, insulin, and hyperthyroidism on the rapid intravenous glucose tolerance test. J Clin Invest 1954;33:97

83. Kreines K, Jett M, Knowles HC. Observations in hyperthyroidism of abnormal glucose tolerance and other traits related to diabetes mellitus. Diabetes 1965;14:740

84. Joslin EP, Lahey FH. Diabetes and hyperthyroidism. Am J Med Sci 1928;119:2527

85. Kozak GP, Cooppan R. Diabetes and other endocrinologic disorders. In: Marble A, Krall LP, Bradley RF, et al, eds. Joslin's diabetes mellitus. 12th ed. Philadelphia: Lea & Febiger, 1985:784

86. Foss MC, Paccola GM, Saad MJ, et al. Peripheral glucose metabolism in human hyperthyroidism. J Clin Endocrinol Metab 1990;70:1167

87. Weinstein SP, Watts J, Haber RS. Thyroid hormone increases muscle/fat glucose transporter gene expression in rat skeletal muscle. Endocrinology 1991;129:455

88. Sandler MP, Robinson RP, Rabin D, et al. The effect of thyroid hormones on gluconeogenesis and forearm metabolism in man. J Clin Endocrinol Metab 1983;56:479

89. Marchesini G, Fabbri A, Bianchi GP, et al. Hepatic conversion of amino-nitrogen to urea in thyroid diseases. II. A study in hyperthyroid patients. Metab Clin Exp 1994;43:1023

90. Müller MJ, Burger AG, Ferrannini E, et al. Glucoregulatory function of thyroid hormones: role of pancreatic hormones. Am J Physiol 1989;256:E101

91. Dimitriadis G, Baker B, Marsh H, et al. Effect of thyroid hormone excess on action, secretion, and metabolism of insulin in humans. Am J Physiol 1985;248:E593

92. Marecek RL, Feldman JM. Effect of hyperthyroidism on insulin and glucose dynamics in rabbits. Endocrinology 1973;92:1604

93. O'Meara MN, Blackman JD, Sturis J, Polonsky KS. Alterations in the kinetics of C-peptide and insulin secretion in hyperthyroidism. J Clin Endocrinol Metab 1993;76:79

94. Arner P, Bolinder J, Wennlund A, Ostman J. Influence of thyroid hormone level on insulin action in human adipose tissue. Diabetes 1984;33:369

95. DeRuyter H, Burman KD, Wartofsky L, Taylor SI. Effects of thyroid hormone on the insulin receptor in rat liver membranes. Endocrinology 1982;110:1922

96. Gordon A, Schwartz H, Gross J. The stimulation of sugar transport in heart cells grown in a serum-free medium by picomolar concentrations of thyroid hormones: the effects of insulin and hydrocortisone. Endocrinology 1986;118:52

97. Yoshizato K, Kikuyama S, Shioya N. Stimulation of glucose utilization and lactate production in cultured human fibroblasts by thyroid hormone. Biochim Biophys Acta 1980;627:23

98. Segal J, Ingbar SH. In vivo stimulation of sugar uptake in rat thymocytes: an extranuclear action of 3,5,3'-triiodothyronine. J Clin Invest 1985;76:1575

99. Weinstein SP, Watts J, Graves PN, Haber RS. Stimulation of glucose transport by thyroid hormone in ARL 15 cells: increased

abundance of glucose transporter protein and messenger ribonucleic acid. Endocrinology 1990;126:1421

100. Segal J, Ingbar SH. Stimulation of 2-deoxy-D-glucose uptake in rat thymocytes in vitro by physiologic concentrations of triiodothyronine, insulin, or epinephrine. Endocrinology 1980;107:1354

101. Kuruvilla AK, Perez C, Ismail-Beigi F, Loeb JN. Regulation of glucose transport in Clone 9 cells by thyroid hormone. Biochim Biophys Acta 1991;1094:300

102. Du Bois EF. Basal metabolism in health and disease. 3rd ed. Philadelphia: Lea & Febiger, 1936:333

103. Fink CW, Ferguson JL, Smiley JD. Effect of hyperthyroidism and hypothyroidism on collagen metabolism. J Lab Clin Med 1967;69:950

104. Roodyn DB, Freeman KB, Tata JR. The stimulation by treatment in vivo with triiodothyronine of amino acid incorporation into protein by isolated rat liver mitochondria. Biochem J 1965;94:628

105. Sokoloff L, Kaufman E. Thyroxine stimulation of amino acid incorporation into protein. J Biol Chem 1961;236:795

106. Bronk JR. The nature of the energy requirement for amino acid incorporation by isolated mitochondria and its significance for thyroid hormone action. Proc Natl Acad Sci USA 1963;50:524

107. Gross NJ. Control of mitochondrial turnover under the influence of thyroid hormone. J Cell Biol 1971;48:29

108. Pugsley LI, Anderson E. The effect of desiccated thyroid, irradiated ergosterol, and ammonium chloride on the excretion of calcium in rats. Biochem J 1934;28:754

109. Ruzicka FJ, Rose DP. The influence of thyroidal status on rat hepatic NADH duroquinone reductase. Endocrinology 1981; 109:664

110. Woeber KA, Sobel RJ, Ingbar SH, Sterling K. The peripheral metabolism of triiodothyronine in normal subjects and in patients with hyperthyroidism. J Clin Invest 1970;49:643

111. Oppenheimer JH, Silva E, Schwartz HL, Surks MI. Stimulation of hepatic mitochondrial α-glycerophosphate dehydrogenase and malic enzyme by L-triiodothyronine. J Clin Invest 1977;59:517

112. Aub JC, Bauer W, Heath C, Ropes M. Studies of calcium and phosphorus metabolism. III. The effects of the thyroid hormone and thyroid disease. J Clin Invest 1929;7:97

113. Krane SM, Brownell GL, Stanbury JB, Corrigan H. The effect of thyroid disease on calcium metabolism in man. J Clin Invest 1956;35:874

114. Haldimann B, Kaptein EM, Singer FR, et al. Intestinal calcium absorption in patients with hyperthyroidism. J Clin Endocrinol Metab 1980;51:995

115. Baxter JD, Bondy PK. Hypercalcemia of thyrotoxicosis. Ann Intern Med 1966;65:429

116. Croxson MS, Ibbertson HK. Serum digoxin in patients with thyroid disease. BMJ 1975;3:566

117. Conney AH, Garren LD. Contrasting effects of thyroxin on zoxazolamine and hexobarbital metabolism. Biochem Pharmacol 1961;6:257

118. Kato R, Takahashi A. Thyroid hormone and activities of drug-metabolizing enzymes and electron transport systems of rat liver microsomes. Mol Pharmacol 1968;4:109

119. Kellett HA, Sawers JSA, Boulton FE, et al. Problems of anticoagulation with warfarin in hyperthyroidism. Q J Med 1986;58:43

120. Lowenthal J, Fisher LM. The effect of thyroid function on the prothrombin time response to warfarin in rats. Experientia 1957;13:253

121. Finkelstein JW, Boyar RM, Hellman L. Growth hormone secretion in hyperthyroidism. J Clin Endocrinol Metab 1974;38:635

122. Ingbar SH, Freinkel N. Simultaneous estimation of rates of thyroxine degradation and thyroid hormone synthesis. J Clin Invest 1955;34:808

123. Nicoloff JT, Low JC, Dussault JH, Fisher DA. Simultaneous measurement of thyroxine and triiodothyronine peripheral turnover kinetics in man. J Clin Invest 1972;51:473

124. Bianchi R, Zucchelli GC, Giannessi D, et al. Evaluation of triiodothyronine (T_3) kinetics in normal subjects, in hypothyroid, and hyperthyroid patients using specific antiserum for the determination of labeled T_3 in plasma. J Clin Endocrinol Metab 1978;46:203

125. Fish LH, Schwartz HL, Cavanaugh J, et al. Replacement dose, metabolism, and bioavailability of levothyroxine in the treatment of hypothyroidism: role of triiodothyronine in pituitary feedback in humans. N Engl J Med 1987;316:764

126. Cullen MJ, Doherty GF, Ingbar SH. The effect of hypothyroidism and thyrotoxicosis on thyroxine metabolism in the rat. Endocrinology 1973;92:1028

127. Nisula BC, Galton VA, Ingbar SH. A new method for the assessment of thyroxine metabolism in the rat. Endocrinology 1977;100:1432

128. Smallridge RC, Wartofsky L, Desjardins RE, Burman KD. Metabolic clearance and production rates of 3,3',5'-triiodothyronine in hyperthyroid, euthyroid, and hypothyroid subjects. J Clin Endocrinol Metab 1978;47:345

129. Smallridge RC, Burman KD, Smith CE, et al. Metabolic clearance and production rates of 3',5'-diiodothyronine in hyperthyroidism and hypothyroidism in man: comparison of infusions using radiolabeled versus unlabeled iodothyronine. J Clin Endocrinol Metab 1981;52:722

130. Kaplan MM, Utiger RD. Iodothyronine metabolism in liver and kidney homogenates from hyperthyroid and hypothyroid rats. Endocrinology 1978;103:156

131. Kaplan MM. Changes in the particulate subcellular component of hepatic thyroxine-5'-monodeiodinase in hyperthyroid and hypothyroid rats. Endocrinology 1979;105:548

VITAMIN METABOLISM IN THYROTOXICOSIS

Richard S. Rivlin

Many vitamins, particularly the B vitamins, function as coenzymes in enzymatic reactions that are widely distributed throughout the body.[1] Thyrotoxicosis may exert subtle, often insufficiently appreciated effects on vitamin metabolism that, in turn, disrupt critical aspects of intermediary metabolism. Vitamin A and thyroid hormones both affect differentiation, growth and development, and many important metabolic processes. Furthermore, thyroid hormone receptors interact with retinoic acid receptors, suggesting that either can affect the action of the other.[2]

VITAMIN A

Thyrotoxicosis influences the metabolism of vitamin A in several ways. Serum concentrations of vitamin A tend to be reduced,[3] and diminished dark adaptation has been detected in some patients.[4]

The most direct relationship between thyroid hormones and vitamin A relates to their sharing a common serum transport protein, transthyretin, formerly called thyroxine-binding prealbumin (see chap 6). Retinol-binding protein (RBP) forms a one-to-one complex with transthyretin. The molar ratios of RBP and transthyretin and of RBP and vitamin A are similar in normal and thyrotoxic subjects.[5] In response to fasting, serum transthyretin concentrations in animals fall, as do both serum vitamin A and thyroxine (T_4) concentrations.[6] Fasting also decreases the fraction of T_4 binding to transthyretin in vitro.

VITAMIN D

Disturbances in metabolism of calcium and vitamin D are well-recognized features of thyrotoxicosis. Thyroid hormones directly stimulate bone resorption, and hypercalcemia occurs in occasional patients with severe thyrotoxicosis (see chap 48). Serum parathyroid hormone (PTH) concentrations are low and the conversion of 25-hydroxyvitamin D (25[OH]D) to 1,25-dihydroxyvitamin D (1,25[OH]$_2$D) is diminished, resulting in lowered serum concentrations of the latter.[7] Diminished intestinal absorption of calcium is reflected in enhanced fecal excretion and is likely attributable to the diminished production of 1,25(OH$_2$)D. Urinary excretion of calcium is increased, because of increased bone resorption and inhibition of PTH secretion. Calcium balance thus becomes negative as a result of decreased intestinal absorption and increased urinary calcium loss. The clinical importance of these observations is given emphasis by the finding that doses of thyroid hormone only slightly above the usual replacement range for hypothyroid patients have been associated with osteoporosis[8] (see chap 88).

VITAMIN E (α-TOCOPHEROL)

The serum concentrations of vitamin E tend to be low in patients with thyrotoxicosis.[9] To some extent this decrease may be secondary to generalized disturbances in lipid metabolism because the serum concentrations of the high- and low-density lipoproteins in which vitamin E is incorporated are decreased. There are suggestive findings that therapeutic doses of vitamin E may protect the heart of thyrotoxic animals against the effects of oxidative stress, that is, enhanced lipid peroxidation.[10]

RIBOFLAVIN (VITAMIN B₂)

Physiologic doses of thyroid hormones regulate the conversion of dietary riboflavin into its two active flavin coenzymes, riboflavin-5'-phosphate, formerly called flavin mononucleotide (FMN), and flavin adenine dinucleotide (FAD), and into flavins bound covalently to tissue proteins (Fig 49-1). The activity of flavokinase, the enzyme that converts riboflavin to FMN, is increased twofold by thyroid hormones, as are the activities of a wide variety of enzymes that require FMN or FAD as a coenzyme.[11]

Of particular importance is that thyroid hormones regulate riboflavin metabolism during development. The increased hepatic synthesis of FAD stimulated by thyroid hormones occurs in animals of any age, but in brain FAD synthesis is increased only in newborn animals. The stimulation of tadpole metamorphosis induced by thyroid hormones can be blunted by structural analogues of riboflavin.[12]

Evidence that riboflavin metabolism is regulated by thyroid hormones in humans is provided by studies of erythrocyte glutathione reductase, an FAD-containing enzyme, the activity coefficient of which is widely used as an index of the riboflavin-deficient state. Treatment of hypothyroid patients with 50 μg of T_4 for 2 weeks without changing dietary intake converts the elevated activity coefficient from the riboflavin-deficient range to normal.[13]

OTHER VITAMINS

Disturbances in the metabolism at vitamin K are not prominent in thyrotoxicosis. However, treatment with large doses of thyroid hormones has been reported to potentiate the action of anticoagulant drugs.

Thiamine deficiency is well recognized as a cause of high output cardiac failure but has not been clearly implicated in thyrotoxic heart disease. Studies in animals suggest that thiamine may have some benefit as an adjunct in the therapy of thyrotoxicosis.

In experimental animals, T_4 decreases the hepatic concentrations of niacin-dependent coenzymes (nicotinamide adenine dinucleotide, nicotinamide adenine dinucleotide phosphate and its reduced form), but the clinical importance of these findings is unknown. Preliminary evidence has been

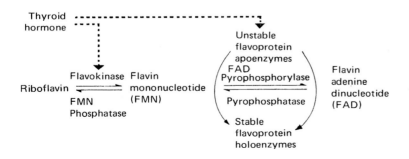

FIGURE 49-1. Enzymatic conversion of riboflavin to FMN and FAD, and stabilization of flavoprotein apoenzymes by their appropriate coenzymes. The postulated role of thyroid hormone in regulating this sequence is shown by dashed lines. An arrow points to flavokinase, the only enzyme shown that undergoes a decrease in activity in hypothyroidism and that increases twofold in thyrotoxicosis. Lesser increases are observed in the activities of FMN phosphatase and FAD pyrophosphorylase. The effect of thyroid hormone on pyrophosphatase in unknown. (Reproduced from Rivlin RS. Medical aspects of vitamin B₂. In: Miller F. ed. Chemistry and biochemistry of flavins. Boca Raton, FL: CRC Press, 1991:201)

obtained in support of vitamin B_6 (pyridoxal phosphate) deficiency in thyrotoxicosis.

Serum concentrations of vitamin B_{12} and folic acid tend to be either normal or low in patients with thyrotoxicosis (see chap 42). The prevalence of pernicious anemia is increased and the turnover of folic acid is accelerated in thyrotoxicosis caused by Graves' disease. Anemia in thyrotoxicosis may less commonly be due primarily to high serum thyroid hormone concentrations alone, independent of the cause.[14]

References

1. Rivlin RS. Disorders of vitamin metabolism: deficiencies, metabolic abnormality and excesses. In: Wyngarden JH, Smith LH Jr, Bennett JC, Plum F, eds. Cecil textbook of medicine. 19th ed. Philadelphia: WB Saunders, 1991:1170
2. Zhang XK, Pfahl M. Hetero- and homodimeric receptors in thyroid hormone and vitamin A action. Receptor 1993;3:183
3. Marrocco W, Adonencecchi L, Suraci C, et al. Comportamento della vitamin A, del B-carotene, della proteina leganta it retinolo e dela prealbumina nel plasma di soggetta ipo ed ipertiroidei. Boll Soc Ital Biol Sper 1984;60:769
4. Walton KW, Scott PJ, Dykes PW, Davies JWC. The significance of alterations in serum lipids in thyroid dysfunction. II. Alterations of the metabolism and turnover of ^{131}I-low-density lipoproteins in hypothyroidism and thyrotoxicosis. Clin Sci 1968;29:217
5. Olson JA. Vitamin A. In: Machlin LJ, ed. Handbook of vitamins. 2nd ed. New York: Marcel Dekker, 1990:1
6. Spear PA, Higueret P, Garcin H. Effects of fasting and 3,3′,4,4′,5,5′-hexabromobiphenyl on plasma transport of thyroxine and retinol: fasting reverses elevation of retinol. J Toxicol Environ Health 1994;42:173
7. Bouillon R, Muls E, DeMoor P. Influence of thyroid function on the serum concentration of 1,25-dihydroxyvitamin D. J Clin Endocrinol Metab 1980;51:793
8. Ross DS. Hyperthyroidism, thyroid hormone therapy, and bone. Thyroid 1994;4:319
9. Krishnamurthy S, Prasanna D. Serum vitamin E and lipid peroxides in malnutrition, hyper- and hypothyroidism. Acta Vitaminol Enzymol 1984;6:17
10. Asayama K, Dobashi K, Hayashibe H, Kato K. Vitamin E protects against thyroxine-induced acceleration of lipid peroxidation in cardiac and skeletal muscle of rats. J Nutr Sci Vitaminol (Tokyo) 1989;35:407
11. Rivlin RS. Medical aspects of vitamin B_2. In: Miller F, ed. Chemistry and biochemistry of flavins. Boca Raton, FL: CRC Press, 1991:201
12. Rivlin RS. Riboflavin. In: Ziegler EE, Filer LJ Jr, eds. Present knowledge in nutrition. Washington, DC: ILSI Press 1996; in press
13. Cimino JA, Jhangiani S, Schwartz E, Cooperman JM. Riboflavin metabolism in the hypothyroid human adult. Proc Soc Exp Biol Med 1987;184:151
14. Fein H, Rivlin RS. Anemia in thyroid diseases. Med Clin North Am 1975;59:1133

Werner and Ingbar's The Thyroid, Seventh Edition,
edited by Lewis E. Braverman and Robert D. Utiger.
Lippincott–Raven Publishers, Philadelphia, © 1996

50

Behavioral and Psychiatric Aspects of Thyrotoxicosis

Peter C. Whybrow

HISTORICAL PERSPECTIVE

When Caleb Parry first described the syndrome of hyperfunction of the thyroid gland in 1825, he attributed the disorder he observed in his young female patient to the fear she had experienced when caught in a runaway wheelchair.[1] In his classic description of the syndrome in 1835, Graves also focused on the nervous dysfunction, suggesting a relation of the thyroid gland to the syndrome of globus hystericus.[2] In 1840, Basedow[3] provided the first description of the associated psychosis. It was not until 1886 that Mobius clearly distinguished a thyrotoxic syndrome of endocrine origin from the group of neuroses.[4]

NEUROPSYCHIATRIC MANIFESTATIONS OF THYROTOXICOSIS

The neurobehavioral and psychological changes associated with thyrotoxicosis are multiple and varied.[5–7] Patients complain of subjective anxiety and dysphoria, emotional lability, insomnia, and at times, intellectual dysfunction. Concentration is particularly impaired; indeed, this may be the earliest subjective disturbance, associated with a growing restlessness and tremulousness. Such people appear irritable, jittery, and easily moved to anger; some may express ideas of reference and frank paranoia. Thoughts and words can come rapidly and are disjointed at times, suggesting a thought disorder.

Motor activity is increased but usually associated with agitation; although this may mimic manic behavior, the fully developed psychiatric syndrome of mania is surprisingly rare in association with thyrotoxicosis. Sleep disturbances including vivid dreams and nightmares are common, but energy levels often are decreased. This latter feature is an important distinction from mania, in which increased energy, irritability, and decreased sleep form the common presentation. When true mania and hypomania have been reported in uncomplicated thyrotoxicosis,[8–12] these patients typically have a previous diagnosis of bipolar disorder or a strong family history of the illness.

Episodic anxiety, frequently in association with subjective awareness of tachycardia or arrhythmia, is a common complaint in thyrotoxicosis. Indeed, some of these diffuse dysphoric feelings have been reported in normal subjects given high doses of thyroid hormone.[13]

In rare instances, the behavioral dysfunction may progress to a nonspecific psychotic illness with bizarre delusional thoughts, usually of a paranoid nature. A careful mental status examination in such people usually reveals associated cognitive clouding, suggesting that the psychotic phenomena are directly correlated with this evidence of delirium.[7,13] Electroencephalographic recordings support these observations; the few studies that have been conducted found abnormal slow activity admixed with paroxysmal fast waves and an augmented response to photic stimulation.[14,15] With the onset of thyrotoxic storm (now a rare phenomenon), delirium, restlessness, and agitation can appear acutely.[16,17]

In contrast to this picture is the mental state of apathetic thyrotoxicosis.[18] Although an uncommon form of presentation of thyrotoxicosis, its recognition is particularly important in the elderly, in whom it may masquerade as a depressive disorder.[19] The apathy, lethargy, pseudodementia, weight loss, and depressed mood frequently are first diagnosed as melancholia. The true diagnosis is easily overlooked because of the minimal elevation of pulse rate, cool skin, and no hyperphagia. Stare and other common manifestations of thyrotoxicosis including goiter may also be absent.[20] Thus, special vigilance for this type of thyrotoxic syndrome should be maintained, especially in patients who present with atypical depressive disturbances later in life.

The true incidence of neuropsychiatric symptoms in patients with thyrotoxicosis is difficult to estimate because no definitive study using objective diagnostic criteria exists. From nine studies of unselected patients, however, certain trends emerge.[6,7,21–27] Some behavioral change, perhaps best characterized as a tense dysphoria, appears ubiquitous; a subjective awareness of diminished intellectual function is also common. In comparison, frank psychiatric symptoms are rare, probably on the order of 10%.[6,21]

OBJECTIVE BEHAVIORAL ASSESSMENT

During the past 25 years, several groups of investigators have sought to quantify the behavioral changes in thyrotoxicosis, both by comparing patients with matched normal subjects and by studying patients during their illness and after recovery.[7,24,26–29] In general, the studies confirm the clinical descriptions reviewed earlier.

In an early study of 7 women and 3 men with thyrotoxicosis evaluated before and after treatment, and various matched control groups, the patients' performance when thyrotoxic most closely approximated the control group with proven structural or physiologic disturbances of the brain; after treatment, the results were similar to those of normal people.[29] In a study in which 16 patients seen in a medical clinic were studied using the Clyde mood scale to document affective changes, more than half the patients reported depression of mood, but the Clyde score did not deviate from the normal mean.[27] The patients' jittery score was increased and corresponded with consistent reports of anxiety, bouts of tachycardia, and restlessness. The score for clear thinking was reduced, reflecting subjective disorganization of cognition.

A thorough psychological study of middle class Turkish women with thyrotoxicosis revealed multiple abnormalities.[28] The range of educational background of the study and control groups was broad, some being illiterate and some having had 12 years of schooling; the groups were well matched for this variable and for age and socioeconomic status. Of the 23 patients, 10 were retested after treatment. Before treatment, the patients' responses to visual stimuli were slow, with recovery occurring after treatment. The auditory reaction times were also slow but did not return to normal after treatment. The patients' visual motor coordination was less accurate, less steady, slower, and more readily fatigued as compared with the normal subjects, and they made more mistakes on mirror drawing tests.

This documentation of impaired cognition, directly correlated with the thyrotoxic state, also was reported in two subsequent studies. In these studies, thyrotoxic patients performed poorly in the Porteus maze and trail-making tests,[7] and performance on those tasks that require concentration and memory was impaired in proportion to the degree of elevation in their serum thyroxine concentrations.[24]

In both of these studies the Minnesota Multiphasic Personality Inventory (MMPI) was used as part of the assessment. The mean corrected raw scores for the clinical scales of so-

matic distress, depression, anxiety, and schizophrenia were all elevated, although not extraordinarily so. With treatment, the scores declined, but the profile of the test results did not change. Of the 19 women with thyrotoxicosis in the second study, all complained of nervousness, 16 of jumpiness, and 15 of restlessness and tension. More than half registered anxiety and irritability. This constellation of symptoms, which perhaps is best described as tense dysphoria, appears characteristic of the affective state of thyrotoxicosis. These findings were recently confirmed in a study of 15 patients with thyrotoxicosis caused by Graves' disease. Treatment resulted in improvement of the dysphoric mood and cognitive ability.[30] The patients reported being more relaxed and less anxious after treatment, had better comprehension, and were more capable of abstraction.

Depressive affect does occur in thyrotoxicosis, but usually it is intermixed with the more common complaint of anxiety; this is an important distinction from hypothyroidism in which the depressive symptoms are dominant, more florid, and may merge into the melancholic syndrome.[7] Unfortunately, there has been no careful study of the mental state in apathetic thyrotoxicosis, in which depressive mood disturbance does appear to dominate.

BEHAVIORAL SYNDROMES THAT MAY MIMIC THYROTOXICOSIS

In most patients, the diagnosis of thyrotoxicosis presents little difficulty. Problems may arise, however, in older patients who are apathetic and have cardiac arrhythmia, congestive failure, cognitive disturbances, and perhaps depressed mood. Such patients may be erroneously thought to have primary cardiovascular disease. In other patients in whom behavioral and psychological symptoms and signs (i.e., anxiety, agitation, lowered attentiveness, irritability, depressed mood with poorly defined ideas of persecution, insomnia, or depression) are foremost, the picture may be misdiagnosed as an agitated major depression or involutional paranoid psychosis if other indications of thyrotoxicosis are overlooked.

The most frequent misdiagnosis is one of anxiety state or neurosis. The differentiation between thyrotoxicosis and an anxiety state may not be easy, especially in the early stages of either disorder.[31] Unlike thyrotoxicosis, which is usually progressive, the intensity of anxiety states tends to vary over time. There may also be an extended history of other adjustment difficulties, and the anxiety state itself may be associated with specific fears of objects or situations.

Panic attacks may present a particular difficulty in differential diagnosis, especially because of the rapid heart rate and palpitations that accompany them. People with panic attacks often awake in the middle of the night with these symptoms. Their resting pulse rates, however, usually are not elevated as in thyrotoxicosis; also the hands and feet are usually cold and clammy, whereas thyrotoxic patients have warm moist hands and feet. Also, although both anxious and thyrotoxic patients may have difficulty sleeping and may eat more than usual, the former usually do not lose weight or complain of heat intolerance; nor do they have the progressive disturbances of memory, calculation, and problem-solving ability that characterize thyrotoxicosis.

The relationship of thyrotoxic states to mania is complex. Motor acceleration, pressure of speech, and disorganization of thought content frequently are found in the psychoses associated with thyrotoxicosis; however, the constellation of symptoms that is necessary to fulfill the criteria for secondary mania[32] is far less common[9,12]; it usually is not a diagnostic problem. Initiation of thyroid hormone therapy with high doses in hypothyroid patients can undoubtedly precipitate classic mania,[33] especially in patients with a family history of affective illness. This possibility should be considered in a patient who exhibits bizarre or hyperactive behavior while receiving thyroid hormone.

THE ROLE OF PSYCHOLOGICAL FACTORS IN THE PATHOGENESIS OF THYROTOXICOSIS

The role of psychosocial strain and trauma in the precipitation of Graves' disease, which is the most common cause of thyrotoxicosis, has been the subject of debate. Although anecdotal reports and a considerable body of clinical opinion seem to support an association, objective evidence remains elusive. One problem in the assessment of the temporal association is determining the precise onset of thyrotoxicosis. The rapidity of onset is variable, and the disorder is probably subclinical for weeks or months, so that the thyrotoxicosis may have already begun by the time of the supposed precipitating event. Similarly, the reaction to the event may be a reflection of an already disturbed psychophysiology. Information distinguishing these points is difficult to obtain in a retrospective format.

Prospective study undoubtedly would offer better information, but it is difficult to conduct. However, in one such study, subjects from the general population who had "thyroid hot spots"—areas of the thyroid gland found on screening to concentrate radioactive iodine avidly—were followed carefully over time. The psychological and thyroid evaluations were independent of each other. In a 12-year follow-up study of 239 women, the hot spots appeared to wax and wane in a direct relation with life stress, and some women developed clinical thyrotoxicosis during conditions of severe or prolonged life strain.[34,35]

Two recent studies have explored the onset of Graves' disease, using a controlled retrospective methodology. In a case-controlled study patients developing Graves' thyrotoxicosis reported more negative life events, such as divorce, bereavement, and educational and occupational failure, than did the control subjects.[36] Similar results were obtained in a consecutive sample of 70 patients attending an endocrine clinic and matched for age and sex with control subjects.[37] In this study the patients had greater life change, both positive and negative, in the year preceding the diagnosis of Graves' thyrotoxicosis than did the control subjects; however, raters unaware of the subjects' study group judged only negative life events to be significantly greater in the patients than in the control subjects.

There is also some support for the notion that environmental stress plays a role in the exacerbations and relapses of established thyrotoxicosis. In a longitudinal study of patients receiving antithyroid drug therapy, the course of thyrotoxicosis seemed to be related to the person's ability to cope with life stress psychologically, especially when confronted with loss (such as financial difficulty) or bereavement.[38] If successful solutions were found, the illness subsided; if not, the exacerbation progressed. Individual case reports provide supporting evidence.[39] For example, in a patient with Graves' disease, surgical biopsy for a benign breast tumor was followed by a rapid increase in thyroid secretion. In another instance, a woman who had been treated successfully for Graves' thyrotoxicosis had a recurrence within 2 months after the death of two young members of her family.

In summary, psychological stress may be associated with the onset of symptoms of thyrotoxicosis and may influence its clinical course.

FACTORS MEDIATING THE PATHOPHYSIOLOGY OF THYROTOXICOSIS

Family studies suggest a strong although complex contribution of genetic factors to Graves' disease[40–42] (see chap 27). However, how psychosocial stressors or anticipation of psychological challenge is linked to the development of thyrotoxicosis, even in genetically predisposed people, is not known.

Many studies have explored the response of the brain-thyroid axis to environmental challenge, but most were conducted before modern techniques of thyroid hormone and thyrotropin (TSH) assay were available. For example, in a study of serum protein-bound iodine (PBI) in five euthyroid and seven treated thyrotoxic persons before and after the viewing of an emotionally disturbing film, the concentrations in all groups were higher during the film than while viewing a travelogue. In both the normal subjects and treated patients, the concentrations fell after the film ended, but in the thyrotoxic patients, they remained high for the next 24 hours.[43]

Serum PBI concentrations increase in response to the challenge of restraint and the avoidance of foot shock in primates.[44] Thyroid hormones and catecholamines are intimately involved in response to cold in animals[45] and serum TSH concentrations rapidly increase in response to cold and other challenges in humans.[46–48] Although these changes may be of adaptive significance and important in the understanding of brain mechanisms in some psychiatric syndromes[49]—and possibly even in the exacerbation of clinical symptomatology in thyrotoxicosis—it appears unlikely that they play a major role in the genesis of thyrotoxicosis.

It seems more probable that the mediating mechanisms in thyrotoxicosis, whereby loss, bereavement, and perhaps the subsequent depression may help precipitate the disorder, lie in a complex interaction between the genetics of the immune system and the general neuroendocrine response to stress.[50]

In Graves' disease, TSH-receptor antibodies cause the thyroid hyperfunction (see section on pathogenesis of Graves' disease in chap 30). These antibodies may be produced as a result of a defect in immunologic surveillance.[50] A reduction in the activity of suppressor lymphocytes secondary to environmental stress is one proposed mechanism whereby the genetic propensity for Graves' disease may be expressed.[50,51] Bereaved and particularly depressed people frequently have sustained elevations of serum cortisol concentrations, reflecting a disturbance of the regulation of the brain-adrenocortical axis.[52–54] A reduction of lymphocyte function in bereaved people also has been described.[55,56] A rapidly expanding body of knowledge now suggests intimate links among immune function, the brain, and the hypothalamic-pituitary-adrenal axis, so that hormones of the pituitary and adrenal glands may exert control over immune function, and vice versa.[57,58] Most recently, inhibition of adrenocorticotropin secretion by thyrotropin-releasing hormone prohormone segment 178–199 has been described in rats.[59] It is these fragments of information that at present form the basis for any speculation that may link genetics, the environment, and the onset of thyrotoxicosis.

Once the thyrotoxic state is established, interactions between biogenic amines, particularly catecholamines, and thyroid hormones clearly have an important role in determining mental state. Catecholamines and thyroid hormones share the amino acid tyrosine as parent and have synergistic action in many metabolic processes, including those in the brain.[49] Animals with thyrotoxicosis have increased adrenergic activity and are especially vulnerable to the toxic effects of drugs, including psychoactive drugs, that enhance catecholamine metabolism.[60] The turnover of catecholamines is decreased, but the β-adrenergic receptor number is increased.[49] These changes may underlie the increased activity, sleeplessness, and anxiety that occur in thyrotoxic patients. The reduction of these symptoms by a β-adrenergic antagonist drug such as propranolol supports this contention. Similarly, the synergism of thyroid hormones and catecholamines may explain the development of mania in predisposed people.[49]

TREATMENT AND OUTCOME

Successful treatment of thyrotoxicosis usually leads to resolution of the major mental disturbances associated with it. Treatment consistently reduced nervousness, anxiety, emotional withdrawal, and motor tension.[7] Those patients who had cognitive difficulty improved. The results of MMPI testing also improved, but there was no change in personality constellation.[7]

Treatment with an adrenergic antagonist drug such as propranolol can be useful in controlling anxiety. In acutely psychotic patients dopamine blockade may reduce excitement. Haloperidol or chlorpromazine can be used, although the latter may increase tachycardia, and there is one report of haloperidol precipitating thyrotoxic storm.[61]

Particularly important is an awareness that if the patient's thyrotoxicosis was misdiagnosed and treated as psychosis or an affective state of other origin, some psychotropic medications may be harmful. In the rare thyrotoxic patient who has psychiatric symptoms simulating bipolar mania, lithium carbonate may be given with subsequent masking of the thyrotoxic state.[62] Lithium has antithyroid actions,[63] and its administration can result in transient symptomatic improvement of thyrotoxicosis,[64] but with exacerbation of thyrotoxicosis and also ophthalmopathy when the lithium is discontinued.[11,65,66]

Also when the thyrotoxicosis is apathetic, mimicking depression, administration of a tricyclic antidepressant drug can be hazardous.[67] The sensitivity to both the anticholinergic and adrenergic effects of these drugs is increased in patients with thyrotoxicosis and serious cardiotoxic effects may occur, especially in elderly patients.

Conversely, in rare instances, successful treatment of thyrotoxicosis may reveal a depressive illness, which in turn requires intervention. In one depressed patient, whenever the thyrotoxicosis was treated, remissions induced by imipramine were negated.[68]

This synergism of the adrenergic and thyroid systems has been successfully used in the treatment of depression.[69] In some depressed patients, especially women, and those who are poorly responsive to antidepressant drug therapy, administration of thyroid hormone may substantially improve the efficacy of the antidepressant drug.[70,71]

References

1. Parry CH. Collections from the unpublished writings of the late C. H. Parry. Vol 2. London: Underwoods, 1825:
2. Graves RJ. Newly observed affection of the thyroid gland in females. Lon Med Surg J 1835;7:516
3. Major RH. Classic descriptions of disease. Springfield, IL: Charles C Thomas, 1959:45
4. Philippopoulos GS. Thyrotoxicosis and its psychosomatic approach. J Nerv Ment Dis 1959;128:415
5. Bennett AW, Cambor CG. Clinical study of hyperthyroidism. Arch Gen Psychiatry 1961;4:160
6. Lidz T, Whitehorn JC. Psychiatric problems in the thyroid clinic. JAMA 1949;139:698
7. Whybrow PC, Prange AJ, Treadway CR. Mental changes accompanying thyroid gland dysfunction. Arch Gen Psychiatry 1969;20:48
8. Checkley SA. Thyrotoxicosis and the course of manic depressive illness. Br J Psychiatry 1978;133:219
9. Corn TH, Checkley SA. A case of recurrent mania with recurrent hyperthyroidism. Br J Psychiatry 1983;143:74
10. Hasan MK, Mooney RP. Mania and thyrotoxicosis. J Family Pract 1981;13:113
11. Reus VI, Gold P, Post R. Lithium-induced thyrotoxicosis. Am J Psychiatry 1979;136:724
12. Villani S, Weitzel WD. Secondary mania. Arch Gen Psychiatry 1979;36:1031
13. Beierwaltes W, Ruff G. Thyroxine and triiodothyronine in excessive dosage to euthyroid humans. Arch Intern Med 1958;101:569
14. Olsen P, Starer M, Siersback-Nielson K, et al. Electroencephalographic findings in hyperthyroidism. Electroencephalogr Clin Neurophysiol 1972;32:171
15. Wilson W, Johnson J. Thyroid hormone and brain function (parts I and II). Electroencephalogr Clin Neurophysiol 1964;16:321
16. Greer S, Parsons V. Schizophrenia-like psychosis in thyroid crisis. Br J Psychiatry 1968;114:1357
17. Ingbar SH. Thyrotoxic storm. N Engl J Med 1966;274:1252
18. Lahey FH. Apathetic thyroidism. Ann Surg 1931;93:1026
19. Taylor JW. Depression in thyrotoxicosis. Am J Psychiatry 1975;132:552
20. Peake RL. Recurrent apathetic hyperthyroidism. Arch Intern Med 1981;141:258
21. Bursten B. Psychoses associated with thyrotoxicosis. Arch Gen Psychiatry 1961;6:267
22. Hermann HT, Quarton GC. Psychological changes and psychogenesis in thyroid hormone disorders. J Clin Endocrinol 1965;25:327
23. Kleinschmidt H, Waxenberg S. Psychophysiology and psychiatric management of thyrotoxicosis: a two year follow up study. Mt Sinai J Med (NY) 1956;23:131

24. MacCrimmon DJ, Wallace JE, Goldberg WM, Steiner DL. Emotional disturbance and cognitive deficits in hyperthyroidism. Psychosom Med 1979;41:331

25. Mandelbrote B, Wittkower E. Emotional factors in Graves' disease. Psychosom Med 1955;17:109

26. Rockey P, Griep R. Behavioral dysfunction in hyperthyroidism: improvement with treatment. Arch Intern Med 1980;140:1194

27. Wilson WP, Johnson JE, Smith RB. Affective change in thyrotoxicosis and experimental hypermetabolism. In: Masserman JM, Wortis J, eds. Recent advances in biological psychiatry. New York: Plenum Press, 1962:234

28. Artunkel S, Togrol S. Psychological studies in hyperthyroidism in brain thyroid relationships. Boston: Little, Brown, 1964:93

29. Robbins LR, Vinson DB. Objective psychological assessment of the thyrotoxic patient and the response to treatment. J Clin Endocrinol 1960;20:120

30. Freedman M, Sala M, Faraj G, Niepomniszcze H. Psychological changes during thyrotoxicosis. Thyroidology 1993;5:25

31. Greer S, Ramsey I, Bagley C. Neurotic and thyrotoxic anxiety: clinical, psychological and physiological measurements. Br J Psychiatry 1973;122:549

32. Krauthammer C, Klerman GL. Secondary mania. Arch Gen Psychiatry 1978;35:1333

33. Josephson AM, Mackenzie TB. Thyroid induced mania in hypothyroid patients. Br J Psychiatry 1980;137:222

34. Voth HM, Holzman PS, Katz JB, Wallerstein RS. Thyroid hot spots: their relationship to life stress. Psychosom Med 1970;32:561

35. Wallerstein RS, Holzman PS, Voth HM, Urh N. Thyroid hot spots: a psychophysiological study. Psychosom Med 1965;27:508

36. Winsa B, Adami H-O, Bergstrom R, et al. Stressful life events and Graves' disease. Lancet 1991;338:1475

37. Sonino N, Girelli ME, Boscaro M, Fallo F, Busnardo B, Fava GA. Life events in the pathogenesis of Graves' disease. A controlled study. Acta Endocrinol 1993;128:293

38. Ferguson-Rayport SM. The relation of emotional factors to recurrence of thyrotoxicosis. Can Med Assoc J 1956;15:993

39. Cushman P. Recurrent hyperthyroidism after normal response to triiodothyronine. JAMA 1967;199:588

40. Carey C, Skosey C, Pinnamaneni KM, et al. Thyroid abnormalities in children of parents who have Graves' disease; possible preGraves' disease. Metabolism 1980;29:369

41. DeGroot LJ, Quintans J. The causes of autoimmune thyroid disease. Endocr Rev 1989;10:537

42. Zaino EC, Guerra W. Hashimoto's disease in identical twins. Arch Intern Med 1964;113:70

43. Flagg GW, Clemens TL, Michael EA. A psychophysiological investigation of hyperthyroidism. Psychosom Med 1965;27:497

44. Mason JW, Lougey EN, Brady JV. Thyroid (PBI) responses to 72 hour avoidance sessions in the monkey. Psychsom Med 1968;30:682

45. Sato T, Imura E, Murata A, Igarashi N. Thyroid hormone-catecholamine interrelationship during cold acclimatization in rats. Compensatory role of catecholamine for altered thyroid states. Acta Endocrinol 1986;113:536

46. Beck U, Reinhardt H, Kendel K, Schmidt-Kessen W. Temperature and endocrine activity during sleep in man. Arch Psychiatr Nerve 1976;222:245

47. Kotchen TA, Mason JW, Hartley LH, et al. Thyroid responses to the anticipation of exhaustive muscular exercise. Psychosom Med 1972;34:473

48. Zuckerman M, Persky H, Hopkins TR, et al. Comparison of stress effects of perceptual and social isolation. Arch Gen Psychiatry 1966;14:348

49. Whybrow PC, Prange AJ. A hypothesis of thyroid-catecholamine receptor interaction: its relevance to affective illness. Arch Gen Psychiatry 1981;38:106

50. Volpe R, Farid NR, Von Westarp C, Row VV. The pathogenesis of Graves' disease and Hashimoto's thyroiditis. Clin Endocrinol 1974;3:239

51. Morillo E, Gardner LI. Bereavement as an antecedent factor in thyrotoxicosis of childhood: four case studies with a survey of possible metabolic pathways. Psychosom Med 1979;41:545

52. Carroll BJ. Neuroendocrine function in psychiatric disorders. In: Lipton MA, DiMascio A, Killam KF, eds. Psychopharmacology: a generation of progress. New York: Raven Press, 1978:487

53. Stein M, Keller SE, Schleifer SJ. Stress and immunomodulation: the role of depression and neuroendocrine function. J Immunol 1985;135:827

54. Wolff CT, Friedman SB, Hofer MA, Mason JW. Relationship between psychological defenses and mean urinary 17-hydroxycorticosteroid excretion rates: a predictive study of parents of fatally ill children. Psychosom Med 1964;26:576

55. Bartop RW, Luckhurst E, Lazarus L, et al. Depressed lymphocyte function after bereavement. Lancet 1977;1:834

56. Syvalahti E. Psychoendocrine and immune systems in depression and stress. Psychiatrica Fennica (suppl) 1986;97

57. Bateman A, Singh A, Kral T, Solomon S. The immune- hypothalamic-pituitary adrenal axis. Endocr Rev 1989;10:92

58. Fessler R, Schaunstein K, Kremer G, et al. Elevation of corticosteroid binding globulin in obese strain chickens: possible implications for disturbed immunoregulation and the development of spontaneous autoimmune thyroiditis. J Immunol 1986;136:36

59. Redei E, Hilderbrand H, Aird F. Corticotropin release inhibiting factor is encoded within prepro-TRH. Endocrinology 1995;136:1813

60. Coville PF, Telford JM. The effect of thyroid hormones on the action of some centrally active drugs. Br J Pharmacol 1970;40:747

61. Hoffman WH, Chodoroff G, Piggott LR. Haloperidol and thyroid storm. Am J Psychiatry 1978;135:484

62. Wharton RN. Accidental lithium carbonate treatment of thyrotoxicosis as mania. Am J Psychiatry 1980;137:747

63. Rogers M, Whybrow PC. Clinical hyperthyroidism occurring during lithium treatment: two case histories and a review of thyroid function in 19 patients. Am J Psychiatry 1971;128:158

64. Lazarus JH, Richard AR, Addison GM. Treatment of thyrotoxicosis with lithium carbonate. Lancet 1974;2:1160

65. Rosser R. Thyrotoxicosis and lithium. Br J Psychiatry 1976;128:61

66. Segal RL, Rosenblatt S, Eliasoph I. Endocrine exophthalmos during lithium therapy of manic-depressive disease. N Engl J Med 1973;289:136

67. Folks DG, Petrie WM. Thyrotoxicosis presenting as depression. Br J Psychiatry 1982;140:432

68. Swartz CM. The dependency of tricyclic antidepressant efficacy on the thyroid hormone potentiation: case studies. J Nerv Ment Dis 1982;170:50

69. Prange AJ Jr, Wilson IC, Rabon AM, Lipton MA. Enhancement of imipramine antidepressant activity by thyroid hormone. Am J Psychiatry 1969;126:457

70. Joffe R, Singer W. Thyroid hormone potentiation of antidepressants. In: Amsterdam J, ed. Advances in neuropsychiatry and psychopathology. Vol 2. Refractory depression. New York: Raven Press, 1991:185

71. Joffe RT, Levitt AJ, Bagby RM, MacDonald C, Singer W. Predictors of response to lithium and triiodothyronine augmentation of antidepressants in tricyclic non-responders. Br J Psychiatry 1993;163:574

Werner and Ingbar's The Thyroid, Seventh Edition,
edited by Lewis E. Braverman and Robert D. Utiger.
Lippincott–Raven Publishers, Philadelphia, © 1996

51

Thyrotoxic Storm

Leonard Wartofsky

Thyrotoxic storm or *crisis* is a relatively rare but life-threatening syndrome characterized by exaggerated manifestations of thyrotoxicosis. Because there may be considerable variation in the criteria for its diagnosis as well as in clinical presentation, it is difficult to obtain an accurate estimation of its incidence; it is clear, however, that the syndrome is much less common today than it was in years past for several reasons, and its incidence may approximate 1% to 2% of hospital admissions for thyrotoxicosis. On the basis of routine function tests, most patients with thyrotoxic storm are indistinguishable from those with uncomplicated thyrotoxicosis. Hence the diagnosis is largely a clinical one, based on determination of the presence of decompensation of a number of organ systems in a thyrotoxic patient. Cardinal manifestations include fever (temperature usually >38.5°C), tachycardia (out of proportion to the fever), gastrointestinal dysfunction (including nausea, vomiting, diarrhea, and, in severe cases, jaundice), and central nervous system (CNS) signs, varying from confusion to apathy and even coma. Despite its relative rarity, early diagnosis and vigorous therapy are required to avoid a fatal outcome; mortality rates of hospitalized patients have ranged from 10% to 75%.[1–3]

CLINICAL FEATURES

Although thyrotoxic storm may occur in a patient with masked or "apathetic" thyrotoxicosis,[4] most patients have rather obvious signs and symptoms of thyrotoxicosis, including goiter and, in the presence of Graves' disease, ophthalmopathy. There may be a history of partially treated thyrotoxicosis, and a large number of events have been associated with the precipitation of thyrotoxic crisis in such patients, including:

Infection
Surgery
Trauma
Iodinated contrast dyes
Hypoglycemia
Parturition
Vigorous palpation of thyroid
Emotional stress
Withdrawal of antithyroid drug therapy
Iodine-131 (^{131}I) therapy
Diabetic ketoacidosis
Pulmonary thromboembolism
Cerebrovascular accident

Before the availability of pharmacologic agents to inhibit thyroid hormone synthesis and release, thyrotoxic storm often was seen in the immediate postoperative setting after thyroidectomy. Presumably, this was the result of augmented hormonal release secondary to surgical manipulation, compounded by other effects of the surgical stress. With improved medical therapy of thyrotoxicosis, this presentation is now rare, although several types of nonthyroid surgery or other trauma have precipitated crisis in patients with previously undiagnosed thyrotoxicosis. The most commonly associated precipitating event today probably is infection, and the physician may have a difficult time determining whether the hyperpyrexia and tachycardia accompanying infection in a patient with thyrotoxicosis herald impending crisis or merely reflect the infection. Excessive diaphoresis with high fever out of apparent proportion to the infection at hand may be the best clue to this complication and signals the need for vigorous treatment. Indeed, when crisis is not recognized and treated, the fever may reach an extremely high and life-threatening level. The appearance of CNS symptoms, with a metabolic encephalopathic picture that may include lability, restlessness, agitation, confusion, psychosis, and coma,[4–7] may be an important further clue to the diagnosis. In one case, thyroid storm was associated with bilateral basal ganglia infarction.[8] In difficult diagnostic cases, it may be most prudent to treat as if the patient had thyrotoxic storm (see section on treatment) and then withdraw therapy as the patient recovers from the infection.

In addition to the sinus tachycardia already mentioned, other tachyarrhythmias may be present, as may signs and symptoms of congestive heart failure. Although the latter are more likely to occur in elderly patients with underlying rheumatic or arteriosclerotic heart disease, cardiac decompensation also may be seen in relatively young or middle-aged patients with no known antecedent (or subsequently demonstrable) heart disease. Systolic hypertension with widened pulse pressure is likely to be noted in most patients, at least initially, although postural hypotension may be demonstrable, particularly in the setting of volume depletion due to vomiting or diarrhea, and vascular collapse with frank shock may supervene. Mortality in the latter patients may be almost inevitable. Other gastrointestinal manifestations include diffuse abdominal pain, hepatomegaly, splenomegaly, and various abnormalities in liver function tests. The liver may be tender, possibly as a result of either congestive failure or hepatic necrosis. The presence of jaundice is another poor prognostic sign and warrants immediate and vigorous therapy.

LABORATORY FINDINGS

Values for serum total thyroxine (T_4) and triiodothyronine (T_3), T_3-resin uptake, and 24-hour radioiodine uptake are elevated above the normal range, but they are not particularly different from the values in uncomplicated thyrotoxicosis.[9] In certain patients, serum T_3 levels may be within normal limits,[10] and in sick patients such as those with diabetic ketoacidosis[11,12] and other causes of the low T_3 syndrome due to systemic illness,[13,14] the decreased (or normal) serum T_3 may obscure a diagnosis of *coexistent thyrotoxicosis* until thyrotoxic storm becomes clinically apparent. In a patient with previously undiagnosed thyrotoxicosis, the most rapid confirmation of the diagnosis may be obtained by performance of a 2-hour radioiodine uptake, although it should be feasible to obtain the result of serum T_4 determination within a few hours on an emergency basis in many hospitals. In any event, given the mortality of untreated thyrotoxic storm, the presence of goiter with a thrill and bruit or ophthalmopathy in the clinical setting described earlier should be considered as sufficient support for the diagnosis of *thyrotoxic crisis* to warrant therapy.

Mild-to-moderate hyperglycemia may occur in the absence of diabetes mellitus, probably as a result of augmented glycogenolysis and catecholamine-mediated inhibition of insulin release. A leukocytosis with a mild shift to the left is common, even in the absence of infection, whereas other hematologic values tend to be normal. Serum electrolyte levels usually are normal as well, whereas calcium levels often are slightly elevated as a result of both hemoconcentration and the known effects of thyroid hormone on bone resorption. Serum lactate dehydrogenase, glutamic oxaloacetate transaminase (aspartate aminotransferase), and bilirubin levels are increased as a result of hepatic dysfunction, whereas elevated alkaline phosphatase levels appear to result primarily from increased osteoblastic bone activity in response to the previously mentioned augmentation of bone resorption. Because serum cortisol levels should be elevated in thyrotoxic storm—as in any other acute stressful situation—a normal value may be interpreted as being inappropriately low. If serum is obtained and sent for cortisol determination before the administration of corticosteroid, those patients with impaired adrenal reserve may be identified. Adrenal insufficiency on an autoimmune basis occurs with greater frequency in Graves' disease and might have a major role in the pathogenesis of the decompensation. Even in the absence of adrenal insufficiency, adrenal reserve may be exceeded in thyrotoxic crisis because of the inability of the adrenal gland to meet the demand placed on it as a result of the accelerated turnover and disposal of glucocorticoids that occur in thyrotoxicosis.

PATHOGENESIS

The precise mechanism by which certain events may precipitate thyrotoxic crisis is incompletely understood, and it is likely that a number of factors could be important. The magnitude alone of serum hormone levels does not appear to be critical because storm does not accompany the astronomically high serum T_4 and T_3 concentrations that may be found after accidental ingestion of T_4 by children.[15] Thus an acute increase in release of T_4 or T_3 from the thyroid usually is not held to be important in the pathogenesis of storm, but this mechanism must play a role in those cases that have been reported after vigorous palpation of the thyroid, after ^{131}I therapy,[2] after the increased hormonal synthesis related to the withdrawal of propylthiouracil (PTU), or after administration of lithium,[16] iodine, or iodinated contrast dyes.[10] Moreover, there may be dramatic improvement after abrupt decrements in hormone levels, such as may be achieved with peritoneal dialysis or plasmapheresis.[17–19] Nevertheless, serum concentrations of total T_4 and T_3 do not differ significantly from those in otherwise uncomplicated thyrotoxicosis although the levels in an affected person could be higher than the values before the precipitating event.[20] An alteration in hormone binding with a relative increase in the percentage and absolute concentration of free hormone is another potential factor that could apply, particularly with underlying conditions such as surgery, stress, infection, and ketoacidosis,[13] in which decreases in binding affinity may be due to circulating inhibitors.[21] Reduced protein binding with increases in free hormone concentrations may be seen transiently early in thyroid storm,[22] and increases in both the percentage of dialyzable free T_4 and absolute concentration of free T_4 have been observed in thyrotoxic storm.[23] The role of decreased binding and high free T_4 in sick patients also may be relevant to the review by McDermott and associates[2] of 15 well-documented cases of ^{131}I-induced storm and the conclusion that the most ill patients were predisposed to develop this complication. Because all of the patients reviewed had some significant acute or chronic systemic illness in addition to severe thyrotoxicosis, the authors described and recommended a more cautious approach to radioiodine therapy in such patients to avoid thyrotoxic crisis.

Because many of the signs and symptoms of severe thyrotoxicosis may be due to either catecholamines or the interaction between the adrenergic system and excessive circulating thyroid hormone,[24,25] there is some likelihood for an important role of the sympathetic nervous system in the pathogenesis of thyrotoxic storm. Although normal serum catecholamine levels and urinary excretion rates mitigate against the concept of augmented adrenergic activity per se, there is little doubt that dramatic clinical improvement follows the use of agents that either deplete tissue catecholamines, such as reserpine,[26] or block β-adrenergic receptors, such as propranolol. Indeed, the availability and use of propranolol may be responsible for the improvement in survival statistics reported in more recent series of patients with thyrotoxic storm although some workers have cautioned that customarily used doses of this drug may not prevent the occurrence of storm.[27] Reserpine may be effective in a patient refractory to propranolol.[28]

Another phenomenon that has been postulated to play a role in the pathogenesis of storm relates to the apparent augmentation of peripheral cellular responses to thyroid hormone, and this may be relevant to those patients with a "common denominator" of tissue hypoxia, ketoacidosis, lactic acidosis, and infection. Conceivably, partial uncoupling of oxidative phosphorylation could result in excessive generation of free fatty acids from increased lipolysis. Oxidation and metabolism of the free fatty acids could be responsible for the increased oxygen consumption, calorigenesis, and hyperthermia of thyrotoxic storm by way of the production of thermal energy rather than adenosine triphosphate. The organism attempts to dissipate the excess generated heat by increased sweating and cutaneous vasodilatation, which are common in severe thyrotoxicosis. Despite its plausibility, this hypothesis remains speculative and little supported by any experimental observations.

TREATMENT

Table 51-1 outlines possible treatment approaches for thyrotoxic storm. The therapy of thyrotoxic crisis may be considered in terms of four components and the relative importance of each for survival varies in a given patient.[29] First, specific antithyroid drugs must be used to decrease the increased thyroid production and release of T_4 and T_3. Second, the systemic decompensation characterized by fever, congestive failure, shock, and so on must be vigorously attacked with specific therapies for each problem. Third, an attempt should be made to block the effects of the excessive circulating concentrations of free T_4 and T_3 in promoting this decompensation in conjunction with heightened adrenergic activity. Last, but equally as important, any underlying precipitating illness such as infection or ketoacidosis must be treated. In view of the serious implications of thyrotoxic storm, no one component of this therapeutic approach should be overlooked.

Therapy Directed Against the Thyroid Gland

The thionamide antithyroid drugs, PTU or methimazole (tapazole), are given to block new hormone synthesis.

No parenteral preparations of these compounds are available, and they must, therefore, be given by mouth, or by nasogastric tube, if necessary, in the comatose or uncooperative patient. Either methimazole or PTU has been administered per rectum and appears to be absorbed satisfactorily,[30,31] although

TABLE 51-1.
Management of Thyroid Crisis

THERAPY DIRECTED AGAINST THE THYROID GLAND

Inhibition of new hormone synthesis
    Antithyroid drugs of thionamide type (PTU, methimazole)
    Lithium carbonate (?)
Inhibition of hormone secretion
    Iodine
        Oral: potassium iodide (SSKI), Lugol's solution, ipodate
        Intravenous: sodium iodide
    Lithium carbonate

THERAPY TO AVOID DECOMPENSATION OF NORMAL HOMEOSTATIC MECHANISMS

Treatment of hyperthermia
    Acetaminophen
    Cooling
Correction of dehydration and poor nutrition
    Fluids and electrolytes
    Glucose (calories)
    Vitamins
Supportive therapy
    Oxygen
    Vasopressors
    Treatment of congestive heart failure, if present (digoxin, diuretics)
    Corticosteroids

THERAPY DIRECTED AGAINST THYROID HORMONE ACTION IN THE PERIPHERY

Inhibition of T_4-to-T_3 conversion
    Ipodate, iopanoate, amiodarone (?)
    Corticosteroids
    Propranolol
    PTU
β-Adrenergic blockade
    Propranolol
    Selective $β_1$-blocking agents
Removal of excess circulating hormone
    Plasmapheresis
    Dialysis
    Hemoperfusion adsorption (?)
    Cholestyramine (?)

TREATMENT DIRECTED AGAINST A PRECIPITATING OR COEXISTENT ILLNESS

diarrhea, when present, would make this problematic. PTU should be started in a dose of 1200 to 1500 mg/d, given as 200 to 250 mg every 4 hours. Methimazole in a daily dose of 120 mg should suffice (given as 20 mg every 4 hours), but PTU has the additional advantage of inhibiting conversion of T_4 to T_3, a property not shared by methimazole. As a consequence, more rapid amelioration of symptoms is possible with PTU. The major effect of both drugs is on new hormone synthesis; thyroid release of preformed glandular stores of hormone is not reduced. Consequently separate treatment must be administered to inhibit proteolysis of colloid and release of T_4 and T_3 into the blood. For this purpose, either inorganic iodine or lithium carbonate[32] may be used. There is considerably more experience with the use of iodides,[33] which may be given either orally as Lugol's solution or as a saturated solution of potassium iodide (8 drops every 6 hours). An earlier mainstay of therapy, the use of an intravenous infusion of sodium iodide (0.5–1 g every 12 hours) has not been feasible recently because of nonavailability of sterile sodium iodide for intravenous use. However, a sterile intravenous preparation could be prepared by a hospital pharmacy.

An important aspect of this combined therapeutic approach to the thyroid is to remember to administer the antithyroid drug before the initiation of iodine therapy. Use of iodine alone is to be avoided because the absence of concomitant antithyroid drug blockade of new hormone synthesis allows enrichment of hormone stores within the gland, thereby generating the potential for further exaggeration of thyrotoxicosis by virtue of further release of hormone. In this unfortunate situation, further use of iodine to inhibit hormonal release is questionable. Even without this complication, the increased glandular stores of hormone resulting from therapy with iodine alone will complicate future management by any modality because ultimate efficacy of antithyroid drug will be delayed, surgical risk will be increased, and use of radioiodine will be substantially delayed, pending clearance of the stable iodine load. Thyrotoxic storm has occurred in patients who were treated with iodine alone and who deteriorated weeks to months after their initial improvement. Iodine has been used as a sole agent to prepare patients for thyroidectomy, and exaggerated thyrotoxicosis became evident when surgery was postponed for various reasons. Because of this propensity for crisis to develop, iodine as sole therapy in thyrotoxicosis should be viewed as potentially hazardous and should not be recommended. When iodine is administered in conjunction with full doses of antithyroid drugs, dramatic, rapid decreases in serum T_4 are seen, with values approaching the normal range within 4 or 5 days.[33]

Other agents that may be used in this manner are the radiographic contrast dyes ipodate (Oragrafin) and iopanoate (Telepaque). These drugs decrease hepatic uptake of T_4 and the percentage of free T_4 and T_3 in serum, and their use can be associated with remarkable clinical improvement.[34] Much of this improvement is probably due to the fall in serum T_3 concentration, which results from decreased peripheral conversion of T_4 to T_3, but some of the improvement may be due to decreased thyroid hormone release as a consequence of the high iodine content (1851 mg iodine per 3-g dose) of these agents. Binding of both T_3 and T_4 to cellular receptors may be inhibited by ipodate. After a loading dose of 3 g, ipodate may be administered as 1 g orally on a daily basis, and preferably should be used (like iodine) only with simultaneous thyroid blockade with PTU or methimazole, to avoid the enrichment of glandular iodine stores that would otherwise occur. Amiodarone, an antiarrhythmic and antianginal drug, also is rich in iodine, and is a potent inhibitor of the peripheral conversion of T_4 to T_3. A similar and perhaps greater potential hazard exists for amiodarone because of its prolonged half-life, with subsequent release of iodine over many months.

In patients who may be allergic to iodine, lithium carbonate may be used as an alternative agent to inhibit hormonal release,[32,35] although some caution has been raised in regard to its use in the setting of storm.[16] This drug also may be used in thyrotoxic patients who are known to have serious toxic reactions to the thionamides. Minor allergic reactions to PTU or methimazole, such as rash, should not interdict their use in a critical situation such as thyrotoxic crisis, but a history of agranulocytosis would warrant alternative therapy such as lithium carbonate. Lithium should be administered initially as 300 mg every 6 hours, with subsequent adjustment of dosage as necessary to maintain serum lithium levels at about 1 mEq/L.

Therapy Directed Against Systemic Decompensation

Fever should be promptly treated with antipyretics, preferably acetaminophen rather than salicylates, because the latter might theoretically temporarily worsen the clinical situation because of an increase in free hormone resulting from displacement of T_4 from serum binding sites. External cooling with alcohol sponging, ice packs, or a hypothermia blanket also may be used. Fluid losses caused by the hyperpyrexia and diaphoresis, as well as by vomiting or diarrhea, when present, must be vigorously replaced to avoid vascular collapse. Cautious replacement of fluids is necessary in the elderly patient with congestive heart failure or other potential cardiac compromise. Intravenous fluids that contain 10% dextrose in addition to electrolytes aid restoration of depleted hepatic glycogen stores. Hypercalcemia, if present, usually is reversed by hydration. Vitamin supplements may be added to the intravenous fluids to replace probable coexistent deficiency. Use of the skeletal muscle relaxant dantrolene was associated with clinical improvement in one case,[36] but the significant risks associated with its use preclude recommending it at this time.

Congestive heart failure may be treated with the usual measures, including digoxin and diuretics, although somewhat greater than usual doses may be required for initial digitalization as well as for maintenance doses in the patient with severe thyrotoxicosis. Therapy for specific arrhythmias also may be indicated, as well as pressor therapy in the event of hypotension not readily reversed by adequate hydration. Large doses of glucocorticoids have been given on empirical grounds for several decades on the basis of postulated relative adrenal insufficiency. This indication notwithstanding, the ability of steroids such as dexamethasone and hydrocortisone to inhibit T_4-to-T_3 conversion is additional justification for their use. An initial dose of 300 mg hydrocortisone followed by 100 mg every 8 hours during the acute phase of this syndrome should be adequate. In one case, thyroid storm returned when steroids had been discontinued after initial clinical improvement.[37]

Therapy Directed Against Ongoing Effects of Thyroid Hormone in the Periphery

Some workers have attempted to reduce the burden of excessive circulating concentrations of the thyroid hormones by either peritoneal dialysis or plasmapheresis.[17–19,38] Hemoperfusion through a resin bed that removes T_4 and T_3 has been demonstrated to be effective experimentally,[39] and charcoal columns may be similarly used.[40] Perhaps related to the relative additional difficulty attending these procedures, most physicians rely on more traditional measures, although such aggressive management should be considered in a severe case. Some removal of T_4 and T_3 may be effected safely by the use of cholestyramine resin.[41] This agent binds thyroid hormone entering the gut via enterohepatic recirculation.

The use of β-adrenergic receptor blockade to ameliorate the manifestations of thyroid hormone excess evolved from the earlier demonstration that agents such as reserpine and guanethidine could blunt the apparently enhanced sympathetic activity in thyrotoxic patients. Hughes[42] was the first to treat successfully a patient with thyrotoxic storm using a β-adrenergic blocker, and other reports followed soon thereafter.[43–45] Propranolol is the agent most commonly used today, at least in the United States. The oral dosage of 20 to 40 mg every 6 hours, which is customary for most thyrotoxic patients, may have to be increased to 60 to 120 mg every 6 hours in crisis or impending crisis.[46,47] Indeed, because of the more rapid metabolism of the drug in severe thyrotoxicosis, even larger oral doses, or preferably intravenous doses, should be given. A plasma propranolol level in excess of 50 ng/mL may have to be maintained to establish clinical response.[45,46] When used intravenously, an initial dose of 0.5 to 1 mg should be given cautiously while the patient's cardiac rhythm is continuously monitored. Subsequent doses of 2 to 3 mg may be given intravenously over 10 to 15 minutes every several hours, while one awaits the effect of the orally administered drug.[48] Although it has been assumed for many years that the primary role of propranolol was to attenuate the effects of catecholamines, this drug also inhibits the conversion of T_4 to T_3, albeit weakly, and it may help to ameliorate the thyrotoxicosis on this basis.

The most dramatic effects of β-adrenergic blockade are manifest in the cardiovascular system, with rapid onset of reduction in heart rate, cardiac work, and cardiac output. Patients who previously seemed refractory to the effects of digoxin and diuretics may respond rapidly after initiation of propranolol therapy. If there is underlying intrinsic cardiac disease, the drug may have the adverse effect of neutralizing the little remaining sympathetic drive to the myocardium. Hence, use of propranolol usually is contraindicated in patients with moderate to severe congestive heart failure, but it may be judiciously used in those patients with minor degrees of cardiac compromise related to their thyrotoxicosis.[49] Any patient with thyrotoxic storm, particularly with cardiac decompensation, deserves to be managed in an intensive care setting. Serious consideration for the insertion of a Swan-Ganz catheter to monitor central hemodynamics also is recommended in patients receiving high-dose propranolol, pressors, digoxin, diuretics, and fluids. Other beneficial effects of propranolol in thyrotoxic storm include improvement in agitation, convulsions, psychotic behavior, tremor, diarrhea, fever, and diaphoresis. In selected patients, there may be relative risks or contraindications to the use of this agent. Because propranolol may obscure some of the important signs and symptoms of hypoglycemia (which are mediated by catecholamines), the drug must be used with caution and plasma glucose must be carefully monitored in diabetic patients receiving insulin or oral sulfonylureas. Propranolol also is contraindicated in patients with bronchospasm or a history of asthma; in such patients, therapy with reserpine or guanethidine should be considered instead. Rather than propranolol, it should be possible, theoretically, to safely use selective $β_1$-blocking agents in patients with asthma, but considerable risk of bronchospasm may still exist with high doses of these newer compounds. A very short-acting β-adrenergic blocker, esmolol, has also been used in thyroid storm with success. An initial loading dose of 0.25 to 0.5 mg/kg is followed by continuous infusion of 0.05 to 0.1 mg/kg per minute.[50,51] Untoward bradycardia caused by propranolol may be reversed by administration of atropine, and isoproterenol should be given to counteract bronchospasm or failing left ventricular function. Reserpine, 2.5 to 5 mg intramuscularly every 4 hours (a 1-mg test dose should be given first and blood pressure carefully monitored), or guanethidine, 30 to 40 mg orally every 6 hours, may be given, but neither of these agents should be used in the presence of shock or cardiovascular collapse. Both agents also may produce hypotension and diarrhea. Although reserpine may have an additional beneficial effect in agitated or psychotic patients, it is not a desirable agent in the patient with apathy, stupor, or coma, in view of its depressant effects on the CNS. The patient whose thyrotoxic storm arises in the operating room or who may require emergency surgery after major trauma may be successfully managed with propranolol, but shock would be more likely to supervene during anesthesia were reserpine or guanethidine used.

Therapy Directed Against the Precipitating Illness

Although the therapies outlined in the three preceding sections may be clearly lifesaving, a careful search for and early treatment of the underlying illness that may have precipitated the thyrotoxic crisis also is important. This is not problematic in the care of readily apparent causes, such as trauma, surgery, or labor; these require no additional management after the primary event has elapsed. On the other hand, patients with enhanced thyroid secretion caused by withdrawal of thiourea therapy or the administration of iodine, iodinated contrast dyes, or ^{131}I require some special concern. The need for continuing effective blockade of hormone biosynthesis and release beyond the period of immediate improvement must be recognized because premature withdrawal of treatment could result in an exacerbation of thyrotoxicosis. Once treatment with antithyroid drugs is instituted, measures such as diuresis and dialysis, designed to deplete iodine in the patient with iodine-induced thyrotoxicosis, are no longer necessary. Patients with thyrotoxic storm related to hypoglycemia, ketoacidosis, pulmonary thromboembolism, or stroke require the same vigorous management ordinarily indicated for each respective specific event. It is important to be alert to the fact that these conditions may underlie thyrotoxic crisis, particularly in the obtunded or psychotic patient, because the dramatic manifestations of severe thyrotoxicosis may overshadow the clinical presentation of these disorders.

In the patient with thyrotoxic crisis in whom none of the latter precipitating factors is apparent, a diligent search for some focus of infection must be carried out. The routine acquisition of cultures of urine, blood, and sputum can readily be defended in the febrile thyrotoxic patient, and cultures of other sites may be warranted. The use of broad-spectrum antibiotic coverage on an empirical basis cannot be recommended unless there is fairly good evidence of infection, and such therapy is viewed as temporary while results of cultures and sensitivity testing are awaited. In most patients who recover, clinical improvement is dramatic and demonstrable within 12 or 24 hours. Defervescence and improvement in agitation, psychosis, or coma herald continued progressive recovery, which will be observed over the subsequent 72 to 96 hours. During this interval, some of the supportive therapy, such as corticosteroids, antipyretics, and intravenous fluids, may be tapered and gradually withdrawn on the basis of stability and continuing improvement.

After the crisis has been resolved, attention may be turned to consideration of future short- and long-term management of the patient's thyrotoxicosis. Because inorganic iodine is likely to have been used in virtually all cases of storm, the choice of ^{131}I as ablative therapy is precluded, except at some future date. If this therapy should be desired, antithyroid drug therapy (without iodine) should be continued, with careful periodic measurement of serum T_4 levels to confirm continued improvement. Surgical thyroidectomy might constitute a more expedient definitive therapy than radioiodine, but care must be taken to ensure that the thyrotoxicosis has been adequately treated beforehand, to obviate any likelihood of another episode of crisis during induction of anesthesia or the surgery itself, or in the immediate postoperative period. Some thyrotoxic patients have been operated on successfully with no preparation other than propranolol.[52,53] Although such perioperative management is not recommended, these results have emphasized the utility of β-adrenergic blockade during surgery in most patients.[54] Consequently, after the acute crisis has subsided and stability has been attained, the continuation of propranolol therapy may allow surgery to be considered and performed at an earlier date. Medical therapy with antithyroid drugs alone in the hope of the patient's sustaining a spontaneous remission also is a possibility. Certain clinical criteria may make a given patient less likely to achieve a successful outcome with these drugs (see chap 53), but many physicians would be more disposed to select an ablative and therefore more definitive form of therapy in a patient with a recent history of thyrotoxic storm.

References

1. Ingbar SH. Thyrotoxic storm. N Engl J Med 1966;274:1252
2. McDermott MT, Kidd GS, Dodson LE, Hofeldt FD. Radioiodine-induced thyroid storm. Am J Med 1983;75:353
3. Roth RN, McAuliffe MJ. Hyperthyroidism and thyroid storm. Emerg Med Clin North Am 1989;7:873
4. Serri O, Gagnon R-M, Goulet Y, Somma M. Coma secondary to apathetic thyrotoxicosis. Can Med Assoc J 1978;119:605
5. Aiello DP, DuPlessis Aj, Pattishall EG III, Kulin HE. Thyroid storm presenting with coma and seizures. Clin Pediatr (Phila) 1989;28:571
6. Howton JC. Thyroid storm presenting as coma. Ann Emerg Med 1988;17:343
7. Modignani RL, Venegoni M, Beretta F, Fassina S. Thyroid storm with encephalopathic symptoms due to Graves' disease and inappropriate secretion of thyrotropin. Ann Ital Med Int 1992;7:250
8. Page SR, Scott AR. Thyroid storm in a young woman resulting in bilateral basal ganglia infarction. Postgrad Med J 1993;69:813
9. Brooks MH, Waldstein SS, Bronsky D, Sterling K. Serum triiodothyronine concentrations in thyroid storm. J Clin Endocrinol Metab 1975;40:339
10. Shimura H, Takazawa K, Endo T, et al. T4-thyroid storm after CT-scan with iodinated contrast medium. J Endocrinol Invest 1990;13:73
11. Ahmad N, Cohen MP. Thyroid storm with normal serum triiodothyronine level during diabetic ketoacidosis. JAMA 1981;245:2516
12. Mayfield RK, Sagel J, Colwell JA. Thyrotoxicosis without elevated serum triiodothyronine during diabetic ketoacidosis. Arch Intern Med 1980;140:408
13. Wartofsky L, Burman KD. Alterations in thyroid function in patients with systemic illness: the "euthyroid sick syndrome." Endocr Rev 1982;3:164
14. Wartofsky L. The low T3 or "sick euthyroid syndrome:" update 1994. In: Braverman LE, Refetoff S, eds. Endocrine reviews monographs. 3. Clinical and molecular aspects of diseases of the thyroid. Bethesda, Maryland. The Endocrine Society 1994:248
15. Mandel SH, Magnusson AR, Burton BT, Swanson JR. Massive levothyroxine ingestion: conservative management. Clin Pediatr (Phila) 1989;28:374
16. Reed J, Bradley EL III. Postoperative thyroid storm after lithium preparation. Surgery 1985;98:983
17. Ashkar FS, Katims RB, Smoak WM, Gilson AJ. Thyroid storm treatment with blood exchange and plasmapheresis. JAMA 1970;214:1275
18. Herrmann J, Hilger P, Kruskemper HL. Plasmapheresis in the treatment of thyrotoxic crisis (measurement of half-concentration tissues for free and total T3 and T4). Acta Endocrinol [Suppl] (Copenh) 1973;173:22
19. Herrman NJ, Kruskemper HL, Grosser KD. Peritoneal-dialyse in der behandlung der thyreotoxischen krise. Dtsch Med Woschenschr 1971;96:742
20. Jacobs HS, Mackie DB, Eastman CJ, et al. Total and free triiodothyronine and thyroxine levels in thyroid storm and recurrent hyperthyroidism. Lancet 1973;2:236
21. Chopra IJ, Solomon DH, Chua Teco GN, Eisenberg JB. An inhibitor of the binding of thyroid hormones to serum proteins is present in extrathyroidal tissues. Science 1982;215:407
22. Colebunders R, Bordoux P, Bekaert J, et al. Determination of free thyroid hormones and their binding proteins in a patient with severe hyperthyroidism (thyroid storm?) and thyroid encephalopathy. J Endocrinol Invest 1984;7:389
23. Brooks MH, Waldstein SS. Free thyroxine concentrations in thyroid storm. Ann Intern Med 1980;93:694
24. Landsberg L. Catecholamines and hyperthyroidism. Clin Endocrinol Metab 1977;6:697
25. Wilson BE, Hobbs WN. Pseudoephedrine-associated thyroid storm: thyroid hormone-catecholamine interactions. Am J Med Sci 1993;306:317
26. Dillon PT, Baba J, Meloni CR, Canary JJ. Reserpine in thyrotoxic crisis. N Engl J Med 1970;283:1020
27. Eriksson MA, Rubenfeld S, Garber AJ, Kohler PO. Propranolol does not prevent thyroid storm. N Engl J Med 1977;296:263
28. Anaissie E, Tohme JF. Reserpine in propranolol resistant thyroid storm. Arch Intern Med 1985;145:2248
29. Burch HB, Wartofsky L. Life-threatening thyrotoxicosis: thyroid storm. Endocrinol Metab Clin North Am 1993;22:263
30. Walter RM Jr, Bartle WR. Rectal administration of propylthiouracil in the treatment of Graves' disease. Am J Med 1990;88:69

31. Nareem N, Miner DJ, Amatruda JM. Methimazole: an alternative route of administration. J Clin Endocrinol Metab 1982;54:180

32. Lazarus JH, Addison GM, Richards AR, Owen GM. Treatment of thyrotoxicosis with lithium carbonate. Lancet 1974;2:1160

33. Wartofsky L, Ransil BJ, Ingbar SH. Inhibition by iodine of the release of thyroxine from the thyroid glands of patients with thyrotoxicosis. J Clin Invest 1970;49:78

34. Wu S-Y, Chopra IJ, Solomon DH, Johnson DE. The effect of repeated administration of ipodate (Oragrafin) in hyperthyroidism. J Clin Endocrinol Metab 1978;47:1358

35. Boehm TM, Burman KD, Barnes S, Wartofsky L. Lithium and iodine combination therapy for thyrotoxicosis. Acta Endocrinol (Copenh) 1980;94:174

36. Bennett MH, Wainwright AP. Acute thyroid crisis on induction of anesthesia. Anaesthesia 1989;44:28

37. Kidess AJ, Caplan RH, Reynertson MD, Wickus G. Recurrence of 131-I induced thyroid storm after discontinuing glucocorticoid therapy. Wis Med J 1991;90:463

38. Tajiri J, Katsuya H, Kiyokaya T, et al. Successful treatment of thyrotoxic crisis with plasma exchange. Crit Care Med 1984;12:536

39. Burman KD, Yeager HC, Briggs WA, et al. Resin hemoperfusion: a method of removing circulating thyroid hormones. J Clin Endocrinol Metab 1976;42:70

40. Candrina R, DiStefano O, Spandrio S, et al. Treatment of thyrotoxic storm by charcoal plasmaperfusion. J Endocrinol Invest 1989;12:133

41. Solomon BL, Wartofsky L, Burman KD. Adjunctive cholestyramine therapy for thyrotoxicosis. Clin Endocrinol (Oxf) 1993;38:39

42. Hughes G. Management of thyrotoxic crisis with a beta-adrenergic blocking agent (pronethalol). Br J Clin Pract 1966;20:579

43. Buckle RM. Treatment of thyroid crisis by beta-adrenergic blockade. Acta Endocrinol (Copenh) 1968;57:168

44. Galaburda M, Rosman NP, Haddow JE. Thyroid storm in an 11-year old boy managed by propranolol. Pediatrics 1974;53:920

45. Hellman R, Kelly KL, Mason WD. Propranolol for thyroid storm. N Engl J Med 1977;297:671

46. Feely J, Forrest A, Gunn A, et al. Propranolol dosage in thyrotoxicosis. J Clin Endocrinol Metab 1980;51:658

47. Rubenfeld S, Silverman VE, Welch KMA, et al. Variable plasma propranolol levels in thyrotoxicosis. N Engl J Med 1979;300:353

48. Das G, Krieger M. Treatment of thyrotoxic storm with intravenous administration of propranolol. Ann Intern Med 1969;70:985

49. Ikram H. Haemodynamic effects of beta-adrenergic blockade in hyperthyroid patients with and without heart failure. Br Med J [Clin Res] 1977;1:1505

50. Brunette DD, Rothong C. Emergency department management of thyrotoxic crisis with esmolol. Am J Emerg Med 1991;9:232

51. Isley WL, Dahl S, Gibbs H. Use of esmolol in managing a thyrotoxic patient needing emergency surgery. Am J Med 1990;89:122

52. Toft AD, Irvine WJ, Sinclair I, et al. Thyroid function after surgical treatment of thyrotoxicosis: a report of 100 cases treated with propranolol before operation. N Engl J Med 1978;298:643

53. Zonszein J, Santangelo RP, Mackin JF, et al. Propranolol therapy in thyrotoxicosis: a review of 84 patients undergoing surgery. Am J Med 1979;66:411

54. Jamison MH, Done HJ. Post-operative thyrotoxic crisis in a patient prepared for thyroidectomy with propranolol. Br J Clin Pract 1979;33:82

Werner and Ingbar's The Thyroid, Seventh Edition,
edited by Lewis E. Braverman and Robert D. Utiger.
Lippincott–Raven Publishers, Philadelphia, © 1996

Section D
Management of Thyrotoxicosis

52

Diagnosis of Thyrotoxicosis

Paul W. Ladenson

Thyrotoxicosis often presents as a distinctive clinical syndrome readily confirmed by the findings of high serum thyroid hormone concentrations and low serum thyrotropin (TSH) concentrations. Nonetheless, there are challenges in both the clinical and laboratory diagnosis of the disorder, including recognizing atypical and occult clinical presentations, differentiating thyrotoxicosis from other conditions causing real and apparent elevations in serum thyroid hormone concentrations,[1] and accurately distinguishing among its different causes so that the most appropriate treatment is used.

CLINICAL DIAGNOSIS

The symptoms and signs of overt thyrotoxicosis often result in a virtually pathognomonic clinical picture. Clinical diagnostic indexes based on these symptoms and signs accurately identify most patients with overt thyrotoxicosis,[2] but they have not been prospectively applied to primary care populations and correlate poorly with its biochemical severity.[3] There is considerable variability among patients in particular clinical features and their severity. For example, although weight loss despite good appetite is a classic manifestation of thyrotoxicosis, some patients gain weight and others are anorectic.[4] Furthermore, elderly patients may have few of the usual symptoms and signs of thyrotoxicosis,[4] but instead have mostly cardiovascular problems or weight loss, a syndrome termed apathetic thyrotoxicosis. Certain other syndromes, such as atrial fibrillation and systolic hypertension, or hypercalcemia, nephrolithiasis and osteoporosis, or persistent vomiting and hyperdefecation, should also suggest thyrotoxicosis.

Severe thyrotoxicosis may mimic febrile illnesses, heart failure due to primary cardiac disease, or toxic delirium. Thus, the clinical manifestations of thyrotoxicosis vary considerably, and it must be suspected clinically before it can be established or excluded by biochemical studies.

In most patients, the cause is Graves' disease, which is often accompanied by ophthalmopathy; rare patients have localized myxedema or thyroid acropachy (see the sections on ophthalmopathy and localized myxedema and thyroid acropachy in chap 30). The presence of exophthalmos, whether symmetric or not, or other extrathyroidal signs of Graves' disease should prompt laboratory assessment for thyrotoxicosis. Furthermore, certain groups have an increased risk for Graves' disease, including women in the third through sixth decade of life, patients with a family history of autoimmune thyroid disease, and those with certain other disorders that have an autoimmune pathogenesis (e.g., pernicious anemia, insulin-dependent diabetes mellitus, and myasthenia gravis).

Clinical features may also identify patients with less common forms of thyrotoxicosis. Patients with thyrotoxicosis caused by subacute (de Quervain's) thyroiditis have thyroid pain and tenderness and constitutional complaints, including fever and malaise. Those with toxic nodular goiter are usually older, and their thyrotoxicosis may have been provoked by recent exposure to iodine-containing medications (e.g., amiodarone or radiographic contrast agents). Detection of a thyroid nodule or multinodular goiter warrants screening for overt or subclinical thyrotoxicosis. Silent (painless) thyroiditis most often affects women 2 to 6 months postpartum (see chap 89). Factitious thyrotoxicosis is most likely to occur in health care workers or persons with access to thyroid hormone preparations, for example, those with a family member who is taking thyroid hormone.

Clues From Routine Laboratory Tests

Certain abnormalities detected by routine biochemical screening may also suggest the presence of thyrotoxicosis. These include hypercalcemia, elevated serum alkaline phosphatase concentrations, and low serum cholesterol concentrations. Similarly, the presence of thyrotoxicosis may be suggested by atrial arrhythmias detected by electrocardiography.

LABORATORY TESTING

Biochemical confirmation of thyrotoxicosis has traditionally been based on detection of elevated serum (or plasma) total and free thyroxine (T_4) and triiodothyronine (T_3) concentrations.[5] Most patients have high serum concentrations of both hormones, but some have isolated increases in either T_4 or T_3. Although serum thyroid hormone measurements are useful for detecting thyrotoxicosis and monitoring treatment of it, they have two limitations. First, there are other causes of high serum T_4 or T_3 concentrations. Second, some clinically thyrotoxic patients have serum T_4 and T_3 concentrations within the upper portion of the normal range. The development of sensitive assays for serum TSH has greatly simplified the diagnostic approach to thyrotoxicosis. These assays have in addition expanded the spectrum of thyrotoxicosis to include subclinical thyrotoxicosis (see chaps 18 and 88).

Serum Thyroxine Determinations

The serum total T_4 concentration can be measured accurately by competitive protein-binding assays using either anti-T_4 antibodies or serum thyroid hormone-binding proteins. Because most (99.97%) of the T_4 in serum is bound to thyroxine-binding globulin (TBG), transthyretin (TTR, or thyroxine-binding prealbumin), or albumin, an increase in any of these serum proteins, especially TBG, can cause a high serum total T_4 concentration (hyperthyroxinemia), which can be misconstrued as thyrotoxicosis (Table 52-1). Conversely, decreased T_4 binding by serum proteins may mask excess thyroid hormone production.

Estimation of the serum free T_4 concentration resolves most potential pitfalls associated with increased serum protein binding of T_4. Although equilibrium dialysis and ultrafiltration are the most accurate techniques for serum free T_4 measurement, the serum free T_4 index and serum free T_4 radioimmunoassays readily differentiate thyrotoxicosis from the most common cause of hyperthyroxinemia, which is TBG excess. Furthermore, the serum free T_4 index and free T_4 radioimmunoassays are simpler, quicker, and less costly. The former is the product of the serum total T_4 and the thyroid hormone-binding ratio (THBR; also known as the T_3 resin uptake).[6] The serum free T_4 radioimmunoassays, some of which use an analogue of T_4 that does not bind to thyroid hormone-binding proteins, usually yield comparable values. These assays are discussed in detail in chapter 18.

Other conditions that cause euthyroid hyperthyroxinemia may be more difficult to differentiate from thyrotoxicosis. Pa-

TABLE 52-1.
Causes of Elevated Serum Thyroxine Concentrations

Thyrotoxicosis
Increased serum protein binding
  Increased serum thyroxine-binding globulin concentrations
    Inherited
    Estrogen: pregnancy, exogenous, tumoral production
    Hepatitis, hepatoma
    HIV infection
    Drugs: methadone, heroin, clofibrate, 5-fluorouracil
  Familial dysalbuminemic hyperthyroxinemia
  Increased serum transthyretin concentrations
    Inherited
    Carcinoma of pancreas, hepatoma
Psychiatric and medical illness
Drugs
  Propranolol
  Amiodarone
  Radiographic contrast agents used for cholecystography
Anti-T_4 immunoglobulins

tients with familial dysalbuminemic hyperthyroxinemia produce a mutated form of albumin that binds T_4 with increased affinity, increasing the serum total serum T_4 concentration.[7,8] Because the mutated albumin binds T_3 poorly, THBR values are normal, and therefore serum free T_4 index values are high. Serum free T_4 analogue radioimmunoassay methods may also yield falsely elevated values in this condition. Similarly, increased TTR binding of T_4, which occurs as both an inherited trait[9] and in patients with carcinoma of the pancreas or liver,[10] causes an increased serum total T_4 concentration. Thyroid hormone-binding antibodies, which may be present in patients with chronic autoimmune thyroiditis or other autoimmune disorders, may cause spurious elevations in serum T_4 (or T_3) concentrations.[11]

Hyperthyroxinemia also may occur as a result of disorders that transiently increase the secretion of TSH (or chorionic gonadotropin) or disorders and medications that reduce T_4 clearance. For example, in one study of patients admitted to an inpatient medical service, modest elevations in serum total T_4 and free T_4 index values were found in 4% and 12%, respectively.[12] Two disorders—acute psychosis[13,14] and hyperemesis gravidarum[15]—have been associated with a substantial prevalence of euthyroid hyperthyroxinemia. Propranolol, when given in high doses (e.g., >160 mg/day[16]), and amiodarone[17] impair T_4 clearance, causing euthyroid hyperthyroxinemia (see section on the effects of pharmacologic agents on thyroid hormone metabolism in chap 14). Even though they have no clinical evidence of thyrotoxicosis, some patients receiving T_4 therapy have modest hyperthyroxinemia. Finally, patients with generalized thyroid hormone resistance typically have elevated serum total and free T_4 and T_3 concentrations and normal or slightly raised TSH concentrations[18] (see chap 90).

Therefore, hyperthyroxinemia is not a pathognomonic manifestation of thyrotoxicosis. The differential diagnosis is often obvious, based on clinical information (i.e., symptoms and signs of thyrotoxicosis or the other conditions associated with hyperthyroxinemia). Serum TSH measurements are valuable in distinguishing euthyroid hyperthyroxinemia, in which serum TSH usually is normal, from all common forms of thyrotoxicosis, in which serum TSH is low.

Serum Triiodothyronine Determinations

Serum total and free T_3 concentrations are high in most patients with thyrotoxicosis. The high values are attributable to both increased thyroidal T_3 production and increased extrathyroidal conversion of T_4 to T_3. About 2% of thyrotoxic patients in the United States have T_3 thyrotoxicosis, that is, they are clinically thyrotoxic and have high serum T_3 but normal T_4 concentrations. The diagnostic sensitivity of serum T_3 determinations alone is limited because some thyrotoxic patients have T_4 thyrotoxicosis.[19] The latter occurs primarily in patients who have both thyrotoxicosis and a severe nonthyroidal illness and in those with amiodarone-induced thyrotoxicosis; in both situations extrathyroidal T_3 production from T_4 is inhibited. Although serum T_3 concentrations are high in patients who have elevated serum TBG concentrations, the lower affinity of TBG for T_3 leads to a lesser rise in serum T_3 than T_4. Serum T_3 concentrations may be spuriously elevated in the rare patients with T_3-binding antibodies.[11] Consequently, an elevated serum total T_3 concentration is only relatively specific for thyrotoxicosis. With the availability of sensitive serum TSH assays, the diagnostic utility of serum T_3 measurements—never great— has declined further. However, they are occasionally useful in monitoring treatment in patients with thyrotoxicosis, in whom antithyroid drug or radioactive iodine therapy may have discordant effects on serum T_4 and T_3 concentrations, for example, the serum T_3 concentration may remain elevated despite a normal or low serum T_4.[20]

Serum Thyrotropin Determinations

The sensitivity of TSH secretion to inhibition by thyroid hormone makes measurement of the serum TSH concentration a remarkably accurate test for diagnosis of all common forms of thyrotoxicosis. TSH assays with detection limits of 0.1 mU/L or lower readily differentiate between these patients and normal subjects.[21] These assays have rendered thyrotropin-releasing hormone (TRH) stimulation tests obsolete, except possibly in the investigation of very sick hospitalized patients, who may have very low serum TSH concentrations[22,23] (see the section on nonthyroidal illness in chap 14). Although a sensitive indicator of thyrotoxicosis in general, serum TSH concentrations are normal or even elevated in the rare patients with TSH-induced thyrotoxicosis (see chap 31).

Screening, Case-Finding and Diagnosis

Based on the infrequency of thyrotoxicosis (see chap 26), and the relative ease with which it can be recognized clinically, biochemical screening for thyrotoxicosis among healthy persons is unjustified. Case-finding, that is, the identification of thyrotoxicosis in patients with vague symptoms or signs that could indicate the presence of thyrotoxicosis or in persons with special risk of thyrotoxicosis, however, can be done reliably by measurement of either the serum free T_4 index or serum TSH concentration.[24] The sensitivity of the former test is good, particularly if the cut-off value for the diagnosis is arbitrarily set at a value somewhat below the upper limit of the normal reference range, for example, 10.5 for an assay with a normal range of 5 to 12, which is comparable to a serum total T_4 concentration of 10.5 µg/dL (135 nmol/L) in a patient with normal serum thyroid hormone-binding proteins. Using this approach, only thyrotoxic patients with small increases in serum T_3 concentrations or low serum TBG concentrations would be overlooked. Falsely elevated serum free T_4 index values may be encountered in patients with familial dysalbuminemic hyperthyroxinemia and those with certain nonthyroidal illnesses or in those receiving several drugs, as noted previously.

A second, more sensitive method for case-finding is determination of the serum TSH concentration. Virtually all patients with thyrotoxicosis have low or undetectable serum TSH concentrations; only the rare patient with TSH-induced thyrotoxicosis will be missed by this approach. Therefore, a normal serum TSH concentration is strong evidence that the patient is euthyroid. However, low (i.e., 0.1 to 0.5 mU/L) or even undetectable (0.1 mU/L or less, depending on assay sensitivity) serum TSH values do not necessarily indicate the presence of thyrotoxicosis. Other causes of low values are subclinical thyrotoxicosis, nonthyroidal illness, and central hypothyroidism. Among older outpatients, the former is common, occurring in about 5%.[25–27] (see chap 88). Patients with nonthyroidal illness who have low serum TSH values are usually although not invariably acutely ill and in the hospital[23,28] (see section on nonthyroidal illness in chap 14). Central hypothyroidism is unlikely to be encountered in a case-finding study for thyrotoxicosis because it is rare and most patients have some clinical manifestations of hypothalamic or pituitary disease.

Whichever test is done for case-finding, any patient having an abnormal result should have the other test before any conclusion is drawn or any intervention is undertaken.

Among patients suspected clinically of having thyrotoxicosis, serum TSH and free T_4 should be measured (Fig 52-1). If the serum TSH value is low and the serum free T_4 value is high, the diagnosis is confirmed. If the serum TSH value is low and the serum free T_4 value is normal, the patient has either T_3 thyrotoxicosis, subclinical thyrotoxicosis, or nonthyroidal illness. Patients in either of the first two groups tend to have serum free T_4 values in the upper portion of the normal range and can be distinguished biochemically from one another by measurement of the serum T_3 concentration. If the serum TSH value is normal or high and the serum free T_4 value is high, then the patient should be evaluated for TSH-induced thyrotoxicosis; other explanations for these results are generalized resistance to thyroid hormone, or, if serum free T_4 was determined by a THBR method, familial dysalbuminemic hyperthyroxinemia. Patients with nonthyroidal illness have low-normal or low serum free T_4 values and also can usually be identified by the context in which they are encountered.

Diagnosis of the Cause of Thyrotoxicosis

Because the various causes of thyrotoxicosis require different therapies, it is essential that diagnosis of thyroid hormone excess be followed by definition of the underlying cause. In

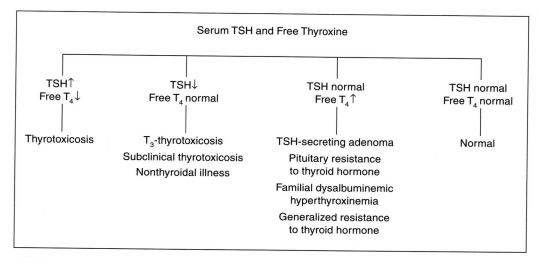

FIGURE 52-1. Diagnostic scheme for evaluating patients suspected of having thyrotoxicosis, subdivided according to combinations of normal or low serum TSH concentrations and normal or high serum fee thyroxine (T_4) values. Serum free thyroxine (T_4) can be measured either directly or indirectly as the serum free T_4 index (only the serum free T_4 index is high in patients with familial dysalbuminemic hyperthyroxinemia).

many patients, the history and physical examination alone are sufficient (e.g., a thyrotoxic woman with diffuse goiter and exophthalmos, indicating Graves' disease, and a thyrotoxic patient with neck pain and tenderness, indicating subacute thyroiditis). In other patients, additional laboratory or in vivo radionuclide studies may be needed to establish the cause and guide therapeutic decision-making (e.g., a woman with postpartum thyrotoxicosis, who could have painless [postpartum] thyroiditis, Graves' disease, or even factitious thyrotoxicosis).

The relative elevations of serum T_3 and T_4 concentrations may provide a clue to the cause of thyrotoxicosis. Exuberant T_3 production is common in Graves' hyperthyroidism and toxic nodular goiter (i.e., a serum T_3:T_4 [ng/dL:µg/dL] ratio > 20.) T_4-predominant thyrotoxicosis (i.e., a serum T_3:T_4 ratio < 15) suggests that thyroiditis (subacute or silent), iodine-induced thyrotoxicosis, or exogenous T_4 ingestion may be the

cause. Measurements of thyroidal uptake of radioactive iodine or pertechnetate or thyroid imaging are needed for differential diagnosis in only a minority of patients (Table 52-2). Thyrotoxicosis caused by excessive thyroid secretion is typically accompanied by increased uptake in functioning tissue, whereas thyroid inflammation and exogenous T_4 ingestion are associated with low thyroidal uptake.

The clinical utility of assays for antibodies directed against the TSH receptor in Graves' disease is limited. These assays measure the ability of the patient's serum (or immunoglobulin fraction) either to inhibit the binding of TSH to its receptor (TSH receptor-binding inhibitory antibodies) or to stimulate thyroid tissue in some way (e.g., adenylyl cyclase activity [thyroid-stimulating antibodies]) (see chap 21). Tests for these antibodies may be used to diagnose Graves' disease in clinically and biochemically euthyroid patients with ophthalmopathy,

TABLE 52-2.
Thyroidal Radioiodine Uptake and Imaging in the Differential Diagnosis of Causes of Thyrotoxicosis

Cause of Thyrotoxicosis	Fractional Uptake in 24 hours (%)	Pattern of Distribution of Radionuclide in Thyroid
Graves' disease	35–95	Homogenous
Toxic nodular goiter (uni- or multinodular)	20–60	Restricted to regions of autonomy
Subacute thyroiditis	0–2	Little or no uptake
Silent thyroiditis	0–2	Little or no uptake
Iodine-induced thyrotoxicosis	0–50	Heterogeneous or no uptake
Factitious or iatrogenic thyrotoxicosis	0–2	Little or no uptake
Struma ovarii*	0–2	Uptake in ovary
Follicular carcinoma	0–5	Uptake in tumor metastases
TSH-induced thyrotoxicosis	30–80	Homogeneous

Autonomously functioning thyroid tissue in an ovarian teratoma.

and in unusual cases when differentiation of Graves' disease from toxic multinodular goiter is otherwise difficult and therapeutically important, but the tests are relatively expensive.

Certain tests are useful in the diagnosis of other forms of thyrotoxicosis. Most patients with subacute thyroiditis have an elevated erythrocyte sedimentation rate, but those with silent thyroiditis do not. Serum thyroglobulin concentrations are high in patients with thyrotoxicosis caused by thyroid hypersecretion or inflammation, but not in those with factitious or iatrogenic thyrotoxicosis (see chap 20). Measurements of the serum glycoprotein hormone alpha-subunit concentration may be of value in confirming a diagnosis of TSH-secreting pituitary adenoma (see chap 31).

References

1. Bartalena L, Robbins. Variations in thyroid hormone transport proteins and their clinical implications. Thyroid 1992;2:237
2. Crooks J, Murray IPC, Wayne EL. Statistical methods applied to the clinical diagnosis of thyrotoxicosis. Q J Med 1959;28:211
3. Trzepacz PT, Klein I, Roberts M, et al. Graves' disease: an analysis of thyroid hormone levels and hyperthyroid signs and symptoms. Am J Med 1989;87:558
4. Nordyke RA, Gilbert FI Jr, Harada AS. Graves' disease. Influence of age on clinical findings. Arch Intern Med 1988;248:626
5. Surks MI, Chopra IJ, Mariash CN, et al. American Thyroid Association guidelines for use of laboratory tests in thyroid disorders. JAMA 1990;263:1529
6. Larsen PR, Alexander NM, Chopra IJ, et al. Revised nomenclature for tests of thyroid hormones and thyroid-related proteins in serum. J Clin Endocrinol Metab 1987;64:1089
7. Heufelder AE, Klee GG, Wynne AG, Gharib H. Familial dysalbuminemic hyperthyroxinemia: cumulative experience in 29 consecutive patients. Endocr Practice 1995;1:4
8. Rushbrook JI, Becker E, Schussler GC, Divino CM. Identification of a human serum albumin species associated with familial dysalbuminemic hyperthyroxinemia. J Clin Endocrinol Metab 1995;80:461
9. Moses AC, Rosen HN, Moller DE, et al. A point mutation in transthyretin increases affinity for thyroxine and produces euthyroid hyperthyroxinemia. J Clin Invest 1990;86:2025
10. Rajatanavin R, Liberman C, Lawrence GD, et al. Euthyroid hyperthyroxinemia and thyroxine-binding prealbumin excess in islet cell carcinoma. J Clin Endocrinol Metab 1985;61:17
11. Sakata S. Autoimmunity against thyroid hormones. Crit Rev Immunol 1994;14:157
12. Gooch BR, Isley WL, Utiger, RD. Abnormalities in thyroid function tests in patients admitted to a medical service. Arch Intern Med 1982;142:1801
13. Spratt DI, Pont A, Miller MB, et al. Hyperthyroxinemia in patients with acute psychiatric disorders. Am J Med 1982;73:41
14. Chopra IJ, Solomon DH, Huang T-S. Serum thyrotropin in hospitalized psychiatric patients: evidence for hyperthyrotropinemia as measured by an ultrasensitive thyrotropin assay. Metabolism 1990;39:538
15. Goodwin TM, Montoro M, Mestman JH, et al. The role of chorionic gonadotropin in transient hyperthyroidism of hyperemesis gravidarum. J Clin Endocrinol Metab 1992;75:1333
16. Cooper DS, Daniels GH, Ladenson PW, Ridgway EC. Hyperthyroxinemia in patients with high-dose propranolol. Am J Med 1982;73:867
17. Figge HL, Figge J. The effect of amiodarone on thyroid hormone function: a review of physiology and clinical manifestations. J Clin Pharmacol 1990;30:588
18. Refetoff S, Usala SJ. The syndromes of resistance to thyroid hormones. Endocr Rev 1993;14:348
19. Caplan RH, Pagliara AS, Wickus G. Thyroxine toxicosis: a common variant of hyperthyroidism. JAMA 1980;244:1934
20. Chen JJ, Ladenson PW. Discordant hypothyroxinemia and hypertriiodothyroninemia in treated patients with hyperthyroid Graves' disease. J Clin Endocrinol Metab 1986;63:102
21. Klee GG, Hay ID. Assessment of sensitive thyrotropin assays for an expanded role in thyroid function testing: proposed criteria for analytic performance and clinical utility. J Clin Endocrinol Metab 1987;64:461
22. Spencer CA, LoPresti JS, Patel A, et al. Applications of a new chemiluminescent thyrotropin assay to subnormal measurement. J Clin Endocrinol Metab 1990;70:453
23. Franklyn JA, Black EG, Betteridge J, Sheppard MC. Comparison of second and third generation methods for measurement of serum thyrotropin in patients with overt hyperthyroidism, patients receiving thyroxine therapy, and those with nonthyroidal illness. J Clin Endocrinol Metab 1994;78:1368
24. de los Santos ET, Stanch GH, Mazzaferri EL. Sensitivity, specificity and cost-effectiveness of the sensitive thyrotropin assay in the diagnosis of thyroid disease in ambulatory patients. Arch Intern Med 1989;149:526
25. Sawin CT, Geller A, Kaplan MM, et al. Low serum thyrotropin (thyroid-stimulating hormone) in older persons without hyperthyroidism. Arch Intern Med 1991;151:165
26. Parle JV, Franklyn JA, Cross KW, et al. Prevalence and follow-up of abnormal thyrotrophin (TSH) concentrations in the elderly in the United Kingdom. Clin Endocrinol 1991;34:77
27. Sawin CT, Geller A, Wolf PA, et al. Low serum thyrotropin concentrations as a risk factor for atrial fibrillation in older persons. N Engl J Med 1994;331:1249
28. Eggertsen R, Petersen K, Lundberg P-A, et al. Screening for thyroid disease in a primary care unit with a thyroid stimulating hormone assay with a low detection limit. BMJ 1988;297:1586

Werner and Ingbar's The Thyroid, Seventh Edition,
edited by Lewis E. Braverman and Robert D. Utiger.
Lippincott–Raven Publishers, Philadelphia, © 1996

53

Treatment of Thyrotoxicosis

David S. Cooper

The ideal treatment of thyrotoxicosis would be directed at its cause. This is possible in only a few patients, for example, those with exogenous thyrotoxicosis or thyrotropin (TSH)-secreting pituitary adenomas. In patients with thyrotoxicosis due to its more common causes, especially Graves' disease, autonomously functioning thyroid adenoma (toxic adenoma), and multinodular goiter, the fundamental causes are not known. Therapy is, therefore, directed to destroying thyroid tissue, pharmacologically inhibiting thyroidal thyroxine (T_4) and triiodothyronine (T_3) synthesis and release, and ameliorating the impact of T_4 and T_3 on peripheral tissues, alone or in combination. There are several means of accomplishing these goals, and their efficacy depends to some extent on the cause of the thyrotoxicosis. Because this is so, an attempt should be made to determine the cause; this usually can be achieved by history and physical examination, aided by selected laboratory tests such as measurements of thyroid radioiodine uptake and thyroid radioisotope imaging (see chap 52 and the several chapters [chaps 30–35] in which the different causes of thyrotoxicosis are discussed).

This chapter considers the several forms of treatment of thyrotoxicosis—antithyroid drugs, radioactive iodine, and thyroidectomy—that are in wide use now. The emphasis is on treatment of the thyroid hyperactivity (hyperthyroidism) caused by Graves' disease because it is the most common cause of thyrotoxicosis, and it is the area in which the relative merits of the three treatments are most vigorously debated. When appropriate, the treatment of some of the other causes of thyrotoxicosis and of special patients (e.g., children, pregnant women, and patients with thyrotoxic storm) are mentioned. Information about treatment of some of the less common causes of the disorder can be found in the chapters dealing with those disorders.

THYROTOXICOSIS CAUSED BY GRAVES' DISEASE

Graves' disease is characterized by thyrotoxicosis caused by diffuse hyperplasia and hypersecretion of the thyroid, infiltrative ophthalmopathy, and localized myxedema. Although the cause is far from certain, Graves' disease is clearly autoimmune in nature and is probably caused by an abnormal population of autoreactive T cells.[1] The consequence is the production of thyroid-stimulating antibodies (TSab), which are antibodies to the TSH receptor on the thyroid follicular cell (thyrocyte) membrane. These antibodies activate the TSH receptor in a manner analogous to TSH itself, causing increased thyroid hormone synthesis and release as well as growth of the thyroid gland. The large body of information about the pathogenesis of Graves' disease is reviewed in the section on pathogenesis in chapter 30.

Autoimmune diseases are well known for their tendency to wax and wane in severity over time, and Graves' disease is no exception. Although spontaneous remissions occur without therapy, Graves' disease—or rather the thyrotoxicosis that results—is now virtually always treated. This is because spontaneous remissions are unusual and because the resulting thyrotoxicosis can have deleterious effects on multiple organ systems, as well as the psyche. In addition, there are a variety of therapies from which to choose, and although all of them have certain drawbacks, treatment usually is effective and safe. Which therapy is best is a matter of debate, and opinions vary from country to country and from continent to continent.[2,3] No treatment is "best" and the final choice depends on a number of factors, not the least of which are the physician's experience and the patient's preferences. In some situations (e.g., in pregnant women and in the elderly), the therapeutic options are more limited.

The chief therapeutic objective is to alleviate the patient's thyrotoxicosis. Pharmacologic therapy, usually with an antithyroid drug, produces a euthyroid state by interfering with thyroid hormone production. Whether the remissions that sometimes occur during such therapy are spontaneous or are associated with drug-related effects on the immune system is a matter of debate and is discussed later in more detail. In contrast, the ablative forms of treatment, surgery and radioiodine, reduce the mass of thyroid tissue but are not thought to alter the underlying pathogenetic mechanisms, except possibly by removing intrathyroidal lymphocytes, a source of TSab. Hypothyroidism usually follows these latter two treatments but also may occur during or after drug therapy,[4,5] possibly because of continuing autoimmune destruction of the thyroid.[6,7] Thus, the end result may be the same, regardless of the form of therapy the patient receives.

PHARMACOLOGIC THERAPY OF THYROTOXICOSIS CAUSED BY GRAVES' DISEASE

Antithyroid Drugs

Antithyroid drugs have been a mainstay of treatment since their introduction in the mid-1940s.[8,9] They can be used in the treatment of patients with other forms of thyrotoxicosis (e.g., toxic nodular goiter), but they usually are not primary modes of therapy for these conditions. These drugs inhibit the synthesis of thyroid hormone, leading to gradual reduction in serum thyroid hormone concentrations. After several weeks or a few months, the dosage usually can be reduced, and ultimately the medication can be discontinued altogether, and the patient may remain euthyroid for months or years. These remissions, usually defined as being euthyroid for at least 1 year, occur in about half the patients. They may not be durable,[10] but may last for many years or be permanent[11] (Fig 53-1).

The antithyroid drugs to be considered here are five- or six-membered heterocyclic compounds known as thionamides that contain the thioureylene moiety within the ring structure

(Fig 53-2). There are two basic classes of antithyroid drugs: the thiouracils and the imidazoles. The thiouracils have six-membered rings, the prototype of which is thiouracil itself; propylthiouracil (6-propyl-2-thiouracil; PTU) is the only member of this class in use today. The imidazoles have five-membered rings, with methimazole (1-methyl 2-mercaptoimidazole; MMI; Tapazole) in use in North America and Japan and a related compound, carbimazole (1-methyl-2-thio-3 carbethoxy-imidazole), used mainly in Europe. Because carbimazole is rapidly metabolized to MMI[12] and has no properties not shared by MMI, the two drugs can be considered as one.

The origin of antithyroid drugs dates back to the early 1940s, with the serendipitous observations of two groups working independently at Johns Hopkins Medical School. Richter and Clisby, who were studying taste preferences in laboratory animals, noted that the bitter substance phenylthiocarbamide caused goiter in rats.[13] The MacKenzies,[14] who were studying the gut flora of guinea pigs, recognized that the nonabsorbable antibiotic sulfaguanidine also caused goiter. They[15] and Astwood[16] subsequently determined that the cause of the goiter was stimulation of the thyroid by the pituitary gland, consequent to the pharmacologic inhibition of thyroid hormone production. Indeed, the elucidation of this seminal aspect of endocrine physiology hinged on the discovery and availability of these goitrogenic compounds. Within 18 months after the observation that sulfaguanidine and thiourea caused goiter, Astwood[8,9] had proposed that goitrogens could be used to treat thyrotoxicosis, had screened a large number of potentially useful compounds using a bioassay system, and had even conducted clinical trials with thiourea and thiouracil. Indeed, he coined the term *antithyroid drug*.[17]

MECHANISM OF ACTION

The actions of the antithyroid compounds can be divided into those effects that are *intrathyroidal* and those that are primarily *extrathyroidal*. The chief intrathyroidal actions are: inhibition of iodine oxidation and organification, inhibition of iodotyrosine coupling, possible alteration of the structure of thyroglobulin, and possible inhibition of thyroglobulin biosyn-

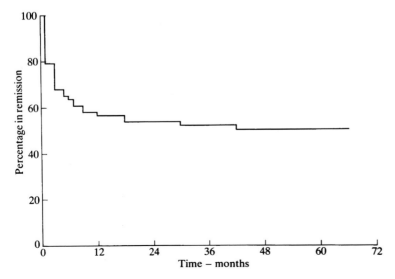

FIGURE 53-1. The percentage of patients with Graves' hyperthyroidism remaining in remission after discontinuation of antithyroid drug therapy. (Young ET, Steel NR, Talor JJ, et al. Prediction of remission after antithyroid drug treatment in Graves' disease. Q J Med 1988;250:175)

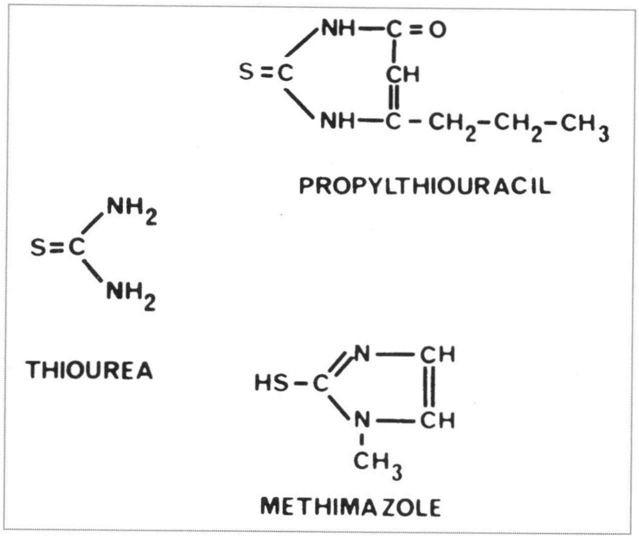

FIGURE 53-2. The structure of the thionamide antithyroid drugs.

thesis. Extrathyroidal actions include: inhibition of conversion of T_4 to T_3 (PTU and other thiouracils, but not MMI) and possible immunosuppressive effects (which are probably intrathyroidal as well).

Intrathyroidal Effects. Detailed descriptions of antithyroid drug pharmacology can be found in chapter 4 and in the section on antithyroid compounds in chapter 14. Antithyroid drugs are actively trapped by the thyroid gland[18–20] by way of a pathway that is similar but probably not identical to the iodide transport system.[21] These compounds do not inhibit iodide transport or block the release of stored thyroid hormone. Their most important actions are interference with thyroid peroxidase (TPO)-mediated iodide oxidation and organification and with iodothyronine coupling. The mechanisms by which these actions occur are far from certain. In the presence of iodine, which is present in high concentrations within the thyroid, the drugs compete with tyrosyl residues in thyroglobulin for oxidized iodine.[22,23] In so doing, they divert the oxidized iodine away from the thyroid hormone biosynthetic process. The drugs themselves ultimately are oxidized and degraded. Antithyroid drugs also interfere with the TPO-catalyzed coupling process by which iodotyrosine residues are combined to form T_4 and T_3; the drug concentrations required to inhibit coupling are less than those required to inhibit iodine organification.[24]

In addition to the important effects on iodine oxidation and organification and on the coupling reaction, autoradiographic studies suggest that antithyroid drugs bind to thyroglobulin after they have been oxidized.[25] Such binding could change the conformation of the thyroglobulin molecule, perhaps rendering it more resistant to subsequent iodination or to hydrolysis. Several other in vitro intrathyroidal actions of antithyroid drugs deserve mention: they may inhibit the biosynthesis of thyroglobulin,[26] although the concentrations required are probably higher (10^{-3} mol/L) than achieved in

vivo in humans,[27] and they may inhibit thyroid follicular cell function and growth.[28,29]

Extrathyroidal Effects. PTU, but not MMI, blocks the conversion of T_4 to T_3 in peripheral tissues (and the thyroid) by inhibiting the activity of type 1 T_4-5′ (outer ring)-deiodinase (see chap 8). The mechanism is uncertain but may involve competition between the drug and the essential cofactor for the reaction, reduced sulfhydryl groups.[30] In addition, PTU and other thiouracil derivatives may bind covalently to the deiodinase enzyme via a selenosulfide bond,[31] thereby inactivating it.[32] MMI is not an inhibitor of this reaction, probably because of the methyl substitution at the N1 position; other imidazole derivatives do inhibit T_4-to-T_3 conversion in vitro.[33] The clinical importance of the ability of PTU to block T_4-to-T_3 conversion is discussed later.

Effects on the Immune System. The possible immunosuppressive effects of the antithyroid drugs have attracted a great deal of attention in recent years.[34–36] Although for the purpose of classification these putative effects are extrathyroidal, they almost certainly involve actions on intrathyroidal immune function as well. The central question is whether the effects are caused primarily by the antithyroid drugs' actions on the immune system itself, or whether the abatement of autoimmune phenomena is simply the result of deactivation of the immune system concomitant with the decline in thyroid secretion. In studies describing in vitro drug effects, the observed activity can be directly ascribed to the drug. In most in vivo studies, however, the distinction between direct and indirect effects is ambiguous.

Despite some negative data,[37] numerous in vitro studies have documented an effect of antithyroid compounds on various arms of the immune system. Antithyroid drugs can inhibit lymphocyte transformation in vitro,[38] and they may have other inhibitory[39–41] (as well as stimulatory[39–41]) effects on lymphocyte, monocyte,[39] and neutrophil[39,42] function and on formation of soluble mediators such as interleukin-2.[43] The formation of free radicals, which may be important in T-cell responsiveness and in complement-mediated thyroid cell injury, may be inhibited by MMI.[44] In addition, the expression of major histocompatibility complex (MHC) class II (HLA-DR) molecules on thyroid cells may be important for the initiation or maintenance of Graves' disease,[45] and antithyroid drugs may reduce HLA-DR expression either directly[46] or by inhibiting secretion of the class II molecule inducer, γ-interferon, by T cells.[47] Recently, MMI was found to reduce MHC class I mRNA concentrations in cultured thyroid cells (FRTL-5 cells) directly.[48]

There is also strong in vivo evidence, albeit circumstantial, for an immunologic effect of antithyroid drugs. The thyroid glands of hyperthyroid patients who had been prepared for thyroidectomy with an antithyroid drug are depleted of lymphocytes, compared with patients who had been prepared only with the β-adrenergic receptor antagonist propranolol.[49] In addition, the serum concentrations of TSab, whether measured by bioassay or receptor assay, and other antithyroid antibodies decline during antithyroid drug therapy.[50,51] The effects appear to be specific for thyroid-related autoantibodies, because the concentrations of antiparietal cell antibodies did not change[52] in patients with coexisting autoimmune gastritis.

Furthermore, antithyroid drug treatment results in changes in cell-mediated immunity in patients with Graves' disease. For example, an increase (normalization) in suppressor T-cell number during treatment was found in several[53-55] but not all[56] studies, and helper T-cell[54] and natural killer-cell activity decrease.[57] Also, MMI decreases the number of activated T cells within the thyroid itself, compared with the pretreatment number,[54] although HLA-DR expression does not change.

Despite the evidence for an immunomodulatory effect of antithyroid drugs, a number of caveats are necessary. With regard to the in vitro data, most studies have documented effects at drug concentrations in the range of 10^{-4} to 10^{-5} mol/L, whereas intrathyroidal concentrations in vivo are unlikely to exceed 5×10^{-5} mol/L,[27,58] thus casting some doubt on the pharmacologic relevance of the observed effects. The changes in autoantibody titers and in T-cell subsets do not occur in all patients, and the changes that do occur are variable. The reasons for this are unclear; they relate to the question of whether remissions of Graves' disease are spontaneous, or whether they are induced by the antithyroid drug (see later discussion). Finally, any changes in immune response markers that may be provoked by antithyroid drug therapy inevitably occur in a setting wherein the thyrotoxic state has been ameliorated, at least to some degree.[34] Thus, if the thyrotoxic state is responsible, at least in part, for perpetuation of the altered immunity, then its correction would tend to reduce the activity of the immune system. Thus, therapy for thyrotoxicosis caused by Graves' disease with potassium perchlorate leads to a decline in serum TSab concentrations in a manner similar to that which occurs during antithyroid drug treatment.[59] However, perchlorate may also have immunosuppressive effects.[60]

Despite these reservations, additional in vivo data indicate an immunosuppressive effect of thionamide derivatives. First, in rats, administration of MMI causes serologic and histologic attenuation of experimental[61,62] and iodine-induced autoimmune thyroiditis.[63] Second, in one study of euthyroid patients with chronic autoimmune (Hashimoto's) thyroiditis, administration of carbimazole caused a decline in antithyroid peroxidase antibody titers,[51] a result not confirmed, however, by two other, more carefully controlled studies.[64,65] Finally, MMI, but not glucocorticoids, blocks the rise in serum TSab concentrations that occurs in patients treated with radioiodine therapy for thyrotoxicosis caused by Graves' disease (see later discussion), suggesting that an organ-specific effect, rather than generalized immunosuppression, is of primary importance.[66] In another study, patients treated with either PTU or carbimazole had identical decrements in serum thyroid hormone concentrations, but the carbimazole-treated patients had greater decreases in serum TSab concentrations and increases in the number of suppressor T cells, suggesting, indirectly, an effect on the immune system independent of thyroid function.[67]

To summarize, antithyroid drugs can inhibit immune function in vitro, but the concentrations of drug required may be higher than are attained within the thyroid gland during treatment. Changes in antithyroid antibodies, TSab, and T-cell subsets occur in patients receiving chronic antithyroid drug therapy, but changes in thyroid function occur concomitantly, making it impossible to distinguish cause and effect satisfactorily.

CLINICAL PHARMACOLOGY OF THE ANTITHYROID DRUGS

Methimazole. MMI is almost completely absorbed from the gastrointestinal tract.[68,69] Peak serum concentrations occur 1 to 2 hours after ingestion and are in the range of 300 ng/mL (2.6 μmol/L) after a 15-mg oral dose[69] (Table 53-1). The serum concentrations are dose related and correlate with effects on iodine organification.[70] Carbimazole is rapidly converted to MMI in the serum: 10 mg carbimazole yields about 6 mg MMI.[12] The relatively long 6- to 8-hour serum half-life of MMI is somewhat surprising because little is bound to serum proteins.[69,71] The serum half-life of MMI is unchanged in patients with thyrotoxicosis[69,71] although MMI clearance may be more rapid in patients who fail to respond to the drug clinically.[72] Drug clearance is unchanged in patients with renal disease[68] but is prolonged in those with hepatic disease.[71] The practical consequence of the latter is uncertain. Intrathyroidal MMI concentrations are about 500 to 2000 ng/g (about 5×10^{-5} mol/L).[27,58] The intrathyroidal turnover of MMI is slow, with concentrations 17 to 20 hours after ingestion similar to those 3 to 6 hours after ingestion,[27] which may account for the longer duration of action of MMI. The effects of MMI dissipated within 24 hours in one study,[73] in contrast to older data suggesting a longer duration of action.[74] The excretion products of MMI are poorly defined although little unchanged drug appears in the urine.[75] Because it is not protein bound[71] and is lipid soluble, MMI freely crosses membranes (e.g., placenta[76] and breast epithelium[71]). Because of its relatively long serum (and intrathyroidal) half-life, as well as its long duration of action, MMI is effective when given as a single daily dose.[77-80]

Although the potency of MMI is commonly regarded as being about 10 times that of PTU, it is almost surely greater and may be up to 50 times more potent.[70] Indeed, thyrotoxicosis can be controlled in most patients with doses of MMI that are less, for example, 10 to 15 mg daily, than those traditionally thought to be necessary.[79,80] The difference in potency between MMI and PTU is probably not due to an actual difference at the biochemical level, but rather to differences in

TABLE 53-1.
Selected Pharmacologic Features of Antithyroid Drugs

	Propylthiouracil	Methimazole
Serum protein binding	~75%	Nil
Serum half-life	75 min	~4–6 h
Volume of distribution	~20 L	~40 L
Metabolism of drug during illness		
Severe liver disease	Normal	Decreased
Severe kidney disease	Normal	Normal
Transplacental passage	Low	Higher
Levels in breast milk	Low	Higher

From references 83, 86, 87, and 120

uptake into and metabolism within the thyroid gland because in vitro studies do not show MMI to be a significantly more potent inhibitor of TPO-catalyzed reactions.[23]

Propylthiouracil. After oral ingestion, PTU is almost completely absorbed. Peak serum concentrations occur about 1 hour after ingestion and are are dose dependent, with peak concentrations of about 3 µg/mL (18 µmol/L) after a 150-mg oral dose[81] (see Table 53-1). Serum PTU concentrations correlate with the drug's effects on iodine oxidation and organification and with inhibition of T_4-5′– deiodinase activity.[81] Data on intrathyroidal concentrations, which are most relevant to efficacy and duration of action, are extremely limited.[20] The serum half-life of PTU is in the range of 1 to 2 hours, and it is not altered in patients with thyrotoxicosis[81] or hepatic[82] or renal failure,[83] or in children[84] and the elderly.[85] The drug is heavily (80–90%) protein bound,[86] largely to serum albumin,[87] and is ionized at physiologic pH.[88] This has important implications for PTU therapy in pregnant and lactating women (see later discussion) because free (i.e., unbound) drug concentrations are low and ionized drug does not freely cross membranes. The primary route of PTU excretion is renal, after formation of the glucuronide derivative in the liver.[76]

The duration of action of PTU is about 12 to 24 hours[74,89] and probably depends on a variety of factors, including the rates at which the drug is concentrated and degraded within the thyroid. Clearly, the duration of action is longer than the serum half-life. This has important implications for therapy because a longer duration of action permits less frequent dosing, and therefore improved compliance. Although PTU can sometimes be given satisfactorily as a single daily dose,[90] it usually is given every 6 to 8 hours,[91] at least when therapy is initiated. With time, the frequency and total daily dose often can be decreased.[89]

CLINICAL CONSIDERATIONS IN THE USE OF ANTITHYROID DRUGS

The thionamide antithyroid drugs are chiefly used for the long-term management of patients with thyrotoxicosis caused by Graves' disease, with the expectation—or at least the hope—that a remission of the Graves' disease will occur. In recent surveys, radioiodine, not an antithyroid drug, was the preferred treatment for these patients in the United States except in children, adolescents, and younger adults.[2,3] In contrast, an antithyroid drug is the treatment of choice in much of the rest of the world, including Europe and Japan.[2] The clinical factors that influence the choice of therapy and the likelihood of remission are discussed later. Antithyroid drugs also are used in several other settings: during pregnancy, which is discussed separately; as a prelude to surgery or radioiodine therapy; and in neonatal Graves' disease, which is usually a transient condition.

Both MMI and PTU are extremely (at least 90%) effective in controlling thyrotoxicosis due to Graves' disease, and to some extent, the choice between the two drugs is a matter of personal preference. In fact, in a survey of practicing thyroidologists in the United States, PTU was preferred over MMI by a margin of more than 2:1.[3] One explanation for this is the fact that PTU was introduced 5 years before MMI, so that experience with it is greater. Another reason is the ability of PTU to inhibit T_4-to-T_3 conversion, a property not shared by MMI. Serum T_3 concentrations do decline more rapidly after the initiation of PTU therapy, but there is no evidence that the more rapid decline is clinically important, except perhaps in the case of severe or life-threatening thyrotoxicosis (thyrotoxic storm).[92,93] In fact, for most patients, MMI therapy results in more rapid normalization of serum T_4 and T_3 concentrations than does PTU therapy.[94] This may be related to the increased potency or the longer duration of action of MMI, as discussed earlier.

Propylthiouracil is available in 50-mg tablets and MMI in either 5- or 10-mg tablets. The usual starting dose of PTU is 100 mg three times daily. The starting dosage of MMI has been 20 to 30 mg daily, often in divided doses, but it is now clear that smaller doses given once daily are adequate for most patients.[95] In a recent prospective multicenter trial from Europe, 10 mg/d was nearly as effective as 40 mg/d;[96] serum T_4 and T_3 concentrations were normal in 6 weeks in 85% of the patients given 10 mg/d and 92% of those given 40 mg/d. Patients living in areas of relative iodine deficiency had a more rapid response, an effect that has been noted previously.[97] There is little additional benefit of even higher doses.[98] For both drugs, an increase in dosage is required if thyroid function fails to improve within 4 to 6 weeks. Doses of PTU as high as 2000 mg daily have been used in patients thought to be resistant to the drug, but in most instances the problem was poor compliance.[99] Assuming that thyroid function improves during the ensuing weeks to months, the dose of antithyroid drug often can be decreased substantially, for example, to 50 to 100 mg PTU daily, or 2.5 to 5 mg MMI daily or even every other day. Other factors that determine the speed of recovery include disease activity, the initial degree of thyroid hyperfunction, and the intrathyroidal hormonal stores. The ability to reduce the dose with continuing treatment probably reflects waning of disease activity, possibly reflected by a decline in TSab production and also because the goal of therapy changes, from complete to partial inhibition of thyroid hormone synthesis.

If large doses of drug should continue to be required for control, remission is unlikely, and ablative therapy usually is selected. Some authors have argued that continuous high-dose antithyroid drug therapy is preferable to the strategy of reducing the dose to maintain thyroid function within normal limits because rates of remission may be higher as a result of greater putative immunosuppressive effects. Such therapy has not been widely used because it requires concomitant T_4 therapy to prevent iatrogenic hypothyroidism and because the frequency of serious side effects may be greater with high doses.[96,100,101] However, combined therapy may enhance the chances of remission,[102] as discussed below.

The choice of antithyroid drug is an individual matter, based mainly on the physician's personal preferences and experience. There are a number of reasons why MMI might be selected over PTU.[103] First, the likelihood of compliance with once-a-day MMI is a clear advantage; whether PTU can be given, at least initially, in a single daily dose is uncertain.[90,91] Second, MMI is less expensive than PTU. Third, patients treated with MMI become euthyroid more quickly.[94] Finally, low doses of MMI may be safer than PTU,[104] at least in terms of the most important side effect of these drugs, which is agranulocytosis (see later discussion). In some special circumstances—pregnancy, lactation, and thyrotoxic storm—PTU is preferable.

SIDE EFFECTS OF ANTITHYROID DRUGS

The side effects of antithyroid drugs are varied (Table 53-2), but most fall into a category that would be considered to be allergic. Fever, rash, urticaria, and arthralgia occur in 1% to 5% of patients treated with these drugs,[105,106] the rates of these minor reactions being more common in patients treated with larger doses.[96,107] A transient asymptomatic rise in serum aminotransferase concentrations may occur in one-third of patients within 2 months of starting PTU therapy,[108] but routine monitoring of liver function is not recommended. The more serious, and rarer, toxic reactions (major side effects) are agranulocytosis, aplastic anemia, a lupus-like syndrome,[109] hepatitis,[110] polyarthritis,[111] and vasculitis,[112,113] all of which, with the exception of agranulocytosis, are more common with PTU. Agranulocytosis, the most feared problem, probably occurs with equal frequency with both drugs (about 0.2–0.5%); the other reactions are less common. Elderly patients may be more susceptible to agranulocytosis.[104,114] Most side effects occur within the first 1 to 3 months after initiation of therapy,[114] but there are well documented cases of serious toxicity developing after 1 year of treatment.[100] Antithyroid drug therapy is commonly intermittent; many patients take a drug for 1 or 2 years, discontinue it for weeks or months, even years, only to resume therapy at a later date if a relapse occurs. In this situation, drug reactions are as likely, or perhaps even more likely to occur,[45] even if the first course of therapy was uneventful.

Agranulocytosis is the most frequent major side effect of antithyroid drug therapy. It is an immunologic phenomenon, with evidence of lymphocyte sensitization in affected patients, but not in those merely exposed to antithyroid compounds.[115] In addition, antibodies to granulocytes and granulocytic progenitor cells are found in the serum of patients during the acute episode.[116,117] Although the mechanisms responsible for the agranulocytosis are unclear, it also is a complication of therapy with other sulfhydryl-containing drugs (e.g., phenothiazines, angiotensin-converting enzyme inhibitors, and sulfonamides).

Agranulocytosis, defined as a granulocyte count less than 250×10^9 cells/L, usually develops so suddenly that routine monitoring of the leukocyte count has been thought to be of little use. A recent report suggested that some patients with severe granulocytopenia, defined as a granulocyte count less than 500×10^9 cells/L, but greater than 250×10^9 cells/L, may be asymptomatic, and that they can be detected by routine monitoring of leukocyte count.[114] In these patients, prompt discontinuation of therapy led to resolution of the granulocytopenia, without progression to agranulocytosis. If this observation is confirmed, periodic surveillance of the leukocyte count would be reasonable, at least during the first 3 months of therapy, when almost all reported cases of agranulocytosis have occurred. However, due to the low frequency of this side effect, the cost effectiveness of routine monitoring must be questioned.

Agranulocytosis typically presents with fever and evidence of infection, usually of the oropharynx. Patients should, therefore, be warned of the possible symptoms and given written instructions that the medication should be discontinued and a physician contacted immediately if the symptoms or fever develop. One must distinguish agranulocytosis from the transient, mild granulocytopenia (granulocyte count below 1.5 $\times 10^9$/L), that occurs in up to 10% of antithyroid drug-treated patients, as well as that occasionally present in patients with thyrotoxicosis or in otherwise healthy black people. It is difficult to know whether a low granulocyte count is transient or whether it will decline further to dangerously low levels. It seems reasonable, therefore, to obtain baseline leukocyte and differential counts before initiation of therapy; if the granulocyte count is normal, and if a subsequent granulocyte count is below 1.5 $\times 10^9$/L, discontinuation of the drug would be prudent. If the drug is not discontinued, the leukocyte count should be repeated at weekly intervals until it is clear that the count is stable or rising.

In addition to prompt discontinuation of the antithyroid drug, the treatment of agranulocytosis typically involves the administration of broad-spectrum antibiotics and implementation of supportive measures. The granulocyte count usually begins to return within several days but may not normalize for 10 to 14 days. Recent reports suggest that granulocyte colony-stimulating factor may be helpful in shortening the duration of agranulocytosis (Fig 53–3), but it seems to be less useful in severe cases.[118] Glucocorticoid therapy is probably ineffective in this situation.[118]

In the case of minor drug-related side effects, one antithyroid drug may be substituted for the other, with the possibility

---

TABLE 53-2.
Side Effects of Antithyroid Drugs

MINOR

COMMON (1%–5%)
  Rash
  Urticaria
  Arthralgia
  Fever
  Transient leukopenia
RARE
  Gastrointestinal
  Abnormalities of taste and smell
  Arthritis

MAJOR

RARE (0.2%–0.5%)
  Agranulocytosis
VERY RARE
  Aplastic anemia
  Thrombocytopenia
  Hepatitis (PTU)
  Cholestatic hepatitis (methimazole)
  Vasculitis, systemic lupus-like syndrome
  Hypoprothrombinemia
  Hypoglycemia (due to antiinsulin antibodies)

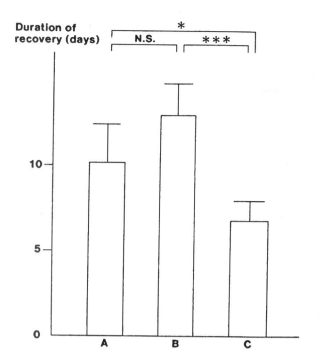

FIGURE 53-3. Mean (± SE) days required for granulocyte counts to increase from less than 0.5×10^9/L to more than 1.0×10^9/L in patients with Graves' hyperthyroidism who had methimazole-induced agranulocytosis. (A) 11 patients treated with antibiotics alone. (B) 11 patients treated with antibiotics and glucocorticoids. (C) 12 patients treated with antibiotics and recombinant human granulocyte colony-stimulating factor (75 µg daily). *$P < 0.05$. ***$P < 0.001$. (Tamai H, Mukuta T, Matsubayashi S, et al. Treatment of methimazole-induced agranulocytosis using recombinant human granulocyte colony-inducing factor [rhG-CSF]. J Clin Endocrinol Metab 1993;77:1356)

that the second drug may be taken without sequelae. Alternatively, minor rashes often are transient (days to 1 week), and sometimes can be treated with an antihistamine without discontinuation of the drug. Substitution should not be attempted in the case of agranulocytosis or the other major side effects because cross reactivity has been reported.

Patients with agranulocytosis who have had their antithyroid drug discontinued are almost always still thyrotoxic. Because antithyroid durg therapy is no longer an option, the patient should be treated with a β-adrenergic blocking drug and other drugs (e.g., an iodinated contrast agent, iodine, and lithium) if radioactive iodine therapy cannot be given promptly.

Other rare side effects include hypoglycemia, caused by the development of anti-insulin antibodies (the insulin-autoimmune syndrome),[119] cholestatic hepatitis (most often with MMI),[110] and a decreased sense of taste.[105]

FOLLOW-UP OF PATIENTS TAKING ANTITHYROID DRUGS FOR GRAVES' DISEASE

Once MMI or PTU therapy has been initiated, the patient should be seen every 4 to 6 weeks until clinical and biochemical euthyroidism has been achieved. This usually occurs within 6 weeks with MMI, but it may take up to 12 weeks with PTU.[94] As the thyrotoxicosis comes under control, the antithyroid drug dose can be lowered, often repeatedly. Hypothyroidism may develop if patients are not monitored and the dosage of drug is not decreased. The frequency of follow-up visits can be later be decreased to every 2 to 3 months and then every 6 months. The usual biochemical tests of thyroid function may be misleading early in the course of antithyroid drug therapy. For example, the serum TSH concentration may remain low for several months despite normalization of the serum T_4 and T_3 concentrations. Some patients remain thyrotoxic despite having a normal or even low serum T_4 concentration; they have persistently elevated serum T_3 concentrations, indicating the need for an increase, rather than a decrease, in antithyroid drug dosage.[120,121] This failure of the serum T_3 to normalize, so-called T_3-predominant thyrotoxicosis, is associated with a relatively poor chance of remission.[122] In addition, although an enlarging thyroid gland may indicate that hypothyroidism has developed, it also may be indicative of persistent TSab production and a poor chance for remission.[120,121]

Remissions and Antithyroid Drug Therapy. The primary goal of antithyroid drug therapy is to render the patient euthyroid. However, a commitment to a lengthy course of drug therapy is usually predicated on the hope that an eventual remission of Graves' disease will occur. The ability to predict which patients are most likely to have remissions is poor. Certain clinical characteristics, however, do seem to be associated with improved odds of long-term (i.e., more than 1 year) remission. They are a small goiter and mild biochemical thyrotoxicosis[123] (Fig 53-4). Older patients may have a higher remission rate, possibly due to the presence of milder disease.[124] Patients with certain HLA haplotypes (especially HLA-DR3) may be less likely,[125] whereas HLA-DR4-positive patients may be more likely, to have remission[126]; others have not found HLA typing to be useful.[123,127] Likewise, a negative family history of Graves' disease may[128] or may not[127] be associated with an increased likelihood of remission. In general, there does not seem to be a relationship between the likelihood of remission and the age or sex of the patient, the presence of ophthalmopathy, or the duration of disease before the initiation of therapy. Thus the low predictive value of any clinical finding makes it difficult to know a priori which patients will have a remission and which will not.

Although most experts recommend that an antithyroid drug be given for 1 to 2 years before it is discontinued, some patients have a remission after courses of therapy ranging from weeks to months.[129,130] In general, longer courses of therapy are preferable, despite one report to the contrary[131]; indeed, there are convincing data, particularly in children,[132] that the longer the drug is given, the more likely the patient is to have a remission once the drug is stopped.[133,134] Combined antithyroid drug plus T_4 therapy may hasten the onset of remission; in a recent randomized study of combined therapy the 1-year remission rates in patients treated for 6 or 12 months were comparable.[135] In a recent Japanese study, the rate of remission in patients receiving combined therapy followed by prolonged (3 years) treatment with T_4 alone was over 90%.[102] Serum TSab concentrations were lower in those patients as compared with patients receiving only MMI (in whom the remission rate was 65%), a finding noted in another

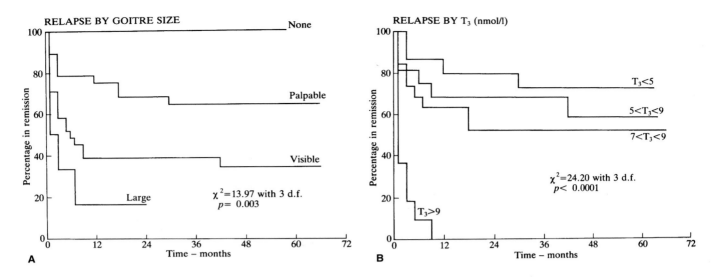

FIGURE 53-4. Likelihood of remission of Graves' hyperthyroidism during antithyroid drug therapy as a function of (*A*) goiter size and (*B*) serum triiodothyronine (T_3) concentration at the beginning of therapy. Therapy was discontinued at time 0. To convert serum T_3 values to ng/dL, multiply by 65.1 (Young ET, Steel NR, Taylor JJ, et al. Prediction of remission after antithyroid drug treatment in Graves' disease. Q J Med 1988;20:175)

report.[136] The authors postulated that a T_4-induced decrease in serum TSH attenuated TSH receptor expression by thyroid cells. This very high remission rate was not confirmed in a similar study done in Scotland.[136a]

Features during therapy that suggest that a patient may be entering remission include a decrease in goiter size,[137,138] the ability to control the thyrotoxicosis with small doses of drug, and normalization of the serum T_4:T_3 ratio.[121] Numerous tests have been devised to ascertain whether a patient has had a remission and therefore will remain euthyroid after withdrawal of antithyroid drug therapy, but none has the requisite sensitivity and specificity to be useful in individual patients.[139,140] The most well-studied biochemical test is the measurement of TSab.[141] Serum TSab concentrations tend to decrease during antithyroid drug therapy because of either an immunosuppressive effect of the drug, amelioration of thyrotoxicosis, spontaneous remission, or a combination of these factors. The failure of TSab to disappear from the serum during antithyroid drug therapy signifies almost certain relapse after drug discontinuation.[123,142] If TSab do disappear, there is still a 20% to 50% chance of relapse. Thus the presence of continuing TSab activity has prognostic value, but its absence is not useful as a prognostic indicator (see chap 21).

Other tests studied as possible predictors of relapse or remission in patients treated with an antithyroid drug include T_3 suppression testing as an index of thyroidal autonomy,[143] thyrotropin-releasing hormone (TRH) testing,[144] and measurements of antithyroid peroxidase antibodies[145] and serum thyroglobulin concentrations.[146] Although each test has its proponents, a large multicenter study involving 451 patients[140] did not find any of these tests of value in individual patients although normal T_3 suppression or TRH stimulation tests were predictive of remission in the group as a whole. Indeed, the combination of both tests had a high sensitivity (0.94), but the specificity was too low (0.13) to be useful (Fig 53-5).

Continued thyroid enlargement, a continuing requirement for large doses of drug, and T_3-predominant disease during therapy all portend a poor outcome. In practice, it is reasonable to reduce gradually and then discontinue the antithyroid drug and follow the patient clinically and with serial thyroid function tests. If a relapse is destined to occur, it usually does so within 3 to 6 months after therapy is discontinued[137] (see Fig 53-1). Characteristically, as relapse occurs, serum T_3 concentrations rise before serum T_4 concentrations. Many remissions are not lifelong. In the older literature, about 60% of patients were still in remission after 4 years,[137] but this was before our current ability to assess thyroid function accurately. More recent studies suggest that the rate of recurrent thyrotoxicosis plateaus at about 50% at 5 years.[10,11,123,147] Relapse may be particularly likely in the postpartum period; in one study, almost 50% of women who were in remission before becoming pregnant developed recurrent thyrotoxicosis after delivery.[148] A recent controlled trial suggested that this high rate of relapse might be lowered by T_4 therapy during pregnancy.[149] Because relapses can occur at any time in a patient's life and because hypothyroidism also can develop many years after antithyroid drug therapy, lifelong follow-up is recommended for all patients with Graves' disease.

The physician should have in mind a treatment strategy that can be implemented if and when a relapse occurs. In children, a second course of antithyroid drug therapy usually is advised. In young adults, either a second course of antithyroid drug therapy or radioiodine therapy is acceptable, although the chances for remission with another course of antithyroid drug therapy are low. In older adults, radioiodine is generally recommended. Long-term administration of an antithyroid drug is safe, and some patients may prefer to take a small daily dose of either MMI or PTU for decades rather than undergo ablative therapy.[150]

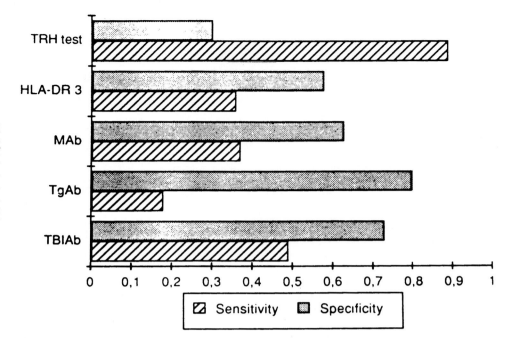

FIGURE 53-5. The sensitivity and specificity of various tests as predictors of a 1-year remission at the end of treatment with an antithyroid drug for 1 year. TRH, thyrotropin-releasing hormone; MAb, antithyroid microsomal antibodies; TgAb, antithyroglobulin antibodies; TBIAb, thyrotropin-binding inhibitory antibodies. (Benker G, Esser J, Kahaly G, Reinwein D. New therapeutic approaches in thyroidal autoimmune diseases. Klin Wochenschr 1990; 68:44. Based on data in Schleusner H, Schwander J, Fischer C, et al. Prospective multicentre study on the prediction of relapse after antithyroid drug treatment in patients with Graves' disease. Acta Endocrinol 1989;120:689)

Other Drugs Used in the Treatment of Thyrotoxicosis Caused by Graves' Disease

INORGANIC IODIDE

The effects of iodide on thyroid function are complex and are discussed in detail in the section on the effects of excess iodide in chapter 14. The major actions of iodide are to decrease iodide transport, to decrease iodide oxidation and organification (the Wolff-Chaikoff effect), and to rapidly block the release of T_4 and T_3 from the thyroid by inhibiting thyroglobulin proteolysis. Patients with thyrotoxicosis caused by Graves' disease are more sensitive to the inhibitory effects of iodide on iodine organification than are normal subjects.[151]

Unfortunately, iodide is not useful as primary therapy because of rapid escape from its inhibitory effects after 10 to 14 days. Indeed, most patients do not have normalization of thyroid function before escape occurs,[152,153] and thyrotoxicosis may worsen after withdrawal of the drug as a result of acceleration of thyroid hormone release. However, occasional patients with mild disease can be controlled for prolonged periods with potassium iodide, given as Lugol's solution (8 mg iodide per drop) or as a saturated solution (SSKI, 35–50 mg iodide per drop).[154] Typical doses for this and other indications are 3 to 5 drops of Lugol's solution three times a day or 1 drop of SSKI three times a day. These doses have been empirically derived, but smaller doses in the range of 5 to 10 mg/d would probably suffice.[154]

The three major uses of iodide today are in the preparation of patients for surgery, in the management of thyrotoxic storm, and as an adjunct after radioiodine therapy. To prepare patients for surgery, iodide usually is given for 10 days. In patients previously untreated or treated with an antithyroid drug, the addition of iodide has been thought to decrease the vascularity of the thyroid.[155] However, in a controlled study, iodide was not more effective than placebo in reducing operative blood loss or making thyroid gland manipulation easier.[156] In patients previously treated only with a β-adrenergic receptor antagonist drug, iodide reduces thyroid function and also thyroid gland blood flow. Patients so treated may have fewer perioperative complications, compared with patients who receive a β-adrenergic antagonist drug alone.[157] Thyroid surgery as therapy for thyrotoxicosis is discussed in detail later.

Iodide also is used in the management of severe thyrotoxicosis because of its ability to block thyroid hormone release acutely (see chap 51). Finally, iodide has been used with mixed success in conjunction with radioiodine,[158,159] and, more rarely, an antithyroid drug,[160] to hasten the return of the euthyroid state. In the case of radioiodine, iodide therapy should be started 1 week after administration of the dose of radioiodine, so as not to interfere with the efficacy of the radioiodine itself. Close follow-up is important because hypothyroidism can develop quickly; for reasons that are not clear, patients treated previously with radioiodine or surgery are less likely to escape from the inhibitory effects of iodide on iodine oxidation and organification,[161] and therefore are more likely to have a sustained antithyroid response. Thus, iodide also can be used to treat patients with recurrent thyrotoxicosis after surgery or after radioiodine therapy. The combination of iodide and MMI does not result in more rapid lowering of serum thyroid hormone concentrations than MMI alone.[162]

Iodide cannot be given with impunity. In patients with toxic nodular goiter, there is the potential for worsening of the thyrotoxicosis. Even patients with thyrotoxicosis caused by Graves' disease may have an exacerbation because of augmentation of thyroid hormone synthesis stimulated by an increased supply of iodide. In addition, although rare, sensitivity to iodine does exist in the form of acneiform eruptions (iodism), sialoadenitis, and vasculitis.

IODINATED RADIOGRAPHIC CONTRAST AGENTS

Oral cholecystographic agents (e.g., sodium iopanoate and sodium ipodate) are triiodoaniline derivatives that inhibit T_4-5′-deiodinase in vivo and in vitro, thereby acutely lowering serum T_3 concentrations.[163,164] Additionally, the inorganic iodide formed as these compounds are deiodinated in vivo inhibits thyroid hormone release. A direct effect of these compounds on thyroid hormone synthesis also has been described.[165] In normal subjects, serum T_4 concentrations may actually rise, probably as a result of a fall in T_4 clearance and perhaps also a decrease in cellular T_4 uptake[166] (see section on effect of pharmacologic agents on thyroid hormone metabolism in chap 14). Although early reports suggested that these agents might be useful as primary therapy of Graves' disease,[167] they have limited value in long-term therapy[168,169] because of the ultimate escape of thyroid hormone synthesis from the effect of iodide. In addition, prior use of these agents may make subsequent control with an antithyroid drug more difficult, presumably because of the large iodine load.[168]

Because of its rapid effect on serum T_3 concentrations, sodium ipodate, the most potent compound in terms of inhibition of T_4 deiodination, has been used in conjunction with PTU[170] to decrease thyroid function in patients with thyrotoxic storm or those who require rapid, short-term control of their disease (e.g., in preparation for thyroidectomy).[171] The usual dose of sodium iopanoate or sodium ipodate is 1 g daily. Because clear evidence of additional benefit beyond that provided by iodide alone is lacking, the use of iodinated contrast agents in thyrotoxic patients should be considered to be an unproven therapy.

POTASSIUM PERCHLORATE

The perchlorate anion (ClO_4^-) is a competitive inhibitor of thyroidal iodide transport. It was used in the past as therapy for thyrotoxicosis but was abandoned because of its side effects (aplastic anemia, gastric ulceration) and because of the advent of PTU and MMI. Potassium perchlorate has recently been used again to treat thyrotoxicosis with success[60] and no toxicity, in doses of 40 to 120 mg/d. The drug also has been used in combination with an antithyroid drug in the management of iodine-induced thyrotoxicosis; blockade of iodine uptake by perchlorate would seem to be a reasonable adjunct in such patients, who are notoriously resistant to therapy with an antithyroid drug alone.[172]

LITHIUM

The antithyroid effects of lithium on thyroid function have been recognized for almost three decades, but the precise mechanisms of its inhibitory actions are still not understood. Many of its actions are similar to those of iodine. Lithium is concentrated by the thyroid,[173] probably by active transport. Its primary effect appears to be blockade of thyroid hormone release, a process that is stimulated by TSH and mediated by cyclic adenosine monophosphate.[174–176] There may be additional effects on thyroid hormone biosynthesis.[174,175] As with iodide therapy, there is a tendency for the thyroid gland to escape from the inhibitory actions of lithium, and its usefulness as a reliable long-term agent in the management of thyrotoxicosis caused by Graves' disease is, therefore, limited.

A study comparing lithium and MMI noted no advantage for lithium,[177] and the risk of side effects of lithium was high. Therefore, there is little indication for lithium in the treatment of thyrotoxicosis, except in the unusual circumstance of severe thyrotoxicosis in a patient who is allergic to iodide. The dose of lithium is 300 to 450 mg orally every 8 hours, the goal being to maintain serum lithium concentrations in the range of 1 mEq/L.

β-ADRENERGIC ANTAGONIST DRUGS

β-Adrenergic antagonist drugs have become an integral part of the management of thyrotoxicosis.[178] Many of the manifestations of thyrotoxicosis mimic a hyperadrenergic state,[179] and blockade of adrenergic receptors provides patients with considerable relief from symptoms such as tremor, palpitation, anxiety, and heat intolerance. Although these effects are not due to changes in thyroid function, small, clinically unimportant decrements in serum T_3 concentrations occur in patients treated with some β-adrenergic antagonist drugs because of inhibition of extrathyroidal conversion of T_4 to T_3.[180]

Although these drugs improve the negative nitrogen balance[181] and decrease heart rate,[182] cardiac output,[183] and oxygen consumption[184] in thyrotoxicosis, these measurements seldom become normal,[185] except in the mildest cases. Hence, these drugs are useful as primary therapy only in patients with self-limited forms of thyrotoxicosis (e.g., the various forms of thyroiditis). On the other hand, they are useful as adjunctive therapy in alleviating symptoms during diagnostic evaluation or while awaiting the results of ablative therapy.

Although propranolol is the drug that was originally used for thyrotoxicosis, and is still used most widely, a number of newer drugs of this class have a longer duration of action (long-acting propranolol, atenolol, metoprolol, and nadolol) or are more cardioselective (atenolol and metoprolol). The usual starting dose of propranolol is in the range of 80 to 160 mg/d; similar effects are produced by 50 to 200 mg/d of atenolol or metoprolol or 40 to 80 mg/d of nadolol. Large doses (e.g., 360 to 480 mg/d of propranolol) sometimes are necessary to control symptoms and slow the heart rate, possibly because of accelerated propranolol clearance.[186] Propranolol and a newer cardioselective agent, esmolol, can be given intravenously to patients who are acutely ill (see later discussion of thyrotoxic storm).

In general, β-adrenergic antagonist drugs are well tolerated. Common side effects include nausea, headache, fatigue, insomnia, and depression. Rash, fever, agranulocytosis, and thrombocytopenia are rare. Complications related to the β-adrenergic antagonist effects are far more common. Patients with a clear history of asthma should not receive these drugs, although a cardioselective drug could be used cautiously in patients with mild asthma. Patients with a history of congestive heart failure should not receive a β-adrenergic blocking drug, except when the heart failure is clearly rate-related or caused by atrial fibrillation.[187] Even then, the drug should be given cautiously, preferably with digoxin. They also are relatively contraindicated in insulin-treated diabetic patients, in whom hypoglycemic symptoms may be masked, and should not be given to patients with bradyarrhythmias or Raynaud's phenomenon, or to patients being treated with a monoamine oxidase inhibitor.

Several studies have examined the potential usefulness of calcium channel blocking drugs in thyrotoxicosis. In one report, diltiazem reduced resting heart rate by 17%, comparable to what can be achieved with a β-adrenergic antagonist drug.[188] Whether calcium channel blockers will attain the importance of propranolol and related drugs in the management of thyrotoxicosis remains to be seen, but they should be considered if the latter are contraindicated.

RADIOACTIVE IODINE THERAPY FOR THYROTOXICOSIS

Since its introduction in the mid-1940s, radioiodine therapy has become the most widely used treatment for adults with thyrotoxicosis caused by Graves' disease in the United States.[2] Aside from the time required for radioiodine to work, it is in many ways an ideal form of therapy because it is effective, safe, and relatively inexpensive. Other isotopes of iodine (e.g., iodine-125), offer no clinical advantage, and iodine-131 (^{131}I) has been and will continue to be the agent of choice. Radioiodine is administered orally as a capsule or in water. It is rapidly and completely absorbed and quickly concentrated, oxidized, and organified by thyroid follicular cells. Although ^{131}I emits both beta and gamma irradiation, destruction of thyroid cells occurs because of the ionizing effects of the beta particles, which have a path length of only 1 to 2 mm. Because this exceeds the diameter of a thyroid cell, cells are irradiated even if they do not trap the radioiodine.

Initially, radioiodine causes cellular necrosis that provokes an inflammatory response. Indeed, mild thyroidal tenderness occasionally occurs, as does transient worsening of thyroid function, as a result of leakage into the bloodstream of stored hormone from disrupted follicles.[189] Histologically, cellular necrosis and inflammation are seen, as are bizarre nuclear changes reminiscent of carcinoma[190]; the latter can persist for years. Over time there is atrophy and fibrosis and an associated chronic inflammatory response that ultimately and perhaps inevitably results in hypothyroidism. Some patients have relatively normal thyroid function for years or even decades, but they are in the minority.

Practical Therapeutic Considerations

Although there is a vast worldwide experience in the use of radioiodine, no unanimity of opinion exists concerning the optimal radioiodine dose or the most satisfactory method of dose calculation. In general, a dose that will deliver about 5000 to 15,000 rad (50 to 150 Gy) to the thyroid will be effective in ameliorating the hyperthyroidism in Graves' disease although higher doses are required in patients with toxic nodular goiter. To achieve doses in this range, various factors must be considered, including thyroid size, the avidity of the gland for iodine (i.e., the 24-hour radioiodine uptake), the turnover of radioiodine within the gland, the physical half-life of the isotope (8 days in the case of ^{131}I), and prior or planned antithyroid drug therapy, which may necessitate larger doses (see later discussion). When an antithyroid drug is given before radioiodine therapy, it should be discontinued for at least 2 to 3 days, lest it interfere with radioiodine organification or

possibly act as a free radical scavenger,[191] thereby diminishing the radiation effect.

Although estimations of gland size by physical examination are unreliable, a recent report in which gland volume was measured by ultrasonography showed no apparent improvement in outcome.[192] Calculation of the biologic half-life of radioiodine is time consuming and often inaccurate. Thus a number of less quantitative methods for determining radioiodine dosage have been proposed, including giving all patients the same dose. One common approach[193] is to use the following formula, in which the administered dose is (in millicuries)

$$\frac{80 - 20 \ \mu Ci \ ^{131}I/g \ of \ thyroid \ x \ estimated \ thyroid \ gland \ weight \ (grams)}{24\text{-hour radioiodine uptake}}$$

Using this formula, typical doses are in the range of 5 to 15 mCi (185–555 MBq). In general, the use of 80 to 120 μCi/g (3.0 to 4.4 mBq/g) yields a radiation dose of 5000 to 10,000 rad (50–100 Gy). The choice of microcuries per gram of thyroid tissue is empiric, and larger doses are reasonable in patients with a relatively low radioiodine uptake (<50%), large goiters, and severe thyrotoxicosis (associated with more rapid intraglandular iodine turnover), and in patients with a toxic nodular goiter. The dose should also be increased by 25% in patients treated with an antithyroid drug before or who will be treated with one after radioiodine administration.[194] It also seems sensible to give larger doses to patients who require a second dose of radioiodine and to those patients in whom persistent disease should be avoided, such as the elderly or those with cardiac disease. Some have suggested that large doses should be given to most patients and that the inevitability of hypothyroidism should be accepted as a desired consequence, rather than as a side effect, of therapy.[195,196] Most patients become euthyroid, regardless of how the dose is determined[197] and ultimately develop hypothyroidism; attempts to reduce the rate of this complication by lowering the dose simply results in the delay or failure to cure the thyrotoxicosis,[198] necessitates additional therapy, and only delays hypothyroidism.[199,200]

Thyroid function gradually declines within weeks to months after radioiodine treatment. Symptoms can be controlled during this interval with a β-adrenergic antagonist drug, if necessary; occasional patients may benefit from antithyroid drug or potassium iodide therapy, as discussed earlier. If either is given, it should be discontinued after several months to determine the effectiveness of the radioiodine. The rate at which improvement occurs depends on factors that are poorly understood, but almost certainly include the initial level of thyroid function, the size of the thyroid, and the rate of intrathyroidal radioiodine turnover, as well as the radioiodine dose. Underlying disease activity, as assessed by TSab assay, probably does not play a role.[201] Indeed, in one study, the *absence* of TSH-receptor antibodies was associated with relative resistance to radioiodine therapy.[202]

In general, 50% to 75% of patients have normal thyroid function and some shrinkage of goiter within 6 to 8 weeks after radioiodine therapy.[203] Overall, over 80% to 90% of patients become euthyroid after one dose of radioiodine (given according to the formula above), 10% to 20% require a second dose, and a rare patient needs a third dose.[203] The figures will vary if other treatment philosophies are used. The decision to give a second or additional dose usually is not made for 6 to 12 months after radioiodine administration.

Complications and Potential Risks of Radioiodine Therapy

HYPOTHYROIDISM

Hypothyroidism may be considered an inevitable consequence of radioiodine therapy rather than a side effect.[204] In the past two or three decades its frequency has increased and it has appeared sooner after therapy,[205–207] probably because of the use of larger doses, as well as the increased ease of detection of hypothyroidism using serum TSH determinations. Hypothyroidism may develop in as many as 90% of patients within the first year after therapy,[205] with a continuing rate of 2% to 3% per year thereafter. The rapidity with which hypothyroidism develops may relate not only to the dose of radioactive iodine given but also to immunologic factors; for example, patients with high titers of antithyroid antibodies have a higher frequency of hypothyroidism.[208] Therapy with an antithyroid drug, initiated soon after radioiodine treatment, appears to lessen the rate of hypothyroidism, but also may increase the risk of persistent thyrotoxicosis.[209–211]

In addition to permanent hypothyroidism, up to one-third of patients develop transient hypothyroidism,[212,213] possibly due to transient thyroid injury, persistent TSH suppression, or both. If hypothyroidism develops in the first 2 months after radioiodine therapy, particularly if there is persistence of goiter, therapy with T_4 may be withheld for 1 to 2 months, unless the patient is unacceptably symptomatic. If hypothyroidism persists for longer than 2 months, it is likely to be permanent.

THYROID AND OTHER TUMORS

Despite the advantages of radioiodine therapy, it continues to be a controversial form of treatment, particularly in children and young adults.[214,215] The major concern has been the possible carcinogenic effects of ionizing radiation, particularly late effects that might not be detected for decades. It is clear that external head and neck irradiation is associated with an increased rate of thyroid carcinoma (see section on pathogenesis in chap 80), but, case reports notwithstanding,[216] there is no documented epidemiologic association between radioiodine therapy for thyrotoxicosis and the subsequent development of thyroid cancer. Indeed, because the question has such great implications, there have been several studies, all of which failed to show such a relationship.[217–219] Similarly, there is no evidence for increased mortality from any form of cancer,[219–221] including leukemia.[222]

Long-term follow-up data on radioiodine therapy in children and adolescents are difficult to find. In one study,[217] thyroid adenomas appeared to be more frequent in patients who received radioiodine therapy as children or adolescents. In the three largest series dealing exclusively with children,[223–225] the longest of which had a 14-year follow-up,[225] the incidence of thyroid cancer, leukemia, or other cancers was not increased, nor was there evidence of abnormal reproductive histories in females. In a smaller study, 3 of 18 children treated with radioiodine developed thyroid nodules, one of which was a low-grade follicular carcinoma.[226] Thus, because extensive

long-term follow-up data are not available in children, most are treated with an antithyroid drug. Radioiodine has gained increasing acceptability as a first-choice therapy in adolescents. A more complete discussion of the treatment of thyrotoxicosis in children can be found at the end of this section and in chapter 86.

TERATOGENICITY AND CHROMOSOMAL DAMAGE

Pregnancy, or the possibility of pregnancy, is an absolute contraindication to radioiodine therapy. Thus, a history of recent menses or a pregnancy test must be obtained in all sexually active women before the administration of radioiodine. In those rare instances in which radioiodine was given inadvertently before the 10th week of pregnancy, there is reassuring evidence that the outcome will be normal.[227] If the radioiodine is given later than the 10th to 12th gestational week, the fetal thyroid may be damaged, with consequent fetal hypothyroidism. Because there are no proven methods to identify or treat fetal hypothyroidism, candid discussion with the parents is required in this unfortunate circumstance, and individualized recommendations concerning the available options are necessary. These options include fetal blood sampling, maternal or intra-amniotic T_4 therapy, and careful follow-up with immediate evaluation at the time of birth.

A more far-reaching question is that of possible genetic damage from radioiodine, with consequent deleterious health effects on the offspring of treated patients. Several studies have documented leukocyte chromosomal abnormalities in patients who received therapeutic doses of radioiodine[228,229] and minor abnormalities in those who received as little as 20 μCi (740 Bq),[230] but the clinical importance of these findings is uncertain. The whole body is exposed to radiation after radioiodine therapy, with gonadal radiation of particular concern because of gamma irradiation from radioiodine in the urinary bladder. The estimates of the gonadal (ovarian) radiation dose after radioiodine therapy have varied more than 10-fold.[231] A rough estimate of the dose is about 0.2 rad/mCi (0.054 Gy/Bq) of administered radioiodine,[231] so that the dose to the ovaries would be 1 to 3 rad (0.01 to 0.03 Gy) for a woman receiving a usual therapeutic dose of 10 mCi (370 MBq). This dose is similar to that from several commonly performed radiologic procedures (e.g., barium enema and intravenous pyelography). It also can be calculated that the increased genetic risk of radioiodine therapy is far less than the spontaneous rate of genetic abnormalities (0.003% or less versus 0.8%).[231] These estimates are borne out by the negative clinical data that are available.[223,224,232] Thus, Safa and colleagues[224] noted no increase in congenital abnormalities in 86 children of 43 women who received radioiodine therapy as children. In a related study, none of 33 children of women who received radioiodine had cytogenetic abnormalities.[233] In summary, there is no evidence that radioiodine therapy for thyrotoxicosis has adverse effects on the health of the offspring of treated patients. It seems reasonable, however, to advise that pregnancy be avoided for 3 months after radioiodine therapy and until thyroid function is stable.

Despite these reassuring data, unnecessary exposure to radioiodine by family members, particularly children, should be minimized. Minor exposure as a result of environmental contamination is almost impossible to avoid.[234] Because most of the radioactivity is excreted in the urine, patients should be instructed to use appropriate hygienic measures. Small amounts of radioiodine appear in the saliva, so that recently treated patients should not share food or drink with others and should avoid kissing them for several days after therapy. Because the thyroid is a source of gamma radiation, parents are usually instructed not to hug their children for several days, and close contact with pregnant women should be avoided for a similar time period.[234] Intimate physical contact should probably be avoided for several days.[234]

Lactation is also an absolute contraindication to radioiodine therapy because iodine is secreted into milk.

MISCELLANEOUS SIDE EFFECTS

There are no allergic reactions to radioiodine, even in people who are sensitive to iodide or iodinated contrast agents, because the mass of iodine in a typical radioiodine dose is only 1 μg.[202] Occasional patients note nausea, possibly caused by radiation gastritis. Mild anterior neck pain, caused by radiation thyroiditis, occurs rarely, and is easily managed with salicylates. Occasional transient exacerbation of thyrotoxicosis[189] and even rare instances of thyrotoxic storm[235] have been reported as a result of release of stored hormone from the damaged thyroid follicles, but the transient rise in serum thyroid hormone concentrations usually is clinically silent, particularly when the patient is being treated with a β-adrenergic antagonist drug. Because MMI and PTU block the synthesis but not the release of T_4 and T_3, their use results in the depletion of hormonal stores within the thyroid. In patients with severe thyrotoxicosis, the elderly, and patients with cardiac disease, pretreatment with these drugs is prudent, not only because they reduce thyroid secretion more rapidly, but also to minimize the risk of aggravation of thyrotoxicosis after radioiodine therapy. This pretreatment is not necessary in most young patients with thyrotoxicosis who are treated with radioiodine.

The relationship of radioiodine therapy to the subsequent development or worsening of ophthalmopathy is an area of continuing controversy.[236] Two large retrospective studies both failed to document a relationship between the type of therapy for Graves' disease (an antithyroid drug, radioiodine, or surgery) and subsequent changes in eye findings.[237,238] Other studies have suggested that radioiodine therapy may lead to the development or worsening of ophthalmopathy,[239,240] possibly because of the release of thyroid antigens and the increase in serum TSab concentrations after therapy.[201,241] Such a mechanism has been refuted by others, however.[242]

In a recent prospective controlled trial, twice as many patients treated with radioiodine developed or had worsening of preexisting eye disease, as compared with similar patients treated with MMI or surgery.[243] The baseline serum T_3 concentration was a significant independent risk factor for the occurrence or worsening of eye disease in patients who received any of the three forms of therapy. Unfortunately, the patients receiving radioiodine were permitted to become hypothyroid before T_4 replacement therapy was initiated, whereas the drug and surgery groups were not hypothyroid at any time. In a recent retrospective study comparing radioiodine-treated patients receiving early T_4 therapy with those who became hypothyroid, the rate of eye disease was higher in the latter

group,[244] raising the possibility that it was the posttherapy hypothyroidism rather than the radioiodine therapy per se that was responsible for the increased risk of ophthalmopathy in the prospective study. Other data also support the notion that hypothyroidism after radioiodine therapy is associated with an increased risk of development or exacerbation of ophthalmopathy.[242] The use of antithyroid agents after radioiodine to block the posttherapy rise in TSAb titers did not prevent the development of eye problems.[242] However, posttherapy worsening may be preventable by glucocorticoid therapy (0.4–0.5 mg/kg prednisone per day) beginning immediately after radioiodine administration and continued for 1 month, with tapering and discontinuation by 3 months.[239]

Other rare associations with radioiodine, not necessarily complications, include hypoparathyroidism, hyperparathyroidism, and vocal cord palsy.[202]

Indications for Radioiodine Therapy

The indications for radioiodine therapy are somewhat controversial. In North America, radioiodine has become the treatment of choice for adults, whereas an antithyroid drug is the treatment of choice, even in older patients, in Europe and Japan.[2,3] Although children and adolescents are being treated with radioiodine with increasing frequency, an antithyroid drug is usually preferred in this age group.[2] Although some believe that all patients with thyrotoxicosis caused by Graves' disease should be given a trial of antithyroid drug therapy, in the hope that a remission will occur, many thyroidologists recommend radioiodine therapy, even in young adults.

SURGICAL THERAPY FOR THYROTOXICOSIS

Subtotal thyroidectomy is the oldest form of therapy for thyrotoxicosis. Although the Nobel prize was awarded to Kocher in 1909 for his innovations in thyroid surgery, it was not until the introduction of iodide, and later antithyroid drugs, as preparation for surgery that the risks of surgery became acceptable. Although surgery represented the only form of therapy for many decades, nowadays it is performed only in special circumstances: children, adolescents, and pregnant women who are allergic to or noncompliant with antithyroid drugs, patients with large goiters, and patients who prefer ablative therapy but are apprehensive about radioiodine therapy.[245]

Subtotal thyroidectomy usually is defined as a procedure that removes the bulk of the thyroid gland, leaving a rim of a few grams of each lobe posteriorly.[246] Although the mortality of subtotal thyroidectomy now is close to zero,[246,247] two worrisome complications of surgery can occur, albeit rarely (1–2%), even in the most expert hands: recurrent laryngeal nerve damage and hypoparathyroidism. Either can result in lifelong disability. Furthermore, transient hypocalcemia, postoperative bleeding, wound infection, keloid formation, and unsightly scars may develop. Although the skill of the surgeon is of paramount importance in avoiding perioperative morbidity, the number of surgeons experienced in doing subtotal thyroidectomies is decreasing as other therapies increasingly dominate the treatment of thyrotoxicosis.

Hypothyroidism occurs in the first year after surgery in 12% to 80% of patients,[245,248,249] with late-onset hypothyroidism developing in an additional 1% to 3% per year,[248] possibly reflecting the natural history of Graves' disease. The development of hypothyroidism depends on a number of factors, most importantly the size of the thyroid remnant, but also the presence of antithyroid antibodies, perhaps reflecting autoimmune destruction of the remnant,[250] and the duration of follow-up. In addition, and most unfortunately, recurrent thyrotoxicosis develops in at least 5% of patients.[246,247,251,252] Recurrences may develop many years after surgery; in one study,[253] 43% of recurrences developed more than 5 years after surgery. Radioiodine is the treatment of choice in this situation.

Preparation for subtotal thyroidectomy has changed in recent years. Although an antithyroid drug in combination with iodide was standard therapy for several decades, preparation with a β-adrenergic antagonist drug, with or without iodide, has lately been in vogue in some centers.[157,249,254] The latter regimen enables surgery to be done sooner than would ordinarily be possible if one waited the usual 4 to 6 weeks for the antithyroid drug to have its optimal effect. Propranolol or a similar drug is given for several weeks before surgery, in doses sufficient to lower the resting pulse rate to less than 80 beats/min. Patients treated with propranolol are not biochemically euthyroid when operated on, including many of those who also received iodide[255]; because the half-life of T_4 is about 7 days, patients may be hyperthyroxinemic postoperatively and require continued propranolol therapy. Furthermore, more postoperative problems (e.g., fever and tachycardia) occur in patients treated in this manner, especially in those with severe thyrotoxicosis.[254—256] Therefore, unless surgery must be performed quickly for some reason, it seems wiser to treat the patient in the traditional manner with an antithyroid drug until the euthyroid state has been achieved. If surgery must be performed urgently, preparation for 5 days with a β-adrenergic antagonist (propranolol 40 mg every 6 hours), high-dose glucocorticoids (betamethasone 0.5 mg every 6 hours), and sodium iopanoate (500 mg every 6 hours) has been reported to be safe and effective.[171]

The addition of iodide (1–3 drops of SSKI daily) to the traditional antithyroid drug regimen 10 days before surgery is controversial because of the lack of controlled data supporting a decrease in blood loss at the time of surgery,[156] despite studies demonstrating a decrease in thyroidal blood flow.[155,257] Nevertheless, it is a commonly recommended practice.[246]

SPECIAL CONSIDERATIONS IN THE MANAGEMENT OF THYROTOXICOSIS

Treatment of Children and Adolescents

Although radioiodine has been used in this age group, most prefer to use an antithyroid drug as initial therapy[2,3] (see chap 86). MMI is the drug of choice because of the ease of once-a-day administration. If antithyroid drugs are unsatisfactory or unsuitable, either radioiodine therapy or surgery is appropriate. Although radioiodine has obvious advantages over surgery, not the least being cost, because of lingering doubts about carcinogenesis and genetic damage, surgery is still an acceptable alternative.

Because antithyroid drug therapy in children and adolescents usually is given for a protracted period of time, data on remission rates as a function of treatment duration are available.[132,258] These data confirm the generally held impression that longer periods of therapy are associated with more frequent remission; more than 75% of patients were in remission after treatment for about 11 years. On the other hand, many children and adolescents ultimately require radioiodine because of drug side effects (which may be more common in children and adolescents), noncompliance, or failure to achieve long-term remission.[259]

Treatment of Elderly Patients

Elderly patients respond well to antithyroid drug therapy and may have a higher remission rate than younger patients.[124] Nevertheless, most are treated with radioiodine[2]; pretreatment with an antithyroid drug to reduce the risk of exacerbation of thyrotoxicosis after radioiodine therapy seems prudent[260] despite concerns about increases in serum thyroid hormone concentrations after antithyroid drug withdrawal.[261] Antithyroid drug therapy is often resumed after radioiodine administration to ensure continuing euthyroidism while the radioiodine is taking effect.[262] In patients with mild thyrotoxicosis, a β-adrenergic antagonist drug can be used as sole adjunctive therapy, both before and after radioiodine, with the usual caveats about these drugs in patients with underlying cardiopulmonary disease or diabetes. With regard to the radioiodine dose, it should be high enough to ensure prompt resolution of the thyrotoxicosis, with a minimum chance for recurrence.

Although most elderly thyrotoxic patients have Graves' disease,[263] the frequency of solitary toxic adenoma and toxic multinodular goiter as a cause is higher than in young patients (see later discussion). In patients with nodular disease, higher doses of radioiodine are required, particularly because the goiters may be large and the radioiodine uptake relatively low.[264]In the United States, the patient must be hospitalized if the dose to be given is greater than 30 mCi (1110 MBq); in many European countries the dose necessitating hospitalization is considerably lower. Patients with toxic multinodular goiter should not receive potassium iodide after radioiodine therapy or in preparation for surgery, for fear of exacerbating the thyrotoxicosis.

Thyrotoxicosis in Pregnancy and Lactation

PREGNANCY

A full discussion of this topic is beyond the scope of this chapter; additional information can be found in chapter 89 and in recent reviews.[265,266] Because radioiodine therapy is contraindicated, antithyroid drugs are the treatment of choice in this situation. PTU usually is preferred because it crosses the placental barrier poorly[76] and because a minor birth defect (aplasia cutis) may be associated with MMI.[267] MMI is an acceptable alternative, and in fact, it is used as the drug of first choice in pregnant women in many parts of the world.

Antithyroid drugs are not teratogens,[268] but neonatal thyroid function can be affected by their transplacental passage.

Fetal wastage and maternal morbidity are important problems in pregnant women with untreated or inadequately treated thyrotoxicosis,[269] but to minimize fetal exposure to the antithyroid drug the dose should be just adequate to control the disease, keeping the serum free T_4 value in the upper part of the normal range or slightly elevated.[270] Fortunately, thyrotoxicosis, which in pregnant women is nearly always caused by Graves' disease, often spontaneously improves in the later months of pregnancy, permitting the dose of drug to be lowered or even discontinued.[270] Doses of PTU below 150 mg/d are seldom associated with fetal thyroid dysfunction.[271] Also, even if affected, neonatal thyroid function usually is only mildly depressed,[272] it recovers quickly after delivery, and children exposed to an antithyroid drug in utero have no developmental or intellectual deficits.[273,274] Combined antithyroid drug and T_4 therapy is not recommended because it does not prevent neonatal hypothyroidism and because it may result in the administration of doses of the antithyroid drug that are higher than are necessary. After delivery, there often is an exacerbation of mild thyrotoxicosis.[148]

Other drugs may be used in the management of the pregnant woman with thyrotoxicosis. A β-adrenergic antagonist drug can be used to alleviate bothersome symptoms and usually is considered to be safe in pregnancy.[265] It also can be used for preoperative therapy, if that should become necessary because the patient is allergic to or noncompliant with antithyroid drug therapy. Potassium iodide also could be given for 7 to 10 days preoperatively, but the long-term use of iodide in pregnancy is contraindicated because of the risk of development of fetal goiter. In a recent Japanese study, however, potassium iodide was used as single-agent therapy in pregnant women with mild thyrotoxicosis, starting as early as 11 weeks of gestation, without sequelae in the neonate.[275]

LACTATION

In the past, antithyroid drug therapy was proscribed in lactating women. It is, however, probably safe,[88,276–278] based on recent measurements of drug concentrations in milk. Although the concentration of MMI in milk is higher than that of PTU, deleterious effects on neonatal thyroid function, even including increased serum TSH concentrations, have not been documented with either drug. It seems reasonable to permit breast-feeding in women who desire to do so, particularly given the advantages of breast-feeding, but it would be prudent to monitor thyroid function periodically in their infants.

Thyrotoxic Storm

Thyrotoxic storm is a rare condition characterized by uncompensated thyrotoxicosis, with fever, tachycardia or tachyarrhythmia, and altered mental status. It is almost always precipitated by an event such as infection, surgery, or trauma in a previously untreated or poorly controlled patient. Thyrotoxic storm is considered in detail in chapter 51 and elsewhere[92,93]; therefore, only a few general principles of management are outlined here. In addition to supportive measures (e.g., intravenous fluid administration, cooling blankets, mild sedation), a large dose of an antithyroid drug should be given to block thyroid hormone synthesis completely. Doses of PTU of 200 to 300 mg every 6 hours or MMI 10 to 15 mg

every 8 hours usually are recommended; PTU is preferred because it has the theoretical advantage of inhibiting extrathyroidal conversion of T_4 to T_3. Either drug can be given by nasogastric tube and even by rectal administration, if necessary.[279,280] In addition to an antithyroid drug, iodide is given to block release of thyroid hormone from the gland. Potassium iodide must be given orally (SSKI, 5 drops three or four times a day), because sodium iodide for intravenous administration is no longer available. Iodide should be given only after the first dose of antithyroid drug to avoid enriching the thyroid gland with iodine and possibly accelerating hormonal synthesis. Because of its dual actions as an inhibitor of thyroid secretion and of extrathyroidal T_3 production (see earlier), sodium ipodate or sodium iopanoate, administered for the short term in a dose of 1 g daily, might also be useful in this setting.

β-Adrenergic antagonist drugs are a cornerstone of therapy for thyrotoxic storm. Intravenous propranolol (2–5 mg every 4 hours or as an infusion at a rate of 5–10 mg/h)[93] or oral propranolol, in doses of 160 to 480 mg/24 h, usually controls tachyarrhythmia and other catecholamine-mediated effects. Esmolol also can be used in this setting, especially if there is a history of pulmonary disease; the dose is 50 to 100 μg/kg per minute intravenously. Stress doses of glucocorticoids usually are recommended; such doses inhibit T_4-to-T_3 conversion and may help to stabilize the circulation. They also may have a direct antithyroid effect in patients with Graves' disease. If conventional therapy fails, thyrotoxic storm also can be treated by plasmapheresis[281] or peritoneal dialysis.[282]

THYROTOXICOSIS DUE TO TOXIC ADENOMA AND MULTINODULAR GOITER

Toxic adenoma and multinodular goiter are unusual causes of thyrotoxicosis in young adults, but the latter may account for a significant minority of cases in older patients. Treatment is rather straightforward; because the problem is intrinsic thyroid autonomy, rather than external stimulation, an antithyroid drug is never the treatment of choice, except as preparation for ablative therapy with radioiodine or surgery.[283,284] Most toxic adenomas can be destroyed by radioiodine therapy, and postablative hypothyroidism is uncommon because the radioiodine is not concentrated by the suppressed, normal paranodular tissue.[285,286] The nodule may not completely disappear after therapy.[287]

Theoretical arguments have been presented suggesting that the paranodular tissue receives potentially carcinogenic doses of gamma radiation from the large doses of radioiodine sometimes required to treat these patients,[288] but contralateral thyroid cancer in this situation has only rarely been reported[289] and may be coincidental.[216] The morbidity of radioiodine is clearly less than that of surgery. Large doses of radioiodine may be needed to treat toxic adenomas, but one recent study noted a 90% cure rate with a mean ^{131}I dose of 10 mCi (370 MBq).[285] On the other hand, surgery would be reasonable in a young patient with a large (>5 cm) nodule.

Most patients with toxic multinodular goiters are over age 50 years and they often have other, nonthyroidal illnesses. Particular care must be used in managing these patients; large and often multiple doses of radioiodine are required.[290] Most patients should be treated initially with an antithyroid drug to reduce thyroid function quickly and to minimize the risk of exacerbation after radioiodine therapy. Even if the thyrotoxicosis is cured, there may be little change in thyroid size because of the presence of intrathyroidal calcifications, fibrosis, and large areas of relatively poorly functioning tissue. Thus, surgery may be a better option in the patient with a very large goiter, especially if there is evidence of substernal extension, because radioiodine could cause thyroidal swelling and jeopardize the airway. Indeed, functional airway compromise from a goiter, substernal or otherwise, is an indication for surgery. Postsurgical hypothyroidism is common because of the need to remove as much tissue as possible.[291]

References

1. Martin A, Davis TF. T cells and human autoimmune thyroid disease: emerging data show lack of need to invoke suppressor T cell problems. Thyroid 1992;2:247

2. Solomon B, Glinoer D, Lagasse R, Wartofsky L. Current trends in the management of Graves' disease. J Clin Endocrinol Metab 1990;70:1518

3. Wartofsky L, Glinoer D, Solomon B, et al. Differences and similarities in the diagnosis and treatment of Graves' disease in Europe, Japan, and the United States. Thyroid 1991;1:129

4. Hirota Y, Tamai H, Hayashi Y, et al. Thyroid function and histology in forty-five patients with hyperthyroid Graves' disease in clinical remission more than ten years after thionamide drug treatment. J Clin Endocrinol Metab 1986;62:165

5. Wood LC, Ingbar SH. Hypothyroidism as a late sequela in patients with Graves' disease treated with antithyroid agents. J Clin Invest 1979;64:1429

6. Tamai H, Hirota Y, Kasagi K, et al. The mechanism of spontaneous hypothyroidism in patients with Graves' disease after antithyroid drug treatment. J Clin Endocrinol Metab 1987;64:718

7. Tamai H, Kasagi K, Takaichi Y, et al. Development of spontaneous hypothyroidism in patients with Graves' disease treated with antithyroidal drugs: clinical, immunological, and histological findings in 26 patients. J Clin Endocrinol Metab 1989;69:49

8. Astwood EB. Treatment of hyperthyroidism with thiourea and thiouracil. JAMA 1943;122:78

9. Astwood EB. Chemotherapy of hyperthyroidism. Harvey Lect 1944;40:195

10. Sugrue D, McEvoy M, Feely J, Drury MI. Hyperthyroidism in the land of Graves: results of treatment by surgery, radio-iodine and carbimazole in 837 cases. Q J Med 1980;49:51

11. Hedley AJ, Young RE, Jones SJ, et al. Antithyroid drugs in the treatment of hyperthyroidism of Graves' disease: long-term follow up of 434 patients. Clin Endocrinol 1989;31:209

12. Jansson R, Dahlberg PA, Lindstrom B. Comparative bioavailability of carbimazole and methimazole. J Clin Pharm Ther Toxicol 1983;21:505

13. Richter CR, Clisby KH. Toxic effects of the bitter tasting phenylthiocarbamide. Arch Pathol 1942;33:46

14. MacKenzie JB, MacKenzie CG, McCollum EV. The effect of sulfanilylguanidine on the thyroid of the rat. Science 1941;94:518

15. MacKenzie CG, MacKenzie JB. Effect of sulfonamides and thioureas on the thyroid gland and basal metabolism. Endocrinology 1943;32:185

16. Astwood EB, Sullivan J, Bissell A, et al. Action of certain sulfonamides and of thiourea upon the function of the thyroid gland of the rat. Endocrinology 1943;32:210

17. Vanderlaan WP. Antithyroid drugs in hyperthyroidism. In: Van Middlesworth L, ed. The thyroid gland. Chicago: Year Book Medical Publishers, 1986:333

18. Lazarus JH, Marchant B, Alexander WD, Clark DH. 35S-antithyroid drug concentration and organic binding of iodine in the human thyroid. Clin Endocrinol 1975;4:609

19. Marchant B, Alexander WD. The thyroid accumulation, oxidation and metabolic rate of 35 S-methimazole in the rat. Endocrinology 1972;91:747

20. Marchant B, Alexander WD, Robertson JWK, Lazarus JH. Concentration of 35S-propylthiouracil by the thyroid gland and its relationship to anion trapping mechanism. Metabolism 1971;20:989

21. Connell JMC, Ferguson MM, Chang DSC, Alexander WD. Influence of sodium perchlorate on thioureylene antithyroid drug accumulation in mice. J Endocrinol 1983;98

22. Davidson B, Soodak M, Neary JT, et al. The irreversible inactivation of thyroid peroxidase by methylmercaptoimidazole, thiouracil, and propylthiouracil in vitro and its relationship to in vivo findings. Endocrinology 1978;103:871

23. Taurog A, Dorris M. A reexamination of the proposed inactivation of thyroid peroxidase in the rat thyroid by propylthiouracil. Endocrinology 1989;124:3038

24. Engler H, Taurog A, Dorris ML. Preferential inhibition of thyroxine and 3,5,3'-triiodothyronine formation by propylthiouracil and methylmercaptoimidazole in thyroid peroxidase-catalyzed iodination of thyroglobulin. Endocrinology 1982;110:190

25. Papapetrou PD, Mothon S, Alexander WD. Binding of the 35-S of 35S-propylthiouracil by follicular thyroglobulin in vivo and in vitro. Acta Endocrinol 1975;79:248

26. Monaco F, Santolamazza C, DeRos I, Andreoli. Effects of propylthiouracil and methylmercaptoimidazole on thyroglobulin synthesis. Acta Endocrinol 1980;93:32

27. Jansson R, Dahlberg PA, Johansson H, Lindstrom B. Intrathyroidal concentrations of methimazole in patients with Graves' disease. J Clin Endocrinol Metab 1983;57:129

28. Taniguchi S, Yoshida A, Mashiba H. Direct effect of methimazole on rat thyroidal cell growth induced by thyrotropin and insulin-like growth factor I. Endocrinology 1989;124:2046

29. Korytkowski M, Cooper D. Antithyroid drug effects on function and growth of FRTL-5 cells. Thyroid 1992;2:345

30. Leonard JL, Rosenberg IN. Thyroxine 5'-deiodinase activity of rat kidney: observations on activation by thiols and inhibition by propylthiouracil. Endocrinology 1978;103:2137

31. Berry MJ, Kieffer JD, Harney JW, Larsen PR. Selenocysteine confers the biochemical properties characteristic of the type I iodothyronine deiodinase. J Biol Chem 1991;266:14155

32. Visser TJ, Overmeeren EV. Binding of radioiodinated propylthiouracil to rat liver microsomal fractions. Biochem J 1979;183:167

33. Visser TJ, Overmeeren E, Fekkes D, et al. Inhibition of iodothyronine 5'-deiodinase by thioureylenes: structure-activity relationship. FEBS Lett 1979;103:314

34. Volpe R. Evidence that the immunosuppressive effects of antithyroid drug are mediated through actions on the thyroid cell, modulating thyrocyte-immunocyte signaling. Thyroid 1994;4:217

35. Wartofsky L. Has the use of antithyroid drugs of Graves' disease become obsolete? Thyroid 1993;3:335

36. Weetman AP, McGregor AM, Hall R. Evidence for an effect of antithyroid drugs on the natural history of Graves' disease. Clin Endocrinol 1984;24:163

37. Bagnasco M, Venuti D, Ciprandi G, et al. The effect of methimazole on the immune system is unlikely to operate directly on T lymphocytes. J Endocrinol Invest 1990;13:493

38. Wall JR, Manwar GL, Greenwood DM, Walters BA. The in vitro suppression of lectin induced 3H-thymidine incorporation into DNA of peripheral blood lymphocytes after the addition of propylthiouracil. J Clin Endocrinol Metab 1976;43:1406

39. Balazs C, Kiss E, Leovey A, Farid NR. The immunosuppressive effect of methimazole on cell-mediated immunity is mediated by

its capacity to inhibit peroxidase and to scavenge free oxygen radicals. Clin Endocrinol 1986;25:7

40. Hallengren B, Forsgren A, Melander A. Effects of antithyroid drugs on lymphocyte function in vitro. J Clin Endocrinol Metab 1980;51:298

41. Weiss I, Davies TF. Inhibition of immunoglobulin secreting cells by antithyroid drugs. J Clin Endocrinol Metab 1981;53:1223

42. Imamura M, Aoki N, Saito T, et al. Inhibitory effects of antithyroid drugs on oxygen radical formation in human neutrophils. Acta Endocrinol 1986;112:210

43. Weetman AP. Effect of the anti-thyroid drug methimazole on interleukin-1 and interleukin-2 levels in vitro. Clin Endocrinol 1986;25:133

44. Weetman AP, Tandon N, Morgan BP. Antithyroid drugs and release of inflammatory mediators by complement-attacked thyroid cells. Lancet 1992;340:633

45. Volpe R. Graves' disease. In: Burrow GN, Oppenheimer JH, Volpe R, eds. Thyroid function and disease. Philadelphia: WB Saunders, 1989:214

46. Bodolay E, Suranyi P, Juhasz F, et al. Methimazole blocks Graves' IgG but not interferon-HLA-DR expression by thyroid cells. Immunol Lett 1988;18:167

47. Davies TF, Yang C, Platzer M. The influence of antithyroid drugs and iodine on thyroid cell MHC class II antigen expression. Clin Endocrinol 1989;31:125

48. Saji M, Moriarty J, Ban T, Singer DS, Kohn LD. Major histocompatibility complex class I gene expression in rat thyroid cell is regulated by hormones, methimazole, and iodide as well as interferon. J Clin Endocrinol Metab 1992;75:871

49. Beck JS, Young RJ, Simpson JG, et al. Lymphoid tissue in the thyroid gland and thymus of patients with primary thyrotoxicosis. Br J Surg 1973;60:769

50. Hardisty CA, Fowles A, Munro DS. The effect of radioiodine and thyroid drugs on serum long acting thyroid stimulator protector (LATS-P). A three year prospective study. Clin Endocrinol 1984;20:547

51. McGregor AM, Petersen MM, McLachlan SM, et al. Carbimazole and the autoimmune response in Graves' disease. N Engl J Med 1980;303:302

52. McGregor AM, Rees-Smith B, Hall R, et al. Specificity of the immunosuppressive action of carbimazole in Graves' disease. BMJ 1982;284:1750

53. Madec AM, Allannic H, Genetet N, et al. T lymphocyte subsets at various stages of hyperthyroid Graves' disease: effect of carbimazole treatment and relationship with thyroid-stimulating antibody levels or HLA status. J Clin Endocrinol Metab 1986;62:117

54. Totterman TH, Karlsson FA, Bengtsson M, Mendel-Hartvig I. Induction of circulating activated suppressor-like T cells by methimazole therapy for Graves' disease. N Engl J Med 1987;316:15

55. Ohashi H, Okugawa T, Itoh M. Circulating active T cell subsets in autoimmune thyroid diseases: differences between untreated and treated patients. Acta Endocrinol 1991;125:502

56. Charreire J, Karsenty G, Bouchard P, Schaison G. Effect of carbimazole treatment on specific and nonspecific immunological parameters in patients with Graves' disease. Clin Exp Immunol 1984;57:633

57. Wang PW, Luo SF, Huang BY, et al. Depressed natural killer in Graves' disease and during antithyroid medication. Clin Endocrinol 1988;28:205

58. Okuno A, Yano K, Inyaku F, et al. Pharmakokinetics of methimazole in children and adolescents with Graves' disease. Acta Endocrinol 1987;115:112

59. Wenzel KW, Lente JR. Similar effects of antithyroid drugs and perchlorate on thyroid stimulating immunoglobulins in Graves' disease: evidence against an immunosuppressive effect of antithyroid drugs. J Clin Endocrinol Metab 1984;58:62

60. Weetman AP, Gunn C, Hall R, McGregor A. Immunosuppression by perchlorate. Lancet 1984;1:906

61. Davies TF, Weiss I, Gerber M. Influence of methimazole on murine thyroiditis. J Clin Invest 1984;73:397

62. Rennie DP, McGregor AM, Keast D, et al. The influence of methimazole on thyroglobulin-induced autoimmune thyroiditis in the rat. Endocrinology 1983;112:326

63. Reinhardt W, Appel MC, Alex S, et al. The inhibitory effect of large doses of methimazole on iodine induced lymphocytic thyroiditis and serum anti-thyroglobulin antibody titers in BB/Wor rats. J Endocrinol Invest 1989;12:559

64. Jansson R, Karlsson A, Dahlberg PA. Thyroxine, methimazole, and thyroid microsomal autoantibody titres in hypothyroid Hashimoto's thyroiditis. BMJ 1985;290:11

65. Romaldini JH, Werner MC, Rodriques HF, et al. Graves' disease and Hashimoto's thyroiditis: effects of high doses of antithyroid drugs on thyroid autoantibody levels. J Endocrinol Invest 1986;9:233

66. Gamstedt A, Wadman B, Karlsson A. Methimazole, but not betamethasone, prevents ^{131}I treatment-induced rises in thyrotropin receptor autoantibodies in hyperthyroid Graves' disease. J Clin Endocrinol Metab 1986;62:773

67. Wilson R, McKillop JH, Pearson C, et al. Differential immunosuppressive action of carbimazole and propylthiouracil. Clin Exp Immunol 1988;73:312

68. Jansson R, Lindstrom B, Dahlberg PA. Pharmacokinetic properties and bioavailability of methimazole. Clin Pharmacokinet 1985;10:443

69. Okamura Y, Shigemasa C, Tatsulhara T. Pharmacokinetics of methimazole in normal subjects and hyperthyroid patients. Endocrinol Jpn 1986;33:605

70. Low LCK, McCruden DC, Alexander WD. Intrathyroidal iodide binding rates and plasma methimazole concentrations in hyperthyroid patients on small doses of carbimazole. Br J Clin Pharmacol 1981;12:315

71. Cooper DS, Bode HH, Nath B, et al. Methimazole pharmacology in man: studies using a newly developed radioimmunoassay for methimazole. J Clin Endocrinol Metab 1984;58:473

72. Syrenicz A, Gawronska-Szklarz B, Wojcicki J, Czekalski S. Pharmacokinetic parameters of thiamazole in hyperthyroid patients responding rapidly and slowly to the treatment. Pol J Pharmacol Pharm 1991;43:207

73. McCruden DC, Hilditch TE, Connell JMC, et al. Duration of antithyroid action of methimazole estimated with an intravenous perchlorate discharge test. Clin Endocrinol 1987;26:33

74. Wartofsky L, Ingbar SH. A method for assessing the latency, potency and duration of action of antithyroid agents in man. In: Fellinger K, Hofer R, eds. Further advances in thyroid research. Wien: Verlag der Wiener Medizinischen Akademia 1971;121

75. Taurog A, Dorris ML. Propylthiouracil and methimazole display contrasting pathways of peripheral metabolism in both rat and human. Endocrinology 1988;122:592

76. Marchant B, Brownlie BEW, Hart DM, Horton PW, Alexander WD. The placental transfer of propylthiouracil, methimazole and carbimazole. J Clin Endocrinol Metab 1977;45:1187

77. MacFarlane IA, Davies D, Longson D, et al. Single daily dose short term carbimazole therapy for hyperthyroid Graves' disease. Clin Endocrinol 1983;18:557

78. Messina M, Milani P, Gentile L, et al. Initial treatment of thyrotoxic Graves' disease with methimazole: a randomized trial comparing different dosages. J Endocrinol Invest 1987;10:291

79. Roti E, Gardini E, Minelli R, et al. Methimazole and serum thyroid hormone concentrations in hyperthyroid patients: effects of single and multiple daily doses. Ann Intern Med 1989;111:181

80. Shiroozu A, Okamura K, Ikenoue H, et al. Treatment of hyperthyroidism with a small single daily dose of methimazole. J Clin Endocrinol Metab 1986;63:125

81. Cooper DS, Saxe VC, Meskell M, et al. Acute effects of propylthiouracil (PTU) on thyroidal iodine organification and peripheral iodothyronine deiodination: correlation with serum PTU levels measured by radioimmunoassay. J Clin Endocrinol Metab 1982;54:101

82. Giles HG, Roberts EA, Orrego H, Sellers EM. Determination of free propylthiouracil clearance and single sample prediction of steady state. J Pharm Pharmacol 1982;34:62

83. Cooper DS, Steigerwalt S, Migdal S. Pharmacology of propylthiouracil in thyrotoxicosis and chronic renal failure. Arch Intern Med 1987;147:785

84. Hoffman WH, Miceli JN. Pharmacokinetics of propylthiouracil in children and adolescents with Graves' disease in the hyperthyroid and euthyroid states. Dev Pharmacol Ther 1988;11:73

85. Kampmann JP, Mortenson HB, Back D, et al. Kinetics of propylthiouracil in the elderly. Acta Med Scand 1979;624:93

86. Kampmann JP, Hansen JEM. Serum protein binding of propylthiouracil. Br J Clin Pharmacol 1983;16:549

87. Zaton A, Martinez A, DeGandarias JM. The binding of thioureylene compounds to human serum albumin. Biochem Pharmacol 1988;37:3127

88. Kampmann JP, Hansen IM, Johansen K, Helweg J. Propylthiouracil in human milk. Lancet 1980;2:736

89. Barnes HV, Bledsoe T. A simple test for selecting the thioamide schedule in thyrotoxicosis. J Clin Endocrinol Metab 1972;35:250

90. Greer MA, Meihoff WC, Studer H. Treatment of hyperthyroidism with a single daily dose of propylthiouracil. N Engl J Med 1965;272:888

91. Gwinup G. Prospective randomized comparison of propylthiouracil. JAMA 1978;239:2457

92. Burch HB, Wartofsky L. Life-threatening thyrotoxicosis. Endocrinol Metab Clin North Am 1993;22:263

93. Nicoloff JT. Thyroid storm and myxedema coma. Med Clin North Am 1985;69:1005

94. Okamura K, Ikenoue H, Shiroozu A, et al. Reevaluation of the effects of methylmercaptoimidazole and propylthiouracil in patients with Graves' hyperthyroidism. J Clin Endocrinol Metab 1987;65:719

95. Mashio Y, Beniko M, Ikota A, et al. Treatment of hyperthyroidism with a small single daily dose of methimazole. Acta Endocrinol 1988;119:139

96. Reinwein D, Benker G, Lazarus JH, et al. A prospective randomized trial of antithyroid drug dose in Graves' disease therapy. J Clin Endocrinol Metab 1993;76:1516

97. Azizi F. Environmental iodine intake affects the response to methimazole in patients with diffuse toxic goiter. J Clin Endocrinol Metab 1985;61:374

98. O'Malley BP, Rosenthal FD, Northover BJ, Jennings PE, Woods KL. Higher than conventional doses of carbimazole in the treatment of thyrotoxicosis. Clin Endocrinol 1988;29:281

99. Cooper DS. Propylthiouracil levels in hyperthyroid patients unresponsive to large doses. Ann Intern Med 1985;102:328

100. Cooper DS. Antithyroid drugs. N Engl J Med 1984;311:1353

101. Wiberg JJ, Nuttall FQ. Methimazole toxicity from high doses. Ann Intern Med 1972;77:414

102. Hashizume K, Ichikawa I, Sakurai A, et al. Administration of thyroxine in treated Graves' Disease. N Engl J Med 1991;324:947

103. Cooper DS. Which antithyroid drug? Am J Med 1986;80:1165

104. Cooper DS, Goldminz D, Levin AA, et al. Agranulocytosis associated with antithyroid drugs. Ann Intern Med 1983;98:26

105. Ducornet B, Duprey J. Effects secondaires des antithyroidiens de synthese. Ann Med Interne 1988;139:410

106. Meyer-Gessner M, Benker G, Olbricht T, et al. Nebenwirkungen der antithyreoidalen therapie der hyperthyreose. Dtsch Med Wochenschr 1989;114:166

107. Meyer-Gessner M, Benker G, Lederbogen S, et al. Antithyroid drug-induced agranulocytosis: clinical experience with ten patients at one institution and review of the literature. J Endocrinol Invest 1994;17:29

108. Liaw Y-F, Huang M-J, Fan K-D, et al. Hepatic injury during propylthiouracil therapy in patients with hyperthyroidism. Ann Intern Med 1993;118:424

109. Wing SS, Fantus IG. Adverse immunologic effects of antithyroid drugs. Can Med Assoc J 1987;136:121

110. Vitug AC, Goldman JM. Hepatotoxicity from antithyroid drugs. Horm Res 1985;21:229

111. Shabtai R, Shapiro MS, Orenstein D, et al. The antithyroid arthritis syndrome reviewed. Arthritis Rheum 1984;27:227

112. Dolman KM, Gans RO, Vervaat TJ, et al. Vasculitis and antineutrophil cytoplasmic autoantibodies associated with propylthiouracil therapy. Lancet 1993;342:651

113. Vogt BA, Kim Y, Jennette CJ, et al. Antineutrophil cytoplasmic autoantibody-positive crescentic glomerulonephritis as a complication of treatment with propylthiouracil in children. J Pediatr 1994;124:986

114. Tajiri J, Noguehi S, Murakami T, Murakami N. Antithyroid drug-induced agranulocytosis. Arch Intern Med 1990;150:621

115. Wall JR, Fang SL, Kuroki T, et al. In vitro immunoreactivity to propylthiouracil, methimazole, and carbimazole in patients with Graves' disease: a possible cause of antithyroid drug-induced agranulocytosis. J Clin Endocrinol Metab 1984;58:868

116. Fibbe WE, Claas FHJ, Star-Dijkstra WVD, et al. Agranulocytosis induced by propylthiouracil: evidence of a drug dependent antibody reacting with granulocytes, monocytes and haematopoietic progenitor cells. Br J Haematol 1986;64:363

117. Toth EL, Mant MJ, Shivji S, Ginsberg J. Propylthiouracil-induced agranulocytosis: an unusual presentation and a possible mechanism. Am J Med 1988;85:725

118. Tamai H, Mukuta T, Matsubayashi S, et al. Treatment of methimazole-induced agranulocytosis using recombinant human granulocyte colony stimulating factor (rhG-CSF). J Clin Endocrinol Metab 1993;77:1356

119. Hirota Y, Tominaga M, Ito J, Noguchi A. Spontaneous hypoglycemia with insulin autoimmunity in Graves' disease. Ann Intern Med 1974;81:214

120. Hegedus L, Hansen JM, Bech K, et al. Thyroid stimulating immunoglobulins in Graves' disease with goitre growth, low thyroxine and increasing triiodothyronine during PTU treatment. Acta Endocrinol 1984;107:482

121. Wenzel KW, Lente JR. Syndrome of persisting thyroid stimulating immunoglobulins and growth promotion of goiter combined with low thyroxine and high triiodothyronine serum levels in drug treated Graves' disease. J Endocrinol Invest 1983;6:389

122. Takamatsu J, Sugawara M, Kuma K, et al. Ratio of serum triiodothyronine to thyroxine and the prognosis of triiodothyronine-predominant Graves' disease. Ann Intern Med 1984;100:372

123. Young ET, Steel NR, Talor JJ, et al. Prediction of remission after antithyroid drug treatment in Graves' disease. Q J Med 1988;250:175

124. Yamada T, Aizawa T, Koizumi Y, et al. Age-related therapeutic response to antithyroid drug in patients with hyperthyroid Graves' disease. J Am Geriatr Soc 1994;42:513

125. McGregor AM, Smith BR, Hall R, et al. Prediction of relapse in hyperthyroid Graves' disease. Lancet 1980;1:1101

126. DeBruin TWA, Blk JH, Bussemaker JK, et al. Graves' disease: immunological and immunogenetic indicators of relapse. BMJ 1988;296:1292

127. Allannic H, Fauchet R, Lorcy Y, et al. A prospective study of the relationship between relapse of hyperthyroid Graves' disease after antithyroid drugs and HLA haplotype. J Clin Endocrinol Metab 1983;57:719

128. Eshoj O, Kvetny J, Mogensen EF, et al. Prediction of the course of Graves' disease after medical antithyroid treatment. Acta Med Scand 1985;217:225

129. Bing RF, Rosenthal FD. Early remission in thyrotoxicosis produced by short courses of treatment. Acta Endocrinol 1982;100:221

130. Greer MA, Kammer H, Bouma DJ. Short-term antithyroid drug therapy for the thyrotoxicosis of Graves' disease. N Engl J Med 1977;297:173

131. Garcia-Mayor RVG, Paramo C, Luna-Cano R, et al. Antithyroid drug and Graves' hyperthyroidism. Significance of treatment duration and TRAb determination on lasting remission. J Endocrinol Invest 1992;15:815

132. Lippe BM, Landaw EM, Kaplan SA. Hyperthyroidism in children treated with long term medical therapy: twenty-five percent remission every two years. J Clin Endocrinol Metab 1987;64:1241

133. Allannic H, Fauchet R, Orgiazzi J, et al. Antithyroid drugs and Graves' disease: a prospective randomized evaluation of the efficacy of treatment duration. J Clin Endocrinol Metab 1990;70:675

134. Tamai H, Nakagawa T, Fukino O, et al. Thionamide therapy in Graves' disease: relation of relapse rate to duration of therapy. Ann Intern Med 1980;92:488

135. Weetman AP, Pickerill AP, Watson P, et al. Treatment of Graves' disease with the block-replace regimen of antithyroid drugs: the effect of treatment duration and immunogenetic susceptibility on relapse. Q J Med 1994;87:337

136. Kuo S-W, Huang W-S, Hu C-A, et al. Effect of thyroxine administration on serum thyrotropin receptor antibody and thyroglobulin levels in patients with Graves' hyperthyroidism during antithyroid drug therapy. Eur J Endocrinol 1994;131:125

136a. McIver B, Rae P, Beckett G, Wilkinson E, Gold A, Toft A. Lack of effect of thyroxine in patients with Graves' hyperthyroidism treated with an antithyroid drug. N Engl J Med 1996;334:220

137. Hershman JM, Givens JR, Cassidy CE, Astwood EB. Long-term outcome of hyperthyroidism treated with antithyroid drugs. J Clin Endocrinol Metab 1966;26:803

138. Solomon DH, Beck JC, Vanderlaan WP, Astwood EB. Prognosis of hyperthyroidism treatment with antithyroid drugs. JAMA 1953;152:201

139. Benker G, Esser J, Kahaly G, Reinwein D. New therapeutic approaches in thyroidal autoimmune diseases. Klin Wochenschr 1990;68:44

140. Schleusner H, Schwander J, Fischer C, et al. Prospective multicentre study on the prediction of relapse after antithyroid drug treatment in patients with Graves' disease. Acta Endocrinol 1989;120:689

141. Feldt-Rasmussen U, Schleusener H, Carayon P. Meta-analysis evaluation of the impact of thyrotropin receptor antibodies on long term remission after medical therapy of Graves' disease. J Clin Endocrinol Metab 1994;78:98

142. Teng CS, Yeung RTT. Changes in thyroid-stimulating antibody activity in Graves' disease treated with antithyroid drug and its relationship to relapse: a prospective study. J Clin Endocrinol Metab 41980;50:144

143. Yamada T, Koizumi Y, Sato A, et al. Reappraisal of the 3,5,3'-triiodothyronine suppression test in the prediction of long term outcome of antithyroid drug therapy in patients with hyperthyroid Graves' disease. J Clin Endocrinol Metab 1984;58:676

144. Dahlberg PA, Karlsson FA, Jansson R, Wide L. Thyrotropin-releasing hormone testing during antithyroid drug treatment of Graves' disease as an indicator of remission. J Clin Endocrinol Metab 1985;61:1100

145. Hamada N, Ito K, Mimura T, et al. Retrospective evaluation of the significance of thyroid microsomal antibody in the treatment of Graves' disease. Acta Endocrinol 1987;114:328

146. Aizawa T, Ishiham M, Koizumi Y, et al. Serum thyroglobulin concentration as an indicator for assessing thyroid stimulation in patients with Graves' disease during antithyroid drug therapy. Am J Med 1990;89:175

147. Berglund J, Christensen SB, Dymling JF, Hallengren B. The incidence of recurrence and hypothyroidism following treatment with antithyroid drugs, surgery or radioiodine in all patients with thyrotoxicosis in Malmö during the period 1970–1974. J Intern Med 1991;229:435

148. Amino N, Tanizawa O, Mori H, et al. Aggravation of thyrotoxicosis in early pregnancy and after delivery in Graves' disease. J Clin Endocrinol Metab 1982;55:108

149. Hashizume K, Ichikawa K, Nishii Y, et al. Effect of administration of thyroxine on the risk of postpartum recurrence of hyperthyroid Graves' disease. J Clin Endocrinol Metab 1992;75:6

150. Slingerland DW, Burrows BA. Long-term antithyroid treatment in hyperthyroidism. JAMA 1979;242:2408

151. Stewart RDH, Murray IPC. Effect of small doses of carrier iodide upon the organic binding of radioactive iodine by the human thyroid gland. J Clin Endocrinol 1967;27:500

152. Emerson CH, Anderson AJ, Howard WJ, Utiger RD. Serum thyroxine and triiodothyronine concentrations during iodide treatment of hyperthyroidism. J Clin Endocrinol Metab 1975;40:33

153. Philippou G, Koutras DA, Piperingos G, et al. The effect of iodide on serum thyroid hormone levels in normal persons, in hyperthyroid patients, and in hypothyroid patients on thyroxine replacement. Clin Endocrinol 1992;36:573

154. Thompson WO, Thompson PK, Brailey AG, Cohen AC. Prolonged treatment of exophthalmic goiter by iodine alone. Arch Intern Med 1930;45:481

155. Chang DCS, Wheeler MH, Woodcock JP, et al. The effect of preoperative Lugol's iodine on thyroid blood flow in patients with Graves' hyperthyroidism. Surgery 1987;102:1055

156. Coyle PJ, Mitchell JE. Thyroidectomy: is Lugol's iodine necessary? Ann R Coll Surg Engl 1982;64:334

157. Peden NR, Gunn A, Browning MCK, et al. Nadolol and potassium iodide in the surgical treatment of thyrotoxicosis. Br J Surg 1982;69:638

158. Ross DS, Daniels GH, DeStefano P, et al. Use of adjunctive potassium iodide after radioactive iodine (^{131}I) treatment of Graves' hyperthyroidism. J Clin Endocrinol Metab 1983;57:250

159. Schimmel M, Utiger RD. Acute effect of inorganic iodide after ^{131}I therapy for hyperthyroidism. Clin Endocrinol 1977;6:329

160. Kasai K, Suzuki H, Shimoda SI. Effects of propylthiouracil and relatively small doses of iodide on early phase treatment of hyperthyroidism. Acta Endocrinol 1980;93:315

161. Braverman LE, Woeber KA, Ingbar SH. Induction of myxedema by iodide in patients euthyroid after radioiodine or surgical treatment of diffuse toxic goiter. N Engl J Med 1969;281:816

162. Roti E, Robuschi G, Gardini E, et al. Comparison of methimazole, methimazole and sodium ipodate, and methimazole and saturated solution of potassium iodide in the early treatment of hyperthyroid Graves' disease. Clin Endocrinol 1988;28:305

163. Burgi H, Wimpfheimer C, Burger A, et al. Changes of circulating thyroxine, triiodothyronine and reverse triiodothyronine after radiographic contrast agents. J Clin Endocrinol Metab 1976;43:1203

164. Wu SY, Chopra IJ, Solomon DH, Bennett LR. Changes in circulating iodothyronines in euthyroid and hyperthyroid subjects given ipodate (Oragrafin), an agent for oral cholecystography. J Clin Endocrinol Metab 1978;46:691

165. Laurberg P. Multisite inhibition by ipodate of iodothyronine secretion from perfused dog thyroid lobes. Endocrinology 1985;117:1639

166. Fellicetta JV, Green WL, Nelp WB. Inhibition of hepatic binding of thyroxine by cholecystographic agents. J Clin Endocrinol Metab 1980;65:1032

167. Wu SY, Shyh TP, Chopra IJ, et al. Comparison of sodium ipodate (Oragrafin) and propylthiouracil in early treatment of hyperthyroidism. J Clin Endocrinol Metab 1982;54:630

168. Martino E, Balzano S, Bartalena L, et al. Therapy of Graves' disease with sodium ipodate is associated with a high recurrence rate of hyperthyroidism. J Endocrinol Invest 1991;14:847

169. Roti E, Gardini E, Minelli R, et al. Sodium ipodate and methimazole in the long-term treatment of hyperthyroid Graves' disease. Metabolism 1993;42:403

170. Sharp B, Reed AW, Tamagna EI, Geffner DL, Hershman JM. Treatment of hyperthyroidism with sodium ipodate (Oragrafin) in addition to propylthiouracil and propranolol. J Clin Endocrinol Metab 1981;53:622

171. Baeza A, Aguayo M, Barria M, Pineda G. Rapid preoperative preparation in hyperthyroidism. Clin Endocrinol 1991;35:439

172. Martino E, Lombardi-Aghini F, Mariotti S, et al. Treatment of amiodarone associated thyrotoxicosis by simultaneous administration of potassium perchlorate and methimazole. J Endocrinol Invest 1986;9:201

173. Berens SC, Wolff J, Murphy DL. Lithium concentration by the thyroid. J Endocrinol 1970;87:1085

174. Berens SC, Bernstein RS, Robbins J, Wolff J. Antithyroid effects of lithium. J Clin Invest 1970;49:1357

175. Burrow G, Burke WR, Himmelhoch JM, et al. Effect of lithium on thyroid function. J Clin Endocrinol Metab 1971;32:647

176. Williams JA, Berens SC, Wolff J. Thyroid secretion in vitro: inhibition of TSH and dibutyryl cyclic-AMP stimulated ^{131}I release by Li. Endocrinology 1971;88:1385

177. Kristenson O, Andersen HH, Pallisgaard G. Lithium carbonate in the treatment of thyrotoxicosis. Lancet 1976;1:603

178. Geffner DL, Hershman JM. Beta-adrenergic blockade for the treatment of hyperthyroidism. Am J Med 1992;93:61

179. Ginsberg AM, Clutter WE, Shah SD, Cryer PE. Triiodothyronine-induced thyrotoxicosis increases mononuclear leukocyte beta-adrenergic receptor density in man. J Clin Invest 1981;67:1785

180. Cooper DS, Daniels GH, Ladenson PW, Ridgway EC. Hyperthyroxinemia in patients treated with high-dose propranolol. Am J Med 1982;73:867

181. Georges LP, Santangelo RP, Mackin JF, Canary JJ. Metabolic effects of propranolol in thyrotoxicosis. I. Nitrogen, calcium and hydroxyproline. Metabolism 1975;24:11

182. Valcavi R, Menozzi C, Roti E, et al. Sinus node function in hyperthyroid patients. J Clin Endocrinol Metab 1992;75:239

183. Grossman W, Robin NI, Johnson LW, et al. Effects of beta blockade on the peripheral manifestations of thyrotoxcosis. Ann Intern Med 1971;74:875

184. Saunders J, Hall SEH, Crowther A, et al. The effect of propanolol on thyroid hormones and oxygen consumption in thyrotoxicosis. Clin Endocrinol 1978;9:67

185. O'Malley BP, Abbott RJ, Barnett DB, et al. Propranolol versus carbimazole as the sole treatment for thyrotoxicosis. A consideration of circulating thyroid hormone levels and tissue thyroid function. Clin Endocrinol 1982;16:545

186. Feely J, Stevenson IH, Crooks J. Increased clearance of propranolol in thyrotoxicosis. Ann Intern Med 1981;94:472

187. Ikram H. The nature and prognosis of thyrotoxic heart disease. Q J Med 1985;54:19

188. Roti E, Montermini M, Roti S, et al. The effect of diltiazem, a calcium channel-blocking drug, on cardiac rate and rhythm in hyperthyroid patients. Arch Intern Med 1988;148:1919

189. Tamagna E, Levine GA, Hershman JM. Thyroid hormone concentrations after radioiodine therapy for hyperthyroidism. J Nucl Med 1979;20:387

190. Dobyns BM, Vickery AL, Maloof F, Chapman EM. Functional and histologic effects of therapeutic doses of radioactive iodine on the thyroid of man. J Clin Endocrinol Metab 1953;13:548

191. Connell JMC, Hilditch TE, Alexander WD. Treatment of hyperthyroidism with radioiodine. Lancet 1988;2:165

192. Tsuruta M, Nagayama Y, Yokoyama N, et al. Long-term follow-up studies on iodine-131 treatment of hyperthyroid Graves' disease based on the measurement of thyroid gland volume by ultrasonography. Ann Nucl Med 1993;7:193

193. Beierwaltes WH. The treatment of hyperthyroidism with iodine-131. Semin Nucl Med 1978;8:95

194. Crooks J, Buchanan WW, Wayne EJ, MacDonald E. Effect of pretreatment with methylthiouracil on results of 131-I therapy. BMJ 1960;1:151

195. Erikson E, Erikson K, Wahlberg P. Treatment of hyperthyroidism with standard doses of radioiodine aiming at ablation. Acta Med Scand 1985;214:55

196. Safa AM, Skillern PG. Treatment of hyperthyroidism with a large initial dose of sodium iodide I^{131}. Arch Intern Med 1975;135:673

197. Franklyn JA, Daykin J, Droic Z, et al. Long-term follow-up of treatment of thyrotoxicosis by three different methods. Clin Endocrinol 1991;34:71

198. Nordyke RA, Gilbert FI. Optimal iodine-131 dose for eliminating hyperthyroidism in Graves' disease. J Nucl Med 1991;32:411

199. Cevallos JL, Hagen GA, Maloof F, Chapman EM. Low-dose ^{131}I therapy of thyrotoxicosis (diffuse goiter). N Engl J Med 1974;290:141

200. Sridama V, McCormick M, Kaplan EL, et al. Long-term follow-up study of compensated low-dose ^{131}I therapy for Graves' disease. N Engl J Med 1984;311:426

201. Teng CS, Yeung RTT, Khoo RKK, Alagaratnam TT. A prospective study of the changes in thyrotropin binding inhibitory immunoglobulins in Graves' disease treated by subtotal thyroidectomy or radioactive iodine. J Clin Endocrinol Metab 1980;50:1005

202. Davies TF, Platzer M, Farid NR. Prediction of therapeutic response to radioiodine in Graves' disease using TSH-receptor antibodies and HLA-status. Clin Endocrinol 1982;16:183

203. Holm LE, Lundell G, Dahlqvist I, Israelsson A. Cure rate after ^{131}I therapy for hyperthyroidism. Acta Radiol 1981;20:161

204. Graham GD, Burman KD. Radioiodine treatment of Graves' disease. Ann Intern Med 1986;105:900

205. Cunnien AJ, Hay ID, Gorman CA, et al. Radioiodine-induced hypothyroidism in Graves' disease: factors associated with the increasing incidence. J Nucl Med 1982;23:978

206. Holm LE. Changing annual incidence of hypothyroidism after iodine-131 therapy for hyperthyroidism, 1951–1975. J Nucl Med 1982;23:108

207. Peden NR, Hart IR. The early development of transient and permanent hypothyroidism following radioiodine therapy for hyperthyroid Graves' disease. Can Med Assoc J 1984;130:1141

208. Lundell G, Holm LE. Hypothyroidism following ^{131}I therapy for hyperthyroidism in relation to immunologic parameters. Acta Radiol Oncol 1980;19:449

209. Steinbach JJ, Donoghue GD, Goldman JK. Simultaneous treatment of toxic diffuse goiter with I-131 and antithyroid drugs: a prospective study. J Nucl Med 1979;20:1263

210. Marcocci C, Gianchecchi D, Masini I, et al. A reappraisal of the role of methimazole and other factors on the efficacy and outcome of radioiodine therapy of Graves' hyperthyroidism. J Endocrinol Invest 1990;13:513

211. Velkeniers B, Vanhaelst L, Cytryn R, Jonckheer MH. Treatment of hyperthyroidism with radioiodine: adjunctive therapy with antithyroid drugs reconsidered. Lancet 1988;2:1127

212. Connell JM, Hilditch TE, McCruden DC, Alexander WD. Transient hypothyroidism following radioiodine therapy for thyrotoxicosis. Br J Radiol 1983;56:309

213. Sawers JSA, Toft AD, Irvine WJ, et al. Transient hypothyroidism after iodine-131 treatment of thyrotoxicosis. J Clin Endocrinol Metab 1980;50:226

214. Halnan KE. Risks from radioiodine treatment of thyrotoxicosis. BMJ 1983;287:1821

215. Henneman G, Krenning EP, Sankaranarayanan K. Place of radioactive iodine in treatment of thyrotoxicosis. Lancet 1986; 1:1369

216. Wiener JD, Thijs LG, Meijer S. Thyroid carcinoma after ^{131}I treatment for hyperthyroidism. Acta Med Scand 1975;198:329

217. Dobyns BM, Sheline GE, Workman JB, et al. Malignant and benign neoplasms of the thyroid in patients treated for hyperthyroidism: a report of the cooperative thyrotoxicosis therapy follow-up study. J Clin Endocrinol Metab 1974;38:976

218. Holm LE, Dahlqvist I, Israelsson A, Lundell G. Malignant thyroid tumors after iodine-131 therapy. N Engl J Med 1980;303:188

219. Hoffman DA, McConahey WM, Diamond EL, Kurland LT. Mortality in women treated with hyperthyroidism. Am J Epidemiol 1982;115:243

220. Goldman MB, Maloof F, Monson RR, et al. Radioactive iodine therapy and breast cancer. Am J Epidemiol 1988;127:969

221. Hall P, Lundell G, Holm LE. Mortality in patients treated for hyperthyroidism with iodine-131. Acta Endocrinol 1993;128:230

222. Hall P, Boice JD Jr, Berg G, et al. Leukaemia incidence after iodine-131 exposure. Lancet 1992;340:1

223. Hayek A, Chapman EM, Crawford JD. Long-term results of treatment of thyrotoxicosis in children and adolescents with radioactive iodine. N Engl J Med 1970;283:949

224. Safa AM, Schumacher OP, Rodriguez-Antunez A. Long-term follow-up results in children and adolescents treated with radioactive iodine (^{131}I) for hyperthyroidism. N Engl J Med 1975;292:167

225. Freitas JE, Swanson DP, Gross MD, Sisson JC. Iodine-131: optimal therapy for hyperthyroidism in children and adolescents? J Nucl Med 1979;20:847

226. Sheline GE, Lindsay S, Bell HG. Occurrence of thyroid nodules in children following therapy with radioiodine for hyperthyroidism. J Clin Endocrinol Metab 1959;19:127

227. Stoffer SS, Hamburger JI. Inadvertent ^{131}I therapy for hyperthyroidism in the first trimester of pregnancy. J Nucl Med 1976; 17:146

228. Cantolino SJ, Schmickel RD, Ba UM, Cisar CF. Persistent chromosomal aberrations following radioiodine therapy for thyrotoxicosis. N Engl J Med 1966;275:739

229. Nofal MM, Beierwaltes WH. Persistent chromosomal aberrations following radioiodine therapy. J Nucl Med 1964;5:840

230. Vormittag W, Ring F, Kunze-Muhl E, Weissel M. Structural chromosomal aberrations before and after administration of 20 μCi iodine-131. Mutat Res 1982;105:333

231. Robertson JS, Gorman CA. Gonadal radiation dose and its genetic significance in radioiodine therapy of hyperthyroidism. J Nucl Med 1976;17:826

232. Sarkar SD, Beierwaltes WH, Gill SP, Cowley BJ. Subsequent fertility and birth histories of children and adolescents treated with ^{131}I for thyroid cancer. J Nucl Med 1976;17:460

233. Einhorn J, Hulten M, Lindsten J, et al. Clinical and cytogenetic investigation in children of parents treated with radioiodine. Acta Radiol 1972;11:193

234. Culver C, Dworkin HJ. Radiation safety considerations for post-iodine-131 hyperthyroid therapy. J Nucl Med 1991;32:169

235. McDermott MT, Kidd GS, Dodson LE, Hofeldt FD. Radioiodine-induced thyroid storm. Am J Med 1983;75:353

236. Marcocci C, Bartalena L, Bogazzi F, et al. Relationship between Graves' ophthalmopathy and type of treatment of Graves' hyperthyroidism. Thyroid 1992;2:171

237. Gwinup G, Elias AN, Ascher MS. Effect on exophthalmos of various methods of treatment of Graves' disease. JAMA 1982; 247:2135

238. Sridama V, DeGroot LJ. Treatment of Graves' disease and the course of ophthalmopathy. Am J Med 1989;87:70

239. Bartalena L, Marcocci C, Bogazzi F, et al. Use of corticosteroids to prevent progression of Graves' ophthalmopathy after radioiodine therapy for hyperthyroidism. N Engl J Med 1989; 321:1349

240. Vestergaard H, Laurberg P. Radioiodine and aggravation of Graves' ophthalmopathy. Lancet 1989;1:47

241. Atkinson S, McGregor AM, Kendall-Taylor P, et al. Effect of radioiodine on stimulatory activity of Graves' immunoglobulins. Clin Endocrinol 1982;16:537

242. Kung WC, Yau CC, Cheng A. The incidence of ophthalmopathy after radioiodine therapy for Graves' disease: prognostic factors and the role of methimazole. J Clin Endocrinol Metab 1994;79:542

243. Tallstedt L, Lundell G, Torring O, et al. Occurrence of ophthalmopathy after treatment For Graves' hyperthyroidism. N Engl J Med 1992;326:1733

244. Tallstedt L, Lundell G, Blomgren H, Bring J. Does early administration of thyroxine reduce the development of Graves' ophthalmopathy after radioiodine treatment? Eur J Endocrinol 1994;130:494

245. Parwardhan NA, Moront M, Rao S, et al. Surgery still has a role in Graves' hyperthyroidism. Surgery 1993;114:1108

246. Klementschitsch P, Shen K, Kaplan EL. Reemergence of thyroidectomy as treatment for Graves' disease. Surg Clin North Am 1979;59:35

247. Maier WP, Derrick BM, Marks AD, et al. Long-term follow-up of patients with Graves' disease treated by subtotal thyroidectomy. Am J Surg 1984;147:267

248. Hedley AJ, Bewsher PD, Jones SJ, et al. Late onset hypothyroidism after subtotal thyroidectomy for hyperthyroidism: implications for long term follow-up. Br J Surg 1983;70:740

249. Lee TC, Coffey RJ, Currier BM, et al. Propranolol and thyroidectomy in the treatment of thyrotoxicosis. Ann Surg 1982;195:766

250. Reid DJ. Hyperthyroidism and hypothyroidism complicating the treatment of thyrotoxicosis. Br J Surg 1987;74:1060

251. Sugrue D, Drury MI, McEvoy M, et al. Long term follow-up of hyperthyroid patients treated by subtotal thyroidectomy. Br J Surg 1983;70:408

252. Harada T, Shimaoka K, Arita S, Nakaniski Y. Follow up evaluation of thyroid function after thyroidectomy for thyrotoxicosis. World J Surg 1984;8:444

253. Kalk WJ, Durbach D, Kantor S, Levin J. Postthyroidectomy thyrotoxicosis. Lancet 1978;1:2911

254. Lennquist S, Jortso E, Anderberg BO, Smeds S. Beta blockers compared with antithyroid drugs as preoperative treatment in hyperthyroidism: drug tolerance, complications, and postoperative thyroid function. Surgery 1985;98:1141

255. Peden NR, Browning MCK, Feely J, et al. The clinical and metabolic responses to early surgical treatment for hyperthyroid Graves' disease: a comparison of three preoperative treatment regimens. Q J Med 1985;221:579

256. Feely J, Crooks J, Forrest AL, et al. Propranolol in the surgical treatment of hyperthyroidism, including severely thyrotoxic patients. Br J Surg 1981;68:865

257. Marigold JH, Morgan AK, Earle DJ, et al. Lugol's iodine: its effect on thyroid blood flow in patients with thyrotoxicosis. Br J Surg 1985;72:45

258. Buckingham BA, Costin G, Roe TF, et al. Hyperthyroidism in children. Am J Dis Child 1981;135:112

259. Hamburger JI. Management of hyperthyroidism in children and adolescents. J Clin Endocrinol Metab 1985;60:1019

260. Cooper DS. Antithyroid drugs and radioiodine therapy: a grain of (iodized) salt. Ann Intern Med 1994;121:612

261. Burch HB, Solomon BL, Wartofsky L, Burman KD. Discontinuing antithyroid drug therapy before ablation with radioiodine in Graves' Disease. Ann Intern Med 1994;121:553

262. Aro A, Huttunen JK, Lamberg B-A, et al. Comparison of propranolol and carbimazole as adjuncts to iodine-131 therapy of hyperthyroidism. Acta Endocrinol 1981;96:321

263. Ronnov-Jessen V, Kirkegaard C. Hyperthyroidism: a disease of old age? BMJ 1973;1:41

264. Hamburger JI, Paul S. When and how to use higher ^{131}I doses for hyperthyroidism. N Engl J Med 1968;279:1361

265. Burrow GN. Thyroid function and hyperfunction during gestation. Endocr Rev 1993;14:194

266. Hamburger JI. Diagnosis and management of Graves' disease in pregnancy. Thyroid 1992;2:219

267. Mandel SJ, Brent GA, Larsen PR. Review of antithyroid drug use during pregnancy and report of a case of aplasia cutis. Thyroid 1994;4:129

268. Momotani N, Ito K, Hamada N, et al. Maternal hyperthyroidism and congenital malformation in the offspring. Clin Endocrinol (Oxf) 1984;20:695

269. Davis LE, Lucas MJ, Hankins GDV, et al. Thyrotoxicosis complicating pregnancy. Am J Obstet Gynecol 1989;160:63

270. Momotani N, Noh J, Oyanagi H, et al. Antithyroid drug therapy for Graves' disease during pregnancy. N Engl J Med 1986;315:24

271. Gardner DF, Cruikshank DP, Hays PM, Cooper DS. Pharmacology of propylthiouracil (PTU) in pregnant hyperthyroid women: correlation of maternal PTU concentrations with cord serum thyroid function tests. J Clin Endocrinol Metab 1986;62:277

272. Cheron RG, Kaplan MM, Larsen PR, et al. Neonatal thyroid function after propylthiouracil therapy for maternal Graves' disease. N Engl J Med 1981;304:525

273. Messer PM, Hauffa BP, Olbricht T, et al. Antithyroid drug treatment of Graves' disease in pregnancy: long-term effects on somatic growth, intellectual development and thyroid function of the offspring. Acta Endocrinol 1990;123:311

274. Eisenstein Z, Weiss M, Katz Y, Bank H. Intellectual capacity of subjects exposed to methimazole or propylthiouracil in utero. Eur J Pediatr 1992;151:558

275. Momotani N, Hisaokat, Noh J, et al. Effects of iodine on thyroid status of fetus versus mother in treatment of Graves' disease complicated by pregnancy. J Clin Endocrinol Metab 1992;75:738

276. Lamberg BA, Ikonen E, Osterlung K, et al. Antithyroid treatment of maternal hyperthyroidism during lactation. Clin Endocrinol 1984;21:81

277. Cooper DS. Antithyroid drugs: to breast-feed or not to breast-feed. Am J Obstet Gynecol 1987;157:234

278. Momotani N, Yamashita R, Yoshimoto M, et al. Recovery from foetal hypothyroidism: evidence for the safety of breast-feeding while taking propylthiouracil. Clin Endocrinol 1989;31:591

279. Walter MR, Bartlett WR. Rectal administration of propylthiouracil in the treatment of Graves' disease. Am J Med 1990;88:69

280. Nabil N, Miner DJ, Amatruda M. Methimazole: an alternative route of administration. J Clin Endocrinol Metab 1982;54:180

281. Ashkar FS, Katimus RB, Smoak WM, Gilson AJ. Thyroid storm treatment with blood exchange and plasmapheresis. JAMA 1970;214:1275

282. Herrmann J, Kruskemper JL, Grosser DK, et al. Peritonealdialyse in der thyreotoxischen krise. Dtsch Med Wochenschr 1972;95:742

283. Cooke ST, Ratcliffe G, Fogelman I, Maisey M. Prevalence of inappropriate drug treatment in patients with hyperthyroidism. BMJ 1985;291:1491

284. Van Soestbergen MJM, Van der Vijver JCM, Graafland AD. Recurrence of hyperthyroidism in multinodular goiter after long-term drug therapy: a comparison with Graves' disease. J Endocrinol Invest 1992;15:797

285. Ross DS, Ridgway EC, Daniels GH. Successful treatment of solitary toxic thyroid nodules with relatively low-dose iodine-131, with low prevalence of hypothyroidism. Ann Intern Med 1984;101:488

286. Huysmans DA, Corstens FH, Kloppenborg PW. Long-term follow-up in toxic solitary autonomous thyroid nodules treated with radioactive iodine. J Nucl Med 1991;32:27

287. Goldstein R, Hart IA. Follow-up of solitary autonomous thyroid nodules treated with [131]I. N Engl J Med 1983;309:1473

288. Gorman CA, Robertson JS. Radiation dose in the selection of ^{131}I or surgical treatment for toxic thyroid adenoma. Ann Intern Med 1978;89:85

289. Hamburger JI, Meier DA. Cancer following treatment of an autonomously functioning thyroid nodule with sodium iodide I[131]. Arch Surg 1971;103:763

290. Hamburger JI, Hamburger SW. Diagnosis and management of large toxic multinodular goiters. J Nucl Med 1985;26:888

291. Thomas CG Jr, Croom RD. Current management of the patient with autonomously functioning nodular goiter. Surg Clin North Am 1987;67:315

FIVE

Thyroid Diseases: Hypothyroidism

Werner and Ingbar's The Thyroid, Seventh Edition,
edited by Lewis E. Braverman and Robert D. Utiger.
Lippincott–Raven Publishers, Philadelphia, © 1996

Section A
Introduction

54

Introduction to Hypothyroidism

Lewis E. Braverman
Robert D. Utiger

Hypothyroidism is undoubtedly the most common disorder of thyroid function. It is most often caused by some disorder of the thyroid gland that causes decreased thyroid hormone production and secretion, which is referred to as primary or thyroidal hypothyroidism and is invariably accompanied by increased thyrotropin (TSH) secretion. Much less often it is caused by decreased thyroidal stimulation by TSH, which is referred to as central, hypothyrotropic, or secondary hypothyroidism. Central hypothyroidism may be caused by either pituitary or hypothalamic disease, the latter causing deficiency of thyrotropin-releasing hormone (TRH). It is usually accompanied by low or inappropriately normal serum TSH concentrations, but a few patients have increased secretion of immunoreactive but bioinactive TSH. Although most of the daily production of triiodothyronine (T_3) occurs in extrathyroidal tissue, and extrathyroidal T_3 production is impaired in patients with nonthyroidal illness, the decrease in T_3 production in these patients is accompanied by few if any clinical manifestations of hypothyroidism (see section on nonthyroidal illness in chap 14). The rare patients with generalized resistance to thyroid hormone may have some residual signs of past hypothyroidism, but usually there are few if any symptoms or signs of hypothyroidism when the condition is recognized (see chap 90).

Hypothyroidism is sometimes referred to as myxedema, but the two terms are not interchangeable. Myxedema is the nonpitting edema caused by the accumulation of glycosaminoglycans in subcutaneous and other interstitial tissue that occurs in hypothyroid patients. It is most often present in long-standing or severe primary hypothyroidism.

Primary hypothyroidism may result from diseases or treatments that destroy thyroid tissue or interfere with thyroid hormone biosynthesis (Table 54-1). Worldwide, iodine deficiency is the most common cause of hypothyroidism. In areas where iodine intake is adequate, the most common causes are chronic autoimmune thyroiditis, which occurs in both goitrous and atrophic forms, and radiation-induced hypothyroidism. The latter may be caused either by radioactive iodine treatment of thyrotoxicosis or external radiation therapy directed to the neck in patients with lymphoma or head and neck cancer. Although central hypothyroidism is rare, some of its causes, such as pituitary or hypothalamic tumors, may have disabling and even potentially fatal effects independent of the thyroid deficiency. For this reason and because primary hypothyroidism may not be due to permanent thyroid destruction, an attempt should always be made to determine the cause of hypothyroidism in an individual patient.

The clinical manifestations of hypothyroidism are largely independent of its cause. It affects persons of both sexes and all ages. It may be overt or subclinical; the latter is defined as increased serum TSH and normal free thyroxine (T_4) and T_3 concentrations in a patient who has few or no clinical mani-

TABLE 54-1.
Causes of Hypothyroidism

PRIMARY HYPOTHYROIDISM

Destruction of thyroid tissue
  Chronic autoimmune thyroiditis: atrophic and goitrous forms
  Radiation: ^{131}I therapy for thyrotoxicosis, external radiotherapy
    to the neck for lymphoma or head and neck cancer
  Subtotal and total thyroidectomy
  Infiltrative diseases of the thyroid (amyloidosis, scleroderma)
  Defective thyroid hormone biosynthesis
  Iodine deficiency
  Drugs with antithyroid actions: lithium, iodine, iodine-containing
    drugs, and iodine-containing radiographic contrast agents

CENTRAL HYPOTHYROIDISM

Pituitary disease
Hypothalamic disease

TRANSIENT HYPOTHYROIDISM

Silent thyroiditis*
Subacute thyroiditis
After withdrawal of thyroid hormone therapy in euthyroid patients

Including postpartum thyroiditis.

TABLE 54-2.
Clinical Manifestations of Hypothyroidism

SYMPTOMS

Fatigue
Lethargy
Sleepiness
Mental impairment
Depression
Cold intolerance
Hoarseness
Dry skin
Decreased perspiration
Weight gain
Decreased appetite
Constipation
Menstrual disturbances
Arthralgia
Paresthesia

SIGNS

Slow movements
Slow speech
Hoarseness
Bradycardia
Dry skin
Nonpitting edema (myxedema)
Hyporeflexia
Delayed relaxation of reflexes

SYMPTOMS AND SIGNS ASSOCIATED WITH SPECIFIC CAUSES OF HYPOTHYROIDISM

Diffuse or nodular goiter
Symptoms and signs of pituitary or hypothalamic tumor
  Headache
  Visual impairment
  Deficiency or excess of pituitary hormones other than TSH

festations of hypothyroidism[1] (see chap 87). Even among patients with overt hypothyroidism, the severity is variable. At one extreme are patients who have few symptoms and signs of hypothyroidism; at the other extreme are those with myxedema coma (see chap 75). Some of the more common symptoms and signs of hypothyroidism are listed in Table 54-2[2,3]; these and others are discussed in the chapters on the effects of hypothyroidism on different organ systems.

The clinical manifestations of hypothyroidism are influenced by the age of the patient,[4] the presence of other disease, and the rate at which hypothyroidism develops. In very young infants, hypothyroidism can result in irreversible mental and physical retardation unless treatment is initiated within weeks after birth, whereas in children and adults its effects, though they may be profound, are reversible. In general, patients who develop hypothyroidism rapidly have more symptoms than those in whom it develops slowly. Older patients tend to have fewer symptoms and signs of hypothyroidism, and those the patients have tend to be less specific.[5] In some patients, particularly those with chronic autoimmune thyroiditis, hypothyroidism may remain subclinical for many years, probably even decades, before becoming overt, testimony both to the indolent nature of the process and the ability of the compensatory increase in TSH secretion to maintain near-normal thyroid secretion if the thyroid gland is not seriously damaged.

We now have excellent tools to confirm the presence of hypothyroidism and to determine whether it is caused by thyroid or hypothalamic-pituitary disease in an individual patient. Determining its cause is less easy, but usually possible on the basis of history, physical examination, and tests for thyroid autoantibodies. The major product of the thyroid, T_4, can be easily replaced, but it is important to understand that, as shown in Table 54-1, hypothyroidism is not always due to thyroid de-

struction and that in such patients the proper treatment is not to provide T_4 but to remedy the underlying disorder that led to decreased thyroid hormone synthesis, such as iodine deficiency or excess.

References

1. Staub J-J, Althaus BU, Engler H, et al. Spectrum of subclinical and overt hypothyroidism: effect on thyrotropin, prolactin, and thyroid reserve, and metabolic impact on peripheral tissues. Am J Med 1992;92:621
2. Billewicz WZ, Chapman RS, Crooks J, et al. Statistical methods applied to the diagnosis of hypothyroidism. Q J Med 1969;38:255-66
3. Oddie TH, Boyd CM, Fisher DA, Hales IR. Incidence of signs and symptoms in thyroid disease. Med J Aust 1972;2:981
4. Griffin JE. Hypothyroidism in the elderly. Am J Med Sci 1990;299:334
5. Doucet J, Trivalle C, Chassagne P, et al. Does age play a role in clinical presentation of hypothyroidism? J Am Geriatr Soc 1994;42:984

Werner and Ingbar's The Thyroid, Seventh Edition,
edited by Lewis E. Braverman and Robert D. Utiger.
Lippincott–Raven Publishers, Philadelphia, © 1996

Section B
Causes of Hypothyroidism

55

Chronic Autoimmune Thyroiditis

Anthony P. Weetman

Chronic autoimmune thyroiditis is the original paradigm for autoimmune diseases in general. Only foreign proteins were considered true antigens until Witebsky and Rose demonstrated that rabbits immunized with a saline extract of homologous thyroid tissue and Freund's adjuvant produced thyroid autoantibodies and had lymphocytic infiltration in the target organ.[1] In the same year, 1956, Doniach and Roitt reported that thyroglobulin (Tg) was a major autoantigen stimulating autoantibody formation in chronic goitrous (Hashimoto's) thyroiditis.[2] A year later a second autoantigen was identified in the microsomal fraction of thyroid homogenates; it is now known to be thyroid peroxidase (TPO).[3]

The term autoimmune thyroiditis encompasses a number of different entities (Table 55-1) whose interrelationships remain unclear; the most important are chronic goitrous thyroiditis and chronic atrophic thyroiditis. The pathology of these disorders, considered in detail in chapter 28, consists of varying degrees of lymphocytic infiltration, fibrosis, and loss of follicular epithelium. Repeat biopsies, taken at intervals up to 20 years, show little alteration in thyroid histology, even in patients treated with thyroxine (T_4).[4] There is no good evidence that goitrous thyroiditis precedes atrophic thyroiditis,

although among hypothyroid patients the severity of fibrosis correlates with age.[5] Distinct mechanisms (considered below) may give rise to these variants, but they share many features.

EXPERIMENTAL AUTOIMMUNE THYROIDITIS

Major insights into the etiology and pathogenesis of autoimmune thyroiditis have been obtained from studies of various types of experimental autoimmune thyroiditis (EAT) although none is completely satisfactory as a model of human chronic thyroiditis. Immunization of mice with Tg and an adjuvant causes transient thyroiditis, but its severity correlates only moderately well with Tg antibody production[6] and there is little change in thyroid function. Genetic susceptibility is determined predominantly by class I and II major histocompatibility complex (MHC) genes.[6] Iodide may influence the disease because iodine-deficient Tg fails to induce thyroiditis in this model.[7] A critical T-cell epitope in Tg contains T_4, and stimulation of thyroiditis-inducing T cells is curtailed by replacement of T_4 in the epitope with non-iodinated residues.[8]

TABLE 55-1.
Types of Autoimmune Thyroiditis

	Course	Features
Goitrous (Hashimoto's) thyroiditis	Chronic	Goiter, lymphocytic infiltration, fibrosis, thyroid cell hyperplasia
Atrophic thyroiditis (primary myxedema)	Chronic	Atrophy, fibrosis
Juvenile thyroiditis	Chronic	Usually lymphocytic infiltration
Postpartum thyroiditis	Transient; may progress to chronic thyroiditis	Small goiter, some lymphocytic infiltration
Silent thyroiditis	Transient	Small goiter, some lymphocytic infiltration
Focal thyroiditis	Progressive in some patients	Present in 20% of thyroid glands at autopsy

Pathogenic T cells in immunization-induced EAT are controlled by small changes in circulating Tg concentrations that affect both CD4 and CD8 regulatory T cells.[9] Cytotoxic T cells are an important effector mechanism in this form of EAT.[6] However, a role for Tg autoantibodies has been suggested; in situ perfusion with these antibodies alone can result in follicular destruction and fibrosis, most likely via complement activation.[10]

Modulating the T-cell repertoire of mice or rats, for example by thymectomy with or without sublethal irradiation, causes many organ-specific, genetically determined autoimmune diseases, including EAT.[11,12] Disease can be transferred by CD4 cells, but a subfraction of normal CD4 cells prevents EAT, either directly or by inducing regulatory (suppressor) T cells.[13] At least two explanations are offered for the etiology of this type of EAT, related to different mechanisms for maintaining self-tolerance (Table 55-2). One possibility is that autoreactive T cells escape tolerance because they do not encounter thyroid autoantigen in the appropriate setting in the athymic animal. However, intrathymic tolerance is never complete, and other mechanisms are required to prevent autoimmunity, such as T cell–mediated suppression. Thymectomy could therefore induce EAT if performed at a stage of T-cell development when autoreactive, effector T cells have left the thymus for the periphery but the suppressor-inducer (or suppressor) cells have not.

Chronic thyroiditis occurs spontaneously in several animal species. A low proportion of female Buffalo strain rats develops chronic thyroiditis and Tg antibodies, and the proportion can be increased by thymectomy or administration of methylcholanthrene.[14] About 50% of Biobreeding (BB) rats develop Tg antibodies and thyroid lymphocytic accumulation, in addition to diabetes mellitus, but thyroid follicular destruction does not occur; this strain may be a model of euthyroid goiter caused by growth-stimulating immunoglobulins.[15] The incidence of chronic thyroiditis and thyroid autoantibodies is even higher in non-obese diabetic mice;[16] in neither model is there a female preponderance of disease.

Chronic thyroiditis in Obese strain (OS) chickens is perhaps the most like chronic goitrous thyroiditis because these animals develop overt hypothyroidism as well as appropriate immunologic abnormalities.[17] The MHC contributes slightly in determining susceptibility, but the major contribution is from uncharacterized immunoregulatory genes outside the MHC that increase interleukin-2 responsiveness and control Tg antibody production. Additional genes enhance the susceptibility of the thyroid to autoimmune damage although no analogous genetic influence is apparent in other forms of EAT. Finally, genetic and environmental factors affecting control of glucocorticoid and sex hormone secretion are also important.[18]

PREDISPOSITION TO CHRONIC AUTOIMMUNE THYROIDITIS

Autoimmune diseases generally occur when there is a failure of T-cell tolerance as a result of a combination of genetic and nongenetic factors (Table 55-3). The detailed genetics of chronic goitrous and chronic atrophic thyroiditis are considered in chapter 27. Nongenetic factors may be endogenous or exogenous. The increased female prevalence of chronic autoimmune thyroiditis is related to the effects of sex hormones and is best demonstrated by manipulation of estrogen and androgen concentrations in EAT.[6,18] Postpartum thyroiditis (see chap 89) may also result from hormonal effects on the immune system and is an important predictor of subsequent hypothyroidism.[19] A role for stress is not apparent in chronic autoimmune thyroiditis, possibly because the disease evolves over such a long period, but stress-related variations in circulating cortisol concentrations could affect susceptibility, as suggested by observations in the OS chicken.[18] Finally, birth weight correlates inversely with the prevalence of thyroid autoantibodies in women.[20] This effect is modest and of uncer-

TABLE 55-2.
Mechanisms Involved in Immunologic Self-Tolerance

Intrathymic (central) deletion of autoreactive T cells

Intrathymic (central) anergy due to autoantigen presentation in the absence of a co-stimulatory signal

Peripheral tolerance, usually by anergy, but deletion may occur

Active suppression of T-helper cells by several possible pathways

Sequestration of autoantigen

Absence of the activated CD4 cells required for expansion of CD8 cells

TABLE 55-3.
Roles of Genetic and Nongenetic Factors in Autoimmunity

Factor	Effect
MHC class II genes	Encode products that delete autoreactive T cells, select for presentation of autoantigenic peptides, or activate suppressor T cells
Other MHC genes	Diverse potential effects on antigen presentation; the cytokine tumor necrosis factor is also encoded in the MHC
Cytokine regulatory genes	Control cytokine production
T-cell receptor and immunoglobulin genes	Uncertain—some reports of association with autoimmunity
Infectious agents	May release autoantigens, alter expression of surface molecules, directly affect the immune system, or contain immunogenic sequences that mimic autoantigens
Dietary factors	Diverse potential effects; for example, iodide may enhance the immunogenicity of thyroglobulin and alter thyroid cell function
Toxins, pollutants	Diverse potential effects; for example, methylcholanthrene enhances thyroiditis in Buffalo strain rats
Hormones	Diverse potential effects; estrogens generally enhance immune responses, whereas glucocorticoids and androgens are suppressive
Stress	May alter neuroendocrine interactions with the immune system

MHC, major histocompatibility complex.

tain importance for the development of chronic autoimmune thyroiditis, but it demonstrates the potential effect of early nutritional and hormonal factors.

Infection and iodide uptake are the two exogenous susceptibility factors that have received the most attention. Despite the plausibility of infectious agents causing autoimmunity via tissue damage or molecular mimicry, there is little evidence that infection plays a major role in chronic autoimmune thyroiditis, partly because it is difficult to prove the influence of any environmental agent that may operate only at the beginning of what is a long preclinical course of disease. Normal gut microflora are required for the appearance of EAT after thymectomy and irradiation in rats although the mechanism is unclear.[21] Polyclonal activation or molecular mimicry are both possible. A unique avian retrovirus has been associated with thyroiditis in OS chickens, but direct involvement has not been proved.[22] There is a clear increase in thyroid autoimmunity in patients with the congenital rubella syndrome,[23] and recently hepatitis C virus infection has been associated with chronic goitrous thyroiditis.[24] However, typical chronic autoimmune thyroiditis is not a sequela of subacute thyroiditis, which is probably caused by a variety of viruses, so any effects of infection are more complex than simple tissue damage.[25]

Observations in EAT provide the most compelling evidence that excessive dietary iodide intake can exacerbate thyroid autoimmunity. A high iodide intake increases the frequency of spontaneous thyroiditis in rats and OS chickens, as does a normal amount given after a period of iodine restriction.[26–28] The antigenicity of Tg, the main autoantigen in these models, is increased when it is iodide rich, and iodide is a critical constituent of a major T-cell epitope of Tg in murine EAT induced by immunization.[8] Iodide may also interact with reactive oxygen metabolites to produce highly reactive forms of iodine

with inflammatory potential, as shown in OS chickens.[29]

Similar effects in chronic autoimmune thyroiditis in humans are suggested by epidemiologic studies showing a higher frequency of thyroid autoantibodies in residents of iodide-sufficient areas as compared with residents of iodide-deficient areas.[30] Iodide prophylaxis has been associated with a marked increase in lymphocytic thyroiditis in thyroid glands resected for papillary carcinoma,[31] and a modest but significant increase in TPO antibodies in serum was found in patients with Graves' disease who had been treated with an antithyroid drug and were then given pharmacologic doses of potassium iodide.[32] Furthermore, in another study,[33] lymphocytic thyroiditis was present in thyroid biopsies from 14 of 28 patients with iodide-induced hypothyroidism. However, it is possible that it was the presence of chronic autoimmune thyroiditis that caused this effect of iodide, rather than vice versa. Iodide has a direct toxic effect on cultured human thyroid cells,[34] possibly due to free radical attack; this could trigger or exacerbate autoimmune thyroiditis by providing excess autoantigen in a modified and thus more immunogenic form. Finally, iodide in vitro enhances production of heat shock proteins by stressed thyroid cells.[35] This is an additional mechanism by which iodide excess may lead to disease exacerbation because heat shock proteins have a number of immunomodulatory effects that could exacerbate chronic autoimmune thyroiditis.[36]

In patients with cancer or chronic hepatitis who have subclinical chronic autoimmune thyroiditis, treatment with α-interferon, interleukin-2, or granulocyte-macrophage colony-stimulating factor worsens the autoimmune process and may cause overt hypothyroidism.[37–39] The frequency of chronic autoimmune thyroiditis is also increased in atomic bomb survivors.[40] These findings may have little to do with the ordinary clinical development of chronic autoimmune thyroiditis, but demonstrate that diverse, nongenetic factors can exacerbate or perhaps even cause the disorder.

PATHOGENESIS OF CHRONIC AUTOIMMUNE THYROIDITIS

Antigen Presentation

This is the initial event in the autoimmune process, in which an antigen is taken up, processed into peptide epitopes, and then presented to T-cell antigen receptors on CD4 cells by forming bimolecular complexes with MHC class II molecules (Fig 55-1).[41] The binding of these complexes to T-cell antigen receptors leads to T-cell activation and the release of cytokines that can, for instance, provide help for B cells to make antibodies. To stimulate certain T cells, particularly those not previously exposed to antigen, co-stimulatory signals are required, the best characterized of which is a family of ligands called B7 on the antigen-presenting cell.[42] These ligands bind to CD28 and CTLA-4 receptors on T cells and ensure activation. Other co-stimulatory signals exist, including cytokines like interleukin-1.

Most antigen-presenting cells (e.g., macrophages and dendritic cells) constitutively express MHC class II molecules and co-stimulatory molecules. Normal thyroid cells do not express class II molecules, but those from patients with chronic autoimmune thyroiditis do. The appearance of class II molecules on thyroid cells could be the initiating factor in chronic autoimmune thyroiditis.[43] A close spatial correlation exists between the presence of class II molecules on thyroid cells and γ-interferon–containing T cells in thyroid tissue,[44] and this T cell-derived cytokine is the only known initiator of class II expression by normal thyroid cells in vitro.[45] MHC class II expression is, therefore, probably the consequence rather than the cause of thyroid autoimmunity. This is supported by observations in thymectomy-induced and spontaneous EAT because class II-positive thyroid cells only appear late in disease, after T-cell infiltration.[15,46]

Nonetheless, antigen presentation by thyroid cells could be important in the perpetuation of the autoimmune response. Class II-positive thyroid cells can stimulate T cells, but it is unclear whether the thyroid cells also express co-stimulators and it is difficult to exclude an effect of contaminating macrophages and dendritic cells.[47] Class II–positive thyroid cells only weakly stimulate the allogeneic mixed lymphocyte response by T cells, but phorbol esters induce an unknown co-stimulator on thyroid cells that promotes alloreactivity, indicating that the signals necessary for this response can be induced under in vitro conditions.[48] The co-stimulator is not B7, which is undetectable on thyroid cells in vitro or in vivo.[49] In the absence of B7, it seems unlikely that thyroid cells could stimulate naive, autoreactive T cells. Instead, tolerance to such T cells might actually be acquired through the operation of anergy, which can be viewed as a protective mechanism (see Table 55-2). Once T cells have encountered appropriately presented antigen, they are less dependent on co-stimulation for subsequent activation and therefore could respond to class II–positive thyroid cells.

Thus, the extent of antigen presentation by thyroid cells in autoimmune thyroiditis will depend at least in part on the timing of the appearance of class II molecules on these cells. Prompt appearance of class II molecules on thyroid cells, for example in response to a viral infection, could be an important protective mechanism because this might render potentially autoreactive T cells anergic (Fig 55-2). However, in chronic autoimmune thyroiditis, such T cells are presumably first activated by macrophages and dendritic cells and may then be further expanded by class II–expressing thyroid cells, depending on their requirement for co-stimulation.

T-Cell Responses

Phenotypic changes in peripheral blood and thyroid-infiltrating T cells provide only indirect information on T-cell function in chronic autoimmune thyroiditis. In one recent study, circulating CD8 cells were decreased only during an aggravated phase of thyroid gland damage.[50] Similar decreases in CD8 cells have been reported in several autoimmune disorders, but the meaning of these alterations is unclear. Of more direct relevance is the phenotype of T cells infiltrating the thyroid, which are mainly CD4 and express activation markers such as MHC class II molecules.[51,52]

The clonality of these T cells is of major interest because in some animal models of autoimmune disease there is a clonally restricted T-cell response in the early phase of the disease, marked by the utilization of particular α- or β-variable (V) region genes encoding the T-cell antigen receptor of pathogenic T cells.[53,54] Unfortunately, detecting such restriction in human autoimmune disease has been difficult.[55] The prolonged nat-

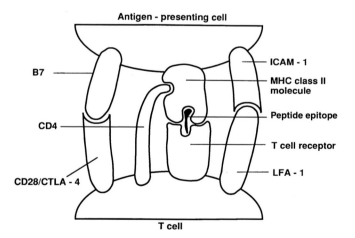

FIGURE 55-1. Major molecular interactions in antigen presentation. Protein antigen is processed into a peptide epitope of around 12 to 20 amino acids that binds to the polymorphic region of a major histocompatibility complex (MHC) class II molecule. This is recognized by the heterodimeric T-cell receptor, composed of an α and β chain, and the interaction is stabilized by CD4 that binds to a nonpolymorphic region of the class II molecule. Full activation of the T cell may also require the interaction of adhesion molecules on both the antigen-presenting cells and T-cells, an example of which is the binding of intercellular adhesion molecule-1 (ICAM-1) to lymphocyte function-associated antigen-1 (LFA-1), and a co-stimulatory signal, such as that supplied by B7 through CD28 or CTLA-4.

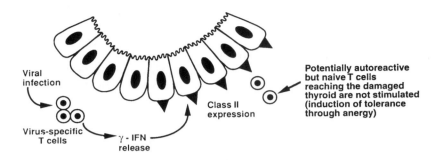

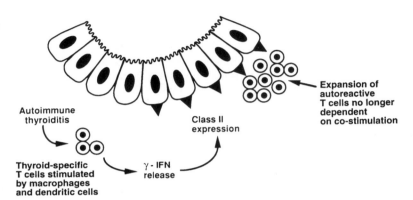

FIGURE 55-2. Alternative outcomes after expression of major histocompatibility complex (MHC) class II molecules by thyroid cells. Naive T cells undergo peripheral tolerance through anergy because the thyroid follicular cells do not supply co-stimulatory signals. However, T cells that have already encountered autoantigen presented by a macrophage or dendritic cell may be stimulated in the absence of further co-stimulation, exacerbating the autoimmune response.

ural history of these conditions, in particular chronic autoimmune thyroiditis, means that the immune response has had a chance to spread and involve many determinants within autoantigens, which are recognized by multiple T-cell receptors, by the time of diagnosis.[56]

Striking restriction of Vα gene usage has been found among T cells infiltrating the thyroid gland in patients with Graves' disease and chronic autoimmune thyroiditis, with an average of only 4 to 5 of 18 Vα gene families used.[57,58] Subsequent studies in chronic autoimmune thyroiditis using tissue obtained by fine-needle aspiration biopsy failed to find such marked restriction, with an average of 12 Vα and 17 Vβ families being used,[59] and we found no evidence for restriction of Vα gene usage by interleukin-2 receptor-positive, recently activated intrathyroidal lymphocytes from patients with Graves' disease[60] or chronic autoimmune thyroiditis (unpublished observations). Therefore, in most patients with chronic autoimmune thyroiditis, the T-cell response is polyclonal by the time of diagnosis. Moreover, in EAT in non-obese mice, marked restriction in V gene usage is not apparent even in early thyroiditis, with 10 of 17 Vβ families used,[61] and considerable heterogeneity of Vβ usage has also been found in EAT induced by T-cell depletion.[62]

There is general agreement that circulating and intrathyroidal T cells from patients with chronic autoimmune thyroiditis are weakly stimulated by Tg and TPO. Attempts have been made using synthetic peptides or recombinant fusion proteins to identify the T-cell epitopes within TPO. Although some regions of the molecule, particularly between residues 415–589, contain epitopes, the overall responses are heterogeneous,

with patients responding to one or several TPO fragments and with marked variation between patients.[63–66] This is compatible with a polyclonal T-cell response that has spread to involve a number of determinants, some of which are "cryptic" in the sense that they only become exposed to recognition by the immune system during the course of an autoimmune response.[56] Further study of T-cell responses will be facilitated by using Epstein-Barr virus-transformed B-cell lines transfected with expression plasmids encoding thyroid autoantigen cDNA to present antigen; impressive T-cell responses to TPO have recently been reported using this technique.[67]

The effector function of T cells in chronic autoimmune thyroiditis is considered further below, but another important role for the T-cell population is to regulate the immune response. An impairment in T cell–mediated immune suppression has been proposed to play a major role in the pathogenesis of this condition.[68] A number of different in vitro techniques have been used to identify such a defect, including the migration inhibition assay and mitogen-dependent autoantibody production.[69,70] The results suggest that some population of circulating T cells from normal subjects is capable of inhibiting the function of T cells from patients with chronic autoimmune thyroiditis, and that these cells are lacking in the patients, but the physiologic relevance of these assay systems has been questioned, not least because they involve coculture of allogeneic cells and because such effects are not always antigen specific.[71]

It is most likely that T cell–mediated suppression of autoreactive T cells is one of several back-up systems used to control those few cells escaping central tolerance during development (see Table 55-2). Nonetheless, there is little doubt from studies of EAT that some form of antigen-specific T cell–mediated suppression can be critical in determining the outcome of an immune response; how such T cells mediate this effect is unclear.[9,13] The profile of cytokines released by antigen-stimulated T–helper cell subsets may confer suppressor function, with the products of the T_H1 subset suppressing T_H2 cells and vice versa.[72] On this basis, genetically determined differences in cytokine production could result in disordered immunoregulation and contribute to autoimmune disease. There are several other explanations for suppressor-like effects, including idiotypic interaction between T-cell receptors, direct cytotoxicity, and secretion of antigen-specific suppressor factors.[73] With such complexity, it is not surprising that there remain questions regarding the specificity and time of appearance of any suppressor defect in chronic autoimmune thyroiditis in humans.

B-Cell Responses

The production of Tg, TPO, and other thyroid antibodies in patients with chronic autoimmune thyroiditis is considered in detail in chapter 21. The heavy and light chain composition of Tg and TPO autoantibodies indicates that these are the result of a polyclonal B cell response.[74] However, there is a relatively restricted range of heavy and light chain combinations used by B cells producing TPO antibodies,[75] which could relate to the genetic control of thyroid antibody production noted previously. The thyroid is an important source of thyroid antibodies in autoimmune thyroid disease although there are also contributions from the parathyroidal lymph nodes and bone marrow.[76] Intrathyroidal B cells are generally polyclonal, but when B-cell lymphoma arises as a complication of chronic autoimmune thyroiditis, immunoglobulin gene rearrangements reveal a monoclonal B cell population.[77]

Effector Mechanisms

Both humoral and cell-mediated effector mechanisms cause tissue injury in chronic autoimmune thyroiditis (Fig 55-3). Intrathyroidal complement fixation by thyroid antibodies is revealed by the presence of terminal complement complexes around the thyroid follicles in chronic autoimmune thyroiditis; complexes are also found in the circulation.[78] Although TPO

antibodies can activate complement, there is incomplete correlation between complement fixation and TPO antibody concentrations, indicating the presence of additional complement-fixing antibodies in patients with chronic autoimmune thyroiditis.[79] Thyroid cells are not necessarily lysed by complement attack because they are protected by a number of regulators of complement activation.[80] Nonlethal complement attack may lead to metabolic impairment, such as impaired responsiveness to thyrotropin (TSH),[81] and the release of a number of proinflammatory molecules including interleukin-1, interleukin-6, prostaglandin E_2, and reactive oxygen metabolites, all of which could exacerbate the autoimmune response.[82] Nonetheless, sustained complement attack will ultimately kill thyroid cells and contribute to the development of hypothyroidism.[79] Transplacental passage of complement-fixing antibodies does not affect the fetal thyroid.

Autoantibodies play a key role in the process of antibody-dependent cell-mediated cytotoxicity, in which natural killer (NK) cells kill thyroid cells because the latter have autoantibodies bound to their surface that engage the immunoglobulin Fc receptors of the NK cells. Both TPO and Tg antibodies can mediate antibody-dependent cell-mediated cytotoxicity in experimental systems, and other uncharacterized thyroid autoantibodies also may be involved.[83] The importance of this mechanism in vivo is unclear, although intrathyroidal NK cells can be detected in patients with chronic autoimmune thyroiditis.[52]

In addition, autoantibodies may have direct functional effects, considered in detail in chapter 21. TPO antibodies may impair the activity of the enzyme.[84] Blocking antibodies, directed against unique determinants on the TSH receptor,[85] can cause hypothyroidism, although the relative contribution of this mechanism, as compared with the others described in this section, has not been established. In Japan and Korea, these antibodies are present in 20% to 75% of hypothyroid patients with atrophic thyroiditis.[86,87] In whites, TSH receptor–blocking antibodies are found less often, and the frequency is similar in goitrous and atrophic thyroiditis.[88,89] The existence of growth-promoting and growth-blocking antibodies, operating independently of the TSH receptor, has been suggested to account for these two different types of chronic autoimmune thyroiditis.[90] Transplacental passage of TSH receptor-blocking antibodies may cause neonatal hypothyroidism.

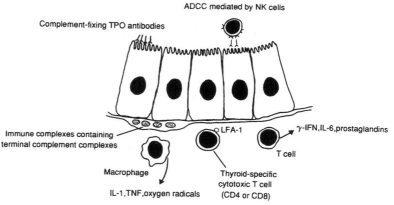

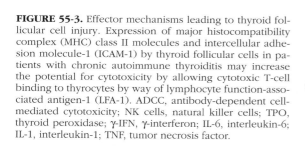

FIGURE 55-3. Effector mechanisms leading to thyroid follicular cell injury. Expression of major histocompatibility complex (MHC) class II molecules and intercellular adhesion molecule-1 (ICAM-1) by thyroid follicular cells in patients with chronic autoimmune thyroiditis may increase the potential for cytotoxicity by allowing cytotoxic T-cell binding to thyrocytes by way of lymphocyte function-associated antigen-1 (LFA-1). ADCC, antibody-dependent cell-mediated cytotoxicity; NK cells, natural killer cells; TPO, thyroid peroxidase; γ-IFN, γ-interferon; IL-6, interleukin-6; IL-1, interleukin-1; TNF, tumor necrosis factor.

T cell–mediated cytotoxicity is demonstrable in EAT[6] and seems likely to be important in chronic autoimmune thyroiditis in humans. One CD8 cell clone established from a patient with chronic autoimmune thyroiditis killed thyroid cells in vitro, but the nature of the thyroid antigen recognized was not established.[91] CD4 cells may also be cytotoxic, and theoretically these could kill class II–positive thyroid cells. Expansion of the infiltrating T cells with interleukin-2 usually leads to the development of lymphokine-activated killer cells, which have no target specificity.[92,93]

The infiltrating T cells also release a wide array of cytokines, including γ-interferon, interleukin-2, interleukin-6, tumor necrosis factor, and transforming growth factor.[93,94] Although direct injury of thyroid cells has been difficult to detect in vitro,[95] these cytokines (plus those derived from macrophages and the thyroid cells themselves) may impair the functional responses of thyroid cells, and therefore contribute to the development of hypothyroidism (Table 55-4).[96] One important consequence of intrathyroidal cytokine production is the expression of intercellular adhesion molecule-1 on thyroid cells.[97] This increases the ability of T cells to bind to thyroid cells by lymphocyte function–associated antigen-1, a receptor for intercellular adhesion molecule-1, and enhances T cell–mediated cytotoxicity.[98]

The mechanisms involved in thyroid injury are therefore diverse. It is likely that quantitative differences in their contributions, rather than simply the presence or absence of a particular antibody or cytokine, account for the different clinical types of autoimmune thyroiditis (see Table 55-1). The participation of the thyroid cells themselves in the autoimmune response is of particular interest because these cells express cytokines and cell surface molecules with the potential to promote or protect against autoimmune damage.[99] Genetic or environmentally induced alterations in these responses could be important in the progression of autoimmune thyroiditis.

CLINICAL ASPECTS

Patients with chronic autoimmune thyroiditis may present with clinical features of hypothyroidism, accompanied in some by painless goiter. However, the widespread use of thyroid tests reveals many patients with subclinical chronic autoimmune thyroiditis (e.g., positive tests for anti-TPO antibodies), some of whom also have increased serum TSH concentrations (subclinical hypothyroidism), goiter, or both (see chap 26).

When present, the goiter is usually firm, with size varying from small to very large, and is often lobulated, these characteristics sometimes giving rise to the suspicion of a multinodular goiter or even cancer. The presence of pain suggests the development of lymphoma although pain may also occur rarely in uncomplicated cases.[100] Fine-needle aspiration biopsy or even surgical biopsy may be needed to distinguish between these conditions. Biopsy is also warranted if there is a dominant nodule or rapid change in goiter size. In the majority of patients, however, biopsy is not indicated, the diagnosis being made on clinical and biochemical grounds and supported by the presence of positive tests for TPO (or Tg) antibodies in serum. Ophthalmopathy occurs in a small proportion of patients, and there is evidence of chronic autoimmune thyroiditis in a large percentage of the patients with euthyroid (ophthalmic) Graves' disease, who represent between 5% and 10% of cases of Graves' ophthalmopathy.[101] Localized myxedema is extremely rare in chronic autoimmune thyroiditis.[102]

In atrophic thyroiditis, patients usually present with hypothyroidism. The rate of decline in thyroid secretion in this subgroup of patients with chronic autoimmune thyroiditis is uncertain, but the presence of focal chronic thyroiditis in about 40% of white American women aged more than 20 years,[103] the majority of whom do not have a goiter, suggests that progression to thyroid failure is slow and occurs only in a minority of subjects. In about 25% of adolescent subjects with goitrous thyroiditis, there is spontaneous resolution over a 20-year period, although 33% had become hypothyroid during this time.[104] Postpartum thyroiditis may be associated with the subsequent development of chronic autoimmune thyroiditis in up to a quarter of patients over a 4-year period.

Among a group of hypothyroid patients with goitrous thyroiditis, therapy with T_4 for 2 years led to a 32% reduction in thyroid volume (as determined by ultrasonography).[105] Serum TPO antibody concentrations may decrease[106,107] or not

TABLE 55-4.
Effect of Cytokines on Thyroid Cell Function

Cytokine	Effect
γ-Interferon	Increased expression of major histocompatibility complex (MHC) class I and II molecules, complement regulatory proteins and intercellular adhesion molecule-1 (ICAM-1); growth inhibition; enhanced iodide uptake; decreased thyroglobulin (T_g) and thyroid hormone synthesis; increased interleukin-6 synthesis
Interleukin-1	Increased expression of complement regulatory proteins and ICAM-1; inhibition of cAMP, Tg, and thyroid peroxidase (TPO) production; enhanced growth; increased interleukin-6 and interleukin-8 synthesis
Interleukin-6	Decreased cAMP and TPO production
Tumor necrosis factor	Increased expression of MHC class I molecules; enhanced effect of γ-interferon on MHC class II expression; increased production of interleukin-6 and complement regulatory proteins; growth inhibition; decreased thyroid hormone release

---

TABLE 55-5.
Autoimmune Disorders Occurring With Increased Frequency in Patients With Chronic Autoimmune Thyroiditis

---

TYPE 2 AUTOIMMUNE POLYGLANDULAR SYNDROME

The presence of two or more of the following disorders: autoimmune thyroid disease, insulin-dependent diabetes mellitus, Addison's disease, premature ovarian failure, myasthenia gravis, celiac disease; alopecia, hypophysitis, vitiligo, serositis, and pernicious anemia also occur

RHEUMATOLOGIC DISORDERS

Rheumatoid arthritis, systemic lupus erythematosus, Sjögren's syndrome, polymyalgia rheumatica, temporal arteritis, relapsing polychondritis, and systemic sclerosis

OTHERS

Chronic active hepatitis, primary biliary cirrhosis, dermatitis herpetiformis

---

change[105] during T_4 therapy. In a serial study of 21 Japanese patients with TSH receptor-blocking antibodies, T_4 treatment for 4 to 8 years was associated with disappearance of these antibodies in 71% of patients, and over 50% of these patients remained euthyroid after therapy was discontinued.[108] However, the possibility of remission in patients without TSH receptor antibodies was not assessed. In Japanese children with atrophic thyroiditis, hypothyroidism is irreversible, but thyroid function may return to normal in goitrous thyroiditis during T_4 treatment.[109] T_4 may directly affect the autoimmune process or, more likely, suppression of TSH secretion decreases thyroid cell expression of autoantigens.

The permanence of such remissions is presently unclear and, although the concentration of TSH receptor–blocking antibodies decreased in French patients with goitrous thyroiditis treated with T_4 for 1 year, no patient remained euthyroid after T_4 was discontinued.[107] Thus, genetic and environmental effects are likely to influence outcome. Withdrawal of T_4 for a month is the only practical method of assessing whether hypothyroidism is persistent,[110] but at present there is little justification for this because of the low frequency of remission among unselected patients.

ASSOCIATED DISORDERS

Graves' disease may precede or follow chronic autoimmune thyroiditis in the same patient, presumably related to the similar autoimmune processes in the two disorders. This is highlighted by observations in five patients with Graves' ophthalmopathy and biopsy evidence of chronic goitrous thyroiditis in whom TSH receptor–stimulating antibodies characteristic of Graves' disease were detected.[111] These patients had a fluctuating clinical course thought to be due to changes in the balance between antibody-mediated TSH receptor stimulation and the effector mechanisms discussed above. Hypothyroidism, due to chronic autoimmune thyroiditis, ultimately supervenes in about 20% of patients with Graves' thyrotoxicosis treated with antithyroid

drugs; TSH receptor–blocking antibodies contribute to the hypothyroidism in about one-third of cases.[112]

There is a clear association between chronic autoimmune thyroiditis and primary B-cell lymphoma of the thyroid; in one recent series of 119 patients, this tumor occurred only in the presence of chronic autoimmune thyroiditis.[113] Presumably, prolonged stimulation of intrathyroidal B cells ultimately results in the emergence of a malignant clone. The frequency of other thyroid tumors is not increased in chronic autoimmune thyroiditis although cancer may be overlooked in patients with irregular goiters caused by thyroiditis.[114] Riedel's thyroiditis has recently been suggested to have an autoimmune etiology because many patients have thyroid antibodies and a lymphocytic infiltrate composed of CD4 and CD8 cells,[115] but the relationship of this condition to chronic autoimmune thyroiditis is unclear.

Chronic autoimmune thyroiditis is a well-recognized component of the type 2 autoimmune polyglandular syndrome[116] and occurs with increased prevalence in a variety of other disorders (Table 55-5). These associations are due, at least in part, to shared immunogenetic susceptibility. Some evidence suggests that the pattern of islet-cell autoreactivity in patients with insulin-dependent diabetes mellitus differs between patients with and without autoimmune thyroid disease, indicating a qualitative or quantitative difference in autoreactivity in the type 2 syndrome.[117,118] In addition to the conditions listed in Table 55-5, in small numbers of patients chronic autoimmune thyroiditis has been associated with several other potentially autoimmune conditions, including primary pulmonary hypertension,[119] lymphocytic interstitial pneumonitis,[120] Tolosa-Hunt syndrome,[121] and sclerosing lymphocytic lobulitis of the breast.[122]

References

1. Rose NR, Witebsky E. Studies in organ specificity. V. Changes in the thyroid glands of rabbits following active immunization with rabbit thyroid extracts. J Immunol 1956;76:417
2. Roitt IM, Doniach D, Campbell PN, Vaughan Hudson R. Autoantibodies in Hashimoto's disease (lymphadenoid goitre). Lancet 1956;2:820
3. Trotter WR, Belyavin G, Wadhams A. Precipitating and complement-fixing antibodies in Hashimoto's disease. Proc R Soc Med 1957;50:961
4. Mizukami Y, Michigishi T, Kawato M, et al. Thyroid function and histologic correlations in 601 cases. Hum Pathol 1991;23:980
5. Hayashi Y, Tamai H, Fukata S, et al. A long term clinical, immunological, and histological follow-up study of patients with goitrous chronic lymphocytic thyroiditis. J Clin Endocrinol Metab 1985;61:1172
6. Charreire J. Immune mechanisms in autoimmune thyroiditis. Adv Immunol 1989;46:263
7. Champion B, Rayner DC, Byfield PGH, et al. Critical role of iodination for T cell recognition of thyroglobulin in experimental murine thyroid autoimmunity. J Immunol 1987;139:3665
8. Champion BR, Page KR, Parish N, et al. Identification of a thyroxine-containing self-epitope of thyroglobulin which triggers thyroid autoreactive T cells. J Exp Med 1991;174:363
9. Nabozny GH, Flynn JC, Kong Y-CM. Synergism between mouse thyroglobulin- and vaccination-induced suppressor mechanisms in murine experimental autoimmune thyroiditis. Cell Immunol 1991;136:340

10. Inoue K, Niesen N, Milgrom F, Albini B. Transfer of experimental autoimmune thyroiditis by in situ perfusion of thyroids with immune sera. Clin Immunol Immunopathol 1993;66:11

11. Sakaguchi S, Sakaguchi N. Organ-specific disease induced in mice by elimination of T cell subsets. J Immunol 1989;142:471

12. Smith H, Chen I-M, Kubo R, Tung KS. Neonatal thymectomy results in a repertoire enriched in T cells deleted in adult thymus. Science 1989;245:749

13. Sugihara S, Izumi Y, Yoshioka T, et al. Autoimmune thyroiditis induced in mice depleted of particular T cell subsets. I. Requirement of Lyt-1 dull L3T4 bright normal T cells for the induction of thyroiditis. J Immunol 1988;141:105

14. Cohen SB, Weetman AP. Characterization of different types of experimental autoimmune thyroiditis in the Buffalo strain rat. Clin Exp Immunol 1987;69:25

15. Voorby HAM, Van Der Gaag RD, Jeucken PHM, et al. The goitre of the BB/O rat: an animal model for studying the role of immunoglobulins stimulating growth of thyroid cells. Clin Exp Immunol 1989;76:290

16. Bernard NF, Ertug F, Margolese H. High incidence of thyroiditis and anti-thyroid autoantibodies in NOD mice. Diabetes 1991;41:40

17. Wick G, Brezinschek HP, Hala K, et al. The Obese strain of chickens: an animal model with spontaneous autoimmune thyroiditis. Adv Immunol 1989;47:433

18. Wick G, Hu Y, Schwarz S, Kroemer G. Immunoendocrine communication via the hypothalamo-pituitary-adrenal axis in autoimmune diseases. Endocr Rev 1993;14:539

19. Othman S, Phillips DIW, Parkes AB, et al. A long-term follow-up of postpartum thyroiditis. Clin Endocrinol 1990;32:559

20. Phillips DIW, Cooper C, Fall C, et al. Fetal growth and autoimmune thyroid disease. Q J Med 1993;86:247

21. Penhale WJ, Young PR. The influence of the normal microbial flora on the susceptibility of rats to experimental autoimmune thyroiditis. Clin Exp Immunol 1988;72:288

22. Ziemiecki A, Kromer G, Mueller RG, et al. ev22, a new endogenous avian leukosis virus locus found in chickens with spontaneous autoimmune thyroiditis. Arch Viol 1988;100:267

23. Clarke WL, Shaver KA, Bright GM, et al. Autoimmunity in congenital rubella syndrome. J Pediatr 1984;104:370

24. Tran A, Quaranta JF, Beusnel C, et al. Hepatitis C virus and Hashimoto's thyroiditis. Eur J Med 1992;1:116

25. Tomer Y, Davies TF. Infection, thyroid disease, and autoimmunity. Endocr Rev 1993;14:107

26. Cohen SB, Weetman AP. The effect of iodine depletion and supplementation in the Buffalo strain rat. J Endocrinol Invest 1988;11:625

27. Ebner SA, Lueprasitsakul W, Alex S, et al. Iodine content of rat thyroglobulin affects its antigenicity in inducing lymphocytic thyroiditis in the BB/Wor rat. Autoimmunity 1992;13:209

28. Sundick RS, Herdegen DM, Brown TR, Bagchi N. The incorporation of dietary iodine into thyroglobulin increases its immunogenicity. Endocrinology 1987;120:2078

29. Bagchi N, Brown TR, Urdanivia E, Sundick RS. Induction of autoimmune thyroiditis in chickens by dietary iodine. Endocrinology 1990;230:325

30. Reinwein D, Benker G, König MP, et al. Hyperthyroidism in Europe: clinical and laboratory data of a prospective multicentre survey. J Endocrinol Invest 1986;9:1

31. Harach HR, Escalante DA, Onativia A, et al. Thyroid carcinoma and thyroiditis in an endemic goitre region before and after iodine prophylaxis. Acta Endocrinol 1985;108:55

32. Roti E, Gardini E, Minelli R, et al. Effects of chronic iodine administration on thyroid status in euthyroid subjects previously treated with antithyroid drugs for Graves' hyperthyroidism. J Clin Endocrinol Metab 1993;76:928

33. Mizukami Y, Michigishi T, Nonomura A, et al. Iodine-induced hypothyroidism: a clinical and histological study of 28 patients. J Clin Endocrinol Metab 1993;76:466

34. Many MC, Mestdagh C, Van Den Hove MF, Denef JF. In vitro study of acute toxic effects of high iodide doses in human thyroid follicles. Endocrinology 1992;131:621

35. Sztankay A, Trieb K, Lucciarini P, et al. Interferon gamma and iodide increase the inducibility of the 72kD heat shock protein in cultured human thyroid epithelial cells. J Autoimmun 1994;7:219

36. Heufelder AE, Goellner JR, Wenzel BE, Bahn RS. Immunohistochemical detection and localization of a 72-kilodalton heat shock protein in autoimmune thyroid disease. J Clin Endocrinol Metab 1991;74:724

37. Gisslinger H, Gilly B, Woloszczuk W, et al. Thyroid autoimmunity and hypothyroidism during long-term treatment with recombinant interferon-alpha. Clin Exp Immunol 1992;90:363

38. Van Liessum PA, De Mulder PHM, Mattijssen EJM, et al. Hypothyroidism and goitre during interleukin-2 therapy without LAK cells. Lancet 1989;1:224

39. Hoekman K, Von Blomberg-Van Der Flier BME, Wagstaff J, et al. Reversible thyroid dysfunction during treatment with GM-CSF. Lancet 1991;338:541

40. Nagataki S, Shibata Y, Inou S, et al. Thyroid diseases amongst atomic bomb survivors in Nagasaki. JAMA 1994;272:364

41. Germain RN. MHC-dependent antigen processing and peptide presentation: providing ligands for T lymphocyte activation. Cell 1994;76:287

42. Janeway CA, Bottomly K. Signals and signs for lymphocyte responses. Cell 1994;76:275

43. Bottazzo GF, Pujol-Borrell R, Hanafusa T, Feldmann M. Role of aberrant HLA-DR expression and antigen presentation in induction of endocrine autoimmunity. Lancet 1983;2:1115

44. Hamilton F, Black M, Farquharson MA, et al. Spatial correlation between thyroid epithelial cells expressing class II MHC molecules and interferon-gamma-containing lymphocytes in human thyroid autoimmune disease. Clin Exp Immunol 1991;83:64

45. Weetman AP, Volkman DJ, Burman KD, et al. The in vitro regulation of human thyrocyte HLA-DR antigen expression. J Clin Endocrinol Metab 1985;61:817

46. Cohen SB, Dijkstra CD, Weetman AP. Sequential analysis of experimental autoimmune thyroiditis induced by neonatal thymectomy in the Buffalo strain rat. Cell Immunol 1988;114:126

47. Weetman AP. Antigen presentation in the pathogenesis of autoimmune endocrine diseases. J Autoimmun 1995;8:305

48. Tandon N, Weetman AP. Thyroid cells in Graves' disease and Hashimoto's thyroiditis stimulate allogeneic T cells when pretreated with phorbol ester. Clin Endocrinol 1992;37:274

49. Tandon N, Metcalfe RA, Barnett D, Weetman AP. Expression of the costimulatory molecule B7/BB1 in autoimmune thyroid disease. Q J Med 1994;87:231

50. Iwatani Y, Amino N, Hidaka Y, et al. Decreases in $\alpha\beta$ T cell receptor negative T cells and CD8 cells, and an increase in CD4$^+$ CD8$^+$ cells in active Hashimoto's disease and subacute thyroiditis. Clin Exp Immunol 1992;87:444

51. Jansson R, Karlsson A, Forsum U. Intrathyroidal HLA-DR expression and T lymphocyte phenotypes in Graves' thyrotoxicosis, Hashimoto's thyroiditis and nodular colloid goitre. Clin Exp Immunol 1984;58:264

52. Aichinger G, Fill H, Wick G. In situ immune complexes, lymphocyte subpopulations, and HLA-DR positive epithelial cells in Hashimoto's thyroiditis. Lab Invest 1985;52:132

53. Moss PAH, Rosenberg WMC, Bell JI. The human T cell receptor in health and disease. Annu Rev Immunol 1992;10:71

54. Brostoff SW, Howell MD. T cell receptors, immunoregulation and autoimmunity. Clin Immunol Immunopathol 1992;62:1

55. Navarrete C, Bottazzo GF. In search of TCR restriction in autoreactive T cell in human autoimmunity: why is it so elusive? Clin Exp Immunol 1993;91:189

56. Lehmann PV, Sercarz EE, Forsthuber T, et al. Determinant spreading and the dynamics of the autoimmune T-cell repertoire. Immunol Today 1993;14:203

57. Davies TF, Martin A, Concepcion ES, et al. Evidence of limited variability of antigen receptors on intrathyroidal T cells in autoimmune thyroid disease. N Engl J Med 1991;325:238

58. Davies TF, Martin A, Concepcion ES, et al. Evidence for selective accumulation of intrathyroidal T lymphocytes in human autoimmune thyroid disease based on T cell receptor V gene usage. J Clin Invest 1992;89:157

59. Davies TF, Concepcion ES, Ben-Nun A, et al. T-cell receptor V gene use in autoimmune thyroid disease: direct assessment by thyroid aspiration. J Clin Endocrinol Metab 1993;76:660

60. McIntosh RS, Tandon N, Pickerill AP, et al. IL-2 receptor-positive intrathyroidal lymphocytes in Graves' disease: analysis of Vα transcript microheterogeneity. J Immunol 1993;151:3884

61. Matsuoka N, Unger P, Ben-Nun A, et al. Thyroglobulin-induced murine thyroiditis assessed by intrathyroidal T cell receptor sequencing. J Immunol 1994;152:2562

62. Sugihara S, Fujiwara H, Shearer GM. Autoimmune thyroiditis induced in mice depleted of particular T cell subsets. J Immunol 1993;150:683

63. Fukuma N, McLachlan SM, Rapoport B, et al. Thyroid antigens and human T cell responses. Clin Exp Immunol 1990;82:275

64. Tandon N, Freeman M, Weetman AP. T cell responses to synthetic thyroid peroxidase peptides in autoimmune thyroid disease. Clin Exp Immunol 1991;86:56

65. Dayan CM, Londei M, Corcoran AE, et al. Autoantigen recognition by thyroid-infiltrating T cells in Graves' disease. Proc Natl Acad Sci U S A 1991;88:8294

66. Ewins CL, Barnett PS, Ratanachaiyavong S, et al. Antigen-specific T cell recognition of affinity-purified and recombinant thyroid peroxidase in autoimmune thyroid disease. Clin Exp Immunol 1992;90:93

67. Mullins RJ, Chernajovsky Y, Dayan C, et al. Transfection of thyroid autoantigens into EBV-transformed B cell lines. J Immunol 1994;152:5572

68. Volpe R. Suppressor T lymphocyte dysfunction is important in the pathogenesis of autoimmune thyroid disease: a perspective. Thyroid 1993;3:345

69. Okita N, Topliss D, Lewis M, et al. T-lymphocyte sensitization in Graves' and Hashimoto's diseases confirmed by an indirect migration inhibition factor test. J Clin Endocrinol Metab 1981;52:523

70. Iitaka M, Aguayo JF, Iwatani Y, et al. Studies of the effect of suppressor T lymphocytes on the induction of antithyroid microsomal antibody-secreting cells in autoimmune thyroid disease. J Clin Endocrinol Metab 1988;66:708

71. Davies TF, Platzer M. The T cell suppressor defect in autoimmune thyroiditis: evidence for a high set "autoimmunostat." Clin Exp Immunol 1985;63:73

72. Fowell D, Mason D. Evidence that the T cell repertoire of normal rats contains cells with the potential to cause diabetes. Characterization of the CD4+ T cell subset that inhibits this autoimmune potential. J Exp Med 1993;177:627

73. Bloom BR, Salgame P, Diamond B. Revisiting and revising suppressor T cells. Immunol Today 1992;13:131

74. Weetman AP, Black CM, Cohen SB, et al. Affinity purification of IgG subclasses and the distribution of thyroid autoantibody reactivity in Hashimoto's thyroiditis. Scand J Immunol 1989;30:73

75. Chazenbalk GD, Portolano S, Russo D, et al. Human organ-specific autoimmune disease. Molecular cloning and expression of an autoantibody gene repertoire for a major autoantigen reveals an antigenic immunodominant region and restricted immunoglobulin gene usage in the target organ. J Clin Invest 1993;92:62

76. Weetman AP, McGregor AM, Wheeler MH, Hall R. Extrathyroidal sites of autoantibody synthesis in Graves' disease. Clin Exp Immunol 1984;56:330

77. Katzin WE, Fishleder AJ, Tubbs R. Investigation of the clonality of lymphocytes in Hashimoto's thyroiditis using immunoglobulin and T-cell receptor gene probes. Clin Immunol Immunopathol 1989;51:264

78. Weetman AP, Cohen SB, Oleesky DA, Morgan BP. Terminal complement complexes and C1/C1 inhibitor complexes in autoimmune thyroid disease. Clin Exp Immunol 1989;77:25

79. Chiovato L, Bassi P, Santini F, et al. Antibodies producing complement-mediated thyroid cytotoxicity in patients with atrophic or goitrous autoimmune thyroiditis. J Clin Endocrinol Metab 1993;77:1700

80. Tandon N, Yan SL, Morgan BP, Weetman AP. Expression and function of multiple regulators of complement activation in autoimmune thyroid disease. Immunology 1994;81:643

81. Weetman AP, Freeman MA, Morgan BP. Thyroid follicular cell function after non-lethal complement membrane attack. Clin Exp Immunol 1990;82:69

82. Weetman AP, Tandon N, Morgan BP. Antithyroid drugs and release of inflammatory mediators by complement-attacked thyroid cells. Lancet 1992;340:633

83. Bogner U, Kotulla P, Peters H, Schleusener H. Thyroid peroxidase/microsomal antibodies are not identical with thyroid cytotoxic antibodies in autoimmune thyroiditis. Acta Endocrinol 1990;123:431

84. Banga JP, Barnett PS, McGregor AM. Immunological and molecular characteristics of the thyroid peroxidase autoantigen. Autoimmunity 1991;8:335

85. Kosugi S, Ban T, Akamizu T, et al. Use of thyrotropin receptor (TSHR) mutants to detect stimulating TSHR antibodies in hypothyroid patients with idiopathic myxedema, who have blocking TSHR antibodies. J Clin Endocrinol Metab 1993;77:19

86. Arikawa K, Ichikawa Y, Yoshida T, et al. Blocking type antithyrotropin receptor antibody in patients with nongoitrous hypothyroidism: its incidence and characteristics of action. J Clin Endocrinol Metab 1985;60:953

87. Cho BY, Shong YK, Lee HK, et al. Inhibition of thyrotrophin-stimulated adenylate cyclase activation and growth of rat thyroid cells, FRTL-5, by immunoglobulin G from patients with primary myxedema: comparison with activities of thyrotrophin-binding inhibitor immunoglobulins. Acta Endocrinol 1989;120:99

88. Steel NR, Weightman DR, Taylor JJ, Kendall-Taylor P. Blocking activity to action of thyroid stimulating hormone in serum from patients with primary hypothyroidism. BMJ 1984;288:1559

89. Kraiem Z, Lahat N, Glaser B, et al. Thyrotropin receptor blocking antibodies: incidence, characterization and in vivo synthesis. Clin Endocrinol 1987;27:409

90. Doniach D. Hashimoto's thyroiditis and primary myxoedema viewed as separate entities. Eur J Clin Invest 1981;11:245

91. MacKenzie WA, Schwartz AE, Friedman EW, Davies TF. Intrathyroidal T cell clones from patients with autoimmune thyroid disease. J Clin Endocrinol Metab 1987;64:818

92. Del Prete GF, Vercelli D, Tiri A, et al. In vivo activated cytotoxic T cells in the thyroid infiltrate of patients with Hashimoto's thyroiditis. Clin Exp Immunol 1986;65:140

93. Del Prete GF, Tiri A, Mariotti S, et al. Enhanced production of γ-interferon by thyroid-derived T cell clones from patients with Hashimoto's thyroiditis. Clin Exp Immunol 1987;69:323

94. Grubeck-Loebenstein B, Turner M, Pirich K, et al. CD4+ T-cell clones from autoimmune thyroid tissue cannot be classified according to their lymphokine production. Scand J Immunol 1990;32:433

95. McLachlan SM, Taverne J, Atherton MC, et al. Cytokines, thyroid autoantibody synthesis and thyroid cell survival in culture. Clin Exp Immunol 1990;79:175

96. Mariotti S, Del Prete GF, Chiovato L, et al. Cytokines and thyroid autoimmunity. Int J Immunopathol Pharmacol 1992;5:103

97. Weetman AP, Cohen SB, Makgoba MW, Borysiewicz LK. Expression of an intercellular adhesion molecule, ICAM-1, by human thyroid cells. J Endocrinol 1989;122:185

98. Weetman AP, Freeman MA, Borysiewicz LK, Makgoba MW. Functional analysis of intercellular adhesion molecule-1-expressing human thyroid cells. Eur J Immunol 1990;20:271

99. Weetman AP. The potential immunological role of the thyroid cell in autoimmune thyroid disease. Thyroid 1994;4:493

100. Shigemasa C, Ueta Y, Mitani Y, et al. Chronic thyroiditis with painful tender thyroid enlargement and transient thyrotoxicosis. J Clin Endocrinol Metab 1990;70:385

101. Burch HB, Wartofsky L. Graves' ophthalmopathy: current concepts regarding pathogenesis and management. Endocr Rev 1993;14:747

102. Fatourechi V, Pajouhi M, Fransway AF. Dermopathy of Graves disease (pretibial myxedema). Review of 150 cases. Medicine 1994;73:1

103. Ikayasu I, Hara Y, Nakamura K, et al. Racial and age-related differences in incidence and severity of focal autoimmune thyroiditis. Am J Clin Pathol 1994;101:698

104. Rallison ML, Dobyns BM, Meikle AW, et al. Natural history of thyroid abnormalities: prevalence, incidence, and regression of thyroid diseases in adolescents and young adults. Am J Med 1991;91:363

105. Hegedüs L, Hansen JM, Feldt-Rasmussen U, et al. Influence of thyroxine treatment on thyroid size and anti-thyroid peroxidase antibodies in Hashimoto's thyroiditis. Clin Endocrinol 1991;35:235

106. Mariotti S, Caturegli P, Piccolo P, et al. Antithyroid peroxidase autoantibodies in thyroid diseases. J Clin Endocrinol Metab 1990;71:661

107. Rieu M, Richard A, Rosilio M, et al. Effects of thyroid status on thyroid autoimmunity expression in euthyroid and hypothyroid patients with Hashimoto's thyroiditis. Clin Endocrinol 1994;40:529

108. Takasu N, Yamada T, Takasu M, et al. Disappearance of thyrotropin-blocking antibodies and spontaneous recovery from hypothyroidism in autoimmune thyroiditis. N Engl J Med 1992;326:513

109. Okamura K, Sato K, Ikenoue H, et al. Primary hypothyroidism manifested in childhood with special reference to various types of reversible hypothyroidism. Eur J Endocrinol 1994;131:131

110. Utiger RD. Vanishing hypothyroidism. N Engl J Med 1992;326:562

111. Kasagi K, Hidaka A, Nakamura H, et al. Thyrotropin receptor antibodies in hypothyroid Graves' disease. J Clin Endocrinol Metab 1993;75:504

112. Tamai H, Kasagi K, Takaichi Y, et al. Development of spontaneous hypothyroidism in patients with Graves' disease treated with antithyroidal drugs: clinical, immunological, and histological findings in 26 patients. J Clin Endocrinol Metab 1989;69:49

113. Matsuzuka F, Miyauchi A, Katayama S, et al. Clinical aspects of primary thyroid lymphoma: diagnosis and treatment based on our experience of 119 cases. Thyroid 1993;3:93

114. McKee RF, Krukowski ZH, Matheson NA. Thyroid neoplasia coexistent with chronic lymphocytic thyroiditis. Br J Surg 1993;80:1303

115. Schwaegerle SY, Bauer TW, Esselstyn CB. Riedel's thyroiditis. Am J Clin Pathol 1988;90:715

116. Eisenbarth GS, Jackson RA. The immunoendocrinopathy syndromes. In: Wilson JD, Foster DW eds. Williams' textbook of endocrinology. 8th ed. Philadelphia: WB Saunders, 1992;1555

117. Betterle C, Presotto F, Magrin L, et al. The natural history of pretype 1 (insulin-dependent) diabetes mellitus in patients with autoimmune endocrine diseases. Diabetologia 1994;37:95

118. Kawasaki E, Takino H, Yano M, et al. Autoantibodies to glutamic acid decarboxylase in patients with IDDM and autoimmune thyroid disease. Diabetes 1994;43:80

119. Badesch DB, Wynne K, Bonvallet S, et al. Hypothyroidism and primary pulmonary hypertension: an autoimmune pathogenetic link? Ann Intern Med 1993;119:44

120. Khardori R, Eagleton LE, Soler NG, McConnachie PR. Lymphocytic interstitial pneumonitis in autoimmune thyroid disease. Am J Med 1991;90:649

121. Vailati A, Marena C, Comis S, et al. Hashimoto's thyroiditis in association with Tolosa Hunt syndrome: a case report. Thyroid 1993;3:125

122. Lammie GA, Bobrow LG, Staunton MDM, et al. Sclerosing lymphocytic lobulitis of the breast—evidence for an autoimmune pathogenesis. Histopathology 1991;19:13

Werner and Ingbar's The Thyroid, Seventh Edition,
edited by Lewis E. Braverman and Robert D. Utiger.
Lippincott–Raven Publishers, Philadelphia, © 1996

56

Hereditary Metabolic Disorders Causing Hypothyroidism

Jan J. M. de Vijlder

Thomas Vulsma

Most hereditary disorders of thyroid hormone synthesis result in hypothyroidism and, as a result of the thyroid growth-stimulating actions of the thyrotropin (TSH) secreted in response, also in goitrogenesis. Accordingly, goitrogenesis and familial occurrence of hypothyroidism were formerly the major clues to the detection of abnormalities in thyroid hormonogenesis. Now, however, in many countries most patients with these disorders are identified by neonatal screening (see chap 85). This early diagnosis, usually before the onset of clinical manifestations, raises the need for etiologic classification at a very young age, both for specific management and for genetic counseling. Thus, later progeny can be treated immediately after birth or even prenatally. Because adequate early treatment prevents excessive thyroid growth, thyroidectomy has become obsolete, making it unethical to obtain thyroid tissue for in vitro study. Furthermore, diagnostic procedures have to be adapted to the very young age of the patients. The contribution of molecular biology to classification of hereditary congenital hypothyroidism is increasing rapidly,[1,2] but for the present it is still often necessary to perform in vivo studies with radioiodine (^{123}I), together with sensitive immuno- and bioassays and thyroid imaging techniques (Table 56-1). The results provide information about the step in the pathway of thyroid hormone biosynthesis that is defective and therefore is responsible for the patient's congenital hypothyroidism, which is a requirement for detection of the causal gene mutation(s).

We now recognize that hypothyroidism can be caused by inherited defects in thyroid stimulation (TSH biosynthesis and TSH action) as well as by intrathyroidal defects in thyroid hormone synthesis. Patients with the latter, but not the former

types of defects, will gradually develop goiter if not treated soon after birth. At birth, however, infants with hereditary thyroid disorders rarely have a goiter or other conspicuous symptoms, presumably because there is substantial maternal–fetal transfer of thyroxine (T_4).[3]

The heredity of the disorders discussed in this chapter is mendelian in character and follows, with a few exceptions, an autosomal recessive pattern (see Table 56-1). For children at risk it is advisable to detect hypothyroidism even before the usual date of neonatal screening, preferably by measuring TSH and iodothyronines in cord serum, because advancing the start of treatment by a few weeks may further diminish impairment in motor and cognitive development.[4]

DEFECTS IN THYROTROPIN SYNTHESIS

Hereditary pituitary disorders limited to defects in the synthesis of TSH have been described only occasionally. Spitz and colleagues[5] described a patient with high serum concentrations of an aberrant TSH that had impaired biologic activity. This patient was euthyroid, demonstrating that diminished activation of the transducing system can be compensated completely by increased TSH secretion. Hayashizaki and coworkers[6] reported three probably related patients with congenital hypothyroidism whose TSH was totally inactive as a result of a glycine-to-arginine substitution in the so-called [cys.ala.gly.tyr.cys] region of the TSH β-subunit that is involved in the association with the α-subunit. Other patients have had a single base mutation[7] and a deletion,[8] respectively, in the gene encoding the β-subunit of

TABLE 56-1.
Etiologic Classification of Hereditary Metabolic Disorders Causing Hypothyroidism*

Diagnostic Determinant†	Serum Free T₄‡	Serum Thyroglobulin	Urinary Excretion of Low-Molecular-Weight Iodopeptides	Ultrasound or Radioiodide Imaging	Radioiodide Uptake in the Thyroid Gland§	Radioiodide Discharge‖	Saliva/Blood Ratio of Radioiodide¶	Mode of Inheritance#
TSH synthesis defect	Low	Probably (very) low	Unknown	Normal or hypoplasia	Low or very low	Unknown	Normal	Autosomal recessive
TSH hyporesponsiveness	Variable	Low or absent	Unknown	Normal or hypoplasia	Low	Absent	Normal	Autosomal recessive
Stimulating G-protein deficiency	Variable	Low	Absent	Normal	Low	Absent	Unknown	Autosomal dominant
Total iodide transport defect**	Very low	Very high	Absent	Goiter or normal	Absent	Absent	Unity	Autosomal recessive
Total iodide organification defect	Very low	Very high	Absent	Goiter or normal	High	Total	Normal	Autosomal recessive
Partial iodide organification defect	Variable	High	Low or absent	Goiter or normal	High	Partial	Normal	Autosomal recessive
Thyroglobulin synthesis defect	Variable	Low or absent	High	Goiter or normal	High or very high	Absent	Normal	Autosomal recessive or dominant
Iodotyrosine deiodinase defect	Variable	High or very high	Increased MIT and DIT	Goiter or normal	High or very high	Absent	Normal	Autosomal recessive
TSH hyperresponsiveness	High	High	Unknown	Goiter	Probably high	Unknown	Normal	Autosomal dominant
Thyroid dysgenesis	Variable	Variable	Low or absent	Dystrophic remnant	Low	Low or absent	Normal	Sporadic
Thyroid agenesis	Very low	Absent	Absent	Absent	Absent	Absent	Normal	Sporadic

*In comparison with the classification of sporadic congenital hypothyroidism.

†The hereditary thyroid disorders have in common that serum TSH concentrations are elevated, at least relative to the serum free T₄ concentration, certain subtypes of TSH synthesis defects excluded.

‡In case a newborn infant cannot produce any T₄, maternal–fetal transfer is responsible for T₄ concentrations of 2.7–5.4 µg/dL (35–70 nmol/L) in cord serum, which disappear with a half-life of 2.7–5.3 d.[3]

§In general, the radioiodide uptake is a function of the amount of thyroid tissue and the degree of stimulation by TSH. The height of the uptake is expressed in relation to the serum TSH concentration during the test.

‖Discharge of thyroidal radioiodide 1 h after intravenous administration of sodium perchlorate; < 10% is normal; 10%–20% is borderline; > 20% is abnormal. Two hours after IV injection of Na¹²⁵I (1 MBq [27 µCi] for infants younger than 1 y and 2 MBq [54 µCi] for older children), NaClO₄ is administered IV (100 mg for infants younger than 1 y, 200 mg for infants of 1–9 y, and 400 mg J for older children).

¶For neonates, a radioiodide saliva/serum ratio > 10 is normal, 3–10 is borderline, < 3 is abnormal.[16,22] The saliva/blood ratio is 1.17 times the saliva/blood ratio (95% confidence interval, 1.15–1.19).[16]

#When the full-blown disease has an autosomal recessive pattern of inheritance, some heterozygous relatives have mild abnormalities in the relevant tests.[61,62]

**Partial iodide transport defect is an ill-defined condition; if it exists, the diagnostic determinants entirely depend on the iodine intake, which varies greatly worldwide.

MIT, monoiodotyrosine; DIT, diiodotyrosine.

TSH that introduced premature termination signals. All of these patients with totally inactive TSH were severely hypothyroid.

HYPORESPONSIVENESS TO THYROTROPIN

Thyrotropin exerts its biologic activity by binding to the TSH receptor, a glycoprotein containing an extracellular domain, seven transmembrane domains, and an intracellular domain[9] (see chap 11).

Thyrotropin hyporesponsiveness was first demonstrated in *hyt/hyt* mice,[10] in which there is a single nucleotide mutation in the gene for the TSH receptor that leads to substitution of a highly conserved proline residue in the fourth transmembrane domain by leucine. A recent report described a family in which the parents had slightly high serum TSH concentrations, and their three daughters had much higher serum TSH concentrations, but all were clinically euthyroid and none had a goiter.[11] Sequencing revealed a different point mutation in each allele of the daughters' TSH receptor gene. Both mutations, one inherited from each parent, were located in the region encoding the extracellular domain of the receptor and probably decrease its affinity for TSH. The mutated paternal allele, when transfected in Cos cells, had almost no TSH-inducible activity, whereas transfaction of the mutated maternal allele caused a 10-fold reduction in activity. Cotransfection of both parental alleles indicated that a 20-fold elevation of the TSH concentration was needed to equal the activity of the transfected wild-type allele. Indeed, the daughters' serum TSH concentrations were increased to about this magnitude, indicating that residual TSH receptor activity can be activated normally by increased TSH secretion.

A different type of TSH hyporesponsiveness may be found in patients with pseudohypoparathyroidism type Ia (Albright's hereditary osteodystrophy),[12,13] a variably expressed disorder with autosomal dominant inheritance.[14] These patients have an approximately 50% reduction in the activity of the stimulatory guanine nucleotide-binding protein (Gs). In them, multiple different mutations have been found in the gene that encodes the α-subunit of Gs, on chromosome 20q13. Most of the patients have hyporesponsiveness to TSH, with slightly elevated serum TSH concentrations and low-normal or slightly decreased serum T_4 concentrations. Hypothyroidism due to this type of TSH hyporesponsiveness is usually not completely compensated. The reason is that Gs-mediated signal transduction may be reduced not only in thyroid tissue but also in the thyrotrophs, because thyrotropin-releasing hormone also acts via Gs-coupled receptors. Detection of patients with pseudohypoparathyroidism type Ia by neonatal thyroid screening has been reported,[15,16] but it is likely that most affected patients will be missed because their blood TSH and T_4 concentrations will not reach the cut-off levels used in screening programs.

DEFECTS IN IODIDE TRANSPORT

Accumulation of iodide is not confined to the thyroid gland but also occurs in the salivary glands, gastric and small intestinal mucosa, choroid plexus, ciliary body, uterus, mammary tissue, and placenta. The thyroid is unique, however, in that its ability to transport iodide is regulated by TSH. Iodide transport is mediated by membrane-bound Na^+/I^- symporter that is able to increase the intrathyroidal iodide concentration up to 10 to 100 times the concentration in the circulation. The mRNA coding for the symporter is 2.8 to 4.2 kb in size,[17] and the cDNA was recently cloned.[17a]

Hereditary defects in the thyroidal transport of iodide had been postulated[18] before patients with goiters that could not be visualized with radioiodide were described.[19,20] To date, 35 patients with a genetic defect in thyroidal iodide transport have been described.[21,22] These patients (female:male ratio of 1:0.75) originated from 21 families from all over the world. Vertical transmission has never been reported and in some cases the parents were consanguineous, making autosomal recessive inheritance most likely. The exact nature of the defect(s) is unknown, but the consequence is intrathyroidal iodine deficiency. The patients have in common gradual goiter formation, a low or very low serum T_4 concentration, absent radioiodide uptake by the thyroid, and a radioiodide saliva/blood ratio around unity (see Table 56-1). The clinical features, including the neurodevelopmental level, vary considerably, probably as a result of variation in dietary iodine intake. These patients can be treated with large doses of iodine, but therapy with T_4 is preferable.

DEFECTS IN IODINATION OF THYROGLOBULIN

Iodide transported into the thyroid gland is oxidized by hydrogen peroxide (H_2O_2) and bound to tyrosine residues in thyroglobulin (Tg). Subsequently, some of the iodotyrosine residues couple to form iodothyronine residues. Both iodination and coupling are catalyzed by thyroid peroxidase (TPO; EC 1.11.1.8) at the apical border of the thyroid follicular cells (see chap 4). Normally, iodide entering the thyroid is rapidly oxidized and bound to protein, mainly Tg, and the concentration of iodide is very low. In patients with iodination defects, little or no iodide is oxidized and bound to protein. Accumulation of iodide in the thyroid gland will continue until a steady state is reached between active influx, protein binding, and efflux, which occurs mainly by diffusion. The influx and efflux can be followed by administration of tracer amounts of radioiodide. Competitive inhibition of the (radio)iodide uptake by anions of similar molecular size and charge, such as perchlorate or thiocyanate, allows identification of the efflux of accumulated iodide into the circulation. Depending on the degree to which iodide can be organified, the defect will be partial or total. Total iodide organification defects are characterized by discharge of greater than 90% of the (radio)iodide taken up by the gland within 1 hour after administration of sodium perchlorate, which is usually given 2 hours after the radioiodide (see Table 56-1), and with complete loss of the thyroid image on the scintiscan. Partial organification defects are characterized by discharge of more than 20% of the accumulated radioiodide.

Iodide organification defects can be the result of abnormalities of TPO or the H_2O_2 generating system.[1,2,23,24] TPO abnormalities have been attributed to completely absent or diminished TPO activity, defects in its heme or substrate binding site, the presence of an inhibitor, and abnormalities in the distribution of TPO in the thyroid. Positive perchlorate discharge tests have also been reported in patients with defects in Tg, probably because of an imbalance between the amount of Tg present in the thyroid and a relatively high dietary iodine intake. This phenomenon has been recognized in a strain of Dutch goats that has a defect in Tg synthesis. Giving affected goats 1 mg iodide per day per animal (normal intake 50–100 µg/d) for 1 month resulted in a partial iodide organification defect.[25]

Because the structure of the TPO gene is known, iodide organification defects have been approached with the aid of recombinant DNA technology. The human TPO gene is located on chromosome 2p24→p25[26–28] and spans about 150 kb of DNA, divided into 17 exons.[29,30] The full length of the mRNA encoding TPO has 3048 bp.[30–32] From studies in thyroid tissue and from DNA linkage studies a number of organification defects have been related to abnormalities in the TPO gene. They are transmitted as autosomal recessive traits.[23]

In thyroid tissue from a severely hypothyroid goitrous patient, very little peroxidase activity was found and no iodinated Tg was detected. DNA studies revealed that this patient was homozygous for a GGCC insertion in exon 8 of the TPO gene that introduced a premature termination signal by a shift in the reading frame. The presence of an alternative acceptor splice site could theoretically result in synthesis of an aberrant TPO molecule that might have some residual activity.[33]

Recently, a total iodide organification defect was identified in 13 Dutch families (see Table 56-1). Thyroid tissue was available from three unrelated patients, all born in the prescreening era. Their concentrations of TPO mRNA ranged from undetectable to high as compared with values in normal thyroid tissue, but in all three patients TPO activity was undetectable and Tg was not iodinated. To search for mutations, genomic DNA was isolated from white blood cells of members of the 13 families and the TPO gene was screened by denaturating gradient gel electrophoresis and, if aberrant, subsequently sequenced.[34] Eight different mutations were detected, including the GGCC insertion described above.[33] In 2 families the patients were homozygous and in 3 other families the patients were compound heterozygous for this insertion. Figure 56-1 shows an overview of the various TPO mutations that have been found.

A remarkable variant of a partial organification defect is Pendred's syndrome, which is characterized by overt or subclinical hypothyroidism, goiter, and moderate-to-severe sensorineural hearing impairment.[35] Several hundred patients have been reported since Pendred's original report in 1896.[36,37]

Both the cause of the sensorineural hearing loss and the metabolic basis of the thyroid dyshormonogenesis are still unknown. The heredity appears to be autosomal recessive, but the expression of the defect(s) is variable. The hearing abnormality is usually bilateral, is often associated with malformation of the cochlea, and affects predominantly the higher sound frequencies. Deafness is usually detected in infancy, but may not become evident until later in childhood. Goiter is usually detected after the hearing problem, often in the second or third decade, because thyroid hormone synthesis is only mildly decreased. Not surprisingly, therefore, few patients with Pendred's syndrome are detected by neonatal thyroid screening.[16,38] On the other hand, recognition of the hearing problem at an early age provides an opportunity for early detection of thyroid dysfunction. The incidence of Pendred's syndrome is estimated to be 1 in 25,000 newborn infants, suggesting that it is the most common hereditary metabolic disorder causing hypothyroidism.[37] In general, the discharge of radioiodide after administration of perchlorate is increased (> 20%), indicating a partial organification defect. The results of measurements of TPO activities in thyroid tissue from affected patients have varied. In one family, no mutations in the TPO gene were found,[39] suggesting that if the defect is homogeneous the disorder is not caused by impairment of TPO.

DEFECTS IN THYROGLOBULIN SYNTHESIS

Thyroglobulin synthesis occurs exclusively in the thyroid gland (see reviews[1,2] and chap 5). The human Tg gene is greater than 300,000 bp in size and located on chromosome 8q24. The coding sequence of 8244 bp is divided into 42 exons, each of about 200 bp in size, except that exons 9 and 10 contain 1101 bp and 588 bp, respectively. Tg is a homodimer with subunits of 330,000 Da containing several repeated amino acid sequences and 10% carbohydrate residues.[40,41] The exceptional size of the Tg gene has made investigation of defects at the molecular level difficult.

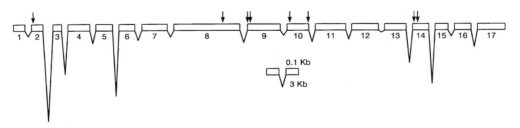

FIGURE 56-1. Mutations in the TPO gene cosegregating with total iodide organification defects.[34] The mutations were determined in the genomic DNA of patients from 13 unrelated families. Eight different mutations (indicated by ↓) were detected. Three were frame shifting mutations: one a 20 bp duplication in exon 2;[66] one a 4 bp mutation in exon 8, and the third, an insertion of a single nucleotide (C) in exon 14 (right-sided ↓). Five mutations were single nucleotide substitutions: one at the intron 8/exon 9 border; one in exon 9, causing a Tyr → Asp substitution in a highly conserved region in several peroxidases; one in exon 10 (left-sided ↓) leading to a termination codon; one at the exon 10/intron 10 border causing a Gly → Ser substitution or giving rise to alternative splicing; and one in exon 14 causing a Glu → Lys substitution in a conserved region of TPO.

Thyroglobulin synthesis defects occur in humans with an incidence of about 1 in 80,000 to 100,000 newborns.[16] Most are inherited as autosomal recessive traits, as demonstrated by restriction fragment length polymorphism (RFLP) studies, but in 1 family the mode of inheritance was proven to be autosomal dominant.[42] Affected patients are moderately to severely hypothyroid.[1,2,16] Usually, the serum Tg concentration is low, but there are exceptions, as for example a patient who had a high serum concentration of Tg of low molecular weight.[43] These patients often have abnormal iodoproteins, mainly iodinated albumin, in their serum and they excrete iodopeptides of low molecular weight in the urine.[44,45] Effective formation of T_4 and triiodothyronine (T_3) does not occur when Tg structure is abnormal, even though Tg synthesis and also iodide uptake, oxicdation and organification are increased. The result is called a coupling defect. As a consequence we do not consider defective coupling as a separate disorder (see chap 4).

Three Tg synthesis defects in humans have been elucidated at the molecular level. In one consanguineous family in which the affected patients were severely hypothyroid and had low serum Tg concentrations, exon 4 of Tg mRNA, which encodes a peptide fragment containing tyrosine 130 and one of the repeated sequences, was missing.[46] Iodinated tyrosine 130 has been proposed to be involved in iodothyronine synthesis,[47,48] while the repeated sequences may be important determinants of the quaternary structure of the Tg dimer. In another patient, a single base mutation in the Tg gene created a premature termination signal, leading to a truncated Tg molecule. However, alternative splicing could result in a formation of Tg mRNA lacking 171 nucleotides but having an intact reading frame, giving a Tg molecule missing 57 amino acid residues.[49] The third Tg synthetic defect was caused by low expression of the thyroid-specific transcription factor TTF1, which resulted in poor Tg synthesis and very low serum Tg concentrations.[49a]

Defects in Tg synthesis also have been found in cattle,[50] sheep,[51] mice,[52] goats,[53] and antelopes.[54] In all these species the mode of inheritance is autosomal recessive, based on studies of large pedigrees and by RFLP studies.[51,55,56]

In goitrous Afrikander cattle the goiter tissue contained two Tg mRNAs, one of 8.4 kb (normal size) containing a termination codon in exon 9, and one of 7.3 kb lacking exon 9 as a result of alternative splicing. Translation of goiter RNA yielded Tg polypeptides of 75,000 and 250,000 Da, suggesting that both mRNAs were translated.[57] In a strain of goitrous Dutch goats the goiter tissue contained very low concentrations of normal-size Tg mRNA.[58] In the aberrant Tg gene a point mutation in exon 8 gave rise to a termination signal. Accordingly, in vitro translation produced an N-terminal Tg polypeptide of 35,000 Da.[59] In vivo, adequate amounts of T_4, and T_3 could be produced in this Tg fragment if iodine intake was sufficiently high.[25]

DEFECTS IN IODOTYROSINE DEIODINATION

Before T_4 and T_3 are secreted into the circulation, Tg has to be taken up from the follicular lumen into the thyroid follicular cells and then hydrolyzed in the lysosomes. The hydrolysate includes monoiodotyrosine (MIT) and diiodotyrosine (DIT) in addition to T_4 and T_3. Subsequently MIT and DIT are deiodinated by specific dehalogenase(s) found not only in the thyroid but also in many peripheral tissues. Hereditary disorders in this deiodinating system lead to excessive renal loss of iodine, in the form of MIT and DIT, mimicking hypothyroidism due to iodine deficiency.[60–63]

Patients with iodotyrosine dehalogenase deficiency have a high to very high initial radioiodide uptake, followed by a relatively rapid decline of the radioiodine content. Administration of perchlorate does not result in discharge, and much of the radioiodine is in the form of radiolabeled MIT and DIT.[60] The MIT and DIT formed by hydrolysis of Tg are not deiodinated, but released into the circulation. The wasting of tyrosine-bound iodine from the thyroid, enhanced by increased TSH secretion, leads to an extremely low thyroidal iodine content.[61] Since the enzyme(s) is also deficient in peripheral tissue (especially liver and kidney), the MIT and DIT are excreted as such in the urine.

Although the inheritance must be considered as autosomal recessive, some features of the disorder are expressed in heterozygous relatives, for example, goiter, a relatively high radioiodide uptake, and increased urinary DIT excretion.[63] The clinical expression will strongly depend on the iodine content of the diet, which might explain why autosomal dominant inheritance has been suggested.[64]

DIAGNOSIS

The great majority of patients with congenital hypothyroidism detected by neonatal screening have a thyroid malformation (see chap 85). Therefore, the first step in classification should be an imaging procedure, either ultrasonography or ^{123}I scintigraphy. If the infant has a normally shaped and located thyroid gland, irrespective of its size, further studies with ^{123}I will provide information about the thyroidal uptake of iodide, the response to perchlorate, and the saliva/blood ratio of radioiodine. Measurements of serum Tg and low molecular weight iodopeptides in the urine help to discriminate between the various types of defects (see Table 56-1), and measurement of the total urinary iodine excretion helps to differentiate inborn errors from acquired, transient forms of hypothyroidism due to iodine deficiency or iodine excess. Because it is essential to treat the affected newborn infant without delay, blood and urine samples must be obtained immediately after referral. In an infant with severe hypothyroidism the radioiodide study may be done after T_4 therapy is started, so long as the patient's serum TSH concentration is high. However, if the infant has only a slightly low serum free T_4 concentration, the ^{123}I study should be performed either before the start of the treatment or several years later after interruption of T_4 therapy for at least 4 weeks. The scheme shown in Table 56-1 is helpful in identifying the most likely etiology, but absolute proof may not be obtained. A definite determination of the underlying cause depends on elucidation of the responsible mutation in the genetic code.

TREATMENT

In general, treatment of patients with hereditary defects in thyroid hormone secretion is the same as for any other hypothyroid patient of the same age and sex (see chaps 77 and

85). Irrespective of the cause of congenital hypothyroidism, early treatment is mandatory to prevent cerebral damage. Therefore, the patient should be given sufficient T_4 to maintain normal serum TSH concentrations,[65] so that not only will growth and development be normal but also goiter will be prevented. In most of the inherited disorders the thyroid will eventually become hyperplastic and nodular if serum TSH concentrations are even only slightly elevated. However, if T_4 therapy is started at a very young age, and serum TSH concentrations are maintained within the normal range, goiter should not occur. In patients who have elevated serum Tg concentrations initially, maintaining them within the normal range will help to minimize thyroid growth. In patients with TSH deficiency or Gs-deficiency, the optimal dose of T_4 must be based on determinations of the serum (free) T_4 concentration. In exceptional patients, like those with partial TSH hyporesponsiveness, hypothyroidism may be completely compensated and goiter does not occur. Yet, because establishing the correct etiologic diagnosis will take several weeks or longer, initially these patients should be treated immediately like any other infant with congenital hypothyroidism.

References

1. Dumont JE, Vassart G, Refetoff S. Thyroid disorders. In: Scriver CR, Beaudet AL, Sly WS, Valle D, eds. The metabolic basis of inherited disease. 6th ed. New York: McGraw-Hill, 1989;1843

2. DeGroot LJ. Congenital defects in thyroid hormone formation and action. In: DeGroot, LJ, ed. Endocrinology. 3rd ed. Philadelphia: WB Saunders, 1995;871

3. Vulsma T, Gons MH, de Vijlder JJM. Maternal–fetal transfer of thyroxine in congenital hypothyroidism due to a total organification defect or thyroid agenesis. N Engl J Med 1989;321:13

4. Kooistra L, Laane C, Vulsma T, Schellekens JMH, van der Meere JJ, Kalverboer AF. Motor and cognitive development in congenital hypothyroidism: a long-term evaluation of the effects of neonatal treatment. J Pediatr 1994;124:903

5. Spitz IM, Le Roith D, Hirsch H, et al. Increased high-molecular-weight thyrotropin with impaired biologic activity in a euthyroid man. N Eng J Med 1981;304:278

6. Hayashizaki Y, Hiraoka Y, Tatsumi K, et al. Deoxyribonucleic acid analyses of five families with familial inherited thyroid stimulating hormone deficiency. J Clin Endocrinol Metab 1990;71:792

7. Dacou-Voutetakis C, Feltquate DM, Drakopoulou M, et al. Familial hypothyroidism caused by a nonsense mutation in the thyroid-stimulating hormone beta-subunit gene. Am J Hum Genet 1990;46:988

8. Rajan SG, Kommareddi S, Nations M, et al. Familial hypothyroidism caused by a frameshift mutation in the thyrotropin beta-subunit gene: evidence for a bioinactive molecule. Thyroid 1992;2(Suppl 2):S68

9. Parmentier M, Libert F, Maenhaut, et al. Molecular cloning of the thyrotropin receptor. Science 1989;246:1620

10. Stein SA, Oates EL, Hall CR, et al. Identification of a point mutation in the thyrotropin receptor of the *hyt/hyt* hypothyroid mouse. Mol Endocrinol 1994;8:129

11. Sunthornthepvarakul T, Gottschalk ME, Hayashi Y, Refetoff S. Resistance to thyrotropin caused by mutations in the thyrotropin receptor gene. N Engl J Med 1995;332:155

12. Albright F, Burnett CH, Smith PH, Parson W. Pseudohypoparathyroidism an example of "Seabright-Bantam syndrome." Report of three cases. Endocrinology 1942;30:922

13. Levine MA, Schwindinger WF, Downs RW Jr, Moses AM. Pseudohypoparathyroidism. In: Bilezikian JP, Levine MA, Marcus R, eds. The parathyroids. New York: Raven Press, 1994:781

14. Davies SJ, Hughes HE. Imprinting in Albright's hereditary osteodystrophy. J Med Genet 1993;30:101

15. Levine MA, Jap T-S, Hung W. Infantile hypothyroidism in two sibs: an unusual presentation of pseudohypoparathyroidism type Ia. J Pediatr 1985;107:919

16. Vulsma T. Etiology and pathogenesis of congenital hypothyroidism (Thesis). Amsterdam, University of Amsterdam, 1991

17. Vilijn F, Carrasco N. Expression of the thyroid sodium/iodide symporter in *Xenopus laevis* oocytes. J Biol Chem 1989;264:11901

17a. Levy O, Dai G, Carrasco N. Characterisation of the sodium/iodide symporter of the thyroid gland. Thyroid 1995;5(Suppl 1):S67.

18. Stanbury JB, Querido A. Genetic and environmental factors in cretinism: a classification. J Clin Endocrinol Metab 1956;16:1522

19. Federman D, Robbins J, Rall JE. Some observations on cretinism and its treatment. N Engl J Med 1958;259:610

20. Stanbury JB, Chapman EM. Congenital hypothyroidism with goitre. Absence of an iodide-concentrating mechanism. Lancet 1960;1:1162

21. Wolff J. Congenital goiter with defective iodide transport. Endocr Rev 1983;4:240

22. Vulsma T, Rammeloo JA, Gons MH, de Vijlder JJ. The role of serum thyroglobulin concentration and thyroid ultrasound imaging in the detection of iodide transport defects in infants. Acta Endocrinol 1991;124:405

23. Medeiros-Neto GA, Billerbeck AE, Wajchenberg BL, Targovnik HM. Defective organification of iodide causing hereditary goitrous hypothyroidism. Thyroid 1993;3:143

24. Niepomniszcze H, Targovnik HM, Gluzman BE, Curutchet P. Abnormal H_2O_2 supply in the thyroid of a patient with goiter and iodine organification defect. J Clin Endocrinol Metab 1987;65:344

25. van Voorthuizen WF, de Vijlder JJ, van Dijk JE, Tegelaers WHH. Euthyroidism via iodide supplementation in hereditary congenital goiter with thyroglobulin deficiency. Endocrinology 1978;103:2105

26. Kimura S, Kotani T, McBride OW, et al. Human thyroid peroxidase: complete cDNA and protein sequence, chromosome mapping and identification of two alternately spliced mRNAs. Proc Natl Acad Sci U S A 1987;84:5555

27. de Vijlder JJ, Dinsart C, Libert F, et al. Regional localization of the gene for thyroid peroxidase to human chromosome 2pterp12. Cytogenet Cell Genet 1988;47:170

28. Barnett PS, Jones TA, McGregor AM, et al. Regional sublocalization of the human peroxidase gene (TPO) by tritium and fluorescence in situ hybridization to chromosome 2p25p24. Cytogenet Cell Genet 1993;62:88

29. Bikker H, Dinsart C, de Vijlder JJ. TPO cDNA detects a VNTR polymorphism and reveals that the TPO gene is ≤ 140 kb. Ann Endocrinol 1992;15:40

30. Kimura S, Hong YS, Kotani T, et al. Structure of the human thyroid peroxidase gene: comparison and relationship to the human myeloperoxidase gene. Biochemistry 1989;28:4481

31. Libert F, Ruel J, Ludgate M, et al. Thyroperoxidase, an autogen with a mosaic structure made of nuclear and mitochondrial gene modules. EMBO J 1987;6:4193

32. Seto P, Hirayu H, Magnusson RP, et al. Isolation of a complementary DNA clone for thyroid microsomal antigen. Homology with the gene for thyroid peroxidase. J Clin Invest 1987; 80:1205

33. Abramowicz MJ, Targovnik HM, Varela V, et al. Identification of a mutation in the coding sequence of the human thyroid peroxidase gene causing congenital goiter. J Clin Invest 1992;90:1200

34. Bikker H, Vulsma T, Baas F, de Vijlder JJ. Identification of five novel inactivating mutations in the human thyroid peroxidase

gene by denaturating gradient gel electrophoresis. Hum Mutations 1995;6:9

35. Pendred V. Deaf mutism and goitre. Lancet 1896;2:532
36. Fraser GR. Association of congenital deafness with goitre (Pendred's syndrome): a study of 207 families. Ann Hum Genet 1965;28:201
37. Deramaeker R. Congenital deafness and goiter. Am J Hum Genet 1956;8:253
38. Coakley JC, Keir EH, Connelly JF. The association of thyroid dyshormonogenesis and deafness (Pendred syndrome): experience of the Victorian Neonatal Thyroid Screening Programme. J Paediatr Child Health 1992;28:398
39. Billerbeck AEC, Cavaliere H, Goldberg AC, et al. Clinical and molecular genetics studies in Pendred's syndrome. Thyroid 1994;4:279
40. Malthiery Y, Lissitzky S. Primary structure of human thyroglobulin deduced from the sequence of its 8431-base complementary DNA. Eur J Biochem 1987;165:491
41. Mercken L, Simons MJ, Swillens S, Massaer M, Vassart G. Primary structure of bovine thyroglobulin deduced from the sequence of its 8431-base complementary DNA. Nature 1985;316:647
42. Baas F, Bikker H, van Ommen GJB, de Vijlder JJ. Unusual scarcity of restriction site polymorphism in the human thyroglobulin gene. A linkage study suggesting autosomal dominance of a defective thyroglobulin allele. Hum Genet 1984;67:301
43. Enrique J, Santelices R, Hishihara M, Schneider A. Low molecular weight thyroglobulin leading to a goiter in a 12 year old girl. J Clin Endocrinol Metab 1984;58:526
44. de Vijlder JJM, Veenboer GJM, van Dijk JE. Thyroid albumin originates from blood. Endocrinology 1992;131:578
45. Gons MH, Kok JH, Tegelaers WHH, de Vijlder JJM. Concentration of plasma thyroglobulin and urinary excretion of iodinated material in the diagnosis of thyroid disorders in congenital hypothyroidism. Acta Endocrinol 1983;104:27
46. Ieiri T, Cochaux P, Targovnik HM, et al. A 3′ splice mutation in the thyroglobulin gene responsible for congenital goiter with hypothyroidism. J Clin Invest 1991;88:1901
47. Marriq C, Lejeune PJ, Venot N, Vinet L. Hormone synthesis in human thyroglobulin: possible cleavage of the polypeptide chain at the tyrosine donor site. FEBS Lett 1989;242:414
48. Den Hartog MT, Sijmons CC, Bakker O, Ris-Stalpers C, de Vijlder JJ. Importance of the content and localization of tyrosine residues for thyroxine formation within the N-terminal part of human thyroglobulin. Eur J Endocrinol 1995;132:611
49. Targovnik HM, Medeiros-Neto G, Varela V, Cochaux P, Wajchenberg BL. A nonsense mutation causes human hereditary congenital goiter with preferential production of a 171 nt-deleted thyroglobulin RNA messenger. J Clin Endocrinol Metab 1993;77:210
49a. Acebron A, Aza-Blanc P, Rossi DL, Lamas L, Santisteban P. Congenital human thyroglobulin defect due to low expression of the thyroid-specific transcription factor. J Clin Invest 1995;96:781

50. Ricketts MH, Simons MJ, Parma J, et al. A nonsense mutation caused hereditary goitre in the Afrikander cattle and unmasks alternative splicing of thyroglobulin transcripts. Proc Natl Acad Sci U S A 1987;165:491
51. Mayo GME, Mulhearn CJ. Inheritance of congenital goitre due to a thyroid defect in Merino sheep. Aust J Agric Res 1969; 20:533
52. Beamer WG, Maltais LJ, De Baets MH, Eicher EM. Inherited congenital goiter in mice. Endocrinology 1987;120:838
53. Veenboer GJM, de Vijlder. Molecular bases of the thyroglobulin synthesis defect in Dutch goats. Endocrinology 1993;132:377
54. Doi S, Shifrin S, Santisteban P, et al. Familial goiter in bongo antelope (*Tragelaphus eurycerus*). Endocrinology 1990;127:857
55. Ricketts MH, Schultz K, van Zyl, A et al. Autosomal recessive inheritance of congenital goiter in Afrikander cattle. J Hered 1985;76:12
56. Kok K, van Dijk JE, Sterk A, et al. Autosomal recessive inheritance of goiter in Dutch goats. J Hered 1987;78:298
57. Tassi VNP, Di Lauro R, Van Jaarsveld P, Alvino CG. Two abnormal thyroglobulin-like polypeptides are produced from Afrikander cattle congenital goiter mRNA. J Biol Chem 1984; 259:10507
58. Van Voorthuizen WF, Dinsart C, Flavell RA, et al. Abnormal cellular localization of thyroglobulin mRNA associated with hereditary congenital goiter and thyroglobulin deficiency. Proc Natl Acad Sci U S A 1978;75:74
59. Sterk A, Van Dijk JE, Veenboer GJM, et al. Normal sized thyroglobulin mRNA in Dutch goats with a thyroglobulin synthesis defect is translated into a 35,000 molecular weight N-terminal fragment. Endocrinology 1989;124:477
60. Stanbury JB, Kassenaar AAH, Meijer JWA, Terpstra J. The occurrence of mono- and di-iodotyrosine in the blood of a patient with congenital goiter. J Clin Endocrinol Metab 1955;15:1216
61. Choufour JC, Kassenaar AAH, Querido A. The syndrome of congenital hypothyroidism with defective dehalogenation of iodotyrosines. Further observations and a discussion of the pathophysiology. J Clin Endocrinol Metab 1960;20:983
62. Hutchison JH, McGirr EM. Hypothyroidism as an inborn error of metabolism. J Clin Endocrinol Metab 1954;14:869
63. McGirr EM, Hutchison JH, Clement WE. Sporadic goitrous cretinism. Dehalogenase deficiency in the thyroid gland of a goitrous cretin and in heterozygous carriers. Lancet 1959;2:823
64. Ismail-Beigi F, Rahimifar M. A variant of iodotyrosine-dehalogenase deficiency. J Clin Endocrinol Metab 1977;44:499
65. Alemzadeh R, Friedman S, Fort P, et al. Is there compensated hypothyroidism in infancy? Pediatrics 1992;90:207
66. Bikker H, den Hartog MT, Baas F, Gons MH, Vulsma T, de Vijlder JJ. A 20 basepair duplication in the human thyroid peroxidase gene results in a total iodide organification defect and congenital hypothyroidism. J Clin Endocrinol Metab 1994;79:248

Werner and Ingbar's The Thyroid, Seventh Edition,
edited by Lewis E. Braverman and Robert D. Utiger.
Lippincott–Raven Publishers, Philadelphia, © 1996

57

Endemic Cretinism

François M. Delange

In severe endemic goiter, an abnormally high number of individuals exhibit irreversible anomalies of intellectual and physical development. These anomalies are extremely polymorphous and have been grouped under the general heading of endemic cretinism. The prevalence of the disease may reach 5% to 15% of the population. It is by far the most serious complication of endemic goiter and represents a veritable scourge, both medically and socially.[1–3]

The pathogenesis of endemic cretinism is only partly understood and information on its pathology is scanty.[4–6] For these reasons, the diagnosis of the condition is mostly descriptive and made on epidemiologic grounds. In 1986, a study group of the Pan American Health Organization (PAHO) formulated the following definition of endemic cretinism[7]:

> The condition of endemic cretinism is defined by three major features:
>
> A. Epidemiology. It is associated with endemic goiter and severe iodine deficiency.
> B. Clinical manifestations. These comprise mental deficiency, together with either:
>   1. A predominant neurological syndrome including defects of hearing and speech and characteristic disorders of stance and gait of varying degree; or
>   2. Predominant hypothyroidism and stunted growth.
>   Although in some regions one of the two types may predominate, in other areas a mixture of the two syndromes will occur.
> C. Prevention. In areas where adequate correction of iodine deficiency has been achieved, endemic cretinism has been prevented.

This chapter summarizes the current knowledge on the epidemiology and clinical manifestations, laboratory data, pathogenesis, therapy, and prevention of endemic cretinism. A comprehensive bibliography, including the historical aspects, is available in more extensive reviews on the topic.[1–6,8–12]

EPIDEMIOLOGY, CLINICAL MANIFESTATIONS, AND LABORATORY DATA

The clinical manifestations of endemic cretinism summarized in the PAHO definition correspond to the two extreme types of endemic cretinism initially defined in the pioneer work of McCarrison in 1908[13] in the Himalayas and subsequently reported in the studies of endemic goiter and cretinism carried out in other parts of the world, namely New Guinea[14,15] and Zaire[16–23]: the first type is marked by dominant neurological disorders (neurologic cretinism) and the second by symptoms of severe thyroid insufficiency (myxedematous cretinism).

Figure 57-1 illustrates the typical picture of neurologic cretinism as seen in New Guinea[14,15]: the cretins in this endemia are extremely mentally retarded and most of them are reduced to a vegetative existence. Almost all are deaf-mutes and are afflicted with the following neurologic defects: (1) impaired voluntary motor activity, usually involving paresis or paralysis of pyramidal origin, chiefly in the lower limbs, with hypertonia and clonus and plantar cutaneous reflexes in extension; extrapyramidal signs are occasional; (2) spastic or ataxic gait; walking or even standing is impossible in the severest cases; and (3) strabismus.

The prevalence of goiter in neurologic cretins is as high as in the noncretin population of the area and they are clinically euthyroid. Thyroid function is usually normal,[14,15] but subclinical hypothyroidism with elevated basal TSH or exaggerated TSH response to TRH may occur.[24,25]

Figure 57-2 shows the clinical aspects of myxedematous endemic cretinism as most typically seen in Zaire.[3,8,16–23] These cretins show less mental retardation than the neurologic cretins; they are often capable of performing simple manual tasks. All exhibit major clinical symptoms of long-standing hypothyroidism: dwarfism, myxedema, dry skin, sparseness of

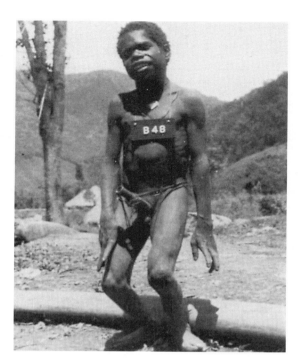

FIGURE 57-1. Fourteen-year-old boy with neurologic endemic cretinism in Mulia Valley, Western New Guinea. The boy has severe mental retardation, deaf-mutism, spastic diplegia, and strabismus. There are no clinical signs of hypothyroidism. (Photograph courtesy of Professor A. Querido, Leiden)

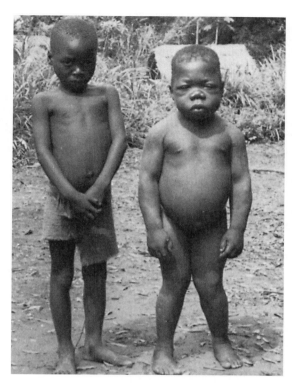

FIGURE 57-2. Myxedematous endemic cretinism in children in Ubangi, Northwestern Zaire. On the left, a clinical euthyroid 6-year-old girl with a height of 105 cm (50th percentile for age for the local population). On the right, a 17-year-old girl with a height of 100 cm, severe mental retardation, myxedema, markedly delayed puberty, flat and broad nose, hypoplastic mandible, dry and scaly skin, dry and brittle hair, and prominent abdomen. Pseudomuscular hypertrophy, muscular weakness, flat feet, and genu valgum are present; no deaf-mutism. The thyroid gland was not palpable. The 17-year-old had a serum concentration of TSH of 288 µU/mL, T_4 of 1.29 nmol/L, and T_3 of 0.153 nmol/L.

hair and nails, retarded sexual development, and retarded maturation of body proportions and of nasoorbital configuration. The initial reports from Zaire indicated that myxedematous cretins occasionally exhibited neurologic signs including spasticity of the lower limbs, jerky movements, Babinski's sign, and shifting gait.

The prevalence of goiter in the myxedematous cretins is much lower than in the noncretin population. Many of them have nonpalpable thyroid tissue, although thyroid scintigrams show small residues of thyroid tissue located in the normal position,[18,23] precluding thyroid dysgenesis (agenesis, ectopic thyroid) as the cause of hypothyroidism.

The clinical diagnosis of hypothyroidism in myxedematous cretins is confirmed by a biochemical picture of thyroid failure with almost undetectable serum concentrations of thyroxine (T_4) and triiodothyronine (T_3) and extremely elevated serum levels of thyrotropin (TSH) (Table 57-1). The iodine pool of the thyroid is drastically reduced, and a particularly fast turnover rate of iodine is indicated by elevated serum radiolabeled protein-bound iodine (PB[131]I). The diagnosis of severe and long-standing hypothyroidism is further confirmed by a very significant retardation in bone maturation; epiphyseal dysgenesis, which indicates hypothyroidism of perinatal onset; and characteristic changes in the electrocardiogram.[23]

The review of the world literature on endemic cretinism up to the late 1970s indicated that the frequency distribution of the two extreme types of endemic cretinism varied markedly from one endemic area to another. In most areas the neurologic type predominated, but in some, especially in

Zaire, myxedematous endemic cretinism was most frequently encountered. The reasons for these geographic variations in the epidemiologic pattern of endemic cretinism were unknown. It was also agreed that, between the two extreme types of cretinism, there were a number of mixed forms characterized by dominant neurologic disorders or dominant hypothyroidism in the same individual.[9,14–23,26–36]

It was consequently considered that neurologic and myxedematous endemic cretinism, in fact, constituted the extreme aspects of a continuous spectrum of developmental abnormalities made up of numerous intermediate forms.[8,9,37] A similar variability in the geographic pattern of endemic cretinism has been reported from China: neurologic cretinism has been found in almost all the cretin endemias of China; the myxedematous type was seen less frequently and principally in northwestern China.[38–40]

The results of subsequent detailed studies of cretinism in Ecuador,[41–43] China,[44–47] and Indonesia[48] vigorously challenged this concept of a continuous spectrum of developmental abnormalities in endemic cretinism. In studies in China and Indonesia, Halpern and colleagues reported an identical pattern of intensity of neurologic, intellectual, and audiometric deficits in all cretins examined, regardless of type (myxedematous or

TABLE 57-1.
Thyroid Function Tests: Clinical and Radiologic Data in Hypothyroid Endemic Cretins in Zaire, China, and Indonesia*

Variables	Belgian controls (N = 12–255)	Noncretin Iodine-deficient Adults (Zaire) (N = 30–358)	Hypothyroid Endemic Cretins		
			ZAIRE: IDJWI-UBANGI (N = 6–120)	CHINA: QINGHAI (N = 25)	INDONESIA: BANDUNG (N = 3)
Thyroid function tests					
Serum concentration of:					
T_4 (nmol/l)	104.2 ± 1.3	63.1 ± 2.6	6.4 ± 0.1	53.9 ± 7.1	
FT_4 (pmol/l)				8.4 ± 1.3	11.2
T_3 (nmol/l)	2.21 ± 0.05	2.55 ± 0.04	0.70 ± 0.05	2.1 ± 0.2	
TSH (μU/ml)	1.7 ± 0.1	18.6 ± 2.1	303 ± 20	123.8 ± 23.0	40.1
Protein bound ^{131}I (% dose/l)	0.06 ± 0.01	0.17 ± 0.02	1.09 ± 0.18		
24-h ^{131}I thyroid uptake (% dose)	46.4 ± 1.1	65.2 ± 0.9	28.3 ± 2.6		
Thyroid organic iodine pool (mg)	15.8 ± 3.5	1.60 ± 0.3	0.01 – 0.1		
Clinical and radiologic data					
Age (yr)			16.8	31.6	33.3
Clinical myxedema (%)			100	54	
Height (cm)			103	131	144
Bone maturation (yr)			2.8	26.2	
Epiphyseal dysgenesis			+++	±	±
Mental development versus euthyroid cretins			Higher	Equal	Equal

*Values recorded as mean ± SEM. The number of patients is shown in brackets.
Data are from references 18, 20, 44, 48, 107, 108, and 118.

neurologic) and current thyroid function.[44,48] The neurologic aspects of both euthyroid and hypothyroid cretins were polymorphous and varied widely from one subject to another. In the 139 subjects investigated in China and Indonesia, Halpern and coworkers[48] reported significant pyramidal dysfunction in a proximal distribution and exaggeration of the tendon reflexes, which were more commonly encountered in the lower limbs than in the upper. The posture was typical with hips and knees flexed and the trunk tilted forward. The gait was broad-based and knock-kneed. The arms were held with the shoulders abducted and the elbows flexed. These signs indicated extrapyramidal features. All of the subjects had severe intellectual impairment with a mean IQ of about 29%. About half the patients had impaired hearing and nearly one-third had a squint. Musculoskeletal abnormalities were common and predominantly involved the weight-bearing joints with excessive laxity of the hips, feet, and ankles. There were no signs of cerebellar dysfunction.

In another study, in an attempt to better define the underlying pathology in the nervous system causing the functional deficits and to determine the developmental timing of the critical neurologic events, Delong and colleagues[47] identified five patterns of neurologic involvement in these defective subjects:

1. "Typical" pattern with hearing and speech deficit, proximal spastic rigid motor disorder, and mental retardation
2. "Thalamic" posturing with undermost limbs extended and uppermost limbs flexed, together with severe mental retardation; marked microcephaly; inability to sit, stand, or walk; and primitive facial reflexes including a marked suck or rooting reflex elicited by bringing an object into the visual field near the face
3. An autistic pattern with severe mental deficiency aggravated by deaf-mutism and an almost total disregard of the surroundings and absence of purposeful activity
4. A cerebellar pattern with marked abnormalities in standing, walking, and sitting; hypotonic truncal tone, tremor, and dysmetria that are typical of cerebellar dysfunction
5. A hypotonic pattern with marked truncal hypotonia and delayed sitting, standing, and walking

The hypothesis was proposed that the typical pattern may represent an insult during the third trimester of pregnancy; that the severe thalamic form may represent a longer period of insult, including the second trimester; that the cerebellar form may result from a postnatal insult; and that the autistic form may depend on a severe insult to the cerebral cortex as well as the hippocampus, both pre- and postnatally.

In contrast to the exhaustive clinical descriptions of the nervous system defects in cretins and the diversity and severity of these deficits, information on brain pathology is scant and does not elucidate entirely the anatomic locations of the injury. Computed tomographic (CT) scans of cretins from Ecuador demonstrated widespread atrophy that included the cerebral cortex and subcortical structures of the brainstem, with corresponding enlargement of the basal cisternae, the lateral ventricles, and the sulci over the surface of the cerebral cortex.[49] Basal ganglia calcifications and cerebral atrophy were occasionally observed by Halpern and colleagues,[48] but there was no correlation between the CT scan abnormalities and the clinical signs. Magnetic resonance imaging in three cretins from China overall appeared remarkably normal.[47]

On the basis of the observations performed in China and Indonesia, the concept was proposed that all cretins, including the so-called myxedematous form, belong to the neurologic type.[44,48] The reason for the discrepancy between this concept and that of a spectrum between two extreme types is unclear. One possible explanation could be an underevaluation or misinterpretation of the neurologic signs in myxedematous cretins in Zaire by the different Belgian and Zairian teams which investigated the Uele, Idjwi Island, and Ubangi areas during the past 30 years.[16–23] If so, the same mistakes were also done by the team from Washington, which recently again investigated the Uele area and obtained exactly the same epidemiologic findings.[50] It has to be recognized that at least some of the neurologic signs found in the myxedematous cretins of Zaire, including flat feet, knock-knees, hyperreflexia, ataxia, strabismus, nystagmus, and hearing defects have been occasionally reported in the past in unrecognized and consequently untreated children with sporadic congenital hypothyroidism.[51]

Another possible explanation of the difference between the two concepts could be that the term "myxedematous cretinism" has been applied in China to patients with predominantly neurologic cretinism and postnatally acquired hypothyroidism with a biochemical picture of moderate impairment of thyroid function, similar to that found in neurologic cretinism in other parts of the world and in noncretin, severely iodine-deficient adults (Table 57-1). There is no doubt that the degree of hypothyroidism reported in the hypothyroid cretins in China and Indonesia is usually milder than the severe degree of hypothyroidism observed in Africa. The difference in severity is reflected by the results obtained from the biochemical tests and could explain that retardation in height and especially in bone maturation is much less marked in hypothyroid cretins in China than in Zaire, where hypothyroidism is of perinatal onset, and that only half of the myxedematous cretins in China are clinically myxedematous whereas, by definition, all of them are in Zaire.

The most probable explanation for the discrepancy between the two concepts, however, is that, although severe iodine deficiency is a common cause of all types of cretinism, additional causes, varying from place to place, may modulate the clinical expression of the disorder (see section on etiology). Further discussion of the neurologic effects of endemic iodine deficiency is given in chapter 67.

ENDEMIC MENTAL RETARDATION IN SEVERE ENDEMIC GOITER

The statement that "feeble mindedness, apart of cretinism, arises distinctly in areas of endemic goiter"[52] has been rather difficult to appreciate on an objective basis, in particular because of major technical limitations in the assessment of intelligence in preindustrialized societies.[6,53]

Table 57-2 summarizes the data available in the literature on the neuromotor and intellectual development in noncretinous individuals in areas with severe endemic goiter and cretinism. The same tests, optimally with no or as little as possible "cultural bias," were administered to two groups of noncretinous individuals living in the same environmental conditions except for the goitrogenic factors: a test group was exposed to these factors while a control group either was given iodine prophylaxis or had never been exposed to these factors. Table 57-2 indicates that in severe endemic goiter, neuromotor and intellectual deficits are frequently observed in individuals who do not present any of the other signs of endemic cretinism.

Thus, endemic cretinism only constitutes the extreme expression of a spectrum of abnormalities in physical and intellectual development and in the functional capacities of the thyroid gland observed in the inhabitants of severe endemic goiter areas.

ETIOLOGY

Iodine Deficiency

Iodine deficiency is fundamental in the etiology of endemic cretinism. This conclusion rests on (1) the correlation between the degree of iodine deficiency and the frequency of cretinism[3,9,12]; (2) the prophylactic action of iodine on the incidence of cretinism (see section on prevention); and (3) the emergence of cretinism in previously unaffected populations as a consequence of iodine deficiency of recent onset, as observed in the Jimi valley in New Guinea after replacement of natural rock salt rich in iodine with low-iodine industrial salt.[54]

In addition, iodine deficiency during gestation in animals results in thyroid deficiency in the offspring. All of the models used mimic the myxedematous type of cretinism; none was able to reproduce the neurologic type.[55–57]

Naturally Occurring Goitrogens

The additional role played by naturally occurring goitrogens (see chap 14) in the etiology of endemic cretinism has been established for a cyanogenic glucoside (linamarin) present in cassava, a staple food in many tropical areas.[19,20] Linamarin yields cyanide on hydrolysis. This is metabolized to thiocyanate (SCN), which is well known for its goitrogenic effects. The role of SCN in the etiology of endemic cretinism in Africa has been proposed from the observation that people in areas with severe but uniform iodine deficiency exhibit cretinism only when a certain critical threshold in the dietary supply of SCN is reached.[58] It has been shown experimentally in the rat that SCN affects the development of the central nervous system during fetal life.[20] The action of SCN is entirely due to an aggravation of iodine deficiency resulting in fetal hypothyroidism.

Thyroid Autoimmunity

Boyages and colleagues[59] showed that purified IgG fractions of serum from patients with myxedematous endemic cretinism inhibited thyrotropin-induced DNA synthesis and, conse-

TABLE 57-2.
Intellectual, Cognitive, and Neurologic Deficits in Noncretins in Severe Endemic Goiter Regions

Regions	Tests	Findings	References
Ecuador	Goodenough Draw-A-Man Stanford-Binet Gesell Leiter Bender-Gestalt	Low DQ, IQ, and visual–motor performances	53, 115, 119–121
Bolivia	Stanford-Binet Bender Gestalt	Low IQ and visual–motor performances	122
Chile	Wechsler Bender Kopitz	Low IQ	123
Papua–New Guinea	Motor performances	Low motor skill	82, 124, 125
Zaire	Brunet-Lezine	Low DQ	126
Java–Spain	Locally adapted "culture-free" intelligence tests Wechsler Catell Raven Ozeretsky	Low IQ Low perceptual and neuromotor abilities	127
China	Griffith Hiskey-Nebraska	Low IQ; relationship between IQ and nerve deafness and abnormal neurologic signs	48, 128, 129
India	Bhatia Malin Bender-Gestalt	Low IQ	130

quently, thyroid growth in guinea pig thyroid segments in a sensitive cytochemical assay. In contrast, no growth-blocking effect was observed with IgG fractions from euthyroid subjects or neurologic cretins from the same area. It was concluded that the IgG fractions identified specifically in myxedematous cretinism were responsible for the condition because they inhibited thyroid growth. These IgG fractions, often called *thyroid growth-blocking immunoglobulins* (TGBI), are similar to the ones found by the same authors in sporadic congenital hypothyroidism.[60] The antigenic stimulus is unknown, nor is the timing of appearance in action of these IgG fractions in the course of pregnancy and fetal or postnatal life. Serum TGBI were also identified using the FRTL-5 system in cretins in Brazil with atrophic thyroids.[61] However, TGBI could not be found in sporadic congenital hypothyroidism or myxedematous endemic cretinism in Peru and Italy by other authors[62,63,63a] so that, consequently, the possible role of thyroid autoimmunity in the etiology of endemic cretinism remains controversial.

Trace Elements

One stimulating new concept in the etiology of both myxedematous and neurologic endemic cretinism is the role of combined iodine and selenium deficiencies.[64–66] In Zaire, myxedematous cretinism is found only in severely iodine-deficient areas, which are also deficient in selenium.[67,68] Selenium is present in high concentrations (0.72 $\mu g/g$) in the normal thyroid.[69] It is present in glutathione peroxidase (GPX) and super-

oxide dismutase, the enzymes of the thyroid responsible for the detoxification of toxic derivates of oxygen (H_2O_2 and perhaps O_2-).[70] It is also present in the type I iodothyronine 5'-deiodinase responsible for the peripheral conversion of T_4 to T_3.[71]

The following scheme has been proposed to explain the frequency of myxedematous cretinism and the relative rarity of neurologic cretinism in areas such as Zaire where both iodine and selenium are deficient[64–68] (Fig 57-3): Iodine deficiency results in hyperstimulation of the thyroid by TSH and consequently in increased production of H_2O_2 within the cells. Selenium deficiency results in GPX deficit and consequently in accumulation of H_2O_2. Excess H_2O_2 could induce thyroid cell destruction and finally thyroid fibrosis, resulting in myxedematous cretinism. The recent observation that the necrotizing effect of a high dose of iodide on the thyroid cells is much greater in selenium-deficient than in selenium-supplemented rats is consistent with this hypothesis, suggesting that the selenium-deficient thyroid gland is more sensitive to oxidative stress.[72]

On the other hand, deficiency in the selenoenzyme iodothyronine 5'-deiodinase in pregnant mothers induced by selenium deficiency causes decreased catabolism of T_4 to T_3 and thus increased availability of maternal T_4 for the fetus and its brain. This mechanism could prevent the development of neurologic cretinism. Combined iodine and selenium deficiencies in Zaire could thus explain the large predominance of the myxedematous type of endemic cretinism, rather than the neurologic type, as seen typically in this area.

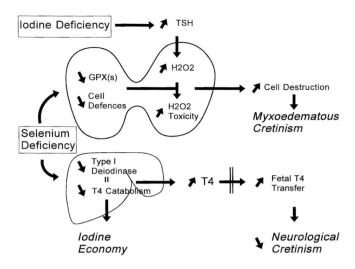

FIGURE 57-3. Effects of selenium deficiency on thyroid function and thyroxine metabolism in the presence of severe iodine deficiency. GPX, gluatathione peroxidase. (From Contempré B, et al. Interaction between two trace elements: selenium and iodine. Implications of both deficiencies. In: Stanbury JB, ed. The damaged brain and iodine deficiency. New York: Cognizant Communication, 1994:133)

PATHOGENESIS

Endemic cretinism results from an insufficient supply of thyroid hormones to the developing brain. The concept that these hormones are supplied only by the fetal thyroid[73] is now challenged by a series of experimental and clinical data and it is accepted that thyroid hormones of maternal origin contribute.[74,75] Thyroid hormone receptors have been detected in the human brain by 9 weeks of pregnancy,[76] and thyroid hormones are available to the embryo at least from the second trimester of pregnancy.[74] The fetal thyroid gland is believed to actively secrete thyroid hormones only from 20 to 22 weeks of gestation.[77] Before that time, the contribution of maternal thyroid hormones to the fetus could be important.[74]

Maternal and Fetal Hypothyroidism Before Efficient Fetal Thyroid Function (20 Weeks)

Despite the independence of maternal and fetal hypothalamus-pituitary-thyroid feedback mechanisms in physiologic conditions,[73] the possibility arises that in severe endemic goiter, maternal thyroid status could be involved in the development and in the thyroid function of the fetus. Maternal hypothyroxinemia is rare in nonendemic areas and can result in impaired neurointellectual development in the offspring.[5,78,79] In contrast, maternal hypothyroxinemia is extremely frequent in endemic areas.[80–84] It is associated with increased mortality and morbidity in offspring[83–86] and increased incidence of hypothyroidism in neonates.[80,87,88] In addition, data collected in rats showed that maternal hypothyroxinemia results in lack of thyroid hormones in fetal tissues during early pregnancy, even before the onset of fetal thyroid function, and also later during fetal development

when maternal hypothyroxinemia is due to iodine deficiency.[89–92] These data indicate that in rats, there is a substantial transfer of thyroid hormones from mother to fetus during early gestation, which plays a role in fetal development, especially of the brain. In humans, the classic concept that there is no or only minimal transfer[73,93] has been recently challenged by the observation that infants born without any thyroid (thyroid agenesis) or with nonfunctioning thyroids (dyshormonogenesis) still have detectable but low serum concentrations of thyroid hormones at birth (cord blood), which rapidly decrease thereafter.[94,95]

A unifying concept has been proposed that the neurologic defect present in all cretins is due to maternal or fetal hypothyroxinemia.[48] This would account for the picture of cretinism as found in China and Indonesia. In Africa, as indicated earlier, brain damage during early fetal life could be mitigated by concomitant selenium deficiency, which impairs peripheral conversion of T_4 to T_3 and consequently increases the availability of the prohormone T_4 to the fetal brain.

Fetal and Neonatal Hypothyroidism After Onset of Active Fetal Thyroid Function

Even a moderate degree of iodine deficiency during pregnancy, as seen in Western Europe, can be accompanied by indices of hyperstimulation of the thyroid in the neonate, as indicated by elevated serum levels of TSH and thyroglobulin (Tg) and by a slight enlargement of the thyroid. These anomalies are prevented by the daily administration of a physiologic dose of iodide to the pregnant woman throughout pregnancy.[96] This is an indication of the particular sensitivity of the neonatal thyroid to the effects of iodine deficiency.

Several observations clearly demonstrate that myxedematous endemic cretinism results from severe thyroid failure occurring during late fetal or early postnatal life. Chinese data have indicated that hypothyroidism is present in human fetuses from the fourth month of gestation in regions of severe iodine deficiency and myxedematous endemic cretinism.[97] Thyroid failure at birth due to iodine deficiency occurs in several endemic areas with myxedematous endemic cretinism such as Zaire,[87,88] India,[98] Algeria,[99] and even in some parts of Europe such as Sicily.[100] The most dramatic picture of neonatal hypothyroidism has been reported from Zaire (Fig 57-4) where the frequency of myxedematous endemic cretinism is the highest: in this area, about 10% of unselected newborns and young infants aged 1 to 24 months have both serum TSH above 100 μU/mL and T_4 below 40 nmol/L[80,88,101]—that is, a biochemical picture characteristic of congenital hypothyroidism in Western countries.[102,103] About 10% of infants aged less than 12 months are clinically hypothyroid, and nearly half have a marked delay in bone maturation, which is directly correlated to serum TSH and inversely correlated to serum T_4.[87] Finally, correction of iodine deficiency in pregnant women by injections of iodized oil results in a complete normalization of the biochemical and radiologic indices in newborns and infants.[87,88,104]

The presence of epiphyseal dysgenesis in x-ray studies of the knees (see Fig 57-4B) of some adult myxedematous endemic cretins with clinical, biochemical, and radiologic signs of long-standing hypothyroidism suggests that hypothyroidism

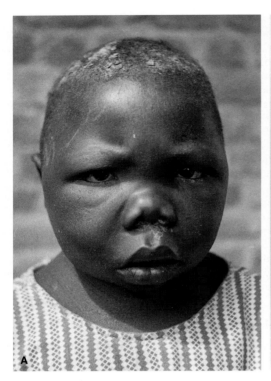

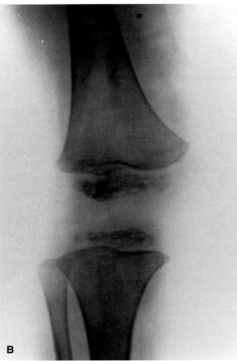

FIGURE 57-4. (*A*) Clinical appearance and (*B*) knee x-ray film of a 17-year-old myxedematous cretin of Idjwi Island, Zaire, with a height of 87.5 cm (56% of normal for the local population) and a serum protein-bound iodine (PBI) of 1.0 μg/dL. Bone maturation is estimated at 2 to 5 years; the x-ray film shows failure of modelling, and tibial and femoral epiphyseal dysgenesis. The immaturity of the naso-orbital configuration, the mandibular hypoplasia, and the epiphyseal dysgenesis indicate hypothyroidism of pre- or perinatal onset.

was present before or around birth[105]; this provides indirect evidence of perinatal hypothyroidism (see Fig. 57-3). Also, the direct correlations observed in these cretins between mental retardation and both height retardation and retardation in bone maturation indicate that hypothyroidism present in early life could account for the mental deficiency of these dwarfs.[17]

In some young infants in the Ubangi area in Zaire, the biochemical signs of thyroid failure disappeared spontaneously within 6 to 10 weeks of life.[106] The hypothesis has been proposed that permanent thyroid failure from birth results in myxedematous endemic cretinism, whereas transient hypothyroxinemia occurring during the critical period of brain development could at least partly explain the endemic mental retardation observed in this population.[107]

The cause of fetal hypothyroidism in Zaire is most likely the combined action of iodine deficiency and thiocyanate (SCN) overload. The latter results from the chronic consumption of cassava, which aggravates the effects of iodine deficiency.[19,20] SCN freely crosses the placenta[93] and its concentration in cord blood is three times higher in Ubangi than in Brussels.[80] The role played by this SCN overload in the impairment of thyroid function of the newborn is strongly suggested by the observation that, in severely iodine-deficient pregnant women, elevated urinary SCN values are accompanied by a further increase of TSH and decrease of T_4 levels in cord blood.[80] The hypersensitivity of the newborn to the antithyroid action of SCN probably results from the fact that this ion interferes with the trapping of iodide by the placenta and by the thyroid gland of the newborn. These two factors probably critically reduce the buildup of iodine stores within the thyroid gland during fetal and early postnatal life.

This mechanism is consistent with the very low iodine content of the thyroid gland reported in myxedematous cretins[108] (see Table 57-1).

As discussed earlier (in the section on etiology), selenium deficiency could further aggravate thyroid failure during the late-fetal and neonatal periods by damaging the hyperstimulated gland through the accumulation of H_2O_2 derivatives. This process, called *exhaustion atrophy*, would explain the usual absence of goiter or even of palpable thyroid tissue in the myxedematous cretins in Zaire. Another possible but controversial mechanism of thyroid damage is the action of TGBI.

In addition, iodine deficiency can induce thyroid failure at any time, including after brain development, resulting in infantile hypothyroidism without the irreversible brain damage characteristic of cretinism.[109,110]

This unifying view on the pathogenesis of endemic cretinism would account for the differences in the epidemiologic and clinical aspects of cretinism seen around the world: in all cases, iodine deficiency is a prerequisite. When present during early gestation before onset of fetal thyroid function, it would account for the neurologic aspects of cretinism caused by maternal and fetal hypothyroxinemia. Additional selenium deficiency could mitigate the neurologic picture by increasing the availability of the prohormone T_4 to the developing brain. Severe iodine deficiency aggravated by SCN overload occurring during late pregnancy, after the onset of active fetal thyroid function, would account for the myxedematous component of cretinism. Additionally, selenium deficiency could induce irreversible damage of the thyroid.

It thus appears that the particular situation reported in Zaire of less neurologic damage and severe thyroid failure could be explained by a combination of severe degrees of iodine and selenium deficiencies complicated by SCN overload. The damaging consequences of these three conditions can be prevented by the correction of iodine deficiency in the pregnant mother.

THERAPY

There is no specific therapy for neurologic endemic cretinism. These patients need rehabilitation as patients with cerebral palsy do in Western countries. Some authors have reported that thyroid function improved by iodine supplementation in myxedematous cretins aged less than 4 years but not in older patients, suggesting that in this type of cretinism, the atrophic thyroid progressively loses its functional capacities.[111,112] Other authors, however, recently reported significant improvement in neuromotor and physical appearance even in 30- to 40-year-old myxedematous endemic cretins treated by injections of iodized oil.[50]

PREVENTION

Endemic cretinism is prevented when iodine deficiency has been corrected.[3,9,12,113] Wespi reported that iodization of salt was introduced independently in various Swiss cantons be-

tween 1922 and 1925 and that the decline of endemic deaf-mutism in these cantons could be correlated with the extent of salt iodination.[114] However, it must be pointed out that in Switzerland endemic cretinism started to diminish about 10 years before the introduction of iodine prophylaxis,[5] probably because of improved socioeconomic conditions and communication, resulting in a "silent iodine prophylaxis."

Table 57-3 summarizes the results of the controlled trials conducted during the past 20 years on the effect of iodine prophylaxis on the incidence of endemic cretinism. In Ecuador, in an attempt to study the effectiveness of iodine supplementation in early fetal life, pregnant women in the test village (Tocachi) were given iodine supplementation. Mothers who were in the sixth, seventh, eighth, and ninth months of pregnancy at the time of iodization were excluded. There have been no new cases of endemic cretinism among the infants investigated in the treated village, while six instances of severe and persistent mental and neuromotor deficiencies have appeared in the control village.[115] The data of Pharoah and colleagues[116] indicate that iodized oil injections prevent neurologic endemic cretinism in offspring only if administered before pregnancy, indicating that the damage occurs during early fetal life.

The data from Zaire show that correction of iodine deficiency prevents myxedematous endemic cretinism in the offspring, even if administered during pregnancy.[88] Subsequent studies have showed that correction of iodine deficiency in

TABLE 57-3.
Prevention of Endemic Cretinism by Injections of Iodized Oil

Regions	Methods	Findings	References
NEUROLOGIC CRETINISM			
Ecuador	One village injected (Tocachi); One village not injected (La Esperanza); follow-up of the children born in the two villages up to 60 mo of age	No cretin in the 205 children born in the treated village, 6 neurologic cretins in the 447 children born in the untreated village	115
Papua–New Guinea	Families injected or not injected at random; follow-up of the children up to 60 mo of age	6 neurologic cretins in the 687 children in the treated group—in 5 of the 6, the mother was pregnant at the time of injection; 31 cretins in the 688 children in the untreated group	116
MYXEDEMATOUS CRETINISM			
Zaire			
Idjwi Island	Two villages injected; one village not injected, surveys after 1, 3.5, and 5 y in the treated villages and after 5 y in the untreated village	No cretin born in the treated villages; 3 myxedematous cretins in the untreated village during the 5 y of the investigation	131
Ubangi	Pregnant women injected at random between the 20th and 36th wk of gestation (mean, 28th wk)		87, 88, 104
	Follow-up of 99 infants aged 1.5–15 mo (mean, 6.5 mo)	1 myxedematous cretin of 44 children in the treated group (mother injected during the last month of gestation); 4 myxedematous cretins of 45 in the untreated group	
	Follow-up of 671 infants and children aged 0–7 y	In infants aged 0–2 y, myxedematous cretinism in 1 of 192 in the treated group and 10 of 109 in the untreated group (p < 0.01); the difference disappeared in children aged 3–7 y	

pregnant mothers does not protect the infants against hypothyroidism for more than 2 or 3 years.[104] The possibility that, in some children, hypothyroidism could start after the age of 3 years is consistent with the observation of Goslings and colleagues[28] that hypothyroid patients in areas of severe endemic goiter are not necessarily affected by severe and irreversible mental retardation, and that of Boyages and colleagues[44] that cretins with thyroid failure may have only moderate retardation in height and bone maturation (see Table 57-1).

CONCLUSION

The epidemiology, pathogenesis, and prevention of endemic cretinism are only partly understood. Consequently, an attempt to "rationalize the problem and to arrive at a simplified conceptual framework in which the varied observations can be placed"[117] is still difficult. Iodine deficiency appears to be a necessary factor and, if severe enough, may be the sole factor in its causation. The spectrum of severity of each of the several clinical manifestations may relate to differences in the degree, timing, or duration of this deficiency. The additional role of thiocyanate has been demonstrated. It aggravates the effects of iodine deficiency, and, as a consequence, its action is also corrected by iodine supplementation. The possible roles of additional autoimmune, and environmental factors such as selenium deficiency remain to be clarified. Nevertheless, because of the gravity of endemic cretinism and the well-established preventive action of iodine, an efficient iodine prophylaxis is urgently needed in areas affected by endemic goiter and cretinism.

References

1. Stanbury JB, Ermans AM, Hetzel BS, Pretell EA, Querido A. Endemic goitre and cretinism: public health significance and prevention. WHO Chron 1974;28:220
2. Hetzel BS, Dunn JT, Stanbury JB. The prevention and control of iodine deficiency disorders. Amsterdam: Elsevier, 1987
3. Delange F. Endemic cretinism. An overview. In: Delong GR, Robbins J, Condliffe PG, eds. Iodine and the brain. New York: Plenum Press, 1989:219
4. De Quervain F, Wegelin C. Der Endemische Kretinismus. Berlin: Springer Verlag, 1936
5. König MP. Die Kongenitale Hypothyreose und der Endemische Kretinismus. Berlin: Springer Verlag, 1968
6. Stanbury JB. The damaged brain of iodine deficiency. New York: Cognizant Communication, 1994:1
7. Delange F, Bastani S, Benmiloud M, et al. Definitions of endemic goiter and cretinism, classification of goiter size and severity of endemias, and survey techniques. In: Dunn JT, Pretell E, Daza CH, Viteri FE, eds. Towards the eradication of endemic goiter, cretinism and iodine deficiency. No 502. Washington, DC: Pan American Health Organization, 1986:373
8. Dumont JE, Delange F, Ermans AM. Endemic cretinism. In: Stanbury JB, ed. Endemic goiter. No 193. Washington, DC: Pan American Health Organization 1969:91
9. Pharoah P, Delange F, Fierro-Benitez R, Stanbury JB. Endemic cretinism. In: Stanbury JB, Hetzel BS, eds. Endemic goiter and endemic cretinism. Iodine nutrition in health and disease. New York: John Wiley, 1980:395
10. Hetzel BS, Querido A. Iodine deficiency, thyroid function, and brain development. In: Stanbury JB, Hetzel BS, eds. Endemic goiter and endemic cretinism. New York: John Wiley 1980:461
11. Hetzel BS. The story of iodine deficiency. Oxford: Oxford University Press, 1989
12. Querido A. History of iodine prophylaxis with regard to cretinism and deaf-mutism. In: Stanbury JB, Kroc RL, eds. Human development and the thyroid gland. Relation to endemic cretinism. New York: Plenum Press, 1972:191
13. McCarrison R. Observations on endemic cretinism in the Chitral and Gilgit valleys. Lancet 1908;ii:1275
14. Choufoer JC, Van Rhijn M, Querido A. Endemic goiter in Western New Guinea. II. Clinical picture, incidence and pathogenesis of endemic cretinism. J Clin Endocrinol Metab 1965;25:385
15. Buttfield IH, Hetzel BS. Endemic cretinism in Eastern New Guinea. Aust Ann Med 1969;18:217
16. Bastenie PA, Ermans AM, Thys O, Beckers C, Van den Schrieck HG, de Visscher M. Endemic goiter in the Uele region. III. Endemic cretinism. J Clin Endocrinol Metab 1962;22:187
17. Dumont JE, Ermans AM, Bastenie PA. Thyroidal function in a goiter endemic. IV. Hypothyroidism and endemic cretinism. J Clin Endocrinol Metab 1963;23:325
18. Delange F, Ermans AM, Vis HL, Stanbury JB. Endemic cretinism in Idjwi Island (Kivu Lake, Republic of the Congo). J Clin Endocrinol Metab 1972;34:1059
19. Ermans AM, Mbulamoko NM, Delange F, Ahluwalia R. Role of cassava in the etiology of endemic goitre and cretinism. Ottawa: International Development Research Centre, 1980
20. Delange F, Iteke FB, Ermans AM. Nutritional factors involved in the goitrogenic action of cassava. Ottawa: International Development Research Centre, 1982
21. Vanderpas JB, Rivera-Vanderpas MT, Bourdoux P, et al. Reversibility of severe hypothyroidism with supplementary iodine in patients with endemic cretinism. N Engl J Med 1986;315:791
22. Vanderpas JB, Contempré B, Duale NL, et al. Iodine and selenium deficiency associated with cretinism in Northern Zaire. Am J Clin Nutr 1990;52:1087
23. Delange F. Endemic goitre and thyroid function in Central Africa. Monographs in paediatrics. Vol 2. Basel: S. Karger, 1974
24. Shenkman L, Medeiros-Neto GA, Mitsuma T, et al. Evidence for hypothyroidism in endemic cretinism in Brazil. Lancet 1973;ii:67
25. Zhu XY. Endemic goiter and cretinism in China with special reference to changes of iodine metabolism and pituitary-thyroid function two years after iodine prophylaxis in Gui-Zhou. In: Ui N, Torizuka K, Nagataki S, Miyai K, eds. Current problems in thyroid research. Amsterdam: Excerpta Medical, 1983:13
26. Fierro-Benitez R, Ramirez I, Garces J, Jaramillo C, Moncayo F, Stanbury JB. The clinical pattern of cretinism as seen in Highland Ecuador. Am J Clin Nutr 1974;27:531
27. Lobo LCG, Pompeu F, Rosenthal D. Endemic cretinism in Goiaz, Brazil. J Clin Endocrinol Metab 1963;23:407
28. Goslings BM, Djokomoeljanto R, Doctor R, et al. Hypothyroidism in an area of endemic goiter and cretinism in Central Java, Indonesia. J Clin Endocrinol 1977;44:481
29. Costa A, Cottino F, Mortara M, Vogliazzo U. Endemic cretinism in Piedmont. Panminerva Med 1964;6:250
30. Squatrito S, Delange F, Trimarchi F, Lisi E, Vigneri R. Endemic cretinism in Sicily. J Endocrinol Invest 1981;4:295
31. Delange F, Valeix P, Bourdoux P, et al. Comparison of the epidemiological and clinical aspects of endemic cretinism in Central Africa and in the Himalayas. In: Hetzel BS, Smith RM, eds. Fetal brain disorders. Recent approaches to the problem of mental deficiency. Amsterdam: Elsevier North Holland, 1981;243
32. Ibbertson HK, Tait JM, Pearl M, Lim T, McKinnon JR, Gill MB. Himalayan cretinism. In: Stanbury JB, Kroc RL, eds. Human devel-

opment and the thyroid gland. Relation to endemic cretinism. New York: Plenum Press, 1972:51

33. Stanbury JB, Fierro-Benitez R, Estrella E, Milutinovic PS, Tellez MU, Refetoff S. Endemic goiter with hypothyroidism in three generations. J Clin Endocrinol Metab 1969;29:1596

34. Lagasse R, Roger G, Delange F, et al. Continuous spectrum of physical and intellectual disorders in severe endemic goitre. In: Ermans AM, Mbulamoko NM, Delange F, Ahluwalia R, eds. Role of cassava in the etiology of endemic goitre and cretinism. Ottawa: International Development Research Centre, 1980:135

35. Trimarchi F, Vermiglio F, Finocchrio MD, et al. Epidemiology and clinical characteristics of endemic cretinism in Sicily. J Endocrinol Invest 1990;13:543

36. Donati L, Antonelli A, Bertoni F, et al. Clinical picture of endemic cretinism in Central Apennines (Montefeltro). Thyroid 1992;2:283

37. Delange F, Costa A, Ermans AM, Ibbertson HK, Querido A, Stanbury JB. Clinical and metabolic patterns of endemic cretinism. In: Stanbury JB, Kroc RL, eds. Human development and the thyroid gland. Relation to endemic cretinism. New York: Plenum Press, 1972:175

38. Wang HM, Ma T, Li XT, et al. A comparative study of endemic myxedematous and neurological cretinism in Hetian and Luopu, China. In: Ui N, Torizuka K, Nagataki S, Miyai K, eds. Current problems in thyroid research. Amsterdam: Excerpta Medica, 1983:349

39. Shi ZF, Zeng GH, Zhang JX, et al. Endemic goiter and cretinism in GuiZhou. Clinical analysis of 247 cretins. Chinese Med J 1984;97:689

40. Ma T, Lu TZ, Tan YB, Chen BZ. Neurological cretinism in China. In: Kochupillai N, Karmakar MG, Ramalingaswami V, eds. Iodine nutrition, thyroxine and brain development. New Delhi: Tata McGraw-Hill, 1986:28

41. DeLong GR, Stanbury JB, Fierro-Benitez R. Neurological signs in congenital iodine-deficiency disorder (endemic cretinism). Dev Med Child Neurol 1985;27:317

42. DeLong GR. Observations on the neurology of endemic cretinism. In: DeLong GR, Robbins J, Condliffe PG, eds. Iodine and the brain. New York: Plenum Press, 1989:231

43. DeLong GR. Neurological involvment in iodine deficiency disorders. In: Hetzel BS. Dunn JT, Stanbury JB, eds. The prevention and control of iodine deficiency disorders. Amsterdam: Elsevier, 1987:49

44. Boyages SC, Halpern JP, Maberly GF, et al. A comparative study of neurological and myxedematous endemic cretinism in Western China. J Clin Endocrinol Metab 1988;67:1262

45. Halpern JP, Morris JGL, Boyages S, et al. Neurological aspects of cretinism in Qinghai Province. In: DeLong GR, Robbins J, Condliffe PG, eds. Iodine and the brain. New York: Plenum Press, 1989:239

46. Boyages SC. Iodine deficiency disorders. J Clin Endocrinol Metab 1993;77:587

47. Delong GR, Ma Tai, Cao Xue-Ui, et al. The neuromotor deficit in endemic cretinism. In: Stanbury JB, ed. The damaged brain of iodine deficiency. New York: Cognizant Communication, 1994:9

48. Halpern JP, Boyages SC, Maberly GF, Collins JK, Eastman CJ, Morris JGL. The neurology of endemic cretinism. Brain 1991;114:825

49. Ramirez I, Cruz M, Varea J. Endemic cretinism in the Andean region: New methodological approaches. In: Delange F, Ahluwalia R, eds. Cassava toxicity and thyroid: research and public health issues. Ottawa: International Development Research Centre, 1983:73

50. Downing D, Geel Hoed GW. Goiter and cretinism in the Uele Zaire endemia: studies of an iodine deficient popula-

tion with changes following intervention. II. Functional and behavioral aspects. In: Stanbury JB, ed. The damaged brain of iodine deficiency. New York: Cognizant Communication, 1994:233

51. Smith DW, Blizzard RM, Wilkins L. The mental prognosis in hypothyroidism of infancy and childhood. A review of 128 cases. Pediatrics 1957;19:1011

52. Raman G, Beierwaltes WH. Correlation of goiter, deafmutism and mental retardation with serum thyroid hormone levels in non-cretinous inhabitants of a severe endemic goiter area in India. J Clin Endocrinol Metab 1959;19:228

53. Trowbridge FL. Intellectual assessment in primitive societies, with a preliminary report of a study of the effects of early iodine supplementation on intelligence. In: Stanbury JB, Kroc RL, eds. Human development and the thyroid gland. Relation to endemic cretinism. New York: Plenum Press, 1972:137

54. Pharoah POD, Hornabrook RW. Endemic cretinism of recent onset in New Guinea. Lancet 1973;ii:1038

55. Hetzel BS, Hay ID. Thyroid function, iodine nutrition and fetal brain development. Clin Endocrinol 1979;11:445

56. Smith RM. Thyroid hormones and brain development. In: Hetzel BS, Smith RM, eds. Fetal brain disorders. Recent approaches to the problem of mental deficiency. Amsterdam: Elsevier/North Holland Biomedical Press, 1981:149

57. Potter BJ, McIntosh, Hetzel BS. The effect of iodine deficiency on fetal brain development in the sheep. In: Hetzel BS, Smith RM, eds. Fetal brain disorders. Recent approaches to the problem of mental deficiency. Amsterdam: Elsevier/North Holland Biomedical Press, 1981:119

58. Courtois P, Bourdoux P, Lagasse R, Ermans AM, Delange F. Role of the balance between the dietary supplies of iodine and thiocyanate in the etiology of endemic goitre in the Ubangi area. In: Delange F, Iteke FB, Ermans AM, eds. Nutritional factors involved in the goitrogenic action of cassava. Ottawa: International Development Research Centre, 1982:65

59. Boyages SC, Maberly GF, Chen J, et al. Endemic cretinism: possible role for thyroid autoimmunity. Lancet 1989;ii:529

60. Boyages SC, Lens JW, Van Der Gaag RD, Maberly GF, Eastman CJ, Maberly HA. Sporadic and endemic congenital hypothyroidism: evidence for autosensitization. In: Delange F, Fisher DA, Glinoer D, eds. Research in congenital hypothyroidism. New York: Plenum Press, 1989:123

61. Medeiros-Neto G, Tsuboi K, Lima N. Thyroid autoimmunity and endemic cretinism. Lancet 1989;i:111

62. Brown RS, Keating P, Mitchell E. Maternal thyroid-blocking immunoglobulins in congenital hypothyroidism. J Clin Endocrinol Metab 1990;70:1341

63. Chiovato L, Vitti P, Marcocci C, et al. TSH-blocking antibodies and congenital hypothyroidism. In: Delange F, Fisher DA, Glinoer D, eds. Research in congenital hypothyroidism. New York: Plenum Press, 1989:141

63a. Chiovato L, Vitti P, Bendinelli G, et al. Humoral thyroid autoimmunity is not involved in the pathogenesis of myxedematous endemic cretinism. J Clin Endocrinol Metab, 1995; 80:1509.

64. Corvilain B, Contempré B, Longombe AO, et al. Selenium and the thyroid: how the relationship was established. Am J Clin Nutr Suppl 1993;57:244S

65. Contempré B, Many MC, Vanderpas J, Dumont JE. Interaction between two trace elements: selenium and iodine. Implications of both deficiencies. In: Stanbury JB, ed. The damaged brain and iodine deficiency. New York: Cognizant Communication, 1994:133

66. Dumont JE, Corvilain B, Contempré B. Endemic cretinism: the myxedematous and neurologic forms of a disease caused by severe iodine deficiency. In: Stanbury JB, ed. The damaged brain and iodine deficiency. New York: Cognizant Communication, 1994:133

67. Goyens P, Golstein J, Nsombola B, Vis H, Dumont JE. Selenium deficiency as possible factor in the pathogenesis of myxedematous endemic cretinism. Acta Endocrinol 1987;114:497

68. Vanderpas JB, Contempré B, Duale NL, et al. Iodine and selenium deficiency associated with cretinism in Northern Zaire. Am J Clin Nutr 1990;52:1087

69. Aaseth J, Frey H, Glattre E, Norheim G, Ringstad J, Thomassen Y. Selenium concentrations in the human thyroid. Biol Trace Elem Res 1990;24:147

70. Dumont JE. The action of thyrotropin on thyroid metabolism. Vitam Horm 1971;29:287

71. Arthur JR, Nicol F, Beckett GJ. Hepatic iodothyronine 5'-deiodinase. The role of selenium. Biochem J 1990;272:537

72. Contempré B, Denef JF, Dumont JE, Many MC. Selenium deficiency aggravates the necrotizing effects of a high iodide dose in iodine deficient rats. Endocrinology 1993;132:1866

73. Fisher DA, Klein AH. Thyroid development and disorders of thyroid function in the newborn. N Engl J Med 1981;304:702

74. Morreale de Escobar G, Escobar del Rey F. Thyroid physiology in utero and neonatally. In: Rubery E, Smales E, eds. Iodine prophylaxis following nuclear accidents. Oxford: Pergamon Press, 1990:3

75. Morreale de Escobar G, Obregon MJ, Escobar del Rey F. Hormone nurturing of the developing brain: the rat model. In: Stanbury JB, ed. The damaged brain of iodine deficiency. New York: Cognizant Communication, 1994:103

76. Bernal J, Pekonen F. Ontogenesis of the nuclear 3,5,3'-triiodothyronine receptor in the human fetal brain. Endocrinology 1984;114:677

77. Thorpe-Beeston JG, Nicolaides KH, Felton CV, Butler J, McGregor AM. Maturation of the secretion of thyroid hormone and thyroid-stimulating hormone in the fetus. N Engl J Med 1991; 324:532

78. Man EB, Jones WS, Holden RH, Hellits ED. Thyroid function in human pregnancy. VIII. Retardation of progeny aged 7 years; relationship to maternal age and maternal thyroid function. Am J Obstet Gynecol 1971;111:905

79. Matsuura N, Konishi J. Transient hypothyroidism in infants born to mothers with chronic thyroiditis. A nationwide study of twenty-three cases. Endocrinol Japon 1990;37:369

80. Delange F, Thilly C, Bourdoux P, Hennart P, Ermans AM. Influence of dietary goitrogens during pregnancy in humans on thyroid function of the newborn. In: Delange F, Iteke FB, Ermans AM, eds. Nutritional factors involved in the goitrogenic action of cassava. Ottawa: International Development Research Centre, 1982:40

81. Stanbury JB. Cretinism and fetal-maternal relationship. In: Stanbury JB, Kroc RL, eds. Human development and the thyroid gland. Relation to endemic cretinism. New York: Plenum Press, 1972:487

82. Pharoah POD, Connolly KJ, Ekins RP, Harding AG. Maternal thyroid hormone levels in pregnancy and the subsequent cognitive and motor performance of the children. Clin Endocrinol 1984; 21:265

83. Pharoah POD, Ellis SM, Ekins RP, Williams ES. Maternal thyroid function, iodine deficiency and fetal development. Clin Endocrinol 1976;5:159

84. Pharoah POD, Connolly KJ. Iodine deficiency in Papua, New Guinea. In: Stanbury JB, ed. The damaged brain of iodine deficiency. New York: Cognizant Communication, 1994:299

85. Thilly C, Lagasse R, Roger G, Bourdoux P, Ermans AM. Impaired fetal and postnatal development and high perinatal death-rate in a severe iodine deficient area. In: Stockigt JR, Nagataki S, Meldrum E, Barlow JW, Harding PE, eds. Thyroid research VIII. Canberra: Australian Academy of Sciences, 1980:20

86. Thilly CH, Swennen B, Moreno-Reyes R, Hindlet JY, Bourdoux P, Vanderpas JB. Maternal, fetal and juvenile hypothyroidism. Birth

weight, and infant mortality in the etiopathogenesis of the IDD spectrum in Zaire and Malawi. In: Stanbury JB, ed. The damaged brain of iodine deficiency. New York: Cognizant Communication, 1994:241

87. Delange F, Thilly C, Camus M, et al. Evidence for fetal hypothyroidism in severe endemic goiter. In: Robbins J, Braverman LE, eds. Thyroid research. Amsterdam: Excerpta Medica, 1976:493

88. Thilly CH, Delange F, Lagasse R, et al. Fetal hypothyroidism and maternal thyroid status in severe endemic goiter. J Clin Endocrinol Metab 1978;47:354

89. Woods RJ, Sinha AK, Ekins R. Uptake and metabolism of thyroid hormones by the rat fetus in early pregnancy. Clin Sci 1984; 67:359

90. Morreale de Escobar G, Pastor R, Obregon MJ, Escobar del Rey F. Effect of maternal hypothyroidism on the weight and thyroid hormone content of rat embryonic tissues, before and after onset of fetal thyroid function. Endocrinology 1985;117:1890

91. Potter BJ, McIntosh GH, Mano MT, et al. The effect of maternal thyroidectomy prior to conception on foetal brain development in sheep. Acta Endocrinol 1986;112:93

92. Escobar del Rey F, Pastor R, Mallol J, Morreale de Escobar G. Effects of maternal iodine deficiency on the L-thyroxine and 3,5,3'-triiodo-L-thyroxine contents of rat embryonic tissues before and after onset of fetal thyroid function. Endocrinology 1986; 118:1259

93. Braverman LE. Placental transfer for substances from mother to fetus affecting fetal pituitary-thyroid function. In: Delange F, Fisher DA, Glinoer D, eds. Research in congenital hypothyroidism. New York: Plenum Press, 1989:3

94. Vulsma T, Gons MH, De Vijlder JJM. Maternal-fetal transfer of thyroxine in congenital hypothyroidism due to a total organification defect or thyroid agenesis. N Engl J Med 1989;321:13

95. Delange F, De Vijlder J, Morreale de Escobar G, Rochiccioli P, Varrone S. Significance of early diagnostic data in congenital hypothyroidism: report of the Subcommittee on Neonatal Hypothyroidism of the European Thyroid Association. In: Delange F, Fisher DA, Glinoer D, eds. Research in congenital hypothyroidism. New York: Plenum Press, 1989:225

96. Glinoer D, De Nayer P, Delange F, et al. A randomized trial for the treatment of excessive thyroidal stimulation in pregnancy: maternal and neonatal effects. J Clin Endocrinol Metab 1995; 80:258

97. Liu JL, Tan YB, Zuang ZL, Zhu XY, Chen BZ. Morphologic study of development of cerebral cortex of therapeutically aborted fetuses in endemic goiter region, Gui-Zhou Province, China. In: Ui N, Torizuka K, Nagataki S Miyai K, eds. Current problems in thyroid research. Amsterdam: Excerpta Medica, 1983:390

98. Kochupillai N, Pandav CS. Neonatal chemical hypothyroidism in iodine-deficient environments. In: Hetzel BS, Dunn JT, Stanbury JB, eds. The prevention and control of iodine deficiency disorders. Amsterdam: Elsevier, 1987:85

99. Chaouki ML, Delange F, Maoui R, Ermans AM. Endemic cretinism and congenital hypothyroidism in endemic goiter in Algeria. In: Meideiros-Neto GA, Gaitan E, eds. Frontiers of thyroidology. New York: Plenum Press, 1986:1055

100. Sava L, Delange F, Belfiore, Purello F, Vigneri R. Transient impairment of thyroid function in newborn from an area of endemic goiter. J Clin Endocrinol Metab 1984;59:90

101. Lagasse R, Bourdoux P, Courtois P, et al. Influence of the dietary balance of iodine/thiocyanate and protein on thyroid function in adults and young infants. In: Delange F, Iteke FB, Ermans AM, eds. Nutritional factors involved in the goitrogenic action of cassava. Ottawa: International Development Researc Centre, 1982:34

102. Delange F, Beckers C, Höfer R, König MP, Monaco F, Varrone S. Progress report on neonatal screening for congenital hypothyroidism in Europe. In: Burrow GN, Dussault JH, eds. Neonatal thyroid screening. New York: Raven Press, 1980:107

103. Dussault JH, Mitchell ML, La Franchi S, Murphey WH. Regional screening for congenital hypothyroidism: results of screening one million North American infants with filter paper spot T_4-TSH. In: Burrow GN, Dussault JH, eds. Neonatal thyroid screening. New York: Raven Press, 1980:155

104. Thilly C, Vanderpas J, Bourdoux P, et al. Prevention of myxedematous cretinism with iodized oil during pregnancy. In: Ui N, Torizuka K, Nagataki S, Miyai K, eds. Current problems in thyroid research. Amsterdam: Excerpta Medica, 1983:386

105. Wilkins L. Epiphyseal dysgenesis associated with hypothyroidism. Am J Dis Child 1941;61:13

106. Courtois P, Delange F, Bourdoux P, Ermans AM. Significance of neonatal thyroid screening tests in severe endemic goiter (Abstract no 81). Ann Endocrinol 1982;43:51a

107. Delange F. Adaptation to iodine deficiency during growth: etiopathogenesis of endemic goiter and cretinism. In: Delange F, Fisher D, Malvaux P, eds. Pediatric thyroidology. Basel: Karger, 1985:295

108. Dumont JE, Ermans AM, Bastenie PA. Thyroid function in a goiter endemic. V. Mechanism of thyroid failure in the Uele endemic cretins. J Clin Endocrinol Metab 1963;23:847

109. Vanderpas J, Bourdoux P, Lagasse R, et al. Endemic infantile hypothyroidism in a severe endemic goitre area of Central Africa. Clin Endocrinol 1984;20:327

110. Moreno-Reyes R, Boelaert M, El Badawi S, Eltom M, Vanderpas JB. Endemic juvenile hypothyroidism in a severe endemic goitre area in Sudan. Clin Endocrinol 1993;38:19

111. Vanderpas JB, Rivera-Vanderpas MT, Bourdoux P, et al. Reversibility of severe hypothyroidism with supplementary iodine in patients with endemic cretinism. N Engl J Med 1986;315:791

112. Boyages SC, Halpern JP, Maberly GF, et al. Supplementary iodine fails to reverse hypothyroidism in adolescents and adults with endemic cretinism. J Clin Endocrinol Metab 1990;70:336

113. Hetzel BS, Thilly CH, Fierro-Benitez R, Pretell EA, Buttfield IH, Stanbury JB. Iodized oil in the prevention of endemic goiter and cretinism. In: Stanbury JB, Hetzel BS, eds. Endemic goiter and endemic cretinism. New York: John Wiley, 1980:513

114. Wespi HJ. Abnahme der Taubstumnheit in der Schweiz als Folge der Kropfprophylaxe mit iodertem Kochsalz. Schweiz Med Wochenschr 1945;75:625

115. Ramirez I, Fierro-Benitez R, Estrella E, et al. The results of prophylaxis of endemic cretinism with iodized oil in rural Andean Ecuador. In: Stanbury JB, Kroc RL, eds. Human development and the thyroid gland. Relation to endemic cretinism. New York: Plenum Press, 1972:223

116. Pharoah POB, Buttfield IH, Hetzel BS. Neurological damage to the fetus resulting from severe iodine deficiency during pregnancy. Lancet 1971;i:308

117. Stanbury JB. The pathogenesis of endemic retardation associated with endemic goiter. In: Reinwein D, Klein E, Beysel D, eds. Diminished thyroid hormone formation. Possible causes and clinical aspects. Stuttgart: Schattauer Verlag, 1982:80

118. Ermans AM, Kinthaert J, Delcroix C, Collard J. Metabolism of intrathyroidal iodine in normal men. J Clin Endocrinol Metab 1968;28:169

119. Fierro-Benitez R, Ramirez I, Estrella E, Stanbury JB. The role of iodine deficiency in intellectual development in an area of endemic goiter. In: Dunn JT, Medeiros-Neto GA, eds. Endemic goiter and cretinism: continuing threats to world health. No 292. Washington, DC: Pan American Health Organization, 1974:135

120. Dodge PR, Palkes H, Fierro-Benitez R, Ramirez I. Effect on intelligence of iodine in oil administered to young Andean children. A preliminary report. In: Stanbury JB, ed. Endemic goiter. No 193. Washington, DC: Pan American Health Organization, 1969:378

121. Greene LS. Physical growth and development, neurological maturation and behavioral functioning in two Andean communities in which goiter is endemic. Am J Phys Anthropol 1973;38:119

122. Bautista A, Barker PA, Dunn JT, Sanchez M, Kaiser D. The effects of oral iodized oil on intelligence, thyroid status, and somatic growth in school-age children from an area of endemic goiter. Am J Clin Nutr 1982;35:127

123. Muzzo S, Leiva L, Carrasco D. Possible etiological factors and consequences of a moderate iodine deficiency on intellectual coefficient of school-age children. In: Meideiros-Neto GA, Gaitan E, eds. Frontiers of thyroidology. New York: Plenum Press, 1985:1001

124. Connolly KJ, Pharoah POD, Hetzel BS. Fetal iodine deficiency and motor performance during childhood. Lancet 1979;ii:1149

125. Pharoah POD, Connolly K, Hetzel B, Ekins R. Maternal thyroid function and motor competence in the child. Dev Med Child Neurol 1981;23:76

126. Thilly CH, Roger G, Lagasse R, et al. Fetomaternal relationship, fetal hypothyroidism, and psychomotor retardation. In: Ermans AM, Mbulamoko NM, Delange F, Ahluwalia R, eds. Role of cassava in the etiology of endemic goitre and cretinism. Ottawa: International Development Research Centre, 1980:111

127. Bleichrodt N, Garcia I, Rubio C, Morreale de Escobar G, Escobar del Rey F. Developmental disorders associated with severe iodine deficiency. In: Hetzel BS, Dunn JT, Stanbury JB, eds. The prevention and control of iodine deficiency disorders. Amsterdam: Elsevier, 1987:65

128. Boyages SC, Collins JK, Maberly GF, Jupp JJ, Morris J, Eastman CJ. Iodine deficiency impairs intellectual and neuromotor development in apparently normal persons. Med J Aust 1989;150:676

129. Ma T, Wang YY, Wang D, Chen ZP, Chi SP. Neuropsychological studies in iodine deficiency areas in China. In: DeLong GR, Robbins J, Condliffe PG, eds. Iodine and the brain. New York: Plenum Press, 1989:259

130. Kochupillai N, Pandav CS, Godbole MM, Metha M, Ahuja MMS. Iodine deficiency and neonatal hypothyroidism. Bull WHO 1986;64:547

131. Thilly CH, Delange F, Golstein-Golaire J, Ermans AM. Endemic goiter prophylaxia by iodized oil: a reassessment. J Clin Endocrinol Metab 1973;36:1196

Werner and Ingbar's The Thyroid, Seventh Edition,
edited by Lewis E. Braverman and Robert D. Utiger.
Lippincott–Raven Publishers, Philadelphia, © 1996

58

Other Forms of Primary Hypothyroidism

Charles P. Barsano

Primary hypothyroidism occurs as a consequence of, or concomitant with, numerous disorders, therapies, and chemical exposures. Chronic autoimmune thyroiditis and iodine deficiency are probably the most common causes worldwide and are discussed in detail in chapters 55 and 57, respectively. Less common causes of hypothyroidism include dyshormonogenetic defects of the thyroid (chap 56) and the transient hypothyroidism that occurs during recovery in patients with subacute thyroiditis, silent (painless) thyroiditis (chap 34), and postpartum thyroiditis (chap 89). Congenital causes of hypothyroidism that nearly always appear in infancy or childhood, such as thyroid ectopy, are discussed in chapter 85. This chapter primarily addresses the other forms of hypothyroidism, both common and rare, as outlined in Table 58-1.

INFILTRATIVE DISEASES OF THE THYROID

Various systemic disorders may cause primary hypothyroidism by progressive infiltration, destruction, and replacement of normal thyroid tissue. Several disorders characterized by abnormal tissue infiltrations are also associated with chronic autoimmune thyroiditis. These disorders thus cause thyroid dysfunction by dual mechanisms.

Riedel's Thyroiditis (Invasive Fibrous Thyroiditis)

Fewer than 200 cases of Riedel's thyroiditis have been reported since the disorder was recognized 100 years ago (reviewed in references 1 to 3). The disorder predominantly affects middle-aged women.[3] The presenting complaints include pressure in the anterior neck, dysphagia, dyspnea secondary to tracheal compression, and goiter. The thyroid is usually enlarged but is most remarkable for its very hard consistency and attachment to surrounding structures in the neck.

In this disorder, the thyroid parenchyma is gradually replaced by dense fibrous tissue that may penetrate the capsule and infiltrate the adjacent muscle and soft tissues. The thyroid initially is infiltrated by plasma cells, lymphocytes, and other inflammatory cells, but fibrosis and destruction of thyroid follicles predominate later. The histology of Riedel's thyroiditis is distinct from silent thyroiditis and subacute thyroiditis but may be similar to the fibrosing variant of goitrous autoimmune thyroiditis. Because of the histologic similarities, the frequent presence of antithyroid antibodies, and the sometimes favorable response to corticosteroid therapy, Riedel's thyroiditis may be a variant form of goitrous autoimmune thyroiditis.[4–6]

Hypothyroidism occurs in 30% to 40% of patients and is attributed to loss of thyroid parenchyma. Many patients also have retroperitoneal fibrosis. Less commonly, they have fibrosis in the mediastinum, liver, lungs, or retroorbital tissue.[7,8] Hypoparathyroidism has also been described in a few patients.[1,9–11] Riedel's thyroiditis may therefore be one component of a generalized disorder of fibrous tissue proliferation.[1,12]

The diagnosis of Riedel's thyroiditis generally requires surgical biopsy to rule out carcinoma, and at least partial thyroidectomy may be necessary to relieve symptoms of tracheal compression.[7,8,13] Magnetic resonance imaging may be diagnostically helpful.[14] Treatment with corticosteroids may help stabilize the fibrosis,[6,13,15,16] and thyroxine (T$_4$) replacement therapy is indicated for treatment of concomitant hypothyroidism.

Cystinosis (Cystine Storage Disease)

Cystinosis is an autosomal recessive disorder characterized by an abnormal intracellular accumulation of cystine crystals that

TABLE 58-1.
Other Forms of Primary Hypothyroidism

Infiltrative diseases of the thyroid
    Riedel's thyroiditis (invasive fibrous thyroiditis)
    Cystinosis (cystine storage disease)
    Hemochromatosis
    Progressive systemic sclerosis (scleroderma)
    Sarcoidosis
    Amyloidosis
    Chondrocalcinosis
Thyroid irradiation
    External radiotherapy
    Radioiodine therapy
Postoperative hypothyroidism
Drug-induced hypothyroidism
    Lithium
    Interferon-α and interleukin-2
    Other drugs
Industrial and environmental chemicals
Thyroid ectopy

typically results in end-stage renal disease in childhood. Many affected children also have hypothyroidism.[17–21] The thyroid glands of children with fatal cystinosis may show intracellular cystine crystals, fibrosis, or atrophy.[21,22] The incidence of hypothyroidism in patients who survive into adulthood because of successful renal transplantation is high—86% in one survey.[23]

Hemochromatosis

Hereditary hemochromatosis is a rare metabolic disorder in which excessive iron accumulates in multiple tissues, including the thyroid, causing parenchymal damage and fibrosis.[24–27] In one study, 3 of 34 men with hemochromatosis had primary hypothyroidism[24]; each also had high serum titers of antithyroid peroxidase antibodies. The (nongoitrous) thyroid tissue of one patient contained some lymphocytic infiltration, fibrosis, and atrophic thyroid follicular cells laden with iron. Iron was also demonstrable in the pituitary, but there was no evidence of pituitary atrophy or damage. Iron accumulation in the thyroid probably damages the follicular epithelium, resulting in the release of thyroidal antigens, generation of antibodies to these antigens, thyroid inflammation, and eventual hypothyroidism. Primary hypothyroidism associated with iron-laden thyroid tissue has also been demonstrated in acquired hemochromatosis resulting from repeated blood transfusions[28,29] or severe hemolytic anemia.[30] Hemochromatosis also can cause central hypothyroidism (see chap 59).

Progressive Systemic Sclerosis (Scleroderma)

Progressive systemic sclerosis is a connective tissue disorder with features of autoimmunity characterized by sclerosis of the skin, subcutaneous tissue, and multiple visceral organs. Multi-

ple case studies suggest an association between systemic sclerosis and hypothyroidism of an autoimmune origin,[31–34] although thyroid dysfunction secondary to a nonimmune infiltrative process may also occur. In one study of thyroid tissue from 70 fatal cases and age- and sex-matched control subjects, severe fibrosis was seen in the thyroid in 14% of the patients with systemic sclerosis but in only 2% of the control subjects.[35] Evaluation of stored serum samples from 27 of the patients with systemic sclerosis revealed low serum T_4 and elevated serum thyrotropin (TSH) concentrations in seven patients. Three of the seven patients had clinical hypothyroidism.

In a similar, more recent study of 39 patients with this disorder, seven had subclinical hypothyroidism (high serum TSH and normal serum T_4 values) and two had overt hypothyroidism.[36] Four of the nine patients had high serum antithyroid antibody titers. The increased frequency of antithyroid antibodies in patients with systemic sclerosis, with or without concomitant hypothyroidism, was confirmed in another survey[37] in which 14 of 43 patients had high antithyroid antibody titers.

Sarcoidosis

About 5% of patients with sarcoidosis have evidence of thyroidal involvement at autopsy.[38–40] Clinically evident hypothyroidism as a result of sarcoidosis is rare, although sarcoid goiters have been recognized.[41–43]

Amyloidosis

Amyloid is found in the thyroid glands of patients with either primary[44] or secondary amyloidosis, including amyloidosis associated with tuberculosis,[45,46] rheumatoid arthritis,[46] multiple myeloma,[47] and inflammatory bowel disease.[48] The infiltration is usually diffuse but may present as multiple nodules.[49]

A minority of patients with thyroid amyloidosis have a goiter.[45] Some amyloid goiters, however, are large (130 g) and firm to hard in consistency. In a survey of 376 thyroidectomy specimens in Papua New Guinea between 1980 and 1990, amyloid goiters represented 1.9% of the specimens.[50] Ultrasonography and other techniques such as fine-needle aspiration may be helpful in diagnosing amyloid goiters.[51–54]

The thyroid parenchyma of amyloid goiters is atrophic, but hypothyroidism is rare. The composition of the amyloid depends on the nature of the associated systemic disorder. In familial amyloidotic neuropathy, variant transthyretins with single amino acid substitutions (e.g., a methionine substitution for valine in position[30]) have been identified.[55,56] Lambda light chains,[47,57] cytoskeletal proteins,[58,59] and other proteins have also been described as components of amyloid deposits.

Chondrocalcinosis

Chondrocalcinosis is a disorder resulting from the deposition of calcium pyrophosphate crystals in cartilage. If symptomatic, it usually causes a chronic arthropathy or an acute synovitis. The results of surveys of the prevalence of hypothyroidism among patients with chondrocalcinosis or the prevalence of chondrocalcinosis among hypothyroid patients, are conflicting,[60–64] but a comprehensive statistical survey has suggested a small association.[65] In a recent study the prevalence of chondrocalcinosis was 17% in a group of hypothyroid patients and only 10% in control patients, but no evidence of a cause–effect relationship could be identified.[66] If there is an association between chondrocalcinosis and hypothyroidism, the cause of the hypothyroidism is not clear.

THYROIDAL IRRADIATION

External Radiotherapy

External radiotherapy to the neck in patients with Hodgkin's or non-Hodgkin's lymphomas causes hypothyroidism in about 25% to 50% of patients.[67–71] In many patients, the hypothyroidism is initially subclinical but gradually becomes overt; in others overt hypothyroidism appears rapidly.[72–75] The interval between radiotherapy and the onset of hypothyroidism in most patients ranges from 2 to 7 years,[72,76–80] although it may occur sooner.[75,76,80] Higher doses of radiation are associated with higher frequencies of hypothyroidism.[72,81,82] Anterior shielding of the thyroid during mantle field irradiation may decrease radiation-induced hypothyroidism.[83]

Chemotherapy without adjunctive radiotherapy also causes hypothyroidism, but much less often than radiotherapy.[84,85] The combination of radiotherapy and chemotherapy was associated with a higher rate of hypothyroidism than radiotherapy alone in some[73,84,86] but not all studies.[85] Similarly, lymphangiography with iodine-containing contrast agents increased the vulnerability of the thyroid to radiation in some[78–80,82,87] but not all studies.[85]

Overt or subclinical hypothyroidism (27% and 14%, respectively) is common in patients with primary thyroid lymphomas before treatment, presumably as a consequence of the chronic autoimmune thyroiditis that very often precedes thyroid lymphoma.[88–90] The frequency of hypothyroidism increases after radiotherapy, as in patients with nonthyroid lymphoma treated with radiation (see also chap 82).

External radiotherapy in patients with tumors of the head and neck also results in hypothyroidism in approximately 10% to 50% of patients.[75,91–95] In about two-thirds, the hypothyroidism is subclinical.[96,97] Most cases of hypothyroidism become evident within 1 year.[98,99] Radiotherapy combined with partial thyroidectomy for head and neck cancer presents a distinctly greater risk for hypothyroidism than radiotherapy alone.[75,94,96,98,99] Craniospinal irradiation, more than limited cranial irradiation, is also a risk factor for hypothyroidism.[92,100] Whether concurrent chemotherapy is an additional risk factor is disputed.[92,96]

Approximately one-fourth of patients receiving total body irradiation followed by bone marrow transplantation for acute leukemia or aplastic anemia develop hypothyroidism.[93,101–103] Most of these patients have subclinical hypothyroidism.[101,104] The median onset is approximately 1 year after transplantation,[93,104] and the hypothyroidism is transient in about half of the patients. Total body irradiation delivered in one dose is much more likely to cause hypothyroidism than irradiation given in 6 to 8 fractions.[102,103]

Radioiodine Therapy

When relatively high doses of radioiodine (^{131}I) in the order of ≥10 mCi (370 MBq) ^{131}I or ≥150 μCi (5.6 MBq) ^{131}I per gram of thyroid tissue are administered, about 50% of patients with Graves' hyperthyroidism become hypothyroid within 1 year, and about 70% are hypothyroid 10 years later[105–109] (see chap 53). Lower dose regimens (e.g., 40–70 μCi [1.5–2.6 MBq]/g tissue retained at 24 hours) are less likely to result in early hypothyroidism (e.g., 12% after 1 year in one study[110]) but increase the likelihood of persistent hyperthyroidism (33% in the same study). Although lower doses of ^{131}I are associated with less hypothyroidism soon (about 1 year) after treatment as compared with higher doses, the difference in the frequency of hypothyroidism is substantially smaller 10 years later.[110] When the cumulative frequency of hypothyroidism after any effective dose is plotted as a function of time after therapy, it can be projected that virtually all patients will eventually become hypothyroid.[107,108,111–115]

The likelihood and time of onset of hypothyroidism after ^{131}I therapy in patients with Graves' hyperthyroidism cannot be accurately predicted when usual doses of ^{131}I are given. Goiter size, percent of ^{131}I uptake at 24 hours, and postdosage retention of ^{131}I are regarded as factors relevant to the total exposure and the ultimate effect of the radiation on the thyroid. Whether administration of an antithyroid drug before or after ^{131}I treatment limits the efficacy of ^{131}I therapy or reduces the frequency of hypothyroidism is debated.[116–120]

Overt hypothyroidism in patients who have received ^{131}I therapy is often preceded by subclinical hypothyroidism, which may become apparent within 2 to 4 months after ^{131}I therapy.[121,122] Approximately one-half of patients with subclinical hypothyroidism to develop overt hypothyroidism within 3 months to 2 years,[74] but it may persist for many years or resolve.

Radioiodine-induced hypothyroidism is generally less frequent after treatment for toxic multinodular goiters. In two studies, hypothyroidism occurred in 6% of patients one year after a 15 mCi (555 MBq) dose of ^{131}I[106] and in 7% 4 to 5 years after a similar dose.[123] In contrast with patients with Graves' hyperthyroidism, patients with toxic multinodular goiters would be expected to have some suppressed thyroid tissue and thereby should be less susceptible to ^{131}I-induced hypothyroidism. Presumably for the same reason, hypothyroidism after ^{131}I therapy in patients with an autonomously functioning thyroid adenoma is also unusual, with rates of 13% 1 year after administration of 15 mCi (555 MBq) ^{131}I[106] and 6% 10 years after administration of 20 mCi (740 MBq).[124]

Treatment of patients with large, nontoxic, multinodular goiters with ^{131}I for the purpose of decreasing goiter size causes hypothyroidism more often than does treatment of patients with toxic multinodular goiters.[125–128] High doses of ^{131}I (20–50 mCi [740–1850 MBq]) induce hypothyrodism in 30% of patients after 2 years and in all patients after 8 years.[127] In patients treated with a lower dosage (0.1 mCi [3.7 MBq]/g of thyroid tissue), the cumulative risk of hypothyroidism after 5 years was 22%.[126]

POSTOPERATIVE HYPOTHYROIDISM

The frequency of hypothyroidism after subtotal thyroidectomy for Graves' hyperthyroidism varies from 3% to 75%,[129–134] although 25% to 45% is probably a more representative range. The risk of postoperative hypothyroidism depends largely on the mass of remaining thyroid tissue. The optimal balance between postoperative hypothyroidism and recurrent hyperthyroidism is when from 4 to 8 g of thyroid is left.[135–140] Hypothyroidism can, however, be associated with relatively large remnants (>10 g) and, conversely, recurrent thyrotoxicosis can occur in patients in whom the remnant is small (<5 g). The risk of postoperative hypothyroidism after bilateral subtotal thyroidectomy is somewhat less than that after total lobectomy with contralateral subtotal lobectomy.[141,142]

Most patients who become hypothyroid after subtotal thyroidectomy do so within 1 year.[108,110,139,143] Thereafter, the cumulative incidence of hypothyroidism increases by only 1% to 2% per year. Subclinical hypothyroidism has been estimated to occur in one-fourth to one-half of patients and may be transient.[140,144,145] In most patients, it is evident 3 months after surgery and resolves by 6 months. Lymphocytic infiltration of the thyroid tissue[146–148] or exposure to iodine[149] appears to increase the risk of hypothyroidism. The presence of TSH-receptor antibodies, however, does not decrease the risk.[150] Postoperative hypothyroidism may also be more likely in patients living in areas of low or marginally adequate iodine intake,[151] in older patients,[137] and in children,[135] or it may be independent of age.[138,152]

Partial thyroidectomy for nontoxic multinodular goiter[153–156] is associated with a much lower risk of postoperative hypothyroidism (<15%) than is subtotal thyroidectomy for Graves' hyperthyroidism.[153,157–160] When postoperative hypothyroidism occurs in patients with nontoxic multinodular goiters, chronic autoimmune thyroiditis is often present in the resected thyroid tissue.[158,159] The risk of hypothyroidism after partial thyroidectomy for toxic multinodular goiter is similarly low.[152,161]

As would be expected, hemithyroidectomy for solitary nodules is not associated with permanent hypothyroidism, although some patients have transient subclinical hypothyroidism postoperatively.[162] Conversely, total thyroidectomy for carcinoma of the thyroid always results in hypothyroidism, even though postoperative ^{131}I scans often reveal some remaining thyroid tissue.

DRUG-INDUCED HYPOTHYROIDISM

Primary hypothyroidism has been implicated as a side-effect of many drugs. Those used to treat hyperthyroidism (propylthiouracil, methimazole, carbimazole, and perchlorate) are discussed in the section on antithyroid drugs in chapter 14 and chapter 53. The antithyroid effects of iodide and other iodine-containing drugs such as amiodarone are discussed in the section on effect of excess iodide in chapter 14.

Lithium

Lithium inhibits thyroidal iodide transport and release of T_4 and T_3 and may also induce chronic autoimmune thyroiditis.[163] All of these actions would be expected to predispose to, if not directly induce, hypothyroidism. In practice, the frequency of hypothyroidism in lithium-treated patients is about 20% to 30%.[164–168] In most patients the hypothyroidism is subclinical, although overt hypothyroidism does occur occasionally.[169–170] The frequency of goiter in lithium-treated patients is approxi-

mately 50%.[149,165,166] The goiter sometimes occurs in the absence of elevated serum TSH concentrations and is typically small and diffuse. Lithium-induced hypothyroidism or goiter usually develops during the first 2 years of therapy, and may or may not persist.[164,171,172]

It is unclear whether lithium is capable of inducing clinically important hypothyroidism in patients without preexisting thyroid disease.[173,174] The prevalence of antithyroid antibodies is higher in hypothyroid lithium-treated patients than in euthyroid lithium-treated patients.[164,170,175] Lithium-induced increases in serum TSH are often transient in patients who do not have antithyroid antibodies.[171] The observation that depressed patients treated with lithium more often have antithyroid antibodies than depressed patients whose therapy does not include lithium also suggests that lithium may directly induce the generation of antithyroid antibodies.[163] Conversely, however, some patients with lithium-induced hypothyroidism do not have goiter or antithyroid antibodies.[165] Regardless of the potential for lithium to induce hypothyroidism in patients with a normal thyroid gland, those patients with subclinical thyroid disease are prone to develop goiter or clinically apparent hypothyroidism when given lithium.

Interferon-α and Interleukin-2

Treatment with interferon-α (IFN) for malignant disease or chronic hepatitis B or C is known to induce various autoantibodies, including, in 10% to 20% of patients, antithyroglobulin, antithyroid peroxidase, and TSH receptor antibodies.[176,177] These antibodies often disappear after discontinuation of treatment. Hypothyroidism, thyrotoxicosis, and the biphasic thyrotoxicosis-hypothyroidism pattern of silent thyroiditis[178] are often associated with the development of IFN-induced thyroid autoimmunity. The presence of thyroid autoimmunity before the initiation of IFN treatment increases the risk of thyroid dysfunction during treatment.[179] The induction of antithyroid antibodies and associated hypothyroidism, thyrotoxicosis, or biphasic thyrotoxicosis-hypothyroidism has also been reported in cancer patients receiving interleukin-2 therapy.[180–184]

Other Drugs

Many other drugs have been reported to cause hypothyroidism in occasional patients.[185] Patients treated with carbamazepine or phenytoin (see section on effects of pharmacologic agents on thyroid hormone metabolism in chap 14) may have biochemical features of secondary hypothyroidism, that is, low serum total and free T_4 concentrations and normal serum TSH concentrations.[186–188] Most of these patients have no other evidence of hypothyroidism,[189–190] but rare cases of hypothyroidism caused by carbamazepine in combination with phenytoin or lithium have been reported.[166,171,192,193]

Aminoglutethimide therapy for seizures, breast carcinoma, or prostate carcinoma causes goiter and hypothyroidism in some patients.[194–197]

Other drugs reported to induce hypothyroidism include sulfonamides,[198–201] sulfonylureas,[202] ethionamide,[203] *p*-aminosalicylic acid,[204] dimercaprol (BAL),[205] phenylbutazone,[206] nicardipine[186,198] and tumor necrosis factor-α.[207] Because of

TABLE 58-2.
Industrial and Environmental Chemicals With Goitrogenic or Antithyroid Effects

Compounds	Humans	Animals	In Vitro
SULFURATED ORGANIC COMPOUNDS*			
Thiocyanate (SCN)	+	+	+
Isothiocyanates	NT	+	+
L-5-vinyl-2-thiooxazolidone (goitrin)†	+	+	+
Disulfides (R-S-S-R)	NT	+	?+
FLAVONOIDS (POLYPHENOLS)†			
Glycosides	NT	+	+
Aglycones	NT	+	+
C-ring fission metabolites (phloroglucinols and phenolic acids)	NT	+	+
POLYHYDROXYPHENOLS AND PHENOL DERIVATIVES†			
Phenol	NT	NT	+
Catechol (1,2-dihydroxybenzene)	NT	NT	+
Resorcinol (1,3-dihydroxybenzene)	+	+	+
Hydroquinone (1,4-dihydroxybenzene)	NT	NT	+
m-Dihydroxyacetophenones	NT	NT	+
2-Methylresorcinol	NT	+	+
5-Methylresorcinol (orcinol)	NT	+	+
4-Methylcatechol	NT	NT	+
Pyrogallic acid (1,2,3-trihydroxybenzene)	NT	+	+
Phloroglucinol (1,3,5-trihydroxybenzene)	NT	+	+
4-Chlororesorcinol	NT	+	+
3-Chloro-4-hydroxybenzoic acid	NT	NT	+
2,4-Dinitrophenol‡	+	+	0
PYRIDINES†			
3-Hydroxypyridine	NT	NT	+
Dihydroxypyridines	NT	+	+
PHTHALATE ESTERS AND METABOLITES†			
Diisobutyl phthalate	NT	NT	0
Dioctyl phthalate	NT	NT	0
o-Phthalic acid	NT	NT	0
m-Phthalic acid	NT	NT	0
3,4-Dihydroxybenzoic acid (DHBA)	NT	NT	+
3,5-Dihydroxybenzoic acid	NT	NT	+
POLYCHLORINATED (PCB) AND POLYBROMINATED (PBB) BIPHENYLS§			
PCBs (Aroclor)	NT	+	NT
PBBs and PBB oxides	+	+	NT
OTHER ORGANOCHLORINES§			
Dichlorodiphenyltrichloroethane (*p,p'*-DDT)	NT	+	NT
Dichlorodiphenyldichloroethane (*p,p'*-DDE) and dieldrin	NT	+	NT
2,3,7,8-Tetrachlorodibenzo-*p*-dioxin (TCDD)	NT	+	NT
POLYCYCLIC AROMATIC HYDROCARBONS (PAH)§			
3,4-Benzpyrene (BaP)	NT	?+	NT
3-Methylcolanthrene (MCA)	NT	+	NT
7,12-Dimethylbenzanthracene (DMBA)	NT	+	NT
INORGANIC ATOMS‖			
Excess iodine	+	+	+
Lithium	+	+	+

*Impairs uptake and retention of inorganic iodide.
†Impairs organification of iodine by its inhibition of thyroid peroxidase.
‡Interferes with protein-binding of serum T_4 and accelerates the disappearance of T_4 from the circulation.
§Enhances biliary losses of thyroid hormones by induction of hepatic microsomal enzymes.
‖Blocks release of thyroid hormones from the thyroid.
NT, not tested; +, some effects; 0, no effect.
Adapted from reference 213.

the very low potential of these drugs for causing hypothyroidism, the more common causes of hypothyroidism should be seriously considered before attributing hypothyroidism to any of these drugs.

INDUSTRIAL AND ENVIRONMENTAL CHEMICALS

A large number of synthetic and naturally occurring compounds other than drugs are known to interfere with thyroid hormone metabolism. Many are goitrogenic and a few may be capable of inducing hypothyroidism under certain circumstances, such as concurrent iodine deficiency or preexisting thyroid disease. The concentrations of resorcinol in the watersheds of coal- and shale-rich regions of Colombia and Kentucky correlated positively with the regional prevalence of goiter.[208] Surveys of people accidentally exposed to polybrominated biphenyls have revealed reductions in serum T_4 or elevations of serum TSH indicative of an antithyroid effect.[209–212] Many other compounds, and their suspected mechanisms of action, are listed in Table 58-2.[213] Several general reviews on this topic have been published.[186,198,214–217]

THYROID ECTOPY

As discussed in the section on congenital hypothyroidism in chapter 85, thyroid dysplasia (ectopy, hypoplasia, or aplasia) is a common cause of congenital hypothyroidism. Essentially all cases of thyroid aplasia and most cases of thyroid ectopy become clinically evident in infancy or childhood. In some patients, however, a lingual thyroid secretes adequate quantities of hormone during childhood but is associated with hypothyroidism in adolescence or adulthood.[218,219]

References

1. DeLange WE, Freling NJM, Molenaar WM, Doorenbos H. Invasive fibrous thyroiditis (Riedel's struma): a manifestation of multifocal fibrosclerosis? A case report with review of the literature. Q J Med 1989;72:709

2. Girod DA, Bigler SA, Coltrera MD. Riedel's thyroiditis: report of a lethal case and review of the literature. Otolaryngol Head Neck Surg 1992;107:591

3. Schwaegerle SM, Bauer TW, Esselstyn CB, Jr. Riedel's thyroiditis. Am J Clin Pathol 1988;90:715

4. Ross DS. Riedel's thyroiditis associated with Hashimoto's thyroiditis. J Endocrinol Invest 1992;15:479

5. Taubenberger JK, Merino MJ, Medeiros LJ. A thyroid biopsy with histologic features of both Riedel's thyroiditis and the fibrosing variant of Hashimoto's thyroiditis. Hum Pathol 1992;23:1072

6. Zimmermann-Belsing T, Feldt-Rasmussen U. Riedel's thyroiditis: an autoimmune or primary fibrotic disease? J Intern Med 1994;235:271

7. al-Hilaly MA, Koshi PD, Nasr AN, Cheryan JK, al-Manee MS. Riedel's thyroiditis. Case report. Acta Chir Scand 1990;156:237

8. Malotte MJ, Chonkich GD, Zuppan CW. Riedel's thyroiditis. Arch Otolaryngol Head Neck Surg 1991;117:214

9. Best TB, Munro RE, Burwell S, Volpe R. Riedel's thyroiditis associated with Hashimoto's thyroiditis, hypoparathyroidism, and retroperitoneal fibrosis. J Endocrinol Invest 1991;14:767

10. Chopra D, Wool MS, Crosson A, Sawin CT. Riedel's struma associated with subacute thyroiditis, hypothyroidism, and hypoparathyroidism. J Clin Endocrinol Metab 1978;46:869

11. McRorie ER, Chalmers J, Campbell IW. Riedel's thyroiditis complicated by hypoparathyroidism and hypothyroidism. Scott Med J 1993;38:27

12. Mitchinson MJ. The pathology of idiopathic retroperitoneal fibrosis. J Clin Pathol 1970;23:681

13. Laitt RD, Hubscher SG, Buckels JA, Darby S, Elias E. Sclerosing cholangitis associated with multifocal fibrosis: a case report. Gut 1992;33:1430

14. Perez-Fontan FJ, Cordido-Carballido F, Pombo-Felipe F, Mosquera-Oses J, Villalba-Martin C. Riedel thyroiditis: US, CT, and MR evaluation. J Comput Assist Tomogr 1993;17:324

15. Brady OH, Hehir DJ, Heffernan SJ. Riedel's thyroiditis—case report and literature review. Ir J Med Sci 1994;163;176

16. Frankenthaler R, Batsakis JG, Suarez PA. Tumefactive fibroinflammatory lesions of the head and neck. Ann Otol Rhinol Laryngol 1993;102:481

17. Almond PS, Matas AJ, Nakhleh RE, et al. Renal transplantation for infantile cystinosis: long-term follow-up. J Pediatr Surg 1993;28:232

18. Ehrich JH, Brodehl, Byrd DI, et al. Renal transplantation in 22 children with nephropathic cystinosis. Pediatr Nephrol 1991; 5:708

19. Schneider JA, Katz B, Melles RB. Update on nephropathic cystinosis. Pediatr Nephrol 1990;4:645

20. Tobias JD. Anaesthetic implications of cystinosis. Can J Anaesth 1993;40:518

21. Vogel DG, Malekzadeh MH, Cornford ME, Schneider JA, Shields WD, Vinters HV. Central nervous system involvement in nephropathic cystinosis. J Neuropathol Exp Neurol 1990;49:591

22. Chan AM, Lynch MJG, Bailey JD, Ezrin C, Fraser D. Hypothyroidism in cystinosis. Am J Med 1970;48:678

23. Theodoropoulos DS, Krasnewich D, Kaiser-Kupfer MI, Gahl WA. Classic nephropathic cystinosis as an adult disease. JAMA 1993; 270:2200

24. Edwards CQ, Kelly TM, Ellwein G, Kushner JP. Thyroid disease in hemochromatosis. Arch Intern Med 1983;143:1890

25. MacDonald RA, Mallory GK. Hemochromatosis and hemosiderosis. Arch Intern Med 1960;105:686

26. Moerman P, Pauwels P, Vandenberghe K, et al. Neonatal haemochromatosis. Histopathology 1990;17:345

27. Schneider BL, Setchell KD, Whitington PF, Neilson KA, Suchy FJ. Delta 4-3-oxosteroid 5 beta-reductase deficiency causing neonatal liver failure and hemochromatosis. J Pediatr 1994; 124:234

28. Oerter KE, Kamp GA, Munson PJ, Nienhuis AW, Cassorla FG, Manasco PK. Multiple hormone deficiencies in children with hemochromatosis. J Clin Endocrinol Metab 1993;76:357

29. Shirota T, Shinoda T, Aizawa T, et al. Primary hypothyroidism and multiple endocrine failure in association with hemochromatosis in a long-term hemodialysis patient. Clin Nephrol 1992; 38:105

30. Nagai H, Takazakura E, Oda H, et al. An autopsy case of pyruvate kinase deficiency anemia associated with severe hemochromatosis. Intern Med 1994;33:56

31. Clemson BS, Miller WR, Luck JC, Feriss JA. Acute myocarditis in fulminant systemic sclerosis. Chest 1992;101:872

32. Horita M, Takahashi N, Seike M, Nasu S, Takaki R. A case of primary biliary cirrhosis associated with Hashimoto's thyroiditis, scleroderm and Sjogren's syndrome. Intern Med 1992; 31:418

33. Schmid AH, Meltzer BR. Psychotic episodes in an elderly woman with an anticentromere-positive scleroderma variant. J Geriatr Psychiatry Neurol 1994;7:93

34. Sheehan NJ, Stanton-King K. Polyautoimmunity in a young woman. Br J Rheumatol 1993;32:254

35. Gordon MB, Klein I, Dekker A, Rodnan GP, Medsger TA. Thyroid disease in progressive systemic sclerosis: increased frequency of glandular fibrosis and hypothyroidism. Ann Intern Med 1981;95:431

36. DeKeyser L, Narhi DC, Furst DE, et al. Thyroid dysfunction in a prospectively followed series of patients with progressive systemic sclerosis. J Endocrinol Invest 1990;13:161

37. Molnar I, Balazs C, Szabo E, Czirjak L. Evaluation of thyroid function and anti-thyroid autoantibodies in systemic sclerosis. Acta Derm Venereol 1992;72:112

38. Bell NH. Endocrine complications of sarcoidosis. Endocrinol Metab Clin North Am 1991;20:645

39. Harach HR, Williams ED. The pathology of granulomatous diseases of the thyroid gland. Sarcoidosis 1990;7:19

40. Winnacker JL, Becker KL, Katz S. Endocrine aspects of sarcoidosis. N Engl J Med 1968;278:483

41. Buckle RM. Sarcoid goitre. Proc R Soc Med 1954;56:611

42. Hemmings IL, Jr, McLean DC. Thyroid involvement in systemic sarcoidosis. J Pediat 1971;78:131

43. Karlish AJ, MacGregor GA. Sarcoidosis, thyroiditis, and Addison's disease. Lancet 1970;2:330

44. Duhra P, Cassar J. Thyroid function tests in amyloid goitre. Postgrad Med J 1990;66:304

45. James PD. Amyloid goitre. J Clin Path 1972;25:683

46. Kennedy JS, Thomson JA, Buchanan WM. Amyloid in the thyroid. Q J Med 1974;43:127

47. Hirota S, Miyamoto M, Kasugai T, Kitamura Y, Morimura Y. Crystalline light-chain deposition and amyloidosis in the thyroid gland and kidneys of a patient with myeloma. Arch Pathol Lab Med 1990;114:429

48. Greenstein AJ, Sachar DB, Panday AK, et al. Amyloidosis and inflammatory bowel disease. A 50-year experience with 25 patients. Medicine 1992;71:261

49. Moriuchi A, Yokoyama S, Kashima K, Andoh T, Nakayama I, Noguchi S. Localized primary amyloid tumor of the thyroid developing in the course of Hashimoto's thyroiditis. Acta Pathol Jpn 1992;42:210

50. Sinha SN, Sengupta SK. Surgical thyroid disease in Papua New Guinea. Aust N Z J Surg 1993;63:878

51. Butler SL, Oertel YC. Lipomas of anterior neck simulating thyroid nodules: diagnosis by fine-needle aspiration. Diagn Cytopathol 1992;8:528

52. el Reshaid K, al Tamami M, Johny KV, Madda JP, Hakim A. Amyloidosis of the thyroid gland: role of ultrasonography. J Clin Ultrasound 1994;22:239

53. Mache CJ, Schwingshandl J, Riccabona M, et al. Ultrasound and MRI findings in a case of childhood amyloid goiter. Pediatr Radiol 1993;23:565

54. Perez-Fontan FJ, Mosquera-Oses J, Pombo-Felipe F, Rodriguez-Sanchez I, Arnaiz-Pena S. Amyloid goiter in a child—US, CT and MR evaluation. Pediatr Radiol 1992;22:393

55. Alves IL, Divino CM, Schussler GC, et al. Thyroxine binding in a TTR Met 119 kindred. J Clin Endocrinol Metab 1993;77:484

56. Takahashi K, Yi S, Kimura Y, Araki S. Familial amyloidotic polyneuropathy type 1 in Kumamoto, Japan: a clinicopathologic, histochemical, immunohistochemical, and ultrastructural study. Hum Pathol 1991;22:519

57. Fukuzawa M, Maejima T, Sano K, Ito M, Hotchi M, Muramatsu A. Immunohistochemical, electron microscopic, and immunoelectron microscopic features of plasmacytoma of the thyroid with amyloid disposition. Ultrastruct Pathol 1993;17:681

58. Loeffler KU, Edward DP, Tso MO. An immunohistochemical study of gelsolin immunoreactivity in corneal amyloidosis. Am J Ophthalmol 1992;113:546

59. Maury CP. Immunohistochemical localization of amyloid in Finnish hereditary amyloidosis with antibodies to gelsolin peptides. Lab Invest 1991;64:400

60. Alexander GM, Dieppe, PA, Doherty M, et al. Pyrophosphate arthropathy: a study of metabolic associations and laboratory data. Ann Rheum Dis 1982;41:377

61. Dorwart BB, Schumacher HR. Joint effusions, chondrocalcinosis and other rheumatic manifestations in hypothyroidism. Am J Med 1975;59:780

62. Komatireddy GR, Ellman MH, Brown NL. Lack of association between hypothyroidism and chondrocalcinosis. J Rheumatol 1989;16:807

63. Smith MD. Lack of association between hypothyroidism and chondrocalcinosis. J Rheumatol 1990;17:272

64. Visinoni RA, Ferraz MB, Furlanetto RP, Fernandes AR, Oliveira HC, Atra E. Hypothyroidism and chondrocalcinosis: new evidence for lack of association between the 2 pathologies. J Rheumatol 1993;20:1991

65. Jones AC, Chuck AJ, Arie EA, Green DJ, Doherty M. Diseases associated with calcium pyrophosphate deposition disease. Semin Arthritis Rheum 1992;22:188

66. Job-Deslandre C, Menkas CJ, Guinot M, Luton JP. Does hypothyroidism increase the prevalence of chondrocalcinosis? Br J Rheumatol 1993;32:197

67. Behar RA, Hoppe RT. Radiation therapy in the management of bulky mediastinal Hodgkin's disease. Cancer 1990;66:75

68. Brusamolino E, Lazzarino M, Orlandi E, et al. Early-stage Hodgkin's disease: long-term results with radiotherapy alone or combined radiotherapy and chemotherapy. Ann Oncol 1994; 5(Suppl 2):101

69. DeGroot LJ. Effects of irradiation on the thyroid gland. Endocrinol Metab Clin North Am 1993;22:607

70. Hubbard SM, Longo DL. Treatment-related morbidity in patients with lymphoma. Curr Opin Oncol 1991;3:852

71. Peerboom PF, Hassink EA, Melkert R, DeWit L, Nooijen WJ, Bruning PF. Thyroid function 10–18 years after mantle field irradiation for Hodgkin's disease. Eur J Cancer 1992; 28A:1716

72. Constine LS, Donaldson SS, McDougall IR, Cox RS, Link MP, Kaplan HS. Thyroid dysfunction after radiotherapy in children with Hodgkin's disease. Cancer 1984;53:878

73. Hancock SL, Cox RS, McDougall IR. Thyroid diseases after treatment of Hodgkin's disease. N Engl J Med 1991;325:599

74. Kabadi UM. `Subclinical hypothyroidism'. Natural course of the syndrome during a prolonged follow-up study. Arch Intern Med 1993;153:957

75. Shafer RB, Nuttall FQ, Pollak K, Kuisk, H. Thyroid function after radiation and surgery for head and neck cancer. Arch Intern Med 1975;135:843

76. Nelson DF, Reddy KV, O'Mara RE, Rubin P. Thyroid abnormalities following neck irradiation for Hodgkin's disease. Cancer 1978;42:2553

77. Schimpff SC, Diggs CH, Wiswell JG, Salvatore PC, Wiernik PH. Radiation-related thyroid dysfunction: implications for the treatment of Hodgkin's disease. Ann Intern Med 1980;92:91

78. Shalet SM, Rosenstock JD, Beardwell CG, Pearson D, Morris Jones PH. Thyroid dysfunction following external irradiation to the neck for Hodgkin's disease in childhood. Clin Radiol 1977;28:511

79. Smith RE Jr, Adler RA, Clark P, Brinck-Johnsen T, Tulloh ME, Colton T. Thyroid function after mantle irradiation in Hodgkin's disease. JAMA 1981;245:46

80. Glatstein E, McHardy-Young S, Brast N, Eltringham JR, Kriss JP. Alterations in serum thyrotropin (TSH) and thyroid function following radiotherapy in patients with malignant lymphoma. J Clin Endocrinol 1971;32:833

81. deVathaire F, Fragu P, Francois P, et al. Long-term effects on the thyroid of irradiation for skin angiomas in childhood. Radiat Res 1993;133:381

82. Kaplan MM, Garnick MB, Gelber R, et al. Risk factors for thyroid abnormalities after neck irradiation for childhood cancer. Am J Med 1983;74:272

83. Marcial-Vega VA, Order SE, Lastner G, Cole PD, LaFrance N, O'Neill M. Prevention of hypothyroidism related to mantle irradiation for Hodgkin's disease: preparative phantom study. Int J Radiat Oncol Biol Phys 1990;18:613

84. Pasqualini T, Iorcansky S, Gruneiro L, et al. Thyroid dysfunction in Hodgkin's disease. Cancer 1989;63:335

85. Tamura K, Shimaoka K, Friedman M. Thyroid abnormalities associated with treatment of malignant lymphoma. Cancer 1981;47:2704

86. Devney RB, Sklar CA, Nesbit ME, Jr, et al. Serial thyroid function measurements in children with Hodgkin disease. J Pediatr 1984;105:223

87. Feyerabent T, Kapp B, Richter E, Becker W, Reiners C. Incidence of hypothyroidism after irradiation of the neck with special reference to lymphoma patients. A retrospective and prospective analysis. Acta Oncol 1990;29:597

88. Brownlie BE, Fitzharris BM, Abdelaal AS, Hay NM, Bremner JM, Hamer JW. Primary thyroid lymphoma: clinical features, treatment and outcome: a report of 8 cases. N Z Med J 1994; 107:301

89. Matsuzuka F, Miyauchi A, Katayama S, et al. Clinical aspects of primary thyroid lymphoma: diagnosis and treatment based on our experience of 119 cases. Thyroid 1993;3:93

90. Scholefield JH, Quayle AR, Harris SC, Talbot CH. Primary lymphoma of the thyroid, the association with Hashimoto's thyroiditis. Eur J Surg Oncol 1992;18:89

91. Gaspar LE, Dawson DJ, Tilley-Gulliford SA, Banerjee P. Medulloblastoma: long-term follow-up of patients treated with electron irradiation of the spinal field. Radiology 1991;180:867

92. Livesey EA, Brook CGD. Thyroid dysfunction after radiotherapy and chemotherapy of brain tumours. Arch Dis Chld 1989;64:593

93. Sklar CA, Kim TH, Ramsay NKC. Thyroid dysfunction among long-term survivors of bone marrow transplantation. Am J Med 1982;73:688

94. Tami TA, Gomez P, Parker GS, Gupta MB, Frassica DA. Thyroid dysfunction after radiation therapy in head and neck cancer patients. Am J Otolaryngol 1992; 13:357

95. Zamboni C, Olmi P, Cellai E, Forti G. Endocrine status in 29 patients treated by curative radiation therapy for nasopharyngeal carcinoma. Tumori 1991;77:44

96. Grande C. Hypothyroidism following radiotherapy for head and neck cancer: multivariate analysis of risk factors. Radiother Oncol 1992;25:31

97. Liening DA, Duncan NO, Blakeslee DB, Smith DB. Hypothyroidism following radiotherapy for head and neck cancer. Otolaryngol Head Neck Surg 1990;103:10

98. Buisset E, Leclerc L, Lefebvre JL, et al. Hypothyroidism following combined treatment for hypopharyngeal and laryngeal carcinoma. Am J Surg 1991;162:345

99. Weissler MC, Berry BW. Thyroid-stimulating hormone levels after radiotherapy and combined therapy for head and neck cancer. Head Neck 1991;13:420

100. Pasqualini T, McCalla J, Berg S, et al. Subtle primary hypothyroidism in patients treated for acute lymphoblastic leukemia. Acta Endocrinol 1991;124:375

101. Carlson K, Lonnerholm G, Smedmyr B, Oberg G, Simonsson B. Thyroid function after autologous bone marrow transplantation. Bone Marrow Transplant 1992;10:123

102. Locatelli F, Giorgiani G, Pession A, Bozzola M. Late effects in children after bone marrow transplantation: a review. Haematologica 1993;78:319

103. Thomas BC, Stanhope R, Plowman PN, Leiper AD. Endocrine function following single fraction and fractionated total body irradiation for bone marrow transplantation in childhood. Acta Endocrinol 1993;128:508

104. Katsanis E, Shapiro RS, Robison LL, et al. Thyroid dysfunction following bone marrow transplantation: long-term follow-up of 80 pediatric patients. Bone Marrow Transplant 1990;5:335

105. Berglund J, Christensen SB, Dymling JF, Hallengren B. The incidence of recurrence and hypothyroidism following treatment with antithyroid drugs, surgery or radioiodine in all patients with thyrotoxicosis in Malmo during the period 1970–1974. J Intern Med 1991;229:435

106. Bertelsen J, Herskind AM, Sprogoe-Jakobsen U, Hegedus L. Is standard 555 MBq ^{131}I-therapy of hyperthyroidism ablative? Thyroidol Clin Exp 1992;4:103

107. Cunnien AJ, Hay ID, Gorman CA, Offord KP, Scanlon PW. Radioiodine-induced hypothyroidism in Graves' disease: factors associated with the increasing incidence. J Nucl Med 1982; 23:978

108. Nofal MM, Beierwaltes WH, Patno ME. Treatment of hyperthyroidism with sodium iodide I-131. A 16-year experience. JAMA 1966;197:605

109. Roudebush CP, Hoye KE, DeGroot LJ. Compensated low-dose ^{131}I therapy of Graves' disease. Ann Intern Med 1977;87:441

110. Sridama V, McCormick M, Kaplan EL, Fauchet R, DeGroot LJ. Long-term follow-up study of compensated low-dose ^{131}I therapy for Graves' disease. N Engl J Med 1984;311:426

111. Bronsky D, Kiamko RT, Waldstein SS. Posttherapeutic myxedema. Arch Intern Med 1968;121:113

112. Dunn JT, Chapman EM. Rising incidence of hypothyroidism after radioactive-iodine therapy in thyrotoxicosis. N Engl J Med 1964;271:1037

113. Greig WR. Radioactive iodine therapy for thyrotoxicosis. Br J Surg 1973;60:758

114. Holm L-E. Changing annual incidence of hypothyroidism after iodine-131 therapy for hyperthyroidism, 1951-1975. J Nucl Med 1982;23:108

115. Holm L-E, Lundell G, Israelsson A, Dahlqvist I. Incidence of hypothyroidism occurring long after iodine-131 therapy for hyperthyroidism. J Nucl Med 1982;23:103

116. Bazzi MN, Bagchi N. Adjunctive treatment with propylthiouracil or iodine following radioiodine therapy for Graves' disease. Thyroid 1993;3:269

117. Clerc J, Izembart M, Dagousset F, et al. Influence of dose selection on absorbed dose profiles in radioiodine treatment of diffuse toxic goiters in patients receiving or not receiving carbimazole. J Nucl Med 1993;34:387

118. DeGroot LJ, Manglabruks A, McCormick M. Comparison of RA ^{131}I treatment protocols for Graves' disease. J Endocrinol Invest 1990;13:111

119. Gamstedt A, Karlsson A. Pretreatment with betamethasone of patients with Graves' disease given radioiodine therapy: thyroid autoantibody responses and outcome of therapy. J Clin Endocrinol Metab 1991;73:125

120. Kung AW, Pun KK, Lam KS, Choi P, Wang C, Yeung RT. Long-term results following ^{131}I treatment for Graves' disease in Hong Kong Chinese—discriminant factors predicting hypothyroidism. Q J Med 1990;76:961

121. Hagen GA, Ouellette RP, Chapman EM. Comparison of high and low dosage levels of ^{131}I in the treatment of thyrotoxicosis. N Engl J Med 1967;277:559

122. Peden NR, Hart IR. The early development of transient and permanent hypothyroidism following radioiodine therapy for hyperthyroid Graves' disease. Can Med Assoc J 1984;130:1141

123. Huysmans DA, Hermus AR, Corstens FH, Kloppenborg PW. Long-term results of two schedules of radioiodine treatment for toxic multinodular goitre. Eur J Nucl Med 1993;20:1056

124. Huysmans DA, Corstens FH, Kloppenborg PW. Long-term follow-up in toxic solitary autonomous thyroid nodules treated with radioactive iodine. J Nucl Med 1991;32:27

125. Jarlov AE, Faber J, Hegedus L, Hansen JM. Subtle changes in serum thyrotrophin (TSH) and sex-hormone-binding globulin (SHBG) levels during long-term follow-up after radioactive iodine in multinodular non-toxic goitre. Clin Endocrinol 1992;37:335

126. Nygaard B, Hegedus L, Gervil M, Hjalgrim H, Soe-Jensen P, Hansen JM. Radioiodine treatment of multinodular non-toxic goitre. BMJ 1993;307:828

127. Verelst J, Bonnyns M, Glinoer D. Radioiodine therapy in voluminous multinodular non-toxic goitre. Acta Endocrinol 1990;18:613

128. Wiersinga WM. Determinants of outcome in sporadic nontoxic goiter. Thyroidol Clin Exp 1992;4:41

129. Csaky G, Balazs G, Bako G, Ilyes I, Kalman K, Szabo J. Late results of thyroid surgery for hyperthyroidism performed in childhood. Prog Pediatr Surg 1991;26:31

130. Hedley AJ, Flemming CJ, Chesters MI, Michie W, Crooks J. Surgical treatment of thyrotoxicosis. BMJ 1970;1:519

131. Kahky MP, Weber RS. Complications of surgery of the thyroid and parathyroid glands. Surg Clin North Am 1993;73:307

132. Leese GP, Jung RT, Scott A, Waugh N, Browning MC. Long term follow-up of treated hyperthyroid and hypothyroid patients. Health Bull Edinb 1993;51:177

133. Sugrue D. McEvoy M, Feely J, Drury MI. Hyperthyroidism in the land of Graves: results of treatment by surgery, radio-iodine and carbimazole in 837 cases. Q J Med 1980;49:51

134. Taylor JD, Radcliffe SN, Basu PK, Atkins P. Iodine therapy for thyroidectomy patients exhibiting high thyroid-stimulating hormone values: a randomised study. Ann R Coll Surg Engl 1993;75:168

135. Farnell MB, van Heerden JA, McConahey WM, Carpenter HA, Wolff LH, Jr. Hypothyroidism after thyroidectomy for Graves' disease. Am J Surg 1981;142:535

136. Kasuga Y, Sugenoya A, Kobayashi S, et al. Clinical evaluation of the response to surgical treatment of Graves' disease. Surg Gynecol Obstet 1990;170:327

137. Maier WP, Derrick BM, Marks AD, Channick BJ, Au FC, Caswell HT. Long-term follow-up of patients with Graves' disease treated by subtotal thyroidectomy. Am J Surg 1984;147:266

138. Michie W, Pegg CAS, Bewsher PD. Prediction of hypothyroidism after partial thyroidectomy for thyrotoxicosis. BMJ 1972;1:13

139. Patwardhan NA, Moront M, Rao S, Rossi S, Braverman LE. Surgery still has a role in Graves' hyperthyroidism. Surgery 1993;114:1108

140. Toft AD, Irvine WJ, Sinclair I, McIntosh D, Seth J, Cameron EHD. Thyroid function after surgical treatment of thyrotoxicosis. N Engl J Med 1978;298:643

141. Andaker L, Johansson K, Smeds S, Lennquist S. Surgery for hyperthyroidism: hemithyroidectomy plus contralateral resection or bilateral resection? A prospective randomized study of postoperative complications and long-term results. World J Surg 1992;16:765

142. Menegaux F, Ruprecht T, Chigot JP. The surgical treatment of Graves' disease. Surg Gynecol Obstet 1993;176:277

143. Olsen WR, Nishiyama RH, Graber LW. Thyroidectomy for hyperthyroidism. Arch Surg 1970;101:175

144. Kuma K, Matsuzuka F, Kobayashi A, et al. Natural course of Graves' disease after subtotal thyroidectomy and management of patients with postoperative thyroid dysfunction. Am J Med Sci 1991;302:8

145. Sugino K, Mimura T, Toshima K, et al. Follow-up evaluation of patients with Graves' disease treated by subtotal thyroidectomy and risk factor analysis for post-operative thyroid dysfunction. J Endocrinol Invest 1993;16:195

146. Green M, Wilson GM. Thyrotoxicosis treated by surgery or iodine-131. With special reference to development of hypothyroidism. BMJ 1964;1:1005

147. Okamoto T, Fujimoto Y, Obara T, Ito Y, Aiba M. Retrospective analysis of prognostic factors affecting the thyroid functional status after subtotal thyroidectomy for Graves' disease. World J Surg 1992;16:690

148. Van Welsum M, Feltkamp TE, De Vries MJ, Doctor R, Van Zijl J, Hennemann G. Hypothyroidism after thyroidectomy for Graves' disease: a search for an explanation. BMJ 1974;4:755

149. Clark OH, Moser C, Cavalierri RR, Hammond ME, Ingbar SH. Iodide sensitivity in the hemithyroidectomized patient. In: Robbins J, Braverman LE, eds. Thyroid research. New York: American Elsevier, 1976:477

150. Mori Y, Matoba N, Miura S, Sakai N, Taira Y. Clinical course and thyroid stimulating hormone (TSH) receptor antibodies during surgical treatment of Graves' disease. World J Surg 1992;16:647

151. Thjodleifsson B, Hedley AJ, Donald D, et al. Outcome of subtotal thyroidectomy for thyrotoxicosis in Iceland and northeast Scotland. Clin Endocrinol 1977;7:367

152. Palestini N. Valori MR, Carlin R, Iannucci P. Mortality, morbidity and long-term results in surgically treated hyperthyroid patients. Acta Chir Scand 1985;151:509

153. Geerdsen JP, Frolund L. Recurrence of nontoxic goitre with and without postoperative thyroxine medication. Clin Endocrinol 1984;21:529

154. Geerdsen JP, Frolund L. Thyroid function after surgical treatment of nontoxic goitre. Acta Med Scand 1986;220:341

155. Geerdsen JP, Hee P. Nontoxic goitre. I. Surgical complications and longterm prognosis. Acta Chir Scand 1982;148:221

156. Hegedus L, Hansen JM, Veiergang D, Karstrup S. Does prophylactic thyroxine treatment after operation for non-toxic goitre influence thyroid size? BMJ 1987;294:801

157. Berghout A, Wiersinga WM, Drexhage HA, et al. The long-term outcome of thyroidectomy for sporadic non-toxic goitre. Clin Endocrinol 1989;31:193

158. Berglund J, Bondeson L, Christensen SB, Larsson AS, Tibblin S. Indications for thyroxine therapy after surgery for nontoxic benign goitre. Acta Chir Scand 1990;156:433

159. Berglund J, Bondeson L, Christensen SB, Tibblin S. The influence of different degrees of chronic lymphocytic thyroiditis on thyroid function after surgery for benign, non-toxic goitre. Eur J Surg 1991;157:257

160. Geerdsen JP, Hee P. Nontoxic goitre. II. A study of the pituitary-thyroid axis in 14 recurrent cases. Acta Chir Scand 1982;148:225

161. Blichert-Toft M, Jorgensen SJ, Hansen JB, Watt-Boolsen S, Christiansen C, Ibsen J. Long-term observation of thyroid function after surgical treatment of thyrotoxicosis. Acta Chir Scand 1977;143:221

162. Matte R, Ste-Marie LG, Comtois R, et al. The pituitary-thyroid axis after hemithyroidectomy in euthyroid man. J Clin Endocrinol Metab 1981;53:377

163. Wilson R, McKillop JH, Crocket GT, et al. The effect of lithium therapy on parameters thought to be involved in the development of autoimmune thyroid disease. Clin Endocrinol 1991;34:357

164. Emerson CH, Dyson WL, Utiger RD. Serum thyrotropin and thyroxine concentrations in patients receiving lithium carbonate. J Clin Endocrinol Metab 1973;36:338

165. Perrild H, Hegedus L, Baastrup PC, Kayser L, Kastberg S. Thyroid function and ultrasonically determined thyroid size in patients receiving long-term lithium treatment. Am J Psychiatry 1990;147:1518

166. Bocchetta A, Bernardi F, Pedditzi M, et al. Thyroid abnormalities during lithium treatment. Acta Psychiatr Scand 1991;83:193

167. Lee S, Chow CC, Wing YK, Shek CC. Thyroid abnormalities during chronic lithium treatment in Hong Kong Chinese: a controlled study. J Affect Disord 1992;26:173

168. Vincent A, Baruch P, Vincent P. Early onset of lithium-associated hypothyroidism. J Psychiatry Neurosci 1993;18:74

169. Schou M. Lithium prophylaxis: myths and realities. Am J Psychiatry 1989;146:573

170. Lindstedt G, Nilsson L-A, Walinder J, Skott A, Ohman R. On the prevalence, diagnosis and management of lithium-induced hypothyroidism in psychiatric patients. Br J Psychiatry 1977;130:452

171. Bocchetta A, Bernardi F, Burrai C, et al. The course of thyroid abnormalities during lithium treatment: a two-year follow-up study. Acta Psychiatr Scand 1992;86:38

172. Bartalena L, Pellegrini L, Meschi M, et al. Evaluation of thyroid function in patients with rapid-cycling and non-rapid-cycling bipolar disorder. Psychiatry Res 1990;34:13

173. Bagchi N, Brown TR, Mack RE. Studies on the mechanism of inhibition of thyroid function by lithium. Biochim Biophys Acta 1978;542:163

174. Berens SC, Bernstein RS, Robbins J, Wolff J. Antithyroid effects of lithium. J Clin Invest 1970;49:1357

175. Myers DH, Carter RA, Burns BH, Armond A, Hussain SB, Chengapa VK. A prospective study of the effects of lithium on thyroid function and on the prevalence of antithyroid antibodies. Psychol Med 1985;15:55

176. Baudin E, Marcellin P, Pouteau M, et al. Reversibility of thyroid dysfunction induced by recombinant alpha interferon in chronic hepatitis C. Clin Endocrinol 1993;39:657

177. Gisslinger H, Gilly B, Woloszczuk W, et al. Thyroid autoimmunity and hypothyroidism during long-term treatment with recombinant interferon-alpha. Clin Exp Immunol 1992;90:363

178. Vassilopoulou-Sellin R, Sella A, Dexeus FH, Theriault RL, Pololoff DA. Acute thyroid dysfunction (thyroiditis) after therapy with interleukin-2. Horm Metab Res 1992;24:434

179. Watanabe U, Hashimoto E, Hisamitsu T, Obata H, Hayashi N. The risk factor for development of thyroid disease during interferon-alpha therapy for chronic hepatitis C. Am J Gastroenterol 1994;89:399

180. Schwartzentruber DJ, White DE, Zweig MH, Weintraub BD, Rosenberg SA. Thyroid dysfunction associated with immunotherapy for patients with cancer. Cancer 1991;68:2384

181. Kroemer G, Francese C, Martinez C. The role of interleukin 2 in the development of autoimmune thyroiditis. Int Rev Immunol 1992;9:107

182. Vial T, Descotes J. Clinical toxicity of interleukin-2. Drug Saf 1992;7:417

183. Vialettes B, Guillerand MA, Viens P, et al. Incidence rate and risk factors for thyroid dysfunction during recombinant interleukin-2 therapy in advanced malignancies. Acta Endocrinol 1993;129:31

184. Weijl NI, Van der Harst D, Brand A, et al. Hypothyroidism during immunotherapy with interleukin-2 is associated with antithyroid antibodies and response to treatment. J Clin Oncol 1993;11:1376

185. Kaplan MM. Interactions between drugs and thyroid hormones. Thyroid Today 1981;4:1

186. Curran PG, DeGroot LJ. The effect of hepatic enzyme-inducing drugs on thyroid hormones and the thyroid gland. Endocr Rev 1991;12:135

187. Liewendahl K, Tikanoja S, Helenius T, Majuri H. Free thyroxin and free triiodothyronine as measured by equilibrium dialysis and analog radioimmunoassay in serum of patients taking phenytoin and carbamazepine. Clin Chem 1985;31:1993

188. Surks MI, Smith PJ. Multiple effects of 5,5'-diphenylhydantoin on the thyroid hormone system. Endocr Rev 1984;5:514

189. Herman R, Obarzanek E, Mikalauskas KM, Post RM, Jimerson DC. The effects of carbamazepine on resting metabolic rate and thyroid function in depressed patients. Biol Psychiatry 1991;29:779

190. Isojarvi JI, Airaksinen KE, Repo M, Pakarinen AJ, Salmela P, Myllyla VV. Carbamazepine, serum thyroid hormones and myocardial function in epileptic patients. J Neurol Neurosurg Psychiatry 1993;56:710

191. Aanderud S, Strandjord RE. Hypothyroidism induced by antiepileptic therapy. Acta Neurol Scand 1980;61:330

192. Strandjord RE, Aanderud S, Myking OL, Johannessen SI. Influence of carbamazepine on serum thyroxine and triiodothyronine in patients with epilepsy. Acta Neurol Scandinav 1981;63:111

193. Kramlinger KG, Post RM. Addition of lithium carbonate to carbamazepine: hematological and thyroid effects. Am J Psychiatry 1990;147:615

194. Pittman JA, Brown RW. Antithyroid and antiadrenocortical activity of aminoglutethimide. J Clin Endocrinol Metab 1966;26:1014

195. Rallison ML, Kumagai LF, Tyler FH. Goitrous hypothyroidism induced by amino-glutethimide, anticonvulsant drug. J Clin Endocr 1967;27:265

196. Dowsett M, Mehta A, Cantwell BM, Harris AL. Low-dose aminoglutethimide in postmenopausal breast cancer: effects on adrenal and thyroid hormone secretion. Eur J Cancer 1991;27:846

197. Figg WD, Thibault A, Sartor AO, et al. Hypothyroidism associated with aminoglutethimide in patients with prostate cancer. Arch Intern Med 1994;154:1023

198. Capen CC. Pathophysiology of chemical injury of the thyroid gland. Toxicol Lett 1992;64/65:381

199. Doerge DR, Decker CJ. Inhibition of peroxidase-catalyzed reactions by arylamines: mechanism for the anti-thyroid action of sulfamethazine. Chem Res Toxicol 1994;7:164

200. Gupta A, Eggo MC, Uetrecht JP, et al. Drug-induced hypothyroidism: the thyroid as a target organ in hypersensitivity reactions to anticonvulsants and sulfonamides. Clin Pharmacol Ther 1992;51:56

201. Krieger DT, Moses A, Ziffer H, Gabrilove JL, Soffer LJ. Effect of acetazoleamide on thyroid metabolism. Am J Physiol 1959;196:291

202. Hunton RB, Wells MV, Skipper EW. Hypothyroidism in diabetics treated with sulphonylurea. Lancet 1965;2:449

203. Drucker D, Eggo MC, Salit IE, Burrow GN. Ethionamide-induced goitrous hypothyroidism. Ann Intern Med 1984;100:837

204. Christensen K. The metabolic effect of p-aminosalicylic acid. Acta Endocrinol 1959;31:608

205. Current JV, Hales IB, Dobyns BM. The effect of 2,3-dimercaptopropanol (BAL) on thyroid function. J Clin Endocrinol 1960;20:13

206. Linsk JA, Paton BC, Persky M, Isaacs M, Kupperman HS. The effect of phenylbutazone and a related analogue (G25671) upon thyroid function. J Clin Endocrinol 1957;17:416

207. Miyakoshi H, Ohsawa K, Yokoyama H, Nagai Y, Bando YIY, Kobayashi K. Exacerbation of hypothyroidism following tumor necrosis factor-α infusion. Intern Med 1992;31:200

208. Jolley RL, Gaitan E, Douglas EC, Felker LK. Identification of organic pollutants in drinking waters from areas with endemic thyroid disorders and potential pollutants of drinking water sources associated with coal processing areas. Am Chem Soc Environ Chem 1986;26:59

209. Bahn AK, Mills JL, Snyder PJ, et al. Hypothyroidism in workers exposed to polybrominated biphenyls. N Engl J Med 1980;302:31

210. Barsano CP. Polyhalogenated and polycyclic aromatic hydrocarbons. In: Gaitan E, ed. Environmental goitrogenesis. Boca Raton: CRC Press, 1989;115

211. Kreiss K, Roberts C, Humphreys HEB. Serial PBB levels, PCB levels, and clinical chemistries in Michigan's PBB cohort. Arch Environ Health 1982;37:141

212. Stross JK. Hypothyroidism and polybrominated biphenyls. N Engl J Med 1980;302:1421

213. Gaitan E, Cooksey RC. General concepts of environmental goitrogenesis. In: Gaitan E, ed. Environmental goitrogenesis. Boca Raton: CRC Press, 1989:3

214. Barsano CP. Environmental factors altering thyroid function and their assessment. Environ Health Perspect 1981;38:71

215. Barsano CP, Thomas JA. Endocrine disorders of occupational and environmental origin. In: Shusterman DJ, Blanc PD, eds. Occupational medicine: state of the art reviews—unusual occupational diseases. Philadelphia: Hanley & Belfus, 1992:479

216. Gaitan E, ed. Environmental goitrogenesis. Boca Raton: CRC Press, 1989

217. Gaitan E, Cooksey RC, Legan J, Cruse JM, Lindsay RH, Hill J. Antithyroid and goitrogenic effects of coal-water extracts from iodine-sufficient goiter areas. Thyroid 1993; 3:49

218. Ahuja MMS, Chopra IJ, Sridhar CB. Sporadic cretinism and juvenile hypothyroidism. Metabolism 1969;18:488

219. Neinas FW, Gorman CA, Devine KD, Woolner LB. Lingual thyroid. Clinical characteristics of 15 cases. Ann Intern Med 1973;79:205

Werner and Ingbar's The Thyroid, Seventh Edition,
edited by Lewis E. Braverman and Robert D. Utiger.
Lippincott–Raven Publishers, Philadelphia, © 1996

59

Central Hypothyroidism

Enio Martino

Luigi Bartalena

Giovanni Faglia

Aldo Pinchera

Central hypothyroidism is defined as reduced thyroid hormone secretion due to deficient stimulation of an intrinsically normal thyroid gland by thyroid-stimulating hormone (thyrotropin; TSH). This condition can be the consequence of an anatomic or functional disorder of the pituitary gland, the hypothalamus, or both. Since in both cases the final result is deficient TSH secretion, the formerly employed terms *secondary* hypothyroidism of pituitary origin, and *tertiary* hypothyroidism of hypothalamic origin due to absent or insufficient TSH stimulation by TSH-releasing hormone (TRH), are no longer recommended. In addition, a clear-cut distinction between pituitary and hypothalamic forms of central hypothyroidism cannot easily be made on the basis of the TSH response to exogenous TRH administration, as suggested in the past. It had been stated that a rise in serum TSH after TRH administration is suggestive of hypothalamic hypothyroidism, while the lack of a TSH response suggests pituitary hypothyroidism. It is now established that considerable overlap exists between the profile of TSH responses to TRH in the two conditions. Finally, TSH secretion can be impaired not only quantitatively, but also qualitatively, due to secretion of a TSH that is biologically inactive.[1-3] For these reasons, the term *central hypothyroidism* is now preferred because it includes both quantitative and qualitative abnormalities of TSH secretion, irrespective of the hypothalamic or pituitary origin of the disorder.

Central hypothyroidism is rarely an isolated defect, most often being part of a more complex deficit in pituitary hormone secretion, *hypopituitarism*, which can also affect gonadotropin, adrenocorticotropin (ACTH), and growth hormone (GH) secretion. In this respect, hypothyroidism may be mild and overshadowed by the clinical features of other pituitary hormone defects, or may be so severe as to dominate the clinical picture. Isolated TSH deficiency can occur as an autosomal recessive trait due to a TSH-β subunit gene abnormality.[4-6]

The precise prevalence of central hypothyroidism is unknown, but it is much rarer than primary hypothyroidism. The latter is found in approximately 1% to 2% of the general population. Based on the prevalence of pituitary tumors, central hypothyroidism has indirectly been estimated to occur in 0.0002% of the general population,[7] but the true prevalence is probably higher, since pituitary tumors are not the only cause of this disorder. In our experience, the frequency of central hypothyroidism in the general population is approximately 0.005%. Central hypothyroidism is equally distributed among the sexes, with an age peak in childhood for the idiopathic and genetic forms, and between 30 to 60 years of age for cases due to lesions of the pituitary and hypothalamus.

Although central hypothyroidism is rare, from a clinical standpoint it is important to recognize because it is often associated with defects of other pituitary hormones, and correction of hypothyroidism by L-thyroxine (L-T$_4$) alone can precipitate acute adrenocortical insufficiency.

ETIOLOGY

Table 59-1 illustrates the different causes of central hypothyroidism, which are subdivided according to the main location of the lesion. Because several of these conditions can affect both the hypothalamus and the pituitary either simultaneously or sequentially, it is often impossible to locate the precise

TABLE 59-1.
Causes of Central Hypothyroidism

PITUITARY DISORDERS	HYPOTHALAMIC DISORDERS
Tumors	Tumors
Pituitary adenomas (functioning and nonfunctioning)	Suprasellar extension of pituitary adenomas
Craniopharyngiomas	Craniopharyngiomas
Meningiomas	Meningiomas
Dysgerminomas	Gliomas and other brain tumors
Metastatic tumors	Metastatic tumors
Ischemic necrosis	Traumas
Postpartum (Sheehan's syndrome)	Ischemic necrosis
Severe shock	Iatrogenic
Diabetes mellitus	Radiation therapy
Aneurysm of internal carotid artery	Surgery
Iatrogenic	Infections
Radiation therapy	Abscesses
Surgery	Tuberculosis
Infectious diseases	Syphilis
Abscesses	Toxoplasmosis
Tuberculosis	Sarcoidosis
Syphilis	Histiocytosis
Toxoplasmosis	Congenital malformations
Sarcoidosis	Basal encephalocele
Histiocytosis (Hand-Schüller-Christian)	Septooptic dysplasia
Hemosiderosis	Idiopathic
Chronic lymphocytic hypophysitis	
Pituitary aplasia or hypoplasia	
Genetic abnormality in TSH synthesis	
Idiopathic	

anatomic site of the hormone deficiency. For example, in the presence of a large pituitary tumor, an intrinsic deficiency of the pituitary thyrotrophs can be associated with interruption of the hypothalamic TRH input.

Pituitary adenoma is the most frequent cause of central hypothyroidism, accounting for more than half the cases.[8] The tumor may be nonfunctioning or secrete GH, prolactin, or both, and less frequently, ACTH or gonadotropins. Varying degrees of hypopituitarism may result from compression of the nontumorous portion of the pituitary. The pituitary stalk and the hypothalamus may also be involved by suprasellar extension of the tumor. Interference with the adenohypophyseal blood flow is an additional factor. Rarely, hypopituitarism may result from hemorrhage within a pituitary adenoma, leading to pituitary apoplexy.[8,9]

Primary extrasellar brain tumors can be responsible for central hypothyroidism.[10] Metastatic tumors of the hypothalamic-pituitary region arising from carcinomas of the breast, lung, and occasionally other sites are infrequent and usually reflect the presence of advanced neoplastic disease. Hypopituitarism is rare because of the limited survival of the patients and, when present, is usually preceded or accompanied by diabetes insipidus.

Craniopharyngioma is a relatively frequent cause of central hypothyroidism, especially in the younger age group.[11] Meningiomas, gliomas, and nontumorous mass lesions are rare causes of central hypothyroidism.

Postpartum pituitary necrosis (Sheehan's syndrome) is now rare in developed countries owing to improved health care, but it remains a relatively common cause of adult panhypopituitarism.[8,12,13] Pituitary insufficiency does not occur unless most of the anterior pituitary is affected.

Although less frequent, pituitary necrosis may also occur in patients with severe shock due to nonobstetric conditions, as in patients with diabetes mellitus and traumatic head injury, in association with cerebrovascular accidents, increased intracranial pressure, or epidemic hemorrhagic fever,[8] and in patients with various diseases who are maintained on mechanical respirators before death.[14] Other rare disorders that lead to central hypothyroidism include vasculitis, aneurysms of the internal carotid artery, and rupture of an aneurysm of the circle of Willis. Hypothalamic rather than pituitary lesions that lead to central hypothyroidism have also been reported in patients with severe head injury, whether associated with prolonged coma or not.[12,15–17] Indeed, the first case of documented hypothalamic hypothyroidism was ascribed to a lesion in the hypothalamus resulting from head trauma.[18]

External radiotherapy for tumors of the head and neck can affect the hypothalamus, the pituitary, and the thyroid, and hypothyroidism often results from damage of one or more of these structures. Hypothyroidism due to pituitary or hypothalamic dysfunction has been observed in 20% to 53% of patients irradiated for nasopharyngeal or paranasal sinus tumors,[19,20] and more recently in 65% of patients, both children and adults, irradiated for brain tumors.[21] TSH deficiency can also result from direct irradiation of the pituitary, either by conventional external radiotherapy[8] or by α-particle radiotherapy[22] for GH-secreting adenomas or other pituitary tumors.

If not present initially, central hypothyroidism may result from surgical therapy of pituitary tumors. Radical excision of large pituitary tumors induces hypothyroidism in about 10% of patients, but selective removal of microadenomas is rarely followed by impaired TSH secretion.

Purulent hypophysitis may occur in patients with septicemia or by direct extension of infection from neighboring areas.[23] Abscesses may also develop in pituitary tumors or craniopharyngiomas.[8] Granulomatous lesions of diverse etiology, including tuberculosis, syphilis, and giant-cell granuloma, are rare causes of pituitary insufficiency.[8] Persistent hypothalamic-pituitary insufficiency after viral meningoencephalitis has been described.[24–26] Pituitary sarcoidosis is often associated with granulomatous lesions in the neurohypophysis and the hypothalamus.[27] Histiocytosis (Hand-Schüller-Christian disease) may involve the pituitary and result in varying degrees of hypopituitarism.[8] The neurohypophysis is also affected in most patients, leading to diabetes insipidus. In hemochromatosis, iron pigment accumulates in the cytoplasm of anterior pituitary cells and can lead to fibrosis of the anterior pituitary and hypopituitarism.[28] Central hypothyroidism may also occur in thalassemia patients treated with frequent blood transfusions.[29] Chronic lymphocytic hypophysitis has been described with or without pituitary insufficiency in association with autoimmune thyroiditis or adrenalitis.[8] Hypothalamic atrophy with gradually evolving hypopituitarism has been described in an adolescent girl.

Pituitary aplasia or hypoplasia is a rare congenital defect, usually associated with other severe malformations.[8,30] These infants usually die shortly after birth, and evidence of multiple endocrine failure is found at autopsy. Isolated pituitary aplasia may also occur, and dwarfism with hypothyroidism, hypogonadism, and hypoadrenalism has been found in the few patients surviving beyond infancy.[31]

Rare cases of hereditary panhypopituitarism have been reported in association with a small but normally shaped sella turcica.[32] The occurrence of a familial form of hypopituitarism with deficiency of GH and TSH was described in three siblings with short stature and an enlarged sella turcica.[33]

Idiopathic hypopituitarism indicates deficiency of one or more of the anterior pituitary hormones in the absence of any demonstrable pathology. Idiopathic TSH deficiency usually occurs in association with GH deficiency,[34] but secretion of other pituitary hormones may also be deficient.[35] The finding of a normal, exaggerated, or delayed TSH response to TRH in most of these patients suggests the presence of a hypothalamic lesion.[17,35–37] Birth trauma has been implicated as the etiologic factor secondary to the use of vacuum extraction or breech delivery in the histories of many of these patients.[38]

Some cases of isolated TSH deficiency have been reported in patients with a pituitary tumor[20,39] or diabetes mellitus,[40] but in most instances no apparent cause has been identified and the anatomic site of the lesion remains largely elusive.[41,42] A few of these patients had an increased TSH response to TRH, but most had no change in serum TSH, suggesting that the defect was at the level of the pituitary.[43] The defect may be partial rather than complete, and therapy with thyroid hormone may facilitate the release of small amounts of TSH after TRH administration.[41] Although more common in adults, isolated TSH deficiency also occurs in children and may result in a secondary impairment of GH secretion, simulating primary deficiency of TSH and GH.[8] In these patients GH secretion is restored after initiation of L-T$_4$ therapy.

Inherited isolated TSH deficiency is an autosomal recessive disease that results in congenital central hypothyroidism and has been described in a few families.[4–6] It is related to single-base substitution or to nonsense mutation in the TSH-β subunit gene,[5,6,44] although recently defects in a pituitary specific transcription factor (Pit 1/GHF-1) have been described[45–47] (see following).

PATHOGENESIS

Impairment of TSH secretion in central hypothyroidism may result from a variety of mechanisms. Hyposecretion of TSH in pituitary hypothyroidism may be ascribed to a reduced mass of functioning thyrotrophs as a consequence of various lesions, including mechanical compression by tumor, destruction by vascular, inflammatory, or physical injuries, aplasia, or hypoplasia. In these patients, low serum TSH levels and no response to TRH are the expected findings.

Several explanations are possible for idiopathic isolated TSH deficiency. Provided that the thyrotrophs are present and morphologically intact, the abnormality could reside in the TRH receptor or at some subsequent step in the transmission of the hypothalamic message, in the process of TSH synthesis, or in the mechanism of TSH release. Any abnormality in the TRH receptor does not involve the prolactin-secreting cells because the prolactin response to TRH is normal in these patients.[1,15] Isolated TSH deficiency in children has been found in association with pseudohypoparathyroidism,[48–50] but in other pseudohypoparathyroid patients, primary hypothyroidism has also been described.[51]

In inherited TSH deficiency due to an abnormal TSH-β subunit gene, a few families have been described with a single-base mutation in nucleotide 145 of exon 2 of the gene with substitution of glycine for arginine in the 29th amino acid. This substitution causes a conformational change of TSH-β that hampers its dimerization with the α-subunit to form a complete TSH molecule. In two families, the molecular abnormality has been found to be a nonsense mutation in nucleotide 94 of exon 2, leading to premature termination of TSH-β synthesis at amino acid 11.[5,6,52] Recently, central hypothyroidism has also been related to a nonsense mutation in the pituitary specific transcription activator, Pit 1/GHF-1, in the context of multiple pituitary hormone deficiencies.[45–47]

Hypothalamic hypothyroidism is commonly attributed to TRH deficiency, whether due to acquired or congenital abnormalities of the hypothalamus. These patients have low or normal serum TSH levels that increase after the administration of TRH. No evidence directly supports the concept of TRH deficiency as the cause of hypothalamic hypothyroidism because of the interference of various serum components in the available TRH radioimmunoassays, the rapid degradation of TRH by serum, and the uncertain origin of TRH in the peripheral blood. Indeed, most of TRH is derived from extrahypothalamic sources.[53] Indirect evidence favoring TRH deficiency as the cause of hypothyroidism in these patients has come from the demonstration that their hypothyroidism can be corrected by the repetitive administration of exogenous TRH.[54] The reasons for such TRH deficiency are unknown, but this might be related to reduced TRH synthesis resulting from some destructive lesions of the hypophysiotropic areas of the hypothalamus.

Reduced stimulation of the pituitary by TRH may also be due to suprasellar lesions preventing hypothalamic TRH from reaching the anterior pituitary, as in tumorous or vascular lesions involving the pituitary stalk. The delayed TSH response to TRH frequently seen in these patients could be explained by the fact that TRH reaches the pituitary through the systemic circulation and not through the hypothalamic-pituitary portal system.

A possible explanation for idiopathic hypothalamic hypothyroidism is the excessive production of substances, such as dopamine or somatostatin, that inhibit TSH secretion.[55-57] Some indirect support for this concept has been provided by the demonstration that naloxone pretreatment resulted in the normalization of a subnormal TSH response to TRH in a patient with hypothyroidism.[58] The effect of naloxone might be related to the experimental evidence indicating that opiates inhibit TSH secretion by increasing production of a hypothalamic TSH inhibitory factor, such as dopamine.[59,60]

Recent data indicate that in central hypothyroidism, irrespective of the underlying lesion, the nocturnal surge of serum TSH that occurs in normal subjects[61,62] is reduced or abolished,[62-64] although this finding may be equivocal in some patients.[65] This loss is due to diminished TSH pulse amplitude with relatively preserved pulse frequency and daytime amplitude. The loss of the nocturnal surge in TSH secretion may contribute to thyroid hypofunction, since it appears that the thyroid is most stimulated at night after the nocturnal surge.

Administration of GH to children with idiopathic GH deficiency may result in central hypothyroidism.[66,67] It has been postulated that GH administration leads to increased secretion of somatostatin, thereby blocking TSH release.[66] It should be mentioned that other studies have documented a subnormal nocturnal TSH surge in GH-deficient children prior to GH therapy, with no further changes in the pituitary-thyroid axis function after GH administration.[68] GH therapy also increases peripheral conversion of T_4 to triiodothyronine (T_3), which may result in biochemical changes that mimic central hypothyroidism, such as low serum T_4 concentration and impaired TSH secretion.[69-71]

Biologically Inactive TSH

Secretion of biologically inactive TSH accounts for some cases of central hypothyroidism. The association of low serum thyroid hormone levels with normal or slightly elevated serum TSH concentrations has often been observed in patients with pituitary or hypothalamic disorders.[55,56,72-77] This finding could not be explained by the coexistence of primary thyroid failure, since the patients had an adequate thyroidal response to exogenous TSH[72,73] and no evidence of thyroid autoimmune disease.[72] Nevertheless, the thyroid appeared to be unresponsive to endogenous TSH because the administration of TRH produced a normal or even an exaggerated serum TSH response that was followed by an inadequate thyroidal release of T_3.[2,38] This suggested that the immunoreactive TSH secreted in these patients might have reduced or absent biologic activity. This possibility has been documented by evaluating the biologic activity of circulating TSH by a cytochemical assay,[72] or by an adenylyl cyclase stimulation assay in thyroid plasma membranes, rat FRTL-5 cells,[79-81] or, more recently, in Chinese hamster ovary cells transfected with the recombinant human TSH receptor (CHO-R cells).[82] These studies have shown that the biologic activity of serum TSH and the ratio between biologic and immunoreactive TSH (B/I) is reduced in basal conditions in some patients with central hypothyroidism.

Interestingly, although the acute intravenous administration of TRH did not substantially modify the biologic activity of TSH, chronic oral TRH treatment (40 mg/d for 4 weeks) was associated with an increase in both the biologic and receptor-binding activities of TSH.[1,82] These observations suggest that TRH is required to produce TSH with full biologic potency.[1,73] Thus, the reduced TSH biologic activity might be due to TRH deficiency. The hypothalamic hormone might regulate not only TSH release but also the structural features of the pituitary hormone needed for appropriate receptor binding and adenylyl cyclase stimulation. In rats with hypothalamic hypothyroidism due to paraventricular nuclear lesions, an altered TSH carbohydrate structure has been demonstrated, which could be corrected by TRH administration in parallel with the normalization of serum TSH levels.[83] Abnormal TSH glycosylation, as assessed by ricin and lentil lectin affinity chromatography,[84] has also been reported in patients with central hypothyroidism[85] and reduced TSH biologic activity, with prevalent hybrid, high-mannose type and biantennary oligosaccharide moieties and a reduced degree of sialylation.[86] It is, therefore, likely that the correct glycosylation of the molecule is essential for the expression of TSH biologic activity.

The secretion of TSH-β and TSH-α-subunits may be altered in patients with central hypothyroidism. An excess of circulating TSH-β has been reported in five patients with idiopathic central hypothyroidism,[54] but whether this has any relevance for the assembly of an inactive molecule of TSH remains to be determined.

Differences in the molecular size of TSH, as assessed by gel chromatography, have been found when the TSH of some patients with central hypothyroidism was compared with normal TSH[9,87]; normalization of the chromatographic pattern occurred after chronic oral TRH administration.[79] In one patient with idiopathic central hypothyroidism, a TSH-β-subunit of large molecular size was found.[54] The interpretation of these observations is uncertain, since immunoreactive TSH of greater than normal molecular size has been found in pituitary extracts from patients with long-standing primary hypothyroidism. So far, defects in the primary amino acid sequence of

TSH have been found only in patients with familial TSH deficiency, but not in those with central hypothyroidism associated with bioinactive TSH.

Functional Abnormalities in TSH Secretion

Functional abnormalities of TSH secretion associated with concomitant variations in serum thyroid hormone concentrations resembling those found in central hypothyroidism due to hypothalamic and/or pituitary lesions can be observed in several pathophysiologic conditions (Table 59-2). Transient hypothyroidism due to functional TSH deficiency is found in euthyroid subjects after withdrawal of long-term L-T$_4$ suppressive therapy for nontoxic goiter.[88–90] The features of pituitary hypothyroidism, including low serum thyroid hormone and TSH concentrations and subnormal or absent serum TSH responses to TRH, are observed shortly after the abrupt cessation of thyroid hormone therapy. Complete recovery of TSH secretory function and normalization of serum thyroid hormone concentrations usually requires 4 to 6 weeks. A similar biochemical situation is commonly observed in hyperthyroid patients shortly after radioactive iodine administration or the institution of antithyroid drug treatment: serum thyroid hormone concentrations decrease, but the compensatory rise in serum TSH concentrations is delayed.[8] Likewise, the initial recovery phase of subacute thyroiditis that follows the thyrotoxic phase due to a thyroidal destructive process is associated with a functional suppression of TSH secretion in spite of the low/normal serum thyroid hormone concentrations. This type of abnormality of the hypothalamic-pituitary-thyroid axis does not require any treatment because of its temporary nature.

TABLE 59-2.
Functional Abnormalities of TSH Secretion

Use of drugs inhibiting TSH secretion
  L-Thyroxine withdrawal syndrome
  Glucocorticoids
  Dopamine
  Growth hormone (?)
Suppressed TSH secretion after hyperthyroidism or thyrotoxicosis
  Antithyroid drug treatment
  Radioactive iodine therapy
  Subacute thyroiditis
Nonthyroidal illnesses
  Major surgery
  Bone marrow transplantation
  Chronic renal failure
  Burns and traumas
  Decompensated diabetes mellitus
  AIDS (?)
  Depressive disorder
  Anorexia nervosa and bulimia
  Fasting
Aging

An impaired serum TSH response to TRH is frequently found in patients with Cushing's syndrome or during prolonged glucocorticoid administration,[91–93] but clinical hypothyroidism does not occur. Patients with Cushing's syndrome do not have the normal nocturnal surge in TSH secretion.[91] This occurs in association with both ACTH-secreting pituitary adenomas and adrenal tumors, suggesting that the abnormal TSH secretory pattern is due to hypercortisolism itself.[91] Increased cortisol secretion may also account for the deficient nocturnal surge of TSH that can be observed for several days after major surgical procedures.[94]

Patients with acromegaly who have no clinical or biochemical evidence of hypothyroidism often have no serum TSH response to TRH,[8] while an exaggerated or delayed serum TSH response is frequently found in children with idiopathic GH deficiency.[38,95] Administration of therapeutic doses of GH to children with pituitary dwarfism has occasionally been associated with reversible central hypothyroidism,[67] although other studies have failed to confirm this finding.[96,97] Thus, GH might have a suppressive effect on TSH secretion, mediated by an increase in somatostatin secretion, but this remains to be clarified. Dopamine causes inhibition of TSH secretion,[59] and withdrawal of the drug is followed by a prompt increase in serum TSH and thyroid hormone concentrations.[57]

In patients with nonthyroidal illness (NTI) (Table 59-2), serum TSH concentrations are frequently low or normal despite the reduction in serum T$_3$, and in most severe cases also T$_4$, concentrations.[98,99] Indeed, many patients with NTI have suppressed TSH and/or an attenuated or abolished nocturnal TSH surge.[100–103] The latter finding has been related to a loss of the usual nocturnal increase of TSH pulse amplitude rather than in the TSH pulse frequency.[104] Studies carried out in NTI patients have demonstrated that circulating TSH has a normal or slightly increased biologic activity as compared to controls. Although subnormal serum TSH responses to TRH have been reported, most NTI patients have normal TRH tests. The functional abnormalities of the hypothalamic-pituitary-thyroid axis just described and resembling those found in central hypothyroidism due to hypothalamic and/or pituitary lesions are frequently encountered in chronic renal failure treated with regular maintenance hemodialysis,[91,97] decompensated diabetes mellitus,[40,100] burns and trauma,[105] after bone marrow transplantation,[103] and in other serious illnesses. These functional abnormalities are particularly frequent in patients with depressive disorders,[106] anorexia nervosa, and bulimia. The abnormalities of TSH secretion observed in patients with endogenous depression might be accounted for, at least in part, by the increased cortisol secretion.[106] An increased concentration of TRH in the cerebrospinal fluid has been found in depressed patients,[107] suggesting the presence of some hypothalamic abnormalities. Recently, interleukin-6 (IL-6) and other cytokines have been reported to affect pituitary-thyroid function both in animals and in man, causing a reduction in serum thyroid hormone and TSH concentrations.[108] Increased serum IL-6 levels have been found in NTI patients.[109,110] Whether this increase merely represents an epiphenomenon of NTI or plays a role in the pathogenesis of abnormalities of pituitary-thyroid function found in these patients remains to be elucidated.

In AIDS patients, during the terminal phase of the disease, serum thyroid hormone concentrations are reduced and serum TSH is normal or low, similar to patients with other causes of severe NTI.[111] However, in HIV-positive patients who are either asymptomatic or with less severe disease, mean 24-hour TSH levels are higher, owing to an increase in TSH pulse amplitude that is associated with an increased TSH responsiveness to TRH and a normal nocturnal TSH surge.[112]

Aging is associated with a variety of hypothalamic-pituitary-thyroid axis changes, but in many instances these are related to concomitant NTI, drug administration, or the increased prevalence of primary hypothyroidism in the elderly. In male Fisher rats, aging has been found to be associated with a decreased synthesis of hypothalamic TRH and consequently with decreased pituitary TSH-β mRNA levels and TSH content, suggesting a defect at the hypothalamic level.[113] Recently, evaluation of the pituitary-thyroid axis in healthy elderly subjects, including centenarians, has shown a complex derangement of thyroid function probably resulting from a combination of defective peripheral metabolism of thyroid hormones and of decreased thyroid hormone secretion of central origin; as a consequence, a slight, but progressive decrease in serum TSH concentration was observed with age in these healthy subjects; this might be related to a resetting of the pituitary threshold of TSH suppression.[114]

CLINICAL FEATURES

The clinical picture of central hypothyroidism varies widely depending on the severity of the thyroid failure, the extent of the associated hormone deficiencies, the age of the patients at the time of onset, and the nature of the underlying lesion.[115]

The clinical features of thyroid insufficiency resulting from TSH deficiency are similar to those of primary hypothyroidism, although generally less pronounced. The patients may complain of cold intolerance, constipation, fatigue, lethargy, and mental dullness. Physical findings include bradycardia, hypothermia, slow speech, and a prolonged relaxation phase of the deep tendon reflexes. Children may present with stunted growth and delay in sexual maturation and bone development. Dwarfism and cretinism occur in the rare patient with familial inherited TSH deficiency.[43] Several differentiating features largely related to the hyposecretion of other pituitary hormones help to distinguish central hypothyroidism from primary hypothyroidism. The skin is pale and cool, but not as coarse and dry as in primary hypothyroidism. The face is characteristically covered with fine wrinkles, but periorbital and peripheral edema are uncommon in patients with central hypothyroidism (Fig 59-1). Loss of axillary, pubic, and facial hair and thinning of the lateral eyebrows are usually more pronounced, and the texture of the remaining hair is thinner than in primary hypothyroidism. The tongue is not enlarged, and hoarseness of the voice is not prominent in patients with central hypothyroidism. The heart tends to be small, and blood pressure is low. Pericardial, pleural, and peritoneal effusions are rare in these patients but are occasionally encountered.[116] Atrophic breasts and amenorrhea, rather than metrorrhagia, are found in premenopausal women. Body weight is more likely to be reduced than increased. The severity of the hypothyroid state ranges from mild to severe, but, in general, is mild. Although residual hormone secretion from the unstimulated thy-

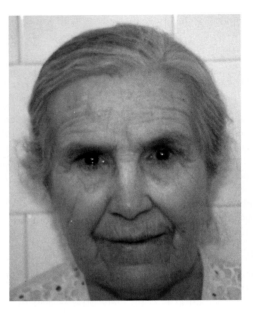

FIGURE 59-1. Patient with central hypothyroidism due to a nonfunctioning pituitary tumor. The patient had low serum thyroid hormone and TSH concentrations, no serum TSH response to TRH, and ACTH, GH, and gonadotropin deficiency.

roid gland may account for the mild degree of hypothyroidism in most patients, early recognition is also an important factor. In fact, most patients have other endocrine and non-endocrine manifestations of the disease that lead them to seek medical attention before their hypothyroidism becomes severe.

Defects in GH and gonadotropin secretion usually precede TSH insufficiency as hypopituitarism develops, and ACTH secretion is usually the last to be affected. Growth failure with delayed skeletal maturation is the result of GH deficiency in children, but it has few manifestations in adults. Hypoglycemia may occur, especially if hypocortisolism is also present. In diabetic patients, GH deficiency decreases insulin requirements. Gonadotropin insufficiency results in impotence, loss of libido, diminished beard growth, and testicular atrophy in men; amenorrhea, infertility, and atrophy of the breasts in women; and loss of pubic and axillary hair in both sexes. Delayed sexual maturation is the result of gonadotropin insufficiency in children. ACTH deficiency leads to weakness, postural hypotension, and depigmentation of the areolae and other normally pigmented areas of the skin. Dangerous and potentially lethal adrenal crisis may be precipitated by trauma, intercurrent infection, or surgery.

Symptoms and signs that arise directly from the hypothalamic or pituitary lesion may precede, accompany, and even obscure the manifestations of the pituitary failure. Headache and visual field defects are often the presenting symptoms in patients with nonfunctioning pituitary adenomas that extend beyond the sella turcica. As a rule, hormone-secreting adenomas manifest themselves through the consequences of pituitary hormone hypersecretion before symptoms of pituitary insufficiency become apparent. This may not be the case, however, in men with prolactin-secreting adenomas. In addition to headache and visual loss, diabetes insipidus occurs frequently in patients with craniopharyngioma, in association with growth failure in children and hypogonadism in adults. Diabetes insipidus is also a prominent feature of histiocytosis and of sarcoidosis involving the hypothalamus. In patients with tumors arising in the hypothalamus or in the region of the third ventricle, meningeal signs may occur early in the course of the disease. Rarely , hypothalamic lesions may cause obesity and abnormal temperature regulation. Patients with postpartum pituitary necrosis have a history of hemorrhage and shock after delivery, followed by deficient lactation, persistent amenorrhea, and other signs of hypogonadism. Severe headache is usually the predominant symptom of pituitary apoplexy, whereas a sudden decrease in insulin requirement may be the first indication of pituitary infarction in a diabetic patient. In other cases, a history of head injury, pituitary surgery, or radiation to the head or neck suggests the underlying lesion. Patients with idiopathic hypopituitarism may have a history of breech delivery or birth by vacuum extraction.

The rate of progression and the degree of central hypothyroidism are markedly influenced by the nature of the underlying disease. Clinical features of thyroid failure are usually detectable within 1 month after hypophysectomy. The development of hypothyroidism is less abrupt in Sheehan's syndrome, but in most instances it is relatively rapid when compared with the slow and insidious onset of primary hypothyroidism due to atrophic autoimmune thyroiditis. It is not infrequent, however, that several years elapse after a postpartum hemorrhage before hypothyroidism, adrenal insufficiency, and hypogonadism become clinically apparent. A long latent period may also occur in patients who develop central hypothyroidism after receiving a head injury or radiation. In patients with pituitary or hypothalamic tumors, the course and the severity of hypopituitarism depend on the rate of tumor growth and the degree of compression of adjacent structures. Overt manifestations of central hypothyroidism are rare in patients with metastatic pituitary tumors or in infants with pituitary aplasia or hypoplasia because of the short life span.

Central hypothyroidism that results from prolonged thyroid hormone therapy is characteristically transient and is usually more evident at the biochemical than the clinical level. Similarly, clinical evidence of central hypothyroidism is rare in patients with other functional abnormalities of TSH secretion, such as endogenous depression and endogenous or exogenous hypercortisolism.

DIAGNOSIS AND LABORATORY TESTS

Central hypothyroidism must be suspected when symptoms and signs of hypothyroidism are associated with manifestations of other hormonal deficiencies or pituitary mass lesions. Because the clinical expression of thyroid insufficiency may be obscured by the features of other hormonal deficiencies or by features arising directly from the underlying disease, thyroid function should be evaluated in any patient suspected of having a hypothalamic or pituitary disorder. The possibility of central hypothyroidism should also be considered in hypothyroid patients with no evidence of pituitary failure because it may be difficult, if not impossible, to distinguish clinically central from primary hypothyroidism.

The diagnosis of central hypothyroidism is based on the demonstration of low serum thyroid hormone concentrations in the presence of inappropriately low serum TSH values. Laboratory evaluation of this condition should include assessment of (1) serum thyroid hormone concentrations and TSH secretion, (2) the secretion of the other pituitary hormones, and (3) the anatomy of the hypothalamic or pituitary region.

Serum Thyroid Hormone Concentrations and TSH Secretion

The prerequisite for the diagnosis of central hypothyroidism is the finding of low serum total and free T_4 concentrations. Measurements of serum total and free T_3 concentrations are much less useful because they are frequently within the normal range. The reduction of serum thyroid hormone concentrations in central hypothyroidism is usually less pronounced than in primary hypothyroidism, although very low concentrations are found occasionally in patients with severe, long-standing central hypothyroidism.

Basal serum TSH values are inappropriately low with respect to the decreased serum thyroid hormone concentrations and are either undetectable or within the normal range in most patients.[8,117,118] Serum TSH may be slightly elevated in some patients,[55,56,72,75-77,119] but not to the levels commonly found in patients with primary hypothyroidism who have a comparable reduction of serum T_4. This finding may be explained by the secretion of immunoreactive but biologically inactive TSH, as discussed previously.[3,72,73,79,80,82] Considerable overlap exists in basal serum TSH values between the two types of central hypothyroidism. Thus, determination of basal serum TSH is essential for the differentiation between primary and central hypothyroidism but does not allow the distinction between hypothalamic and pituitary hypothyroidism.

Measurements of the serum TSH response to TRH (200–500 μg or 5 μg/kg IV) have been used in an attempt to identify the site of the primary lesion. On the basis of the classic concept of the control mechanism of TSH secretion, it was anticipated that the serum TSH response to TRH would be impaired in pituitary hypothyroidism but preserved in hypothalamic hypothyroidism. Several studies have shown, however, that serum TSH responses to TRH differ little in patients with hypothalamic or pituitary disorders. As shown in Table 59-3 and Figure 59-2, serum TSH responses to TRH may be subdivided into several categories according to the magnitude of the increase in serum TSH after TRH administration and the pattern of the response curve.[55] Although absent and impaired responses have been more frequently encountered in hypothyroid patients who have pituitary lesions,[55] they have also been found in some patients with hypothalamic disorders who have no apparent pituitary involvement.[56] Conversely, normal or even exaggerated serum TSH responses with a prolonged or delayed pattern are found in some hypothyroid patients with hypothalamic disorders[44,55,75,120] and in occasional patients with documented primary pituitary disease with no apparent hypothalamic involvement.[11,55,56,76] Thus, it appears that the pattern of the serum TSH response to TRH does not distinguish hypothalamic from pituitary lesions reliably. For this reason, an analysis of the entire clinical picture and the results of other tests of pituitary function is required. It should be

TABLE 59-3.
Patterns of TSH Responses to TRH*

Patterns of Response	Net increase (mU/L)
MAGNITUDE OF RESPONSE	
Normal	
Females	6–22
Males	4–15
Absent	<1
Impaired	
Females	>1–<6
Males	>1–<4
Exaggerated	
Females	>22
Males	>15
RESPONSE CURVE	
Normal	Peak at 20 or 30 min
	60 min value <20 min
	60 min after the peak,
	TSH falls below
	40% of the peak value
Delayed	60 min value > 20 min
Prolonged	60 min after the peak TSH is more
	than 40% of the peak value

*200 μg IV of thyrotropin-releasing hormone.

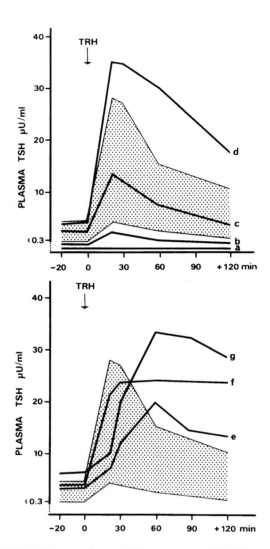

FIGURE 59-2. Patterns of serum TSH response to TRH (200 mg IV) in patients with central hypothyroidism. Magnitude of TSH response (*upper panel*): (a) absent, (b) impaired, (c) normal, (d) exaggerated. Response curve (*lower panel*); (e) delayed, (f) prolonged, (g) delayed and prolonged (and exaggerated). The shaded area represents the normal response.

noted that some euthyroid patients with hypothalamic-pituitary disorders (e.g., empty sella) also have abnormal serum TSH responses to TRH, for which there is no satisfactory explanation. The question of whether these abnormalities may be predictive of the subsequent development of central hypothyroidism remains to be clarified.[20,55] In normal subjects, TSH secretion is characterized by a nocturnal surge that begins in the evening and reaches a peak at the time of onset of sleep.[61–63,121] This surge does not occur in central hypothyroidism. A reasonable assessment of the nocturnal surge of TSH may be obtained by measuring serum TSH in samples taken every 30 minutes from 11:00 PM to 2:00 AM.[61,62] Evaluation of the nocturnal TSH peak has been found to be a more reliable test for confirming the diagnosis of central hypothyroidism than the TRH test.[61]

Biologic Assay of Serum TSH

The paradoxical finding of measurable and even slightly elevated serum immunoreactive TSH concentrations in patients with central hypothyroidism (see previous discussion) has stimulated the study of the biologic activity of circulating TSH in this condition. Bioassayable serum TSH may be determined by cytochemical assay, based on the ability of TSH to increase lysosomal membrane permeability in thyroid follicular cells.[72,79] Less sensitive, but more feasible assays are based on the stimulation of adenylate cyclase activity in human thyroid membranes or cells,[80,82] and in continuously cultured thyroid

rat cells (FRTL-5)[81,82] or CHO-R cells.[82] These assays require preliminary concentration and purification of serum TSH by immunoaffinity chromatography. Using these techniques, reduced biologic activity of immunoreactive serum TSH has been documented in several patients with central hypothyroidism.[1,3,72] These tests, although important for the assessment of TSH biologic activity, are not widely available.

Serum T₃ Response to TRH

The release of T_3 from the thyroid in response to the rise in serum TSH that follows TRH administration may provide an indirect assessment of the bioactivity of endogenous TSH. In normal subjects, serum T_3 concentrations increase from 30% to 100% above the baseline values 120 to 180 minutes after the intravenous injection of 200 μg of TRH. An impaired or absent serum T_3 response is indicative of central hypothyroidism, provided that a primary thyroid lesion has been excluded.[2,75] The coexistence of a normal or exaggerated serum immunoreactive TSH response with an abnormally low serum T_3 response suggests the secretion of bioinactive TSH.[2,72]

Measurement of TRH

Attempts to measure serum or urine TRH by radioimmunoassay have been made by several authors.[118,122] TRH is widely distributed throughout extrahypothalamic brain and several other tissues, which suggests that most of the TRH in peripheral blood is derived from nonhypothalamic sources.[60,118] Thus, measurement of serum or urinary TRH cannot be used as a reliable test for the evaluation of the hypothalamic-pituitary-thyroid axis.

Other Tests

Circulating antibodies to thyroglobulin and thyroid peroxidase are present in a high proportion of patients with primary hypothyroidism[123] due to autoimmune thyroiditis, but they are usually undetectable in patients with central hypothyroidism.[72]

Routine laboratory tests are of little value in the differentiation between primary and central hypothyroidism. Hypercholesterolemia is commonly regarded as characteristic of primary hypothyroidism, but mild to moderate elevations of serum cholesterol occur in some patients with central hypothyroidism.[124]

In the rare forms of inherited TSH deficiency, recently developed molecular biology methodology allows identification of the affected subjects, identification of the mutated gene carriers, and prenatal diagnosis in at-risk pregnancies, which is of the greatest value for the early institution of L-T_4 replacement therapy.

Tests of Other Pituitary Hormones

In hypothyroid patients with impaired TSH secretion, deficiency of other pituitary hormones should be sought by specific tests for each hormone. Evaluation of GH and prolactin secretion under basal conditions and after appropriate stimulation, as well as tests of the pituitary-adrenal and pituitary-gonadal axes, should be performed. Abnormalities of various degrees in these tests are common in patients with central hypothyroidism. Caution should be used, however, in the interpretation of the results, because some of these abnormalities may be due to thyroid insufficiency itself. Diminished serum GH concentration with a blunted GH response to hypoglycemia are frequent findings in central hypothyroidism but may also occur in patients with primary hypothyroidism . In the latter condition, as in patients with isolated TSH deficiency, GH secretion is restored to normal by L-T_4 therapy. Elevated basal serum prolactin concentrations with an increased response to TRH are frequently associated with hypothalamic-pituitary disorders, but they too may occur in primary hypothyroidism.[125] Serum follicle-stimulating hormone and luteinizing hormone concentrations are decreased in most patients with central hypothyroidism, but some reduction and an impaired response to gonadotropin-releasing hormone are found in patients with primary hypothyroidism. In postmenopausal women with primary hypothyroidism, however, serum gonadotropin concentrations remain elevated.

Serum cortisol concentrations are characteristically reduced in hypopituitarism and are usually normal in primary hypothyroidism. Measurements of serum cortisol concentration may help differentiate the hypothyroxinemia of central hypothyroidism (low/normal cortisol) from the low T_4 state due to nonthyroidal illness, which is generally associated with increased serum cortisol values.[126] The response to metyrapone is frequently subnormal in hypopituitarism, reflecting diminished ACTH reserve. The response is usually normal in primary hypothyroidism, although delayed or subnormal responses occur in some patients. Similarly, the serum cortisol response to insulin-induced hypoglycemia may be impaired in hypopituitarism as well as in some patients with primary hypothyroidism.[125]

Location of the Hypothalamic–Pituitary Lesion

Various imaging techniques may be used to identify lesions in the hypothalamic and pituitary region. Skull radiography and tomography have been largely replaced by more sensitive procedures, such as computed tomography (CT) and magnetic resonance imaging (MRI). Indirect signs of pituitary neoplasms detectable by the older techniques include enlargement of the sella, erosion of its floor, and erosion or elevation of the anterior clinoid processes. The presence of soft tissue densities within the sphenoid sinus suggests the presence of extrasellar extension of a pituitary tumor. Suprasellar calcification is a common finding in craniopharyngioma. Long-standing primary hypothyroidism may also be associated with enlargement of the pituitary gland that can be reversed by L-T_4 therapy.[39,127] Normal or small sella turcicae are found in patients with central hypothyroidism due to nontumorous lesions.[128] CT and MRI have the advantage of visualizing the pituitary gland directly and therefore may provide direct evidence of pituitary tumors or other abnormalities, such as an empty sella turcica. CT and MRI are especially useful in the evaluation of extrasellar extension of pituitary tumors.

Carotid angiography, cavernous sinus venography, and pneumoencephalography have virtually been abandoned since CT and MRI became available. Angiography can be a valuable tool in the detection of aneurysms of the internal carotid artery, which may cause hypopituitarism.

THERAPY

Therapy of central hypothyroidism should be directed toward restoring and maintaining euthyroidism. In addition, hypofunction of other endocrine glands resulting from pituitary hormone deficiencies should be corrected and the pituitary or hypothalamic cause of the central hypothyroidism treated appropriately.

Patients with central hypothyroidism should be treated with L-T_4 in the same way as patients with primary hypothyroidism, except when there is coexisting ACTH deficiency. Before L-T_4 therapy is initiated, pituitary-adrenal function should be evaluated by measurement of serum cortisol and assessment of ACTH reserve. If ACTH deficiency is present, adrenal steroid replacement should be initiated before any L-T$_4$ is given because of the risk of precipitating an adrenal crisis. In addition, if gonadotropin, GH (in children), and antidiuretic hormone deficiencies are present, appropriate replacement therapy should be instituted after the adrenal steroid and L-T$_4$ are given. Patients with isolated TSH deficiency require only L-T$_4$ therapy but should be carefully evaluated at least twice a year to detect further loss of pituitary function. Transient functional TSH deficiency usually does not require any treatment.

Although other thyroid preparations can be used, L-T$_4$ is the preparation of choice. The initial dose of L-T$_4$ should be based on the age and cardiovascular status of the patient. In young adults who do not have ACTH deficiency, therapy may be initiated at a daily dose of 1.4 to 16 µg/kg L-T$_4$ for 4 to 6 weeks; the dose may then be adjusted on the basis of its peripheral effects. In patients with cardiovascular disease or ACTH deficiency and in elderly patients, therapy should be begun with 0.3 to 0.7 µg/kg/d L-T$_4$; after 3 to 4 weeks, the amount of L-T$_4$ can be progressively increased until an optimal effect is achieved. In infants and children, the dose of L-T$_4$ should be relatively higher, because T$_4$ clearance is more rapid and underreplacement may result in mental retardation and impaired physical growth.

Serum TSH measurements cannot be used as in primary hypothyroidism to determine the adequacy of L-T$_4$ therapy. Instead, the correct dosage should be determined by clinical response and by measurements of serum total and free T$_4$ concentrations.

References

1. Beck-Peccoz P, Amr S, Menezes-Ferreira NM, Faglia G, Weintraub BD. Decreased receptor binding of biologically inactive thyrotropin in central hypothyroidism: effect of treatment with thyrotropin-releasing hormone. N Engl J Med 1985; 312:1085

2. Faglia G, Ferrari C, Paracchi A, Spada A, Beck-Peccoz P. Triiodothyronine response to thyrotropin releasing hormone in patients with hypothalamic-pituitary disorders. Clin Endocrinol (Oxf) 1975;4:585

3. Petersen VV, McGregor AM, Belchetz PE, Elkeles RS, Hall R. The secretion of thyrotropin with impaired biological activity in patients with hypothalamic-pituitary disease. Clin Endocrinol (Oxf) 1978;8:397

4. Dacou-Votetakis C, Felquate DM, Drakopoulos M, Kourides IA, Dracopoli NC. Familial hypothyroidism caused by a nonsense mutation in thyroid-stimulating hormone beta subunit gene. Am J Human Genet 1990;46:988

5. Hayashizaky J, Hiraoka Y, Endo Y, Miyai K, Matsubara K. Thyroid-stimulating hormone (TSH) deficiency caused by a single base substitution in the Cagyc region of the B-subunit . EMBO J 1989;8:2291

6. Hayashizaky J, Hiraoka Y, Tatsumi K, et al. DNA analysis of five families with familial inherited thyroid stimulating hormone (TSH) deficiency. J Clin Endocrinol Metab 1990;71:792

7. Hershman JH. Hypothalamic and pituitary hypothyroidism. In: Bastenie TA, Bonnyns M, Vanhaelst L. eds. Recent progress in diagnosis and treatment of hypothyroidism condition. Amsterdam: Excerpta Medica, 1980:40

8. Samuels MH, Ridgway EC. Central hypothyroidism. Endocrinol Metabol Clin North Am 1992;21:903

9. Spitz IM, LeRoit D, Hirsh H, et al. Increased high-molecular-weight thyrotropin with impaired thyrotropin activity in an euthyroid man. N Engl J Med 1981;304:278

10. Rivarola MA, Mendilaharzou H, Warman M, et al. Endocrine disorders in 66 suprasellar and pineal tumors of patients with prepubertal and pubertal ages. Horm Res 1992;37:1

11. Jenkins JS, Gilbert CG, Ang V. Hypothalamic-pituitary function in patients with craniopharyngiomas. J Clin Endocrinol Metab 1976;43:394

12. Leiba S, Schindel B, Weinstein R, Lidor I, Friedman S, Matz S. Spontaneous post-partum regression of pituitary mass with return of function. JAMA 1986;255:230

13. Sheehan HL, Davis JC. Pituitary necrosis. Br Med Bull 1968;24:59

14. Daniel PM, Spicer EJF, Treip CS. Pituitary necrosis in patients maintained on mechanical respirators. J Pathol 1973;111:135

15. Rudman D, Fleisher AS, Kutner MH, Raggio JF. Suprahypophysial hypogonadism and hypothyroidism during prolonged coma after head trauma. J Clin Endocrinol Metab 1977;45:747

16. Valenta LJ, DeFeo DR. Post-traumatic hypopituitarism due to a hypothalamic lesion. Am J Med 1980;68:614

17. Woolf PD. Hypothyroidism and amenorrhea due to hypothalamic insufficiency. A study in four young women. Am J Med 1977;63:343

18. Pittman JA Jr, Haigler ED, Hershman JM, Pittman CS. Hypothalamic hypothyroidism. N Engl J Med 1971;285:844

19. Samaan NA, Cangir A, Maor MH, Sampiere VA, Jesse RH. Effect of irradiation on the hypothalamic, pituitary and thyroid function in patients with tumors of the head and neck. In: Linfoot JA, ed. Recent advances in the diagnosis and treatment of pituitary tumors. New York: Raven Press, 1979:148

20. Sawin CT, McHugh JE. Isolated lack of thyrotropin in man. J Clin Endocrinol Metab 1966;26:955

21. Constine LS, Woolf PD, Cann D, et al. Hypothalamic-pituitary dysfunction after radiation for brain tumors. N Engl J Med 1993;328:87

22. Linfoot JA. Alpha particle pituitary irradiation in the primary and postsurgical management of pituitary microadenoma. In: Faglia G, Giovannelli MA, Mac Leod RM, eds. Pituitary microadenomas. New York: Academic Press, 1980:515

23. Dominique JN, Wilson CB. Pituitary abscesses: report of seven cases and review of the literature. J Neurosug 1977;46:601

24. Hagg E, Astrom L, Tenn L. Persistent hypothalamic pituitary insufficiency following acute meningo-encephalitis. Acta Med Scand 1978;203:231

25. Kupari M, Pelkonen R., Valtonen V. Post encephalitic hypothalamic-pituitary insufficiency. Acta Endocrinol (Copenh) 1980; 94:433.

26. Lichtenstein MJ, Tilley WS, Sandler MP. The syndrome of hypothalamic hypopituitarism complicating viral meningoencephalitis. J Endocrinol Invest 1982;5:11

27. Bell NH. Endocrine complications of sarcoidosis. Endocrinol Metabol Clin North Am 1991;20:645

28. Peillon F, Racadot J. Modifications histopathologiques de l'hypophyse dans six cas d'hèmochromatose. Ann Endocrinol (Paris) 1972;30:800

29. Lai ME, Balzano S., Murtas ML, et al. High incidence of primary not autoimmune hypothyroidism in adult thalassemia major patients. In: Nagataki S, Torizuka K, eds. The Thyroid. Amsterdam: Excerpta Medica, 1988:487

30. Salazar H, MacAulay MA, Charles D, Pardo M. The human hypophysis in anencephaly. Arch Pathol 1969;87:201

31. Steiner MW, Boggs JD. Absence of pituitary gland, hypothyroidism, hypoadrenalism and hypogonadism in a 17-year-old dwarf. J Clin Endocrinol Metab 1965;25:1591

32. Schimke RN, Spaulding JJ, Hollowell JB. X-linked congenital panhypopituitarism. Birth Defects 1971;7:21

33. Parks JM, Tenore A, Bongiovanni AM, Kirkland RT. Familial hypopituitarism with large sella turcica. N Engl J Med 1978;298:698

34. Gharib H, Abboud CF. Primary idiopathic hypothalamic hypothyroidism. Am J Med 1987;83:171

35. Streja D, Corenblum B, Ezrin C. Hypothalamic hypopituitarism presenting as galactorrhea-amenorrhea. JAMA 1978;239:1783

36. Martin LG, Martul P, Connor TB, Wiswell JG. Hypothalamic origin of idiopathic hypopituitarism. Metabolism 1972;21:143

37. Proulx F, Weber ML, Collu R, Lelievre M, Larbrisseau A, Delisle M. Hypothalamic dysfunction in a child: a distinct syndrome. Eur J Pediatr 1993;152:526

38. Andler W, Stolecke H, Kohns U. Thyroid function in children with growth hormone deficiency, either idiopathic or caused by diseases of the central nervous system. Eur J Pediatr 1978; 128:273

39. Lawrence AM, Wilbert JF, Hagen TC. The pituitary and primary hypothyroidism. Arch Intern Med 1973;132:327

40. Chandra M, Lifshitz F, Fort P, Derosas FJ, Kantrow A. Isolated thyrotropin deficiency in diabetes mellitus. Acta Endocrinol (Copenh) 1977;84:80

41. Boehm TM, Dimond RC, Wartofsky L. Isolated thyrotropin deficiency with thyrotropin releasing hormone induced TSH secretion and thyroidal reserve. J Clin Endocrinol Metab 1976;43:1041

42. Nygren A, Rojdmark S. Isolated thyrotropin deficiency in a man with narcoleptic attacks. Acta Med Scan 1982;212:175

43. Miyai K, Azukizawa M, Onishi T, et al. Familial isolated thyrotropin deficiency. In: James WHT, ed. Endocrinologica. Vol 2. Amsterdam: Excerpta Medica, 1977:345

44. Suter SN, Kaplan SL, Aubert ML, Grumbach MM. Plasma prolactin and thyrotropin and the response to thyrotropin-releasing factor in children with primary and hypothalamic hypothyroidism. J Clin Endocrinol Metab 1978;47:1015

45. Pfaffle RW, Di Mattia GE, Parks JS, et al. Mutation of the POU-specific domain of Pit 1 and hypopituitarism without pituitary hypoplasia. Science 1992;257:1118

46. Pfaffle RW, Parks JS, Brown MR, Heinemann G. Pit 1 and pituitary function. J Pediatr Endocrinol 1993;6:229

47. Tatsumi K, Miyai K, Notomi T, et al. Cretinism with combined hormone deficiency caused by a mutation in the Pit 1 gene. Nature Genet 1992;1:56

48. Spiegel AM, Levine MA, Marx SJ, Aurbach GD. Pseudohypoparathyroidism: the molecular basis for hormone resistance. A retrospective. N Engl J Med 1982;307:679

49. Winnacker JL, Becker KL, Moore CF. Pseudohypoparathyroidism and selective deficiency in thyrotropin: an interesting association. Metabolism 1967;16:644

50. Zisman E, Lotz M, Jenkins ME, Bartter FC. Studies in pseudohypoparathyroidism: two new cases with a probable selective deficiency of thyrotropin. Am J Med 1969;46:464

51. Mallet E, Caryon P, Amr S, et al. Coupling defects of thyrotropin receptor and adenylate cyclase in pseudohypoparathyroid patients. J Clin Endocrinol Metab 1982;54:1028

52. Tatsumi K, Hayashizaki Y, Hiraoka Y, Miyai K, Matsubara K. The structure of the thyrotropin B-subunit gene. 1988;73:489

53. Martino E, Bartalena L, Gasperi M. Extrapituitary effects of thyrotropin-releasing hormone. In: Monaco F, Satta MA, Shapiro BS, Troncone L, eds. Thyroid diseases. Clinical fundamentals and therapy. Boca Raton: CRC Press, 1993:595

54. Faglia G, Beck-Peccoz P, Ballabio M, Nava C. Excess of beta-subunit of thyrotropin in patients with idiopathic central hypothyroidism due to the secretion of TSH with reduced biological activity. J Clin Endocrinol Metab 1983;56:908

55. Faglia G, Beck-Peccoz P, Ferrari C, et al. Plasma thyrotropin response to thyrotropin releasing hormone in patients with pituitary and hypothalamic disorders. J Clin Endocrinol Metab 1973;37:595

56. Snyder PJ, Jacobs LS, Rabello MM, et al. Diagnostic value of thyrotropin-releasing hormone in pituitary and hypothalamic disorders. Ann Intern Med 1974;81:751

57. Van den Berghe G, De Zegher F, Lauwers P. Dopamine and the sick euthyroid syndrome in critical illness. Clin Endocrinol (Oxf) 1994;41:731

58. Dunger DB, Leonard JW, Wolff OH, Preece MA. Effect of naloxone in a previously undescribed hypothalamic syndrome. Lancet 1980;1:1277

59. Kaptein EM, Spencer CA, Kamiel MB, Nicoloff JP. Prolonged dopamine administration and thyroid economy in normal and critically ill subjects. J Clin Endocrinol Metab 1980;51:387

60. Morley JE. Neuroendocrine control of thyrotropin secretion. Endocr Rev 1981;2:396

61. Bartalena L, Martino E, Falcone M, et al. Evaluation of the nocturnal serum thyrotropin (TSH) surge, as assessed by TSH ultrasensitive assay, in patients receiving long term L-thyroxine suppression therapy and in patients with various thyroid disorders. J Clin Endocrinol Metab 1987;65:1265

62. Caron PJ, Lynette KN, Rose SR, Nisula BC. Deficient nocturnal surge of thyrotropin in central hypothyroidism. J Clin Endocrinol Metab 1986;62:969

63. Rose SR, Manasco PK, Pearce S, Nisula BC. Hypothyroidism and deficiency of the nocturnal thyrotropin surge in children with hypothalamic pituitary disorders. J Clin Endocrinol Metab 1990;70:1750

64. Samuels MH, Lillehei K, Kleinschmidt-Demasters BK, Stears J, Ridgway EC. Patterns of pulsatile pituitary glycoprotein secretion in central hypothyroidism and hypogonadism. J Clin Endocrinol Metab 1990;70:391

65. Adriaanse R, Romijn JA, Endert E, Wiersinga WM. The nocturnal thyroid-stimulating hormone surge is absent in overt, present in mild primary and equivocal in central hypothyroidism. Acta Endocrinol (Copenh) 1992;126:206

66. Lippe BM, Van Herle AJ, La Franchi SH, Uller RP, Lavin N, Kaplan SA. Reversible hypothyroidism in growth hormone-deficient children treated with human growth hormone. J Clin Endocrinol Metab 1975;40:612

67. Porter BA, Refetoff S, Rosenfield RL, Degroot LJ, Fang VS, Stark BA. Abnormal Thyroxine metabolism in hyposomatrophic dwarfism and inhibition of responsiveness to TRH during GH therapy. Pediatrics 1973;51:668

68. Maghnie M, Triulzi F, Larizza D, et al. Hypothalamic-pituitary dysfunction in growth hormone-deficient patients with pituitary abnormalities. J Clin Endocrinol Metab 1991;73:79

69. Cobb WE, Reichlin S, Jackson IMD. Growth hormone secretory status is a determinant of the thyrotropin response to thyrotropin-releasing hormone in euthyroid patients with hypothalamic pituitary disease. J Clin Endocrinol Metab 1981;52:324

70. Jorgensen JOL, Pedersen FA, Lauerberg P, Weeke J, Skakkebaek NE, Christiansen JS. Effects of growth hormone therapy on thyroid function of growth hormone deficient adults with and without concomitant thyroxine substituted central hypothyroidism. J Clin Endocrinol Metab 1989;69:1127

71. Sato T, Suzuki Y, Taketani T, et al. Enhanced peripheral conversion of thyroxine to triiodothyronine during hCG therapy in GH deficient children. J Clin Endocrinol Metab 1977;45:324

72. Faglia G, Bitensky L, Pinchera A, et al. Thyrotropin secretion in patients with central hypothyroidism: evidence for reduced biological activity of immunoreactive thyrotropin. J Clin Endocrinol Metab 1979;48:989

73. Illig R, Krawczynka M, Torresani T, Prader A. Elevated plasma TSH and hypothyroidism in children with hypothalamic hypothyroidism. J Clin Endocrinol Metab 1975;41:722

74. Krieger DT. Glandular and organ deficiency associated with secretion of biologically inactive pituitary peptides. J Clin Endocrinol Metab.1974;38:964

75. Mitsuma T, Shenkman L, Suphavai A, Hollander CS. Hypothalamic hypothyroidism: diminished thyroidal response to thyrotropin-releasing hormone. Am J Med Sci 1973;265:315

76. Patel YG, Burger HG. Serum thyrotropin (TSH) in pituitary and/or hypothalamic hypothyroidism: normal or elevated basal levels and paradoxical response to thyrotropin-releasing hormone. Clin Endocrinol Metab 1973;37:190

77. Woolf PD, Jacobs LS, Donofrio R, Burday SZ, Schalch DS. Secondary hypopituitarism: evidence for continuing regulation of hormone release. J Clin Endocrinol Metab 1974;38:71

78. Lee HB, Faiman C. Isolated thyrotropin deficiency due to a pituitary tumor. Can Med Assoc J 1977;116:520

79. Beck-Peccoz P, Persani L. Variable biological activity of thyroid-stimulating hormone. Eur J Endocrinol 1994;131:331

80. Persani L, Asteria C, Beck-Peccoz P. Dissociation between immunological and biological activities of circulating TSH. Exp Clin Endocrinol 1994;102:38

81. Vitti P, Valente WA, Ambesi-Impiombato FS, Fenzi GF, Pinchera A, Kohn LD. Graves' IgG stimulation of continuously cultured rat thyroid cells: a sensitive and potentially useful clinical assay. J Endocrinol Invest 1982;5:179

82. Persani L, Tonacchera M, Beck-Peccoz P, et al. Measurement of cAMP accumulation in Chinese hamster ovary cells transfected with the recombinant human TSH receptor (CHO-R); a new bioassay for human thyrotropin. J Endocrinol Invest 1993;16:511

83. Taylor T, Weintraub BD. Altered thyrotropin (TSH) carbohydrate structures in hypothalamic hypothyroidism created by paraventricular nuclear lesions are corrected by in vivo TSH-releasing hormone administration. Endocrinology 1989;125:2189

84. Magner J, Klibanski A, Fein H, et al. Ricin and lentil lectin affinity chromatography reveals oligosaccharide heterogeneity of thyrotropin secreted by 12 human pituitary tumors. Metabolism 1992;41:1109

85. Miura Y, Perkel VS, Papenberg KA, Johnson MJ, Magner JA. Concanavalin-A, lentil, and ricin lectin affinity binding characteristic of human thyrotropin: differences in the sialylation of thyrotropin in sera of euthyroid, primary, and central hypothyroid patients. J Clin Endocrinol Metab 1989;69:985

86. Papandreou MJ, Persani L, Asteria C, Ronin C, Beck-Peccoz P. Variable carbohydrate structures of circulating thyrotropin as studied by lectin affinity chromatography in different clinical conditions. J Clin Endocrinol Metab 1993;77:393

87. Faglia G, Beck-Peccoz P. Thyrotropin, thyrotropin beta and alpha-subunit secretion in central hypothyroidism. In: Motta M, Zanisi M, Piva F, eds. Pituitary hormones and related peptides. London: Academic Press, 1982:353

88. Krugman LC, Hershman JM, Chopra IJ, et al. Patterns of recovery of hypothalamic-pituitary-thyroid axis in patients taken off chronic thyroid therapy. J Clin Endocrinol Metab 1975;41:70

89. Singer PA, Nicoloff JT, stein RB, Jaramillo J. Transient TRH deficiency after prolonged thyroid hormone therapy. J Clin Endocrinol Metab 1978;47:512

90. Vagenakis AG, Braverman LE, Azizi F, Portnay GI, Ingbar SH. Recovery of pituitary thyrotropic function after withdrawal of prolonged thyroid-suppression therapy. N Engl J Med 1975;293:681

91. Bartalena L, Martino E, Petrini L, et al. The nocturnal serum thyrotropin surge is abolished in patients with ACTH-dependent or ACTH-independent Cushing's syndrome. J Clin Endocrinol Metab 1991;72:1203

92. Benker G, Raida M, Olbright T, Wagner R, Reinhardt W, Reinwein D. TSH secretion in Cushing's syndrome: relation to glucocorticoid excess, diabetes, goiter, and the "sick euthyroid syndrome". Clin Endocrinol (Oxf) 1990:33:777

93. Berlinger FG, Ruder HJ, Wilbert JF. Cushing's syndrome associated with galactorrhea, amenorrhea, and hypothyroidism: a primary hypothalamic disorder. J Clin Endocrinol Metab 1977;45:1205

94. Bartalena L, Martino E, Brandi LS, et al. Lack of nocturnal serum thyrotropin surge after surgery. J Clin Endocrinol Metab 1990;70:293

95. Okada Y, Onishi T, Tanaka K, et al. Prolactin and TSH responses to TRH, chlorpromazine and L-dopa in children with human growth hormone deficiency. Acta Endocrinol (Copenh) 1978;88:217

96. Municchi G, Malozowski S, Nisula BC, Cristiano A, Rose SR. Nocturnal thyrotropin surge in growth hormone-deficient children. J Pediatr 1992;121:214

97. Pasqualini T, Zantleifer D, Balzaretti M, et al. Evidence of hypothalamic-pituitary thyroid abnormalities in children with end-stage renal disease. J Pediatr 1991;118:873

98. Cavalieri RR. The effect of nonthyroid disease and drugs on thyroid function tests. Med Clin North Am 1991;75:27

99. Docter R, Krenning EP, De Jong M, Hennemann G. The sick euthyroid syndrome: changes in thyroid hormone serum parameters and hormone metabolism. Clin Endocrinol (Oxf) 1993;39:499

100. Bartalena L, Cossu E, Grasso L, et al. Relationship between nocturnal serum thyrotropin peak and metabolic control in diabetic patients. J Clin Endocrinol Metab 1993;76:983

101. Bartalena L, Pacchiarotti A, Palla R, et al. Lack of nocturnal serum thyrotropin (TSH) surge in patients with chronic renal failure undergoing regular maintenance hemofiltration: a case of central hypothyroidism. Clin Nephrol 1990;34:30

102. Custro N, Scafidi V, Gallo S, Notarbartolo A. Deficient pulsatile thyrotropin secretion in the low-thyroid-hormone state of severe non-thyroidal illness. Eur J Endocrinol 1994;130:132

103. Wehmann RE, Gregerman RI, Burns WH, Sarla R, Santos GW. Suppression of thyrotropin in the low-thyroxine state of severe nonthyroid illness. N Engl J Med 1985;312:546

104. Adriaanse R, Romijn JA, Brabant G, Endert E, Wiersinga WM. Pulsatile thyrotropin secretion in nonthyroidal illness. J Clin Endocrinol Metab 1993;77:1313

105. Vaughan GM, Pruitt BA. Thyroid function in critical illness and burn injury. Sem Nephrol 1993;13:359

106. Bartalena L, Martino E, Placidi GF, et al. Nocturnal serum thyrotropin (TSH) and the TSH response to TSH-releasing hormone: dissociated behavior in untreated depressives. J Clin Endocrinol Metab 1990;71:650

107. Kirkegaaard C, Faber J, Hummer C, Rogowski P. Increased levels of TRH in cerebrospinal fluid from patients with endogenous depression. Psychoneuroendocrinology 1979;4:227

108. Bartalena L, Brogioni S, Grasso L, Martino E. Interleukin-6 and the thyroid. Eur J Endocrinol 1995;132:386

109. Bartalena L, Brogioni S, Grasso L, Velluzzi F, Martino E. Relationship of the increased serum interleukin-6 to changes of thyroid function in nonthyroidal illness. J Endocrinol Invest 1994;17:269

110. Boelen A, Platvoet-ter Schiphorst MC, Wiersinga WM. Association between serum interleukin-6 and serum 3,5,3'-triiodothyronine in nonthyroidal illness. J Clin Endocrinol Metab 1993;77:1695

111. Merenich JA. Hypothalamic and pituitary function in AIDS. Bailliere's Clin Endocrinol Metab 1994;8:757

112. Lambert M. Thyroid dysfunction in HIV infection. Bailliere's Clin Endocrinol Metab 1994;8:825

113. Cizza G, Brady LS, Calogero AE, et al. Central hypothyroidism is associated with advanced age in male Fisher 344/N rats: in vivo and in vitro studies. Endocrinology 1992;131:2672

114. Mariotti S, Barbesino G, Caturegli P, et al. Complex alteration of thyroid function in healthy centenarians. J Clin Endocrinol Metab 1993;77:1130

115. Braverman LE, Vagenakis AG. Endocrine manifestations of systemic disease: the thyroid. Clin Endocrinol Metab 1970;8:621

116. Parker DR, Shabourry AH. Central hypothyroidism presenting with pericardial and pleural effusions. J Intern Med 1993; 234:429

117. Ehrman DA, Weinberg N, Sarne DH. Limitations to the use of a sensitive assay for serum thyrotropin in the assessment of thyroid status. Arch Intern Med 1989;149:369

118. Martino E, Bambini G, Bartalena L, et al. Human serum thyrotropin measurement by ultrasensitive immunoradiometric assay as first line test in the evaluation of thyroid function. Clin Endocrinol (Oxf) 1986;24:599

119. Spencer CA. Schwarzbein D, Guttler RB, Lo Presti JS, Nicoloff JT. Thyrotropin (TSH)-releasing hormone stimulation test responses employing third and fourth generation TSH assays. J Clin Endocrinol Metab 1993:76:494

120. Mills GH, Ellis RD, Beck PR. Exaggerated and prolonged thyrotrophin-releasing hormone (TRH) test responses in tertiary hypothyroidism. J Clin Pathol 1991;44:522

121. Brabant G, Prank K, Hoang-vu C, Hesch RD, Von zur Muhlen A. Hypothalamic regulation of pulsatile thyrotropin secretion. J Clin Endocrinol Metab 1991;72:145

122. Engler D, Scanlon MF, Jackson IMD. Thyrotropin-releasing hormone in the systemic circulation of the neonatal rat is derived from the pancreas and other extraneural tissues. J Clin Invest 1981;67:800

123. Mariotti S, Caturegli P, Piccolo P, Barbesino G, Pinchera A. Antithyroid peroxidase autoantibodies in thyroid disease. J Clin Endocrinol Metab 1990;71:661

124. O'Brien T, Dinneem SF, O'Brien PC, Palumbo PJ. Hyperlipidemia in patients with primary and secondary hypothyroidism. Mayo Clin Proc 1993;68:860

125. Bigos ST, Ridgway EC, Kourides IA, Maloof F. Spectrum of pituitary alterations with mild and severe thyroid impairment. J Clin Endocrinol Metab 1978;46:317

126. Rosen HN, Greenspan SL, Landsberg L, Faix JD. Distinguishing hypothyroxinemia due to euthyroid sick syndrome from pituitary insufficiency. Isr J Med Sci 1994;30:746

127. Vagenakis AG, Dole K, Braverman LE. Pituitary enlargement, pituitary failure and primary hypothyroidism. Ann Intern Med 1976;85:195

128. Meador CK, Worrel JL. The sella turcica in postpartum pituitary necrosis (Sheehan's syndrome). Ann Intern Med 1966;65:259

Werner and Ingbar's The Thyroid, Seventh Edition,
edited by Lewis E. Braverman and Robert D. Utiger.
Lippincott–Raven Publishers, Philadelphia, © 1996

Section C
Organ System Manifestations of Hypothyroidism

60

The Skin in Hypothyroidism

Jeffrey D. Bernhard
Irwin M. Freedberg
Louis N. Vogel

The cutaneous changes of hypothyroidism were recognized by Gull and Ord in the late 1800s and were subsequently well documented in the classic study by the Clinical Society of London.[1-3] More than a century later, Ord's accurate and concise description warrants repetition:

> The skin of the face and particularly of the eyelids, becoming thick, semi-transparent, and waxy....The face was generally pale, but had the delicate blush on the cheeks. The eyelids were swollen and ridged...[and they]...hang down flaccidly on the cheeks. [They] did not pit on being squeezed...The skin....was singularly dry...it was harsh and rough to the touch: the hairs were feebly developed, and no trace of fatty secretion could be found. [Within] two years the complexion was pale yellow. The pathology...is...a jelly-like state of the fibrillar or white element of the connective tisue...well seen in the corium genrally, but most clearly in the investments of glands and of hair sacs, and in the coats of vessels.

Subsequent reports have confirmed these observations and have indicated that cutaneous signs and symptoms are extremely prevalent and often important in the diagnosis of hypothyroidism.[4,5] These cutaneous abnormalities and estimates of their frequencies are catalogued in Table 60-1. Although other important symptoms or signs of hypothyroidism may be present, it is remarkable that changes in the skin may be the single most important factor in a patient's decision to seek medical attention. In one example, a 27-year-old woman with menstrual irregularities, severe constipation, and lethargy finally sought medical attention because of progressive yellowing of her skin.[6]

EPIDERMAL CHANGES

The epidermis and its appendages, targets for the action of many hormones,[7] show distinct changes in patients with hypothyroidism and in those with virtually all other endocrine diseases. In over 80% of patients with primary hypothyroidism, the epidermis is dry, rough, and covered with fine superficial scales. The skin may have a finely wrinkled, parchment-like character.[8] Inflammatory changes may be present.[9] These gross changes are histologically represented by

TABLE 60-1.
Cutaneous Signs and Symptoms of Hypothyroidism

Cutaneous Manifestation	Approximate Frequency (%)
Cold intolerance	50–95
Nail abnormality (thin, brittle, striated)	90
Thickening and dryness of hair and skin	80–90
Edema of hands, face, and eyelids	70–85
Change in shape of face	70
Malar flush	50
Nonpitting or dependent edema	30
Alopecia (loss or thinning of hair)	30–40
Eyebrows	25
Scalp	20
Pallor	25–60
Yellowish discoloration of skin	25–50
Decrease or loss of sweat secretion	10–70

Compiled from various references cited in the text.

thinning of the epidermis and hyperkeratosis of the stratum corneum. When hypothyroidism occurs secondary to pituitary disease, the abnormalities are much less frequent, occurring in less than 10% of patients.[10] These patients' skin is wrinkled, with less mucin deposition.[11] Etiologically, the clinical changes may be attributed to the well-documented effects of thyroid hormones on cell division and protein synthesis.

DERMAL CHANGES

The dermal pathologic findings in patients with hypothyroidism are clinically manifested by nonpitting swelling or puffiness, most marked around the eyes and hands—that is, *myxedema*. This is related to infiltration of the tissue with a metachromatic staining material, which disappears within several weeks after appropriate replacement therapy and reappears within about the same time after discontinuation of therapy.[12] The material has been identified as a mixture of the mucopolysaccharides hyaluronic acid and chondroitin sulfate. It is found predominantly in the papillary dermis, is localized around vessels and cutaneous appendages, and is associated with a perivascular lymphocytic infiltrate.[13,14] The histogenesis of the material remains a point of dispute. Although most investigators believe it to be secreted by fibroblasts, another investigator has concluded that it is a product of dermal mast cells.[15]

The elastic fibers of skin are decreased in hypothyroidism, and there are qualitative changes in staining characteristics as well.[16]

The occurrence of multiple cutaneous focal mucinoses has been reported with hypothyroidism: a woman aged 54 years with myxedema had hundreds of discrete, cutaneous, mucinous papules that both clinically and histologically resembled focal mucinosis. With appropriate replacement thy-

roxine therapy, most of the smaller cutaneous papules disappeared, and the contents of the larger papules became resorbed, leaving flat, light-brown macules.[17]

An additional cause of the dermal swelling has been suggested on the basis of observations concerning sodium in patients with myxedema, namely the decrease in serum sodium and increase in tissue sodium space.[18] It has been postulated that the high osmotic pressure of the ground substance leads to loss of sodium and water from the intravascular compartment of the extracellular space. The initial cutaneous swelling from mucopolysaccharides would thus be enhanced by the addition of water.

The accumulation of fluid and macromolecules in the dermis, which occurs in both primary and secondary hypothyroidism, is accompanied by an alteration in dermal collagen. This change may also contribute to the clinical abnormalities, including slow wound healing. In hypothyroid animals, rates of both collagen synthesis and degradation are decreased, and the free and total hydroxyproline contents of the dermis are lowered.[19,20] Urinary hydroxyproline is decreased in hypothyroidism,[21] a finding consistent with the experimental animal data.

Mucin is present in the dermis in several dermatologic diseases in which no evidence of a pathologic condition of the thyroid exists. There are localized papular or follicular mucinoses that offer no difficulty in differential diagnosis,[22,23] but nosologic problems arise when the infiltration is diffuse. Hyaluronic acid and chondroitin sulfate are found in the dermis, usually associated with fibroblastic proliferation. In true myxedema, the degree of separation and replacement of collagen by mucopolysaccharides is usually not as great as that seen in other processes,[24] but differential diagnosis may be extremely difficult.[25]

SKIN COLOR

The cause of the prominent malar flush that occurs in over half of hypothyroid patients has never been ascertained. In contrast, the diffuse pallor and pale waxy surface color can be attributed to at least two pathophysiologic mechanisms. First, vasoconstriction occurs, perhaps as a homeostatic response, to preserve basal temperature in the face of decreased metabolism. Second, the excess fluid and mucopolysaccharides in the dermis may physically compress small vessels to create blanching as well as interference with the transmission of color from the deeper vessels. Anemia may also contribute to the pallor.

Yellowish discoloration of the skin, most notably the palms, soles, and nasolabial folds, occurs in patients with hypothyroidism of relatively long duration. It is caused by elevation of serum and tissue carotene concentrations[26] and is due to a block in the metabolic pathway from carotene to vitamin A. Diffuse yellowing of the skin may occur; scleral sparing is a clue to hypercarotenemia as opposed to jaundice.[6]

HAIR FOLLICLES

Definite effects on hair follicle function have been described in hypothyroidism, and hair loss has been noted in up to half of hypothyroid patients. The hair is dull, coarse, and brittle, in part due to diminished sebum secretion. Loss of scalp, genital, and beard hair occurs. Inhibition of the initiation of the actively growing phase of the hair cycle leads to diffuse hair loss in hypothyroid animals.[27] The finding of a similar decrease in the percentage of growing hairs in two hypothyroid patients with hair loss suggests that this change in the growth cycle is the cause of alopecia in human hypothyroidism as well.[28] Other workers who studied a larger number of patients, however, were unable to document an abnormality in the hair growth cycle.[29] They did demonstrate fragility of the internal root sheath in hypothyroid subjects, but the relation between this observation and the clinical changes is not clear. Increased telogen counts have been documented in hypothyroid patients,[30] and the effects may be on initiation and duration of the hair cycle.

The growth of long, terminal dark hairs on the back and extremities of several children with hypothyroidism has been described. After thyroid replacement therapy, this hair completely disappeared.[31] The loss of the lateral third of the eyebrows, described as common in hypothyroidism, is actually seen in many older euthyroid patients and in association with several types of cutaneous disease, including atopic dermatitis, Hansen's disease, thallium toxicity, lupus erythematosus, and seborrheic dermatitis.

NAILS

Nail deformities are reported in as many as 90% of patients with myxedema.[32] The nails are thin, brittle, and striated, with both longitudinal and transverse grooves. Their size and rate of growth may be markedly decreased.[33]

SWEAT GLANDS

The dry skin of hypothyroidism, dependent in part on the direct effect of thyroid hormone deficiency on epidermal metabolism, is also related to decreased eccrine gland secretion. A decrease has been documented in the insensible cutaneous water loss in patients with myxedema that cannot be attributed to changes in the metabolic rate.[34] The eccrine glands themselves are atrophic, perhaps secondary to pressure from the mucinous, periappendageal infiltrates discussed previously.

In the eccrine sweat glands, periodic acid-Schiff-positive, nonglycogen, nonmucin inclusions have been observed in the large pale cells of the glandular secretory coil. These inclusions occurred in over 75% of hypothyroid patients.[35,36] The genesis of the material is unknown, and its concentration does not correlate with the degree of hypothyroidism.

MISCELLANEOUS CUTANEOUS CHANGES AND ASSOCIATIONS

An increased frequency of hypothyroidism is seen in patients with progressive systemic sclerosis, and this appears to be autoimmune in nature.[37] The prevalence of thyroid abnormalities is reportedly increased in patients with vitiligo, alopecia

areata, and dermatitis herpetiformis.[5,38] Hypothyroidism is also part of a distinctive type of hypohidrotic ectodermal dysplasia that is also associated with alopecia, nail dystrophy, and freckles, as well as gastrointestinal, ophthalmologic, and pulmonary changes.[39]

Although dry skin may itch, pruritus is not a cardinal feature of hypothyroidism, in contrast with thyrotoxicosis, in which it may be an important presenting symptom.[40]

The coexistence or possible association of a number of other disorders that may involve the skin and the thyroid gland is discussed in reference 5.

References

1. Gull WW. On a cretinoid state supervening in adult life in women. Trans Clin Soc (Lond) 1874;7:180
2. Ord WM. On myxoedema. A term proposed to be applied to an essential condition in the "cretinoid" affection occasionally observed in middle-aged women. Med Chir Trans 1878;61:57
3. Report of a committee of the clinical society of London to investigate the subject of myxoedema. Trans Clin Soc (Lond) [Suppl] 1838:21
4. Rosen T, Kleman GA. Thyroid and skin. In: Callen JP, Jorizzo JL, Greer KE, et al, eds. Dermatological signs of internal disease, 2nd ed. Philadelphia: WB Saunders, 1994:189
5. Heymann WR. Cutaneous manifestations of thyroid disease. J Am Acad Dermatol 1992;26:885
6. Al-Jubouri MA, Coombes EJ, Young RM, et al. Xanthoderma: an unusual presentation of hypothyroidism. J Clin Pathol 1994;47:850
7. Ebling FJG, Hale PA, Randall VA. Hormones and hair growth. In: Goldsmith LA, ed. Physiology, biochemistry, and molecular biology of the skin, 2nd ed. New York: Oxford University Press, 1991:660
8. Freinkel RK. Cutaneous manifestations of endocrine diseases. In: Fitzpatrick TB, Eisen AZ, Wolff K, et al, eds. Dermatology in general medicine, 4th ed. New York: McGraw-Hill, 1993:2113
9. Warin AP. Eczema craquelé as a presenting feature of myxedema. Br J Dermatol 1973;89:289
10. Wayne EJ. Clinical and metabolic studies in thyroid disease. Br Med J 1960;1:78
11. Holt PJA, Lazarus J, Marks R. The epidermis in thyroid disease. Br J Dermatol 1976;95:513
12. Gabrilove JL, Ludwig AW. The histogenesis of myxedema. J Clin Endocrinol Metab 1957;17:925
13. Feingold KR, Elias PM. Endocrine skin interactions. J Am Acad Dermatol 1987;17:921
14. Reuter MJ. Histopathology of the skin in myxedema. Arch Dermatol Syph 1931;24:55
15. Asboe-Hansen G. The intercellular substance of the connective tissue in myxedema. J Invest Dermatol 1950;15:25
16. Matsuoka LY, Wortsman J, Uitto J, et al. Altered skin elastic fibers in hypothyroid myxedema and pretibial myxedema. Arch Intern Med 1985;145:117
17. Jakubovic HR, Saloma SSS, Rosenthal D. Multiple cutaneous focal mucinoses with hypothyroidism. Ann Intern Med 1982;96:56
18. Aikawa JK. The nature of myxedema. Ann Intern Med 1956;44:30
19. Kivirikko KI, Laitinen O, Aer J, et al. Metabolism of collagen in experimental hyperthyroidism and hypothyroidism in the rat. Endocrinology 1967;80:1051
20. Fink CW, Ferguson JL, Smiley JD. Effect of hyperthyroidism and hypothyroidism on collagen metabolism. J Lab Clin Med 1967;69:950

21. Keiser HR, Sjoerdsma A. Effect of thyroid hormone on collagen metabolism. J Clin Invest 11962;41:1371

22. Johnson WC, Helwig EB. Cutaneous focal mucinosis: a clinico-pathological and histochemical study. Arch Dermatol 1966; 93:13

23. Montgomery H, Underwood LJ. Lichen myxedematosus (differentiation from cutaneous myxedema or mucoid states). J Invest Dermatol 1953;20:213

24. Bloomer HA, Kyle LH. Myxedema. Arch Intern Med 1969; 104:234

25. Reed RJ, Clark WH Jr, Mihm MC. The cutaneous mucinoses. Hum Pathol 1973;4:201

26. Escamilla RF. Carotenemia in myxedema: explanation of the typical slightly icteric tint. J Clin Endocrinol Metab 1942;2:33

27. Mohn MP. The effects of different hormonal states on the growth of hair in rats. In: Montagna W, Ellis RA, eds. The biology of hair growth. New York: Academic Press, 1958:335

28. Rook A. Endocrine influences on hair growth. Br Med J 1965;1:609

29. Smith JG, Weinstein GD, Burr JM. Hair roots of the human scalp in thyroid disease. J Invest Dermatol 1959;32:35

30. Freinkel RK, Freinkel N. Hair growth and alopecia in hypothyroidism. Arch Dermatol 1972;106:349

31. Perloff WH. Hirsutism: a manifestation of juvenile hypothyroidism. JAMA 1955;157:651

32. Barrett AM. Hereditary occurrence of hypothyroidism with dystrophies of the nails and hair. Arch Neurol 1919;2:628

33. Tosti A, Baran R, Dawber RPR. The nail in systemic diseases and drug-induced changes. In: Baran R, Dawber RPR, eds. Diseases of the nails and their management, 2nd ed. Oxford: Blackwell Scientific Publications, 1994:175

34. Gilligan DR, Edsall G. The relationship between insensible water loss and heat production in patients with hypothyroidism compared with normal subjects. J Clin Invest 1935;14:659

35. Dobson RL, Abele DC. Cytological changes in the eccrine sweat gland in hypothyroidism. J Invest Dermatol 1961;37:457

36. Means MA, Dobson RL. Cytological changes in the sweat gland in hypothyroidism. JAMA 1965;186:113

37. DeKeyser L, Narhi DC, Furst DE, et al. Thyroid dysfunction in a prospectively followed series of patients with progressive systemic sclerosis. J Endocrinol Invest 1990;13:161

38. Cunningham MJ, Zone JJ. Thyroid abnormalities in dermatitis herpetiformis: prevalence of clinical thyroid disease and thyroid autoantibodies. Ann Intern Med 1985;102:194

39. Pike-Michael G, Baraitser M, Dinwiddle R, et al. A distinctive type of hypohidrotic ectodermal dysplasia featuring hypothyroidism. J Pediatr 1986;108:109

40. Bernhard JD. Endocrine itches. In: Bernhard JD, ed. Itch: Mechanisms and management of pruritus. New York: McGraw-Hill, 1994:251

Werner and Ingbar's The Thyroid, Seventh Edition,
edited by Lewis E. Braverman and Robert D. Utiger.
Lippincott–Raven Publishers, Philadelphia, © 1996

61

Connective Tissue in Hypothyroidism

Terry J. Smith

William Ord in 1878[1] first described the pathologic process of myxedema associated with long-standing dysfunction of the thyroid gland. Reuter,[2] some 50 years later, published a detailed histopathologic description of a skin biopsy from a hypothyroid (myxedenatous) patient. He wrote:

> Evidence was found of moderate, uniform, relative and absolute hyperkeratosis, with distinct atrophy and almost complete flattening of the rete ridges. The epithelial cells varied considerably in staining; some of the nuclei took a heavy basic stain. In many of the cells of the rete there was also perinuclear vacuolization. In areas there appeared to be merging of the cytoplasm of the basal cells with the cutis; the cytoplasm stained faintly with eosin, and the nuclei lay at the upper poles of the cells. The corium was definitely thickened. In the upper layer of the corium there was homogenization of the collagen fibers, a tendency to take a basophilic stain with hematoxylin, sparse, perivascular infiltration with lymphocytes, and slight dilation of the blood and lymph vessels. The upper and middle portions of the corium were edematous, and the collagen and elastic fibers were spread apart and fragmented. The connective tissue cells appeared to be slightly increased in number. Sections stained with the mucicarmine stain revealed the presence of material that stained red, which extended in a bandlike form throughout the upper part of the cutis, and which lay over and between the bundles of collagen. There was mucicarmine staining material in the deeper parts of the cutis. Under oil immersion, this substance appeared to be composed of fine threads and granules. This material was also especially prominent about the blood vessels and to some extent about the sweat glands. Evidence of collastin (a degenerative combination product of collagen and elacin) was lacking, as it was impossible to demonstrate any tinctorial change with the acid orcein and neutral orcein stains.

Although this description clearly defines the histopathology of generalized myxedema, elucidation of the biochemical nature of that process awaited development of techniques to isolate glycosaminoglycans from human and animal tissue. Trotter and Eden[3] attempted to establish criteria for differentiating between the biochemical abnormalities responsible for the localized myxedema associated with Graves' disease and those responsible for generalized myxedema. They were unsuccessful in establishing clear differences between the two lesions, and they concluded that hyaluronan (hyaluronic acid) appeared to be a major constituent of the substance accumulating in both. Watson and Pearce[4] were among the first to explore the chemical composition of myxedema using semiquantitative and reasonably specific assays. Analyzing specimens from lesions of localized myxedema, they identified the glycosaminoglycans in acid-alcohol extracts as hyaluronan and chondroitin sulfate. (See chap 37 for a detailed discussion of connective tissue metabolism.)

CLINICAL PRESENTATION

Generalized myxedema develops in people who have severe long-standing hypothyroidism. The features of myxedema are attributable to accumulation of glycosaminoglycan in soft tissues. Because of the large volume occupied by the hydrated glycosaminoglycan molecules, the affected skin becomes edematous. Unlike cardiogenic or nephrotic edema, myxedema does not pit and is not rapidly resorbed during recumbency. Prominent among the clinical manifestations are facial fullness, especially periorbital edema (Fig 61-1), and edema of the hands and feet. Other cutaneous signs of hypothyroidism are nearly always present; the skin is coarse and dry, and the hair is brittle.

The phenomenon of myxedema is not limited to the subcutaneous tissue. In a fatal case of long-standing hypothyroidism, the intestine, lung, myocardium, tongue, and kidney contained an increased amount of hyaluronan.[5] In contrast, the abundance of chondroitin sulfate, heparan sulfate, and dermatan sulfate was similar to that in age- and

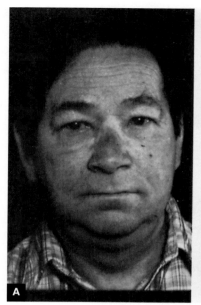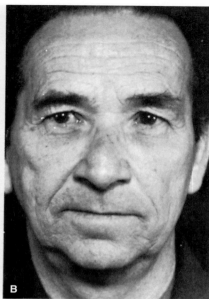

FIGURE 61-1. Photograph of a hypothyroid patient with myxedema before (*A*) and after (*B*) treatment. (Reproduced from Smith TJ, Bahn RS, Gorman CA Connective tissue, glycosaminoglycans and diseases of the thyroid. Endocr Rev 1989;10:366)

sex-matched euthyroid patients. A classic finding in patients with severe hypothyroidism is a pericardial effusion that contains high concentrations of cholesterol and glycosaminoglycans.[6] Histologic examination of the myocardium reveals interstitial fibrosis, edema and interstitial glycosaminoglycan accumulation. The characteristic microscopic changes of myxedema also are seen in renal biopsies. The functional effects of the changes in the heart and kidneys are uncertain, but the intestinal dilatation, atony, and pseudo-obstruction associated with hypothyroidism also could be related to the deposition of glycosaminoglycans in the gut wall (see chap 65).

In addition to glycosaminoglycan accumulation in many tissues, patients with myxedema also have an increased plasma volume, a decreased serum albumin concentration, and a normal intravascular albumin mass. The extravascular albumin mass is, however, increased because the rate of transcapillary escape of albumin is increased due to increased vascular permeability.[7]

Patients with hypothyroidism typically have hypercholesterolemia and so may be at increased risk for developing coronary artery disease (see chap 73). They have a defect of the low-density lipoprotein receptor that is similar to that in homozygous familial hypercholesterolemia,[8] but that is reversed with adequate thyroxine (T_4) therapy.

The myxedematous changes in the connective tissue disappear after the attainment of adequate serum and tissue concentrations of thyroid hormone. The interval between the initiation of therapy and complete resolution of the physical abnormalities is variable and is influenced by factors such as age, the patient's general state of health, and the duration of hypothyroidism. Some improvement may be evident within a week; however, in elderly patients some abnormalities may persist for several months after therapy is initiated.

PATHOGENESIS OF GENERALIZED MYXEDEMA

Early investigators believed the myxedematous changes of hypothyroidism were due to a stimulatory effect of thyrotropin (TSH) on affected tissues.[9] They reasoned that the elevated serum TSH concentrations in patients with primary hypothyroidism directly stimulated glycosaminoglycan synthesis in extrathyroidal tissues. Asboe-Hansen[10] hypothesized that mast cells were the ultimate target of the hormones that influenced the hyaluronan content of extracellular tissue, a theory that was consistent with the increased numbers of subcutaneous mast cells in hypothyroidism. The hypothesis was ruled out when the skin of hypophysectomized rats was found to have a pattern of glycosaminoglycan deposition similar to that in thyroidectomized animals. Direct evidence that thyroid hormone deficiency per se stimulates the accumulation of glycosaminoglycan derives from the observations that fibroblasts incubated in medium depleted of thyroid hormone synthesize hyaluronan at an increased rate.[11] In addition, TSH does not affect the rate of hyaluronan synthesis in fibroblast cultures.

Experimental studies in rats have provided some of the best evidence that hyaluronan is an important constituent of myxedema.[12] In iodine-deficient, propylthiouracil-treated rats, the half-life of hyaluronan in tissues was 7.3 days, as compared with 4.2 days in normal rats and 3.8 days in hypothyroid rats treated with T_4. The effects of hypothyroidism on chondroitin sulfate in these studies were complex. Whereas the turnover rate of chondroitin sulfate was slower in hypothyroid rats than in those receiving T_4, the skin concentration of sulfated glycosaminoglycans was lower in hypothyroid rats. These results suggest that the accumulation of hyaluronan in hypothyroid rats results from a diminished rate of degradation.

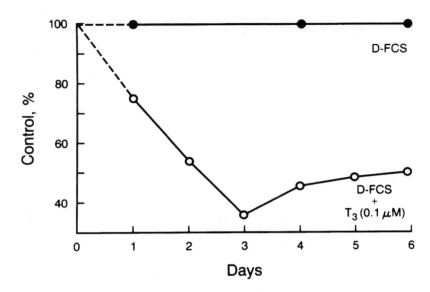

FIGURE 61-2. Time course of T_3-induced inhibition of [^{3}H]-glycosaminoglycan accumulation in fibroblast cultures. Confluent cultures were shifted to a medium enriched with serum that had been depleted of thyroid hormone (D-FCS) to which T_3 (○) or diluent (●) was added. (From Smith TJ, et al. Regulation of glycosaminoglycan synthesis by thyroid hormone in vitro. J Clin Invest 1982;70:1066)

More recent studies of cultured human skin fibroblasts suggest that changes in hyaluronan degradation may not account fully for the tissue accumulation of hyaluronan in hypothyroidism. Skin fibroblasts cultured in medium containing thyroid hormone–deficient serum accumulated hyaluronan at a faster rate than did cultures incubated with T_4 or triiodothyronine (T_3).[11,13,14] The T_3 concentration that elicited maximal inhibition of hyaluronan accumulation was comparable to that in normal serum; the effect took about 3 days to become maximal[11] (Fig 61-2). Pulse-labeling of cultures with [^{3}H]acetate followed by addition of unlabeled acetate to the medium revealed no detectable degradation of hyaluronan during the course of the studies (up to 96 hours),[11] consistent with earlier studies.[15] Moreover, the activity of hyaluronan synthetase in whole-cell sonicates was increased in cultures deprived of thyroid hormone. Thus, the inhibition by T_3 of hyaluronan accumulation in cultured human skin fibroblasts probably involves an alteration of the rate of hyaluronan synthesis.

Extrapolating from these results to human disease may be problematic. Nevertheless, it appears that thyroid hormone inhibits the synthesis of hyaluronan and stimulates its degradation. The relative contribution of increased synthesis and decreased degradation to the formation of myxedema in vivo will be known only when whole-body hyaluronan turnover studies are performed in humans.

References

1. Ord WM. On myxoedema, a term proposed to be applied to an essential condition in the "cretinoid" affection occasionally observed in middle-aged women. Med Chir Trans Lord 1878;61:57
2. Reuter MJ. Histopathology of the skin in myxedema. Arch Dermatol Syph 1931;24:55
3. Trotter WR, Eden KC. Localized pretibial myxoedema in association with toxic goitre. Q J Med 1942;11:229
4. Watson EM, Pearce RH. The mucopolysaccharide content of the skin in localized (pretibial) myxedema. Am J Clin Pathol 1947;17:507
5. Parving H-H, Helin G, Garbarsch C, et al. Acid glycosaminoglycans in myxoedema. Clin Endocrinol 1982;16:207
6. Davis PJ, Jacobson S. Myxedema with cardiac tamponade and pericardial effusion of "gold paint" appearance. Arch Intern Med 1967;120:615
7. Parving H-H, Hansen JM, Nielsen SL, Rossing N, Munck O, Lassen NA. Mechanisms of edema formation in myxedema—increased protein extravasation and relatively slow lymphatic drainage. N Engl J Med 1979;301:460
8. Thompson GR, Soutar AK, Spengel FA, Jadhav A, Gauigan SJP, Myant ND. Defects of receptor-mediated low density lipoprotein catabolism in homozygous familial hypercholesterolemia and hypothyroidism in vivo. Proc Natl Acad Sci U S A 1981;78:2591
9. Asboe-Hansen G. The variability in the hyaluronic acid content of the dermal connective tissue under the influence of thyroid hormone: mast cells—the peripheral transmitters of hormone action. Acta Derm Venereol 1950;30:221
10. Asboe-Hansen G. The intercellular substance of the connective tissue in myxedema. J Invest Dermatol 1950;15:25
11. Smith TJ, Murata Y, Horwitz AL, Philipson L, Refetoff S. Regulation of glycosaminoglycan synthesis by thyroid hormone in vitro. J Clin Invest 1982;70:1066
12. Schiller S, Slover GA, Dorfman A. Effect of the thyroid gland on metabolism of acid mucopolysaccharides in skin. Biochim Biophys Acta 1962;58:27
13. Smith TJ, Horwitz AL, Refetoff S. The effect of thyroid hormone on glycosaminoglycan accumulation in human skin fibroblasts. Endocrinology 1981;108:2397
14. Smith TJ. Dexamethasone regulation of glycosaminoglycan synthesis in cultured human skin fibroblasts. Similar effects of glucocorticoid and thyroid hormones. J Clin Invest 1984;74:2157
15. Arbogast B, Hopwood JJ, Dorfman A. Absence of hyaluronidase in cultured human skin fibroblasts. Biochem Biophys Res Commun 1975;67:376

Werner and Ingbar's The Thyroid, Seventh Edition,
edited by Lewis E. Braverman and Robert D. Utiger.
Lippincott–Raven Publishers, Philadelphia, © 1996

62

The Cardiovascular System in Hypothyroidism

Irwin Klein

Kaie Ojamaa

The cardiovascular changes that occur in patients with hypothyroidism are opposite to those of thyrotoxicosis.[1] However, in contrast to the prominent cardiovascular symptoms and signs that often occur in thyrotoxicosis, those that accompany hypothyroidism tend to be more subtle.[2] In this chapter we will review the pathophysiologic basis for the cardiac findings of hypothyroidism, including impaired ventricular contractile performance, cardiomegaly, hypertension, and the potential for accelerated atherosclerosis.

CARDIOVASCULAR HEMODYNAMICS OF HYPOTHYROIDISM

The hemodynamic changes associated with hypothyroidism are listed in Table 62-1. Most patients with hypothyroidism have an increase in systemic vascular resistance and a decrease in tissue perfusion, as well as a decrease in peripheral oxygen consumption. As compared with normal subjects, patients with hypothyroidism have increases of 50% to 60% in peripheral vascular resistance and decreases of 30% to 50% in cardiac output.[3–5] The net effect of the decreases in blood flow and tissue oxygen consumption is that arteriovenous oxygen extraction across major organs is not different in hypothyroid patients and normal subjects.[3] The mechanism underlying the increase in systemic vascular resistance is not understood. Thyroid hormone, specifically triiodothyronine (T_3), may act as a vasodilator, and in its absence vascular smooth muscle tone and systemic vascular resistance may rise.[4] The roles of the endothelium and of vasoactive substances including endothelium-derived relaxing factor (EDRF, nitric oxide) are unknown.[6]

All measurements of left ventricular performance are decreased in patients with either short-term and long-term hypothyroidism.[7–12] Cardiac output (index) is decreased as a result of decreases in both stroke volume and, to a lesser extent, heart rate.[7,8] The duration of both the pre-ejection time and isovolumic contraction time is prolonged as compared with normal subjects, and these times decrease in response to thyroid hormone replacement therapy.[10] Conversely, the rate of ventricular relaxation during diastole is slower and diastolic filling and compliance are impaired.[12] The rate of diastolic filling may decrease from normal values of 400 mL/sec to less than 300 mL/sec. The mechanisms underlying the impaired ventricular performance in patients with hypothyroidism are multifactorial. As noted in chapter 38 the expression of many cardiac genes is modulated by thyroid hormone, and in experimental animals lowering the serum concentrations of thyroxine (T_4) and T_3 alters the expression of myocyte-specific genes and the distribution of the heavy-chain isoforms of sarcomeric myosin and of the calcium regulatory proteins.[13,14]

The rate of tension development during cardiac systole is determined in part by the rate at which the myosin molecule catalyzes ATP hydrolysis.[13] Of the two myosin-heavy chain isoforms expressed in cardiac myocytes, the slower catalytic beta-myosin heavy chain is preferentially expressed in hypothyroidism and the fast alpha-myosin heavy chain in euthyroidism.[15] Although the transcriptional regulation of myosin heavy-chain gene expression in the heart of animals is one of the best studied examples of the nuclear action of T_3,[16] the hormone does not have this action in the human myocardium.[13] The beta-myosin heavy chain predominates in human ventricular tissue, and it is unaltered in thyroid disease or by thyroid hormone treatment. In one hypothyroid patient

Table 62-1.
Cardiovascular Hemodynamics in Hypothyroidism

	Finding	Comments
Systemic vascular resistance	↑	50%–60% higher
Cardiac output	↓	50% decreased
Blood pressure		
Systolic	↓ or normal	Narrowed pulse pressure
Diastolic	↑ or normal	20% prevalence of diastolic hypertension
Heart rate	↓ or normal	
Cardiac contractility	↓	Systolic and diastolic function both subnormal
Cardiac mass	↓	Pericardial effusion may suggest cardiomegaly
Blood volume	↓	

with severe left ventricular dysfunction given thyroid hormone, there was only a minor increase in alpha-myosin heavy chain content, and beta-myosin heavy chain remained the predominant isoform.[17] Left ventricular contractile function improved during treatment, most probably a result of improved calcium handling in cardiac muscle cells[18] and through changes in systemic vascular resistance.[1,3]

In hypothyroidism, both diastolic and systolic performance of the heart is subnormal,[9] suggesting that alterations in myocyte calcium uptake and release are responsible for the changes in inotropic state.[14] The activities of several enzymes involved in regulating calcium fluxes in the heart are controlled by thyroid hormone. These include calcium-activated ATPase of the sarcoplasmic reticulum and phospholamban.[18] Transcription of the genes coding for these proteins is regulated by nuclear thyroid hormone receptors.[14]

As a result of the increase in systemic vascular resistance and decrease in cardiac output in hypothyroidism, mean blood pressure is largely unaltered.[3,19] There may be an increase in diastolic pressure and a fall in systolic pressure, so that pulse pressure is low. Hypothyroid patients may have diastolic hypertension (see later) that responds to T_4 replacement with improvement or normalization of blood pressure as well as a return to normal systemic vascular resistance.[19,20]

Blood volume is decreased in hypothyroid patients,[5] an unexpected finding because some of the patients have both pitting as well as nonpitting edema suggestive of fluid overload. The mechanism of edema formation in hypothyroidism is an increase in protein (albumin) distribution in the extravascular extracellular space, at least in part due to an increase in capillary permeability.[21] This increase occurs in the pleural, pericardial, cerebrospinal, peritoneal, scrotal, and middle ear spaces, as well as in the extracellular space of the legs and sacrum.[21,22] Whereas total body fluid and albumin content may rise, blood volume is lowered in parallel with the decrease in basal metabolic rate.[5] Despite this decrease in blood volume, right atrial pressures are unchanged.[3]

CARDIOVASCULAR PATHOPHYSIOLOGY

The cardiovascular manifestations of hypothyroidism are the result of decreased action of thyroid hormone on both the heart and the peripheral circulation.[1,10,13,14]

Cardiac Effects

Thyroid hormone deficiency can alter cardiac muscle function by decreasing the expression of several contractile proteins in myocytes. Myocyte nuclei contain T_3 receptors that bind to specific DNA sequences of several genes, which suggests that regulation by T_3 occurs at the level of gene transcription.[14–16,23] The inherent delay in a process that requires gene transcription and protein translation before changes in physiologic function occur is consistent with the observation that the cardiovascular responses to intravenous T_3 administration occur over a period of hours to several days.[24] Genomic changes in the expression of sarcoplasmic reticulum calcium ATPase, phospholamban, Na^+,K^+-ATPase, malic enzyme, and β-adrenergic receptors may all play a role in the impaired left ventricular contractility of patients with hypothyroidism[14,23] (see chaps 9 and 38).

Thyroid hormone also can effect the contractile performance of the heart in an acute nongenomic manner.[6,25] In patients with ischemic heart disease undergoing cardiac surgery and in hypothyroid and euthyroid animals, the acute administration of T_3 can rapidly increase cardiac contractility and lower systemic vascular resistance.[25,26] This increase may involve changes in sodium and calcium transport by the plasma membrane, an increase in sarcoplasmic reticulum calcium fluxes, or an increase in high energy phosphate generation and mitochondrial function.[25] Notwithstanding those results, the reluctance to administer thyroid hormone therapeutically to increase cardiac contractility and output in certain clinical situations is warranted by concerns of increased myocardial oxygen consumption and the potential to precipitate myocardial ischemia.[8,10] There is also concern regarding the use of thyroid hormone to treat patients with hypothyroidism who have coronary artery disease (see later). In both of these settings the potential for improvement in cardiac performance must be balanced against the possibility of worsening myocardial ischemia due to coronary artery disease.

Peripheral Circulatory Effects

Systemic vascular resistance is consistently increased in hypothyroidism.[3,5,8,19] The decrease in tissue oxygen and substrate utilization in hypothyroidism reflects diminished blood flow, which is mediated through increased vascular tone.[4] A high systemic vascular resistance increases cardiac afterload, which lowers cardiac output while maintaining mean arterial pressure. Reflex changes in cardiac function, including a small decrease in heart rate and a decrease in the left ventricular ejection fraction, form the basis for the decrease in cardiac output that is characteristic of hypothyroidism.

The response of hypothyroid patients to exercise supports the hypothesis that peripheral circulatory changes mediate many of the changes in cardiac performance. Exercise lowers systemic vascular resistance in hypothyroid patients, causing an increase in cardiac index, heart rate, and stroke volume to 85% to 90% of the responses in euthyroid subjects.[27] These observations indicate that the reduced left ventricular function in hypothyroid patients at rest is at least in part the result of a decrease in hemodynamic loading rather than inherent changes in left ventricular contractility.[1,27]

One of the earliest responses to acute thyroid hormone administration in hypothyroid animals and humans is a fall in systemic vascular resistance.[4,28–30] Although the exact mechanism for this change remains to be determined, T_3 may act directly on vascular smooth muscle or endothelial cells either alone or in concert with adrenergic, cholinergic, and other vasoactive agents.[4,30]

Blood flow to the kidneys is decreased in hypothyroidism, resulting in a fall in renal perfusion and in glomerular filtration rate.[31] Renin and aldosterone production are decreased.[32] Cold intolerance results because of decreased blood flow to the skin and extremities, despite normal core body temperature.

Thyroid Hormone–Catecholamine Interactions

Many of the hemodynamic characteristics of hypothyroidism suggest a decrease in adrenergic tone. However, plasma catecholamine concentrations in hypothyroid patients are increased[33] (see chap 70). Various hypotheses have been put forward to explain this apparent paradox, including a decrease in β-adrenergic receptor number, an increase in the adenylate cyclase inhibitory G-protein, adenylyl, or changes in other cellular signaling pathways that can diminish β-adrenergic sensitivity.[34,35]

CLINICAL MANIFESTATIONS

Most hypothyroid patients have few symptoms directly referable to the cardiovascular system.[36–38] Although exertional dyspnea and exercise intolerance have been attributed to impaired cardiac performance, they are more likely to be related to skeletal muscle dysfunction.[22,39] Whether or not congestive heart failure with orthopnea and paroxysmal nocturnal dyspnea occur solely as a result of hypothyroidism will be discussed later in this chapter.[40] Complaints of anginal-like pain in some hypothyroid patients suggest that coronary heart disease may be more prevalent in these patients.[37,41] An occasional patient with normal coronary arteries established by angiography has angina that resolves with thyroid hormone therapy.[37] One report described an increased prevalence of asymmetric septal hypertrophy in patients with hypothyroidism and suggested that various forms of atypical chest pain may occur in this setting,[40] but more recent studies have questioned this association.[42]

Physical Examination

Certain findings on physical examination of the cardiovascular system suggest the presence of hypothyroidism (Table 62-1). The heart rate is variably lowered, the pulse pressure is often narrowed, and the carotid upstroke and left ventricular apical impulse are diminished.[1–3,8,12] The heart sounds are often diminished, consistent with either decreased left ventricular contractility or the presence of a pericardial effusion.[10,43,44]

From 20% to 40% of hypothyroid patients have a diastolic blood pressure greater than 90 mm Hg.[19,20] The characteristic nonpitting myxedema occurs with long-standing hypothyroidism, and pitting edema of the lower extremities or presacral region may occur because of an increase in albumin content of extracellular fluid.[21] Cold extremities and delayed capillary filling result from the decreased blood flow to the skin and muscles.

Laboratory Tests

Hypothyroidism can alter many of the tests commonly used in the evaluation of patients with known or suspected heart disease.[39] Hemoglobin and hematocrit values may be slightly low.[22] The partial thromboplastin time and other measures of coagulation may be prolonged, owing to a decrease in serum concentrations of factor VIII.[22,45] Serum total, low-density lipoprotein (LDL), and very–low–density lipoprotein (VLDL)[46] cholesterol concentrations tend to be high in hypothyroidism. These increases have been related to a reduced expression of the LDL receptor.[47]

Serum creatine kinase activity is high in as many as 30% of patients.[39] Whereas the increase may reflect myocardial necrosis, in most patients the isoenzyme distribution is almost completely MM, indicating its source is skeletal rather than cardiac muscle.[39,48] Further evidence that the elevated serum creatine kinase concentrations are of skeletal muscle origin includes the concomitant increase in serum and urine myoglobin. A prolongation of the half-life of creatine kinase in the circulation contributes to the elevated serum concentration. The serum concentrations of other muscle-specific enzymes such as aldolase may also be increased, and occasionally serum aminotransferase concentrations are raised.

Electrocardiography

Hypothyroidism has classically been associated with bradycardia, but the degree of heart rate slowing is often modest.[49,50] In contrast to thyrotoxicosis, in which atrial tachyarrhythmias are common and ventricular arrhythmias rare, in hypothyroidism the atrial pacemaker function is normal and atrial ectopy is rare, but ventricular premature beats and occasionally ventricular tachycardia occur. The syndrome of torsades de pointes with a long QT interval and ventricular tachycardia can occur with hypothyroidism, and resolve with T_4 therapy alone.[51] Electrocardiograms may demonstrate low voltage and nonspecific ST wave changes.[22,49] Although occasionally suggestive of myocardial ischemia, these waveform changes often disappear during T_4 therapy but rarely during anti-anginal therapy.[37] The low voltage is more often a result of pericardial effusion rather than altered myocyte ion conduction or cardiac atrophy.

Noninvasive Evaluation

All measures of left ventricular contractility and cardiac workload are decreased in patients with hypothyroidism.[9,52–54] These include systolic time intervals[10] as well as diastolic performance measures such as isovolumic filling and compliance.[12,43,54] Whereas cardiac contractility and work are impaired at rest, they increase appropriately during exercise,[27] suggesting that the inherent inotropic state of the heart is not as abnormal as suggested by the resting measures of function.[52] Even mild degrees of hypothyroidism of short duration are associated with predictable prolongation in the isovolumic relaxation time,[12] thus diastolic relaxation appears to be a very sensitive and specific measurement of the cardiovascular response to the biologic actions of thyroid hormone.[13]

Some patients have been reported to have asymmetric hypertrophy of the intraventricular septum by echocardiography that resolves with T_4 therapy,[40,55] but a recent study failed to demonstrate septal hypertrophy in any hypothyroid patient studied.[42] Asymmetric septal hypertrophy is unlikely to be responsible for the abnormalities in left ventricular function that occur in hypothyroidism, because the abnormalities often occur in the absence of cardiac morphologic changes.[54] Whether these anatomic changes are responsible for the occasional anginal-like pain[37] or syncopal episodes reported to occur in hypothyroidism remains to be determined.[40]

Pericardial effusions occur in approximately one-third to one-half of patients with overt hypothyroidism.[44] The effusions are more common and their volume is greater in patients with long-standing, severe disease.[22,44] The protein content of the pericardial fluid tends to be high, most likely due to an increase in albumin transudation similar to that in other serous cavities.[21] The fluid also has a high cholesterol concentration and is often viscous.[22] The clearing of pericardial effusions in response to T_4 therapy may require 6 to 9 months.[44,56] Cardiac tamponade is a very rare complication; most patients have no hemodynamic alterations,even those with very large volumes of pericardial fluid.[56,57]

Hypertension

As noted before, many hypothyroid patients have hypertension caused by the increase in systemic vascular resistance.[19] In large series of hypertensive patients, varying degrees of hypothyroidism may be a contributing factor in approximately 3% to 5%.[20,44] This is a low renin form of hypertension[32] that may occur early in the course of the hypothyroidism.[58] The identification of coexistent thyroid disease is useful therapeutically, because many hyperthyroid patients with hypertension respond to T_4 treatment with either an improvement or normalization of their blood pressure.[19,20] The possibility that T_3 is a vasodilator and that in its absence smooth muscle contraction increases has been suggested.[4,6] Accelerated atherosclerosis of the large arteries or arterioles may occur in hypothyroidism and decrease the compliance of the arterial bed.[41]

HEART FAILURE

The pathophysiologic consequences of impaired left ventricular contractility, diastolic hypertension, increased systemic vascular resistance, and peripheral edema suggest that heart failure could arise in the setting of hypothyroidism.[1,3,17,19,54,57] However, documentation of hypothyroidism as the sole cause

of congestive heart failure is rare.[17] Arteriovenous oxygen extraction is normal in hypothyroid patients, whereas it is increased in patients with organic heart disease and heart failure.[3] Patients with hypothyroidism can increase their cardiac output or decrease systemic vascular resistance in response to exercise, for example, unlike patients with heart failure.[3,27] In contrast to patients with heart failure, hypothyroid patients are able to excrete a sodium load[31,58] and do not develop signs of pulmonary fluid overload characteristic of organic heart disease.

Histologic changes in the hearts of patients dying of hypothyroidism include myocyte swelling and mucinous edema.[59,60]

TREATMENT

All of the changes in cardiovascular function in patients with hypothyroidism respond to T_4 therapy. In most patients, the symptoms are chronic and hemodynamic performance is not sufficiently impaired to require urgent therapy.[42,43,61] Oral T_4 replacement therapy starting with low doses and progressing through step-wise increments in time leads to a normalization of cardiac output and left ventricular contractile performance[10,43] (see chap 77). In young patients, full replacement therapy can be instituted without untoward cardiovascular effects. In patients with severe hypothyroidism treated with large doses of T_4, cardiovascular performance improves within 48 to 96 hours.[30]

Thyroid hormone replacement in chronically hypothyroid patients causes a decline in serum cholesterol, a lowering of diastolic blood pressure, and a return to normal of the elevated serum creatine kinase, aldolase, and myoglobin concentrations.[19,20,39,46]

ADDITIONAL CLINICAL CONSIDERATIONS

Thyroid Hormone Therapy and Coronary Heart Disease

Several points need to be considered in the management of hypothyroid patients with known or suspected coronary heart disease. The first is whether there is an increase in the prevalence of coronary disease in hypothyroid patients.[19,39,62,63] The elevation in serum LDL cholesterol that occurs in hypothyroidism is, at least in other settings, an important risk factor for the development of coronary disease.[46] In one study, an association between serum markers of autoimmune thyroid disease and an increased prevalence of coronary disease in women was reported.[62] Hypertension is a well-established risk factor for the development of coronary disease, and it is a frequent finding in hypothyroidism. Lastly, both coronary disease and hypothyroidism tend to be more prevalent with increasing age. In a case-controlled autopsy series it was found that coronary disease was more prevalent in hypothyroid patients with coexistent hypertension, but not normotensive hypothyroid patients, as compared with euthyroid patients.[63]

In hypothyroidism the decrease in cardiac work and in oxygen demand could lead to better toleration of decreases in myocardial blood flow. These considerations have led some clinicians to avoid or limit the dose of T_4 therapy in patients with known or suspected coronary artery disease.[37] However, hypothyroid animals tolerate myocardial ischemia less well than do euthyroid animals, and in hypothyroid animals myocardial damage is more extensive and lethal ventricular arrhythmias are more common after experimentally-induced myocardial infarction than in normal animals.[64] In view of the important effects of thyroid hormone on the entire cardiovascular system, the possible benefit of thyroid hormone therapy in this clinical setting should be reevaluated.[19,65]

With regard to pectoris angina, the effects of thyroid hormone treatment are mostly beneficial. In the largest study of this issue 1503 hypothyroid patients received thyroid hormone replacement therapy and subsequently were evaluated for angina pectoris and myocardial infarction.[65] Of the 55 patients with known symptomatic coronary disease, 38% improved with treatment, 46% had no change, and only 16% had more symptoms. Thirty-five patients had chest pain after thyroid hormone replacement was begun, but in two-thirds of them the pain began more than 1 year after initiation of treatment. When considering the demographics of the overall study group it can be estimated that approximately 400 to 450 patients were at risk for coronary disease; thus, the overall incidence of problems attributable to coronary disease after initiation of thyroid therapy was low. From these results it seems clear that the beneficial effects of thyroid hormone on the heart and cardiovascular system in hypothyroid patients justifies T_4 therapy, and when necessary treating the associated or developing anginal symptoms with conventional medical therapy. In this way the potential for T_4 to decrease afterload and optimize myocardial work and cardiac output can be realized.[19] Whether or not the cholesterol-lowering effects of T_4 treatment leads to a reduction in the progression of coronary atherosclerosis is not known.

Occasional hypothyroid patients have sufficiently extensive coronary disease to justify coronary artery bypass surgery before or soon after T_4 therapy is initiated.[66] In these patients surgery can be performed safely and without untoward morbidity.[66,67]

THYROID HORMONE THERAPY AND CARDIOPULMONARY BYPASS SURGERY

Serum total and free T_3 concentrations decline in euthyroid patients during and soon after cardiopulmonary bypass, reaching a nadir 24 hours after surgery.[68] This observation of a low T_3 syndrome after bypass surgery and the marked effects of thyroid hormone on cardiac contractility provided the rationale for using T_3 as a potential positive inotropic agent in these patients. The results of short-term, T_3 administration in this setting suggest that T_3 may augment cardiac output and decrease systemic vascular resistance, but it does not affect postoperative morbidity or mortality.[25,26,28,69]

References

1. Klein I. Thyroid hormone and the cardiovascular system. Am J Med 1990;88:631

2. Watanakunakorn C, Hodges RE, Evans TC. Myxedema—a study of 400 cases. Arch Intern Med 1965;116:183

3. Graettinger JS, Muenster JJ, Checchia CS, et al. A correlation of clinical and hemodynamic studies in patients with hypothyroidism. J Clin Invest 1957;37:502

4. Ojamaa K, Balkman C, Klein I. Acute effects of triiodothyronine on arterial smooth muscle cells. Ann Thorac Surg 1993;56:S61

5. Anthonisen P, Holst E, Thomsen AA. Determination of cardiac output and other hemodynamic data in patients with hyper- and hypothyroidism, using dye dilution technique. Scand J Clin Lab Invest 1960;12:472

6. Klein I, Ojamaa K, Powell S. Potential clinical applications for parenteral thyroid hormone therapy. Hosp Form 1993;28:848

7. Klein I, Ojamaa K. Cardiovascular manifestations of endocrine disease. J Clin Endocrinol Metab 1992;75:339

8. Polikar R, Albert G, Urs S, Nicod P. The thyroid and the heart. Circulation 1993;87:1435

9. Amidi M, Leon DF, DeGroot LJ, et al. Effect of the thyroid state on myocardial contractility and ventricular ejection rate in man. Circulation 1968;38:229

10. Crowley WF Jr Ridgway EC, Bough EW, et al. Non-invasive evaluation of cardiac function in hypothyroidism. N Engl J Med 1977;296:1

11. Tseng K, Walfish P, Persaud J, Gilbert B. Concurrent aortic and mitral valve echocardiography permits measurement of systolic time intervals as an index of peripheral tissue thyroid functional status. J Clin Endocrinol Metab 1989;69:633

12. Wieshammer S, Keck F, Waitzinger J, et al. Acute hypothyroidism slows the rate of left ventricular diastolic relaxation. Can J Physiol Pharmacol 1988;67:1007

13. Klein I, Ojamaa K. Thyroid hormone and the cardiovascular system: from theory to practice. J Clin Endocrinol Metab 1994;78:1026

14. Dillmann WH. Biochemical basis of thyroid hormone action in the heart. Am J Med 1990;88:626

15. Ojamaa K, Klein I. In vivo regulation of recombinant cardiac myosin heavy chain gene expression by thyroid hormone. Endocrinology 1993;132:1002

16. Ojamaa K, Klemperer JD, MacGilroy SS, Klein I, Samarel A. Thyroid hormone and hemodynamic regulation of β-myosin heavy chain promoter in the heart. Endocrinology 1996;137:in press

17. Ladenson PW, Sherman SI, Baughman KL, et al. Reversible alterations in myocardial gene expression in a young man with dilated cardiomyopathy and hypothyroidism. Proc Natl Acad Sci 1992;89:5251

18. Rohrer D, Dillmann WH. Thyroid hormone markedly increases the mRNA coding for sarcoplasmic reticulum Ca^{2+}-ATPase in the rat heart. J Biol Chem 1988;263:6941

19. Klein I, Ojamaa K. Thyroid hormone and blood pressure regulation. In: Laragh J, Brenner B, eds. Hypertension. 2nd ed. New York: Raven Press, 1995:2247

20. Streeten DHP, Anderson GH Jr, Howland T, et al. Effects of thyroid function on blood pressure: recognition of hypothyroid hypertension. Hypertension 1988;11:78

21. Parving HH, Hansen JM, Nielsen SL, et al. Mechanism of edema formation in myxedema: increased protein extravasation and relatively slow lymphatic drainage. N Engl J Med 1979;301:460

22. Klein I, Levey GS. Unusual manifestations of hypothyroidism. Arch Intern Med 1984;144:123

23. Balkman C, Ojamaa K, Klein I. Time course of the effects of thyroid hormone on cardiac gene expression. Endocrinology 1992;130:2001

24. Ladenson AW, Goldenheim PD, Ridgway EC. Rapid pituitary and peripheral tissue responses to intravenous L-triiodothyronine in hypothyroidism. J Clin Endocrinol Metab 1983;56:1252

25. Salter DR, Dyke CM, Wechsler AS. Triiodothyronine (T_3) and cardiovascular therapeutics: a review. J Cardiac Surg 1992;7:363

26. Klemperer JD, Gomez M, etal. Thyroid hormone treatment after coronary-artery bypass surgery. N Engl J Med 1995; 333:1522

27. Wieshammer S, Keck FS, Waitzinger J, et al. Left ventricular function at rest and during exercise in acute hypothyroidism. Br Heart J 1988;60:204

28. Vavouranakis I, Sanoudos G, Manios A, et al. Triiodothyronine administration in coronary artery bypass surgery: effect on hemodynamics. J Cardiovasc Surg 1994;35:383

29. Kapitola J, Vilimovska D. Inhibition of the early circulatory effects of triiodothyronine in rats by propranolol. Physiol Bohemoslov 1981;30:347

30. Kaptein EM, Quion-Verde H, Swinney RS, et al. Acute hemodynamic effects of levothyroxine loading in critically ill hypothyroid patients. Arch Intern Med 1986;146:662

31. DeRubertis FR Jr, Michelis MF, Bloom ME, et al. Impaired water excretion in myxedema. Am J Med 1971;51:41

32. Saruta T, Kitajima W, Hayashi, et al. Renin and aldosterone in hypothyroidism: relation to excretion of sodium and potassium. Clin Endocrinol 1980;12:483

33. Polikar R, Kennedy B, Ziegler M, et al. Plasma norepinephrine kinetics, dopamine beta-hydroxylase and chromogranin A in hypothyroid patients before and following replacement therapy. J Clin Endocrinol Metab 1990;70:277

34. Levine MA, Feldman AM, Robishaw JD. Influence of thyroid hormone status on expression of genes encoding G protein subunits in the rat heart. J Biol Chem 1990;25:3553

35. Bilezikian JP, Loeb JN. The influence of hyperthyroidism and hypothyroidism on the alpha and beta-adrenergic receptor systems and adrenergic receptor systems and adrenergic responsiveness. Endocr Rev 1983;4:378

36. Cooper DS, Halpern R, Wood LC, et al. L-thyroxine therapy in subclinical hypothyroidism: a double-blind, placebo-controlled trial. Ann Intern Med 1984;101:18

37. Myerowitz P, Kamienski R, Swanson D, et al. Diagnosis and management of the hypothyroid patient with chest pain. J Thorac Cardiovasc Surg 1983;86:57

38. Billewicz WZ, Chapman RS, Crooks J, et al. Statistical methods applied to the diagnosis of hypothyroidism. Q J Med 1969;38:255

39. Klein I, Mantell P, Parker M, Levey GS. Resolution of abnormal muscle enzymes in hypothyroidism. Am J Med Sci 1980;279:159

40. Santos AD, Miller RP, Puthenpurakal, KM. Echocardiographic characterization of the reversible cardiomyopathy of hypothyroidism. Am J Med 1980;68:675

41. Tunbridge WMG, Evered DC, Hall R, et al. Lipid profiles and cardiovascular disease in the Whickham area with particular reference to thyroid failure. Clin Endocrinol 1977;7:495

42. Bernstein R, Muller C, Midtbo K, et al. Coronary dysfunction in severe hypothyroidism. In: Braverman LE, Eber O, Langsteger W, eds. Heart and thyroid. Vienna: Blackwell, 1994:154

43. Bough EW, Crowley WF, Ridgway E, et al. Myocardial function in hypothyroidism. Arch Intern Med 1978;138:1476

44. Kabadi UM, Kumar SP. Pericardial effusion in primary hypothyroidism. Am Heart J 1990;120:1393

45. Attivissimo LA, Lichtman SM, Klein I. Acquired von Willebrand's syndrome causing a hemorrhagic diathesis in a patient with hypothyroidism. Thyroid 1995;5:399

46. Friis T, Pedersen LR. Serum lipids in hyper and hypothyroidism before and after treatment. Clin Chim Acta 1987;162:155

47. Thompson GR, Soutar AK, Spengel FA. Defects in receptor-mediated low density lipoprotein catabolism in homozygous familial hypercholesterolemia and hypothyroidism. Proc Natl Acad Sci USA 1981;78:2591

48. LeMar H Jr, West SG, Garrett CR, Hofeldt FD. Covert hypothyroidism presenting as a cardiovascular event. Am J Med 1991;92:549

49. Sawin CT. Hypothyroidism. Med Clin North Am 1985;69:989

50. Staub JJ, Althaus BU, Engler H, et al. Spectrum of subclinical and overt hypothyroidism: Effect on thyrotropin, prolactin and thyroid reserve and metabolic impact on peripheral target tissues. Am J Med 1992;92:631

51. Fredlund B, Olsson SB. Long QT interval and ventricular tachycardia of "Torsade de Pointe" type in hypothyroidism. Acta Med Scand 1983;213:231

52. Buccino RA, Spann JF, Pool PE, et al. Influence of the thyroid state on the intrinsic contractile properties and energy stores of the myocardium. J Clin Invest 1967;46:1669

53. Vora J, O'Malley B, Petersen S, et al. Reversible abnormalities of myocardial relaxation in hypothyroidism. J Clin Endocrinol Metab 1985;61:269

54. Bernstein R, Muller C, Midtbo K, et al. Cardiac left ventricular function before and during early thyroxine treatment in severe hypothyroidism. J Intern Med 1991;230:493

55. Shenoy MM, Goldman JM. Hypothyroid cardiomyopathy. Echocardiographic documentation of reversibility. Am J Med Sci 1987;294:1

56. Kerber RE, Sherman B. Echocardiographic evaluation of pericardial effusion in myxedema. Circulation 1975;52:823

57. Manolis A, Varriale P, Ostrowski R. Hypothyroid cardiac tamponade. Arch Intern Med 1987;147:1167

58. Resnick LM, Laragh JH. Plasma renin activity in syndromes of thyroid hormone excess and deficiency. Life Sci 1982;30:585

59. LaDue JS. Myxedema heart: a pathological and therapeutic study. Ann Intern Med 1943;18:332

60. Higgins WH. The heart in myxedema: correlation of physical and post-mortem findings. Am J Med Sci 1936;191:80

61. Klein I, Levey GS. Thyroid emergencies: thyroid storm and myxedema coma. Top Emerg Med 1984:5;33

62. Bastenie PA, Bonnyns M, Neve P, Vanhaelst L. Asymptomatic atrophic thyroiditis in coronary heart disease. Lancet 1972;1:1072

63. Steinberg AD. Myxedema and coronary artery disease: a comparative autopsy study. Ann Intern Med 1968;68:338

64. Karlsberg RA, Friscia DA, Aronow WS, Sekhon SS. Deleterious influence of hypothyroidism on evolving myocardial infarction in conscious dogs. J Clin Invest 1981;67:1024

65. Keating FR Jr, Parkin TW, Selby JB, et al. Treatment of heart disease associated with myxedema. Prog Cardiovasc Dis 1961;3:364

66. Drucker DJ, Burrow GD. Cardiovascular surgery in the hypothyroid patient. Arch Intern Med 1985;145:1585

67. Ladenson PW, Levin AA, Ridgway EC, Daniels GH. Complications of surgery in hypothyroid patients. Am J Med 1984;77:261

68. Holland FW II, Brown PS Jr, Weintraub BD, Clark RE. Cardiopulmonary bypass and thyroid function: A "euthyroid sick syndrome." Ann Thorac Surg 1991;52:46

69. Novitzky D, Cooper DK, Barton CI, et al. Triiodothyronine as an inotropic agent after open heart surgery. J Thorac Cardiovasc Surg 1989;98:972

Werner and Ingbar's The Thyroid, Seventh Edition,
edited by Lewis E. Braverman and Robert D. Utiger.
Lippincott–Raven Publishers, Philadelphia, © 1996

63

The Respiratory System in Hypothyroidism

David H. Ingbar

Respiratory manifestations are seldom the major complaint of the patient with hypothyroidism; nonetheless, the pulmonary system may be affected in many ways. Fatigue and dyspnea on exertion are frequent symptoms.[1] Occasionally, pulmonary involvement is major and life-threatening, as in the patient with myxedema coma and CO_2 retention.

Recently, neonatologists and thyroidologists have been very interested in the role of thyroid hormone in lung development and regulation of ventilation. Pulmonologists have paid increasing attention to airway obstruction, especially during sleep, and to neuromuscular function during breathing. All these subjects are brought together in the patient with hypothyroidism. This chapter examines the various ways in which the respiratory system can be affected in the hypothyroid patient.

The pulmonary consequences of hypothyroidism can be categorized as those that directly affect the lung or that result from changes in the function of other organ systems. Table 63-1 classifies these consequences.

ALTERATIONS IN PULMONARY FUNCTION IN ADULTS

Pulmonary Function Tests and Gas Exchange

Analysis of changes in pulmonary function is complicated by an increased frequency of obesity in hypothyroid patients. Abnormalities attributed in the literature to hypothyroidism may have been due to obesity, which by itself frequently decreases the diffusing capacity for carbon monoxide (DLCO) and in the lung volumes, including decreases in vital capacity (VC), total lung capacity (TLC), functional residual capacity, and espe-

cially expiratory reserve volume. In the individual patient, all these abnormalities do not necessarily occur together.

Wilson and Bedell[2] contrasted patients with either myxedema alone or myxedema accompanied by obesity. The 16 patients with myxedema alone had normal lung volumes and arterial blood gases (ABG), with decreased DLCO. After replacement with thyroid hormone, the patients lost a mean of 6 kg from their initial mean weight of 71 kg, and the DLCO returned to normal. Pretherapy, patients with myxedema and obesity (mean weight was 136 kg) had diminished lung volumes, DLCO, peak expiratory flow rate, and maximal voluntary ventilation. ABG analysis revealed arterial CO_2 retention to 55 mm Hg and resting hypoxemia (83% oxygen saturation). After hormone replacement and a mean weight loss of 32 kg, DLCO, $PaCO_2$, and the lung volumes returned to normal.

Summarizing the relatively few studies, there is little abnormality of resting pulmonary function in most non-obese patients with hypothyroidism. Some patients may exhibit a decrease of VC, probably due to muscular weakness (discussed later). Overall oxygen transfer may be slightly decreased, as evidenced by a decreased PaO_2, possibly a decreased DLCO corrected for hemoglobin, and a widened alveolar-arterial (A-a) DO_2 gradient. Proposed explanations for these changes include a diffusion defect, an increase in ventilation perfusion mismatching, or an opening of anatomic shunts. Several older studies of patients with hypothyroidism have shown increased capillary wall thickness in the skin; however, no morphologic studies of lung capillaries have been published. Some authors propose that microatelectasis that is not radiographically visualized exists and that this results from either respiratory muscle weakness or a deficiency of surfactant. However, no definite evidence shows altered muscle function, abnormal surfactant production, or an opening of anatomic shunts in the lung.

DIRECT EFFECTS

Altered pulmonary function tests

    Increased (A-a) O_2 gradient

    Decreased DLCO (?)

    Decreased maximal exercise capacity

Depressed ventilatory drives

Pleural effusions

Decreased surfactant production in the neonate

Upper airway obstruction (goiter, enlarged tongue, or pharyngeal muscle dysfunction)

Sleep apnea syndrome, obstructive >> central type

INDIRECT EFFECTS

Phrenic nerve paralysis

Neuromuscular weakness or dyscoordination (?)

Obesity causing atelectasis

Congestive heart failure causing pulmonary edema

Difficulty in weaning from mechanical ventilation

Tendency toward theophylline intoxication

Exercise Capacity

Many patients with hypothyroidism complain of fatigue and exercise intolerance. These subjective sensations could arise from limited pulmonary reserve, limited cardiac reserve, decreased muscle strength, or increased ease of muscle fatigue. Analysis of the effects of hypothyroidism on exercise performance is hampered by the limited number of clinical studies.

The most detailed study of exercise in hypothyroid patients suggested that the primary problem is cardiac limitation resulting from an inability to increase stroke volume.[3] The maximal oxygen consumption and work loads achieved were significantly diminished, and arterial lactate levels rose more than normal. There also may be abnormalities of blood flow distribution, especially to muscles, but these are not well established. On return to euthyroid status, some, but not all, exercise parameters returned to normal. For example, the (A-a) O_2 gradient worsened, and the lactate levels remained high.[3]

Experimental studies on hypothyroid rats[4] found that muscle oxidation of pyruvate and palmitate decreased with more rapid use of glycogen stores and diminished fatty acid mobilization, reducing endurance. Hypothyroidism increased activity of enzymes of glycolysis, the tricarboxylic acid cycle, and fatty acid oxidation of resting rat diaphragm muscle.[5]

Several poorly documented reports have indicated that hypothyroidism may reduce the severity of dyspnea in patients with severe chronic obstructive pulmonary disease (COPD). In one study,[6] 7 of 10 patients with COPD performed greater activity after induction of hypothyroidism with either methimazole or ^{131}I. Hurst[7] claimed in the mid-1950s that 10 of 24 patients with COPD had increased exercise tolerance, appetite, and sense of well-being after ^{131}I treatment. Neither of these reports provides information on changes in pulmonary

functions, ABG, responses to exercise, or ventilatory drives. One patient[8] with severe emphysema and hypothyroidism had increased dyspnea after thyroxine (T_4) replacement therapy, accompanied by increases in both rest and exercise oxygen consumption, while $PaCO_2$ decreased. Discontinuation of T_4 therapy led to improvement in the 12-minute walking distance. These studies are reminiscent of Blumgart's induction of hypothyroidism in patients with coronary artery disease as a treatment for angina. However, another study of 10 euthyroid COPD patients treated with carbimazole in a double-blind crossover trial found no effect on ABG, dyspnea, 12-minute walking distance, or resting minute ventilation.[9]

These reports do not differentiate between two possible mechanisms by which an increase in thyroid hormone may increase dyspnea. First, increased oxygen consumption may necessitate higher minute ventilation and alveolar ventilation, thereby increasing the work of breathing. This poses a special problem for patients with COPD, who waste much of their ventilation on an increased physiologic dead space. Second, the patient may not be capable of increasing ventilation to match the increase of ventilatory drive (discussed later). This mismatch may cause the subjective sensation of dyspnea. Other interventions known to decrease ventilatory drive, such as ethanol or codeine, also may increase the sense of well-being in some patients with COPD and decrease their dyspnea.

In summary, the limited data suggest that decreased stroke volume and cardiac output play a greater role than pulmonary dysfunction in limiting the exercise capacity of hypothyroid patients. The roles of abnormal muscle function, blood flow distribution, and energy metabolism are not yet well defined. Some patients with severe lung disease may have increased dyspnea upon correction of hypothyroidism as a result of increases in either oxygen consumption or ventilatory drive.

Ventilatory Control

In the late 1950s and early 1960s, patients with myxedema coma were noted to retain CO_2.[10] In the mid-1960s, some of these patients had diminished ventilatory response to hypercapnia, which improved after thyroid hormone replacement therapy.[11,22] This finding led to the investigation of ventilatory control in hypothyroid patients without myxedema coma.

Ventilatory drive represents the net output of the respiratory centers in response to a given physiologic stimulus. Drive is measured indirectly by examining the change in function of the pulmonary system when the respiratory center input is changed. Most studies of ventilatory drive measure the response to either progressive hypercapnia (HCVR) or isocapneic hypoxia (HVR) as the stimulus and minute ventilation as the measured response. Newer indices, such as transdiaphragmatic pressure (P_{di}), percentage of inspiratory time per respiratory cycle, diaphragmatic electromyogram (EMG), and inspiratory mouth occlusion pressure in the first 0.1 second ($P_{0.1}$), have not yet been widely applied. There are several limitations to interpreting changes in these measurements. First, the normal drive response varies widely from person to person, probably because of a strong genetic influence. Second, the response to differing stimuli may not be quantitatively or qualitatively similar. Finally, pulmonary abnormalities may limit the measured response. For example, an extremely obese patient might have a normal neural output response to progressive hypercapnia but be unable to increase minute ventilation to a normal extent because of the high mechanical work load of breathing.

Patients with either primary or iatrogenic (postoperative or postirradiation) hypothyroidism have depressed HVR and HCVR.[13] In one study, the HVR was more severely depressed in the former group but both the HVR and HCVR rapidly returned to normal with therapy. After therapy for 3 to 9 months in the iatrogenic group, the HVR—but not the HCVR—increased significantly but did not return to normal. Neither group had significant improvements in lung volumes or ABG with therapy, and muscle weakness was not assessed. A possible explanation for the difference between the two groups is that those patients with primary hypothyroidism had never been treated for hypothyroidism, whereas the iatrogenic group comprised patients previously receiving hormone replacement whose treatment was stopped for 3 weeks before initial testing.

The largest study of ventilatory drive in hypothyroid patients found decreases in 34% of 38 hypothyroid patients.[14] Depressed responses to hypercapnia or hypoxia often did not occur in the same patients. The best predictors were female sex and very high TSH levels (>90 mU/L). Almost all these patients normalized their ventilatory drives after 1 week of replacement therapy, and HVR often returned more rapidly.

A recent detailed study[15] of 13 patients with severe hypothyroidism found that there were two subsets of patients. Seven patients had normal ventilatory drives, but 4 of them had decreased maximal inspiratory pressures (MIP). The other 6 patients had decreased HCVR assessed by minute ventilation and diaphragmatic EMG, while only 2 of these 6 had diminished MIP. The HCVR increased after thyroid hormone replacement, but MIP did not increase in patients with low pretreatment values. These results suggest that the low HCVR in some patients is not due to impaired respiratory muscle function, but is more likely a central nervous system effect. The lack of correlation between respiratory muscle strength and ventilatory drive indicates that these abnormalities occur independently and are not directly related.

In summary, some patients with hypothyroidism have depressed HVR and HCVR. There usually is rapid reversibility of at least the hypercapneic component during hormone replacement. The mechanism by which thyroid hormone influences ventilatory drive is unknown. It also is unclear why these changes occur only in some patients.

Pulmonary Function in Myxedema Coma

The role of pulmonary dysfunction due to hypothyroidism in causing myxedema coma is not clearly defined and remains controversial. Not only is coma a rare complication of myxedema, but the analysis of cause and effect is difficult, since coma of any cause can result in hypoventilation and CO_2 retention. There also are many other precipitants of coma in hypothyroidism, including decreased cerebral oxygen delivery, sedative and respiratory depressant medications, hyponatremia, adrenal insufficiency, infection, heart failure, hypoglycemia, and hypothermia.[16–18] Because many of these factors occur together in the very ill patient, it is difficult to ascribe causality to an individual factor. In 1960, Nordqvist[10] reported on two patients with CO_2 retention and myxedema coma. Unfortunately, both had multiple possible causes of CO_2 retention.

Either the obesity-hypoventilation syndrome or CO_2 retention can depress ventilatory drive. In the former, it is not clear whether this is a primary or secondary phenomenon. As discussed later, myxedema can cause sleep apnea, and at least some patients with sleep apnea have depressed ventilatory drives.

Patients with myxedema coma almost always have at least one other factor causing hypoventilation, such as lung disease, central nervous system disease, neuromuscular weakness, obesity, kyphoscoliosis, or pleural restrictive disease.[12,19]

In summary, all reported cases of myxedema coma with severe CO_2 retention have had at least one additional potential cause for hypoventilation. Some of the other causes of hypoventilation, such as respiratory depressant medications, are avoidable, but most are not. It seems likely that hypothyroidism contributes to coma in some of these patients by decreasing the HVR and HCVR. It alone, however, probably is not sufficient to cause CO_2 retention and thereby precipitate myxedema coma. Thus, a careful review of all potential contributing causes of an elevated $PaCO_2$ is worthwhile in the patient with respiratory failure and myxedema coma.

Pleural Effusions

Effusions may occur at many sites in patients with hypothyroidism. Most common among these is the pericardial space, but peritoneal, pleural, middle ear, and uveal effusions have been reported.[20–22] Pericardial effusions are frequently rich in protein, and some authors[22] believe that most of the effusions of myxedema are exudates. In the few well-characterized cases reported in which myxedema was the sole cause of the effusion, however, pleural effusions were either transudates or exudates.[23] In most patients, congestive heart failure, pericardial effusion, or transdiaphragmatic passage of ascitic fluid may have caused the pleural effusions.[23] There is consensus that the pleural fluid in patients with hypothyroidism may be either bilateral or unilateral, usually is small, and usually does not cause clinical symptoms.[23,24] Rare case reports suggest that chylous effusions may occur in myxedema.

The reason that effusions occur in patients with hypothyroidism is not well established, but changes in the capillaries may be involved. Capillary structure is altered in patients with hypothyroidism, with a probable decrease in number, a narrowed diameter,[25] and an increase in permeability as assessed by a low-molecular-weight fluorescein dye.[26] There have been no histopathologic studies of the pulmonary arterial or bronchial capillary beds in patients with hypothyroidism. Further study and documentation of pleural effusions are necessary, both to clarify their nature and to better understand their pathogenesis.

Sleep Apnea and Obesity-Hypoventilation Syndromes

Sleep apnea syndrome and obesity-hypoventilation syndrome have generated great interest over the last decade, but confusion remains about their relation to each other, to simple obesity, and to other conditions of diminished respiratory drive. Both conditions are associated with hypothyroidism.

Patients with obesity-hypoventilation syndrome, and also probably most patients with sleep apnea syndrome, have decreased ventilatory drive. In the case of obesity-hypoventilation syndrome, it is not clear if diminished drive is a primary pathogenic factor or is an acquired defect secondary to a rise in $PaCO_2$, neurologic dysfunction, hypoxemia, or the increased work of breathing against an increased ventilatory load. By definition, all patients with obesity-hypoventilation syndrome have an elevated $PaCO_2$ while awake and resting.

Sleep apnea syndrome is divided into three types: (1) a pure obstructive form, (2) a central type caused by the absence of respiratory efforts, and (3) a mixed type, with both obstructive and neurologic abnormalities.

How are these two disorders related to hypothyroidism? Many of the patients with myxedema coma described in the 1960s were obese and probably had obesity-hypoventilation syndrome. It is not surprising that the increased work of breathing and increased CO_2 production rate found in obese patients will combine with the diminished HCVR in patients with myxedema to cause CO_2 retention.

Hypothyroidism is a well-recognized cause of obstructive sleep apnea.[27-29] Most patients described have had enlarged tongues. In all reported cases, the patient's sleep apnea responded to hormone therapy or weight loss. The apneic episode of one patient with mild hypothyroidism disappeared without weight change after 1 month of treatment with either medroxyprogesterone or T_4.[30] Orr and colleagues[27] thought it unlikely that the improvement in this group of patients was due solely to weight loss, since the weight change in their patients was only moderate. In another study,[29] 9 of 11 consecutive patients newly diagnosed with hypothyroidism had sleep apnea. The severity of the sleep apnea was much worse in the 6 patients who were obese. All patients had significant improvement, with a sixfold reduction in sleep apnea after T_4 replacement, without weight loss. Ventilatory drive also increased after therapy. A recent study[30] of 26 consecutive Finnish patients with hypothyroidism who underwent sleep studies revealed nocturnal breathing abnormalities in 50% and severe obstructive apnea in 7.7% of the group. However, multivariate analysis found that hypothyroidism was not as strong an independent predictor of nocturnal breathing abnormalities as male gender or obesity.

Hypothyroidism may predispose to upper airway obstruction by several mechanisms: increased size of the tongue and other pharyngeal skeletal muscles; a slow and sustained pharyngeal muscle contraction pattern; or diminished neural output of the respiratory center. Clearly, the first of these mechanisms is significant. In addition, the favorable response to medroxyprogesterone alone is surprising and lends support to a role for decreased neural output, at least in some patients.[28] One hypothyroid patient with purely central sleep apnea has been reported.[31]

Upper Airway Effects

A variety of minor complaints referable to the upper airway, ear, nose, and throat are common in hypothyroidism. Patients frequently experience nasal stuffiness, recurrent colds, voice change, foreign body sensation, and discomfort or dryness of the throat.[32] It is not clearly established, however, that these complaints truly occur more often in hypothyroidism, and their cause is uncertain. Nasal mucus secretion may be increased, and 20% of patients have tonsillar enlargement. Although there has been speculation concerning the role of myxedematous thickening of the vocal cords or stretching of the recurrent laryngeal nerves by an enlarging thyroid gland, there is little evidence to support either theory. It also has been suggested that laryngeal muscle function may be altered by myxedematous infiltration.

Neuromuscular Dysfunction

Hypothyroid myopathy can occur in either children or adults, as discussed in chapter 67. In adults, it may be accompanied by an increased muscle volume and then is known as Hoffman's syndrome. Hypothyroid myopathy may involve the respiratory muscles and the diaphragm, slowing contraction and relaxation and decreasing maximal power.

Respiratory muscle dysfunction clinically manifests as hypoventilation, atelectasis, or easy fatigability. Values for many classic pulmonary function tests usually decrease: peak expiratory flow, compliance, DLCO, MIP, and all of the lung volumes except residual volume (RV). The RV/TLC ratio increases, and the $PaCO_2$ might be elevated. The most sensitive readily available test of diaphragmatic function is measurement of maximal static inspiratory and expiratory pressures (Pi_{max} and Pe_{max}, respectively). The P_{di} and diaphragmatic EMG are noninvasive methods for early detection of myopathy.

In the 1980s, four patients with diaphragm dysfunction due to hypothyroidism were reported.[33,34] The abnormalities returned toward or to normal with thyroid replacement therapy, although there also was an average 7-kg weight loss. A more recent study in Greece examined respiratory muscle function in 43 hypothyroid patients.[35] Although the mean pretreatment values for VC, FVC, and FEVI were within the normal range, each variable increased significantly after hormone replacement therapy. Before treatment both the maximal inspiratory and expiratory pressures were reduced. After 3 months of treatment, there was almost a 50% increase in both pressures, even though only half the patients were euthyroid by TSH level and there was almost no mean weight change. Since it is not clear from the study how many patients were screened out in the selection process, it is difficult to estimate the prevalence of respiratory muscle dysfunction in hypothyroidism, but this recent study[35] suggests it may be common. Other respiratory system abnormalities (obesity, ventilatory drive) need to be carefully looked for in these patients, since they also generate a restrictive physiologic pattern and predispose to hypoventilation and a shallow, rapid respiratory pattern.

The mechanism of thyroid myopathy remains undefined. Some investigators have found a decrease in the activity of muscle 1,4-glucosidase (acid maltase). This enzyme also is deficient in the rare, recessively inherited disease of generalized glycogenolysis, Pompe's disease, which is a slowly progressive chronic myopathy without glycogen accumulation in the heart, liver, or brain. Interestingly, some of these patients present with acute hypercapneic respiratory failure.[36]

Two patients with orthopnea and dyspnea on exertion had bilateral phrenic nerve paralysis due to hypothyroidism.[37] Lack of diaphragm function was demonstrated by supine fluoroscopy. Percutaneous phrenic nerve conduction studies showed greatly slowed conduction in one patient and nonexcitability in the other. One patient had return of normal phrenic nerve function after 4 months of thyroid hormone replacement therapy. The other patient died in an accident; autopsy revealed demyelination and fibrosis of the phrenic nerves.

Miscellaneous Pulmonary Consequences of Hypothyroidism

Hypothyroidism can decelerate theophylline metabolism and predispose patients to theophylline intoxication if they are given usual daily doses.[38] Hypothyroidism may limit weaning patients from mechanical ventilation by a combination of the mechanisms discussed previously—decreased VC, respiratory muscle weakness, decreased ventilatory drive, and pleural effusions. Screening of 121 ventilator-dependent patients in a long-term ventilator care unit found 4 hypothyroid patients.[39] The weaning of 3 of these patients was facilitated by treatment of their hypothyroidism. Finally, the response to sepsis may be altered by hypothyroidism. Rats with hypothyroidism and sepsis had decreased survival compared with euthyroid septic rats (30% vs. 65% survival), possibly related to decreases in oxygen consumption[40] or to improvements in pulmonary edema.[41]

LUNG MATURATION AND SURFACTANT PRODUCTION

Studies in the early 1970s[42,43] first demonstrated that thyroid hormone accelerates surfactant production and fetal lung maturation. These studies followed the pioneering discovery that glucocorticoids accelerated surfactant production by type II pneumocytes. The role of the thyroid hormones in lung development is discussed in chapter 39.

Injection of T_4 into rabbit fetuses in utero led to an earlier appearance of both surface active material in lung washes and lamellar bodies in type II pneumocytes.[43] Exogenous T_4 given subcutaneously to adult rats for 14 days increased type II cell size, lamellar body size and number, and surfactant per unit wet weight of lung.[42] Hypothyroid adult rats showed the converse changes. The cellular biochemistry of the interaction of thyroid hormones with the type II pneumocyte is discussed in chapter 39.

Further studies confirmed these early results. Acceleration of fetal lung maturation and surfactant production has been shown in many in vitro model systems, including fetal rat lung explants, cultures of mixed fetal rabbit lung cells, and culture of fetal type II cells.[44,45] However, one problem in relating these models to in vivo development is that the ability of triiodothyronine (T_3), T_4, or TSH to cross the placenta in different species remains controversial.[46] It is not clear whether it is fetal or maternal hormone that may be physiologically important in normal development, or whether T_3 and T_4 are involved. A T_3 analogue that readily crosses the placenta, 3,5-dimethyl-3′-isopropyl-L-thyronine, increases fetal rabbit phosphatidylcholine synthesis.[47] Exogenous thyrotropin-releasing hormone also crosses the placenta. Lung lavage from the fetuses of mothers given thyrotropin-releasing hormone displayed increases in phosphatidylcholine, total phospholipids, and phosphatidylcholine/sphingomyelin ratio.[45] The lung tissue itself did not reveal a change in any of these variables, suggesting an effect on surfactant release but not synthesis. Studies using in utero injection of hormone require careful experimental control, since the stress of in utero injection, by itself, can increase the rate of fetal lung maturation, probably by increasing the release of corticosteroids.[48] Whether or not thyroid hormones affect the production of any of the surfactant apoproteins is uncertain.

In addition to promoting early alveolar development before birth, thyroid hormones also modulate postnatal alveolar development. Rat pups given exogenous T_3 postnatally increase their alveolar gas exchange surface area and the surface/volume ratio more than normal, whereas postnatal propylthiouracil (PTU) has the opposite effect.[49]

Other hormones that influence lung development may act by interacting with thyroid hormones. Thyroid hormones may potentiate the promotion of surfactant and lung maturation by glucocorticoids.[50–53] In fetal sheep, the β-adrenergic–induced increase in lung liquid resorption that normally occurs before birth is inhibited by fetal thyroidectomy.[54] In vitro, dexamethasone, T_3, and theophylline synergistically promote phospholipid release in organ cultures of fetal rat lung explants,[55,56] human lung explants,[55,56] and fetal rats in vitro.[50] This combined effect is faster and greater than the impact of glucocorticoids alone.[52]

Many aspects of thyroid hormone effects on development are uncertain. Although thyroid hormones can affect lung lipid biosynthesis, their physiologic role in normal lung maturation and surfactant synthesis is not clear and may differ at different ages. The responsible form of the hormone also is uncertain. In the adult, this is likely to be T_3 rather than T_4, because high-affinity nuclear receptors for T_3 exist in lung cells.[48,57] The biochemical loci at which thyroid hormones alter phospholipid synthesis or release are not defined. Finally, the effects of thyroid hormones could be exerted directly or indirectly. For example, thyroid hormone may be a permissive factor in the regulation of lung β-adrenergic receptors[58] or may potentiate the action of glucocorticoids or fibroblast-pneumocyte factor. It is likely that multiple steps in type II pneumocyte development and surfactant synthesis are regulated in a complex and interactive fashion by different hormones, including thyroid hormones.

In summary, there is good in vitro evidence for a stimulatory effect of thyroid hormones on type II pneumocyte differentiation and function in the fetus and adult. The in vivo physiologic significance of thyroid hormones in this role, however, apart from any interactions with glucocorticoids, is not yet clear for any age group. Their significance may depend on the stage of lung development.

Respiratory Distress Syndrome of the Newborn

The stimulation of surfactant production by type II pneumocytes by thyroid hormones raises the question of whether hypothyroidism in utero or in the early postnatal period contributes to the pathogenesis of respiratory distress syndrome (RDS) in the premature newborn.

Early studies supported an association of hypothyroidism with an increased frequency of RDS. Cord serum values for total T_4 and free T_4 index were lower in premature infants with RDS than in premature infants without RDS.[59] TSH and T_3 levels were not measured. Cuestas compared 120 premature infants with and without RDS. No difference in thyroid status was observed in the infants born at less than 33 weeks of gestation.[60] In infants born at 33 to 37 weeks, those with RDS had lower values for serum T_4, T_3, and free T_3 index; the serum TSH levels and the T_4/T_3 ratio were increased, but the free T_4 index was unchanged. These differences persisted even after infants with other conditions associated with RDS were excluded. The same investigators reconfirmed these results, except that the postnatal TSH surge in infants with RDS was less than that seen in control infants of the same gestational age.[61]

Klein and colleagues confirmed these findings but questioned their physiologic significance.[62,63] The initial cord serum TSH levels and the rises in TSH after birth were the same in RDS and normal premature infants, although the rise was less than that seen in mature-term infants. The reverse T_3 level gradually rose after birth only in the infants with RDS. A later case control study[64] showed a lower cord serum T_3 level at birth in the infants with RDS but no difference in total reverse T_3 or TSH levels. The incidence of RDS has not been explained as a function of maternal thyroid status. Lower fetal and neonatal T_3 levels may have been due to altered peripheral thyroid hormone metabolism associated with nonthyroidal illness, rather than hypothyroidism, since the lack of an elevated serum TSH level was evidence against fetal or postnatal hypothyroidism.

Treatment with thyroid hormone for prevention of RDS in high-risk premature infants has undergone nonrandomized testing in a small number of infants.[64] Intraamniotic injection of 200 µg of T_4 was performed in 8 mothers with 9 fetuses at high-risk for RDS who required early delivery. In 7 of the 8 cases, repeat amniocentesis yielded fluid with improved parameters of fetal lung maturity. None of the 9 fetuses developed RDS. Since no adequate control group was included in this study, and in view of the lack of reported complications, a larger randomized trial would be worthwhile. Eighteen mothers with serious toxemia of pregnancy received intraamniotic injections of T_4 due to immature amniotic lipid profiles.[65] Within 24 hours, the L/S ratios of the amniotic fluid increased at least twofold in all cases. Only one child died, and none of the others had RDS.

Another important question is whether there is an additive or synergistic effect on lung maturation when thyroid hormone and glucocorticoids are given in combination. In vitro studies suggest that there may be little additive benefit in midgestation. Thyroid hormone slows the rise in glycogen content due to corticosteroids[66] by inhibition of fatty acid synthase[67] and suppresses the development of lung antioxidant enzymes,[68] so it may also have adverse effects. However, the experimental in vitro and in vivo data suggest that combined use of thyroid hormone and glucocorticoids accelerates lung epithelial maturation, surfactant production, and surfactant release. Two recent randomized clinical trials used maternal antenatal treatment with TRH combined with corticosteroids. Combined therapy reduced adverse outcomes, including ventilator days and bronchopulmonary dysplasia.[69,70] Additional randomized trials are under way.

References

1. Hall R, Scanlon MF. Hypothyroidism: clinical features and complications. Clin Endocrinol Metab 1979;8:29
2. Wilson WR, Bedell GN. The pulmonary abnormalities in myxedema. J Clin Invest 1960;39:42
3. Burack R, Edwards RHT, Green M, et al. The response to exercise before and after treatment of myxedema with thyroxine. J Pharm Exp Ther 1971;176:212
4. Baldwin KM, Hooker AM, Herrick RE, et al. Respiratory capacity and glycogen depletion in thyroid deficient muscle. J Appl Physiol 1980;49:102
5. Ianuzzo CD, Chen V, O'Brien P, et al. Effect of experimental dysthyroidism on the enzymatic character of the diaphragm. J Appl Physiol 1984;56:117
6. Bercu BA, Mandell HN. Radioactive iodine for chronic lung disease. [Abstract]. J Clin Invest 1954;33:917
7. Hurst A, Levine MH, Rich DR. Radioactive iodine in the management of patients with severe emphysema. Ann Allergy 1955;13:393
8. Butland RJA, Pang JA, Geddes DM. Thyroxine and dyspnea in emphysema. Br J Dis Chest 1981;75:96
9. Butland RJA, Pang JA, Geddes DM. Carbimazole and exercise tolerance in chronic airflow obstruction. Thorax 1982;37:64
10. Nordqvist P, Dhuner KG, Stenberg K, et al. Myxedema coma and CO_2 retention. Acta Med Scand 1960;166:189
11. Massumi RA, Winnacker JL. Severe depression of the respiratory center in myxedema. Am J Med 1964;36:876
12. Weg JG, Calverly JR, Johnson C. Hypothyroidism and alveolar hypoventilation. Arch Intern Med 1965;115:302
13. Zwillich CW, Pierson DJ, Hofeldt FD, et al. Ventilatory control in myxedema and hypothyroidism. N Engl J Med 1975;292:662
14. Ladenson PW, Goldenheim PD, Ridgway EC. Prediction and reversal of blunted ventilatory responsiveness in patients with hypothyroidism. Am J Med 1988;84:877
15. Duranti R, Gheri RG, Gorini M, et al. Control of breathing in patients with severe hypothyroidism. Am J Med 1993;95:29
16. Blum M. Myxedema coma. Am J Med Sci 1972;264:432
17. Forester CF. Coma in myxedema. Arch Intern Med 1963;111:100
18. Royce PC. Severely impaired consciousness in myxedema: a review. Am J Med Sci 1971;261:46
19. Domm BM, Vassallo CL. Myxedema coma with respiratory failure. Am Rev Respir Dis 1973;107:842
20. Marzullo ER, Franco S. Myxedema with multiple serous effusions and cardiac involvement (myxedema heart). Am Heart J 1939;17:360
21. Schneierson SJ, Katz M. Solitary pleural effusion due to myxedema. JAMA 1958;168:1003
22. Sachdev Y, Hall R. Effusions into body cavities in hypothyroidism. Lancet 1975;1:564
23. Gottehrer A, Roa J, Stanford G, et al. Hypothyroidism and pleural effusions. Chest 1990;98:1130
24. Brown SD, Brashear RE, Schnute RB. Pleural effusion in a young woman with myxedema. Arch Intern Med 1983;143:1458
25. Zondek H, Michael M, Kaatz A. The capillaries in myxedema. Am J Med Sci 1941;202:435

26. Lange K. Capillary permeability in myxedema. Am J Med Sci 1944;208:5

27. Orr WC, Males JL, Imes NK. Myxedema and obstructive sleep apnea. Am J Med 1981;70:1061

28. Skatrud J, Iber C, Ewart R, et al. Disordered breathing during sleep in hypothyroidism. Am Rev Respir Dis 1981;124:325

29. Rajagopal KR, Albrecht PH, Derderian SS, et al. Obstructive sleep apnea in hypothyroidism. Ann Intern Med 1984;101:491

30. Pelttari L, Rauhala E, Polo O, et al. Upper airway obstruction in hypothyroidism. J Intern Med 1994;236:177

31. Millman RP, Bevilacqua J, Peterson DD, et al. Central sleep apnea in hypothyroidism. Am Rev Respir Dis 1983;127:504

32. Gupta OP, Bhatia PL, Agarwal MK, et al. Nasal, pharyngeal, and laryngeal manifestations of hypothyroidism. Ear Nose Throat J 1977;56:349

33. Laroche CM, Cairns T, Moxham J, et al. Hypothyroidism presenting with respiratory muscle weakness. Am Rev Respir Dis 1988;138:472

34. Martinez FJ, Bermudez-Gomez M, Celli BR. Hypothyroidism: a reversible cause of diaphragmatic dysfunction. Chest 1989; 96:1059

35. Siafakas NM, Salesiotou V, Filaditaki V. Respiratory muscle strength in hypothyroidism. Chest 1992;102:189

36. Rosenow EC, Engel AG. Acid maltase deficiency in adults presenting as respiratory failure. Am J Med 1978;64:485

37. Hamly FH, Timms RM, Mihn VD, et al. Bilateral phrenic paralysis in myxedema [Abstract]. Am Rev Respir Dis 1975;111:911

38. Aderka D, Shavit G, Garfinkel D, et al. Life-threatening theophylline intoxication in a hypothyroid patient. Respiration 1985;44:77

39. Pandya K, Lal C, Scheinhorn D, et al. Hypothyroidism and ventilator dependency. Arch Intern Med 1989;149:2115

40. Moley JR, Ohkawa M, Chaudry IH, Clemens MG, Baue AE. Hypothyroidism abolishes the hyperdymanic phase and increases susceptibility to sepsis. J Surg Res 1984;36:265

41. Dulchavsky SA, Hendrick SR, Dutta S. Pulmonary biophysical effects of triiodothyronine augmentation during sepsis-induced hypothyroidism. J Trauma 1993;35:104

42. Redding RA, Douglas WHJ, Stein M. Thyroid hormone influence on lung surfactant metabolism. Science 1972;175:994

43. Wu B, Kikkawa Y, Drzaleski MM, et al. The effect of thyroxine on the maturation of fetal rabbit lungs. Biol Neonate 1973; 22:161

44. Ballard PL, Hovey ML, Gonzales LK. Thyroid hormone stimulation of phosphatidylcholine synthesis in cultured fetal rabbit lung. J Clin Invest 1984;74:898

45. Rooney SA, Marino PA, Bogran LI, Cross I, Warshaw JB. Thyrotropin-releasing hormone increases the amount of surfactant in lung lavage from fetal rabbits. Pediatr Res 1979;13:623

46. Burrow GN, Fisher DA, Larsen PR. Maternal and fetal thyroid function. N Engl J Med 1994;331:1072

47. Ballard PL, Benson BJ, Bichjen A, et al. Transplacental stimulation of lung development in the fetal rabbits by 3,5-dimethyl, 3'-isopropyl-L-thyronine. J Clin Invest 1980;65:1407

48. Hitchcock KR. Hormones and the lung. I. Thyroid hormones and glucocorticoids in lung development. Anat Rec 1979;194:15

49. Massaro D, Teich N, Massaro GD. Postnatal development of pulmonary alveoli: modulation in rats by thyroid hormones. Am J Physiol 1986;250:R51

50. Gross I, Dynia DW, Wilson CM, et al. Glucocorticoid-thyroid hormone interactions in fetal rat lung. Pediatr Res 1984;18:191

51. Smith BT, Sabry K. Glucocorticoid-thyroid synergism in lung maturation: a mechanism involving epithelial-mesenchymal interaction. Proc Natl Acad Sci USA 1983;80:1951

52. Ballard PL. Combined hormonal treatment and lung maturation. Semin Perinatol 1984;8:283

53. Gonzales LW, et al. Glucocorticoids and thyroid hormone stimulate biochemical and morphological differentiation of human fetal lung in organ culture. J Clin Endocrinol Metab 1986;62:687

54. Barker PM, Brown MJ, Ramsden CA, Strang LB, Walters DV. The effect of thyroidectomy in the fetal sheep on lung liquid reabsorption induced by adrenaline or cyclic AMP. J Physiol 1988;407:373

55. Gross I, Wilson CM, Ingleson LD, et al. Fetal lung in organ culture. III. Comparison of dexamethasone, thyroxine, and methylxanthines. J Appl Physiol 1980;48:872

56. Gross I, Wilson CM. Fetal lung in organ culture. IV. Supra-additive hormone interactions. J Appl Physiol 1982;52:1421

57. Gonzales VW, Ballard PL. Identification and characterizations of nuclear T_3-binding sites in fetal human lung. J Clin Endocrinol Metab 1981;53:21

58. Whitsett J, Darovec-Beckerman C, Manton M, et al. Thyroid dependent maturation of adrenergic receptors in the rat lung. Biochem Biophys Res Commun 1980;97:913

59. Redding RA, Pereira C. Thyroid function in respiratory distress syndrome of the newborn. Pediatrics 1974;54:423

60. Cuestas RA, Lindall A, Engel RR. Low thyroid hormones and respiratory distress syndrome of the newborn: studies on cord blood. N Engl J Med 1976;295:297

61. Cuestas RA, Engel RR. Thyroid function in preterm infants with respiratory distress syndrome. J Pediatr 1979;94:643

62. Klein AH, Stinson D, Foley B, et al. Thyroid function studies in perterm infants recovering from the respiratory distress syndrome. J Pediatr 1977;91:261

63. Klein AH, Foley B, Foley TP, MacDonald HM, Fisher DA. Thyroid function studies in cord blood from premature infants with and without respiratory distress syndrome. J Pediatr 1981;98:818

64. Mashiach S, Barkai G, Sack J, et al. Enchancement of fetal lung maturity by intraamniotic administration of thyroid hormone. Am J Obstet Gynecol 1979;130:289

65. Veszelovszky I, Nagy ZB, Bodis L. Effects of intraamniotically administered thyroxine on acceleration of fetal pulmonary maturity in preeclamptic toxemia. J Perinatol Med 1986;14:227

66. Rooney SA, Gobran LI, Chu AJ. Thyroid hormone opposes some glucocorticoid effects on glycogen content and lipid synthesis in developing fetal rat lung. Pediatr Res 1986;20:545

67. Pope TS, Rooney SA. Effects of glucocorticoid and thyroid hormones on regulatory enzymes of fatty acid synthesis and glycogen metabolism in developing fetal rat lung. Biochim Biophys Acta 1987;918:141

68. Sosenko IRS, Frank L. Thyroid inhibition and developmental increases in fetal rat lung antioxidant enzymes. Am J Physiol 1989;257:L94

69. NIH Consensus Panel. Effect of corticosteroids for fetal maturation on perinatal outcomes. JAMA 1995;273:413

70. Moya FR, Gross I. Combined hormonal therapy for the prevention of respiratory distress syndrome and its consequences. Semin Perinatol 1993;17:267

Werner and Ingbar's The Thyroid, Seventh Edition,
edited by Lewis E. Braverman and Robert D. Utiger.
Lippincott–Raven Publishers, Philadelphia, © 1996

64

The Kidneys and Electrolyte Metabolism in Hypothyroidism

Arnold M. Moses
Steven J. Scheinman

RENAL HEMODYNAMICS AND TUBULAR FUNCTION

Hypothyroid patients often have generalized vascular constriction, but little is known about its cause. This vascular constriction leads to increased systemic vascular resistance and diastolic hypertension, despite low cardiac output and hypovolemia. In a study of 688 patients with hypertension, 3.6% had previously unrecognized hypothyroidism.[1] Stimulated plasma renin activity was low in 52% of the hypothyroid patients, but the importance of the latter finding is unknown, because many normotensive patients with hypothyroidism have low plasma renin activity.[2] In a group of patients with hypothyroidism induced by radioiodine treatment of thyrotoxicosis, the diastolic blood pressure was above 90 mm Hg in 40%.[1] Thyroid replacement therapy reduced the diastolic blood pressure to below 90 mm Hg in all the patients who were younger than 45 years of age but in only 23% of the patients aged 50 to 69 years.[3] Since most of the older hypothyroid patients remained hypertensive after restoration of euthyroidism, their hypertension was probably not induced by hypothyroidism.

The generalized vascular constriction and increased systemic vascular resistance that occurs in hypothyroidism (see chap 62) cause a proportionate decrease in glomerular filtration rate (GFR) and renal plasma flow. Other factors that decrease the GFR are intrarenal vasoconstriction and thickening of the glomerular basement membrane. In patients with severe hypothyroidism, the GFR may decrease by as much as 20% to 30%. Micropuncture studies have demonstrated a marked reduction in single-nephron GFR in thyroidectomized rats, caused by a decrease in renal plasma flow, an increase in vascular resistance of both the afferent and efferent arterioles, and a reduction in the glomerular ultrafiltration coefficient, all of which are reversed with inhibition of generation of angiotensin II.[4]

Tubular transport capacity measured by Diodrast or para-aminohippurate (PAH) excretion is below normal in hypothyroid patients and animals. Another abnormality of renal tubular function is decreased urinary urate excretion, which may result in hyperuricemia.

Thyroid hormone induces de novo synthesis of both the alpha and beta subunits of Na^+,K^+-ATPase by increasing their mRNA content in target cells.[5] Thyroid deficiency, conversely, decreases the activity of this enzyme in the kidney, particularly in the proximal tubules.[6] This decrease, in turn, impairs sodium transport. Na^+–H^+ exchange activity (amiloride-sensitive Na^+ and H^+ flux) in renal proximal tubular brush border membrane vesicles also is decreased in hypothyroid rats,[7] further decreasing sodium reabsorption.

Hypothyroid rats have other defects of renal tubular function. For example, renal responsiveness to vasopressin is decreased, primarily in the medullary thick ascending limbs of the loops of Henle.[8,9] As a result, generation of a hypertonic medullary interstitium is impaired.[9] This, in turn, impairs generation of free water and reduces maximal urine concentrating ability. These defects are corrected by thyroid replacement therapy.[8-11] Patients with hypothyroidism also have diminished renal responses to parathyroid hormone.[12] The inability of hypothyroid patients to concentrate urine maximally and their renal resistance to parathyroid hormone are of little clinical importance. In contrast, the impaired ability to generate free water may be clinically important (see later).

In general, alterations in renal hemodynamics and tubular function seldom are clinically important in patients with mild to moderate hypothyroidism. For example, there is rarely an increase in serum urea or creatinine concentration. This lack of change results from balanced reduction in both function and homeostatic demand, because the hypometabolic state decreases the rate of generation of nitrogenous wastes that counterbalances any decrease in renal function.[11,13]

HORMONES AFFECTING WATER AND ELECTROLYTE METABOLISM

Under normal conditions the amount of sodium and water filtered through the glomeruli far exceeds the urinary excretion of these substances because of tubular reabsorption. In the proximal tubules, water is reabsorbed passively as a consequence of the active transport of solute across the tubular epithelial cells. In the thick ascending limbs of the tubules, sodium and chloride, but little water, are reabsorbed. In this way free water is created. Sodium and water reabsorption in the distal tubules and collecting ducts are under the influence of aldosterone and arginine vasopressin (AVP), respectively.

Hypothyroid rats and sheep have increased plasma AVP concentrations,[9,14] and AVP production rates in thyroidectomized sheep are increased.[14] Some hypothyroid patients also have increased plasma AVP concentrations. For instance, in a study of 20 hypothyroid patients who had serum sodium concentrations of 130 to 142 mEq/L, 15 had elevated plasma AVP concentrations that failed to suppress normally after water ingestion.[15] Other patients in the study had a non-AVP–mediated defect in water excretion. The rapidity of recovery was demonstrated in two patients with myxedema coma and hyponatremia who had elevated plasma AVP concentrations and in whom T_4 treatment resulted in restoration of normal serum sodium and plasma AVP concentrations in days, even before the patients improved in other ways.[16] Apparently AVP secretion is not normally inhibited by hypotonicity in these patients. However, osmotic regulation of AVP secretion was normal in eight patients with severe primary hypothyroidism who were infused with hypertonic saline,[17] in that the rise in plasma AVP concentrations with rising plasma osmolality was normal or nearly so in all patients.[17] The general belief is that increases in random plasma AVP values in hypothyroid patients, when they occur, are due to a non-osmotic stimulus, namely hypovolemia,[18,19] thereby resulting in urine concentration even when the plasma is hypotonic. This helps to maintain intravascular volume, even at the expense of tonicity. Our understanding of the metabolism of AVP in hypothyroidism will be improved when well-designed studies of the release of AVP in response to non-osmotic stimuli and of urinary and metabolic clearance of AVP are carried out.

The major threats to sodium balance are changes in glomerular filtration, and hence in the filtered load of sodium, and changes in sodium intake. These changes are normally counteracted by appropriate alterations in glomerulotubular balance, autoregulation of the glomerular filtration rate (GFR), changes in production of renin, angiotensin and aldosterone, and redistribution of blood flow to individual nephrons.

Hypothyroid rats have decreased plasma renin activity and plasma angiotensin and aldosterone concentrations.[20] Similarly, patients with hypothyroidism often have low plasma renin activity and plasma aldosterone concentrations.[2,21] These abnormalities correct quickly after treatment of the hypothyroidism. Perhaps as a result of these hormonal changes, or because of decreased sodium reabsorption related to defects in sodium transport, hypothyroid animals and patients have an impaired ability to conserve sodium during rigid sodium restriction.[4,10,22,23] Plasma atrial natriuretic peptide concentrations are decreased,[24] and therefore this hormone does not contribute to the sodium-losing tendency. This tendency towards sodium loss has no clinical importance, and does not cause the hyponatremia that occurs in some hypothyroid patients (see below). The role of aldosterone deficiency in hypothyroid patients is unknown.

HYPONATREMIA

The incidence and magnitude of hyponatremia in patients with hypothyroidism is a function of the severity of the hypothyroidism. It is most common in patients with myxedema coma. The hypothyroidism is almost always primary; with rare exceptions,[25] the hyponatremia that occurs in patients with anterior pituitary disease is associated with ACTH deficiency and is corrected by glucocorticoid—not thyroid— replacement therapy. Despite the impaired sodium conservation in hypothyroidism,[4,10,22,23] the hyponatremia is attributed to water retention because there is an increase in total body sodium.[26] Patients with hypothyroidism, whether or not hyponatremic, have diminished ability to excrete free water, fail to achieve maximum urinary dilution, and have delayed excretion of a water load.[15] The two major postulated causes for the abnormal water retention of hypothyroidism are decreased renal blood flow and GFR and excessive AVP secretion in response to non-osmotic stimuli. Occasionally, hyponatremia may be due in part to binding of sodium to glycosaminoglycans in the extracellular space.

In both normal rats and rats with congenital hypothalamic diabetes insipidus, hypothyroidism impairs free water excretion.[27] The hypothyroid rats have reduced clearances of inulin, free water, and sodium. When distal delivery of sodium is augmented by an intravenous infusion of a carbonic anhydrase inhibitor or by removal of one kidney, free water clearance is greatly increased. These results suggest that the major cause of the diminished water excretion is a reduction in GFR, which limits the delivery of glomerular filtrate to the distal diluting segment and thus impairs the ability to create and excrete free water. In a study of hypothyroid patients, normal subjects, and patients with mild chronic renal failure whose GFRs were similar to those of the hypothyroid patients, the hypothyroid patients and those with chronic renal failure had decreased proximal tubular sodium reabsorption and increased distal tubular sodium reabsorption (beyond the loop of Henle), as compared with the normal subjects.[28] The maximal urinary flow rate and free water clearance were similarly reduced in both groups of patients. Proximal sodium reabsorption and maximal urinary volume were directly correlated with the GFR, and distal sodium reabsorption was proportionate to delivery of sodium from the proximal tubule. These results suggest that the abnormalities in sodium and water handling in hypothyroidism are comparable with those in patients with a similar degree of renal insufficiency, and may be a direct consequence of the decrease in GFR.

Some hypothyroid patients with hyponatremia fulfill all of the diagnostic criteria for the syndrome of inappropriate antidiuresis, and in these patients ethanol, a known inhibitor of AVP secretion, may cause transient dilution of the urine. However, this effect of ethanol cannot always be demonstrated. There is a poor correlation between plasma AVP concentrations and the efficiency with which a water load is excreted in hypothyroid patients. Also, inappropriate antidiuresis is not invariably present, even in patients with severe hypothyroidism, and not all investigators find elevated plasma AVP concentrations in patients with hypothyroidism who have hyponatremia.[17,25,29] Plasma AVP concentrations may decline appropriately during water loading, even in patients who have hyponatremia and mild diluting defects during water loading.[17] All told, the evidence supporting an important causative role for AVP in the hyponatremia of hypothyroidism is not very persuasive. The role of elevated plasma AVP concentrations in hyponatremic patients with hypothyroidism will be more clearly defined when these patients can be studied with specific antagonists of the vasopressin-V2 receptors, the receptors that mediate the antidiuretic action of AVP.[30]

We conclude that water retention and hyponatremia in hypothyroidism results from AVP-independent and -dependent mechanisms. In some hypothyroid patients with an excess of AVP, the AVP may have little or nothing to do with the predisposition to water retention and hyponatremia. Regardless, when these patients are treated with thyroid hormone, renal plasma flow and GFR increase toward normal, plasma AVP concentrations decrease, a brisk diuresis of water and sodium occurs, and serum sodium concentrations rise.

Hypothyroidism does not cause abnormal serum potassium concentrations. When hyperkalemia is associated with hypothyroidism, adrenal insufficiency should be suspected.

EDEMA

Edema is a common manifestation of hypothyroidism and is related to the severity of the hypothyroidism. It may be present in early thyroid failure when the only biochemical abnormality is a modest increase in serum thyrotropin (TSH) concentration. The pathogenesis of the fluid retention in the absence of heart failure is still not clear. Protein-rich fluid accumulates most commonly in subcutaneous tissues, but at times as a pericardial effusion or ascites.[31] Using radioactive albumin as a tracer, Parving and coworkers found large extravascular accumulations of albumin, and presumably other proteins, in patients with hypothyroidism.[19] They concluded that the interstitial fluid of the skin and muscle was the major

site of albumin accumulation, possibly due to decreased barrier function of endothelial cells leading to an increase in the transcapillary escape rate of albumin.[19,32] A second abnormality, peculiar to hypothyroidism, is an absence of a compensatory increase in lymph flow.[19] Thus, the edema of hypothyroidism and the accumulation of cavitary fluid may represent generalized lymphedema. The problem may be aggravated by increased renal tubular reabsorption of water and electrolytes. When thyroid hormone therapy is administered, there is a diuresis of water and solutes and a restoration of normal plasma volume.

MINERAL METABOLISM

Serum calcium and phosphorus concentrations are nearly always normal in patients with hypothyroidism. In contrast to the increased bone resorption that occurs in patients with thyrotoxicosis, hypothyroidism is associated with decreased bone turnover, which tends to lower serum calcium concentrations. However, normocalcemia is maintained by a small increase in serum parathyroid hormone concentrations and the subsequent increase in serum 1,25-dihydroxyvitamin D concentrations.[33,34] Urinary calcium excretion is frequently decreased in hypothyroid patients, reflecting the decreased filtered load of calcium and the effects of increased parathyroid hormone secretion (see chap 72).

Even though hypothyroidism does not cause hypocalcemia, the two conditions are occasionally found in association. For example, hypoparathyroidism may be a complication of thyroidectomy. In the absence of a history of thyroid surgery, the presence of primary hypothyroidism in a patient with hypocalcemia suggests the possibility of pseudohypoparathyroidism, type 1a,[35] which is caused by deficient activity of guanine nucleotide-binding stimulatory protein (Gs).[36] As a consequence, peptide hormone receptors become uncoupled from adenylyl cyclase, resulting in impaired production of cAMP in many tissues. Few of these patients have overt hypothyroidism, but subclinical hypothyroidism or at least an excessive serum TSH response to thyrotropin-releasing hormone (TRH) indicative of very mild hypothyroidism are common.[35]

Although hypercalcemia is rare in patients with hypothyroidism, it can occur if calcium intake is high or if hypocalciuria is marked and parathyroid hormone secretion is not normally suppressible.[37,38] Infants with congenital hypothyroidism also may have mild hypercalcemia.[39] Other situations in which hypercalcemia may occur in a patient with hypothyroidism are primary hyperparathyroidism associated with radioactive iodine therapy,[40] sarcoidosis (increased 1,25-dihydroxyvitamin D production) with concomitant TSH or TRH deficiency,[41] and lithium therapy.[42]

Plasma and erythrocyte magnesium concentrations may be slightly elevated in hypothyroid patients, perhaps because of reduced renal clearance of magnesium.[43] In a series of 84 patients with a variety of thyroid diseases, both serum and erythrocyte magnesium concentrations were negatively correlated with serum thyroid hormone concentrations. Serum and urinary zinc concentrations are low in hypothyroidism.[44] The clinical implications of these alterations in magnesium and zinc metabolism are not known.

References

1. Streeten DHP, Anderson GH Jr, Howland T, Chiang R, Smulyan H. Effects of thyroid function on blood pressure. Recognition of hypothyroid hypertension. Hypertension 1988;11:78

2. Hauger-Klevene JH, Brown H, Zavaleta J. Plasma renin activity in hyper- and hypothyroidism: effect of adrenergic blocking agents. J Clin Endocrinol Metab 1972;34:625

3. Streeten DHP, Anderson GH Jr, Elias MF. Prevalence of secondary hypertension and unusual aspects of the treatment of hypertension in elderly individuals. Geriatr Nephrol Urol 1992;2:91

4. Gillum DM, Falk SA, Hammond WS, Conger JD. Glomerular dynamics in the hypothyroid rat and the role of the renin-angiotensin system. Am J Physiol 1987;253:F170

5. McDonough AA, Brown TA, Horowitz B, et al. Thyroid hormone coordinately regulates Na+-K+-ATPase alpha- and beta-subunit mRNA levels in kidney. Am J Physiol 1988;254:C323

6. Garg LC, Tisher CC. Effects of thyroid hormone on Na-K- adenosine triphosphatase activity along the rat nephron. J Lab Clin Med 1985;106:568

7. Kinsella J, Sacktor B. Thyroid hormones increase Na+-H+ exchange activity in renal brush border membranes. Proc Natl Acad Sci U S A 1985;82:3606

8. Harkcom TM, Kim JK, Palumbo PJ, et al. Modulatory effect of thyroid function on enzymes of the vasopressin-sensitive adenosine 3',5'-monophosphate system in renal medulla. Endocrinology 1978;102:1475

9. Kim JK, Summer SN, Schrier RW. Cellular action of arginine vasopressin in the isolated renal tubules of hypothyroid rats. Am J Physiol 1987;253:F104

10. Vaamonde CA, Michael UF, Oster JR, et al. Impaired renal concentrating ability in hypothyroid man. Nephron 1976;17:382

11. Bradley SE, Stephan F, Coelho JB, Reville P. The thyroid and the kidney. Kidney Int 1974;6:346

12. Fraser WD, Logue FC, MacRitchie K, et al. Intact parathyroid hormone concentration and cyclic AMP metabolism in thyroid disease. Acta Endocrinol 1991;124:652

13. Emmanouel DS, Katz AI. Kidney-thyroid interactions. Kidney 1980;13:7

14. Skowsky WR, Fisher DA. Arginine vasopressin secretion in thyroidectomized sheep. Endocrinology 1977;100:1022

15. Skowsky WR, Kikuchi TA. The role of vasopressin in the impaired water excretion of myxedema. Am J Med 1978;64:613

16. Archambeaud-Mouveroux F, Dejax C, Jadaud JM, et al. Coma myxoedemateux avec hypervasopressinisme. Ann Med Interne 1987;138:114

17. Iwasaki Y, Oiso Y, Yamauchi K, et al. Osmoregulation of plasma vasopressin in myxedema. J Clin Endocrinol Metab 1990;70:534

18. Schrier RW, Goldberg JP. The physiology of vasopressin release and the pathogenesis of impaired water excretion in adrenal, thyroid, and edematous disorders. Yale J Biol Med 1980;53:525

19. Parving HH, Hansen JM, Nielsen SL, Rossing N, Munck O, Lassen NA. Mechanisms of edema formation in myxedema-increased protein extravasation and relatively slow lymphatic drainage. N Engl J Med 1979;301:460

20. Marchant C, Brown L, Sernia C. Renin-angiotensin system in thyroid dysfunction in rats. J Cardiovasc Pharmacol 1993;22:449

21. Resnick LM, Laragh JH. Plasma renin activity in syndromes of thyroid hormone excess and deficiency. Life Sci 1982;30:585

22. Katz AI, Lindheimer MD. Renal sodium- and potassium-activated adenosine triphosphate and sodium reabsorption in the hypothyroid rat. J Clin Invest 1973;52:796

23. Katz AI, Emmanouel DS, Lindheimer MD. Thyroid hormone and the kidney. Nephron 1975;15:223

24. Rolandi E, Santaniello B, Bagnasco M, et al. Thyroid hormones and atrial natriuretic hormone secretion: study in hyper- and hypothyroid patients. Acta Endocrinol 1992;127:23

25. Macaron C, Famuyiwa O. Hyponatremia of hypothyroidism: appropriate suppression of antidiuretic hormone levels. Arch Intern Med 1978;138:820

26. Aikawa JK. The nature of myxedema: Alterations in the serum electrolyte concentrations and radiosodium space and in the exchangeable sodium and potassium contents. Ann Intern Med 1956;44:30

27. Emmanouel DS, Lindheimer MD, Katz AI. Mechanism of impaired water excretion in the hypothyroid rat. J Clin Invest 1974;54:926

28. Allon M, Harrow A, Pasque CB, Rodriquez M. Renal sodium and water handling in hypothyroid patients: the role of renal insufficiency. J Am Soc Nephrol 1990;1:205

29. Koide Y, Oda K, Shimizu K, et al. Hyponatremia without inappropriate secretion of vasopressin in a case of myxedema coma. Endocrinol Jpn 1982;29:363

30. Ohnishi A, Orita Y, Okahara R, et al. Potent aquaretic agent. A novel nonpeptide selective vasopressin 2 antagonist (OPC-31260) in men. J Clin Invest 1993;92:2653

31. Sachdev Y, Hall R. Effusions into body cavities in hypothyroidism. Lancet 1975;1:564

32. Wheatley T, Edwards OM. Mild hypothyroidism and oedema: evidence for increased capillary permeability to protein. Clin Endocrinol 1983;18:627

33. Castro JH, Genuth SM, Klein L. Comparative response to parathyroid hormone in hyperthyroidism and hypothyroidism. Metabolism 1975;24:839

34. Bouillon R, De Moor P. Influence of thyroid function on the serum concentration of 1,25-dihydroxyvitamin D3. J Clin Endocrinol Metab 1980;51:793

35. Levine MA, Downs RW Jr, Moses AM, et al. Resistance to multiple hormones in patients with pseudohypoparathyroidism. Association with deficient activity of guanine nucleotide regulatory protein. Am J Med 1983;74:545

36. Levine MA, Schwindinger WF, Downs RW Jr, Moses AM. Pseudohypoparathyroidism: clinical, biochemical, and molecular features. In: Bilezikian JP, Marcus R, Levine MA, eds. The parathyroids: basic and clinical concepts. New York: Raven Press, 1994:781

37. Lowe CE, Bird ED, Thomas WC. Hypercalcemia in myxedema. J Clin Endocrinol Metab 1962;22:261

38. Zaloga GP, Eil C, O'Brian JT. Reversible hypocalciuric hypercalcemia associated with hypothyroidism. Am J Med 1984;77:1101

39. Tau C, Garabedian M, Farriaux JP, Czernichow P, Pomarede R, Balsan S. Hypercalcemia in infants with congenital hypothyroidism and its relation to vitamin D and thyroid hormones. J Pediatr 1986;109:808

40. Bondeson AG, Bondeson L, Thompson NW. Hyperparathyroidism after treatment with radioactive iodine: not only a coincidence? Surgery 1989;106:1025

41. Bell NH. Endocrine complications of sarcoidosis. Endocrinol Metab Clin North Am 1991;20:645

42. Salata R, Klein I. Effects of lithium on the endocrine system: a review. J Lab Clin Med 1987;110:130

43. Shibutani Y, Yokota T, Iijima S, Fujioka A, Katsuno S, Sakamoto K. Plasma and erythrocyte magnesium concentrations in thyroid disease: relation to thyroid function and the duration of illness. Jpn J Med 1989;28:496

44. Dolev E, Deuster PA, Solomon B, Trostmann UH, Wartofsky L, Burman KD. Alterations in magnesium and zinc metabolism in thyroid disease. Metabolism 1988;37:61

Werner and Ingbar's The Thyroid, Seventh Edition,
edited by Lewis E. Braverman and Robert D. Utiger.
Lippincott–Raven Publishers, Philadelphia, © 1996

65

The Gastrointestinal Tract and Liver in Hypothyroidism

Rena Vassilopoulou-Sellin

Joseph H. Sellin

The sluggish and slow response that is characteristic of the myxedematous patient in general marks the major gastrointestinal (GI) manifestations of hypothyroidism: sluggish intestinal motility ranging from mild obstipation to paralytic ileus and intestinal pseudo-obstruction. Spontaneous hypothyroidism most often afflicts the elderly, who frequently discount the significance of an insidious decrease of bowel movements. Severe constipation unresponsive to laxatives may, therefore, be a prominent finding at the time of diagnosis. Younger patients with iatrogenic hypothyroidism secondary to treatment for thyrotoxicosis or thyroid cancer frequently gain weight because of decreased physical activity coupled with unchanged food intake. In infants, the observation of infrequent hard stools should serve as a prompt clue to the diagnosis so that the serious neurologic sequelae of unrecognized myxedema can be prevented.

Hypothyroidism affects the GI tract in several additional ways. As with thyrotoxicosis, atrophic gastritis and pernicious anemia may be associated with myxedema. Therefore, prompt investigation of gastric histology and vitamin B_{12} metabolism should follow the discovery of megaloblastic anemia in the hypothyroid patient. Although there may be a specific hepatic lesion of hypothyroidism, associated autoimmune liver disease is probably more common. In the myxedematous patient with liver function abnormalities, particular diagnostic efforts should be directed toward the possibility of primary biliary cirrhosis or chronic active hepatitis.

INTESTINAL MOTILITY IN MYXEDEMA

Although most patients with hypothyroidism average one bowel movement daily, about one-eighth have less than three motions weekly; these patients also show a significant increase in laxative use.[1] Insidious symptoms of vague abdominal pain and distention may be present and often are diagnosed as functional bowel disease. Unusual GI manifestations, such as a gastric phytobezoar[2] or a lesion mimicking carcinoma of the sigmoid colon,[3] have been reported. Rectal prolapse and sigmoid volvulus are occasionally seen. Severe cases may present with intestinal atony and ileus,[4] often misinterpreted as intestinal obstruction. With earlier diagnosis of hypothyroidism, fewer cases have progressed to pseudo-obstruction in recent years. In myxedema, radiologic studies reveal generalized dilatation of the GI tract, especially the colon. Pathologic examination of the hypothyroid intestine has demonstrated a thickened, pale, leathery colon, generally lengthened; microscopically, myxedematous and round cell infiltration of the submucosal and muscle layers is evident. A decrease in colonic crypts suggests mucosal atrophy.

The motility of the GI tract may be assessed using several different methods (see chap 41). Studies of hypothyroid humans and dogs have demonstrated a decrease in the electrical and motor activity of the esophagus, stomach, small intestine, and colon.[5–7] Dysphagia is not uncommon in hypothyroidism and may be related to esophageal motility abnormalities, including decreases in amplitude and velocity of peristalsis and a decrease in lower esophageal sphincter pressure. These abnormalities correct with thyroid replacement.[5] Gastric emptying, as measured with a liquid meal of glucose, is prolonged in hypothyroidism and returns to normal with therapy.[8] The neuropeptide TRH has a central effect on gastric emptying; injected into the cerebrospinal fluid, TRH increases phasic motor activity of the stomach, mediated by TRH receptors on postsynaptic vagal neurons.[9] Orocecal (intestinal) transit time, as measured by a lactulose-hydrogen breath test, decreased significantly in one study when hypothyroid patients received thyroid hormone replacement therapy[10] but, in another study, was normal in the hypothyroid state and was not significantly altered by thyroid hormone replacement therapy.[11] The relative importance of the small bowel and colon in the "sluggish gut" of hypothyroidism remains to be determined. In the sigmoid colon and rectum, the number and amplitude of muscular contractions are decreased. Several theories have been proposed to explain the changes of the hypothyroid intestine, including autonomic neuropathy, altered impulse transmission at the myoneural junction, intestinal ischemia, and intestinal myopathy.

ABSORPTION IN MYXEDEMA

In most patients, intestinal absorption is normal. The malabsorption occasionally reported in severely hypothyroid patients remains poorly understood but has been attributed to myxedematous infiltration of the mucosa, altered intestinal motility, or associated autoimmune phenomena. Intestinal handling of D-xylose is normal, although renal clearance after both intravenous and oral administration is lower due to a decrease in glomerular filtration rate. In addition, glucose absorption is overall normal whereas net transmural transport is enhanced, in part because of decreased glucose utilization.[12] Hypercalcemia may occur owing to increased absorption of dietary calcium in conjunction with a decrease in calcium incorporation into bone.[13] Pancreatic function is generally normal in hypothyroidism; hypothermia associated with severe myxedema may occasionally result in hyperamylasemia, probably secondary to pancreatitis.[14] The hypothyroid intestinal epithelium may be less responsive to secretory stimuli such as vasoactive intestinal peptide, suggesting a possible pathophysiologic mechanism for some of the intestinal alterations of hypothyroidism.[15] In hypothyroid patients who receive thyroid hormone replacement therapy, the addition of other pharmacologic agents (such as bile acid sequestrants, sucralfate, ferrous sulfate, or aluminum hydroxide) may impair thyroxine absorption and complicate their management.[16–17]

THYROID FUNCTION IN MALABSORPTION AND INTESTINAL DISEASE

An enterohepatic circulation of thyroid hormone has been described[18] in which thyroid hormone secreted into bile is delivered into the intestinal lumen, reabsorbed, and delivered back to the liver (see chap 41). This system is similar to that described for other hormones, such as vitamin D and estrogens. Interactions of the gut with thyroid hormone, the potential role of the intestine both as a reservoir for thyroid hormones and as a regulator of hormone activity,[19] and the presence of enterohepatic circulation raise several interesting questions: Does intraluminal thyroid hormone affect intestinal function? Does thyroid hormone delivered to the liver through the enterohepatic circulation and portal vein in relatively high concentrations have an effect on hepatic function? Given the ability of intestinal bacteria to bind and degrade thyroid hor-

mones,[20] is there a clinically significant, although indirect, effect of intestinal hypomotility on thyroid hormone economy?

Significant adaptation in fecal losses of hormone takes place in hypothyroidism,[21] both through decreased excretion and increased absorption. Nevertheless, intestinal diseases and malabsorption may affect the metabolism of thyroid hormone. Increased fecal thyroxine losses may occur in pancreatic steatorrhea, celiac sprue,[22] and inflammatory bowel disease.[23] In addition, autoimmune thyroid disease (hypothyroidism more frequently than thyrotoxicosis) may be more prevalent in patients with celiac disease.[24] Malabsorption of oral thyroid medication is seen after jejunoileal bypass.[25,26] In balance, the euthyroid patient is generally capable of compensating for intestinal losses with increased endogenous thyroid secretion, whereas the hypothyroid patient may require adjustment of thyroid hormone replacement dosage.

THYROID HORMONE AND TRANSPORT

The role of thyroid hormone in thermogenesis has been linked to a stimulation of $Na^+,-K^+$-ATPase activity in both liver and intestine.[27,28] Thyroid hormone stimulation of hepatic $Na^+,-K^+$-ATPase is associated with an increase in bile salt–independent bile flow.[29]

The effect of thyroid hormone on intestinal transport is less clear-cut. An increase in jejunal secretion of fluid, amylase, invertase (sucrase), and mucoprotein was suggested in early studies, but more recently animal studies have demonstrated complex and conflicting effects on active (electrogenic) transfer of amino acids and sugars.[30,31] Hypothyroidism is associated with changes in colonic epithelial membrane lipid composition and fluidity.[32] In the colon, thyroid hormone alone does not have an independent effect on the electrical parameters of transport, but it appears to have a permissive role in mineralocorticoid-stimulated absorption of sodium and water.[33,34]

Therefore, although thyroid hormone alters several different transport systems in the GI tract, there does not appear to be a consistent pattern. Understanding the impact of these effects in clinical myxedema requires further study.

GUT AND LIVER DEVELOPMENT

Intestinal growth and development is physiologically regulated by thyroid hormone at multiple levels.[35–37] In humans, fetal hypothyroidism does not appear to seriously affect the gut; in young animals, however, hypothyroidism results in decreased mucosal thickness and villous height, weight, and protein content of the small intestine[38] and in abnormal gut peptide content and binding properties.[15,39,40] Understanding the role of thyroid hormone in intestinal development has been complicated because (1) manipulation of thyroid status is associated with changes in glucocorticoids and (2) most studies have employed pharmacologic rather than physiologic replacement of thyroid hormone. Thyroid hormone regulates rat gut brush border enzyme gene expression[41] as well as lactose ontogenesis.[42] Overall, it appears that thyroid hormone alone has little effect on intestinal maturation, but when combined with glucocorticoids may have a synergistic effect on the developmental profile of multiple intestinal enzymes including sucrase, maltase, and alkaline phosphatase. This effect is, however, not universally found with all intestinal enzymes.[43–45] Experimental thyrotoxicosis in developing animals has been associated with mucosal hypertrophy and epithelial hyperplasia of the jejunum, with increased villous height, microvillous-enzymatic activity, and protein content of the whole small intestine. It is not clear whether the changes seen with thyroid excess or deprivation are direct tissue effects of the hormone or secondary to associated changes in food intake and gut motility. The observation, in tissue culture, that thyroxine increases cell enzymatic activity in embryonic duodenum[46] indicates that there is, at least in part, a direct effect. Thyroid deprivation alters secretion of gastric mucus,[47] an action of unknown clinical importance. Thyroid hormone affects hepatic enzymatic maturation as well as mitochondrial metabolism[48,49] and plays an important role in hepatic regeneration after resection.

GASTRIC FUNCTION IN MYXEDEMA

Immune gastritis coexists with hypothyroidism in about 11% of patients. This association is probably due to the propensity of such patients for autoimmune disease.[50] As with thyrotoxicosis, abnormalities of B_{12} metabolism without overt anemia, antiparietal cell antibodies, and hypochlorhydria or achlorhydria have been much more commonly reported. Similarly, there is a high incidence of thyroid antibodies in patients with pernicious anemia.[51] The mechanism of gastric acid secretory dysfunction is also not clear. The observation that hyperthyroidism is associated with hypergastrinemia[52,53] whereas patients with hypothyroidism have subnormal serum gastrin[54] implies that the pathophysiology of achlorhydria differs in the two conditions. The embryologic similarity between thyroid and gastric tissue, their mutual iodine concentrating ability, and their similar histologic abnormalities have led many investigators to consider that thyrogastric autoimmune disorders are linked pathophysiologically; no HLA association has been found to date.

LIVER IN HYPOTHYROIDISM

An assocation exists between Hashimoto's thyroiditis and hypothyroidism with autoimmune liver diseases such as chronic active hepatitis[55,56] and primary biliary cirrhosis.[57,58] Liver, gastric, and thyroid dysfunction in autoimmune disease may comprise a constellation of coexisting abnormalities (see chap 41 for a discussion of thyroid and liver interactions). Thyroid hormones have significant impact in the regulation of hepatic mitochondrial metabolism.[59,60] Hypothyroid animals have decreased resting metabolic rate with decreased hepatocyte oxygen consumption.[61] A specific hypothyroid hepatic lesion of central congestive fibrosis without myxedematous infiltration has been reported.[62] Persistent hyperbilirubinemia in the newborn may suggest the diagnosis of congenital hypothyroidism.

Myxedema ascites is a rare and poorly understood complication of severe hypothyroidism[62,63] and consists of a yellow and gelatinous peritoneal exudate. It has been suggested that myxedema ascites is related to congestive heart failure, enhanced capillary permeability, or the inappropriate secretion of antidiuretic hormone associated with hypothyroidism; however, no firm evidence indicates its etiology.

Reversible abnormalities of liver function tests, although usually mild, are common in hypothyroidism. In addition, there is abnormal fuel use, with significant decrease in gluconeogenesis.[64] Hypothyroid patients show specific defects in hepatic handling of amino acids that result in decreased urea nitrogen generation.[65]

Thyroid status clearly affects bile flow and composition. In experimental models of hypothyroidism, decrease in bile flow primarily is due to a decrease in the bile salt–independent component.[29] Additionally, the biliary excretion of bilirubin is diminished, in association with some subtle alterations of hepatic bilirubin metabolism.[66] In hypothyroidism, the fraction of bile acids conjugated with glycine is increased; this may be a result of decreased availability of dietary taurine to the hepatic conjugating system. Thyroidectomy in rats affects several key enzymes in the pathways of cholesterol and bile acid synthesis. Both HMG-CoA reductase and cholesterol-7 α-hydroxylase are reduced; the latter responds more promptly to thyroid replacement.[51,67] In addition, thyroid hormone modifies lipoprotein metabolism in the liver.[68–74] It is unclear whether this is a direct thyroid effect on liver enzymes or secondary to altered intestinal handling of cholesterol and bile acids.[75,76] The changes in enzyme activities, the hypercholesterolemia of myxedema, and the hypotonia of the gallbladder seen in hypothyroidism suggest the possibility of increased cholesterol saturation of bile[69] and a higher incidence of gallstones. However, direct measurements of the lithogenicity of hypothyroid bile are not available.

SUMMARY

Hypothyroidism appears to affect the GI tract more profoundly than thyroid excess. Hypomotility with constipation is a fairly frequent, although usually mild, manifestation of hypothyroidism. Associated gastric, liver, and thyroid dysfunctions are often due to systemic autoimmune diseases. Although the clinical picture of myxedema has been well characterized, the mechanims of thyroid action on the gut and liver remain poorly understood.

References

1. Baker JT, Harvey RF. Bowel habits in thyrotoxicosis and hypothyroidism. Br Med J 1971;1:322
2. Kaplan LR. Hypothyroidism presenting as a gastric phytobezoar. Am J Gastroenterol 1980;74:168
3. Duks S, Pitlik S, Rosenfeld JB. Hypothyroidism mimicking a tumor of the sigmoid colon. Mayo Clin Proc 1979;54:623
4. Abbasi AA, Douglass RC, Bissel GW, Chen Y. Myxedema Ileus. JAMA 1975;234:181
5. Eastwood GL, Braverman LG, White EM, et al: Reversal of lower esophageal sphincter hypotension and esophageal aperistalsis after treatment for hypothyroidism. J Clin Gastroenterol 1982; 4:307

6. Karaus M, Wienbeck M, Grussendorf M, Erckenbrecht JF, Strohmeyer G. Intestinal motor activity in experimental hyperthyroidism in conscious dogs. Gastroenterol 1989;97:911

7. Kowalewski K, Kolodej A. Myoelectrical and mechanical activity of stomach and intestine in hypothyroid dogs. Am J Digest Dis 1977;22;235

8. Holdsworth DC, Besser GM. Influence of gastric emptying rates and of insulin response on oral glucose tolerance in thyroid disease. Lancet 1968;ii:700

9. Raybould HE, Jacobsen LJ, Tache J: TRH stimulation and L-glutamic acid inhibition of proximal gastric motor activity in the rat dorsal vagal complex. Brain Res 1989;49:319

10. Shafer RB, Prentiss RA, Bond JH. Gastrointestinal transit in thyroid disease. Gastroenterol 1994;86:852

11. Tobin MV, Fisken RA, Diggory RT, Morris AI, Gilmore IT. Orocecal transit time in health and disease. Gut 1989;30:26

12. Khoja SM, Kellett GL. Effects of hypothyroidism on glucose transport and metabolism in rat small intestine. Bioch Biophys Acta 1993;1179:76

13. Lekkerkerker JF, Van Woudenberg F, Beekhuis H, Doorenbos H. Enhancement of calcium absorption in hypothyroidism. Isr J Med Sci 1971;7:399

14. Maclean D, Murison J, Griffiths PD. Acute pancreatitis and diabetic ketoacidosis in accidental hypothermia and hypothermic myxoedema. Br Med J 1973;4:757

15. Molinero P, Calvo JR, Jimenez J, Goberna R, Guerrero JM. Decreased binding of vasoactive intestinal peptide to intestinal epithelial cells from hypothyroid rats. Biochem Biophys Res Commun 1989;162:701

16. Shakir KM, Michaels RD, Hays JH, Potter BB. The use of bile acid sequestrants to lower serum thyroid hormones in iactrogenic hyperthyroidism. Ann Intern Med 1993;118:112

17. Sherman SI, Tielens ET, Ladenson RW. Sucralfate causes malabsorption of L-thyroxine. Am J Med 1994;96:531

18. Miller JL, Gorman CA, Go VLM. Thyroid-gut interrelationships. Gastroenterol 1978;75:901

19. Hays MT. Thyroid hormone and the gut. Endocr Res 1988;14:203

20. Distefano III JJ, De Luze A, Nguyen TT. Binding and degradation of 3,5,3'-triiodothyronine and thyroxine by rat intestinal bacteria. Am J Physiol 1993;264:E966

21. Distefano JJ III, Morris WL, Nguyen TT, Van Herle AJ, Florrsheim W. Enterohepatic regulation and metabolism of 3,5,3'-triiodothyronine in hypothyroid rats. Endocrinology 1993;132:1665

22. Vanderschuren-Lodeweyckx M, Eggermont E, Cornette C, Beckers C, Malvaux P, Eeckels R. Decreased serum thyroid hormone levels and increased TSH response to TRH in infants with coeliac disease. Clin Endocrinol 1977;6:361

23. Janerot G, Kagedal B, Von Schenk H, Truelove SC. The thyroid in ulcerative colitis and Crohn's disease. Acta Med Scand 1976;199:229

24. Counsell CE, Taha A, Rudell WJJ. Coeliac disease and autoimmune thyroid disease. Gut 1994;35:844

25. Azisi F, Belur R, Albano J. Malabsorption of thyroid hormones after jejunoileal bypass for obesity. Ann Intern Med 1979;90:941

26. Topliss DJ, Wright JA, Volpe R. Increased requirements for thyroid hormone after a jejuno-ileal bypass operation. Can Med Assoc J 1978;123:765

27. Edelman IS, Ismail-Beigi F. Thyroid thermogenesis and active sodium transport. Rec Prog Horm Res 1974;30:235

28. Giannella RA, Orlowski J, Jump ML, Lingrel JB. Na$^+$,-K$^+$-ATPase gene expression in rat intestine Caco-2 cells: response to thyroid hormone. Am J Physiol 1993;265:G775

29. Layden TJ, Boyer JL. Effect of thyroid hormone on bile-salt-independent bile flow and Na$^+$,-K$^+$-ATPase activity in liver plasma membrane enriched bile canaliculi. J Clin Invest 1976;57:1009

30. Levin RJ, Syme G. Differential changes in the "apparent Km" and maximum potential differences of the hexose and amino acid electrogenic transfer mechanisms of the small intestine, induced by fasting and hypothyroidism. J Physiol 1971;213:46

31. Syme G, Levin RJ. The effects of hypothyroidism and fasting on electrogenic amino acid transfer. Biochim Biophys Acta 1977;464:620

32. Brasitus TA, Dudeja PH. Effect of hypothyroidism on the lipid composition and fluidity of rat colonic apical membranes. Biochim Biophys Acta 1988;939:189

33. Edmonds CJ, Thompson BD. Interrelationship of the effects of aldosterone and thyroid hormones on sodium transport and electrical properties of rat colon. J Endocrinol 1970;48:189

34. Edmonds CJ, Willis CJ. Aldosterone and thyroid hormone interaction on the sodium and potassium transport pathways of rat colonic epithelium. J Endocrinol 1990;124:47

35. Galton VA, McCarthy PT, St. Germain DL. The ontogeny of iodothyronine deiodinase systems in liver and intestine of the rat. Endocrinology 1991;128:1717

36. Henning JJ. Permissive role of thyroxine in the ontogeny of jejunal sucrase. Endocrinol 1978:102:9

37. Hodin RA, Meng S, Chamberlain SM. Thyroid hormone responsiveness is developmentally regulated in the rat small intestine: a possible role for the α-2 receptor variant. Endocrinology 1994;135:564

38. Blanes A, Martinez A, Bujan J, Junquera SRC, Carballido SM. Intestinal mucosal changes following induced hypothryroidism in the developing rat. Virchows Arch (A) 1977;375:233

39. Shi YN, Hayes WP. Thyroid hormone-dependent regulation of the intestinal fatty acid-binding protein gene during amphibian metamorphosis. Dev Biol 1994;161:48

40. Zheng B, Eng J, Yalow RS. Cholecystokinin and vasoactive intestinal peptide in brain and gut of the hypothyroid neonatal rat. Horm Metab Res 1989;21:127

41. Hodin RA, Chamberlain SM, Uptan MP. Thyroid hormone differentially regulates rat intestinal brush border enzyme gene expression. Gastroenterol 1992;103:1529

42. Liu T, Reisenaner AM, Castillo RO. Ontogeny of intestinal lactose: post translational regulation by thyroxine. Am J Physiol 1992;263:G538

43. Brewer LM, Betz TW. Thyroxine and duodenal development in chicken embryos. Can J Zool 1979;57:416

44. Henning SJ. Rubin DC, Shulman RJ: Ontogeny of the intestinal mucosa. In: Johnson LR, ed. Physiology of the gastrointestinal tract. New York: Raven Press, 1994:586

45. Mood F. Endocrine influences on the functional differentiation of the small intestine. J Animal Sci 1979;49:239

46. Black BL. Morphological development of the epithelium of the embryonic chick intestine in culture: influence of thyroxine and hydrocortisone. Am J Anat 1978;151:573

47. Kowalewski K, Pachkowski T, Secord DC. Gastric mucinous secretion under various conditions of stimulation in hypothyroid dogs. Pharmacology 1977;15:348

48. Goglia F, Liverini G, Lanni A, Barletta A. Mitochondrial DNA, RNA and protein synthesis in normal, hypothyroid and mildly hyperthyroid rat liver during cold exposure. Mol Cell Endocrinol 1988;55:141

49. Lippolis R, Altamura N, Landriscina C. Ketone-body metabolism in hyperthyroid rats: reduced activity of D-3-hydroxybutyrate dehydrogenase in both liver and heart and of succinyl-coenzyme A: 3-oxacid coenzyme A-transferase in heart. Arch Biochem Biophys 1988;260:94

50. Irvine WJ. The association of atrophic gastritis with autoimmune thyroid disease. J Clin Endocrinol Metab 1975;4:351

51. Markson JL, Moore JM. Thyroid auto-antibodies in pernicious anemia. Br Med J 1962;2:1352

52. Muller MK, Pederson R, Olbricht T, Goebell H. Increased release of gastrin in hyperthyroid rats in vitro. Horm Metab Res 1986;18:675

53. Noll B, Goke B, Printz H, Gerberding J, Keim V, Arnold R. Influence of experimental hyperthyroidism on the adult rat pancreas, small intestine, and blood gastrin levels. Z Gastroenterol 1988;26:331

54. Seino Y, Matsukura S, Inoue Y, Kadowaki S, Mori K, Imura H. Hypogastrinemia in hypothyroidism. Digest Dis 1978;23;189

55. Doniach D, Roitt IM, Walkers JG, Sherlock S. Tissue antibodies in primary biliary cirrhosis, active chronic hepatitis, cryptogenic cirrhosis. Clin Exp Immunol 1966;237:262

56. Tran A, Quaranta HF, Benzaken S, et al. High prevalence of thyroid autoantibodies in a prospective series of patients with chronic hepatitis C before interferon therapy. Hepatology 1993;18:253

57. Crowe JP, Christensen E, Butler J, Et al. Primary biliary cirrhosis: prevalence of hypothyroidism and its relationship to thyroid antibodies. Gastroenterology 1980;78:1437

58. Culp KS, Fleming CR, Duffy J, Baldus WP, Dickson ER. Autoimmune association in primary biliary cirrhosis. Mayo Clin Proc 1982;57:365

59. Paradies G, Ruggiero FM, Dinoi P. The Influence of hypothyroidism on the transport of phosphate and on the lipid composition in rat-liver mitochondria. Bioch Biophys Acta 1991;1070:180

60. Sobol S. Long-term and short-term changes in mitochondrial parameters by thyroid hormones. Biochem Soc Trans 1993;21:799

61. Liverini G, Iossa S, Barletta A. Relationship between resting metabolism and hepatic metabolism: Effect of hypothyroidism and 24 hour fasting. Horm Res 1992;38:154

62. Baker A, Kaplan M, Wolfe H. Central congestive fibrosis of the liver in myxedema ascites. Ann Intern Med 1972;77:927

63. Clancy RL, MacKay IR. Myxoedematous ascites. Med J Aust 1979;ii:415

64. Comte B, Vidal H, Laville M, Riou J-P. Influence of thyroid hormones on gluconeogenesis from glycerol in rat hepatocytes: a dose-response study. Metabolism 1990:39:259

65. Marchesini G, Fabbri A, Bianchi GP, et al. Hepatic conversion of amino nitrogen to urea nitrogen in hypothyroid patients and upon L-thyroxine therapy. Metabolism 1993:42:1263

66. Van Steenbergen W, Fevery J, DeVos R, Leyten R, Heirwegh KPM, DeGroot J. Thyroid hormones and the hepatic handling of bilirubin. Hepatology 1989;9:314

67. Balasubramaniam S, Mitropoulous KA, Myant NB. Hormonal control of the activities of cholesterol-7 a-hydroxylase and hydroxy methylglutaryl-CoA reductase in rats. In: Matern S, Hachenschmidt J, Back P, Gerok W, Eds. Advances in bile acid research. Stuttgart: Schattauer Verlag, 1975:61

68. Caro JF, Cecchin F, Folli F, Marchini C, Sinha MK. Effect of T_3 on insulin action, insulin binding, and insulin receptor kinase activity in primary cultures of rat hepatocytes. Horm Metab Res 1988;20:327

69. Dang AQ, Fass FH, Carter WJ. Effects of experimental hypo- and hyperthyroidism on hepatic long-chain fatty Acyl-CoA synthetase and hydrolase. Metabol Res 1989;21:359

70. Davidson NO, Carlos RC, Drewek MJ, Parmer TG. Apolipoprotein gene expression in the rat is regulated in a tissue-specific manner by thyroid hormone. J Lipid Res 1988;29:1511

71. Hoogenbrugge v.d. Linden H, Jansen H, Hulsmann WC, Birkenhager C. Relationship between insulin-like growth factor-I and low density lipoprotein cholesterol levels in primary hypothyroidism in women. J Endocrinol 1989;123:341

72. Lin-Lee YC, Strobl W, Soyal S, et al. Role of thyroid hormone in the expression of apolipoprotein A-IV and C-III genes in rat liver. J Lipid Res 1993;34:249

73. Staels B, Tol AV, Chan L, Wil H, Verhoeven G, Auwerx J. Alterations in thyroid status modulate apolipoprotein, hepatic tryglyceride lipase, and low density lipoprotein receptor in rats. Endocrinology 1990:127:1144

74. Strobl W, Gorder NL, Lin-Lee YC, Gotto AM, Patsch W. Role of thyroid hormones in apolipoprotein A-I gene expression in rat liver. J Clin Invest 1990;85:659

75. Gebhart RL, Stone BG, Andreini JP, Duane WC, Evans CD, Prigge W. Thyroid hormone differentially augments biliary sterol secretion in the rat. I. The isolated-perfused liver model. J Lipid Res 1992;33:1459

76. Goldfarb S. Regulation of hepatic cholesterogenesis. In: Javitt NB, ed. Liver and biliary tract. Physiology I. Baltimore: University Park Press, 1980

Werner and Ingbar's The Thyroid, Seventh Edition,
edited by Lewis E. Braverman and Robert D. Utiger.
Lippincott–Raven Publishers, Philadelphia, © 1996

66

The Blood in Hypothyroidism

Jack E. Ansell

Hematologic changes, especially anemia, are common and well characterized in hypothyroidism. Reports date back to the late 1800s when first Charcot and then Kocher recognized the occurrence of anemia in cretins or in patients after thyroidectomy.[1] As in thyrotoxicosis, the major hematologic changes occur in red blood cells, with clinically insignificant alterations in leukocyte and platelet counts and only minor changes in coagulation proteins or platelet function. This chapter highlights the physiologic changes of the formed elements of the blood that result from a deficiency of thyroid hormone and then places these findings in a clinical context (Table 66-1). For additional insight into the effect of thyroid hormone on the blood, see chapter 42.

PHYSIOLOGIC EFFECTS OF DEFICIENT THYROID HORMONE

Erythrocytes

Many of the erythropoietic effects in hypothyroidism mirror those alterations seen in thyrotoxicosis, but in the opposite direction. Erythropoiesis is diminished, as reflected by a reduction in total blood volume,[2] red blood cell mass,[3,4] ^{59}Fe turnover and clearance,[3,5–7] ^{3}H-thymidine-labeling index,[7] and serum erythropoietin[3,7] and by hypocellularity of bone marrow tissue.[7,8] As discussed in chapter 42, the thyroid hormone stimulatory effect on erythropoiesis is mediated in part by erythropoietin, the concentration of which increases in response to greater oxygen requirements and relative degrees of tissue hypoxia[3,4,8,8a] and by a direct effect of thyroid hormone on erythroid precursors.[9–17] When thyroid hormone is deficient, erythropoiesis diminishes and often leads to a simple, mild anemia that can be thought of as a normal physiologic response.[18]

2,3-Diphosphoglycerate (2,3-DPG), the molecule that regulates the affinity of hemoglobin for O_2, was originally thought to be reduced in hypothyroidism;[19] Zaroulis and coworkers,[20] however, reported no differences in 2,3-DPG levels in hypothyroid patients compared with normal subjects.

Glucose-6-phosphate dehydrogenase (G-6-PD) activity is elevated in some thyrotoxic subjects, accompanying a reduction in red blood cell osmotic fragility.[21] In hypothyroidism, however, G-6-PD activity is only mildly reduced and still within the normal range.[22] Osmotic fragility is presumably normal.

Although thyrotoxicosis is associated with a shortened red blood cell survival,[3,23] red blood cells seem to survive normally in hypothyroidism.[3,6,23]

Once again, in contradistinction to thyrotoxicosis, hemoglobin A_2 levels appear to be minimally reduced compared with normal subjects,[24] presumably because of an absolute decrease in hemoglobin δ-chain synthesis. The explanation for this remains unclear.

Leukocytes

Alterations in lymphocyte or granulocyte counts are even less common in hypothyroidism than in thyrotoxicosis. Reports are contradictory on the relative numbers of T- and B-lymphocytes in Hashimoto's thyroiditis,[25–27] and in general, any alterations seem mild at best. Reports have been made of increased natural killer cell activity early in the course of Hashimoto's thyroiditis.[25] A significant reduction in leukocyte counts should alert the physician to the possibility of an associated problem, such as vitamin B_{12} or folic acid deficiency. Reports of disturbances in basophil counts in the old literature have not held up, based on more recent evaluation of basophil numbers in hypothyroid states.[28]

Hemostasis

Thrombocytopenia is a well-characterized phenomenon in thyrotoxicosis and is usually due to immune destruction of platelets.[29] Hypothyroid states, however, are associated with few quantitative changes in platelet counts,[30] although an in-

TABLE 66-1.
Clinical Hematologic Features of Thyroid Hormone Deficiency

Blood Cell	Clinical Effect	Comment
Red blood cell	Anemia	Common in hypothyroidism. Often a physiologic response to a decrease in oxygen requirement resulting in a decrease in erythropoietin and a decrease in erythropoiesis. Bone marrow shows erythroid hypoplasia. Anemia also may be due to deficiency of specific nutrients
	Microcytic anemia	Seen in up to 15% of cases. Most likely due to iron deficiency
	Normocytic anemia	Typical morphology in the physiologic anemia of hypothyroidism
	Macrocytic anemia	The most common morphologic abnormality. May be seen with the physiologic anemia of hypothyroidism but also may reflect a deficiency of vitamin B_{12} or folic acid
White blood cell	No important effect	If leukopenia occurs, consider other causes such as vitamin B_{12} or folic acid deficiency
Platelets	Occasional mild bleeding	Platelet counts are usually normal, but qualitative defects in platelet function may occur and predispose to bleeding. Coagulation factor deficiencies of questionable importance

crease in platelet count associated with a reduction in mean platelet volume[31] has been reported, as well as with an increase in mean platelet volume.[32] Qualitative changes in platelet function are more likely to be encountered. Thus, investigators have noted patients with prolonged bleeding times[33,34] or excessive elevations in the bleeding time in response to aspirin challenge.[35] Decreased platelet adhesiveness[33] and a syndrome of easy bruising[36] associated with increased platelet-associated immunoglobulin have also been described. Factor VIII coagulant activity may be depressed,[33,34,37,38] and this finding, often associated with a prolonged bleeding time or partial thromboplastin time,[33,34,38] has raised the question of a von Willebrand's-like defect. Palareti and coworkers[39] have implicated impaired platelet aggregation to epinephrine, collagen, and ristocetin due to reduced levels of factor VIII and von Willebrand's factor found in patients post-thyroidectomy who were taken off thyroid replacement therapy. Most of these abnormalities tend to revert to normal after thyroid hormone replacement therapy.

Investigators have noted a depression of other factors (VII, IX, XI) in hypothyroidism[33,38,40]; clearance rates of factors II, VII, IX, and X from plasma are also reduced.[40,41] The reduced factor levels have been attributed to a generalized decrease in protein synthesis.[38] Increased fibrinolytic activity, as determined by increased plasminogen[42] or shortened euglobulin lysis time,[43] has also been noted.

CLINICAL CORRELATES AND ASSOCIATED HEMATOLOGIC ABNORMALITIES

Red Blood Cells

In contrast to thyrotoxicosis, anemia is a frequent concomitant of hypothyroidism, occurring in perhaps one-third of patients, although higher frequencies have been reported.[18,44,45,46] Children may be more likely to develop anemia.[47] About one-quarter of such patients have a decrease in red blood cell mass,

presumably due to a decrease in O_2 requirements, and eventually to a reduction in erythropoietin. Because of a simultaneous fall in plasma volume, this physiologic anemia is less noticeable than it would be otherwise.[2,4,18,46] The red blood cells are usually normocytic, normochromic, or occasionally macrocytic. Other red blood cell shape abnormalities, such as burr cells, have also been described.[48] The bone marrow generally shows mild hypoplasia of all elements,[7,8] especially of erythroid precursors,[44] with an increase in fatty marrow. This anemia is slowly correctable by thyroid hormone replacement therapy and usually does not call for any other specific intervention or therapy.

Microcytic hypochromic anemias can be seen in 2% to 15% of hypothyroid subjects.[45,46] Iron deficiency may be responsible for this anemia in some but not all cases.[45,46] Patients with hypothyroidism may be at greater risk for iron deficiency because of reduced iron absorption or increased blood loss.[18] Iron parameters suggestive of iron deficiency, however, may reflect changes in iron turnover due to diminished erythropoiesis as demonstrated experimentally in hypothyroid rats by Seven et al.[49] Iron requires an acid gastric environment for normal absorption. Since reduced acid secretion (hypochlorhydria or achlorhydria) occurs in as many as half of patients with hypothyroidism,[50] such patients may be at greater risk of iron malabsorption. Hypothyroidism is also associated with menorrhagia, providing another potential for reduced iron stores and iron deficiency in women. The coagulation or platelet dysfunction occasionally seen in hypothyroidism provides a final mechanism for the development of iron deficiency by means of a greater likelihood of blood loss.

Iron deficiency in hypothyroidism responds to oral iron therapy as it does in other conditions, even without thyroid hormone replacement therapy.[46] As in any patient, however, the presence of iron deficiency should trigger a search for a source of blood loss, since that is often the most likely cause. If the underlying condition is not resolved, then iron deficiency is likely to recur once therapy is discontinued. A recent study cautions against the simultaneous ingestion of ferrous sulfate and thyroxine medication, which can lead to poor absorption of thyroxine, possibly by precipitation of the hormone when in contact with ferrous sulfate.[51]

Macrocytosis is probably the most common morphologic red cell abnormality associated with hypothyroidism, occurring in 38% of subjects in one series.[45] It may be secondary to vitamin B_{12} or folic acid deficiency, or it may have no apparent cause. The latter case usually represents the simple anemia of hypothyroidism, reversible by thyroid hormone replacement therapy.[18] Abnormalities in lipid metabolism with excess red blood cell membrane cholesterol and phospholipid may be responsible for the macrocytosis[18] in this condition.

Hypothyroidism is often an autoimmune disease, and it is not surprising that a strong association exists with pernicious anemia, another autoimmune illness. As discussed in chapter 42, thyroid and gastric tissue share a common embryonic origin; the latter tissue is the source of intrinsic factor secretion necessary for vitamin B_{12} absorption. Antibodies to one tissue or the other are often present when either is diseased.[52] Gastric tissue antibodies occur in 27% of patients with hypothyroidism[53] and in 20% of their relatives.[52] Similarly, patients with pernicious anemia and their relatives have a high frequency of thyroid antibodies.[52] Intrinsic factor antibodies are also present in hypothyroidism, but to a lesser degree (3 of 47 patients, or 6% in one study).[54] As previously mentioned, achlorhydria is a common finding in hypothyroid patients,[50] and various degrees of atrophic gastritis are often present.[55]

Pernicious anemia and hypothyroidism share a high concordance rate. Tudhope and Wilson[46,50] noted that 7% to 12% of patients with hypothyroidism also have pernicious anemia and that an additional 10% have latent pernicious anemia.[50] Carmel and Spencer[56] found that 11.7% of subjects with pernicious anemia were overtly hypothyroid (another 8.6% were thyrotoxic); this association increased to 14.7% when thyroid-stimulating hormone levels were used as the diagnostic test. Thus, pernicious anemia may present years before overt thyroid disease.[57]

Folate deficiency has been reported in patients with hypothyroidism,[58] perhaps because of malabsorption or anorexia, but other studies have reported no difference in folate levels in newly diagnosed hypothyroid or thyrotoxic patients.[59]

The evaluation of patients with vitamin B_{12} or folic acid deficiency in the presence of hypothyroidism is no different than if thyroid disease were not present. The cause of malabsorption of vitamin or of dietary inadequacy in the case of folic acid must be sought through appropriate history-taking and diagnostic tests. In either vitamin B_{12} or folic acid deficiency, the thyroid disease should be corrected, since folic acid and thyroid hormone enhances vitamin B_{12} absorption.[60] Thus, in hypothyroidism and associated pernicious anemia, neither thyroid hormone nor vitamin B_{12} alone corrects the anemia.[44] One might also be alert to the presence of other endocrine or inflammatory disorders that might be present in the setting of pernicious anemia and hypothyroidism.[61]

Leukocytes

Hypothyroidism alone does not produce any clinically significant alterations in white blood cells. Response to infection appears normal in both qualitative and quantitative respects.

Associated problems, however, such as folic acid or vitamin B_{12} deficiency, may lead to a reduction in leukocytes; therefore, such problems should be considered if leukopenia is observed. As in thyrotoxicosis, reports of myeloid neoplasia have been described in association with hypothyroidism, but this relationship may be coincidental.[62]

Hemostasis

As already discussed, quantitative changes in platelet count are unusual in hypothyroidism, although one recent report found a reduction in mean platelet volume and an elevated count in 12 hypothyroid subjects (post-thyroidectomy).[31] More significant alterations seem to affect platelet function. A number of investigators have reported the presence of clinical bleeding attributable to qualitative platelet disorders in hypothyroidism.[33–36] A specific abnormality, however, has not been identified, although Hymes and coworkers[36] found elevated levels of platelet-associated immunoglobulin in most patients with bruising. They suggested that a qualitative platelet defect might be caused by that immunoglobulin.

Fibrinolytic activity seems to be increased in hypothyroidism as determined by increased plasminogen, decreased plasminogen-activator inhibitor,[42,43] and a shortened euglobulin lysis assay.[43] However, this finding and the mild reduction in certain coagulation factors seem to have little clinical relevance. The possibility of a hypercoagulable state in hypothyroidism has even been raised by Marongiu and colleagues,[63] based on findings of an increase in prothrombin activation vis à vis plasminogen activation. However, the clinical significance of this remains unknown.

SUMMARY

Hypothyroidism is frequently associated with anemia, but few changes in the other cellular elements of the blood occur. Erythropoiesis is diminished in the presence of reduced thyroid hormone owing to a slowing of the metabolic rate, a decrease in oxygen requirement, and a drop in erythropoietin levels. Other changes in red blood cell metabolism are of questionable significance. A reduction in thyroid hormone has little impact on leukocyte or platelet counts, but a mild defect in platelet function may occur, possibly related to increased immunoglobulin deposited on the platelet membrane.

Anemia may be present in 30% to 40% of patients with hypothyroidism. In many instances, this anemia is due to a physiologic reduction in erythropoiesis that returns to normal with treatment of the thyroid disease. The red blood cells are often normocytic or macrocytic in appearance. Microcytic, hypochromic anemias do occur in some patients and are probably related to iron deficiency that can occur from excessive blood loss as well as decreased iron absorption.

Macrocytosis is the most common red cell morphologic abnormality encountered. Associated vitamin B_{12} or folic acid deficiencies are important causes in addition to the physiologic anemia discussed earlier. Patients with hypothyroidism secondary to autoimmune thyroid disease have a high incidence of pernicious anemia and an even higher frequency of gastric acid secretory dysfunction and parietal cell or intrinsic factor antibodies.

Neither leukocyte nor platelet counts are altered to a significant degree, but a hemorrhagic tendency has been attributed to a qualitative defect in platelet function that is reversible with correction of the thyroid disease in some patients.

References

1. Erslev AJ. Anemia of endocrine disorders. In: Williams WJ, Beutler E, Erslev AJ, Lichtman MA, eds. Hematology. 4th ed. New York: McGraw-Hill, 1990
2. Gibson JG, Harris AW. Clinical studies of the blood volume. V. Hyperthyroidism and myxedema. J Clin Invest 1939;18:59
3. Das KC, Mukherjee M, Sarkar TK, Dash RJ, Rastogi GK. Erythropoiesis and erythropoietin in hypo- and hyperthyroidism. J Clin Endocrinol Metab 1975;40:211
4. Muldowney FP, Crooks J, Wayne EJ. The total red cell mass in thyrotoxicosis and myxedema. Clin Sci 1957;16:309
5. Donati RM, Fletcher JW, Warnecke MA, Gallagher NI. Erythropoiesis in hypothyroidism. Proc Soc Exp Biol Med 1973;144:78
6. Kiely JM, Purnell DC, Owen CA. Erythrokinetics in myxedema. Ann Intern Med 1967;67:533
7. Nakao K, Maekawa T, Shirabura T, Yaginama M. Anemia due to hypothyroidism. Isr J Med Sci 1965;1:742
8. Axelrod AR, Berman L. The bone marrow in hyperthyroidism and hypothyroidism. Blood 1951;6:436
8a. Peschle C, Zanjani ED, Gidari AS, McLaurin WD, Gordon AS. Mechanism of thyroxin action on erythropoiesis. Endocrinology 1971;89:609
9. Boussios T, McIntyre WR, Gordon AS, Bertles JF. Receptors specific for thyroid hormones in nuclei of mammalian erythroid cells: involvement in erythroid cell proliferation. Br J Haematol 1982;51:99
10. Brenner B, Fandrey J, Jelkmann W. Serum immunoreactive erythropoietin in hyper- and hypothyroidism: Clinical observations related to cell culture studies. Eur J Haematol 1994;53:6
11. Dainiak N, Hoffman R, Maffei LA, Forget BG. Potentiation of human erythropoiesis in vitro by thyroid hormone. Nature 1978;272:260
12. Donati RM, Warnecke MA, Gallagher NI. Effect of triiodothyronine administration on erythrocyte radioiron incorporation in rats. Proc Soc Exp Biol Med 1964;115:405
13. Fandrey J, Pagel H, Frede S, Wolff M, Jelkmann W. Thyroid hormones enhance hypoxia-induced erythropoietin production in vitro. Exp Hematol 1994;22:272
14. Golde DW, Beroch N, Chopra IJ, Cline MJ. Thyroid hormones stimulate erythropoiesis in vitro. Br J Haematol 1977;37:173
15. Meineke HA, Crafts RC. Evidence for noncalorigenic effect of thyroxin on erythropoiesis as judged by radioiron utilization. Proc Soc Exp Biol Med 1964;117:520
16. Popovic WJ, Brown JE, Adamson JW. The influence of thyroid hormones on in vitro erythropoiesis. J Clin Invest 1977;60:907
17. Shirakura T, Azuma M, Malkawa T. A study on the erythropoiesis stimulating effect of the thyroid hormone. Blut 1970;21:240
18. Green ST, Ng JP. Hypothyroidism and anemia. Biomed Pharmacother 1986;40:326
19. Grosz HJ, Farmer BB. Reduction-oxidation potential of blood determined by oxygen releasing factor in thyroid disorders. Nature 1969;222:875
20. Zaroulis CG, Kourides IA, Valeri CR. Red cell 2,3-diphosphoglycerate and oxygen affinity of hemoglobin in patients with thyroid disorders. Blood 1978;52:181
21. Baikie AG, Lawson N. Glucose-6-phosphate dehydrogenase activity and an osmotic abnormality of erythrocytes in thyrotoxicosis. Lancet 1965;1:86
22. Viherkoski M, Lamberg BA. The glucose-6-phosphate dehydrogenase activity of the red blood cells in hyperthyroidism and hypothyroidism. Scand J Clin Lab Invest 1970;25:137
23. McClellan JE, Donegan C, Thorup OA, Leavell BS. Survival time of the erythrocyte in myxedema and hyperthyroidism. J Lab Clin Med 1958;51:91
24. Kuhn JM, Rieu M, Rochette J, et al. Influence of thyroid status on hemoglobin A$_2$ expression. J Clin Endocrinol Metab 1983;57:344
25. Calder EA, Irvine WJ, Davidson McD, Wu F. T, B and K cells in autoimmune thyroid disease. Clin Exp Immunol 1976;25:17
26. Farid NR, Munro RE, Row VV, Volpe R. Peripheral thymus dependent (T) lymphocytes in Graves' disease and Hashimoto's thyroiditis. N Engl J Med 1973;228:1313
27. Urbaniak SJ, Penhale WJ, Irvine WJ. Peripheral blood T and B lymphocytes in patients with thyrotoxicosis and Hashimoto's thyroiditis and in normal subjects. Clin Exp Immunol 1974;18:449
28. Petrasch SG, Mlynek-Kersjes ML, Haase R, et al. Basophilic leukocytes in hypothyroidism. Clin Investig 1993;71:27
29. Herman J, Resnitzky P, Fink A. Association between thyrotoxicosis and thrombocytopenia. Isr J Med Sci 1978;14:469
30. Endo Y. Relationship between thyroid function and platelet counts. Acta Haematol 1985;74:58
31. van Doormaal JJ, van der Meer J, Oosten HR, Halie MR, Doorenbos H. Hypothyroidism leads to more small-sized platelets in circulation. Thromb Haemost 1987;58:964
32. Marongiu F, Conti M, Murtas ML, Mameli G, Sorano FF, Martino E. What causes the increase in platelet mean volume in thyroid pathological conditions? Thromb Haemost 1990;63:323
33. Edson JR, Fecher DR, Doe RP. Low platelet adhesiveness and other hemostatic abnormalities in hypothyroidism. Ann Intern Med 1975;82:342
34. Egeberg O. Influence of thyroid function on the blood clotting system. Scand J Clin Lab Invest 1963;15:1
35. Zeigler ZR, Hasiba U, Lewis JH, Vagnucci AH, West VA, Bezek EA. Hemostatic defects in response to aspirin challenge in hypothyroidism. Am J Hematol 1986;23:391
36. Hymes K, Blum M, Lackner H, Karpatkin S. Easy bruising, thrombocytopenia, and elevated platelet immunoglobulin G in Graves' disease and Hashimoto's thyroiditis. Ann Intern Med 1981;94:27
37. Farid NR, Griffiths BL, Collins JR, Marshall WH, Ingram DW. Blood coagulation and fibrinolysis in thyroid disease. Thromb Haemost 1976;35:415
38. Simone JV, Abilgaard CF, Schulman I. Blood coagulation in thyroid dysfunction. N Engl J Med 1965;273:1057
39. Palareti G, Biagi G, Legnani C, et al. Association of reduced factor VIII with impaired platelet reactivity to adrenalin and collagen after total thyroidectomy. Thromb Haemost 1989;62:1053
40. van Oesterom AT, Kerkhoven P, Veltkamp JJ. Metabolism of the coagulation factors of the prothrombin complex in hypothyroidism in man. Thromb Haemost 1979;41:273
41. Loeliger EA, van der Esch B, Mattern MJ, Hemker HC. The biological disappearance rate of prothrombin, factor VII, IX, X from plasma in hypothyroidism, hyperthyroidism, and during fever. Thromb Diath Hemorrh 1964;10:267
42. Bennett NB, Ogston CM, McAndrew GM. The thyroid and fibrinolysis. Br Med J 1967;4:147
43. Rennie JAN, Bewsher PD, Murchison LE, Ogston D. Coagulation and fibrinolysis in thyroid disease. Acta Haematol 1978;59:171
44. Fein HG, Rivlin RS. Anemia in thyroid diseases. Med Clin North Am 1975;59:1133

45. Horton L, Coburn RJ, England JM, Hinesworth RL. The hematology of hypothyroidism. Q J Med 1975;45:101

46. Tudhope GR, Wilson GM. Anemia in hypothyroidism. Q J Med 1960;29:513

47. Chu JY, Monteleone JA, Peden VH, Graviss ER, Vernava AM. Anemia in children and adolescents with hypothyroidism. Clin Pediatr 1981;20:696

48. Wardrop C, Hutchison HE. Red cell shape in hypothyroidism. Lancet 1969;1:1243

49. Seven A, Toktamis N, Hacibekiroglu M, et al. Fe parameters and erythrocytic parameters in experimental hypothyroidism. Biochem Soc Trans 1993;21:224S

50. Tudhope GR, Wilson GM. Deficiency of vitamin B_{12} in hypothyroidism. Lancet 1962;1:703

51. Campbell NRC, Hasinoff BB, Stalts H, Rao B, Wong NCW. Ferrous sulfate reduces thyroxine efficacy in patients with hypothyroidism. Ann Intern Med 1992;117:1010

52. Doniach D, Roitt IM, Taylor KB. Autoimmunity in pernicious anemia and thyroiditis: a family study. Ann NY Acad Sci 1965;124:605

53. Doniach D, Roitt IM, Taylor KB. Autoimmune phenomena in pernicious anemia. Br Med J 1963;1:1374

54. Ardeman S, Chanarin I, Krafchik B, Singer W. Addisonian pernicious anemia and intrinsic factor antibodies in thyroid disorders. Q J Med 1966;35:421

55. Bock OAA, Witts LL. Gastric acidity and gastric biopsy in thyrotoxicosis. Br Med J 1963;2:20

56. Carmel R, Spencer CA. Clinical and subclinical thyroid disorders associated with pernicious anemia. Arch Intern Med 1982; 142:1465

57. Forssell J, Halonen PI. Thyroid function and pernicious anemia. Acta Med Scand 1958;162:61

58. Hines JD, Halsted CH, Griggs RC, Harris JW. Megaloblastic anemia secondary to folate deficiency associated with hypothyroidism. Ann Intern Med 1968;68:792

59. Caplan RH, Dairs K, Bengston B, Smith MJ. Serum folate and vitamin B_{12} levels in hypothyroid and hyperthyroid patients. Arch Intern Med 1975;135:701

60. Okuda K, Chow BF. The thyroid and absorption of vitamin B_{12} in rats. Endocrinology 1961;68:607

61. Govindarajan R, Galpin OP. Coexistence of Addison's disease, ulcerative colitis, hypothyroidism and pernicious anemia. J Clin Gastroenterol 1992;15:82

62. Boonen AL, Lefebvre Ch. Lambert M, Ferrant A, Michaux JL, Coche E. Hypothyroidism associated with myeloid neoplasia: About 2 cases. Acta Clin Belg 1992;47:397

63. Marongiu F, Biondi F, Conti M, et al. Is a hypercoagulable state present in hypothyroidism? Thromb Haemost 1992; 67:729

Werner and Ingbar's The Thyroid, Seventh Edition,
edited by Lewis E. Braverman and Robert D. Utiger.
Lippincott–Raven Publishers, Philadelphia, © 1996

67

The Neuromuscular System and Brain in Hypothyroidism

G. Robert DeLong

This chapter discusses the clinical effects of deprivation of thyroid hormone. Some of these effects are the opposite of those induced by thyrotoxicosis (see chap 43); others involve changes that are unique to hypothyroidism.

MYOPATHIC DISORDERS

Clinical Observations

In patients with hypothyroidism, disordered muscle function often is the predominating feature of the clinical syndrome. Muscular abnormality with long-standing hypothyroidism in adults is known as Hoffman's syndrome,[1] and when it is associated with hypothyroidism in childhood, it is known as Kocher-Debré-Sémélaigne syndrome,[2] in acknowledgment of the early and complete descriptions by these physicians. The most severe involvement has been observed in childhood, but hypothyroidism at all ages may be associated with this disorder of musculature.

Increased volume of muscle and slowness of contraction constitute the muscular syndrome. The typical patient presents with firm, large, well-developed muscles, like those of an athlete. The entire musculature is affected to some extent, but the most obvious enlargement is in the tongue, arms, and legs. Entrapment syndromes may ensue.[3] In one woman, the biceps had become so thick that she could no longer touch her fingertips to her shoulders, and the increase in size of thenar and hypothenar muscles prevented apposition of thumb and little finger. The patient appeared muscle-bound. In women, the enlargement imparts a masculine appearance, although secondary sexual characteristics are not altered; in the infant, it suggests precocious physical development.

A sense of stiffness and even slight discomfort in the large muscles are frequent complaints, and movement may even be mildly painful. These are probably expressions of the basic slowness of contraction. Hoffman's[1] original patient had difficulty opening the mouth after biting; another patient, a 3-year-old boy, had difficulty releasing the hand grip. A relative deficiency in muscle α-glucosidase (acid maltase) has been suggested as a basis for the muscle cramps and aching in hypothyroidism.[4] Acute exertional rhabdomyolysis was described in two adults with hypothyroidism; one had no rise in serum lactate after an ischemic exercise test. After thyroid replacement, his ischemic exercise test was normal.[4a]

Speech is often dysarthric. The gait may be clumsy and slow, particularly the first steps. This tardiness of movement is especially troublesome in cold weather. All voluntary movements are slowed, and the tendon reflexes are characteristically prolonged. A review of 20 patients with primary hypothyroidism found 70% of the patients had muscular weakness, which was severe in 40%, involving scapular and pelvic muscles, with no atrophy or hypertrophy. All cases with weakness showed electromyographic alterations. Histologic findings showed alterations of the fiber subtypes in 90% of cases; the type I fibers had sarcolemmal and mitochondrial accumulations in 85%, and 70% had areas without oxidative activity ("cores"). The authors found no correlation between the evolution time of hypothyroidism, thyroid hormone levels, creatine phosphokinase (CPK) increase, and muscular weakness.[5] After treatment, CPK and EMG changes improved within 1 to 8 weeks; histopathologic changes of muscle also improved but over a longer time course.[6]

Physiologic Studies

In 115 patients with hypothyroidism, the mean duration of ankle jerk, as measured by the half-relaxation time, was 0.53 seconds, whereas the mean of 280 normal subjects was 0.34 seconds. The interval between the tap on the tendon and the action potential that marks the beginning of the muscle contraction was between 0.03 and 0.04 seconds in thyrotoxic, hypothyroid, and normal subjects, showing that there is no change in transmission of the nervous impulse along nerves or through nerve-muscle synapses.

Because there is generally poor correlation between the duration of the ankle jerk and the patient's thyroid function, as determined biochemically, measurement of Achilles reflex time is of limited diagnostic value in thyroid diseases.[7]

In 16 of 20 consecutive patients with frank hypothyroidism, two or more of the following abnormalities were found on EMG: (1) polyphasic action potentials, (2) hyperirritability, (3) repetitive discharge after reflex motion, and (4) low-voltage, short-duration motor unit potentials.[8] The typical EMG of myotonia has not been recorded in patients with hypothyroidism. Quinine, which lessens myotonia, has only equivocal effect on the stiffness of hypothyroidism.

Biochemical Studies

Plasma skeletal creatine kinase activity markedly increased in hypothyroidism and correlates with its severity.[9] In a subgroup of hypothyroid patients with serous effusions, myopathy, and abnormal findings on muscle biopsies, the mean plasma creatine kinase activity was 1339 IU/L, compared with 679 IU/L for the entire hypothyroid group and 10 to 120 IU/L for normal subjects.[10] Serum cardiac muscle creatine kinase levels may also be elevated when measured by a sensitive assay and may remain elevated during the first few weeks of L-thyroxine therapy.[12] With treatment, these patients' creatine kinase levels rapidly became normal, although weakness was slow to disappear.[11]

Pathologic Studies

The histopathology of skeletal muscle in patients with hypothyroidism has been extensively described.[5,10,13,14] The explanation of the enlargement of muscle has eluded all clinical investigators.

A histochemical and ultrastructural study of skeletal muscle in a 3-year-old girl with the Kocher-Debré-Sémélaigne syndrome showed type I fiber atrophy, pronounced alterations in oxidative enzyme activity, abnormal collections of glycogen, peripheral crescents, and distention of the sarcoplasmic reticulum. After treatment with thyroid hormone, the child's skeletal muscle bulk decreased to normal size, and the skeletal muscle changes (none of which is specific for hypothyroidism) disappeared.[15] Muscle biopsy in a 72-year-old man with hypothyroidism accompanied by marked hypertrophy and stiffness of skeletal musculature disclosed histologic evidence of a vacuolar myopathy. With correction of the patient's hypothyroid state, his muscles reduced considerably, and their consistency became normal.[16]

The most common abnormality on light microscopy was type II fiber atrophy, found in 8 of 11 patients.[13] Others have found variable type I or type II atrophy or hypertrophy.[14,17] Moderate fiber atrophy, increased central nuclear counts and glycogen accumulation, central cores without oxidative activity in type I fibers, and occasional vacuolar changes have been seen by light microscopy in hypothyroid myopathy.[5,11,13] Ultrastructural alterations include focal myofibrillar disorganization, in some instances with nemaline rods; mitochondrial accumulations; and occasional basophilic degeneration.[18] The latter is deposits of polysaccharide material, seen in both cardiac and skeletal muscle in patients with severe hypothyroidism; their pathogenesis is unknown but may be related to impaired glycogenolysis in hypothyroidism.[18] Cretinous muscle shows no definite abnormalities.[19]

Clinical Diagnosis

The diagnosis of these syndromes in infants and young children can present some difficulty. Enlargement of muscles, slowness of movement, and retarded mental development are observed in both cretinism and in mentally defective children who exhibit spasticity or rigidity of the limbs as part of an extrapyramidal motor disturbance (de Lange's syndrome).

Dystonia in the early stages of extrapyramidal disease may also simulate the muscular picture of hypothyroidism. The typical biochemical features of hypothyroidism—elevated serum thyroid-stimulating hormone and low serum thyroxine (T_4)—should lead to the correct diagnosis in most patients. There may be some difficulty in distinguishing the muscular syndrome of hypothyroidism from the true muscular hypertrophy and the myotonia of myotonia congenita.

NEUROLOGIC DISORDERS

Peripheral Neuropathy

Mononeuropathies occur in hypothyroidism, as attested to by the high incidence of carpal tunnel syndrome (i.e., compression of the median nerve at the wrist).[20] Nocturnal paresthesia and pain in a median nerve distribution in one or both hands is the usual manifestation of this condition. Exceptionally, muscle weakness and atrophy and sensory loss are added; they become permanent if the carpal ligament is not incised. Thickening of connective tissue of tendon sheaths allegedly entraps the nerve. Facial weakness from involvement of the facial nerve in the tight fallopian canal of the temporal bone has also been listed as a rare hypothyroid symptom.[21] Slowed conduction velocities also have been demonstrated in the ulnar and posterior tibial nerves of children with untreated congenital hypothyroidism.[22]

As to more diffuse involvement of the peripheral nervous system, a recent study of 39 consecutive patients with primary hypothyroidism found subjective complaints of polyneuropathy (mainly paraesthesia) in 64%, objective findings of polyneuropathy in 33%, and a definite diagnosis by electrophysiologic criteria in 72%.[23] Sural nerve biopsies in cases of polyneuropathy have shown axonal degeneration.[24] Symptoms and neurophysiologic parameters uniformly improve after treatment with thyroid medication; in severe cases improvement in neuropathic symptoms may require 2 years, and in myopathy longer.[25]

Cerebellar Ataxia

Although reference to an unsteady gait may be found in the earliest medical discussions of adult hypothyroidism, Soederbergh, in 1910,[26] seems to have been the first to focus attention on it as a true cerebellar ataxia. Most of the published examples have concerned middle-aged or elderly people whose gait had become ataxic over months or years, sometimes to the point where they could not stand or walk without assistance. The difficulty in locomotion results in shuffling steps rather than reeling. Arm movements are disturbed to lesser degree, and all the limbs exhibit the phenomena of intention tremor, slowness in alternating movements, dysmetria, and general incoordination. The speech may be dysarthric.

The ataxia is not simply a reflection of psychomotor retardation and lethargy. Several of the patients have been mentally alert when the ataxia was prominent. Moreover, the signs are typical of cerebellar deficit. Treatment with T_4 has restored motor function to normal or nearly normal.

The importance in selecting the patient with hypothyroid disease from the larger group of patients with late-life cerebellar ataxia thus becomes obvious. Diagnosis proves to be not always easy, since a number of the patients do not appear mentally deteriorated, and the clinical and laboratory test results do not always provide a clear answer. Some patients did not appear to be myxedematous. It is of interest that relatively pure cerebellar ataxia has not been a feature of cretinism or childhood hypothyroidism.

The pathologic basis of the state remains uncertain. The reversibility of part of the cerebellar deficit with thyroid treatment would suggest a subcellular or molecular type of lesion. In a postmortem examination of a 57-year-old hypothyroid woman who had had a cerebellar ataxia mainly affecting the lower limbs, there was a cerebellar atrophy that was most marked in the anterosuperior vermis and atrophy of the ventral pons, transverse pontine fibers, and middle and superior cerebellar peduncles.[27] The topography of these cerebellar changes was remarkably similar to those shown to underlie the gait ataxia of alcoholic cerebellar degeneration.

Sleep Apnea

There is a high incidence of sleep apnea in patients with hypothyroidism.[28,29] Hypothyroid myopathy involving the upper airway[28] or respiratory muscles, including the diaphragm,[30] is a potential mechanism of sleep apnea in hypothyroidism. In a related study, chronic alveolar hypoventilation was documented in two of three patients with diaphragmatic dysfunction in hypothyroidism. Treatment with L-T_4 often improves sleep apnea in these hypothyroid patients.

Myxedematous Dementia

Myxedematous dementia involves a serious deterioration of cerebral function under conditions of extreme hypothy-

roidism. The clinical state, in bold outline, is essentially one of impairment of all sensory, psychic, and motor functions. The patient takes little notice of surroundings, and motor activity, as manifested in speech and movement, is reduced. All psychic activity is impoverished. Bizarre behavior and abnormal ideation (psychosis) may develop (see chap 74).

Probably of particular significance is extreme somnolence. The number of hours per day when the patient lies inert, either asleep or drowsy, is greatly increased. One of our patients slept 21 or 22 hours each day and had to be prodded even to eat. His state approached myxedematous coma, yet more detailed neurologic examination disclosed no other abnormality. The movements of such patients are usually well coordinated, and the plantar reflexes are of flexor type. The tendon reflexes are slowed in most cases. Often there is hypothermia.

The electroencephalogram, as a rule, substantiates the impairment of cerebral function. Most of these patients have an absence of alpha rhythm, with appearance of slow waves of a frequency of 3 to 6 per second.[31,32] These abnormalities are said to be more pronounced in children than in adults.

The pathologic basis of this condition is unknown. Since the dementia can be reversed by thyroid therapy, one would hardly expect visible abnormalities at a cellular level. Cerebral metabolism and blood flow are reduced in hypothyroidism,[33] but this does not reveal itself in ischemic cortical lesions.

Differential diagnosis may be difficult if the signs of hypothyroidism are absent. The neurologic picture, except possibly for the extreme somnolence, bears considerable resemblance to that of low-pressure hydrocephalus, chronic subdural hematoma, chronic bromidism, nutritional depletion syndrome (e.g., pellagra), and possibly Alzheimer's disease.

An important and complex relationship exists between hypothyroidism and psychiatric disorders, which is discussed further in chapter 74. In most, if not all, hypothyroid patients, the psychiatric symptoms of depression or psychosis will improve after treatment with T_4, unless endogenous psychiatric disease is present.[34,35]

Myxedema Coma

Severe myxedema may progress, perhaps precipitated by intercurrent illness, to extreme lethargy, unresponsiveness, hypothermia, and hypoventilation, described as *myxedema coma*. Treatment includes support of respiration and vital functions, T_4, and treatment of intercurrent illness (see chap 75).

Psychoeducational Consequences of Hypothyroidism

The question of psychologic and educational consequences to children as a result of juvenile hypothyroidism has received little attention heretofore, although clinicians have been aware of such problems. In a recent study, 23 children and adolescents with a new diagnosis of juvenile acquired hypothyroidism underwent a battery of psychoeducational tests before and after replacement therapy. Adverse behavioral reaction and learning problems were relatively rare in these children, although symptoms of juvenile acquired hypothyroidism were associated with increased distractibility, hyperactivity, and poorer achievement in about 25% of the children, who represented the most severe cases at diagnosis. Achievement improved after treatment, with the best psychologic outcome in those who achieved euthyroidism more slowly.[36]

CRETINISM

The similarities and differences between sporadic and endemic cretinism have been summarized by Stanbury and Hetzel[37] and elsewhere in this book (see chap 57 and the subchapter on congenital hypothyroidism in chap 85). Thus, the discussion that follows is limited to specific features of neurologic interest.

Thyroid hormone is a principal hormonal determinant of the normal growth and development of the human central nervous system. Lack of thyroid hormone during brain development causes cretinism in one of three forms. *Sporadic cretinism,* caused by defective thyroid gland function in the fetus and infant, is characterized by retardation of physical and mental development that is preventable by treatment with thyroid hormone starting in early infancy. *Endemic cretinism* is geographically associated with environmental iodine deficiency and endemic goiter, and is preventable by correction of iodine deficiency. It includes two reasonably distinct clinical entities: (1) neurologic cretinism, characterized by mental deficiency, deaf-mutism, and a spastic-rigid disorder of gait and motility, without clinical hypothyroidism; (2) hypothyroid or myxedematous cretinism, seen in its most exaggerated form in Zaire, typified neurologically by modestly retarded psychomotor development and slow psychomotor activity but not by deaf-mutism or notable motor spasticity or rigidity. These cretins have severe stunting of growth, coarse facial features, and severe hypothyroidism, and they commonly have musculoskeletal disorders, including bone maldevelopment and hypotrophic muscles.[38–41]

Descriptive Neurology of Endemic Cretinism

In neurologic endemic cretinism, several patterns of neurologic involvement are identifiable.[42,43] The "typical" pattern is that of hearing and speech deficits—often amounting to deaf-mutism—with a proximal spastic-rigid motor disorder and mental deficiency. Commonly associated with this picture are slowness and either masking or disinhibition of facial expression, and at times strabismus. The mental deficiency is severe for abstraction and intellectual efforts, but with relative preservation of personality. Even if the involvement is mild, this same pattern is usually discernible.

A second pattern is that characterized by "thalamic" posturing: the subjects show severe motor deficits and exhibit characteristic postures: when laid on their side, the undermost limbs extend and the uppermost limbs flex. We have encountered a few cretins who demonstrate this posturing. They also show very severe retardation; marked microcephaly; inability to sit, stand, or walk; and floridly exaggerated primitive facial reflexes including most notably "visual suck"—a marked suck or rooting reflex elicited by bringing an object into the visual field near the face. Facial defensive reflexes are equally exag-

gerated, for instance, blepharospasm and wincing elicited by glabellar tap. This pattern suggests a severe forebrain deficit.

A third pattern is "autistic." These children also have very severe mental deficiency, exacerbated by deaf-mutism, but also with very poor visual attention, almost total disregard of their surroundings, and an absence of purposeful (or any) activity. Such children typically stand with a narrow base and can walk usually a step or two if propelled.

A fourth pattern was recently encountered for the first time: a "cerebellar" pattern. In general, we and others[42–44] have commented on the absence of noteworthy cerebellar deficits: gait and station are generally preserved in cretins, and dysmetria or cerebellar tremor is not seen. To some extent, tremor may be submerged in the predominant rigidity; but nevertheless, the preservation of gait, station, and reasonably skilled use of the hands (e.g., drawing without marked tremor or dysmetria) argues for preservation of cerebellar function in most cases. In Hotien, China, however, we encountered 2 children with marked abnormalities of standing, walking, and sitting which are most typical of cerebellar dysfunction. Their truncal tone was typically hypotonic instead of rigid. Their attempts to reach and to draw revealed tremor and dysmetria. In other respects they were typical cretins.

A final pattern is hypotonia. These children exhibit marked truncal hypotonia and delayed sitting, standing, and walking. In other respects they are not severely deficient. They do not demonstrate evident gait ataxia as do the cerebellar group.

The mildest degree may be represented by children without evident signs of cretinism, in iodine-deficient areas, who have significant deficits in perceptual and neuromotor abilities and in school performance. Such children, so-called "subclinical cretins," are fivefold more common than frank cretins in endemic areas of iodine deficiency.[45]

A point to emphasize is the degree of microcephaly shown by these various groups in our studies in China.[44] Mild typical cretins had a mean head circumference approximating American norms. Severe typical cretins had a mean head circumference three standard deviations (SD) below the mean. The "thalamic" group, the most severely affected motorially, had severe microcephaly. In the other groups, the degree of microcephaly was intermediate. Pure myxedematous cretin subjects had normal neurologic findings and near-normal head circumferences, suggesting that early brain development was spared.

PATHOLOGY

Cretin brains are generally smaller than normal; in severe cases they may weigh one-half to two-thirds of normal. The macroscopic form and gyral patterns are normally developed. Histologic study shows small neuronal cell bodies with increased cell packing density, decreased neuropil, decreased amounts of myelin, and gliosis.[46] Neuroimaging studies of cretins have expanded this picture: CT scans of adult cretins have shown widespread brain atrophy, particularly of the brain stem and perisylvian regions.[43,47] The cerebellum, which matures postnatally during the first year, has generally been spared. Magnetic resonance images of three neurologic cretin adults showed an overall normal appearance except for prominent changes, consistent with gliosis, in the substantia nigra and globus pallidus; this finding fits with the proximal rigidity found to be a prominent feature in neurologic cretins.[48]

PATHOGENESIS

Endemic cretinism occurs only in areas of severe iodine deficiency, with iodine intake of 20 μg/day or less. It can be prevented by iodine supplementation (using iodized oil) before conception.[49] How iodine deficiency interacts with brain development has been a subject of much interest.

Early brain development appears not to depend on thyroid hormone. Thyroid hormone receptors can be detected in human fetal brain after 9 weeks' gestation, but their functional role is unclear.[50] The fetal thyroid gland begins to accumulate colloid at 12 weeks, and in conditions of iodine deficiency, fetal thyroid hypertrophy has been documented in the fifth fetal month.[51] Studies supplying iodine to severely iodine-deficient women at specific times in pregnancy have shown that if iodine treatment occurred by the end of the second trimester, normal neurologic development and brain growth ensued; whereas iodine treatment later in pregnancy or postnatally did not prevent neurologic abnormality, mental retardation, or impaired brain growth.[44,52] Treatment in the third trimester or neonatal period did, however, produce some improvement in mental development and head growth at age 2 years, compared to untreated infants. These findings suggest a definitive requirement for thyroid hormone for normal human brain development beginning at the end of the second trimester and in the neonatal period and early infancy. This timing corresponds with the normal increase in fetal T_4 production, which shows a ramp-like increase throughout the third trimester; and with the period of rapid increase in brain weight and protein content corresponding with the time of neuronal differentiation, major outgrowth of neuronal axons and dendrites, and synaptogenesis. It also corresponds to the postnatal period in the rat (in whom much experimental work has been done; see later) when neuronal differentiation and neurite formation occur, at the same time that brain T_3 receptors increase 40-fold and that thyroid hormone critically affects brain development.

Studies of a sheep model of iodine deficiency have yielded comparable findings.[53,54] In the human fetus, cells of Corti's organ are generated during the period of 10 to 18 weeks' gestation,[55] and the neurons of the cerebral cortex and basal ganglia are generated during weeks 12 through 18.[56]

The foregoing observations suggest that thyroid hormone has its primary effect on the later parts of central nervous system development, that is, differentiation, formation of neuritic processes, synaptogenesis, and myelination, and indeed this is the pattern shown by experimental work. Thyroid hormone appears not to affect embryogenesis of the brain (cretin brains are well formed overall). It has effects on neuronal proliferation in some instances, but its principal effect is on later differentiation and growth. The developmental failure occurring at the beginning of the third trimester under conditions of iodine deficiency, which results in neurologic cretinism, may be likened to failure of metamorphosis in the amphibian: a major developmental transformation of the brain fails and results in severe mental and motor deficiency. If the failure of thyroid hormone is deferred until the postnatal period, as in sporadic congenital hypothyroidism, the result is a milder deficit of neural development, manifested as moderate mental retardation but without deaf-mutism or severe motor disorder.

Congenital Hypothyroidism (Sporadic Cretinism)

This subject is fully covered in chapter 85. Here only some important neurologic aspects are discussed. It has been firmly established that if treatment of congenital hypothyroidism is begun during the first months of life, the intellectual potential of these children is improved dramatically. In a valuable study, Wolter and colleagues,[57] on the basis of data from the literature, compared IQ scores of infants treated before the age of 1 month and those treated between 1 and 3 months. IQ was within the normal range in all cases in the first group but only in 75% in the second. Thus, any delay in treatment, even during the first weeks of life, may result in lower mental capacity. The same authors also showed that if the starting age of hypothyroidism was prenatal (as judged by bone age), IQ score progressively decreased as a function of age at onset of therapy. In those with neonatal onset of hypothyroidism, their IQ score was normal even if treatment was delayed several months.

Neurologic sequelae of congenital hypothyroidism were seen in some infants in the prenatal group treated after 7 months of age; these included cerebellar ataxia and strabismus but not spasticity or gross motor defect. Neuropsychologic sequelae were frequent in these infants, independent of mental retardation, and included short attention span, fine motor incoordination, impaired spatial orientation, slow ideation, and slow motor performance. These neuropsychologic sequelae were present in 50% to 75% of the prenatal onset group even though they were treated before the age of 1 month and had normal IQ scores. This work demonstrates that assessment of bone age at time of diagnosis has important prognostic value.

Also valuable are reports on the abnormalities in children and adults with congenital hypothyroidism who did not receive early screening and treatment. In England, 73 children and 43 adults were studied[58]; mean IQ scores were 1 to 2 standard deviations (SD) below scores of normals, and mean motor scores were reduced 1 to 2 SD in the children and 1 to 3 SD in adults. It was noted that behavioral and personality problems were common and persisted into adult life. Another study[59] of 18 such patients reached similar conclusions: 44% had mental retardation (IQ < 70), and typically the patients had neurotic personality patterns.

Although much has been written on the mental deficiency accompanying sporadic cretinism, little attention has been paid to the presence and nature of any coexisting neurologic signs. The accompanying motor syndrome has been subject to comment[60] in an excellent article on the mental prognosis in early-life hypothyroidism. In 26 of 79 patients with severe hypothyroidism, mainly of the agoitrous type, a neurologic abnormality was prominent and took the form of one or more of the following: spasticity, shuffling gait, incoordination (which was most striking in precise volitional movements), awkwardness, jerky movements, coarse tremor, and increased tendon reflexes. Five patients also had seizures.

EFFECTS OF THYROID ON BRAIN DEVELOPMENT

The effects of thyroid hormones on brain development have been extensively studied in the experimental animal, usually the rat.[61,62] In the neonatally thyroidectomized rat,[63] brain weight is significantly diminished, the brain retains an infantile configuration, and cortical neurons are reduced in size and are more closely spaced. Biochemical data have also been consistent with a decrease in the size of neurons in the cerebral cortex of the hypothyroid rat (determined by increased DNA concentration with lowered RNA per unit of tissue).[64] The cerebral cortex of the cretinous rat also contains fewer capillaries[65] and fewer axons,[66] the dendritic arborization of neurons is severely retarded in the cerebral cortex,[67] and the number of nerve terminals per nerve cell is reduced.[68] Using morphologic and biochemical techniques, it has been shown that brains of hypothyroid rats contain less myelin than controls and manifest a delay in the sequential development of all myelinated fiber tracts.[69] The same workers have studied purified myelin isolated from cretinoid rats and have shown that brain myelin in hypothyroidism is structurally and biochemically unaltered.[70] They also have shown that in the later stages of development, the hypothyroid rat has the capacity to increase synthesis of brain myelin so that myelin yields approach those of the control animals.[71]

Because body growth is reduced in hypothyroidism and since a number of the brain alterations of hypothyroidism also occur in malnutrition,[66,72] the specificity of these changes must be called into question. According to data cited earlier,[69] there are only quantitative differences—the disturbance in myelinogenesis of experimental malnutrition being intermediate between that of control rats and the more pronounced disturbance of hypothyroidism. The degree of retardation in the former state, however, was never found to approach that of neonatal hypothyroidism; hence, thyroid lack has a specific effect on development.

Impaired histogenesis of the cerebellar cortex has been demonstrated in the neonatally thyroidectomized rat. Inward migration of external granular cells, which cross the molecular layer to form the internal granular layer, is retarded, with delay in the disappearance of the external granular layer.[73] Dendritic arborization of Purkinje's cells is severely retarded,[74] there is a marked reduction in the numbers of basket cells in the cerebellar cortex,[75] and synaptogenesis is reduced significantly.[76,77] Morphologic changes in the cerebella of hypothyroid animals have been reversed by treatment with thyroid hormone.[78]

Thyroid hormone is necessary for brain growth, particularly during the peak growth period, which in rats occurs after birth. Rat pups subjected to intrauterine and postnatal iodine deficiency had normal body and brain weight at birth.[79] By 21 days, however, brain weight was significantly decreased (7.9%), with biochemical evidence of decreased myelination and decreased cell size. These changes were most marked in the cerebellum. In another study, hypothyroidism and thyrotoxicosis in neonatal rats decreased growth of the cerebellum.[80] In the early phase, protein/DNA and RNA/DNA ratios were higher in both groups of animals, suggesting a primary failure of cell proliferation. By 35 days, however, these ratios were lower than normal, implying a failure of cell maturation.

Brain uptake of exogenous T_4 is threefold greater in the rat pup, and thyroid hormone content in brain tissue and in isolated cortical neurons is five times greater at 10 days (during peak brain growth) than at maturity.[81] Evidence suggests that brain growth does not parallel growth hormone availability but may more closely parallel thyroid hormone levels during peak growth.[82] Available data indicate that T_4 is taken up by the brain during development and locally monodeiodinated to T_3, which is then bound to brain cell nuclear receptors. Thus, T_4 and its local conversion to T_3 is essential for normal brain development.

Increased or decreased availability of thyroid hormone alters the rate and completeness of evolution of the innate development program in the brain. Thyrotoxicosis accelerates cell multiplication early in postnatal development (e.g., in the external granule cell layer of the cerebellum) but produces premature termination of cell division and ultimately a deficit in cell number.[83] Hypothyroidism decreases cell proliferation postnatally (e.g., in the hippocampus) and also results ultimately in a deficit in cell number.

Excess thyroid hormone accelerates and hypothyroidism retards many histogenic processes in the brain. Those most studied are in the cerebellum, hippocampus, and cerebral cortex. In the cerebellum, postnatal hypothyroidism delays the deposition of external granule cells and the maturation of Bergmann's glia, causes hypoplasia of Purkinje-cell dendritic arborizations, and retards development of parallel fibers; the retardation in synaptogenesis between parallel fibers and Purkinje-cell dendritic spines is secondary to this retardation in growth and branching of neuronal processes.[84]

Sustained hypothyroidism not only retards myelinogenesis but also leads to a decrease in the total amount of myelin in the brain. In thyrotoxic rats, myelin accumulation is accelerated but also terminates earlier than normal, and final brain myelin weight is decreased.[85]

Neonatal thyrotoxicosis in rats stimulates increased growth and extension of the mossy fiber projection that synapses on the basal dendrites of hippocampal pyramidal cells. The extent of this projection has been inversely correlated with the rate of learning of a two-way avoidance task. In neonatally-treated animals as adults, the learning rate correlated with the extent of mossy fiber projection induced by thyrotoxicosis.[86] This suggests a direct correlation between a manipulable neuroanatomic feature and learning performance.

The development of nerve cell connections strongly depends on thyroid status. Examples from the cerebellum and hippocampus were described earlier. In the cerebral cortex, severe hypothyroidism in suckling rats causes a decrease in the number of spines on apical shafts of pyramidal cells of visual[87] and auditory cortex.[88]

T_4 was necessary for formation of nerve fiber outgrowth from explants of locus ceruleus grafted to the iris.[89] This corroborates other evidence that T_4 plays a crucial role in tubulin assembly and thus presumably in the ability of neurons to form processes.[90,91]

The preceding experimental studies of the effect of thyroid hormone on the brain have established several fundamental facts:

1. T_4, not T_3, is the primary form of the hormone taken up by brain; thus normal thyroid hormone–dependent brain development depends on the availability of thyroxine, not T_3. T_4 is deiodinated intracellularly in the brain to T_3, a process which is already established in the fetal brain.[92] T_3 then binds to the nuclear T_3-receptors, which in turn control thyroid-sensitive gene expression. The brain contains a specific T_3-receptor type: the beta-form, whereas all tissues contain the alpha-form.

2. Thyroid hormone has some effects on cell proliferation, but has a more important and pervasive effect on post-proliferation events including differentiation, neurite growth, synaptogenesis, and myelination. Thyroid hormone acts on the T_3-nuclear receptor, which controls gene expression by acting on thyroid-responsive elements in the promoter region of thyroid-sensitive genes to enhance transcription. This process is described in detail elsewhere. There is also evidence of thyroid hormone effects on translation and post-translational events.

3. Thyroid hormone controls the developmental timing and modifies the pace of some developmental events in the brain. Thyrotoxicosis may accelerate, and hypothyroidism retard, the time of onset and/or the rate of developmental events. In either case, the final result is generally disordered.

4. Thyroid hormone acts only on certain genes in the brain. Its actions are complex and are specific temporally, regionally, and in respect to specific cell types and neural systems. A full picture of its actions on brain development is not yet available.

It is beyond the scope of this chapter to detail the known effects of thyroid hormone on brain development, primarily in experimental animals (most commonly the rat) and brain cell culture systems. Some effects may be on timing of specific events and some on rate, and thyroid hormone actions vary by developmental time, brain region, cell type, and specific molecule or gene regulated. Most events are genomic, although non-nuclear effects of thyroid hormone also occur. These thyroid hormone–mediated effects are discussed in chapter 9.

In brief, thyroid hormone action on the brain affects gene expression,[93–98] growth factors,[99] cell proliferation,[100,101] cell migration,[102] neuronal differentiation,[103–109] myelin,[110–114] neurotransmitters,[111,115–117] actin polymerization,[118] type II 5'-deiodinase,[123] and tau transcripts.[107]

References

1. Hetzel BS, Potter BJ, Dulberg EM. The iodine deficiency disorders: nature, pathogenesis, and epidemiology. In: Bourne GH, ed. Aspects of some vitamins, minerals and enzymes in health and disease. World Rev Nutr Diet 1990;62:59

2. Debré R, Sémélaigne G. Syndrome of diffuse muscular hypertrophy in infants causing athletic appearance. Am J Dis Child 1935;50:1351

3. Soled M. Simple clues to diagnosis of hypothyroidism. Postgrad Med 1994;95:35

4. Hurwitz LJ, McCormick D, Allen IV. Reduced muscle, alpha-glucosidase (acid-maltase) activity in hypothyroid myopathy. Lancet 1970;1:67

4a. Riggs JE. Acute exertional rhabdomyolysis in hypothyroidism: the result of a reverse defect in glycogenolysis? Milit Med 1990;155:171

5. del Palacio A, Trueba JL, Cabello A, Gutierrez E, Moya I, Fernandez Miranda C, Garcia Albea E, Ricoy JR. Miopatia hipotiroidea. Estudio clinico-patologico de 20 casos. Anales Medicina Interna 1990;7:115

6. del Palacio A, Trueba JL, Cabello A, Gutierrez E, Moya I, Fernandez Miranda C, Garcia Albea E, Ricoy JR. Miopatia tiroidea. Efecto del tratimiento con hormonas tiroideas. Anales de Medicina Interna 1990;7:120

7. Costin G, Kaplan SA, Ling SM. The Achilles reflex time in thyroid disorders. J Pediatr 1970;76:277

8. Waldstein SS, Bronsky D, Shrifter H, Dester Y. The electromyogram in myxedema. Arch Intern Med 1958;101:97

9. Burnett JR, Crooke MJ, Delahunt JW, Feek CM. Serum enzymes in hypothyroidism. New Zealand Med J 1994:107:355

10. Khaleeli AA, Griffith DG, Edwards RH. The clinical presentation of hypothyroid myopathy and its relationships to abnormalities in structure and function of skeletal muscle. Clin Endocrinol (Oxf) 1983;19:365

11. Khaleeli AA, Edwards RH. Effect of treatment on skeletal muscle dysfunction in hypothyroidism. Clin Sci 1984;66:63

12. Miyamoto T, Nagasaka A, Kato K, Masunaga R, Kotake M, Kawabe T, Nakai A, Mokuno T, Sawai Y, Oda N, Mano T, Nishida Y. Immunoreactive creatine kinase-MB and creatine kinase isozyme concentrations during treatment of hypothyroid patients. Eur J Clin Chem Clin Biochem 1994;32:589

13. Khaleeli AA, Gohil K, McPhail G, et al. Muscle morphology and metabolism in hypothyroid myopathy: effects of treatment. J Clin Pathol 1983;36:510

14. Mastaglia FL, Ojeda VJ, Sarnat HB, et al. Myopathies associated with hypothyroidism: a review based upon 13 cases. Aust N Z J Med 1988;18:799

15. Spiro AJ, Kirano A, Beilin RL, Finkelstein JW. Cretinism with muscular hypertrophy (Kocher-Debré-Sémélaigne syndrome). Arch Neurol 1970;23:340

16. Pearce J, Aziz H. The neuromyopathy of hypothyroidism: some new observations. J Neurol Sci 1969;9:243

17. Ono S, Inouye K, Mannen T. Myopathology of hypothyroid myopathy. Some new observations. J Neurol Sci 1987;77:237

18. Ho KL. Basophilic degeneration of skeletal muscle in hypothyroid myopathy. Arch Pathol Lab Med 1984;108:239

19. Vickery AL, Fierro-Benitez R, Kakulas BA. Skeletal muscle structure in endemic cretinism. Am J Pathol 1966;49:193

20. Phalen GS. The carpal-tunnel syndrome: 17 years experience in diagnosis and treatment of 654 hands. J Bone Joint Surg (Am) 1966;48:211

21. Earll JM, Kolb FO. Facial paralysis occurring with hypothyroidism. A report of two cases. Calif Med 1967;106:56

22. Moosa A, Dubowitz V. Slow nerve conduction velocity in cretins. Arch Dis Child 1971;46:852

23. Beghi E, Delodovici ML, Bogliun G, et al. Hypothyroidism and polyneuropathy. J Neurol Neurosurg Psychiatry 1989;52:1420

24. Nemni R, Bottacchi E, Fazio R, et al. Polyneuropathy in hypothyroidism: clinical, electrophysiological and morphological findings in four cases. J Neurol Neurosurg Psychiatry 1987;50:1454

25. Torres CF, Moxley RT. Hypothyroid neuropathy and myopathy: clinical and electrodiagnostic longitudinal findings. J Neurol 1990;237:271

26. Soederbergh G. Faut-il attribuer à une perturbation des fonctions cérébelleuses certain troubles moteur du myxoedème? Rev Neurol (Paris) 1910;2:487

27. Barnard RO, Campbell MJ, McDonald WI. Pathological findings in a case of hypothyroidism with ataxia. J Neurol Neurosurg Psychiatry 1971;34:755

28. Grunstein RR, Sullivan CE. Sleep apnea and hypothyroidism: mechanisms and management. Am J Med 1988;85:775

29. VanDyck P, Chadband R, Chaudhary B, Stachura M. Sleep apnea, sleep disorders and hypothyroidism. Am J Med Sci 1989;298:119

30. Martinez FJ, Bermudez-Gomez M, Celli BR. Hypothyroidism: a reversible cause of diaphragmatic dysfunction. Chest 1989; 96:1059

31. Harris R, Della Rovere M, Prior PF. Electroencephalographic studies in infants and children with hypothyroidism. Arch Dis Child (Chicago) 1965;40:612

32. Hermann HT, Quarton GC. Changes in alpha frequency with change in thyroid hormone level. Electroenceph Clin Neurophysiol 1964;16:515

33. Scheinberg P, Stead EA, Brannon ES, Warren JV. Correlative observations on cerebral metabolism and cardiac output in myxedema. J Clin Invest 1950;29:1139

34. Darko DF, Krull A, Dickerson M, et al. The diagnostic dilemma of myxedema and madness, axis I and axis II: a longitudinal case report. Int J Psychiatry Med 1988;18:263

35. Haggerty JJ Jr, Evans DL, Prange AJ Jr. Organic brain syndrome associated with marginal hypothyroidism. Am J Psychiatry 1986; 143:785

36. Rovet JF, Daneman D, Bailey JD. Psychologic and psychoeducational consequences of thyroxine therapy for juvenile acquired hypothyroidism. J Pediatrics 1993;122:543

37. Stanbury JB, Hetzel BS, eds. Endemic goiter and cretinism. New York: John Wiley & Sons, 1980

38. Ermans AM, Mbulamoko NM, Delange F, Ahluwalia R, eds. Role of cassava in the etiology of endemic goitre and cretinism. Ottawa: International Development Research Center, 1980

39. Vanderpas J, Contempra B, Duale NL, et al. Selenium deficiency mitigates hypothyroxinemia in iodine deficient subjects. Am J Clin Nutr 1993;57:2715

40. Stanbury JB, Fierro-Benitez R, Estrella E, et al. Endemic goiter hypothyroidism in three generations. J Clin Endocrinol Metab 1969;29:1596

41. Vulsma T, Gons MT, De Viglder JJM. Maternal-fetal transfer of thyroxine in congenital hypothyroidism due to a total organification defect or thyroid agenesis. N Engl J Med 1989;321:13

42. DeLong R. Neurological involvement in iodine deficiency disorders. In: Hetzel BS, Dunn JT, Stanbury JB, eds. The prevention and control of iodine deficiency disorder. Amsterdam: Elsevier, 1987:49

43. Halpern J-P, Boyages SC, Maberly GF, Collins JK, Eastman CJ, Morris JGL. The neurology of endemic cretinism: a study of two endemias. Brain 1991;114:1825

44. DeLong GR, Ma T, Cao XY, Jiang XM, Dou ZH, Murdon AR, Zhang ML, Heinz ER. The neuromotor deficit in endemic cretinism. In: Stanbury JB, ed. The damaged brain of iodine deficiency. New York: Cognizant Communication, 1994:9

45. Ma T, Wang D, Chen ZP. Mental retardation other than typical cretinism in IDD endemias in China. In: Stanbury JB, ed. The damaged brain of iodine deficiency. New York: Cognizant Communications, 1994:265.

46. Lotmar F. Histopathologische Befunde in Gehirnen von kongenitales Myxödem (thyreoaplasie), und Kachexia thyreopriva. Monatschr Neurol Psychiatry 1929;119:491

47. Cruz M, Canelos P, Utreras A, Malo L. Guia de tomografia axial computerizada. Ecuador: Quito, 1984

48. Ma T, Lian ZC, Qi SP, Heinz ER, DeLong GR. Magnetic resonance imaging of brain and the neuromotor disorder in endemic cretinism. Ann Neurology 1993;34:91

49. Pharoah POD, Buttfield IH, Hetzel BS. Neurological damage to the fetus resulting from severe iodine deficiency during pregnancy. Lancet 1971;1:308

50. Bernal J, Pekonen F. Ontogenesis of the nuclear 3,5,3'-triiodothyronine receptor in the human fetal brain. Endocrinology 1984; 114:677

51. Liu J-L, Tan Y-B, Zhuang Z-J, Shi Z-F, Chen B-Z, Zhang J-X. Influence of iodine deficiency on human fetal thyroid gland and brain. In: DeLong GR, Robbins J, Condliffe PD, eds. Iodine and the brain. New York: Plenum Press, 1989:249

52. Cao XY, Jiang XM, Dou ZH, Murdon AR, Zhang ML, O'Donnell K, Ma T, Kareem A, DeLong N, DeLong GR. Timing of vulnerability of the brain to iodine deficiency in endemic cretinism. N Engl J Med 1994;331:1739

53. Hetzel BS, Mano MT. A review of experimental studies of iodine deficiency during fetal development. J Nutr 1989;119:145

54. Potter BJ, Mano MT, Belling GB, et al. Restoration of brain growth in fetal sheep after iodized oil administration to pregnancy iodine-deficient ewes. J Neurol Sci 1984;66:15

55. Konig MP, Neiger M. The pathology of the ear in endemic cretinism. In: Stanbury JB, Kroc RL, eds. Human development and the thyroid gland: relation to endemic cretinism. New York: Plenum Press, 1972:325

56. Davison AN, Dobbing J. The developing brain. In: Davison AN, Dobbing J, eds. Applied neurochemistry. Oxford: Blackwell Scientific, 1968:253

57. Wolter R, Noel P, Craen M, et al. Neuropsychological study in treated thyroid dysgenesis. Acta Paediatr Scand Suppl 1979; 227:41

58. Frost GJ, Parkin JM. A comparison between the neurological and intellectual abnormalities in children and adults with congenital Hypothyroidism. Eur J Pediatr 1986;145:480

59. Mendorla G, Sava L, Calaciura F, et al. Personality traits and mental prognosis in patients with congenital hypothyroidism not treated from early life. J Endocrinol Invest 1988;11:289

60. Smith DW, Blizzard RM, Wilkins L. The mental prognosis in hypothyroidism of infancy and childhood. J Pediatr 1957; 19:1011

61. Stein SA. Molecular and neuroanatomical substrates of motor and cerebral cortex abnormalities in fetal thyroid hormone disorders. In: Stanbury JB, ed. The damaged brain of iodine deficiency. New York: Cognizant Communications, 1994:67

62. DeLong GR, Robbins J, Condliffe P, eds. Iodine and the brain. New York: Plenum Press, 1989:379

63. Eayrs JT, Taylor SH. The effect of thyroid deficiency induced by methyl thiouracil on the maturation of the central nervous system. J Anat 1951;85:350

64. Geel SE, Timiras PS. The influence of neonatal hypothyroidism and of thyroxine on the ribonucleic acid and deoxyribo-nucleic acid concentrations of rat cerebral cortex. Brain Res 1967;4:135

65. Eayrs JT. The vascularity of the cerebral cortex in normal and cretinous rats. J Anat 1954;88:164

66. Eayrs JT, Horn G. The development of cerebral cortex in hypothyroid and starved rats. Anat Rec 1955;121:53

67. Eayrs JT. The cerebral cortex of normal and hypothyroid rats. Acta Anat (Basel) 1955;25:160

68. Cragg BG. Synapses and membranous structures in experimental hypothyroidism. Brain Res 1970;18:297

69. Rosman NP, Malone MJ, Helfenstein M, Kraft E. The effect of thyroid deficiency on myelination of brain. Neurology 1972;22:99

70. Malone MJ, Rosman NP, Szoke M, Davis D. Myelination of brain in experimental hypothyroidism: an electron microscopic and biochemical study of purified myelin isolates. J Neurol Sci 1975;26:1

71. Rosman NP, Malone MJ, Szoke M. Reversal of delayed myelinogenesis in experimental hypothyroidism. J Neurol Sci 1975; 26:159

72. Horn G. Thyroid deficiency in inanition. Anat Rec 1955;121:63

73. Hamburgh M, Lynn E, Weiss EP. Analysis of the influence of thyroid hormone on prenatal and postnatal maturation of the rat. Anat Rec 1964;150:147

74. Legrand J. Analyse de l'action morphogénétique des hormones thyroidiennes sur le cervelet des jeunes rats. Arch Anat Microsc Morphol Exp 1967;56:205

75. Clos J, Legrand J. Effects of thyroid deficiency on the different cell populations of the cerebellum in the young rat. Brain Res 1973;63:450

76. Nicholson JL, Altman J. The effects of early hypo- and hyperthyroidism on the development of rat cerebellar cortex. II. Synaptogenesis in the molecular layer. Brain Res 1972;44:25

77. Nicholson JL, Altman J. Synaptogenesis in the rat cerebellum: effects of early hypo- and hyperthyroidism. Science 1972;176:530

78. Legrand J. Maturation du cervelet et déficience thyroidienne données chronologique. Arch Anat Microsc Morphol Exp 1963; 52:205

79. McIntosh GH, Howard DA, Mano MT, et al. Iodine deficiency and brain development in the rat. Anat J Biol Sci 1981;34:427

80. Dainat J, Rebiere A. Correction of the biochemical effects of neonatal hypothyroidism by daily low doses of thyroxine: comparative effects of hyperthyroidism and these corrections. Acta Neurol Scand 1978;58:167

81. Vigouroux E, Clos J, Legrand J. Uptake and metabolism of exogenous and endogenous thyroxine in the brain of young rats. Horm Metab Res 1979;11:228

82. Pascual-Leone AM, Garcia MD, Hervas F. Changes in parameters of growth hormone and thyrotrophic hormone and of thyroid function, during the early post-natal period in the rat. Rev Esp Fisiol 1978;34:301

83. Seress L. Divergent responses to thyroid hormone treatment of the different secondary germinal layers in the postnatal rat brain. J Hirnforsch 1978;19:395

84. Vincent J, Legrand C, Rabie A, et al. Effects of thyroid hormone on synaptogenesis in the molecular layer of the developing rat cerebellum. J Physiol (Paris) 1982/1983;78:729

85. Walters SN, Morell P. Effects of altered thyroid states on myelinogenesis. J Neurochem 1981;36:1792

86. Lipp HP, Schwegler H, Driscoll P. Postnatal modification of hippocampal circuitry alters avoidance learning in adult rats. Science 1984;225:80

87. Ruiz-Marcos A, Sanchez-Toscano F, Escobar del-Rey F, Morrele de Escobar G. Severe hypothyroidism and the maturation of the rat cerebral cortex. Brain Res 1979;162:315

88. Ruiz-Marcos A, Salas J, Sanchez-Toscano F, et al. Effect of neonatal and adult-onset hypothyroidism on pyramidal cells of the rat auditory cortex. Brain Res 1983;285:205

89. Seiger A, Granholm AC. Thyroxin dependency of the developing locus coeruleus: evidence from intraocular grafting experiments. Cell Tissue Res 1981;220:1

90. Fellous A, Lennon AM, Francon J, et al. Thyroid hormones and neurotubule assembly in vitro during brain development. Eur J Biochem 1979;101:365

91. Takahashi T. Transplacental effects of 3,5-dimethyl-3-isopropyl-L-thyronine on tubulin content in fetal brains in rats. Jpn J Physiol 1984;34:365

92. Morreale de Escobar G, Obregon MJ, Calvo R, Escobar del Rey F. Effects of iodine deficiency on thyroid hormone metabolism and the brain in fetal rats: the role of the maternal transfer of thyroxine. Am J Clin Nutr 1993;57(Suppl):280S

93. Garcia-Fernandez LF, Iniguez MA, Rodriguez-Pena A, Munoz A, Bernal J. Brain-specific prostaglandin D2 synthetase mRNA is dependent on thyroid hormone during rat brain development. Biochem Biophys Res Commun 1993;196:396

94. Mellstrom B, Pipaon C, Naranjo JR, Perez-Castillo A, Santos A. Differential effect of thyroid hormone on NGFI-A gene expression in developing rat brain. Endocrinology 1994;135:583

95. Pipaon C, Santos A, Perez-Castillo A. Thyroid hormone up-regulates NGFI-A gene expression in rat brain during development. J Biol Chem 1992;267:21

96. Iniguez MA, Rodriguez-Pena A, Ibarrola N, Aguilera M, Munoz A, Bernal J. Thyroid hormone regulation of RC3, a brain-specific gene encoding a protein kinase-c substrate. Endocrinology 1993;133:467

97. Strait KA, Schwartz HL, Perez-Castillo A, Oppenheimer JH. Relationship of c-erbA mRNA content to tissue triiodothyronine nuclear binding capacity and function in developing and adult rats. J Biol Chem 1990;265:10514

98. Li J, Chow SY. Subcellular distribution of carbonic anhydrase and Na$^+$,K($^+$)-ATPase in the brain of the hyt/hyt hypothyroid mice. Neurochem Res 1994;19:83

99. Hendrich CE, Porterfield SP. Serum growth hormone levels in hypothyroid and GH-treated thyroidectomized rats and their progenies. Proc Soc Exp Biol Med 1992;201:296

100. Madeira MD, Cadete-Leite A, Andrade JP, Paula-Barbosa MM. Effects of hypothyroidism upon the granular layer of the dentate gyrus in male and female adult rats: a morphometric study. J Comp Neurol 1991;314:80

101. Madeira MD, Pereira A, Cadete-Leite A, Paula-Barbosa MM. Estimates of volumes and pyramidal cell numbers in the prelimbic subarea of the prefrontal cortex in experimental hypothyroid rats. J Anatomy 1990;171:41

102. Chakraborty M, Lahiri P, Chatterjee D. Thyroidal influence on the cell surface GM1 of granule cells: its significance in cell migration during rat brain development. Cell Mol Neurobiol 1992;12:589

103. Madeira MD, Paula-Barbosa MM. Reorganization of mossy fiber synapses in male and female hypothyroid rats: a stereological study. J Comp Neurol 1993;337:334

104. Madeira MD, Sousa N, Lima-Andrade MT, Calheiros F, Cadete-Leite A, Paula-Barbosa MM. Selective vulnerability of the hippocampal pyramidal neurons to hypothyroidism in male and female rats. J Comp Neurol 1992;322:501

105. Pickard MR, Sinha AK, Ogilvie L, Ekins RP. The influence of the maternal thyroid hormone environment during pregnancy on the ontogenesis of brain and placental ornithine decarboxylase activity in the rat. J Endocrinology 1993;139:205

106. Aniello F, Couchie D, Gripois D, Nunez J. Regulation of five tubulin isotypes by thyroid hormone curing brain development. J Neurochem 1991;57:1781

107. Anniello F, Couchie D, Bridoux AM, Gripois D, Nunez J. Splicing of juvenile and adult tau mRNA variants is regulated by thyroid hormone. Proc Natl Acad Sci U S A 1991;88:4035

108. Madeira MD, Cadete-Leite A, Sousa N, Paula-Barbosa MM. The supraoptic nucleus in hypothyroid and undernourished rats: an experimental morphometric study. Neuroscience 1991;41:827

109. Zou L, Hagen SG, Strait KA, Oppenheimer JH. Identification of thyroid hormone response elements in rodent Pcp-2, a developmentally regulated gene of cerebellar Purkinje cells. J Biol Chem 1994;269:13346

110. Noguchi T. Retarded cerebral growth of hormone-deficient mice. Comp Biochem Physiol (C) 1991;98:239

111. Virgili M, Saverino O, Vaccari M, Barnabei O, Contestabile A. Temporal, regional and cellular selectivity of neonatal alteration of the thyroid state on neurochemical maturation in the rat. Exp Brain Res 1991;83:555

112. Farsetti A, Mitsuhashi T, Desvergne B, Robbins J, Nikodem VM. Molecular basis of thyroid hormone regulation of myelin basic protein gene expression in rodent brain. J Biol Chem 1991; 266:23226

113. Rodriguez-Pena A, Ibarrola N, Iniguez MA, Munoz A, Bernal J. Neonatal hypothyroidism affects the timely expression of

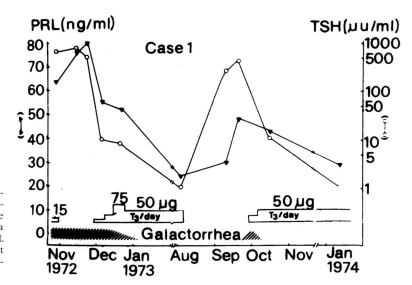

FIGURE 68-4. Serum prolactin (PRL) and TSH concentrations in a woman who presented with galactorrhea and primary hypothyroidism. When she was treated with T_3, the serum PRL and TSH concentrations fell and the galactorrhea disappeared. When treatment was discontinued, serum PRL and TSH concentrations both rose again. When treatment was resumed, both fell again. (Onishi T et al. Primary hypothyroidism and galactorrhea. Am J Med 1977;63:373)

been normal to mildly supranormal.[19–21] Even when the serum PRL concentrations in hypothyroidism are supranormal, however, they are usually less than 100 ng/mL, so a higher value should raise the suspicion of a PRL-secreting adenoma. In one study of serum PRL concentrations in hypothyroid men, the values were normal in magnitude, pulsatility, and circadian pattern,[22] suggesting that hypothyroidism alone is not sufficient to cause hyperprolactinemia, but requires another stimulus such as estrogen. The strongest case for concluding that hypothyroidism is the cause of the hyperprolactinemia in patients who are both hypothyroid and hyperprolactinemic is that the serum PRL concentration falls to normal when they are treated with thyroid hormone (Fig 68-4).[14,15,23,24]

The mechanism by which hypothyroidism causes hyperprolactinemia is not known, but it is probably due to a direct effect on the pituitary gland. Patients who are hypothyroid have greater than normal serum PRL responses to thyrotropin-releasing hormone (TRH), and the responses decrease to normal during thyroid hormone therapy.[16,17] Thyroid hormone may also influence PRL secretion through an effect on TRH secretion, because T_3 decreases the expression of the mRNA for the TRH precursor in the hypothalamus.[25]

References

1. Katz HP, Youltan R, Kaplan SL, et al. Growth and growth hormone. III. Growth hormone release in children with primary hypothyroidism and thyrotoxicosis. J Clin Endocrinol Metab 1969;29:346

2. MacGillivray MH, Aceto T, Frohman LA. Plasma growth hormone responses and growth retardation in hypothyroidism. Am J Dis Child 1968;115:273

3. Root AW, Rosenfeld RL, Bongiovanni AM, Eberlein WR. The plasma growth hormone response to insulin-induced hypoglycemia in children with retardation of growth. Pediatrics 1967;39:844

4. Chernausek SD, Turner R. Attenuation of spontaneous, nocturnal growth hormone secretion in children with hypothyroidism and its correlation with plasma insulin-like growth factor I concentrations. Pediatr 1989;114:968

5. Valcavi R, Dieguez C, Preece M, Taylor A, Portioli I, Scanlon MF. Effect of thyroxine replacement therapy on plasma insulin-like growth factor I levels and growth hormone responses to growth hormone releasing factor in hypothyroid patients. Clin Endocrinol 1987;27:85

6. Williams T, Maxon H, Thorner MO, Frohman LA. Blunted growth hormone (GH) response to GH-releasing hormone in hypothyroidism resolves in the euthyroid state. J Clin Endocrinol Metab 1985;61:454

7. Chernausek SD, Underwood LE, Utiger RD, Van Wyk JJ. Growth hormone secretion and plasma somatomedin-C in primary hypothyroidism. Clin Endocrinol 1983;19:337

8. Brent GA, Harney JW, Moore DD, Larsen PR. Multihormonal regulation of the human, rat, and bovine growth hormone promoters: differential effects of 3',5' cyclic adenosine monophosphate, thyroid hormone, and glucocorticoids. Mol Endocrinol 1988;2:792

9. Katakami H, Downs TR, Frohman LA. Decreased hypothalamic growth hormone–releasing hormone content and pituitary responsiveness in hypothyroidism. J Clin Invest 1987;77:1704

10. Downs TR, Chomczynski P, Frohman LA. Effects of thyroid hormone deficiency and replacement on rat hypothalamic growth hormone (GH)-releasing hormone gene expression in vivo are mediated by GH. Mol Endocrinol 1990;4:402

11. Amit T, Hertz P, Ish-Shalom S, et al. Effects of hypo- or hyperthyroidism on growth hormone-binding protein. Clin Endocrinol 1991;35:159

12. Miell JP, Taylor AM, Zini M, Maheshwari HG, Ross RJ, Valcavi R. Effects of hypothyroidism and hyperthyroidism on insulin-like growth factors (IGFs) and growth hormone- and IGF-binding proteins. J Clin Endocrinol Metab 1993;76:950

13. Contreras P, Generini G, Michelsen H, Pumarino H, Campino C. Hyperprolactinemia and galactorrhea: spontaneous versus iatrogenic hypothyroidism. J Clin Endocrinol Metab 1981;53:1036

14. Groff TR, Shulkin BL, Utiger RD, Talbert LM. Amenorrhea-galactorrhea, hyperprolactinemia, and suprasellar pituitary enlargement as presenting features of primary hypothyroidism. Obstet Gynecol 1984;63:865

15. Grubb MR, Chakeres D, Malarkey WB. Patients with primary hypothyroidism presenting as prolactinomas. Am J Med 1987; 83:765

16. Refetoff S, Fang VS, Rapoport B, Friesen HG. Interrelationships in the regulation of TSH and prolactin secretion: effects of L-dopa, TRH and thyroid hormone in various combinations. J Clin Endocrinol Metab 1974;38:450

17. Snyder PJ, Jacobs LS, Utiger RD, Daughaday WH. Thyroid hormone inhibition of the prolactin response to thyrotropin-releasing hormone. J Clin Invest 1973;52:2324

18. Gibbi KS, Van Herle AJ, Kellett KA. Serum prolactin levels in untreated primary hypothyroidism. Am J Med 1978; 64:782

19. Gomez F, Reyes Fl, Faiman C. Nonpuerperal galactorrhea and hyperprolactinemia. Am J Med 1977;62:648

20. Kleinberg DL, Noel GL, Frantz AG. Galactorrhea: a study of 235 cases, including 48 with pituitary tumors. N Engl J Med 1977; 296:589

21. Tolis G, Somma M, Van Campenhout J, Friesen H. Prolactin secretion in sixty-five patients with galactorrhea. Am J Obstet Gynecol 1974;118:91

22. Iranmanesh A, Lizarralde G, Veldhuis JD. Robustness of the male lactotropic axis to the hyperprolactinemic stimulus of primary thyroidal failure. J Clin Endocrinol Metab 1992; 74:559

23. Boroditsky RS, Faiman C. Galactorrhea-amenorrhea due to primary hypothyroidism. Am J Obstet Gynecol 1973;116:661

24. Onishi T, Miyai K, Aono T, et al. Primary hypothyroidism and galactorrhea. Am J Med 1977;63:373

25. Dyess EM, Segerson TP, Liposits Z, et al. Triiodothyronine exerts direct cell-specific regulation of thyrotropin releasing hormone gene expression in the hypothalamic paraventricular nucleus. Endocrinology 1988;123:2291

Werner and Ingbar's The Thyroid, Seventh Edition,
edited by Lewis E. Braverman and Robert D. Utiger.
Lippincott–Raven Publishers, Philadelphia, © 1996

69

The Adrenal Cortex in Hypothyroidism

Robert G. Dluhy

Physicians and physiologists have long known of a connection between hypothyroidism and adrenocortical dysfunction. A potentially important interrelationship was recognized more than 50 years ago in patients with central (secondary) hypothyroidism due to pituitary insufficiency. Treatment of such patients with thyroxine (T_4) without the simultaneous administration of cortisol could exaggerate unrecognized and therefore untreated secondary adrenocortical failure and could result in adrenal crisis if a major stress such as surgery or sepsis supervened.[1] This observation is best explained by thyroid hormone–induced stimulation of the metabolism of cortisol and other adrenocortical steroids[2,3] (see chap 45). If the cortisol pool is small and the pituitary-adrenal system is atrophic, then compensation may be inadequate.

EFFECTS OF HYPOTHYROIDISM ON CORTISOL PRODUCTION AND CLEARANCE

Cortisol secretion and metabolism are decreased in patients with both primary and secondary hypothyroidism. As a result, their serum cortisol concentrations and urinary cortisol excretion are normal.[4] In contrast, the urinary excretion of cortisol metabolites and of 17-ketosteroids is low, reflecting the decreased hepatic clearance of cortisol and adrenal androgens.[2,3] Treatment with T_4 increases the hepatic clearance of these steroids to normal. As cortisol clearance increases and serum cortisol concentrations decline, adrenocorticotropin (ACTH) secretion increases, resulting in increases in steroid production. The serum concentrations of cortisol and other adrenal steroids remain normal, owing to the intact feedback relationship.

EFFECTS OF HYPOTHYROIDISM ON PITUITARY-ADRENAL FUNCTION

Pituitary-adrenal responses to administration of metyrapone or insulin-induced hypoglycemia are normal or slightly decreased in patients with primary hypothyroidism,[5] the responses tending to be more abnormal in patients with more severe hypothyroidism.[6] Similarly, the adrenal response to exogenous ACTH is normal or reduced. In a study of the dynamics of 24-hour cortisol secretion in patients with primary hypothyroidism, the mean 24-hour serum cortisol concentration was slightly elevated, the circadian rhythmicity of serum cortisol was normal, and cortisol clearance was slowed; the calculated endogenous production rate of cortisol was normal.[4] Serum corticosteroid-binding globulin (CBG) concentrations also were normal in these patients. Most of the abnormalities were not fully reversed after T_4 therapy for 6 months, but many of the patients still had high serum thyrotropin (TSH) concentrations at that time. The mild hypercortisolemia in these hypothyroid patients in the setting of normal endogenous cortisol production is consistent with a decrease in the negative feedback effect of cortisol on corticotropin-releasing hormone (CRH) or ACTH secretion. Other evidence of hypothalamic dysfunction in hypothyroidism is the finding of an exaggerated ACTH response to ovine CRH.[7]

In sum, patients with primary hypothyroidism have subtle abnormalities of pituitary-adrenal function that may be correlated with the severity and duration of their hypothyroidism. However, while cortisol is secreted and disposed of at a rate that is slower than normal, the quantity available to peripheral tissues is normal. Thus, basal pituitary-adrenal function and the adrenocortical response to stress are normal.

This formulation explains the usual absence of signs of adrenocortical insufficiency in patients with primary hypothyroidism. The theoretic possibility has been raised that vigorous T_4 treatment in the setting of severe hypothyroidism might induce adrenocortical insufficiency.[2,3] In practice, this does not occur unless severe secondary adrenal deficiency is also present.[1]

EFFECTS OF HYPOTHYROIDISM ON THE RENIN-ANGIOTENSIN-ALDOSTERONE SYSTEM

Thyroid hormone affects most components of the renin-angiotensin-aldosterone system including the secretion of renin,[9,10] the hepatic production of angiotensinogen,[11] serum angiotensin-converting enzyme activity,[12] and the adrenal production and metabolism of aldosterone.[13,14] The dominant effect is on the hepatic degradation of aldosterone, similar to that described for cortisol (see earlier); this decrease in the hepatic clearance of aldosterone results in an increase in its plasma half-life.[2,13–15] The reduced rate of clearance of aldosterone is balanced by a lower secretion rate, so that serum aldosterone concentrations are normal and there is no clinical evidence of hyperaldosteronism. Independently, angiotensinogen production by the liver is decreased,[11] as are serum angiotensin-converting enzyme concentrations[12] and plasma renin activity.[10] In spite of these multiple effects of hypothyroidism, its overall effects on the renin-angiotensin-aldosterone system are minimal and are not responsible for alterations in sodium and potassium homeostasis[9] or the hypertension that occurs in some hypothyroid patients (see chaps 62 and 64).

POLYGLANDULAR AUTOIMMUNE SYNDROMES

Schmidt's Syndrome

In 1926, Schmidt reported two patients who died of Addison's disease and were found at autopsy to have bilateral nontuberculous atrophy of the adrenal cortex and lymphocytic infiltration of the thyroid with a normal pituitary gland.[16] Neither patient was deemed hypothyroid, but Schmidt believed that both would have become hypothyroid if they had survived long enough. He based this speculation on what he thought to be the progressive character of the thyroid lesion, which resembled what is now known as chronic autoimmune thyroiditis, and his paper emphasizes his conviction that the pathologic nature of the lesions in the thyroid and adrenal was the same.[16]

Many reports subsequently documented the coincidence of primary adrenocortical insufficiency and primary hypothyroidism, and the combination has come to be known as Schmidt's syndrome.[17,18] This syndrome is more common in women, most of whom are in the age range of 20 to 50 years; there is strong evidence for a genetic predisposition to and an autoimmune basis for this syndrome.[17–22] For example, thyroid involvement occurs nine times more often in patients with idiopathic (autoimmune) Addison's disease than in those with tuberculous Addison's disease,[18] and the histopathologic features of the thyroid and adrenal lesions in Schmidt's syndrome resemble those of experimental autoimmune thyroiditis and

adrenalitis. However, because the syndrome often occurs with other autoimmune endocrine deficits, such as insulin-dependent diabetes mellitus and primary ovarian failure,[20,21] it probably should be viewed as one phenotype within the type-II polyglandular failure syndrome (see following).

Some patients with idiopathic Addison's disease have slightly high serum TSH concentrations and serologic evidence of chronic autoimmune thyroiditis. In them, glucocorticoid replacement therapy results in normalization of TSH secretion,[23,24] probably because even normal amounts of glucocorticoid reduce the intensity of chronic autoimmune thyroiditis and allow an increase in thyroid secretion. The clinical importance of this phenomenon is that a patient presenting with idiopathic Addison's disease and a slightly high serum TSH concentration before T_4 therapy is initiated should be treated with adrenal replacement therapy alone, with subsequent reassessment of thyroid function. However, if the patient has symptoms and signs of hypothyroidism, a higher serum TSH concentration (>20 µU/mL) and a low serum T_4 concentration, a diagnosis of Schmidt's syndrome is presumed and both thyroid and adrenal replacement therapy should be instituted at the outset.

Type-I and Type-II Polyglandular Autoimmune Syndromes

Two distinct polyglandular autoimmune syndromes have been described.[25–29] The type-I syndrome consists of at least two of the triad of Addison's disease, hypoparathyroidism, and chronic mucocutaneous candidiasis; associated autoimmune disorders, such as chronic autoimmune thyroiditis, pernicious anemia, malabsorption, and alopecia universalis, may also be present. This rare syndrome usually presents with persistent candidiasis during infancy, with the associated autoimmune disorders usually appearing before puberty. The more common type-II syndrome consists of Addison's disease with chronic autoimmune thyroiditis (Schmidt's syndrome), insulin-dependent diabetes mellitus, primary hypogonadism (especially in women), and several other autoimmune diseases, but no hypoparathyroidism or candidiasis. In contrast to the type-I syndrome, the type-II syndrome usually occurs in young or middle-aged women.

The range of autoimmune disorders that have been reported in association with Addison's disease is shown in Table 69-1, and the differences between the type-I and type-II forms of polyglandular autoimmune disease are shown in Table 69-2. There is considerable genetic heterogeneity in both disorders. The type-I syndrome can occur in both sporadic and familial (autosomal recessive) forms; there is no association with any specific HLA antigens. The type-II syndrome is most often familial (autosomal dominant) and has distinct HLA associations (Table 69-2). The humoral autoantibodies that occur in many patients with either syndrome may themselves have cytotoxic properties, or they may inhibit tropic hormone actions on their target glands.[26,27,29–32]

The clinical importance of these findings is clear. If a single autoimmune endocrine disease is discovered, another may appear later. Antibodies in serum may precede the onset of clinical disease. Thus, the clinician should monitor patients with hypothyroidism caused by chronic autoimmune thyroiditis for these other disorders, especially if there is a family history of endocrine deficiency.

TABLE 69-1.

Associated Autoimmune Disorders in 295 Patients* with Type I or Type II Polyglandular Autoimmune Syndrome Who Had Addison's Disease

Associated Entity	No.	%	Females	Males	Female/Male Ratio
Chronic autoimmune thyroiditis	162	55	112	50	2.2
Insulin-dependent diabetes mellitus	118	40	66	52	1.3
Hypoparathyroidism	54	18	33	21	1.6
Chronic mucocutaneous candidiasis	52	15	29	23	1.3
Alopecia	24	8	14	10	1.4
Primary hypogonadism	20	7	15	5	3.0
Vitiligo	16	5	8	8	1.0
Intestinal malabsorption	16	5	6	10	0.6
Pernicious anemia	10	3	4	6	0.7
Chronic active hepatitis	9	3	6	3	2.0

*183 females and 112 males.
From reference 29.

GLUCOCORTICOIDS, THYROID DISEASE, AND THYROID FUNCTION

When replacement doses of a glucocorticoid are given to patients with primary or secondary hypothyroidism, signs of Cushing's syndrome may appear[33,34] because of the hypothyroidism-induced decrease in cortisol clearance.[2] This finding explains the observation that patients with hypothyroidism are more susceptible than euthyroid subjects to the untoward effects of glucocorticoid therapy. This clinical state of relative hyperadrenocorticism abates when thyroid hormone is given

TABLE 69-2.

Clinical Characteristics of Patients with Type I and Type II Polyglandular Autoimmune Syndrome

	Type I	Type II
Age at onset	Childhood	Adult life
Female/male ratio	1.4–1.7	1.8
HLA associations	None	B8, Dw3, DR3
Disease components (% of patients)		
Addison's disease	100	60–67
Chronic autoimmune thyroiditis	10–12	70
Diabetes mellitus	2–4	50–52
Primary hypogonadism	5–50	12–45
Pernicious anemia	1	13–16
Vitiligo	4–9	4.5
Hypoparathyroidism	82–89	None
Chronic mucocutaneous candidiasis	73–78	None
Alopecia	20–32	Undetermined
Chronic active hepatitis	11–13	None
Malabsorption syndrome	22–25	None
Myasthenia gravis	None	Undetermined

From reference 26.

and the normal rate of metabolism of not only cortisol but also synthetic glucocorticoids is restored.[2,33,34]

Hyperadrenocorticism

Patients with either endogenous or exogenous Cushing's syndrome have multiple abnormalities in pituitary-thyroid function (see below). These changes are more biochemically evident than clinically important, and they disappear after the Cushing's syndrome is treated or the exogenous glucocorticoid is discontinued. Glucocorticoid excess may also suppress chronic autoimmune thyroiditis, and it may become evident as hypothyroidism or goiter after reversal of the glucocorticoid excess.[35] In addition, pharmacologic doses of glucocorticoids ameliorate thyrotoxicosis in patients with silent thyroiditis or Graves' disease. In summary, the anti-inflammatory or immunosuppressive actions of glucocorticoids can ameliorate both thyrotoxicosis and hypothyroidism when the underlying cause is thyroid autoimmune disease.

Effects of Glucocorticoids on Thyroid Function

Pharmacologic amounts of glucocorticoids have multiple reversible effects on pituitary-thyroid function. They include inhibition of TSH secretion[36]; decreased serum thyroxine-binding globulin (TBG) concentrations[37]; inhibition of extrathyroidal conversion of T_4 to triiodothyronine (T_3)[38,39]; and an increase in the renal clearance of iodide[40] (Table 69-3). Thus, serum TSH, TBG, T_4, and T_3 concentrations are slightly decreased, albeit usually within the respective ranges of normal; serum free T_4 values are normal. With respect to TSH secretion, the effect of glucocorticoids is to decrease the amplitude of TSH pulses, probably by inhibiting the secretion of thyrotropin-releasing hormone (TRH)[41] (see also chap 12). There is in time escape from glucocorticoid-induced suppression of TSH secretion, which is why patients with either exogenous or endogenous Cushing's syndrome have serum free T_4 concentrations within

TABLE 69-3.
Effects of Glucocorticoids on Pituitary–thyroid Function

Inhibition of TSH secretion

Decrease in serum thyroxine-binding globulin concentrations

Inhibition of extrathyroidal conversion of T_4 to T_3

Increase in renal iodide clearance

the normal range. The increase in renal clearance of iodide is modest and does not materially affect iodide availability unless dietary intake is limited.

References

1. Means JH, Hertz S, Lerman J. The pituitary type of myxedema or Simmonds' disease masquerading as myxedema. Trans Assoc Am Physicians 1940;55:32

2. Peterson RE. The influence of the thyroid on adrenal cortical function. J Clin Invest 1958;37:736

3. Peterson RE. The miscible pool and turnover rate of adrenocortical steroids in man. Recent Prog Horm Res 1959;15:231

4. Iranmanesh A, Lizarralde G, Johnson ML, Veldhuis JD. Dynamics of 24-hour endogenous cortisol secretion and clearance in primary hypothyroidism assessed before and after partial thyroid hormone replacement. J Clin Endocrinol Metab 1990;70:155

5. Ridgway EC, McCammon JA, Benotti J, Maloof F. Acute metabolic responses in myxedema to large doses of intravenous L-thyroxine. Ann Intern Med 1972;77:549

6. Bigos ST, Ridgway EC, Kourides IA, Maloof F. Spectrum of pituitary alterations with mild and severe thyroid impairment. J Clin Endocrinol Metab 1978;46:317

7. Kamilaris TC, DeBold CR, Pavlou SN, et al. Effect of altered thyroid hormone levels on hypothalamic-pituitary adrenal function. J Clin Endocrinol Metab 1987;65:994

8. Turnbridge WMG, Marshall JC, Burke CW. Primary hypothyroidism presenting as pituitary failure. BMJ 1973;1:153

9. Cain JP, Dluhy, RG, Williams GH, Selenkow HA, Milech A, Richmond S. Control of aldosterone secretion in hyperthyroidism. J Clin Endocrinol Metab 1973;36:365

10. Resnick LM, Laragh JH. Plasma renin activity in syndromes of thyroid hormone excess and deficiency. Life Sci 1982;30:585

11. Deschepper CF, Hong-Brown LQ. Hormonal regulation of the angiotensinogen gene in liver and other tissues. In: Raizada MK, Phillips MI, Sumners C. eds. Cellular and molecular biology of renin-angiotensin system. Boca Raton, FL: CRC Press, 1993;152

12. Brent GA, Hershman JM, Reed AW, Sastre A, Lieberman J. Serum angiotensin-converting enzyme in severe nonthyroidal illnesses associated with low serum thyroxine concentration. Ann Intern Med 1984;100:680

13. Luetscher JA Jr, Camargo CA, Cohen AP, et al. Observations on metabolism of aldosterone in man. Ann Intern Med 1963;59:1

14. Luetscher JA Jr, Lieberman AH. Aldosterone. Arch Intern Med 1958;102:314

15. Peterson RE. Metabolism of adrenocorticoids in man. Ann NY Acad Sci 1959;82:846

16. Schmidt MB. Eine biglandulare Erkrankung (Nebennieren und Schild-druse) bei Morbus Addisonii. Verh Dtsch Ges Pathol 1926;21:212

17. Bloodworth JMB Jr, Kirkendall WM, Carr TL. Addison's disease associated with thyroid insufficiency and atrophy (Schmidt syndrome). J Clin Endocrinol Metab 1954;14:540

18. Carpenter CCJ, Solomon N, Silverberg SG, et al. Schmidt's syndrome (thyroid and adrenal insufficiency): a review of the litera-ture and a report of fifteen new cases including ten instances of co-existent diabetes mellitus. Medicine 1964;43:153

19. Blizzard RM, Kyle M. Studies of the adrenal antigens and antibodies in Addison's disease. J Clin Invest 1963;42:1653

20. Edmonds M, Lamki L, Killinger DW, Volpe R. Autoimmune thyroiditis, adrenalitis, and oophoritis. Am J Med 1973;54:782

21. Spinner MW, Blizzard RM, Childs B. Clinical and genetic heterogeneity in idiopathic Addison's disease and hypoparathyroidism. J Clin Endocrinol Metab 1968;28:795

22. Strakosch CR, Wenzel BE, Row VV, Volpe R. Immunology of autoimmune thyroid diseases. N Engl J Med 1982;307:1499

23. Gharib H, Hodgson SF, Gastineau CF, et al. Reversible hypothyroidism in Addison's disease. Lancet 1972;2:734

24. Topliss DJ, White EL, Stockigt JR. Significance of thyrotropin excess in untreated primary adrenal insufficiency. J Clin Endocrinol Metab 1980;50:52

25. Ahonen P, Myllaruiemi DDS, Sipila I, Perheentupa J. Clinical variation of autoimmune polyendocrinopathy-candidiasis-ectodermal dystrophy (APECED) in a series of 68 patients. N Engl J Med 1990;322:1829

26. Leor J, Levartowsky D, Sharon C. Polyglandular autoimmune syndrome, Type 2. South Med J 1989;82:374

27. Meyerson J, Lechuga-Gomez EE, Bigazzi PE, Walfish PG. Polyglandular autoimmune syndrome: current concepts. Can Med Assoc J 1988;138:605

28. Neufeld M, Maclaren NK, Blizzard RM. Autoimmune polyglandular syndrome. Pediatr Ann 1980;9:154

29. Neufeld M, Maclaren NK, Blizzard RM. Two types of autoimmune Addison's disease associated with different polyglandular autoimmune (PGA) syndromes. Medicine 1981;60:355

30. Bigazzi PE. Autoimmune thyroid disease. In: Rose NR, Mackey IR, eds. The autoimmune diseases. New York: Academic Press, 1985:161

31. Bigazzi PE. Autoimmunity of the adrenals. In: Volpe R, ed. Autoimmunity and endocrine diseases. New York: Marcel Dekker, 1985:345

32. Volpe R. The role of autoimmunity in hypoendocrine and hyperendocrine function. Ann Intern Med 1977;87:86

33. Howard JE, Migeon CJ. Cushing's syndrome produced by normal replacement doses of cortisone in a patient with defective mechanism for steroid degradation. Am J Med Sci 1958;235:387

34. Parfitt AM. Cushing's syndrome with normal replacement dose of cortisone in pituitary hypothyroidism. J Clin Endocrinol Metab 1964;24:560

35. Takasu N, Komiya I, Nagasawa Y, Asawa T, Yamada T. Exacerbation of autoimmune thyroid dysfunction after unilateral adrenalectomy in patients with Cushing's syndrome due to an adrenocortical adenoma. N Engl J Med 1990;322:1708

36. Re RN, Kourides IA, Ridgway EC, et al. The effect of glucocorticoid administration on human pituitary secretion of thyrotropin and prolactin. J Clin Endocrinol Metab 1976;43:338

37. Gamstedt A, Jarnerot G, Kagedal B. Dose related effects of betamethasone on iodothyronines and thyroid hormone-binding proteins in serum. Acta Endocrinol 1981;96:484

38. Chopra IJ, Williams DE, Orgiazzi J, Solomon DH. Opposite effects of dexamethasone on serum concentrations of $3,3'.5'$-triiodothyronine (reverse T_3) and $3,3'.5$-triiodothyronine (T_3). J Clin Endocrinol Metab 1975;41:911

39. Duick DS, Warren DW, Nicoloff JT, et al. Effect of a single dose of dexamethasone on the concentration of serum triiodothyronine in man. J Clin Endocrinol Metab 1974;39:1151

40. Ingbar SH. Effect of cortisone on the thyroidal and renal metabolism of iodine. Endocrinology 1953;53:171

41. Adriaanse R, Brabant G, Endert E, Wiersinga WM. Pulsatile thyrotropin secretion in patients with Cushing's syndrome. Metabolism 1994;43:782

Werner and Ingbar's The Thyroid, Seventh Edition,
edited by Lewis E. Braverman and Robert D. Utiger.
Lippincott–Raven Publishers, Philadelphia, © 1996

70

Catecholamines and the Sympathoadrenal System in Hypothyroidism

J. Enrique Silva

The interactions of thyroid hormones and the sympathoadrenal system have been considered at length in chapter 46. This discussion briefly summarizes those aspects that relate specifically to catecholamines and hypothyroidism.

Hypothyroidism influences the sympathetic nervous system basically in a direction opposite to that of thyrotoxicosis. At the cell and tissue levels, the responses to catecholamines are reduced, whereas the central sympathetic output reaching the tissues is in general enhanced. The mechanisms leading to decreased responsiveness or sensitivity to catecholamines vary according to tissue and species. These mechanisms include: reduced number of β- and increased number of α-adrenergic receptors[1]; enhanced inhibitory responses to adenosine,[2–4] probably related to increases in $G_a i$- or G_β-protein subunits[5–8]; enhanced phosphodiesterase activity[9]; and lack of triiodothyronine (T_3) potentiation of cAMP effects at the gene level.[10–12] A novel β-adrenergic receptor, the β_3-receptor, is receiving much attention (see reference 13 for review). This receptor is coupled to adenylyl cyclase via Gs proteins, as are its β_1 and β_2 counterparts, and is abundantly expressed in brown adipose tissue and less so in white adipose tissue. This receptor and its mRNA are increased in brown adipose tissue of hypothyroid rats and are rapidly reduced by T_3,[14] adding another bit of complexity to the intricate thyroid-adrenergic interactions. The α_2-adrenergic pathway, which causes inhibition of cAMP production by coupling to G_i proteins, is little affected by thyroid dysfunction.[15,16]

In hypothyroidism, in contrast to the overall depression of the adrenergic responses at the peripheral level, there is an increase in efferent sympathetic activity reaching virtually every tissue.[17–22] The clearance of norepinephrine is not altered, and the overall production rate of norepinephrine is higher than normal.[18,23] Accordingly, plasma norepinephrine concentrations are elevated in hypothyroid patients.[24–27] Furthermore, the increase in production rate is selective for norepinephrine; epinephrine production is not affected.[28] The increase in sympathetic activity appears to be compensatory in nature, and may come about in response to the deficient peripheral responses to catecholamines, the thermal stress derived from the lack of the calorigenic effect of thyroid hormone, the reduction in cardiac output, or from the lack of T_3 in critical regulatory centers of the central nervous system. Some of the abnormalities in the norepinephrine signal pathway in hypothyroidism may not be directly caused by the lack of thyroid hormone in the tissues but by the increased sympathetic tone; that is, they may represent desensitization. Thus, the reduced β_1- and β_2-adrenergic receptors in brown adipose tissue are normalized in athyreotic rats when sympathetic activity is ameliorated by placing them at 30°C, whereas the number of these receptors decreases in euthyroid rats placed at 4°C.[29] Desensitization at a post-receptor level has also been described in brown adipose tissue in cold-exposed hamsters.[30]

Severely hypothyroid patients may develop hypothermia and myxedema coma after exposure to low environmental temperatures or medications that compromise heat conservation. Thermogenesis is markedly reduced in these patients: obligatory thermogenesis because of the slow rate of metabolism,[31] and facultative thermogenesis because of the diminished response to catecholamines and limited substrate availability ensuing from the lack of thyroid hormone. In hypothyroid rats, brown adipose tissue, the main site of facultative thermogenesis, does not respond to cold exposure, exogenous norepinephrine, or nerve stimulation.[32–37] In humans with hypothyroidism, the metabolic responses to adrenergic stimulation involved in facultative thermogenesis, such as glycogenolysis, lipolysis, gluconeogenesis, and intracellular calcium mobilization, are reduced.[31,38–42] Reduced heat loss through the skin becomes an essential mechanism for hypothyroid patients to maintain their body temperature. These patients have intense skin and subcutaneous tissue vasoconstriction[43] probably caused by elevated sympathetic tone[44] and increased α_1-adrenergic receptors,[1] but the vascular response to exogenous catecholamines or nerve stimulation is reduced.[45,46] This suggests that peripheral vasculature is maximally stimulated, although post-receptor defects in the α-adrenergic pathway may be a contributory factor.[40] In the clinical situation of severe, profound hypothyroidism, therefore, it would seem more prudent to treat the thyroid insufficiency as aggressively as possible, provide glucose and other supportive treatment, and not to rely on catecholamines to improve hemodynamic status or thermogenesis.

In addition to the depressed peripheral vascular response to α_1-adrenergic agonists, the responsiveness of the heart to catecholamines is markedly reduced in hypothyroidism. Although this is caused primarily by a reduced number of β-adrenergic receptors in the myocardium,[1] there is evidence to indicate important post-receptor defects as well.[4,7,47,48] Even though sympathetic stimulation of the heart is increased in hypothyroidism,[20,22] the contractility[49] and functional reserve of the heart[45] are severely compromised because of both the direct biochemical consequences of the lack of thyroid hormone and the reduced sympathetic responsiveness. This condition can easily become clinically important if there is bleeding, contraction of the extracellular volume, or a decrease in peripheral vascular resistance, as may occur when patients with severe hypothyroidism are rapidly rewarmed. Likewise, volume or pressure overloads may precipitate congestive heart failure. The solutions to such problems are to avoid situations that require important hemodynamic adjustments and to provide thyroid hormone as rapidly as possible. Since the heart has little thyroxine (T_4)-5′-deiodinase activity, and since T_4 to T_3 conversion by type-I T_4-5′-deiodinase is generally reduced in hypothyroidism (see chaps 7 and 8), hypothyroid patients with severely depressed myocardial function may need to be given small doses of T_3 in addition to T_4 to accelerate the recovery of the heart (see chap 75).

A number of metabolic abnormalities are also caused by the negative effect of hypothyroidism in several signal transduction pathways. Lipolytic responses to catecholamines and glucagon are decreased, largely because of post-receptor defects in the cAMP cascade in both animals and humans.[8,41,50,51] Muscle and liver glycogenolysis are also reduced, in part because of defects in the β-adrenergic-cAMP pathway and Ca^{2+} mobilization.[40,52] Insulin secretory responses are diminished, owing in part to defects in the cAMP signaling pathway.[53,54] Gluconeogenic responses to glucagon and epinephrine are also limited in hypothyroidism, because of defects in the cAMP cascade and because of the lack of thyroid hormone action at the level of the phosphoenolpyruvate carboxykinase gene.[11,55] Regardless of its importance as a site of thermogenesis in adult humans, brown adipose tissue has been a good model to unravel adrenergic-thyroid interactions. As mentioned previously, brown adipose tissue is under maximal adrenergic stimulation in hypothyroid rats, yet its responses are dramatically depressed.[10,37,56,57] The lipolytic, respiratory,[58] and uncoupling protein responses to catecholamines and cAMP are also decreased in brown adipocytes from hypothyroid rats.[59] In spite of a clear reduction in β_1 and β_2-adrenergic receptors[60] and in cAMP accumulation,[29,61] these defects do not seem to account for much of the reduced uncoupling protein responses since, by the time thyroid hormone administration has completely restored the response of this protein to norepinephrine, neither the receptor number nor cAMP production has been normalized.[10,29,37] Rather, the dominant defect in thermogenic responses to adrenergic stimulation in brown adipose tissue of hypothyroid rats seems to be distal to the generation of cAMP.[10,12,58]

Thyroid hormone is also important for the development of the sympathetic nervous system. Congenital hypothyroidism results in numerous and ubiquitous abnormalities of the sympathoadrenal system. These include the receptors and signaling pathways as well as enzymes involved in the synthesis of catecholamines.[62–66]

References

1. Bilezikian JP, Loeb JN. The influence of hyperthyroidism and hyperthyroidism on α- and β-adrenergic receptor systems and adrenergic responsiveness. Endocr Rev 1983;4:378

2. Bumgarner JR, Ramkumar V, Stiles GL. Altered thyroid status regulates the adipocyte A_1 adenosine receptor-adenylate cyclase system. Life Sci 1989;44:1705

3. Woodward JA, Saggerson ED. Effect of adenosine deaminase, N6-phenylisopropyladenosine and hypothyroidism on the responsiveness of rat brown adipocytes to noradrenaline. Biochem J 1986;238:395

4. Kaasik A, Seppet EK, Ohisalo JJ. Enhanced negative inotropic effect of an adenosine A1-receptor agonist in rat left atria in hypothyroidism. J Mol Cell Cardiol 1994;26:509

5. Michel-Reher MB, Gross G, Jasper JR, et al. Tissue- and subunit-specific regulation of G-protein expression by hypo- and hyperthyroidism. Biochem Pharmacol 1993;45:1417

6. Orford MR, Leung FCL, Milligan G, Saggerson ED. Treatment with triiodothyronine decreases the abundance of the α-subunits of G_i1 and G_i2 in the cerebral cortex. J Neurol Sci 1992;112:34

7. Levine MA, Feldman AM, Robishaw JD, et al. Influence of thyroid hormone status on expression of genes encoding G protein subunits in rat heart. J Biol Chem 1990;265:3553

8. Rapiejko PJ, Watkins DC, Ros M, Malbon CC. Thyroid hormones regulate G-protein β-subunit mRNA expression in vivo. J Biol Chem 1989;264:16183

9. Goswami A, Rosenberg IN. Effects of thyroid status on membrane-bound low K_m cyclic nucleotide phosphodiesterase activities in rat adipocytes. J Biol Chem 1985;260:82

10. Bianco AC, Sheng X, Silva JE. Triiodothyronine amplifies norepinephrine stimulation of uncoupling protein gene transcription by a mechanism not requiring protein synthesis. J Biol Chem 1988;263:18168

11. Giralt M, Park EA, Gurney AL, Liu J, Hakimi P, Hanson RW. Identification of a thyroid hormone response element in the phosphoenolpyruvate carboxykinase (GTP) gene. Evidence for synergistic interaction between thyroid hormone and cAMP cis-regulatory elements. J Biol Chem 1991;266:21991

12. Rabelo R, Schifman A, Rubio A, Sheng X, Silva JE. Delineation of thyroid hormone responsive sequences within a critical en-

hancer in the rat uncoupling protein gene. Endocrinology 1995;136:1003

13. Emorine LJ, Feve B, Pairault J, et al. Structural basis for functional diversity of β_1-, β_2-, and β_3-adrenergic receptors. Biochem Pharmacol 1991;41:853

14. Rubio A, Raasmaja A, Silva JE. Thyroid hormone and norepinephrine signaling in brown adipose tissue: differential effects of thyroid hormone on β_3-adrenergic receptors in brown and white adipose tissue. Endocrinology 1995;136:3277

15. Del Rio G, Zizzo G, Marrama P, Venneri MG, Della Casa L, Velardo A. Alpha 2-adrenergic activity is normal in patients with thyroid disease. Clin Endocrinol 1994;40:235

16. Richelsen B, Sorensen NS. Alpha 2- and beta-adrenergic receptor binding and action in gluteal adipocytes from patients with hypothyroidism and hyperthyroidism. Metabolism 1987;36:1031

17. Gross G, Lues I. Thyroid-dependent alterations of myocardial adrenoceptors and adrenoceptor-mediated responses in the rat. Naunyn Schmiedebergs Arch Pharmacol 1985;329:427

18. Polikar R, Kennedy B, Ziegler M, O'Connor DT, Smith J, Nicod P. Plasma norepinephrine kinetics, dopamine-beta-hydroxylase, and chromogranin-A in hypothyroid patients before and following replacement therapy. J Clin Endocrinol Metab 1990;70:277

19. Gripois D, Valens M. Uptake and turnover rate of norepinephrine in interscapular brown adipose tissue of the young rat. Influence of hypothyroidism. Biol Neonate 1982;42:113

20. Tu T, Nash CW. The influence of prolonged hyper- and hypothyroid states on the noradrenaline content of rat tissues and on the accumulation and efflux rates of tritiated noradrenaline. Can J Physiol Pharmacol 1975;53:74

21. Matsukawa T, Mano T, Gotoh E, Minamisawa K, Ishii M. Altered muscle sympathetic nerve activity in hyperthyroidism and hypothyroidism. J Auton Nerv Syst 1993;42:171

22. Landsberg L, Axelrod J. Influence of pituitary, thyroid and adrenal hormones on norepinephrine turnover and metabolism in the rat heart. Circ Res 1968;22:559

23. Coulombe P, Dussault JH. Catecholamine metabolism in thyroid disease. II. Norepinephrine secretion rate in hyperthyroidism and hypothyroidism. J Clin Endocrinol Metab 1977;44:1185

24. Christensen NJ. Plasma noradrenaline and adrenaline in patients with thyrotoxicosis and myxoedema. Clin Sci 1973;45:163

25. Manhem P, Bramnert M, Hallengren B, Lecerof H, Werner R. Increased arterial and venous plasma noradrenaline levels in patients with primary hypothyroidism during hypothyroid as compared to euthyroid state. J Endocrinol Invest 1992;15:763

26. Brown RT, Lakshmanan MC, Baucom CE, Polinsky RJ. Changes in blood pressure and plasma noradrenaline in short-term hypothyroidism. Clin Endocrinol 1989;30:635

27. Coulombe P, Dussault JH, Walker P. Plasma catecholamine concentrations in hyperthyroidism and hypothyroidism. Metabolism 1976;25:973

28. Coulombe P, Dussault JH, Letarte J, Simard SJ. Catecholamine metabolism in thyroid diseases. I. Epinephrine secretion rate in hyperthyroidism and hypothyroidism. J Clin Endocrinol Metab 1976;42:125

29. Rubio A, Raasmaja A, Maia AL, Kim KR, Silva JE. Effects of thyroid hormone on norepinephrine signaling in brown adipose tissue. I. B_1-and B_2 adrenergic receptors and cyclic adenosine 3′ 5′-monophosphate generation. Endocrinology 1995;136:3267

30. Svoboda P, Unelius L, Cannon B, Nedergaard J. Attenuation of $G_s\alpha$ coupling efficiency in brown-adipose-tissue plasma membranes from cold-acclimated hamsters. Biochem J 1993;295:655

31. Sestoft L. Metabolic aspects of the calorigenic effect of thyroid hormone in mammals. Clin Endocrinol 1980;13:489

32. Seydoux J, Giacobino J, Girardier L. Impaired metabolic response to nerve stimulation in brown adipose tissue of hypothyroid rats. Mol Cell Endocrinol 1982;25:213

33. Triandafillou J, Gwilliam C, Himms-Hagen J. Role of thyroid hormone in cold-induced changes in rat brown adipose tissue mitochondria. Can J Biochem 1982;60:530

34. Mory G, Ricquier D, Pesquies P, Hemon P. Effects of hypothyroidism on the brown adipose tissue of adult rats: comparison with the effects of adaptation to the cold. J Endocrinol 1981;91:515

35. Carvalho SD, Kimura ET, Bianco AC, Silva JE. Central role of brown adipose tissue thyroxine 5′-deiodinase on thyroid hormone-dependent thermogenic response to cold. Endocrinology 1991;128:2149

36. Bianco AC, Silva JE. Intracellular conversion of thyroxine to triiodothyronine is required for the optimal thermogenic function of brown adipose tissue. J Clin Invest 1987;79:295

37. Silva JE. Full expression of uncoupling protein gene requires the concurrence of norepinephrine and triiodothyronine. Mol Endocrinol 1988;2:706

38. Clausen T, van Hardeveld C, Everts ME. Significance of cation transport in control of energy metabolism and thermogenesis. Physiol Rev 1991;71:733

39. Leijendeckker WJ, van Hardeveld C, Elzinga G. Heat production during contraction in skeletal muscle of hypothyroid mice. Am J Physiol 1987;253:E124

40. Storm H, van Hardeveld C. Effect of thyroid hormone on intracellular Ca^{2+} mobilization by noradrenaline and vasopressin in relation to glycogenolysis in rat liver. Biochim Biophys Acta 1985;846:275

41. Wahrenberg H, Wennlund A, Arner P. Adrenergic regulation of lipolysis in fat cells from hyperthyroid and hypothyroid patients. J Clin Endocrinol Metab 1994;78:898

42. McCulloch AJ, Johnston DG, Baylis PH, et al. Evidence that thyroid hormones regulate gluconeogenesis from glycerol in man. Clin Endocrinol 1983;19:67

43. Vagn Nielsen H, Hasselstrom K, Feldt-Rasmussen U, et al. Increased sympathetic tone in forearm subcutaneous tissue in primary hypothyroidism. Clin Physiol 1987;7:297

44. Fagius J, Westermark K, Karlsson A. Baroreflex-governed sympathetic outflow to muscle vasculature is increased in hypothyroidism. Clin Endocrinol 1990;33:177

45. Bramnert M, Hallengren B, Lecerof H, Werner R, Manhem P. Decreased blood pressure response to infused noradrenaline in normotensive as compared to hypertensive patients with primary hypothyroidism. Clin Endocrinol 1994;40:317

46. Polikar R, Kennedy B, Ziegler M, Smith J, Nicod P. Decreased sensitivity to alpha-adrenergic stimulation in hypothyroid patients. J Clin Endocrinol Metab 1990;70:1761

47. Beekman RE, van Hardeveld C, Simonides WS. On the mechanism of the reduction by thyroid hormone of beta-adrenergic relaxation rate stimulation in rat heart. Biochem J 1989;259:229

48. Daly MJ, Dhalla NS. Alterations in the cardiac adenylate cyclase activity in hypothyroid rat. Can J Cardiol 1985;1:288

49. Buccino RA, Spann JF Jr, Pool PE, Sonneblick EH, Braunwald E. Influence of the thyroid state on the intrinsic contractile properties and energy stores of the myocardium. J Clin Invest 1967;46:1669

50. Milligan G, Saggerson ED. Concurrent up-regulation of guanine-nucleotide-binding proteins G_i1 alpha, G_i2 alpha and G_i3 alpha in adipocytes of hypothyroid rats. Biochem J 1990;270:765

51. Saggerson ED. Sensitivity of adipocyte lipolysis to stimulatory and inhibitory agonists in hypothyroidism and starvation. Biochem J 1986;238:387

52. Chu DT, Shikama H, Khatra BS, Exton JH. Effects of altered thyroid status on beta-adrenergic actions on skeletal muscle glycogen metabolism. J Biol Chem 1985;260:9994

53. Diaz GB, Paladini AA, Garcia ME, Gagliardino JJ. Changes induced by hypothyroidism in insulin secretion and in the proper-

ties of islet plasma membranes. Arch Int Physiol Biochim Biophys 1993;101:263

54. Young JB, Landsberg L. Catecholamines and the regulation of hormone secretion. Clin Endocrinol Metab 1977;6:657

55. Hoppner W, Sussmuth W, Seitz HJ. Effect of thyroid state on cyclic AMP-mediated induction of hepatic phosphoenolpyruvate carboxykinase. Biochem J 1985;226:67

56. Arieli A, Chinet A. Brown adipose tissue heat production in heat acclimated and perchlorate treated rats. Horm Metab Res 1985;17:12

57. Ilyes I, Stock MJ. Thermogenic responses to selective and nonselective beta-adrenergic agonists in hypothyroidism of Sprague-Dawley rats. Acta Physiol Hung 1991;78:293

58. Sundin U, Mills I, Fain JN. Thyroid-catecholamine interactions in isolated brown adipocytes. Metabolism 1984;33:1028

59. Bianco AC, Kieffer JD, Silva JE. Adenosine 3′,5′-monophosphate and thyroid hormone control of uncoupling protein messenger ribonucleic acid in freshly dispersed brown adipocytes. Endocrinology 1992;130:2625

60. Revelli J, Pescini R, Muzzin P, et al. Changes in β_1- and β_2-adrenergic receptor mRNA levels in brown adipose tissue and heart of hypothyroid rats. Biochem J 1991;277:625

61. Raasmaja A, Larsen PR. α_1- and β-Adrenergic agents cause synergistic stimulation of the iodothyronine deiodinase in rat brown adipocytes. Endocrinology 1989;125:2502

62. Pracyk JB, Slotkin TA. Thyroid hormone regulates ontogeny of *beta* adrenergic receptors and adenylate cyclase in rat heart and kidney: Effects of propylthiouracil-induced perinatal hypothyroidism. J Pharmacol Exp Ther 1992;261:951

63. Blouquit MF, Gripois D. Norepinephrine and dopamine content in the brown adipose tissue of developing eu- and hypothyroid rats. Horm Metab Res 1991;23:326

64. Blouquit MF, Gripois D. Activity of enzymes involved in norepinephrine biosynthesis in the brown adipose tissue of the developing rat. Influence of hypothyroidism. Horm Metab Res 1990;22:423

65. Diarra A, Lefauconnier JM, Valens M, Georges P, Gripois D. Tyrosine content, influx and accumulation rate, and catecholamine biosynthesis measured in vivo, in the central nervous system and in peripheral organs of the young rat. Influence of neonatal hypo- and hyperthyroidism. Arch Int Physiol Biochim 1989;97:317

66. Gripois D, Valens M, Richter P, Genermont J. Adrenal dopamine content of the developing rat. Influence of the thyroid status and insulin-hypoglycaemia. J Auton Nerv Syst 1987;21:181

Werner and Ingbar's The Thyroid, Seventh Edition,
edited by Lewis E. Braverman and Robert D. Utiger.
Lippincott–Raven Publishers, Philadelphia, © 1996

71

The Male and Female Reproductive Systems in Hypothyroidism

Christopher Longcope

HYPOTHYROIDISM IN THE FEMALE REPRODUCTIVE SYSTEM

Hypothyroidism seems to affect the reproductive system in women more than in men. A review of the normal development and physiology of the female reproductive system has been given in chapter 47.

Animal Studies

In sheep, fetal hypothyroidism does not affect reproductive tract development but does result in prolonged gestation despite maternal euthyroidism.[1] However, in the rat, fetal hypothyroidism results in small ovaries deficient in lipid and cholesterol.[2] Thyroidectomy of sexually immature rats results in delayed vaginal opening and sexual maturation; smaller ovaries and follicles than in controls[3,4]; and uteri and vaginas that are not well developed.[5]

When adult female rats are rendered hypothyroid their estrous cycles become irregular and their ovaries become atrophic.[6] There is an enhanced response to HCG with the development of large cystic ovaries in hypothyroid rats.[7] Hypothyroidism in hamsters and cows is associated with abnormal estrous cycles,[8,9] and in hypothyroid hens there is a decrease in egg production.[9]

In the mature female rat, hypothyroidism apparently does not result in sterility but does interfere with gestation, especially in the first half of pregnancy,[10] with resorption of the embryo and subsequent reduction in litter size and an increase in stillbirths.[11]

In hypothyroid sheep, the uterus shows endometrial hyperplasia and smooth muscle hypertrophy, perhaps related to the prolonged estrous noted in hypothyroid ewes.[12] Ruh and coworkers[13] reported increased estradiol binding in uteri of hypothyroid rats, but Kirkland and coworkers[14] found a decrease in the uterine response to estrogen in hypothyroid rats.

Hypothyroidism inhibits the photoperiod responses and seasonal breeding patterns in sheep and birds.[15,16]

Human Studies and Clinical Aspects

The reproductive tract appears to develop normally in cretins; thus, hypothyroidism during fetal life does not appear to affect the normal development of the reproductive tract. Hypothyroidism in prepubertal years generally leads to short stature and may lead to a delay in sexual maturity.[4] However, an interesting syndrome described by Kendle[17] and Van Wyk and Grumbach[18] occurs not infrequently: it is characterized by precocious menstruation, galactorrhea, and sella enlargement in girls with juvenile hypothyroidism. The cause is thought to be an overlap in the pituitary production of TSH and gonadotropins, with the latter causing early ovarian secretion of estrogens and subsequent endometrial stimulation with vaginal bleeding. Prolactin levels are elevated, leading to galactorrhea. However, there is no pubertal increase in the adrenal production of androgen precursors, so that axillary and pubic hair are usually not apparent.[18] Therapy with thyroxine in proper dosage results in prompt alleviation of the symptomatology.

In adult women, hypothyroidism results in changes in cycle length and amount of bleeding[19–21] and has been reported

849

in association with the ovarian hyperstimulation syndrome.[22] Menorrhagia is a frequent complaint and is probably due to estrogen breakthrough bleeding secondary to anovulation, which is frequent in severe hypothyroidism.[19] The anovulation is reflected in the frequent finding of a proliferative endometrium on endometrial biopsy.[23] TRα-1 and TRβ-1 receptors have been found in human granulosa cells and both triiodothyronine and thyroxine have been found in follicular fluid.[24] Earlier work indicated that thyroxine enhanced the action of gonadotropins on luteinization and progestin secretion by cultured granulosa cells,[25] and it has recently been noted that in a group of infertile women, those with elevated TSH levels had a higher incidence of out-of-phase biopsies than women with normal TSH.[26] Ovulation and conception can occur in mild hypothyroidism, but in the past those pregnancies that did occur were often associated with abortions in the first trimester, stillbirths, or prematurity.[19,27] Recent studies indicate these events may be less common but that gestational hypertension occurs often in pregnant women with untreated hypothyroidism.[28] Pregnancy occurring in women with myxedema has been reported to be uncommon,[27] but this is somewhat hard to document and may be the result of anovulation. The use of L-thyroxine is not helpful in treating euthyroid patients for infertility, menstrual irregularity, or the premenstrual syndrome.[29,30]

In evaluating the thyroid status of the pregnant woman, the level of TSH is probably the best indicator of changes in thyroid function. Because radioiodine will readily cross the placenta and can cause fetal hypothyroidism, tests involving radioiodine administration to the mother are contraindicated in pregnancy.[19] When hypothyroidism is diagnosed during pregnancy, L-thyroxine therapy should be instituted promptly to increase the chances for a normal pregnancy. Although it has been thought that little L-thyroxine would cross the placenta,[19] it appears that L-thyroxine will cross the placenta in modest amounts,[31] at least early in pregnancy. Women who have required thyroid hormone therapy prior to pregnancy should continue with such therapy throughout the pregnancy. However, recent evidence indicates that the hormone dose needs to be increased during pregnancy, even though adequate replacement had been given before conception.[31] It is advisable to monitor the serum TSH concentration at least once during each trimester to ensure that an adequate dose is received. Thyroid disease during and after pregnancy is discussed in detail in chapter 89.

Some myxedematous women will present with amenorrhea and galactorrhea and elevated serum prolactin concentrations.[19] Thus, thyroid evaluation should be an essential part of the work-up in any person with galactorrhea. If hypothyroidism is the cause, the amenorrhea and galactorrhea and elevated serum prolactin will disappear promptly with thyroxine therapy.[32]

There is an increased incidence of Hashimoto's thyroiditis in individuals with Turner's syndrome,[33] and, although a chromosomal linkage between autoimmune disease and the X-chromosome has been suggested, this has not been confirmed.[34] Inherited abnormalities in serum thyroxine-binding globulin (TBG) are X-linked, and patients with Turner's syndrome may have low serum TBG values.[35]

Women with hypothyroidism have decreased metabolic clearance rates of androstenedione and estrone and increased peripheral aromatization.[36] The ratio of 5α/5β metabolites of androgens is decreased in hypothyroid women, and there is an increase in the excretion of estriol and a decrease in the excretion of 2-oxygenated estrogens.[37]

In summary, hypothyroidism in girls can cause alterations in the pubertal process; this is usually a delay, but occasionally it can result in pseudoprecocious puberty. In mature women, hypothyroidism usually is associated with abnormal menstrual cycles, especially anovulatory cycles, and an increase in fetal wastage.

HYPOTHYROIDISM IN THE MALE REPRODUCTIVE SYSTEM

The normal development and physiology of the male reproductive system has been described in chapter 47. Although less common in men than in women, hypothyroidism, induced or spontaneous, affects the male reproductive tract in a number of ways depending, in part, on the age of onset.

Animal Studies

The fetal thyroid starts functioning about the same time as the gonads.[38] Although thyroid hormones play a role in sex differentiation and gonadal maturation in fish and amphibians,[39] they do not appear to be necessary for the normal development of the reproductive tract in mammals.[1]

However, hypothyroidism, induced or occurring soon after birth, is associated with a marked delay in sexual maturation and development.[40] When rats are made hypothyroid with propylthiouracil administered from birth to 24 to 26 days of age, testicular size is decreased, Sertoli cell differentiation is retarded, and the time of Sertoli cell proliferation is prolonged.[41,42] As these rats become older and euthyroid, then the testis size, Sertoli cell number, and sperm production are all increased.[41,42] Leydig cell numbers are increased but testosterone secretion per cell is decreased, although total testosterone secretion remains the same as controls.[43] FSH and LH levels tend to remain low throughout treatment and recovery periods, whereas inhibin levels are elevated.[41]

However, if hypothyroidism persists untreated, there is an arrest of sexual maturity with absent libido and ejaculate.[44] The interstitial cells of the testis are reduced in number and the arrested growth of the accessory male sex organs indicates a decrease in the production of testosterone.[44] The longer the hypothyroidism persists, the greater the degree of damage to the testes,[44] although genetically induced hypothyroidism in male mice is associated with normal fertility.[45]

In the adult ram, hypothyroidism is associated with a decrease in testosterone concentration but normal spermatogenesis.[46] In the mature male rat, the induction of hypothyroidism has little effect on the pathology of the testes, spermatogenesis, or serum testosterone concentrations.[47] Thus, it would appear that hypothyroidism can affect the immature, but not the mature, testis.

Human Studies and Clinical Aspects

The development of hypothyroidism in the male fetus does not appear to affect the reproductive system. Cretins are usually born with a normally developed reproductive tract. The presence of hypothyroidism in the prepubescent years usually results in a delay of sexual maturation and of the whole pre-pubertal process, which can be overcome by the administration of adequate doses of thyroxine. However, in some instances, hypothyroidism can result in precocious pseudopuberty marked by the early development of external genitalia, but without the appearance of axillary and pubic hair.[48] This syndrome probably results from an increased secretion of gonadotropins along with TSH from the enlarged pituitary.[48]

In men, hypothyroidism has been suggested as a cause of infertility,[49] but there is considerable disagreement with this suggestion.[50] If an infertile man is found to be hypothyroid, one should suspect secondary hypothyroidism and pituitary disease rather than primary myxedema, and there is no reason to treat infertile euthyroid men with thyroid hormone.[50]

In hypothyroid men, testicular size and potency may be normal and, despite early reports of defective spermatogenesis in hypothyroidism,[51] semen analysis is usually normal.[52] Wortsman and colleagues reported that myxedema was often associated with infertility and impotence, but in this report the impotence did not improve when the men became euthyroid.[49] In addition, there was a decrease in serum testosterone and free testosterone and, in the men who were not overweight, an increase in sex hormone-binding globulin. It should be noted that sex hormone-binding globulin levels have also been reported as both decreased[53] and normal[54] in hypothyroid men. Many men with hypothyroidism do note a decrease in libido, but this is probably a nonspecific disease-related complaint, which disappears when the euthyroid state is achieved with thyroid replacement therapy.

Variations in testis size and histology have been noted in autopsy material,[55,56] and De La Balze and coworkers[51] noted Leydig cell hyperplasia and tubular hyalinization. There is a marked decrease in the $5\alpha/5\beta$ ratio of the metabolites of androstenedione and testosterone, which is the reverse of that seen in hyperthyroidism.[37]

In summary, although hypothyroidism in boys frequently interferes with the normal pubertal process, the development of hypothyroidism in men has a less clear-cut effect on the reproductive system.

References

1. Hopkins PS, Thorburn GD. The effects of foetal thyroidectomy on the development of the ovine foetus. J Endocrinol 1972;54:55
2. Leathem JH. Extragonadal factors in reproduction. In: Lloyd CW, ed. Recent progress in the endocrinology of reproduction. New York: Academic Press, 1959:179
3. Leathem JH. Role of the thyroid. In: Balin H, Glasser S, eds. Reproductive biology. Amsterdam: Excerpta Medica, 1972:23
4. Hayles AB, Cloutire MD. Clinical hypothyroidism in the young—a second look. Symp Endocr Disorders 1972:56:871
5. Scow RO, Simpson ME. Thyroidectomy in the newborn rat. Anat Rec 1945;91:209
6. Ortega E, Rodriguez E, Ruiz E. Activity of the hypothalamo-pituitary ovarian axis in hypothyroid rats with or without tri-iodothyronine replacement. Life Sci 1990;46:391
7. Takacs-Jarrett M, Bruot BC. Steroid secretion by follicles and cysts from the hypothyroid, hCG-treated rat. Soc Experimental Biol Med 1994;207:62
8. Vriend J, Bertalanffy FD, Ralcewicz TA. The effects of melatonin and hypothyroidism on estradiol and gonadotropin levels in female Syrian hamsters. Biol Reprod 1987;36:719
9. Maqsood M. Thyroid functions in relation to reproduction of mammals and birds. Biol Rev 1952;27:281
10. Bonet B, Herrera E. Maternal hypothyroidism during the first half of gestation compromises normal catabolic adaptations of late gestation in the rat. Endocrinology 1991;129:210
11. Rao PM, Panda JN. Uterine enzyme changes in thyroidectomized rats at parturition. J Reprod Fertil 1981;61:109
12. Nesbitt REL, Abdul-Karim RW, Prior JT, Shelley TF, Rourke JE. Study of the effect of experimentally induced endocrine insults upon pregnant and nonpregnant ewes. III. ACTH and propylthiouracil administration and the production of polycystic ovaries. Fertil Steril 1967;18:739
13. Ruh MF, Ruh TS, Klitgaard HM. Uptake and retention of estrogens by uteri from rats in various thyroid states. Proc Soc Biol Med 1970;134:558
14. Kirkland JL, Gardner RM, Mukku VR, Akhtar M, Stancel GM. Hormonal control of uterine growth: The effect of hypothyroidism on estrogen-stimulated cell division. Endocrinology 1981;108:2346
15. Moenter SM, Woodfill CJI, Karsch FJ. Role of the thyroid gland in seasonal reproduction: Thyroidectomy blocks seasonal suppression of reproductive neuroendocrine activity in ewes. Endocrinology 1991;128:1337
16. Dawson A. Thyroidectomy progressively renders the reproductive system of starlings (*Sturnus* vulgaris) unresponsive to changes in daylength. J Endocrinol 1993;139:51
17. Kendle F. Case of precocious puberty in a female cretin. Br Med J 1905;1:246
18. Van Wyk J, Grumbach MM. Syndrome of precocious menstruation and galactorrhea in juvenile hypothyroidism: an example of hormonal overlap pituitary feedback. J Pediatr 1960;57:416
19. Thomas R, Reid RL. Thyroid disease and reproductive dysfunction: a review. Obstet Gynecol 1987;70:789
20. Wilansky DL, Greisman B. Early hypothyroidism in patients with menorrhagia. Am J Obstet Gynecol 1989;160:673
21. Higham JM, Shaw RW. The effect of thyroxine replacement on menstrual blood loss in a hypothyroid patient. Br J Obstet Gynaecol 1992;99:695
22. Rotmensch S, Scommegna A. Spontaneous ovarian hyperstimulation syndrome associated with hypothyroidism. Am J Obstet Gynecol 1989;160:1220
23. Goldsmith RE, Sturgis SH, Lerman J, Stanbury JB. The menstrual pattern in thyroid disease. J Clin Endocrinol Metab 1952;12:846
24. Wakim AN, Polizotto SL, Buffo ML, Marrero MA, Burholt DR. Thyroid hormones in human follicular fluid and thyroid hormone receptors in human granulosa cells. Fertil Steril 1993;59:1187
25. Channing CP, Tsai V, Sachs D. Role of insulin, thyroxine and cortisol in luteinization of porcine granulosa cells grown in chemically defined media. Biol Reprod 1976;15:235
26. Gerhard I, Becker T, Eggert-Kruse W, Klinga K, Runnebaum B. Thyroid and ovarian function in infertile women. Hum Reprod 1991;6:338
27. Davis LE, Leveno KJ, Cunningham FG. Hypothyroidism complicating pregnancy. Obstet Gynecol 1988;72:108
28. Leung AS, Millar LK, Koonings PP, Montoro M, Mestman JH. Perinatal outcome in hypothyroid pregnancies. Obstet Gynecol 1993;81:349
29. Nikolai TF, Mulligan GM, Gribble RK, Harkins PG, Meier PR, Roberts RC. Thyroid function and treatment in premenstrual syndrome. J Clin Endocrinol Metab 1990;70:1108
30. Roti E, Minelli R, Gardini E, Braverman LE. The use and misuse of thyroid hormone. Endocr Rev 1993;14:401

31. Burrow GN, Fisher DA, Larsen PR. Maternal and fetal thyroid function. N Engl J Med 1994;331:1072

32. Edwards CRW, Forsyth IA, Besser GM. Amenorrhea, galactorrhea and primary hypothyroidism with high circulating levels of prolactin. Br Med J 1971;3:462

33. Van Campenhout J, Van J, Antaki A, Rasio E. Diabetes mellitus and thyroid autoimmunity in gonadal dysgenesis. Fertil Steril 1973;24:1

34. Vallotton MB, Forbes AP. Autoimmunity in gonadal dysgenesis and Klinefelter's syndrome. Lancet 1967;1:648

35. Refetoff S, Selenkow HA. Familial thyroxine-binding globulin deficiency in a patient with Turner's syndrome (XO). N Engl J Med 1968;278:1081

36. Longcope C, Abend S, Braverman LE, Emerson CH. Androstenedione and estrone dynamics in hypothyroid women. J Clin Endocrinol Metab 1990;70:903

37. Gallagher TF, Fukushima DK, Noguchi S, et al. Recent studies in steroid hormone metabolism in man. Recent Prog Horm Res 1966;22:283

38. Saenger P. Abnormal sex differentiation. J Pediatr 1984;104:1

39. Lynn WG. The thyroid gland and reproduction in cold blooded vertebrates. Proceedings of the Fifth Mid-West Conference Thyroid 1969;17

40. Palmero S, de Marchis M, Gallo G, Fugassa E. Thyroid hormone affects the development of Sertoli cell function in the rat. J Endocrinol 1989;123:105

41. Kirby JD, Jetton AE, Cooke PS, et al. Developmental hormonal profiles accompanying the neonatal hypothyroidism-induced increase in adult testicular size and sperm production in the rat. Endocrinology 1992;131:559

42. Van Haaster LH, de Jong FH, Docter R, De Rooij DG. The effect of hypothyroidism on Sertoli cell proliferation and differentiation and hormone levels during testicular development in the rat. Endocrinology 1992;131:1574

43. Hardy MP, Kirby JD, Hess RA, Cooke PS. Leydig cells increase their numbers but decline in steroidogenic function in the adult rat after neonatal hypothyroidism. Endocrinology 1993;132:2417

44. Gomes WR. Metabolic and regulatory hormones influencing testis function. In: Johnson AD, Gomes WR, Vandemark NL, eds. The testis. Vol III. Influencing factors. New York: Academic Press, 1970:67

45. Chubb C, Henry L. The fertility of hypothyroid male mice. J Reprod Fertil 1988;83:819

46. Chandrasekhar Y, Holland MK, D'Occhio MJ, Setchell BP. Spermatogenesis, seminal characteristics and reproductive hormone levels in mature rams with induced hypothyroidism and hyperthyroidism. J Endocrinol 1985;105:39

47. Weiss SR, Burns JM. The effect of acute treatment with two goitrogens on plasma thyroid hormones, testosterone and testicular morphology in adult male rats. Comp Biochem Physiol (A) 1988;90A:449

48. Castro-Magana M, Angulo M, Canas A, Sharp A, Fuentes B. Hypothalamic-pituitary gonadal axis in boys with primary hypothyroidism and macroorchidism. J Pediatr 1988;112:397

49. Wortsman J, Rosner W, Dufau ML. Abnormal testicular function in men with primary hypothyroidism. Am J Med 1987;82:207

50. Steinberger E. The thyroid gland in male infertility. In: Garcia C-R, Mastroianni L Jr, Amelar R, Dubin L, eds. Current therapy of infertility 1982—1983. St Louis: CV Mosby, 1982:15

51. De La Balze FA, Arrilloga F, Mancini RE. Male hypogonadism in hypothyroidism: a study of six cases. J Clin Endocrinol Metab 1962;22:212

52. Griboff S. Semen analysis in myxedema. Fertil Steril 1962;13:436

53. Cavaliere H, Abelin N, Medeiros-Neto G. Serum levels of total testosterone and sex hormone binding globulin in hypothyroid patients and normal subjects treated with incremental doses of L-T_4 or L-T_3. J Androl 1988;9:215

54. De Nayer P, Lambot MP, Desmons MC, Rennotte B, Malvaux P, Beckers C. Sex hormone-binding protein in hyperthyroxinemic patients. A discriminator for thyroid status in thyroid hormone resistance and familial dysalbuminemic hyperthyroxinemia. J Clin Endocrinol Metab 1986;62:1309

55. Douglass RC, Jacobson SD. Pathologic changes in adult myxedema: survey of 10 necropsies. J Clin Endocrinol Metab 1957;17:1354

56. Marine D. Changes in the interstitial cells of the testis in Gull's disease. Arch Pathol 1939;28:65

Werner and Ingbar's The Thyroid, Seventh Edition,
edited by Lewis E. Braverman and Robert D. Utiger.
Lippincott–Raven Publishers, Philadelphia, © 1996

72

The Skeletal System in Hypothyroidism

Daniel T. Baran

Thyroid hormone is important for normal skeletal development. Growth and maturation of the skeleton are complex events and are the result of interaction between nutritional, genetic, and hormonal factors. Deficient thyroid hormone production in utero and in the neonate retards growth and delays skeletal maturation. Growth retardation in the thyroid-deficient neonate may be due in part to deficient growth hormone (GH) and insulin-like growth factor I (IGF-I) production, as well as to impaired nutrition.[1] In the adult skeleton, thyroid hormone deficiency decreases recruitment, maturation, and the activity of bone cells, leading to decreased remodeling, which is especially reflected in the impaired function of the osteoclasts.[2] These effects of thyroid hormone on the recruitment and maturation of bone cells in the developing and adult skeleton emphasize that the actions of thyroid hormone are not only the stimulation of catabolic processes.

ALTERATIONS IN SKELETAL GROWTH AND MATURATION IN HYPOTHYROIDISM

Skeletal growth is the result of a complex interplay of nutritional, genetic, and hormonal factors. Decreased skeletal growth in thyroid-deficient animals may be due in part to decreased production of GH.[3–5] Growth stimulation is minimal in the hypophysectomized animal given thyroid hormone alone.[6,7] This is in contrast to the stimulation of growth in the thyroid hormone–deficient animal by GH alone,[7] although GH exerts a greater effect on skeletal growth when thyroid hormone is present.[8–10] The two hormones appear to potentiate each other's effect on skeletal growth in rats[6,7,9] and in humans.[8,10] The doses of thyroxine that induce endochondral osteogenesis in the thyroidectomized rat also increase GH content.

Many studies suggest that the effects of thyroid hormone on bone and cartilage may be mediated in part through stimulation of IGF-I production. IGF-I levels are decreased in hypothyroidism.[11–19] It is unclear, however, whether the decreased IGF-I levels are related to thyroid hormone deficiency per se or to the frequently associated GH deficiency. Studies in animals and humans are conflicting, suggesting that thyroid hormone alone may increase IGF-I levels, or that thyroid hormone may have a synergistic effect on GH-mediated IGF-I synthesis. GH response to stimulation in hypothyroid patients is diminished, suggesting that the low IGF-I levels in hypothyroidism reflect decreased GH secretion.[20–22]

In contrast, thyroxine treatment of hypophysectomized male rats increases somatomedin activity to normal, despite the absence of GH. Treatment of genetically hypopituitary dwarf mice with thyroxine (T_4) increases somatomedin activity.[23] In hypothyroid patients treated with T_4, there is a positive correlation between free triiodothyronine (T_3) and IGF-I levels after treatment.[17] No correlation was found between IGF-I levels and GH response to GH-releasing factor.[17]

The complexity of the events involved in IGF-I synthesis has been demonstrated in the hypophysectomized rat.[24] Thyroid hormones have relatively little direct effect on hepatic IGF-I mRNA but can have major effects on GH-stimulated IGF-I synthesis and secretion. The pattern of these effects depends on the integrity of the pituitary gland, prior exposure of the liver to GH and/or thyroid hormone, and the temporal relationship between GH and thyroid hormone administration.[24] These molecular studies confirm previous studies demonstrating that thyroid hormone has a synergistic or additive effect on GH-stimulated IGF-I production.[12,25]

Body weight also has an effect on IGF-I levels and may confound the interpretation of the effects of thyroid hormone. IGF-I levels are positively correlated with birth weight,[1,26,27] and this relationship is confounded by serum total T_4 levels.[1] Impaired nutritional state in children[28–30] and adults[18,31] is the most likely explanation for the association between IGF-I and T_3 in nonthyroidal illness.

Skeletal maturation, defined as the appearance of secondary centers of ossification, depends largely on the presence of thyroid hormone. There is a delay in the appearance of all secondary centers of ossification in rats made hypothyroid from birth with propylthiouracil.[32] T_3 alone increases the rate of skeletal differentiation in immature rats.[33] T_4 and T_3 increase the maturation of isolated chick limb bones in tissue culture.[34] Incubation of growth plate cartilage from fetal pig scapulae[35] or embryonic chick pelvis[36] with T_3 increases amino acid and sulfate incorporation into protein and proteoglycans and stimulates the chondrocytes. Histologic examination shows that T_3 increases the width of the maturation zone, suggesting a direct effect on cartilage growth and maturation, primarily by stimulating chondrocytes.

The retardation of skeletal maturation in childhood hypothyroidism manifests itself as a delay in ossification at epiphyseal centers. When ossification does occur in the untreated hypothyroid child, the pattern is irregular and mottled, with multiple foci that coalesce to give a porous or fragmented appearance known as *epiphyseal dysgenesis*[37,38] (Fig 72-1). These changes are most frequently noted in large cartilaginous centers, such as the head of the femur and the tarsal navicular bone. Changes in the upper lumbar vertebrae result in wedge-shaped anterior margins, which appear between the ages of 6 months and 2 years, and may lead to spondylolisthesis.[39]

The onset of thyroid deficiency can be determined by the presence of epiphyseal dysgenesis at an ossification site. Absence of osseous retardation excludes the diagnosis of hypothyroidism unless thyroid deficiency is a recent occurrence.[38] Since the various epiphyseal centers begin to ossify at different times during childhood, the presence of epiphyseal dysgenesis at a particular site will date the onset of thyroid deficiency. For ex-

ample, the presence of stippled epiphyses in the femoral head of a 6-year-old child indicates that thyroid deficiency began before the 9th to 12th month, the age when these centers usually ossify. Likewise, the presence of dysgenesis in centers that ossify before birth suggests prenatal hypothyroidism. The observation that dysgenesis occurs in athyreotic cretins whose mothers had normal thyroid function during pregnancy indicates that the maternal thyroid is not able to protect the fetal skeleton against hypothyroidism. Normal infants born of hypothyroid mothers do not show retardation of ossification.

These alterations in bone growth and maturation are also noted in dental structures. In rats, thyroidectomy[40] and thyroid deficiency induced by propylthiouracil decrease rates of tooth eruption and tooth size. In contrast, excess doses of T_4 increase the rate of eruption of the incisor teeth in rats.[41] In human cretins, the growth of roots is slowed, dental enamel is thinned, and loss of deciduous teeth is delayed.[42–44]

ALTERATIONS IN CALCIUM METABOLISM IN HYPOTHYROIDISM

Serum calcium levels are usually normal in patients with hypothyroidism.[45] However, hypothyroid patients have a greater decrease in serum calcium levels after ethylenediaminetetraacetic acid infusion and recover from the hypocalcemia more slowly than do normal subjects.[46] The blunted response to hypocalcemia in hypothyroidism is presumably due to decreased renal and bone sensitivity to parathyroid hormone (PTH),[47] since PTH levels are increased in hypothyroidism.[46,47] The increased levels of PTH result in elevated levels of 1α,25-dihydroxyvitamin D_3,[48] which in turn increases intestinal calcium absorption.[49]

Biochemical markers of bone metabolism suggest that skeletal turnover is decreased in hypothyroidism. Calcium losses in the urine and feces are decreased.[45] ^{45}Ca-specific ac-

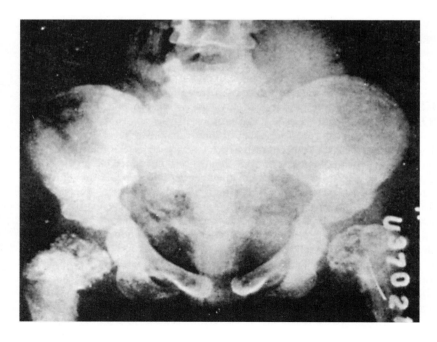

FIGURE 72-1. Roentgenogram of the hips of an untreated case of cretinism in a 24-year-old patient. (Sokoloff L, Francis CM, Campbell PL. Thyroxine stimulation of amino acid incorporation into protein independent of any action on messenger RNA synthesis. Proc Natl Acad Sci USA 1964;52:728)

tivity decreases more slowly after intravenous injection into hypothyroid subjects.[50] Serum alkaline phosphatase levels are often decreased[50–53] as are serum osteocalcin levels.[51,53] Urinary excretion of hydroxyproline is also decreased in both adults and children with hypothyroidism.[53–56] Although any condition that decreases growth rate may be associated with decreased hydroxyproline excretion, the observation that such decreases are also found in adult myxedematous subjects in whom longitudinal growth has ceased suggests that this finding is due to hypothyroidism. Although overall calcium balance is unaffected by hypothyroidism, the decreased osteoclastic activity results in a decreased bone resorption rate compared with normals.[57] This decreased release of calcium from bone presumably alters the steady-state levels of PTH, resulting in the previously described elevated levels of the hormone in hypothyroid subjects.

ALTERATIONS IN SKELETAL METABOLISM IN HYPOTHYROIDISM

Hypothyroidism decreases recruitment, maturation, and activity of bone cells, leading to decreased bone resorption and bone formation.[2] Despite this decrease in osteoclastic activity, trabecular bone volume[2] and bone mineral density[58] appear to be comparable to age-matched normals, presumably because of the corresponding decrease in osteoblastic activity. Studies have demonstrated that moderate doses of exogenous thyroid hormone replacement may predispose to bone loss and osteoporosis[59,60] (Fig 72-2). Histomorphometric studies have documented that exogenous thyroid hormone administration in doses of 0.1 to 0.4 mg/d leads to a marked osteoclastosis of both trabecular and cortical bone within the first month of treatment, which persists throughout therapy and leads to a decrease in bone mass.[61,62] The bone sites most adversely affected by thyroid hormone replacement therapy remain unclear. Finally, the effects of replacement or TSH suppressive doses of L-T$_4$ on the induction of osteoporosis remains somewhat controversial and is discussed in detail in chapter 48.

The role of calcitonin deficiency in the bone loss following thyroid hormone replacement therapy in hypothyroid patients has not been defined. Although there is a diminution of the calcitonin secretory capacity in hypothyroid subjects,[63,64] there is no evidence that calcitonin deficiency per se decreases bone mass. Hypothyroid patients do not show a decrease in bone mass prior to thyroid hormone replacement therapy despite calcitonin deficiency.[58] Although calcitonin deficiency could render the skeleton more sensitive to thyroid hormone replacement, the use of excessive doses of thyroid hormone has not been excluded.[58,61,63,65,66]

ARTHROPATHIES ASSOCIATED WITH HYPOTHYROIDISM

Patients with hypothyroidism often complain of articular and muscular pains and stiffness of the extremities.[67] The symptoms are usually worse after immobilization and are also exacerbated by cold or dampness, all of which are characteristic of rheumatoid arthritis. Morning stiffness is not remarkable.[68]

Patients may exhibit joint effusions involving the knees and small joints of the hands and feet.[69,70] Biopsies from patients with effusions show synovial membrane thickening and a noninflammatory effusion. The synovial fluid tends to be viscous because of the increased hyaluronic acid concentration. Calcium pyrophosphate dihydrate (CPPD) crystals are present in the effusions,[69] often resulting in the general diagnosis of chronic pseudo-gout.[71]

Carpal tunnel syndrome occurs commonly in patients with hypothyroidism. Several series have reported a 6.7% to 10% incidence of hypothyroidism in patients with carpal tunnel syndrome.[72] Compression of the median nerve resulting from the accumulation of viscous material has been suggested as the cause of the nerve entrapment.[68] Other causes of pain or paresthesia in the fingers, such as tenosynovitis, should also be considered.[72]

Avascular necrosis of the hip has been reported to occur more frequently in patients with hypothyroidism.[73] The elevated levels of serum cholesterol that often occur in hypothy-

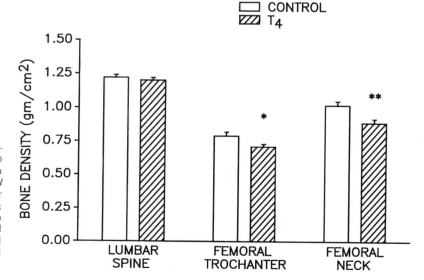

FIGURE 72-2. Bone density measured at three sites in premenopausal women. Femoral neck bone density (12.8%) and femoral trochanter bone density (10.1%) are lower in women receiving long-term L-thyroxine therapy (*hatched bars*) compared with control women (*open bars*). Lumbar spine bone density is not significantly different. *, $P < 0.02$; **, $P < 0.0002$. (Paul TL, Kerrigan J, Kelly AM, Braverman LE, Baran DT. Long-term L-thyroxine therapy is associated with decreased hip bone density in premenopausal women. JAMA 1988;259:3138. © 1988, American Medical Association)

roid patients have been implicated as a contributing factor to the development of the osteonecrosis.[74,75]

Hypothyroidism may present with proximal muscle pain and stiffness. Weakness is usually not a presenting symptom.[76-78] The myopathy suggests either polymyalgia rheumatica or polymyositis. The dramatic reversal of the rheumatic manifestation with T_4 therapy emphasizes the importance of including hypothyroidism in the differential diagnosis.[68] Recent studies strongly suggest an association between autoimmune thyroiditis with or without hypothyroidism in patients with rheumatoid arthritis[79] and other connective tissue diseases.[80] Laboratory and clinical features of Sjögren's syndrome may be observed in younger women with previous postpartum thyroiditis.[81]

References

1. Mitchell ML, Hermos RJ, Feingold M, Moses AC. The relationship of insulin-like growth factor-I to total thyroxine in normal and low birth weight infants. Pediatr Res 1989;25:336

2. Eriksen EF, Mosekilde L, Melsen F. Kinetics of trabecular bone resorption and formation in hypothyroidism: evidence for a positive balance per remodeling cycle. Bone 1986;7:101

3. Dieguez C, Jordan V, Harris P, et al. Growth hormone responses to growth hormone-releasing factor (1-29) in euthyroid, hypothyroid, and hyperthyroid rats. J Endocrinol 1986;109:53

4. Katakami H, Downs TR, Frohman LA. Decreased hypothalamic growth hormone-releasing hormone content and pituitary responsiveness in hypothyroidism. J Clin Invest 1986; 77:1704

5. Martin D, Epelbaum J, Bluet-Pajot M-T, Prelot M, Kordon C, Durand D. Thyroidectomy abolishes pulsatile growth hormone secretion without affecting hypothalamic somatostatin. Neuroendocrinology 1985;41:476

6. Scow RO. Effect of growth hormone and thyroxine on growth and chemical composition of muscle, bone, and other tissues in the thyroidectomized-hypophysectomized rats. Am J Physiol 1959;196:859

7. Thorngren K-G, Hansson LI. Effect of thyroxine and growth hormone on longitudinal bone growth in the hypophysectomized rat. Acta Endocrinol (Copenh) 1973;74:24

8. Harada Y, Okada Y, Hikita T, Ninomiya T, Ishihara Y. Comparison of growth acceleration of pituitary dwarfs treated with anabolic steroid and thyroid hormone with normal growth spurt. Acta Endocrinol (Copenh) 1973;74:237

9. Levenson D, Bialik GM, Ochberg Z. Differential effects of hypothyroidism on the cartilage and the osteogenic process in the mandibular condyle: recovery by growth hormone and thyroxine. Endocrinology 1994;135:1504

10. Van den Brande JL, Van Wyk JJ, French FS, Strickland AL, Radcliffe WB. Advancement of skeletal age of hypopituitary children treated with thyroid hormone plus cortisone. J Pediatr 1973;82:22

11. Burstein PJ, Draznin B, Johnson CJ, Schalch DS. The effect of hypothyroidism on growth, serum growth hormone, the growth hormone-dependent somatomedin, insulin-like growth factor, and its carrier protein in rats. Endocrinology 1979;104:1107

12. Cavaliere H, Knobel M, Medeiros-Neto G. Effect of thyroid hormone therapy on plasma insulin-like growth factor I levels in normal subjects, hypothyroid patients and endemic cretins. Horm Res 1987;25:132

13. Chernausek SD, Turner R. Attenuation of spontaneous, nocturnal growth hormone secretion in children with hypothyroidism and its correlation with plasma insulin-like growth factor I concentrations. J Pediatr 1989;114:968

14. Draznin B, Burstein PJ, Heinrich UE, Johnson CB, Emler CA, Schalch DS. Insulin-like growth factor and its carrier protein in

15. Hoogerbrugge-v.d. N, Linden N, Jansen H, Hulsmann WC, Birkenhager JC. Relationship between insulin-like growth factor-I and low-density lipoprotein cholesterol levels in primary hypothyroidism in women. J Endocrinol 1989;123:341

16. Ren SG, Malozowski S, Simoni C, et al. Dose-response relationship between thyroid hormone and growth velocity in cynomolgus monkeys. J Clin Endocrinol Metab 1988;66:1010

17. Valcavi R, Dieguez C, Preece M, Taylor A, Portioli I, Scanlon MF. Effect of thyroxine replacement therapy on plasma insulin-like growth factor 1 levels and growth hormone responses to growth hormone releasing factor in hypothyroid patients. Clin Endocrinol (Oxf) 1987;27:85

18. Valimaki M, Liewendahl, Karonen S-L, Helenius T, Suikkari A-M. Concentrations of somatomedin-C and triiodothyronine in patients with thyroid dysfunction and nonthyroidal illnesses. J Endocrinol Invest 1990;13:155

19. Westermark K, Alm J, Skottner A, Karlsson A. Growth factors and the thyroid: effects of treatment for hyper- and hypothyroidism on serum IGF-I and urinary epidermal growth factor concentrations. Acta Endocrinol (Copenh) 1988;118:415

20. Chernausek SD, Underwood LE, Utiger RD, Van Wyk JJ. Growth hormone secretion and plasma somatomedin-C in primary hypothyroidism. Clin Endocrinol (Oxf) 1983;19:337

21. Clemmons DR, Van Wyk JJ. Factors controlling blood concentration of somatomedin C. Clin Endocrinol Metab 1984; 13:113

22. Williams T, Maxon H, Thorner MO, Frohman LA. Blunted growth hormone (GH) response to GH-releasing hormone in hypothyroidism resolves in the euthyroid state. J Clin Endocrinol Metab 1985;61:454

23. Blows JA, Morrell DJ, Taylor AM, Holden AT. The effects of thyroid hormones on incorporation of sulphate into costal cartilage from dwarf mice and rats. IRCS J Med Sci 1984;12:759

24. Wolf M, Ingbar SH, Moses AC. Thyroid hormone and growth hormone interact to regulate insulin-like growth factor-I messenger ribonucleic acid and circulating levels in the rat. Endocrinology 1989;125:2905

25. Gaspard T, Wondergem R, Hamandzic M, Klitgaard HM. Serum somatomedin stimulation in thyroxine-treated hypophysectomized rats. Endocrinology 1978;102:606

26. Bennett A, Wilson DM, Liu F, Nagashima R, Rosenfeld RG, Hintz RL. Levels of insulin-like growth factors I and II in human cord blood. J Clin Endocrinol Metab 1983;57:609

27. Cassio A, Capelli M, Cacciari E, et al. Somatomedin-C levels related to gestational age, birth weight and day of life. Eur J Pediatr 1986;145:187

28. Grant DB, Hambley J, Becker D, Pimstone BL. Reduced sulphation factor in undernourished children. Arch Dis Child 1973;48:596

29. Hintz RL, Suskind R, Amatayakul K, Thanangkul O, Olsen R. Plasma somatomedin and growth hormone values in children with protein-caloric malnutrition. J Pediatr 1978;92:153

30. Zucker AR, Chernow B, Fields AI, Hung W, Burman KD. Thyroid function in critically ill children. J Pediatr 1985;107:552

31. Clemmons DR, Klibanski A, Underwood LE, et al. Reduction of plasma immunoreactive somatomedin C during fasting in humans. J Clin Endocrinol Metab 1981;53:1247

32. Hamburgh M. An analysis of the action of thyroid hormone on development based on in vivo and in vitro studies. Gen Comp Endocrinol 1968;10:198

33. Walker DG. An assay of the skeletogenic effect of L-triiodothyronine and its acetic acid analogue in immature rats. Johns Hopkins Med J 1957;101:101

34. Fell HB, Mellanby E. The effect of L-triiodothyronine on the growth and development of embryonic chick limb-bones in tissue culture. J Physiol (Lond) 1956;133:89

35. Burch WM, Lebovitz HE. Triiodothyronine stimulates maturation of porcine growth-plate cartilage in vitro. J Clin Invest 1982; 70:496

36. Burch WM, Lebovitz HE. Triiodothyronine stimulation of in vitro growth and maturation of embryonic chick cartilage. Endocrinology 1982;111:462

37. Edeiken J, Hodes PJ. Skeletal maturation. In: Robbins, LL, ed. Roentgen diagnosis of diseases of bone. Baltimore: Williams & Wilkins, 1973:8

38. Wilkins LW. Hormonal influences on skeletal growth. Ann N Y Acad Sci 1955;60:763

39. Fourman P, Royer P, Levell MJ, Morgan DB. Calcium metabolism and the bone. Philadelphia: FA Davis, 1968:388

40. Baume LJ, Becks H, Evans HM. Hormonal control of tooth eruption: 1. The effect of thyroidectomy on the upper rat incisor and the response to growth hormone, thyroxine, or the combination of both. J Dent Res 1954;33:80

41. Karnofsky D, Cronkite EP. Effect of thyroxine on eruption of teeth in newborn rats. Proc Soc Exp Biol Med 1939;40:568

42. Garn SM, Lewis AB, Blizzard RM. Endocrine factors in dental development. J Dent Res 1965;44:243

43. Hinrichs EH Jr. Dental changes in juvenile hypothyroidism. J Dent Child 1966;33:167

44. Jenkins GN. The physiology of the mouth. Philadelphia: F A Davis, 1966:199

45. Aub JC, Bauer W, Heath C, Ropes M. Studies of calcium and phosphorus metabolism: III. The effects of thyroid hormone and thyroid disease. J Clin Invest 1929;7:97

46. Bouillon R, De Moor P. Parathyroid function in patients with hyper- and hypothyroidism. J Clin Endocrinol Metab 1974; 38:999

47. Castro JH, Genuth SM, Klein L. Comparative response to parathyroid hormone in hyperthyroidism and hypothyroidism. Metabolism 1975;24:839

48. Bouillon R, Muls E, De Moor P. Influence of thyroid function on the serum concentration of 1,25-dihydroxyvitamin D_3. J Clin Endocrinol Metab 1980;51:793

49. Lekkerkerker JFF, Doorenbos H. The influence of thyroid hormone on calcium absorption from the gut in relation to urinary calcium excretion. Acta Endocrinol (Copenh) 1973;73:672

50. Krane SM, Brownell GL, Stanbury JB, Corrigan H. The effect of thyroid disease on calcium metabolism in man. J Clin Invest 1956;35:874

51. Brixen K, Nielsen HK, Eriksen EF, Charles P, Mosekilde L. Efficacy of wheat germ lectin-precipitated alkaline phosphatase in serum as an estimator of bone mineralization rate: comparison to serum total alkaline phosphatase and serum bone Gla-protein. Calcif Tissue Int 1989;44:93

52. Cassar J, Joseph S. Alkaline phosphatase levels in thyroid disease. Clin Chim Acta 1969;23:33

53. Charles P, Poser JW, Mosekilde L, Jensen FT. Estimation of bone turnover evaluated by ^{47}Ca-kinetics: efficiency of serum bone gamma-carboxyglutamic acid-containing protein, serum alkaline phosphatase, and urinary hydroxyproline excretion. J Clin Invest 1985;76:2254

54. Kivirikko KI. Urinary excretion of hydroxyproline in health and disease. Int Rev Connect Tissue Res 1970;5:93

55. Kivirikko KI, Laitinen O, Lamberg B-A. Value of urine and serum hydroxyproline in the diagnosis of thyroid disease. J Clin Endocrinol Metab 1965;25:1347

56. Siersbaek-Nielsen K, Skovsted L, Hansen JM, Kristensen M, Christensen LK. Hydroxyproline excretion in the urine and calcium metabolism during long-term treatment of thyrotoxicosis with propylthiouracil. Acta Med Scand 1971;189:485

57. Mosekilde L, Eriksen EF, Charles P. Effects of thyroid hormones on bone and mineral metabolism. Endocrinol Metab Clin North Am 1990;19:35

58. Krolner B, Jorgensen JV, Nielsen SP. Spinal bone mineral content in myxoedema and thyrotoxicosis. Effects of thyroid hormone(s) and antithyroid treatment. Clin Endocrinol (Oxf) 1983;18:439

59. Franklyn JA, Sheppard MC. Thyroxine replacement treatment and osteoporosis. Br Med J 1990;300:693

60. Perry HM III. Thyroid replacement and osteoporosis. Arch Intern Med 1986;146:41

61. Coindre J-M, David J-P, Riviere L, et al. Bone loss in hypothyroidism with hormone replacement: a histomorphometric study. Arch Intern Med 1986;146:48

62. Fallon MD, Perry HM III, Bergfeld M, Droke D, Teitelbaum SL, Avioli LV. Exogenous hyperthyroidism with osteoporosis. Arch Intern Med 1983;143:442

63. Demeester-Mirkine N, Bergmann P, Body J-J, Corvilain J. Calcitonin and bone mass status in congenital hypothyroidism. Calcif Tissue Int 1990;46:222

64. Body J-J, Demeester-Mirkine N, Borkowski A, Suciu S, Corvilain J. Calcitonin deficiency in primary hypothyroidism. J Clin Endocrinol Metab 1986;62:700

65. Ribot C, Tremollieres F, Pouilles JM, Louvet JP. Bone mineral density and thyroid hormone therapy. Clin Endocrinol (Oxf) 1990;33:143

66. Lakatos P, Tarjan G, Foldes J, Krasznai I, Hollo I. The effect of thyroid hormone treatment on bone mineral content in patients with hypothyroidism and euthyroid benign adenoma. In: Christiansen C, Johansen JS, Riis BJ, eds. Osteoporosis 1987. Viborg, Denmark: Norhaven A/S, 1987:452

67. Hill SR JR, Holley HL. The role of the endocrine glands in rheumatic diseases. In: Hollander JL, ed. Arthritis and allied conditions. 7th ed. Philadelphia: Lea & Febiger, 1966:597

68. McGuire JL. Arthropathies associated with endocrine disorders. In: Kelley WN, Harris ED Jr, Ruddy S, Sledge CB. Textbook of rheuamtology. Philadelphia: WB Saunders, 1989:1648

69. Bland JM, Frymoyer JW. Rheumatic syndromes of myxedema. N Engl J Med 1970;282:1171

70. Golding DN. Hypothyroidism presenting with musculoskeletal symptoms. Ann Rheum Dis 1970;29:10

71. Alexander GM, Scott DG, Dieppe PA, Doherty M. Pyrophosphate arthropathy: a study of metabolic associations and laboratory data. Ann Rheum Dis 1982;4:377

72. Frymoyer JW, Bland J. Carpal-tunnel syndrome in patients with myxedematous arthropathy. J Bone Joint Surg [Am] 1973; 55A:78

73. Seedat YK, Randeree M. Avascular necrosis of the hip joints in hypothyroidism. South Afr Med J 1975;49:2071

74. Rubinstein HM, Brooks MH. Aseptic necrosis of bone in myxedema. Ann Intern Med 1977;87:580

75. Siegelman SS, Schlossberg I, Becker NH, Sachs BA. Hyperlipoproteinemia with skeletal lesions. Clin Orthop 1972;87:228

76. Fessel WJ. Myopathy of hypothyroidism. Ann Rheum Dis 1968;27:590

77. Goldman J, Matz R, Mortimer R, Freeman R. High elevations of creatinine phosphokinase in hypothyroidism: an isoenzyme analysis. JAMA 1977;238:325

78. Hochberg MC, Koppes GM, Edwards CQ, Barnes HV, Arnette FC Jr. Hypothyroidism presenting as a polymyositis-like syndrome. Arthritis Rheum 1976;19:1363

79. Shiroky JB, Cohen M, Ballachey M-L, Neville C. Thyroid dysfunction in rheumatoid arthritis: a controlled prospective study. Ann Rheum Dis 1993;52:454

80. Arnaout MA, Nasrallah NS, El-Khateeb MS. Prevalence of abnormal thyroid function tests in connective tissue disease. Scand J Rheumatol 1994;23:128

81. Gudbjörnsson B, Karlsson-Parra A, Karlsson E, Hällgren R, Kämpe O. Clinical and laboratory features of Sjögren's syndrome in young women with previous postpartum thyroiditis. J Rheumatol 1994;21:215

Werner and Ingbar's The Thyroid, Seventh Edition,
edited by Lewis E. Braverman and Robert D. Utiger.
Lippincott–Raven Publishers, Philadelphia, © 1996

73

Metabolic Changes in Hypothyroidism

METABOLIC CHANGES IN HYPOTHYROIDISM

John N. Loeb

BASAL METABOLIC RATE AND CALORIGENESIS

In hypothyroidism the slowing of a wide variety of energy-requiring reactions is reflected in a decreased rate of oxygen consumption per unit of body surface area and a decrease in the rate of heat production.[1] The clinical reflections of these changes include a fall in the basal metabolic rate (although rarely by more than 40%[2]), cold intolerance, and some degree of weight gain (despite a decrease in appetite). Although weight gain of 15 pounds or more or the presence of obesity has been reported in approximately 50% of patients with hypothyroidism,[2] such patients are only rarely markedly obese.

In the absence of sufficient thyroid hormone, mitochondrial oxygen consumption and adenosine triphosphate (ATP) formation are both slowed, but the coupling of oxidative phosphorylation (i.e., the number of molecules of ATP generated per molecule of oxygen consumed) is normal.[3] A substantial fraction of basal oxygen consumption and ATP formation in the euthyroid state may be used to provide energy for the sodium-potassium pump (Na^+-K^+ pump; Na^+,K^+-ATPase), whose function is to maintain normal intracellular-to-extracellular sodium and potassium ion gradients,[4] although the importance of the contribution of active Na^+-K^+ transport to overall tissue oxygen consumption has been questioned.[5–9] In the hypothyroid state the rate of Na^+ extrusion from cells is reduced, and in some instances Na^+ and K^+ gradients across the plasma membrane may decrease.[10] Administration of thyroid hormone to hypothyroid animals restores both oxygen consumption and the functioning of the Na^+-K^+ pump to normal, and an increase in the activity of the pump may account for some of the calorigenic effect of the hormone.[11,12] Exposure of cultured hepatocytes to thyroid hormone likewise has a thermogenic effect,[13] and treatment with triiodothyronine (T_3) stimulates both active and passive monovalent cation fluxes in rat-liver cell lines in vitro.[14,15]

In brown adipose tissue, a specialized tissue that plays a major role in cold adaptation in several species,[16] an additional calorigenic effect of thyroid hormone is attributable to the local deiodination of thyroxine (T_4) to T_3[17,18] and the action of the latter (more potent) hormone to uncouple mitochondrial oxidative phosphorylation in this tissue. The generation of T_3 from T_4 is mediated by a T_4-5′-deiodinase isoform (type 2), whose activity in brown adipose tissue is enhanced by sympathetic stimulation.[19,20] The local generation of T_3 induces a rise in the level of an uncoupling protein (UCP) that appears to be unique to brown adipose tissue and that is located in the inner mitochondrial membrane. Basal levels of UCP are markedly reduced in brown adipose tissue of hypothyroid rats and can be restored to normal by the administration of replacement doses of T_4 but not of T_3.[21,22] The effects of thyroid hormone and catecholamines on brown adipose tissue in vivo can likewise be demonstrated in freshly dispersed brown adipocytes in vitro[23] as well as in long-term cultures of fetal rat brown adipocytes[24] (see also chap 70).

FAT METABOLISM

Carcasses of hypothyroid rats contain proportionately more fat than those of normal rats,[25] reflecting a preponderance of lipid synthesis over degradation. Both synthesis and degradation, however, are slowed in hypothyroidism. The biosynthesis of fatty acids by both adipose tissue and liver is depressed,[26–28] and the rates of catabolism of triglyceride and fatty acids are similarly less than normal. Synthesis of long-chain fatty acids in vitro from a number of different precursors is reduced in adipose tissue from hypothyroid rats, and there is a decrease in the rate of glycerol production and palmitate oxidation.[26] Lipolysis in response to catecholamines and other lipolytic agents is retarded in fat cells from both humans and rats with hypothyroidism.[29–32] Although the lipolytic sensitivity to catecholamines in white fat cells from hypothyroid rats is blunted, the number of β-adrenergic receptors per cell, as well as the response to a maximally stimulating concentration of epinephrine, are unaltered.[33]

A variety of abnormalities in plasma lipid concentrations occur in hypothyroidism. Plasma free fatty acid concentrations are normal[34] or slightly decreased[35]; in contrast, plasma concentrations of triglycerides, phospholipids, and low-density lipoprotein cholesterol are all elevated. The rate of synthesis of plasma triglycerides is normal in hypothyroidism, but their fractional removal rate is markedly reduced, which accounts for the increased plasma concentrations.[35] The decrease in plasma triglyceride removal rate in hypothyroidism has been ascribed in part to a decrease in plasma post-heparin lipolytic activity,[35,36] and indeed both abnormalities are corrected by administration of T_4.[36] Hypercholesterolemia (plasma cholesterol concentrations above 250 mg/dL [6.5 mmol/L] is present in the majority of patients with overt hypothyroidism. Despite a probable decrease in the rate of cholesterol biosynthesis, hypercholesterolemia is accompanied, at least in rats, by a marked diminution in the rate of cholesterol secretion into the bile.[37] A fall in cholesterol excretion, as well as a several-fold increase in the concentration of low-density cholesterol-carrying apolipoproteins (reflecting decreased catabolism and turnover[38]), account for the hypercholesterolemia in human hypothyroidism. The observation that patients with primary hypothyroidism more often have hypercholesterolemia than do those with central hypothyroidism may be explained at least in part by the fact that hypothyroidism in the former group is frequently more profound.

CARBOHYDRATE METABOLISM

In hypothyroidism, absorption of glucose from the gastrointestinal tract is slowed[39,40] and peripheral glucose assimilation is retarded.[41] At the same time, glycerol release from adipose tissue is slowed,[26] and the availability of amino acids[26] and glycerol[32,42] for gluconeogenesis is decreased. Plasma insulin concentrations in hypothyroid rats are somewhat low,[43] and, because the plasma half-life of the hormone is prolonged,[44,45] the rate of insulin synthesis is probably reduced. The insulin content of pancreatic slices from thyroidectomized rats is normal, but insulin release in vitro is diminished.[46] Peak plasma insulin responses to an intraperitoneal glucose load are lower

in hypothyroid than in euthyroid rats, even though the rise in plasma glucose is similar in both groups.[41] Fat cells from hypothyroid rats oxidize glucose at a normal rate despite a concurrent reduction in their capacity to oxidize palmitate.[26]

Insulin-stimulated glucose utilization by isolated adipocytes and soleus muscle from hypothyroid rats is decreased.[47] In hypothyroid humans, however, insulin sensitivity within the physiologic range of plasma glucose concentrations is normal, and the rate of fall in plasma glucose after a standard insulin challenge is nearly normal.[48,49] As in experimental hypothyroidism,[50] however, the maximal rate of glucose utilization after a large intravenous glucose load may be decreased in hypothyroid humans,[51] even after injection of appreciable doses of insulin.[52] The retarded uptake of glucose under these conditions may represent a diminished capacity of hypothyroid tissues to assimilate glucose because of a metabolic block distal to the site of action of insulin rather than insulin insensitivity per se. The number of insulin receptors in adipocytes from hypothyroid human is increased[53] but is unchanged in liver membranes from hypothyroid rats.[54]

Adult brain is one of the few tissues in which oxygen consumption is not stimulated by thyroid hormone.[55] In hypothyroid humans cerebral extraction of both glucose and oxygen from the arterial circulation is normal.[56]

Despite the easily demonstrable abnormalities in carbohydrate metabolism in hypothyroidism, clinical manifestations of these abnormalities are seldom conspicuous. Patients with hypothyroidism may have a decreased rate of glucose absorption from the gastrointestinal tract and flattened oral glucose tolerance curves despite the concomitant reduction in peripheral glucose assimilation. Although hypoglycemia is sometimes listed as a manifestation of hypothyroidism, it is rarely a sign of isolated thyroid hormone deficiency, and the presence of hypoglycemia in a patient with hypothyroidism should suggest the presence of hypopituitarism. The occurrence of hypothyroidism in a patient with insulin-dependent diabetes mellitus may result in some diminution in exogenous insulin requirement due both to decreased rate of insulin degradation[44,45] and decreased appetite. Such patients, however, may still develop ketoacidosis.[57] Conversely, correction of hypothyroidism in an insulin-dependent diabetic patient usually necessitates an increase in insulin dose.

Thyroidectomy has little effect on the severity of experimentally induced diabetes in cats[58] or dogs[59] but has been reported to reduce the incidence of late diabetes in subtotally pancreatectomized rats.[60]

PROTEIN METABOLISM

In human as well as in experimental hypothyroidism, there is a generalized decrease in both the synthesis[61] and degradation[62–64] of protein that is corrected by replacement with thyroid hormone. The effects of hypothyroidism on growth are discussed later, but it is worth noting here that young thyroidectomized rats force-fed the same amount of food as that consumed by normal rats store large quantities of fat but have far less positive nitrogen balance than do normal rats.[25]

Degradation of tissue proteins is slowed in hypothyroidism,[62,64] and the characteristic rise in plasma amino acid concentrations after evisceration is retarded in hypothyroid rats.[65] In addition to a generalized decrease in protein synthesis, there are specific decreases in a variety of mitochondrial and cytosolic enzymes[66] and substantial increases in several liver enzymes,[67,68] including those involved in urea synthesis.[69] In hypothyroid rats collagen accumulates as a result of a reduction in the rate of collagen breakdown in the face of a near-normal rate of synthesis.[70]

Changes in plasma and other extracellular fluid proteins are prominent in human hypothyroidism. Plasma low-density lipoprotein cholesterol concentrations increase, as noted earlier, because uptake and degradation of low-density lipoprotein by fibroblasts are reduced.[71] Both the synthesis and degradation of albumin are reduced,[72,73] the latter more than the former, so that the total-body albumin pool is increased. Nearly all of the increase is in the extravascular pool[72,73] and is accompanied by increased capillary permeability to albumin.[73] Enhanced capillary permeability may also account for some of the increase in cerebrospinal fluid protein concentration in hypothyroidism,[74] as well as for the increased albumin concentrations in interstitial fluid and for the various serous effusions that sometimes occur in hypothyroid patients. The mechanisms responsible for the widespread deposition of glycosaminoglycans material so typical of severe hypothyroidism[75] remain obscure; the major carbohydrate components of this material consist of hyaluronan and chondroitan sulfate, whose rate of synthesis by fibroblasts appears to be increased in hypothyroidism[76,77] (see chap 61).

MINERAL METABOLISM

The rates of excretion of calcium and phosphorus in both urine and feces are decreased in adults with hypothyroidism.[78] Nevertheless, there may be a mild net negative calcium balance, and the rate of calcium deposition in bone is characteristically reduced.[79] Serum calcium concentrations are usually normal. Abnormalities of calcium and phosphorus metabolism in hypothyroidism are discussed in detail in chapter 72.

GROWTH AND DEVELOPMENT

Perhaps the most dramatic consequences of an insufficiency of thyroid hormone occur in amphibians, in which the absence of thyroid hormone results in complete inhibition of metamorphosis. Replacement of thyroid hormone permits the normal orderly sequence of metamorphosis from tadpoles to frogs.[80] Resorption of the tadpole tail is induced, and limb buds sprout and develop into miniature legs within a few days after the onset of hormone treatment.[81] Thyroid hormone also has striking effects on the growth and maturation of cartilage.[82] T_3 promotes the growth of embryonic chick cartilage in large part by sensitizing this tissue to the stimulatory effects of insulin-like growth factor-I (IGF-I).[83] In contrast, the acceleration of cartilage maturation in the presence of T_3 appears to be independent of effects of IGF-I and to reflect a direct effect of thyroid hormone on cell differentiation.[83]

In postnatal but still immature mammals, the most conspicuous effect of thyroid hormone deficiency is growth failure. Both bone growth and bone maturation are delayed, and

the resumption of growth after administration of thyroid hormone is one of the most sensitive responses of hypothyroid animals to replacement therapy.[84] In rats, hypothyroidism also decreases growth hormone secretion[85]; in this species the thyroid hormones probably exert their growth-promoting effects by restoring growth hormone secretion and independently promoting growth in peripheral tissues.[86,87] In children with hypothyroidism, both linear growth and skeletal maturation are impaired as a result of decreased skeletal effects of thyroid hormone as well as decreased growth hormone and IGF-I production (see chaps 68 and 85).

DRUG AND HORMONE METABOLISM

Consonant with the slowing of a wide variety of metabolic processes, the metabolism of many drugs and hormones is retarded in hypothyroidism. As an example, in one study the daily administration of 0.5 mg of digoxin for a week was found in one study to result in a mean plasma drug concentration of 1.5 ng/mL (19 nmol/L), whereas the same dose in patients with thyrotoxicosis resulted in a mean concentration of only 0.7 ng/mL.[88] The plasma half-life of digoxin was prolonged because of both a reduction in glomerular filtration rate and a decrease in the rate of peripheral metabolism. The rate of metabolism of many other drugs is similarly slowed, a finding perhaps related to the observation that thyroidectomy in experimental animals results in a decrease in the activities of many, although not all, cytosolic and mitochondrial enzymes.[66–68,89]

The maintenance dose of many drugs is decreased, and the sensitivity to a loading dose may be heightened. As an example, the exquisite sensitivity of patients with hypothyroidism to even very small doses of morphine is unlikely to be due solely to a decrease in the rate of morphine metabolism. Such a decrease, while perhaps accounting for a reduction in maintenance dose, does not explain the profound respiratory depression that may follow the administration of a single small dose of morphine to a hypothyroid patient.

An apparent exception is the observation that patients with hypothyroidism may be resistant to the anticoagulant effect of warfarin.[90] Hypothyroid rats similarly have decreased sensitivity to warfarin initially,[91,92] but they may have enhanced sensitivity during more prolonged administration.[92] The mechanisms underlying these changes are uncertain, but the most likely explanation for the results in hypothyroid humans is slower-than-normal clearance of vitamin K–dependent coagulation factors.

The turnover, and consequently the output, of a variety of hormones are decreased in hypothyroidism. The plasma half-life of insulin is increased,[44,45] and the rate of secretion required to sustain a reduced[43] or even normal plasma insulin concentration is diminished. Hypothyroidism in rats leads to reductions in both plasma and pituitary growth hormone concentrations,[45,85,93] but the values in humans are more variable. Changes in prolactin secretion and adrenal steroid and catecholamine metabolism are discussed in chapters 68, 69, and 70, respectively.

The turnover of T_4 and T_3 themselves is slowed in hypothyroidism, and there are corresponding increases in the plasma half-lives of both hormones.[94,95] In hypothyroid rats, total T_4 clearance rate is decreased as a result of decreases in both fecal and deiodinative clearances.[96] The metabolic clearance and production of 3,3',5'-triiodothyronine[97] and of 3',5'-diiodothyronine[98] are decreased as well. The rate of conversion of T_4 to T_3 in vitro is substantially reduced in liver from hypothyroid rats,[99,100] a reduction in large part attributable to a decrease in type-1 T_4-5'-deiodinase activity.[101,102]

References

1. Du Bois EF. Basal metabolism in health and disease. 3rd ed. Philadelphia: Lea & Febiger, 1936:333

2. Watanakunakorn C, Hodges RE, Evans TC. Myxedema. Arch Intern Med 1965;116:183

3. Bronk JR, Bronk MS. The influence of thyroxine on oxidative phosphorylation in mitochondria from thyroidectomized rats. J Biol Chem 1962;237:897

4. Whittam R. The interdependence of metabolism and active transport. In: Hoffman JF, ed. The cellular functions of membrane transport. Englewood Cliffs, NJ: Prentice-Hall, 1964:139

5. Chinet A, Clausen T, Girardier L. Microcalorimetric determination of energy expenditure due to active sodium-potassium transport in the soleus muscle and brown adipose tissue of the rat. J Physiol 1977;265:43

6. Folke M, Sestoft L. Thyroid calorigenesis in perfused rat liver: Minor role of active sodium-potassium transport. J Physiol (Lond) 1977;269:407

7. Biron R, Burger A, Chinet A, Clausen T, Dubois-Ferrière R. Thyroid hormones and the energetics of active sodium-potassium transport in mammalian skeletal muscle. J Physiol 1979;297:47

8. van Hardeveld C, Kassenaar AAH. Evidence that the thyroid state influences Ca^{++}-mediated processes in perfused skeletal muscle. Horm Metab Res 1981;13:33

9. Haber RS, Loeb JN. Early enhancement of passive potassium efflux from rat liver by thyroid hormone: relation to induction of Na,K-ATPase. Endocrinology 1984;115:291

10. Ismail-Beigi F, Edelman IS. Effects of thyroid status on electrolyte distribution in rat tissues. Am J Physiol 1973;225:1172

11. Edelman IS. Thyroid thermogenesis. N Engl J Med 1974;290:1303

12. Fain JN, Rosenthal JW. Calorigenic action of triiodothyronine on white fat cells: effects of ouabain, oligomycin, and catecholamines. Endocrinology 1971;89:1205

13. Ismail-Beigi F, Bissell DM, Edelman IS. Thyroid thermogenesis in adult rat hepatocytes in primary monolayer culture: direct action of thyroid hormone in vitro. J Gen Physiol 1979;73:369

14. Ismail-Beigi F, Haber RS, Loeb JN. Stimulation of active Na^+ and K^+ transport by thyroid hormone in a rat liver cell line: role of enhanced Na^+ entry. Endocrinology 1986;119:2527

15. Haber RS, Ismail-Beigi F, Loeb JN. Time course of Na,K transport and other metabolic responses to thyroid hormone in Clone 9 cells. Endocrinology 1988;123:238

16. Himms-Hagen J. Brown adipose tissue metabolism and thermogenesis. Annu Rev Nutr 1985;5:69

17. Reiter RJ, Klaus S, Ebbinghaus C, et al. Inhibition of 5'-deiodination of thyroxine suppresses the cold-induced increase in brown adipose tissue messenger ribonucleic acid for mitochondrial uncoupling protein without influencing lipoprotein lipase activity. Endocrinology 1990;126:2550

18. Carvalho SD, Kimura ET, Bianco AC, Silva JE. Central role of brown adipose tissue thyroxine 5'-deiodinase on thyroid hormone-dependent thermogenic response to cold. Endocrinology 1991;128:2149

19. Silva JE, Larsen PR. Adrenergic activation of triiodothyronine production in brown adipose tissue. Nature (Lond) 1983;305:712

20. Silva JE, Larsen PR. Potential of brown adipose tissue type II thyroxine 5'-deiodinase as a local and systemic source of triiodothyronine in rats. J Clin Invest 1985;76:2296

21. Bianco AC, Silva JE. Intracellular conversion of thyroxine to triiodothyronine is required for the optimal thermogenic function of brown adipose tissue. J Clin Invest 1987;79:295

22. Bianco AC, Silva JE. Cold exposure rapidly induces virtual saturation of brown adipose tissue nuclear T_3 receptors. Am J Physiol 1988;255:E496

23. Bianco AC, Kieffer JD, Silva JE. Adenosine 3',5'-monophosphate and thyroid hormone control by uncoupling protein in freshly dispersed brown adipocytes. Endocrinology 1992;130:2625

24. Guerra C, Porras A, Roncero C, Benito M, Fernandez M. Triiodothyronine induces the expression of the uncoupling protein in long term fetal rat brown adipocyte primary cultures: role of nuclear thyroid hormone receptor expression. Endocrinology 1994;134:1067

25. Scow RO. Development of obesity in force fed young thyroidectomized rats. Endocrinology 1951;49:522

26. Bray GA, Goodman HM. Metabolism of adipose tissue from normal and hypothyroid rats. Endocrinology 1968;82:860

27. Freake HC, Schwartz HL, Oppenheimer JH. The regulation of lipogenesis by thyroid hormone and its contribution to thermogenesis. Endocrinology 1989;125:2868

28. Blennemann B, Moon YK, Freake HC. Tissue-specific regulation of fatty acid synthesis by thyroid hormone. Endocrinology 1992;130:637

29. Rosenqvist U. Noradrenaline-induced lipolysis in subcutaneous adipose tissue from hypothyroid subjects. Acta Med Scand 1972;192:361

30. Wahrenberg H, Wennlund A, Arner P. Adrenergic regulation of lipolysis in fat cells from hyperthyroid and hypothyroid patients. J Clin Endocrinol Metab 1994;78:898

31. Deykin D, Vaughan M. Release of free fatty acids by adipose tissue from rats treated with triiodothyronine or propylthiouracil. J Lipid Res 1963;4:200

32. Goodman HM, Bray GA. Role of thyroid hormones in lipolysis. Am J Physiol 1966;210:1053

33. Malbon CC, Moreno FJ, Cabelli RJ, Fain JN. Fat cell adenylate cyclase and β-adrenergic receptors in altered thyroid states. J Biol Chem 1978;253:671

34. Hamburger J, Smith RW Jr, Miller JM. Effects of epinephrine on free fatty acid mobilization in hyperthyroid and hypothyroid subjects. Metabolism 1963;12:821

35. Nikkilä EA, Kekki M. Plasma triglyceride metabolism in thyroid disease. J Clin Invest 1972;51:2103

36. Porte D Jr, O'Hara DD, Williams RH. The relation between postheparin lipolytic activity and plasma triglyceride in myxedema. Metabolism 1966;15:107

37. Friedman M, Byers SO, Rosenman RH. Changes in excretion of intestinal cholesterol and sterol digitonides in hyper- and hypothyroidism. Circulation 1952;5:657

38. Walton KW, Scott PJ, Dykes PW, Davies JWL. The significance of alterations in serum lipids in thyroid dysfunction. II. Alterations of the metabolism and turnover of ^{131}I-low-density lipoproteins in hypothyroidism and thyrotoxicosis. Clin Sci 1965;29:217

39. Althausen TL, Stockholm M. Influence of thyroid gland on absorption in the digestive tract. Am J Physiol 1938;123:577

40. Althausen TL. Hormonal and vitamin factors in intestinal absorption. Gastroenterology 1949;12:467

41. Jolín T, Montes A. The different effects of thyroidectomy, $KClO_4$, and propylthiouracil on insulin secretion and glucose uptake in the rat. Endocrinology 1974;94:1502

42. Fisher JN, Ball EG. Studies on the metabolism of adipose tissue. XX. The effect of thyroid status upon oxygen consumption and lipolysis. Biochemistry 1967;6:637

43. Jolín T, Morreale de Escobar G, Escobar del Rey F. Differential effects in the rat of thyroidectomy, propylthiouracil and other goitrogens on plasma insulin and thyroid weight. Endocrinology 1970;87:99

44. Elgee NJ, Williams RH. Effects of thyroid function on insulin-^{131}I degradation. Am J Physiol 1955;180:13

45. Cohen AM. Interrelation of insulin activity and thyroid function. Am J Physiol 1957;188:287

46. Malaisse WJ, Malaisse-Lagae F, McCraw EF. Effects of thyroid function upon insulin secretion. Diabetes 1967;16:643

47. Czech MP, Malbon CC, Kerman K, Gitomer W, Pilch PF. Effect of thyroid status on insulin action in rat adipocytes and skeletal muscle. J Clin Invest 1980;66:574

48. Iwatsubo H, Omori K, Okada Y, et al. Human growth hormone secretion in primary hypothyroidism before and after treatment. J Clin Endocrinol Metab 1967;27:1751

49. Brauman H, Corvilain J. Growth hormone response to hypoglycemia in myxedema. J Clin Endocrinol Metab 1968;28:301

50. Scow RO, Cornfield J. Effect of thyroidectomy and food intake on oral and intravenous glucose tolerances in rats. Am J Physiol 1954;179:39

51. Lamberg B-A. Glucose metabolism in thyroid disease. Acta Med Scand 1965;178:351

52. Elrick H, Hlad CH Jr, Arai Y. Influence of thyroid function on carbohydrate metabolism and a new method for assessing response to insulin. J Clin Endocrinol Metab 1961;21:387

53. Arner P, Bolinder J, Wennlund A, Ostman J. Influence of thyroid hormone level on insulin action in human adipose tissue. Diabetes 1984;33:369

54. DeRuyter H, Burman KD, Wartofsky L, Taylor SI. Effects of thyroid hormone on the insulin receptor in rat liver membranes. Endocrinology 1982;110:1922

55. Barker SB, Klitgaard HM. Metabolism of tissues excised from thyroxine-injected rats. Am J Physiol 1952;170:81

56. Sensenbach W, Madison L, Eisenberg S, Ochs L. The cerebral circulation and metabolism in hyperthyroidism and myxedema. J Clin Invest 1954;33:1434

57. Kozak GP, Cooppan R. Diabetes and other endocrinologic disorders. In: Marble A, Krall LP, Bradley RF, Christlieb AR, Soeldner JS, eds. Joslin's diabetes mellitus. 12th ed. Philadelphia: Lea & Febiger, 1985:784

58. Dohan FC, Lukens FDW. The effect of thyroidectomy upon pancreatic diabetes in the cat. Am J Physiol 1938;122:367

59. DeFinis ML, Houssay BA. Tiroides y diabetes en el perro. Rev Soc Argent Biol 1943;19:94

60. Houssay BA. The thyroid and diabetes. Vitam Horm 1946; 4:188

61. Crispell KR, Parson W, Hollifield G. A study of the rate of protein synthesis before and during the administration of L-triiodothyronine to patients with myxedema and healthy volunteers using N-15 glycine. J Clin Invest 1956;35:164

62. Hoberman HD, Graff J. Influence of thyroxine on the metabolism of amino acids and proteins during fasting. Yale J Biol Med 1950/1951;23:195

63. Burini R, Santidrian S, Moreyra M, Brown P, Munro HN, Young VR. Interaction of thyroid status and diet on muscle protein breakdown in the rat, as measured by N[7]-methylhistidine excretion. Metabolism 1981;30:679

64. Marchesini G, Fabbri A, Bianchi GP, et al. Hepatic conversion of amino nitrogen to urea nitrogen in hypothyroid patients and upon L-thyroxine therapy. Metabolism 1993;42:1263

65. Bondy PK. The effect of the adrenal and thyroid glands upon the rise of plasma amino acids in the eviscerated rat. Endocrinology 1949;45:605

66. Pitot HC, Yatvin MB. Interrelationships of mammalian hormones and enzyme levels in vivo. Physiol Rev 1973;53:228

67. Chatagner F, Jollès-Bergeret B. Effects of thyroid hormones on different types of pyridoxal phosphate-dependent enzymes of rat liver. In: Snell EE, Fasella PM, Braunstein A, Rossi Fanelli A, eds. Symposium on chemical and biological aspects of pyridoxal catalysis. New York: Pergamon, 1963:477

68. Chatagner F, Durieu-Trautmann O. Effects of pyridoxine deficiency on the adaptation of rat liver cystathionase to DL-ethionine and to thyroidectomy. Nature 1965;207:1390

69. Marti J, Portoles M, Jimenez-Nacher I, Cabo J, Jorda A. Effect of thyroid hormones on urea biosynthesis and related processes in rat liver. Endocrinology 1988;123:2167

70. Fink CW, Ferguson JL, Smiley JD. Effect of hyperthyroidism and hypothyroidism on collagen metabolism. J Lab Clin Med 1967;69:950

71. Chait A, Bierman EL, Albers JJ. Regulatory role of triiodothyronine in the degradation of low density lipoprotein by cultured skin fibroblasts. J Clin Endocrinol Metab 1979;48:887

72. Schwartz E. The effect of thyroid hormone upon the degradation rate and miscible pool of radioiodinated human serum albumin in myxedema. J Lab Clin Med 1955;45:340

73. Lewallen CG, Rall JE, Berman M. Studies of iodoalbumin metabolism. II. The effects of thyroid hormone. J Clin Invest 1959;38:88

74. Bronsky D, Shrifter H, De la Huerga J, Dubin A, Waldstein SS. Cerebrospinal fluid proteins in myxedema, with special reference to electrophoretic partition. J Clin Endocrinol Metab 1958;18:470

75. Gabrilove JL, Ludwig AW. The histogenesis of myxedema. J Clin Endocrinol Metab 1957;17:925

76. Smith TJ, Horwitz AL, Refetoff S. The effect of thyroid hormone on glycosaminoglycan accumulation in human skin fibroblasts. Endocrinology 1981;108:2397

77. Smith TJ, Murata Y, Horwitz AL, Philipson L, Refetoff S. Regulation of glycosaminoglycan synthesis by thyroid hormone in vitro. J Clin Invest 1982;70:1066

78. Aub JC, Bauer W, Heath C, Ropes M. Studies of calcium and phosphorus metabolism. III. The effects of the thyroid hormone and thyroid disease. J Clin Invest 1929;7:97

79. Krane SM, Brownell GL, Stanbury JB, Corrigan H. The effect of thyroid disease on calcium metabolism in man. J Clin Invest 1956;35:874

80. Gudernatsch JF. Feeding experiments on tadpoles. I. The influence of specific organs given as food on growth and differentiation. Arch Entwicklungsmechanik Organ 1912;35:457

81. Frieden E. Thyroid hormones and the biochemistry of amphibian metamorphosis. Rec Progr Horm Res 1967;23:139

82. Burch WM, Lebovitz HE. Triiodothyronine stimulation of in vitro growth and maturation of embryonic chick cartilage. Endocrinology 1982;111:462

83. Burch WM, Van Wyk JJ. Triiodothyronine stimulates cartilage growth and maturation by different mechanisms. Am J Physiol 1987;252:E176

84. Evans ES, Rosenberg LL, Simpson ME. Relative sensitivity of different biological responses to thyroxine. Endocrinology 1960;66:433

85. Peake GT, Birge CA, Daughaday WH. Alterations of radioimmunoassayable growth hormone and prolactin during hypothyroidism. Endocrinology 1973;92:487

86. Thorngren K-G, Hansson LI. Effect of thyroxine and growth hormone on longitudinal bone growth in the hypophysectomized rat. Acta Endocrinol 1973;74:24

87. Coiro V, Braverman LE, Christianson D, Fang S-L, Goodman HM. Effect of hypothyroidism and thyroxine replacement on growth hormone in the rat. Endocrinology 1979;105:641

88. Croxson MS, Ibbertson HK. Serum digoxin in patients with thyroid disease. BMJ 1975;3:566

89. Ruzicka FJ, Rose DP. The influence of thyroidal status on rat hepatic NADH duroquinone reductase. Endocrinology 1981;109:664

90. Stephens MA, Self TH, Lancaster D, Nash T. Hypothyroidism: effect on warfarin anticoagulation. South Med J 1989;82:1585

91. Lowenthal J, Fisher LM. The effect of thyroid function on the prothrombin time response to warfarin in rats. Experientia 1957;13:253

92. McIntosh TJ, Wilson WR, Waters L, Fouts JR. Response to warfarin in hypothyroid rats. Eur J Pharmacol 1971;14:176

93. Daughaday WH, Peake GT, Birge CA, Mariz IK. The influence of endocrine factors on the concentration of growth hormone in rat pituitary. In: Pecile A, Müller EE, eds. Growth hormone. Proceedings of the First International Symposium, International Congress Series No. 158. Amsterdam: Excerpta Medica, 1968:238

94. Nicoloff JT, Low JC, Dussault JH, Fisher DA. Simultaneous measurement of thyroxine and triiodothyronine peripheral turnover kinetics in man. J Clin Invest 1972;51:473

95. Bianchi R, Zucchelli GC, Giannessi D, et al. Evaluation of triiodothyronine (T_3) kinetics in normal subjects, in hypothyroid, and hyperthyroid patients using specific antiserum for the determination of labeled T_3 in plasma. J Clin Endocrinol Metab 1978;46:203

96. Cullen MJ, Doherty GF, Ingbar SH. The effect of hypothyroidism and thyrotoxicosis on thyroxine metabolism in the rat. Endocrinology 1973;92:1028

97. Smallridge RC, Wartofsky L, Desjardins RE, Burman KD. Metabolic clearance and production rates of 3,3′,5′-triiodothyronine in hyperthyroid, euthyroid, and hypothyroid subjects. J Clin Endocrinol Metab 1978;47:345

98. Smallridge RC, Burman KD, Smith CE, Latham KR, Wright FD, Wartofsky L. Metabolic clearance and production rates of 3′,5′-diiodothyronine in hyperthyroidism and hypothyroidism in man: comparison of infusions using radiolabeled versus unlabeled iodothyronine. J Clin Endocrinol Metab 1981;52:722

99. Balsam A, Sexton F, Ingbar SH. The effect of thyroidectomy, hypophysectomy, and hormone replacement on the formation of triiodothyronine from thyroxine in rat liver and kidney. Endocrinology 1978;103:1759

100. Kaplan MM, Utiger RD. Iodothyronine metabolism in liver and kidney homogenates from hyperthyroid and hypothyroid rats. Endocrinology 1978;103:156

101. Balsam A, Sexton F, Ingbar SH. On the mechanism of impaired in vitro generation of 3,5,3′-triiodothyronine from thyroxine in the livers of hypothyroid rats. Endocrinology 1979;105:1115

102. Kaplan MM. Changes in the particulate subcellular component of hepatic thyroxine-5′-monodeiodinase in hyperthyroid and hypothyroid rats. Endocrinology 1979;105:548

Vitamin Metabolism in Hypothyroidism

Richard S. Rivlin

A number of the clinical features of hypothyroidism, such as weakness, anemia, pallor, carotenemia, behavioral abnormalities, and night blindness, may be attributable, at least in part, to disturbances in vitamin metabolism.

VITAMIN A

Vitamin A is the most easily recognized example of disturbed vitamin metabolism in hypothyroidism. Hypothyroid patients may have a characteristic orange-yellow pigmentation of the skin that makes them look sallow and tends to exaggerate their pale appearance if they are also anemic. This discoloration is due to deposition in the skin of carotenes, the plant-derived substances that are the dietary precursors of vitamin A. The sclerae are not involved in carotenemia, an observation that enables the clinician to distinguish the condition from jaundice.

Vitamin A metabolism is probably disturbed at several sites in hypothyroidism. Conversion of carotenes to vitamin A is diminished. Intestinal absorption of carotenes may be inhibited, and the binding capacity of cellular retinol-binding protein for retinol may be decreased.[1]

One of the most important metabolic effects of hypothyroidism is on serum concentrations of lipoproteins (see preceding section). Both serum cholesterol and triglyceride concentrations may be increased.[2] After cholesterol feeding, there is a marked increase in serum concentrations of so-called remnant lipoproteins. The relevance of these effects to vitamin A metabolism is that carotene, lycopene, and other carotenoids are transported by serum lipoproteins, and elevated serum carotene concentrations reflect overall increases in serum lipoprotein concentrations.

In serum, vitamin A (as retinol) is bound to a specific protein, retinol-binding protein (RBP), and the latter forms a one-to-one complex with transthyretin, formerly designated thyroxine-binding prealbumin (see chap 6). Vitamin A and thyroxine (T_4) transport are therefore related; in addition, thyroid hormone receptors and retinoic acid receptors interact with one another at the molecular level[3] (see chap 9). In hypothyroid patients serum concentrations of vitamin A tend to be elevated, and those of RBP and transthyretin are generally normal.[4]

Disturbances of vitamin A metabolism may account for the diminished darkness adaptation that occurs in hypothyroid patients. Those who drink ethanol to excess would be particularly vulnerable to night blindness, inasmuch as alcohol also has deleterious effects on vitamin A utilization.

VITAMIN D

Hypothyroidism results in a decrease in the rate of bone turnover and in the size of the exchangeable pool of calcium, and usually low to normal serum calcium concentrations (see chap 72). In response to calcium loading, serum calcium concentrations increase more in hypothyroid patients than in normal subjects. Furthermore, hypothyroid patients tend to have elevated serum parathyroid hormone (PTH) and 1,25-dihydroxyvitamin D concentrations.[5]

As a result of decreased bone turnover and elevated serum PTH concentrations, serum phosphate concentrations tend be low. Low serum phosphate, high PTH, and low-normal calcium concentrations favor increased synthesis of 1,25-dihydroxyvitamin D which, in turn, may stimulate increased intestinal absorption of calcium. With this postulated sequence of events, plus the decrease in bone turnover, it is not surprising that bone mass may be increased in patients with hypothyroidism.[5]

VITAMIN E

Serum vitamin E concentrations may be elevated in patients with hypothyroidism, at least in part as a result of an overall increase in serum concentrations of lipoproteins, especially low-density lipoprotein (LDL). Vitamin E is incorporated into LDL and also high-density lipoproteins (HDL). The serum vitamin E concentration should therefore be interpreted in relation to the patient's serum LDL and HDL cholesterol values.

THIAMINE (VITAMIN B_1)

Thiamine directly inhibits the synthesis of monoiodotyrosine (MIT) and diiodotyrosine (DIT) in calf thyroid slices.[7] There is no evidence, however, to suggest that large doses of thiamine inhibit thyroid function or cause hypothyroidism in humans.

RIBOFLAVIN (VITAMIN B_2)

Hypothyroidism in experimental animals causes a number of disturbances in riboflavin metabolism. Hepatic concentrations of the two riboflavin-derived coenzymes, riboflavin-5′-phosphate, formerly called flavin mononucleotide (FMN), and flavin adenine dinucleotide (FAD), are reduced and can be restored to normal by physiologic doses of thyroid hormones. The reduced hepatic FMN and FAD concentrations are likely due to diminished conversion from riboflavin by flavokinase, because the activity of this enzyme is reduced by half in hypothyroidism.[7]

In addition, the activities of a wide variety of FMN- and FAD- requiring enzymes, such as xanthine oxidase, are decreased in hypothyroidism. In fact, dietary riboflavin deficiency and hypothyroidism share a number of similar biochemical abnormalities: decreases in tissue FMN and FAD concentrations, decreases in the activities of FMN- and FAD-requiring enzymes, and usually similar alterations of activities of enzymes involved in riboflavin metabolism.

Further evidence of disturbed riboflavin metabolism in hypothyroidism is provided by measurements of erythrocyte glutathione reductase (Fig 73-1). The magnitude of increase in activity of this FAD-requiring enzyme after incubation with FAD in vitro (activity coefficient) is greater in erythrocytes from hypothyroid than from normal rats. These findings indicate less saturation of the apoenzyme with its coenzyme, reflecting a state of relative riboflavin deficiency in hypothyroidism.[8]

In hypothyroid patients, the erythrocyte glutathione reductase activity coefficient is similarly elevated above normal, and can be corrected by T_4 treatment.[9]

Chlorpromazine markedly inhibits the biosynthesis of FAD and blocks covalent binding of flavins to tissue proteins. This drug also inhibits the stimulatory effects of T_4 on FAD biosynthesis.[7] A number of female psychiatric patients have

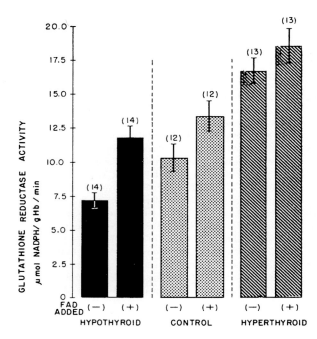

FIGURE 73-1. Glutathione reductase activity in erythrocyte hemolysates from hypothyroid, control, and thyrotoxic animals. Assays were performed with and without incubation of erythrocyte hemolysates with flavin adenine dinucleotide (*FAD*) in vitro, at 37°C for 20 minutes. Data are shown as means ± SE. Figures in parentheses refer to numbers of animals in each group. *NADPH*, reduced nicotinamide adenine dinucleotide phosphate. (Adapted from Menendez CE, Hacker P, Sonnenfeld M, McConnell R, Rivlin RS. Thyroid hormone control of glutathione reductase activity in rat erythrocytes and liver. Am J Physiol 1974;266:1480)

been reported who had both hypothyroidism and riboflavin deficiency,[10] suggesting that decreased FAD synthesis may be a sensitive index of hypothyroidism in this group.

VITAMIN B_{12} AND FOLIC ACID

Some patients with hypothyroidism have macrocytic anemia (see chap 66). A high prevalence (20%) of folic acid deficiency was found in some but not other studies of hypothyroidism.[11] In other hypothyroid patients, macrocytic anemia is due to deficiency of vitamin B_{12}. The incidence of true pernicious anemia is about 8% in patients with primary hypothyroidism caused by chronic autoimmune thyroiditis. A similar percentage appears to have latent B_{12} deficiency with reduced serum vitamin B_{12} concentrations, histamine-fast achlorhydria, and an abnormal Schilling test.[12] Studies in experimental animals suggest that hypothyroidism may lead to diminished utilization of vitamin B_{12} and, in addition, to an increased proportion of tetrahydrofolate relative to methyltetrahydrofolate in the liver.[13]

OTHER VITAMINS

Thyroidectomy raises serum pyridoxal phosphate (vitamin B_6) concentrations and raises activities of enzymes utilizing this coenzyme in experimental animals. There is no information as to possible disturbances of pyridoxine metabolism in hypothyroid humans.

Thyroidectomized rats have decreased liver and kidney concentrations of both ascorbic acid and dehydroascorbic acid, but the clinical importance of the decreases is uncertain.

References

1. Rajguru S, Nahavandi M, Ahluwalia B. Facilitory role of thyroid hormone in vitamin A uptake in the rat testes. Int J Vit Min Res 1989;59:107

2. Walton KW, Campbell DA, Tonks EL. The significance of alterations in serum lipids in thyroid dysfunction. I. The relation between serum lipoproteins, carotenoids and vitamin A in hypothyroidism and thyrotoxicosis. Clin Sci 1965;29:199

3. Zhang XK, Pfahl M. Hetero- and homodimeric receptors in thyroid hormone and vitamin A action. Receptor 1993;3:183

4. Smith FR, Goodman DS. The effects of diseases of the liver, thyroid and kidneys on the transport of vitamin A in human plasma. J Clin Invest 1971;50:2426

5. Bouillon R, Muls E, DeMoor P. Influence of thyroid function on the serum concentration of 1,25-dihydroxyvitamin D. J Clin Endocrinol Metab 1980;51:793

6. Slingerland DW, Sullivan JJ. An antithyroid effect of thiamine. Endocrinology 1968;82:895

7. Rivlin RS. Medical aspects of vitamin B_2. In: Muller F, ed. Chemistry and biochemistry of flavins. Boca Raton, FL: CRC Press. 1991:201

8. Menendez CE, Hacker P, Sonnenfeld P, McConnell R, Rivlin RS. Thyroid hormone control of glutathione reductase activity in rat erythrocytes and liver. Am J Physiol 1974;226:1480

9. Cimino JA, Jhangiani S, Schwartz E, Cooperman JM. Riboflavin metabolism in the hypothyroid human adult. Proc Soc Exp Biol Med 1987;184:151

10. Bell IR, Morrow FD, Read M, Berkes S, Perrone G. Low thyroxine levels in female psychiatric inpatients with riboflavin deficiency: implications for folate-dependent methylation. Acta Psychiatr Scand 1992;85:360

11. Das KC, Mukherjee M, Sarkar TK, et al. Erythropoiesis and erythropoietin in hypo- and hyperthyroidism. J Clin Endocrinol Metab 1975;40:211

12. Tudhope GR, Wilson GM. Anaemia in hypothyroidism. Q J Med 1960;64:513

13. Chan MMS, Stokstad ELR. Metabolic responses of folic acid and related compounds to thyroxine in rats. Biochim Biophys Acta 1980;632:244

Werner and Ingbar's The Thyroid, Seventh Edition,
edited by Lewis E. Braverman and Robert D. Utiger.
Lippincott–Raven Publishers, Philadelphia, © 1996

74

Behavioral and Psychiatric Aspects of Hypothyroidism

Peter C. Whybrow

HISTORICAL PERSPECTIVE

The prevalence, nature, and clinical course of the behavioral and psychologic changes that occur in adults with primary hypothyroidism were first described in the latter half of the 19th century.[1–4] In 1888, the Clinical Society of London described myxedematous (hypothyroid) patients, most of whom had some mental disturbance, ranging from irritability and agoraphobia to dementia and melancholia.[3] Subsequently, it became generally accepted that hypofunction of the thyroid gland had severe effects on brain function and could irreversibly damage the developing brain. In hypothyroid adults, the subtle behavioral and psychologic changes, especially during the early stages of the illness, confounded the clinical diagnosis, and people with "myxedematous madness" were commonly found on careful screening of mental hospital patients.[5] Objective laboratory tests have improved this situation enormously, but isolated case reports of hypothyroid patients presenting with severe mental disturbance continue to appear, and it remains important that the clinician be aware of the wide range of behavioral disturbances that hypothyroidism can induce.[6–8]

NEUROPSYCHIATRIC FEATURES

The initial behavioral and psychologic changes in adults with primary hypothyroidism are nonspecific and ill-defined complaints (e.g., weakness) and disturbances in cognition. The latter include inattentiveness, inability to concentrate, slowing of thought processes, and inability to calculate and to understand complex questions. Memory for recent events is frequently poor, and eventually memory for remote events may also be-

come impoverished. Ability to perform everyday, routine tasks is decreased. The patient becomes less concerned and responsive to others, less interested in their surroundings, and less capable of learning and performing new tasks. There is a paucity of speech, frequently with perseveration. Motor functions are slowed. Alterations in the accuracy of perception with an increased tendency to illusion formation may appear; still later, visual and other hallucinatory distortions may occur that result in bizarre behavior and paranoid ideas. We know from historical descriptions that as hypothyroidism becomes more severe, progressive drowsiness, with lethargy and difficulty in arousal, occurs. The patient may sleep for long periods during the day and, finally, may lapse into stupor and even coma.[9] Convulsions also can occur.[10]

Because of slowing of thought and speech, decreased attentiveness, poor concentration, and diminished interest in and responsiveness to others, the diagnosis initially may be confused with that of a depressive mood state. Indeed, hypothyroidism may induce a specific melancholic disorder in some patients,[11] with crying, loss of appetite, constipation, insomnia, delusions of self-reproach, and suicidal ideation.[7,12–14] The picture is not consistently one of depression; a disorganized agitated state also has been described. In case vignettes of hypothyroid patients with psychosis,[5,15–17] insomnia, hyperactivity, irritability, anger, and both auditory and visual hallucinations are reported. Other patients became fearful, suspicious, and delusional. Hence, although depressed mood seems to predominate, the specific mental state and thought content varies with the individual patient. Cognitive changes, however, with alterations in attention, concentration, perception, and speed of thought, appear to be the most common of the clinical manifestations.

OBJECTIVE BEHAVIORAL ASSESSMENT

These clinical observations are confirmed by the few objective studies of behavior that have been conducted. Taken together, the symptoms and signs are diverse, and the mental state of hypothyroid patients thus has much in common with other organic syndromes of brain dysfunction. The results of electroencephalographic (EEG) studies reflect this, with low voltage Θ- and δ-waves predominating.[18,19] Stages 3 and 4 of the sleep EEG may be reduced,[13] and evoked responses are also slowed[20–22]. The changes in the EEG can be correlated with the mental status examination and particularly with tests of cognitive function, such as mental arithmetic or short-term memory and attention.[23] Objective psychologic testing has consistently revealed intellectual impairment that improves with treatment.[14,24–27]

Few behavioral studies have been conducted in hypothyroid patients unselected for psychiatric disorder, and hence the incidence of psychosis in hypothyroidism is difficult to estimate. In the untreated group studied in 1888, it was about 15%.[3] A study in the 1920s described hallucinations in 26% of patients.[28] The improvements in laboratory tests that aid in the early diagnosis of hypothyroidism have reduced the incidence enormously, probably to less than 5%. Subjective mental change in both mood and cognition is profound, however, in some hypothyroid patients. Furthermore, some patients with prolonged hypothyroidism have residual intellectual dysfunction after treatment. Without objective antemorbid data, however, these reports are difficult to assess.

ASSOCIATED PSYCHIATRIC SYNDROMES: DIAGNOSTIC CONSIDERATIONS

Schizophrenic and Affective Psychoses

The psychoses that occur in hypothyroidism are nonspecific, representing a final common path of neurobiologic disorganization. Thus, they may mimic schizophrenic, paranoid, and affective psychoses. Although a careful history and physical examination usually reveal at least a few stigmata of hypothyroidism, the florid and acute nature of the psychotic disturbance may distract the physician or preclude such detailed clinical examination. Of special importance in clarifying the differential diagnosis is the impairment of cognitive function that is found in hypothyroidism. Even though confusion occurs in acute schizophrenia, together with distractibility that may masquerade as poor memory, visual hallucination with profound and persistent cognitive disturbance (including memory and orientation) is rare. Thus, formal neuropsychologic testing can be helpful. The very low amplitude EEG waves that occur in patients with severe hypothyroidism suggest an underlying delirium,[18] but the EEG cannot be considered a reliable differential diagnostic procedure.

In the affective psychoses, cognitive impairment or pseudodementia is more common, especially in the elderly, in whom it may be dismissed as the dementia of old age. Indeed, the symptoms of hypothyroid psychosis may so closely mimic those of the severely psychotic affective states that routine thyroid screening should be done in all patients over 60 years of age who present with the clinical syndrome of affective psychosis and intellectual impairment.

Depressive Syndrome

A number of metabolic and behavioral disturbances are common to hypothyroidism and affective illness, even in the absence of psychosis, suggesting that changes in pituitary-thyroid secretion may play an important role in the modulation of mood.[29,30]

Patients with depression have a spectrum of abnormalities in thyroid test results, the most common of which is a mild elevation of serum total thyroxine (T_4) concentrations.[29,31] A decline in the increased serum T_4 concentrations correlates with clinical response to pharmacologic intervention.[31,32] The serum thyrotropin (TSH) response to thyrotropin-releasing hormone (TRH) is blunted in approximately 25% of depressed patients, even though their serum T_4 concentrations are within normal limits.[33]

Hypothyroidism is a graded phenomenon, and changes in serum T_4 and especially TSH concentrations can be detected before any clinical evidence of hypothyroidism appears. Approximately 10% of 250 consecutive patients referred to a psychiatric hospital for treatment of depression or anergia had evidence of subclinical or overt hypothyroidism.[34] Furthermore, triiodothyronine (T_3) given as an adjunct to tricyclic antidepressant drug treatment speeds recovery in some patients with depression,[35] especially women.[32] These findings suggest that some of these patients may have subclinical hypothyroidism.[36] Also, depressed patients resistant to therapeutic doses of tricyclic antidepressant drugs may respond when T_3 is added to the therapeutic regimen.[37–39] Finally, as part of the disturbed circadian endocrine profile, the nocturnal surge in serum TSH is lost in depression[40] but returns with recovery.

Among women with postpartum depression, some also have postpartum thyroiditis, which occurs in about 6% of postpartum women (see chap 89). Each of these disorders can occur separately, but patients with serologic evidence of postpartum thyroiditis may be more likely to be depressed. In a study of 145 women with positive thyroid-antibody tests 6 weeks postpartum, 47% had significant depressive symptoms, as compared with 32% of women with negative tests.[41]

Thyroid dysfunction is particularly important in the clinical course of bipolar illness, especially rapid cycling disease, a malignant form of the illness. Patients with rapid cycling disease, 85% of whom are women, by definition suffer more than four episodes of illness per year.[42] They have a much higher incidence (about 25%–50%) of grade I hypothyroidism (defined as supranormal serum TSH concentrations, an exaggerated serum TSH response to TRH, and normal serum T_4 concentrations) than depressed patients in general (2%–5%) or those taking lithium carbonate (9%).[43,44] High doses of T_4 added to the established treatment with lithium and other psychotropic drugs can reverse this rapid cycling pattern.[45]

Lithium carbonate, a standard treatment for bipolar illness, is a weak antithyroid agent[46] that may also inhibit brain and pituitary T_4-5′-deiodinase activity.[47] Tricyclic antidepressant drugs, which can precipitate rapid cycling disease,[48] also alter thyroid hormone metabolism in the brain.[49] Hence, the treatment of bipolar illness may iatrogenically impair brain thyroid economy and thus complicate the clinical course of the mood disturbance itself.[42] Conversely, in some hypothyroid patients with a family history of bipolar affective illness, rapid replacement with T_4 can induce mania.[50]

Taken together, these studies suggest that thyroid abnormalities, including overt and subclinical hypothyroidism, may contribute to psychiatric disability. Thyroid screening by determination of serum TSH seems warranted in all patients with resistant syndromes of affective illness, especially women, and in those with atypical psychoses with significant cognitive disorder.

PATHOPHYSIOLOGY OF BEHAVIORAL DYSFUNCTION IN HYPOTHYROIDISM

The specific pathophysiology responsible for the behavioral disturbances of hypothyroidism is unknown. It is probable that the general decline in cognitive and behavioral function is an integral part of the hypometabolic state characteristic of the syndrome.

It has long been recognized that thyroid hormone is essential for the normal development of the central nervous system[51] (see chap 67). T_4 is taken up avidly by the developing rat brain, and brain T_3 content in those animals is five times that of mature animals.[10] During development, T_4 and T_3 determine the rate and completeness of neuronal cell division and the activity of many enzyme systems, by exerting major effects on both nucleic acid and protein synthesis in the brain.[52]

In a study of adults with hypothyroidism, cerebral blood flow was reduced (38% below normal), as were oxygen and glucose consumption (27% below normal), and cerebrovascular resistance was increased twofold.[53] All of the patients in this study had evidence of cognitive impairment. The three patients studied after treatment had normal values for those measurements. These changes, coupled with the EEG disturbances noted earlier,[13,18,20–22] suggest delirium as the nonspecific final common path to mental dysfunction.

T_4 and T_3 regulate cellular function in most organs, including the brain.[54] T_3 nuclear receptors are prominent in brain tissue, particularly in neurons, and are regionally distributed; high concentrations are found in amygdala and hippocampus and low concentrations in brain stem and cerebellum.[55] T_3-receptor complexes regulate expression of various proteins[54] and, in the brain, T_3-receptor binding is exquisitely sensitive to the local thyroid hormone economy.[56] (A complete discussion of thyroid hormone action at the molecular level can be found in chap 9.)

About half of the nuclear T_3 in brain is produced within the neuron itself by the deiodination of T_4, a reaction catalyzed by type II T_4-5′-deiodinase[56] (see chap 8). The activity of this enzyme is increased in hypothyroidism and decreased in thyrotoxicosis. This precise autoregulatory mechanism not only underscores the importance of T_4 and its deiodination to optimum brain function, but also suggests that minor changes in local thyroid homeostasis may lead to major changes in metabolism and behavior.[57] Thus, in hypothyroidism, intracerebral generation of T_3 from T_4 increases as serum T_4 declines, so that intracellular T_3 concentrations decline little until serum T_4 is virtually exhausted.[58]

Are changes of this central thyroid economy important to the aberrant behavior of patients with hypothyroidism and psychiatric disease? Until the thyroid economy of the brain can be quantified in vivo, this question cannot be answered. However, strong clinical evidence in support of such speculation exists: the role of mild hypothyroidism in depressive illness and in postpartum depressive states associated with thyroiditis; the association of the rapid cycling variant of bipolar illness with hypothyroidism; the adjunctive therapeutic role of thyroid hormones in both depression and rapid-cycling bipolar illness; and the profound disturbances that are found in hypothyroidism.

The depressive mood disturbances in clinical hypothyroidism are of great interest to the psychiatrist because they suggest the possibility of a common pathophysiology in the affective disorders and thyroid disease. In this, the biogenic amines, putatively disturbed in both disorders, may form a linkage.[30] The interaction of thyroid state and sympathetic nervous system activity has been recognized for many years.[59,60] The biochemical activity of noradrenergic neurons and thyroid function are inversely related. For example, in hypothyroid rats norepinephrine is synthesized from tyrosine at an accelerated rate in heart, spleen, and adrenal tissue.[61] Conversely, in rats given T_4 for 10 days norepinephrine synthesis in the heart and brain is decreased by 30% and 15%, respectively.[62] The activity of the enzyme dopamine β-hydroxylase changes similarly in animals and humans.[63]

This paradox, by which the biochemical activity of the adrenergic nervous system is apparently inversely related to thyroid state whereas physiologic activity is directly related, is possibly explained by changes in adrenergic receptor function. In heart and adipose tissue, increasing thyroid activity increases β-adrenergic receptor number, whereas α-adrenergic receptor numbers decline; and decreasing thyroid hormone availability leads to the reverse.[64] In rat brain, both the serotonergic (5-HT) and noradrenergic (NA) receptor systems are responsive to changes in hypothalamic-pituitary-thyroid function.[65,66] Thyroidectomy causes a decrease in ligand binding to β- and α_2-adrenoreceptors in the limbic regions of the brain, and increases ligand binding to 5-HT$_{1A}$ receptors in the cortex and hippocampus. T_4 replacement therapy causes the receptors to return to control levels. These results suggest that there is a neuromodulatory link between serotonergic and adrenergic receptors and the thyroid state. Also, the sensitivity of Purkinje neurons in hypothyroid rat cerebellum to iontophoretically applied norepinephrine is decreased. This decreased sensitivity was associated with decreased adenylyl cyclase activity and returned to normal after the administration of T_3.[67] Whether these changes induced in adrenergic brain mechanisms by hypothyroidism cause the melancholic symptoms that commonly occur in hypothyroid patients remains speculative but intriguing.

TREATMENT AND OUTCOME

The behavioral disturbances of hypothyroidism in adults respond to adequate T_4 replacement unless there is underlying depression unrelated to the hypothyroidism, in which case cognition may improve but the depressed mood persists.[17] Exacerbation of the psychosis may occur soon after T_4 treatment is initiated[18] and thus, ideally, severely disturbed patients should be hospitalized. Therapy with a major tranquilizing drug may be necessary in a few patients, but the drug should be given with great caution and in conjunction with T_4 therapy to avoid precipitating myxedema coma. Haloperidol and the phenothiazines are the drugs most frequently used. Because of the cardiovascular changes in severe hypothyroidism, the patient should be monitored carefully for arrhythmia, especially those patients treated with a phenothiazine. There is a case report of cardiac arrest in such a situation.[68]

When a hypothyroid patient has a strong family history of affective disturbance, especially bipolar in character, the initiation of treatment may precipitate manic excitement.[50] In such patients, it may be necessary to add lithium or a phenothiazine to the treatment regimen. Conversely, patients receiving lithium who develop a severe depressive state, cognitive confusion, and anergy, including those who have a serum lithium concentration below the therapeutic range, should always be carefully examined for the symptoms and signs of hypothyroidism.

When the hypothyroidism is mild and complicating a predominantly depressive syndrome, the therapeutic goal is to provide sufficient T_4 to reduce the serum TSH concentration to normal; however, the amount may not be sufficient to reverse the melancholia. In such cases, antidepressant drugs or even electroconvulsive therapy may be necessary. In other instances, severe depressive illness even without evidence of hypothyroidism may be aided by the addition of T_3 (25–50 μg daily for 2–4 weeks) to the regimen. Empirically, this strategy appears to be particularly helpful in women and some patients with drug-resistant depression.[31,37–39]

References

1. Gull WW. On a cretinoid state supervening in adult life in women. Trans Clin Soc (Lond) 1873;7:180
2. Inglis T. Two cases of myxoedema. Lancet 1880;2:496
3. Report of a committee of the Clinical Society of London. Report on myxedema. Trans Clin Soc (Suppl) (Lond) 1888;21:18
4. Savage GH. Myxoedema and its nervous symptoms. J Ment Sci 1880;25:417
5. Asher R. Myxoedematous madness. BMJ 1949;2:555
6. Granet RB, Kalman JP. Hypothyroidism and psychosis: a case illustration of the diagnostic dilemma in psychiatry. J Clin Psychiatry 1978;39:260
7. McNamara ME, Southwick SM, Fogel BS. Sleep apnea and hypothyroidism presenting as depression in 2 patients. J Clin Psychiatry 1987;48:164
8. Vieweg WV, Yank GR, Steckler TL, Clayton MT. Grades 1 and 2 hypothyroidism in a state mental hospital: risk factors and clinical findings. Psychiatr Q 1987;58:135
9. Levin ME, Daughaday WH. Fatal coma due to myxedema. Am J Med 1955;18:1017
10. Jellinek EH. Fits, faints, coma and dementia in myxoedema. Lancet 1962;2:1010
11. Shaw C. Case of myxedema with restless melancholia treated by injections of thyroid juice. BMJ 1892;2:451
12. Jain V. A psychiatric study of hypothyroidism. Psychiatr Clin 1972;5:121
13. Kales A, Henze G, Jacobson A, et al. All night sleep studies in hypothyroid patients before and after treatment. J Clin Endocrinol Metab 1967;27:1593
14. Whybrow PC, Prange AJ, Treadway CR. Mental changes accompanying thyroid gland dysfunction. Arch Gen Psychiatry 1969;20:48
15. Easson WM. Myxedema with psychosis. Arch Gen Psychiatry 1966;14:277
16. Karnosh LJ, Stout RE. Psychoses of myxoedema. Am J Psychiatry 1934;91:1263
17. Treadway CR, Prange AJ, Duehne EF, Edens CJ, Whybrow PC. Myxedema psychosis: clinical and biochemical changes during recovery. J Psychiatr Res 1967;5:289
18. Browning TB, Atkins RW, Weiner H. Cerebral metabolic disturbances in hypothyroidism: clinical and electroencephalographic studies in the psychosis of myxoedema and hypothyroidism. Arch Intern Med 1954;93:938
19. Neiman EA. The electroencephalogram in myxoedema coma: clinical and electroencephalographic study of three cases. BMJ 1959;1:1204
20. Himelfarb MZ, Lakretz T, Gold S, Shanon E. Auditory brain stem responses in thyroid dysfunction. J Laryngol Otol 1981;95:679
21. Huang TS, Chang YC, Lee SH, Chen FW. Evoked potential abnormalities in thyroid disorders. In: Nagataki S, Torizuka K, eds. The thyroid. Amsterdam: Elsevier, 1988:411
22. Ladenson PW, Stakes JW, Ridgway EC. Reversible alteration of the visual evoked potential in hypothyroidism. Am J Med 1984;77:1010
23. Logothetis J. Psychotic behavior as the initial indicator of adult myxoedema. J Nerv Ment Dis 1963;36: 561
24. Crown S. Notes on an experimental study of intellectual deterioration. BMJ 1949;ii:684
25. Reitan RM. Intellectual functions in myxoedema. Arch Neurol Psychiatry 1953;69:436
26. Schon M, Sutherland AM, Rawson RW. Hormones and neuroses—the psychological effects of thyroid deficiency. Vol 2. Proceedings of the Third World Congress of Psychiatry. Montreal, Canada: McGill University Press/University of Toronto Press, 1961:835
27. Haggerty JJ Jr., Garbutt JC, Evans DL, et al. Subclinical hypothyroidism: a review of neuropsychiatric aspects. Int J Psychiatry Med 1990;20:193
28. Beck HG. The hallucinations of myxedema. Med Times 1926;54:201
29. Bauer MS, Whybrow PC. Thyroid hormones and the central nervous system in affective illness: interactions that may have clinical significance. Integr Psychiatry 1988;6:75
30. Whybrow PC, Prange AJ. A hypothesis of thyroid-catecholamine-receptor interaction: its relevance to affective illness. Arch Gen Psychiatry 1981;38:106
31. Whybrow PC, Coppen A, Prange AJ Jr, Noguera R, Bailey JE. Thyroid function and the response of L-liothyronine in depression. Arch Gen Psychiatry 1972;26:242
32. Coppen A, Whybrow PC, Noguera R, Maggs R, Prange AJ. The comparative antidepressant value of L-tryptophan and imipramine with and without attempted potentiation by liothyronine. Arch Gen Psychiatry 1972;26:234
33. Hein MD, Jackson IMD. Thyroid function in psychiatric illness. Gen Hosp Psychiatry 1990;12:232
34. Gold MS, Pottash ALC, Extein I. Hypothyroidism and depression: evidence from complete thyroid function evaluation. JAMA 1981;245:1919
35. Prange AJ Jr, Wilson IC, Rabon AMN, Lipton MA. Enhancement of imipramine antidepressant activity by thyroid hormone. Am J Psychiatry 1969;126:457
36. Howland RH. Thyroid Dysfunction in refractory depression: implications for pathophysiology and treatment. J Clin Psychiatry 1993;54:47

37. Goodwin FK, Prange AJ Jr, Post RM, Muscettola G, Lipton MA. Potentiation of antidepressant effects by triiodothyronine in tricyclic nonresponders. Am J Psychiatry 1982;139:34

38. Joffe R, Singer W. Thyroid hormone potentiation of antidepressants. In: Amsterdam J, ed. Advances in neuropsychiatry and psychopathology, Vol 2: Refractory depression. New York: Raven Press, 1991:185

39. Joffe R, Levitt A, Bagby R, MacDonald C, Singer W. Predictors of response to lithium and triiodothyronine augmentation of antidepressantst in tricyclic non-responders. Br J Psychiatry 1993;163:574

40. Bartalena L, Placidi GF, Martino E, et al. Nocturnal serum thyrotropin (TSH) surge and the TSH response to TSH-releasing hormone: Disssociated behavior in untreated depressives. J Clin Endocrinol Metab 1990;71:650

41. Harris B, Othman S, Davies JA, et al. Association between postpartum thyroid dysfunction and thyroid antibodies and depression. BMJ 1992;305:152

42. Bauer M, Whybrow P. Rapid cycling bipolar disorder: clinical features, treatment and etiology. In: Amsterdam J, ed. Refractory depression: frontiers in research and treatment. New York: Raven Press, 1991:191

43. Bauer MS, Whybrow PC, Winokur A. Rapid cycling bipolar affective disorder. I. Association with grade I hypothyroidism. Arch Gen Psychiatry 1990;47:427

44. Cowdry RW, Wehr TA, Zis AP, Goodwin FK. Thyroid abnormalities associated with rapid cycling bipolar illness. Arch Gen Psychiatry 1983;40:414

45. Bauer MS, Whybrow PC. Rapid cycling bipolar affective disorder. II. Treatment of refractory rapid cycling with high dose levothyroxine: a preliminary study. Arch Gen Psychiatry 1990; 4:435

46. Rogers M, Whybrow PC. Clinical hypothyroidism occurring during lithium treatment: two case histories and a review of thyroid function in 19 patients. Am J Psychiatry 1971;128:158

47. St Germain D. Regulatory effect of lithium on thyroxine metabolism in murine neural and anterior pituitary tissue. Endocrinology 1987;120:1430

48. Wehr TA, Goodwin FK. Rapid cycling in manic-depressives induced by tricyclic antidepressants. Arch Gen Psychiatry 1979;36:555

49. Dratman M, Crutchfield F. Thyroid hormones and adrenergic neurotransmittors. In: Usdin E, Kopin I, eds. Catecholamines basic and clinical. Fourth International Catecholamine Symposium. Elmsford, NY: Pergamon Press, 1978:1155

50. Josephson AM, McKenzie TB. Thyroid induced manias in hypothyroid patients. Br J Psychiatry 1980;137:222

51. Timiras PS. Thyroid hormones and nervous system development. Biol Neonate 1989;55:376

52. Berti CN, Sato C, Gomez CL, et al. Thyroid hormone effects on RNA synthesis in brain and liver of neonatal hypothyroid rats. Horm Metab Res 1981;13:691

53. Scheinberg P, Stead EA Jr, Brannon ES, Warren JV. Correlative observations on cerebral metabolism and cardiac output in myxedema. J Clin Invest 1950;29:1139

54. Oppenheimer JH, Schwartz HL, Mariash CN, Kinlaw WB, Wong NEW, Freake HC. Advances in our understanding of thyroid hormone action at the cellular level. Endocr Rev 1987; 8:288

55. Ruel J, Faure R, Dussault JH. Regional distribution of nuclear T_3 receptors in rat brain and evidence for preferential localization in neurons. J Endocrinol Invest 1985;8:343

56. Larsen PR. Thyroid hormone metabolism in the central nervous system. Proceedings of the 2nd Thyroid Symposium: Peripheral thyroid hormone metabolism, Graz, Austria. Acta Med Austriaca 1988;15:5

57. Dratman MB, Crutchfield FL, Gordon JT, Jennings A. Iodothyronine homeostasis in rat brain during hypo- and hyperthyroidism. Am J Physiol 1983;245:R185

58. Dratman MB, Crutchfield FL. Interactions of adrenergic and thyroergic systems in the development of the low T_3 syndrome. In: Hesch R, ed. The low T_3 syndrome. London: Academic Press, 1981:115

59. Goetsch E. New methods in the diagnosis of thyroid disorders: pathological and clinical. NY State Med J 1918;18:257

60. Harrison TS. Adrenal medullary and thyroid relationships. Physiol Rev 1964;44:161

61. Lipton MA, Prange AJ, Dairman W. Increased rate of norepinephrine biosynthesis in hypothyroid rats. Fed Proc 1968; 27:399

62. Prange AJ Jr, Meek JL, Lipton MA. Catecholamines: diminished rate of norepinephrine biosynthesis in rat brain and heart after thyroxine pretreatment. Life Sci 1970;9:901

63. Stolk JM, Whybrow PC. Clinical and experimental interrelationships between sympathetic nervous activity and pituitary thyroid function. Proceedings of the Academiai Kiado Symposium of the International Society of Psychoneuroendocrinology. Budapest: Hungarian Academy of Sciences, 1976:273

64. Scarpace P, Abrass I. Thyroid hormone regulations of rat heart, lymphocyte and lung β-adrenergic receptors. Endocrinology 1981;108:1007

65. Tejani-Butt SM, Yang J, Kaviani A. Time course of altered thyroid states on 5-HT$_{1A}$ receptors and 5-HT uptake sites in rat brain: An autoradiographic analysis. Neuroendocrinology 1993; 57:1011

66. Tejani-Butt SM, Yang J. A time course of altered thyroid states on the noradrenergic system in rat brain by quantitative autoradiography. Neuroendocrinology 1994;59:235

67. Marwaha J, Prasad KN. Hypothyroidism elicits electrophysiological noradrenergic subsensitivity in rat cerebellum. Science 1981; 214:675

68. Gomez ST. Hypothyroidism, psychotropic drugs and cardiotoxicity. Br J Psychiatry 1980;136:89

Werner and Ingbar's The Thyroid, Seventh Edition,
edited by Lewis E. Braverman and Robert D. Utiger.
Lippincott–Raven Publishers, Philadelphia, © 1996

75

Myxedema Coma

Leonard Wartofsky

Myxedema coma is a rare syndrome that represents the extreme expression of severe hypothyroidism. It was probably first reported in 1879 by Ord from the St. Thomas Hospital, London. Two of 12 patients with fatal hypothyroidism described in a report of the Clinical Society of London in 1888 appeared to have died in coma.[1] Amazingly, the next cases did not appear in the literature until 1953,[2,3] and about 200 cases have subsequently been reported. Additional references may be obtained from earlier reviews.[4–6] The syndrome most often is seen in hospitalized, elderly women who have had long-standing hypothyroidism, and the classic features of the disease usually are present. Once considered, the diagnosis should be easy to establish on both clinical and laboratory grounds, but early vigorous therapy may still be associated with a mortality rate as high as 60%.

CLINICAL FEATURES

Precipitating Events

The syndrome most often is encountered during the winter months, which has given rise to speculation that external cold may be an aggravating factor. Other events most commonly reported to be associated with the onset of myxedema coma include pulmonary infections, cerebrovascular accidents, and congestive heart failure (Table 75-1). Pulmonary infection also may occur as a secondary event in the comatose, hypoventilating patient, as can aspiration pneumonia. Similarly, it may be difficult to determine whether other abnormalities, such as hypoglycemia, hyponatremia, hypercapnia, and hypoxemia, which often are associated with myxedema coma, may have contributed to the precipitation of the coma or are secondary consequences. Drugs often can be incriminated as being responsible for initiating or compounding the downward spiral of the hypothyroid patient into coma. In this regard, the common culprits include anesthetics, narcotics, sedatives, antide-

pressants, and tranquilizers, and the mechanism appears to be related to depression of respiratory center drive.

General Description

Two of the cardinal features of myxedema coma are hypothermia and unconsciousness. It is not unusual for the syndrome to present in patients with previously undiagnosed hypothyroidism whose illness has become complicated by infection or other systemic disease. There may be a history of antecedent thyroid disease, thyroid hormone replacement therapy that was discontinued for no apparent reason, or therapy with radioactive iodine. Examination of the neck may reveal a surgical scar and no palpable thyroid tissue, or a goiter. Fewer than 10% of patients have hypothalamic or pituitary disease as the basis for their hypothyroidism. The course often is one of lethargy progressing to stupor and then coma, which may be hastened by the use of sedatives or narcotics, leading to respiratory failure and CO_2 retention. The usual features of dry, coarse, and scaly skin, delayed deep-tendon reflexes, sparse or coarse hair, carotenemic pallor, puffy facies, large tongue, and hoarseness may be present, as well as moderate to profound (80°F) hypothermia. It also is conceivable that coma could be precipitated by an overwhelming systemic process in a patient with a milder clinical hypothyroidism who has few of these more dramatic signs of the disease.

Respiratory System

The most important factor underlying the ventilatory abnormality in myxedema is a depression of the hypoxic respiratory drive, which may be accompanied by a depressed ventilatory response to hypercapnia, albeit of lesser pathophysiologic significance.[7] The resulting decrease in alveolar ventilation leads to progressive CO_2 narcosis and coma, and impaired respiratory muscle function may compound the hypoventilation.[8] Wilson and Bedell[9] suggested that the bellows action of the

TABLE 75-1.
Myxedema Coma: Precipitating Factors

Cerebrovascular accidents

Hypothermia

Infection

Congestive heart failure

Drugs

    Anesthetics

    Sedatives

    Tranquilizers

    Narcotics

    Lithium carbonate[31]

    Amiodarone[32]

Trauma

Gastrointestinal bleeding

Metabolic disturbances compounding obtundation

    Hypoglycemia

    Hyponatremia

    Hypercapnia

    Acidosis

chest was impaired in hypothyroidism, and it also was proposed that obesity might favor hypoventilation. Studies of two patients by Massumi and Winnacker[10] indicated that obesity was not a significant factor, but that a depressed ventilatory response to CO_2 was central to the pathophysiology of coma.[11] Careful studies in an additional patient by Domm and Vassallo[12] further incriminated depression of the respiratory center response to CO_2 as the key element in coma. Although these early reports[9,10,12] noted some improvement in the response to CO_2 with thyroid hormone therapy, this was not found to be the case in a larger, well-studied series of patients reported more recently by Zwillich and coworkers.[7] They noted that maximum voluntary ventilation was preserved in hypothyroidism, with only minimal reduction in spirometric measurements of lung function. In contrast to a dramatic improvement in hypoxic ventilatory reserve with thyroid hormone treatment, they observed little change in mechanical ventilatory function or in hypercapneic ventilatory response with hormone replacement.[7] Regardless of the cause, mechanical function in myxedema coma usually is reduced enough to require mechanically assisted ventilation, especially if narcotic or sedative drugs may be playing a role in the depressed ventilation. Several other physical or anatomic factors may impede ventilation in the hypothyroid patient, such as the presence of pleural effusions or ascites. In addition, swelling of the tongue and tissue of the upper respiratory tract with a myxedematous infiltrate can cause partial obstruction that can become more complete with superimposed infection (e.g., laryngeal obstruction caused by marked edema of the vocal cords), leading to an acute respiratory emergency. Recovery from respiratory failure may be delayed,[13] despite apparently adequate therapy.

Cardiovascular Manifestations

The findings considered typical of hypothyroid heart disease also are found in myxedema coma, and include enlargement of the cardiac silhouette, bradycardia, decreased quality and intensity of the heart sounds, and minor electrocardiographic abnormalities. The latter consist of varying degrees of block, low voltage, prolonged QT interval, and flattened or inverted T waves. Although enlargement of the cardiac silhouette may be partly due to some ventricular dilatation, it largely is the result of pericardial effusion secondary to accumulation of fluid rich in mucopolysaccharide. This fluid tends to accumulate over a long time, and as a consequence, cardiac tamponade is rare. Optimal diagnosis of pericardial effusion would be achieved by echocardiography, and confirmation by angiocardiography is seldom needed.

Although stroke volume and cardiac output are reduced on the basis of impaired cardiac contractility, frank congestive heart failure is very rare. The abnormalities in left ventricular function and the pericardial effusions return progressively toward normal with thyroxine (T_4) replacement therapy.[14] Myocardial infarction may be present or occur with thyroid treatment because of underlying coronary atherosclerosis. Although the hypercholesterolemia of myxedema has been suspected as playing a causative role in the latter, concomitant hypertension has been a more specific contributory factor.[15] The lactate dehydrogenase isoenzyme pattern in severe hypothyroidism may mimic that of myocardial infarction,[16] and creatine kinase levels also are elevated.[17] To add to the potential confusion, patients with hypothyroidism are at risk of sustaining myocardial infarction with injudicious thyroid hormone replacement. Nevertheless, the high mortality of untreated myxedema coma demands vigorous treatment with thyroid hormone, as will be discussed.

Although total body water and extracellular fluid volume may be increased, intravascular volume is reduced, and this contributes to the propensity for hypotension. Improvement in the hypotension regularly follows replacement with thyroid hormone. Cardiovascular collapse and shock may supervene in myxedema coma before there is adequate time for thyroid hormone to act, in which case the use of pressors is mandatory. It has been repeatedly observed that combined therapy with pressor amines and thyroid is required in shock. This situation is fraught with an extremely high potential for fatal arrhythmias and demands careful monitoring of such patients in an intensive care unit.

Gastrointestinal Manifestations

Decreased intestinal motility is common in hypothyroidism, and its severest manifestation, paralytic ileus, is frequent in myxedema coma. Impaired peristalsis may be due to both neuropathic changes related to thyroid deficiency and myxedematous infiltration of the muscularis of the gut. Accompanying problems include constipation and obstipation, both of which improve with replacement therapy. The differential diagnosis of paralytic ileus may include mechanical obstruction necessitating consideration of surgical intervention, which could itself be fatal in myxedema coma. Hence, conservative decompression and temporization are desirable until the response to thyroid hormone can be assessed. Gastric atony in myxedema coma is a particularly troublesome problem because absorption of oral medications is affected. Because of this, parenteral administration of T_4 or triiodothyronine (T_3) may be preferable (see later).

Renal and Electrolyte Manifestations

Abnormalities that have been noted in severe hypothyroidism include increased body water, decreased plasma volume, decreased serum sodium and osmolality, increased urine sodium and osmolality, and reduced glomerular filtration rate and renal plasma flow. Similar to the reduced intestinal tone described earlier, bladder atony with retention of large residual urine volumes is not unusual. The hyponatremia is probably secondary to impaired water diuresis caused by reduced delivery of water to the distal nephron[18] and in part to elevated levels of antidiuretic hormone.[19] Hyponatremia, if present, is likely to compound the patient's mental confusion, and when severe, it may be largely responsible for precipitating the comatose state. Treatment with thyroid hormone promotes water diuresis, with a resultant decrease in edema and total body water and an increase in serum sodium.

Neuropsychiatric Manifestations

The patient with the full-blown syndrome of myxedema coma manifests or complains of few neuropsychiatric signs or symptoms other than the coma itself. There may be a history of disorientation, depression, paranoia, or hallucinations ("myxedema madness"). The subjects demonstrate poor memory to frank amnesia, varying degrees of somnolence and lethargy progressing into coma, and cerebellar signs, such as clumsy movements of the hands and feet, ataxia, and adiadochokinesia. The electroencephalogram is abnormal, with low amplitude and a decreased rate of alpha activity.[20] Minor seizures or frank convulsions have occurred in about 25% of patients with myxedema coma, but hyponatremia may be responsible for most of these. In these usually elderly patients, decreased cardiac output combined with arteriosclerotic cerebrovascular disease is likely to produce decreased perfusion and cerebral hypoxia. Improvement in all of the functional parameters occurs gradually with thyroid hormone replacement.

Infections

The possibility of occult pneumonia leading to a worsening of the respiratory status has been mentioned. Overall prognosis also may be reduced as a consequence of delays in the diagnosis of other infections because of the absence of fever and other clues to infection, such as diaphoresis and tachycardia. Respiratory tract infection may be more common because of the risk of aspiration in a stuporous patient, particularly when complicated by seizures related to hyponatremia.[21] Because of these considerations and the fear that undiscovered infection might lead inexorably to vascular collapse and death, some authors have advocated the routine use of antibiotics in patients with myxedema coma.[22] This approach might be most defensible if limited to the period of delicate prognostic balance during the initial 24 to 48 hours of management. Rather,

it may be more prudent to keep alert to the possibility of infection, especially in the presence of hypothermia, and vigorously seek any potential source of infection, instituting specific antibiotic therapy only when indicated on the basis of appropriate specimen smears and cultures.

Hypothermia

Hypothermia is present in about three-fourths of patients, often is dramatic (<80°F), and may be the first clinical clue to the diagnosis of myxedema coma. Similarly, the diagnosis should seriously be considered in any unconscious patient with a known infectious process who does not have an elevation in temperature. A careful history and physical examination usually serve to confirm the diagnosis or render it unlikely enough to justify awaiting the results of serum T_4 and thyrotropin (TSH) determinations before the initiation of treatment. Patients with core temperatures less than 90°F tend to have the worst prognosis. Underlying hypoglycemia may serve to further decrease body temperature. In those hospitals still using oral or rectal thermometers, the temperature recorded may be inaccurately high, because the mercury column has not been shaken to a sufficiently low reading. Moreover, because these older clinical thermometers do not record below 94°F, true temperature may be either missed or discounted as an error. Modern electronic thermometers are not a problem in this regard. The presence of any appreciable hypothermia implies a poor prognosis, and the immediate initiation of thyroid hormone therapy is mandatory. With treatment, the hypothermia gradually improves in parallel with increments in serum T_4 and T_3 levels.

DIAGNOSIS

The importance of making the diagnosis cannot be stressed strongly enough, because the unnecessary administration of relatively large doses of thyroid hormone to an elderly euthyroid patient clearly may provoke an early demise. On the other hand, when there is a reasonably high index of suspicion, treatment should not be delayed to await laboratory confirmation. It may be difficult to distinguish severe fatigue and somnolence in an uncomplicated hypothyroid patient from true myxedema coma. Although overzealous treatment in such a patient is discouraged, diagnostic aggressiveness is mandatory to determine whether CO_2 retention, hypoxia, hyponatremia, or infection is present. These derangements can then be treated promptly, thereby obviating the development of myxedema coma.

Of great interest is the observation that coma frequently has supervened in hypothyroid patients while they were hospitalized for other problems or for diagnostic studies. It well may have been the stress of the diagnostic procedures, the administration of intravenous fluids, or, more importantly, the all-too-common routine hospital use of sedative and hypnotic drugs that precipitated decline of the patient into the comatose state. Other causes of coma need to be ruled out.

As previously mentioned, the typical patient is a woman in her seventies who presents during the winter, commonly with a history of thyroid disease or possibly of taking depressant medications. Physical findings often include bradycardia, macroglossia, hoarseness, delayed reflexes, dry skin, general cachexia, hypoventilation, and hypothermia, commonly without shivering. The routine laboratory evaluation may indicate anemia, hyponatremia, hypercholesterolemia, and increased serum lactate dehydrogenase and creatine kinase. A lumbar puncture performed during the evaluation of coma reveals increased pressure and cerebrospinal fluid with a high protein content. The electrocardiogram and chest radiograph may demonstrate the characteristic findings described earlier.

In many patients, the clinical features may be so overwhelming as to render the measurement of thyroid-function tests necessary only for confirmation of the diagnosis. The urgency of the diagnosis should be stressed to the laboratory, which often can perform a serum T_4 determination in 3 to 6 hours and a TSH determination in 6 to 8 hours. Although an elevated serum TSH concentration is the most important laboratory evidence of the diagnosis, the presence of severe, complicating systemic illness may serve to reduce the elevation in TSH levels.[23,24] Also, one must be alert to the possibility of a pituitary cause for the hypothyroidism, in which case an increased TSH would not be found. The clinical features that are more characteristic of secondary (pituitary) hypothyroidism have been reviewed in chapter 59. The latter cause of myxedema coma has different implications for the initial treatment of the syndrome, and this is discussed later. Moreover, the finding of a low serum T_4 and a normal serum TSH could indicate that the patient is not hypothyroid, but rather has severe nonthyroidal illness. This differential diagnosis has been discussed elsewhere.[24] If the latter appears unlikely in a patient with a decreased serum T_4 level and the serum TSH is low-normal or undetectable, then pituitary insufficiency must be ruled out and further workup is indicated. Until the absence of pituitary disease is demonstrated, corticosteroid therapy is required in addition to thyroid hormone.

THERAPY

In view of the extremely high mortality anticipated in untreated patients with myxedema coma, it is essential that treatment be instituted promptly and vigorously as soon as the diagnosis is made. Because it is likely that physiologic and metabolic derangement in many (if not all) of the various organ systems described earlier may be contributing to the comatose state, a multifaceted approach is required for effective therapy. The entire treatment team should be made aware that they are dealing with a true medical emergency, and meticulous care in a critical care setting with modern electronic monitoring equipment is essential.

Ventilatory Support

Hypoventilation due to a number of factors may be present and may result in CO_2 retention, respiratory acidosis, and aggravation of the comatose state. The possibility of complicating pneumonitis in these patients also has been discussed, and appropriate diagnostic and therapeutic measures must be instituted for any suspicious infiltrate seen on chest radiography, with the recognition that fever and cough may not be prominent. Death caused by respiratory failure is not unusual, and hence the maintenance of an adequate airway and the prevention of hypoxemia is the single most important supportive measure required to avoid catastrophe. Mechanical ventilatory support usually is mandatory during the first 48 hours, particularly if the hypoventilation is due in part to drug-related respiratory depression. Although the patient may become alert by the 2nd or 3rd day of therapy, complicated cases may require assisted or controlled ventilation for as long as 2 to 3 weeks.[13]

Arterial blood gases need to be monitored regularly until the patient is fully recovered. The physician should not hesitate to insert an endotracheal tube or to perform a tracheostomy, if necessary, as dictated by a worsening in blood gases. Numerous reports have cited the danger of relapse with premature withdrawal of the endotracheal tube. Hence, this should be attempted cautiously, with close attention to possible worsening of blood gases, and it should never be attempted until the patient is fully conscious.

Hyponatremia

Total-body sodium is probably normal to increased, and impaired water excretion is the major underlying reason for hyponatremia. Serum sodium levels low enough to induce a semicomatose state and seizures in otherwise euthyroid patients may be found in myxedema coma. Hence, such severe hyponatremia (105–120 mEq/L) is likely to contribute substantially to the coma in these patients. Therapy with intravenous fluids in general, and saline in particular, must be approached cautiously, because some element of decreased cardiac reserve is likely in many of these patients. If hypoglycemia is present, sodium chloride should be added to any fluids given to correct the low blood glucose, or a concentrated glucose solution should be used. Otherwise, fluid restriction may be all that is necessary to correct hyponatremia, especially if it is mild (120–130 mEq/L). If severe hyponatremia is present, it may be appropriate to administer a small amount of hypertonic saline (50–100 mL of 5% sodium chloride) early in the course of treatment, and this can be followed by an intravenous bolus dose of 40 to 120 mg of furosemide to promote a water diuresis.[25] A central venous pressure line should be used to monitor any fluid or saline therapy that is administered, and placement of a Swan-Ganz catheter is justifiable in the presence of significant cardiovascular decompensation.

Hypothermia

Administration of thyroid hormone ultimately is essential to restore body temperature to normal. Until that effect is achieved, some physical means of keeping the patient warm may be advisable; ordinary blankets or increasing room temperature can be used, but great caution must be exercised in the use of measures for external warming. The use of electric warming blankets can cause vasodilation and provide too precipitous a fall in peripheral vascular resistance. The resultant augmentation in peripheral blood flow is accompanied by increased oxygen consumption, and this may lead to aggravated hypotension or even vascular collapse.

Hypotension

Like the hypothermia, hypotension also should be correctable by specific treatment with thyroid hormone. Because this may take several days or longer, profound hypotension requires additional therapy. Initially, fluids may be cautiously administered as 5% to 10% glucose in half-normal sodium chloride, or as isotonic sodium chloride if hyponatremia is present. Administration of hydrocortisone (100 mg IV every 8 hours) may be justified until the tendency toward hypotension is corrected. A rare patient may require pressor agents to maintain a blood pressure sufficient to sustain adequate perfusion. Indeed, hypotension in these patients may be due in part to a reduction in the normal physiologic synergism between circulating catecholamines and thyroid hormones. As a consequence, both thyroid hormone and pressor agents may have to be given, while recognizing the possibility of inducing dangerous ventricular tachyarrhythmias, because these patients have a high incidence of underlying ischemic heart disease. An agent such as dopamine might be preferable to metaraminol or norepinephrine to maintain coronary blood flow, but in any event, an effort should be made to taper the dosage and wean the patient from any pressor agent as soon as possible. Although an adverse interaction between administered catecholamine and thyroid hormone is possible, the physician must weigh this risk against the known high mortality in myxedema coma of hypotension that proves unresponsive to the initial therapy.

Adrenal Steroids

The coexistence of adrenal insufficiency in patients with myxedema coma may be suggested by the presence of hypotension, hypothermia, hypoglycemia, hyponatremia, and hyperkalemia. Indeed, decreased adrenal reserve has been found in 5% to 10% of patients on the basis of either hypopituitarism or primary adrenal failure accompanying Hashimoto's disease (Schmidt's syndrome). Serum cortisol levels and the adrenal response to adrenocorticotropic hormone (ACTH) infusion are normal in hypothyroidism and in myxedema coma. It is believed, however, that ACTH reserve or the ACTH response to stress is impaired in these patients, although definitive studies on this point remain to be done. Moreover, given the potential risk to the patient undergoing the stress of acute illness versus the relative safety of short-term steroid therapy, there should be no reluctance to administer hydrocortisone or a comparable compound until the patient is stable and the integrity of the pituitary-adrenal axis is determined. With the institution of thyroid hormone therapy, there is an additional theoretic basis for supplemental corticosteroids, in view of the sluggish response of the pituitary-adrenal axis in hypothyroidism to the accelerated metabolism of cortisol that follows T_4 replacement. Hydrocortisone usually is given in a dosage of 50 to 100 mg every 6 to 8 hours during the first 7 to 10 days and is then tapered on the basis of clinical response and plans for further diagnostic evaluation.

Thyroid Hormone Therapy

Perhaps the most controversial aspect of the management of myxedema coma relates to the technique for restoring the low serum and tissue thyroid hormone concentrations. The differences of opinion largely relate to whether to administer T_4 and allow the patient to convert it to T_3, or to give T_3 itself. Secondary issues include dose, frequency, and route of administration (of either compound). Different approaches to management are based on balancing concerns for the high mortality of the untreated disease and the obvious need for attaining effective thyroid hormone levels against the risks of precipitating a fatal tachyarrhythmia or myocardial infarction. Because of the relative rarity of this condition and the consequent paucity of reported treatment results, as well as the difficulties inherent in performing any controlled study, the optimum mode of therapy remains uncertain.

Those who advocate T_4 as the therapeutic choice point out that it provides a steady, smooth onset of action with less risk of adverse effects. Although monitoring of therapeutic efficacy was formerly easier when T_4 rather than T_3 was given because of the ubiquity of assays for T_4 in serum, this may no longer apply, since most hospitals can perform a serum T_3 assay in a comparably short turnaround time. TSH levels may be monitored with the use of either preparation.

There are now parenteral preparations of either T_4 or T_3 available for intravenous administration. Although oral forms of either T_3 or T_4 can be given by nasogastric tube, this route is fraught with risks of aspiration and uncertain absorption, particularly because gastric atony may be present. Preparations of T_4 for parenteral use are available in ampules of 100 and 500 μg. The latter dose, as a single intravenous bolus, was popularized by reports[26] suggesting that replacement of the entire estimated pool of extrathyroidal T_4 (usually 300–600 μg) was desirable to restore near-normal hormonal status as rapidly as possible. Although the importance of T_4 conversion to T_3 was not fully appreciated when this therapeutic regimen was proposed, the approach proved efficacious. After the initial loading dose, a daily maintenance dose of 50 to 100 μg is given (intravenously, or by mouth when the patient becomes alert). This method is attended by increases in serum T_4 to within the normal range within 24 hours and by significant decrements in serum TSH. Larger doses of T_4 probably have no advantage and may, in fact, be more dangerous.[27] The 300 to 600 μg doses of T_4 should result in progressive increases in serum T_3, as have been described by Ridgway and coworkers.[27]

There is one real and important potential drawback to the total reliance on generation of T_3 from T_4. It is now well known that the rate of conversion of T_4 to T_3 is reduced in a wide variety of systemic illnesses (the low T_3 syndrome),[24] and hence T_3 generation may be reduced in myxedema coma as a consequence of an associated illness.[25] In such a patient, measured increases in serum T_4 might not be accompanied by clinical improvement, and serum TSH might not fall. In view of this potential problem, it would appear that at least small supplements of T_3 should be given along with T_4 during the initial few days of therapy, especially if obvious associated illness is present. Experimentally in baboons, T_3 crosses the blood–brain barrier more readily than does T_4.[28] Regardless of which type of therapy is selected, all patients should have continuous electrocardiographic monitoring so that thyroid hormone dosage can be reduced if arrhythmias or ischemic changes are detected.

In addition to the problem with T_3 generation from T_4 in the sick patient, advocates of T_3 as the choice for therapy point out that it has a much quicker onset of action. T_3 for intravenous use (Triostat; SmithKline Beecham) is available in 1 ml vials containing 10 μg/mL. Therapy with T_3 alone may be given as a 20-μg bolus followed by 10 μg every 4 hours for the first 24 hours, dropping to 10 μg every 6 hours for the second and third days, by which time oral administration should be feasible. Increases in body temperature and oxygen consumption may occur 2 to 3 hours after intravenous T_3, compared with 8 to 14 hours after intravenous T_4. Because the mortality rate in myxedema coma is high, advocates for T_3 therapy argue that the more rapid onset of action could make the difference between life and death. But as alluded to initially, one also must accept a greater risk of complications along with the benefits of the more rapid onset of action. As a consequence, it is difficult to justify the high risk/benefit ratio of a regimen that uses rapid replacement with relatively large doses of intravenous T_3 alone. Such treatment would be marked by large and unpredictable fluctuations in serum T_3 levels and a significantly greater risk of a dangerous cardiac event. Indeed, in addition to advanced age, high serum T_3 levels during treatment with thyroid hormone have been associated with fatal outcome.[29] Again, perhaps some compromise (i.e., combined therapy with both T_4 and T_3) may be a rational approach until more adequate data are available.

Consequently our approach to therapy uses both thyroid hormones. Rather than administer 300 to 500 μg of T_4 intravenously initially, a dose of 4 μg/kg lean body weight (or about 200–300 μg) is given, and an additional 100 μg is given 24 hours later. By the third day, the dose is reduced to a daily maintenance dose of 50 μg, which can be given by mouth as soon as the patient is stable and conscious. This dose subsequently is adjusted on the basis of clinical and laboratory results, as in any other hypothyroid patient. Simultaneously with the initial dose of T_4, a bolus of 20 μg of T_3 is given and intravenous T_3 is continued at a dosage of 10 μg/8 hours until the patient is conscious and taking maintenance T_4. Sensitivity to thyroid hormone in terms of cardiac risk varies, depending on age, cardiac medications, and the presence of underlying hypoxemia, coronary artery disease, congestive failure, and electrolyte imbalance. Even a single dose of only 2.5 μg of T_3 may be associated with clinical improvement.[30] No general guide to management can take all of these factors into account, and hence it is wise to carefully monitor the patient for any untoward effects of therapy before administering each dose of thyroid hormone.

In addition to the specific therapies outlined, general supportive measures are indicated as in treatment of any other elderly, cachectic patient. This includes the treatment of any underlying problems with specific medications (e.g., digoxin for congestive heart failure), recognizing that the dosage of such drugs may need to be modified based on their altered distribution and metabolism in myxedema. Finally, the prognosis for myxedema coma remains grim even with apparently vigorous therapy, and patients with severe hypothermia and hypotension seem to do the worst. Perhaps further elucidation of thyroid economy in health and disease will provide approaches to therapy that will result in an improved prognosis. Until then, early recognition and treatment, with meticulous attention to the details of management during the first 48 hours, remain critical for the avoidance of a fatal outcome.

References

1. Report of a committee of the Clinical Society of London to investigate the subject of myxedema. Trans Clin Soc (Lond) (Suppl) 1888:21
2. LeMarquand HS, Hausmann W, Hemstead EH. Myxedema as a cause of death. Br Med J [Clin Res] 1953;1:704
3. Summers VK. Myxedema coma. Br Med J [Clin Res] 1953;2:336
4. Blum M. Myxedema coma. Am J Med Sci 1972;264:432
5. Royce PC. Severely impaired consciousness in myxedema: a review. Am J Med Sci 1971;261:46
6. Nicoloff JT, LoPresti JS. Myxedema coma: A form of decompensated hypothyroidism. Endocrin Metab Clin North Am 1993;22:279
7. Zwillich CW, Pierson DJ, Hofeldt FD, Lufkin EG, Weil JV. Ventilatory control in myxedema and hypothyroidism. N Engl J Med 1975;292:662
8. Martinez FJ, Bermudez-Gomez M, Celli BR. Hypothyroidism: a reversible cause of diaphragmatic dysfunction. Chest 1989;96:1059
9. Wilson WR, Bedell GM. The pulmonary abnormalities in myxedema. J Clin Invest 1960;39:42
10. Massumi RA, Winnacker JL. Severe depression of the respiratory center in myxedema. Am J Med 1964;36:876
11. Ladenson PW, Goldenheim PD, Ridgway EC. Prediction of reversal of blunted respiratory responsiveness in patients with hypothyroidism. Am J Med 1988;84:877
12. Domm BB, Vassallo CL. Myxedema coma with respiratory failure. Am Rev Respir Dis 1973;107:842
13. Yamamoto T. Delayed respiratory failure during the treatment of myxedema coma. Endocrinol Jpn 1984;31:769
14. Crowley WF, Ridgway EC, Bough EW, et al. Noninvasive evaluation of cardiac function in hypothyroidism. N Engl J Med 1977;296:1
15. Steinberg AD. Myxedema and coronary artery disease: a comparative autopsy study. Ann Intern Med 1968;68:338
16. Aber CP, Noble RL, Thomson GS, Wyn-Jones E. Serum lactic dehydrogenase isoenzymes in "myxedema heart disease." Br Heart J 1966;28:663
17. Nee PA, Scane SC, Lavelle PH, Fellows IW, Hill PG. Hypothermic myxedema coma erroneously diagnosed as myocardial infarction because of increased creatine kinase MB. Clin Chem 1987;33:1083
18. DeRubertis FR Jr, Michelis MF, Bloom MG, et al. Impaired water excretion in myxedema. Am J Med 1971;51:41
19. Skowsky RW, Kikuchi TA. The role of vasopressin in the impaired water excretion of myxedema. Am J Med 1978;64:613
20. Sanders V. Neurologic manifestations of myxedema. N Engl J Med 1962;266:547
21. Senior RM, Birge SJ. The recognition and management of myxedema coma. JAMA 1971;217:61
22. Lindberger K. Myxoedema coma. Acta Med Scand 1975;198:87
23. Hooper MJ. Diminished TSH secretion during acute non-thyroidal illness in untreated primary hypothyroidism. Lancet 1976;1:48
24. Wartofsky L, Burman KD. Alterations in thyroid function in patients with systemic illness: the "euthyroid sick syndrome." Endocr Rev 1982;3:164
25. Pereira VG, Haron ES, Lima-Neto N, Medeiros-Neto GA. Management of myxedema coma: report on three successfully treated cases with nasogastric or intravenous administration of triiodothyronine. J Endocrinol Invest 1982;5:331

26. Holvey DN, Goodner CJ, Nicoloff JT, Dowling JT. Treatment of myxedema coma with intravenous thyroxine. Arch Intern Med 1964;113:89

27. Ridgway EC, McCammon JA, Benotti J, et al. Metabolic responses of patients with myxedema to large doses of intravenous L-thyroxine. Ann Intern Med 1972;77:549

28. Chernow B, Burman KD, Johnson DL, et al. T_3 may be a better agent than T_4 in the critically ill hypothyroid patient: evaluation of transport across the blood-brain barrier in a primate model. Crit Care Med 1983;11:99

29. Hylander B, Rosenqvist U. Treatment of myxoedema coma: factors associated with fatal outcome. Acta Endocrinol (Copeh) 1985;108:65

30. McCulloch W, Price P, Hinds CJ, Wass JA. Effects of low dose oral triiodothyronine in myxoedema coma. Intensive Care Med 1985;11:259

31. Waldman SA, Park D. Myxedema coma associated with lithium therapy. Am J Med 1989;87:355

32. Mazonson PD, Williams ML, Cantley LK, et al. Myxedema coma during long-term amiodarone therapy. Am J Med 1984;77:751

Werner and Ingbar's The Thyroid, Seventh Edition,
edited by Lewis E. Braverman and Robert D. Utiger.
Lippincott–Raven Publishers, Philadelphia, © 1996

Section D
Management of Hypothyroidism

76

Diagnosis of Hypothyroidism

Paul W. Ladenson

Since the syndrome of myxedema was described more than a century ago, the criteria for diagnosis of hypothyroidism have changed from clinical observation to bioassays, increasingly specific measurements of thyroid hormones in serum, and quantitation of endogenous thyrotropin (TSH) production. Accurate diagnosis of hypothyroidism requires awareness of the clinical features that define a patient's risk for thyroid hormone deficiency and proper use of the two tests usually required to confirm the disorder: serum TSH and free thyroxine (T_4). These sensitive and specific measures of thyroid function have largely resolved the inaccuracy associated with the clinical diagnosis of hypothyroidism. However, they have also introduced new diagnostic challenges. First, we now appreciate that there are many patients with few clinical manifestations of hypothyroidism and mild thyroid hormone deficiency that is revealed only by serum TSH measurements—a disorder defined as subclinical hypothyroidism.[1] Second, thyroid test abnormalities are common in patients with nonthyroidal illness.[2] Consequently, clinicians must still integrate clinical observations with laboratory test results to diagnose and manage patients with hypothyroidism properly.

CLINICAL DIAGNOSIS

Three types of clinical evidence suggest hypothyroidism: symptoms and signs consistent with thyroid hormone defi-

ciency; evidence of disease, previous treatment, or exposure known to cause thyroid or pituitary failure; and the presence of disorders associated with increased risk of chronic autoimmune thyroiditis.

Clinical Manifestations

Thyroid hormone deficiency may present as an obvious clinical syndrome (e.g., cretinism or myxedema). Clinical manifestations usually provide clues to the presence of hypothyroidism, but they are too insensitive and nonspecific for definitive diagnosis.[3] Even in patients with overt biochemical hypothyroidism, symptoms and signs may be minimal or absent. Several factors account for the subtlety with which hypothyroidism can present: its insidious onset, the presence of mild thyroid hormone deficiency, and the passivity that characterizes hypothyroidism in many patients. Furthermore, many of the symptoms of hypothyroidism are nonspecific (e.g., fatigue and constipation), as are several of the physical findings (e.g., dry skin and weight gain). Among patients with symptoms potentially attributable to hypothyroidism in a primary care setting, the diagnosis is established in only 1% to 4%.[4,5] Moreover, hypothyroidism has age- and sex-specific presentations (e.g., impaired growth in children, menorrhagia in menstruating women, and dementia in the elderly).

Predisposition to Hypothyroidism

Hypothyroidism should be suspected when there is evidence of an underlying thyroid, pituitary, or hypothalamic disorder known to cause thyroid failure, or when some previous treatment has destroyed thyroid, pituitary, or hypothalamic tissue. For example, the presence of a diffuse goiter, a common manifestation of chronic autoimmune thyroiditis, should prompt laboratory evaluation for hypothyroidism (see chap 55). A history of previous thyroid surgery or radioactive iodine therapy likewise suggests possible primary hypothyroidism, which can occur both soon or many years after either treatment. This is particularly true in patients with Graves' disease, who may eventually become hypothyroid even in the absence of destructive therapy.[6] Neck surgery and external radiation therapy for lymphoma and head and neck cancer also frequently cause hypothyroidism (see chap 58).

Clinical evidence of hypothalamic or pituitary disease should raise suspicion of central hypothyroidism, also known as secondary or hypothyrotropic hypothyroidism (see chap 59). Hypothalamic disorders that can cause thyrotropin-releasing hormone (TRH) deficiency include tumors and granulomatous diseases. The pituitary is affected principally by endocrine and other tumors, or treatment for them. Therefore, evidence of hypopituitarism, such as growth failure, hypogonadism, adrenal insufficiency, or diabetes insipidus; an expanding sellar mass lesion (e.g., headache, bitemporal hemianopsia); or a pituitary tumor secreting hormones other than TSH should prompt evaluation for hypothyroidism.

Risk factors for hypothyroidism include a variety of drugs, of which lithium carbonate is the most commonly used[7] (see chap 58). Iodine in pharmacologic quantities can cause hypothyroidism in patients with underlying thyroid disease by interfering with thyroid hormone synthesis and release (see subchapter on the effect of excess iodide in chap 14). Phenytoin, carbamazepine, and rifampin, which increase the clearance of T_4, can cause hypothyroidism in patients with limited thyroid reserve[8] (see subchapter on effects of pharmacologic agents on thyroid hormone metabolism in chap 14).

Chronic Autoimmune Thyroiditis and Hypothyroidism

The family and personal history and the presence of a goiter on physical examination may provide clues to the presence of chronic autoimmune thyroiditis and therefore the presence of hypothyroidism. Because of the genetic predisposition to chronic autoimmune thyroiditis, patients with affected family members are at increased risk of having hypothyroidism. Certain other endocrine deficiencies believed to have an autoimmune pathogenesis also are associated with chronic autoimmune thyroiditis, including idiopathic adrenal insufficiency, insulin-dependent diabetes mellitus, hypoparathyroidism, and primary ovarian failure (see chap 69).

LABORATORY TESTING

Several laboratory test abnormalities may suggest hypothyroidism, but are not tests for it. They include hypercholesterolemia, hyperprolactinemia, anemia, and hyponatremia. Other abnormalities that may indicate the presence of hypothyroidism are x-ray or echocardiographic evidence of pericardial effusion or impaired cardiac contractility.

Failure of thyroid hormone production causes a decline in serum (or plasma) T_4 concentrations. Serum T_3 concentrations also decline, but not until the hypothyroidism is severe. Most patients with overt hypothyroidism have primary thyroid disease, which results in low serum T_4 and high serum TSH concentrations. In contrast, the infrequent patients with central hypothyroidism have low serum T_4 concentrations and low or normal serum TSH concentrations. However, these biochemical findings are not entirely specific for either primary or central hypothyroidism. Abnormal serum thyroid hormone-binding protein concentrations may mask or falsely suggest hypothyroidism (see next section). Serum TSH concentrations may be elevated despite normal serum T_4 concentrations when hypothyroidism is mild (subclinical hypothyroidism), and a few patients with central hypothyroidism have slightly elevated serum TSH concentrations due to secretion of TSH that is immunoreactive but bioinactive.[9]

Serum Thyroxine Determinations

The serum total T_4 concentration can be measured accurately by competitive protein-binding assays that use either anti-T_4 antibodies or serum thyroid hormone-binding proteins (see chap 18). Because most (99.97%) of the T_4 in serum is bound to thyroxine-binding globulin (TBG), transthyretin (TTR, or thyroxine-binding prealbumin), and albumin, low concentrations of one or more of these serum proteins and drug-induced inhibition of T_4 binding to them result in low serum total T_4 concentrations (hypothyroxinemia) that can be misconstrued as indicating hypothyroidism (Table 76-1). Conversely, increased serum protein binding of T_4 may mask hypothyroidism.

Measurement of serum free T_4 resolves most of these problems. Although equilibrium dialysis and ultrafiltration are the most accurate methods for determining serum free T_4, the serum free T_4 index and serum free T_4 radioimmunoassays are adequate for this purpose in most circumstances, and they are simpler, quicker, and less costly. The serum free T_4 index is the product of the serum total T_4 and the thyroid hormone-binding ratio (THBR, also known as the T_3-resin uptake)[10] (see chap 18). Serum free T_4 assay techniques usually yield comparable values. The THBR value, however, can provide additional useful information in patients with nonthyroidal illness, in whom the values are often normal or high despite low calculated serum free T_4 index values and free T_4 concentrations; in contrast, THBR values are low in most patients with hypothyroidism.[11]

Almost all serum free T_4 assays have excellent sensitivity for detection of hypothyroidism in symptomatic patients. In fact, when patients who are clinically screened for abnormal serum TBG concentrations (e.g., those receiving estrogen or oral contraceptive therapy and those who are pregnant) are excluded, the sensitivity of even the serum total T_4 assay as a test for hypothyroidism is greater than 90%. This is particularly true if the cut-off value for the diagnosis is arbitrarily set 2 to 3 μg/dL (26 to 39 nmol/L) above the lower limit of the normal reference range.[4]

MIMICKING CONDITIONS—HYPOTHYROXINEMIA

Decreased serum thyroxine-binding globulin (TBG) concentrations

    Inherited

    Drugs: androgens, glucocorticoids

    Nephrotic syndrome

Competitive inhibition of T_4 binding

    Drugs: salicylate, furosemide

    Nonthyroidal illness

MASKING CONDITIONS

Increased serum TBG concentrations

    Inherited

    Estrogen: pregnancy, exogenous, tumoral production

    Hepatitis, hepatoma

    HIV infection

    Drugs: methadone, heroin, clofibrate, 5-fluorouracil

Familial dysalbuminemic hyperthyroxinemia

Increased transthyretin binding

    Inherited

    Pancreatic and hepatic tumors

The principal shortcoming of serum T_4 determinations is the frequency of low values in hospitalized patients with nonthyroidal illness. For example, in one study about 20% and 12% of patients admitted to an inpatient medical service had low serum total T_4 concentrations and free T_4 index values, respectively.[12]

Serum TSH Determinations

Assay of serum TSH is an exquisitely sensitive test for identifying patients with any degree of primary hypothyroidism. As thyroid hormone production decreases in patients with any form of thyroid injury, serum TSH increases. The decrease in thyroid secretion may be small and not sufficient to reduce the serum total or free T_4 concentration to below the normal range. Because an elevated serum TSH concentration identifies primary hypothyroidism, the analytic sensitivity of the TSH assay (i.e., the least detectable TSH concentration) is not important in using this test to study patients suspected of having hypothyroidism.

The combination of an elevated serum TSH with a normal free T_4 value defines subclinical hypothyroidism. Some of these patients have symptoms or hypercholesterolemia that responds to T_4 therapy,[1,13] but others do not. Therefore, the importance of subclinical hypothyroidism is controversial (see chap 87).

Serum TSH measurements alone do not identify all patients with hypothyroidism. Some patients with central hypothyroidism have normal serum TSH concentrations, although in others they are low. Furthermore, serum TSH con-centrations may be high in conjunction with high total and free serum T_4 concentrations in patients with two unusual conditions: generalized thyroid hormone resistance and TSH-induced thyrotoxicosis.[14,15] However, this combination of results is most often due to erratic ingestion of large doses of T_4 in hypothyroid patients.[16] Serum TSH concentrations may also be transiently elevated during recovery from nonthyroidal illness[17] (see subchapter on nonthyroidal illness in chap 14).

Serum TSH concentrations are often low in patients with nonthyroidal illness,[18] but low TSH secretion seldom, if ever, masks primary hypothyroidism. The exception to this rule may be the hypothyroid patient who has a severe nonthyroidal illness and who is receiving dopamine or glucocorticoid therapy, either of which inhibits TSH secretion. Differentiating the hypothyroxinemia of nonthyroidal illness from central hypothyroidism requires careful consideration of clinical and laboratory evidence suggesting hypothalamic or pituitary disease (e.g., low serum cortisol concentrations, atrophic testes in men, or lack of elevated serum follicle-stimulating hormone concentrations in postmenopausal women) and cranial imaging, but serial testing of thyroid function is usually more informative.

Other Measures of Thyroid Hormone Action

A variety of physiologic measures and serum constituents have been used to quantify thyroid hormone action in peripheral tissues (see chap 19), among them determinations of serum cholesterol, ankle reflex time, and cardiac contractility. However, none of these tests is sufficiently sensitive or specific for hypothyroidism to be useful clinically. Similarly, measurement of basal body temperature is a very poor diagnostic test for hypothyroidism.

SCREENING, CASE-FINDING, AND DIAGNOSIS

Two strategies may be used in screening or case-finding: measurement of serum free T_4 or TSH. The choice should be based on the pretest probability of hypothyroidism, the potential for confounding influences in assay interpretation, and cost. Screening adults for hypothyroidism has not been considered cost effective.[19] However, in a recent study, the cost effectiveness of periodically screening women and men over age 65 years was $829 and $3182 per quality-adjusted life-year respectively, considerably less than the amounts widely considered reasonable for detection of other conditions (e.g., screening for mild hypertension in women over 40 years costs $28,103 per quality-adjusted life-year).[20]

With respect to case-finding, patients can be categorized as having low, moderate, or high risk of hypothyroidism based on published studies of patients with different conditions (Table 76-2). In patients with low risk for hypothyroidism, only one test should be used. The serum free T_4 index is less expensive than the serum TSH, but the latter is preferable even in low-risk patients when detection of subclinical hypothyroidism is important, when coexisting nonthy-

TABLE 76-2.
Screening and Case Finding for Hypothyroidism in Various Patients and Conditions

PATIENTS OR CONDITIONS WITH LOW RISK (PREVALENCE, <2%)

Adults and children at routine visits

Dementia

Psychiatric patients

Elderly patients

Hypercholesterolemia

Sleep apnea

PATIENTS OR CONDITIONS WITH MODERATE RISK (PREVALENCE, 3%–10%)

Goiter or thyroid nodular disease

Lithium carbonate therapy

Associated autoimmune diseases, such as pernicious anemia

Graves' ophthalmopathy

Postpartum women

PATIENTS OR CONDITIONS WITH HIGH RISK (PREVALENCE, >10%)

Chronic autoimmune thyroiditis

Previous treatment for thyrotoxicosis

Previous high-dose neck radiation therapy

Suspected hypopituitarism

Amiodarone therapy

roidal illness may cause hypothyroxinemia, or when both hypothyroidism and thyrotoxicosis must be excluded. No matter which test is done initially, the other test should be done before any intervention is undertaken.

In patients at moderate or high risk of hypothyroidism or those who have symptoms or signs of hypothyroidism in the absence of any of the risk factors listed in Table 76-2, serum TSH and free T_4 should both be measured (Fig. 76-1). A high serum TSH value and a low serum free T_4 value nearly always confirm the diagnosis of primary hypothyroidism; the rare exception is a patient who has central hypothyroidism and is producing bioactive TSH.[9] A high serum TSH value—albeit

usually less than 25 mU/L—and a normal serum free T_4 value are diagnostic of subclinical hypothyroidism. If the serum TSH is low or normal and the serum free T_4 is low, the diagnosis is central hypothyroidism or nonthyroidal illness. The distinction between these two possibilities must be based on the context in which the patient is encountered, the presence of other manifestations of hypothalamic or pituitary disease, and the results of follow-up determinations.

DIAGNOSIS OF DIFFERENT CAUSES OF HYPOTHYROIDISM

Clinical findings suggest the cause of hypothyroidism in most patients, but it is crucial that these be supported by serum TSH assay to exclude those with central hypothyroidism. These latter patients may be endangered by the failure to recognize and treat other consequences of hypopituitarism, particularly adrenal insufficiency, and pituitary mass lesions. The apparent paradox of normal and occasionally even minimally increased serum TSH concentrations in some hypothyroid patients with hypothalamic or pituitary disease is attributable to secretion of TSH with diminished bioactivity.

Antithyroid peroxidase (microsomal) or antithyroglobulin antibodies are present in more than 90% of patients with chronic autoimmune thyroiditis. Although detection of these antibodies indicates that this disorder is the probable cause of primary hypothyroidism, the practical value of these assays is greater in other settings, for example, in predicting the likelihood of progression of subclinical hypothyroidism,[13] in increasing suspicion of underlying thyroid disease in hypothyroxinemic patients with nonthyroidal illness, and in predicting postpartum thyroiditis.[21]

Several tests have little or no value in diagnosing or defining the cause of hypothyroidism, or are outmoded. Serum T_3 measurements are insensitive, because the values are normal in about one-third of overtly hypothyroid patients, and they are nonspecific, because the values are subnormal in many patients with nonthyroidal illness (see subchapter on nonthyroidal illness in chap 14). TRH stimulation testing is no more useful than basal serum TSH measurements in identifying subclinical hypothyroidism. TRH tests also fail to distinguish reliably between hypothalamic and pituitary hypothyroidism, and between these two disorders and nonthyroidal illness.[2]

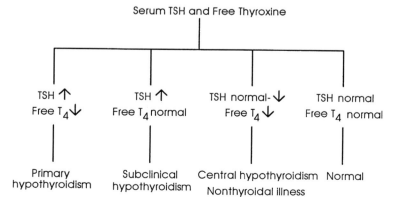

FIGURE 76-1. Diagnostic scheme for evaluating patients at moderate or high risk of hypothyroidism or clinically suspected to have hypothyroidism. Serum free thyroxine (T_4) can be measured either directly or indirectly as the serum free T_4 index.

FUTURE ADVANCES IN LABORATORY ASSESSMENT

Despite the several sensitive and usually specific tests for accurate evaluation of patients with potential hypothyroidism, certain clinical problems occasionally remain unresolved. The evaluation of hypothyroxinemic patients with nonthyroidal illness would be aided by more practical techniques to quantify the biologically active free thyroid hormone fractions in serum and tissues. Simple methods of quantifying tissue thyroid hormone responsiveness—in addition to serum TSH assay—would be very useful, but all foreseeable approaches are nonspecific and, like serum TSH, are unlikely to be generalizable beyond the organ system assessed. A second major need is for tests that more accurately predict the occurrence and prognosis of thyroid autoimmune disease.

References

1. Staub JJ, Althaus BU, Engler H, et al. Spectrum of subclinical an overt hypothyroidism: effect on thyrotropin, prolactin, and thyroid reserve, and metabolic impact in target tissues. Am J Med 1992;92:631
2. Docter R, Krenning EP, deJong M, Hennemann G. The sick euthyroid syndrome: changes in serum thyroid hormone parameters and hormone metabolism. Clin Endocrinol 1993;39:499
3. Seshadri MS, Samuel BU, Kanagasabapathy AS, Cherian AM. Clinical scoring system for hypothyroidism: is it useful? J Gen Intern Med 1989;4:490
4. Goldstein BJ, Mushlin AL. Use of a single thyroxine test to evaluate ambulatory patients for suspected hypothyroidism. J Gen Intern Med 1987;2:20
5. Schectman JM, Kallenberg GA, Shumacher RJ, Hirsh RP. Yield of hypothyroidism in symptomatic primary care patients. Arch Intern Med 1989;149:861
6. Murakami M, Koizumi Y, Aizawa T, et al. Studies of thyroid function and immune parameters in patients with hyperthyroid Graves' disease in remission. J Clin Endocrinol Metab 1988;66:103
7. Myers DH, Carter RA, Burns BH, Armond A, Hussain SB, Chengapa VK. A prospective study of the effect of lithium on thyroid function and on the prevalence of antithyroid antibodies. Psychol Med 1985;15:55
8. Curran PG, De Groot LJ. The effect of hepatic enzyme-inducing drugs on thyroid hormones and the thyroid gland. Endocr Rev 1991;12:135
9. Horimoto M, Nishikawa M, Ishihara T, Yoshikawa N, Yoshimura M, Inada M. Bioactivity of thyrotropin (TSH) in patients with central hypothyroidism: comparison between the in vivo 3,5,3′-triiodothyronine response to TSH and in vitro bioactivity of TSH. J Clin Endocrinol Metab 1995;80:1124
10. Larsen PR, Alexander NM, Chopra IJ, et al. Revised nomenclature for tests of thyroid hormones and thyroid related proteins in serum. J Clin Endocrinol Metab 1987;64:1089
11. Kaptein EM, MacIntyre SS, Weiner JM, Spencer CA, Nicoloff JT. Free thyroxine estimates in nonthyroidal illness: comparison of eight methods. J Clin Endocrinol Metab 1981;52:1073
12. Gooch BR, Isley WL, Utiger, RD. Abnormalities in thyroid function tests in patients admitted to a medical service. Arch Intern Med 1982;142:1801
13. Vanderpump MPJ, Tunbridge WMG, French JM, et al. The incidence of thyroid disorders in the community: a twenty-year follow-up of the Whickham Survey. Clin Endocrinol 1995;43:55
14. Refetoff S, Usala SJ. The syndromes of resistance to thyroid hormones. Endocr Rev 1993;14:348
15. Gesundheit N, Petrick PA, Nissim M, et al. Thyrotropin-secreting pituitary adenomas: clinical and biochemical heterogeneity. Case reports and follow-up of nine patients. Ann Intern Med 1989;111:827
16. England ML, Hershman JM. Serum TSH concentration as an aid to monitoring compliance with thyroid hormone therapy in hypothyroidism. Am J Med Sci 1986;292:264
17. Hamblin PS, Dyer SA, Mohr VS, et al. Relation between serum thyrotropin and thyroxine changes during recovery from severe hypothyroxinemia of critical illness. J Clin Endocrinol Metab 1986;62:717
18. Spencer CA, Eigen A, Shen D, et al. Specificity of sensitive assays of thyrotropin (TSH) used to screen for thyroid disease in hospitalized patients. Clin Chem 1987;33:1391
19. Helfand M, Crapo LM. Screening for thyroid disease. Ann Intern Med 1990;112:840
20. Danese MD, Powe NR, Nathe AS, Ladenson PW. Cost-effectiveness of detecting and treating subclinical hypothyroidism: relative dependence of TSH assay cost and L-thyroxine efficacy and cost.[Abstract]. Program of the 77th Meeting of the Endocrine Society 1995:61
21. Hayslip CC, Fein HG, O'Donnell VM, Friedman DS, Klein TA, Smallridge RC. The value of serum antimicrosomal antibody testing in screening for symptomatic postpartum thyroid dysfunction. Am J Obstet Gynecol 1988;159:203

Werner and Ingbar's The Thyroid, Seventh Edition,
edited by Lewis E. Braverman and Robert D. Utiger.
Lippincott–Raven Publishers, Philadelphia, © 1996

77

Treatment of Hypothyroidism

Gregory A. Brent

P. Reed Larsen

Hypothyroidism was the first endocrine disorder treated by supplementation of the deficient hormone, in the form of extracts of animal thyroid glands. Subsequently, the development of purified thyroid hormone preparations and greater understanding of thyroid physiology has made it possible to closely replicate the function of the normal thyroid gland with thyroid hormone replacement therapy.[1–3] Thyroid hormone treatment is safe and well tolerated by most patients. However, there are a number of clinical situations and drugs that can influence the absorption, metabolism, and action of exogenous thyroid hormone and therefore may necessitate adjustment of therapy. The range of modern dose preparations that are available now and the ability to monitor therapy with measurements of serum thyrotropin (TSH) allow the clinician to provide adequate therapy while minimizing toxicity. In this chapter we discuss the treatment of adults with hypothyroidism. The treatment of infants and children with hypothyroidism is discussed in chapter 85 and the treatment of patients with myxedema coma in chapter 75.

PHARMACOLOGY OF THYROID HORMONE PREPARATIONS

A variety of thyroid hormone preparations are available for the treatment of hypothyroidism, including levothyroxine (T_4), liothyronine (triiodothyronine, T_3), liotrix (a combination of synthetic T_3 and T_4), and thyroid USP (desiccated animal thyroid containing T_3 and T_4 in the form of thyroglobulin). Thyroid hormone replacement utilized thyroid extracts containing both hormones until synthetic combination preparations were introduced. Subsequent studies in humans[4] and animals[5] revealed that the majority of circulating T_3 (about 80%) is produced in peripheral tissues from deiodination of T_4, and that administration of T_4 alone produced adequate serum and tissue concentrations of T_3 and replicated normal thyroid physiology.

The most widely used and the preferred preparation for treatment of hypothyroidism is synthetic T_4. T_4 is absorbed throughout the small intestine, although about two-thirds of the absorption takes place in the proximal portion.[6] Overall, about 70% to 80% of ingested T_4 is absorbed, in contrast to almost 100% of T_3. The advantages of T_4 include its long half-life (approximately 7 days), ease of absorption, reliable measurement of serum concentration, small (<15%) fluctuation in serum T_4 concentrations between single daily doses, and the ability for a precise dose to be titrated based on multiple available tablet strengths. Although the fraction of patients receiving T_4 has increased steadily during the last 30 years, 30% of the patients receiving thyroid products in 1991 were taking thyroid extract or combinations of synthetic T_4 and T_3.[7]

The T_4 content of tablets is standardized by high-pressure liquid chromatography and must be between 90% and 110% of the stated amount. Before 1982, the standard was based on iodine content, and therefore included not only authentic T_4 but also biologically inactive degradation products. T_4 preparations may lose potency if they are exposed to moisture, light, or air. Tablets are available now from several manufacturers in North America in multiple sizes ranging from 25 to 300 µg, which allows most patients to be correctly regulated with a single daily tablet.

There are a number of drawbacks to administration of T_3 or T_3-containing preparations in comparison with administration of T_4. T_3 is rapidly absorbed, with peak T_3 concentrations being reached 2 to 4 hours after oral T_3 administration. Penetration into its large volume of distribution is slow, so that doses of as little as 25 µg result in elevated serum T_3 concentrations for 6 to 8 hours. As compared with T_4, the circulating half-life is much shorter (approximately 1 day). As a result of these characteristics of T_3 absorption and metabolism, serum T_3 concentrations vary widely according to the time of the most recent dose.

THERAPEUTIC APPROACH TO HYPOTHYROIDISM

The goal of treatment of hypothyroidism is to normalize thyroid status in peripheral tissues and is generally independent of its cause. Since it is difficult to measure accurately thyroid hormone action in many tissues, the usual approach is to normalize the serum TSH concentration.[8] By this means the clinician can identify patients who are receiving too much T_4 (serum TSH concentration below the normal range) as well as those who are receiving too little (serum TSH concentration above the normal range). Additionally, the serum TSH value reflects a sensitive thyroid hormone-regulated process at the tissue level, that is, the synthesis and release of TSH.

Excessive T_4 replacement has been associated with accelerated bone loss in postmenopausal women,[9,10] as well as increases in heart rate and left ventricular wall thickness and contractility.[11] Conversely, inadequate replacement will not correct the manifestations of hypothyroidism. In T_4-treated hypothyroid patients who have normal serum TSH concentrations, serum total and free T_4 concentrations are usually in the upper portion of the normal range or slightly elevated, and serum T_3 concentrations are normal. These patients lack the 20% of the serum T_3 contributed by direct thyroidal secretion, and since both T_4 and T_3 contribute to the regulation of TSH secretion, a serum T_4 concentration slightly higher than normal is usually required to maintain normal serum T_3 and TSH concentrations.

Patients who have taken thyroid extract or combined T_4 and T_3 preparations for many years may be reluctant to change to T_4 despite its advantages (better standardization, more constant absorption, more stable serum T_4 and T_3 concentrations). If they do agree to change, the activity of a 60 mg (1 grain) tablet of desiccated thyroid can be considered approximately equivalent to 80 µg of T_4.[12] However, thyroid extracts or combination preparations can be continued as long as serum TSH—not serum T_4 or T_3—measurements are used to monitor treatment.

The serum TSH value is not an accurate reflection of thyroid status in patients with central hypothyroidism. In these patients some estimate of serum free T_4 should be used as the indicator of thyroid status and to monitor treatment. A similar strategy should be used in patients recently treated for thyrotoxicosis in whom serum TSH concentrations may remain low for several months due to the slow recovery of the pituitary from prolonged suppression.

INITIATION OF THERAPY

The initial dose of T_4 should be based on the age of the patient, the severity and duration of hypothyroidism, and the presence of any other associated disorders. The mean T_4 dose to restore euthyroidism has diminished in the last decade, due to both increased bioavailability of the T_4 in the tablets[13] and the ability to identify patients receiving excessive T_4 replacement by measurements of serum TSH. Healthy patients under the age of 60 years, with no history of cardiac or respiratory disease, can be started on a full replacement dose of T_4, 1.6 to 1.8 µg/kg ideal body weight/day (usually 75 to 125 µg in

women and 125 to 200 µg in men).[2] These doses must be given for 4 to 8 weeks before their tissue effects and serum T_4 and TSH concentrations reach a steady state.

Elderly patients require 20% to 30% less T_4.[14,15] It is prudent to start with no more than 50 µg/day in them, increasing the dose by 25 µg at intervals of at least 6 weeks. The underlying cause of thyroid disease can also influence the dose requirement. For example, patients with primary hypothyroidism caused by chronic autoimmune thyroiditis or who have had a total thyroidectomy require slightly higher doses of T_4 than patients with Graves' hyperthyroidism who are hypothyroid as a result of radioactive iodine or surgical therapy. Among those with Graves' hyperthyroidism in the past, the replacement dose can vary as a function of not only the extent of antithyroid treatment but also the time since treatment.[16,17]

Hypothyroid patients who are unable to take oral medication for a brief period of time (several days) do not need parenteral therapy, owing to the long half-life of T_4. For those patients unable to absorb T_4 orally, an intravenous preparation is available and should be given daily calculated at 70% to 80% of the usual oral dose, based on the fraction of an oral dose that is absorbed.[18]

THYROXINE THERAPY IN PATIENTS WITH UNDERLYING CARDIAC DISEASE

The majority of hypothyroid patients with ischemic or other cardiac disease have no change, or improvement, in their cardiac disease after T_4 therapy is initiated. T_4 can improve cardiac performance by reducing systemic vascular resistance, reducing end-diastolic volume, increasing the strength of contraction, and improving cardiac output.[19] Among a large group of hypothyroid patients treated with thyroid hormone, only 2% developed new-onset angina pectoris. Among those patients with preexisting angina, 38% improved, 46% had no change, and only 16% worsened.[20] Despite this generally favorable response, however, the consequences of worsening ischemic heart disease can be serious and dictate a cautious approach to T_4 replacement in affected patients. Furthermore, even if the patient has no clinical manifestations of ischemic heart disease, the presence of risk factors for it should raise concern, because of the possibility that hypothyroidism masked its effects (or the patient does not remember having had cardiac symptoms in the past). If cardiac disease is present or suspected, there is little harm in delaying T_4 therapy until evaluation, and in some cases until treatment, is completed. For example, patients with angina and hypothyroidism should in most instances have appropriate evaluation of underlying coronary artery disease and treatment of their coronary artery disease, if necessary, before or concomitant with initiation of T_4 treatment.[21,22]

MONITORING THYROXINE THERAPY

The approach to monitoring T_4 therapy is dependent on the severity of hypothyroidism and the clinical context. For those patients initially given what is estimated to be a full replacement dose, the patient should be reevaluated and the serum TSH concentration should be measured in about 8 weeks. The dose of T_4 should be increased if the serum TSH concentration is elevated, or decreased if it is low. Dose increments of 12 to 25 µg are usually sufficient when making an adjustment, depending on the deviation of serum TSH. If the dose is not changed, the patient should be reevaluated and serum TSH measured again in 4 to 6 months, because the clearance of T_4 can be increased after the euthyroid state is established. If a dose change is necessary, the patient should be reevaluated and serum TSH measured 6 to 8 weeks later. If, as a consequence of the change in dose, the serum TSH concentration is abnormal at the other extreme, tablets are available which are 12-µg increments between the commonly used doses of 75, 100, 125, and 150 µg. Smaller increments for doses less than 75 µg or greater than 150 µg can be achieved with a combination of tablets of different content. Given the availability of tablets with 12-µg increments, there is no need for alternate-day dosing schedules, which are difficult for patients to follow.

The relationship between serum TSH and T_4 concentrations is log-linear, so that a small reduction in serum T_4 concentration results in a large increase in the serum TSH concentration, as demonstrated in a study of patients receiving a stable dose of T_4 who had normal serum TSH concentrations in whom the dose then was increased or decreased in increments of 25 µg[23] (Fig. 77-1). Once the appropriate dose of T_4 is determined, annual reevaluation and serum TSH measurement are recommended. Most patients can be treated with the same dose until the seventh to eighth decade, when the dose needed usually decreases by about 20%.[14,15] There are a number of drugs and conditions, however, that can alter the requirement for T_4 (see later).

TREATMENT OF CENTRAL HYPOTHYROIDISM

Patients with central (secondary) hypothyroidism also should be treated with T_4, but as noted earlier, serum TSH measurements are not useful for monitoring therapy. Instead, serum free T_4 concentrations or serum free T_4 index values should be used, the goal being values in the middle or upper end of the normal range for the test used. It is important that other aspects of pituitary function be assessed, especially pituitary-adrenal function. Patients with both hypothyroidism and hypocortisolism may have only symptoms of hypothyroidism, but then develop symptoms of hypocortisolism when T_4 therapy is begun, because the metabolic clearance of cortisol is reduced in hypothyroidism (see chap 69). For this reason, if there is any question of the adequacy of adrenal reserve, both T_4 and hydrocortisone should be given until hypothalamic-pituitary-adrenal function can be evaluated.

RESPONSE TO THYROXINE TREATMENT

The response to T_4 therapy should be assessed both clinically and biochemically. Normalization of clinical and biochemical manifestations of hypothyroidism, however, occurs at different

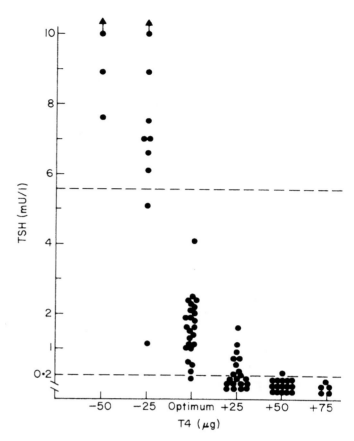

FIGURE 77-1. Changes in serum TSH concentrations in hypothyroid patients receiving a stable optimal dose of T_4 (defined as a normal serum TSH concentration) in whom the dose was increased or decreased by the amounts shown. The upper horizontal dashed line indicates the upper limit of the normal range for the serum TSH assay and the lower horizontal dashed line indicates the lower limit of detection of the assay. Each dot represents an individual patient. (From Carr D, McLeod DT, Parry G, Thornes HM. Fine adjustment of thyroxine replacement of dosage: comparison of the thyrotrophin releasing hormone test using a sensitive thyrotrophin assay with measurement of free thyroid hormones and clinical assessment. Clin Endocrinol 1988;28:325, with permission from Blackwell Scientific Ltd.)

times and varies among patients. The earliest change usually is normalization of the serum T_4 concentration, which occurs after several weeks of treatment. Normalization of the serum TSH may require up to 8 weeks, depending on the magnitude of the initial elevation. Most patients note improvement of symptoms in several weeks, but complete recovery usually requires several months. A substantial fraction of patients with hypothyroidism complain of weight gain and have an expectation of weight loss when they are treated. Most of the weight that is lost, however, is body fluid that is mobilized, and the decrease in weight does not usually exceed 10% of body weight.[24]

CONDITIONS ASSOCIATED WITH ALTERED THYROXINE REQUIREMENTS

A number of conditions as well as drugs can alter T_4 requirements (Table 77-1). Aging patients, especially those in their 70s, need less T_4,[14,15] perhaps due to a decrease in T_4 clearance. Hypothyroid patients receiving T_4 replacement who are treated with an androgen also need less T_4,[25] which may be due to a reduction in the T_4 pool as a result of a decrease in serum thyroxine-binding globulin (TBG) or a decrease in T_4 clearance.

More often an increase in the dose of T_4 is needed. Most hypothyroid women require an increase in T_4 dose during pregnancy.[26] The magnitude of the increase averages 50%, but it is variable and is related to the amount of residual thyroid tissue[27] (see chap 89). A greater increase in dose is needed in those women whose hypothyroidism is caused by previous radioiodine treatment or thyroidectomy, as compared with those who have chronic autoimmune thyroiditis. The prepregnancy dose of T_4 can be resumed immediately after delivery. Patients who undergo bowel resection or have intestinal disease may malabsorb T_4, and hence need a larger dose.[28] Similarly, several drugs cause malabsorption of T_4, including sucralfate,[29] aluminum hydroxide,[30] ferrous sulfate,[31] cholestyramine,[32] and possibly sodium polystyrene sulfonate,[33] and lovastatin.[34] For most of these drugs, separation of the times at which the T_4 and the drug are taken by several hours eliminates the effect. Rifampin,[35] carbamazepine,[36] and phenytoin[37,38] which increase T_4 clearance, and amiodarone, which inhibits T_4 to T_3 conversion, may increase the need for T_4.[39]

ADVERSE EFFECTS OF THYROXINE THERAPY

Excessive T_4 treatment has some adverse effects, mostly on

TABLE 77-1.
Circumstances Associated With Altered T_4 Requirements

REDUCED REQUIREMENT

Elderly (older than 65)
Women receiving androgen therapy

INCREASED REQUIREMENT

Pregnancy
Malabsorption
   Mucosal disease (eg, sprue)
   Short bowel (eg, postjejunoileal bypass)
Pharmacologic agents or dietary supplements
   Reduced absorption
     Sucralfate
     Aluminum hydroxide
     Ferrous sulfate
     Cholestyramine
     ? Sodium polystyrene sulfonate (Kayexalate)
     ? Lovastatin
   Increased clearance
     Rifampin
     Carbamazepine
     Phenytoin
   Reduced T_4 to T_3 conversion
     Amiodarone
     Selenium deficiency

bone and the heart (see chap 88). The results of studies of bone density in T_4-treated patients are conflicting. In general, however, accelerated bone loss does not occur when the serum TSH concentration is maintained in the normal range, but may occur in postmenopausal women who receive sufficient T_4 to reduce TSH secretion below normal.[9,10] As noted above, patients receiving larger doses of T_4 who have low serum TSH concentrations may have increased pulse rates and increased cardiac wall thickness and contractility,[11] and elderly patients have an increased risk of atrial fibrillation.[40]

TREATMENT FAILURES

Persistently Elevated Serum TSH Concentrations

In some patients the serum TSH concentration remains high despite a T_4 dose that should be adequate. Poor compliance is the most common reason for this finding and should be suspected in patients receiving excessive doses of T_4 for their size, or in those with widely varying thyroid function studies while taking the same prescribed dose.[41] In patients who take multiple daily doses just before a follow-up visit, the serum free T_4 index may be high or normal and the serum TSH high.

A persistent elevation in serum TSH despite good compliance may be the result of one of the conditions that increases the need for T_4 listed in Table 77-1. In the absence of one of the factors listed in the table, changing the brand of T_4 can result in improved absorption. Despite the identical content of T_4 in different brands, there is enough variation in the dissolution time among them that absorption of some brands may be decreased in patients with rapid intestinal transit.[13,42] T_3 can also be used in refractory patients because of its greater absorption. Finally, there are a very small number of patients who have persistently elevated serum TSH and T_4 concentrations. These patients should be evaluated for resistance to the action of thyroid hormone[43] (see chap 90), particularly if they have undergone thyroidectomy or received radioactive iodine therapy for a mistaken diagnosis of hyperthyroidism in the past. A single patient with isolated peripheral thyroid resistance has been reported in whom the serum TSH concentration was low despite peripheral hypothyroidism;[44] this diagnosis requires rigorous demonstration that the end organ effects of thyroid hormone are reduced relative to the serum T_4 concentration.

Hypothyroid Symptoms Despite Normal Thyroid Function Studies

Hypothyroid patients may complain of persistent symptoms despite adequate T_4 therapy. This is especially true of those previously given excessive doses of T_4. Given the potential complications of excessive doses, it is important to educate the patient to the fact that a normal serum TSH concentration is the best goal for T_4 treatment. Since T_4 has such varied effects, it is not unusual for patients to attribute a broad range of symptoms to inadequate therapy, and some will titrate their own dose of T_4 based on their symptoms. Because of the long half-life of T_4 and the unreliability of the subjective assessment of thyroid hormone-related symptoms, this practice is ineffective and even dangerous, and should be discouraged. Many patients are responsive to education about thyroid hormone testing and monitoring of therapy, along with reassurance. If symptoms persist, other causes for the complaints should be investigated.

References

1. Roti E, Minelli R, Gardini E, Braverman LE. The use and misuse of thyroid hormone. Endocr Rev 1993;14:401
2. Mandel SJ, Brent GA, Larsen PR. Levothyroxine therapy in patients with thyroid disease. Ann Intern Med 1993;119:492
3. Toft AD. Thyroxine therapy. N Engl J Med 1994;331:174
4. Braverman LE, Ingbar SH, Sterling K. Conversion of thyroxine (T_4) to triiodothyronine (T_3) in athyreotic subjects. J Clin Invest 1970;49:855
5. Oppenheimer JH, Schwartz HL, Surks MI. Propylthiouracil inhibits the conversion of L-thyroxine to L-triiodothyronine: an explanation of the antithyroxine effect of propylthiouracil and evidence supporting the concept that triiodothyronine is the active thyroid hormone. J Clin Invest 1972;51:2493
6. Hays MT. Localization of human thyroxine absorption. Thyroid 1991;3:241
7. Kaufman SC, Gross TP, Kennedy DL. Thyroid hormone use: trends in the United States from 1960 through 1988. Thyroid 1991;1:285
8. Gow SM, Caldwell G, Toft AD, Seth J, Hussey AJ, Sweeting VM. Relationship between pituitary and other target organ responsiveness in hypothyroid patients receiving thyroxine replacement. J Clin Endocrinol Metab 1987;64:364
9. Stall GM, Harris S, Sokoll LF, Dawson-Hughes B. Accelerated bone loss in hypothyroid patients overtreated with L-thyroxine. Ann Intern Med 1990;113:265
10. Adlin EV, Maurer AH, Marks AD, Channick BJ. Bone mineral density in postmenopausal women treated with L-thyroxine. Am J Med 1991;90:360
11. Biondi B, Fazio S, Carella C, et al. Cardiac effects of long term thyrotropin-suppressive therapy with levothyroxine. J Clin Endocrinol Metab 1993;77:334
12. Blumberg KR, Mayer WJ, Parikh DK, Schnell LA. Liothyronine and levothyroxine in Armour thyroid. J Pharm Sci 1993;76:346
13. Fish LH, Schwartz HL, Cavanaugh J, Steffes MW, Bantle JP, Oppenheimer JH. Replacement dose, metabolism, and bioavailability of levothyroxine in the treatment of hypothyroidism. N Engl J Med 1987;316:764
14. Rosenbaum RL, Barzel US. Levothyroxine replacement dose for primary hypothyroidism decreases with age. Ann Intern Med 1982;96:53
15. Sawin CT, Geller A, Hershman JM, Castelli W, Bacharach P. The aging thyroid: the use of thyroid hormone in older persons. JAMA 1989;261:2653
16. Bearcroft CP, Toms GC, Williams SJ, Noonan K, Monson JP. Thyroxine replacement in post-radioiodine hypothyroidism. Clin Endocrinol 1991;34:115
17. Davies P, Franklyn JA, Daykin J, Sheppard MC. The significance of TSH values measured in a sensitive assay in the follow-up of hyperthyroid patients treated with radioiodine. J Clin Endocrinol Metab 1992;74:1189
18. Hays MT, Nielsen KRK. Human thyroxine absorption: age effects and methodological analyses. Thyroid 1994;4:55
19. Klein I, Ojamaa K. Cardiovascular manifestations of endocrine disease. J Clin Endocrinol Metab 1992;75:339
20. Keating FR, Parkin TW, Selby JB, Dickinson LS. Treatment of heart disease associated with myxedema. Prog Cardiovasc Dis 1961;3:364
21. Hay ID, Duick DS, Vlietstra RE, Maloney JD, Pluth JR. Thyroxine therapy in hypothyroid patients undergoing coronary revascularization: a retrospective analysis. Ann Intern Med 1981;95:456
22. Ladenson PW, Levin AA, Ridgway EC, Daniels GH. Complications of surgery in hypothyroid patients. Am J Med 1984;77:261
23. Carr K, McLeod DT, Parry G, Thornes HM. Fine adjustment of thyroxine replacement dosage: comparison of the thyrotrophin releasing hormone tests using a sensitive thyrotrophin assay with measurement of free thyroid hormones and clinical assessment. Clin Endocrinol 1988;28:325
24. Hoogwerf BJ, Nuttall FQ. Long-term weight regulation in treated hyperthyroid and hypothyroid subjects. Am J Med 1984;76:963
25. Arafah BM. Decreased levothyroxine requirement in women with hypothyroidism during androgen therapy for breast cancer. Ann Intern Med 1994;121:247
26. Mandel SJ, Larsen PR, Seely EW, Brent GA. Increased need for thyroxine during pregnancy in women with primary hypothyroidism. N Engl J Med 1990;323:91
27. Kaplan MM. Monitoring thyroxine treatment during pregnancy. Thyroid 1992;2:147
28. Stone E, Leiter LA, Lambert JR, Silverberg JDH, Jeejeebhoy KN, Burrow GN. L-Thyroxine absorption in patients with short bowel. J Clin Endocrinol Metab 1984;59:139
29. Havrankova J, Lahaie R. Levothyroxine binding by sucralfate. Ann Intern Med 1992;117:445
30. Sperber AD, Liel Y. Evidence for interference with the intestinal absorption of levothyroxine sodium by aluminum hydroxide. Arch Intern Med 1992;152:183
31. Campbell NRC, Hasinoff BB, Stalts H, Rao B, Wong NCW. Ferrous sulfate reduces thyroxine efficacy in patients with hypothyroidism. Ann Intern Med 1992;117:1010
32. Harmon SM, Seifert CF. Levothyroxine-cholestyramine interaction reemphasized. Ann Intern Med 1991;115:658
33. McLean M, Kirkwood I, Epstein M, Jones B, Hall C. Cation-exchange resin and inhibition of intestinal absorption of thyroxine. Lancet 1993;341:1286
34. Demke DM. Drug interaction between thyroxine and lovastatin. N Engl J Med 1989;321:1341
35. Isley WL. Effect of rifampin therapy on thyroid function tests in a hypothyroid patient on replacement L-thyroxine. Ann Intern Med 1987;107:517
36. DeLuca F, Arrigo T, Pandullo E, Siracusano MF, Benvenga S, Trimarchi F. Changes in thyroid function tests induced by 2 month carbamazepine treatment in L-thyroxine-substituted hypothyroid children. Eur J Pediatr 1986;145:77
37. Hegedus L, Hansen JM, Luhdorf K, Perrild H, Feldt-Rasmussen U, Kampmann JP. Increased frequency of goitre in epileptic patients on long-term phenytoin or carbamazepine treatment. Clin Endocrinol 1985;23:423
38. Backshear JL, Schultz AL, Napier JS, Stuart DD. Thyroxine replacement requirements in hypothyroid patients receiving phenytoin. Ann Intern Med 1983;99:341
39. Figge J, Dluhy RG. Amiodarone-induced elevation of thyroid stimulating hormone in patients receiving levothyroxine for primary hypothyroidism. Ann Intern Med 1990;113:553
40. Sawin CT, Geller A, Wolf PA, et al. Low serum thyrotropin concentrations as a risk factor for atrial fibrillation in older persons. N Engl J Med 1994;331:1249
41. Ain KB, Refetoff S, Fein HG, Weintraub BD. Pseudomalabsorption of levothyroxine. JAMA 1991;266:2118
42. LeBoff MS, Kaplan MM, Silva JE, Larsen PR. Bioavailability of thyroid hormones from oral replacement preparations. Metabolism 1982;31:900
43. Refetoff S, Weiss RE, Usala SJ. The syndromes of resistance to thyroid hormone. Endocr Rev 1993;14:348
44. Kaplan MM, Swartz SL, Larsen PR. Partial peripheral resistance to thyroid hormone. Am J Med 1981;70:1115

SIX

Thyroid Diseases: Nontoxic Diffuse and Multinodular Goiter

Werner and Ingbar's The Thyroid, Seventh Edition,
edited by Lewis E. Braverman and Robert D. Utiger.
Lippincott–Raven Publishers, Philadelphia, © 1996

78

Pathogenesis of Nontoxic Diffuse and Nodular Goiter

Hans Jakob Peter

Ulrich Bürgi

Hans Gerber

MORPHOLOGIC ASPECTS

The basic process in the pathogenesis of diffuse as well as of nodular goiters is the proliferation of follicular epithelial cells resulting in the formation of new follicles.[1–6] The increase in thyroid volume leading to goiter formation is mainly the result of this increased number of thyroid follicles.[1–6] An accumulation of interstitial tissue and follicular colloid usually accounts for only a minor fraction of total goiter growth.[1,7]

Whereas diffuse goiter and normal thyroid tissue are almost indistinguishable on light microscopic examination, multinodular goiters display marked morphologic heterogeneity[1–6]: follicular size, colloid content, and follicular cell morphology vary not only between different goiter regions or nodules but also within nodules (Figs. 78-1 and 78-2). Differences in follicular cell morphology, with flat cells alternating with cuboidal or columnar cells, may be seen even within individual follicles.[1–6]

Similar variations are also found with respect to the presence of a connective tissue capsule around nodules in multinodular goiters. Whereas some nodules are completely separated from adjacent tissue by a well developed fibrous capsule and may display a distinct morphologic pattern which clearly distinguishes them from the surrounding thyroid tissue, other nodules are only partly encapsulated and may show a smooth histologic transition from nodular to apparently normal thyroid tissue.[1–4,7,8] Nodules in multinodular goiters therefore do not display a single distinct histologic pattern. However, analyses of clonality have shown that independent of the presence of histologic homogeneity or heterogeneity, some of the nodules in human multinodular goiters represent true monoclonal adenomas (see chap 28).[9–13]

A variety of cellular alterations related to the control of proliferation including enhanced expression of protooncogenes (e.g., *ras, myc, fos*) are observed in nodular areas of multinodular goiters.[14–17] Their pathogenic significance, however, has so far not been firmly established.

FUNCTIONAL ASPECTS

A functional aspect well known to all clinicians is the characteristic irregular patchy pattern of radionucleotide uptake invariably found in scintiscans of nodular goiters. If high resolution scintigraphic methods are used, even diffuse goiters often display such a patchy pattern (see chap 17). Depending on the type of radionucleotide used (^{99m}Tc or ^{123}I or ^{131}I), the patchy pattern results from regional variations in radioisotope uptake, that is, regional differences in the activity of the iodine pump or of iodine organification,[18] and reflects an important functional characteristic of nodular goiters, namely the heterogeneity of iodine metabolism (Figs 78-1 and 78-2).[1–6,18]

It is of particular clinical relevance that the patchy scintigraphic patterns of multinodular goiters are often not superimposable onto the nodular patterns found on physical or ultrasonographic examination; the boundaries of the scintigraphic areas of increased or decreased radioisotope uptake do not necessarily correspond to the anatomic boundaries of the thyroid nodules.[1,2]

Comparison of morphology and function at the level of individual follicles by radioiodine labeling prior to thyroidectomy and subsequent autoradiographic assessment of radioiodine organification on histologic sections reveals that the

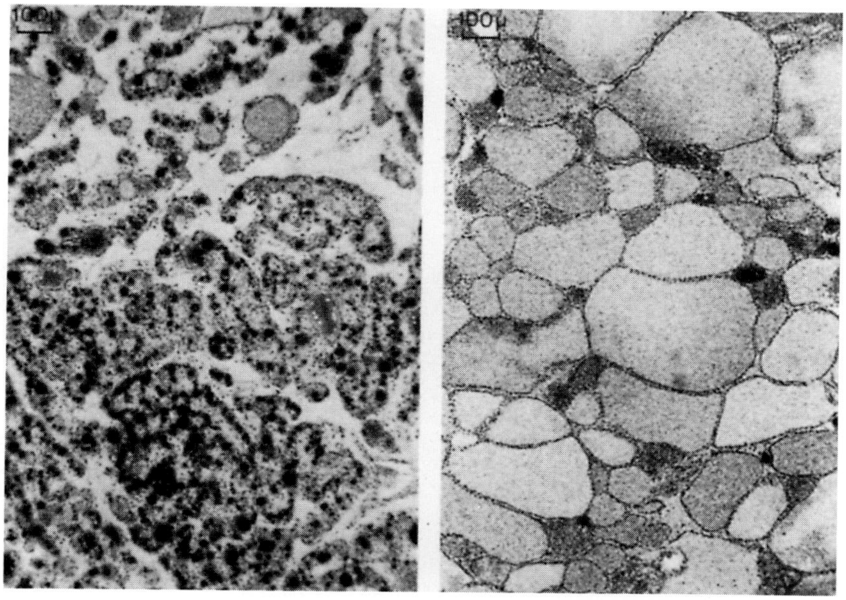

FIGURE 78-1. Variability of follicle morphology and iodine turnover in different areas of the same goiter. Autoradiographs are of a multinodular goiter in a 28-year-old euthyroid woman with decreased TSH secretion. Entirely different growth patterns of the thyroid tissue are shown at two different sites of the same goiter. All follicles have an appreciable autonomous (i.e., TSH-independent) ^{125}I uptake. Although darkening of the follicles is roughly inversely proportional to their size in most follicles, as in normal glands, there are many exceptions to this rule in the right panel, indicating considerable heterogeneity of iodine metabolism. All follicles in the right panel are lined by a flat epithelium lacking all morphologic signs of stimulation. (Courtesy of Prof. H. Studer, Berne)

functional activity varies widely between different follicles or even between single cells within the same follicle in human and animal goiters (Figs. 78-1 and 78-2).[1–6,8,18–22,22a]

When analyzed at the follicular or cellular level, the clinical entity known as diffuse or nodular nontoxic goiter thus comprises a large spectrum of morphologic and functional variations.

Autonomy of Function

It is of particular clinical significance that iodine metabolism in some of the follicles in nodular goiters may remain highly active even when TSH secretion becomes suppressed by increasing endogenous thyroid hormone production or by exogenous thyroxine administration.[1–6,23] Such follicles are said to display a high degree of functional autonomy.

An increase in the total mass of these thyroid follicles with a high autonomous iodine metabolism during goiter growth explains why a patient with an originally euthyroid goiter can become subclinically or even overtly hyperthyroid. Since goiter growth is usually slow, hyperthyroidism in these patients often develops insidiously over years (see chap 32).[1–6] Follicles with a high autonomous iodine metabolism are also the origin of thyrotoxicosis that may occur when formerly nontoxic goiter patients (particularly patients in iodine-deficient areas) are exposed to excessive amounts of iodine (see chap 14).

MECHANISMS OF GOITER GROWTH AND NODULAR TRANSFORMATION

As pointed out, the common pathogenetic mechanism of diffuse and nodular goiter formation is, irrespective of the underlying etiologic factors, the generation of new follicles (Fig. 78-3).

Nontoxic diffuse and nodular goiter growth is probably initiated by a low or moderate goitrogenic stimulus. A crucial point for the understanding of the role of follicular neoformation and its implications in the pathogenesis of nontoxic diffuse and nodular goiter is the fact that the follicular cells, even of the normal thyroid gland, are not identical among themselves with respect to their growth potential and their functional activity.[1–6,19,24,27] The growth potential of individual follicular cells differs in two respects:

> Sensitivity to goitrogenic stimulation, resulting in mitosis
> Ability to divide repeatedly upon chronic stimulation

As a consequence of the unequal growth potentials of different follicular cells, a low or moderate goitrogenic stimulation induces only a small fraction of follicular cells (namely those with a high growth potential) to enter the mitotic cycle.[1–6,24,25] Upon chronic stimulation, some preferentially dividing cells which are able to undergo several cell divisions may repeatedly enter the cycle of follicular neoformation and thereby eventually cause enlargement of the thyroid. This type of slow thyroid growth contrasts with the rapid diffuse growth of the thyroid caused by a massive growth stimulus such as thyroid stimulating immunoglobulins (TSI) in Graves' disease (see below).

Autonomy of Growth

As a second consequence of the unequal growth potential of different thyroid follicular cells, long-term growth stimulation increases the fraction of dividing follicular cells within the goiter, thus enhancing the propensity of a goiter to grow with time. Ultimately, proliferation of follicular cells may continue even if the initial stimulus that triggered goiter development declines or entirely ceases to be active.[1–6] Goiter growth then becomes truly autonomous. This can be observed in endemic and in sporadic goiter areas, where a negative correlation exists between goiter size and TSH levels,[28,29] and in multinodular goiters growing despite TSH suppression by T_4 treatment (see chap 79).

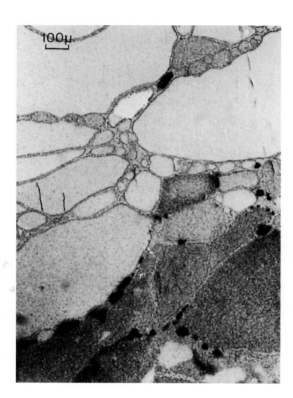

FIGURE 78-2. There is heterogeneity of size and function between follicles adjacent to one another as seen in an autoradiograph of a multinodular goiter from a 36-year-old euthyroid woman with decreased TSH secretion. Any ^{125}I uptake (17 hours), therefore, represents autonomous function. Follicles with identical size may have an entirely different iodine turnover. There is no correlation between follicle size and ^{125}I uptake. Also, follicular cells are uniformly flat, illustrating the impossibility of correlating function and morphology. (Courtesy of Prof. H. Studer, Berne)

Goiter growth varies regionally, because, as pointed out before, preferentially proliferating follicular cells entering the mitotic cycle under low goitrogenic stimulation are not evenly distributed within the thyroid. Therefore, if growth stimulation lasts for a long enough period of time, nodular transformation of the thyroid will ultimately result.

To understand the pathogenesis of nontoxic diffuse and nodular goiter one must realize that growth potential and iodine metabolism in individual follicular cells are not necessarily related. Thus, although newly formed thyroid follicles are preferentially generated from follicular cells with a high growth potential, the activity of the iodine metabolism of these newly generated follicles may vary widely (Fig. 78-3).[1–6] If a group of follicles generated in this way grows large enough, it may become visible as a hot or cold nodule on a scintiscan depending on the degree of activity of its iodine metabolism (see chap 17).

Mechanisms similar to those described above also apply to the physiologic turnover of follicular cells in the normal thyroid. This explains the nodular transformation of normal thyroid glands with age, even in people not exposed to recognizable goitrogenic stimuli.[30,31]

In contrast to a mild or moderate goitrogenic stimulus, acute and intense stimulation of the normal thyroid gland

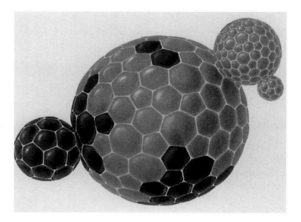

FIGURE 78-3. Diagram of the pathogenesis of functional and morphologic heterogeneity of diffuse nontoxic nodular goiter. The mother follicle is composed of cells with either high (*black*) or low (*gray*) peroxidase activity at the apical cell membrane. Moreover, two families of cells, one black and the other gray, are endowed with a high intrinsic growth capacity that is passed on to the offspring. Therefore, they have generated two daughter follicles with widely differing iodination activity. Instead of iodination activity, other individual and heritable cell traits such as thyroglobulin synthesis, endocytotic capacity, iodide transport, and phenotype may be sent into the diagram to illustrate the mechanisms generating the characteristic morphologic and functional diversity among the goiter follicles shown in Figures 78-1 and 78-2. (Courtesy of Prof. H. Studer, Berne)

(e.g., by TSI in Graves' disease, see chaps 21 and 30) induces a large fraction of follicular cells to proliferate, and causes at least initially diffuse thyroid enlargement. However, if the stimulation continues over a long enough period of time, diffuse goiters also almost invariably become nodular.

Nodular transformation of primarily diffuse goiters has been extensively studied in experimental animal models[1–4,13,31a] and is also a well known clinical feature in longstanding Graves' goiter, juvenile goiters, and endemic goiters of children and adults in iodine-deficient areas.[1–4,31b]

A variety of cellular alterations related to the control of cell proliferation (e.g., expression of protooncogenes) has been observed in nodular areas of goiter tissue.[14–16] However, it has not yet been established to what extent these changes are of pathogenic significance or whether they merely represent secondary events.

Specific gain-of-function mutations of the TSH-receptor (such as those found in some toxic adenomas,[32,33,33a,33b] nonautoimmune hereditary hyperthyroidism,[33a,34] and sporadic congenital non-autoimmune hyperthyroidism[33a,35]) have so far not been identified in nodules of multinodular goiters.

FACTORS MODULATING GOITER GROWTH

TSH

The role of TSH as a regulator of follicular cell function and proliferation has long been a subject of intensive debate (see chap 11).[36–39] Since the elucidation of the structure of the TSH-receptor and of the intracellular mechanisms of TSH-action by

G-proteins and IP3/cAMP pathways and of the links between the cAMP cascade and the intracellular effector systems of the IGF-receptor family,[37] a significant pathogenic role of TSH in the development of many goiters is now widely accepted.[36,37] This concept of a TSH-mediated regulation of thyroid function and growth by modulation of the effects of other growth factors such as IGF-I,[37,40] FGF,[41,42,42a] and EGF[37,43] on follicular cells now largely explains goiter growth in states associated with elevated TSH levels, such as severe iodine deficiency (see chap 14) or defects in hormone biosynthesis (see chap 56).

The negative correlation of goiter size and TSH levels found in euthyroid goiters from areas with only moderate iodine deficiency or sufficient iodine supply[28,29] and the clinical observations that nontoxic goiters may grow despite suppressive T_4-treatment indicate that mechanisms other than those based on TSH stimulation are also involved in goiter growth. It has also been postulated that T_4 itself affects proliferation of thyroid follicular cells.[37]

Iodine

Low iodine levels are known to enhance directly thyroid sensitivity toward growth stimuli. This effect is possibly mediated by organic iodocompounds such as iodolipids[35,36,44] and is independent of an iodine deficiency–induced increase of TSH levels.

IGF-I

IGF-I may well be involved in both thyroid follicular cell proliferation and nodular transformation,[36,37,45] since IGF-I and IGF-I receptors (depicted by immunohistochemical and in situ hybridization methods) show uneven distribution patterns in multinodular goiters. Such a pathogenic role for IGF-I in goitrogenesis is supported by the finding that patients with acromegaly who have elevated IGF-I levels develop multinodular goiters,[46] whereas pygmies in whom IGF levels are decreased have a low goiter prevalence even in states of severe iodine deficiency (Merimee T, personal communication).[47]

Thyroid Growth Stimulating Immunoglobulins

In contrast to the firmly established role of thyroid stimulating immunoglobulins (TSI) in the pathogenesis of Graves' disease, no clear evidence exists for an etiologic role for specific thyroid growth stimulating immunoglobulins (TGI) in nontoxic goiter.[48–50,50a]

Various Growth Factors

A large number of experimental studies using various species suggest that additional modulators of follicular cell proliferation such as EGF, TGFs, PDGF, FGF, and cytokines are also involved in the control of goiter growth (see also chap 11).* However, their effects may vary in different species and experimental systems[37] and their relevance to goitrogenesis in humans remains to be established. Therefore, at present they do not play a role in the clinical diagnostic assessment or the therapeutic management of goiter patients.

CLINICAL IMPLICATIONS

The fact that functional activity of follicular cells or of a given area of goiter tissue does not necessarily parallel the growth potential suggests that the functional activity of a given goiter area or nodule, as depicted on a scintiscan, does not allow any predictions about its prospective growth behavior.

Thus, successful surgical management of a multinodular goiter depends on the removal of all potentially growing goiter tissue, and the extent of the surgery cannot be based on the scintigraphic appearance of the goiter in question (see chap 79).[54]

The effectiveness of medical treatment of nontoxic goiters by TSH suppression through thyroxine administration depends on the size of the autonomously growing follicular cell fraction. Thyroid hormone treatment may thus be effective in smaller diffuse goiters in which the fraction of autonomously growing cells is relatively low. It will usually fail in cases of larger multinodular goiters in which this fraction is high (see chap 79).

References

1. Studer H, Ramelli F. Simple goiter and its variants: euthyroid and hyperthyroid multinodular goiters. Endocr Rev 1982;3:40
2. Studer H, Gerber H, Peter HJ. Natural heterogeneity of thyroid cells: the basis for understanding thyroid function and nodular goiter growth. Endocr Rev 1989;10:125
3. Studer H, Gerber H. Nontoxic goiter. In: Greer MA, ed. The thyroid gland. Comprehensive endocrinology. New York: Raven Press, 1990:391
4. Studer H, Gerber H. Multinodular goiter. In: De Groot LJ, ed. Endocrinology. 3rd ed. Philadelphia: WB Saunders, 1994:769
5. Peter HJ, Studer H, Groscurth P. Autonomous growth, but not autonomous function, in embryonic human thyroids: a clue to understanding autonomous goiter growth. J Clin Endocrinol Metab 1988;66:968
6. Peter HJ, Gerber H, Studer H, Smeds S. Pathogenesis of heterogeneity in human multinodular goiter: a study on growth and function of thyroid tissue transplanted onto nude mice. J Clin Invest 1985;76:1992
7. Ramelli F, Burgi U, Siebenhuner L, Kohler H, Studer H. A disproportionate accumulation of fibrous tissue is not a causal factor in human goiter growth. Acta Endocrinol (Copenh) 1987;116:502
8. Peter HJ, Gerber H, Studer H, Becker DV, Peterson ME. Autonomy of growth and of iodine metabolism in hyperthyroid feline goiters transplanted onto nude mice. J Clin Invest 1987;80:491
9. Hicks DG, LiVolsi VA, Neidich JA, Puck JM, Kant JA. Clonal analysis of solitary follicular nodules in the thyroid. Am J Pathol 1990;137:553
10. Fey M, Peter HJ, Hinds HL, et al. Clonal analysis of human tumours with M27beta, a highly informative polymorphic X-chromosomal probe. J Clin Invest 1992;89:1438
11. Bamberger AM, Bamberger CM, Barth J, et al. Clonal analysis of thyroid nodules from patients with multinodular goiters: determination by x-chromosome inactivation analysis using the highly polymorphic M27beta probe. [Abstract]. Proceedings of

---

*See references 1–4, 36, 37, 40–43a, and 51–53.

the 75th Annual Meeting of the Endocrine Society, Las Vegas, June 1993;157

12. Kopp P, Kimura EET, Aeschimann S, et al. Polyclonal and monoclonal thyroid nodules coexist within human multinodular goiters. J Clin Endocrinol Metab 1994;79:134

13. Gerber H, B rgi U, Peter HJ. Etiology and pathogenesis of thyroid nodules. 1993;100:9

14. Studer H, Gerber H, Zbären J, Peter HJ. Histomorphological and immunohistochemical evidence that human nodular goiters grow by episodic replication of multiple clusters of thyroid follicular cells. J Clin Endocrinol Metab 1992;75:1151

15. Mizukami Y, Nonomura A, Hashimoto T, et al. Immunohistochemical demonstration of ras p21 oncogene product in normal, benign and malignant human thyroid tissues. Cancer 1988; 61:873

16. Johnson TL, Lloyd RV, Thor A. Expression of ras oncogene p21 antigen in normal and proliferative thyroid tissues. Am J Pathol 1987;127:6

17. Wallin G, Brönnegard M, Grimelius L, McGuire J, Törring O. Expression of the thyroid hormone receptor, the oncogenes c-myc and H-ras, and the 90 kD heat shock protein in normal, hyperplastic and neoplastic thyroid tissue. Thyroid 1992;2:307

18. Sch rch M, Peter HJ, Gerber H, Studer H. Cold follicles in a multinodular human goiter arise partly from a failing iodine pump and partly from deficient iodine organification. J Clin Endocrinol Metab 1990;71:1224

19. Bergé-Lefrance JL, Cartouzou G, Bignon C, Lissitzky S. Quantitative in situ hybridization of 3 H-labeled complementary deoxyribonucleic acid (cDNA) to the messenger ribonucleic acid of thyroglobulin in human thyroid tissues. J Clin Endocrinol Metab 1983;57:470

20. Gerber H, Peter HJ, Bachmeier C, Kaempf J, Studer H. Progressive recruitment of follicular cells with graded secretory responsiveness during stimulation of the thyroid gland by thyrotropin. Endocrinology 1987;120:91

21. Gerber H, Peter HJ, Studer H. Age related failure of endocytosis may be the pathogenetic mechanism responsible for "cold" follicle formation in the aging mouse thyroid. Endocrinology 1987;120:1758

22. Many MC, Denef JF, Hamudi S, Haumont S. Increased follicular heterogeneity in experimental colloid goiter produced by refeeding iodine excess after thyroid hyperplasia. Endocrinology 1986;118:637

22a. Aeschimann S, Gerber H, von Gr nigen C, Oestreicher M, Studer H. The degree of inhibition of thyroid follicular cell proliferation by iodide is a highly individual characteristic of each cell and differs profoundly in vitro and in vivo. Europ J Endocrinol 1994;130:595

23. Miller JM. Hyperthyoidism form the thyroid follicle with autonomous function. Clin Endocrinol Metab 1978;7:177

24. Smeds S, Peter HJ, Jörtsö H, Gerber H, Studer H. Naturally occurring clones of cells with high intrinsic proliferation potential within the follicular epithelium of mouse thyroids. Cancer Res 1987;47:1646

25. Huber G, Derwahl M, Kaempf J, Peter HJ, Gerber H, Studer H. Generation of intercellular heterogeneity of growth and function in cloned rat thyroid cells (FRTL-5). Endocrinology 1990; 126:1639

26. Groch KM, Clifton KH. The plateau phase rat goiter contains a sub-population of TSH responsive follicular cells capable of proliferation following transplantation. Acta Endocrinol (Copenh) 1992;126:85

27. Baptist M, Roger RR. Assessment of heterogeneity of proliferative responses of thyrocytes in primary cultures. Demonstration of a mechanism generating heterogeneity. [Abstract]. Annales d'endocrinologie 1991;52:86

28. Fenzi GF, Ceccarelli C, Macchia E, et al. Reciprocal changes of serum thyroglobulin and TSH in residents of a moderate endemic goiter area. Clin Endocrinol 1985;23:115

29. Berghout A, Wiersinga WM, Smits NJ, Touber JL. Interrelationships between age, thyroid volume, thyroid nodularity, and thyroid function in patients with sporadic nontoxic goiter. Am J Med 1990;89:602

30. Mortensen JD, Woolner LB, Bennet WA. Gross and microscopic findings in clinically normal thyroid glands. J Clin Endocrinol Metab 1955;15:1270

31. Horlocker TT, Hay JE, James EM, Reading CC, Charboneau JW. Prevalence of incidental nodular thyroid disease detected during high- resolution parathyroid ultrasonography. In: Medeiros-Neto Ga, Gaitan E, eds. Frontiers in thyroidology. Proceedings of the 9th International Thyroid Conference, Sao Paulo, 1985. New York: Plenum Publishing, 1986:1309

31a. Ledent C, Marcotte A, Dumont JE, Vassart G, Parmentier M. Differentiated carcinomas develop as a consequence of the thyroid specific expression of a thyroglobulin-human papillomavirus type 16 E7 transgene. Oncogene 1995;10:1789

31b. Baltisbereger BL, Minder CE, B rgi H. Decrease of incidence of toxic nodular goiter in a region of Switzerland after full correction of mild iodine deficiency. Europ J Endocrinol 1995;132:546

32. Parma J, Duprez L, van Sande J, et al. Somatic mutations in the thyrotropin receptor gene cause hyperfunctioning thyroid adenomas. Nature 1993;365:649

33. Porcellini A, Ilaria C, Laviola L, et al. Novel mutations of thyrotropin receptor gene in thyroid hyperfunctioning adenomas. J Clin Endocrinol Metab 1994;79:657

33a. Ledent C, Parma J, Dumont JE, Vassart G, Targovnik H. Molecular genetics of thyroid diseases. Europ J Endocrinol 1994;130:8

33b. Russo D, Arturi F, Wicker R, et al. Genetic alterations in thyroid hyperfunctioning adenomas. J Clin Endocrinol Metab 1995; 80:1347

34. Duprez L, Parma J, van Sande J, et al. Germline mutations in the thyrotropin receptor gene cause non autoimmune autosomal dominant hyperthyroidism. Nature Genetics 1994;7:396

35. Kopp P, van Sande J, Parma J, et al. Congenital hyperthyroidism caused by neomutation in the thyrotropin receptor gene. N Engl J Med. 1995;332:150

36. Dumont JE, Lamy F, Roger P, Maenhaut C. Physiological and pathological regulation of thyroid cell proliferation and differentiation by thyrotropin and other factors. Physiol Rev 1991;72:667

37. Dumont JE, Maenhaut C, Pirson I. Growth factors controlling the thyroid gland. Baillière's Clin Endocrinol Metab 1991;5:727

38. Roger PP, Dumont JE. Thyrotropin is a potent growth factor for normal human thyroid cells in primary culture. Biochem Biophys Res Commun 1987;146:707

39. Roger PP, Taton M, Van Sande J, Dumont JE. Mitogenic effects of thyrotropin and cyclic AMP in differentiated human thyroid cells in vitro. J Clin Endocrinol Metab 1988;66:1158

40. Tramontano D, Moses AC, Veneziani BM, Ingbar SH. Adenosine $3',5'$-monophospate mediates both the mitogenic effect of thyrotropin and its ability to amplify the response to insulin-like growth factor I in FRTL-5 cells. Endocrinology 1988; 122:127

41. DeVito WJ, Chanoine JP, Alex S, et al. Effect of in vivo administration of recombinant acidic-fibroblast growth factor on thyroid function in the rat: induction of colloid goiter. Endocrinology 1992;131:729

42. Chanoine JP, Stein GS, Braverman LE, et al. Acidic fibroblast growth factor modulates gene expression in the rat thyroid in vivo. J Cell Biochem 1992;50:392

42a. Eggo MC, Hopkins JM, Franklyn JA, et al. Expression of fibroblast growth factors in thyroid cancer. J Clin Endocrinol Metab 1995;80:1006

43. Westermark K, Karlsson FA, Westermark B. Epidermal growth factor modulates thyroid growth and function in culture. Endocrinology 1983;112:1680

43a. Asmis l, Gerber H, Kaempf J, Studer H. EGF stimulates cell proliferation and inhibits iodide uptake of FRTL-5 cells in vitro. J Endocrinol 1995;145:513

44. Dugrillon A, Gärtner R. The role of iodine and thyroid cell growth. Thyroidology 1992;4:31

45. Thomas GA, Williams ED. Aetiology of simple goiter. Baillière's Clin Endocrinol Metab 1988;2:703

46. Megumi M, Motoyasu S, Toshio T, Kae W, Kazuo S. Thyroid volume and serum thyroglobulin levels in patients with acromegaly: Correlation with plasma insulin-like growth factor I levels. J Clin Endocrinol Metab 1988;67:973

47. Dormitzer PR, Ellison PT, Bode HH. Anomalously low endemic goiter prevalence among Efe pygmies. Am J Phys Anthropol 1989;78:527

48. Dumont JE, Roger PP, Ludgate M. Assays for thyroid growth immunoglobulins and their clinical implications: methods, concepts, and misconceptions. Endocr Rev 1987;8:448

49. Zakarija M, McKenzie JM. Do thyroid growth-promoting immunoglobulins exist? J Clin Endocrinol Metab 1990;70:308

50. Vitti P, Chiovato L, Tonacchera M, et al. Failure to detect thyroid growth promoting activity in immunoglobulin G of patients with endemic goiter. J Clin Endocrinol Metab 1994;78:1020

50a. Brown RS. Immunoglobulins affecting thyroid growth: a continuing controversy. J Clin Endocrinol Netab 1995;80:1506

51. Grubeck-Loebenstein B, Buchan G, Chantry D, et al. Analysis of intrathyroidal cytokine production in thyroid autoimmune disease: thyroid follicular cells produce interleukin-1a and interleukin-6. Clin Exp Immunol 1989;77:324

52. Zheng RQH, Abney E, Chu CG, et al. Detection of interleukin-6 and interleukin-1 production in human thyroid epithelial cells by non-radioactive in situ hybridization and immunohistochemical methods. Clin Exp Immunol 1991;83:314

53. Weetman AP, Bennett GL, Wong WLT. Thyroid follicular cells produce interleukin-8. J Clin Endocrinol Metab 1992;75:328

54. Teuscher J, Peter HJ, Gerber H, Berchtold R, Studer H. Pathogenesis of nodular goiter and its implications for surgical management. Surgery 1988;103:87

Werner and Ingbar's The Thyroid, Seventh Edition,
edited by Lewis E. Braverman and Robert D. Utiger.
Lippincott–Raven Publishers, Philadelphia, © 1996

79

Clinical Manifestations and Management of Nontoxic Diffuse and Nodular Goiter

Ulrich Bürgi

Hans Jakob Peter

Hans Gerber

DEFINITION OF NONTOXIC DIFFUSE AND NODULAR GOITER

Nontoxic diffuse and nodular goiter (NDNG) is sometimes also described as "simple goiter." It is defined as an enlargement of the thyroid not caused by thyroid autoimmune disease, thyroiditis, or thyroid malignant neoplasia (although these may coexist) and not associated with clinical or laboratory evidence of thyroid dysfunction. Potential etiologies of and pathogenic mechanisms leading to NDNG are discussed in chapter 78. The extent to which a thyroid gland must be enlarged to be considered a goiter may vary somewhat from country to country; in countries with an adequate dietary iodine intake, thyroid glands larger than 25 g in men and 18 g in women qualify as goiters.[1,2]

CLINICAL MANIFESTATIONS OF NDNG

Many small NDNGs do not produce any clinical symptoms at all and patients with NDNGs, by definition, do not display any symptoms or signs of thyroid dysfunction.

The clinical manifestations of NDNG are those of an anterior cervical or substernal space-occupying lesion. Symptoms and signs range from a sensation of fullness or of a (growing) tumor in the neck to esthetic disfigurement as well as to inspiratory stridor, disturbances of deglutition, or cervical venous

congestion because of compression of the trachea, the esophagus, or cervical veins, respectively.

Hoarseness is a rare symptom of NDNG and, when present, should alert the clinician to the possibility of a malignant thyroid tumor encroaching on the recurrent laryngeal nerve.

As the name implies, NDNGs can be diffuse or nodular. The diffuse and the nodular variants are not different pathologic entities but merely represent different stages of the same disease. Smaller goiters more often tend to be diffuse on clinical examination, but larger goiters, which have grown over many years, have almost invariably become nodular[3–7] (for mechanisms leading to the formation of thyroid nodules, see chap 78). However, on sonographic or histologic examination, even goiters that seem diffuse on palpation usually have undergone nodular transformation.[8–11]

DIAGNOSIS OF NDNG

When a goiter is discovered in a patient, usually by inspection or palpation (for palpation technique, see chap 25), laboratory studies (see chap 18) are required to decide whether this goiter is a NDNG or not.

Thyroid Hormone and Thyrotropin Measurements.
In any patient with a goiter, thyroid function should be assessed by at least measuring the serum thyrotropin (TSH) con-

centration. Because patients with NDNG are euthyroid by definition, their TSH concentration is normal. Although thyrotoxicosis and primary hypothyroidism, which can be associated with goiters, are readily diagnosed by determination of the serum TSH concentration alone, the extent of the thyroid dysfunction can only be judged by the additional measurements of free thyroxine (T_4) and free triiodothyronine (T_3) in suspected thyrotoxic patients or free T_4 in suspected hypothyroid patients. As discussed in chapters 87 and 88, subclinical thyrotoxicosis or hypothyroidism, as defined by a low or elevated serum TSH concentration, respectively, and normal serum total and free T_4 and T_3 concentrations, is not infrequently associated with a goiter.

Thyroid Antibodies. Serum antithyroid peroxidase and antithyroglobulin antibodies are almost always normal in the sera of patients with NDNG. Elevated levels of thyroid-stimulating immunoglobulins, typical of Graves' disease, are not found in patients with NDNG (except in the rare cases in which NDNG and Graves' disease coexist).

Serum Thyroglobulin. An elevated serum thyroglobulin (Tg) concentration is a nonspecific finding that can be associated with any thyroid disease. Serum Tg is often, sometimes even considerably, elevated in patients with NDNG, especially in iodine-deficient regions.[12–15] The extent of the elevation of the serum Tg does not permit the differentiation of benign from malignant goiters. Measuring serum Tg concentration is, therefore, not helpful in making the diagnosis of NDNG.

Fine-Needle Aspiration Biopsy. Fine-needle biopsy (FNB) of every nodule of a nontoxic multinodular goiter is neither practical nor warranted. The main indication for FNB is the exclusion of a malignant thyroid tumor. FNB is indicated in every growing or solitary thyroid nodule, especially those that are hypofunctioning on thyroid scintigraphy.[11,16,17] Because thyroid nodules in young patients or in patients with a history of radiation therapy to the neck have an increased risk of being malignant, the procedure also needs to be considered in these cases.

Imaging. Imaging procedures (see also chaps 17 and 22) are not usually required to diagnose NDNG, but they may provide information useful for the choice of therapy of these goiters:

- *Ultrasonography* is the most readily available method to determine the dimensions of a goiter and its nodules and to differentiate solid nodules from thyroid cysts. Serial ultrasonography provides a means to precisely assess growth of a goiter and its individual nodules or the response to L-T_4 suppression therapy. Ultrasonographic control facilitates accurate FNB in the nodules that are more difficult to define clinically.
- *Conventional radiography* of the neck and upper thorax can provide information on tracheal compression by a goiter.
- *Computed tomography and magnetic resonance imaging* aid in the visualization of the thyroid gland. Both methods are particularly useful in goiters that extend

into the retrosternal space and, therefore, cannot be completely visualized by ultrasonography.

Scintigraphy typically shows a NDNG composed of intermingled areas of different radioiodine uptake and size. In the majority of patients with NDNG, scintigraphy is not necessary (see chaps 17 and 78). Scintigraphy is not a good method for assessing goiter size because marginal areas of the goiter, which may not take up radioactive tracer, are not visualized. However, thyroid scintigraphy is indicated in uninodular goiters because its result (hot/cold single nodule) influences the therapeutic approach.

NATURAL HISTORY OF NDNG

The natural history of NDNG with respect to goiter growth and function varies and is difficult to predict in a given patient.

Goiter Growth. NDNGs can remain stable in size or grow very slowly over many years. However, rapid growth of one or several nodules is also possible[5,6,11,16–23] (see chaps 78 and 83). Unfortunately, no specific parameter exists that can accurately predict the growth behavior of NDNG. The most convenient way to assess growth in such goiters is by serial measurements (usually every 6 months or yearly) of the size of the entire goiter and individual nodules by ultrasonography.

Development of Thyroid Carcinoma. NDNGs are usually not associated with a significantly increased risk for the development of malignant thyroid tumors. However, any fast-growing goiter or thyroid nodule is suspect of harboring a malignancy and should be biopsied or removed.[5,6,11,16–23] Furthermore, a dominant nodule in a patient with a nontoxic goiter should probably be investigated with a thyroid scan. If the dominant nodule is hypofunctioning, FNB should be done. Although FNB revealing malignant cells is proof of the presence of a thyroid malignancy, a negative FNB result does not exclude cancer.

Painful Nodules. These are usually the result of a hemorrhage into a nodule or a cyst in the nontoxic goiter. The diagnosis is readily made by ultrasonographic examination and FNB. It should be emphasized that a growing, painful nodule in a patient with NDNG may also represent thyroid malignancy.

Development of Thyroid Dysfunction. Although patients with NDNGs are, by definition, euthyroid, they can become thyrotoxic or, less commonly, hypothyroid. However, thyrotoxicosis or hypothyroidism usually develops only after the nontoxic goiter has existed for many years.

Thyrotoxicosis in such patients often develops insidiously, in contrast to the abrupt onset of thyrotoxicosis in Graves' disease or lymphocytic painless thyroiditis. It often begins with a prolonged period of subclinical thyrotoxicosis characterized by low serum TSH and normal serum free T_4 and T_3 concentrations[3–6,24,25] (see chap 88). The development of thyrotoxicosis in a patient with a NDNG is the consequence of goiter growth and an associated increase in the mass of autonomously hormone-producing thyroid cells[3,6,7,12] (see chaps

32 and 78). Thyrotoxicosis can also result from an increase in iodine intake from iodine-containing drugs such as disinfectants and amiodarone or radiographic contrast agents, which, in a goiter with increased autonomous iodine metabolism, leads to the production of excessive amounts of thyroid hormones (see chap 14).

Development of *hypothyroidism* in a patient with a NDNG is rarer. It is difficult to explain because goiters in such patients usually contain considerable amounts of iodine.[3–6,26,27] One must assume that there is some acquired disturbance of thyroid hormone biosynthesis in these goiters. Such an acquired defect may resemble that found in some thyroid follicles of aging mice[28,29] and in experimental rat goiters.[30,31]

MANAGEMENT OF NDNG

Although NDNG is not uncommon (see chap 26), many of these goiters never produce any significant symptoms. Therefore, not every patient with an NDNG requires treatment.

Treatment is unquestionably indicated in the following clinical situations:

1. Progressive growth of the entire goiter or individual nodules
2. Compression of the trachea, esophagus, recurrent laryngeal nerve, or cervical veins by the goiter causing inspiratory stridor, disturbances of deglutition, hoarseness, or marked cervical venous congestion
3. Development of thyrotoxicosis or hypothyroidism
4. Significant esthetic disfigurement

In other clinical situations, the decision whether or not to treat a patient with a NDNG can be more difficult (see below).

Therapeutic Options

Various therapeutic options are available.

1. *Surgery* is the treatment of choice for growing and large goiters or individual nodules within the goiter[32–38] (see chap 80). The main advantage of thyroidectomy is its immediate effectiveness. Disadvantages include the general risks and side effects of a surgical procedure and the small (1–2%) specific risks of postoperative hypoparathyroidism and recurrent laryngeal nerve damage. The classical surgical procedure is a bilateral subtotal thyroidectomy,[32,34,36,38] removing, at the least, all nodular tissue.[32,34] Recently, more radical removal of goiter tissue has been advocated by some.[38] This more aggressive surgical approach reduces goiter recurrence rate without increasing the number of peri- and postoperative complications, providing that the surgeon is experienced in the thyroid operations.
2. *Thyroid hormone treatment* (usually T_4) can reduce goiter size[5,6,13,17,33,39–43] by suppressing pituitary TSH secretion, thereby eliminating the TSH-mediated stimulation of goiter growth. Thyroid hormone treatment can thus only inhibit TSH-dependent goiter growth but does not affect TSH-independent, autonomous growth of goiter nodules (see chap 32).

The goal of thyroid hormone therapy is to decrease the serum TSH to the lowest normal or slightly below normal value to eliminate the TSH-mediated stimulation of goiter growth without inducing thyrotoxicosis with its undesired side effects. This goal is usually achieved with a daily T_4 dose of 0.1 to 0.15 mg. Some endocrinologists advocate the use of a combination of T_3 and T_4 or of iodine and thyroid hormones instead of treatment with T_4 alone in areas of mild iodine deficiency.[44] Assessment of the serum TSH concentration should be carried out approximately 6 weeks after instituting T_4 therapy. A thyroid scan may be done at the same time to rule out autonomously functioning goiter tissue.

Thyroid hormone therapy is contraindicated in patients with a NDNG who are already subclinically thyrotoxic (i.e., serum TSH concentration is suppressed while serum T_3 and T_4 levels are still normal) because of the risk of the development of iatrogenic thyrotoxicosis.

Thyroid hormone treatment may be used to reduce the size of NDNGs that are not growing rapidly and do not contain nodules with a diameter greater than 2 to 3 cm because such nodules virtually never disappear with thyroid hormone therapy and are not likely to contain a malignant tumor.

The effect of a course of thyroid hormone therapy should be documented by serial ultrasonographic measurements (usually every 6 months) of the size of the goiter and—if present—its individual nodules. If there is no satisfactory response to thyroid hormone treatment after 6 months, it should be discontinued.

It has been hypothesized that a serum Tg concentration that is persistently elevated during thyroid hormone treatment characterizes patients in whom thyroid hormone therapy fails.[13–15] However, definite proof of the validity of this hypothesis and, therefore, of the value of serum Tg measurements during thyroid hormone treatment has not been provided.

Thyroid hormone therapy of NDNGs rarely gives satisfactory long-term results.[5,6,13,17,33,37–43] It is potentially dangerous in elderly patients who may develop tachyarrhythmias, congestive heart failure, angina, and myocardial infarctions due to iatrogenic thyrotoxicosis (this is especially common when individual goiter nodules are not suppressible with thyroid hormone treatment). Even if the size of a nontoxic nodular goiter decreases initially during a course of thyroid hormone treatment, it may only be because the TSH-responsive tissue between the nodules shrinks while the autonomous nodules are unchanged in size or even continue to grow. However, significant reduction of goiter volume by thyroid hormone treatment is sometimes achieved in diffuse nontoxic goiters.

3. *Radioiodine* can be used to treat patients with nontoxic diffuse or nodular goiters in whom hyperthyroidism has developed (see chaps 16, 32 and 53). Although radioiodine uptake is in general too low for radioiodine treatment to significantly decrease goiter size in patients with NDNGs, a few reports suggest that radioiodine goiter therapy can reduce NDNG size.[6,45–48] The availability

of recombinant human TSH in the future may be efficacious in such patients by increasing the radioiodine uptake, especially in quiescent tissue.

4. *Antithyroid drugs* are used in patients with NDNG who have become thyrotoxic and who need to be rendered euthyroid before thyroidectomy or radioactive iodine therapy.

Management of Specific Clinical Situations

All nontoxic goiters containing nodules suspected or proven to harbor cancer should be treated surgically. The probability that a thyroid nodule is malignant is increased in rapidly growing nodules (unless the rapid growth is caused by a hemorrhage), in single nodules, in nodules in young patients, in nodules in males, in nodules that are scintigraphically cold, and in nodules in patients with a history of neck irradiation.[5,6,11,16–23] However, definite proof that a thyroid malignancy is present can only be obtained before surgery by a positive FNB or cutting-needle biopsy.

Large NDNGs that cause inspiratory stridor, disturbances of deglutition, hoarseness, or significant cervical venous congestion by compression of the trachea, the esophagus, the recurrent laryngeal nerve, or cervical veins should be removed surgically provided that the patient is well enough and the surgeon is skilled. Thyroid hormone treatment of such goiters causes partial regression of their size at best because large nontoxic goiters frequently contain nodules whose autonomous growth is TSH independent and, therefore, not suppressed by thyroid hormone therapy.[3–6,13,17,33,39–43] Radioiodine treatment may be effective if the radioiodine uptake is sufficient. Thyroid hormone or radioiodine therapy of large nontoxic goiters causing compression symptoms should, therefore, only be considered in patients who are unable to undergo surgery.

The therapeutic approach is more complex for small or moderate-sized NDNGs that, based on the patient's history and physical examination, have shown little or no growth over a prolonged period of time and do not produce symptoms related to compression of neighboring structures.

In elderly patients with such goiters, aggressive (i.e., surgical) treatment is not warranted. However, yearly visits including physical examination of the neck (to exclude significant goiter growth) and thyroid hormone measurements to exclude the development of subclinical or overt hyperthyroidism are indicated. Recognition of subclinical or overt hyperthyroidism is of particular importance in elderly patients because of their increased risk of developing thyrotoxicosis-associated cardiac tachyarrhythmias.[24,25] Thyroid sonography should perhaps be done once in elderly patients to obtain exact information about the size of the goiter and prominent nodules for later comparison.

In middle-aged patients with such goiters thyroid sonography is important for making decisions on therapy and follow-up. In patients with goiters that do not contain nodules with a diameter greater than 2 to 3 cm on sonography and that do not show an increase in size on two sonograms done 6 months to a year apart, a therapeutic trial with thyroid hormone or simple follow-up with yearly clinical evaluation and examination of the thyroid and thyroid hormone measurements is adequate. A sonogram is done in addition whenever growth of the entire goiter or individual nodules is suspected but cannot be proven clinically. However, if the clinical examination or two thyroid sonograms done 6 months to a year apart show a definite increase in goiter size, surgery is the treatment of choice. Surgical treatment should also be considered in patients with a thyroid nodule with a diameter greater than 2 to 3 cm because nodules of that size practically never regress spontaneously or with thyroid hormone treatment and may require a time-consuming follow-up with frequent clinical, ultrasonographic, FNB, and laboratory tests, which can be expensive and difficult for the patient. However, clinical evaluation and examination of the thyroid and thyroid function tests yearly may be sufficient in many such patients, in whom there is no clinically detectable growth of the thyroid nodule, especially in countries where cost-conscious medicine has become the rule.

A therapeutic trial with thyroid hormones is justified in young patients with clinically diffuse nontoxic goiters and may prevent the later development of nodular goiter. Young patients with nodular nontoxic goiters, especially if there are nodules with a diameter greater than 2 to 3 cm on ultrasound, are surgical candidates, but conservative management with appropriate isotopic imaging and FNB may be an alternative approach.

References

1. Gutekunst R, Smolarek H, Hasenpusch U, et al. Goitre epidemiology: thyroid volume, thyroglobulin and thyrotropin in Germany and Sweden. Acta Endocrinol (Copenh) 1986; 112:494

2. Berghout A, Wiersinga M, Smits NJ, et al. Determinants of thyroid volume as measured by ultrasonography in healthy adults in a non-iodine deficient area. Clin Endocrinol 1987;26:273

3. Studer H, Ramelli F. Simple goiter and its variants: euthyroid and hyperthyroid multinodular goiters. Endocr Rev 1982;3:40

4. Studer H, Peter HJ, Gerber H. Natural heterogeneity of thyroid cells: the basis for understanding thyroid function and nodular goiter growth. Endocr Rev 1989;10:125

5. Studer H, Gerber H. Non-toxic goiter. In: Greer MA, ed. The thyroid gland. Comprehensive endocrinology. New York: Raven Press, 1990:391

6. Studer H, Gerber H. Multinodular goiter. In: DeGroot LJ, ed. Endocrinology. 3rd ed. Philadelphia: WB Saunders, 1994:769

7. Berghout A, Wiersinga WM, Smits NJ, Touber JL. Interrelationships between age, thyroid volume, thyroid nodularity, and thyroid function in patients with sporadic nontoxic goiter. Am J Med 1990;89:602

8. Mortensen JD, Woolner LB, Bennet WA. Gross and microscopic findings in clinically normal thyroid glands. J Clin Endocrinol Metab 1955;15:1270

9. Horlocker TT, Hay JE, James EM, et al. Prevalence of incidental nodular thyroid disease detected during high-resolution parathyroid ultrasonography. In: Medeiros-Neto GA, Gaitan E, eds. Frontiers in thyroidology. Proceedings of the 9th International Thyroid Conference, Sao Paulo, 1985. New York: Plenum Press, 1986:1309

10. Brander A, Viikinkoski P, Nickels, Kivisaari L. Thyroid gland: US screening in a random adult population. Radiology 1991;181:683

11. Gharib H. Current evaluation of thyroid nodules. Trends Endocrinol Metab 1994;5:365

12. Fenzi GF, Ceccarelli C, Macchia E, et al. Reciprocal changes of serum thyroglobulin and TSH in residents of a moderate endemic goiter area. Clin Endocrinol 1985;23:115

13. Bürgi U, Scazziga BR, Rosselet PO, et al. Can serum thyroglobulin predict the effect of thyroid hormone therapy on goiter growth? Acta Endocrinol (Copenh) 1988;119:118

14. Gebel F, Ramelli F, Bürgi U, et al. The site of leakage of intrafollicular thyroglobulin into the blood stream in simple human goiter. J Clin Endocrinol Metab 1983;57:915

15. Bürgi U, Gebel F. Die diagnostische Bedeutung der Thyreoglobulinbestimmung im Blut. Schweiz Med Wochenschr 1984; 114:365

16. Ashcraft MW, Van Herle AJ. Management of thyroid nodules. I. History and physical examination, blood tests, x-ray tests, and ultrasonography. Head Neck Surg 1981;3:216

17. Ashcraft MW, Van Herle AJ. Management of thyroid nodules. II. Scanning techniques, thyroid suppressive therapy, and fine needle aspiration. Head Neck Surg 1981;3:297

18. Molitch M, Beck R, Dreisman M, et al. The cold thyroid nodule: an analysis of diagnostic and therapeutic options. Endocr Rev 1984;5:185

19. Rojeski MT, Gharib H. Nodular thyroid disease. Evaluation and management. N Engl J Med 1985;313:428

20. Franklyn JA, Sheppard MC. Thyroid nodules and thyroid cancer-diagnostic aspects. Baillières Clin Endocrinol Metab 1988;2:761

21. Ross DS. Evaluation of the thyroid nodule. J Nucl Med 1991; 32:2181

22. Ridgway EC. Clinician's evaluation of a solitary thyroid nodule. J Clin Endocrinol Metab 1992;74:231

23. Mazzaferri E. Management of a solitary thyroid nodule. N Engl J Med 1993;328:553

24. Gemsenjäger E, Staub JJ Girard J, Heitz PH. Preclinical hyperthyroidism in multinodular goiter. J Clin Endocrinol Metab 1976; 43:810

25. Sawin C, Geller A, Wolf P, et al. Low serum thyrotropin concentrations as a risk factor for atrial fibrillation in older persons. N Engl J Med 1994;331:1249

26. Studer H, Gerber H. Intrathyroidal iodine. Heterogeneity of iodocompounds and kinetic compartmentalization. Trends Endocrinol Metab 1991;2:29

27. Aeschimann S, Bürgi U, Wagner HE, et al. Low intrathyroidal iodine concentration in non-enedmic human goiters: a consequence rather than a cause of autonomous goiter growth. J Endocrinol 1994;140:155

28. Studer H, Forster R, Conti A, et al. Transformation of normal follicles into thyrotropin-refractory "cold" follicles in the aging mouse thyroid gland. Endocrinology 1978;102:1576

29. Gerber H, Peter HJ, Studer H. Age-related failure of endocytosis may be the pathogenetic mechanism responsible for "cold" follicle formation in the aging mouse thyroid. Endocrinology 1987; 120:1758

30. van Middlesworth L. Thiocyanate feeding with low iodine diet causes chronic iodine retention in thyroids of mice. Endocrinology 1985;116:665

31. Gerber H, Huber G, Peter HJ, et al. Transformation of normal thyroids into colloid goiters in rats and mice by diphenylthiohydantoin. Endocrinology 1994.;135:2688

32. Gemsenjäger E, Heitz PU, Staub JJ, et al. Surgical aspects of thyroid autonomy in multinodular goiter. World J Surg 1983;7:363

33. Westermark K, Peter C, Persson A, et al. Nodular goiter: effects of surgery and thyroxine medication. World J Surg 1986;10:481

34. Teuscher J, Peter HJ, Gerber H, et al. Pathogenesis of nodular goiter and its implications for surgical management. Surgery 1988;103:87

35. Gemsenjäger E, Girard J, Martina B. Prae- and postoperative Thyreoglobulingabe in das Blut bei Knotenstruma. Schweiz Med Wochenschr 1984;114:826

36. Röher HD, Goretzki PE. Management of goiter and thyroid nodules in an area of endemic goiter. Surg Clin North Am 1987; 67:233

37. Wagner H, Seiler Ch. Indikationen und Resultate der Rezidiveingriffe an der Schilddrüse. Schweiz Med Wochenschr 1994; 124:1222

38. Kaplan EL, Shukla M, Hara H, Ito K. Surgery of the thyroid. In: DeGroot LJ, ed. Endocrinology. 3rd ed. Philadelphia: WB Saunders, 1994:900

39. Perrild H, Hansen JM, Hegedüs L, et al. Triiodothyronine and thyroxine treatment of diffuse non-toxic goitre evaluated by ultrasonic scanning. Acta Endocrinol (Copenh) 1982;100:382

40. Feldt-Ramussen U, Hegedüs L, Hansen JM, Perrild H. Relationship between thyroid volume and serum thyroglobulin during long-term suppression with triiodothyronine in patients with diffuse non-toxic goitre. Acta Endocrinol (Copenh) 1984; 105:184

41. Morita T, Tamai H, Ohshima A, et al. Changes in serum thyroid hormone, thyrotropin and thyroglobulin concentrations during thyroxine therapy in patients with solitary thyroid nodules. J Clin Endocrinol Metab 1989;69:227

42. Berghout A, Wiersinga WM, Drexhage HA, et al. Comparison of placebo with L-thyroxine alone or with carbimazole for treatment of sporadic non-toxic goitre. Lancet 1990;336:193

43. Toft A. Thyroxine therapy. N Engl J Med 1994;331:174

44. Olbricht TH, Hoff HG, Benker G, et al. Sonographische Volumetrie der Schilddrüse zur Verlaufskontrolle bei der Thyroxin- und Jodidbehandlung der blanden Struma. Dtsch Med Wochenschr 1985;110:863

45. Kay T, d'Emden M, Andrews J, Martin F. Treatment of nontoxic multinodular goiter with radioactive iodine. Am J Med 1988; 84:19

46. Hegedüs L, Hansen BM, Knudsen N, Hansen JM. Reduction of size of thyroid with radioactive iodine in multinodular non-toxic goiter. BMJ 1988;297:661

47. Verelst J, Bonnyns M, Glinoer D. Radioiodine therapy in voluminous multinodular non-toxic goitre. Acta Endocrinol (Copenh) 1990;122:417

48. Huysmans DA, Hermus AR, Corstens FH, et al. Large, compressive goiters treated with radioiodine. Ann Intern Med 1994; 121:757

SEVEN

Thyroid Diseases:
Tumors

Werner and Ingbar's The Thyroid, Seventh Edition,
edited by Lewis E. Braverman and Robert D. Utiger.
Lippincott–Raven Publishers, Philadelphia, © 1996

80

Carcinoma of Follicular Epithelium

PATHOGENESIS

Arthur B. Schneider
Elaine Ron

The thyroid gland is an uncommon site of cancer, accounting for only 0.6% and 1.6% of cancers among men and women, respectively, in the United States. Because of its good prognosis, thyroid cancer causes an even lower percentage of cancer deaths, 0.16% and 0.24% for men and women, respectively.[1] During the past several decades, the incidence of thyroid carcinoma has been increasing, particularly among women, whereas mortality from thyroid carcinoma has decreased among both women and men.[2] In part, the increased incidence is due to improved diagnosis, whereas the reduced mortality is due to earlier detection, improved treatment, and a decline in anaplastic thyroid carcinoma. The increase in incidence of thyroid carcinoma in Connecticut from 1935 to 1975 corresponds to the years that would be expected if the increase were associated with radiation treatment to the head and neck area of children, which is the only proven thyroid carcinogen.[3] However, studies from Sweden,[4] Switzerland,[5] and Norway,[6] where childhood radiation treatment was never widely used, suggest that other factors may be important as well. In some countries the incidence of thyroid carcinoma is no longer increasing,[7,8] but U.S. data from 1973 to 1991 still show an increase.[2]

Thyroid carcinoma is more common in women than in men.[2,9] The reason for this difference, including whether specific hormonal factors are involved, is not known. Environmental factors have been considered potential causes of thyroid carcinoma. Many of them are thought to operate through the action of thyrotropin (TSH). Considerable evidence from animal experiments indicates that prolonged TSH stimulation can cause thyroid carcinoma, but the evidence with respect to humans is not as clear.[10,11]

The genetic and cellular mechanisms giving rise to benign and malignant thyroid tumors are receiving a great deal of attention, with recent work implicating alterations in particular cellular oncogenes and tumor suppressor genes (see the next section). As yet, it is not known whether these genes are targets for the factors that cause thyroid carcinoma. Inherited genetic factors are related to thyroid carcinoma in Gardner's syndrome, Cowden's disease, and possibly in other familial occurrences of thyroid carcinoma.

EXTERNAL RADIATION

The distinction between factors that act as initiators of thyroid carcinoma and those that act as promoters may be clinically important. Radiation initiates thyroid carcinoma, but additional factors are probably required before it becomes clinically evident. Factors that cause TSH hypersecretion may not be sufficient to cause thyroid carcinoma but may stimulate its growth once it is present. Thus, giving thyroid hormone to an irradiated patient may prevent the development of clinically important thyroid tumors of all types.

Evidence That Radiation Causes Thyroid Carcinoma

The relationship between radiation and thyroid carcinoma was first recognized by Duffy and Fitzgerald in 1950.[12] They found that an unusually large fraction of their pediatric patients with thyroid carcinoma had a history of radiation therapy. This relationship was subsequently confirmed by many studies.[13,14] Ron and colleagues[15] recently reported an analysis of radiation exposure and thyroid carcinoma, combining the observations from seven large studies in which individual thyroid doses were estimated. Their analysis of childhood exposure, which included nearly 500 patients with thyroid carcinoma, demonstrated a strong association between radiation and thyroid carcinoma. Based on an excess relative risk model (i.e., risk increases multiplicatively with dose) a linear dose-response relationship fit the data well. There was little evidence for a radiation effect among persons exposed after age 20 years.

Two major difficulties arise in studying the relationship between radiation and thyroid carcinoma. One is the fact that many people are unaware of or uncertain about prior radiation exposure because this usually occurred at a young age (recall bias). The other is that the diagnosis of thyroid tumors depends on the extent of the diagnostic procedures used to look for them (diagnostic bias). The cumulative evidence shown in Table 80-1 is especially strong because individual studies minimize each of these problems. In the case-control studies, the cases had thyroid carcinoma and were identified by their entry into a tumor registry or by their admission to a hospital. The control subjects were comparable subjects without thyroid carcinoma. Information on risk factors, such as radiation exposure, was obtained and the distribution in the two groups compared. Therefore, in these case-control studies, diagnostic bias was minimized, but recall bias could have been important. In the cohort studies, exposure to radiation was generally documented, and often the amount of exposure was known. The frequency of thyroid carcinoma in the radiation-exposed group was compared with a group of similar subjects who were not exposed. Therefore, in cohort studies, recall bias was minimized, but diagnostic bias could have been important. A consistent and strong relationship between radiation exposure, possibly at doses as low as 0.1 Gy (10 rads), and thyroid carcinoma has been found in both types of studies.[13–15] At doses below 0.1 Gy (10 rads), the results have been equivocal, but a linear no-threshold dose response fits the data from most studies very well.

In contrast to external radiation, there is little evidence to suggest that internal radiation from iodine-131 (^{131}I) used for therapeutic or diagnostic medical purposes causes thyroid carcinoma in humans[27–30] (see chap 16). The reason for the difference between external and internal radiation is not known, but the lower dose rate of ^{131}I may allow repair of radiation damage. Observations on brief, generally high-dose exposures to ^{131}I, as occurs in the medical setting, may not provide data applicable to the prolonged, generally low-dose radiation received by people accidentally exposed to nuclear fallout or living near nuclear production facilities.

The question of internal radiation, however, is not completely resolved. Some people living on some of the Marshall Islands who were exposed to fallout from a nuclear test explosion in 1954 subsequently developed thyroid tumors, including carcinomas.[22,31,32] However, their radiation exposure came from a combination of ^{131}I, other more rapidly decaying isotopes of iodine, and external gamma radiation. A new study of children exposed to nuclear fallout from weapons testing at the Nevada Test Site found a significant association between all thyroid nodules and dose, but not for thyroid carcinoma separately.[24] Although there was no increase in thyroid neoplasia among persons living in areas contaminated by the Chernobyl accident in 1986,[33] there have been recent reports of a large increase the incidence of thyroid carcinoma among children living in Belarus and the Ukraine.[34–36]

TABLE 80-1.
Selected Epidemiologic Studies of the Relation Between External Radiation and Thyroid Carcinoma

Locations and References	Study Population		Comments
COHORT STUDIES*	EXPOSED (N)	NONEXPOSED (N)	
Boston, tonsils[16]	1,192	1,063	Elevated risk for nodules, not carcinoma
Chicago, tonsils[17]	2,643	0	ERR/Gy = 2.5
China, background radiation[18]	1,001	1,005	No effects
China, radiology workers[19]	27,000	26,000	Doses unknown, rel. risk = 2.1
Israel, tinea capitis[20]	10,834	16,226	ERR/Gy = 32.5
Japan, atomic bomb[21]	41,234	38,738	ERR/Gy = 4.7 (children), 0.4 (adults)
		(< 0.01 Sv)	
Marshall Islands, fallout[22]	250	600	ERR/Gy = 0.3 (children), 0.5 (adults)
New York City, tinea capitis[13]	2,200	1,400	ERR/Gy = 7.7 (not significant)
Rochester NY, thymus[23]	2,475	4,991	ERR/Gy = 9.1
Utah-Nevada-Arizona, fallout[24]	1,055	1,418	ERR/Gy = 7 for neoplasms, carcinoma not significant
		(< 0.05 Gy)	
NESTED CASE-CONTROL STUDIES*	CASES (N)	CONTROLS (N)	
International, cervical cancer[25]	43	81	ERR/Gy = 34.9
International, childhood cancer[26]	22	82	ERR/Gy = 1.1

In the cohort studies, dose response was evaluated. In the nested case-control studies, case patients had thyroid carcinoma and control subjects did not. In the two case-control studies, the cases were derived from 150,000 patients treated for carcinoma of the uterine cervix and 9170 children treated for carcinoma, respectively.
EER, excess relative risk. All of the estimates of ERR are taken from reference 15 except for the Marshall Island study[22] and for the Utah-Nevada-Arizona study.[24]

Evaluation of Irradiated Patients

An essential part of evaluating a person with a history of irradiation is determining the type of radiation, the site or sites treated, the age at treatment, and the dose. Among the potential risk factors, the dose received by the thyroid is the most important. The patient's age at the time of therapy is an independent risk factor, with younger age associated with greater risk. The dose schedule may be a risk factor, with fractionation reducing the risk. There is a greater spontaneous risk for women, but the effect of gender on radiation-induced thyroid carcinoma is still not clear.[13–15]

External irradiation formerly was used to treat a wide range of benign conditions during childhood. These included enlargement of the thymus, tonsils, adenoids, and cervical lymph nodes; pertussis; asthma; bronchitis; tinea capitis; and acne. For acne it is important to distinguish between ultraviolet therapy and radiation therapy and then to distinguish superficial (grenz rays) from conventional radiation therapy. Another commonly used form of therapy was the local application of radioactive plaques to treat hemangiomas, other localized lesions, and enlarged tonsils. The dose received by the thyroid as a result of these therapies is probably less than with external radiation therapy. External radiation of the neck for malignant conditions such as Hodgkin's disease and carcinoma of the larynx continues in wide use. Such treatment often results in subclinical or overt hypothyroidism[37–39] and sometimes in nodular thyroid disease and thyroid carcinoma.[40,41] It is important to obtain the best radiation history possible because it is needed to decide whether further evaluation, particularly thyroid radionuclide imaging, should be performed.

Much has been written about the value of thyroid radionuclide imaging in screening.[42] The discussion has been generated, in part, by the observation that many people with nodular thyroid disease were discovered solely by imaging, with no corresponding palpable abnormalities.[43] Some clinicians believe that even if imaging discloses otherwise undetectable nodules, they are too small to be of clinical importance and can be safely disregarded until they become evident by palpation. Thyroid ultrasonography is an alternative to radionuclide imaging of irradiated patients. Ultrasonography does not expose the thyroid to radiation and is more sensitive, but it is associated with considerable observer variation and may be too sensitive, because approximately one-third of adult women have ultrasonographically detectable thyroid nodules.[44,45] Whether nonpalpable nodules are clinically important is not known. For a patient with a small nodule, the benefit of careful follow-up and thyroid suppression is likely to outweigh any risk from radionuclide imaging.

Determining the serum thyroglobulin (Tg) concentration in patients who received radiation treatment may be of some clinical value. Many patients with nodular thyroid disease have increased serum Tg concentrations, but the test is not sufficiently reliable to be used as the sole means of screening irradiated patients. When nodular thyroid disease is detected, the serum Tg value does not distinguish between malignant and benign disease; however, patients who appear to be normal but have elevated serum Tg concentrations may be at greater risk for developing nodular disease in the future.[46]

There is no evidence that subclinical or overt hypothyroidism or thyrotoxicosis results from the doses of radiation used to treat benign childhood conditions.[47] The evaluation and treatment of patients with nodular disease is discussed further in chapters 79 and 83 and in the next section of this chapter.

Other tumors may arise in patients exposed to radiation to the head and neck during childhood, some of which can have equal or greater clinical importance for the patient than thyroid tumors. Parathyroid adenomas have been reported in people who received radiation therapy. The Michael Reese Hospital study of tonsillar radiation, a Japanese study of atomic bomb survivors, and a study of radiation treatment for tuberculous cervical adenitis all demonstrated a significant dose-response relationship for hyperparathyroidism.[48–50] Salivary gland tumors most commonly occur in the parotid glands.[51–53] These tumors usually are readily evident to the patient. About one-third are malignant, and most of these are of the mixed-cell variety. They can occur many years after radiation therapy and are continuing to occur. Neural tumors also occur after radiation exposure. In a large group of children treated for tinea capitis by radiation epilation, more brain tumors occurred than in a control group.[54] Benign neural tumors, such as neurilemomas and acoustic neuromas, also were more common in people who received childhood radiation therapy.[55] Finally, an association between thymic irradiation in childhood and the subsequent occurrence of breast cancer in adult women was found in one study.[56] Of less clinical importance is the finding of an elevated risk of nonmelanoma skin cancer among several of the groups studied.[21,57,58]

Clinical Features of Radiation-Related Thyroid Tumors

A history of radiation exposure has two major clinical implications: the increased risk of developing thyroid nodules and the increased risk of a thyroid nodule being malignant. In the Michael Reese Hospital study, more than one-third of the patients exposed to radiation who had thyroidectomies had a thyroid carcinoma.[52]

Follow-up studies indicate that radiation-related thyroid carcinomas behave the same as other thyroid carcinomas in children and adults.[59–61] Therefore, therapy and follow-up probably should be the same as that provided to other patients with thyroid carcinoma. The thyroid carcinomas that arise in relation to radiation treatment are almost all well-differentiated papillary or papillary-follicular carcinomas. Case reports of anaplastic thyroid carcinoma occurring after radiation treatment have appeared but are rare.[62] There is no evidence that the well-differentiated thyroid carcinomas found in patients who received radiation therapy are more likely to undergo transition to more aggressive or less differentiated forms. It is possible, however, that as the population ages, more aggressive carcinomas will be seen, as occurs in the general population.[63]

All irradiated patients who have had nodular thyroid disease treated by thyroidectomy should receive thyroid hormone treatment, even if enough of the gland remains to maintain normal thyroid hormone secretion. This recommendation is based on the observation that nodules continue to occur in these patients with equal or greater frequency compared with patients who did not have surgery. When thyroid hormone therapy is given after thyroidectomy, the frequency of recurrence is reduced.[64]

Patients with a currently normal thyroid and a history of irradiation should be examined periodically. Radiation-related nodular disease continues to occur for as long as it has been possible to study patients irradiated from 1939 to 1962.[17,46,52] Patients at especially high risk should have thyroid radionuclide (^{99m}Tc-pertechnetate or ^{123}I-iodide) or ultrasound imaging as part of their follow-up examination. The results of ultrasonography should be interpreted with caution because of the high prevalence of abnormalities found in the adult population. Examples of high-risk patients are those with one or more of the factors listed in Table 80-2. An examination interval of 1 to 2 years and an imaging interval of 3 to 5 years, continued indefinitely, seem prudent.

Prophylactic therapy to prevent the occurrence of nodular thyroid disease should be considered in patients who received radiation treatment.[65,66] Further studies are needed to confirm one report that demonstrated the effectiveness of thyroid hormone therapy in preventing the appearance of nodules in irradiated patients.[67] In patients at high risk, thyroxine (T_4) therapy has potential benefits that probably outweigh its risks. In this instance a reasonable definition of high risk is more than one of the factors listed in Table 80-2. Also, an abnormal or equivocal thyroid imaging finding, such as a nodule seen by ultrasonography that is too small to aspirate, would contribute to the classification as high risk. Even if only benign nodules occur less frequently in T_4-treated patients, reducing anxiety and the likelihood of surgery are important.

Radiation and Cellular Oncogenes

Because radiation is a mutagen, it is reasonable to expect genetic changes in radiation-induced thyroid carcinomas. In one study, mutations were found in codon 61 of the K-*ras* gene, a locus that is rarely mutated in other thyroid carcinomas.[68] In an early study from the Chernobyl area, mutations were found in the *ret* oncogene in papillary thyroid carcinomas.[69] Whether these or any other mutations cause radiation-induced thyroid carcinoma or are specific for radiation-induced thyroid carcinoma remains to be seen.

PREEXISTING THYROID DISEASE

Thyroid carcinoma is often preceded by other thyroid abnormalities, including endemic and sporadic goiter, benign thy-

---

TABLE 80-2.
Risk Factors Associated With Radiation-Induced Thyroid Tumors

---

High dose of radiation

Young age at exposure

High serum thyroglobulin concentration

Other radiation-related tumor

First-degree relative with radiation-related tumor

---

roid nodules, chronic autoimmune thyroiditis, and Graves' disease, all of which are common. Whether patients with them should be considered at increased risk of developing thyroid carcinoma is uncertain. Despite considerable efforts to resolve this question, the results remain inconclusive. Many case-control studies of thyroid carcinoma have revealed more preexisting benign thyroid nodules and goiter in the carcinoma patients than in the control subjects.[70-76] The risks generally have been high, especially for nodules. In addition, in a recent prospective study of women with benign thyroid conditions in Boston, there was a significant excess of thyroid carcinoma mortality among patients with thyroid adenomas.[77] Interpreting the findings is difficult because of potential ascertainment bias (one thyroid disorder could draw attention to another), the large difference between the frequency of thyroid carcinoma discovered by histologic examination and that discovered by clinical examination, and the failure to categorize thyroid carcinoma by histologic type. Thus, even though there is much published evidence that favors a relationship between preexisting thyroid conditions and thyroid carcinoma, the clinical implications of these findings are not clear.

Recent genetic data suggest that thyroid tumors may progress from benign tumors to well-differentiated carcinomas to anaplastic carcinomas as somatic mutations accumulate (see next section). The epidemiologic data relating previous nodular thyroid disease to thyroid carcinoma are consistent with this model.

HORMONAL AND REPRODUCTIVE FACTORS

Thyroid carcinoma, like most other thyroid diseases, occurs more frequently in women than men, suggesting that hormonal factors are involved in its pathogenesis. In England and Wales, the female/male ratio was highest at the time of puberty. From puberty to menopause the difference between females and males declined consistently.[9] This finding suggests that hormonal events occurring at puberty might be most important in influencing the development of thyroid carcinoma, but a significant relationship between age at menarche and thyroid carcinoma has not been found in most studies. Even the direction of the difference has not been consistent across studies.[70,73–76,78–81] In Switzerland, the female/male ratio at puberty for papillary carcinoma was very high, but for follicular carcinoma the ratio was highest between the ages of 25 and 44 years.[5]

Results from some, but not all, epidemiologic studies indicate that parity may increase the risk of thyroid carcinoma.[70,73–75,82] The most convincing data come from a prospective study of 1.1 million Norwegian women of reproductive age. Based on almost 1000 thyroid carcinomas, a significant trend for increasing risk with increasing parity was demonstrated.[82] To determine whether this trend was related to life-style or environmental exposures, the influence of number of children on the thyroid carcinoma risk in males was studied.[83] No trend was found, which led the authors to conclude that the effect was due to biologic changes during pregnancy. In some studies, thyroid carcinoma occurred more often among women having a late age at first pregnancy.[23,78] Other data indicate that women with a history of spontaneous or induced abortion, particularly during the first pregnancy, have an enhanced risk of thyroid carcinoma,[23,73,75,80,81] and the risk of thyroid carcinoma was increased in two studies of women seeking medical care for fertility problems.[84,85]

Other suggested risk factors for thyroid carcinoma in women are exogenous estrogen, including oral contraceptives,[73,74,86] lactation suppressant drugs,[86] postmenopausal estrogen therapy,[86] and fertility drugs.[80] The associations were usually fairly weak and not dose dependent. Although positive associations between hormonal and reproductive factors and the incidence of thyroid carcinoma have been found in many studies, the results were not always consistent among the different studies. However, the elevated serum concentrations of thyroid stimulators during pregnancy and oral contraceptive therapy provide a possible mechanism for some of these observations.[87,88]

DIETARY FACTORS

Iodine

A relationship between iodine-deficient endemic goiter and thyroid carcinoma has been suspected since Wegelin[89] reported more thyroid carcinoma at autopsy in Bern, Switzerland, compared with Berlin, Germany, an endemic goiter versus a nonendemic goiter area. Since then, attempts to compare the frequency of thyroid carcinoma in geographic areas with and without endemic goiter have provided ambiguous results,[70,90] and the results of studies of the effects of iodine supplementation have been inconsistent. In Switzerland, thyroid carcinoma mortality fell after the introduction of iodized salt,[91] but it did not in Italy or the United States.[90,92]

Clarification of the effects of iodine comes, in part, from observations on the histologic types of thyroid carcinomas that occur in relationship to iodine intake. In endemic goiter areas, follicular and, perhaps, anaplastic thyroid carcinoma predominate. When iodine supplementation is introduced, the proportion of papillary carcinomas increases and that of follicular carcinomas decrease.[11] In Hawaii, where iodine intake is high, the proportion of papillary carcinoma is also high.[80] In Sweden, the risk of follicular carcinoma was higher in iodine-deficient areas than in iodine-sufficient areas, whereas the pattern was opposite for papillary carcinoma.[4] Similar findings were reported in Sicily.[93] These data suggest that follicular carcinomas are related to iodine deficiency and prolonged TSH stimulation.

There are a few studies in which iodine consumption was evaluated. In a case-control study in Hawaii in which iodine intake from food sources and supplements was quantitated, iodine intake was higher in the patients with thyroid carcinoma than in the control subjects.[80] There have been seven case-control studies in which fish and shellfish intake was examined as a surrogate measure of iodine intake. In all but the Hawaiian study the dietary data were extremely limited and, therefore, the findings should be interpreted with caution. Because shellfish generally have a higher iodine content than fish, they are a better indication of high iodine intake. Although the results were not always statistically significant, fish or shellfish consumption was reported more frequently among case patients than control subjects in four studies.[74,75,80,94] In contrast, results from Northern Italy and Vaud, Switzerland indicated a protective effect of fish.[95] In a study conducted in northern Sweden, the results were equivocal: consumption of fish was associated with a slightly decreased risk of thyroid carcinoma and shellfish intake with a higher risk.[79]

Other Dietary Factors

Attempts to determine if there are other dietary factors related to thyroid carcinoma have yielded one consistent finding. Vegetables, particularly cruciferous ones, are associated with a reduced risk of thyroid carcinoma.[75,80,95] This is a somewhat surprising finding because these vegetables contain natural goitrogens. However, cruciferous vegetables also contain several constituents that could reduce tumor risk.[96–98] In a pooled analysis of Italian and Swiss studies, pasta, bread, pastry, and potatoes were associated with an increased risk,[95] but other studies failed to confirm these findings. In the Hawaiian study, the case patients reported eating more fat, protein, and carbohydrates than the control subjects. The higher total calorie intake among cases is consistent with overweight found in the Hawaiian study,[80] as well as two other epidemiologic studies.[75,86] Finally, in a small study conducted in Greece, coffee consumption protected against thyroid carcinoma.[99]

PHARMACEUTICAL AGENTS AND TOXINS

Although no pharmaceutical agent or toxin has been proved to cause thyroid carcinoma in humans, there is reason to remain open to this possibility. Drugs such as lithium and phenobarbital may cause goiter and increased serum TSH concentrations, making it reasonable to suspect that certain drugs could cause or promote the growth of thyroid carcinoma. In laboratory animals, agents that increase TSH secretion may cause thyroid carcinoma.[100]

Patients with congenital goiter have thyroid glands that are subjected to intense TSH stimulation until appropriate treatment is given. Rare patients with congenital goiter who have developed thyroid carcinoma have been reported, supporting the possibility that prolonged intense TSH stimulation alone is sufficient to cause thyroid carcinoma in humans.[101]

FAMILIAL THYROID CARCINOMA

The existence of two uncommon familial syndromes that include carcinoma of thyroid follicular cell origin among their manifestations supports the existence of genetic factors in the pathogenesis of thyroid carcinoma. One is Gardner's syndrome, a dominantly inherited form of familial polyposis of the large intestine, which sometimes is accompanied by thyroid carcinoma.[102] As in other genetic diseases, the thyroid carcinomas that occur in conjunction with polyposis coli are usually diagnosed before age 35 years. The other syndrome is Cowden's disease, an autosomal dominant disorder characterized by the development of multiple hamartomas in several organs, including the thyroid, as well as a high incidence of carcinoma in the same organs.[103]

There have been reports of family aggregates of papillary thyroid carcinoma.[104] In a clinical study, 6% of 226 patients with papillary carcinoma reported having at least one relative who also had the same tumor.[105] An increased frequency of thyroid carcinoma in close relatives of patients with non-medullary thyroid carcinoma was found in one of the case-control studies.[75] The role of genetic factors in these or other cases of thyroid carcinoma remains to be determined.

There are probably genetic factors related to the possibility of developing radiation-induced thyroid tumors. Patients with one radiation-induced tumor (thyroid, salivary, or benign neural) are more likely to develop another tumor than are patients with comparable risk factors exposed to the same amount of radiation.[55,106] Further, in sibling pairs in which both members were irradiated, thyroid tumor development was concordant more often than would be expected by chance.[107] These findings are limited by the possibility that other unknown risk factors rather than radiation susceptibility might account for the observations.

SUMMARY

Besides radiation, no other risk factors have been proven to cause thyroid carcinoma in humans. One of the major problems in understanding the pathogenesis of thyroid carcinoma is the need to consider histology. The four major histologic types of thyroid carcinoma appear to have different risk factors and the rarity of the disease makes it extremely difficult to study the histologic types separately. Just as pooling data from several studies of radiation-induced thyroid carcinoma has helped resolve many questions regarding the shape of the dose-response curve and effect modification, pooling data from studies of the etiology of thyroid carcinoma may be necessary to determine the role of previous thyroid diseases, iodine and other dietary intake, reproductive and hormonal factors, and genetics.

References

1. Boring CC, Squires TS, Tong T. Cancer statistics, 1993. CA Cancer J Clin 1993;43:7
2. Ries LAG, Miller BA, Hankey BF, et al. SEER cancer statistics review, 1973–1991: tables and graphs. National Cancer Institute. NIH Pub. No. 94-2789. Bethesda, MD: 1994
3. Pottern LM, Stone BJ, Day NE, et al. Thyroid cancer in Connecticut, 1935–1975: an analysis by cell type. Am J Epidemiol 1980; 112:764
4. Pettersson B, Adami H-O, Wilander E, Coleman MP. Trends in thyroid cancer incidence in Sweden, 1958–1981, by histopathologic type. Int J Cancer 1991;48:28
5. Levi F, Franceschi S, Te VC, et al. Descriptive epidemiology of thyroid cancer in the Swiss canton of Vaud. J Cancer Res Clin Oncol 1990;116:639
6. Akslen LA, Haldorsen T, Thoresen S, Glattre E. Incidence pattern of thyroid cancer in Norway: influence of birth cohort and time period. Int J Cancer 1993;53:183
7. Glattre E, Akslen LA, Thoresen S, Haldorsen T. Geographic patterns and trends in the incidence of thyroid cancer in Norway 1970–1986. Cancer Detect Prev 1990;14:625
8. Hrafnkelsson J, Jonasson JG, Sigurdsson G, et al. Thyroid cancer in Iceland 1955–1984. Acta Endocrinol 1988;118:566

9. dos Santos Silva I, Swerdlow AJ. Sex differences in the risks of hormone-dependent cancers. Am J Epidemiol 1993;138:10
10. Henderson BE, Ross RK, Pike MC, Casagrande JT. Endogenous hormones as a major factor in human cancer. Cancer Res 1982; 42:3232
11. Williams ED. TSH and thyroid cancer. Horm Metabol Res 1990; 23(Suppl):72
12. Duffy BJ Jr, Fitzgerald PJ. Cancer of the thyroid in children: a report of 28 cases. J Clin Endocrinol Metab 1950;10:1296
13. Shore RE. Issues and epidemiological evidence regarding radiation-induced thyroid cancer. Radiat Res 1992;131:98
14. UNSCEAR (United Nations Scientific Committee on the Effects of Atomic Radiation). Sources and effects of ionizing radiation. Publ. E94.IX.11. New York: United Nations, 1994
15. Ron E, Lubin JH, Shore RE, et al. Thyroid cancer after exposure to external radiation: a pooled analysis of seven studies. Radiat Res 1995;141:259
16. Pottern LM, Kaplan MM, Larsen PR, et al. Thyroid modularity after childhood irradiation for lymphoid hyperplasia: a comparison of questionnaire and clinical findings. J Clin Epidemiol 1990;43:449
17. Schneider AB, Ron E, Lubin J, et al. Dose-response relationships for radiation-induced thyroid cancer and thyroid nodules: evidence for the prolonged effects of radiation on the thyroid. J Clin Endocrinol Metab 1993;77:362
18. Wang Z, Boice JD Jr, Wei L, et al. Thyroid nodularity and chromosome aberrations among women in areas of high background radiation in China. J Natl Cancer Inst 1990;82:478
19. Wang JX, Boice JD Jr, Li BX, et al. Cancer among medical diagnostic x-ray workers in China. J Natl Cancer Inst 1988;80:344
20. Ron E, Modan B, Preston D, Alfandary E, Stovall M, Boice JD Jr. Thyroid neoplasia following low-dose radiation in childhood. Radiat Res 1989;120:516
21. Thompson DE, Mabuchi K, Ron E, et al. Cancer incidence in atomic bomb survivors. Part II: solid tumors, 1958–1987. Radiat Res 1994;137(Suppl):S17
22. Robbins J, Adams WH. Radiation effects in the Marshall Islands. In: Nagataki S, ed. Radiation and the thyroid. Amsterdam: Excerpta Medica, 1989:11
23. Shore RE, Hildreth N, Dvoretsky E, et al. Thyroid cancer among persons given x-ray treatment in infancy for an enlarged thymus gland. Am J Epidemiol 1993;137:1068
24. Kerber RA, Till JE, Simon SL, et al. A cohort study of thyroid disease in relation to fallout from nuclear weapons testing. JAMA 1993;270:2076
25. Boice JD Jr, Engholm G, Kleinerman RA, et al. Radiation dose and second cancer risk in patients treated for cancer of the cervix. Radiat Res 1988;116:3
26. Tucker MA, Morris-Jones PH, Boice JD Jr, et al. Therapeutic radiation at a young age is linked to secondary thyroid cancer. Cancer Res 1991;51:2885
27. Dobyns BM, Sheline GE, Workman JB, et al. Malignant and benign neoplasms of the thyroid in patients treated for hyperthyroidism: a report of the cooperative thyrotoxicosis therapy follow-up study. J Clin Endocrinol Metab 1974;38:976
28. Hall P, Berg G, Bjelkengren G, et al. Cancer mortality after iodine-131 therapy for hyperthyroidism. Int J Cancer 1992;50:886
29. Hall P, Holm L-E, Lundell G, et al. Cancer risks in thyroid-cancer patients. Br J Cancer 1991;64:159
30. Holm LE, Wiklund KE, Lundell GE, et al. Thyroid cancer after diagnostic doses of iodine-131: a retrospective cohort study. J Natl Cancer Inst 1988;80:1131
31. Conard RA. Late radiation effects in Marshall Islanders exposed to fallout 28 years ago. In: Boice JD Jr, Fraumeni JR, eds. Radiation carcinogenesis: epidemiology and biological significance. New York: Raven Press, 1984:57
32. Hamilton T, van Belle G, LoGerfo JP. Thyroid neoplasia in Marshall Islanders exposed to nuclear fallout. JAMA 1987;258:629

33. Mettler FA, Williamson MR, Royal HD, et al. Thyroid nodules in the population living around Chernobyl. JAMA 1992;268:616

34. Kazakov VS, Demidchik EP, Astakhova LN. Thyroid cancer after Chernobyl. Nature 1992;359:21

35. Stsjazhko VA, Tsyb AF, Tronko ND, Souchkevitch G, Baverstock KF. Childhood thyroid cancer since accident at Chernobyl. BMJ 1995;310:801

36. Williams D. Chernobyl, eight years on. Nature 1994;371:556

37. Fleming ID, Black TL, Thompson EI, et al. Thyroid dysfunction and neoplasia in children receiving neck irradiation for cancer. Cancer 1985;55:1190

38. Kaplan MM, Garnick MB, Gelber R, et al. Risk factors for thyroid abnormalities after neck irradiation for childhood cancer. Am J Med 1983;74:272

39. Pasqualini T, Iorcansky S, Gruneiro L, et al. Thyroid dysfunction in Hodgkin's disease. Cancer 1989;63:335

40. Schneider AB. Cancer therapy and endocrine disease: radiation-induced thyroid tumours. In: Sheaves R, Jenkins PJ, Wass JAH, eds. Clinical endocrine oncology. Oxford: Blackwell, 1996. In press

41. Hancock SL, Cox RS, McDougall IR. Thyroid disease after treatment of Hodgkin's disease. N Engl J Med 1991;325:599

42. Stockwell RM, Barry M, Davidoff F. Managing thyroid abnormalities in adults exposed to upper body irradiation in childhood: a decision analysis. J Clin Endocrinol Metab 1984;58:804

43. Favus MJ, Schneider AB, Stachura ME, et al. Thyroid cancer occurring as a late consequence of head and neck irradiation. N Engl J Med 1976;294:1019

44. Brander A, Vikinkoski P, Nickels J, Kivisaari L. Thyroid gland: US screening in middle-aged women with no previous thyroid disease. Radiology 1989;173:507

45. Jarlov AE, Karstrup B, Hegedüs L, et al. Observer variation in ultrasound assessment of the thyroid gland. Br J Radiol 1993;66:625

46. Schneider AB, Bekerman C, Favus M, et al. Continuing occurrence of thyroid nodules after head and neck irradiation: relation to plasma thyroglobulin concentration. Ann Intern Med 1981;94:176

47. Schneider AB, Favus MJ, Stachura ME, et al. Plasma thyroglobulin in detecting thyroid carcinoma after childhood head and neck irradiation. Ann Intern Med 1977;86:29

48. Schneider AB, Gierlowski T, Shore-Freedman E, et al. Dose-response relationships for radiation-induced hyperparathyroidism. J Clin Endocrinol Metab 1995;80:245

49. Fujiwara S, Sposto R, Ezaki H, et al. Hyperparathyroidism among atomic bomb survivors in Hiroshima. Radiat Res 1992;130:363

50. Tisell LE, Carlsson S, Fjalling M, et al. Hyperparathyroidism subsequent to neck irradiation. Cancer 1985;56:1529

51. Schneider AB, Favus MJ, Stachura ME, et al. Salivary gland neoplasms as a late consequence of head and neck irradiation. Ann Intern Med 1977;87:160

52. Schneider AB, Shore-Freedman E, Ryo UY, et al. Radiation-induced tumors of the head and neck following childhood irradiation. Medicine 1985;64:1

53. Shore-Freedman E, Abrahams C, Recant W, Schneider AB. Neurilemomas and salivary gland tumors of the head and neck following childhood irradiation. Cancer 1983;51:2159

54. Ron E, Modan B, Boice JD Jr, et al. Tumors of the brain and nervous system after radio therapy in childhood. N Engl J Med 1988;319:1033

55. Schneider AB, Shore-Freedman E, Weinstein RA. Radiation-induced thyroid and other head and neck tumors: occurrence of multiple tumors and analysis of risk factors. J Clin Endocrinol Metab 1986;63:107

56. Hildreth NG, Shore RE, Dvoretsky PM. The risk of breast cancer after irradiation of the thymus in infancy. N Engl J Med 1989;321:1281

57. Ron E, Modan B, Preston DL, et al. Radiation-induced skin carcinoma of the head and neck. Radiat Res 1991;125:318

58. Shore RE, Albert RE, Reed M, et al. Skin cancer incidence among children irradiated for ringworm of the scalp. Radiat Res 1984;100:192

59. Samaan NA, Schultz PN, Ordonez NG, et al. A comparison of thyroid carcinoma in those who have and have not had neck irradiation in childhood. J Clin Endocrinol Metab 1987;64:219

60. Schneider AB, Recant W, Pinsky SM, et al. Radiation-induced thyroid carcinoma. Ann Intern Med 1986;105:405

61. Viswanathan K, Gierlowski TC, Schneider AB. Childhood thyroid cancer: characteristics and long-term outcome in children irradiated for benign conditions of the head and neck. Arch Pediatr Adolesc Med 1994;148:260

62. Shimaoka K, Getaz EP, Rao U. Anaplastic carcinoma of thyroid. N Y State J Med 1979;79:874

63. Mazzaferri EL, Young RL. Papillary thyroid carcinoma: a 10 year follow-up report of the impact of therapy in 576 patients. Am J Med 1981;70:511

64. Fogelfeld L, Wiviott MBT, Shore-Freedman E, et al. Recurrence of thyroid nodules after surgical removal in patients irradiated in childhood for benign conditions. N Engl J Med 1989;320:835

65. Kaplan MM. Thyroid hormone prophylaxis after radiation exposure. In: Robbins J, ed. Treatment of thyroid cancer in childhood. Springfield, VA: U.S. Department of Commerce, 1994:143

66. Robbins J. Thyroid suppression therapy for prevention of thyroid tumors after radiation exposure. In: DeGroot LJ, Frohman LA, Kaplan EL, Refetoff S, eds. Radiation-associated thyroid carcinoma. New York: Grune & Stratton, 1976;419

67. Murphy ED, Scanlon EF, Garces RM, et al. Thyroid hormone administration in irradiated patients. J Surg Oncol 1986;31:214

68. Wright PA, Williams ED, Lemoine NR, Wynford-Thomas D. Radiation-associated and `spontaneous' human thyroid carcinomas show a different pattern of *ras* oncogene mutation. Oncogene 1991;6:471

69. Ito T, Seyama T, Iwamoto KS, et al. Activated RET oncogene in thyroid cancers of children from areas contaminated by Chernobyl accident. Lancet 1994;344:259

70. Franceschi S, Fassina A, Talamini R, et al. Risk factors for thyroid cancer in northern Italy. lnt J Epidemiol 1989;18:578

71. Levi F, Franceschi S, La Vecchia C, et al. Previous thyroid disease and risk of thyroid cancer in Switzerland. Eur J Cancer 1991;27:85

72. McTiernan AM, Weiss NS, Daling JR. Incidence of thyroid cancer in women in relation to previous exposure to radiation therapy and history of thyroid disease. J Natl Cancer Inst 1984;73:575

73. Preston-Martin S, Bernstein L, Pike MC, et al. Thyroid cancer among young women related to prior thyroid disease and pregnancy history. Br J Cancer 1987;55:191

74. Preston-Martin S, Jin F, Duda MJ, Mack WJ. A case-control study of thyroid cancer in women under age 55 in Shanghai (People's Republic of China). Cancer Causes Control 1993;4:431

75. Ron E, Kleinerman RA, Boice JD Jr, et al. A population-based case-control study of thyroid cancer. J Natl Cancer Inst 1987;79:1

76. Wingren G, Hatschek T, Axelson O. Determinants of papillary cancer of the thyroid. Am J Epidemiol 1993;138:482

77. Goldman MB, Monson RR, Maloof F. Cancer mortality in women with thyroid disease. Cancer Res 1990;50:2283

78. Akslen LA, Nilssen S, Kvåle G. Reproductive factors and risk of thyroid cancer. A prospective study of 63,090 women from Norway. Br J Cancer 1992;65:772

79. Hallquist A, Hardell L, Degerman A, Boquist L. Thyroid cancer: reproductive factors, previous thyroid diseases, drug intake, family history and diet. A case-control study. Eur J Cancer Prev 1994;3:481

80. Kolonel LN, Hankin JH, Wilkens LR, et al. An epidemiologic study of thyroid cancer in Hawaii. Cancer Causes Control 1990 ;1:223

81. Levi F, Franceschi S, Gulie C, et al. Female thyroid cancer: the role of reproductive and hormonal factors in Switzerland. Oncology 1993;50:309

82. Kravdal O, Glattre E, Haldorsen T. Positive correlation between parity and incidence of thyroid cancer: new evidence based on complete Norwegian birth cohorts. Int J Cancer 1991; 49:831

83. Glattre E, Kravdal O. Male and female parity and risk of thyroid cancer. Int J Cancer 1994;58:616

84. Brinton LA, Melton J, Malkasian GD Jr, et al. Cancer risk after evaluation for infertility. Am J Epidemiol 1989;129:712

85. Ron E, Lunenfeld B, Menczer J, et al. Cancer incidence in a cohort of infertile women. Am J Epidemiol 1987;125:780

86. McTiernan AM, Weiss NS, Daling JR. Incidence of thyroid cancer in women in relation to reproductive and hormonal factors. Am J Epidemiol 1984;120:423

87. Chan V, Paraskevaides CA, Hale JF. Assessment of thyroid function during pregnancy. Br J Obstet Gynaecol 1975;82:137

88. Weeke J, Hansen AP. Serum TSH and serum T_3 levels during normal menstrual cycles and during cycles on oral contraceptives. Acta Endocrinol 1975;79:431

89. Wegelin C. Malignant disease of the thyroid gland and its relation to goiter in men and animals. Cancer Rev 1928;3:297

90. Franceschi S, Talamini R, Fassina A, Bidoli E. Diet and epithelial cancer of the thyroid gland. Tumori 1990;76:331

91. Wynder EL. Some practical aspects of cancer prevention (concluded). N Engl J Med 1952;246:573

92. Pendergrast WJ, Milmore BK, Marcus SC. Thyroid cancer and thyrotoxicosis in the United States: their relation to endemic goiter. J Chronic Dis 1961;13:22

93. Belfiore A, La Rosa GL, Padova G, et al. The frequency of cold thyroid nodules and thyroid malignancies in patients from an iodine-deficient area. Cancer 1987;60:3096

94. Glattre E, Haldorsen T, Berg JP, et al. Norwegian case-control study testing the hypothesis that seafood increases the risk of thyroid cancer. Cancer Causes Control 1993;4:11

95. Franceschi S, Levi F, Negri E, et al. Diet and thyroid cancer: a pooled analysis of four European case-control studies. Int J Cancer 1991;48:395

96. NAS (National Academy of Sciences): Committee on Diet, Nutrition, and Cancer. Diet, nutrition, and cancer: interim dietary guidelines. J Natl Cancer Inst 1983;70:1151

97. Negri E, La Vecchia C, Franceschi S, et al. Vegetable and fruit consumption and cancer risk. Int J Cancer 1991;48:350

98. Wattenberg LW. Inhibition of neoplasia by minor dietary constituents. Cancer Res 1983;43(Suppl):2448S

99. Linos A, Linos DA, Vgotza N, et al. Does coffee consumption protect against thyroid disease? Acta Chir Scand 1989; 155:317

100. Hill RN, Erdreich LS, Paynter OE, et al. Thyroid follicular cell carcinogenesis. Fundam Appl Toxicol 1989;12:629

101. Cooper DS, Axelrod L, DeGroot LJ, et al. Congenital goiter and the development of metastatic follicular carcinoma with evidence for a leak of nonhormonal iodide: clinical, pathological, kinetic, and biochemical studies and a review of the literature. J Clin Endocrinol Metab 1981;52:294

102. Delamarre J, Capron J-P, Armand A, et al. Thyroid carcinoma in two sisters with familial polyposis of the colon: case reports and review of the literature. J Clin Gastroenterol 1988:10:659

103. Thyresson HN, Doyle JA. Cowden's disease (multiple hamartoma syndrome). Mayo Clin Proc 1981;56:179

104. Kwok Cg, McDougall IR. Familial differentiated carcinoma of the thyroid:report of five pairs of siblings. Thyroid 1995;5:395

105. Stoffer SS, Van Dyke DL, Bach JV, et al. Familial papillary carcinoma of the thyroid. Am J Med Genet 1986;25:775

106. Cohen J, Gierlowski TC, Schneider AB. A prospective study of hyperparathyroidism in individuals exposed to radiation in childhood. JAMA 1990;264:581

107. Perkel VS, Gail MH, Lubin J, et al. Radiation-induced thyroid neoplasms: evidence for familial susceptibility factors. J Clin Endocrinol Metab 1988;66:1316

MOLECULAR PATHOGENESIS

James A. Fagin

Solitary thyroid nodules are found with increasing prevalence throughout life.[1] Although most are benign follicular tumors, a spectrum of phenotypes can be encountered, including well-differentiated papillary and follicular carcinomas. Less frequently, clinically aggressive carcinomas develop, including the rare and invariably fatal anaplastic carcinomas.

This chapter reviews the biologic events and genetic determinants that underlie the formation and progression of human thyroid tumors. In addition, the relationship between thyroid oncogenesis and thyroid follicular cell differentiation is discussed because the disruption of both growth control and thyroid cell-specific functional properties are important in the determination of tumor phenotype and biologic behavior. The subject of medullary thyroid carcinoma is not be covered because this tumor arises from a separate cell type (C cells) and results from a distinct set of genetic abnormalities (see chap 81).

CLONAL COMPOSITION OF THYROID TUMORS

Tumors arise as a result of inherited or acquired mutations that affect the structural integrity of genes involved in the regulation of cell growth or differentiation.[2] A sequence of mutational events is believed to occur, each leading to clonal expansion of the genetically modified cells. Besides conferring cells with a growth advantage, mutations of certain genes (i.e., *ras*, p53) may also render the cells more susceptible to further genetic damage. The degree of genomic instability resulting from these and other molecular defects may eventually lead to major disruptions in the structure and expression of many genes and in the profound phenotypic abnormalities associated with the advanced forms of cancer. These general concepts apply to tumors of the thyroid gland. Both benign and malignant thyroid tumors are monoclonal,[3–5] and many of the mutational events that may lead to thyroid tumor formation and progression have been uncovered.[6–8] Interestingly, some nodules arising within multinodular goiters also are monoclonal.[3,5] Thus, although the primary defect in these goiters may result in thyroid hyperplasia, the more rapidly dividing cells are also subject to mutations of critical genes and generation of monoclonal adenomas (see chap 78).

Based on their mechanism of action, genes subject to mutations in cancer can be classified as either oncogenes or tumor suppressor genes. Oncogenes are proteins that when inappropriately activated through a structural mutation promote cell growth. They usually act in a dominant fashion, that is, mutation of one allele is sufficient to evoke the neoplastic phenotype. In contrast, tumor suppressor genes transform cells by inactivating a protein involved in limiting cell growth. The latter genes are usually recessive, that is, both alleles must be mutated for the loss-of-function phenotype to be fully expressed. These biallelic mutations can occur as acquired somatic events. Alternatively, a mutation of one allele of a tumor suppressor gene may be inherited and the second mutation occur after conception in the target tissue (e.g., retinoblastoma). A third class of cancer genes acts by interfering with the control of programmed cell death. Under physiologic circumstances, cell death is not a random, chaotic event, but a process responding to specific signals and requiring the expression of certain genes. Mutations of the genes involved in the control of cell death can therefore contribute to tumorigenesis by increasing cellular longevity.[9]

FAMILIAL THYROID CARCINOMA

Besides the well-documented families with a high prevalence of papillary carcinomas,[10] thyroid carcinomas occur with higher frequency in other inherited tumor syndromes such as adenomatous polyposis coli (APC)[11] and multiple endocrine neoplasia type I (MEN1) (Table 80-3). Other autosomal dominant disorders causing disseminated gastrointestinal polyposis, such as Cowden's disease (hamartomas, fibrocystic disease of the breast, breast cancer) or Gardner's syndrome (osteomas, fibromas, lipomas, epidermoid cysts), also are associated with an increased prevalence of thyroid carcinoma. These associations may provide a molecular clue as to the origin of at least some familial thyroid cancer syndromes because the gene conferring predisposition to familial APC has recently been identified and mapped to a region on the long arm of chromosome 5.[12,13] The APC gene is believed to function as a tumor suppressor gene and has also been implicated in the progression of sporadic colorectal neoplasms. Recently, sporadic thyroid tumors with APC mutations have also been reported.[14] Whether mutations of this gene predispose patients with familial APC to thyroid carcinoma is not known.

Thyroid tumors are also found with increased prevalence in patients with MEN1. Thyroid tumors from families with this condition have not been examined for defects within the locus of the MEN1 gene, but loss of genetic material at or close to the MEN1 region is found in some sporadic follicular tumors.[15]

EARLY EVENTS IN THYROID TUMOR FORMATION

Eukaryotic DNA is subject to methylation at the 5 position of cytosine in the dinucleotide sequence cytosine-phosphate-guanine (CpG). DNA methylation is controlled enzymatically, and the pattern of methylated sites is transmitted during somatic cell replication. DNA methylation is changed in virally transformed cells and immortalized cell lines[16–18] and in primary human tumors.[19,20] Altered DNA methylation appears to occur early in the progression of colorectal tumors.[20] Also, the prevalence of aberrant methylation patterns of selected genes in benign and malignant thyroid tumors is high.[21] The frequency of these events in adenomatous nodules from multinodular goiters, consisting largely of hyperplastic tissue, is lower. These findings suggest that widespread changes in DNA methylation may be one of the earliest steps in thyroid tumorigenesis and contribute to transformation through changes in DNA conformation, impairment of transcriptional activity of certain genes, or increased instability of fragile sites of genes.

Thyroid adenomas vary in the degree to which they retain differentiated properties, for instance, the ability to accumulate radioiodine (i.e., hyperfunctioning versus hypofunctioning nodules). Recent information on mutational activation of certain oncogenes may help to understand the relationship between transformation and differentiation in thyroid tumors. Mutations of *ras* oncogenes appear to be about equally prevalent in benign and malignant thyroid tumors, suggesting that they may be an early lesion in the process of thyroid cell transformation.[22–25] Many tyrosine kinase receptors, including those for epidermal growth factor, insulin, and nerve growth factor, signal through *ras* proteins. The three *ras* proteins, H-*ras*, K-*ras* and N-*ras*, are anchored to the plasma membrane and exist in two states: a resting state in which they are bound to guanosine diphosphate (GDP) and an active state in which they bind guanosine triphosphate (GTP). Inactivation occurs through hydrolysis of GTP. The most common form of mutational activation of *ras* oncogenes in human tumors is through single base substitutions affecting either the GTP-binding domain (codons 12 and 13) or the GTPase domain (codon 61) of the protein. Thus, mutant *ras* proteins result in constitutive activation of the downstream signaling cascade because their affinity for GTP is increased or their GTPase activity is decreased, so that the protein cannot return to the resting state. In most types of tumors with *ras* mutations in humans only one of the three *ras* genes is mutated: K-*ras* in pancreatic and colon cancers, N-*ras* in hematologic tumors, and H-*ras* in bladder cancer.[26] In contrast, any of the three *ras* genes may be mutated in thyroid tumors.

Besides activating point mutations of *ras*, some thyroid tumors also have *ras* gene amplification. Here, many copies of the gene are arranged in a tandem repeat sequence, presumably leading to overexpression of the mutant protein.[27] Increasing evidence indicates that activating point mutations of *ras* lead to genomic instability, as measured by the capacity to undergo gene amplification.[28,29] The mechanism for this effect

TABLE 80-3.
Syndromes of Familial Thyroid Neoplasia

Syndrome	Gene Conferring Predisposition
Familial papillary carcinoma	Unknown
Familial adenomatous polyposis coli	APC
Multiple endocrine neoplasia type I	Tumor suppressor gene on chromosome 11q13

is not known, but it may involve accelerated traversion through the G_1 phase of the cell cycle, with premature entry into S phase before the DNA damage arising from endogenous sources, such as free radicals or nucleases, can be repaired.[29] Indeed, although mutant *ras* alleles are strongly implicated in human tumorigenesis, their proposed dominance has been questioned.[30] In rat fibroblasts, replacement of a normal H-*ras* gene by an activated mutant H-*ras* under control of its natural promoter by homologous recombination does not by itself modify the cell phenotype. The H-*ras* mutant-containing cells do, however, have a higher rate of spontaneous transformation after serial passage in vitro, and the mutant *ras* allele is amplified in the majority of the transformed cells. These findings suggest that a *ras* allele containing an activating point mutation is not transforming through a dominant mechanism when it is expressed at normal levels, yet predisposes to transformation by distal events, such as amplification and consequently overexpression of the mutant allele. The fact that both *ras* point mutations and *ras* gene amplification are found in thyroid tumors strongly implicates *ras* as an important factor in thyroid tumorigenesis. Although there is agreement that *ras* mutations are at least one of the initial events in the path to thyroid cell transformation, there is some discrepancy as to their overall prevalence (up to 50%) and whether or not *ras* mutations are more commonly found in follicular than in papillary carcinomas.[23,24,31]

Thyroid cells normally express thyroglobulin (Tg) and thyroid peroxidase (TPO), and their growth and ability to concentrate iodine are thyrotropin (TSH) dependent. The expression of Tg, TPO, and TSH receptors is controlled by the interaction of a group of thyroid-specific transcription factors with the respective promoter sequences of these genes. The DNA-binding proteins TTF-1 and Pax-8 are expressed in the thyroid at the onset of organogenesis.[32] TTF-1 is the main regulator of the Tg gene. Pax-8, although able to bind to specific elements on the promoter regions of both the TPO and Tg genes, appears to activate transcription of the TPO gene preferentially.[33] The ability of cancer genes to disrupt cell differentiation ultimately depends on the manner in which they interfere with the transcription of various genes. Transformation of thyroid cells in vitro with viral *ras* or mutant human *ras* cDNA is associated with loss of expression of TPO and Tg and decrease in cellular uptake of iodine.[34] Although the mechanism of *ras*-mediated dedifferentiation is not understood, it may occur in part by exclusion of the catalytic domain of protein kinase A from the nucleus or interference with the expression or activation of TTF-1.[35] In K-*ras*-transformed rat thyroid FRTL-5 cells, TTF-1 mRNA is markedly reduced, and activation of a Tg promoter can be restored by overexpression of TTF-1.[34] However, K-*ras* may also impair TTF-1 binding to its specific binding site on the promoter.[35] Transformation of H-*ras* is associated with impairment in Tg expression without changes in the abundance of TTF-1 and may be caused by dephosphorylation of TTF-1.

Mutant *ras* cooperates with other oncogenes in promoting thyroid transformation in vitro.[36] Thus, adenomas with *ras* mutations are likely to be hypofunctioning. These mutations may promote genomic instability and consequently increase the likelihood of further mutational events and malignant transformation (Fig 80-1). Certain environmental agents may predispose to mutations of specific target genes. For example, thyroid tumors from patients exposed to external radiation to the neck during childhood may have a high prevalence of point mutations of K-*ras*.[37]

PATHOGENESIS OF AUTONOMOUSLY FUNCTIONING THYROID ADENOMAS

Besides functioning as the major regulator of differentiated function of thyroid cells, TSH is also a thyroid growth factor. TSH stimulation of growth of thyroid follicular cells is mediated in part through a cyclic adenosine monophosphate (cAMP)-dependent signal transduction cascade.[38] Proteins along this activation pathway are logical candidate oncogenes if intrinsically activated through somatic mutations. Support for this concept comes from the discovery of mutations in the α subunit of the guanine nucleotide-binding (G) stimulatory protein in a subset of growth hormone-secreting pituitary tumors (*gsp* oncogene), the growth and function of which are also cAMP dependent.[39] Gs is activated after ligand binding to its respective seven-transmembrane domain receptor (the TSH receptor is a member of this receptor family [see chap 11]), and in turn stimulates the activity of adenylyl cyclase. Point mutations that decrease the intrinsic GTPase activity of Gs_α have been found in about 25% of hyperfunctioning thyroid adenomas.[40–42] Cells expressing mutant Gs_α have constitutive activation of adenylyl cyclase (e.g., no stimulatory ligand like TSH is needed), and therefore stimulation of both cell growth and thyroid hormone synthesis and secretion.

Some hyperfunctioning adenomas have constitutive activation of the TSH receptor as a result of somatic mutations affecting the third intracellular loop of the receptor.[43] These mutations cause inappropriate activation of adenylyl cyclase but not of phospholipase C. Other hyperfunctioning adenomas have activating somatic mutations in the sixth transmembrane domain (codons 631, 632, and 633) of the TSH receptor.[44] Thus, mutational activation of several components of the adenylyl cyclase signal transduction cascade (i.e., TSH receptor, Gs_α) explains the stimulation of growth and differentiated properties of many hyperfunctioning thyroid adenomas (see also chap 32). Constitutive overexpression of inhibitory G protein $Gi_{\alpha-1}$ also has been demonstrated in some hyperfunctioning adenomas, probably leading to adenylyl cyclase-independent stimulation of cell growth. Thus, activation of alternative pathways may be involved in the pathogenesis of some of these tumors.[45]

There is little evidence that constitutive activation of the adenylyl cyclase signal transduction cascade leads to malignant transformation (Fig 80-2). Mutational activation of Gs_α is infrequent in thyroid carcinomas, and no mutations of the TSH receptor have been reported so far in non-hyperfunctioning thyroid adenomas or in thyroid carcinomas.[46] In addition, transgenic mice overexpressing mutant Gs_α in thyroid cells (through a transgene coupling the Tg promoter to the *gsp* oncogene) have adenomatous thyroid hyperplasia but not thyroid carcinoma.[47] These results, as well as the clinical evidence that autonomously functioning adenomas are only rarely associated with malignant transformation, indicate that mutations along the adenylyl cyclase signal transduction cascade are not major determining factors in the development of malignant thyroid tumors.

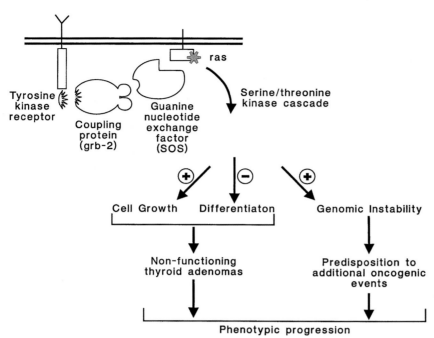

FIGURE 80-1. Mechanisms of thyroid tumor formation after activating mutations of *ras* oncogenes. Under physiologic conditions, many ligand-activated tyrosine kinase receptors bind to the coupling protein grb 2. In turn, grb 2 binds to the carboxy-terminal portion of SOS, a guianine nucleotide-release factor that directly controls *ras* activity by allowing the exchange of GDP for GTP. *Ras* can also be activated through other signalling intermediates. Mutations of *ras* genes result in constitutive activation (asterisk) and unregulated signalling through the serine-threonine kinases raf, map kinase kinase (MAPKK), and a series of intermediates that lead to stimultaion of cell growth and interference with thyroid-specific gene expression. *Ras* point mutations may also result in genomic instability[28,29] and increased susceptibility to other genetic defects that in turn may result in a more aggressive tumor phenotype.

THE *RET* AND *TRK* ONCOGENES AND PAPILLARY CARCINOMAS

Whereas *ras* mutations are found in most thyroid tumor phenotypes, a novel oncogene has been reported that is unique to papillary thyroid carcinomas.[48-58] The PTC/*ret* oncogene arises through an intrachromosomal inversion or translocation that juxtaposes unrelated 5′ sequences of different activating genes to the tyrosine-kinase domain of the *ret* proto-oncogene, a plasma membrane receptor for an as yet unidentified ligand. So far, three different transforming *ret* fusion proteins have been reported.[59] Each has constitutive tyrosine kinase ac-

tivity that is probably responsible for their transforming capability.[60] The prevalence of the PTC/*ret* oncogene in papillary carcinomas is relatively low (about 25% in Italy) although there may be some regional variability.

Other tyrosine kinase oncogenes, such as *trk*, the membrane receptor for nerve growth factor, are also activated in some papillary carcinomas, either through intrachromosomal gene rearrangements or unequal crossovers between the two copies of chromosome 1.[61-63] Whether papillary carcinomas with mutations of PTC/*ret* or *trk* have particular phenotypic characteristics or clinical behavior is not known. The pathogenetic role of tyrosine kinase receptors in papillary thyroid

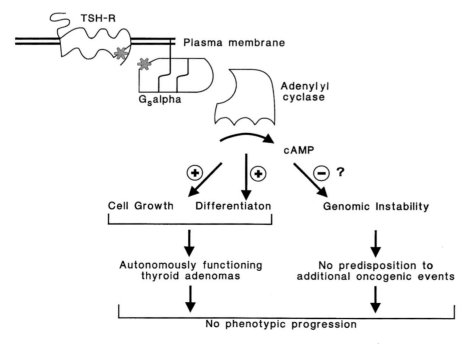

FIGURE 80-2. Growth of thyroid vells is controlled in part by the binding of TSH to its specific receptor. Activating mutations of the TSH receptor or of the α-subunit of the heterotrimeric stimulatory G protein, (Gs$_\alpha$, *asterisks*) results in constitutive stimulation of adenylyl cyclase and increased cell growth and thyroid hormone production. Activation of this cascade probably does not predispose to further genetic damage, explaining the rarity of malignant transformation of autonomously functioning thyroid adenomas.

carcinoma is further suggested by the fact that some of these tumors overexpress the *met* proto-oncogene that codes for the membrane receptor for hepatocyte growth factor.[64]

Rearrangements of *ret* may be important in the pathogenesis of radiation-induced thyroid tumorigenesis, based on preliminary studies of papillary thyroid carcinomas arising in children exposed to radiation after the Chernobyl nuclear reactor accident in 1986.[65] Also, *ret* rearrangements have been documented in thyroid cells exposed to high doses of radiation in vitro.[66] Little is known about the manner in which activating rearrangements of *ret* and *trk* may influence thyroid cell differentiation. However, signal transduction activated by the *ret* tyrosine kinase may not primarily involve *ras* proteins, suggesting that there may be distinct patterns of interference with cell differentiation.[60]

TUMOR SUPPRESSOR GENES IN THYROID NEOPLASMS

Tumor suppressor genes promote tumor formation through loss of function. This functional impairment usually requires mutations in both copies of the gene. One of these alleles is often lost as part of a large chromosomal deletion. Although these events appear to be relatively infrequent in human thyroid tumors, some sporadic follicular, but not papillary, adenomas and carcinomas have loss of part of the long arm of chromosome 11 (11q13).[15] This region is known to contain several genes associated with tumorigenesis, including the putative gene conferring predisposition to MEN1. Although it has not yet been cloned, the MEN1 gene is also believed to act in a recessive manner.[67,68] Indeed, the DNA of the endocrine tumors from patients with MEN1 frequently is lacking one of the 11q13 alleles.[69] This finding suggests that these patients inherit a mutant MEN1 gene on 11q13 and that tumors develop when the function of the normal allele is lost, which often occurs through gene deletion. Loss of function of a gene in the 11q13 locus (perhaps the MEN1 gene) may thus direct progression of sporadic thyroid tumors toward a follicular phenotype.[15]

Whereas this latter defect may be common to benign and malignant follicular tumors, disruption of a putative tumor suppressor gene on chromosome 3p may be specific for follicular carcinomas.[70] The chromosome 3p region affected may contain a tumor suppressor gene important in the development of several types of lung cancer,[71–73] but evidence for a role for this putative tumor suppressor gene in the development of follicular tumors is indirect. Because loss of function of one of the tumor suppressor alleles usually involves a major deletion, it is likely that these lesions occur when the genomic stability of the thyroid tumor cell population is already compromised by an initiating event.

Mutations of the p53 Tumor Suppressor Gene in Undifferentiated Thyroid Carcinoma

Anaplastic carcinomas are the most aggressive form of thyroid cancer. They are rare, have few features of thyroid differentiated tissue, and are invariably fatal. The prevalence of point mutations of the p53 tumor suppressor gene in anaplastic carcinomas is high, whereas among differentiated thyroid carcinomas these mutations are rare.[74–79] Thus, mutational inactivation of the p53 tumor suppressor gene may be the transitional step leading to progression to anaplastic carcinoma. p53 is the most frequently mutated gene in human cancers. It is believed to function as a transcriptional regulator and may function to arrest the cell cycle after environmental insults, presumably to allow DNA repair to occur, or alternatively to activate the pathway toward programmed cell death. Disruption of its function is believed to remove an important protective mechanism for the structural integrity of the genome.[80] As opposed to *ras* mutations, which occur uniquely in two discrete functional domains of the protein, mutations of p53 occur at multiple sites within the evolutionarily conserved regions of the gene. Evidence indicates that loss of the normal function of p53 may completely abrogate the vestiges of thyroid differentiated gene expression still present in the cancer cells and that the paired box domain transcription factor Pax-8 may be involved in mediating the effects of p53 on the transcriptional machinery controlling thyroid-specific gene expression.[81, 82]

OVERVIEW

Information on the relative prevalence of gene defects in the various human thyroid tumor phenotypes provides insights on the sequence of events involved in tumor initiation and progression (Fig 80-3 and Table 80-4). Aberrant methylation patterns of genomic DNA may predispose to structural defects affecting the function of oncogenes or tumor suppressor genes. Mutations of *ras* appear to be an early event because they are common to benign and malignant tumors. Mutational activation of the *ret* and *trk* tyrosine kinase receptor oncogenes is specific for papillary carcinomas. Conversely, loss of function of a gene on chromosome 11q13, possibly the MEN1 gene, may help direct the tumor clone toward a follicular phenotype. Mutational inactivation of a putative tumor suppressor gene on chromosome 3p could be important in the progression from follicular adenoma to follicular carcinoma. Finally, mutations of p53 are highly prevalent in anaplastic carcinomas and may represent the transitional step in the development of these aggressive tumors.

Some of these defects are not highly prevalent and may be representative of only a subset of the respective tumor types. For instance, mutations of *ras* are present in less than half of thyroid tumors. However, recent clarification of the mechanisms of tyrosine kinase receptor signaling holds promise that other gain-of-function mutations along this pathway will be uncovered. Although papillary carcinoma is the most common differentiated thyroid cancer, it is relatively difficult to study because tumor cells are often interspersed with stromal cells, obscuring the clonal nature of any molecular defect.

A major problem in clinical thyroidology is the difficulty in diagnosing follicular carcinoma preoperatively. Furthermore, present strategies to determine prognosis remain unreliable. Many mutated variants of the p53 protein are more stable than the normal p53, so that an increase in immunostaining for p53 is indirect evidence for mutational inactivation. This technique therefore may provide prognostic information in the future.

57. Grieco M, Monzini N, Miozzo M, et al. Characterization of an inversion on the long arm of chromosome 10 juxtaposing D10S170 and RET creating the oncogenic sequence RET/PTC. Proc Natl Acad Sci U S A 1992;89:1616

58. Santoro M, Carlomagno F, Hay ID, et al. *Ret* oncogene activation in human thyroid neoplasms is restricted to the papillary cancer subtype. J Clin Invest 1992;89:1517

59. Bongarzone I, Butti MG, Coronelli S, et al. Frequent activation of *ret* protooncogene by fusion with a new activating gene in papillary thyroid carcinomas. Cancer Res 1994;54:2979

60. Santoro M, Wong WT, Aroca P, et al. An epidermal growth factor receptor/*ret* chimera generates mitogenic and transforming signals: evidence for a *ret*-specific signaling pathway. Mol Cell Biol 1994;14:663

61. Bongarzone I, Pierotti MA, Monzini M, et al. High frequency of activation of tyrosine kinase oncogenes in human papillary thyroid carcinoma. Oncogene 1989;4:1457

62. Greco A, Pierotti MA, Bongarzone I, Pagliardini S, Lanzi C, Della Porta G. TRK-T1 is a novel oncogene formed by the fusion of TPR and TRK genes in human papillary thyroid carcinomas. Oncogene 1992;7:237

63. Santoro M, Melillo KM, Grieco M, et al. The TRK and tyrosine kinase oncogenes cooperate with *ras* in the neoplastic transformation of a rat ligand epithelial line. Cell Growth Differ 1993;4:77

64. De Renzo MF, Narsimhan RP, Olivero M, et al. Expression of the Met/HGF receptor in normal and neoplastic human tissues. Oncogene 1991;6:1997

65. Ito T, Seyama T, Iwamoto KS, et al. Activated *ret* oncogene in thyroid cancers of children contaminated by Chernobyl accident. Lancet 1994:344:259

66. Ito T, Seyama T, Iwamoto KS, et al. In vitro irradiation is able to cause RET oncogene rearrangement. Cancer Res 1993;53:2940

67. Larsson C, Skogseid B, Oberg K, et al. Multiple endocrine neoplasia type I maps to chromosome 11 and is lost in insulinoma. Nature 1988;332:85

68. Bystrom C, Larsson C, Blomberg C, et al. Localization of the MEN1 gene to a small region within chromosome 11q13 by deletion mapping in tumors. Proc Natl Acad Sci U S A 1988;87:1968

69. Bale AE, Norton JA, Wong EL, et al. Allelic loss of chromosome 11 in hereditary and sporadic tumors related to familial multiple endocrine neoplasia type I. Cancer Res 1991;51:1154

70. Herrmann MA, Hay ID, Bartelt DH Jr, et al. Cytogenetic and molecular genetic studies of follicular and papillary thyroid cancers. J Clin Invest 1991;88:1596

71. Naylor SL, Johnson BE, Minna JD, Sakaguchi AY. Loss of heterozygosity of chromosome 3p markers in small cell lung cancer. Nature 1987;329:451

72. Kok K, Osinga J, Carritt B, et al. Deletion of a DNA sequence at the chromosomal region 3p21 in all major types of lung cancer. Nature 1987;330:578

73. Baruch H, Johnson B, Hovis J, et al. The molecular analysis of the short arm of chromosome 3 in small-cell and non-small cell carcinoma of the lung. N Engl J Med 1987;317:1109

74. Fagin JA, Matsuo K, Karmarkar A, et al. High prevalence of mutations of the p53 gene in poorly differentiated human thyroid carcinomas. J Clin Invest 1993;91:179

75. Ito T, Seyama T, Mizuno T, et al. Unique association of p53 mutations with undifferentiated but not with differentiated carcinomas of the tyroid gland. Cancer Res 1992;52:1369

76. Wright PA, Jasani B, Newman GR, et al. p53 immunopositivity is a late event in human thyroid carcinoma development (abstract). J Pathol 1993;169:176

77. Nakamura T, Yana I, Kobayashi T, et al. p53 mutations associated with anaplastic transformation of human thyroid carcinomas. Jpn J Cancer Res 1992;83:1293

78. Donghi R, Longoni A, Pilotti S, et al. Gene p53 mutations are restricted to poorly differentiated and undifferentiated carcinomas of the thyroid gland. J Clin Invest 1993;91:1753

79. Zou M, Shi Y, Farid NR. p53 mutations in all stages of thyroid carcinoma. J Clin Endocrinol Metab 1993;77:1054

80. Lane DP. p53, guardian of the genome. Nature 1992;358:15

81. Fagin JA, Tang SH, Zeki K, et al. Reexpression of thyroid peroxidase in a clonal derivative of an undifferentiated thyroid carcinoma cell line by introduction of wild type p53. Cancer Res 1996:in press

82. Battista S, Martelli ML, Fedele M, et al. A mutated p53 alters thyroid cell differentiation. Oncogene 1995:in press

83. Terrier P, Sheng Z-M, Shlumberger M, et al. Structure and expression of c-*myc* and c-*fos* proto-oncogenes in thyroid carcinomas. Br J Cancer 1988;57:43

Surgical Therapy

Allan E. Siperstein
Orlo H. Clark

Effective therapy for patients with documented or suspected thyroid cancer begins with careful preoperative evaluation and the correct selection of the operation to be performed. Overall, thyroid nodules are common, being present in about 4% of the population. Only 1/1000 of these nodules is actually a clinically recognized thyroid cancer, for an incidence of 40/1,000,000.[1,2] This should not lead to a false sense of security in evaluating thyroid nodules because patients with solitary nodules or those with solitary nodules who are referred for surgical consultation harbor cancer 5% to 10% of the time and even more often in some series.[2,3]

The widespread use and acceptance of fine-needle aspiration biopsy (FNB) has simplified the evaluation of thyroid nodules. The test is fast, minimally invasive, with little discomfort to the patient, and highly reliable when performed by a knowledgeable physician and interpreted by an experienced cytopathologist. Papillary carcinomas, which constitute 80% of thyroid cancers, may be quickly and reliably identified, prompting appropriate surgical therapy.

With the exception of a few highly aggressive lesions, most thyroid carcinomas are effectively treated with surgery. Although the use of FNB has simplified the preoperative evaluation of most patients, a debate exists among even experienced endocrine surgeons over whether total thyroidectomy, near-total thyroidectomy, or lobectomy and isthmusectomy is the operation of choice for most patients with thyroid carcinoma. Unfortunately, no prospective randomized studies exist to answer this question. Most patients do well regardless of the operation chosen. It is difficult not to recommend total thyroidectomy as the treatment of choice for most patients with thyroid cancer because it provides the best long-term results and greatest ease of follow-up. Overall, thyroid surgery is tolerated even in elderly patients; patients are ambulatory and able to take liquids on the evening of surgery and usually are well enough to be discharged on the first or second postoperative day.

EVALUATION OF PATIENTS WITH THYROID NODULES

The reader is referred to chapters 23 and 83 for further discussion and perhaps some disagreement in the evaluation of patients with thyroid nodules.

History

Although few features are pathognomonic of thyroid carcinoma, a careful history helps to identify those patients with thyroid nodules more likely to harbor a carcinoma (Table 80-5). Most patients present with an asymptomatic nodule noticed by the patient, or the nodule is detected on routine physical examination. Pain or tenderness in a nodule, which must be differentiated from thyroiditis, increases the chance of the lesion being malignant. Rapid enlargement of a lesion, especially in a patient over 65 years of age, is worrisome, and rapid localized or diffuse enlargement of the thyroid should alert the clinician to the possibility of a focal or diffuse, infiltrating malignancy. The latter lesions are best detected by FNB. Nodules that continue to enlarge while the patient is receiving thyroid hormone are more likely to be malignant. A thyroid nodule in a man is more likely to be malignant although both benign and malignant lesions are more common in women. Although the peak age for developing papillary carcinoma is about 30 years of age and follicular carcinoma, 45 years of age, a thyroid nodule in a very young or very old patient is more likely to contain carcinoma. A thyroid nodule in a patient under 14 years of age has a 50% chance of being cancerous.[2,4,5]

Most patients with thyroid carcinoma are euthyroid. Patients with Graves' disease or thyroiditis may have a slightly increased risk of clinically apparent thyroid cancer. Most of these

---

TABLE 80-5.
Characteristics of Benign and Malignant Thyroid Nodules

BENIGN

Family history of benign goiter
Diffuse or multinodular goiter
Constant size
Benign by fine-needle aspiration
Simple cyst by sonography
Hyperfunctioning nodule by radioiodine scan
Decreasing size with thyroid hormone replacement

MALIGNANT

Solitary nodule
Hard, fixed
Rapidly enlarging
Hoarseness with vocal cord paralysis
Development of nodule at age <14 or >65 y
Suspicious or malignant by fine-needle aspiration
Cyst >4 cm or complex cyst
Hypofunctioning by radioiodine scan
History of low-dose ionizing radiation
Ipsilateral adenopathy

---

cancers are small or microscopic papillary thyroid cancers that are found incidentally with resection of thyroid, and many are multifocal.[6] Although the association of medullary thyroid cancer with the autosomal dominantly inherited multiple endocrine neoplasia type II is well recognized, certain inherited disorders lead to an increased incidence of thyroid cancer of follicular cell origin. Gardner's syndrome, associated with multiple polyps of the gastrointestinal tract and with colon cancer, also carries an increased risk of papillary thyroid cancer. Cowden's syndrome, referred to as multiple hamartoma syndrome or multiple epithelioma syndrome, is associated with goiters in 40% of patients and with thyroid cancer of follicular cell origin in 10%. These patients have an increased incidence of breast cancer and colon cancer and are identified by multiple skin tags about the face and papules on the tongue.[7-9]

A history of ionizing radiation to the thyroid puts the patient at significant risk of developing thyroid cancer. For patients exposed to low-dose therapeutic radiation (<2000 rad), especially in infancy or childhood, there is up to a 7% incidence of developing thyroid cancer, even higher in children.[10] For patients who present with a history of neck radiation and a thyroid nodule, there is a 40% chance that a cancer is located somewhere within the thyroid gland. Only in 60% of cases is the cancer located in the nodule that brought the patient to clinical attention.[11-13] In the past, low-dose therapeutic radiation was commonly used to treat various conditions, including acne, external otitis, ringworm, and scrofula. It has been documented that the risk of developing thyroid cancer increases linearly with doses of 6.5 to 2000 rad.[10,14] With higher doses, the risk falls back toward baseline because thyroid tissue is destroyed.[15] The distribution of the histologic types of thyroid cancer is similar to that in nonradiated patients. These tumors also appear to behave in a similar manner but are more likely to be multifocal. Because of the high incidence of thyroid cancer in these patients who have thyroid nodules and because of the multifocal nature of their disease, further work-up, including FNBs, usually is not warranted, and the patient should be referred for total or near-total thyroidectomy. Patients treated by thyroid lobectomy have a 20% chance of requiring reoperation because of the development of palpable nodules in the contralateral lobe.[16]

Patients with a history of thyroid cancer are at the highest risk of developing recurrent lesions because of preexistent metastatic disease or an inadequate primary operation.

Physical Examination

Certain features on physical examination lead the clinician to suspect that a thyroid nodule is malignant. Lesions found to be solitary on careful physical examination have a 5% to 10% chance of being malignant, whereas multinodular goiters have only a 1% chance of containing cancer. Lesions that are hard or fixed to the surrounding tissue are more likely to be malignant. Malignancy also is common if the patient presents with hoarseness or is documented to have unilateral vocal cord paralysis. Cervical adenopathy is found in 15% of adults who present with a malignant thyroid nodule and up to 85% of children.[2,17] Patients may present with cervical adenopathy and no palpable thyroid lesion, despite careful examination. At operation, the ipsilateral thyroid lobe virtually always contains a small primary papillary carcinoma although in many cases it is microscopic.

Laboratory Tests

The laboratory test of choice to be done on a patient with a solitary or dominant thyroid nodule is FNB. This procedure is easily done in the office; it is safe and usually causes no more discomfort than a venipuncture. Initial fears that FNB might result in seeding of the needle tract with malignant cells proved unwarranted. For this test to be of value, the slides *must* be reviewed by an experienced cytopathologist. If none is available locally, slides may be mailed to an individual with expertise in their interpretation.

The accuracy and clinical utility of FNB were documented by Lowhagen and associates,[18] who performed the test on 412 patients with thyroid nodules. Because all patients were operated on as part of the study, the authors were able to compare FNB results with histologic results. The FNB aspirates were classified into four categories: cancerous, suspicious, benign, or inadequate. Of 63 lesions diagnosed as being malignant, all proved to be malignant on histologic examination, for a 0% false-positive rate. A realistic false-positive rate in accordance with several other studies is about 1%. There is a 4% false-negative rate, that is, lesions interpreted by FNB to be benign contain cancer on histologic section 4% of the time. This is due to sampling tissue outside of the nodule or misinterpreting the slides. This rate is low enough to warrant follow-up of patients whose FNB is interpreted as benign; if the lesion continues to enlarge or exhibits other worrisome features, another biopsy specimen should be obtained or the lesion should be removed. Of samples interpreted as suspicious, most were follicular lesions, with 20% of them being malignant.[19] Distinguishing between a follicular carcinoma and a follicular adenoma depends on the presence of capsular or vascular invasion on histologic section. This distinction cannot be reliably made by FNB. In addition to technical limitations (i.e., sampling error and the inability to distinguish follicular adenomas from carcinomas), the technique is less reliable in patients with a history of therapeutic radiation to the neck because many of these lesions are multifocal.

When a cyst is encountered in the course of performing FNB, it should be completely drained because 70% of simple cysts are adequately treated by aspiration alone.[20,21] Although the findings are less accurate because of cellular degeneration, the cyst fluid should still be sent for cytologic examination. Cysts greater than 4 cm in diameter and complex cysts (i.e., those that contain both solid and cystic components) have a greater chance of being malignant.[22,23] When a cyst is complex, the solid component should be sampled by FNB after the cystic component has been aspirated.

Ultrasound examination of the thyroid is useful in several settings. For patients with a history of therapeutic radiation to the head and neck, ultrasonography may be useful in the evaluation of the thyroid despite a normal clinical examination. Ultrasonography also provides a noninvasive and relatively inexpensive means to objectively follow the size of suspected benign nodules. This is especially useful when the patient is treated with thyroid hormone, to determine whether the nodule or the surrounding normal thyroid tissue decreases in size.

The differentiation of cystic versus solid lesions also is reliably made by sonography and should be used in the follow-up of patients whose cysts have been treated by FNB. Recurrent or simple cysts without internal echoes can be effectively treated by instillation of tetracycline and lidocaine into the cyst.[24,25]

Before the widespread use of FNB, a thyroid scan using iodine-123 or technetium-99m was the initial test of choice in the evaluation of thyroid nodules. Nodules that trap less iodine than the surrounding thyroid tissue are termed cold or nonfunctional or hypofunctional. Such lesions have a 10% to 25% chance of being malignant. The 5% of lesions that are shown to be warm or hot by thyroid scan are seldom malignant.[2,26]

Although the yield of routine chest radiographs is relatively low, certain findings may be helpful to the clinician. A speckled pattern of calcification within the thyroid indicates the presence of psammoma bodies, suggesting a papillary carcinoma. The appearance of rim or eggshell calcification suggests a benign lesion. Bilateral calcification at the upper lateral portion of the thyroid suggests medullary thyroid carcinoma. Pulmonary metastases may be seen as well as tracheal deviation from a large lesion.

Computed tomographic scanning and magnetic resonance imaging are useful in evaluating patients with suspected aggressive carcinomas. In lesions that are large, fixed, or associated with cervical adenopathy or tracheal deviation, such studies are useful to define the extent of the invasion and adenopathy. They also may be useful in the preoperative evaluation of large benign goiters with substernal extension.

Preoperative Preparation

The preoperative preparation for a patient about to undergo thyroid surgery usually is straightforward and does not fundamentally differ from the preparation for any major operation. Any underlying medical conditions, especially cardiovascular and pulmonary disease, should be evaluated and treated preoperatively. Aspirin or any other medication that might cause the patient to bleed perioperatively should be discontinued 1 week before thyroidectomy. Evaluation of the vocal cords should be performed by direct or indirect laryngoscopy on any patient who has had hoarseness or a change in voice or who has had prior neck surgery. Appropriate informed consent needs to be obtained. The various treatment options should be explained to the patient and, in particular, why surgery is indicated. The patient also should understand, especially in cases in which FNB indicates that a lesion is suspicious for carcinoma, that no cancer may be found. Complications of surgery should be frankly discussed with the patient. The serious long-term complications of permanent hypoparathyroidism or recurrent laryngeal nerve injury should occur less than 2% of the time. Other complications, such as bleeding that necessitates a return to the operating room for evacuation of hematoma, superior laryngeal nerve damage, and keloid formation, also should be discussed.[27] Patients should understand that lifetime thyroid hormone replacement will be necessary when total or near-total thyroidectomy is performed. When a patient is due to undergo a thyroid lobectomy for a suspicious follicular lesion, a total thyroidectomy may be required within the next several days, once the final pathology results are available, because follicular cancer may be difficult to diagnose by frozen section.

CHOICE OF OPERATION

The following surgical procedures have been used in the treatment of thyroid tumors:

Lumpectomy—removal of the nodule alone with minimal surrounding thyroid tissue

Partial thyroidectomy—removal of the nodule with a larger margin of surrounding thyroid tissue

Subtotal thyroidectomy—bilateral removal of more than half the thyroid gland on each side plus the isthmus

Lobectomy or hemithyroidectomy—removal of one thyroid lobe and the isthmus

Near-total thyroidectomy—total lobectomy and isthmusectomy, leaving less than 10% of the posterior lateral portion of the contralateral lobe

Total thyroidectomy—removal of both thyroid lobes and isthmus

Several factors influence the choice of operation for patients with documented or suspected thyroid cancer. All documented or suspected foci of tumor should be removed; this includes any palpable cervical adenopathy. The surgical strategy should be planned to minimize the need for subsequent operations. Scarring created by the previous operation increases the chance of complications. Operations need to be chosen that minimize the risk of recurrent disease and facilitate patient follow-up with serum thyroglobulin determinations and iodine-131 (^{131}I) scanning or ablation. Finally, the surgeon should be experienced in performing thyroid surgery.[28] The benefits of a more extensive operation to minimize recurrence rates and improve survival[29] should not be offset by an unacceptably high rate of permanent hypoparathyroidism or recurrent laryngeal nerve injury.

Some surgeons advocate less aggressive surgery in patients whose tumor may be predicted to have a less aggressive course. The AGES (age, grade, extent, size) classification scheme from the Mayo Clinic[30] predicts a better prognosis if the patient's age is less than 40 years for men and 50 years for women, if the histologic grade of the tumor is well differentiated, if the tumor is confined to the thyroid gland, and if the size of the tumor is less than 5 cm. Other groups, using similar prognostic indicators, have reported different classification systems, including the AMES classification of Cady and Rossi (age, metastases, extent, and size).[31] Patients with tumors that fail to take up radioactive iodine have a worse prognosis, probably because of the less differentiated nature of these tumors and the inability to treat microscopic metastatic disease by iodine ablation. Patients whose tumors have an aneuploid DNA content have a more aggressive course.[32] Studies in our own laboratory have shown that tumors that make less cyclic adenosine monophosphate in response to thyrotropin (TSH) stimulation have a more aggressive course.[33] As our understanding of the biochemical lesions responsible for the aberrant growth of thyroid tissues increases, we may be better able to predict the behavior of individual tumors. Promising factors include abnormalities in TSH receptors, epidermal growth factor receptors, G protein mutations, and the presence of *ras* and other oncogenes.[34]

With the exception of thyroid nodules situated on the isthmus, the minimum operation that should be performed for any patient with a documented or suspected carcinoma is a total lobectomy. Performing a lumpectomy or partial lobectomy should not be considered adequate therapy because these procedures are associated with a higher recurrence rate and shortened survival.[35,36] In addition, the ipsilateral recurrent laryngeal nerve and at least one parathyroid gland need to be identified in the course of the dissection and removal of the entire lobe poses minimal additional risk. Lumpectomy or partial lobectomy also increases the difficulty and complication rate if the remainder of the lobe needs to be removed at a future date. Isthmusectomy and removal of the pyramidal lobe, if present, should be performed in concert with total lobectomy. It adds little to the time or risk of the operation and prevents possible recurrent disease in the isthmus leading to tracheal invasion, a difficult problem to manage. Additionally, compensatory thyroid hypertrophy may lead to an unsightly bulge in the midneck if the isthmus has not been removed.

Lobectomies should be performed with a minimal complication risk. Hypoparathyroidism should never occur because the contralateral parathyroids are not dissected. Although hoarseness may result from ipsilateral recurrent laryngeal nerve damage, the risk of bilateral recurrent laryngeal nerve damage necessitating permanent tracheostomy is avoided. Although recommended to minimize tumor recurrence, thyroid hormone replacement is not needed in these patients to prevent hypothyroidism.[27]

Considerable controversy exists in the literature and among experienced thyroid surgeons as to whether total thyroidectomy or less than total thyroidectomy is the preferable operation for patients with documented thyroid cancer.[28,37,38] Thyroid cancers exhibit a wide spectrum of biologic behavior, and many patients do well regardless of the operation performed. We believe that if total thyroidectomy can be performed with only a minimal increase in complications, it offers substantial benefits to less than total thyroidectomy.[39] Biologically, thyroid cancer tends to be a multifocal disease. Histologic studies of the contralateral lobe in patients with papillary carcinoma have shown microscopic foci of cancer in the contralateral lobe in 30% to 82% of patients. Clinically, recurrences occur after lobectomy in 5% to 24% of patients (with a mean of 7%). Half the patients with recurrent thyroid cancer die of their disease.[40] Total thyroidectomy has been documented to reduce the recurrence of thyroid cancer compared with lesser procedures. Mazzaferri and colleagues[36] studied a group of 576 patients with papillary carcinoma and found that in 10 years of follow-up, the recurrence rate was lowest in patients with total thyroidectomy, radioactive iodine ablation, and thyroid hormone replacement in patients whose tumors were greater than 1.5 cm in diameter. For smaller papillary lesions, the recurrence rate was not statistically different if less than a total thyroidectomy was performed. Mazzaferri offers his current views on this controversial topic in the next section of this chapter. Studies by Massin and coworkers,[41] Schlumberger and associates,[42] and DeGroot and associates[29] also strongly support the use of total thyroidectomy. The study of DeGroot and coworkers is important because patients with what appeared to be nonaggressive papillary thyroid cancers (i.e., thyroid cancers < 2 cm in maximal diameter) benefited from total or near-total thyroidectomy. We also favor total thyroidectomy because foci of differentiated thyroid cancer have the potential to dedifferentiate into undifferentiated cancer, which carries an extremely poor prognosis.

Total thyroidectomy also has advantages for the postoperative follow-up and treatment of patients. After total thyroidectomy, serum thyroglobulin determinations are a more sensitive indicator of recurrent disease, prompting earlier treatment. In addition, normal thyroid tissue has about a 100-fold greater affinity for iodine uptake, making ^{131}I scans much less useful in patients with remaining normal thyroid tissue. Total thyroidectomy also is necessary for the successful use of high-dose ^{131}I for the ablation of microscopic persistent or recurrent disease (Table 80-6).

We therefore believe that the operation of choice for patients with follicular carcinoma (except for those with minimal invasion) or papillary carcinoma (>1.5 cm in diameter) is a total thyroidectomy when this operation can be performed safely. For follicular carcinomas with minimal invasion and for papillary carcinomas less than 1.5 cm in diameter, ipsilateral total lobectomy and isthmusectomy is adequate. In patients with minimally invasive follicular carcinomas, we perform chest radiography and a technetium bone scan to rule out the rare patient with distant metastases to lung and bone, respectively.

A difficult group of patients to deal with are those who have a suspicious follicular neoplasm by FNB. Core-needle biopsies offer little additional help because capsular invasion or angioinvasion must be documented on histologic sections to make the diagnosis of cancer. Additionally, core-needle biopsy carries a higher complication risk, and we do not advocate its use. In the operating room, we perform a total lobectomy and isthmusectomy. Unfortunately, frozen section diagnosis done during surgery is not highly reliable, and in fact, in some cases, it confuses the diagnosis. We, therefore, wait 2 to 3 days after the hemithyroidectomy, until the final histologic diagnosis is made, and if follicular carcinoma is found, the patient undergoes a total thyroidectomy either at this time or after 6 weeks. Unfortunately, with current technology, there usually is no definitive way to make the diagnosis of follicular cancer preoperatively, so that some patients (about 10% of those with follicular tumors) are subjected to the risk of two operations, although there is minimal additional surgical risk. Some surgeons favor a near-total thyroidectomy in patients with follicular tumors to avoid a second operation, should carcinoma be found. We do not agree with this suggestion because all patients must then receive thyroid hormone.

Hürthle cell carcinomas are an aggressive variant of follicular carcinomas and are distinguished by an eosinophilic, mitochondria-rich cytoplasm. As with follicular lesions, the distinction between benign and malignant Hürthle cell lesions is made on the basis of capsular invasion or angioinvasion. Most surgeons believe that a lobectomy and isthmusectomy is adequate treatment for Hürthle call adenomas. Hürthle cell carcinomas differ from follicular carcinomas because regional lymph node involvement is more common and because only about 5% of Hürthle cell carcinomas take up radioactive iodine. We recommend total lobectomy and isthmusectomy for Hürthle cell adenomas and total thyroidectomy with removal of regional nodes for Hürthle cell carcinomas.

The correct strategy in performing a thyroidectomy is to first dissect the lobe containing the lesion. If tumor invasion has necessitated sacrifice of the recurrent laryngeal nerve or removal of parathyroid glands, then it may be safest to perform a near-total thyroidectomy, leaving a small rim of thyroid tissue posterolaterally on the contralateral side to protect the parathyroid blood supply and recurrent laryngeal nerve. If a parathyroid gland is removed at the time of surgery, a frozen section should be obtained to confirm that it is indeed parathyroid tissue and not a lymph node or metastatic cancer. The parathyroid then may be minced into 1-mm cubes and autotransplanted into individual pockets in the sternocleidomastoid muscle.

Lymph node dissections are indicated in the central neck ipsilateral to the nodule in all patients and when metastatic disease is palpable in the lateral neck. Although up to 80% of patients with papillary carcinoma have occult or microscopic metastatic disease, this usually does not become clinically apparent, and occult disease usually is effectively treated by ^{131}I ablation.[35,36] The preferred procedure for patients with palpable nodes in the lateral neck is a modified radical neck dissection, which involves removal of the lymph node-bearing fibrofatty tissue in the lateral neck between the first and third layers of deep cervical fascia. The internal jugular vein and sternocleidomastoid are preserved, unless invaded or adherent to tumor, giving a much better cosmetic result. In addition, nodal tissue in the central neck and upper mediastinum accessible through the cervical incision should be removed. We perform modified neck dissections by making a MacFee lateral extension of the Kocher transverse cervical incision. Vertical incisions on the neck are discouraged.[36] Finally, regional anesthesia is an alternative to general anesthesia in selected patients.[36a,36b]

POSTOPERATIVE MANAGEMENT

At the completion of surgery, a light pressure dressing should be placed over the incision. The patient's head and shoulders are elevated 20° to minimize venous pressure in the wound. The patient should be extubated while still asleep to minimize the chance of coughing, resulting in increased venous pressure and postoperative hemorrhage. Respiratory difficulty or stridor at the completion of the operation should alert the physician to the possibility of a hematoma putting pressure on the trachea, bilateral recurrent laryngeal nerve injury, or vocal cord edema, necessitating immediate evaluation and possible reintubation or opening of the neck wound.

TABLE 80-6.
Advantages of Total Thyroidectomy

Higher survival rate for lesions >1.5 cm in diameter

Lowest recurrent rate

Prevention of recurrence in the contralateral lobe

Improved sensitivity of serum thyroglobulin as a marker for persistent or recurrent disease

Radioactive iodine can be used to detect and treat persistent or recurrent disease

Reduces possibility of residual tumor in contralateral lobe undergoing transformation to anaplastic carcinoma

In the postoperative period, discomfort is usually minimal. Narcotics should be used sparingly because nausea and vomiting may lead to hematoma formation. Any respiratory difficulty should be presumed to be due to a neck hematoma; it requires prompt attention. In urgent situations, the wound may be opened at the bedside, where partial evacuation of the hematoma can be lifesaving. Any patient with a large hematoma should be returned to the operating room for evacuation, to control any bleeding sites.

Serum calcium and phosphorus levels should be measured postoperatively. Transient, symptomatic hypocalcemia usually manifests itself as tetany and circumoral tingling, numbness, or paresthesia in the hands or feet, and usually can be managed with oral calcium supplementation. Intravenous calcium should be used only for marked symptoms and only through a well-functioning intravenous line because extravasation can cause local necrosis and skin loss.

For the best cosmetic results, skin clips can be removed on the first postoperative day and adhesive strips placed on the skin. Drains are needed only when there is a space after the removal of large thyroid lesions or for neck dissections; they usually can be removed on the first or second postoperative day. For cosmetic reasons, drains should be brought out laterally through the cervical incision instead of through a separate stab wound. Most patients are able to take liquids by mouth on the evening of surgery and are taking a regular diet on the first postoperative day. Most patients can be discharged on the first or second postoperative day.

SUMMARY

Thyroid carcinomas of follicular cell origin span a wide spectrum of biologic behavior. Patients with small papillary carcinomas do extremely well with a low rate of recurrence and death. On the other hand, undifferentiated carcinomas, despite aggressive management, have a poor prognosis, with few survivors beyond 1 to 2 years. For most lesions between these two extremes, prompt evaluation and surgical therapy improve outcome. With the increasing use of FNB in the evaluation of thyroid nodules, diagnoses are being made earlier with greater certainty. Debate will continue on how extensive an operation should be for most thyroid cancers. Because most patients with thyroid cancer do well, it would require a large, multicenter, prospective, randomized study to determine the value of the various surgical approaches. Regardless, patient outcome can be optimized by careful preoperative evaluation and by the procedures being performed by surgeons who are experienced in the technique of thyroidectomy.

References

1. Butler SJ, Young JL. Third national cancer survey incidence data, National Cancer Institute. Washington, DC: Department of Health Education and Welfare (NIH), 1975:775
2. Thompson NW, Nishiyama RH, Harness JK. Thyroid carcinoma: current controversies. Curr Probl Surg 1978;15:1
3. Clark OH. Endocrine surgery of thyroid and parathyroid glands. St Louis: CV Mosby, 1985:56
4. Cady B, Sedgwick CE, Meissner WA, et al. Risk factor analysis in differentiated thyroid cancer. Cancer 1979;43:810
5. Woolner LB, Beahrs OH, Black BM, et al. Classification and prognosis of thyroid carcinoma: a study of 885 cases observed in a 30 year period. Am J Surg 1961;102:354
6. Livadas D, Psarras A, Loutras DA. Malignant cold thyroid nodules in hyperthyroidism. Br J Surg 1976;63:726
7. Lee FI, MacKinnon MD. Papillary thyroid carcinoma associated with "polyposis coli": a case of Gardner's syndrome. Am J Gastroenterol 1981;76:138
8. Phade VR, Lawrence WR, Max MH. Familial papillary carcinoma of the thyroid. Arch Surg 1981;116:836
9. Sogol PB, Sugawara M, Gordon HE, et al. Cowden's disease: familial goiter and skin hamartomas. West J Med 1983;139:324
10. Greenspan FS. Radiation exposure and thyroid cancer. JAMA 1977;237:2089
11. Deaconson TF, Wilson SD, Cerletty JM, et al. Total or near total thyroidectomy versus limited resection for radiation-associated thyroid nodules: a twelve year follow-up of patients in a thyroid screening program. Surgery 1986;100:1116
12. Wilson SD, Komorowski R, Cerletty JM, et al. Radiation-associated thyroid tumors: extent of operation and pathology technique influence the apparent incidence of carcinoma. Surgery 1983;94:663
13. Witt TR, Mang RL, Economon SG, Southwick HW. The approach to the irradiated thyroid. Surg Clin North Am 1979;59:45
14. Maxon HR, Thomas SR, Saenger EL, et al. Ionizing irradiation and the induction of clinically significant disease in the human thyroid gland. Am J Med 1977;63:967
15. Pretorius HT, Katikineni M, Kinsella TJ, et al. Thyroid nodules after high-dose radiotherapy: fine needle aspiration cytology in diagnosis and management. JAMA 1982;247:3217
16. Fogelfeld L, Wiviott MB, Shore-Freedman E, et al. Recurrence of thyroid nodules after surgical removal in patients irradiated in childhood for benign conditions. N Engl J Med 1989;320:835
17. Harness JK, Thompson NW, Nishiyama RH. Childhood thyroid carcinoma. Arch Surg 1971;102:278
18. Lowhagen T, Granberg PO, Lundell G, et al. Aspiration biopsy cytology (ABC) in nodules of the thyroid gland suspected to be malignant. Surg Clin North Am 1979;59:3
19. Gharib H, Goelliner JR, Zinsmeister AR, et al. Fine-needle aspiration of the thyroid: a problem of suspicious cytologic findings. Ann Intern Med 1984;101:25
20. Clark OH, Greenspan FS, Coggs GC. Evaluation of solitary cold thyroid nodules by echography and thermography. Am J Surg 1975;130:206
21. Clark OH, Okerlund MD, Cavalieri RR, et al. Diagnosis and treatment of thyroid, parathyroid and thyroglossal duct cysts. J Clin Endocrinol Metab 1979;48:963
22. Blum M, Goldman A, Herskovic A, et al. Clinical applications of thyroid echography. N Engl J Med 1972;207:1164
23. Rosen IB, Provias JP, Walfish PG. Pathologic nature of cystic thyroid nodules selected for surgery by needle aspiration biopsy. Surgery 1986;100:606
24. Goldfarb WB, Bigos ST, Nishiyama RH. Percutaneous tetracycline instillation for sclerosis of recurrent thyroid cysts. Surgery 1987;102:1096
25. Ryan WG, Schwartz TB, Harris J. Sclerosis of thyroid cysts with tetracycline (letter). N Engl J Med 1983;308:157
26. Clark OH. Thyroid nodules and thyroid cancer: surgical aspects. West J Med 1980;133:1
27. Clark OH. Total thyroidectomy: the treatment of choice for patients with differentiated thyroid cancer. Ann Surg 1982;196:361
28. Lennquist S. Surgical strategy in thyroid carcinoma: a clinical review. Acta Chiurgica Scandinavica 1986;152:321

29. DeGroot LJ, Kaplan EL, McCormick M, Straus FH. Natural history, treatment, and course of papillary thyroid carcinoma. J Clin Endocrinol Metab 1990;71:414

30. Hay ID, Taylor WF, McConahey WM. Ipsilateral lobectomy versus bilateral lobar resection in papillary thyroid carcinoma: a retrospective analysis of surgical outcome using a novel prognostic scoring system. Surgery 1987;102:1088

31. Cady B, Rossi R. An expanded view of risk-group definition in differentiated thyroid carcinoma. Surgery 1988;104:947

32. Cohn K, Backdahl M, Gorslund G, et al. Prognostic value of nuclear DNA content in papillary thyroid carcinoma. World J Surg 1984;8:474

33. Siperstein AE, Zeng QH, Gum ET, et al. Adenylate cyclase activity as a predictor of thyroid tumor aggressiveness. World J Surg 1988;12:528

34. Lyons J, Landis CA, Harsh G, et al. Two G protein oncogenes in human endocrine tumors. Science 1990;249:655

35. Mazzaferri EL, Young RL. Papillary thyroid carcinoma: a 10-year follow-up report of the impact of therapy in 576 patients. Am J Med 1981;70:511

36. Mazzaferri EL, Young RL, Oertel JE, et al. Papillary thyroid carcinoma: the impact of therapy in 576 patients. Medicine (Baltimore) 1977;56:171

36a. Logerfo P, Ditkoff BN, Chabot J, Feind C. Thyroid surgery using monitored anesthesia care: an alternative to general anesthesia. Thyroid 1994;4:437.

36b. Kulkarni R, Braverman LE, Patwardhan N. Regional anesthesia for thyroidectomy and parathyroidectomy. Thyroid 1994;4:530

37. Grant CS, Hay ID, Gough IR, et al. Local recurrence in papillary thyroid carcinoma: is extent of surgical resection important? Surgery 1988;104:954

38. Reeve TS, Delbridge K. Thyroid cancers of follicular origin: the place of radical or limited surgery. Progr Surg 1988;19:78

39. Clark OH, Levin K, Zeng QH, et al. Thyroid. cancer: the case for total thyroidectomy. Eur Cancer Clin Oncol 1988;24:305

40. Silverberg SG, Hutter RVP, Foote FWJ. Fatal carcinoma of the thyroid: histology, metastases, and causes of death. Cancer 1970;25:792

41. Massin JP, Savoie JC, Garnier H, et al. Pulmonary metastases in differentiated thyroid carcinoma. Cancer 1984;53:982

42. Schlumberger J, Tubiana M, De Vathaire F, et al. Long-term results of treatment of 283 patients with lung and bone metastasis from differentiated thyroid carcinoma. J Clin Endocrinol Metab 1986;63:960

RADIOIODINE AND OTHER TREATMENTS AND OUTCOMES

Ernest L. Mazzaferri

Differentiated (papillary or follicular) thyroid carcinoma typically presents as a solitary thyroid nodule. About half the time the thyroid nodule is discovered by a physician during a routine physical examination, and the rest of the time it is first noticed by the patient. The diagnosis is usually established by fine-needle or excisional biopsy, often when the tumor is confined to the thyroid or has metastasized only to regional nodes, giving ample opportunity to cure the disease. Thyrotoxicosis is an extremely rare manifestation of the disease and never the presenting one. However, as many as 5% of patients with papillary carcinoma and up to 10% with follicular cancer present with distant metastases or tumor that aggressively invades the neck, which substantially lowers the likelihood of a cure. The choice

of therapy rests on an understanding of the natural history of these tumors and on the premise that prognosis can be altered by early intervention. The treatment of choice is surgery, whenever possible. In most patients this is followed by radioactive iodine (^{131}I) and thyroxine (T_4) therapy, but external radiation and chemotherapy have a role in management of some patients.

Papillary thyroid carcinomas comprise about 80% of all malignant thyroid tumors, follicular carcinomas about 10%, and medullary thyroid carcinomas about 5%; nearly all the remainder are anaplastic carcinomas and lymphomas (see chap 82). Although papillary and follicular carcinomas are distinct pathologic entities, they have similar clinical features and outcomes if they are discovered when confined to the neck. Accordingly, much of the following discussion refers to differentiated thyroid carcinoma because the approach to treatment of either papillary or follicular carcinoma is usually similar. Where there are differences between the two in prognosis or behavior, such as the higher mortality with follicular carcinoma, the differences are highlighted.

CONTEMPORARY VIEWS CONCERNING THERAPY

The prognosis of these tumors is typically so favorable that it is difficult to demonstrate a beneficial effect of therapy unless very large cohorts are studied for several decades. No prospective, randomized clinical trials have been done, so that all views of the efficacy of different treatments are based on retrospective studies.

Therapy should be based on the anticipated clinical behavior of the carcinoma. Two studies shed some light on current practice. At an international symposium held in 1987 in The Netherlands, 160 participants—surgeons, endocrinologists, pathologists, and nuclear medicine specialists—recommended total thyroidectomy followed by postoperative ^{131}I ablation of any remaining thyroid tissue for most patients with differentiated thyroid carcinoma, regardless of their age.[1] Hemithyroidectomy alone was considered sufficient therapy for carcinomas confined to one lobe if they were either papillary carcinomas without or with ipsilateral nodal metastases or follicular carcinomas with minimal capsular invasion. The second study was based on the responses of 157 thyroid experts from around the world to a questionnaire concerning management of a patient with a solitary thyroid nodule.[2] Total or near-total thyroidectomy was recommended for papillary carcinoma by 60% and for follicular carcinoma by 74% of the respondents; most would not alter the extent of surgery in relation to the tumor's histologic type. Ablation of the thyroid remnant with ^{131}I was advised for patients with papillary carcinoma by 81% and for those with follicular carcinoma by 97%. Almost all recommended postoperative suppression of thyrotropin (TSH) secretion with T_4 and determinations of serum thyroglobulin (Tg) during follow-up.

PROGNOSTIC FEATURES

The distinction between aggressive and slow-growing tumors becomes less clear when multiple and opposing prognostic features intermingle to shape the final outcome. Overall, however, the two main features determining prognosis are tumor stage and age at the time of diagnosis. The most disagreement stems from the weight clinicians allocate to these and other variables when planning therapy.

Mortality Rates

Overall 10-year survival rates for middle-aged adults are about 95% for papillary carcinoma and about 90% for follicular carcinoma. The survival rates are higher for children and lower in older patients and among patients with certain histologic variants.[3] In our 1355 patients with differentiated thyroid carcinoma whose mean age at diagnosis was 36 years, the 30-year cancer-specific mortality rate was 8% (Fig 80-4); it was 6% for papillary and 15% for follicular carcinoma (*P<0.001*).

Recurrence Rates

About 30% of patients have recurrences over several decades, depending on the initial therapy (see Fig 80-4).[4-6] About two-thirds of the recurrences occur within the first decade after initial therapy. Although not usually fatal, a recurrence is not a trivial event, and a recurrence in the neck may be the first sign of a lethal outcome.[7-10] In our patients who had local recurrences, 74% were in cervical lymph nodes, 20% were in the thyroid remnant, and 6% were in the trachea or muscle; 7% of this group ultimately died of cancer.[11] The tumors recurred at distant locations in 21%, most often in the lungs alone (63%); half of this group died of cancer. Recurrent tumor caused over half the cancer deaths in our patients; the other deaths were due to persistent disease. Mortality rates are lower when recurrences are detected by ^{131}I scans than by clinical signs.[10]

Tumor Features That Influence Outcome

Features of the tumor often play a major role in decisions regarding therapy. What follows are summaries considered more or less independently of variations in therapy.

TYPICAL PAPILLARY CARCINOMAS

Papillary carcinoma has distinctive cellular features that can be recognized by fine-needle aspiration biopsy (FNB) or frozen section in 95% of cases[12,13] (see chap 28). Most are, in fact, mixed papillary-follicular carcinomas, but a few have a purely papillary pattern, a feature that has no bearing on prognosis. Most also are unencapsulated tumors that are 2 to 3 cm in diameter and tend to infiltrate the thyroid but are confined by its capsule. This tumor has a strong tendency to invade lymphatics and is commonly found in multiple sites within the thyroid and in regional lymph nodes. Those that metastasize to the lung via lymphatics usually appear as diffuse bilateral pulmonary infiltrates on chest x-ray or are visible only by ^{131}I scans. Hematogenous spread to bone, the central nervous system (CNS), and other sites can occur. These features all have important prognostic implications, as noted below.

PAPILLARY CARCINOMA VARIANTS

Survival rates vary considerably among certain subsets of patients with papillary carcinoma.[14] About 10% of papillary carcinomas have a well-defined capsule, which is a particularly favorable prognostic sign.[15,16] Other variants have a more serious prognosis. Anaplastic tumor transformation, a rare event occurring in fewer than 1% of papillary carcinomas, is often associated with p53 oncogene expression and causes death within a year.[17,18] Tall-cell papillary carcinomas, large tumors in older patients that can be identified by FNB, have a 25% 10-year mortality rate.[14,19-21] The outcome is even worse with the columnar variant of papillary carcinoma, which is a rapidly growing tumor with a 90% mortality rate.[14,22] About 2% of papillary carcinomas are diffuse sclerosing variants that infiltrate the entire gland, may cause a diffuse goiter without a palpable nodule, and may be mistaken for goitrous autoimmune thyroiditis.[14,23] Most metastasize to lymph nodes and about 25% of patients have distant metastases. Although mainly affecting younger persons, they are aggressive tumors that may have a poor prognosis.[14,24] Follicular-variant papillary carcinomas are recognized by their follicular architecture and typical papillary cytology; their clinical behavior resembles that of papillary more than follicular carcinoma, but some are aggressive.[3,13,14]

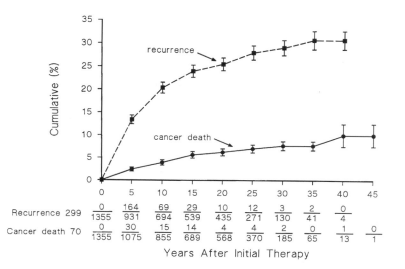

FIGURE 80-4. Tumor recurrence and cancer death (±SE) from differentiated thyroid carcinoma. The vertical bars represent standard errors. The numerators are the number of events during the previous interval and the denominators the number of patients at the end of that interval. (From Mazzaferri EL, Jhiang SM. Long-term impact of initial surgical and medical therapy on papillary and follicular thyroid cancer. Am J Med 1994;97:418. Reproduced with the permission of the publisher.)

FOLLICULAR CARCINOMA HISTOLOGY

Follicular carcinomas are usually solitary encapsulated tumors that may be slightly more aggressive than papillary carcinomas. Follicular carcinomas typically have a microfollicular histologic pattern and are identified as malignant by invasion of the tumor capsule and blood vessels by malignant cells. Widely invasive follicular carcinomas have a poor prognosis and are easily recognized by their aggressive extension into surrounding tissues. Up to 80% of patients with these invasive tumors have metastases and about 20% die of their disease.[25] Most follicular carcinomas, however, are minimally invasive encapsulated tumors that closely resemble follicular adenomas. The distinction can be made only by review of permanent histologic sections, but not by FNB or frozen section study, which poses a serious management predicament at the time of surgery.[12,13] The main diagnostic criteria for carcinoma are cells penetrating the tumor capsule or invading blood vessels. The latter has a worse prognosis than capsular penetration alone.[26] However, few patients with minimally invasive follicular carcinomas, the main type diagnosed in recent years, have distant metastases or die of their disease.[11,25,27,28]

The somewhat poorer prognosis of follicular carcinoma is more closely related to the patient's older age and more advanced tumor stage and larger tumor size at the time of diagnosis than histology alone.[11,29] The survival rates of patients with papillary or follicular carcinomas are similar in patients of comparable age and disease stage.[29–32] Both tumors have an excellent prognosis if they are confined to the thyroid, are small (<1.0 cm) or are minimally invasive.[7,11] Both have poor outcomes if they are widely invasive (papillary carcinoma invading the thyroid capsule and adjacent structures and follicular carcinoma invading blood vessels and the tumor capsule) or are metastatic to distant sites.[31,33]

The 30-year survival rate in our series of 1355 patients was 76% and the cancer-specific death rate was 8%, of whom 79% had papillary and 21% follicular carcinoma.[11] Although the mortality rate in patients with follicular carcinoma was more than twice that of the patients with papillary carcinoma, at the time of diagnosis the patients with follicular carcinoma were older (mean age 38 years) than those with papillary carcinoma (mean age 34 years, P<0.001), they had larger tumors and more advanced local disease, and more of them had distant metastases. Patients with tumors of similar stage had 30-year recurrence and cancer-specific mortality rates that were similar, regardless of the papillary or follicular histology of the tumor.[11]

HÜRTHLE CELL FOLLICULAR VARIANT

Hürthle (oncocytic) cells may constitute most or all of a tumor; such tumors are sometimes classified as Hürthle cell carcinomas although the World Health Organization classification considers them as variants of follicular carcinoma.[34] There is some controversy about the diagnosis and management of this type of tumor, because only about 300 cases have been reported.[34,35] Some consider these to be aggressive and unpredictable tumors with a mortality rate as high as 25% in 30 years,[36] but others find them to be no more aggressive than similarly staged follicular carcinomas without Hürthle cells.[34,37] In two large series, 25% and 35% of patients with Hürthle cell carcinomas had pulmonary metastases, about twice the frequency in patients with follicular carcinoma.[33,38] Hürthle cell variant

papillary carcinoma is even less common but may be associated with higher than usual recurrence and mortality rates.[39]

TUMOR SIZE

Papillary carcinomas smaller than 1 cm, termed microcarcinomas (formerly occult carcinomas), are often found unexpectedly during surgery for benign thyroid conditions and sometimes during routine physical examination. These tumors should be widely excised, but they pose no threat to survival and the patients should not undergo further surgery.[3] In one study, only one cancer death occurred among 454 patients with microcarcinomas.[40] Occasionally, however, papillary carcinomas smaller than 1 cm that are multifocal may become locally invasive and even widely metastatic.[41] Nonetheless, tumors as large as 1.5 cm seldom recur after initial surgery and almost none cause death. In our series, 30-year recurrence rates in patients with papillary and follicular carcinomas smaller than 1.5 cm were one-third those in patients with larger tumors.[11] The small tumors rarely metastasized to distant sites and cancer-specific mortality rates were very low (0.4% versus 7% for tumors ≥ 1.5 cm, P<0.001).[11]

The prognosis is progressively poorer in patients with carcinomas of increasing size. For example, in one study the 20-year cancer-specific mortality rates steadily increased from 6% for papillary carcinomas 2 to 3.9 cm in diameter, to 16% for those 4 to 6.9 cm, and to 50% for tumors 7 cm or larger.[40] The same is true for follicular carcinomas.[28] After a minimum follow-up of 5 years, the cancer-specific mortality rates in one study were 5% for tumors smaller than 5 cm and 39% for larger ones.[42] Distant metastases occurred more often in patients whose primary tumor was larger than 5.0 cm. There is a linear relationship between tumor size and recurrence and cancer-specific mortality for both papillary and follicular carcinomas[11] (Fig 80-5).

MULTIPLE INTRATHYROIDAL TUMORS

Multiple thyroid tumors are generally regarded as intrathyroidal metastases rather than multifocal tumors arising independently although the distinction cannot be made with certainty. Multiple microscopic intraglandular metastases occur in about 20% of patients with papillary carcinoma when the thyroid is examined routinely and in up to 80% if the thyroid is examined with great care.[4,9,43,44] The clinical importance of these metastases is debated. However, their presence, which is not usually apparent until the histologic sections of the tumor have been studied, has a bearing on the need to excise the thyroid remnant or ablate it with [131]I. In patients who have a subtotal lobectomy and then completion of the thyroidectomy, about 30% have one or more foci of carcinoma in the contralateral, clinically normal lobe[27,45–47] (Table 80-7).

Those who find few recurrences in the contralateral thyroid lobe after hemithyroidectomy argue that multiple microscopic tumors are of little clinical consequence.[42,48] Others find that recurrence rates are higher, ranging from 5% to 20%, in patients with large thyroid remnants and that pulmonary metastases occur more frequently after subtotal than total thyroidectomy.[11,49] In one study, patients with multiple intrathyroidal tumors had almost twice the incidence of nodal metastases and three times the incidence of pulmonary and other distant metastases than those with single tumors, and the likelihood of persistent disease was three times more likely in

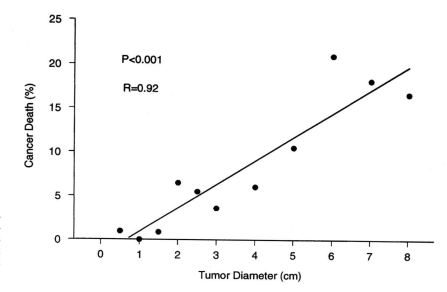

FIGURE 80-5. Tumor size and death from differentiated thyroid carcinoma. (Adapted from data published in Mazzaferri EL, Jhiang SM. Long-term impact of initial surgical and medical therapy on papillary and follicular thyroid cancer. Am J Med 1994;97:418)

those with multiple tumors.[9] The 30-year cancer-specific mortality rate among our patients with multiple tumors was two times that in the patients with a single tumor.[11] Similarly, the 30-year recurrence rate among the 436 patients who had undergone subtotal thyroidectomy was 40%, as compared with 26% among the 698 patients who had undergone total or near-total thyroidectomy (*P*<0.002); the cancer-specific mortality rate was also higher in the subtotal thyroidectomy group (9% versus 6%, *P*=0.02).[11]

LOCAL TUMOR INVASION

About 5% to 10% of tumors grow directly into the surrounding tissues, increasing both morbidity and mortality. Local invasion, which can occur with both papillary and follicular carcinoma, ranges from microscopic to gross tumor invasion.[11,27] The most commonly invaded structures are the neck muscles and vessels, recurrent laryngeal nerves, larynx, pharynx, and esophagus, but tumor can extend into the spinal cord and brachial plexus. The symptoms are usually hoarseness, cough, dysphagia, hemoptysis, and airway insufficiency. Patients with invasive tumors have recurrence rates that are two times higher than patients with noninvasive tumors, and up to one-third die of cancer within the first decade, depending on the extent of invasion.[9,50,51] The tumor was locally inva-

sive in 115 of our patients (8% of those with papillary and 12% of those with follicular carcinoma); their 10-year recurrence rate was 1.5 times and the cancer-specific death rate was five times that of the patients with no local invasion.

LYMPH NODE METASTASES

In one review, nodal metastases were reported in 36% of 8029 adult patients with papillary carcinoma and in 17% of 1540 with follicular carcinoma.[3] They are reported in up to 80% of children with papillary carcinoma.[52,53] The first sign of thyroid carcinoma may be an enlarged cervical lymph node; in such a patient, multiple nodal metastases are usually found at surgery.[54]

The impact of the presence of cervical lymph node metastases on outcome is controversial. Many believe that their presence has little impact on outcome.[9,42,44,55,56] On the other hand, in some studies they were a risk factor for recurrence and cancer-specific mortality,[5,51,57–62] especially if bilateral cervical or mediastinal lymph node metastases were present. In one study, 15% of patients with and none without cervical node metastases died of their disease (*P*<0.02).[59] In another study of patients with distantly metastatic papillary carcinoma, 80% had mediastinal node metastases at the time cancer was diagnosed.[63] We found that patients with papil-

TABLE 80-7.
Residual Carcinoma in Contralateral Thyroid Lobe Found With Completion Thyroidectomy

Investigators	Total No. of Patients	Papillary	Follicular	Hürthle	No. With Residual Cancer (%)
Emerick et al[27]	19	0	19	0	2 (11)
DeGroot et al[62]	26	18	8	0	8 (31)
Rao et al[46]	129	75	54	0	35 (27)
Auguste et al[47]	80	58*	17	5	30 (38)
TOTAL	254	151	98	5	75 (30)

Two were designated as microscopic foci of carcinoma without further description.

lary or follicular carcinoma who had cervical or mediastinal lymph node metastases had significantly higher 30-year cancer-specific mortality rates than those without metastases (10% versus 6%, $P < 0.01$). The most aggressive tumors are locally invasive tumors with cervical lymph node metastases in patients over age 45 years and those with mediastinal node metastases.[11,60]

DISTANT METASTASES

Almost 10% of patients with papillary carcinoma and up to 25% of those with follicular carcinoma have distant metastases at some time; half have them at the time of diagnosis[64] (Table 80-8). Distant metastases occur even more often in patients with Hürthle cell carcinoma (35%) and after age 40 years.[33,38] The sites among 1231 patients reported in 13 studies were lung (49%), bone (25%), both lung and bone (15%), and CNS or other soft tissues (10%).[3]

The outcome in patients with distant metastases is influenced mainly by the patient's age and the tumor's metastatic site(s), ability to concentrate ^{131}I, and morphology on chest x-ray.[33,38,65,66] Although some patients, especially younger ones, survive for decades, about half die within 5 years regardless of tumor histology.[3] Pulmonary metastases are compatible with longer survival, whereas multiple bone and CNS metastases have the most serious prognosis. In one study, when distant metastases were confined to the lung, over half the patients were alive and free of disease at 10 years, whereas no patient with skeletal metastases survived this long.[67] In a study from France, the survival rates were 53% at 5 years, 38% at 10 years, and 30% at 15 years[68]; the rates were much higher in young patients with pulmonary metastases.[66]

Survival is longest with diffuse pulmonary metastases seen only on ^{131}I imaging and not by x-ray.[68,69] Prognosis is much worse when the metastases do not concentrate ^{131}I or appear as large lung nodules and is intermediate when the tumors are small nodular densities that concentrate [131]I.[38,63,68,69] A few adults with distant metastases have survived 30 years or longer with little therapy.[70,71]

THYROGLOSSAL DUCT TUMORS

Small papillary carcinomas that arise in a thyroglossal duct remnant are typically encapsulated by the cyst and usually are not recognized until the permanent histologic sections are re-viewed. Local excision of the cyst is usually adequate therapy because the tumors contained in them rarely metastasize.[72]

Patient Features Influencing Prognosis

AGE

Practically every study shows that the age of the patient at the time of diagnosis is an important prognostic variable. Thyroid carcinoma is more lethal after age 40 years. The risk of cancer death increases with each subsequent decade of life, rising dramatically after age 60 years (Fig 80-6). However, there is a remarkably different pattern of tumor recurrence: rates are highest (40%) at the extremes of life, before age 20 years and after age 60 years[4,11,73–75] (see Fig 80-6).

Despite the clear effect of age on survival, there is considerable disagreement about how it should be factored into the treatment plan, especially in children and young adults. Children commonly present with more advanced disease than adults and have more tumor recurrences after therapy, yet their prognosis for survival is good.[53] Some believe that young age has such a favorable influence on survival that it overshadows the prognosis predicted by the characteristics of the tumor.[42,55] Others, including myself, believe that the tumor stage and histologic differentiation are as important as the patient's age in determining prognosis and management.[11,62,76]

SEX

Men have a less favorable prognosis than women, but the difference is small.[11,30,42] In our study, the risk of death from cancer was about twice as great in men as women.[11] Because of this, men with thyroid carcinoma should be regarded with special concern, especially those over age 50 years.

GRAVES' DISEASE

Thyroid receptor antibodies may promote tumor growth in patients with Graves' hyperthyroidism.[77–79] In one large study, thyroid carcinoma was found in 46% of the palpable nodules in patients with Graves' disease.[80] The carcinomas were larger and displayed more aggressive behavior than usual. Some, but not all, find that thyroid carcinoma occurring in patients with Graves' hyperthyroidism is more often invasive and metastatic to regional lymph nodes, even when the primary tumor is small.[81]

TABLE 80-8.
Regional and Distant Metastases at Diagnosis and After Tumor Recurrence

	Papillary Carcinoma Metastases			**Follicular Carcinoma Metastases**		
	N	NODAL (%)	DISTANT (%)	N	NODAL (%)	DISTANT (%)
Presentation*	7845	36	5	1437	17	13
Recurrence‡	4165	9 (17)†	4	1185	7 (15)†	12

*All patients in 13 series. (data from reference 3).
†In parenthesis are all local recurrences, including those in the contralateral thyroid lobe and other neck structures.
‡All patients in 6 series considered free of cancer after initial therapy.

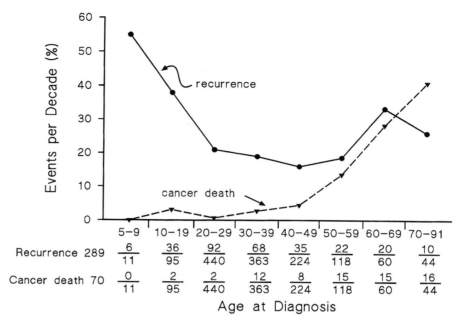

FIGURE 80-6. Effect of patient age at the time of diagnosis on tumor recurrence and death from differentiated thyroid carcinoma. The numerators are the number of events during the previous interval and the denomiators are the number of patients at the end of the interval. (From Mazzaferri EL, Jhiang SM. Long-term impact of initial surgical and medical therapy on papillary and follicular thyroid cancer. Am J Med 1994;97:418. Reproduced with the permission of the publisher.)

Clinical Staging Systems and Prognostic Indexes

Although the patient's age and tumor stage at the time of diagnosis are the most important variables predicting outcome, their relative importance is debated.[3] Several clinical staging and prognostic scoring systems have been proposed that use age over 40 years as a major feature to identify risk. When more weight is assigned to the patient's age, the relative importance of tumor stage tends to be decreased. This concept, however, does not appear to be widely accepted among practicing physicians. At the international consensus conference in 1987, only 5 of 160 participants treated younger patients more conservatively.[1] Similarly, in the international survey of thyroid specialists done in 1988, age was not used by the majority of respondents in their therapeutic decisions.[2]

The seven schemes for clinically staging differentiated thyroid carcinoma are summarized in Table 80-9.[11,40,42,55,62,82,83] When applied to the papillary carcinoma data from the Mayo Clinic, four of the schemes that use age (EORTC, TNM, AMES, AGES) were effective in separating low-risk patients in whom cancer-specific mortality was 1% at 20 years from high-risk patients in whom it was 30% to 40% at 20 years.[40] The 20-year survival rates for patients with MACIS scores less than 6, 6 to 6.99, 7 to 7.99, and 8+ were 99%, 89%, 56%, and 24%, respectively.[55] However, these schemes do not consider tumor recurrence and are inaccurate in predicting recurrence-free survival. Moreover, staging systems derived from multivariate analyses that do not consider the effects of therapy assume that treatment does not alter a tumor's natural behavior. This is likely incorrect.

OHIO STATE UNIVERSITY STAGING SYSTEM

The classification we now use is shown in Tables 80-9 and 80-10. In our recent analysis,[11] stage IV patients were significantly older than the others. After a median follow-up of almost 16 years, tumor recurrence and cancer-specific mortality rates were progressively and significantly greater with each tumor stage (see Table 80-10). Based on regression modeling on 1322 patients, excluding those who presented with distant metastases but including therapy in the remainder, the likelihood of death from thyroid carcinoma was increased in those aged 40 years or older, if the tumor size was 1.5 cm or larger, local tumor invasion or regional lymph node metastases were present, or if therapy had been delayed for 12 or more months. The likelihood of death was reduced in women, by surgery more extensive than lobectomy, and by ^{131}I plus T_4 therapy, and was unaffected by tumor histologic type (Table 80-11).

Regardless of the staging system used, its rigid application in support of conservative treatment for low-risk patients may lead to inadequate initial therapy. There are documented examples of aggressive disease in patients who appear to be at low risk at the time of diagnosis.[11,74,84,85] Strict application of scoring systems that rely heavily on the patient's age at the time of diagnosis may result in undertreatment of some young patients.

THERAPY

Delay in Therapy

The median time from the first detection of the tumor—nearly always a neck mass—to initial therapy in our patients was 4 months, but ranged from less than 1 month to 20 years. Delay in diagnosis correlated with cancer mortality (Fig 80-7). The median delay was 18 months in patients who died of cancer as compared with 4 months in those still living ($P<0.001$). Cancer mortality was 4% in patients who underwent initial therapy within a year as compared with 10% in the others; the 30-year cancer mortality rates in these two groups, respectively, were 6% and 13% ($P<0.001$).

TABLE 80-9.
Staging of Differentiated Thyroid Carcinoma

A. Components of Staging Systems and Rating Schemes for Defining Risk Category in Patients With Differentiated Thyroid Carcinoma

Variable at the Time of Diagnosis	Staging System and Rating Schemes						
	TNM[a,b]	EORTC[b]	AMES[b]	AGES[c]	MACIS[c]	UNIVERSITY OF CHICAGO[c]	OHIO STATE UNIVERSITY[b]
Patient characteristics							
Age	X	X	X	X	X		
Sex	X	X	X				
Tumor characteristics							
Cell type	X	X					
Size	X		X	X	X	X	X
Grade (histologic)				X			
Extension beyond thyroid	X	X	X	X	X	X	X
Lymph node metastases	X[d]					X	X
Distant metastases	X	X	X	X	X	X	X
Therapy characteristics							
Incomplete resection					X		

[a]T, primary tumor; T1, ≤ 1 cm; T2, > 1 cm to ≤ 4 cm; T3, > 4 cm; T4, extension beyond thyroid capsule. N, regional lymph nodes; N1, regional lymph node metastases (cervical and upper mediastinal nodes). M, distant metastases; M0, no distant metastases; M1, distant metastases present.
[b]Both papillary and follicular carcinoma.
[c]Only papillary carcinoma.
[d]Not applied to patients with papillary or follicular carcinoma under age 45 y.

B. Scoring Methods

TNM (American Joint Committee on Cancer. Manual for staging of cancer, ed 4. Philadelphia: JB Lippincott, 1992:53)
Staging varies with cell type and age (see table below). Undifferentiated (anaplastic) carcinomas are stage IV.

TNM Stage	Papillary or Follicular Carcinoma		Medullary Carcinoma
	<45 YEARS	≥45 YEARS	
I	M0	T1	T1
II	M1	T2–3	T2–4
III		T4 or N1	N1
IV		M1	M1

EORTC (European Organization for Research on Treatment of Cancer) (Byar DP, Green SB, Dor P, et al. A prognostic index for thyroid cancer. Eur J Cancer 1979;15:1033); Age in years: + 12 if male, + 10 if medullary, + 10 if poorly differentiated follicular, + 45 if anaplastic, + 10 if extending beyond thyroid, + 15 if one distant metastasis, + 30 if multiple distant metastases.

AMES (Age-Metastasis-Extent-Size). (Cady B, Rossi R. An expanded view of risk group definition in differentiated thyroid carcinoma. Surgery 1988; 104:947) High risk if female older than 50 y, male older than 40 y, tumor ≥ 5 cm (if older age), distant metastases, substantial extension beyond tumor capsule (follicular) or gland capsule (papillary).

AGES .(Age-Grade-Extent-Size). (Hay I. Papillary thyroid carcinoma. Endocrinol Metab Clin North Am 1990;19:545) 0.5 × age in years (if > 40), + 1 (if grade 2), + 3 (if grade 3 or 4), + 1 (if extra thyroidal), + 3 (if distant spread), + 0.2 × maximum tumor diameter.

MACIS (Metastasis-Age-Completeness of Resection, Invasion-Size). (Hay ID, Bergstralh EJ, Goellner JR, et al. Predicting outcome in papillary thyroid carcinoma: development of a reliable prognostic scoring system in a cohort of 1779 patients surgically treated at one institution during 1940 through 1989. Surgery 1993;114:1050) MACIS = 3.1 (if age ≤ 39 y) or 0.08 × age (if age ≥ 40 y), + 0.3 × tumor size (in cm), + 1 (if incompletely resected), + 1 (if locally invasive), + 3 (if distant metastases present).

University of Chicago system for papillary carcinoma. (DeGroot LJ, Kaplan EL, McCormick M, Straus FH. Natural history, treatment, and course of papillary thyroid carcinoma. J Clin Endocrinol Metab 1990;71:414). Staging variables (Part A) not scored quantitatively.

The Ohio State system for papillary or follicular carcinoma (Mazzaferri EL, Jhiang SM. Long-term impact of initial surgical and medical therapy on papillary and follicular thyroid cancer. Am J Med 1994;97:418). Staging variables (Part A) not scored quantitatively.

TABLE 80-10.
Ohio State University Staging of Differentiated Thyroid Carcinoma

Variables	Stage I	Stage II	Stage III	Stage IV
Tumor size (cm)	<1.5	1.5–4.4 (or)	≥4.5 (or)	Any
Cervical metastases	No	Yes*	Any	Any
Multiple thyroidal tumors (>3), any size	No	Yes*	Any	Any
Local tumor invasion	No	No	Yes	Any
Distant metastases	No	No	No	Yes
No. of patients (%)	170 (13)	948 (83)	204 (15)	33 (2)
Age (mean y)	38	34	38	48
P values†	—	0.001	<0.05	0.01
No. of Recurrences (%)‡	10 (8)	210 (31)	59 (36)	10 (62)
P values‡	—	0.001	0.001	NS
No. deaths from cancer (%)‡	0	34 (6)	19 (14)	17 (65)
P values‡	—	0.01	0.001	0.001

*Includes tumors <1.5 cm with cervical metastases and palpable tumors of uncertain size confined to the thyroid; any tumor that fulfills one of the three criteria for size, cervical metastases, or multiple intrathyroidal tumors is considered stage 2.
†Wilcoxon rank-sum test comparing stage with preceding lower stage (left).
‡30-y recurrence or cancer-specific death rate, logrank test comparing stage with preceding lower stage (left).
NS, not significiant.

Extent of Surgery

Surgery for thyroid carcinoma is discussed in detail in a previous section of this chapter. However, the extent of surgery has an impact on the subsequent medical therapy. Recurrence rates are high in patients with large thyroid gland remnants. For example, in a Mayo Clinic study[4] of patients with papillary carcinoma, the tumor recurrence rates during the first 2 years after surgery were about fourfold greater after unilateral lobectomy than after total or near-total thyroidectomy (26% versus 6%, *P*=0.01). In a subsequent report from the same institution, patients with papillary carcinoma whose AGES score was 4 or more had a 25-year cancer mortality rate almost twice as high after lobectomy than after bilateral thyroid resection (65% versus 35%, *P*=0.06). In another study of patients with papillary thyroid carcinoma,[62] near-total thyroidectomy decreased the risk of death from tumors larger than 1 cm and decreased the risk of recurrence as compared with lobectomy or bilateral subtotal thyroidectomy. We found recurrence and cancer death rates were both about 50% lower after near-total or total thyroidectomy as compared with less surgery in patients with stage II and III tumors,[11] and that surgery more extensive than lobectomy was an independent variable that reduced the likelihood of cancer mortality rate by 60% (see Table 80-11). Thus, there is abundant evidence that microscopic residual disease remaining after initial surgery leads to high recurrence and cancer mortality rates.

Thyroxine Therapy

EFFECTS OF THYROTROPIN SUPPRESSION ON TUMOR GROWTH

The idea that TSH stimulates the growth of thyroid carcinoma forms the basis for the wide use of T_4 in treating this dis-

TABLE 80-11.
Hazard Ratios for Recurrence or Death From Differentiated Thyroid Carcinoma in 1322 Patients Without Distant Metastases at the Time of Diagnosis

	Hazard Ratio	95% Confidence Interval	P value
RECURRENCE			
Local tumor invasion*	1.7	1.1–2.4	<0.01
Lymph node metastases†	1.4	1.1–1.8	<0.01
Tumor size‡	1.3	1.2–1.3	<0.001
^{131}I therapy§	0.4	0.3–0.5	<0.001
CANCER DEATHS			
Age‖	2.4	2.0–2.9	<0.001
Time to treatment¶	2.3	1.3–4.2	<0.01
Local tumor invasion	2.0	1.1–4.2	<0.05
Lymph node metastases	1.9	1.1–3.4	<0.05
Tumor size	1.3	1.1–1.5	<0.01
Female#	0.5	0.3–0.9	<0.05
Radioiodine therapy	0.4	0.2–0.9	<0.05
Surgery more than lobectomy**	0.4	0.2–1.0	<0.05

*Local tumor invasion present vs absent.
†Lymph node metastases present vs absent.
‡Tumor diameter stratified into 1 cm increments from tumors smaller than 1 cm to 5 cm or more.
§Any ^{131}I therapy (plus T_4) vs no ^{131}I but including T_4 therapy.
‖Age stratified by 10-y increments.
¶Time to initial treatment ≤12 mo vs more than 12 mo.
#Versus male.
**Versus lobectomy or less than lobectomy.
Data from reference 110.

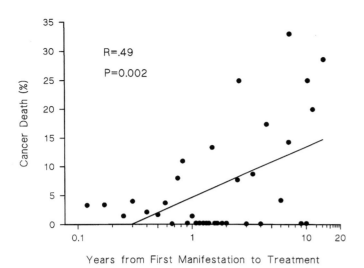

FIGURE 80-7. Time from first manifestation of the tumor to initial treatment. each data point represents one to three patients. (From Mazzaferri EL, Jhiang SM. Long-term impact of initial surgical and medical therapy on papillary and follicular thyroid cancer. Am J Med 1994;97:418. Reproduced with the permission of the publisher.)

ease.[86,87] Like normal thyroid tissue, most differentiated thyroid carcinomas contain functional TSH receptors; they are more abundant in follicular than papillary carcinomas.[78,88] Whether T_4 alone (in addition to surgery) improves survival is controversial.[8,89,90] There have been no prospective trials of T_4 as the only therapy (in addition to surgery) for differentiated thyroid carcinoma, but evidence indicates that TSH stimulates tumor growth. Tumors in patients with Graves' disease may be more aggressive, presumably because the patients have circulating TSH-receptor antibodies.[77,78] Rapid tumor growth sometimes follows T_4 withdrawal in preparation for ^{131}I therapy. Moreover, T_4 given as an adjuvant to surgical and ^{131}I therapy is effective because tumor recurrence rates are higher if T_4 is not given after surgery.[91] After 30 years' follow-up, we found that there were 25% fewer recurrences in patients treated with T_4 as compared with no adjunctive therapy (Fig 80-8; $P<0.01$) and there were fewer cancer deaths in the T_4 group (6% versus 12%, $P<0.001$).[11]

POTENTIAL ADVERSE EFFECTS OF THYROXINE THERAPY

Patients with thyroid carcinoma are usually treated with T_4 in doses sufficient to lower TSH secretion below normal, thereby deliberately causing subclinical thyrotoxicosis (see chap 88) if not overt thyrotoxicosis. One consequence may be osteoporosis, even in children.[92] A comprehensive review of the potential adverse effects of T_4 given to treat patients with thyroid carcinoma, however, concluded that it contributes to osteoporosis mainly in postmenopausal women.[86] A recent meta-analysis reached a similar conclusion.[93]

Cardiovascular abnormalities, well recognized in overt thyrotoxicosis, also occur in patients taking suppressive doses of T_4.[94] Among the cardiovascular problems associated with subclinical thyrotoxicosis are an increased risk of atrial fibrillation,[95] a higher 24-hour heart rate, more atrial premature contractions per day, increased cardiac contractility, and ventricular hypertrophy.[94]

THYROXINE DOSE

Patients with thyroid carcinoma who have undergone total thyroid ablation require more T_4 than those with spontaneously occurring primary hypothyroidism.[96] In a study of 180 patients who had undergone total thyroidectomy and remnant ^{131}I ablation, the average dose of T_4 that resulted in an undetectable basal serum TSH concentration and no increase in serum TSH after thyrotropin-releasing hormone (TRH) was 2.7 ± 0.4 (SD) µg/kg/d. Younger patients needed larger doses than older patients and TSH suppression was more likely when the therapy had been prolonged. In a comparative study of patients with thyroid carcinoma and patients with non-cancer-related hypothyroidism, the dose of T_4 needed to reduce serum TSH concentrations to normal was 2.11 and 1.62 µg/kg/d, respectively.[97] These results suggest that some T_4 is secreted from residual thyroid tissue in patients who have spontaneously occurring hypothyroidism.

As a practical matter, the most appropriate dose of T_4 for most patients with thyroid carcinoma is that which reduces the serum TSH concentration to just below the lower limit of the normal range for the assay being used. Some clinicians prefer greater suppression, for example, serum TSH concentrations between 0.05 to 0.1 µU/mL in low-risk patients and less than 0.01 µU/mL in high-risk patients,[86] and a few advocate the latter target for all patients.[98] There is no evidence that maintaining serum TSH concentrations less than 0.01 µU/mL has benefits, and it does have some risks.

^{131}I Therapy

Therapy with ^{131}I has been used for over 40 years in the treatment of patients with papillary and follicular thyroid carcinoma, both to ablate any remaining normal thyroid tissue and to treat the carcinoma. It has gained wide use because these tumors tend to be infiltrative, locally invasive, and associated with occult regional lymph node metastases. Moreover, recurrence rates are high in patients treated with surgery and T_4 alone. Although effective in both regards, the explicit indications for its use continue to provoke debate.[40]

ABLATION OF RESIDUAL NORMAL THYROID TISSUE

Routine thyroid remnant ablation with ^{131}I, although questioned by some,[99,100] is widely used and has appeal for several reasons.[1,2] First, it may destroy occult microscopic carcinoma within the thyroid remnant because the carcinoma cells receive radiation from ^{131}I taken up by adjacent normal thyroid cells. Second, it eases later detection of recurrent or persistent disease, particularly in the neck, by ^{131}I scanning because no normal thyroid tissue remains. Third, it increases the value of serum Tg measurements during follow-up. Few metastases can be visualized by ^{131}I scanning when appreciable amounts of normal thyroid tissue remain after surgery. Moreover, measurements of serum Tg —the most sensitive marker of recurrent or persistent disease—are less reliable in patients with large thyroid remnants. Accordingly, ^{131}I is often given postoperatively to ablate thyroid gland remnants even in patients without known residual disease who have a very good prognosis.

Although many report lower recurrence rates after ^{131}I ablation of the thyroid remnant, not all find this to be the case.

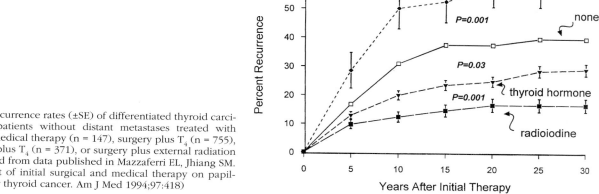

FIGURE 80-8. Recurrence rates (±SE) of differentiated thyroid carcinoma in 1322 patients without distant metastases treated with surgery and no medical therapy (n = 147), surgery plus T$_4$ (n = 755), surgery plus ^{131}I plus T$_4$ (n = 371), or surgery plus external radiation (n = 49). (Adapted from data published in Mazzaferri EL, Jhiang SM. Long-term impact of initial surgical and medical therapy on papillary and follicular thyroid cancer. Am J Med 1994;97:418)

At the Mayo Clinic, the recurrence rates were slightly but not significantly higher in 220 patients treated with surgery and ^{131}I ablation than in 726 patients treated with surgery alone (13% versus 10%); the 10-year cancer-specific mortality rates were 3% and 2% in the two groups, respectively. These results contrast with those reported by most others, who find a more favorable effect of ^{131}I ablation.[86] For example, in one study[62] ablation of residual thyroid tissue with ^{131}I after surgery decreased the risk of recurrence in patients with tumors larger than 1 cm and reduced the risk of death in those with stage 1 or 2 disease who had tumors larger than 1 cm. We studied 138 patients with no obvious residual disease who were given ^{131}I postoperatively to ablate presumably normal thyroid gland remnants. Their 30-year recurrence rate was less than one-third that in patients not given ^{131}I (Fig 80-9), and no patient treated this way has died of thyroid carcinoma (Fig 80-10).

LOW-DOSE 131I FOR THYROID REMNANT ABLATION

The standard ^{131}I dose for remnant ablation was between 75 and 150 mCi (2775 and 5550 MBq) for many years, but now many use 25 to 30 mCi (925–1110 MBq) if the amount of thyroid tissue remaining after surgery is small. This has appeal because hospitalization (in the United States) is not required for safety reasons, the lower cost, and the lower whole body radiation dose. The average whole body radiation exposure after ^{131}I administration for remnant ablation has been estimated to be 6.1 rem for 30 mCi (1110 MBq), 8.5 rem for 50 mCi (1850 MBq), and 12.2 rem for 60 mCi (2220 MBq).[101]

Some have found that larger ^{131}I doses are necessary to ablate normal thyroid tissue (and to treat residual microscopic carcinoma) and suggested that 100 to 149 mCi (3700–5513 MBq) is optimal after finding that a single dose of this amount ablated uptake in 87% of patients.[99] However, in another study, smaller doses (<30 mCi, 1110 MBq) ablated thyroid remnant ^{131}I uptake in 77% of patients (compared with 84% given larger doses); the lower dose was not surprisingly more successful after near-total thyroidectomy than less extensive surgery (90% versus 22%).[102] Stated in different terms, 94% of patients had successful ablation when the surgeon left less than 2 g of thyroid tissue as compared with a 68% success rate

when the remnant was larger. The ^{131}I must deliver about 30,000 rads (300 Gy) to ablate normal thyroid tissue and 8000 rads (80 Gy) to ablate metastatic deposits.[103]

Thus, thyroid uptake can be ablated in about 80% of patients with 25 to 30 mCi (925 to 1110 MBq) ^{131}I, providing the surgeon has left a relatively small thyroid remnant and thyroid ablation is defined as absence of uptake on diagnostic scans that use a 2- to 3-mCi (74–110 MBq) dose of ^{131}I.[101,102,104] The success rates are lower when large scanning doses are used, regardless of the prior therapeutic dose of ^{131}I.[105–107] In a randomized prospective study of this question, the first dose ablated thyroid bed uptake in 81% of patients given 30 mCi (1110 MBq) and in 84% treated with 100 mCi (3700 MBq).[108] However, regardless of the dose, over 40% of patients had elevated serum Tg concentrations at the time of complete scintigraphic ablation. This may not be a true measure of the long-term effects of ablation because serum Tg concentrations decline slowly after ^{131}I ablation.[109]

Tumor recurrence rates are lowered with low-dose ^{131}I remnant ablation. Despite the suggestion that this is not an effective therapeutic strategy on the basis of a 9% recurrence rate in 69 patients given 30 mCi (1110 MBq) doses of ^{131}I,[104] this rate is about one-third the recurrence rate reported from the same institution in a larger group with papillary thyroid carcinoma who did not receive ^{131}I.[4] In a 25-year prospective study, none of 44 patients in whom total ^{131}I ablation was achieved died of cancer; however, 70% died of cancer when total ablation was not possible.[110] Among 831 patients with differentiated thyroid carcinoma in another series, pulmonary metastases developed in 58; they occurred in 11% of patients treated by partial thyroidectomy, 5% of those treated by subtotal thyroidectomy and ^{131}I, and only 1.3% of those treated by total thyroidectomy and ^{131}I.[49] Among 321 patients treated in 13 Canadian hospitals, most of whom had microscopic residual papillary or follicular carcinoma, local disease was controlled significantly more often with either postoperative external radiotherapy or ^{131}I therapy, or both together, than with thyroid hormone alone (*P*<0.001).[8] Survival at 20 years among patients with microscopic residual disease treated by surgery alone was lower (about 40%) than among those treated with either ^{131}I or external radiation (about 90%,

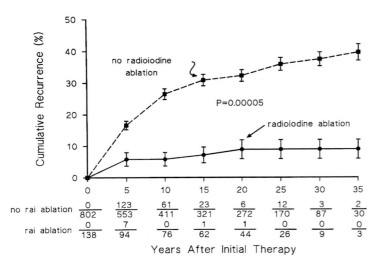

FIGURE 80-9. Recurrence rates (±SE) in 138 patients with stage II or III differentiated thyroid carcinoma treated with ^{131}I to ablate residual thyroid tissue compared with recurrence rates in 802 patients not treated with [131]I. More patients treated with ^{131}I had follicular cancer (*P* < 0.001). The numerators are the number of events during the previous interval and the denominators are the number of patients at the end of that interval. (From Mazzaferri EL, Jhiang SM. Long-term impact of initial surgical and medical therapy on papillary and follicular thyroid cancer. Am J Med 1994;97:418. Reproduced with the permission of the publisher.)

P<0.01), but ^{131}I treatment of patients without obvious residual disease did not increase survival significantly. We found tumor recurrences in 7% of patients given 29 to 50 mCi (1073–1850 MBq) and 9% given 51 to 200 mCi (1887–7400 MBq) [131]I to ablate thyroid remnants. Both rates were significantly lower than that in patients who received no [131]I (see Fig 80-9).

PATIENT PREPARATION

One must closely adhere to a protocol that ensures optimal preparation for ^{131}I scanning and therapy (Fig 80-11). There is a close relationship between adherence to the treatment protocol and the results of therapy.[31] At the time of the scan, the serum TSH concentration should be above 30 μU/mL[111] and the total body iodine pool should be as low as possible.[112]

Triiodothyronine (T_3) is given immediately after surgery. In a young adult the dose is 75 μg/d in divided doses; older patients are given 50 μg/d. T_3 is given for 4 weeks, then discontinued for 2 weeks, at which time the scan is done. Another option is to give no thyroid hormone and simply perform the scan 5 to 6 weeks postoperatively. With either protocol, the serum TSH concentration should rise above 30

μU/mL and may be as high as 200 μU/mL in patients who have undergone total or near-total thyroidectomy. If it is not above 30 μU/mL, the scan should be delayed. Although the protocol that uses T_3 ensures the fewest symptoms of hypothyroidism, most patients do not feel well for at least a week before the scan is done. Rapid tumor growth is rarely stimulated by a brief rise in serum TSH concentration.

Recombinant Human Thyrotropin. Recombinant human TSH should be available for clinical use within a year. In initial studies, recombinant human TSH was as effective as endogenous TSH in raising serum TSH concentrations and inducing ^{131}I uptake in normal thyroid tissue and carcinomas.[114] One or two daily injections of 10 to 20 units stimulates thyroid ^{131}I uptake in patients with low serum TSH concentrations as much as that caused by 2 or 3 weeks of thyroid hormone withdrawal. The side effects appear to be minimal. The initial studies were aimed at demonstrating its efficacy in ^{131}I scanning, but it undoubtedly will be used to prepare patients for ^{131}I therapy.

Low-Iodine Diet. A daily intake of about 50 μg of iodine can raise ^{131}I uptake in normal subjects and can double the

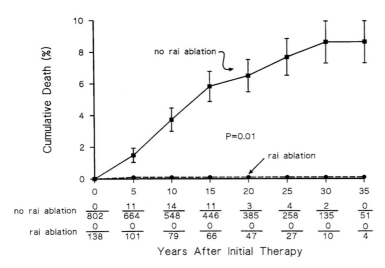

FIGURE 80-10. Cancer mortality rates (±SE) in 138 patients with stage II or III differentiated thyroid carcinoma treated with ^{131}I to ablate thyroid remnants compared with mortality rates in 802 patients not treated with [131]I. More patients treated with ^{131}I had follicular cancer (*P* < 0.001) The numerators are the number of events during the previous interval and the denominators are the number of patients at the end of that interval. (From Mazzaferri EL, Jhiang SM. Long-term impact of initial surgical and medical therapy on papillary and follicular thyroid cancer. Am J Med 1994;97:418. Reproduced with the permission of the publisher.)

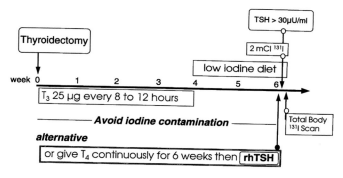

FIGURE 80-11. Protocol for patient preparation for a diagnostic whole body ^{131}I scan after initial thyroidectomy or at yearly follow-up intervals. T_3 is given to prevent symptoms of hypothyroidism. The serum TSH concentration should be above 30 μU/mL before the scan is done. (rhTSH, recombinant human TSH).

thyroid dose in rads (Gy) per 100 mCi (3700 MBq) of ^{131}I administered.[115] However, total body radiation after therapeutic ^{131}I administration may be increased up to 70% as the result of delayed iodine clearance.[116] A daily iodine intake of 50 μg can be achieved by restricting the use of iodized salt, dairy products, eggs, and seafood[112] (Table 80-12). Patients should check the labels of prepared foods for algae derivatives and all breads for iodates, avoid all red-colored foods and medicines, and avoid eating in restaurants if possible. The diet should be started 2 weeks before ^{131}I scanning and continued for several days thereafter. More complex regimens that include diuretics can be used, but they are usually unnecessary unless tumor ^{131}I uptake is very low.[112]

Lithium. This drug enhances tumor ^{131}I retention by reducing release of iodine from normal thyroid and tumor tissue.[117] In a dosage of 400 to 800 mg daily (10 mg/kg) for 7 days, lithium increases ^{131}I uptake in metastatic lesions while only slightly increasing ^{131}I uptake in normal tissue.[117] Serum lithium concentrations should be measured frequently and maintained between 0.8 and 1.2 mmol/L. Radiation of tumors in which the biologic half-life of iodine is short (<6 days) is maximized without increasing that to other organs.

WHOLE BODY ^{131}I SCANS

Whole body scans are most useful in patients with little or no remaining normal thyroid tissue. When there is a large amount of thyroid tissue in the neck, the scan usually shows a starburst effect of high ^{131}I uptake in the remnant that makes visualizing uptake elsewhere impossible. Ideally, scans are done with quantitative radiation dose estimates at 24, 48, and 72 hours after the oral administration of 2 mCi (74 MBq) ^{131}I. A metastatic lesion concentrating 0.02% of this dose per gram will contain 0.4 μCi (0.01 MBq) of ^{131}I per gram of tissue, which can be detected using current imaging techniques. Assuming a 4-day half-life of ^{131}I in the tumor, a subsequent treatment dose of 150 mCi (5550 MBq) ^{131}I will deliver about 1000 rads (10 Gy) to the lesion.[25] Although some prefer to use larger scanning doses, most metastatic lesions amenable to ^{131}I therapy are not likely to be missed in an athyrotic patient using a 2-mCi (74-MBq) diagnostic dose of ^{131}I.[25,99] Also, scanning doses of ^{131}I larger than 2 mCi (74 MBq) may have a sufficiently harmful effect on the tis-

sue that concentrates it to interfere with subsequent uptake of a therapeutic dose of ^{131}I. This effect, referred to as "thyroid stunning," may be more pervasive than heretofore suspected. In one study, diagnostic ^{131}I doses as low as 3 mCi (111 MBq) reduced the subsequent uptake of ^{131}I, particularly in thyroid remnants and cervical lymph nodes.[118] The effect was progressively greater with larger ^{131}I doses. The uptake of therapeutic doses of ^{131}I was not reduced by ^{123}I or 0.3 mCi (11 MBq) ^{131}I scanning doses, but was reduced after 3, 5, and 10 mCi (111, 185, and 370 MBq) ^{131}I, respectively, by 40%, 67%, and 89%. On the other hand, some metastases are visualized only after therapeutic doses of ^{131}I are given (see below).

FALSE-POSITIVE ^{131}I SCANS

False-positive scans may result from body secretions, pathologic transudates and inflammation, nonspecific mediastinal uptake, or tumors of nonthyroidal origin.[119] Misleading scans can be caused by physiologic secretion of ^{131}I from the nasopharynx, salivary and sweat glands, and stomach; from genitourinary excretion or spilling; and from skin contamination with sputum. Pathologic pulmonary transudates and inflammation due to cysts and lung lesions caused by fungal and other inflammatory disease may produce false-positive scans.[119–121] Diffuse physiologic hepatic ^{131}I uptake is seen after scanning and therapeutic doses of ^{131}I.[122]

TUMOR UPTAKE OF ^{131}I

The effect of ^{131}I therapy is related to the tumor's capacity to concentrate iodine. Even after meticulous preparation and large ^{131}I doses, many thyroid carcinomas do not concentrate ^{131}I in amounts sufficient for therapy. This is more common in patients over age 40 years and in those with Hürthle cell tumors. For example, among 101 patients with distant metastases, ^{131}I was concentrated by 60% of papillary, 64% of follicular, and only 36% of Hürthle cell carcinomas.[38] In another series,[123] only half of 123 patients with pulmonary metastases had tumors that concentrated ^{131}I; most patients (80%) with metastases that concentrated ^{131}I were under age 40 years. In a French study[68] two-thirds of 283 patients with lung or bone metastases had tumors that concentrated ^{131}I.

EFFICACY OF ^{131}I THERAPY FOR MACROSCOPIC RESIDUAL OR RECURRENT DISEASE

Therapy with ^{131}I had a favorable effect on outcome in most but not all studies. To summarize several studies in which there was little or no benefit, or even harm: ^{131}I therapy improved survival only in patients over age 50 years[56]; there were more recurrences (14% versus 1%) and deaths (5% versus none) after 7 years' follow-up in patients treated with ^{131}I than in those treated with T_4 alone[124]; and in a comparison of 36 patients studied at the Cleveland Clinic with 28 at the University of Michigan, the authors concluded that patients between the ages of 7 and 45 years with distant metastases from papillary carcinoma can be treated as effectively by subtotal thyroidectomy and T_4 as by total thyroidectomy followed by ^{131}I.[48]

There is, however, considerably more evidence of benefit. Among 1599 patients with differentiated thyroid carcinoma treated at the M.D. Anderson Cancer Center between 1948 and

TABLE 80-12.
Instructions for Low-Iodine Diet

Avoid the following foods for 2 weeks before radioactive iodine test and until thyroid scan and treatment, if needed, are completed:
1. Iodized salt, sea salt
2. Milk or other dairy products, including ice cream, cheese, yogurt, etc.
3. Eggs
4. Seafood, including fish, shellfish, kelp, and seaweed
5. Foods that contain the additives carrageenan, agar-agar, algin, alginate
6. Cured and corned foods (eg, ham, lox, corned beef, sauerkraut)
7. Breads made with iodate dough conditioners
8. Foods and medications containing red food dyes
9. Chocolate
10. Molasses
11. Soy products (eg, soy sauce, soy milk)

Additional guidelines:
- Avoid restaurant foods because there is no reasonable way to determine which restaurants use iodized salt.
- Foods that contain small amounts of milk or eggs may be used.
- Noniodized salt may be used as desired.
- Consult your doctor before discontinuing any red-colored medication.

Sample meal patterns:

BREAKFAST	**LUNCH**	**DINNER**
Orange juice	Turkey sandwich	London broil
Cream of wheat	Lettuce and tomato	Mushroom sauce w/ margarine
Whole wheat toast	Italian dressing	Green beans
Margarine	Fresh apple	Cucumber vinaigrette
Coffee	Graham crackers	Small roll
	Iced tea	Lemon sherbet
		Iced tea

(Pineda JD, Lee T, Robbins J. Treating metastatic thyroid cancer. Endocrinologist 1992;6:433–442)

1989, of whom about half received 100 mCi (3700 MBq) [131]I for ablation or 150 mCi (5550 MBq) for metastatic disease, with repeated doses every 6 to 12 months to achieve complete ablation or until a total dose of 500 mCi (18500 MBq) was reached, ^{131}I therapy was the single most powerful prognostic indicator of increased disease-free survival.[125] Low-risk patients had significantly fewer recurrences and deaths after ^{131}I therapy as compared with those treated with T_4 alone ($P<0.001$). With high-risk patients, ^{131}I therapy conferred a slight advantage.

In our study, the 30-year recurrence rates were 15% after ^{131}I plus T_4 therapy, 30% with T_4 alone, 40% with no medical therapy, and 63% after external radiation plus T_4, ($P<0.001$ between and among the four groups, see Fig 80-8). At 30 years, the cancer-specific death rates were 3% in the ^{131}I group, 6% in those treated with T_4 alone and 12% in the no medical therapy group ($P<0.001$ for all comparisons, but ^{131}I versus T_4 alone $P=0.30$). However, patients treated with ^{131}I had more advanced disease than those treated with T_4 alone. When only patients with stage II or III tumors were considered, those treated with ^{131}I had lower 30-year recurrence rates (16% versus 38%, $P<0.001$) and cancer-specific mortality rates (3% versus 9%, $P=0.03$; Fig 80-12) than those not treated with [131]I.

THERAPEUTIC ^{131}I DOSIMETRY

Of the dosimetry methods available, the most widely used and simplest is to administer a large fixed dose. Most clinics use this method regardless of the percentage uptake of ^{131}I in the remnant or metastatic lesion. Patients with lymph nodes metastases that are not large enough to excise are treated with 100 to 175 mCi (3700–6475 MBq). Carcinoma extending through the thyroid capsule and invading the neck is treated with 150 to 200 mCi (5550–7400 MBq), which should not induce radiation sickness or produce serious damage to other structures. The dose may vary according to the patient's risk category.[126] Patients with distant metastases are usually treated with 200 mCi (7400 MBq) [131]I. Diffuse pulmonary metastases that concentrate 50% or more of the diagnostic dose of ^{131}I, which is uncommon, are treated with 75 mCi (2775 MBq) [131]I to avoid lung injury. Many believe that to eradicate a tumor it must concentrate at least 0.1% of the ^{131}I dose at 24 hours. However, in some patients metastases detected only by high serum Tg concentrations can be treated effectively.[127]

A second approach is to use quantitative dosimetry methods to estimate tumor uptake. This is favored by some because radiation exposure from arbitrarily fixed doses of ^{131}I can vary considerably. If the calculated dose that will be delivered is less than 3500 rads (35 Gy), it is unlikely that the cancer will respond to ^{131}I therapy.[102,103,128] Doses that deliver 50,000 to 60,000 rads (500–600 Gy) to the residual normal tissue and 4000 to 5000 rads (40–50 Gy) to metastatic foci are likely to be effective. To make these calculations, it is necessary to estimate not only uptake but also tumor size, which is difficult to do with deep metastatic deposits. Patients who have metastases that will receive only a few hundred rads from 150- to 200-mCi (5550–7400-MBq) doses of ^{131}I should be considered for surgery, external radiation, or medical therapy.

A third approach is to administer a dose calculated to deliver a maximum of 200 rads (2 Gy) to the blood, keeping the whole body retention less than 120 mCi (4440 MBq) at 48 hours and the amount in the lungs less than 80 mCi (2960 MBq) when there is diffuse pulmonary uptake. The maximum administered dose is kept at 300 mCi (11100 MBq).

When ^{131}I doses of 30 mCi (1110 MBq) or larger are given in the United States, the patient must remain isolated in the hospital until the total body ^{131}I burden falls to less than 30 mCi (1110 MBq). With normal renal function and good hydration, this is ordinarily achieved within 3 days. During this time, oral fluid intake should be large to increase urine output in order to minimize radiation injury to the bladder. Also, the patient should suck on lemon drops to stimulate salivary flow to minimize the risk of radiation-induced sialadenitis. Constipation should be treated with cathartics to reduce gonadal radiation. Radiation safety procedures must be followed carefully to minimize the risk to personnel in contact with the patient and to avoid radiation exposure to family members. T_4 therapy is resumed 24 hours after ^{131}I therapy. However, it may take up to 2 months for serum TSH concentrations to fall to normal or below when T_4 doses of 100 μg are given.[129] TSH suppression may be expedited by giving 300 to 400 μg T_4 daily or 50 to 100 μg T_3 for several days. In the future, scanning after recombinant human TSH stimulation will alleviate this problem because T_4 will not be discontinued.

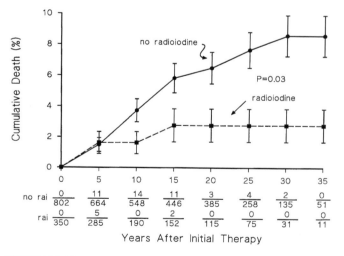

FIGURE 80-12. Cancer mortality rates (±SE) in 350 patients with stage II or III differentiated thyroid carcinoma given ^{131}I for any reason (ablation of thyroid remnant or treatment of carcinoma versus mortality rates in 802 patients not treated with ^{131}I. Of those treated with ^{131}I, more were men (38% versus 30%, *P* = 0.02) and more had lymph node metastases (53% versus 45%, *P* < 0.05) and stage III tumors (23% versus 16%, *P* < 0.01). The two groups were comparable with respect to other risk factors. The numerators are the number of events during the previous interval and the denominators are the number of patients at the end of that interval. (From Mazzaferri EL, Jhiang SM. Long-term impact of initial surgical and medical therapy on papillary and follicular thyroid cancer. Am J Med 1994;97:418. Reproduced with the permission of the publisher.)

CHOICE OF THERAPY

In our clinic therapeutic recommendations are made as summarized in Table 80-13. Patients with tumors of different stages are treated somewhat differently after having been fully informed of the potential risks and benefits.

Stage I Tumors. Patients with small (≤1.5 cm) tumors—single papillary carcinomas that are clearly confined to one lobe or follicular tumors with minimal capsular invasion—may be adequately treated with lobectomy and T_4 alone. When discovered at the time of subtotal thyroidectomy for another thyroid lesion or in the specimen later, we do not routinely advise ^{131}I therapy for stage I carcinomas because there is usually a large thyroid remnant, so that high or multiple doses of ^{131}I are needed for ablation.[130]

However, when the diagnosis is known preoperatively, near-total thyroidectomy is preferred because tumor stage is often not apparent until after the specimen has been studied by the pathologist and ^{131}I scanning has been done. We advise completion thyroidectomy (assuming nodule excision or unilateral lobectomy was the initial operation) and slightly less than 30 mCi (1110 MBq) ^{131}I for patients with the following stage I tumors: papillary variants with known aggressive behavior, more than one primary papillary carcinoma, and most follicular carcinomas, especially in patients over age 45 years, particularly men. In this group, we then maintain serum TSH concentration in the low-normal range. If uptake in the remnant is less than 1% at 48 hours, a second dose of ^{131}I is unlikely to be of further benefit. Even with an uptake above 1%, if there is no evidence of residual thyroid carcinoma when the serum TSH concentration is over 30 μU/mL, another therapeutic dose of ^{131}I need not be given.

Stage II Tumors. For tumors that are 1.5 to 4.4 cm in diameter that are not locally invasive, with or without regional lymph node metastases, we advise total or near-total thyroidectomy with modified neck dissection for lymph node metastases recognized at surgery followed by ^{131}I therapy (see Table 80-13). When the surgeon and pathologist believe the tumor was completely resected, and the diagnostic ^{131}I scan shows no uptake outside the thyroid bed, 30 mCi (1110 MBq) ^{131}I is administered 6 weeks after surgery. Repeat doses of 30 mCi (1110 MBq) may be given 1 year later if uptake in the thyroid bed is above 1% and the serum Tg concentration during T_4 therapy is greater than 5 ng/mL. Patients with tumors that were incompletely resected or bilateral tumors or who have mediastinal lymph node metastases are given larger doses of ^{131}I (from 150 to 175 mCi [3700–5550 MBq]). Then, T_4 is given in a dosage sufficient to maintain the serum TSH concentration just below normal.

Stage III Tumors. For tumors that are large (>4.5 cm) or invading local structures, we advise total thyroidectomy and modified neck dissection for lymph node metastases recognized at surgery followed by ^{131}I therapy (see Table 80-13). If there is any question that residual tumor remains after surgery, as with locally invasive tumors, at least 150 mCi (5550 MBq) ^{131}I should be given, followed by a dose of T_4 sufficient to maintain the serum TSH concentration just below normal. Long-term, serum TSH concentrations are maintained in the

TABLE 80-13.
Suggested Treatment of Papillary and Follicular Thyroid Carcinoma

Clinical Stage	Thyroid Surgery	^{131}I dosage (mCi)	T$_4$ Therapy (Target Serum TSH* and Tg‡ values)
I	Near-total thyroidectomy† (preferred if carcinoma identified at surgery, or if follicular or multiple tumors, or age more than 45 y, or male)	<30 (preferred)	TSH < 0.5 µU/mL Tg < 5 ng/mL
	Subtotal thyroidectomy* (if single tumor <1.5 cm in a young person is detected in a resected specimen, do not complete thyroidectomy)§	None	TSH < 0.5 µU/mL Tg < 10 ng/mL
II	Near-total or total thyroidectomy; modified neck dissection as needed¶	<30 or 150–175‖	TSH < 0.5 µU/mL Tg < 5 ng/mL
III	Near-total or total thyroidectomy; modified neck dissection as needed¶	150–200	TSH < 0.5 µU/mL Tg < 5 ng/mL
IV	Near-total or total thyroidectomy; modified neck dissection as needed¶	200 or more	TSH < 0.1 µU/mL Tg < 10 ng/mL

*Serum TSH is maintained at low-normal values if serum Tg is 5 ng/mL or lower.
†Near-total thyroidectomy is defined as an attempt to remove all thyroid tissue without damage to recurrent laryngeal nerves or parathyroid tissue, usually leaving portions of the posterior thyroid behind on the contralateral side.
‡Serum Tg measured during T$_4$ therapy.
§Subtotal thyroidectomy defined as lobectomy plus contralateral subtotal lobectomy.
‖<30 mCi (1110 MBq) for patients without residual tumor after surgery; larger doses for patients with bilateral cervical or mediastinal node disease or incomplete resection of involved cervical lymph nodes.
¶An en bloc dissection is not done, and an attempt is made to retain the jugular vein and sternocleidomastoid muscles.

same range if the serum Tg concentration remains below 5 ng/mL during T$_4$ therapy.

Stage IV Tumors (Distant Metastases). ^{131}I therapy is most effective in young patients with pulmonary metastases that concentrate the isotope. In a study of 283 patients with distant metastases, the four independent variables that adversely affected survival were extensive metastases, older age at discovery of the metastases, absence of ^{131}I uptake, and moderately differentiated follicular cell type.[68] In another study of 123 patients with distant metastases, ^{131}I uptake was achieved most often and 10-year survival was greatest (80%) in young patients with papillary carcinoma whose chest x-rays showed fine pulmonary metastases.[123] Survival in the others was only 29% at 10 years and 12% at 15 years. The best prognosis—sometimes associated with apparent cure after ^{131}I therapy— is with lung metastases seen only on ^{131}I imaging and not by x-ray or computed tomography (CT). Among 23 patients treated with ^{131}I for diffuse pulmonary metastases detected only by ^{131}I imaging, 87% had no lung uptake on subsequent scans.[131] After ^{131}I therapy, serum Tg became undetectable and CT scans of the lungs showed disappearance of the micronodules in almost half the patients, whereas lung biopsy showed no evidence of disease in two. In other studies, patients considered free of disease after ^{131}I therapy survived three times longer than those with persistent disease,[31] and 65% of 20 patients with only pulmonary metastases had a complete response to ^{131}I therapy; there were no relapses after 4 to 32 years.[67]

We initially treat patients with stage IV disease with total thyroidectomy and modified neck dissection as required, followed by 200 mCi (7400 MBq) ^{131}I when the tumor concentrates ^{131}I. T$_4$ is given in doses sufficient to maintain the serum TSH concentration below normal, often less than 0.1 µU/mL.

Over the long term, however, if the patient's serum Tg concentration remains below 5 ng/mL, the serum TSH concentration is kept in the low-normal range.

Scanning and treatment with ^{131}I are repeated at 6- to 12-month intervals until the tumor no longer concentrates ^{131}I, large cumulative doses are reached, or adverse effects appear. We try to wait a full year between treatments and try to keep the cumulative dose under 500 mCi (18500 MBq) in children and 700 mCi (25900 MBq) in adults. Although there is no specific limit to the cumulative dose that can be administered safely, and more than 2000 mCi (74000 MBq) can be given without long-term adverse effects, such large cumulative doses should be avoided. The whole body radiation doses for each patient should be kept under 200 rads (2 Gy) in most patients or 300 rads (3 Gy) in those with rapidly progressive disease; this allows total cumulative ^{131}I doses of about 450 to 680 mCi (16650–25160 MBq).[132] Total cumulative doses of 1000 mCi (37000 MBq) or more can be given to patients with serious distant metastases, but the frequency of complications rises (see below).[67,133] Moreover, there is an apparent loss of benefit from ^{131}I in patients receiving more than 500 mCi (18500 MBq), although the reason is not known.[134]

TREATMENT OF CHILDREN AND ADOLESCENTS

Treatment of children and adolescents is even more controversial than it is in adults because there are not even any large retrospective studies with a well-defined treatment protocol. Indeed, treatment has been so variable that it is almost impossible to determine its influence on outcome.[53] With this limitation, the following represent the therapeutic options.

Less than 10% of differentiated thyroid carcinomas occur in patients younger than 20 years old.[135] Although children and adolescents commonly present with more advanced disease, their prognosis is excellent. The survival rates at 15 to 20 years in series published since 1981 were over 90%.[136] Some report few or no cancer deaths after three decades of follow-up of patients first treated under age 20.[137,138] Even children with distant metastases respond well to therapy. Only one cancer death occurred among 66 children in one study after an average follow-up of about 15 years although most (84%) had lymph node metastases and many (12%) had pulmonary metastases.[139] Another study reported almost the same results among 54 children treated aggressively and followed for several decades although most (88%) had lymph node metastases and some (19%) had distant metastases at the time of diagnosis.[140] In a third study of 72 children younger than age 16 years, 42% developed distant metastases, mostly to the lungs, but 70% had a complete remission.[66]

Nevertheless, not all authors relate such good survival rates. One study reported that 2 of 29 children died of papillary carcinoma; both had distant metastases at the time of diagnosis. In another study of 11 children under age 16 years, a 5-year-old patient with lung metastases died 1 month after diagnosis.[141] In the most comprehensive study, involving 140 children and adolescents less than age 19 years, total thyroidectomy was performed in 73% and ^{131}I was administered to almost half.[125] Forty percent had recurrences and 19% had distant metastases, most of which (96%) were in the lung. The results suggested that total thyroidectomy was the therapy of choice and that ^{131}I therapy was beneficial. Another study from the same institution reported that nearly 10% of 209 patients under age 25 years had pulmonary metastases at diagnosis.[69] Although most of the lung metastases concentrated ^{131}I, almost half were not seen on x-ray, suggesting that pulmonary metastases may be overlooked unless near-total thyroidectomy is followed by total body ^{131}I scanning in all children with regional lymph node metastases. These observations underscore the need for meticulous treatment of children with this disease and provide evidence that this is not always an indolent disease in the young.

Surgery is the treatment of choice, but as with adults there is no consensus concerning the optimal procedure.[142] Some perform total or near-total thyroidectomy and cervical lymph node dissection if metastases are present, whereas others perform subtotal thyroidectomy.[52,53] Surgical complications occur more frequently in children than in adults, even at large centers.[142] Because the risk of cancer death is so low in children, the risk of complications thus constitutes the major reservation about performing more extensive surgery. There are strong arguments for an aggressive approach in children, including the high incidence of primary tumor multicentricity and metastases, the high recurrence rate, and the fact that life expectancy exceeds 60 years.

Children with multifocal or invasive tumors, or with cervical lymph node metastases, should be treated the same as adults with aggressive tumors.[53] The indications for postoperative ^{131}I are controversial, but many recommend whole body ^{131}I scanning and ablation of the thyroid remnant with 30 mCi (1110 MBq) of [131]I.[52,53,140,143,144] T$_4$ should be given in doses sufficient to maintain the serum TSH concentration in the low-normal range. Excellent results have been reported using this approach.[139,140]

POSTTREATMENT ^{131}I SCANS

Metastases often do not concentrate much ^{131}I or may not concentrate it at all when much normal thyroid tissue is present.[25] A whole body scan should be done 7 to 10 days after treatment to document ^{131}I uptake by the tumor. About 25% of these posttreatment scans show lesions not detected by the diagnostic scan done before therapy, which may or may not be clinically important. In a systematic study of pre- and posttreatment scans, the two differed in 27% of the treatment cycles, but only 10% of the posttreatment scans showed new locations of metastatic disease.[145] Posttreatment scans were most likely to reveal clinically important new information in patients under age 45 years who had received ^{131}I therapy in the past. In older patients and those who had not previously received ^{131}I therapy, the posttreatment scans rarely yielded new information that might have altered the patient's prognosis.[145]

Posttreatment ^{131}I scans are especially likely to yield the most information when diagnostic scans are negative and serum Tg concentrations are very high. In a study of 283 patients, 18 (6%) who had elevated serum Tg concentrations had lung and bone metastases detected after treatment with 100 mCi (3700 MBq) [131]I that had not been detected after 2 mCi (74 MBq) scans.[68] In another study, all but 1 of 17 patients with elevated serum Tg concentrations and negative 5-mCi (185-MBq) diagnostic scans showed ^{131}I uptake after 75 to 140 mCi (2775–5180 MBq) [131]I; more than half had lung metastases.[146]

ACUTE COMPLICATIONS OF ^{131}I THERAPY

Radiation thyroiditis occurs in about 20% of patients, most often in patients with large thyroid remnants given doses of ^{131}I that deliver about 50,000 rads (500 Gy).[147] It usually appears within the first week after ^{131}I administration and is characterized by neck and ear pain, painful swallowing, thyroid swelling and tenderness, and transient mild thyrotoxicosis. Rarely, the thyroid remnant may swell enough to cause airway obstruction. Patients with mild pain can be treated with salicylate or acetaminophen, but those with severe pain or swelling should receive corticosteroid therapy, for example, prednisone 30 mg daily for several days and then tapered over 7 to 10 days.

Painless neck edema within 48 hours after ^{131}I administration is a different and much less common problem than radiation thyroiditis.[148] It occurs after high radiation doses, sometimes rather rapidly and accompanied by stridor, in patients with small as well as large remnants.[149] This is thought to be an allergic response rather than a direct radiation effect, and it responds to corticosteroid therapy.[148]

Radiation sialadenitis occurs after ^{131}I therapy in up to 12% of patients. It may be either transient or chronic and involve either the parotid or submandibular glands.[150] It may begin within 24 hours after therapy and is more likely when a large dose of ^{131}I is given to a patient with little functioning thyroid tissue.[151] Most patients have intermittent painless salivary gland swelling that lasts a few days, reminiscent of a salivary duct stone, require no therapy, and improve spontaneously; a few have chronic xerostomia. Chewing gum, sucking on lemon candies, and hydration may prevent the sialadenitis and xerostomia due to large doses of [131]I. Occasional patients have transient nausea, gastrointestinal discomfort, tongue pain, or reduced taste.[152]

The most important acute complication of ^{131}I therapy is edema or hemorrhage of deposits of tumor. Serious symptoms can occur rapidly when ^{131}I is given to a patient with tumor in a critical location in the central nervous system, spinal cord, or airway. For example, a patient with brain metastases developed cerebral edema, slurred speech, right-sided weakness, and a focal seizure 12 hours after receiving 200 mCi (7400 MBq) [131]I.[153] Pretreatment with prednisone may minimize the hazards of ^{131}I in patients with brain or spinal cord metastases or bulky tumors around the airway. Surgical debulking of spinal or peritracheal lesions may be prudent before ^{131}I is given.

Pain in distant metastases can occur shortly after ^{131}I therapy as a result of radiation-induced inflammation, as can vocal cord paralysis in patients with a large amount of functioning thyroid tissue in close proximity to the vocal cords.[154] Transient peripheral facial nerve palsy was reported in two patients after high-dose ^{131}I therapy, presumably due to radiation of the nerve as it courses through the parotid area.[155]

Acute hematologic changes, especially a slight reduction in platelet and white blood cell counts, may follow ^{131}I therapy, but they are transient and usually cause no symptoms.[152] More severe bone marrow suppression with anemia also occurs but is reversible and does not require transfusion.[152]

LATE COMPLICATIONS OF ^{131}I THERAPY

The main long-term complications of ^{131}I are damage to the gonads, bone marrow, and lungs and the induction of other cancers. In a group of older women, 27% had transient amenorrhea and elevated serum gonadotropin concentrations during the first year after therapy.[156] In men, the problem may be more severe. Young men may develop permanent testicular damage with a reduction in sperm count that is roughly proportional to the ^{131}I dose administered.[157] In 103 men treated with ^{131}I for residual or metastatic disease, the mean serum follicle-stimulating hormone (FSH) concentration was almost threefold higher than in normal men, and 37% had elevated concentrations.[158] In a longitudinal analysis of 21 men, 6 had no change or only a slight increase in serum FSH after ^{131}I therapy while 11 others had a transient rise above normal 6 to 12 months after treatment. Four men treated with several doses of ^{131}I had a progressive increase in serum FSH that eventually became permanent. Semen analysis, performed in a small subgroup of men, showed a consistent reduction in sperm motility. The serum testosterone concentrations in the treated and normal men were similar.

In 33 children treated at an average age of 15 years with a mean ^{131}I dose of 196 mCi (7252 MBq), the frequency of infertility (12%), miscarriage (1%), prematurity (8%), and major congenital anomalies (1%) after an average of almost 19 years of follow-up was not significantly different from the general population.[159] In another study, fertility was normal in 30 women who were 30 years old or less when treated; they had 44 live births.[133] Two men who had received a total of 972 and 1432 mCi (35964 and 52984 MBq) of ^{131}I between ages 10 and 19 years had fathered 2 and 3 children, respectively, up to 13 and 24 years later.

Thus, ^{131}I therapy transiently and occasionally permanently impairs testicular germinal cell function, posing a significant risk of infertility. Young men should consider banking sperm specimens before therapy.

Induction of other tumors and bone marrow damage are the most serious late problems of ^{131}I therapy. Large doses of [131]I (usually >1000 mCi [37000 MBq]) are associated with a small but significant excess of deaths from bladder cancer and leukemia.[133] In a report from Germany, 80% of 35 patients with thyroid carcinoma treated with ^{131}I had bone marrow abnormalities, including 3 with acute myeloid leukemia. The patients with abnormalities of erythrocytes, platelets, and granulocytes had all received more than 1000 mCi (37000 MBq) of [131]I.[132] In 13 large series comprising a total of 2753 patients with thyroid carcinoma, 14 cases of leukemia were detected.[154] The prevalence of about five leukemia cases per 1000 patients is higher than expected in the general population. Acute myeloid leukemia, the type associated with ^{131}I therapy, usually has occurred within 10 years after treatment, most often in patients given ^{131}I every few months and in whom the total blood doses per administration were more than 200 rad (2 Gy). Despite this report, the lifetime risk of leukemia is so small (≤0.3%) that it does not outweigh the benefit of ^{131}I therapy.[160] The absolute risk of life lost because of recurrent thyroid carcinoma exceeds that from leukemia by fourfold to 40-fold, depending on the age at which the patient is treated.[160] When lower total cumulative ^{131}I doses (600–800 mCi [22200–29600 MBq]) are given at widely spaced intervals (12 months), long-term effects on the bone marrow are minimal[152] and few cases of leukemia occur.[161] Furthermore, one large population study did not find an increased risk of leukemia in patients with thyroid carcinoma.[162]

Pulmonary fibrosis occurs rarely in patients with diffuse pulmonary metastases treated with [131]I.[67] It can be avoided by using smaller than usual doses (e.g., 75 mCi [2775 MBq]) of ^{131}I when scans show high uptake of scanning doses in the lungs.

TREATMENT OF RECURRENT DISEASE

Whenever possible, surgery is the treatment of choice for recurrent disease; however, ^{131}I therapy is usually adequate treatment for tumors detectable only by scintigraphy. If the tumor cannot be excised and does not concentrate ^{131}I, external radiation may be effective. The likelihood of dying is less if recurrent or persistent disease is detected by ^{131}I scan than if it is detected by clinical examination.[10]

External Radiation Therapy

External radiation may be beneficial in the initial postoperative management of patients with differentiated thyroid carcinoma.[1,2] Patients with aggressive tumors that fail to concentrate ^{131}I, especially those that have extended beyond the thyroid or are poorly differentiated, should be considered for external beam radiotherapy. Patients with microscopic residual papillary carcinoma after surgery more often remain disease free when external radiotherapy is given (90%) than when it is not (26%).[8] This also is true for patients with microscopically invasive follicular carcinoma, more of whom are disease free when postoperative external radiation is given (53%) than when it is not (38%). Among patients with papillary carcinomas treated with 4500 rads (45 Gy), 20% had recurrence and none died of cancer, but lower doses were not beneficial.[163] Patients with follicular carcinomas treated with higher doses had only a 2% recurrence rate, but external radiation did not alter mortality. In a study of external beam radiotherapy in patients who had incomplete surgical resection of their tumors, the 15- and 25-year survival rates were 57% and 40%, respectively.[164] Although the patients who received radiotherapy had larger and more extensive tumors than those treated with surgery alone, their 15-year local recurrence rate was less than half that of the patients treated with surgery alone (11% versus 23%). In a study of external radiotherapy in 113 patients with differentiated thyroid carcinoma whose tumors failed to concentrate ^{131}I or were inoperable or poorly differentiated, the response rate was 60%. The 10-year survival rates were 81% in patients under age 45 years, but fell to 36% in those aged 45 to 65 years, and were only 6% in patients over age 65 years.[165] We found a very high recurrence rate in a small number of patients with advanced disease who were treated with external radiation[11] (see Fig 80-8).

Chemotherapy

The experience with chemotherapy in patients with differentiated thyroid carcinoma is limited because most recurrent tumors respond so well to surgery, ^{131}I therapy, or external beam radiotherapy.[10,131,164] Its main use is for patients with tumors that are not surgically resectable, are not responsive to ^{131}I, and have been treated with, or are not amenable to, external radiotherapy. Among 49 patients with metastatic differentiated thyroid carcinoma treated with five chemotherapy protocols, only 2 (3%) patients had objective responses.[166] Initial enthusiasm for bleomycin has been limited by its pulmonary toxicity. In a recent review of published series, 38% of patients had a response to doxorubicin, defined as a reduction in tumor mass.[167] The usual effective dose is between 60 and 90 mg/m² every 3 weeks and is limited by cardiac toxicity above a total cumulative dose of 550 mg/m². Doxorubicin at a dose below that used in cancer chemotherapy has been used as adjunctive therapy with external beam radiotherapy, but it may be no better than radiotherapy alone.[168] It is now being tested in a randomized treatment protocol using 10 mg/m² before each ^{131}I dose.[127] Combination chemotherapy is not clearly superior to doxorubicin monotherapy.[3]

FOLLOW-UP

Serum Thyroglobulin

Serum Tg determinations and whole body ^{131}I imaging together will detect recurrent or residual disease in most patients. In general, serum Tg should be measured and whole body ^{131}I scanning done after thyroidectomy and ^{131}I ablation, after T_4 is discontinued. A test for serum anti-Tg antibodies should be done in the sample obtained for serum Tg assay because these antibodies invalidate serum Tg measurements in most assays (see chap 20). Although serum Tg can be measured while the patient is taking T_4, the measurement is more sensitive when T_4 has been stopped and the serum TSH concentration is elevated. Under these circumstances, serum Tg determination has a lower false-negative rate than whole body ^{131}I scanning.

Serum Tg assays, however, have not been well standardized, which accounts at least in part for the variations in values used by different investigators in decision-making. In our clinic we use a serum Tg value of above 5 ng/mL while the patient is taking T_4 as an indication to repeat scanning in patients with no other evidence of disease who have had ^{131}I ablation and a subsequent negative diagnostic whole body ^{131}I scan.

Depending on the stage of the disease, initially the patients are evaluated every 6 to 12 months with both diagnostic ^{131}I scans and serum Tg measurements until the scan shows less than 1% uptake and the serum Tg concentration is less than 10 ng/mL after T_4 has been discontinued. Thereafter, scans can be done less frequently providing the serum Tg value remains low. Follow-up with serum Tg measurements alone seems safe in patients who have undergone near-total or total thyroidectomy and ^{131}I ablation, even when the patient is taking T_4, providing serum Tg concentrations are less than 5 ng/mL (Fig 80-13). If the serum Tg concentration rises above 5 ng/mL or if the patient has suspicious findings on physical examination, ^{131}I imaging is done. When the serum Tg value is above 10 ng/mL during T_4 therapy or above 40 ng/mL after it is discontinued, even if the diagnostic ^{131}I scan is negative (i.e., <1% [131]I uptake), we give a therapeutic dose of [131]I—usually 100 to 150 mCi (3700–5550 MBq)—and perform a posttreatment scan. Others use different cut-off values and different doses of [131]I.

Patients who have not undergone near-total thyroidectomy and ^{131}I ablation who have large thyroid remnants are much more difficult to evaluate (Fig 80-14). When thyroid ablation has not been done, whole body ^{131}I scans are not as sensitive and serum Tg measurements are less reliable.

In a comparison of serum Tg measurements and whole body ^{131}I scans after thyroid hormone withdrawal in 233 patients who had undergone total thyroidectomy with or without ^{131}I therapy, of whom 35% had local or distant metastases, the serum Tg and whole body ^{131}I scanning results were concordant in only 44% of those with local or distant disease.[169] Most had negative whole body scans and positive serum Tg tests; only three had the opposite pattern. The test sensitivities were 96% for serum Tg measurements and 48% for whole body ^{131}I scans. In 374 patients who had previously undergone thyroid ablation and who had serum Tg measurements, ^{131}I whole body scans, CT scans, and high-resolution ultrasonography, 11% had recurrent disease.[170] The sensitivity of serum Tg was 50% before and 83% after T_4 was discontinued. The false-negative serum Tg tests were in patients with small papillary carcinomas with cervical or mediastinal lymph node metastases. The other tests were less sensitive than serum Tg; 43% of the patients who had an elevated serum Tg value had no other evidence of disease and were presumed to have occult metastases. Further evidence of the sensitivity of serum Tg measurements was provided by a study of 27 patients with lung metastases who had been treated with [131]I.[171] All had negative scans after the ^{131}I therapy, but serum Tg values remained elevated for several years. CT scans showed micronodules in 7 of 13 patients with normal chest x-rays; these were thought to be due to fibrosis.

In a study of serum Tg measurements in 180 patients followed up to 18 years, 94% of those patients who had undergone near-total or total thyroidectomy and ^{131}I ablation had

Management Without a Thyroid Remnant

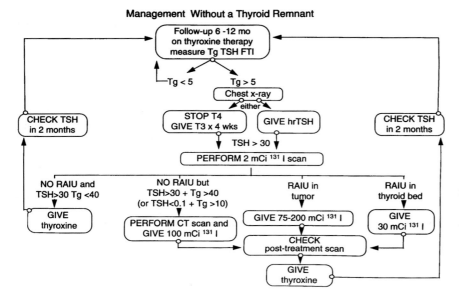

FIGURE 80-13. Follow-up patients with no thyroid remnant after initial therapy. Diagnostic scans are done with 2 mCi (74 MBq) [131]I and treatment with 30 mCi (1110 MBq), 75 mCi (2775 MBq), 100 mCi (3700 MBq), or 200 mCi (7400 MBq) [131]I, depending on the clinical situation (see text). FTI, free T_4 index; rhTSH, recombinant human TSH; RAIU, radioiodine uptake. Units for serum Tg, ng/ml, and for TSH, μU/ml.

serum Tg values less than 5 ng/mL and over 98% had values less than 10 ng/mL during T_4 therapy.[109] A serum Tg value less than 10 ng/mL during T_4 therapy in a patient who had undergone ablative therapy indicated the absence of tumor in over 98%; however, off T_4, the serum Tg value was over 5 ng/mL in 23% and over 10 ng/mL in 10%. Although the sensitivity of serum Tg for detecting recurrent thyroid carcinoma increased after withdrawal of T_4, the rate of false-positive tests also increased and no cut-off value properly categorized all patients. Even in patients who underwent total thyroidectomy and ^{131}I ablation and were considered cured, small foci of thyroid carcinoma that are undetectable by 2 mCi (74 MBq) [131]I scans may exist and produce some Tg, but these residual cells do not have an adverse effect on outcome in most patients. The authors concluded that the results of serum Tg and ^{131}I tests are complementary and that patients who have undergone

near-total or total thyroidectomy and ^{131}I ablation and have had a negative postablation scan and have serum Tg values less than 2 ng/mL while receiving T_4 and 3 ng/mL after it is discontinued rarely have recurrent thyroid carcinoma.

Even in patients with low serum Tg concentrations, very large doses of ^{131}I may reveal tumor metastases. For example, among 224 patients who received 100 to 200 mCi (3700–7400 MBq) [131]I either as an ablation dose or for treatment on the basis of a previous ^{131}I scan in combination with poor prognostic factors, 35% had one or several very low serum Tg values (<3 ng/mL) despite ^{131}I uptake on the posttherapy scans.[172] [131]I uptake was limited to the thyroid bed and regional lymph nodes in over 90%, but 7 patients (9%) had evidence of bone or lung metastases. Using this approach, many patients will be given large doses of ^{131}I with as yet no evidence that it improves outcome.

Management With a Thyroid Remnant

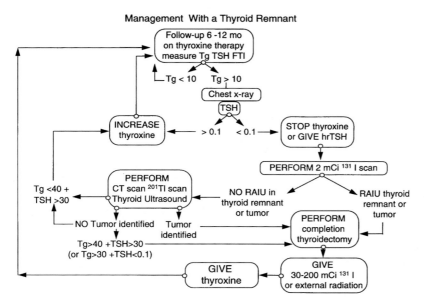

FIGURE 80-14. Follow-up of patients with a thyroid remnant after initial therapy. Diagnostic scans are done with 2 mCi (74 MBq) [131]I and treatment with 30 mCI (1110 MBq) to 200 mCI (7400 MBq) depending on the clinical situation (see text). FTI, free T_4 index; rhTSH, recombinant human TSH; RAIU, radioiodine uptake. Units for serum Tg, ng/ml, and for TSH, μU/ml.

Imaging Studies

Although we prefer whole body ^{131}I scans for follow-up, other imaging studies may be useful. [201]Thallium (^{201}Tl) or the newer agent ^{99m}Tc methoxy-isobutylisonitrate has the advantage that T_4 need not be discontinued; imaging is done immediately after injection of the isotope, and the whole body radiation dose is lower than with [131]I. Some studies suggest that ^{201}Tl scanning is more sensitive but less specific than ^{131}I in detecting thyroid carcinoma, but that ^{131}I detects residual normal thyroid tissue better than [201]Tl. In a comparison of ^{201}Tl and ^{131}I scans in 326 patients who had been treated with total thyroidectomy, scanning with ^{201}Tl was more sensitive (94%) but ^{131}I was more specific (99%).[173] Another study of 52 patients reached similar conclusions.[174] In a comparison of serum Tg and ^{131}I and ^{201}Tl scintigraphy in the postoperative follow-up of patients with differentiated thyroid carcinoma, serum Tg had the highest sensitivity (97%) and specificity (100%) for detecting local tumor or metastases.[175] [131]I scanning, after a therapeutic dose (165 mCi [6105 MBq]), had a sensitivity of 77% and specificity of 98%. After a 5 mCi (185 MBq) diagnostic dose of ^{131}I, the sensitivity was 57% and specificity was 98%; after 2 mCi (74 MBq) ^{201}Tl the respective values were 55% and 91%. The combination of serum Tg assay and ^{131}I scanning had a sensitivity of 100% and a specificity of 98% in detecting persistent or recurrent tumor. [201]Tl scans may be more sensitive in detecting miliary lung metastases and bone metastases. Others report little difference between ^{201}Tl and ^{131}I or report lower diagnostic sensitivity of ^{201}Tl scanning.[176–178]

A tumor's ability to concentrate ^{131}I has important therapeutic implications that may not be the case with [201]Tl. Thallium imaging should be considered for localizing tumor in patients with negative ^{131}I scans and elevated serum Tg concentrations, mainly to determine whether the tumor is amenable to surgical or external beam radiotherapy, and perhaps also to identify patients with lung metastases that might concentrate ^{131}I when a therapeutic dose was given.

Other imaging studies may be used for follow-up. High-resolution real-time ultrasonography can detect cervical lymph node metastases as small as 0.5 cm, but it is difficult to know that such small lymph nodes are infiltrated with tumor. Chest x-rays can be useful for diagnosis and to evaluate the response to treatment of pulmonary metastases, but sensitivity is relatively low.

Scanning with CT and magnetic resonance imaging (MRI) yields high-resolution cross-sectional images of the thyroid bed and neck and is particularly helpful in evaluating the extent of local invasion of a tumor.[176] CT scanning of the lungs may reveal micronodular lesions, but radiographic contrast agents should not be given because their high iodine content interferes with ^{131}I uptake. They are therefore absolutely contraindicated if ^{131}I scanning or therapy is contemplated. MRI offers certain advantages. It can be performed in the transaxial, coronal, and sagittal planes, and vascular structures are well defined without contrast material. MRI can detect micronodular pulmonary and hepatic metastases not revealed by CT. Bone metastases usually are detected with ^{131}I scanning. In a comparison of whole body ^{131}I scans, ^{99m}Tc pyrophosphate bone scans, chest x-rays and skeletal survey x-rays in 108 patients, 29 of whom had known metastatic thyroid carcinoma, most patients' metastases were identified by ^{131}I uptake in the lungs or by chest x-rays.[179] Six patients had bone metastases;

four had positive ^{131}I scans, two had positive ^{99m}Tc pyrophosphate bone scans, and only one had positive skeletal x-rays.

CONCLUSION

Although it is unlikely that controversies regarding management of thyroid carcinoma will be resolved in the near future, it is clear that mortality from thyroid carcinoma has diminished in the past several decades. Data published by the National Cancer Institute indicates that there has been a gradual improvement in 5-year survival rates for thyroid carcinoma of all types.[135] Estimated to be around 83% in 1960–1963, relative 5-year survival rates (the likelihood that a patient will not die of cancer) have increased from 92% in 1974–1976 to 94% in 1981–1986. A number of factors may be responsible for this improvement, but it is likely that early diagnosis and effective management, particularly of differentiated thyroid carcinoma, accounts for much of it.

References

1. Van De Velde CJH, Hamming JF, Goslings BM, et al. Report of the consensus development conference on the management of differentiated thyroid cancer in the Netherlands. Eur J Cancer Clin Oncol 1988;24:287
2. Baldet L, Manderscheid JC, Glinoer D, et al. The management of differentiated thyroid cancer in Europe in 1988. Results of an international survey. Acta Endocrinol 1989;120:547
3. Mazzaferri EL. Thyroid carcinoma: papillary and follicular. In: Mazzaferri EL, Samaan N, eds. Endocrine tumors. Cambridge, MA: Blackwell Scientific, 1993:278
4. McConahey WM, Hay ID, Woolner LB, et al. Papillary thyroid cancer treated at the Mayo Clinic, 1946 through 1970: initial manifestations, pathologic findings, therapy and outcome. Mayo Clin Proc 1986;61:978
5. Rösler H, Birrer A, Lüscher D, Kinser J. Long-term course in differentiated thyroid carcinoma. Schweiz Med Wochenschr 1992;122:1843
6. Ruiz de Almodóvar JM, Ruiz-Garcia J, Olea N, et al. Analysis of risk of death from differentiated thyroid cancer. Radiother Oncol 1994;31:207
7. Crile G Jr. Factors influencing the survival of patients with follicular carcinoma of the thyroid gland. Surg Gynecol Obstet 1985;160:409
8. Simpson WJ, Panzarella T, Carruthers JS, et al. Papillary and follicular thyroid cancer: impact of treatment in 1578 patients. Int J Radiat Oncol Biol Phys 1988;14:1063
9. Carcangiu ML, Zampi G, Pupi A, et al. Papillary carcinoma of the thyroid. A clinicopathologic study of 241 cases treated at the University of Florence, Italy. Cancer 1985;55:805
10. Coburn M, Teates D, Wanebo HJ. Recurrent thyroid cancer: role of surgery versus radioactive iodine (I[131]). Ann Surg 1994; 219:587
11. Mazzaferri EL, Jhiang SM. Long-term impact of initial surgical and medical therapy on papillary and follicular thyroid cancer. Am J Med 1994;97:418
12. Mazzaferri EL. Management of a solitary thyroid nodule. N Engl J Med 1993;328:553
13. Tielens ET, Sherman SI, Hruban RH, Ladenson PW. Follicular variant of papillary thyroid carcinoma: a clinicopathologic study. Cancer 1994;73:424
14. LiVolsi VA. Unusual variants of papillary thyroid carcinoma. Adv Endocrinol Metab 1995;6:39

15. Evans HL. Encapsulated papillary neoplasms of the thyroid. A study of 14 cases followed for a minimum of 10 years. Am J Surg Pathol 1987;11:592

16. Schroder S, Bocker W, Dralle H, et al. The encapsulated papillary carcinoma of the thyroid. A morphologic subtype of the papillary thyroid carcinoma. Cancer 1984;54:90

17. Matias-Guiu X, Cuatrecasas M, Musulen E, Prat J. p53 expression in anaplastic carcinomas arising from thyroid papillary carcinomas. J Clin Pathol 1994;47:337

18. Venkatesh YS, Ordonez NG, Schultz PN, et al. Anaplastic carcinoma of the thyroid. A clinicopathologic study of 121 cases. Cancer 1990;66:321

19. Johnson TL, Lloyd RV, Thompson NW, et al. Prognostic implications of the tall cell variant of papillary thyroid carcinoma. Am J Surg Pathol 1988;12:22

20. Harach HR, Zusman SB. Cytopathology of the tall cell variant of thyroid papillary carcinoma. Acta Cytol 1992;36:895

21. Leung C-S, Hartwick RWJ, Bédard YC. Correlation of cytologic and histologic features in variants of papillary carcinoma of the thyroid. Acta Cytol 1993;37:645

22. Sobrinho-Simoes MA, Nesland JM, Johannessen JV. Columnar-cell carcinoma. Another variant of poorly differentiated carcinoma of the thyroid. Am J Clin Pathol 1988;89:264

23. Fujimoto Y, Obara T, Ito Y, et al. Diffuse sclerosing variant of papillary carcinoma of the thyroid. Clinical importance, surgical treatment, and follow-up study. Cancer 1990;66:2306

24. Mizukami Y, Nonomura A, Michigishi T, et al. Diffuse sclerosing variant of papillary carcinoma of the thyroid. Report of three cases. Acta Pathol Jpn 1990;40:676

25. Lang W, Choritz H, Hundeshagen H. Risk factors in follicular thyroid carcinomas: a retrospective follow-up study covering a 14-year period with emphasis on morphologic findings. Am J Surg Pathol 1986;10:246

26. van Heerden JA, Hay ID, Goellner JR, et al. Follicular thyroid carcinoma with capsular invasion alone: a nonthreatening malignancy. Surgery 1992;112:1130

27. Emerick GT, Duh Q-Y, Siperstein AE, et al. Diagnosis, treatment, and outcome of follicular thyroid carcinoma. Cancer 1993; 72:3287

28. Brennan MD, Bergstralh EJ, van Heerden JA, McConahey WM. Follicular thyroid cancer treated at the Mayo Clinic, 1946 through 1970: initial manifestations, pathologic findings, therapy, and outcome. Mayo Clin Proc 1991;66:11

29. Donohue JH, Goldfien SD, Miller TR, et al. Do the prognoses of papillary and follicular thyroid carcinomas differ? Am J Surg 1984;148:168

30. Tubiana M, Schlumberger M, Rougier P, et al. Long-term results and prognostic factors in patients with differentiated thyroid carcinoma. Cancer 1985;55:794

31. Beierwaltes WH, Nishiyama RH, Thompson NW, et al. Survival time and "cure" in papillary and follicular thyroid carcinoma with distant metastases: statistics following University of Michigan therapy. J Nucl Med 1982;23:561

32. Balan KK, Raouf AH, Critchley M. Outcome of 249 patients attending a nuclear medicine department with well differentiated thyroid cancer: a 23 year review. Br J Radiol 1994;67:283

33. Ruegemer JJ, Hay ID, Bergstralh EJ, et al. Distant metastases in differentiated thyroid carcinoma: a multivariate analysis of prognostic variables. J Clin Endocrinol Metab 1988;67:501

34. Watson RG, Brennan MD, van Heerden JA, et al. Invasive Hürthle cell carcinoma of the thyroid: natural history and management. Mayo Clin Proc 1984;59:851

35. Rosen IB, Luk S, Katz I. Hürthle cell tumor behavior: dilemma and resolution. Surgery 1985;98:777

36. Thompson NW, Dunn EL, Batsakis JG, Nishiyama RH. Hürthle cell lesions of the thyroid gland. Surg Gynecol Obstet 1973; 139:555

37. Arganini M, Behar R, Wu TC, et al. Hürthle cell tumors: a twenty-five-year experience. Surgery 1986;100:1108

38. Samaan NA, Schultz PN, Haynie TP, Ordonez NG. Pulmonary metastasis of differentiated thyroid carcinoma: treatment results in 101 patients. J Clin Endocrinol Metab 1985;60:376

39. Herrera MF, Hay ID, Wu PS, et al. Hürthle cell (oxyphilic) papillary thyroid carcinoma: a variant with more aggressive biologic behavior. World J Surg 1994;16:669

40. Hay ID. Papillary thyroid carcinoma. Endocrinol Metab Clin North Am 1990;19:545

41. Allo MD, Christianson W, Doivunen D. Not all "occult" papillary carcinomas are "minimal." Surgery 1988;104:971

42. Cady B, Rossi R. An expanded view of risk-group definition in differentiated thyroid carcinoma. Surgery 1988;104:947

43. LiVolsi VA. Papillary lesions of the thyroid. In: Surgical pathology of the thyroid. Philadelphia: WB Saunders, 1990:136

44. Mazzaferri EL. Papillary thyroid carcinoma: factors influencing prognosis and current therapy. Semin Oncol 1987; 14:315

45. DeGroot LJ, Kaplan EL. Second operations for "completion" of thyroidectomy in treatment of differentiated thyroid cancer. Surgery 1991;110:936

46. Rao RS, Fakih AR, Mehta AR, et al. Completion thyroidectomy for thyroid carcinoma. Head Neck Surg 1987;9:284

47. Auguste LJ, Attie JN. Completion thyroidectomy for initially misdiagnosed thyroid cancer. Otolaryngol Clin North Am 1990;23:429

48. Crile G Jr, Antunez AR, Esselstyn CB Jr, et al. The advantages of subtotal thyroidectomy and suppression of TSH in the primary treatment of papillary carcinoma of the thyroid. Cancer 1985;55:2691

49. Massin JP, Savoie JC, Garnier H, et al. Pulmonary metastases in differentiated thyroid carcinoma. Study of 58 cases with implications for the primary tumor treatment. Cancer 1984;53:982

50. Cody HS III, Shah JP. Locally invasive, well-differentiated thyroid cancer. 22 years' experience at Memorial Sloan-Kettering Cancer Center. Am J Surg 1981;142:480

51. Salvesen H, Njolstad PR, Akslen LA, et al. Papillary thyroid carcinoma: a multivariate analysis of prognostic factors including an evaluation of the p-TNM staging system. Eur J Surg 1992;158:583

52. Hung W. Well-differentiated thyroid carcinomas in children and adolescents: a review. Endocrinologist 1994;4:117

53. De Keyser LFM, Van Herle AJ. Differentiated thyroid cancer in children. Head Neck Cancer 1985;8:100

54. Attie JN, Setzin M, Klein I. Thyroid carcinoma presenting as an enlarged cervical lymph node. Am J Surg 1993;166:428

55. Hay ID, Bergstralh EJ, Goellner JR, et al. Predicting outcome in papillary thyroid carcinoma: development of a reliable prognostic scoring system in a cohort of 1779 patients surgically treated at one institution during 1940 through 1989. Surgery 1993; 114:1050

56. Cunningham MP, Duda RB, Recant W, et al. Survival discriminants for differentiated thyroid cancer. Am J Surg 1990;160:344

57. Scheumann GFW, Gimm O, Wegener G, et al. Prognostic significance and surgical management of locoregional lymph node metastases in papillary thyroid cancer. World J Surg 1994;18:559

58. Akslen LA, Haldorsen T, Thoresen SO, Glattre E. Survival and causes of death in thyroid cancer: a population-based study of 2479 cases from Norway. Cancer Res 1991;51:1234

59. Sellers M, Beenken S, Blankenship A, et al. Prognostic significance of cervical lymph node metastases in differentiated thyroid cancer. Am J Surg 1992;164:578

60. Coburn MC, Wanebo HJ. Prognostic factors and management considerations in patients with cervical metastases of thyroid cancer. Am J Surg 1992;164:671

61. McHenry CR, Rosen IB, Walfish PG. Prospective management of nodal metastases in differentiated thyroid cancer. Am J Surg 1991;162:353

62. DeGroot LJ, Kaplan EL, McCormick M, Straus FH. Natural history, treatment, and course of papillary thyroid carcinoma. J Clin Endocrinol Metab 1990;71:414

63. Hoie J, Stenwig AE, Kullmann G, Lindegaard M. Distant metastases in papillary thyroid cancer. A review of 91 patients. Cancer 1988;61:1

64. Solan MJ. Multiple primary carcinomas as sequelae of treatment of pulmonary tuberculosis with repeated induced pneumothoraces. Case report and review of the literature. Am J Clin Oncol 1991;14:49

65. Casara D, Rubello D, Saladini G, et al. Different features of pulmonary metastases in differentiated thyroid cancer: natural history and multivariate statistical analysis of prognostic variables. J Nucl Med 1993;34:1626

66. Schlumberger M, De Vathaire F, Travagli JP, et al. Differentiated thyroid carcinoma in childhood: long term follow-up of 72 patients. J Clin Endocrinol Metab 1987;65:1088

67. Brown AP, Greening WP, McCready VR, et al. Radioiodine treatment of metastatic thyroid carcinoma: the Royal Marsden Hospital experience. Br J Radiol 1984;57:323

68. Schlumberger M, Tubiana M, De Vathaire F, et al. Long-term results of treatment of 283 patients with lung and bone metastases from differentiated thyroid carcinoma. J Clin Endocrinol Metab 1986;63:960

69. Vassilopoulou-Sellin R, Klein MJ, Smith TH, et al. Pulmonary metastases in children and young adults with differentiated thyroid cancer. Cancer 1993;71:1348

70. Hurley DL, Sizemore GW, McConahey WM. Prolonged remission of metastatic follicular thyroid carcinoma. Mayo Clin Proc 1993;68:1205

71. Maruyama M, Sugenoya A, Kobayashi S, et al. A case of papillary carcinoma of the thyroid with more than 30 years long-term asymptomatic pulmonary metastases. Clin Endocrinol 1993;38:331

72. Weiss SD, Orlich CC. Primary papillary carcinoma of a thyroglossal duct cyst: report of a case and literature review. Br J Surg 1991;78:87

73. Viswanathan K, Gierlowski TC, Schneider AB. Childhood thyroid cancer: characteristics and long-term outcome in children irradiated for benign conditions of the head and neck. Am J Dis Child 1994;148:260

74. Thoresen S, Akslen LA, Glattre E, Haldorsen T. Thyroid cancer in children in Norway 1953—1987. Eur J Cancer 1993;29A:365

75. Frankenthaler RA, Sellin RV, Cangir A, Goepfert H. Lymph node metastasis from papillary-follicular thyroid carcinoma in young patients. Am J Surg 1990;160:341

76. Tscholl-Ducommun J, Hedinger CE. Papillary thyroid carcinomas: morphology and prognosis. Virchows Arch [Pathol Anat] 1982;396:19

77. Mazzaferri EL. Thyroid cancer and Graves' disease. J Clin Endocrinol Metab 1990;70:826

78. Filetti S, Belfiore A, Amir SM, et al. The role of thyroid-stimulating antibodies of Graves' disease in differentiated thyroid cancer. Thyroid 1988;318:753

79. Ahuja S, Ernst H. Hyperthyroidism and thyroid carcinoma. Acta Endocrinol 1991;24:146

80. Belfiore A, Garofalo MR, Giuffrida D, et al. Increased aggressiveness of thyroid cancer in patients with Graves' disease. J Clin Endocrinol Metab 1990;70:830

81. Ozaki O, Ito K, Kobayashi K, et al. Thyroid carcinoma in Graves' disease (discussion). World J Surg 1990;14:437

82. Byar DP, Green SB, Dor P, et al. A prognostic index for thyroid carcinoma. A study of the E.O.R.T.C. Thyroid Cancer Cooperative Group. Eur J Cancer 1979;15:1033

83. American Joint Committee on Cancer. Head and Neck Tumors. Thyroid Gland. In: Beahrs OH, Henson DE, Hutter RVP, Myers MH, eds. Manual for staging of cancer. 4th ed. Philadelphia: JB Lippincott, 1992:53

84. Rosen IB, Bowden J, Luk SC, Simpson JA. Aggressive thyroid cancer in low-risk age population. Surgery 1987;102:1075

85. Jocham A, Joppich I, Hecker W, et al. Thyroid carcinoma in childhood: management and follow up of 11 cases. Eur J Pediatr 1994;153:17

86. Dulgeroff AJ, Hershman JM. Medical therapy for differentiated thyroid carcinoma. Endocr Rev 1994;15:500

87. Dulgeroff AJ, Geffner ME, Koyal SN, et al. Bromocriptine and triac therapy for hyperthyroidism due to pituitary resistance to thyroid hormone. J Clin Endocrinol Metab 1992;75:1071

88. Carayon P, Guibout M, Lissitzky S. Thyrotropin receptor-adenylate cyclase system in plasma membranes from normal and diseased human thyroid glands. J Endocrinol Invest 1978;1:321

89. Rossi RL, Cady B, Silverman ML, et al. Surgically incurable well-differentiated thyroid carcinoma. Prognostic factors and results of therapy. Arch Surg 1988;123:569

90. Cady B, Cohn K, Rossi RL, et al. The effect of thyroid hormone administration upon survival in patients with differentiated thyroid carcinoma. Surgery 1983;94:978

91. Clark OH. TSH suppression in the management of thyroid nodules and thyroid cancer. World J Surg 1981;5:39

92. Radetti G, Castellan C, Tató L, et al. Bone mineral density in children and adolescent females treated with high doses of L-thyroxine. Horm Res 1993;39:127

93. Faber J, Galloe AM. Changes in bone mass during prolonged subclinical hyperthyroidism due to L-thyroxine treatment: a meta-analysis. Acta Endocrinol 1994;130:350

94. Biondi B, Fazio S, Carella C, et al. Cardiac effects of long term thyrotropin-suppressive therapy with levothyroxine. J Clin Endocrinol Metab 1993;77:334

95. Sawin CT, Geller A, Wolf PA, et al. Low serum thyrotropin concentrations as a risk factor for atrial fibrillation in older persons. N Engl J Med 1994;331:1249

96. Bartalena L, Martino E, Pacchiarotti A, et al. Factors affecting suppression of endogenous thyrotropin secretion by thyroxine treatment: retrospective analysis in athyreotic and goitrous patients. J Clin Endocrinol Metab 1987;64:849

97. Burmeister LA, Goumaz MO, Mariash CN, Oppenheimer JH. Levothyroxine dose requirements for thyrotropin suppression in the treatment of differentiated thyroid cancer. J Clin Endocrinol Metab 1992;75:344

98. Wartofsky L. Use of sensitive TSH assay to determine optimal thyroid hormone therapy and avoid osteoporosis. Annu Rev Med 1991;42:341

99. Beierwaltes WH, Rabbani R, Dmuchowski C, et al. An analysis of "ablation of thyroid remnants" with I-131 in 511 patients from 1947—1984: experience at University of Michigan. J Nucl Med 1984;25:1287

100. Goolden AWG. The indications for ablating normal thyroid tissue with 131-I in differentiated thyroid cancer. Clin Endocrinol 1985;23:81

101. DeGroot LJ, Reilly M. Comparison of 30- and 50-mCi doses of iodine-131 for thyroid ablation. Ann Intern Med 1982;96:51

102. Maxon HR, Englaro EE, Thomas SR, et al. Radioiodine-131 therapy for well-differentiated thyroid cancer—a quantitative radiation dosimetric approach: outcome and validation in 85 patients. J Nucl Med 1992;33:1132

103. Maxon HR, Thomas SR, Hertzberg VS, et al. Relation between effective radiation dose and outcome of radioiodine therapy for thyroid cancer. Thyroid 1983;309:937

104. Snyder J, Gorman C, Scanlon P. Thyroid remnant ablation: questionable pursuit of an ill-defined goal. J Nucl Med 1983;24:659

105. Kuni CC, Klingensmith WC. Failure of low doses of 131-I to ablate residual thyroid tissue following surgery for thyroid cancer. Radiology 1980;137:773

106. Siddiqui AR, Edmondson J, Wellman HN, et al. Feasibility of low doses of I-131 for thyroid ablation in postsurgical patients with thyroid carcinoma. Clin Nucl Med 1981;6:158

107. Ramanna L, Waxman AD, Brachman MB, et al. Evaluation of low-dose radioiodine ablation therapy in postsurgical thyroid cancer patients. Clin Nucl Med 1985;10:791

108. Johansen K, Woodhouse NJ, Odugbesan O. Comparison of 1073 MBq and 3700 MBq iodine-131 in postoperative ablation of residual thyroid tissue in patients with differentiated thyroid cancer. J Nucl Med 1991;32:252

109. Ozata M, Suzuki S, Miyamoto T, et al. Serum thyroglobulin in the follow-up of patients with treated differentiated cancer. J Clin Endocrinol Metab 1994;79:98

110. Krishnamurthy GT, Blahd WH. Radioiodine I-131 therapy in the management of thyroid cancer. A prospective study. Cancer 1977;40:195

111. Edmonds CJ, Hayes S, Kermode JC, Thompson BD. Measurement of serum TSH and thyroid hormones in the management of treatment of thyroid carcinoma with radioiodine. Br J Radiol 1977;50:799

112. Lakshmanan M, Schaffer A, Robbins J, et al. A simplified low iodine diet in I-131 scanning and therapy of thyroid cancer. Clin Nucl Med 1988;2:866

113. Goldman JM, Line BR, Aamodt RL, Robbins J. Influence of triiodothyronine withdrawal time on 131-I uptake postthyroidectomy for thyroid cancer. J Clin Endocrinol Metab 1980;50:734

114. Meier CA, Braverman LE, Ebner SA, et al. Diagnostic use of recombinant human thyrotropin in patients with thyroid carcinoma (phase I/II study). J Clin Endocrinol Metab 1994;78:188

115. Maxon HR, Boehringer TA, Drilling J. Low iodine diet in I-131 ablation of thyroid remnants. Clin Nucl Med 1983;8:123

116. Maruca J, Santner S, Miller K, Santen RJ. Prolonged iodine clearance with a depletion regimen for thyroid carcinoma: concise communication. J Nucl Med 1984;25:1089

117. Pons F, Carrio I, Estorch M, et al. Lithium as an adjuvant of iodine-131 uptake when treating patients with well-differentiated thyroid carcinoma. Clin Nucl Med 1987;8:644

118. Park HM, Perkins OW, Edmondson JW, et al. Influence of diagnostic radioiodines on the uptake of ablative dose of iodine-131. Thyroid 1994;4:49

119. Greenler DP, Klein HA. The scope of false-positive iodine-131 images for thyroid carcinoma. Clin Nucl Med 1989;14:111

120. Brachman MB, Rothman BJ, Ramanna L, et al. False-positive iodine-131 body scan caused by a large renal cyst. Clin Nucl Med 1988;13:416

121. Park HM, Tarver RD, Schauwecker DS, Burt R. Spurious thyroid cancer metastasis: saliva contamination artifact in high dose iodine-131 metastases survey. J Nucl Med 1986;27:634

122. Rosenbaum RC, Johnston GS, Valente WA. Frequency of hepatic visualization during I-131 imaging for metastatic thyroid carcinoma. Clin Nucl Med 1988;13:657

123. Němec J, Zamrazil V, Pohunková D, Röhling S. Radioiodide treatment of pulmonary metastases of differentiated thyroid cancer. Results and prognostic factors. Nuklearmedizin 1979;18:86

124. McHenry C, Jarosz H, Davis M, et al. Selective postoperative radioactive iodine treatment of thyroid carcinoma. Surgery 1989;106:956

125. Samaan NA, Schultz PN, Hickey RC, et al. Well-differentiated thyroid carcinoma and the results of various modalities of treatment. A retrospective review of 1599 patients. J Clin Endocrinol Metab 1992;75:714

126. Beierwaltes WH. Radioiodine therapy of thyroid disease. Int J Radiat Appl Instrum [B] 1987;14:177

127. Pineda JD, Lee T, Robbins J. Treating metastatic thyroid cancer. Endocrinologist 1992;3:433

128. Maxon H III. The role of I-131 in the treatment of thyroid cancer. Thyroid Today 1993;16:1

129. Maini CL, Sciuto R, Tofani A. Delayed thyroid-stimulating hormone suppression by L-thyroxine in the management of differentiated thyroid carcinoma. Eur J Cancer [A] 1993;29A:2071

130. Burmeister LA, duCret RP, Mariash CN. Local reactions to radioiodine in the treatment of thyroid cancer. Am J Med 1991;90:217

131. Schlumberger M, Arcangioli O, Piekarski JD, et al. Detection and treatment of lung metastases of differentiated thyroid carcinoma in patients with normal chest X-rays. J Nucl Med 1988;29:1790

132. Gunter HH, Schober O, Schwarzrock R, Hundeshagen H. Hematologic long-term modifications after radio-iodine therapy in carcinoma of the thyroid gland. II. Modifications of the bone marrow including leukemia. Strahlenther Onkol 1986;163:475

133. Edmonds CJ, Smith T. The long-term hazards of the treatment of thyroid cancer with radioiodine. Br J Radiol 1986;59:45

134. Varma VM, Beierwaltes WH, Nofal MM, et al. Treatment of thyroid cancer: death rates after surgery and after surgery followed by sodium iodide I-131. JAMA 1970;214:1437

135. Cancer statistics review 1973—87. Bethesda, MD: U.S. Department of Health and Human Services, Public Health Service, NIH, 1991:I.39

136. Gorlin JB, Sallan SE. Thyroid cancer in childhood. Endocrinol Metab Clin North Am 1990;19:649

137. Buckwalter JA, Gurll NJ, Thomas CG Jr. Cancer of the thyroid in youth. World J Surg 1981;5:15

138. La Quaglia MP, Corbally MT, Heller G, et al. Recurrence and morbidity in differentiated thyroid carcinoma in children. Surgery 1988;104:1149

139. Goepfert H, Dichtel WJ, Samaan NA. Thryoid cancer in children and teenagers. Arch Otolaryngol 1984;110:72

140. Harness JK, Thompson NW, McLeod MK, et al. Differentiated thyroid carcinoma in children and adolescents. World J Surg 1992;16:547

141. Beaugie JM, Brown CL, Doniach I, Richardson JE. Primary malignant tumours of the thyroid: the relationship between histological classification and clinical behaviour. Br J Surg 1976;63:173

142. Zimmerman D, Hay I, Bergstralh E. Papillary thyroid carcinoma in children. In: Robbins J, ed. Treatment of thryoid cancer in childhood: proceedings of a workshop held September 10—11, 1992, at the NIH in Bethesda, Maryland. DOE/EH-0406, Springfield, VA: U.S. Department of Commerce, 1992:3

143. Ceccarelli C, Pacini F, Lippi F, et al. Thryoid cancer in children and adolescents. Surgery 1988;104:1143

144. Lamberg BA, Karkinen Jaaskelainen M, Franssila KO. Differentiated follicle-derived thyroid carcinoma in children. Acta Paediatr Scand 1989;78:419

145. Sherman SI, Tielens ET, Sostre S, et al. Clinical utility of posttreatment radioiodine scans in the management of patients with thyroid carcinoma. J Clin Endocrinol Metab 1994;78:629

146. Pacini F, Lippi F, Formica N, et al. Therapeutic doses of iodine-131 reveal undiagnosed metastases in thyroid cancer patients with detectable serum thyroglobulin levels. J Nucl Med 1987;28:1888

147. Maxon HR, Thomas SR, Saenger EL, et al. Ionizing irradiation and the induction of clinically significant disease in the human thyroid gland. Am J Med 1977;63:967

148. Goolden AWG, Kam KC, Fitzpatrick ML, Munro AJ. Oedema of the neck after ablation of the thyroid with radioactive iodine. Br J Radiol 1986;59:583

149. Lee TC, Harbert JC, Dejter SW, et al. Vocal cord paralysis following I-131 ablation of a postthyroidectomy remnant. J Nucl Med 1985;26:49

150. Allweiss P, Braunstein GD, Katz A, Waxman A. Sialadenitis following I-131 therapy for thyroid carcinoma: concise communication. J Nucl Med 1984;25:755

151. Goolden AW. The use of radioactive iodine in thyroid carcinoma. Eur J Cancer Clin Oncol 1988;24:339

152. Van Nostrand D, Neutze J, Atkins F. Side effects of "rational dose" iodine-131 therapy for metastatic well-differentiated thyroid carcinoma. J Nucl Med 1986;27:1519

153. Datz FL. Cerebral edema following iodine-131 therapy for thyroid carcinoma metastatic to the brain. J Nucl Med 1986;27:637

154. Maxon H III, Smith HS. Radioiodine-131 in the diagnosis and treatment of metastatic well differentiated thyroid cancer. Endocrinol Metab Clin North Am 1990;19:685

155. Levenson D, Gulec S, Sonenberg M, et al. Peripheral facial nerve palsy after high-dose radioiodine therapy in patients with papillary thyroid carcinoma. Ann Intern Med 1994;120:576

156. Raymond JP, Izembart M, Marliac V, et al. Temporary ovarian failure in thyroid cancer patients after thyroid remnant ablation with radioactive iodine. J Clin Endocrinol Metab 1989;69:186

157. Handelsman DJ, Turtle JR. Testicular damage after radioactive iodine (I-131) therapy for thyroid cancer. Clin Endocrinol 1983;18:465

158. Pacini F, Gasperi M, Fugazzola L, et al. Testicular function in patients with differentiated thyroid carcinoma treated with radioiodine. J Nucl Med 1994;35:1418

159. Sarkar SD, Beierwaltes WH, Gill SP, Cowley BJ. Subsequent fertility and birth histories of children and adolescents treated with ^{131}I for thyroid cancer. J Nucl Med 1976;17:460

160. Wong JB, Kaplan MM, Meyer KB, Pauker SG. Ablative radioactive iodine therapy for apparently localized thyroid carcinoma. A decision analytic perspective. Endocrinol Metab Clin North Am 1990;19:741

161. Bitton R, Sachmechi I, Benegalrao Y, Schneider BS. Leukemia after a small dose of radioiodine for metastatic thyroid cancer. J Clin Endocrinol Metab 1993;77:1423

162. Hall P, Holm LE, Lundell G. Second primary tumors following thyroid cancer. A Swedish record-linkage study. Acta Oncol 1990;29:869

163. Ésik O, Németh G, Eller J. Prophylactic external irradiation in differentiated thyroid cancer: a retrospective study over a 30-year observation period. Oncology 1994;51:372

164. Tubiana M, Haddad E, Schlumberger M, et al. External radiotherapy in thyroid cancers. Cancer 1985;55:2062

165. O'Connell MEA, A'Hern RP, Harmer CL. Results of external beam radiotherapy in differentiated thyroid carcinoma: a retrospective study from the Royal Marsden Hospital. Eur J Cancer 1994;30A:733

166. Droz JP, Schlumberger M, Rougier P, et al. Chemotherapy in metastatic nonanaplastic thyroid cancer: experience at the Institut Gustave-Roussy. Tumori 1990;76:480

167. Ahuja S, Ernst H. Chemotherapy of thyroid carcinoma. J Endocrinol Invest 1987;10:303

168. Kim JH, Leeper RD. Treatment of locally advanced thyroid carcinoma with combination doxorubicin and radiation therapy. Cancer 1987;60:2372

169. Ronga G, Fiorentino A, Fragasso G, et al. Complementary role of whole body scan and serum thyroglobulin determination in the follow-up of differentiated thyroid carcinoma. Ital J Surg Sci 1986;16:11

170. Muller-Gartner HW, Schneider C. Clinical evaluation of tumor characteristics predisposing serum thyroglobulin to be undetectable in patients with differentiated thyroid cancer. Cancer 1988;61:976

171. Piekarski JD, Schlumberger M, Leclere J, et al. Chest computed tomography (CT) in patients with micronodular lung metastases of differentiated thyroid carcinoma. Int J Radiat Oncol Biol Phys 1985;11:1023

172. Brendel AJ, Lambert B, Guyot M, et al. Low levels of serum thyroglobulin after withdrawal of thyroid suppression therapy in the follow up of differentiated thyroid carcinoma. Eur J Nucl Med 1990;16:35

173. Hoefnagel CA, Delprat CC, Marcuse HR, de Vijlder JJ. Role of thallium-201 total-body scintigraphy in follow-up of thyroid carcinoma. J Nucl Med 1986;27:1854

174. Ramanna L, Waxman A, Braunstein G. Thallium-201 scintigraphy in differentiated thyroid cancer: comparison with radioiodine scintigraphy and serum thyroglobulin determinations. J Nucl Med 1991;32:441

175. Van Sorge-van Boxtel RAJ, Van Eck-Smit BLF, Goslings BM. Comparison of serum thyroglobulin, ^{131}I and ^{201}Tl scintigraphy in the postoperative follow-up of differentiated thyroid cancer. Nucl Med Commun 1993;12:365

176. Burman KD, Anderson JH, Wartofsky L, et al. Management of patients with thyroid carcinoma: application of thallium-201 scintigraphy and magnetic resonance imaging. J Nucl Med 1990; 31:1958

177. Brendel AJ, Guyot M, Jeandot R, et al. Thallium-201 imaging in the follow-up of differentiated thyroid carcinoma. J Nucl Med 1988;29:1515

178. Charkes ND, Vitti RA, Brooks K. Thallium-201 SPECT increases detectability of thyroid cancer metastases. J Nucl Med 1990; 31:147

179. DeGroot LJ, Reilly M. Use of isotope bone scans and skeletal survey X-rays in the follow-up of patients with thyroid carcinoma. J Endocrinol Invest 1984;7:175

Werner and Ingbar's The Thyroid, Seventh Edition,
edited by Lewis E. Braverman and Robert D. Utiger.
Lippincott–Raven Publishers, Philadelphia, © 1996

81

Medullary Thyroid Carcinoma

Douglas W. Ball
Stephen B. Baylin
Andree C. de Bustros

Although relatively uncommon, medullary thyroid carcinoma (MTC) is noteworthy for its distinctive biochemical and genetic features and unique clinical associations. MTC offers researchers an important experimental model to study tumorigenesis and tumor evolution. Recent key advances that have elucidated the genetic basis of MTC now hold tremendous promise for improving the diagnosis and treatment of this cancer. In this chapter, we highlight the important landmarks in the history of MTC, offer a perspective on the biology of this disease, and suggest guidelines for the diagnosis and management of MTC patients.

HISTORY

Medullary (or solid) thyroid carcinoma was first recognized as a distinct histologic type of thyroid cancer by Hazzard and associates in 1959.[1] In retrospect, many such patients had previously been classified as having anaplastic or small cell thyroid cancer.[2] In 1961, Sipple[3] reported a high incidence of thyroid cancer in patients with pheochromocytomas. Several investigators subsequently recognized that the thyroid cancers that occurred in these patients resembled the medullary type identified by Hazzard and that these tumors followed an autosomal dominant inheritance pattern along with hyperparathyroidism and, occasionally, multiple mucosal neuromas.[4–7] In 1962, Copp and colleagues[8] identified a circulating hypocalcemic substance in plasma that they termed calcitonin. In 1964, Foster and coworkers[9] suggested that calcitonin was produced by the thyroid parafollicular cells. Pearse[10] subsequently classi-

fied these cells as belonging to the so-called amine precursor uptake and decarboxylation (APUD) cell system. In a landmark study, Williams[11] demonstrated that MTC arises from the parafollicular C cells. Melvin and Tashjian[12] demonstrated in 1968 that high levels of calcitonin were present in tumors and the serum of patients with MTC.

In 1987, two groups of investigators provided initial evidence that a susceptibility locus for inherited MTC resided on human chromosome 10.[13,14] In 1993, Mulligan and colleagues[15] and other groups[16,17] proved conclusively that characteristic mutations of a single gene on chromosome 10, the ret protooncogene, were responsible for the different inherited forms of MTC.

CLASSIFICATION

Medullary thyroid carcinoma is an uncommon thyroid tumor, accounting for 3% to 5% of all thyroid malignancies and a somewhat higher proportion of the deaths from thyroid cancer.[18,19] Most patients with MTC (80%) have no family history of the disease. The remaining 20% inherit MTC as an autosomal dominant trait in one of three distinct clinical syndromes (Table 81-1). The term *multiple endocrine neoplasia type 2* (MEN 2) was suggested by Steiner and colleagues[20] in 1968 to distinguish the syndrome of MTC, pheochromocytoma, and hyperparathyroidism from Wermer's syndrome or MEN 1 (parathyroid, pituitary, and pancreatic islet tumors).[21] MEN 2A is now the preferred term for the syndrome defined by Steiner. MEN 2B refers to a distinct syndrome of MTC, pheochromocy-

TABLE 81-1.
Classification of Medullary Thyroid Carcinoma

Type	Associated Lesions	Ret Gene Mutation	Clinical Behavior
Sporadic	None	Somatic (~33% of tumors) Tyrosine kinase domain	Intermediate
FMTC	None	Germline Extracellular domain	Less aggressive
MEN 2A	Pheochromocytoma Hyperparathyroidism	Germline Extracellular domain	Intermediate
MEN 2B	Pheochromocytoma Ganglioneuromas Marfanoid habitus	Germline Tyrosine kinase domain	Aggressive

FMTC, isolated familial medullary thyroid carcinoma; MEN, multiple endocrine neoplasia.

toma, multiple mucosal neuromas, and a marfanoid body habitus. A syndrome of familial MTC (FMTC) in the absence of other endocrinopathy or neural abnormality was characterized by Farndon and colleagues.[22] Recent molecular genetic studies have confirmed that all three of these syndromes stem from characteristic mutations of the ret tyrosine kinase receptor gene on chromosome 10, detailed below. Finally, two interesting clinical variants of MEN 2A have been described. MEN 2A with cutaneous lichen amyloidosis consists of typical manifestations of MEN 2A plus a characteristic pruritic plaquelike skin rash located over the scapular region.[23,24] MEN 2A with concurrent Hirschsprung's disease, with either partial or extensive colonic aganglionosis, has been tied to a specific subset of the ret gene mutations associated with MEN 2A.[25]

The occurrence of MTC in both sporadic and familial forms makes the clinical approach to this tumor different from other forms of thyroid cancer. First, all patients with MTC should be suspected of having the genetic form of the disease because there is an appreciable prevalence of cryptic heritable disease in the absence of an obvious family history.[26] Second, the potential presence of associated conditions, particularly pheochromocytoma, must be recognized before subjecting patients to thyroidectomy. Third, the clinical course of MTC is highly variable, making it essential to individualize the management of each patient with this cancer. MTC has a predilection for early regional lymph node metastasis, placing a premium on early diagnosis and an appropriate surgical approach.

CELLS OF ORIGIN AND BIOCHEMISTRY

Medullary thyroid carcinoma arises from the upper two-thirds of the thyroid lobes, where the parafollicular C cells reside. Unlike endodermally derived thyroid follicular epithelial cells, the C cells originate in embryonic neural crest and enter the developing thyroid when the ultimobranchial body from the fourth pharyngeal pouch fuses with thyroid epithelium[27,28] (see chap 2). The characteristic secretory product of C cells, and the most useful circulating marker for MTC, is calcitonin, a 32-amino acid peptide. Calcitonin is encoded by a multiexonic gene on chromosome 11p, which yields two distinct messen-

ger RNA (mRNA) species. In addition to calcitonin itself, alternative splicing of the primary calcitonin gene transcript generates calcitonin gene-related peptide (CGRP)[29,30] (Fig 81-1). The resulting mature calcitonin and CGRPs contain both common and unique regions and interact with unique receptors. Production of calcitonin versus CGRP is regulated in a highly tissue-specific fashion. Calcitonin predominates in thyroid C cells, whereas CGRP predominates in the brain and other neural tissues.[29] Many extrathyroidal tissues produce moderate amounts of calcitonin, including pulmonary neuroendocrine cells, adrenal medulla, and gastrointestinal endocrine cells.[31] Other pathologic causes of calcitonin elevation (generally at lower levels than in MTC) include pulmonary inflammatory diseases, small cell lung cancer, gastrinoma, carcinoid tumors, and renal failure.[32,33]

In contrast to normal thyroid C cells, MTC tumors can produce both CGRP and calcitonin mRNAs in significant quantities.[34] Although both hormones may circulate at high levels in the blood of patients with MTC, the CGRP levels are much more variable and frequently lower than are levels of calcitonin.[30,35,36] Whereas plasma calcitonin increases briskly in response to pentagastrin stimulation, CGRP responses are variable.[35,36] The role of CGRP in the pathophysiology of MTC is unclear. As a powerful vasodilator, CGRP may play a role in the flushing observed in certain patients with MTC. MTC tumors also produce katacalcin[37] (also known as C-CAP), a 21-amino acid peptide derived from the carboxyl terminus of the calcitonin propeptide by alternate posttranslational processing (see Fig 81-1). Katacalcin is cosecreted with calcitonin and responds to the same stimuli. Its biologic function, if any, is unknown.

In addition to calcitonin gene products, MTC cells express several biochemical markers that typify secretory cells of the diffuse neuroendocrine system. These biochemical markers include additional small polypeptide hormones such as somatostatin,[38] adrenocorticotropic hormone,[39] and gastrin-releasing peptide.[40] Like several other neural and neuroendocrine cell types, MTC cells express the enzyme L-dopa decarboxylase[41] through which biogenic amines such as serotonin are synthesized. MTC cells produce other neuroendocrine markers such as chromogranin A,[42] neuron-specific enolase,[43,44] and the

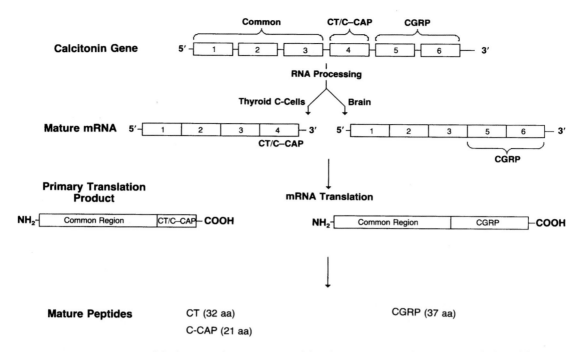

FIGURE 81-1. Diagram of the human calcitonin gene and the alternative RNA splicing pattern. (Adapted from Amara SG, Jonas J, Rosenfeld MG, Ong ES, Evans RM. Alternative RNA processing in calcitonin gene expression generates mRNAs encoding different polypeptide products. Nature 1982; 298:240)

neural cell adhesion molecule (NCAM).[45] Preliminary evidence suggests that the degree of sialic acid modification of NCAM may possibly discriminate between primary (genetic) C-cell hyperplasia and secondary forms of this condition.[45]

Several hormonal products of MTC cells may result in significant clinical manifestations. Elevation of serum calcitonin, per se, appears to have little effect on systemic calcium metabolism or on bone physiology. CGRP release may contribute to episodes of both flushing and diarrhea.[46] Other proposed mediators include vasoactive intestinal peptide,[47] substance P,[48] serotonin,[49] and prostaglandins.[50]

MOLECULAR GENETICS

Recent studies by a number of groups have clarified the molecular etiology of the inherited forms of MTC and provided important insight into the pathogenesis of the more common sporadic form of the disease. The ret proto-oncogene encodes a 150- to 170-kd membrane-associated tyrosine kinase receptor with some resemblance to the epidermal growth factor receptor and related growth factor receptors. The structural domains of ret include an extracellular domain with a cysteine-rich region, a single hydrophobic transmembrane domain, and a carboxyl-terminal tyrosine kinase domain with catalytic and substrate recognition sites (Fig 81-2). To date, both the extracellular ligand(s) and intracellular substrates for the receptor remain obscure. Normal expression of the ret gene in embryonic development is limited to certain neural crest derivatives including the thyroid C cells, adrenal chromaffin cells, enteric ganglia, and to sites in the developing brain, spinal cord, kidney, and urinary tract.[51,52] A subset of calcitonin-positive thyroid C cells and adrenal chromaffin cells continue to express ret after birth.[52] Among tumors, significant ret mRNA expression appears to be limited to MTC, pheochromocytomas, and neuroblastomas.[53,54]

Before the discovery of ret gene mutations in inherited MTC, ret was already known to function as a proto-oncogene, that is, a gene with the potential to promote cancers when activated by specific mutations. Rearrangements of the ret gene, causing deletion of the extracellular and transmembrane portions of the encoded protein, can result in a constitutively active tyrosine kinase with the potential to transform normal cells.[55] In papillary thyroid cancer, a somatic (i.e., tumor-specific) ret gene rearrangement has been detected as a transforming oncogene in 25% of cases[56,57] (the papillary thyroid cancer [PTC] oncogene; see chap 80).

Using a variety of molecular genetic techniques, specific mutations have been discovered for each of the inherited forms of MTC detailed above. In MEN 2A, germline mutations (i.e., in all tissues including germ cells) at five different cysteine residues can be found in the great majority of kindreds.[15,16,58] These mutations originate as single base transitions within exons 10 and 11 of the ret gene. Both the normal and mutated alleles are expressed in the MTC tumor tissue.[15] From a structure-function relationship, it is fascinating that the MEN 2A mutations are confined to a small cluster of cysteine residues located immediately extracellular to the transmembrane domain and that many different amino acid substitutions can be seen (see Fig 81-2). Presumably, disruption of the pattern of cysteine disulfide linkages leads to a critical alteration of normal intramolecular protein folding in the absence of ligand. An important recent study by Santoro and colleagues indicates that these MEN 2A mutations result in

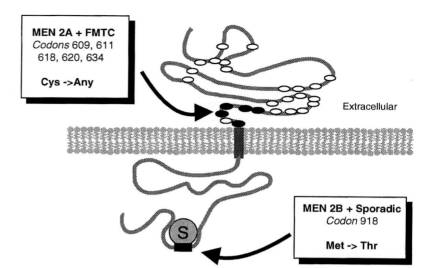

FIGURE 81-2. Diagram of the *ret* protein structure, indicating sites of mutations in hereditary and sporadic MTC. Extracellular cysteine residues are indicated by shaded ovals (sites of known mutations in MEN 2A and FMTC) and unshaded ovals (sites without known mutation). The putative substrate recognition site (mutated in MEN 2B and in some cases of sporadic MTC) is indicated by a shaded rectangle and a substrate molecule by "S." The protein folding pattern represented here is conjectural.

steady-state dimerization and autophosphorylation of the receptor compared to the normal ret protein, which exists as a nonphosphorylated monomer.[59] These findings are hallmarks of ligand-independent activation of the receptor. Unlike the normal receptor, the MEN 2A mutant is capable of causing malignant transformation when it is introduced into cultured fibroblasts, establishing that the mutant receptor functions as an inherited dominant oncogene in these families.[59]

Several groups have linked the prevalence of individual manifestations of the MEN 2A syndrome to specific ret mutation sites. For example, in a recent series, 22 of 30 MEN 2A families with hyperparathyroidism had a specific cysteine 634 mutation (to arginine) versus only 2 of 24 MEN 2A kindreds without hyperparathyroidism.[60] The reason for this association is currently unknown. In the case of isolated FMTC, most, but not all, kindreds have detectable mutations in the same group of cysteine residues that are altered in MEN 2A. Curiously, identical ret mutations may be found both in FMTC kindreds with no history of pheochromocytoma and in MEN 2A kindreds that have a prominent history of pheochromocytoma. Mulligan and associates have observed that mutations located closer to the membrane, especially at cysteine 634, are more commonly associated with MEN 2A, whereas more proximal mutations (cysteine 609, 611, 618, and 620) are more commonly associated with FMTC.[60] In studies to date, a minority of FMTC families have had no detectable ret gene mutation in this region, although by genetic linkage analysis, their disorder maps to the same segment of chromosome 10 as do typical FMTC and MEN 2A.[16,58] Such findings raise the possibility of genetic heterogeneity in FMTC that may interfere with the sensitivity of prospective DNA screening.

In MEN 2B, a single base pair mutation in ret codon 918 within the tyrosine kinase domain results in a substitution of a threonine residue for the normal methionine.[17,61] This specific amino acid substitution may cause a critical change in the substrate specificity of the kinase (see Fig 81-2).[59,61] In comparison with the ret MEN 2A mutations, the MEN 2B mutant form has equivalent potential to transform fibroblast cell lines but exhibits less intense autophosphorylation and little potential to spontaneously dimerize.[59] Perhaps 50% of the MEN 2B mutations are de novo germline mutations with no representation in the DNA of either parent. Strikingly, the vast majority of these de novo germline mutations occur on the allele inherited from the patient's father.[62] Additional studies in progress may help to clarify the oncogenic potency of the ret MEN 2B mutation.

As in the case of several other heritable tumors, the more common sporadic form of MTC occasionally is associated with somatic mutations at the same location as germline mutations in the inherited form. Approximately 33% of sporadic MTC tumors exhibit a ret codon 918 mutation, indistinguishable from the MEN 2B form.[17,63,64] Consistent with the dominant nature of the mutant gene, loss of the corresponding normal ret allele typically is not observed. Such patients do not have ret mutations in their germline leukocytes, confirming that they do not represent new cases of MEN 2B.[63,64] At this point, there is insufficient evidence to suggest that the subset of sporadic MTCs that carry a ret mutation may have a distinct prognosis compared to the majority of sporadic MTCs that lack a ret mutation. To date, somatic ret mutations of the MEN 2A variety have not been reported in sporadic MTC tumors although de novo germline mutations of the MEN 2A type may be encountered rarely in MTC patients with a negative family history.[65] Sporadic pheochromocytoma appears to have a somewhat lower frequency of somatic ret gene mutation than does sporadic MTC, approximately 10% to 20% of cases, with involvement reported for both the MEN 2A and MEN 2B sites.[63,66]

In summary, recent advances in the molecular genetics of MTC now afford a means for DNA-based diagnosis of gene carriers in known families and the potential to clarify the status of individuals with a negative family history. The practical application of these tests is described below.

TUMOR EVOLUTION: BIOCHEMICAL AND MOLECULAR CHANGES

The formation of MTC is distinguished by several well-characterized stages of tumor progression, illustrated in Figure 81-3. In hereditary disease, the initial manifestation is diffuse C-cell hyperplasia, followed by outgrowth of multiple foci of microscopic carcinoma. Each nascent cancer represents a separate clone of tumor cells that has arisen from an individual hyperplastic C cell.[67] Progression from C-cell hyperplasia to microscopic and then gross MTC frequently is accompanied by tumor cell heterogeneity and a variable loss in endocrine markers including calcitonin production.[68,69] Because all thyroid C cells appear to have the potential for hyperplasia in inherited MTC, it is likely that a single activated copy of the ret gene can be sufficient to cause an increase in growth and initiate the hyperplasia process. The role of ret in subsequent tumor progression steps is currently unknown. Also of significant interest is whether mutation of ret is an early or late event in the development of sporadic MTC.

By analogy to the multistage model of colon cancer first proposed by Vogelstein and colleagues[70] and subsequently illustrated in a variety of tumors, it is likely that several subsequent mutational events, involving tumor suppressor genes or oncogenes, are necessary for tumor progression in MTC. An extensive search for evidence of tumor suppressor gene dysfunction in MTC has indicated that a significant percentage of MTC tumors lose genetic material from the short arms of chromosomes 1 and 22 (25% and 20%, respectively).[71] Other studies have shown similar or slightly lower rates of loss.[72,73] Chromosomal losses of this kind, especially when they are fre-

quent in a given tumor type, may indicate the presence of an inactivating mutation of a tumor suppressor gene on the remaining chromosome copy. The identity of any putative suppressor genes on chromosomes 1 and 22 and their actual importance in MTC tumorigenesis remain obscure. Chromosome 1 losses are more frequent in pheochromocytoma, especially in MEN 2A patients.[72] To date, there is no evidence for losses or mutations in MTC among other well-characterized tumor suppressor genes including p53 on chromosome 17, the grouping of suppressor loci including the Von-Hippel Lindau gene on chromosome 3p, and the retinoblastoma gene on chromosome 13.[71,74] Significantly, there is no increased rate of loss of the ret gene site on chromosome 10, consistent with the concept that ret mutations act as dominant, activating mutations rather than as inactivating mutations of a tumor suppressor protein.[75,76]

A second important mechanism for tumor progression is the acquisition of a dominant oncogene function, either by an activating mutation of the normal proto-oncogene (as in the case of ret), or by mechanisms resulting in increased transcription such as amplification of gene copy number, or chromosomal translocation of the proto-oncogene to the site of an active promoter. Ret itself continues to be expressed at high levels in MTC tumors as they progress. In fact, both the normal and mutant ret mRNA species can be detected in tumor

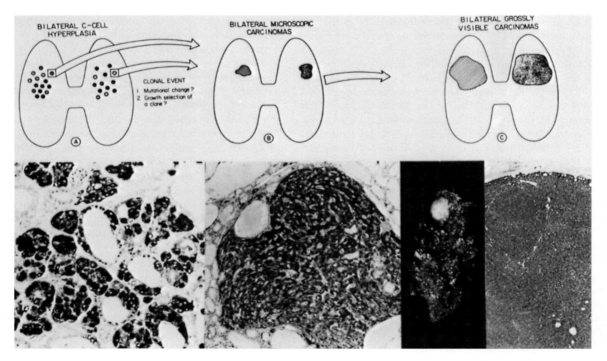

FIGURE 81-3. Stages of MTC evolution. The upper panel shows and diagrammatic representation of C-cell hyperplasia (*A*), microscopic carcinoma (*B*), and frank tumor (*C*). The stippled versus the striped pattern for each C cell in *A* denotes a separate clone, and each tumor in *B* and *C* arises from a separate clone. The lower panel shows calcitonin (CT) immunoperoxidase staining of hyperplastic C cells (*A*), a microscopic tumor (*B*), and of a tumor nodule shown in a very low power photomicrograph (*C*). The dark staining pattern throughout indicates a homogeneous cellular distribution of immunoreactive CT. (Baylin SB, Mendelsohn G. Medullary thyroid carcinoma: a model for the study of human tumor progression and cell heterogeneity. In Owens AH Jr, Coffey DS, Baylin SB, eds. Tumor cell heterogeneity: origins and implications. Vol 4. New York: Academic Press, 1982:12)

tissue from patients with hereditary MTC.[15] Studies are underway to determine whether ret plays an ongoing role in the growth advantage enjoyed by MTC tumors as compared to normal C cells. Conceivably, dysregulation of ret gene expression could contribute to the growth of these tumors.

The role of other oncogenes in MTC including the myc and ras families has been under investigation. High c-myc and N-myc gene expression has been reported in MTC[77]; increased N-myc expression may correlate with an adverse prognosis.[78] Interestingly, ras gene mutations, although frequent in many epithelial cancers, are uncommon in MTC as well as in pheochromocytoma and neuroblastoma, the other tumors that frequently express ret.[79] Indeed, insertion of an activated ras gene into cultured MTC cells[80] or into rodent pheochromocytoma cells[81] leads to slower growth and increased neuroendocrine differentiation. The potential interplay between ras and ret, and between ras and other growth-related receptors, including the neurotrophic growth factor receptors, may provide a fruitful target for understanding the pathobiology of MTC.[82]

PATHOLOGY

Hyperplasia of C cells appears microscopically as increased clusters of C cells, usually visualized only through calcitonin immunostaining, that are interspersed between normal-appearing thyroid follicles. Although initial studies indicated that normal thyroid glands contained fewer than 10 C cells per low power field, more recent studies indicate that some normal glands may contain as many as 50 C cells per low power field.[83] Relative increases in C-cell number are commonly seen in infants and occasionally in healthy elderly adults.[84,85] In C-cell hyperplasia, the increased population of normal-appearing C cells sometimes forms nodular aggregates (see Fig 81-3). C-cell hyperplasia may be difficult to distinguish from normal variation at the lower end of the spectrum and from microscopic MTC at the upper end.[86] Frank C-cell hyperplasia is not specific for hereditary MTC. A moderate degree of C-cell hyperplasia can be recognized in up to 20% of cases of autoimmune thyroiditis,[87] adjacent to follicular adenoma and follicular carcinoma,[88] and in response to chronic hypercalcemia.[89]

In the next stage of MTC development, microscopic carcinomas are characterized by well-demarcated collections of calcitonin-staining cells with variable amounts of interspersed stroma. The small collections of C cells breach the follicular basement membrane and efface the surrounding follicular architecture. Macroscopic MTC lesions are whitish, firm nodules that may appear well demarcated or grossly invasive (see Fig 81-3). Of great clinical importance is the observation that even the smallest visible tumors can be associated with regional lymph node metastasis.

Microscopically, MTCs are highly pleiomorphic in appearance with many variations in pattern, even within individual tumor nodules. The most classic MTC histology consists of nests of polygonal, oval, or spindle-shaped cells separated by variable amounts of fibrous stroma (Fig 81-4). A large number of variants including insular or carcinoid-like, trabecular, papillary, and follicular forms of MTC have been recognized, without clear evidence for altered prognosis.[86] Congo red staining of tumor specimens demonstrates amyloid deposition,

composed of dense parallel fibrils of procalcitonin.[90] Although once considered a reliable criterion for diagnosis for MTC, amyloid is in fact present in only 60% to 80% of tumors.[91] Calcitonin immunohistochemistry is the most useful adjunct to routine histology. The homogeneity of calcitonin staining may reflect the degree of endocrine differentiation in a given tumor and correlates well with long-term survival (Fig 81-5) and prognostic factors (below). Uncommon calcitonin-negative neuroendocrine tumors of the thyroid gland, often with a small cell histology, are often difficult to precisely classify in the absence of a positive family history for MTC or staining for CGRP.[86] Especially tantalizing are rare reports of tumors that stain concurrently for calcitonin and thyroglobulin.[92] Such case reports continue to challenge the dogma of separate lineages for follicular and C cells, by suggesting the possibility of undifferentiated thyroid stem cells capable of both follicular and parafollicular differentiation.[93]

CLINICAL PRESENTATION AND DIAGNOSIS

Sporadic Medullary Thyroid Carcinoma

There are three principle components to the primary diagnosis of MTC: detection, staging, and evaluation for heritable disease. As previously noted, 80% of MTC cases occur sporadically. Patients with this form of MTC most often present with a painless, palpable thyroid nodule, typically in the fifth or sixth decade of life. There is a slight female preponderance of approximately 1.5:1. At the time of presentation with a palpable nodule, at least 50% of patients have detectable cervical lymphadenopathy, whereas the incidence of identifiable distant metastases to lung, liver, or bone is approximately 10% at presentation. Local mass-associated symptoms including dysphagia, stridor, or recurrent laryngeal nerve injury are seen only in a small minority at presentation. Paraneoplastic manifestations including flushing, diarrhea, and the ectopic corticotropin syndrome are also generally confined to advanced disease.

Primary MTC lesions may be visualized as cold nodules on radionuclide imaging and as solid masses on ultrasonography. Occasionally, multiple concurrent MTC tumors can be mistaken in these studies for multinodular goiter. Plain films of the neck sometimes reveal a characteristic dense, coarse calcification pattern, which is distinct from the fine pattern observed with papillary carcinoma. Computed tomography (CT) scans of the lung, mediastinum, or liver may reveal similar calcification at sites of metastatic disease.

Virtually all patients with clinically evident MTC have elevated basal levels of calcitonin. The low prevalence of MTC among patients with thyroid nodules makes serum calcitonin determination an impractical screening approach for the evaluation of thyroid nodules. Rather, fine-needle aspiration biopsy routinely should be used on patients with thyroid nodules. In MTC, aspirates reveal a highly cellular, often heterogeneous pattern that lacks typical papillary or follicular features and is depleted of colloid. Oval, spindle-shaped, or plasmacytoid cytology can be seen.[94] Given an adequate level of suspicion from routine cytologic stains, performance of calcitonin immunohistochemistry on the specimen, combined with a serum calcitonin determination, usually confirms the diagno-

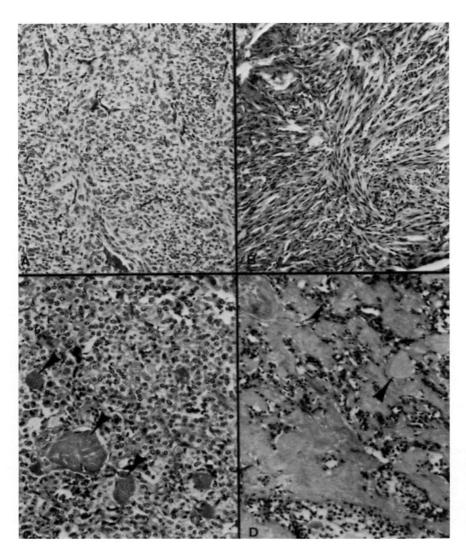

FIGURE 81-4. Histologic features of MTC: (*A*) nests of polygonal cells; (*B*) spindleshaped cells; (*C*) amyloid deposits (*arrows*) and (*D*) large amounts of fibrous stroma with sparse cells and amyloid nodules (*arrows*). (Mendelsohn G, Baylin SB. Medullary thyroid carcinoma: diagnostic and clinical features. Lab Diagn Clin Testing 1983;21:21)

sis. In contrast to cytopathology specimens stained for calcitonin, intraoperative frozen sections have little utility.

After initial detection, the second task in MTC diagnosis is staging. Although there is no consensus regarding an optimal staging work-up, several imaging studies appear to be useful for determining the extent of regional and distant metastatic disease at the time of original diagnosis and in preparation for follow-up surgery. CT, magnetic resonance imaging (MRI), and, in some institutions, ultrasonography are used to screen for lymphadenopathy and evidence of local invasion. CT (or MRI) of the mediastinum and lungs is useful to document whether there is gross metastasis beyond the thyroidectomy field. CT scanning of the liver is insensitive to detect early liver metastasis, which typically occurs in a miliary pattern. Nuclear medicine studies including ^{111}In-octreotide,[95] and to a lesser extent pentavalent dimercaptosuccinic acid[96] and ^{131}I-metaiodobenzylguanidine, appear to have a more limited role in the primary work-up but may be useful in identifying residual disease.

The third task in MTC diagnosis is evaluation for heritable disease. Indications for this testing and available techniques are discussed in the section below. At a minimum, it is prudent to obtain a screening test for pheochromocytoma, either

with urinary catecholamines or metanephrines, before subjecting newly diagnosed patients to thyroidectomy.

The importance of making a preoperative, as opposed to retrospective, diagnosis of MTC has been generally underappreciated. Failure to identify a risk of concurrent pheochromocytoma has occasionally produced avoidable harm. More commonly, patients are exposed to the risks and discomforts associated with follow-up neck explorations after their primary surgical procedure failed to seek out associated lymphadenopathy in the neck and upper mediastinum. Given the high frequency of regional nodal metastases and the absence of truly effective nonsurgical treatment modalities, a well-planned surgical approach necessitates the preoperative differentiation of MTC from other forms of thyroid cancer, as well as careful staging of the disease.

Inherited MTC

The characteristic modes of presentation and natural history of the three forms of inherited MTC are distinctive. MEN 2A is the most common and thoroughly characterized syndrome. C-cell hyperplasia and MTC are the cardinal lesions of MEN 2A, oc-

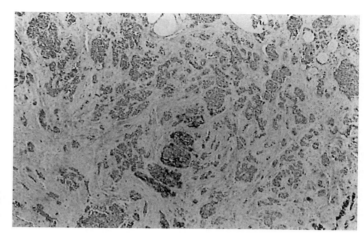

FIGURE 81-5. Calcitonin immunostaining showing marked heterogeneity. This section is from a primary MTC in a patient who died of a very aggressive tumor. Compare this pattern with the homogeneous pattern shown in Fig 81-2*B* and *C.*

curring in greater than 95% of individuals. Pheochromocytoma and hyperparathyroidism are less penetrant with lifetime incidences of 40% to 60% and 10% to 25%, on average. (These incidence rates vary markedly among different kindreds). In more than 80% of affected patients, MTC is the initial manifestation, with pheochromocytoma following at a median age of 29 years.[97] The age-specific prevalence of MTC in MEN 2A depends entirely on the sensitivity of the detection method. The probability that an MEN 2A gene carrier will have presented with clinical features of MTC at a given age has been carefully studied by Ponder and associates.[98] At age 35 years, the likelihood of a clinical presentation with MTC is still only 25% for obligate gene carriers (Fig 81-6*A*). Even at age 70 years, the likelihood is only approximately 60% (Fig 81-6*B*). A more sensitive look at the age-specific penetrance of MTC in MEN 2A has been afforded by serial biochemical screening for early MTC using the calcitonin secretogogues calcium and pentagastrin. Approximately 65% of obligate gene carriers exhibit calcitonin hypersecretion at age 20 years.[98] At age 35 years, fully 95% of gene carriers have a positive screening test. Using prospective germline DNA testing for *ret* mutations, both C-cell hyperplasia and microscopic MTC readily can be detected before conversion to a positive biochemical screening test.[99,100]

For isolated FMTC, comparable age-specific incidence data are not available, owing in part to the relative infrequency of the syndrome. Farndon and colleagues have reported a generally later age of clinical presentation of the MTC and a relatively more favorable prognosis in FMTC as compared to MEN 2A.[22] The incomplete clinical penetrance of FMTC and MEN 2A explains some cases of cryptic heritable disease in individuals with a "negative" family history. Although the majority of FMTC families "breed true," some families classified as FMTC subsequently have one or more members develop pheochromocytoma. In light of the apparent clinical and genetic overlap between these syndromes, it seems prudent to screen all individuals with inherited MTC periodically for development of pheochromocytoma.

Pheochromocytoma, MTC, and the so-called ganglioneuroma phenotype characterize MEN 2B. The presentation and natural history of MEN 2B differ from MEN 2A in several important ways. De novo mutations are relatively common in MEN 2B, accounting for approximately 50% of cases, but are rare in MEN 2A.[62] The thyroid tumors in MEN 2B are usually, though not invariably, aggressive, with widespread metastases at an early age. Pheochromocytomas appear earlier and are almost always bilateral (versus a 50% bilateral incidence in MEN 2A). Hyperparathyroidism is rare in MEN 2B. Patients have a characteristic set of phenotypic abnormalities (Fig 81-7) including mucosal ganglioneuromas (involving the lips, tongue, and entire gastrointestinal tract resulting in achalasia, intestinal hypomotility, and pseudo-obstruction), skeletal deformities (elongated facies, joint hyperextensibility, marfanoid proportions, and pectus excavatum), and thickened corneal nerves. Many of the phenotypic abnormalities, particularly the mucosal neuromas, can be recognized in infancy. Because of the virulent nature of the MTC associated with this syndrome, many investigators recommend prophylactic thyroidectomy before age 3 years in children in whom the syndrome is recognized.

Presymptomatic diagnosis of inherited MTC has historically relied on three different techniques: biochemical screening, family linkage studies, and more recently, germline ret analysis. Biochemical detection, using pentagastrin (0.5 μg/kg) or pentagastrin plus calcium (elemental calcium, 2 mg/kg) over 1 minute to stimulate calcitonin secretion, was the mainstay of diagnosis for over two decades. Yearly screening of individuals at risk beginning at age 6 years can result in the detection of gene carriers at the stage of C-cell hyperplasia or microscopic MTC. Using this procedure, the median age of detection is between 12 and 16 years; subjects are evenly split between those having C-cell hyperplasia alone and those having both hyperplasia and microscopic MTC. Individuals who converted to a positive test over the period of observation have had a low, but detectable, recurrence rate of abnormal calcitonin secretion in follow-up after thyroidectomy.[101] Disadvantages of this screening procedure include the later age of detection of gene carriers compared to DNA-based methods, occasional examples of recurrent postoperative hypercalcitoninemia, the discomfort and inconvenience associated with the yearly infusion, and the appreciable rate of false-positive tests, that is, significant hypercalcitoninemia (often with histopathologic evidence for C-cell hyperplasia) in obligate noncarriers of the ret mutation among families with a known

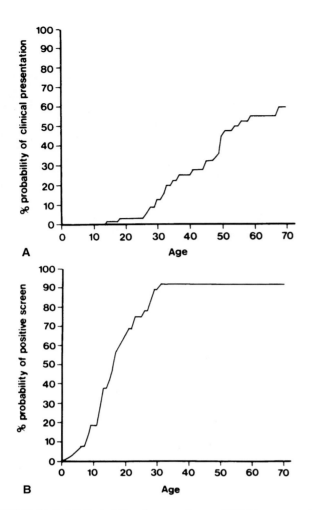

FIGURE 81-6. (*A*) Probability, by age, that an MEN 2A gene carrier will have presented with clinical features of MTC. (*B*) Probability, by age, of a positive calcitonin stimulation test in a person harboring the gene. (Ponder BAJ, Coffey R, Gagel RF, et al. Risk estimation and screening in families of patients with medullary thyroid carcinoma. Lancet 1988;1:397)

mutation.[99,100] Follow-up of such apparently false-positive individuals has revealed no examples of MTC, pheochromocytoma, or recurrent hypercalcitoninemia to date. The explanation for their C-cell hyperplasia remains obscure.

Family linkage studies provided an indirect means of assessing risk of inheritance of MTC before the discovery of pathogenic ret mutations. Linkage studies trace the inheritance pattern from affected parents to their affected and unaffected offspring of a set polymorphic DNA markers, clustering around the disease gene, to determine which patterns correlate with transmission of the disease. Given an adequate family size, it is possible to make accurate predictions about the risk status of additional offspring at an early age. These studies were limited by the need for multigenerational family studies and by the indirect nature of the test. This approach has been superseded by direct detection of ret gene mutations.

The identification of affected individuals in families with inherited MTC is now relatively simple and accurate, using techniques to identify ret gene mutations in the germline (usually white blood cell) DNA. Currently available techniques use polymerase chain reaction (PCR) amplification of the appropriate ret gene exons, usually exons 10, 11, and 16. Several different analysis schemes have been used to detect mutations in these amplified fragments including direct automated DNA sequencing, restriction enzyme analysis, and procedures that detect DNA mismatches on reannealing of normal and mutant strands. Preliminary information regarding the diagnostic accuracy of these procedures indicates that they are highly specific for disease-causing mutations. Sensitivity has also been high. A loss of sensitivity can occur in a subset of cases of FMTC (in which ret mutations have not been detected),[16,58] in rare instances where neutral DNA polymorphisms cause the failure of one ret allele to amplify,[102] or if samples are misidentified or mishandled. A limited number of commercial laboratories in addition to investigative groups currently offer the test.

Prospective studies using ret gene testing in asymptomatic kindred members, beginning at age 6 years, suggest that ret analysis is effective in identifying subjects at risk.[99,100] Among ret mutation-positive individuals undergoing prophylactic thyroidectomy, those with a normal preoperative calcitonin stimulation test were more likely to have C-cell hyperplasia alone without microscopic or macroscopic MTC compared to subjects with a positive calcitonin stimulation test.[99] These early data provide a rationale for advocating prophylactic thyroidectomy in ret mutation-positive individuals beginning at approximately age 6 years, before the development of a positive calcitonin stimulation test. Although an alternative approach of performing more frequent stimulation testing in ret mutation-positive subjects and deferring surgery until later in childhood has also been advocated,[100] most investigators favor earlier treatment based on ret analysis alone. Because MTC can have a more aggressive course in MEN 2B, thyroidectomy is performed earlier in children with a clinical or DNA-based diagnosis of this syndrome.

In MTC patients with a negative family history, the proper role of ret gene analysis has not been clearly established. There is a small but definite rate of cryptic heritable disease in these patients,[98] related in part to incomplete clinical penetrance in MEN 2A and FMTC, and in part to de novo ret mutations. Performing ret analysis in the affected patient offers a distinct advantage in terms of simplicity and diagnostic accuracy compared to performing periodic calcitonin stimulation testing in the patient's siblings, offspring, and parents theoretically at risk. Although a strong argument can be made for doing germline ret analysis in all patients with apparently sporadic MTC,[103] further studies are needed to determine the diagnostic yield and cost effectiveness of such an approach.

TREATMENT

Initial Approach

The primary treatment modality for both the inherited and sporadic forms of MTC is surgery. Patients presenting with

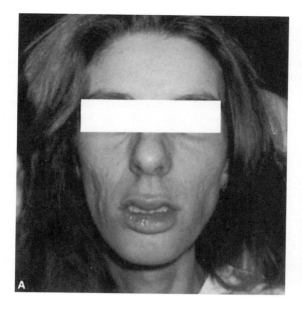

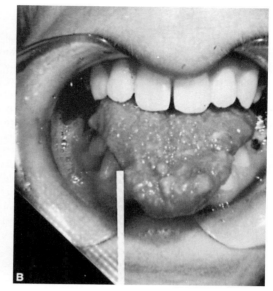

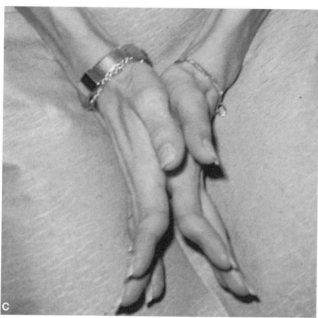

FIGURE 81-7. (*A*) Photograph of a patient with MEN 2B showing the typical facies. (*B*) characteristic musosal neuromas on the tongue. (*C*) Patient's hands, demonstrating the joint hyperextensibility characteristic of the Marfan-like habitus of these patients

palpable disease should undergo a staging work-up as described above, based on the high frequency of nodal metastasis in this setting. Pheochromocytoma must be carefully excluded. For patients presenting with a palpable nodule and no clinical evidence of extrathyroidal disease, the procedure of choice is generally a total (or near-total) thyroidectomy and prophylactic lymph node dissection of the central compartment from the hyoid bone to the innominate veins. The ipsilateral midjugular nodes should be sampled. If they are positive for tumor, a modified neck dissection, with sparing of the sternocleidomastoid muscle, the jugular vein, and the accessory nerve, is frequently indicated. Radical neck dissection can result in significant morbidity and has not been shown to improve prognosis. Patients with known or suspected inherited MTC presenting in adulthood or with a palpable nodule should be considered for bilateral neck exploration. During surgery, the parathyroid glands should be identified and preserved in the absence of clinical hyperparathyroidism and frank parathyroid enlargement.

Residual Disease

In practical terms, a surgical cure of MTC is defined as a normal postoperative calcitonin stimulation test result that persists over time. In fact, young individuals undergoing thyroidectomy based on presymptomatic testing (for whom the chance of cure is presumably high) have postoperative basal and stimulated calcitonin levels that are typically near the lower limit of assay sensitivity (i.e., pproximately 10 pg/mL or less). Levels that are frankly elevated postoperatively or levels that rise progressively through the normal range with repeated testing indicate persistence of disease. Overall, the rate of persistent hypercalcitoninemia is nearly 50% for patients with nonpalpable macroscopic disease and greater than 80% for patients presenting with a palpable MTC.[104] This high frequency of persistent disease is often due to early metastasis to regional lymph nodes. Many of these patients have no abnormalities on neck CT scans, suggesting that these metastatic deposits are microscopic. Other common sites of persistent or recurrent disease include the mediastinum, hilar nodes, liver, and lung. In particular, liver metastases are difficult to detect with typical imaging modalities including CT, MRI, and octreotide scintigraphy. In the absence of extensive adenopathy or overt extranodal disease, the clinical course of MTC is usually marked by gradual progression. A recent Mayo Clinic retrospective series indicated excellent long-term survival in patients with persistent calcitonin elevation but no other evident disease after primary surgery (86% overall survival at 10 years).[105] Similarly, a group at Memorial-Sloan Kettering reported 94% 5-year survival in patients with lymph node metastasis alone versus 41% in patients with extranodal disease.[106]

Given the difficulty of eradicating the MTC with primary surgery, what are the potential indications and outcomes of reoperation? Tisell and colleagues used a microdissection technique in patients with residual calcitonin elevation after primary surgery, normalizing their levels in 4 of 11 cases.[107] More recently, Moley and colleagues reported that 9 of 32 patients (28%) undergoing reexploration for persistent hypercalcitoninemia had initial postoperative stimulated calcitonin values less than 160 pg/mL.[108] Capsular invasion in the primary surgery specimen was a significant predictor of poor response to reoperation. Other centers have reported lower rates of postoperative calcitonin normalization.[106] It is unclear how many of the apparent responders to reoperation will translate into long-term surgical cures. Additional studies, using longer follow-up and sensitive calcitonin assays, are needed before this approach can be recommended more generally.

Apart from reoperation of minimal residual disease with a curative intent, there is a definite role for palliative, debulking surgery in patients with advanced MTC. Special problems include patients with large recurrences in the neck or mediastinum with compression of vital structures or large liver metastases associated with pain or poorly controlled diarrhea and flushing. In the hands of experienced surgeons, repeated surgical debulking can be an effective temporizing measure.

Nonsurgical approaches to MTC treatment have generally met with limited success. Adjuvant postoperative therapy for MTC is not indicated, given currently available treatments. Clearly radioactive iodine ablation does not play a useful role in this form of thyroid cancer.[109] The uptake of iodine by MTC cells is negligible. Furthermore, there is no evidence that neighboring follicular cells that concentrate iodine may actually exert a useful local cytotoxic effect, especially in nodal metastases. The role of external beam radiotherapy is somewhat more controversial. Although most investigators agree that MTC is not generally radiosensitive, some have reported a favorable response in occasional patients. Other studies have failed to show an improvement in outcome of patients treated with adjuvant radiotherapy.[109,110]

Chemotherapy for advanced, metastatic MTC has shown modest response rates in several small scale trials published to date. Several of the regimens with at least limited activity have included the agents doxorubicin or dacarbazine. Five studies using doxorubicin as a single agent demonstrated a combined 30% partial response rate among 46 patients with no stable or complete remissions.[111] Dacarbazine, in combination with cyclophosphamide and vincristine, exhibits significant antitumor activity for malignant pheochromocytoma.[112] A single patient treated with dacarbazine plus 5-fluorouracil had a complete response.[113] In a more recent study of dacarbazine, cyclophosphamide, and vincristine in advanced MTC two of seven patients showed partial biochemical and tumor responses but no complete responses.[114] At the present, combination chemotherapy can be considered in advanced MTC in cases where life-threatening complications appear imminent. In more typical patients with stable or slowly progressing residual tumor, currently available regimens appear to offer little benefit. Additional clinical studies are needed using newer chemotherapy agents, perhaps in combination with the existing agents known to have modest activity.

Biologic response modifiers, such as the long-acting somatostatin analogue octreotide and α-interferon, are effective in some neuroendocrine cancers, especially carcinoid tumors and pancreatic islet cell tumors.[115] Trials of octreotide in MTC to date have shown disappointing antitumor activity and mixed benefits in reducing paraneoplastic flushing and diarrhea.[116,117] Some patients experience a paradoxical worsening of diarrhea.[117] Based on the success of ^{111}In-octreotide as an imaging agent for MTC, limited therapeutic trials are underway using octreotide linked to more potent radioemitters. Other nuclear medicine approaches, for example using monoclonal antibodies to carcinoembryonic antigen (CEA), so far have been largely unsuccessful.

The medical management of diarrhea and flushing, which complicate the course of up to one-third of patients with extensive MTC, remains frustrating. Loperamide and diphenoxylate can be useful for the diarrhea, and histamine-receptor blockers such as diphenhydramine and cimetidine can decrease the intensity and frequency of flushing episodes.

PROGNOSTIC FACTORS

The overall prognosis of MTC is intermediate between well-differentiated papillary or follicular carcinoma and the poorly differentiated variants of thyroid cancer. Patients with inherited MEN 2A and FMTC who are identified in early presymptomatic screening have a high frequency of normal postoperative calcitonin levels and potentially normal life expectancies. For patients with residual disease, several factors have been reported to have prognostic value including genetic background, patient age, factors related to stage of the disease, and histopathologic features such as the intensity and uniformity of calcitonin immunostaining. Patient age does not appear to be an independent predictor when genetic status is controlled for.[110] Although patients with MEN 2A have a significantly higher overall survival rate than patients with sporadic MTC, these differences become nonsignificant when clinical stage (i.e., presence of regional adenopathy or local invasion) is considered.[110]

A comprehensive review of prognostic factors among virtually all patients with MTC in Sweden over a 23-year period showed that several disease features were strong independent predictors of outcome.[118] Patients whose tumors did not exhibit local invasion (i.e., the tumor capsule remained intact) had a 92% relative survival rate at 10 years compared to 67% survival for patients with a nonintact capsule. A second strong predictor of outcome was calcitonin immunostaining (see Fig 81-5). Tumors with greater than 50% of cells staining positive for calcitonin at their original surgery had a 10-year relative survival rate of 87% compared to 60% survival for patients with fewer than 10% of cells staining positive. Presumably, loss of this endocrine differentiation marker correlates with genetic tumor progression events that favor tumor growth and metastasis. Both calcitonin immunostaining and tumor capsule penetration remained independent predictors of survival in a multivariate analysis model.[69] Although the absolute calcitonin level correlates roughly with residual tumor mass and significant rises generally accompany disease progression, the calcitonin level, per se, has not proved to be a useful predictor of survival. Intrinsic biologic variability in calcitonin secretion can lead to calcitonin fluctuations of 30% to 50% over a brief period in patients with clinically stable disease. An additional important prognostic factor in some patients is the CEA level. A rapid doubling of the CEA, particularly in the setting of a stable calcitonin level is an ominous indicator.[118,119]

IMPLICATIONS FOR MANAGEMENT OF PERSISTENT MTC

In summary, although we currently lack an efficient means to treat persistent or recurrent MTC, long-term survival with slow tumor progression is the most typical outcome, owing to the relatively indolent growth pattern of this cancer. Clinical stage at the time of diagnosis (particularly the degree of nodal involvement and the presence of local invasion) and the calcitonin immunostaining pattern are important predictors of outcome. In patients with residual hypercalcitoninemia and no other evidence of recurrence, the choice of whether to pursue reoperation with a curative intent remains controversial, with many centers electing to follow a conservative course. Serum calcitonin, combined with CEA, provides a straightforward means of following these patients. Those who develop accelerated rises in either marker should be reevaluated with imaging studies, including CT or MRI of the neck and chest and possibly octreotide scintigraphy. Individuals with evidence of local invasion, extensive nodal disease, or a calcitonin-poor tumor should be followed carefully with imaging studies. When feasible, debulking procedures may be performed in the hope of preventing further disease progression.

The best opportunity for developing truly effective interventions for patients with persistent MTC will stem from future studies at a molecular level. A principal challenge in the biology of MTC is to incorporate recent findings about tumor initiation in the hereditary setting into a more comprehensive understanding of the mechanisms underlying the growth, metastasis, and invasiveness of this cancer.

References

1. Hazard JB, Hawk WA, Crile G Jr. Medullary (solid) carcinoma of the thyroid: a clinicopathologic entity. J Clin Endocrinol Metab 1959;19:152
2. Frantz VK, Yancopoulos K. Carcinoma of the thyroid: a clinico-pathological study of 216 cases with a ten year follow-up. Advances in thyroid research. New York: Pergamon Press, 1961: 377
3. Sipple JH. The association of pheochromocytoma with carcinoma of the thyroid gland. Am J Med 1961;31:163
4. Cushman P Jr. Familial endocrine tumors. Report of two unrelated kindreds affected with pheochromocytoma, one also with multiple thyroid carcinomas. Am J Med 1962;32:352
5. Manning PC Jr, Molnar GD, Black BM, et al. Pheochromocytoma, hyperparathyroidism, and thyroid carcinoma occurring coincidentally. N Engl J Med 1963;268:68
6. Nourok DS. Familial pheochromocytoma and thyroid carcinoma. Ann Intern Med 1964;60:1028
7. Schimke RN, Hartmann WH, Prout TE, Rimoin DL. Syndrome of bilateral pheochromocytoma, medullary thyroid carcinoma, and multiple neuromas. N Engl J Med 1968;279:1
8. Copp DH, Cameron EC, Cheney BA, et al. Evidence for calcitonin: a new hormone from the parathyroid that lowers blood calcium. Endocrinology 1962;70:638
9. Foster GV, MacIntyre I, Pearse AGE. Calcitonin production and the mitochondrion-rich cells of the dog thyroid. Nature 1964;203:1029
10. Pearse AG. Common cytochemical and ultrastructural characteristics of cells producing polypeptide hormones (the APUD series) and their relevance to thyroid and ultimobranchial C-cells and calcitonin. Proc R Soc Lond [Biol] 1968;170:71
11. Williams ED. Histogenesis of medullary carcinoma of the thyroid. J Clin Pathol 1966;19:114
12. Melvin KEW, Tashjian AH Jr. The syndrome of excessive thyrocalcitonin produced by medullary carcinoma of the thyroid. Proc Natl Acad Sci U S A 1968;59:1216
13. Mathew CGP, Chin KS Easton DF, et al. A linked genetic marker for multiple endocrine neoplasia type 2A on chromosome 10. Nature 1988;328:527
14. Simpson NE, Kidd KK, Goodfellow PJ, et al. Assignment of multiple endocrine neoplasia type 2A to chromosome 10 by linkage. Nature 1988;328:528
15. Mulligan LM, Kwok JBJ, Healey CS, et al. Germline mutations of the ret protooncogene in multiple endocrine neoplasia type 2A. 1993;363:458
16. Donis-Keller H, Dou S, Chi D, et al. Mutations in the ret proto-oncogene are associated with MEN 2A and FMTC. Hum Mol Genet 1993;2:851
17. Hofstra RMW, Landsvater RM, Ceccherini I, et al. A mutation in the ret proto-oncogene associated with multiple endocrine neoplasia type 2B and sporadic medullary thyroid carcinoma. Nature 1994;367:375
18. Franssila K. Value of histologic classification of thyroid cancer. Acta Pathol Microbiol Scanda 1971;(Suppl 225):1
19. Hill CS, Ibanez ML, Samaan NA, et al. Medullary (solid) carcinoma of the thyroid gland: an analysis of the M. D. Anderson

Hospital experience with patients with the tumor, its special features and its histogenesis. Medicine 1973;52:141

20. Steiner AL, Goodman AD, Powers SR. Study of a kindred with pheochromocytoma, medullary thyroid carcinoma, hyperparathyroidism, and Cushing's disease: MEN, type II. Medicine 1968;47:371

21. Wermer P. Genetic aspect of adenomatosis of endocrine glands. Am J Med 1954;16:363

22. Farndon JR, Leight GS, Dilley WG, et al. Familial medullary thyroid carcinoma without associated endocrinopathies: a distinct clinical entity. Br J Surg 1986;73:278

23. Nunziata V, Giannattasio R, di Giovanni G, et al. Hereditary localized pruritis in affected members of a kindred with multiple endocrine neoplasia type 2A (Sipple's syndrome). Clin Endocrinol 1989;30:57

24. Gagel RF, Levy ML, Donovan DT, et al. Multiple endocrine neoplasia type 2a associated with cutaneous lichen amyloidosis. Ann Intern Med 1989;111:802

25. Mulligan LM, Eng C, Attie T, et al. Diverse phenotypes associated with exon 10 mutations of the ret proto-oncogene. Hum Mol Gen 1994;3:2163

26. Ponder BAJ, Ponder MA, Coffey R, et al. Risk estimation and screening in families of patients with medullary thyroid carcinoma. Lancet 1988;1:397

27. LeDouarin N, Le Lievre C. Demonstration de l'origine neurale des cellules a calcitonine du corps ultimobranchial chez l'embryon de poulet. Comptes Rendus des Séances de l'Académie des Sciences (C R Seances Acad Sci) Paris 1970;270:2857

28. Ericson LE, Fredriksson G. Phylogeny and ontogeny of the thyroid gland. In: Greer MA, ed. The thyroid gland. New York: Raven Press, 1990:1

29. Amara SG, Jonas V, Rosenfeld MG, et al. Alternative RNA processing in calcitonin gene expression generates mRNAs encoding different polypeptide products. Nature 1982;298:240

30. Morris MR, Panico M, Etienne T, et al. Isolation and characterization of human calcitonin gene related peptide. Nature 1984;308:746

31. Becker KL, Snider RH, Moore CF, et al. Calcitonin in extra-thyroidal tissues of man. Acta Endocrinol 1979;92:746

32. Becker KL, Nash D, Silva OL, et al. Increased serum and urinary calcitonin in patients with pulmonary disease. Chest 1981;79:211

33. Simmons RE, Hjelle JT, Mahoney C, et al. Renal metabolism of calcitonin. Am J Physiol 1988;254:F593

34. Zajac JD, Penschow J, Mason T, et al. Identification of calcitonin and calcitonin gene-related peptide messenger ribonucleic acid in medullary thyroid carcinomas by hybridization histochemistry. J Clin Endocrinol Metab 1986;62:1037

35. Mason RT, Shulkes A, Zajac JD, et al. Basal and stimulated release of calcitonin gene-related peptide (CGRP) in patients with medullary thyroid carcinoma. Clin Endocrinol (Oxf) 1986;25:675

36. Schifter S. Calcitonin gene related peptide and calcitonin as tumour markers in MEN 2 family screening. Clin Endocrinol (Oxf) 1989;30:263

37. Roos BA, Huber MB, Birnbaum RS, et al. Medullary thyroid carcinomas secrete a noncalcitonin peptide corresponding to the carboxyl-terminal region of pre-procalcitonin. J Clin Endocrinol Metab 1983;56:802

38. Roos BA, Lindall AW, Ells J, et al. Increased plasma and tumor somatostatin-like immunoreactivity in medullary thyroid carcinoma and small cell lung cancer. J Clin Endocrinol Metab 1981;52:187

39. Melvin KEW, Tashjian AH Jr, Cassidy CE, Givens JR. Cushing's syndrome caused by ACTH-and calcitonin-secreting medullary carcinoma of the thyroid. Metabolism 1970;19:831

40. Kameya T, Bessho T, Tsumuraya M, et al. Production of gastrin-releasing peptide by medullary carcinoma of the thyroid. Virchows Arch [A] 1983;401:99

41. Baylin SB, Mendelsohn G. Medullary thyroid carcinoma: a model for the study of human tumor progression and cell heterogeneity. In: Owens AH Jr, Coffey DS, Baylin SB, eds. Tumor cell heterogeneity, origins and implications. New York: Academic Press, 1982:12

42. Deftos LJ, Woloszczuk W, Krisch I, et al. Medullary thyroid carcinomas express chromogranin A and a novel neuroendocrine protein recognized by monoclonal antibody HISL-19. Am J Med 1988;85:780

43. Krisch K, Krisch I, Horvat G, et al. The value of immunohistochemistry in medullary thyroid carcinoma: a systematic study of 30 cases. Histopathology 1985;9:1077

44. Sikri KL, Varndell IM, Hamid QA, et al. Medullary carcinoma of the thyroid. An immunocytochemical and histochemical study of 25 cases using eight separate markers. Cancer 1985;56:2481

45. Komminoth P, Roth J, Saremaslani P, et al. Polysialic acid of the neural cell adhesion molecule in the human thyroid: a marker for medullary thyroid carcinoma and primary C-cell hyperplasia. Am J Surg Pathol 1994;18:399

46. Reasbeck PG, Burns SM, Shulkes A. Calcitonin gene-related peptide: enteric and cardiovascular effects in the dog. Gastroenterology 1988;95:966

47. Said SI. Evidence for secretion of vasoactive intestinal peptide by tumours of pancreas, adrenal medulla, thyroid and lung: support for the unifying APUD concept. Clin Endocrinol 1976;5:201S

48. Skrabanek P, Cannon D, Dempsey J, et al. Substance P in medullary carcinoma of the thyroid. Experientia 1979;35:1259

49. Tamir H, Liu KP, Hsiung SC, et al. Multiple signal transduction mechanisms leading to the secretion of 5-hydroxytryptamine by MTC cells, a neuroectodermally derived cell line. J Neurosci 1990;10:3743

50. Williams ED, Karin SMM, Sandler M. Prostaglandin secretion by medullary carcinoma of the thyroid: a possible cause of the associated diarrhea. Lancet 1968;1:22

51. Pachnis V, Mankoo B, Costantini F. Expression of the c-ret proto-oncogene during mouse embryogenesis. Development 1993;119:1005

52. Tsuzuki T, Takahashi M, Asai N, et al. Spatial and temporal expression of the ret proto-oncogene product in embryonic, infant and adult rat tissues. Oncogene 1995;10:191

53. Santoro M, Rosati R, Grieco M, et al. The ret proto-oncogene is consistently expressed in human pheochromocytomas and thyroid medullary carcinomas. Oncogene 1990;5:1595

54. Ikeda I, Ishizaka Y, Tahira T, et al. Specific expression of the ret proto-oncogene in human neuroblastoma cell lines. Oncogene 1990;5:1291

55. Takahashi M, Ritz J, Cooper GM. Activation of a novel human transforming gene, ret, by DNA rearrangement. Cell 1985;42:581

56. Fusco A, Grieco M, Santoro M, et al. A new oncogene in human thyroid papillary carcinomas and their lymph-nodal metastases. Nature 1987;328:170

57. Grieco M, Santoro MT, Berlingieri M, et al. PTC is a novel rearranged form of the ret proto-oncogene and is frequently detected in vivo in human thyroid papillary carcinomas. Cell 1990;60:557

58. Schuffenecker I, Billaud M, Calender A, et al. Ret proto-oncogene mutations in French MEN 2A and FMTC families. Hum Mol Genet 1994;3:1939

59. Santoro M, Carlomagno F, Romano A, et al. Activation of ret as a dominant transforming gene by germline mutations of MEN2A and MEN2B. Science 1995;267:381

60. Mulligan LM, Eng C, Healey CS, et al. Specific mutations of the ret proto-oncogene are related to disease phenotype in MEN 2A and FMTC. Nature Genet 1994;6:70

61. Carlson KM, Dou S, Chi D, et al. Single missense mutation in the tyrosine kinase catalytic domain of the ret protooncogene is as-

sociated with multiple endocrine neoplasia type 2B. Proc Natl Acad Sci U S A 1994;91:1579

62. Carlson KM, Bracamontes J, Jackson CE, et al. Parent-of-origin effects in multiple endocrine neoplasia type 2B. Am J Hum Genet 1994;55:1076

63. Eng C, Smith DP, Mulligan LM, et al. Point mutation within the tyrosine kinase domain of the ret proto-oncogene in multiple endocrine neoplasia type 2B and related sporadic tumors. Hum Mol Genet 1994;3:237

64. Blaugrund JE, Johns MM, Ebyl YJ, et al. Ret proto-oncogene mutations in inherited and sporadic medullary thyroid cancer. Hum Mol Genet 1994;3:1895

65. Zedenius J, Wallin G, Hamberger B, et al. Somatic and MEN 2A de novo mutations identified in the ret proto-oncogene by screening of sporadic MTCs. Hum Mol Genet 1994;3:1259

66. Lindor NM, Honchel R, Khosla S, Thibodeau SN. Mutations in the ret protooncogene in sporadic pheochromocytomas. J Clin Endocrinol Metab 1995;80:627

67. Baylin SB, Hsu SH, Gann DS. Inherited medullary thyroid carcinoma: the result of a final monoclonal mutation imposed on one of multiple clones of susceptible cells. Science 1978;199:429

68. Lippman SM, Mendelsohn G, Trump DL, et al. The prognostic and biologic significance of cellular heterogeneity in medullary thyroid carcinoma: a study of calcitonin, L-dopa decarboxylase, and histaminase. J Clin Endocrinol Metab 1982;54:233

69. Bergholm U, Adami H-O, Auer G, et al. Histopathologic characteristics and nuclear DNA content as prognostic factors in medullary thyroid carcinoma. Cancer 1989;64:135

70. Fearon ER, Vogelstein B. A genetic model for colorectal tumorigenesis. Cell 1990;61:759

71. Mulligan LM, Gardner E, Smith BA, et al. Genetic events in tumour initiation and progression in multiple endocrine neoplasia type 2. Genes Chromosom Cancer 1993;6:166

72. Moley JF, Brother MB, Fong CT, et al. Consistent association of 1p loss of heterozygosity with pheochromocytoma in patients with multiple endocrine neoplasia type 2 syndromes. Cancer Res 1992;52:770

73. Khosla S, Patel VM, Hay ID, et al. Loss of heterozygosity suggests multiple genetic alterations in pheochromocytomas and medullary thyroid carcinomas. J Clin Invest 1991;87:1691

74. Yana I, Nakamura T, Shin E, et al. Inactivation of the p53 gene is not required for tumorigenesis of medullary thyroid carcinoma or pheochromocytoma. Jpn J Cancer Res 1992;83:1113

75. Nelkin BD, Nakamura Y, White RW, et al. Low incidence of loss of chromosome 10 in sporadic and hereditary human medullary thyroid carcinoma. Cancer Res 1989;49:4114

76. Landsvater RM, Mathew CGP, Smith BA, et al. Development of multiple endocrine neoplasia type 2A does not involve substantial deletions of chromosome 10. Genomics 1989;4:246

77. Boultwood J, Wylie FS, Williams ED, et al. N-myc expression in neoplasia of human thyroid C-cells. Cancer Res 1988;48:4073

78. Roncalli M, Viale G, Grimelius L, et al. Prognostic value of N-myc immunoreactivity in medullary thyroid carcinoma. Cancer 1994;74:134

79. Moley JF, Brother MB, Wells SA, et al. Low frequency of ras gene mutations in neuroblastomas, pheochromocytomas, and medullary thyroid cancers. Cancer Res 1991;51:1596

80. Nakagawa T, Mabry M, de Bustros A, et al. Introduction of Harvey v-ras oncogene induces differentiation of cultured human medullary thyroid carcinoma cells. Proc Natl Acad Sci U S A 1987;84:5923

81. Bar-Sagi D, Feramisco JR. Microinjection of the ras oncogene product into PC-12 cells induces morphological differentiation. Cell 1985;42:841

82. Nelkin BD, Ball DW, Baylin SB. Molecular abnormalities in tumors associated with multiple endocrine neoplasia type 2. Endocrinol Metab Clin N Am 1994;23:187

83. DeLellis RA. The pathology of medullary thyroid carcinoma and its precursors. In: LiVolsi VA, DeLellis RA, eds. Pathobiology of the parathyroid and thyroid glands. Baltimore: Williams and Wilkins, 1993:72

84. O'Toole K, Fenoglio-Preiser C, Pushparaj N. Endocrine changes associated with the human aging process. II. Effect of age on the number of calcitonin immunoreactive cells in the thyroid gland. Hum Pathol 1985;16:991

85. Wolfe HJ, DeLellis RA, Voelkel EF. Distribution of calcitonin containing cells in the normal neonatal human thyroid gland: a correlation of morphology with peptide content. J Clin Endocrinol Metab 1975;41:1076

86. LiVolsi VA. Surgical pathology of the thyroid. Philadelphia: WB Saunders, 1990:223

87. Guyetant S, Wion-Barbot N, Rousellet M-C, et al. C-cell hyperplasia associated with chronic lymphocytic thyroiditis: a retrospective quantitative study of 112 cases. Hum Pathol 1994;25:514

88. Albores-Saavedra J, Montforte H, Nadji M, et al. C-cell hyperplasia in thyroid tissue adjacent to follicular cell tumors. Hum Pathol 1988;19:795

89. LiVolsi VA, Feind CR. Demonstration by immunoperoxidase staining of hyperplasia of parafollicular cells in the thyroid gland in hyperparathyroidism. J Clin Endocrinol Metab 1973;37:550

90. Westermark P, Johnson KH. The polypeptide hormone derived amyloid forms. Acta Pathol Microbiol Scand 1988;96:475

91. Norman T, Johannessen JV, Gautvik KM, et al. Medullary carcinoma of the thyroid. Diagnostic problems. Cancer 1976;38:366

92. Parker LN, Kollin J, Wu S-Y, et al. Carcinoma of the thyroid with a mixed medullary, papillary, follicular, and undifferentiated pattern. Arch Intern Med 1985;145:1507

93. Sobrinho-Simoes M, Nesland JM, Johannessen JV. Farewell to the dual histogenesis of thyroid tumors? (editorial). Ultrastruct Pathol 1985;8:iii

94. Geddie WR, Bedard YC, Strawbridge HTG. Medullary carcinoma of the thyroid in fine needle aspiration biopsies. Am J Clin Pathol 1984;82:552

95. Dorr U, Wurstlin S, Frank-Raue K, et al. Somatostatin receptor scintigraphy and magnetic resonance imaging in recurrent medullary thyroid carcinoma: a comparative study. Horm Metab Res Suppl 1993;27:48

96. Udelsman R, Ball D, Baylin SB, et al. Preoperative localization of occult medullary carcinoma of the thyroid gland with single-photon emission tomography dimercaptosuccinic acid. Surgery 1993;114:1083

97. Howe JR, Norton JA, Wells SA. Prevalence of pheochromocytoma and hyperparathyroidism in multiple endocrine neoplasia type 2A: results of long-term follow-up. Surgery 1993;114:1070

98. Ponder BAJ, Coffey R, Gagel RF, et al. Risk estimation and screening in families of patients with medullary thyroid carcinoma. Lancet 1988;1:397

99. Wells SA, Chi DD, Toshima K, et al. Predictive DNA testing and prophylactic thyroidectomy in patients at risk for multiple endocrine neoplasia type 2A. Ann Surg 1994;220:237

100. Lips CJM, Landsvater RM, Hoppener JWM, et al. Clinical screening as compared with DNA analysis in families with multiple endocrine neoplasia type 2A. N Engl J Med 1994;331:828

101. Gagel RF, Tashjian AH, Cummings T, et al. The clinical outcome of prospective screening for multiple endocrine neoplasia type 2A. N Engl J Med 1988;318:478

102. Bugalho MJM, Cote GJ, Khoran S, et al. Identification of a polymorphism in exon 11 of the ret proto-oncogene. Hum Mol Genet 1994;3:2263

103. Utiger RD. Medullary thyroid carcinoma, genes and the prevention of cancer (editorial). N Engl J Med 1994;331:870

104. Wells SA, Dilley WG, Farndon JA, et al. Early diagnosis and treatment of medullary thyroid carcinoma. Arch Intern Med 1985;145:1248

105. van Heerden JA, Grant CS, Gharib H, et al. Long term course of patients with persistent hypercalcitoninemia after apparent curative primary surgery for medullary thyroid carcinoma. Ann Surg 1990;212:395

106. Ellenhorn JDI, Shah JP, Brennan MF. Impact of therapeutic regional lymph node dissection for medullary carcinoma of the thyroid gland. Surgery 1993;114:1078

107. Tisell LE, Hansson G, Jansson S, Salander H. Reoperation in the treatment of asymptomatic metastasizing medullary thyroid carcinoma. Surgery 1986;99:60

108. Moley JF, Wells SA, Dilley WG, Tisell LE. Reoperation for recurrent or persistent medullary thyroid cancer. Surgery 1993;114:1090

109. Saad MF, Ordonez NA, Rashid RK, et al. Medullary carcinoma of the thyroid: a study of the clinical features and prognostic factors in 161 patients. Medicine 1984;63:319

110. Samaan NA, Schultz PN, Hickey RC. Medullary thyroid carcinoma: prognosis of familial versus sporadic disease and the role of radiotherapy. J Clin Endocrinol Metab 1988;67:801

111. Wu LT, Averbuch SD. Chemotherapy of advanced thyroid cancer. In: Cobin RH, Srota DK, eds. Malignant tumors of the thyroid. New York: Springer-Verlag, 1992:204

112. Averbuch SD, Steakley CS, Young RC, et al. Malignant pheochromocytoma: effective treatment with a combination of cyclophosphamide, vincristine and dacarbazine. Ann Intern Med 1988;109:267

113. Petrusson SR. Metastatic medullary thyroid carcinoma: complete response to combination chemotherapy with dacarbazine and 5-fluorouracil. Cancer 1988;62:1899

114. Wu L-T, Averbuch SD, Ball DW, et al. Treatment of advanced medullary thyroid carcinoma with a combination of cyclophosphamide, vincristine and dacarbazine. Cancer 1994;73:432

115. Kvols LK. Therapy of the malignant carcinoid syndrome and metastatic islet cell carcinoma. In: O'Dorisio TM, ed. Sandostatin in the treatment of GEP tumors. New York: Springer-Verlag 1989:65

116. Modigliani E, Cohen R, Joannidis S, et al. Results of long-term continuous subcutaneous octreotide administration in 14 patients with medullary thyroid carcinoma. Clin Endocrinol 1992;36:183

117. Frank-Raue K, Ziegler R, Raue F. The use of octreotide in the treatment of medullary thyroid carcinoma. Horm Metab Res Suppl 1993;27:44

118. Saad MF, Fritsche HA, Samaan NA. Diagnostic and prognostic values of carcinoembryonic antigen in medullary carcinoma of the thyroid. J Clin Endocrinol Metab 1984;58:889

119. Mendelsohn G, Wells SA, Baylin SB. Relationship of tissue carcinoembryonic antigen and calcitonin to tumor virulence in medullary thyroid carcinoma. Cancer 1984;54:657

Werner and Ingbar's The Thyroid, Seventh Edition,
edited by Lewis E. Braverman and Robert D. Utiger.
Lippincott–Raven Publishers, Philadelphia, © 1996

82

Miscellaneous Tumors of the Thyroid

Martin Schlumberger

Bernard Caillou

Most thyroid carcinomas are well-differentiated carcinomas of thyroid follicular cells or medullary carcinomas (see chaps 80 and 81). There are, however, other types of malignant tumors of the thyroid (Table 82-1).

ANAPLASTIC THYROID CARCINOMA

Anaplastic carcinoma of the thyroid is one of the most aggressive cancers encountered in humans. In most cases, it represents the terminal stage in the dedifferentiation of a follicular or papillary carcinoma. In fact, anaplastic cells do not produce thyroglobulin (Tg), they are not able to transport iodine, and thyrotropin (TSH) receptors are not found in their plasma cell membranes.

Etiology and Pathogenesis

The most common clinical sequence is the long-standing existence of a thyroid tumor, either a benign adenoma or a differentiated carcinoma, in which an anaplastic change occurs. The frequency of this change is unknown, but it is rare because undifferentiated carcinomas represent such a small percentage of thyroid carcinomas.[1–4] Prolonged stimulation by TSH may be responsible for the changes as well as for the higher incidence of anaplastic carcinoma in areas of endemic goiter.[4,5]

A causal relationship between therapeutic radiation and anaplastic carcinoma has been suggested by the occurrence of anaplastic carcinoma in patients who had been treated for a differentiated thyroid carcinoma with radioiodine (^{131}I) or external radiotherapy.[6] However, most patients have never received ^{131}I,[1,2] and no cases of anaplastic carcinoma occurred in several large series of patients with differentiated carcinoma treated with ^{131}I or external beam radiation.[7–9]

The frequency of detection of *ras* oncogene activation in anaplastic carcinoma is high, as in differentiated thyroid tumors[10] (see chap 80). Activation of *ras* is probably an early event in thyroid tumorigenesis. Mutations of p53 are frequently found in anaplastic but not in differentiated thyroid carcinomas, suggesting that p53 mutations play a crucial role in progression from differentiated to undifferentiated carcinoma.[11]

Prevalence

Anaplastic carcinomas are uncommon, representing from less than 5% to 14% of all thyroid cancers.[1,2,4] The incidence is higher in areas of endemic goiter.[4] Nearly all the patients are elderly; the peak incidence is in the seventh decade of life. The male/female ratio is 1:1.5.

Diagnosis

More than one-third of the patients with anaplastic carcinoma have a long-standing goiter. The most common mode of presentation, occurring in two-thirds of the cases, is a rapidly enlarging neck mass. Compressive symptoms including hoarseness, dyspnea, cough, and dysphagia are frequent, and one-third of the patients have neck pain.[1,2]

At initial examination, most patients have a dominant fixed mass of 5 to 10 cm or more in diameter, multiple other nodules in both thyroid lobes, and enlarged lymph nodes. Twenty to 50% of patients have distant metastases, most often in the lungs. A hemorrhage into a benign mass can cause sim-

Anaplastic thyroid carcinoma

Thyroid lymphoma

Histiocytosis X

Mesenchymal tumors

Teratomas

Thyroid metastases of other tumors

ilar symptoms and signs and should be ruled out by ultrasonography and fine-needle biopsy.

Anaplastic carcinomas are solid masses that are hypofunctioning on thyroid scintigraphy. Serum Tg concentrations are frequently elevated because of the preexisting thyroid abnormalities, but serum calcitonin, carcinoembryonic antigen, and neuron-specific enolase concentrations are normal.

The diagnosis of anaplastic carcinoma is established by biopsy or at surgery. The extent of the tumor can be determined using ultrasonography, computed tomography (CT), and endoscopy to search for distant metastases in the lungs, bones, liver, and brain.

Anaplastic carcinomas have a rapidly progressing course. At the time of diagnosis, as noted above, many patients have metastases in cervical lymph nodes and invasion of adjacent organs (trachea, esophagus, vessels, and muscles). Distant metastases ultimately occur in most of the patients, most commonly in the lungs, followed by bones, brain, and liver.

Pathology

The tumor is typically composed of varying proportions of spindle, polygonal, and giant cells[12] (see chap 28), often including squamous cells and sarcomatoid foci. Keratin is the most useful epithelial marker and is present in 40% to 100% of the tumor.[2,13] Many anaplastic carcinomas have a well-differentiated component. Conversely, differentiated carcinomas with small undifferentiated foci should be considered as anaplastic.

Immunohistochemical studies indicate that most tumors previously called small cell undifferentiated carcinomas were in fact primary malignant lymphomas (positive for leukocyte common antigen) or less often medullary thyroid carcinoma (positive for calcitonin and carcinoembryonic antigen), poorly differentiated follicular carcinoma, or a thyroid metastasis from another primary tumor. Some tumors do not react with any antibody; they are considered anaplastic carcinomas and have the same prognosis.[12] Tg is inconsistently detected in anaplastic carcinoma cells. Reactivity for calcitonin has been described in some tumors, but anaplastic forms of medullary thyroid carcinomas are extremely rare.

Treatment

Survival is not altered by treatment with surgery, radiotherapy, or chemotherapy alone. In most patients, death is caused by local tumor invasion. The median survival is 2 to 6 months, and few patients have survived for more than 12 months[1,2,8]

Some therapeutic trials have been carried out. More radical surgery was no more effective than less radical surgery; radiotherapy failed to induce any regression. The most effective single cytotoxic drug against anaplastic carcinomas is doxorubicin, and a few responses have been reported with combined doxorubicin and cisplatin therapy.[14] In fact, only combined multimodality therapy improved the local control rate, thus avoiding death from suffocation.

COMBINATION OF LOW-DOSE DOXORUBICIN, RADIOTHERAPY, AND SURGERY

A combined regimen consisting of once weekly administration of doxorubicin (10 mg/m²) before hyperfractionated radiotherapy (1.6 Gy [160 rads] per treatment, twice a day for 3 days per week to a total dose of 57.6 Gy [5760 rads] in 40 days) was used in 19 patients.[15] There was no unexpected toxicity. The rate of complete neck tumor response was 84% initially and 68% at 2 years. Four patients survived longer than 20 months and the median survival was 1 year, the deaths being due to lung or brain metastases. Patients whose tumor volume exceeded more than 200 cm³ at presentation did not respond, and the patients who survived more than 1 year were those having radical surgery and minimal residual disease at the time of irradiation.

In another group of patients, a combination of hyperfractionated radiotherapy (1 Gy [100 rads] twice a day for 5 days per week to a total dose of 30 Gy [3000 rads]) and doxorubicin (20 mg per week) was followed by surgery after 2 to 3 weeks, when feasible. Then an additional dose of 16 Gy (1600 rads) was given with concomitant doxorubicin and was followed by additional doxorubicin.[16] Among 16 patients, 5 had complete local tumor control and 3 patients survived longer than 20 months. Five patients died from distant metastases and 8 from local growth. Despite the advanced age (>70 years) of most patients, toxicity was moderate and no patients failed to complete the protocol because of treatment-related toxicity.

MULTIMODAL APPROACH WITH AN AGGRESSIVE CYTOTOXIC REGIMEN

A combination of hyperfractionated radiotherapy (1 Gy [100 rads] twice a day for 5 days per week to a total dose of 30 Gy [3000 rads] in 3 weeks) and chemotherapy (bleomycin 5 mg daily, cyclophosphamide 200 mg daily, and 5-fluorouracil 500 mg every second day) was followed by surgery after 2 to 3 weeks, whenever feasible. Then radiotherapy was given with the same protocol to a total dose of 16 Gy (1600 rads) with concomitant chemotherapy and was followed by additional chemotherapy.[17] Severe toxicity occurred in one-third of the patients. Of 20 evaluable patients, 15 had an objective remission and 3 survived for more than a year; 7 patients died of local tumor growth.

A combination of chemotherapy (doxorubicin 60 mg/m² and cisplatin 90 mg/m² every 4 weeks) and radiotherapy was used in 12 patients aged less than 65 years.[18] Radiotherapy was carried out between days 10 and 20 of the first four courses of chemotherapy and delivered 17.5 Gy (1750 rads) in seven fractions to the neck and the upper mediastinum. Severe toxicity occurred in half the patients. Complete tumor control was obtained in 5 patients and 2 patients survived longer than 20 months, all of whom had undergone surgery. None of the patients not operated had complete local control of tumor.

ACCELERATED AND HYPERFRACTIONATED RADIOTHERAPY

Accelerated and hyperfractionated radiotherapy enables the delivery of an efficient radiation dose in a limited period of time and prevents repopulation in rapidly growing tumors. In a Swedish trial the daily fraction was 1.3 Gy (130 rads) twice a day combined with doxorubicin and surgery.[16] Among 17 patients, local control was obtained in 11 patients and death attributable to local failure occurred in 2 patients.

In conclusion, it appears that these treatment modalities are effective in some patients with anaplastic carcinoma. Acute toxicity is high and is the main factor limiting therapy in these elderly patients who are often in poor general condition. At the present time, we advocate a combination of surgery and accelerated and hyperfractionated radiotherapy with one of two protocols of chemotherapy: aggressive chemotherapy (doxorubicin-cisplatin) in patients under 70 years and low-dose doxorubicin in those over 70 years or in poor general condition.

In these series, no response was observed in distant metastases. This underlines the need for treating these patients as soon as possible, before distant metastases appear. Even in patients with metastatic disease, these treatment modalities may be useful because they can avoid death by suffocation caused by local tumor growth. Debulking surgery should be performed whenever possible but should not delay the commencement of the combined protocol of chemotherapy and radiotherapy.

THYROID LYMPHOMA

Prevalence

Primary lymphomas of the thyroid are uncommon tumors constituting approximately 2% of extranodal lymphomas and less than 5% of all malignant thyroid tumors. Most thyroid lymphomas are non-Hodgkin's lymphomas. The peak incidence is in the seventh decade and the male/female ratio is 1:3.[19–22]

Diagnosis

Thyroid lymphomas almost invariably present as a rapidly enlarging, painless neck mass. One-third of patients have compressive symptoms.[19,21] The mass is often fixed to surrounding tissues and half the patients have unilateral or bilateral cervical lymph node enlargement. Clinically evident distant disease is uncommon. About 20% of patients have a preexisting long-standing goiter, and hypothyroidism has been reported in up to 40%. It is due both to coexisting chronic autoimmune thyroiditis and to replacement of normal thyroid tissue by the tumor.

The palpated mass is solid and hypoechoic on ultrasonography, which often shows a characteristic asymmetrical pseudocystic pattern, and its ability to concentrate ^{131}I is lim-

ited. Magnetic resonance imaging (MRI) and CT scanning are similarly effective in determining the extent of the tumor and involvement of lymph nodes.

The majority of primary thyroid lymphomas arise in patients who have chronic autoimmune thyroiditis; most have serum antiperoxidase and anti-Tg antibodies. When peritumor tissues can be examined, nearly all cases have histologic evidence of chronic autoimmune thyroiditis.

Pathology

Primary thyroid lymphomas should be distinguished from generalized lymphomas with thyroid involvement.[22]

Fine-needle aspiration biopsy can be useful to distinguish lymphoid proliferation from epithelial tumors. However, differentiating lymphoma from chronic autoimmune thyroiditis by thyroid cytology may be difficult. Therefore, large-needle biopsy or surgical specimens are almost always needed for histologic diagnosis, immunoglobulin phenotyping, and immunohistochemistry. Immunohistochemical studies identify lymphoid proliferation if positive for leukocyte common antigen.

According to the international "Working Formulation," the majority of cases of thyroid lymphoma are of the diffuse large cell type and of follicular center cell origin. The prognosis is better for follicular tumors than for diffuse large cell or immunoblastic lymphomas. With immunohistochemistry, nearly all of them show B-cell markers. Monoclonality for light chain immunoglobulin is considered a strong indication of malignant lymphoma.

Because chronic autoimmune thyroiditis shows the features of "mucosa-associated lymphoid tissue" (MALT), a distinct subset of thyroid malignant lymphomas can be considered as "mucosa-associated lymphoid tissue" lymphomas (MALT-L). These latter lymphomas are characterized by a low grade of malignancy, slow growth, and a tendency for recurrence in other MALT sites such as the gastrointestinal or respiratory tract, the thymus, or the salivary glands.

Some isolated cases of Hodgkin's disease involving primarily the thyroid gland have been reported. They were of the nodular sclerosis type. Cases of primary plasmocytomas of the thyroid have also been reported.[23]

Treatment

Accurate staging is important for planning treatment. However, these patients are often elderly, are in poor condition, or may require urgent therapy to relieve symptoms, making a full staging investigation before treatment impractical. Staging includes physical examination; complete blood count; serum lactate dehydrogenase and β_2-microglobulin measurements; liver function tests; bone marrow biopsy; CT or MRI of neck, thorax, abdomen, and pelvis; and appropriate biopsies at other sites where tumor is suspected. Involvement of Waldeyer's ring and of the gastrointestinal tract has been associated with thyroid lymphomas, and therefore upper gastrointestinal radiographs or endoscopy should be performed.

Disseminated (stage III or IV) disease requires combined chemotherapy and external radiotherapy. In patients with disease apparently confined to the neck (stage I or II), several therapeutic regimens are available. Small tumors are frequently treated initially as primary thyroid carcinomas. Aggressive surgery to debulk large thyroid lymphomas is neither feasible nor necessary, and all patients should be treated with external radiotherapy and chemotherapy, whatever the extent of surgery.

External radiotherapy should be given in a total dose of 40 Gy (4000 rads) to the neck and mediastinum. About one-third of patients with disease apparently confined to the neck and treated with external radiotherapy alone have a recurrence at distant sites, generally within the first year after treatment. It may be that the patients having a relapse had disseminated disease at the time of diagnosis; even with aggressive staging, distant disease may not be detected. The chemotherapy should be an anthracycline-based regimen. It usually consists of three to six cycles of the CHOP regimen (doxorubicin 50 mg/m^2 on day 1, cyclophosphamide 750 mg/m^2 on day 1, vincristine 1.4 mg/m^2 on day 1, and prednisone 40 mg/m^2/day on days 1–5) every 3 weeks. Most patients with thyroid lymphoma have bulky local disease, which is an adverse risk factor for local control with chemotherapy alone.[21] In some series, the long-term survival rate of combined chemo- and radiotherapy was nearly 100%.[19] This regimen may not be suitable for patients in poor general health or those of advanced age, and external radiotherapy is advised instead.

OTHER UNUSUAL TUMORS OF THE THYROID

Histiocytosis X. Isolated cases of thyroid involvement have been reported in patients with the malignant form of the disease.[24] Chemotherapy with an anthracycline-based regimen induces long-term remission in most of these patients.

Sinus histiocytosis with massive lymphadenopathy (Rosai-Dorfman disease) stimulates chronic autoimmune thyroiditis or a malignant process. S100 protein-positive histiocytes with strong plasma cell reactions are the main histologic features. Most affected patients have an irregular goiter and enlarged cervical lymph nodes. In the majority, spontaneous regression occurs, but the disease may progress and may be lethal.[25] In these latter patients, chemotherapy with an anthracycline-based regimen can be effective.

Mesenchymal Tumors of the Thyroid. Benign mesenchymal tumors of the thyroid such as lipoma and hemangioma are extremely rare. They are usually treated with surgery alone. Primary fibrosarcomas of the thyroid are also rare and can be difficult to distinguish from sarcomatoid forms of anaplastic carcinoma. The same problem arises with angiosarcoma.[26] From a therapeutic viewpoint, all patients with sarcoma-like or angiosarcoma-like malignant tumors of the thyroid should be treated in the same way as are patients with anaplastic thyroid carcinoma.

Teratoma of the Thyroid Gland. There are two different types of thyroid teratomas. In infants, teratomas are often congenital and are composed of mature cystic tissue; they are benign and are treated by total thyroidectomy followed by thyroid hormone replacement therapy.[27] In children and in adults, teratomas are composed of neuroepithelial tissue.[28]

The histogenesis of this proliferation is still controversial. These tumors are highly malignant and metastasize early to lymph nodes and the lungs. They require combined treatment with surgery, external radiotherapy, and chemotherapy.

Other Primary Tumors. Ectopic normal or tumoral parathyroid or thymic tissue can be located inside the thyroid gland, but it should not be confused with a primary thyroid tumor pathologically. The thyroid gland is an unusual site of a primary paraganglioma.[29]

Thyroid Metastases. Microscopic metastases to the thyroid are common findings in autopsies of patients with malignant tumors.[30] A thyroid nodule may rarely be the initial presentation of a tumor arising in a contiguous structure. Such patients ordinarily do not present a diagnostic dilemma. However, the discovery of a squamous or a neuroendocrine tumor of unknown primary origin should dictate a complete work-up including neck CT scan.

Frequently, a thyroid mass is discovered in a patient who has been treated for another cancer, such as carcinoma of the kidney, breast, lung, or colon or a malignant melanoma. The interval between the diagnosis of the primary tumor and the appearance of the thyroid mass may be many years; furthermore, the thyroid mass may be the only known metastatic site. In such patients, fine-needle biopsy may be useful for diagnosis,[31] but surgery is usually performed. Diagnosis may be difficult and require immunohistochemical studies. Negative immunostaining with anti-Tg and anticalcitonin antibodies is a strong argument in favor of the metastatic origin of the thyroid tumor.

References

1. Nel CJC, Van Heerden JA, Goellner JR, et al. Anaplastic carcinoma of the thyroid: a clinicopathologic study of 82 cases. Mayo Clin Proc 1985;60:51
2. Venkatesh YSS, Ordonez NG, Schultz PN, et al. Anaplastic carcinoma of the thyroid. A clinicopathologic study of 121 cases. Cancer 1990;66:321
3. Carcangiu M, Steeper T, Zampi G, Rosai J. Anaplastic thyroid carcinoma. A study of 70 cases. Am J Clin Pathol 1985;83:135
4. Williams ED. Pathologic and natural history of thyroid cancer. Recent results. Cancer Res 1980;73:47
5. Crile G. The endocrine dependency of certain thyroid cancers and the danger that hypothyroidism may stimulate their growth. Cancer 1957;10:1119
6. Baker HW. Anaplastic thyroid cancer twelve years after radioiodine therapy. Cancer 1969;23:885
7. Schlumberger M, Tubiana M, De Vathaire F, et al. Long-term results of treatment of 283 patients with lung and bone metastases from differentiated thyroid carcinoma. J Clin Endocrinol Metab 1986;63:960
8. Tubiana M, Haddad E, Schlumberger M, et al. External radiotherapy in thyroid cancers. Cancer 1985;55:2062
9. Simpson WJ, Panzarella T, Carruthers JS, et al. Papillary and follicular thyroid cancer: impact of treatment in 1578 patients. Int J Radiat Oncol Biol Phys 1988;14:1063
10. Lemoine NR, Mayall ES, Willie FS, et al. Activated *ras* oncogenes in human thyroid cancers. Cancer Res 1988;48:4459
11. Ito T, Seyama T, Mizuno T, et al. Unique association of p53 mutations with undifferentiated but not with differentiated carcinomas of the thyroid gland. Cancer Res 1992;52:1369

12. Hedinger C, Williams ED, Sobin LH. Histological typing of thyroid tumours. International histological classification of tumours. 2nd ed. World Health Organization. Berlin: Springer-Verlag, 1988

13. Livolsi VA, Brooks JJ, Arendash-Durand B. Anaplastic thyroid tumors: immunohistology. Am J Clin Pathol 1987;87:434

14. Shimaoka K, Schoenfeld DA, De Wys WD, et al. A randomized trial of doxorubicin versus doxorubicin plus cisplatin in patients with advanced thyroid carcinoma. Cancer 1985;56:2155

15. Kim JH, Leeper RD. Treatment of locally advanced thyroid carcinoma with combination doxorubicin and radiation therapy. Cancer 1987;60:2372

16. Tennvall J, Lundell G, Hallquist A, Wahlborg P, Wallin G, Tibblin S, and the Swedish Anaplastic Thyroid Cancer Group. Combined doxorubicin, hyperfractionated radiotherapy, and surgery in anaplastic thyroid carcinoma. Report on two protocols. Cancer 1994;74:1348

17. Tallroth E, Wallin G, Lundell G, et al. Multimodality treatment in anaplastic giant cell thyroid carcinoma. Cancer 1987;60:1428

18. Schlumberger M, Parmentier C, Delisle MJ, et al. Combination therapy for anaplastic giant cell thyroid carcinoma. Cancer 1991;67:564

19. Matsuzuka F, Miyauchi A, Katayama S, et al. Clinical aspects of primary thyroid lymphoma: diagnosis and treatment based on our experience of 119 cases. Thyroid 1993;3:93

20. Tsang RW, Gospodarowicz MK, Sutcliffe SB, et al. Non-Hodgkin's lymphoma of the thyroid gland: prognostic factors and treatment outcome. Int J Radiat Oncol Biol Phys 1993; 27:559

21. Doria R, Jekel JF, Cooper DL. Thyroid lymphoma: the case for combined modality therapy. Cancer 1994;73:200

22. Salhany KE, Pietra GG. Extranodal lymphoid disorders. Am J Clin Pathol 1993;99:472

23. Aozasa K, Inoue A, Yoshimura H, et al. Plasmocytoma of the thyroid gland. Cancer 1986;58:105

24. Teja K, Sabio H, Langdon DR, Johanson AJ. Involvement of the thyroid gland in histiocytosis. Hum Pathol 1981;12:1137

25. Foucar E, Rosai J, Dorfman RF. Sinus histocytosis with massive lymphadenopathy: an analysis of 14 deaths occurring in a patient registry. Cancer 1984;54:1834

26. Ruchti C, Gerber HA, Schaffner T. Factor VIII–related antigen in malignant hemangioendotheliomas of the thyroid. Additional evidence for the endothelial origin of the tumor. Am J Clin Pathol 1984;82:474

27. Fisher JE, Cooney DR, Voorhess ML, Jewett TC Jr. Teratoma of thyroid gland in infancy: review of the literature and two case reports. J Surg Oncol 1982;21:135

28. Buckley NJ, Burch WM, Leight GS. Malignant teratoma in the thyroid gland of an adult: a case report and a review of the literature. Surgery 1986;100:932

29. Buss DH, Marshall RB, Baird FG, Myers RT. Paraganglioma of the thyroid gland. Am J Surg Pathol 1980;4:589

30. Ivy HK. Cancer metastatic to the thyroid: a diagnostic problem. Mayo Clin Proc 1984;59:856

31. Smith SA, Gharib H, Goellner JR. Fine-needle aspiration. Usefulness for diagnosis and management of metastatic carcinoma to the thyroid. Arch Intern Med 1987;147:311

Werner and Ingbar's The Thyroid, Seventh Edition,
edited by Lewis E. Braverman and Robert D. Utiger.
Lippincott–Raven Publishers, Philadelphia, © 1996

83

Clinical Evaluation of Solitary Thyroid Nodules

E. Chester Ridgway

The solitary thyroid nodule represents a common and important clinical problem. In the United States, the estimated lifetime risk for developing a nodule is between 5% and 10%.[1] These data were projected by prospective follow-up of 5127 persons in Framingham, Massachusetts. In this cohort, 4.2% had a thyroid nodule when first examined, 6.4% of the women and 1.6% of the men. During a 15-year follow-up period, 67 persons (1.3%) developed new nodules. These population data do not adequately delineate the full problem. In the large autopsy study of Mortenson and colleagues in Minnesota,[2] half the population had either single or multiple thyroid nodules, many of which were small. These results have been corroborated by the use of thyroid ultrasonography in persons not suspected of having thyroid disease.[3,4] It is difficult to estimate the clinical importance of these nodules, but few are thyroid carcinomas.

The natural history of thyroid nodules is poorly understood. In a recent report from Japan, 140 patients with thyroid nodules who had not been treated were reexamined an average of 15 years later.[5] Based on physical examination and ultrasonography, the nodules had increased in size in 13%, not changed in 34%, decreased in 23%, and were no longer palpable in 30%. The nodules that increased in size were originally predominantly solid, whereas those that disappeared were predominantly cystic. Nine of 98 patients (9%) who still had a palpable nodule had a thyroid carcinoma when evaluated by fine-needle aspiration (FNA) and surgery; carcinoma was present in 26% of the nodules that had increased in size, but only 6% and 3% of those unchanged or smaller, respectively. Thus, many nodules (especially cystic nodules) disappear with time, whereas a minority increase (mainly solid nodules). Increasing size has modest but significant predictive power for thyroid carcinoma.

Thus, the critical issue is whether a nodule is benign or malignant. Although thyroid nodules are common, relatively few are carcinomas. As a general rule, between 5% and 10% of clinically detectable solitary hypofunctioning thyroid nodules will prove to be thyroid carcinomas after appropriate evaluation and follow-up.

CLINICAL EVALUATION

Some information that can be obtained by history and physical examination are useful in determining the likelihood that a thyroid nodule is a carcinoma (Table 83-1).

The family history is important because a positive history of goiter in the family suggests the presence of a benign disorder, unless the family history includes medullary thyroid carcinoma, pheochromocytoma, or other components of multiple endocrine neoplasia type 2. Also, several families have been reported in which multiple members had papillary or follicular thyroid carcinoma.

The age of the patient is important. Most benign nodules occur in patients aged 30 to 50 years. In contrast, benign thyroid nodules are less common in children and adolescents, so that a nodule in a patient in these age groups is more likely to be a carcinoma;[6,7] the incidence of carcinoma in patients in these age groups varies from 20% to 73%. Therefore, the diagnostic approach in them should be more aggressive. The same considerations apply to patients over age 60 years.

Similarly, the patient's sex is important. Benign nodules are several-fold more common in women than in men, whereas, the rates of thyroid carcinoma are nearly equal in men and in women. Therefore, a nodule in a man is more likely to be a carcinoma.

A particularly important piece of historical information is whether or not the person received head or neck irradiation in childhood.[8–11] This therapy, which was given between 1940

TABLE 83-1.

Clinical Factors Suggesting the Diagnosis of Thyroid Carcinoma in a Euthyroid Patient With a Solitary Nodule

Family history

Age: <20 or >60 y

Sex: Male > female

History of head and neck irradiation in infancy, childhood, or adolescence

Large, rapidly growing nodule

Pain

Firm or hard texture

Fixation to surrounding structures

Compression symptoms—dysphagia, hoarseness, dypsnea

Lymphadenopathy

Growth during thyroid hormone therapy

and 1960 for thymic enlargement, recurrent tonsillitis, adenoiditis, and other conditions, is known to cause both benign nodules and thyroid carcinomas (see section on pathogenesis in chap 80). Among persons who received head or neck irradiation at an early age, from 10% to 40% will have a thyroid abnormality on physical examination 5 to 30 years later. The abnormality is some type of benign thyroid disease in 70% and carcinoma in 30%. The thyroid carcinomas that occur in patients who received head and neck irradiation are nearly all papillary carcinomas, and most have an excellent prognosis with appropriate therapy. Nonthyroidal lesions, including parathyroid adenomas and parotid tumors, also occur more often in previously irradiated patients.

Useful information also can be obtained by assessing the rate of growth of the thyroid nodule. A nodule that has not changed in size for several years is almost always benign, as is a nodule that appears suddenly; the latter is likely to be a thyroid cyst or a previously undetected thyroid nodule into which a hemorrhage has occurred. In contrast, thyroid carcinomas usually develop over a period of weeks or months. A particularly worrisome feature is enlargement of a nodule while the patient is receiving thyroid hormone therapy.

The presence of certain local symptoms suggests a nodule is a carcinoma. For example, a nodule that causes discomfort in the neck or in the jaw or ear, dysphagia, hoarseness, or dyspnea (indicative of esophageal or tracheal involvement) is likely to be a carcinoma. These symptoms, however, can occur in patients with benign causes of thyroid enlargement, particularly large multinodular goiters.

The functional status of the thyroid is important in determining whether a nodule is benign or malignant. Virtually all patients with thyroid carcinoma are euthyroid. So also are most patients with benign thyroid nodules, but a few have autonomously functioning adenomas that cause thyrotoxicosis and a very few have hypothyroidism caused by chronic autoimmune thyroiditis. Thyroid nodules also may be metastases of carcinomas of the breast, colon, kidney, or other sites (see chap 82).

The physical examination is of great importance in evaluating a patient with a thyroid nodule; the success of the examination is directly related to the skill of the examiner. Nodules smaller than 0.5 cm are difficult to detect by physical examination, whereas most nodules larger than 1 cm in diameter should be detected. The physical examination can give only general clues as to the benign or malignant nature of the nodule. A nodule that is fixed to surrounding structures such as the trachea or strap muscles is probably a carcinoma. Very hard nodules may be carcinomas, but benign nodules also can be hard, especially if they are calcified. Although soft nodules are usually benign, this physical finding does not exclude carcinoma. Paralysis of one of the vocal cords also suggests carcinoma, but large goiters of any type can cause abnormalities of vocal cord function. The presence of ipsilateral lymphadenopathy also suggests the presence of carcinoma. The presence of multiple similar nodules in the thyroid usually indicates a multinodular goiter. Similarly, a thyroid gland that has a palpable nodule but that also feels rubbery and irregular suggests that the underlying process may be chronic autoimmune thyroiditis.

In assessing these clinical factors, some features of the history and physical examination are more suggestive of carcinoma than others. Table 83-2 shows the clinical findings associated with a high, moderate, or low likelihood that a nodule is a carcinoma based on the histology of the resected nodule. If the patient had a single "high-suspicion finding," there was a 71% chance of carcinoma; whereas 14% and 11% of the patients, respectively, with "moderate- or low-suspicion findings" had carcinoma. Furthermore, if a patient had two or

TABLE 83-2.

Occurrence of Carcinoma in 169 Patients With Nodular Thyroid Disease in Relation to Clinical Findings

	No. (%)
High suspicion of carcinoma (n = 31)*	22 (71)
Medullary thyroid cancer (multiple endocrine neoplasia in family)	0 (0)
Rapid nodule growth	5 (100)
Very firm nodule	2 (50)
Fixation to adjacent structures	5 (71)
Vocal cord paralysis (laryngoscopy)	5 (83)
Enlarged regional lymph nodes	12 (71)
Distant metastases (lungs or bones)	4 (100)
Moderate suspicion of carcinoma (n = 64)†	9 (14)
Age <20 y	1 (20)
Age >60 y	4 (16)
History of head and neck irradiation	1 (6)
Male sex and solitary nodule	3 (15)
Dubious fixation	0 (0)
Diameter >4 cm and partially cystic	0 (0)
Low suspicion of carcinoma (n = 74)	8 (11)
All others	8 (11)

*Two or more findings were present in nine patients, all of whom had carcinomas.
†Two or more findings were present in 15 patients, one of whom had a carcinoma.
Data from references 12 and 13.

more high suspicion findings the likelihood of carcinoma was 100%, whereas the presence of two or more findings of moderate or low suspicion did not improve the clinical prediction of carcinoma. These results suggest that some clinical findings have substantial value in assessing the likelihood of carcinoma in a patient with a thyroid nodule. Nevertheless, the results also underscore the lack of specificity and sensitivity of clinical evaluation of patients with solitary thyroid nodules.

LABORATORY EVALUATION

The laboratory evaluation of a patient with a solitary thyroid nodule is shown in Figure 83-1. Serum thyrotropin (TSH) should be measured to determine whether the patient has thyrotoxicosis (caused by an autonomously functioning thyroid adenoma) or hypothyroidism (caused by chronic autoimmune thyroiditis). Nearly all patients with thyroid carcinoma have normal serum TSH concentrations, but so also do most pa-

tients with benign nodules. The finding of a high serum TSH concentration in a patient with a thyroid nodule indicates the presence of hypothyroidism. If the nodule is not obviously part of a thyroid gland affected by chronic autoimmune thyroiditis, then it presumably is unrelated to the hypothyroidism and FNA biopsy should be done. If the serum TSH concentration is low, then a radionuclide scan should be performed. Iodine isotopes are generally preferred because iodine uptake is a measure not only of iodine trapping but also organification. Technetium can also be used, but because it is only trapped but not organified and therefore does not accumulate in the gland, it provides a less complete assessment of the functional integrity of the nodule. For instance, a thyroid nodule may be hyperfunctioning (hot) on a technetium scan but hypofunctioning (cold) on an iodine scan. This distinction is important because hyperfunctioning nodules are benign and carcinomas are usually hypofunctioning. Of the radionuclides used for thyroid scanning, iodine-123, which has a short half-life and low radiation dose, is preferable (see chap 17).

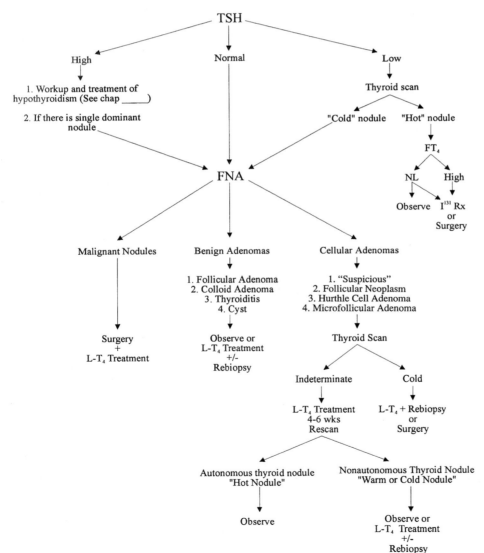

FIGURE 83-1. Evaluation of the patient with a thyroid nodule. The serum TSH concentration is used to define those patients with hypothyroidism or an autonomously functioning thyroid adenoma. Most patients will require fine-needle aspiration (FNA) biopsy.

If the serum TSH concentration is low and the thyroid nodule is hyperfunctioning on a thyroid scan using an iodine isotope, then the patient has an autonomously functioning thyroid adenoma.[14–16] Among patients with these adenomas, about 80% are euthyroid and 20% have thyrotoxicosis. Younger patients usually are euthyroid, whereas older patients have a higher likelihood of having thyrotoxicosis. All of the clinically thyrotoxic and some of the euthyroid patients have low serum TSH concentrations. Serum free thyroxine (T_4) should be measured to confirm or exclude overt thyrotoxicosis if the serum TSH concentration is low. Patients with thyroid adenomas who have thyrotoxicosis should be treated with either radioactive iodine or surgery (see chap 32).[17] Euthyroid patients can be followed, but because they may have an increased risk of cardiac arrhythmia or osteoporosis, a valid argument can be made for treating them with radioactive iodine or surgery also. Ethanol injection of the nodule is a newer alternative to radioactive iodine or surgery.[18–20] If the patient is not treated, adenoma size is an important determinant of the eventual outcome. For instance, patients whose adenomas are greater than 3 cm in size have a 20% chance of developing thyrotoxicosis in a 6-year period, whereas among those with adenomas smaller than 2.5 cm only 2% to 5% become thyrotoxic.[16]

If the serum TSH value is low and the thyroid scan shows that the thyroid nodule is hypofunctioning, FNA biopsy should be performed. In this case, the low serum TSH concentration is unrelated to the thyroid nodule. Possible reasons for the low serum TSH value include thyroid hormone therapy, nonthyroidal illness, coexistent Graves' disease, medications such as glucocorticoids, or very rarely, concomitant hypopituitarism.

If the serum TSH concentration is normal, then a tissue diagnosis should be made. Several methods are available for obtaining tissue for cytologic or histologic examination[21–23] (see chap 23). Among them, the FNA technique is easy to learn and is the most widely used. It involves the use of either a 10- or 25-mL plastic syringe with a 22- to 27-gauge needle. The patient's neck is prepared with the appropriate sterile technique, the overlying skin is anesthetized with lidocaine, and the needle is inserted into the nodule. Suction is applied at various angles, and the cells are withdrawn into the barrel of the needle. This material is then placed on a microscopic slide for subsequent cytologic analysis. Some physicians prefer to use larger needles, including large cutting needles, to obtain more tissue so that histologic analysis, in addition to cytologic analysis, can be performed.[21,23]

When any of these techniques are used for the evaluation of hypofunctioning thyroid nodules, 5% to 15% of the nodules are found to be malignant. These findings contrast with older estimates that 20% to 50% of solitary thyroid nodules are malignant. When the cytologic (or histologic) diagnosis is benign nodule, which will be the result in 60% to 70% of nodules, the nodule is a follicular adenoma, colloid adenoma, thyroiditis, or cyst. Approximately 20% of thyroid aspirates are variously classified as follicular neoplasm, suspicious Hürtle cell tumor, or microfollicular adenoma. These cytologic diagnoses present special difficulties because about 20% of of the nodules in this group prove to be malignant when excised and examined histologically. Depending on the experience of the physician performing the FNA biopsy, up to 10% of aspirates will be in-

determinate or inadequate, meaning that sufficient cells were not obtained for accurate analysis. These nodules should be rebiopsied until a satisfactory sample is obtained.

Patients in whom the aspirate is cellular should undergo radioiodine scanning. If the nodule is hypofunctioning, the patient should be followed carefully for signs of malignancy or the nodule should be excised. If the nodule concentrates some radioiodine, it is variously described as indeterminant or warm. In fact, these nodules may be either hyperfunctioning or hypofunctioning. If the former, the nodule is an autonomously functioning thyroid adenoma but is not secreting enough thyroid hormone to suppress endogenous TSH secretion, and the surrounding paranodular tissue is still functioning normally. A suppression scan may be useful in this circumstance.[24] To do this study, 100 to 200 µg T_4 is given for 4 to 6 weeks, and the thyroid scan is repeated. If the nodule is hyperfunctioning and autonomous, the second scan will reveal uptake by the nodule, but all paranodular tissue will be suppressed (see Fig. 1 in chap 32). This pattern of response proves the nodule is autonomous and hence is benign. In contrast, if T_4 suppresses all uptake, the nodule is considered to be nonautonomous. A patient with such a nodule should be managed like a patient with a hypofunctioning thyroid nodule, with either observation alone, T_4 therapy, or rebiopsy. An example of these various options is shown in Figure 83-2.

An alternative procedure for patients with a solitary nodule that is advocated by many investigators is to perform a FNA biopsy as the first step. If the cytologic examination of the cells reveals a cellular specimen consistent with a follicular neoplasm, Hürthle cell tumor, or microfollicular adenoma, then a radionuclide scan and thyroid function tests are performed to determine the functional status of the nodule. The conceptual framework for this approach is that it eliminates unnecessary biochemical and imaging tests in the initial evaluation of the patient because most patients with a thyroid nodule have normal serum TSH concentrations and hypofunctioning nodules. Both work-up plans discussed in this chapter are more cost effective than the older plan that consisted of a thyroid radionuclide scan and thyroid function tests, followed by FNA biopsy if the nodule was hypofunctioning. The newer plans are less expensive because fewer thyroid scans are performed.

The ultimate value of FNA biopsy in the evaluation of patients with a thyroid nodule has been reviewed extensively.[12,24–29] The sensitivity of the test varies from 83% to 99% and the specificity from 70% to 90%. As noted above, 5% to 15% of nodules are malignant, 60% to 70% are benign, and approximately 20% are cellular specimens variously classified as suspicious or follicular neoplasms and related conditions; about 20% of the latter group prove to be carcinomas.[30] The rates of false-negative and false-positive cytologic diagnosis are 5% and 6%, respectively. In a unique recent study from France, cytologic and histologic findings in 132 patients who had surgery independent of the findings on FNA biopsy were compared.[31] Of 92 nodules considered cytologically to be benign, 91 were confirmed to be benign and only 1 was reclassified as malignant. All 14 nodules considered cytologically to be malignant were confirmed to be malignant. Twenty-one nodules were cytologically classified as suspicious of which 5 were found to be malignant. Thus, FNA biopsy of thyroid nod-

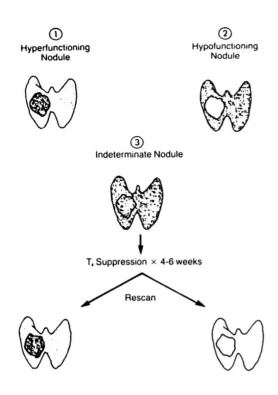

FIGURE 83-2. Possible images obtained by radionuclide scanning of a patient with a solitary thyroid nodule. (1) An autonomously hyperfunctioning thyroid adenoma (hot nodule) with uptake of the radionuclide only in the palpable nodule and decreased or absent uptake in paranodular tissue. (2) A hypofunctioning thyroid nodule (cold nodule) with absent or decreased uptake of the radionuclide in the palpable nodule and normal uptake in the paranodular tissue. (3) An indeterminate nodule in which the distinction between hot and cold is ambiguous. A second radionuclide scan while the patient is taking T_4 is helpful. If the second scan shows a functioning nodule, it is an autonomously functioning thyroid adenoma. If the scan shows no functioning tissue, the nodule is nonautonomous and requires further evaluation.

ules is a reliable test, so widely used and accepted now that the rates of surgery for patients with solitary thyroid nodules have dropped from 90% to 20% to 50%.

Other diagnostic tests also may be used in the evaluation of patients with a thyroid nodule. Thyroid ultrasonography may be useful when a thyroid cyst is suspected by palpation of the thyroid nodule or because a nodule developed rapidly.[32] If a cyst is discovered, then simple aspiration is the treatment of choice. Crystal clear fluid strongly suggests a parathyroid cyst, which is readily confirmed by measuring the concentration of parathyroid hormone in the cyst fluid. Thyroid carcinoma is not excluded by the presence of fluid, particularly if the nodule is large. Therefore, any fluid obtained should be examined cytologically. If the nodule is a mixed solid and cystic nodule, then both regions should be aspirated. Ultrasonography also can be used to determine whether a nodule is solitary or is part of a multinodular goiter, the presence of multiple nodules suggesting the presence of a multinodular goiter. Finally, ultrasonography can help in planning the surgical approach to a malignant nodule. If multiple nodules are found in addition to the malignant or highly suspicious nodule, then a more extensive or complete thyroidectomy is recommended. Thyroid ultrasonography is discussed in more detail in chapter 22.

A number of serum measurements can serve as markers for particular types of thyroid carcinoma. Serum calcitonin, and to a lesser extent, carcinoembryonic antigen measurements are useful as adjunctive diagnostic tests for medullary thyroid carcinoma and even more useful for follow-up and identification of affected family members in families with medullary thyroid carcinoma or multiple endocrine neoplasia type 2. However, the prevalence of medullary thyroid carcinoma among patients with solitary thyroid nodules is so low that recommending these measurements in the initial evaluation of a patient with a thyroid nodule is cost prohibitive. Serum thyroglobulin measurements also have been recommended for the evaluation of patients with thyroid nodules. However, the specificity of elevated serum thyroglobulin concentrations as an indicator of thyroid carcinoma in patients with thyroid nodules is poor because the concentration may be increased in any patient with any type of thyroid nodule (see chap 20).

TREATMENT OF THYROID NODULES

Surgery

All patients with a cytologically malignant thyroid nodule should undergo surgery, and it may be recommended for patients with cytologically suspicious nodules as well (see section on surgical therapy in chap 80). Controversy exists about the extent of the surgical procedure that should be done. If the nodule is small and no other nodules are noted at operation, then either a unilateral lobectomy or a subtotal thyroidectomy is preferred. If the nodule is large or multiple nodules are seen, then a subtotal or near-total thyroidectomy is recommended. To perform a total thyroidectomy in every patient with a malignant nodule is probably excessive, but a simple unilateral lobectomy is too limited an operation for patients with large nodules or multiple nodules. If lymph nodes containing tumor are found at surgery, then local excision without a radical neck dissection commonly is performed. The presence of carcinoma in lymph nodes does not significantly affect the prognosis for survival in most patients. If the thyroid nodule is a medullary or anaplastic thyroid carcinoma, more extensive surgical resection is commonly performed.

Whether the patient has a unilateral lobectomy or a near-total thyroidectomy for the carcinoma, lifelong T_4 therapy is indicated. The dose should be one that inhibits TSH secretion sufficiently that the serum TSH concentration is low. In small, elderly patients, doses of 75 to 125 µg daily usually are sufficient, whereas children and young or middle-aged adults require 100 to 200 µg daily. The purposes of treatment are to minimize the risk of recurrence as well as to treat hypothyroidism caused by the operation. T_4 therapy is also often given after surgical excision of benign thyroid nodules. It is effective in preventing the appearance of new benign nodules in pa-

TABLE 83-3.
Placebo-Controlled Studies of T_4 Treatment of Patients with Thyroid Nodules

Investigators	No. of Patients	T_4 Dose (daily)	Duration (mo)	Palpation*	Ultrasound†	Benefit of T_4‡
Gharib et al[40]	53	3.0 μg/kg	6.0	NS	NS	NS
Cheung et al[41]	74	~150 μg§	18.0	NS	—	NS
Reverter et al[42]	40	2.8 μg/kg	10.6	—	NS	NS
Papini et al[43]	101	2.0 μg/kg	12.0	$P < 0.05$	NS	$P = 0.005$
LaRosa et al[44‖]	80	1.94 μg/kg	12.0	—	$P < 0.001$	$P = 0.004$

*Size assessed by palpation.
†Size assessed by ultrasonography.
‡Comparison of percentage of patients having a decrease in nodule size in the T_4 group with the percentage having a decrease in the control group (NS, P > 0.05).
§Dose not given according to weight.
‖The control group received no treatment rather than placebo.

tients who had surgery for a nodule that appeared after head and neck irradiation,[33] but not in preventing new malignant nodules. Its value in preventing the appearance of new nodules in patients who had not received radiation is controversial.

Medical Therapy

A patient with a cytologically suspicious nodule that is not hyperfunctioning on radionuclide imaging should be treated with T_4 if surgery is not performed. This therapy is designed to reduce TSH secretion and thereby eliminate an important growth factor for thyroid tissue, with the goal of reducing the size of the nodule or at least preventing its further growth. The dose of T_4 should be between 100 and 200 μg daily. In younger patients these doses can be started immediately, whereas in older patients the starting dose should be 50 μg daily and the dose raised gradually to 75 to 150 μg daily. It is important to document that the serum TSH concentration is low and to assess nodule size accurately.[34–37] Unless the nodule decreases substantially in size, FNA biopsy should be repeated to determine if the cytologic characteristics of the nodule have changed. In a study of 217 patients who had a second biopsy an average of 2.4 years after the initial biopsy, 91% of 183 initially benign biopsies remained benign, 6% were suspicious, and 3% were malignant.[38] Of 34 initially suspicious biopsies, 47% remained suspicious, whereas 53% were benign at the second biopsy. These results support a conservative approach to thyroid nodules that are classified as suspicious or a related term as described above. Growth of the nodule during follow-up is an indication for surgery.

Patients with cytologically benign nodules may be treated with T_4 or followed without any therapy, with repeat FNA biopsy at 1- to 5-year intervals.[26,39] The practice of treating all patients with benign nodules with T_4 has recently been challenged by the results of several double-blind, placebo-controlled studies.[40–44] In most of these studies nodule size was measured by ultrasonography (Table 83-3). In three studies, T_4 in doses sufficient to reduce serum TSH concentrations was no more effective than placebo,[40–42] whereas in two recent studies from Italy T_4 was more effective than placebo in reducing nodule size.[43,44] In the most recent study,[44] a daily dose of 1.94

μg/kg T_4 reduced serum TSH concentrations to 0.1 μU/mL and caused a 40% overall reduction in nodule volume, with 39% of the treated patients having a 50% or greater reduction in the volume of their thyroid nodule. These results provide support for the view that patients with a benign nodule should be treated with T_4 in a dose sufficient to lower the serum TSH concentration to the lower limit of normal (approximately 0.5 μU/mL) for 1 year. This dosage recommendation is based on data indicating that larger doses may have adverse effects on the cardiovascular and skeletal systems as well as on bone density measurements.[45–47] If the nodule disappears or decreases substantially in size, therapy should be continued indefinitely. If there is no change, the therapy should be discontinued and the patient followed, perhaps with repeat FNA biopsy for cytologic reevaluation. If the nodule enlarges, repeat FNA biopsy and surgical intervention should be performed.

Patients with a benign thyroid nodule need lifelong follow-up with semiannual or annual reevaluation. The purpose of these visits is to assess nodule size and compliance with T_4 therapy, if prescribed. Serum TSH concentrations should be monitored and nodule size evaluated using calipers and a tape measure. More precise measurements of nodule size can be obtained by ultrasonography, but this test is expensive and is not routinely needed in following patients with a benign condition.

References

1. Vander JB, Gaston EA, Dawber TR. The significance of nontoxic thyroid nodules: final report of a 15 year study of the incidence of thyroid malignancy. Ann Intern Med 1968;69:537
2. Mortenson JD, Woolner LB, Bennett WA. Gross and microscopic findings in clinically normal thyroid glands. J Clin Endocrinol Metab 1955;15:1270
3. Horlocker TT, Hay ID, James EM, et al. Prevalence of incidental nodular thyroid disease detected during high-resolution parathyroid ultrasonography. In: Medeiros-Neto G, Gaitan E, eds. Frontiers of thyroidology. Vol. 2. New York: Plenum Press, 1986:1309
4. Ezzat S, Sarti DA, Cain DR, et al. Thyroid incidentalomas. Prevalence by palpation and ultrasonography. Arch Intern Med 1994;154:1838

5. Kuma K, Matsuzuka F, Kobayashi A, et al. Outcome of long standing solitary thyroid nodules. World J Surg 1992;16:583

6. Scott MD, Crawford JD. Solitary thyroid nodules in childhood: is the incidence of thyroid carcinoma declining? Pediatrics 1976;58:521

7. Silverman SH, Nussbaum M, Rausen AR. Thyroid nodules in children: a ten-year experience at one institution. Mt Sinai J Med 1979;46:460

8. Hempelmann LH. Risk of thyroid neoplasms after irradiation in childhood: studies of populations exposed to radiation in children show a dose-response over a wide dose range. Science 1968;160:159

9. DeGroot LJ, Paloyan E. Thyroid carcinoma and radiation. A Chicago epidemic. JAMA 1973;225:487

10. Refetoff S, Harrison J, Karanfilski BT, et al. Continuing occurrence of thyroid carcinoma after irradiation to the neck in infancy and childhood. N Engl J Med 1975;269:171

11. Favus MJ, Schneider AB, Stachura ME, et al. Thyroid cancer as a late consequence of head-neck irradiation: evaluation of 1056 patients. N Engl J Med 1976;294:1019

12. Caruso D, Mazzaferri EL. Fine needle aspiration biopsy in the management of thyroid nodules. Endocrinologist 1991;1:194

13. Hamming JF, Goslings BM, van Steenis GJ, et al. The value of fine-needle aspiration biopsy in patients with nodular thyroid disease divided into groups of suspicion of malignant neoplasms on clinical grounds. Arch Intern Med 1990;150:113

14. Ridgway EC, Weintraub BD, Cevallos JL, et al. Suppression of pituitary TSH secretion in the patient with a hyperfunctioning thyroid nodule. J Clin Invest 1973;52:2785

15. Hamburger J. Solitary autonomously functioning thyroid lesions: diagnosis, clinical features, and pathogenetic considerations. Am J Med 1975;58:740

16. Hamburger J. Evolution of toxicity in solitary nontoxic autonomously functioning thyroid nodules. J Clin Endocrinol Metab 1980;50:1089

17. O'Brien T, Gharib H, Suman VJ, et al. Treatment of toxic solitary thyroid nodules: surgery versus radioactive iodine. Surgery 1992;112:1166

18. Goletti O, Monzani F, Caraccio N, et al. Percutaneous ethanol injection treatment of autonomously functioning single thyroid nodules: optimization of treatment and short term outcome. World J Surg 1992;16:784

19. Martino E, Murtas ML, Loviselli A, et al. Percutaneous intranodular ethanol injection for treatment of autonomously functioning thyroid nodules. Surgery 1992;112:1161

20. Papini E, Panunzi C, Pacella CM, et al. Percutaneous ultrasound-guided ethanol injection: a new treatment of toxic autonomously functioning thyroid nodules? J Clin Endocrinol Metab 1993;76:411

21. Wang CA, Vickery AL, Maloof F. Needle biopsy of the thyroid. Surg Gynecol Obstet 1976;143:365

22. Gershengorn MC, McClung MA, Chu EW, et al. Fine needle aspiration cytology in the preoperative diagnosis of thyroid nodules. Ann Intern Med 1977;87:265

23. Wang CA, Guyton SP, Vickery AL. A further note on the large needle biopsy of the thyroid gland. Surg Gynecol Obstet 1983;156:508

24. Ridgway ED. Clinician's evaluation of a solitary thyroid nodule. J Clin Endocrinol Metab 1992;74:231

25. Van Herle AJ, Rich P, Britt-Marie EL, et al. The thyroid nodule. Ann Intern Med 1982;96:221

26. Molitch ME, Beck JR, Deisman M, et al. The cold thyroid nodule: an analysis of diagnostic and therapeutic options. Endocr Rev 1984;5:184

27. Grant CS, Hay ID, Gough IR, McCarthy PM, Goellner JR. Long-term follow-up of patients with benign thyroid fine-needle aspiration cytologic diagnoses. Surgery 1989;106:980

28. Gharib H, Goellner JR. Fine-needle aspiration biopsy of the thyroid: an appraisal. Ann Intern Med 1993;118:282

29. Dwarakanathan AA, Staren ED, D'Amore MJ, et al. Importance of repeat fine-needle biopsy in the management of thyroid nodules. Am J Surg 1993;166:350

30. Gharib H, Goellner JR, Zinsmeister AR, et al. Fine needle aspiration biopsy of the thyroid: the problem of suspicious cytological findings. Ann Intern Med 1984;101:25

31. Cochand-Priollet B, Guillausseau PJ, Chagnon S, et al. The diagnostic value of fine-needle aspiration biopsy under ultrasonography in nonfunctional thyroid nodules. A prospective study comparing cytologic and histologic findings. Am J Med 1994;97:152

32. Simeone JF, Daniels GH, Mueller PR, et al. High resolution real time sonography of the thyroid. Radiology 1982;145:431

33. Fogelfeld L, Wiviott MBT, Shore-Freedman E, et al. Recurrence of thyroid nodules after surgical removal in patients irradiated in childhood for benign conditions. N Engl J Med 1989;320:835

34. van Heyningen V, Abbott SR, Daniel SG, Ardisson LJ, Ridgway EC. Development and utility of a monoclonal-antibody-based, highly sensitive immunoradiometric assay of thyrotropin. Clin Chem 1987;33:1387

35. Klee GG, Hay ID. Assessment of sensitive thyrotropin assays for an expanded role in thyroid function testing: proposed criteria for analytic performance and clinical utility. J Clin Endocrinol Metab 1987;64:461

36. Ross DS, Ardrisson LJ, Meskell MJ. Measurement of thyrotropin in clinical and subclinical hyperthyroidism using a new chemiluminescent assay. J Clin Endocrinol Metab 1989;69:684

37. Spencer CA, LoPresti JS, Patel A, et al. Applications of a new chemiluminometric TSH assay to subnormal measurement. J Clin Endocrinol Metab 1990;70:453

38. Hamburger J. Consistency of sequential needle biopsy findings for thyroid nodules. Arch Intern Med 1987;147:97

39. Morita T, Tamai H, Ohshima A, et al. Changes in serum thyroid hormone, thyrotropin and thyroglobulin concentrations during thyroxine therapy in patients with solitary thyroid nodules. J Clin Endocrinol Metab 1989;69:227

40. Gharib H, James EM, Charboneau JW, et al. Suppressive therapy with levothyroxine for solitary thyroid nodules. N Engl J Med 1987;317:70.

41. Cheung PSY, Lee JMH, Boey JH. Thyroxine suppressive therapy of benign solitary thyroid nodules: a prospective randomized study. World J Surg 1989;13:818

42. Reverter JL, Lucas A, Salinas I, et al. Suppressive therapy with levothyroxine for solitary thyroid nodules. Clin Endocrinol 1992;36:25

43. Papini E, Bacci V, Panunzi C, et al. A prospective randomized trial of levothyroxine suppressive therapy for solitary thyroid nodules. Clin Endocrinol 1993;38:507

44. LaRosa GL, Lupo L, Giuffrida D, et al. Levothyroxine and potassium iodide are both effective in treating benign solitary cold nodules of the thyroid. Ann Intern Med 1995;122:1

45. Biondi B, Fazio S, Carella C, et al. Cardiac effects of long term thyrotropin-suppressive therapy with levothyroxine. J Clin Endocrinol Metab 1993;77:334

46. Paul TL, Kerrigan J, Kelly AM, et al. Long-term L-thyroxine therapy is associated with decreased hip bone density in premenopausal women. JAMA 1988;259:3137

47. Ross DS. Subclinical hyperthyroidism: possible danger of overzealous thyroxine replacement therapy. Mayo Clin Proc 1988;63:1223

EIGHT

The Thyroid in Infancy and Childhood

Werner and Ingbar's The Thyroid, Seventh Edition,
edited by Lewis E. Braverman and Robert D. Utiger.
Lippincott–Raven Publishers, Philadelphia, © 1996

84

Thyroid Physiology in the Perinatal Period and During Childhood

Delbert A. Fisher

ONTOGENESIS OF THE THYROID SYSTEM

Role of the Placenta

Fetal development is dependent on the placenta, which regulates substrate supply, provides excretory functions, and synthesizes various polypeptide and steroid hormones that influence aspects of maternal and fetal metabolism.[1,2] With regard to thyroid function, the placenta provides a relative barrier between the maternal and fetal systems. The mammalian placenta is impermeable to thyrotropin (TSH) and relatively impermeable to thyroid hormones. The latter is due, in part, to the presence in the placenta of an iodothyronine inner-ring deiodinase enzyme system that deiodinates thyroxine (T_4) to inactive reverse triiodothyronine (rT_3) and that deiodinates active triiodothyronine (T_3) to inactive diiodothyronine.[3,4] In addition, an inherent placental tissue barrier creates a maternal-fetal gradient of free iodothyronines. There are species variations of placental thyroid hormone permeability; for the species for which most data are available, the order is rat > human > sheep.[5] In rats and humans, there is some, though limited, placental transfer of T_4 and T_3.[6,7] In human infants with thyroid agenesis or a total organification defect, the average cord serum total T_4 concentration is about 4 µg/dL (50 nmol/L), whereas the normal mean concentration in adults is about 11 µg/dL (140 nmol/L).[7]

The placenta is permeable to thyrotropin-releasing hormone (TRH), and evidence suggests that it is capable of TRH synthesis.[8,9] This and fetal extrahypothalamic TRH production lead to a high concentration of TRH in fetal serum.[10,11] The high fetal serum TRH concentration is maintained in part be-

cause of absent or low concentrations of TRH-degrading activity in fetal serum.[10,11] The maternal serum TRH concentration is low and contributes little, if any, TRH to the fetus. The placenta also produces polypeptide hormones with TSH-like bioactivity. Most of this bioactivity is an inherent property of human chorionic gonadotropin; small amounts may be contributed by a separate chorionic thyrotropin.[12,13] This TSH-like bioactivity, which peaks at the end of the first trimester, transiently increases free thyroid hormone concentrations in maternal serum and transiently suppresses maternal TSH secretion, but it has little influence on fetal thyroid function.

Early Development

The fetal hypothalamic-pituitary-thyroid system develops largely free of maternal influence.[4,5] Thyroid embryogenesis is largely complete by 10 to 12 weeks of gestation, by which time the fetal thyroid has developed its characteristic histologic features and is capable of concentrating iodine and synthesizing iodothyronines. By this time, the fetal pituitary gland also is identifiable and contains TSH, which is detectable by bioassay and radioimmunoassay.

Hypothalamic maturation, including the development of the pituitary portal vascular system, proceeds from 6 to 7 weeks through 30 to 35 weeks of gestation.[14,15] The first hypothalamic nuclei and fibers of the supraoptic tract are identifiable by 9 to 10 weeks. TRH is measurable by radioimmunoassay in hypothalamic tissue at 8 to 10 weeks, and the concentrations increase progressively to term in association with continuing histologic maturation. The pituitary portal vascular system develops simultaneously from separate superficial plexuses over the inferior hypothalamus and the developing pituitary gland; the system is immature but functional by 8 to 10 weeks of gestation.[14] By 30 to 35 weeks, the system has matured functionally and comprises an extensive system of hypothalamic vascular channels that communicate through connecting vessels along the pituitary stalk to a second system of capillaries within the substance of the anterior pituitary.

Maturation of the Thyroid System Control

Maturation of control of thyroid hormone secretion is superimposed on a progressive increase in the fetal serum thyroxine-binding globulin (TBG) concentration during the period of 10 to 35 weeks of gestation.[16] The fetal serum TBG concentration increases because of maturation of fetal hepatic TBG synthetic capacity. The secretion of TSH and of thyroid hormones is minimal until midgestation[4,5,17–19] (Fig 84-1). At this time (18–20 weeks of gestation), fetal thyroid gland iodine uptake and serum T_4 concentrations begin to increase. The fetal serum TSH concentration progressively increases from a low value at 16 to 18 weeks, despite progressive increases in serum total and free T_4 concentrations between 20 weeks and term.[5,17,20] Pituitary TSH responsiveness to exogenous TRH is present early in the third trimester; however, maturation of negative feedback control of pituitary TSH secretion develops during the last half of gestation and the first 1 to 2 months of extrauterine life.[5,17,21]

This maturation is reflected in progressive increases in fetal serum TSH and free T_4 concentrations between 20 and 40 weeks of gestation.[19] The full-term fetus in utero has an exaggerated and prolonged TSH response to maternally-administered TRH, a response characteristic of hypothalamic hypothyroidism.[22] Moreover, the serum TSH concentration at birth is relatively high (about 10 mU/L) and the free T_4:TSH ratio is low.[5,14,19] TSH secretion can be inhibited in the human fetus at term by administration of T_4. Klein and associates[23] reported that an intra-amniotic injection of 700 μg of T_4 24 hours before elective cesarean section increased cord serum T_4 concentration from a mean of 15 μg/dL (193 nmol/L) to 27 μg/dL (347 nmol/L) and reduced cord serum TSH concentration from a mean of 12 to 5.5 mU/L without increasing the mean cord serum T_3 concentration. In addition, the elevated cord serum T_4 concentration suppressed the neonatal TSH surge from a mean of 67 to 11 mU/L at 30 minutes of age. This inhibitory effect of T_4 presumably is mediated through pituitary conversion of T_4 to T_3. There are no data on such conversion in the human fetus or newborn, but the neonatal rat pituitary gland converts T_4 to T_3 more actively than does the adult gland.[24]

In the neonatal period, the serum free T_4 concentration increases in response to an early neonatal TSH surge, and there is a marked increase in free T_3 concentration associated with a fall in TSH to the normal adult range by 3 to 5 days[14,17] (see Fig 84-1). The free T_4:TSH and free T_3:TSH concentration ratios approximate adult values by 1 to 2 months of age.[5,17,21] Thus, the human fetus matures from a state of combined primary and hypothalamic-pituitary hypothyroidism during the first trimester, through a period of hypothalamic hypothyroidism during the last half of gestation, to a state of mature function by 1 to 2 months of postnatal life. The increasing serum free T_4:TSH and free T_3:TSH ratios can be viewed as reflecting a progressive in-

crease in the level of tonic TRH stimulation of the fetal pituitary gland during the last trimester of gestation.

Development of Thyroid Gland Responsiveness and Autonomy

The progressive increase in fetal serum free T_4 concentrations during the last half of gestation appears to be due to both increasing fetal serum TSH and progressive maturation of the thyroid follicular cell responsiveness to TSH.[14,19,20] There are no data regarding the thyroid response to TSH for the developing human fetus. Direct data are available, however, from fetal sheep, in which there is a progressive increase in the responses of serum T_4 and the serum T_4:TSH ratio to exogenous TRH during the last trimester of pregnancy.[25]

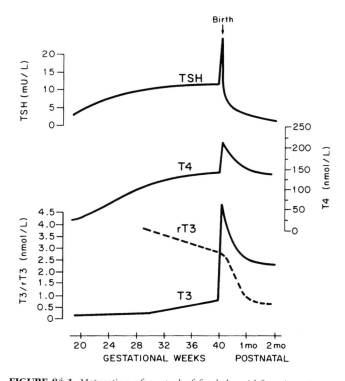

FIGURE 84-1. Maturation of control of fetal thyroid function. A progressive increase in fetal serum TSH occurs during the last half of gestation. This is associated with a progressive increase in serum total thyroxine (T_4) concentration largely caused by an increase in serum thyroxine-binding globulin. A parallel increase occurs in serum free T_4, presumably due to increasing T_4 secretion in response to the increase in serum TSH. Fetal serum triiodothyronine (T_3) concentrations are very low before 30 weeks' gestation and increase modestly near term. Serum reverse T_3 (rT_3) concentrations are relatively high until term. At the time of parturition, there is a marked surge in serum TSH with a peak 30 minutes after birth. This stimulates T_3 and T_4 secretion and increases serum total and free T_3 and T_4 concentrations. The increased T_3 concentration after the TSH surge subsides is due to increased hepatic, renal, and perhaps brown adipose T_4 5'-deiodinase activity and increased T_4-to-T_3 conversion. Serum reverse T_3 concentrations decrease progressively during the first 1 to 2 months of life. To convert serum T_4 to μg/dL, multiply by 0.078. To convert serum T_3 to ng/dL, multiply by 65.1. From Fisher DA, Polk DH. Thyroid disease in the fetus, neonate, and child. In De Groot LJ, ed. Endocrinology. Vol 1, ed 2. Philadelphia:WB Saunders, 1989:734)

Thyroid gland maturation also includes maturation of thyroid autoregulation of iodine transport. The thyroid gland of the adult mammal can modify iodine transport relative to dietary iodine intake and exclusive of variations in serum TSH (see section on autoregulation in chap 13). The developing mammalian thyroid gland lacks this autoregulatory mechanism and is thus susceptible to iodine-induced inhibition of thyroid hormone synthesis.[26,27] The ability of the thyroid gland to defend against the thyroid-blocking effect of excessive iodide does not develop until after 36 to 40 weeks of gestation in the human fetus.[26]

This adaptation presumably involves the capacity of thyroid follicular cells to decrease iodide transport and thus prevent the high intracellular iodide concentrations that cause blockade of hormone synthesis. The responses of thyroid follicular cells to increased iodide concentrations are complex; membrane transport of iodide is inhibited, adenylyl cyclase activity is reduced, and thyroglobulin iodination and turnover are decreased.[28] The membrane autoregulatory mechanism is incompletely characterized, but, in rabbits, failure of the immature thyroid follicular cell to autoregulate iodide transport is associated with the absence or reduced iodination of an 8000 to 10,000 molecular weight protein that is present in adult follicular cells.[29,30]

Maturation of Thyroxine Metabolism

Thyroid hormones undergo several types of biochemical transformation in tissues.[31] These include deiodination, side-chain metabolism, and conjugation (with sulfate or glucuronide). Sequential monodeiodination of the iodothyronines is the most important pathway of thyroid hormone metabolism (see chap 8). Several enzyme activities are involved in this monodeiodination: two types of outer-ring deiodinase (type I and II) activity and an inner-ring iodothyronine deiodinase (type III).[4,17,32–35] Type I deiodinase, predominantly expressed in liver and kidney, is a high-K_m enzyme that is inhibited by propylthiouracil (PTU) and stimulated by thyroid hormone. Type II deiodinase activity, predominantly located in brain, pituitary, and brown adipose tissue, is a low-K_m enzyme that is insensitive to PTU and inhibited by thyroid hormone. Type I activity in liver, kidney, and perhaps muscle accounts for most of the extrathyroidal outer-ring deiodination of T_4 to T_3 and rT_3 to 3,3′-diiodothyronine as well as inner-ring deiodination of T_4 and T_3 sulfate conjugates.

The type II deiodinase probably plays an important role in providing intracellular T_3 to those tissues that are dependent on T_3 during fetal life (pituitary, brain, and brown fat). The inner-ring deiodinase (type III) is present in fetal liver, brain, skin, and placenta.[4,8,34] This enzyme catalyzes the conversion of T_4 to rT_3 and T_3 to 3,3′-diiodothyronine. Studies of deiodination in rodents and sheep have shown a predominance of type III enzyme activity in the fetal period, particularly in placenta and fetal membranes, and this activity accounts for the high concentrations of rT_3 in fetal serum and amniotic fluid.[4,8,34] The persistence of high serum rT_3 concentrations for several weeks in the human newborn indicates that T_4-to-rT_3 conversion in nondecidual tissues also is important to the maintenance of the high rT_3 concentration in the fetus (see Fig 84-1).

The ontogeny of the three deiodinases differs in the developing fetus. The type II and III enzyme activities appear during the second trimester, whereas type I activity appears during the third trimester.[4,17,36] The preterm increase in fetal serum T_3 concentrations is due to an increase in type I deiodinase activity. Serum concentrations of rT_3, T_4 sulfate, T_3 sulfate, and rT_3 sulfate in the umbilical cord at this time are high.[37,38] Sulfated metabolites accumulate in fetal serum as a result of low type I deiodinase activity in fetal tissues and because the sulfated iodothyronines are not substrates for placental type III deiodinase.[39] They represent the predominant thyroid hormone metabolites in the fetus and like rT_3 are not biologically active.[38] The liver, kidney, and brain of adult rats have sulfatase activity, and desulfation of T_3 sulfate to T_3 occurs in the liver and brain of fetal rats, so T_3 sulfate could serve as a local source of T_3 in fetal tissues containing sulfatase.[40,41] The presence of the type II enzyme in critical fetal tissues allows for the possibility of the conversion of T_4 to T_3 by local tissues and the potential for varying local tissue supply of T_3.[4,42] Type II deiodinase activity increases in fetuses with hypothyroidism, whereas the activities of types I and III deiodinase decrease. These changes favor shunting of T_4 to brain tissues, so that even limited placental transfer of maternal T_4 may protect the fetus against thyroid deficiency.

Dramatic changes in the patterns of T_4 deiodination occur in the perinatal period, largely because of changes in deiodinative enzyme activity in various tissues. These changes are reflected in the rises in serum T_3 concentration that occur both before and after parturition. Fetal serum T_3 concentrations are low until about 30 weeks' gestation.[5,14,17] The concentrations increase after this time to a mean value of about 50 ng/dL (0.76 nmol/L) at term, and during the first 4 to 6 hours after birth, the concentrations increase another threefold to sixfold. Fetal serum rT_3 concentrations exceed 250 ng/dL (3.8 nmol/L) early in the last trimester and decrease steadily to term; in contrast to serum T_3 concentrations, serum rT_3 concentrations change little in term infants during the immediate neonatal period, and then gradually fall during the second week of life (see Fig 84-1).

Thus, the prenatal serum T_3 increment occurs over several weeks in human fetuses. The general pattern of this change resembles the perinatal changes in T_3 metabolism in fetal sheep. In this species, fetal serum T_3 concentrations gradually increase during the week immediately preceding parturition (the prenatal T_3 surge) and then abruptly increase during the first 2 to 4 hours after birth (the postnatal surge).[43,44] The prenatal T_3 surge correlates with the prenatal increase in fetal serum cortisol concentrations. Moreover, cortisol administration to premature sheep fetuses increases fetal serum T_3 concentrations over a period of 2 to 3 days, and cortisol administration or the onset of spontaneous labor is associated with a marked increase in the in vitro hepatic conversion of T_4 to T_3.[17,36] In human fetuses, the prenatal increase in serum T_3 between 30 and 40 weeks' gestation (see Fig 84-1) also may be induced by cortisol.[45]

The postnatal T_3 surge occurs during the first 3 to 6 hours of neonatal life. In sheep, this surge is caused by increased T_3 production from thyroid tissue.[46] The serum T_3 concentration remains elevated after the early postnatal increase in serum

TSH abates, and the maintenance of a relatively high serum T_3 concentration in the neonatal period is due to increased conversion of T_4 to T_3 (see Fig 84-1). Liver and brown adipose tissues probably are the major sites of T_3 production, but other tissues may contribute.[32,35]

Ontogenesis of Thyroid Receptors and Actions

There are two genes that code for thyroid hormone (TR) receptors, TRα and TRβ, and alternative splicing of expressed messenger RNA (mRNA) species leads to production of several TR isoforms (see chap 9). The major isoforms, TRα$_1$, TRα$_2$, and TRβ, are present in characteristic concentration ratios in various adult tissues.[47]

There is limited information regarding the maturation of TRs and receptor isoforms and thyroid hormone actions in human fetuses. Most information has been derived from rodents (rats and mice) and sheep. Rats and mice are born relatively immature and poikilothermic. The pattern of thyroid development is analogous to that of humans, except that the late ontogenic events occur after birth.[5,17,36] In these species, hepatic nuclear T_3 receptors mature during the first 3 to 5 weeks of life, a period equivalent to the last trimester of human fetal development.[24,48,49] In contrast to the pattern of T_3 receptor maturation in liver, T_3 nuclear receptor binding in rat pituitary and brain cells develops early.[24,50,51] The TRα isoforms are expressed earlier than the TBβ isoform, which appears during the early postnatal period, when most of the thyroid-dependent maturational events occur in rats.[47] Studies of the timing of thyroid hormone effects on thermogenesis, hepatic enzyme activities, skin and brain maturation, growth hormone metabolism, and growth factor metabolism (insulin-like growth factors, nerve growth factor, epidermal growth factor) indicate that all of these thyroid effects appear during the first 4 weeks postnatally.[17]

The sheep is a precocial species, born homeothermic and with relatively advanced brain maturation.[3,5,46] The pattern of thyroid ontogenesis is comparable to that in rats and humans; in this species, however, most of the events of thyroid maturation occur in utero.[36,52] Thyroid nuclear receptor binding develops in fetal sheep during the latter two-thirds of gestation.[53] Brain receptors are present at midgestation and decrease in number during the first 2 to 3 months after birth. Hepatic thyroid receptor binding matures to the adult level during the last trimester.[53] The timing of appearance of thyroid hormone actions in fetal sheep varies from tissue to tissue. Effects on brain development, carcass and bone growth, skin maturation, hair growth, TSH secretion, and brain iodothyronine deiodinase activity become detectable at midgestation.[17,36,52] Effects on cardiac atrial natriuretic hormone concentrations and cardiac output appear near term; effects on adrenergic receptor in the heart and lung and on hepatic epidermal growth factor receptors appear in the neonatal period.[36]

There is limited information in the human fetus. Low levels of nuclear T_3 binding have been detected in fetal brain at 10 weeks' gestation, with higher levels at 16 to 18 weeks. Liver, heart, and lung receptor binding also have been identified at 16 to 18 weeks.[17] Athyroid infants are born with few, if any, detectable manifestations of thyroid hormone deficiency.

Their serum TSH concentrations are increased, however, and epiphyseal bone maturation can be delayed 6 to 8 weeks in one-third to one-half of such infants.[54–56] Bilirubin clearance also may be impaired.

The classic manifestations of congenital hypothyroidism in human infants appear during the early weeks of life (see also chap 85). These include effects on skin development, gastrointestinal function, linear bone growth, carcass growth, metabolic functions, growth factor metabolism, and brain development.[5,17,52] The mean and range of IQ values in infants with congenital hypothyroidism treated adequately before 45 days of age are similar to those of normal infants.[57,58] However, low-normal or occasionally low IQs have been reported in some children with congenital hypothyroidism who had very low serum T_4 and very high TSH concentrations and delayed bone maturation at birth, suggesting that hypothyroidism in utero may lead to some degree of irreversible retardation; delaying treatment has the same effect on the IQ.[59,60]

Low serum T_4 concentrations during the first year of treatment in infants with congenital hypothyroidism are also associated with lower IQs at 5 to 7 years of age.[59] These results and information obtained from late-treated infants before the advent of newborn screening suggest that newborn infants with severe hypothyroidism, if untreated, lose 3 to 5 points of IQ monthly during the first 6 to 12 months of life.[61] More aggressive early treatment may be beneficial; increasing the dose of T_4 in infants with congenital hypothyroidism from 7 to 9 μg/kg of body weight per day to 8 to 10 μg/kg of body weight per day increased the IQ at the age of 5 to 7 years by 4 to 5 points.[62] These results confirm the thyroid hormone dependency of brain maturation extending in the human infant from several weeks in utero to 2–3 years of age.

Maturation of Brown Fat Thermogenesis

The transition from fetal to neonatal life involves profound metabolic changes. One of the most important is the development of nonshivering thermogenesis. The ability of human infants and selected other homeothermic newborn mammals to maintain body temperature in the immediate extrauterine environment depends on the presence and function of brown adipose tissue.[63,64] In newborn rabbits, cold stress or the administration of exogenous norepinephrine results in an increase in metabolic rate, an increase in temperature over brown adipose tissue storage sites, and release into the circulation of both glycerol and free fatty acids.[65] Surgical removal of brown adipose tissue results in an 80% reduction in the metabolic response to both cold and exogenous catecholamine stimulation.[65] Conversely, direct electrical stimulation of the sympathetic nerves to brown adipose tissue results in an increase in temperature over the brown adipose tissue. In rabbits and sheep, brown adipose tissue is localized to the perirenal, retroperitoneal, subscapular, upper mediastinal, and neck areas.[65,66] The proximity of brown adipose tissue to large blood vessels provides for rapid transfer of heat to the circulating blood.

Brown adipose tissue cells are characterized by high concentrations of mitochondria.[64,66,67] The oxidative degradation of substrate, predominantly lipid, in brown adipose tissue mitochondria as in other mitochondria provides a nicotinamide dehydrogenase-linked supply of electrons to coenzyme Q (ubiquinone) and to the cytochrome system. This respiratory chain maintains a proton gradient across the mitochondrial membrane that provides for the phosphorylation of nucleotides and storage of energy as adenosine triphosphate.[64] Brown adipose tissue mitochondria contain a unique 32,000 molecular weight protein (uncoupling protein or thermogenin) that sits on the inner membrane and uncouples phosphorylation by dissipating the proton gradient created by the respiratory chain[64,66,67] (see also chaps 46 and 70).

Heat production by brown adipose tissue is stimulated by catecholamines by way of β-adrenergic receptors and by thyroid hormones.[64,67] The T_3 in brown adipose tissue is largely generated locally by deiodination of circulating T_4.[68–70] Rat and human brown adipose tissue contains predominantly type II deiodinase, whereas ovine brown adipose tissue contains types I and II deiodinase.[35,36,69,70] T_3 influences brown adipose tissue thermogenesis by way of modulation of the deiodinase activity and stimulation of transcription of thermogenin. Full thermogenin expression in brown adipose tissue requires both catecholamine and T_4 stimulation.[67] The volume and functional activity of brown adipose tissue, including deiodinase activity and thermogenin levels, increase progressively with fetal age so that brown adipose tissue thermogenic activity is maximal in the perinatal period.[63,66,71] Brown adipose tissue disappears in the newborn animal as the capacity for nonshivering thermogenesis develops in other tissues.[66] In lambs within 45 days after birth, the thermogenin concentrations and oxidative capacity of brown adipose tissue are markedly decreased and most of the brown adipose tissue has changed to white fat.[66] The factors that control the appearance and disappearance of brown adipose tissue in fetal and neonatal mammals are not known.

The occurrence of brown adipose tissue in newborn human infants has been well documented, and infants increase their metabolic rate in response to cold stress in the absence of shivering.[65] Moreover, an increase in serum free fatty acid concentrations and in metabolic rate can be produced by the intravenous infusion of norepinephrine. Cold exposure also results in an increase in serum free fatty acid concentrations in association with an increase in urinary catecholamine excretion. The thyroid dependence of human brown adipose tissue thermogenesis is presumed by analogy to rats and sheep.[32,69,72] The dependency of neonatal thermogenesis on thyroid hormone in newborn lambs has been demonstrated by in vitro studies and by fetal thyroidectomy studies.[3,71,72]

THE NEONATAL PERIOD

Term Infants

Exposure of the fetus to the extrauterine environment evokes an acute release of TSH that stimulates a prolonged release of thyroid hormones. Peak serum TSH concentrations occur 30 minutes after birth[5,17,52] (see Fig 84-1), after which they decrease rapidly for 24 hours, with a slower decrease during the next several days. Serum total and free T_4 concentrations gradually increase to peak values at 24 to 36 hours and then slowly

decrease over the first weeks of life. The initial rise in serum TSH appears to be stimulated by cooling in the extrauterine environment.[5,17,52]

An early increase in serum T_3 concentration also occurs (see Fig 84-1). Within 4 hours after birth, serum T_3 concentrations increase threefold to sixfold (the postnatal T_3 surge). In newborn lambs, this early postnatal T_3 surge can be prevented by thyroidectomy.[37,46] In addition, there is an increase in iodothyronine deiodinase activity in the liver, kidney and brown adipose tissue.[3] These observations are consistent with the view that the early (1–4 hours) increase in serum T_3 concentration is due to TSH stimulation of thyroid secretion. A further increase in serum T_3 occurs between 6 and 36 hours of age. This second T_3 peak coincides with the postnatal peak in serum T_4 and is probably due both to increased thyroid gland T_3 secretion in response to the TSH surge and to increased T_4 deiodinase activity in association with increased availability of T_4 substrate for conversion to T_3.[5,17,52] The maintenance of the high serum T_3 concentration after subsidence of the TSH surge is due to increased T_4-to-T_3 conversion mediated by means of increased deiodinase activity.

Premature Infants

Preterm infants are delivered before full maturation of the hypothalamic-pituitary-thyroid system. As indicated in Figures 84-2 and 84-3, they have qualitatively similar but quantitatively decreased changes in serum TSH and iodothyronine concentrations in the neonatal period.[17,52] The serum TSH response to parturition is attenuated, and serum T_4 concentrations remain below those in full-term infants during the first few weeks of life. An abrupt early neonatal (2–4 hours) increase in serum T_3 concentrations also occurs in premature infants, but the increments are smaller and serum T_3 concentrations increase only slowly to the concentrations found in term infants. The decrease in serum rT_3 is similar to that in term infants.[17,52]

Premature infants have tertiary (hypothalamic) hypothyroidism that represents developmental immaturity.[16,52] This is characterized by relatively low serum total and free T_4 concentrations and a normal serum TSH concentration.[16,52] The severity is inversely related to developmental age; infants under 30 weeks' gestational age have a 50% prevalence of hypothyroxinemia (<6 μg/dL [<77 nmol/L]), whereas the prevalence in infants born after 34 to 36 weeks of gestation is about 10%. The condition corrects itself spontaneously in several weeks and does not require therapy.[52,73,74] In addition to their hypothalamic immaturity, premature infants have increased morbidity due to respiratory distress, hypoxia, metabolic dysfunction, undernutrition, infection, trauma, hemorrhage, and tissue necrosis. All of these factors further inhibit T_4 deiodination to T_3 and aggravate the reduction in serum T_3 concentrations.[17,74]

In areas of endemic iodine deficiency, premature infants have a high prevalence of transient primary hypothyroidism during in the early neonatal period. In a Belgian study, 11 of 61 unselected premature infants had transient primary hypothyroidism.[75,76] Screening measurements of T_4 and TSH usually are normal in these infants, but during the first week of life the serum T_4 concentration falls and the TSH concentration increases. In these infants, the available iodine is insuffi-

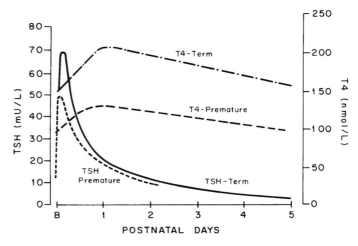

FIGURE 84-2. Changes in serum TSH and T_4 concentrations in full-term and premature infants during the first 5 days of life. The neonatal TSH surge peaks at 30 minutes in both preterm and term infants and is followed by a progressive increase in serum T_4 concentrations, peaking at 24 to 36 hours. Both the TSH and T_4 increments are less in premature infants compared with term infants. To convert serum T_4 to µg/dL, multiply by 0.078. (Modified from Fisher DA, Klein AH. Thyroid development and disorders of thyroid function in the newborn. N Engl J Med 1981:304:702)

cient to provide for the increased thyroid hormone synthesis characteristic of the early neonatal period. The hypothyroid state usually corrects itself spontaneously in a few days to a few weeks and can be promptly corrected with iodine or T_4 treatment.

THYROID FUNCTION DURING INFANCY AND CHILDHOOD

Iodide Metabolism and Thyroid Function

During infancy, the iodide space (on a body weight basis) is larger than in older children, adolescents, or adults, and the thyroid iodide clearance rate is nearly three times that of adults[77,78] (Fig 84-4). The iodide kinetic data shown in Figure 84-4 were derived from a population with relatively low iodine intake in Belgium.[77] Lower values for thyroid clearance and thyroid uptake would be expected in persons living in areas, such as the United States where iodine intake is higher. Renal iodide clearance also is high in infants and decreases

progressively with age. Thus, the progressive decrease in thyroid clearance could be, at least in part, secondary to the change in renal iodide clearance.

During childhood, the growth of the thyroid gland in residents of iodine sufficient areas roughly parallels body growth.[52,78] The gland increases in size from about 1.5 g at birth to a mean of 9 g at 10 years of age (Table 84-1). Thus, thyroid weight is about 0.5 g/kg at birth and 0.3 g/kg after 1 year. Average thyroid iodine content increases from 0.3 mg at

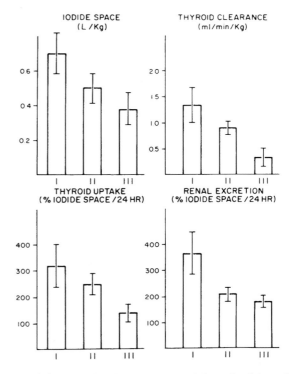

FIGURE 84-4. Iodide distribution space and thyroid iodide and renal iodide clearance rates at different periods of life. Column I represents infants 6 months to 2 years of age; column II, adolescents; and column III, adults. Values are means and SE. (Adapted from Ponchon G, Beckers C, DeVisscher M. Iodide kinetic studies in newborns and infants. J Clin Endocrinol Metab 1966;26:1392)

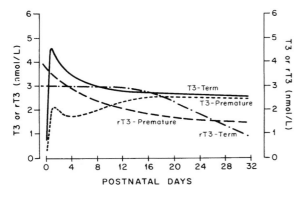

FIGURE 84-3. Changes in serum T_3 and rT_3 concentrations during the first month of life. Values in premature infants vary with gestational age and postnatal morbidity. To convert serum T_3 or rT_3 to ng/dL, multiply by 65.1. (Modified from Fisher DA, Klein AH. Thyroid development and disorders of thyroid function in the newborn. N Engl J Med 1981:304:702)

Variation of Thyroid Weight With Age

Age	Average Thyroid Size (g)	Average Thyroid Weight (g/kg BW)
Birth	1.5	0.5
1 y	2.5	0.25
5 y	6.1	0.34
10 y	8.7	0.30
15 y	15.8	0.43
Adult	20.0	0.30

(Modified from Handmaker H, Lowenstein JM, eds. Nuclear medicine in clinical pediatrics. New York: Society of Nuclear Medicine, 1975;280)

Serum Thyroid Hormone Concentrations and Production Rates

The variations in serum thyroid hormone and TSH concentrations during the first 20 years of life are shown in Figure 84-5. Serum total and free T_4 and T_3 concentrations decrease gradually with age.[79,80] The decreases in serum total T_4 and T_3 result largely from a decrease in serum TBG concentration that is progressive from early childhood through 15 to 16 years of age, when the mean serum TBG concentration is about the same as in adults. Reciprocal changes occur in serum transthyretin concentrations. These changes presumably reflect the effects of gonadal steroids, but other factors may be involved.

Serum free T_4 concentrations decrease modestly during the first decade and plateau during adolescence and then increase slightly.[80] The percentage of iodine-131 labeled protein-bound iodine appearing in blood (percentage of dose per liter per kilogram of body weight) after labeling of the thyroid gland also decreases with age during the first two decades, as does T_4 turnover and production rate on a body weight basis (μg/kg/d) (Fig 84-6; see Table 84-2).[81] Estimated T_4 turnover or production rate values are 5 to 6 μg/kg/d in infants, 4 μg/kg/d at 1 to 3 years, 2 to 3 μg/kg/d at 3 to 9 years, and 1 μg/kg/d in adults.[78,82–84]

The serum concentration of rT_3 remains unchanged or increases slightly during childhood and adolescence (see Fig 84-5).[79] The serum free rT_3 index (total rT_3 × fractional T_3 resin uptake results) remains stable or increases slightly. Because circulating rT_3 is derived almost entirely from peripheral deiodination of T_4, these observations and the fact that the mean calculated ratios of serum rT_3:serum T_4 and free rT_3 index:free T_4 index increase progressively with age suggest that the relative rate of T_4 conversion to rT_3 increases with age during childhood and adolescence.[79] Direct measurements have not been made. The decreases with age in the ratios of serum T_3:serum rT_3 and free T_3 index:free rT_3 index suggest a progressive decrease in the relative conversion of T_4 to T_3 with age during the first 15 years of life.

birth to 16 mg in adolescents and adults.[52] In areas of iodine deficiency, the average thyroid weight in newborn infants approximates 3 g and iodine content may be as low as 40 μg.[52] The iodide space also increases progressively in volume. The relative size (liters per kilogram, expressed as percentage of body weight), however, decreases from about of 50% body weight at birth to 40% in 30-kg children (at about age 10 years). These values can be compared with the 33% body weight values in 65-kg adults.

Data on thyroid radioiodine uptake and clearance in children and adolescents are conflicting. Values have been reported both to decrease progressively with age during the first two decades and to remain relatively stable.[78] This discrepancy is probably caused by variations in iodine intake. The data showing a decrease with age were from areas of low iodine intake in Europe and Australia. A relatively high iodine intake could tend to mask differences in uptake with age. Thyroid iodine clearance (per gram of thyroid tissue) decreases progressively with age, and indicates a decrease in thyroid activity (Table 84-2).

TABLE 84-2.
Variation in Peripheral Thyroxine Metabolism with Age*

Thyroxine Kinetic Parameter	Children (3–9 y)	Adolescents (10–16 y)	Adults (23–26 y)
Half-life (d)	5.0	6.0	6.7
	(0.13)	(0.35)	(0.30)
Fractional clearance†	0.14	0.12	0.11
	(0.005)	(0.008)	(0.004)
Distribution volume (L/kg)	0.16	0.16	0.12
	(0.008)	(0.014)	(0.005)
Thyroxine turnover (μg/kg/d)	1.9	1.5	1.1
	(0.09)	(0.07)	(0.06)

*Data are means and SE.
†Fraction of extrathyroid pool per day.
(Data from Beckers C, Malvaux C, De Visscher M. Quantitative aspects of the secretion and degradation of thyroid hormones during adolescence. J Clin Endocrinol Metab 1966;26:202; Sterling K, Chodos R. Radiothyroxine turnover studies in myxedema, thyrotoxicosis and hypermetabolism without endocrine disease. J Clin Invest 1956;35:806)

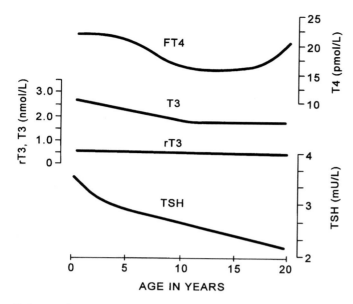

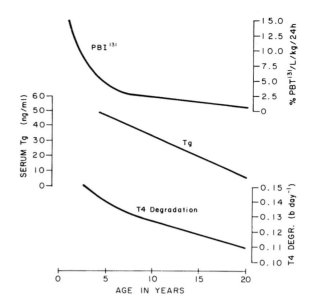

FIGURE 84-5. Variations of serum free T$_4$ (FT$_4$), T$_3$, reverse T$_3$(rT$_3$), and TSH concentrations with age during childhood and adolescence. The trends of mean values are shown. Serum free T$_4$ and T$_3$ concentrations decrease modestly during the first decade and plateau during adolescence. Serum TSH values fall progressively during childhood and adolescence. To convert serum free T$_4$ values to ng/dL multiply by 0.078. To convert serum T$_3$ or rT$_3$ values to ng/dL, multiply by 65.1. Data from Fisher DA, Sack J., Oddie TH, et al. Serum T$_4$, TBG, T$_3$ uptake, T$_3$, reverse T$_3$, and TSH concentrations in children 1 to 15 years of age, J. Clin Endocrinol Metab 1977;45:91; and Nelson JC, Clark SJ, Borut DL, et al, Age related changes in serum free thyroxine during childhood and adolescence, J Pediatrics, 1993;123:899)

FIGURE 84-6. Thyroid function during infancy, childhood, and adolescence. The thyroid gland in the newborn is very active. T$_4$ production amounts to 10 to 15 μg/kg/d relative to an adult value of 1 to 2 μg/kg/d. The trend of mean PBI^{131}/L on a per kilogram of body weight basis decreases progressively. There is a progressive decrease in T$_4$ production per gram of thyroid (not shown), a decreasing T$_4$ degradation rate (as a fraction of the extrathyroidal pool cleared per day [b day$_{-1}$], and a progressive fall in serum thyroglobulin (Tg) concentration. PBI, protein-bound iodine. (Modified from Fisher DA. Thyroid disease in the neonate and childhood. In DeGroot LJ, ed. Endocrinology. Vol 1. 2nd ed. Philadelphia: WB Saunders, 1989:735)

The progressive decrease in serum free T$_4$, T$_4$ turnover, thyroglobulin, and thyroidal radioiodine uptake indicate a progressive relative decrease in thyroid function with age. The decreasing serum TSH concentration with age suggests that these decreases are mediated primarily by reduced TSH secretion. Whether this reflects decreased TRH secretion or non-TRH mechanisms is not clear. A progressive reduction in thyroid gland TSH responsiveness also might be involved.

References

1. Polk DH, Fisher DA. Fetal and neonatal endocrinology. In: DeGroot LJ, ed. Endocrinology. 3rd ed. Philadelphia: WB Saunders, 1995:2239

2. Strauss JF, Gafuels M, King BF. Placental hormones. In: DeGroot LJ, ed. Endocrinology. 3rd ed. Philadelphia: WB Saunders, 1995: 2171

3. Polk DH, Padbury JF, Callegari C, et al. Effect of fetal thyroidectomy on newborn thermogenesis in lambs. Pediatr Res 1987;21:453

4. Burrow GN, Fisher DA, Larsen PR. Maternal and fetal thyroid function. N Engl J Med 1994,331:1072

5. Fisher DA, Dussault JH, Sack J, Chopra IJ. Ontogenesis of hypothalamic-pituitary-thyroid function and metabolism in man, sheep and rat. Recent Prog Horm Res 1977;33:702

6. Morreale de Escobar G, Obregon MJ, Ruiz de Ona C, Escobar Del Rey F. Comparison of maternal to fetal transfer of 3′,5,3′-triiodothyronine versus thyroxine in rats, as assessed from 3,5,5′- triiodothyronine versus thyroxine levels in fetal tissues. Acta Endocrinol 1989;120:20

7. Vulsma T, Gons MH, De Vijlder JJM. Maternal fetal transfer of thyroxine in congenital hypothyroidism due to a total organification defect or thyroid agenesis. N Engl J Med 1989;321:13

8. Roti E, Gnudi A, Braverman LE. The placental transport, synthesis, and metabolism of hormones and drugs which affect thyroid function. Endocr Rev 1983;4:131

9. Polk DH, Reviczky A, Lam RW, Fisher DA. Thyrotropin-releasing hormone in the ovine fetus, ontogeny and effect of thyroid hormone. Am J Physiol 1991;260:E53

10. Engler P, Scanlon MF, Jackson IMD. Thyrotropin releasing hormone in the systemic circulation of the neonatal rat is derived from the pancreas and other extraneural tissues. J Clin Invest 1981;67:800

11. Anderson K, Polk D, Reviczky A, et al. Thyrotropin-releasing hormone and prohormone levels in newborn cord sera. Clin Res 1990;38:169A

12. Ballabio M, Poshyachinda M, Ekins RP. Pregnancy-induced changes in thyroid function: role of human chorionic gonadotropin as putative regulator of maternal thyroid. J Clin Endocrinol Metab 1991,73:824

13. Kennedy RL, Darne J, Cohn M. Human chorionic gonadotropin may not be responsible for thyroid-stimulating activity in normal pregnancy serum. J Clin Endocrinol Metab 1992;74:260

14. Fisher DA. Development of fetal thyroid system control. In: DeLong GR, Robbins J, Condliffe PG, eds. Iodine and the brain. New York: Plenum Publishing, 1989:167

15. Pintar JE, Toran-Allerand CD. Normal development of the hypothalamic-pituitary-thyroid axis. In: Braverman LE, Utiger RD, eds. The thyroid. 6th ed. Philadelphia: JB Lippincott, 1991:7

16. Klein AH, Oddie TH, Parslow M, et al. Developmental changes in pituitary-thyroid function in the human fetus and newborn. Early Hum Dev 1982;6:321

17. Fisher DA, Polk DH. Development of the thyroid. In: Jones CT, ed. Perinatal endocrinology. London: Bailliere-Tindall, 1990:627

18. Polk DH, Wu SY, Wright C, et al. Ontogeny of thyroid hormone effect on tissue 5'-monodeiodinase activity in fetal sheep. Am J Physiol 1988;17:E337

19. Thorpe-Beeston JG, Nicolaides KH, McGregor AM. Fetal thyroid function. Thyroid 1992;2:207

20. Ballabio M, Nicolini U, Jowett T, et al. Maturation of thyroid function in normal human fetuses. Clin Endocrinol 1989;31:565

21. Roti E. Regulation of thyroid-stimulating hormone (TSH) secretion in the fetus and neonate. J Endocrinol Invest 1988;11:145

22. Roti E, Gnudi A, Braverman LE, et al. Human cord blood concentrations of thyrotropin, thyroglobulin and iodothyronines following maternal administration of thyrotropin-releasing hormone. J Clin Endocrinol Metab 1981;53:813

23. Klein AH, Hobel CJ, Sack J, Fisher DA. Effect of intraamniotic fluid thyroxine injection on fetal serum and amniotic fluid iodothyronine concentrations. J Clin Endocrinol Metab 1978;47:1034

24. Coulombe P, Ruel J, Faure R, Dussault JH. Pituitary nuclear triiodothyronine receptors during development in the rat. Am J Physiol 1983;8:E81

25. Klein AH, Fisher DA. Thyrotropin releasing hormone stimulated pituitary and thyroid gland responsiveness and 3,5,3'-triiodothyronine suppression in fetal and neonatal lambs. Endocrinology 1980;106:297

26. Castaing H, Fournet JP, Leger FA, et al. Thyroid of the newborn and postnatal iodine overload. Arch Fr Pediatr 1979;36:356

27. Theodoropoulos T, Braverman LE, Vagenakis AG. Iodide induced hypothyroidism: a potential hazard during perinatal life. Science 1979;205:502

28. Penel C, Rognoni JB, Bastiani P. Thyroid autoregulation: impact of thyroid structure and function in rats. Am J Physiol 1987;16:E165

29. Price DJ, Sherwin JR. Autoregulation of iodide transport in the rabbit: absence of autoregulation in fetal tissue and comparison of maternal and fetal thyroid iodination products. Endocrinology 1986;119:2547

30. Sherwin JR, Price DJ. Autoregulation of thyroid iodide transport: evidence for the mediation of protein synthesis in iodide-induced suppression of iodide transport. Endocrinology 1986;119:2553

31. Burger A. Monodeiodinative pathways of thyroid hormone metabolism. In: Hennemann G, ed. Thyroid hormone metabolism. New York: Marcel Dekker, 1986:255

32. Silva JE, Matthews PS. Thyroid hormone metabolism and the source of plasma triiodothyronine in 2 week old rats: effect of thyroid status. Endocrinology 1984;114:2394

33. Silva JE, Leonard JL. Regulation of rat cerebrocortical and adenohypophyseal type II 5'-deiodinase by thyroxine, triiodothyronine and reverse triiodothyronine. Endocrinology 1985;116:1627

34. Kaplan MM. Regulatory influences on iodothyronine deiodination in animal tissues. In: Hennemann G, ed. Thyroid hormone metabolism. New York: Marcel Dekker, 1986:231

35. Wu SY, Merryfield ML, Polk DH, Fisher DA. Two pathways for thyroxine 5'-monodeiodination in brown adipose tissue in fetal sheep: ontogenesis and divergent responses to hypothyroidism and T$_3$ replacement. Endocrinology 1990;126:1950

36. Fisher DA, Polk DH, Wu SY. Fetal thyroid metabolism: a pluralistic system. Thyroid 1994;4:367

37. Breall JA, Rudolph SM, Heymann MA. Role of thyroid hormone in postnatal circulatory and metabolic adjustments. J Clin Invest 1984;73:1418

38. Polk DH, Reviczky A, Wu SY, et al. Metabolism of sulfoconjugated thyroid hormone derivatives in developing sheep. Am J Physiol 1994;266:E892

39. Santini F, Hurd RE, Chopra IJ. A study of deaminated and sulfoconjugated iodothyronines by rat placental iodothyronine 5'-monodeiodinase. Endocrinology 1992;131:1689

40. Santini F, Hurd RE, Lee B, Chopra IJ. Thyromimetic effects of 3,5,3'-triiodothyronine sulfate in hypothyroid rats. Endocrinology 1993;133:105

41. Santini F, Chopra IJ, Wu SY, et al. Metabolism of 3,5,3'- triiodothyronine sulfate my tissues of the fetal rat: a consideration of the role of desulfation of 3,5,3'-triiodothyronine as a source of T$_3$. Pediatr Res 1992;31:541

42. Calvo R, Obregon MJ, Ruiz de Ona C, et al. Congenital hypothyroidism as studied in rats: crucial role of maternal thyroxine but not of 3,5,3'-triiodothyronine in the protection of the fetal brain. J Clin Invest 1990;86:889

43. Klein AH, Oddie TH, Fisher DA. Effect of parturition on serum iodothyronine concentrations in fetal sheep. Endocrinology 1978;103:1453

44. Nwosu UC, Kaplan MM, Utiger RD, Delivoria-Papadopoulos M. Surge of fetal plasma triiodothyronine before birth in sheep. Am J Obstet Gynecol 1978;132:489

45. Osathanondh R, Chopra IJ, Tulchinsky D. Effects of dexamethasone on fetal and maternal thyroxine, triiodothyronine, reverse triiodothyronine and thyrotropin levels. J Clin Endocrinol Metab 1978;47:1236

46. Polk DH, Wu SY, Fisher DA. Serum thyroid hormone and tissue 5'-monodeiodinase activity in acutely thyroidectomized newborn lambs. Am J Physiol 1986;14:E151

47. Oppenheimer JH, Schwartz HL, Strait KA. Thyroid hormone action 1994: the plot thickens. Eur J Endocrinol 1994;130:15

48. DeGroot LJ, Robertson M, Rue PA. Triiodothyronine receptors during maturation. Endocrinology 1977;100:1511

49. Coulombe P, Ruel J, Dussault JH. Analysis of nuclear 3,5,3'-triiodothyronine binding capacity and tissue response in the liver of neonatal rat. Endocrinology 1979;105:952

50. Naido S, Volcana T, Timiras PS. Thyroid hormone receptors in developing brain. Am Zool 1978;18:545

51. Schwartz HL, Oppenheimer JH. Ontogenesis of 3,5,3'-triiodothyronine receptors in neonatal rat brain: dissociation between receptor concentration and stimulation of oxygen consumption by 3,5,3'-triiodothyronine. Endocrinology 1978;103:943

52. Fisher DA, Polk DH. Development of the fetal thyroid system. In: Thorburn GD, Harding R, eds. Textbook of fetal physiology. Oxford: Oxford University Press, 1994:359

53. Polk DH, Cheromcha D, Reviczky AL, Fisher DA. Nuclear thyroid hormone receptors: ontogeny and thyroid hormone effects in sheep. Am J Physiol 1989;19:E543

54. LaFranchi SH, Hanna CE, Krainz PL, et al. Screening for congenital hypothyroidism with specimen collection at two time periods. Results of the Northwest Regional screening program. Pediatrics 1985;76:734

55. Grant DB, Smith I, Fuggle PW, et al. Congenital hypothyroidism detected by neonatal screening: relationship between biochemical severity and early clinical features. Arch Dis Child 1992;67:87

56. Mori K, Yoshida K, Kraise K, et al. Inhibition of placental thyroxine 5-deiodinase activity decreases amniotic fluid concentration of 3,3',5'-triiodothyronine in rat. Endocr J 1993;40:405

57. Glorieux J, Dussault JH, Morissette J, et al. Follow up at ages 5 and 7 years on mental development in children with hypothyroidism detected by Quebec screening program. J Pediatr 1985;107:913

58. New England Congenital Hypothyroid Collaborative. Neonatal hypothyroidism screening: status of patients at 6 years of age. J Pediatr 1985;107:915

59. Rovet J, Ehrlich R, Sorbara D. Intellectual outcome in children with fetal hypothyroidism. J Pediatr 1987;110:700

60. Glorieux J, Desjardins M, Letarte M, et al. Useful parameters to predict the eventual, mental outcome of hypothyroid children. Pediatr Res 1988;24:6

61. Fisher DA, Foley BL. Early treatment of congenital hypothyroidism. Pediatrics 1989;83:785

62. Dubuis JM, Richer F, Glorieux JM, et al. Should all patients with congenital hypothyroidism be treated with 10–15 μg/kg/day of levothyroxine. Pediatr Res 1994;35:98A

63. Klein AH, Reviczky A, Chou P, et al. Development of brown adipose tissue thermogenesis in the ovine fetus and newborn. Endocrinology 1983;112:1662

64. Himms-Hagen J. Brown adipose tissue metabolism and thermogenesis. Annu Rev Nutr 1985;5:69

65. Polk DH. Thyroid hormone effects on neonatal thermogenesis. Semin Perinatol 1988;12:151

66. Casteilla L, Forest C, Robelin J, et al. Characterization of mitochondrial uncoupling protein in bovine fetus and newborn calf: disappearance in lamb during aging. Am J Physiol 1987;15:E627

67. Silva JE, Matthews PS. Full expression of uncoupling protein gene requires the concurrence of norepinephrine and triiodothyronine. Mol Endocrinol 1988;2:706

68. Silva JE, Larsen PR,. Potential of brown adipose tissue type II thyroxine 5'-deiodinase as a local and systematic source of triiodothyronine in rats. J Clin Invest 1985;76:2296

69. Bianca AC, Silva JE. Intracellular conversion of thyroxine to triiodothyronine is required for the optimal thermogenic function of brown adipose tissue. J Clin Invest 1987;79:295

70. Wu SY, Kim JK, Chopra IJ, et al. Postnatal changes of the two pathways for thyroxine 5'-monodeiodination in brown adipose tissue in the lamb. Am J Physiol 1991;24:E261

71. Hodgkin DD, Gilbert RD, Power GG. In vivo brown fat response to hypothermia and norepinephrine in the ovine fetus. J Dev Physiol 1988;10:383

72. Klein AH, Reviczky A, Padbury JF. Thyroid hormones augment catecholamine-stimulated brown adipose tissue thermogenesis in the ovine fetus. Endocrinology 1984;114:1065

73. Chowdhry P, Scanlon JW, Auerbach R, Abbassi V. Results of controlled double blind study of thyroid replacement in very low birth weight premature infants with hypothyroxinemia. Pediatrics 1984;73:301

74. Fisher DA. Euthyroid low T_4 and T_3 states in premature and sick infants. Pediatr Clin North Am 1990;37:1297

75. Delange F, Dalhem A, Bourdoux P, et al. Increased risk of primary hypothyroidism in preterm infants. J Pediatr 1984; 105:462

76. Delange F, Bourdoux P, Ermans AM. Transient disorders of thyroid function and regulation in preterm infants. In: Delange F, Fisher DA, Malvaux P, eds. Pediatric thyroidology. Basel: Karger, 1985:369

77. Ponchon G, Beckers C, De Visscher M. Iodine kinetic studies in newborns and infants. J Clin Endocrinol Metab 1966;21:1392

78. Fisher DA, Dussault JH. Development of the mammalian thyroid gland. In: Greer MA, Solomon DH, eds. Handbook of physiology. Vol 3. Thyroid. Washington, DC: American Physiological Society, 1974:21

79. Fisher DA, Sack J, Oddie TH, et al. Serum T_4, TBG, T_3 uptake, T_3, reverse T_3 and TSH concentrations in children 1 to 15 years of age. J Clin Endocrinol Metab 1977;45:191

80. Nelson JC, Clark SJ, Borut DL, et al. Age related changes in serum free thyroxine during childhood and adolescence. J Pediatr 1993;123:899

81. Oliner L, Kohlenbrener RM, Fields T, Kunstadter RH. Thyroid function studies in children: normal values for thyroidal I^{131} uptake and PBI^{131} levels up to the age of 18. J Clin Endocrinol Metab 1957;17:67

82. Cottino F, Colombo G, Ferraro GC, Costa A. Investigations on the metabolism of thyroid hormone in children by means of radiothyronine. Minerva Med 1961;52:1317

83. Beckers C, Malvaux C, De Visscher M. Quantitative aspects of the secretion and degradation of thyroid hormones during adolescence. J Clin Endocrinol Metab 1966;26:202

84. Oddie TH, Meade JH Jr, Fisher DA. An analysis of published data on thyroxine turnover in human subjects. J Clin Endocrinol Metab 1966;26:425

Werner and Ingbar's The Thyroid, Seventh Edition,
edited by Lewis E. Braverman and Robert D. Utiger.
Lippincott–Raven Publishers, Philadelphia, © 1996

85

Hypothyroidism in Infants and Children

NEONATAL SCREENING FOR HYPOTHYROIDISM

Robert Z .Klein
Marvin L. Mitchell

The introduction of screening for neonatal hypothyroidism in 1974 revolutionized the prognosis of children with congenital hypothyroidism.[1] The mean intelligence quotient (IQ) of 800 patients with congenital hypothyroidism culled from the pre-screening literature was less than 80.[2] Among 250 of these children, 65% had IQs below 85, 40% had IQs below 70, and over 19% had IQs below 55. The risk of such brain damage was greatest in those children with the least amount of functioning thyroid tissue as indicated by their serum thyroxine (T_4), tri-iodothyronine (T_3), and thyrotropin (TSH) concentrations; thyroid radionuclide imaging; and retardation of bone age.

Neonatal screening was introduced in the hope that earlier treatment would prevent the brain damage of congenital hypothyroidism. This was substantiated in 1981 by the results of a prospective controlled study that demonstrated that the very early treatment afforded by screening was associated with a normal mean IQ score and normal distribution of individual IQ scores.[3] Figure 85-1 shows the distribution of Stanford-Binet IQ scores of 117 children, 3 to 5 years old, with congenital hypothyroidism detected by neonatal screening and promptly treated plotted against the distribution of IQ scores in normal children. These findings were confirmed by Wechsler Intelligence Scale for Children—Revised scores in 72 of the children at 6 to 9 years of age.

Children in the cohort who had been inadequately treated had significantly lower IQ scores than the remainder, but their scores were still within the normal range. Inadequate treatment was indicated by failure of serum T_4 concentrations to rise above 10 μg/dL (130 nmol/L) after 2 to 3 weeks of treatment or by two or more serum T_4 concentrations less than 8.5 μg/dL (110 nmol/L) accompanied by serum TSH concentrations above 15 mU/L during treatment in the first year of life. Adequacy of treatment was the only factor that correlated significantly with IQ scores on stepwise regression analyses. Even with adequate treatment many of the children had lags in the development of fine motor functions that disappeared in about a year.[4]

In later studies, school progress correlated closely with eventual IQ score. Some screening programs have reported less than normal mean IQ scores in children diagnosed as a result of screening although the mean value was higher than that reported before the introduction of screening. The poorer results presumably relate to inadequate treatment due to lack of compliance or to inadequate dosage of T_4 early in the era of screening before proper replacement regimens were established.[4] However, this has not been proven in all instances nor is there documentation of adequate treatment in all programs reporting normal intellectual development. Thus, other as yet undefined factors may play a role in optimal intellectual development.

INITIAL SCREENING

Virtually all industrialized countries now have screening programs for neonatal hypothyroidism that use capillary blood specimens collected on filter paper. Ideal screening for congenital hypothyroidism would entail measurement of both TSH and free T_4. Assay of free T_4, however, is not yet feasible using filter paper blood specimens. Because of financial limitations, screening is presently performed with either assay of blood T_4 (total T_4) followed by assay of TSH in that specimen if the T_4 concentration is less than a given value or, alternatively, blood TSH assay followed by T_4 assay when the TSH concentration is above 20 to 40 mU/L.

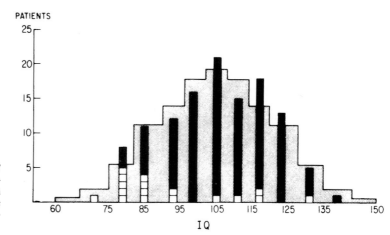

FIGURE 85-1. Distribution of Stanford-Binet IQ scores for 117 children aged 3 to 5 years with permanent congenital hypothyroidism diagnosed as result of neonatal screening. Children who received inadequate treatment are represented by the open squares. The shaded background represents the distribution for 117 normal children (mean ± SD score, 105 ± 15).

A screening program based on a primary TSH assay will not identify infants with secondary hypothyroidism (about 1:100,000 live births), those with low T_4 concentrations but a delayed rise in TSH concentrations (about 10% of hypothyroid infants), and those with deficiency of thyroxine-binding globulin (TBG) (incidence varies widely by geographic area). A primary T_4 program misses infants with elevated TSH but normal T_4 concentrations (10–20% of infants). Both types of programs will miss the rare infant who has normal T_4 and TSH concentrations in the first week of life but then develops high TSH and low T_4 concentrations (<0.5% of infants, chiefly premature infants with transient hypothyroidism). Human error in either type of program adds to the number of diagnoses missed early in any screening program. With experience and automation, the incidence of cases missed due to human error decreases to less than 0.2%. The choice of the type of program to use is generally made on the basis of local laboratory preference because the infants missed by either system tend to be at minimal risk, except for the rare infant with congenital hypopituitarism. Even among the latter group, those infants at major risk usually are a subset with multiple signs and symptoms present in the newborn period when the screening T_4 and TSH concentrations are merely confirmatory of the diagnosis.

The programs that rely primarily on blood T_4 measurements have changed in recent years. Originally, the mean (±SD) for the first week of life was about 12 ± 3 µg/dL (154 ± 39 nmol/L). The indication for a TSH assay from the same filter paper specimen was a T_4 concentration 2 SDs below the mean, 6 µg/dL (77 nmol/L). Because of false-negative results, many programs changed to measuring TSH in specimens in which the T_4 value was in the lowest 5% to 10% of results for the day or were less than 9 µg/dL (116 nmol/L). With adoption of this system, one-third of infants with permanent or transient hypothyroidism have screening T_4 concentrations above 7 µg/dL (90 nmol/L).

The present practice of early discharge from the hospital of healthy full-term infants has led to further modifications of screening. Most screening specimens originally were obtained 3 to 5 days after delivery. In New England, 98% of specimens are now obtained before the infant is 4 days old. The mean (±SD) T_4 concentration obtained before the fourth day is 12.0 ± 1.9 µg/dL (154 ± 24 nmol/L) and that at 4 to 6 days is 11.0 ±

2.5 µg/dL (142 ± 32 nmol/L). In addition, screening on the first day of life has the effect of increasing the chances of finding an elevated TSH concentration as a result of the neonatal surge in TSH secretion. The mean (±SD) TSH concentration decreases from 12 ± 6 mU/L in the first 24 hours to 8 ± 4 mU/L between 24 and 48 hours and to 6 ± 4 between 48 and 72 hours.

FOLLOW-UP EVALUATION

When the screening blood TSH concentration is greater than 40 mU/L, the pediatric caretaker is telephoned and the request is made that the infant be recalled immediately, a blood sample for confirming serum analyses be obtained, and treatment be initiated forthwith. If the serum hormonal assays are normal, the caretaker is then notified to stop therapy.

When the screening blood TSH concentration is 20 to 39 mU/L the caretaker is asked to retest the child immediately but to refrain from initiating treatment until confirmatory values are reported because about 75% of infants with TSH concentrations of 20 to 39 mU/L have concentrations less than 20 mU/L in several weeks after birth.

If the screening blood T_4 concentration in a primary T_4 program is verified to be subnormal but the serum TSH is normal, the most likely causes are deficiency of TBG or diminished protein binding of T_4 characteristic of the newborn. The first is diagnosed by serum TBG assay and the second by finding a normal serum free T_4 concentration. The functional binding defect usually disappears in the first weeks of life but decreased ratios of total T_4 to free T_4 may rarely persist for as long as a year. If the serum free T_4 concentration is low, evidence for hypopituitarism should be sought.

EPIDEMIOLOGY

One of the first discoveries of screening programs was that the incidence of permanent congenital hypothyroidism was higher than anticipated from the clinically determined incidence of 1:6500. In the early 1980s, the reported incidences ranged from 1:3300 in Europe to 1:5700 in Japan, with the incidence in most areas being about 1:4500. Thus, approximately 30% of infants diagnosed as a result of screening would not have been diagnosed clinically until old enough to have been considered to have acquired hypothyroidism or would never have been diagnosed.[2,5] These infants are at negligible risk of mental retardation and their inclusion in follow-up studies of children diagnosed as a result of screening would automatically make the eventual mean IQ score higher.

The incidence figures for permanent congenital hypothyroidism reported around the world ceased to differ much once the infants were followed long enough to exclude cases of transient disease and a higher blood T_4 concentration was adopted as the indication for TSH assay in primary T_4 screening programs.[6] In the United States, for instance, since the adoption of the 10th percentile of blood T_4 as indicating the need for TSH assay, leading to the inclusion of more infants with normal T_4 but elevated TSH concentrations, the incidence of hypothyroidism is 1:3750 live births. This is an increase of 20% from the incidence of 1:4500 reported originally.[6] The low value of 1:5700 in Japan in the 1980s rose dramatically in 1989, and in 1990 it was 1:3900. The highest value was in Europe, 1:3300, but from 1986 to 1990 the incidence there was 1:3770. Despite the apparent similarities, failures in elimination of transient cases still preclude truly accurate comparisons among various screening programs around the world.

Genetic differences do seem to exist, however. The incidence of congenital hypothyroidism in blacks in the United States is about one-half to one-fifth that of the overall population in individual states, whereas the incidence of hypothyroidism in those with Hispanic surnames is nearly twice that of the overall population.

TRANSIENT CONGENITAL HYPOTHYROIDISM

Transient congenital hypothyroidism is defined by diagnostic signs of hypothyroidism at birth that spontaneously and completely disappear in several weeks or months. The minimum diagnostic criterion is a screening blood TSH concentration greater than 40 mU/L. Final diagnosis in an individual infant obviously requires follow-up. The incidence of transient congenital hypothyroidism may be calculated from the percentage of screening blood TSH concentrations greater than 40 mU/L less the percentage of children found to have permanent congenital hypothyroidism. Thus, in New England, 0.05% (1:2000) of screening blood specimens have TSH concentrations above 40 mU/L and the incidence of permanent congenital hypothyroidism is 0.026% (1:3800), leaving an incidence of 0.024% or 1:4200 of transient hypothyroidism.[7]

The incidence of transient congenital hypothyroidism due to maternal iodide deficiency is still as high as 8% in some populations, but it is constantly changing as the disorder slowly approaches elimination. Even in nonendemic goiter areas, the incidence varies markedly depending on definition, method of screening, and age at screening. It is possible that the New England incidence was amplified by the current custom of early postnatal discharge from the hospital, which led to 10% of screening blood specimens being obtained in the

first 24 hours of life when TSH concentrations may still be elevated as a result of the neonatal TSH surge. The adoption of a T_4 concentration below the 10th percentile as the indicator for performing a TSH assay also may have increased the incidence of transient hypothyroidism because patients with normal T_4 and elevated TSH concentrations are more likely to have transient hypothyroidism.

VERY LOW BIRTHWEIGHT (VLBW) INFANTS

Another factor that has introduced complexities into the screening process is the dramatic increase in survival of infants with birthweights under 1500 g (VLBW infants) since the introduction of surfactant. Among just under 400,000 neonates screened in Massachusetts, 0.8% were VLBW infants and 4.8% were low birthweight (LBW) infants weighing 1500 to 2499 g.[7] These infants affect the screening process in two ways. First, the incidence of transient hypothyroidism is 14-fold greater in VLBW infants in Massachusetts than in full-term infants, which would increase the number of T_4 assays in a primary TSH program by 9%. Although the effect of the neonatal TSH surge has not been quantified, it cannot explain the increase in transient hypothyroidism because only 2% of VLBW infants were screened in the first day of life and the neonatal surge is attenuated in these infants.

Second, blood T_4 concentrations are lower in VLBW infants and account for 8% of all TSH assays indicated in a primary T_4 program.[7] The T_4 values are markedly affected by age at screening and by weight. The mean ($\pm$SD) T_4 values in VLBW, LBW, and term infants are 7.8 $\pm$ 3.3, 11.4 $\pm$ 2.5, and 12.0 $\pm$ 1.9 µg/dL (100 $\pm$ 42, 147 $\pm$ 32, and 154 $\pm$ 24 nmol/L), respectively, in the first 3 days of life. There is a positive linear correlation between median T_4 concentrations and median birth weight in 250-g increments up to 2500 g (Fig 85-2). The normal range of T_4 for infants under 1250 g includes unmeasurably low values, that is, less than 0.3 µg/dL (3.9 nmol/L or less). Such values are found in 1.7% of VLBW and 0.1% of LBW infants.

Hospitalization is prolonged in VLBW infants and screening is frequently and needlessly delayed. Blood T_4 concentrations in VLBW infants decrease from a mean of 7.8 µg/dL (100 nmol/L) in the first 3 days to a nadir of 4.0 µg/dL (51 nmol/L) at 2 weeks. The concentrations then rise to their early values by 4 weeks or so of age. Other than to increase the number of TSH, the low total T_4 concentrations have no clinical importance because they are due to diminished thyroid hormone binding in serum and associated with free T_4 concentrations similar to those in full-term infants. Cord blood TBG, T_4, and T_3 concentrations in VLBW infants all are about 60% of those of full-term infants (Table 85-1). Serum free T_4 concentrations and the ratios of T_4 and T_3 to TBG are equivalent in both groups. Free TBG concentrations increase along with serum total and free T_4 concentrations in most VLBW infants by 4 weeks of age.

To avoid increasing the number of TSH assays, separate standards incorporating the effects of weight and the age at screening could be used for VLBW infants or a primary TSH program could be substituted. Although switching to a pri-

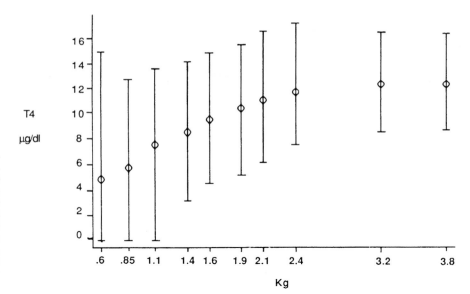

FIGURE 85-2. Median and 2.3 and 97.7 percentile screening capillary blood T_4 concentrations according to birthweight. The 3450 neonates weighing less than 1500 g and the 18,946 neonates weighing 1500 to 2499 g were divided into weight classes of 400 to 750 g and then by 250-g increments to 2499 g. The 9324 full-term infants were divided into two classes of 2500 to 3499 g and 3500 to 5528 g. The T_4 concentrations are plotted against the median weights for each class. To convert the T_4 values to nmol/L multiply by 12.87.

mary TSH system is intellectually the more appealing alternative, it probably makes no practical difference whether it is adopted or the present system is continued.

About 4% of VLBW infants as well as occasional LBW infants with screening TSH values below 20 mU/L are recognized to have transient hypothyroidism at 2 to 6 weeks of life, as manifested by serum TSH concentrations rising to 40 mU/L and sometimes to above 100 mU/L.[2,7,8] How many of these cases are the result of exposure to excess iodide or some other antithyroid agent is not known.

The clinical importance of transient hypothyroidism in VLBW infants is unknown. Transient neonatal hypothyroidism has been associated with brain damage only in endemic cretinism when both mother and fetus are hypothyroid due to iodide deficiency or when the mother has chronic autoimmune thyroiditis with hypothyroidism due to TSH receptor-blocking antibodies, the placental passage of which causes fetal hypothyroidism.[9,10] Studies of the long-term effects of transient congenital hypothyroidism are otherwise limited.[2] Until it is known that late-developing transient hypothyroidism of VLBW infants causes no brain damage, it is recommended that, after initial screening at a week, VLBW infants have repeated screening at 2 and 4 or 6 weeks.

Congenital hypothyroidism is likely to be transient if it is associated with maternal hypothyroidism caused by chronic autoimmune thyroiditis or iodide deficiency or by gestational treatment with iodides or an antithyroid drug. Transient hypothyroidism is associated with pseudohypoparathyroidism, male sex, smaller deviations from normal in serum T_4 and TSH concentrations, a normal-appearing thyroid gland on radionuclide imaging, and, as noted, prematurity.[2] Many infants with transient hypothyroidism cannot be distinguished from those with permanent hypothyroidism because elevation of serum TSH concentrations in the former may persist for several months. Therefore, these infants must be treated until it becomes evident that the dose of T_4 required to maintain the desired TSH concentrations does not need to be increased as the infant grows or until the child is about 4 years old, when it is safe to stop treatment for several weeks and determine if serum TSH and T_4 concentrations remain normal.

TREATMENT

Serum T_4 concentrations should reach 10 µg/dL (129 nmol/L) within 2 weeks after treatment is initiated and then be main-

TABLE 85-1.
Mean Serum Concentrations of T_4, TSH, Free T_4, T_3, and TBG and Ratios of T_4 and T_3 to TBG in Cord Blood of Very-Low-Birthweight (VLBW) and Full-Term Infants*

	T_4 (µg/dL)	TSH (mU/L)	TBG (mg/L)	Free T_4 (ng/dL)	T_3 (ng/dL)	T_4/TBG	T_3/TBG
VLBW	6.5±2.0	7.2±4.1	23±8	1.01±0.25	40±15	0.28±0.07	1.7±0.7
TERM	12±2.2	12±10	38±7	1.02±0.16	70±13	0.32±0.05	1.8±0.7
P	<0.001	>0.05	<0.001	>0.05	<0.001	>0.05	>0.05

Values are means ±SD.
To convert T_4 to nmol/L or free T_4 to pmol/L, multiply by 12.87. To convert T_3 to nmol/L, multiply by 0.015.

tained between 10 and 14.5 μg/dL (129 and 187 nmol/L) for the first year. Eighty to 90% of children so treated will have serum TSH concentrations in the normal range after 2 to 4 weeks of treatment. The serum T_4 concentration may have to be raised to about 17 μg/dL (219 nmol/L) to lower serum TSH to normal in the remaining children. There is no consensus concerning whether this should be done. Some fear that such high serum T_4 concentrations might cause premature closure of cranial sutures with possible increased intracranial pressure and brain damage. Premature craniosynostosis has been reported in three hypothyroid patients. However, they received 200 to 500 μg/d of T_4 for several years.[11] It may still be argued that the achievement of a normal mean IQ score in cohorts in which no attempt was made to normalize serum TSH concentrations obviates the need to do so. On the other hand, noting rising serum TSH concentrations while trying to maintain normal serum TSH concentrations would allow earlier efforts to prevent the effects of waning compliance or other mishaps such as interference in absorption from a change to a soy-based feeding mixture or administration of medications such as iron sulfate that may limit T_4 absorption (see chap 77).

SUMMARY

The results of neonatal screening for hypothyroidism have been dramatic. The most important lesson from screening and follow-up studies is that prompt achievement and maintenance of euthyroidism is critical and that meticulous monitoring is essential to achieve this. Less than a normal mean and distribution of eventual IQ scores in any cohort of hypothyroid children should not be acceptable. With early and optimal treatment, infants with permanent congenital hypothyroidism have the same prospects as their unaffected siblings.

References

1. Dussault JH, Coulombe P, Laberge C, Letarte J, Guyda H, Khoury K. Preliminary report on a mass screening program for neonatal hypothyroidism. J Pediatr 1975;86:670.
2. Klein RZ. Infantile hypothyroidism then and now: the results of neonatal screening. Curr Probl Pediatr 1985;15:5
3. New England Congenital Hypothyroidism Collaborative. Effects of neonatal screening for hypothyroidism: prevention of mental retardation by treatment before clinical manifestations. Lancet 1981;2:1095
4. New England Congenital Hypothyroidism Collaborative. Elementary school performance of children with congenital hypothyroidism. J Pediatr 1990;116:27
5. Larsson A, Hagenfeldt J, Alm J, et al. Incidence of congenital hypothyroidism: a retrospective comparison of neonatal screening and clinical diagnosis. Pediatr Res 1984;18:106
6. Toublanc J-E. Comparison of epidemiological data on congenital hypothyroidism in Europe with those of other parts in the world. Horm Res 1992;138:230
7. Frank JE, Hermos J, Hofman D, et al. Hypothyroidism screening and very low birth-weight infants (VLBW). Pediatr Res 1994;35:99A
8. Mitchell ML, Walraven C, Rojas DA, McIntosh KF, Hermos RJ. Screening very-low-birthweight infants for hypothyroidism. Lancet 1984;343:60
9. Matsuura N, Konishi J, and the Transient Hypothyroidism Study Group in Japan. Transient hypothyroidism in infants born to mothers with chronic thyroiditis—a nationwide study of twenty-three cases. Folia Endocrinol Jpn 1990;37:369
10. Goldsmith RE, McAdams AJ, Larsen PR, et al. Familial autoimmune thyroiditis: maternal fetal relationship and the role of generalized autoimmunity. J Clin Endocrinol Metab 1973;37:265
11. Penfold JL, Simpson DA. Premature craniosynostosis—a complication of thyroid replacement therapy. J Pediatr 1975;86:360

CONGENITAL HYPOTHYROIDISM

Thomas P. Foley, Jr.

HISTORICAL PERSPECTIVES

Congenital hypothyroidism has existed since antiquity, as exemplified by sculptures of goitrous dwarfs in 400 BC in South America and writings about goiter from ancient Rome in the first century, and by the description of mental retardation and goitrous hypothyroidism in a lecture and subsequent publication by Paracelsus in the sixteenth century.[1] Nongoitrous, sporadic congenital hypothyroidism was not reported until the beginning of the Industrial Revolution by Thomas Curling in 1850. Toward the end of the nineteenth century thyroid extract was reported to be effective in congenital hypothyroidism. However, not until the 1970s was it possible for mental retardation caused by congenital hypothyroidism to be virtually eradicated by early treatment as a result of early diagnosis through newborn screening (see preceding section).[2] During the second half of the twentieth century, enzymatic defects in hormonogenesis were defined as causes of the various types of familial goitrous dyshormonogenesis[3] (see chap 56). More recently immune-mediated mechanisms have been proposed as a cause of thyroid dysgenesis although a causative association has not as yet been proven.[4,5]

CLASSIFICATION

Congenital hypothyroidism may be classified as permanent or transient (Table 85-2). The most common cause of congenital hypothyroidism worldwide is iodine deficiency (see chap 57), which can be eradicated by iodine supplementation.[6,7] In iodine-sufficient regions, thyroid dysgenesis is the most common cause of congenital hypothyroidism.[2] This entity presents as athyrosis, which is the absence of detectable thyroid tissue; thyroid ectopia, with thyroid tissue appearing anywhere from the base of the tongue to the anterior mediastinum; or thyroid hypoplasia, a small gland situated in the normal location in the neck. These forms of thyroid dysgenesis are distinguished by radionuclide imaging with ^{123}I-iodine or ^{99m}Tc-pertechnetate.[8,9] In the absence of iodine deficiency, thyroid dysgenesis accounts for 80% to 90% of cases of congenital hypothyroidism[2,8,9] and familial dyshormonogenesis for the remainder. The other causes of permanent congenital hypothyroidism shown in Table 85-2 are rare.

TABLE 85-2.
Classification of Congenital Hypothyroidism

PERMANENT SPORADIC HYPOTHYROIDISM

Thyroid dysgenesis

    Athyrosis (agenesis)

    Ectopia

    Hypoplasia

Iatrogenic

    Maternal exposure to[131]I

Congenital toxoplasmosis

PERMANENT FAMILIAL HYPOTHYROIDISM

Dyshormonogenesis

    TSH receptor defect (TSH unresponsiveness)

    Iodide trapping defect

    Iodide oxidation defects

    Thyroglobulin synthetic defects

    Iodotyrosine deiodinase defect

PERMANENT HYPOTHALAMIC–PITUITARY HYPOTHYROIDISM

Multiple hypothalamic hormone deficiencies

    Idiopathic

    Familial

    Associated with midline CNS anatomic defects

Isolated thyrotropin-releasing hormone deficiency

Isolated TSH deficiency

TRANSIENT HYPOTHYROIDISM

Iodine deficiency

Iatrogenic

    Maternal or neonatal exposure to iodine

    Maternal antithyroid drug therapy

Maternal TSH receptor–blocking antibodies

    Maternal chronic autoimmune thyroiditis

Transient dyshormonogenesis

    Oxidation defect

Congenital nephrosis

Idiopathic hyperthyrotropinemia

    Isolated

    Down's syndrome

Idiopathic primary hypothyroidism

The frequency of transient congenital hypothyroidism in iodine- sufficient regions varies with perinatal and neonatal use of iodine-containing antiseptics or antithyroid drugs[10,11] and the method used for newborn screening for hypothyroidism in the region. A transient defect in iodide oxidation in early infancy presents as familial dyshormonogenesis caused by an oxidation defect, but it cannot be determined to be transient until the child is older and found to have normal thyroid function after discontinuation of thyroxine (T_4) therapy. Primary thyrotropin (TSH) screening will identify more cases of transient primary hypothyroidism than primary T_4 screening because some neonates have elevated blood TSH

but normal T_4 values. Some infants with Down syndrome have serum TSH values greater than the upper limit of normal in infancy, or 8 mU/L, with persistently normal serum free T_4 values for several years, but their serum TSH values then decrease to normal.

Familiarity with classification is important because it dictates the initial diagnostic evaluation, determines the T_4 dosage regimen, and influences the decision to evaluate the patient again at age 3 to 4 years to distinguish between permanent and transient congenital hypothyroidism. For these reasons, thyroid radionuclide imaging at diagnosis is strongly recommended.[12]

ETIOLOGY AND PATHOGENESIS

The cause of thyroid dysgenesis is not known. Antibodies that facilitate cell-mediated cytotoxicity have been found in the serum of some infants with thyroid dysgenesis and their mothers,[5] but their pathogenic role is uncertain. It is puzzling that affected mothers had no other evidence of thyroid disease. Similar comments apply to reports of growth blocking and cytotoxic antibodies in affected infants with sporadic congenital hypothyroidism and their mothers.[4] In cases of familial dyshormonogenesis, specific defects have been reported in virtually all steps of thyroid hormone biosynthesis[13–17] (see chap 56).

Thyrotropin-receptor blocking antibodies (TRAb) are present in infants with transient congenital hypothyroidism born to mothers with chronic autoimmune thyroiditis.[18,19] These maternally derived antibodies gradually disappear so that the infant's hypothyroidism disappears.[20,21] Exposure of a fetus or neonate to inorganic and organic iodine preparations is another cause of transient neonatal hypothyroidism.[10,11]

CLINICAL PRESENTATION

The clinical symptoms and signs of hypothyroidism in neonates and young infants vary according to the cause, severity, and duration of thyroid hormone deficiency before birth[22] (Table 85-3). Most severely affected are infants with prolonged intrauterine hypothyroidism (Fig 85-3). This occurs when high-titer, high-affinity blocking TRAb reach the fetus throughout gestation, in some infants with athyrosis, and in infants with complete thyroid biosynthetic defects. These severely affected infants have hypothermia, poor feeding, bradycardia, and jaundice, the latter caused by unconjugated hyperbilirubinemia.[1,23,24] Most have an enlarged posterior fontanel and many have an umbilical hernia.[24] If hypothyroidism is suspected and the appropriate testing done, treatment may be initiated even earlier than when diagnosis is based on screening.

Most hypothyroid infants, however, have very few or no symptoms and signs before discharge from the nursery[2] and are detected by screening tests.[12] In them, clinical hypothyroidism generally does not appear until 2 to 3 months of age. Rarely an infant with thyroid dysgenesis has normal thyroid function, is not detected by newborn screening,[25] and presents during childhood with an asymptomatic mass in the submental or lateral cervical area or at the foramen cecum of the tongue (Fig 85-4).

TABLE 85-3.
Congenital Hypothyroidism: Symptoms and Signs

EARLY NEONATAL APPEARANCE

Prolonged icterus (>3 d)

   Primary hypothyroidism: unconjugated hyperbilirubinemia

   Hypothalamic–pituitary hypothyroidism: conjugated and
      unconjugated hyperbilirubinemia

Edema

Gestation > 42 wk

Birth weight > 4 kg

Poor feeding

Hypothermia

Abdominal distention

Large posterior fontanel (>5 mm)

ONSET DURING THE FIRST MONTH OF AGE

Peripheral cyanosis and mottling

Respiratory distress

Failure to gain weight and poor sucking ability

Decreased stool frequency

Decreased activity and lethargy

ONSET DURING THE FIRST 3 MONTHS OF AGE

Umbilical hernia

Constipation

Dry and sallow skin

Macroglossia

Generalized myxedema

Hoarse cry

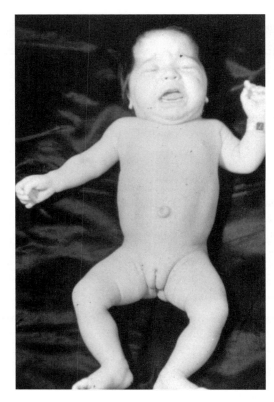

FIGURE 85-3. Photograph of a 6-month-old infant with congenital athyrosis at diagnosis showing pallor, macroglossia, umbilical hernia, and facial edema.

It is important to identify the presence of thyroid enlargement on the initial physical examination because of the information it provides about the cause of the hypothyroidism. The thyroid gland of an infant can be delineated quite easily when the infant is examined with the neck extended. The isthmus is identified by palpation just below the thyroid cartilage and on lateral palpation the lobes may be identified. If no thyroid tissue is palpated, ectopically located thyroid tissue should be sought.

DIAGNOSTIC EVALUATION

To confirm a diagnosis of congenital hypothyroidism suspected on clinical evaluation, complete thyroid function tests and thyroid imaging should be performed as soon as possible.[8,9,24,26,27] If a high blood TSH value is found on routine screening, blood should be collected promptly for measurements of serum TSH, total and free T_4, and thyroglobulin.[24] The former tests, if abnormal, will confirm the diagnosis of primary hypothyroidism, and the serum thyroglobulin value may provide information about the cause of the hypothyroidism[28] (see chap 56). If there is a maternal history of hypothyroidism, serum should be analyzed for the presence of TRAb.[19,21,24]

If the results of newborn screening tests indicate low blood T_4 and normal TSH concentrations, blood should be collected for the measurement of serum TSH, to confirm that it is normal, and total and free T_4, to establish either a diagnosis of a thyroxine-binding protein abnormality, such as thyroxine-binding globulin (TBG) deficiency, or central hypothyroidism, or that the initial test was falsely positive.[24] Serum free T_4 con-

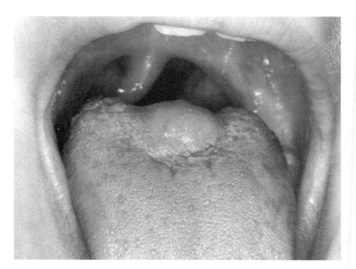

FIGURE 85-4. Photograph of ectopic thyroid tissue underneath the foramen cecum on the anterior surface of the tongue, the location of the embryonic origin of the thyroid. Thyroid function tests were normal when this mass was found at age 12 years.

centration is best measured by equilibrium dialysis.[29] Although T_4 therapy may be initiated before obtaining the results, these tests should be obtained on any infant in whom the diagnosis of hypothalamic-pituitary hypothyroidism is suspected.[30] Serum triiodothyronine concentrations are usually normal,[31] and therefore should not be measured.

Although thyroid radionuclide imaging tests are not absolutely essential, they are strongly recommended for several reasons.[32] If the thyroid gland cannot be palpated, a diagnosis of thyroid dysgenesis can be established within 1 to 2 hours by ^{99m}Tc-pertechnetate imaging. If no thyroid tissue is identified, the infant either has athyrosis (greater than 95% of cases) or the uptake is inhibited by blocking TRAb. In the latter instance, a normal or small thyroid gland can be identified by ultrasonography.[24,32] Ectopic thyroid tissue located anywhere from the foreman cecum to the anterior mediastinum can be identified by imaging (Fig 85-5). If a normal or enlarged thyroid gland is identified on palpation, imaging with ^{123}I-iodine is preferable, because radioiodine imaging not only confirms a

diagnosis of thyroid dysgenesis, but also allows quantitative uptake measurements and tests for iodine transport defects and iodide oxidation defects.

Thyroid radionuclide imaging is important not only because identification of thyroid dysgenesis means that hypothyroidism is permanent, and therefore lifelong T_4 therapy is required, but also because it may establish a diagnosis of familial dyshormonogenesis, so that parents may be counseled about the inheritance of these autosomal recessive diseases. Furthermore, establishing the proper diagnosis in infancy obviates the need for additional studies after temporary discontinuation of T_4 at age 3 to 4 years.

A radiographic examination of the knees and feet to determine bone age can provide information about the age of onset of hypothyroidism because skeletal maturation slows very early in the course of the disorder.[22]

TREATMENT

The goal of treatment is to achieve normal serum T_4 and TSH concentrations rapidly and then maintain them, and thereby achieve normal growth, development, and intellectual function. The treatment of choice for primary hypothyroidism during infancy, childhood, and adolescence is T_4.[27,33,34] It is rapidly converted to metabolically active triiodothyronine (T_3) by several widely distributed deiodinases, so that serum and tissue T_3 concentrations increase soon after T_4 therapy is initiated and in time become normal.

When the results of newborn screening are a blood TSH value greater than 40 mU/L and a T_4 value below 6 μg/dL (77 nmol/L), a blood specimen should be collected for confirmatory tests, imaging performed, and T_4 therapy initiated immediately. An exception might be an infant presumed to have transient hypothyroidism because of maternal antithyroid drug or iodine administration,[8,9,35] because in these infants thyroid function may become normal quickly.

When the screening blood TSH value is greater than 40 mU/L and the T_4 is normal (>6 μg/dL [77 nmol/L]), T_4 therapy can be delayed 1 to 2 days to await the results of serum testing, but, it is preferable to proceed with imaging and initiate T_4 immediately if the thyroid image is in any way abnormal. A similar course of management would be appropriate for the infant less than 2 weeks of age whose screening blood TSH value is mildly elevated (20–40 mU/L) and whose blood T_4 value is normal[24] (Table 85-4).

In infants found to have high serum TSH and low serum T_4 concentrations on reexamination after screening, T_4 therapy should be initiated promptly in a dose of 10 to 15 μg/kg/d.[12,24,27,34] This dose is usually 50 μg/d in an infant who was born at term.[27,34] This dose should be continued for at least 1 week to replenish the deficient T_4 stores in serum and tissue, after which it may be reduced to 37.5 μg/d, depending on the results of thyroid function tests performed on day 7 of treatment. Infants with ectopic thyroid tissue, partial dyshormonogenesis, or elevated serum TSH and normal serum T_4 concentrations can be treated with 10 μg/kg/d, or, in an infant born at term, 37.5 μg/d.[27,34] In an occasional infant the dose will need to be decreased to 25 μg/d if the serum TSH concentration on subsequent testing is low.

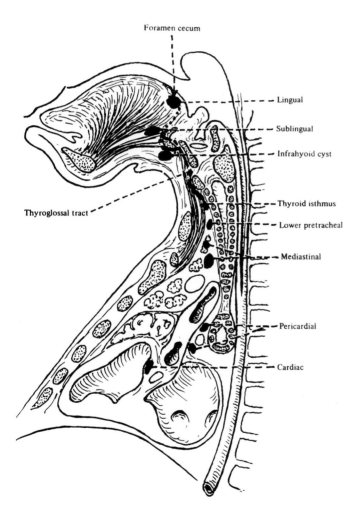

Foramen cecum

Lingual

Sublingual

Infrahyoid cyst

Thyroglossal tract

Thyroid isthmus

Lower pretracheal

Mediastinal

Pericardial

Cardiac

FIGURE 85-5. Diagram of the different locations (shown in black) of ectopic thyroid tissue identified by radionuclide imaging in infants with congenital hypothyroidism. (From Roger WM. Anomalous development of the thyroid. In: Werner SC, Ingbar SH, eds. The Thyroid, 4th ed. Hagerstown, MD. Harper and Row, 1978:419)

TABLE 85-4.
Guidelines for T$_4$ Replacement Therapy

PRIMARY HYPOTHYROIDISM DURING THE FIRST 6 MONTHS OF AGE

ELEVATED SERUM TSH AND LOW SERUM T$_4$ AT DIAGNOSIS

Initial dose in term infant: 50 µg/d

Initial dose in preterm infant: 10–15 µg/kg/d

Maintenance dose after normalization of serum total and free T$_4$

    Term infant: 37.5–50 µg/d

    Preterm infant: 8–10 µg/kg/d

ELEVATED SERUM TSH AND NORMAL SERUM T$_4$ AT DIAGNOSIS

Initial and maintenance dose: 8–10 µg/kg/d

    Term infant: 25–37.5 µg/d

    Preterm infant: 12.5–25 µg/d

HYPOTHALAMIC–PITUITARY HYPOTHYROIDISM DURING THE FIRST 6 MONTHS OF AGE

Initial and maintenance dose: 8–10 µg/kg/d

    Term infant: 25–37.5 µg/d

    Preterm infant: 12.5–25 µg/d

HYPOTHYROIDISM AFTER 6 MONTHS OF AGE

Age 6 to 12 mo	Age 1 to 5 y
50–75 µg/d	75–100 µg/d
6–8 µg/kg/d	5–6 µg/kg/d
Age 6 to 12 y	Age 12 y to adult
75–125 µg/d	100–200 µg/d
4–5 µg/kg/d	1–3 µg/kg/d

Because the dose requirement for an individual infant cannot be predicted, serum TSH and either serum T$_4$ or, preferably, free T$_4$ concentrations should be measured after 7, 14, and 28 days of therapy,[26,27] or until both serum TSH and T$_4$ concentrations are normal. Thereafter, serum TSH and T$_4$ concentrations should be measured at monthly intervals to age 6 months, at 3-month intervals to age 2 years, and annually thereafter.[26] However, if there are symptoms of hypothyroidism or the serum TSH concentration is not in the normal range, dosage adjustments and more frequent testing are indicated until the value is normal.

To achieve consistency in absorption and, therefore, consistency in serum thyroid function tests during treatment, T$_4$ should be given once daily at least 30 minutes before feeding.[24,36,37] The tablet can be crushed in breast milk or other liquid. Dose adjustments can be made by incremental changes of 12.5 µg or by the addition or subtraction of one tablet per week if a very minor adjustment is needed.

If an infant or child receiving T$_4$ has intermittent elevations of serum TSH or an initial decline toward normal and a subsequent rise, the cause in most instances is an insufficient dose of T$_4$.[38] If serum TSH values fluctuate between normal and elevated in an infant taking more than 15 µg/kg/d of T$_4$, the explanation may be parental noncompliance or the ingestion of foods and various medications that interfere with T$_4$ absorption.[39] The latter include soybean formulas and iron-containing medications.[37,39] Whether poor compliance or malabsorption, serum T$_4$ concentrations can be raised to 10 to 12

µg/dL (129–154 nmol/L) by the intramuscular or intravenous administration of T$_4$ in a dose of 50 to 100 µg weekly or biweekly depending on the age and magnitude of T$_4$ deficiency. When this problem occurs during the first 2 years of life, when normal serum T$_4$ concentrations are required for normal brain development, it is essential to measure serum T$_4$ and TSH at least weekly to be sure that therapy is adequate.

In managing infants with hypothyroidism, it is important to remember that serum T$_4$ concentrations during the first years of life in normal infants may be as high as 16 µg/dL (206 nmol/L) and that serum free T$_4$ concentrations are also higher than in older children and adults.[29,38] Therefore, the dose of T$_4$ should not be reduced in infants with seemingly high serum T$_4$ concentrations, unless their serum TSH concentrations are low. An exception would be the occasional infant in whom the serum TSH has never been suppressed into the normal range after starting treatment despite high-normal or elevated serum T$_4$ concentrations in association with symptoms of thyrotoxicosis.[38,40,41] This phenomenon has been reported in infants who had hypothyroidism in utero. In animals, fetal hypothyroidism may result in an abnormality in the set point of TSH secretion such that more T$_4$ than normal is needed to inhibit TSH secretion, analogous to the syndrome of isolated pituitary resistance to thyroid hormone. In patients with congenital hypothyroidism with this type of defect, the dose of T$_4$ needs to be adjusted so that the serum total and free T$_4$ concentrations are in the upper normal range in the absence of symptoms of thyrotoxicosis and despite mild elevations of serum TSH.[38,40,41] This abnormality may disappear during childhood or later.

Whenever thyroid function tests are performed, the length or height and weight of the child should be measured and plotted on a growth chart to ensure that growth is normal.[30] If there is deceleration in linear growth, bone age should be measured.[8,9] Poor weight gain, often in association with symptoms of thyrotoxicosis, may indicate excessive T$_4$ therapy, and should be confirmed by measurements of serum TSH and free T$_4$.

The parents of these infants must understand the necessity for daily T$_4$ therapy if their child is to grow and develop normally. However, intellectual performance, though usually normal and appropriate with respect to parental and sibling achievements, can never be guaranteed. If a dose is missed or if there is uncertainty whether a dose was given, it is preferable to give an additional dose for that day or two doses the next day rather than miss a dose.

INTELLECTUAL AND PSYCHOLOGICAL ACHIEVEMENT

The early recognition and treatment of congenital hypothyroidism made possible by neonatal screening has led to nearly complete disappearance of the mental retardation that was so common in these children in the past. Several studies in North America and Europe have evaluated IQ performance and psychomotor development in infants with congenital hypothyroidism diagnosed by newborn screening.[42–44] There is no doubt that early diagnosis and rapid correction of hypothyroidism results in normal IQ scores of patients as compared with siblings and matched and unmatched normal children. However, on neurodevelopmental evaluations, there may be

subtle residual deficits in neuromotor, language, and cognitive areas in children who have specific risk factors.[33] The latter include greater severity of hypothyroidism at diagnosis, delay in diagnosis, and prolonged inadequate or excessive T_4 therapy. These neurodevelopmental profiles suggest that some children with congenital hypothyroidism may have a mild form of the nonverbal learning disability syndrome. They may also have visual-spatial processing problems such as learning visual numerical sequences, constructing puzzles, and solving mazes. Some attention and memory deficits may be related more to erratic or excessive T_4 therapy than to the primary disease.[33]

At greatest risk are the more severely affected infants, especially those with fetal hypothyroidism who at diagnosis have very low serum T_4 concentrations and retardation of skeletal maturation. In three studies, the IQ deficiencies of these children, as compared with normal children, ranged between 12 and 16 IQ points.[42] Similarly, infants of mothers with hypothyroxinemia from iodine deficiency during the first half of pregnancy have psychomotor developmental impairment as compared with infants born to mothers with normal serum T_4 concentrations during the first half of pregnancy.[7] Some infants with fetal hypothyroidism caused by transplacental passage of maternal TRAb with blocking properties also may have permanent impairment.

A delay in diagnosis and the institution of T_4 therapy beyond 6 weeks of age very likely will be associated with impaired intellectual performance.[45] In a large European study, the age at the start of therapy was negatively correlated with the psychometric score.[42] Lower IQ scores are associated with poor compliance with T_4 therapy and to a lower dose prescribed during infancy. Therefore, the identification and prompt initiation of appropriate T_4 therapy at the earliest possible age, even during intrauterine life in severe cases, is associated with the most favorable outcome of psychomotor development and intellectual achievement. Excessive T_4 therapy also should be avoided to prevent specific adverse behavioral problems during childhood and adolescence.

References

1. Foley TP Jr. Sporadic congenital hypothyroidism. In: Dussault JH, Walker P, eds. Congenital hypothyroidism. New York: Marcel Dekker, 1983:231

2. Fisher DA, Dussault JH, Foley TP Jr, et al. Screening for congenital hypothyroidism: results of screening one million North American infants. J Pediatr 1979;94:700

3. Dumont JE, Vassart G, Refetoff S. Thyroid disorders. In: Scriver CR, Beaudet AL, Sly WS, et al, eds. The metabolic basis of inherited disease. 6th ed. New York: McGraw-Hill, 1989:1843

4. Van der Gaag RO, Drexhage HA, Dussault JH. Role of maternal immunoglobulins blocking TSH-induced thyroid growth in sporadic forms of congenital hypothyroidism. Lancet 1985;1:246

5. Bogner U, Grüters A, Sigle B, et al. Cytotoxic antibodies in congenital hypothyroidism. J Clin Endocrinol Metab 1989;68:671

6. Boyages SC. Iodine deficiency disorders. J Clin Endocrinol Metab 1993;77:587

7. Xue-Yi C, Xin-Min J, Zhi-Hong D, et al. Timing of vulnerability of the brain to iodine deficiency in endemic cretinism. N Engl J Med 1994;331:1739

8. Grüters A. Congenital hypothyroidism. Pediatr Ann 1992;21:15

9. LaFranchi S. Congenital hypothyroidism: a newborn screening success story? Endocrinologist 1994;4:477

10. Lyen KJ, Finegold DN, Orsini R, et al. Transient thyroid suppression associated with topically applied povidone-iodine. Am J Dis Child 1982;136:369

11. Grüters A, l'Allemand D, Heidemann PH, Schurnbrand P. Incidence of iodine contamination in neonatal transient hyper-thyrotropinemia. Eur J Pediatr 1983;140:299

12. Fisher DA. Management of congenital hypothyroidism. J Clin Endocrinol Metab 1991;72:523

13. Sunthornthepvarakul T, Gottschalk ME, Hayashi Y, Refetoff S. Resistance to thyrotropin caused by mutations in the thyrotropin-receptor gene. N Engl J Med 1995;332:155

14. Targovnik HM, Medeiros-Neto G, Varela V, et al. A nonsense mutation causes human hereditary congenital goiter with preferential production of a 171-nucleotide-deleted thyroglobulin ribonucleic acid messenger. J Clin Endocrinol Metab 1993;77:21

15. Mason ME, Dunn AD, Wortsman J, et al. Thyroids from siblings with Pendred's syndrome contain thyroglobulin messenger ribonucleic acid variants. J Clin Endocrinol Metab 1995;80:497

16. Abramowicz MJ, Targovnik HM, Varela V, et al. Identification of a mutation in the coding sequence of the human thyroid peroxidase gene causing congenital goiter. J Clin Invest 1992;90:1200

17. Hayashizaki Y, Hiraoka Y, Endo Y, Matsubara K. Thyroid stimulating hormone (TSH) deficiency caused by a single base substitution in the CAGYC region of the β subunit. EMBO J 1989;8:2291

18. Matsura N, Yamada Y, Nohara Y, et al. Familial, neonatal transient hypothyroidism due to maternal TSH-binding inhibitor immunoglobulins. N Engl J Med 1980;303:738

19. Brown RS, Bellisario RL, Mitchell E, Keating P, Botero D. Detection of thyrotropin binding inhibitory activity in neonatal blood spots. J Clin Endocrinol Metab 1993;77:1005

20. Iseki M, Shimizu M, Oikawa T, et al. Sequential serum measurements of thyrotropin binding inhibiting immunoglobulin G in transient neonatal hypothyroidism. J Clin Endocrinol Metab 1983;57:384

21. Foley TP Jr. Maternally transferred thyroid disease in the infant: recognition and treatment. In: Bercu BB, Shulman DI, eds. Advances in perinatal thyroidology. New York: Plenum Press, 1991:209

22. Grant DB, Smith I, Fuggle PW, et al. Congenital hypothyroidism detected by neonatal screening: relationship between biochemical severity and early clinical features. Arch Dis Child 1992;67:87

23. Sutherland JM, Esselborn VM, Burket RL, et al. Familial nongoitrous cretinism apparently due to maternal antithyroid antibody. N Engl J Med 1960;263:336

24. Foley TP Jr. Congenital hypothyroidism and screening. In: Monaco F, Satta MA, Shapiro B, Troncone L, eds. Thyroid diseases. Boca Raton, FL: CRC Press, 1993:121

25. Fisher DA. Screening for congenital hypothyroidism: prevalence of missed cases. Pediatr Clin N Am 1987;34:881

26. American Academy of Pediatrics. Newborn screening for congenital hypothyroidism: recommended guidelines. Pediatrics 1993;91:1203

27. Germak JA, Foley TP Jr. Longitudinal assessment of L-thyroxine therapy for congenital hypothyroidism. J Pediatr 1990;117:211

28. Czernichow P, Leger J. Thyroglobulin and congenital hypothyroidism. In: Delange F, Fisher DA, Glinoer D, eds. Research in congenital hypothyroidism. New York: Plenum Press, 1989:211

29. Nelson JC, Clark SJ, Borut DL, et al. Age-related changes in serum free thyroxine during childhood and adolescence. J Pediatr 1993;123:899

30. Foley TP Jr, Malvaux P, Blizzard RM. Thyroid disease. In: Kappy MS, Blizzard RM, Migeon CJ, eds. Wilkins' the diagnosis and treatment of endocrine disorders in childhood and adolescence. 4th ed. Springfield, IL: Charles C. Thomas, 1994:457

31. Klein AH, Foley TP Jr, Larsen PR, Augustin AV, Hopwood NJ. Neonatal thyroid function in congenital hypothyroidism. J Pediatr 1976;89:710

32. Muir A, Daneman D, Daneman A, Ehrlich R. Thyroid scanning, ultrasound and serum thyroglobulin in determining the origin of congenital hypothyroidism. Am J Dis Child 1988;142:214

33. Rovet JF, Ehrlich RM, Sorbara DL. Neurodevelopment in infants and preschool children with congenital hypothyroidism: etiological and treatment factors affecting outcome. J Pediatr Psychol 1992;17:187

34. Fisher DA, Foley BL. Early treatment of congenital hypothyroidism. Pediatrics 1989;83:785

35. Cheron RG, Kaplan MM, Larsen PR, et al. Neonatal thyroid function after propylthiouracil therapy for maternal Graves' disease. N Engl J Med 1981;304:525

36. Wenzel KW, Kirschsieper HE. Aspects of the absorption of oral L-thyroxine in normal man. Metabolism 1977;26:1

37. Pinchera A, MacGillivray MH, Crawford JD, et al. Thyroid refractoriness in an athyreotic cretin fed soybean formula. N Engl J Med 1965;273:83

38. Grant DB, Fuggle PW, Smith I. Increased plasma thyroid stimulating hormone in treated congenital hypothyroidism: relation to severity of hypothyroidism, plasma thyroid hormone status, and daily dose of thyroxine. Arch Dis Child 1993;69:55

39. Monaco F. Medical therapy. In: Monaco F, Satta MA, Shapiro B, Troncone L, eds. Thyroid diseases. Boca Raton, FL: CRC Press, 1993;329

40. Sato T, Suzuki Y, Taketani T, et al. Age-related change in pituitary threshold for TSH release during thyroxine replacement therapy for cretinism. J Clin Endocrinol Metab 1977;44:553

41. McCrossin RB, Sheffield LJ, Robertson EF. Persisting abnormality in the pituitary thyroid axis in congenital hypothyroidism. In: Stockigt JR, Nagataki S, eds. Thyroid research VIII. Canberra: Australian Academy of Science, 1980:37

42. Grant DB, Fuggle P, Tokar S, Smith I. Psychomotor development in infants with congenital hypothyroidism diagnosed by newborn screening. Acta Med Austriaca 1992;19:54

43. Glorieux J, Dussault J, Van Vliet G. Intellectual development at age 12 years of children with congenital hypothyroidism diagnosed by newborn screening. J Pediatr 1992;121:581

44. New England Congenital Hypothyroidism Collaborative. Correlation of cognitive test scores and adequacy of treatment in adolescents with congenital hypothyroidism. J Pediatr 1994; 124:383

45. Klein AH, Meltzer S, Kenny FM. Improved prognosis in congenital hypothyroidism treated before age three months. J Pediatr 1972;81:912

Acquired Hypothyroidism During Infancy, Childhood, and Adolescence

Thomas P. Foley, Jr.

The clinical presentation of acquired hypothyroidism in infants and children varies considerably depending primarily on the age at the onset of the disease and the rapidity of its progression. Although the detrimental effect of hypothyroidism on central nervous system (CNS) development is permanent, it is limited to hypothyroidism occurring in the first 2 years of life,[1] whereas its detrimental effects on growth and development occur until puberty is complete, and many of the symptoms and signs of hypothyroidism that occur in adults also occur in children, especially older children and adolescents. This similarity is explained by the generalized effects of thyroid hormone deficiency on intermediary metabolism, oxygen consumption, and control of the metabolic rate as a result of decreased protein synthesis and cellular metabolism.[2] In infancy, many clinical features resemble those of infants with congenital hypothyroidism, probably because of the generalized effects of hypothyroidism during a very rapid period of growth and maturation.[3]

CAUSES OF JUVENILE HYPOTHYROIDISM

Among the causes of juvenile hypothyroidism (Table 85-5), primary hypothyroidism is associated with more severe symptoms and signs of thyroid deficiency than is central (hypothalamic or pituitary) hypothyroidism.[4] In the latter, the clinical features at presentation vary depending on the age of the child, the cause of the pituitary or hypothalamic disorder, the extent of other pituitary hormone deficiencies, and the occurrence of neurologic or other manifestations of that disorder.[4]

TABLE 85-5.
Causes of Acquired Juvenile Hypothyroidism

PRIMARY HYPOTHYROIDISM

Chronic autoimmune thyroiditis

    Goitrous autoimmune thyroiditis

    Atrophic autoimmune thyroiditis

Drug-induced hypothyroidism (iodine, lithium, propylthiouracil, methimazole, carbimazole)

Endemic goiter

Irradiation of the thyroid

    External irradiation of nonthyroid tumors

    Radioiodine therapy

Thyroidectomy

FAMILIAL HYPOTHYROIDISM

Dyshormonogenesis

Generalized resistance to thyroid hormones

CENTRAL (HYPOTHALAMIC–PITUITARY) HYPOTHYROIDISM

Multiple pituitary hormone deficiencies

    Idiopathic

    Familial

    Associated with midline CNS anatomic defects

    Hypothalamic or pituitary tumors

    Treatment of brain and other tumors

        Surgical therapy

        Radiation therapy

Isolated TRH deficiency

Isolated TSH deficiency

The most common cause of primary hypothyroidism worldwide is iodine deficiency[5] (see chap 57); in iodine-sufficient regions it is chronic autoimmune thyroiditis.[6] Several types of chronic autoimmune thyroiditis are recognized during the first two decades of life.[7] The most common is chronic lymphocytic thyroiditis with diffuse goiter, especially in adolescents. The atrophic form of chronic autoimmune thyroiditis occurs at any age and seems to be the most common cause of acquired hypothyroidism in infancy.[3]

With the successful use of external radiation to treat tumors of the neck, such as lymphomas, radiation-induced hypothyroidism is being increasingly recognized.[4,8,9] External radiation therapy for brain tumors, especially those in the posterior fossa, may also cause primary hypothyroidism because of inclusion of the neck in the radiation field.[8,9] Other common causes of hypothyroidism in adults, such as that caused by radioiodine therapy, thyroidectomy, or drugs, are rare in children.

Although most cases of familial hypothyroidism should be identified by newborn screening, mildly affected infants may be missed and present at a later age with goiter.[10] Current screening methods do not identify patients with the thyroid hormone resistance syndromes (see chap 90). Unless the gene for these diseases is known to be present in the family, the diagnosis may be delayed until childhood or later.

Central hypothyroidism, whether caused by thyrotropin-releasing hormone (TRH) or thyrotropin (TSH) deficiency, presents more commonly during childhood and adolescence than infancy. However, cases caused by mutations of the TSH gene may not be identified by newborn screening unless serum free thyroxine (T_4) is measured when an infant who had a low screening blood T_4 value is evaluated.[11] Most often patients with central hypothyroidism have multiple pituitary hormone deficiencies that influence their clinical presentation.[4]

CLINICAL PRESENTATION

Acquired Infantile Hypothyroidism: 6 Months to 3 Years

Infants with acquired hypothyroidism present with symptoms and signs that develop after 6 months of age. In contrast to congenital hypothyroidism, these infants are asymptomatic during the first 6 months of life. However, at diagnosis their clinical presentation is similar to that of infants with congenital hypothyroidism not detected by screening[3] (Table 85-6). The important clinical features are deceleration in linear growth that begins late during the first year (Fig 85-6), evidence of a delay or arrest in developmental milestones, and features of congenital hypothyroidism[3] (see preceding section). If the hypothyroidism begins at about age 2 years there may be some clinical signs characteristic of hypothyroidism during childhood, such as muscular pseudohypertrophy.[12,13] Because hypothyroidism often develops rapidly in these young infants, they may have no delay in skeletal maturation or in eruption of primary teeth when first seen.

Impairment of brain maturation depends on the age at onset of hypothyroidism and its duration.[1] With early diagnosis and treatment after the onset of symptoms, the intellectual

TABLE 85-6.
Symptoms and Signs of Acquired Hypothyroidism

ONSET AFTER 6 MONTHS AND BEFORE 3 YEARS

Deceleration of linear growth

Coarse facial features

Dry, sallow skin

Hoarse cry and macroglossia

Umbilical hernia

Muscular pseudohypertrophy

ONSET DURING CHILDHOOD

Growth retardation with delayed skeletal maturation

Delayed dental development and tooth eruption

Myopathy and muscular pseudohypertrophy

Constipation

Dry, sallow skin

Generalized myxedema

Precocious sexual development

ONSET DURING ADOLESCENCE

Onset of puberty usually delayed

Growth retardation with delayed skeletal maturation

Constipation

Dry, sallow skin

Generalized myxedema

Delayed dental development and tooth eruption

Galactorrhea

and neuropsychological development of these infants should be normal.

Acquired Juvenile Hypothyroidism: 3 Years to Adolescence

Hypothyroidism during childhood is not associated with permanent impairment of CNS function. The important clinical features that suggest the diagnosis are diffuse goiter and deceleration of linear growth.[2] Although some features of congenital hypothyroidism may be evident in younger children,[3] the predominant clinical features are growth retardation, goiter, easy fatigability, and changes in school and athletic performance.[2] Increased fluid retention in the CNS may cause intracranial hypertension (pseudotumor cerebri) either at diagnosis and more often during the first several weeks of therapy.[14] In addition, enlargement of the pituitary gland may be evident by an enlarged sella turcica radiographically mimicking a pituitary adenoma.[15,16] Some children have muscle weakness and muscular pseudohypertrophy, known as the Kocher-Debré-Sémélaigne syndrome,[12,13] (Fig 85-7). Chronic hypothyroidism causes a profound delay in dental and skeletal maturation, often with radiographic evidence of epiphyseal dysgenesis in younger children[17] (Fig 85-8). Some patients present with hip or knee pain and a limp and are found to have a slipped capital femoral epiphysis on radiographic ex-

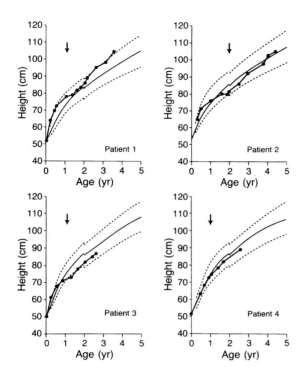

FIGURE 85-6. Growth curves of four infants with acquired primary hypothyroidism caused by autoimmune thyroiditis. (From Foley TP Jr, Abbassi V, Copeland KC, Draznin MB. Hypothyroidism caused by chronic autoimmune thyroiditis in very young infants. N Engl J Med 1993;330:466. Reproduced with permission of the publisher.)

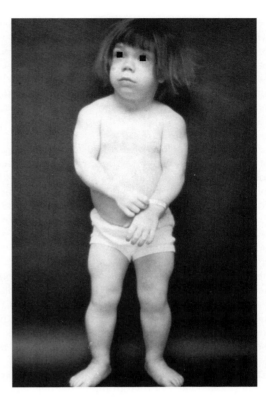

FIGURE 85-7. Photograph of a 7-year-old boy with the Kocher-Debré-Sémélaigne syndrome associated with primary hypothyroidism shows muscular pseudohypertrophy of the extremities and other clinical features of hypothyroidism. (From Foloy TP Jr. Goiters in adolescents. Endocrinol Metab Clin North Am 1993;22:593. Reproduced with permission of the publisher)

amination[18] (Fig 85-9). These children usually have advanced hypothyroidism, with cessation of linear growth and signs of myxedema. Growth hormone secretion is often decreased.[15]

On rare occasions, children with primary hypothyroidism may present with precocious puberty,[12,19,20] which is thought to be caused by TSH activation of gonadal follicle-stimulating hormone (FSH) receptors; gonadotropin secretion is not increased.[21] Although there may be breast development and vaginal bleeding from inappropriate estrogen secretion in girls, sexual hair is characteristically absent. Isolated menarche has been reported.[22] Hyperprolactinemia may be present, and galactorrhea is a rare finding.[19,23] In boys precocious testicular enlargement may occur, but there is little increase in serum testosterone, indicative of activation of FSH but not luteinizing hormone receptors.[21] Rarely there is excess growth of hair over the forehead, back, and lateral aspects of the limbs.[15,24]

Acquired Hypothyroidism During Adolescence

Hypothyroidism during adolescence usually is mild. Most patients have a diffuse goiter.[25] Delayed puberty, severe skeletal and growth retardation, and delayed eruption of permanent teeth are characteristic findings in severe hypothyroidism (see Table 85-6). Other features of hypothyroidism are similar to those that occur in adults. When hypothyroidism develops after the onset of puberty there is maturational arrest, primary amenorrhea, occasionally galactorrhea, and reduction in sexual hair growth, although body hair growth may increase.

Some patients in this age group, however, have few or none of the symptoms and signs of hypothyroidism that occur in adults despite having a goiter and slowing of growth and pubertal development. This poverty of symptomatology relates to the insidious and gradual development of the disease over months or years. School performance may be normal or even advanced as long as rapidity of thought processes and movement, such as typing or completion of timed examinations is not required. These patients may be evaluated initially for the nonspecific complaints that are common during normal adolescence, such as fatigue and excessive sleeping habits, or because of unexplained anemia, headaches, and an enlarged sella turcica, or hip pain associated with a slipped capital femoral epiphysis.[18] Only after several weeks of T_4 therapy do symptoms of hypothyroidism become evident by retrospective comparison.

Acquired Central Hypothyroidism

Although isolated TRH or TSH deficiency may occur, most often central hypothyroidism occurs in association with multiple pituitary hormone deficiencies. During childhood the most common presentation is growth retardation secondary to growth hormone and TSH deficiencies. Adolescents with deficient gonadotropin secretion usually have deficient growth

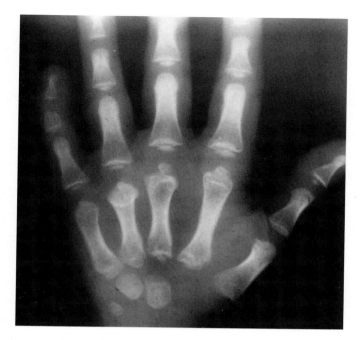

FIGURE 85-8. Radiograph of the hand of 20-year-old man with severe hypothyroidism shows stippled ossification of the epiphyses (epiphyseal dysgenesis) and a bone age of less than one year of age.

hormone and TSH secretion, and present with growth retardation and delayed pubertal development.

The characteristic symptoms and signs of primary hypothyroidism often are minimal or absent in patients with central hypothyroidism, except for growth retardation, and the hypothyroidism usually is mild. The presenting symptoms more often relate to the cause of the hypothalamic or pituitary disease. Patients with pathology in the brain, particularly craniopharyngiomas, often have persistent headaches, impairment

of vision, and abnormal visual field perception.[4] The presence of diabetes insipidus in children with anterior pituitary hormone deficiencies almost invariably indicates a space-occupying lesion in the hypothalamic-pituitary area.[4]

DIAGNOSTIC EVALUATION

Primary Hypothyroidism

In children and adolescents with prominent features of hypothyroidism, the diagnosis should be confirmed by measurements of serum TSH and free T_4 (see chaps 18 and 76). In primary hypothyroidism the serum TSH is usually greater than 50 mU/L and the serum free T_4 is low. The presence of antithyroid peroxidase (formerly microsomal) or thyroglobulin antibodies indicates that chronic autoimmune thyroiditis is the cause of the hypothyroidism. An X-ray of the hand and wrist for determination of bone age can provide useful information. The delay in skeletal maturation often corresponds to the age at the onset of hypothyroidism; the greater the delay in bone age, the better the prognosis for adult height; and epiphyseal dysgenesis may be seen in hypothyroidism with onset during childhood.

Radionuclide imaging studies are rarely indicated. An exception might be a patient with hypothyroidism caused by radiation therapy who has a thyroid nodule, because of the increased risk of carcinoma. The detailed evaluation of patients with inherited defects in thyroid hormonogenesis is discussed in chapter 56. Because the polyglandular autoimmune syndrome[26] may occur in patients with primary hypothyroidism caused by chronic autoimmune thyroiditis, diagnostic tests to identify other deficiencies may be indicated (see chap 69). Similarly, autoimmune thyroid diseases, especially chronic autoimmune thyroiditis and hypothyroidism, occur more often in children with Turner's syndrome[27] and Down's syndrome.[28]

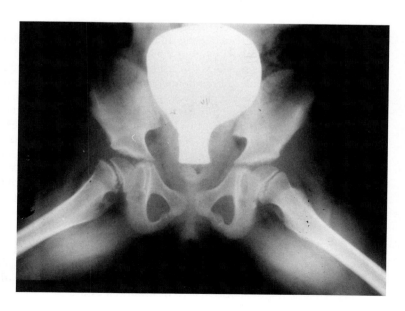

FIGURE 85-9. Radiograph of the pelvis of a 12-year-old girl with hypothyroidism shows slippage of the capital femoral epiphysis.

Central Hypothyroidism

The diagnosis of hypothalamic or pituitary hypothyroidism may be difficult. The characteristic biochemical findings are a normal or low serum TSH concentration and low serum free T_4 values. However, some patients with hypothalamic hypothyroidism have high serum TSH concentrations, as high as 15 or 20 mU/L, because of secretion of bioinactive but immunoreactive TSH.[29] In these patients, a TRH test may be helpful to distinguish primary from hypothalamic hypothyroidism.[30] The characteristic pattern of serum TSH response to TRH in patients with hypothalamic hypothyroidism is a gradual rise in serum TSH with a peak value at 60 minutes or later, whereas in patients with primary hypothyroidism, the peak value is often higher and occurs 15 or 30 minutes after the injection of TRH. In patients with pituitary hypothyroidism, the serum TSH response to TRH characteristically is blunted or absent.

Other pituitary hormones should be measured to identify other pituitary hormone deficiencies. In children with growth hormone deficiency, thyroid function tests may be normal during initial evaluation, but central hypothyroidism may develop during the first 1 to 2 years of growth hormone therapy. Neuroradiologic studies are mandatory in any child with central hypothyroidism.

TREATMENT

Maintenance Thyroxine Therapy

The treatment of choice for hypothyroidism is T_4 given once daily[31]; absorption may be more consistent if the medication is given at least 30 minutes before meals. During infancy, rapid restoration of euthyroidism is essential, as it is for infants with congenital hypothyroidism. Therefore, a full replacement dose of 50 to 75 µg/d (4–8 µg/kg/d) should be given at the outset. Such a dose should promptly restore the serum T_4 concentration to normal without the subsequent development of thyrotoxicosis.[32]

In children and adolescents with chronic hypothyroidism, replacement can be less aggressive. They should be given 25 µg/d (children) or 50 µg/d (adolescents) for 2 to 4 weeks, and the dose increased by 25-µg increments at 4- to 8-week intervals thereafter until the patient's serum TSH concentration is normal.[33,34] Some children may develop a short attention span, restlessness, insomnia, and poor school performance, particularly when full replacement doses are prescribed. Should these symptoms persist despite a reduction in the dose of T_4, some amelioration can be achieved with very low doses of a β-adrenergic antagonist drug.

Excessive T_4 therapy should be avoided at any age. Iatrogenic thyrotoxicosis in infants and children may advance bone maturation, accelerate fontanel and cranial suture closure, reduce bone mineralization, and cause abnormal neurobehavioral development.[35] Occasionally, intracranial hypertension develops soon after initiation of T_4 therapy; it should be suspected if the patient develops headaches, vomiting, or visual symptoms. Skull X-rays may reveal splitting of the sutures and an enlarged sella turcica. When intracranial hypertension occurs, T_4 therapy should be withheld for a few days and then reinstituted at a lower dose. Persistence or recurrence is rare.

The appropriate dose of T_4 is that which ameliorates the clinical manifestations of hypothyroidism and maintains the serum TSH concentration within the normal range. Under these circumstances, most patients have serum T_4 concentrations in the upper half of the normal range for age. Patients with central hypothyroidism should be treated so that their serum T_4 concentrations are in the same range. Once a maintenance dose associated with normal thyroid function tests is achieved, the dose should not be changed unless there is a change in the quality of the medication or the compliance of the patient.

Generally, thyroid function tests need be monitored only at annual visits during childhood and adolescence. If an abnormal result is obtained and the dose of T_4 is changed, reevaluation in 4 to 6 weeks is indicated. If the child remains clinically euthyroid and linear growth is normal, additional assessments such as bone age X-rays are not needed. However, if growth slows, bone age X-rays and thyroid function tests should be done because of the possibility of an inadequate T_4 dose, impaired absorption, or noncompliance. Growth hormone testing may be useful to identify those rare children who develop transient growth hormone deficiency during treatment of hypothyroidism.[36]

Management During Adolescence

The rapid linear growth that normally occurs during adolescence is often attenuated with the development of hypothyroidism. After initiation of T_4 therapy, growth will accelerate and catch-up growth will occur in both children and adolescents. Especially in the latter, the dose often needs to be increased because of increasing body size, and adult doses may be needed before the end of the period of pubertal growth.[33,34] In patients with goitrous autoimmune thyroiditis, the size of the thyroid decreases approximately 75%, but often not to normal.[37]

PROGNOSIS

Growth and Development

In children with chronic hypothyroidism of several years' duration and severe growth retardation at the time of diagnosis, the adult height attained may be less than expected as determined by the growth percentile before the onset of hypothyroidism and the target height for the patient as determined by the height of both parents.[38] Reduction in adult height is most pronounced when treatment is initiated during the adolescent years in a patient who is clinically preadolescent. With restoration of euthyroidism the adolescent-age patient begins puberty without the benefit of one or more years of normal prepubertal growth. Epiphyseal maturation accelerates and fusion with cessation of growth occurs within a few years after initiation of therapy. There is current interest in delaying the onset of puberty in these children by treating them with a gonadotropin-releasing hormone analogue to prevent or at least slow pubertal development, so as to allow additional years of growth before the initiation of puberty.[39] Patients with mild hypothyroidism or hypothyroidism with an onset during early childhood should attain their expected adult height.

Neuropsychological Development

The neuropsychological development of children who develop hypothyroidism after age 3 years and who are treated adequately thereafter is normal. It is too early to determine whether neuropsychological development will be normal in children with acquired hypothyroidism during infancy (age < 2 years). Some impairment was identified in the first few years after diagnosis, but one such child followed for 14 years had normal intellectual function and above average achievement.

References

1. Dobbing J. The later growth of the brain and its vulnerability. Pediatrics 1974;53:2

2. Foley TP Jr, Malvaux P, Blizzard RM. Thyroid disease. In: Kappy MS, Blizzard RM, Migeon CJ, eds. Wilkins the diagnosis and treatment of endocrine disorders in childhood and adolescence. 4th ed. Springfield, IL: Charles C. Thomas, 1994:457

3. Foley TP Jr, Abbassi V, Copeland KC, Draznin MB. Hypothyroidism caused by chronic autoimmune thyroiditis in very young infants. N Engl J Med 1994;330:466

4. Arslanian S, Foley TP Jr, Lee PA. Endocrine and systemic manifestation of brain tumors in children. In: Deutsch M, ed. Management of childhood brain tumors. Boston: Kluwer Academic Publishers, 1990:137

5. Boyages SC. Iodine deficiency disorders. J Clin Endocrinol Metab 1993;77:587

6. LaFranchi S. Thyroiditis and acquired hypothyroidism. Pediatr Ann 1992;21:29

7. Volpe R. The pathology of thyroiditis. Hum Pathol 1978;9:429

8. Maxon HR. Radiation-induced thyroid disease. Med Clin North Am 1985;69:1049

9. Rapaport R, Brauner R. Growth and endocrine disorders secondary to cranial irradiation. Pediatr Res 1989;25:561

10. de Zegher F, Vanderschueren-Lodeweyckx M, Heinrichs C, Van Vliet G. Thyroid dyshormonogenesis: severe hypothyroidism after normal neonatal thyroid stimulating hormone screening. Acta Paediatr 1992;81:274

11. Tatsumi K, Miyai K, Notomi T, et al. Cretinism with combined hormone deficiency caused by a mutation in the PIT1 gene. Nature Genet 1992;1:56

12. Hopwood NJ, Lockhart LH, Bryan GT. Acquired hypothyroidism with muscular hypertrophy and precocious testicular enlargement. J Pediatr 1974;85:233

13. Najjar SS. Muscular hypertrophy in hypothyroid children: the Kocher-Debré-Sémélaigne syndrome. J Pediatr 1974;85:236

14. Foley TP Jr. Effects of the thyroid on gonadal and reproductive function. In: Sanfilippo JS, Muram D, Lee PA, Dewhurst J, eds. Pediatric and adolescent gynecology. Philadelphia: WB Saunders, 1994:139

15. Nishi Y, Hamamoto K, Kajiyama M, et al. Pituitary enlargement, hypertrichosis, and blunted growth hormone secretion in primary hypothyroidism. Acta Paediatr Scand 1989;78:136

16. Atchison JA, Lee PA, Albright AL. Reversible suprasellar pituitary mass secondary to hypothyroidism. JAMA 1989;262:3175

17. Reilly WA, Smyth FS. Stippled epiphyses with congenital hypothyroidism (cretinoid epiphyseal dysgenesis). Am J Roentgenol Radium Therapy 1938;40:675

18. Hirano T, Stamelos S, Harris V, et al. Association of primary hypothyroidism and slipped capital femoral epiphysis. J Pediatr 1978;93:262

19. Van Wyk J, Grumbach M. Syndrome of precocious menstruation and galactorrhea in juvenile hypothyroidism: an example of hormonal overlap in pituitary feedback. J Pediatr 1960;57:416

20. Barnes ND, Hayles AB, Ryan RJ. Sexual maturation in juvenile hypothyroidism. Mayo Clin Proc 1973;48:849

21. Anasti JN, Flack MR, Froehlich J, et al. A potential novel mechanism for precocious puberty in juvenile hypothyroidism. J Clin Endocrinol Metab 1995;80:276

22. Piziak VK, Hahn HB Jr. Isolated menarche in juvenile hypothyroidism. Clin Pediatr 1984;23:177

23. Costin G, Kershnar AK, Kogut MD, Turkington RW. Prolactin activity in juvenile hypothyroidism and precocious puberty. Pediatrics 1972;50:881

24. Stern SR, Kelnan CJ. Hypertrichosis due to primary hypothyroidism. Arch Dis Child 1985;60:763

25. Foley TP Jr. Goiters in adolescents. Endocrinol Metab Clin North Am 1993;22:593

26. Neufeld M, MacLaren N, Blizzard R. Autoimmune polyglandular syndrome. Pediatr Ann 1980;9:154

27. Gruñeiro de Papendieck L, Iorcansky S, Coco R. High incidence of thyroid disturbances in 49 children with Turner syndrome. J Pediatr 1987;111:258

28. Pueschel SM, Pezzallo JC. Thyroid dysfunction in Down syndrome. Am J Dis Child 1985;139:636

29. Illig R, Krawczynska H, Torresani T, Prader A. Elevated plasma TSH and hypothyroidism in children with hypothalamic hypopituitarism. J Clin Endocrinol Metab 1975;41:722

30. Foley TP, Owings J, Hayford JR, Blizzard RM. Serum thyrotropin (TSH) responses to synthetic thyrotropin releasing hormone (TRH) in normal children and hypopituitary patients: a new test to distinguish primary pituitary hormone deficiency. J Clin Invest 1972;51:431

31. Foley TP Jr. Hypothyroidism. In: Hoekelman RA, Friedman SB, Nelson NM, Seidel HM, eds. Primary pediatric care. 2nd ed. St. Louis: CV Mosby, 1992:1292

32. Germak JA, Foley TP Jr. Longitudinal assessment of L-thyroxine therapy in congenital hypothyroidism. J Pediatr 1990;117:211

33. Rezvani I, DiGeorge AM. Reassessment of the daily dose of oral thyroxine for replacement therapy of hypothyroid children. J Pediatr 1977;90:291

34. Abbassi V, Aldige C. Evaluation of sodium L-thyroxine requirement in replacement therapy of hypothyroidism. J Pediatr 1977;90:298

35. Penfold JL, Simpson DA. Premature craniosynostosis: a complication of thyroid replacement therapy. J Pediatr 1975;86:675

36. Dahlem ST, Furlanetto RW, Moshang T Jr, Wiener DE. Transient growth hormone deficiency after treatment of primary hypothyroidism. J Pediatr 1987;111:256

37. Rother KI, Zimmerman D, Schwenk WF. Effect of thyroid hormone treatment of thyromegaly in children and adolescents with Hashimoto disease. J Pediatr 1994;124:599

38. Rivkees SA, Bode HH, Crawford JD. Long-term growth in juvenile acquired hypothyroidism: the failure to achieve normal adult stature. N Engl J Med 1988;318:599.

39. Lee PA, Foley TP. Rapid pubertal progression after primary hypothyroidism therapy: new use of GNRH analogue therapy to salvage height potential (abstract). Recent Developments on Pediatric-Adolescent Gynecology and Endocrinology. Athens, Greece, 1993:102

Werner and Ingbar's The Thyroid, Seventh Edition,
edited by Lewis E. Braverman and Robert D. Utiger.
Lippincott–Raven Publishers, Philadelphia, © 1996

86

Graves' Disease in the Neonatal Period and Childhood

Stephen LaFranchi
Scott H. Mandel

Many aspects of Graves' disease in the neonatal period and childhood are similar to those in adults, but some features are age specific. Neonatal Graves' disease is probably the best example of transient thyroid-stimulating antibody (TSAb)-mediated thyrotoxicosis, a disease that wanes with each half-life of this transplacentally acquired antibody. Some clinical manifestations are unique to the neonate, and appropriate management is important to prevent untoward effects of thyrotoxicosis on the developing central nervous and skeletal systems. In childhood, the autoimmune pathogenesis is similar to that in adults, but thyrotoxicosis has unique effects on growth and skeletal maturation. Graves' ophthalmopathy, although common, seldom is as severe as in adults, and localized myxedema is extremely rare. The differential diagnosis of hyperthyroxinemia is different in childhood; Graves' disease is still the most frequent cause, but generalized resistance to thyroid hormones and binding protein changes are relatively more common causes than in adults. The use of antithyroid drug treatment for indefinite periods is more common in children with thyrotoxicosis caused by Graves' disease although there is growing acceptance of radioiodine treatment at any age. Any form of treatment must be set against the background of a longer life expectancy, and the relative risks of developing hypothyroidism, radiation oncogenesis, and genetic damage must be weighed. This chapter emphasizes the differences between Graves' disease in the neonatal period and childhood, and adult Graves' disease (see subchapter on pathogenesis in chap 30).

NEONATAL GRAVES' DISEASE

Incidence

Neonatal thyrotoxicosis is uncommon, accounting for about 1% of thyrotoxicosis in childhood. There usually is a maternal history of Graves' disease, if not during the pregnancy, then in the more distant past. Neonatal Graves' disease occurs in less than 2% of infants born to mothers who had Graves' thyrotoxicosis during pregnancy,[1] although there may be infants with mild disease who escape clinical detection. Despite the increased female/male sex ratio for Graves' disease in later life, neonatal Graves' disease occurs equally in boys and girls.

Pathogenesis

Most cases of neonatal thyrotoxicosis can be explained by transplacental passage of TSAb.[2–6] Although it is usually associated with active maternal Graves' disease, it also may occur in infants whose mothers have inactive Graves' disease (i.e., mothers who previously had ablative treatment for thyrotoxicosis, or rarely, Hashimoto's thyroiditis). The activity of maternal disease often does not predict neonatal thyroid status, but measurements of maternal TSAb have been useful in predicting the likelihood of neonatal thyrotoxicosis[2,7–10]; thyrotoxicosis is likely in neonates whose mothers have levels of TSAb greater than 500% of control values.[10] The prediction of neonatal thyrotoxicosis is more accurate when both TSAb and thyrotropin (TSH)-binding inhibitory antibodies (TBII) are measured.[7,9] In most infants, neonatal Graves' disease resolves spontaneously in 3 to 12 weeks as the maternal TSAb disappears from the serum of the infants.

A much rarer form of neonatal thyrotoxicosis occurs that is not associated with maternal thyroid disease and persists for a longer period of time than can be explained by transplacental passage of TSAb.[11] Thyrotoxicosis may be very severe in this form of the disease, and it may last for years and have long-term sequelae. Although maternal disease need not be present, there is an increased incidence of thyroid disease in other family members. Recently a mutation in the TSH receptor gene has been described in a child with this condition.[12,13]

Clinical Manifestations

Thyrotoxicosis may be manifested in utero by fetal tachycardia. At birth, the weight of infants with thyrotoxicosis often is low, and birth may be premature (although the thyrotoxic state may influence estimates of fetal maturity[14]). These infants may be microcephalic and may have cerebral ventricular enlargement.[15] They have hyperphagia, but weight gain is poor, despite excessive caloric intake. Thyrotoxic infants are irritable and difficult to console. They may have frontal bossing and triangular facies. Most have exophthalmos and goiter although goiter is not as common as in older children. Rarely, goiter may be large enough to cause tracheal obstruction. Tachycardia and bounding pulses are almost invariably present, and cardiomegaly, congestive heart failure, cardiac arrhythmias, jaundice, hepatosplenomegaly, and thrombocytopenia also may occur.

The onset, severity, and duration of symptoms in neonatal Graves' disease are variable. The fetus of any mother with autoimmune thyroid disease of any type during the pregnancy or in the past should be observed for tachycardia. Measurements of maternal TSAb and TBII may be helpful in predicting which infants may have the disease.[7,9] Symptoms may occur in utero or at birth, or they may be delayed for up to 10 days after birth as maternally transferred antithyroid medication disappears. Rarely, both TSH receptor-blocking antibodies and TSAb are transplacentally acquired from the mother. In one case, the blocking antibodies prevented the effect of the stimulating antibodies for 4 to 6 weeks, thus delaying the onset of thyrotoxicosis.[16]

Diagnosis and Treatment

The diagnosis of neonatal thyrotoxicosis should be confirmed by measurements of serum total and free thyroxine (T_4), and serum TSH (see chap 52). It is important to note that the ranges for serum total and free T_4 (and triiodothyronine [T_3]) are higher in normal neonates than in normal adults (see chap 84). Treatment then should be promptly initiated. Either propylthiouracil (PTU), 5 to 10 mg/kg/d, or methimazole (MMI), 0.5 to 1 mg/kg/d, should be administered every 8 hours to inhibit thyroid hormone synthesis. In severely ill infants, propranolol, 2 mg/kg/d, may be helpful in slowing the pulse rate and reducing hyperactivity. Iodine also has been used to inhibit thyroid hormone synthesis and release. Lugol's solution (126 mg of iodine/mL) may be given in a dose of one drop (8 mg) every 8 hours. Alternatively, iodinated cholecys-

tographic agents, sodium ipodate and iopanoic acid, which also inhibit extrathyroidal conversion of T_4 to T_3 have been used in doses of 100 to 200 mg daily or 500 mg every third day.[17–19] In extremely severe cases, corticosteroids have been used to inhibit thyroid hormone secretion acutely and to decrease peripheral generation of T_3 from T_4. Digoxin may be necessary for treatment of heart failure.

Fetal tachycardia exceeding 160 beats/min after 22 weeks' gestation may be used as evidence of fetal thyrotoxicosis in the at-risk fetus. Treatment may be accomplished by maternal antithyroid medication, which should be adjusted to maintain a fetal heart rate of about 140 beats/min.[20] Fetal blood sampling has been used for diagnostic and therapeutic purposes in two patients in whom maternal and fetal thyroid functions were dissimilar.[21]

Prognosis

In most neonates, improvement is rapid, treatment can be withdrawn over several months, and the infant remains euthyroid. In a few patients, the disease lasts longer than 6 months and it may last many years, suggesting that the disease is endogenous and not due to maternal TSAb.[11] Mortality secondary to prematurity, cardiac failure, and airway obstruction has been estimated to be as high as 25% in the past but is considerably lower now. Long-term morbidity, including retarded growth, craniosynostosis, hyperactivity, and intellectual and developmental impairment, is common.[11,15,22] It may occur even when antithyroid therapy was started early, suggesting that intrauterine thyrotoxicosis affects the developing skeleton and brain. In addition, central (pituitary) hypothyroidism, which may be secondary to prenatal exposure of the hypothalamus and pituitary to excessive thyroid hormone levels during a critical stage of development, has been reported to follow neonatal thyrotoxicosis.[23]

THYROTOXICOSIS IN CHILDHOOD

The vast majority of cases of thyrotoxicosis in children are caused by Graves' disease. Although differences exist in clinical presentation and treatment strategies in children, the pathogenesis of Graves' disease in childhood is the same as that in the adult. Graves' disease may begin in infancy, but it is rare in children under the age of 5 years.[24–26] The incidence progressively increases throughout childhood with a peak incidence in children 11 to 15 years of age.[24–26] Childhood disease is still uncommon, however, accounting for less than 5% of all cases of Graves' disease. The prevalence of Graves' disease in children approximates 0.02%. Outside the neonatal period, girls are more commonly affected than boys, with a female/male ratio of between 3.5 and 6:1.[24–27] Most children with Graves' disease have a positive family history of some type of autoimmune thyroid disease.[26] Other autoimmune endocrine diseases such as diabetes mellitus and Addison's disease may be associated with Graves' disease in childhood.[28] A variety of nonendocrine autoimmune disorders, such as systemic lupus erythematosus, rheumatoid arthritis, myasthenia gravis, vitiligo, idiopathic thrombocytopenic purpura, and pernicious anemia also have been described in children with

Graves' disease.[28] In addition, Graves' disease occurs more commonly in children with trisomy 21.[28]

Clinical Features

The clinical features of thyrotoxicosis in children[24–27] (Table 86-1) are similar to those in adults. Excluding weight loss and atrial fibrillation, the common symptoms and signs of thyrotoxicosis are at least as frequent in children as in adults.[29] Despite the multitude of symptoms and signs that usually are elicited at the time of diagnosis, many children have had some manifestations of thyrotoxicosis for several months to years before diagnosis. The insidious onset of emotional lability and hyperactivity are often attributed to other factors in children, and a small goiter and exophthalmos may go unnoticed.

Diffuse goiter is present in virtually all children with thyrotoxicosis due to Graves' disease. The degree of thyroid enlargement is variable but typically is not great. Thus, thyroid enlargement is usually not the chief complaint, and it is unusual for children outside the neonatal period to have symptoms secondary to thyroid gland enlargement. The gland is nontender, smooth, and firm, and a thyroid bruit may be heard.

Nervousness, behavioral abnormalities, and deteriorating school performance are more likely to bring the child to medical attention. Emotional lability and difficulty concentrating are often noted by a parent or teacher. Children with thyrotoxicosis are restless and have difficulty completing assignments. Referral for evaluation of hyperactivity and possible attention deficit disorder is common. Emotional outbursts, difficulty sleeping, and mood swings may lead to referral to a child psychiatrist or counselor.

TABLE 86-1.
Frequency of Symptoms and Signs of Hyperthyroidism Due to Graves' Disease in Children

Symptom or Sign	Percentage
Goiter	99
Tachycardia	83
Nervousness	80
Increased pulse pressure	77
Hypertension	71
Exophthalmos	66
Tremor	61
Increased appetite	60
Weight loss	54
Thyroid bruit	53
Increased sweating	49
Hyperactivity	44
Heart murmur	43
Palpatations	34
Heat intolerance	33
Fatigue	16
Headache	15
Diarrhea	13

(Compiled from references 24–27.)

Some degree of ophthalmopathy is common in children with Graves' disease, but it seldom is severe. Stare and wide palpebral fissures occur in most children; 50% to 75% have exophthalmos, but only rarely is this the presenting complaint.[30] Asymmetric exophthalmos occurred in 13% of patients, more often in older teenagers, in one series.[31] Severe pain, chemosis, ophthalmoplegia, and diplopia are rare. Although ophthalmopathy may be persistent, it seldom requires treatment in children.[32]

Cardiac findings including tachycardia, a widened pulse pressure, and hyperactive precordium, are common in thyrotoxic children. The child occasionally may complain of heart racing or pounding. Thyrotoxicosis causes a decrease in left ventricular reserve in some children.[33] Arrhythmias and congestive heart failure almost never occur in children outside the neonatal period.

Most children with thyrotoxicosis have an increased appetite. Although weight loss is not as common as in older patients, these children fail to gain weight normally. On the other hand, some children do gain excessive weight. Increased stool frequency occurs in a minority of children, but diarrhea is rare. Once antithyroid treatment is instituted, some of these young patients continue to eat excessively and may become obese.[34] A conscious effort should be made to decrease excessive caloric intake after therapy is initiated.

Acceleration of linear growth is common, so that the patient may increase in height percentiles on the growth chart before treatment. The acceleration in linear growth is accompanied by increased epiphyseal maturation and more rapid advancement in bone age. Thus, epiphyseal closure may occur earlier. There is no increase in adult height.

A fine tremor usually is present, as are brisk deep tendon reflexes. Thyrotoxicosis may result in a decrease in seizure threshold; seizures and coma may be a rare presentation of thyrotoxicosis.[35] Muscle weakness and fatigue are common but seldom severe. Periodic paralysis has been described in children[36] but is probably even rarer than in adults.

Heat intolerance and excessive sweating occur in more than 30% of children. The skin is often warm and moist, and occasionally it is flushed. Localized myxedema and thyroid acropachy are almost unheard of manifestations of Graves' disease in children.

Diagnosis

For the child who presents with classic clinical manifestations of thyrotoxicosis plus features specific for Graves' disease, including diffuse goiter and ophthalmopathy, there is no confusion regarding the diagnosis. In this setting, laboratory tests confirm the presence of thyrotoxicosis, gauge its biochemical severity, and establish a baseline for treatment. Some children, however, may have an insidious onset, unappreciated enlargement of the thyroid gland, and no ophthalmologic findings. Others may have features atypical for Graves' disease, such as painful goiter or a prominent nodule. Another group will have no specific clinical features but will be discovered incidentally to have thyroid function tests compatible with thyrotoxicosis (e.g., the hyperactive child with an elevated serum T_4 concentration or a child with a goiter).

Children with thyrotoxicosis, like adults, have elevated serum total and free T_4 and T_3 levels and low serum TSH concentrations (see chap 52). Measurement of serum TSH before treatment excludes disorders that have been confused with Graves' disease, such as pituitary TSH-secreting adenomas and generalized resistance to thyroid hormone.[37] The introduction of sensitive TSH assays has obviated the need for thyrotropin-releasing hormone (TRH) stimulation tests.

Antithyroid autoantibodies, such as antiperoxidase antibodies and antithyroglobulin antibodies, are detectable in more than 90% of children with Graves' disease, but the titers are not usually as high as in patients with autoimmune thyroiditis. Their measurement usually adds little unless a nonautoimmune disorder is under diagnostic consideration. Similarly, TSH-receptor antibodies (TRAb), either TSAb or TBII, are found in more than 90% of children with Graves' disease.[38,39] Again, their measurement is not necessary for diagnosis although they may be helpful in predicting a relapse at the end of a course of antithyroid drugs[40] (see chap 21).

Measurements of thyroid uptake of iodine-131 or iodine-123 and thyroid scintiscans seldom are needed in children because thyrotoxicosis is nearly always due to Graves' disease. Thyroid radioiodine uptake is low in those few children with silent (painless) thyroiditis, subacute thyroiditis, and factitious thyrotoxicosis. A thyroid radioiodine uptake may be helpful in cases where clinical features are equivocal and serum TSH is low but T_4 and T_3 concentrations are in the normal range. A thyroid scintiscan is indicated in the setting of a single nodule and thyrotoxicosis.

The causes of thyrotoxicosis in children are similar to those in adults and, as in adults, usually can be distinguished by history and physical examination. The frequency of the various causes differs in children and adults; as noted earlier, Graves' disease is more predominant as the cause in children than in adults. Painless or silent thyroiditis is virtually unreported in children,[41] and subacute thyroiditis is rare. Autonomously functioning thyroid adenomas are also uncommon, but they may be part of the McCune-Albright syndrome (café-au-lait pigmentations, precocious puberty, and polyostotic fibrous dysplasia) or result from a mutation in the gene encoding for the TSH receptor, resulting in constitutive activation of the TSH receptor and cyclic adenosine monophosphate production.[42] TSH-secreting pituitary adenomas and factitious thyrotoxicosis are rare in children; occurrence of the latter because of ingestion of thyroid hormone contained in ground beef (hamburger thyrotoxicosis) has been reported.[43] Hereditary thyroid hormone resistance syndromes, often misdiagnosed as Graves' disease, are now increasingly recognized in children[44] (see chap 90). Patients with hyperthyroxinemia due to hereditary T_4-binding globulin excess and familial dysalbuminemic hyperthyroxinemia are euthyroid. The importance of these latter two disorders is that they cause hyperthyroxinemia but not clinical thyrotoxicosis.

Treatment

The same treatment modalities used for adults with Graves' disease—antithyroid drugs, radioiodine, and surgery—have been used successfully in children.[45] Because none corrects the underlying autoimmune abnormality, the goal of each is to decrease the production of thyroid hormone into the normal range. With these three treatment approaches, there are some differences in the time to initial control of the hyperthyroid state, the required degree of patient and family compliance with medication recommendations and follow-up visits, and the short- and long-term risks, including the development of hypothyroidism. In contrast to adults, in whom radioiodine alone or a relatively short course of antithyroid drugs followed by radioiodine if remission does not occur is the most common therapeutic approach,[46] most children with Graves' disease are treated with an antithyroid drug for long periods of time. Although radioiodine has proved to be an effective, safe form of treatment in children, as in adults, some physicians and families still question its long-range potential for radiation oncogenesis in patients who have a 60- to 70-year life span and possible genetic damage in future generations. Subtotal thyroidectomy requires careful medical preparation and experienced anesthesiologists and surgeons to avoid the finite, but definite, operative morbidity. In some centers, radioiodine or surgery is considered preferable initial treatment, but we prefer antithyroid drug treatment until remission of the Graves' disease occurs. Radioiodine is a reasonable second choice if a sustained remission does not occur (see chap 53).

ANTITHYROID DRUG TREATMENT

The antithyroid drugs, PTU, MMI, and carbamizole inhibit thyroid hormone biosynthesis[47] (see chap 4 and subchapter on antithyroid compounds in chap 14). PTU, but not MMI, has the additional property of inhibiting peripheral conversion of T_4 to T_3. In adults, and presumably in children, MMI has a longer serum half-life, roughly 6 hours versus 2 hours for PTU,[48] and its intrathyroidal concentrations, perhaps more important than serum levels, remain high for 16 to 24 hours.[49] The recommended initial dose of PTU is 5 to 10 mg/kg/d (150–300 mg/m²/d) divided into three doses every 8 hours; the equivalent dose of MMI is one-tenth to one-twentieth that of PTU, or 0.25 to 1.0 mg/kg/d, but it can be given one or two times daily. Children who are older, with longer duration of symptoms, larger goiters, and higher serum T_4 and T_3 concentrations, should be given the higher dose. Once a euthyroid state is achieved, PTU can be given twice a day and MMI can be given once a day, a regimen that maximizes compliance. Because compliance can be a problem in children, we have a slight preference for MMI over PTU.

Although the main effect of antithyroid drug therapy is to control overproduction of thyroid hormones until a spontaneous remission occurs, these drugs may have some immunosuppressive effects. MMI treatment is associated with a rise in the percentage of HLA-DR-positive T-suppressor/cytotoxic cells and a decrease in T-helper/inducer cells both in serum[50] and the thyroid gland,[51] changes which might restore immune surveillance; accompanying these changes is a fall in TSAb levels. The practical significance of these changes is unclear, but patients so treated go into remission more frequently than untreated patients or those treated with β-adrenergic antagonist drugs alone.[52] It also is possible that these changes may be due to amelioration of thyrotoxicosis rather than the drug itself.

Antithyroid drugs block new synthesis of thyroid hormones, but there is a lag period between initiation of therapy and achievement of the euthyroid state because of the release of preformed, stored thyroid hormones. The time of depletion of stored hormones is correlated with the size of the goiter, varying from 3 weeks in patients with smaller glands to 3 months in those with larger glands. During this period, adjunctive therapy with a β-adrenergic antagonist may alleviate thyrotoxic symptoms.[53,54] The drug of choice, propranolol, 0.5 to 2.0 mg/kg/d by mouth, given every 8 hours, decreases symptoms such as restlessness, tremor, emotional lability, and palpitations. The use of β-adrenergic antagonist drugs may be dangerous in children with heart failure or asthma.

Table 86-2 summarizes the results of seven reports of antithyroid drug treatment in children with Graves' disease.[24,26,55–59] The success rate of initial control of the thyrotoxic state varied from 87% to 100%. Failure of initial control was attributed to the large size of the gland, greater severity of the disease, and poor compliance; the latter was estimated to occur in 2% to 17% of children in the above series (Table 86-3). When a large dose of antithyroid drug seems ineffective, the explanation usually is poor compliance.[60] For such children, an alternative form of therapy must be selected. If patient compliance with antithyroid drugs is considered an indication for radioiodine or surgical treatment, one should keep in mind the greater risk of hypothyroidism and potential compliance problem with T_4 replacement.

Once a euthyroid state is achieved, either of two treatment strategies may be implemented. One approach is to titrate the antithyroid drug level to the individual clinical and biochemical response to maintain the euthyroid state; the second is to overtreat with antithyroid drugs to produce hypothyroidism and then add T_4 to restore euthyroidism. The first approach requires good clinical judgment, particularly because treatment may lead to low-normal serum T_4 and high-normal T_3 levels, leading to confusion about the need for adjustment of the dose of the drug.[61] Assessment of clinical status and serum TSH determinations should lead to the correct therapeutic decisions. Because prolonged prior thyrotoxicosis may result in persistent TSH suppression, even after a euthyroid state is achieved, serum TSH measurements cannot be relied on to indicate overtreatment for 6 to 8 weeks after a

patient becomes euthyroid.[62] With the second treatment approach, not only is the patient taking two medications when one would suffice, but the presence of thyrotoxicosis may lead to confusion about whether to increase the antithyroid drug or lower the T_4 dose. In addition, patients who receive larger antithyroid drug doses have a greater risk of drug toxicity. Currently, it is our practice to follow the first approach. However, given new information, recently challenged, on possible decreased relapse rates in patients receiving combined MMI and T_4, we are reevaluating this practice (see below).

Antithyroid drug treatment is continued until spontaneous remission occurs, as defined by persistent euthyroidism after withdrawal of therapy; in the series mentioned earlier, 34% to 64% of children had a remission after mean treatment periods of 2 to 4 years. The variation in remission rate appears to be the result of different treatment approaches. Centers that use an arbitrary length of treatment (i.e., 1–2 years) report a lower rate, whereas centers that are willing to treat indefinitely, providing the patient is compliant, report a higher rate. In the patients described in the study by Lippe and associates,[58] the investigators, using a survival method of statistical analysis, found that 25% of patients went into remission every 2 years, with a 50% remission rate by 5 years. In this regard, the titration treatment approach has the advantage that as antithyroid drug dosage is decreased, it is easier to judge when a remission is occurring because the relationship between antithyroid drug action and the activity of the disease is not obscured by exogenous T_4 administration.

Once a remission occurs, relapse of thyrotoxicosis occurs in 3% to 47% of children (see Table 86-2). This wide range reflects the treatment approach and the definition of a relapse. In general, the rate of relapse of thyrotoxicosis has been higher when the duration of treatment was shorter. Relapse of thyrotoxicosis after withdrawal of antithyroid drug therapy takes two general forms. One is relapse a few weeks or few months after cessation of therapy. We consider such early relapses, which occur in up to 47% of patients,[56] to be due to

TABLE 86-2.
Medical Treatment of Hyperthyroid Graves' Disease in Children

Study Location and Reference	No. of Patients	Patients Achieving Control Initially (%)	Duration of Therapy (y)*	Remission (%)†	Relapse (%)‡
Philadelphia[26]	95	87	2–4 (3.2)	40	13
Baltimore[24]	104	100	1–9 (2.9)	61	10
Helsinki[59]	38	100	1.6–6 (3)	50	6
U.S.C.[55]	60	100§	1–7 (2.9)	34	22§
Detroit[57]	182	87	0.5–10 (2)	38	36
U.C.L.A.[58]	63	97	0.4–12.4 (4.3)	25 every 2 y	3
Boston[56]	53	98	0.25–8.7 (2.5)	64	47

Mean is given in parentheses.
†*Percentage of patients remaining euthyroid for a defined period after discontinuation of antithyroid drug therapy. This posttherapy period ranged from 1 to 3 months to 1 or more years in the different studies.*
‡*Percentage of patients who became hyperthyroid after remaining euthyroid for a defined (variable) period after discontinuation of antithyroid drug therapy.*
§*Estimated; results not reported directly.*

TABLE 86-3.
Complications of Medical Treatment of Hyperthyroid Caused by Graves' Disease

Study Locations and References	Poor Compliance (%)	Overall Toxicity (%)	Major Toxicty* (%)	Minor Toxicity		Hypothyroid (%)
				RASH (%)	WBC (%)	
Philadelphia[26]	17	5	0	1	3	8
Baltimore[24]	16	14	6	8	1	NR
Helsinki[59]	5	5	0	1.5	1.5	0
U.S.C.[55]	7	32	14	7.5	9	6
Detroit[57]	9	17	6	8	3	5
U.C.L.A.[58]	2	NR	2	NR	NR	NR
Boston[56]	13	11	4	7	2	11

*Agranulocytosis, collagen vascular syndrome (eg, arthritis, glomerulonephritis, or hepatitis).
WBC, white blood cells; NR, not reported.

dissipation of antithyroid drug action in patients with persistent Graves' disease. True relapses are those that occur many months or years after cessation of therapy. This type of relapse is much less common, for example, occurring in 3% of the patients in one study who had remained euthyroid for 1 year after the cessation of therapy.[58] This latter type of relapse is due to the recurrence of Graves' disease in patients in whom it had disappeared during therapy.

Recent studies have examined the question of whether the addition of T_4 to antithyroid drug therapy will influence the relapse rate of Graves' disease. One study from Japan, where patients received 30 mg MMI daily for 6 months, followed by 10 mg MMI daily combined with 100 μg T_4 or placebo for another 12 months, reported relapse in only 1.7% of the T_4 group versus 34.7% in the placebo group.[63] Further, in the T_4-treated group, TSAb fell from 28% to 10%, whereas it remained unchanged in the placebo group. A subsequent study in Taiwan also reported a fall in TSAb from 38% to 10% in the group treated with MMI and T_4, with no fall in TSAb in the group treated with MMI alone; ultrasound-measured thyroid volume was correlated with the serum TSAb level.[64] It was suggested that suppression of TSH by T_4 resulted in decreased thyroid antigen exposure or presentation to the immune system and decreased TSAb production. Although this treatment approach appears to hold promise for decreasing relapse rates, no studies have been carried out in children; further long-term experience is necessary before clear recommendations can be made. However, two very recent studies found no improvement in the remission rate in adults treated with methimazole and T_4 compared to patients treated with methimazole alone.[64a,64b]

Several clinical and biochemical markers that help to predict whether a relapse is likely to occur when antithyroid drug therapy is discontinued have been examined, but none are completely accurate. Goiter size is the best clinical predictor; the smaller the gland, the less likely a relapse will occur.[65] The most helpful biochemical marker appears to be a TRAb determination at the time therapy is discontinued; in one report, all children who relapsed had positive TRAb tests, whereas 78% of children who subsequently remained in remission had negative tests.[39] Others have found the predictive values of such tests to be much lower.[66]

Toxic effects of antithyroid drug treatment occur in 5% to 32% of children so treated.[24,26,55–59] (see Table 86-3). Most side effects are mild, but some are serious and necessitate changing treatment. The most common minor side effects are skin rashes and transient granulocytopenia (<1500/mm³), occurring in 1% to 9% of children. Other minor toxic reactions include hair loss, nausea, headache, abnormal taste sensation, paresthesias, and arthralgias. The most common skin rashes are a papular or urticarial-like rash. When these occur, the drug should be discontinued for a few days and then treatment with an alternate drug initiated. More resistant cases may require a short course of antihistamine or corticosteroid therapy. Granulocytopenia can occur in untreated patients, as well as after institution of drug therapy; in the latter situation, it appears to be related to the dose of drug.[67] It usually is transient and does not necessitate discontinuation of therapy unless it is persistent (more than a month) or accompanied by clinical features of agranulocytosis. Agranulocytosis (granulocyte < 250/mm³) occurs in 1/500 to 1/1000 children. It usually is accompanied by fever, pharyngitis, buccal ulcerations, and other systemic complaints. We recommend white blood cell counts before initiation of treatment and during treatment if any of the findings mentioned occur, but not routinely. Other serious drug toxic effects include collagen vascular-like symptoms, with a purpuric rash and arthritis, glomerulonephritis, and hepatitis. Appearance of any of these toxic side effects necessitates immediate discontinuation of drug treatment and change to an alternative form of therapy. These side effects, almost always reversible after drug withdrawal,[68] should be explained to parents and patients at the time antithyroid drug treatment is initiated.

RADIOIODINE THERAPY

Radioiodine therapy has proved to be an effective, relatively safe therapy for hyperthyroidism due to Graves' disease in childhood. In some centers, this is the initial treatment of choice, whereas in others, it is the preferred alternate treatment after failure of antithyroid drug treatment. The dose usually is calculated to deliver 50 to 200 μCi of ^{131}I (1.85–7.4 MBq) per gram of thyroid tissue, according to the formula:[69]

$$\text{Estimate thyroid weight in grams} \times \frac{50\text{--}200\ \mu\text{Ci}\ ^{131}\text{I}}{\text{fractional }^{131}\text{I 24-hour uptake}}$$

Younger children with smaller goiters usually require lower doses, whereas children with larger goiters require higher doses. Pretreatment with an antithyroid drug is not necessary. Because the effects of a dose of radioiodine are not complete for several months or more, adjunctive treatment with a β-adrenergic antagonist, as previously described, is recommended. The advantages of radioiodine treatment are its ease of administration (oral), lack of need for an antithyroid drug, and the high rate of permanent amelioration of thyrotoxicosis. Occasional patients do need more than one dose of radioiodine, particularly those given a small initial dose and those with severe disease. In one report in which the standard dose was 200 μCi/g thyroid, 88% of children became euthyroid after one dose of radioiodine, 96% after a second dose, and 97% after a third dose.[57] Thus, only 3% remained thyrotoxic, as compared to 54% when a lower dose, 50 μCi/g thyroid tissue, was used.[70] The major consequence of ^{131}I therapy is hypothyroidism. It occurs in about 10% to 20% of patients in the first year of treatment and about 3%/year thereafter,[38] so that most children become hypothyroid.[71] It appears sooner, and more often, in those children given larger doses of [131]I.[71]

In the past, the main reservations about the use of radioiodine in children centered around radiation oncogenesis and genetic damage. In a national collaborative study of 322 patients who received ^{131}I therapy before age 20, the incidence of benign adenoma increased from an expected 0.6% to 1.9%.[72] This risk appeared to be greater if a smaller dose of ^{131}I had been used. In the same study, the incidence of thyroid carcinoma in adults who received ^{131}I was no different from that in patients who were treated with an antithyroid drug or surgery. It appears that the thyroid glands of infants and young children are more susceptible to the effects of radiation.[73] Hypoparathyroidism and hyperparathyroidism have rarely been reported in a few patients after radioiodine therapy.[69] There is no evidence for an increased risk of leukemia.[74] Studies from Scandinavia report no increased risk for other cancers with the apparent exception of stomach cancer (1.33 increased risk)[75] and breast cancer (1.9 increased risk).[76]

Another potential adverse effect of radioiodine is the development or worsening of ophthalmopathy, reported in some studies but not in others. None of these studies have been carried out in children, and because significant ophthalmopathy is uncommon in children, this potential side effect has not prevented our use of radioiodine when we have chosen this treatment modality.

Studies of offspring born to patients who received ^{131}I therapy for childhood Graves' disease revealed a 3% incidence of congenital anomalies, similar to the general population.[45] On karyotype examination, there was no increase in chromosomal aberrations of the type seen with ionizing radiation.[69] Further, there are no reports of an increase in miscarriage rate or fetal loss because of genetic abnormalities although continued surveillance for this possibility is necessary.

In summary, the reports of patients treated with radioiodine for childhood Graves' disease for over 40 years are reassuring. One must still keep in mind that the life expectancy for children treated with ^{131}I is 60 to 70 years, so surveillance for an increased risk of thyroid and other cancers must continue. When physicians treating childhood Graves' have considered the use of radioiodine in the past, they were particularly hesitant to use it in younger children; the evidence to date shows that it is safe for these youngsters.

SURGERY

Surgery is the oldest treatment modality for these patients and the approach that results in the most rapid resolution of thyrotoxicosis. With appropriate preoperative preparation, the risks are similar to those of other major surgical procedures. Although surgery is the primary treatment choice in some centers, most reserve it for children who have failed medical management and are opposed to radioiodine administration.

To minimize surgical risks, the patient should be treated with an antithyroid drug until euthyroid and then with iodide and the antithyroid drug for 7 to 14 days before surgery. In this setting, the iodide is given not so much for its antithyroid actions as for its ability to decrease thyroid blood flow. It is given as Lugol's solution, 5 to 10 drops three times daily, or as potassium iodide, 2 to 10 drops once daily. β-Adrenergic antagonists may also be used as adjunctive therapy.

The operation of choice is near-total thyroidectomy; experience has shown that when less than 4 g of thyroid tissue remain, the likelihood of recurrent thyrotoxicosis is small.[77–79] The likelihood of recurrence is even smaller after total thyroidectomy, but the morbidity rate is considerably higher. In one summary, one death occurred in 414 operations for childhood Graves' disease.[27] About half developed hypothyroidism. Unilateral recurrent laryngeal nerve damage occurred in 1%, resulting in hoarseness or a change in voice character; no patient had bilateral recurrent laryngeal nerve damage.[80] Transient hypocalcemia occurred in 10% of patients and permanent hypoparathyroidism in 2%.[80] Postoperative hemorrhage or tracheostomy occurred in 0.7%.[80] This summary covered the experience of many years; with thyroidectomy for Graves' disease performed less frequently now, one wonders if the rates of these complications would be as low except in the hands of an experienced thyroid surgeon.

Outcome of Childhood Graves' Disease

Although there are potential complications unique to antithyroid drug, radioiodine, or surgical treatment of Graves' disease, all may result in hypothyroidism to a greater or lesser degree. In children treated with antithyroid drugs[24,26,55–59] (see Table 86-3), follow-up ranging from 8 to 22 years revealed that hypothyroidism eventually occurred in approximately 10%. This is due to the development of chronic autoimmune thyroiditis with destruction of the thyroid or the development of TBII with resulting inhibition of TSH action but not thyroid destruction.[81] As noted earlier, hypothyroidism occurs more commonly in children treated with radioiodine or subtotal thyroidectomy than after medical therapy. Whatever treatment is chosen, the child requires lifelong monitoring for either relapse of thyrotoxicosis or the development of hypothyroidism.

References

1. Ramsay I, Kaur S, Krassas G. Thyrotoxicosis in pregnancy: results of treatment by antithyroid drugs combined with T_4. Clin Endocrinol 1983;18:73

2. Dirmikis SM, Munro DS. Placental transmission of thyroid-stimulating immunoglobulins. BMJ 1975;2:665

3. McKenzie JM. Neonatal Graves' disease. J Clin Endocrinol Metab 1964;24:660

4. McKenzie JM, Zakarija M. Fetal and neonatal hyperthyroidism and hypothyroidism due to maternal TSH receptor antibodies. Thyroid 1992;2:155

5. Smallridge RC, Wartofsky L, Chopra IJ, et al. Neonatal thyrotoxicosis: alterations in serum concentrations of LATS-protector, T_4, T_3, reverse T_3, and 3, 3' T_2. J Pediatr 1978;93:118

6. Sunshine P, Kusumoto H, Kriss JP. Survival time of circulating long-acting thyroid stimulator in neonatal thyrotoxicosis: implications for diagnosis and therapy of the disorder. Pediatrics 1965;36:869

7. Matsura N, Konishi J, Fujieda K, et al. TSH-receptor antibodies in mothers with Graves' disease and outcome in their offspring. Lancet 1988;1:14

8. Munro DS, Dirmikis SM, Humphries H, Smith T. The role of thyroid stimulating immunoglobulins of Graves' disease in neonatal thyrotoxicosis. Br J Obstet Gynaecol 1978;85:837

9. Tamaki H, Amino N, Aozasa M, et al. Universal predictive criteria for neonatal overt thyrotoxicosis requiring treatment. Am J Perinatal 1988;5:152

10. Zakarija M, McKenzie JM. Pregnancy-associated changes in the thyroid-stimulating antibody of Graves' disease and the relationship to neonatal hyperthyroidism. J Clin Endocrinol Metab 1983;57:1036

11. Hollingsworth DR, Mabry CC. Congenital Graves' disease: four familial cases with long-term follow-up and perspective. Am J Dis Child 1976;130:148

12. Kopp P, van Sande J, Parma J, et al. Brief report: congenital hyperthyroidism caused by a mutation in the thyrotropin-receptor gene. N Engl J Med 1995;332:150

13. Duprez L, Parma J, van Sande J, et al. Germline mutations in the thyrotropin receptor gene cause non-autoimmune autosomal dominant hyperthyroidism, Nature Genet 1994;7:396

14. Farrehi C. Accelerated maturity in fetal thyrotoxicosis. Clin Pediatr 1968;7:134

15. Kopelman AE. Delayed cerebral development in twins with congenital hyperthyroidism. Am J Dis Child 1983;137:842

16. Zakarija M, McKenzie JM, Hoffman WH. Prediction and therapy of intrauterine and late-onset neonatal hyperthyroidism. J Clin Endocrinol Metab 1986;62:368

17. Joshi R, Kulin HE. Treatment of neonatal Graves' disease with sodium ipodate. Clin Pediatr 1993;32:181

18. Karpman BA, Rapoport B, Filetti S, Fisher DA. Treatment of neonatal hyperthyroidism due to Graves' disease with sodium ipodate. J Clin Endocrinol Metab 1987;64:119

19. Transue D, Chan J, Kaplan M. Management of neonatal Graves' disease with iopanoic acid. J Pediatr 1992;121:472

20. Cove DH, Johnston P. Fetal hyperthyroidism: experience of treatment in four siblings. Lancet 1985;1:430

21. Wenstrom KD, Weiner CP, Williamson RA, Grant SS. Prenatal diagnosis of fetal hyperthyroidism using funipuncture. Obstet Gynecol 1990;76:513

22. Daneman D, Howard NJ. Neonatal thyrotoxicosis: intellectual impairment and craniosynostosis in later years. J Pediatr 1980;97:257

23. Mandel SH, Hanna CE, LaFranchi SH. Diminished thyroid-stimulating hormone secretion associated with neonatal thyrotoxicosis. J Pediatr 1986;109:662

24. Barnes H, Blizzard RM. Antithyroid drug therapy for toxic diffuse goiter (Graves' disease): thirty years experience in children and adolescents. J Pediatr 1977;91:313

25. Saxena KM, Crawford JD, Talbot NB. Childhood thyrotoxicosis: a long-term perspective. BMJ 1964;2:1153

26. Vaidya VA, Bongiovanni AM, Parks JS, et al. Twenty-two years experience in the medical management of juvenile thyrotoxicosis. Pediatrics 1974;54:565

27. Kogut MD, Kaplan SA, Collip PJ, et al. Treatment of hyperthyroidism in children. N Engl J Med 1965;272:217

28. Friedman JM, Fialkow PJ. The genetics of Graves' disease. Baillieres Clin Endocrinol Metab 1978;7:47

29. Nordyke RA, Gilbert FI, Harada ASM. Graves' disease: influence of age on clinical findings. Arch Intern Med 1988;148:626

30. Bahn RS, Heufelder AE. Pathogenesis of Graves' ophthalmopathy. N Engl J Med 1993; 329:1468

31. Uretsky SH, Kennerdell JS, Gutai JP. Graves' ophthalmopathy in childhood and adolescence. Arch Ophthalmol 1980;98:1963

32. Gorman CA. Temporal relationship between the onset of Graves' ophthalmopathy and the diagnosis of thyrotoxicosis. Mayo Clin Proc 1983;58:515

33. Cavallo A, Casta A, Fawcett HD, et al. Is there a thyrotoxic cardiomyopathy in children? J Pediatr 1985;107:531

34. de la Rosa RE, Hennessey JV, Tucci JR. A longitudinal study of changes in body mass index after I-131 treatment for Graves' disease. Thyroid 1994;4(Suppl 1):S-15

35. Radetti G, Dordi B, Mengarda G, et al. Thyrotoxicosis presenting with seizures and coma in two children. Am J Dis Child 1993; 147:925

36. Drash PW, Money J. Motor impairment and hyperthyroidism in children: report of two cases. Dev Med Child Neurol 1966;8:741

37. Caldwell G, Gow SM, Sweeting VM, et al. Value and limitations of a highly sensitive immunoradiometric assay for thyrotropin in the study of thyrotropin function. Clin Chem 1987;33:303

38. Fisher DA, Pandian MR, Carlton E. Autoimmune thyroid disease: an expanding spectrum. Pediatr Clin North Am 1987;34:907

39. Foley TP Jr, White C, New A. Juvenile Graves' disease: usefulness and limitations of thyrotropin receptor antibody determinations. J Pediatr 1987;110:378

40. McKenzie JM, Zakarija M. The clinical use of thyrotropin receptor antibody measurements. J Clin Endocrinol Metab 1989;69:1093

41. Fisher DA. The thyroid. In: Kaplan SA, ed. Clinical pediatric endocrinology. 2nd ed. Philadelphia: WB Saunders, 1990:110

42. Porcellini A, Ilaria C, Laviola L, et al. Novel mutations of thyrotropin receptor gene in thyroid hyperfunctioning adenomas. J Clin Endocrinol Metab 1994;79:657

43. Hedberg CW, Fishbein DB, Jaussen RS, et al. An outbreak of thyrotoxicosis caused by the consumption of bovine thyroid gland in ground beef. N Engl J Med 1987;316:993

44. Gharib H, Klee GG. Familial euthyroid hyperthyroxinemia secondary to pituitary and peripheral resistance to thyroid hormones. Mayo Clin Proc 1985;60:9

45. Franklyn JA. The management of hyperthyroidism. N Engl J Med 1994;330:1731

46. Wartofsky L, Glinoer D, Solomon B, et al. Differences and similarities in the diagnosis and treatment of Graves' disease in Europe, Japan, and the United States. Thyroid 1991;1:129

47. Cooper DS. Antithyroid drugs. N Engl J Med 1984;311:1353

48. Shirooza A, Okamura K, Ikenoue H, et al. Treatment of hyperthyroidism with a small single daily dose of methimazole. J Clin Endocrinol Metab 1986;63:125

49. Okuno A, Yano K, Inyaku F, et al. Pharmacokinetics of methimazole in children and adolescents with Graves' disease. Studies on plasma and intrathyroidal concentrations. Acta Endocrinol (Copenh) 1987;115:112

50. Totterman TH, Karlsson FA, Bengtsson M, Mendel-Hartrig I. Induction of circulating activated suppressor-like T cells by methimazole therapy for Graves' disease. N Engl J Med 1987; 316:15

51. Ishikawa N, Eguchi K, Otsubo T, et al. Reduction in the suppressor-inducer T cell subset and increase in the helper T cell subset in thyroid tissue from patients with Graves' disease. J Clin Endocrinol Metab 1987;65:17

52. Ratanachaiyavong S, McGregor AM. Immunosuppressive effects of antithyroid drugs. Clin Endocrinol Metab 1985;14:449

53. Codaccioni JL, Orgiazzi J, Blanc P, et al. Lasting remissions in patients treated for Graves' hyperthyroidism with propranolol alone: a pattern of spontaneous evolution of the disease. J Clin Endocrinol Metab 1988;67:656

54. Freely J, Peden N. Use of β-adrenoceptor blocking drugs in hyperthyroidism. Drugs 1984;27:425-426

55. Buckingham BA, Costin G, Roe TF, et al. Hyperthyroidism in children. A reevaluation of treatment. Am J Dis Child 1981; 135:112

56. Gorton C, Sadeghi-Nejad A, Senior B. Remission in children with hyperthyroidism treated with propylthiouracil. Long-term results. Am J Dis Child 1987;141:1084

57. Hamburger JI. Management of hyperthyroidism in children and adolescents. J Clin Endocrinol Metab 1985;60:1019

58. Lippe BM, Landau EM, Kaplan SA. Hyperthyroidism in children treated with long term medical therapy: twenty-five percent remission every two years. J Clin Endocrinol Metab 1987;64:1241

59. Maenpaa J, Kuusi A. Childhood hyperthyroidism. Results of treatment. Acta Paediatr Scand 1980;69:137

60. Cooper DS. Propylthiouracil levels in hyperthyroid patients unresponsive to large doses. Evidence of poor patient compliance. Ann Intern Med 1985;102:328

61. Chen JJS, Ladenson PW. Discordant hypothyroxinemia and hypertriiodothyroninemia in treated patients with hyperthyroid Graves' disease. J Clin Endocrinol Metab 1986;63:102

62. Sills IN, Horlick MNB, Rapaport R. Inappropriate suppression of thyrotropin during medical treatment of Graves' disease in childhood. J Pediatr 1992;121:206

63. Hashizume K, Ichikawa K, Sakurai A, et al. Administration of thyroxine in treated Graves' disease. Effects on the level of antibodies to thyroid-stimulating hormone receptors and on the risk of recurrence of hyperthyroidism. N Engl J Med 1991;324:947

64. Kuo S-W, Huang W-S, Hu C-A, et al. Effect of thyroxine administration on serum thyrotropin receptor antibody and thyroglobulin levels in patients with Graves' hyperthyroidism during antithyroid therapy. Eur J Endocrinol 1994;131:125

64a. Tamai H, Hayaki I, Kawai K, et al. Lack of effect of thyroxine administration on elevated thyroid stimulating hormone receptor antibody levels in treated Graves' disease patients. J Clin Endocrinol Metab 1995;80:1481

64b. McIver B, Rae P, Beckett G. Lack of effect of thyroxine in patients with Graves' hyperthyroidism who are treated with an antithyroid drug. N Engl J Med 1996;334:220

65. Siok-Hoon T, Bee-wah L, Hock-Boon W, Uma R. Relapse markers in childhood thyrotoxicosis. Clin Pediatr 1987;26:136

66. Ikenoue H, Okamura K, Kuroda T, et al. Prediction of relapse in drug-treated Graves' disease using thyroid stimulation indices. Acta Endocrinol 1991;125:643

67. Reinwein D, Benker G, Lazarus JH, Alexander WD, and the European Multicenter Study Group on Antithyroid Drug Treatment. A prospective randomized trial of antithyroid drug dose in Graves' disease therapy. J Clin Endocrinol Metab 1993;6:1516

68. Werner MC, Romaldini JH, Bromberg N, et al. Adverse effects related to thionamide drugs and their dosage regimen. Am J Med Sci 1989;297:216

69. Levy WJ, Schumacher P, Gupta M. Treatment of childhood Graves' disease. A review with emphasis on radioiodine treatment. Cleve Clin J Med 1988;55:373

70. Rapoport B, Caplan R, DeGroot LJ. Low-dose sodium iodide I 131 therapy in Graves' disease. JAMA 1973;244:1610

71. Safa AM, Schumacher OP, Rodriguez-Antunez A. Long-term follow-up results in children and adolescents treated with radioactive iodine for hyperthyroidism. N Engl J Med 1975;292:167

72. Dobyns BM, Sheline GE, Workman JB, et al. Malignant and benign neoplasms of the thyroid in patients treated for hyperthyroidism: a report of the cooperative thyrotoxicosis therapy follow-up study. J Clin Endocrinol Metab 1974;38:976

73. Brill AB, Becker DV. The safety of[131]I treatment of hyperthyroidism. In: Van Middlesworth L, Givins JR, eds. The thyroid, a practical clinical treatise. Chicago: Year Book Medical Publishers, 1986:347

74. Hall P, Boice JD Jr, Berg G, et al. Leukaemia incidence after iodine-131 exposure. Lancet 1992;340:1

75. Holm L-E, Hall P, Wiklund K, et al. Cancer risk after iodine-131 therapy for hyperthyroidism. J Natl Cancer Inst 1991;83:1072

76. Goldman MB, Maloof F, Monson RR, et al. Radioactive iodine therapy and breast cancer. Am J Epidemiol 1988;127:969

77. Andrassy RJ, Buckingham BA, Weitzman JJ. Thyroidectomy for hyperthyroidism in children. J Pediatr Surg 1980;15:501

78. Hayles AB, Chaves-Carballo E, McConahey WM. The treatment of hyperthyroidism (Graves' disease) in children. Mayo Clin Proc 1967;42:218

79. Wesley JR, Buckingham BA, Gahr JA, et al. Surgical treatment of hyperthyroidism in children. Surg Obstet Gynecol 1977;145:343

80. Zimmerman D, Gan-Gaisano M. Hyperthyroidism in children and adolescents. Pediatr Clin North Am 1990;37:1273

81. Tamai H, Kasaqi K, Takaichi Y, et al. Development of spontaneous hypothyroidism in patients with Graves' disease treated with antithyroid drugs: clinical, immunological, and histological findings in 26 patients. J Clin Endocrinol Metab 1989;69:49

N I N E

Special Topics in Thyroidology

Werner and Ingbar's The Thyroid, Seventh Edition,
edited by Lewis E. Braverman and Robert D. Utiger.
Lippincott–Raven Publishers, Philadelphia, © 1996

87

Subclinical Hypothyroidism

Douglas S. Ross

The term *subclinical hypothyroidism* was first introduced in the early 1970s, coincident with the introduction of serum thyrotropin (TSH) measurements, and eventually replaced terms such as preclinical myxedema, compensated euthyroidism, preclinical hypothyroidism, and decreased thyroid reserve. Subclinical hypothyroidism is best defined as a usually asymptomatic state associated with normal serum free thyroxine (T_4) and triiodothyronine (T_3) concentrations and an elevated serum TSH concentration. Some investigators, especially those studying the neuropsychiatric aspects of hypothyroidism, also include patients who have high-normal basal serum TSH concentrations and supranormal serum TSH responses to thyrotropin-releasing hormone (TRH). Table 87-1 defines several grades of hypothyroidism that have been suggested by various authors.[1,2] By definition, patients with subclinical hypothyroidism cannot be identified on the basis of symptoms and signs.[3]

ETIOLOGY

The causes of subclinical hypothyroidism are the same as the causes of overt hypothyroidism (see Part V, Section B), and are listed in Table 87-2. Most patients have chronic autoimmune thyroiditis, as defined by positive tests for serum antithyroid peroxidase (anti-TPO) antibodies. In a Michigan outpatient practice, 54% of patients with subclinical hypothyroidism had chronic autoimmune thyroiditis,[4] and in a community survey in Whickham, England 67% of women and 40% of men with an elevated serum TSH concentration had increased antibody titers.[5] Prior ablative therapy for thyrotoxicosis caused by Graves' disease is the other major cause of subclinical hypothyroidism, accounting for 39% of the cases in the Michigan study.[4] Among clinically euthyroid patients who had received radioiodine therapy for Graves' hyperthyroidism, at least half have elevated serum TSH concentrations,[6,7] and in one survey 65% of clinically euthyroid patients treated surgi-

cally for Graves' hyperthyroidism had elevations in serum TSH concentrations.[8] Several drugs may cause subclinical (or overt) hypothyroidism. They include lithium carbonate, iodide, and iodide-containing medications such as amiodarone. External radiation therapy to the neck may also cause subclinical hypothyroidism. Another important cause of subclinical hypothyroidism is inadequate replacement therapy for overt hypothyroidism. In a community-based study (Framingham, Massachusetts), 37% of older patients taking thyroid hormone preparations for hypothyroidism had elevated serum TSH concentrations.[9] Inadequate thyroid therapy may have been intentional in some patients because of coexistent heart disease, but more often it is caused by poor patient compliance or inadequate monitoring of therapy.

DIFFERENTIAL DIAGNOSIS

Several causes of elevated serum TSH concentrations do not properly fit the definition of subclinical hypothyroidism (see Table 87-2). One is during recovery from nonthyroidal illness, at which time the serum TSH concentration may be transiently elevated. These patients should be reevaluated several weeks after recovery from their illness. Therefore, studies of subclinical hypothyroidism based on serum TSH measurements in hospitalized patients may be invalid because of failure to appreciate this cause of an elevated serum TSH value. An occasional serum TSH determination may exceed the normal reference range because of pulsatile TSH secretion, the nocturnal surge in TSH secretion, or assay variability. Therefore, minimal serum TSH elevations should be confirmed before the diagnosis of subclinical hypothyroidism is accepted. Artifactual increases in serum TSH values may be caused by heterophilic antibodies, which interfere with TSH measurement, although this technical problem has been corrected by most manufacturers of assay materials. Serum TSH concentrations may be transiently increased in patients with adrenal insuffi-

TABLE 87-1.
Grades of Hyperthyroidism

Grade	Clinical Features	Serum T_4	Serum T_3	Serum TSH	Serum TSH Response to Thyrotropin-Releasing Hormone
Overt	Obvious	Low	Usually low	Very high	Supranormal
Mild	Minimal	Low or normal	Normal	Moderately high	Supranormal
Subclinical	None	Normal	Normal	Slightly elevated	Supranormal
Presubclinical	None	Normal	Normal	Normal	Supranormal

ciency and during treatment with metoclopramide or domperidone. Patients with TSH-secreting pituitary adenomas or partial pituitary resistance to thyroid hormone have increased TSH secretion, high serum T_4 and T_3 levels, and clinical thyrotoxicosis, whereas patients with generalized thyroid hormone resistance have slightly elevated serum TSH and elevated serum T_4 concentrations but are clinically euthyroid.

EPIDEMIOLOGY

Several population-based studies have defined the prevalence of subclinical hypothyroidism. In England (the Whickham survey), the prevalence of serum TSH concentrations greater than 6 mU/L in the absence of overt hypothyroidism was 7.5% in women and 2.8% in men.[5] Thyroid antibodies were present in 67% of the women and 40% of the men with elevated serum TSH concentrations. There was an age-dependent increase in serum TSH in women only, which was not found when antibody-positive patients were eliminated from the analysis. In women over the age of 75 years, the prevalence of subclinical hypothyroidism was 17.4%. In a similar study in Detroit the

TABLE 87-2.
Common Causes of Subclinical Hypothyroidism

SUBCLINICAL HYPOTHYROIDISM

Chronic autoimmune thyroiditis
Treated Graves' hyperthyroidism: radioiodine, surgery
Inadequate replacement therapy for overt hypothyroidism
Lithium carbonate therapy
Iodide and iodide-containing medications
External radiotherapy to the neck

SERUM TSH ELEVATIONS NOT ASSOCIATED WITH SUBCLINICAL HYPOTHYROIDISM

Nonthyroidal illness
Pulsatile TSH secretion, nocturnal surge in TSH secretion
Assay variability
Heterophilic anti-TSH antibodies
Therapy with metoclopromide or domperidone
TSH-secreting pituitary adenomas
Thyroid hormone–resistance syndromes

prevalence of serum TSH elevations was 8.5% in women and 4.4% in men.[10] The higher prevalence of subclinical hypothyroidism in elderly patients was confirmed by data from the Framingham study, in which the prevalence of minor elevations in serum TSH in patients over age 60 years was 8.2% in men and 16.9% in women,[11] and by a Dutch study in which the prevalence of subclinical hypothyroidism in a group of women (mean age 55 years) was 4.0%; it was 7.3% in the same group of women 10 years later.[12] In healthy ambulatory subjects in New Mexico, 9.5% of men and 16.2% of women over age 60 years had subclinical hypothyroidism.[13] The prevalence of subclinical hypothyroidism may be lower in extremely old women; in a recent English study the prevalence of subclinical hypothyroidism was 13.7% in women aged 60 to 69 years and 6.2% in women over age 80 years[14] (see also chap 2).

Subclinical hypothyroidism is more prevalent in patients with type I diabetes mellitus[15] and probably in patients with other autoimmune diseases. In a survey of pregnant women in the United States, 2% had subclinical hypothyroidism, 58% of whom had thyroid antibodies.[16]

NATURAL HISTORY

A substantial proportion of patients with subclinical hypothyroidism eventually develop overt hypothyroidism. In the Whickham survey,[17] those persons who had both elevated serum TSH concentrations and thyroid antibodies developed hypothyroidism at a rate of 5% yearly in the following 4 years. No one with an elevated serum TSH concentration and no antibodies became hypothyroid, whereas one woman with antibodies and a normal serum TSH value became hypothyroid. In the New Mexico study of ambulatory subjects older than 60 years,[13] one-third of those with subclinical hypothyroidism developed overt hypothyroidism during 4 years of follow-up; among them were all the subjects whose initial serum TSH concentrations were over 20 mU/L and 80% of those whose anti-TPO antibody titers were 1:1600 or higher (normal ≤ 1:100), but no one with titers less than 1:1600. In an English study of persons with subclinical hypothyroidism who were followed for 1 year, 17.8% developed overt hypothyroidism, 5.5% had normal serum TSH concentrations, and 76.7% had persistent subclinical hypothyroidism.[14] In another study, 53% of patients with subclinical hypothyroidism followed for 8 years became hypothyroid and 47% continued to have subclinical hypothyroidism.[18] The former group included all the patients with autoimmune thyroid disease, prior radioiodine therapy, high-dose external radiotherapy, and long-term lithium therapy, whereas the latter group included patients with thyroid or neck surgery for indications other than hyperthyroidism and external neck radiotherapy during childhood. Thus, the risks of developing overt hypothyroidism are greater with both high serum TSH concentrations and high titers of thyroid antibodies and approach 5% to 10% yearly depending on the population studied.

BIOLOGIC IMPORTANCE

The fundamental clinical question regarding patients with subclinical hypothyroidism is whether they require treatment with thyroid hormone. Based on the natural history of subclinical hypothyroidism alone, one can argue that treatment should be started to prevent the development of overt hypothyroidism. This section summarizes two randomized trials of thyroid hormone, studies that compare various measures of tissue thyroid hormone action in patients with subclinical hypothyroidism with those in normal subjects (Table 87-3), and several uncontrolled treatment studies.

Randomized Trials

The first randomized trial of T_4 therapy in subclinical hypothyroidism was a double-blind study in which patients were treated with T_4 or placebo for 1 year.[19] The dosage was adjusted to normalize serum TSH concentrations. Symptoms were assessed using a standardized hypothyroidism diagnostic index.[20] Before treatment, some patients with subclinical hypothyroidism complained of dry skin, poor energy, and cold intolerance, but there was no increased prevalence of muscle cramps, constipation, or fatigability. The patients assigned to the placebo group had a mean serum TSH concentration of 11.1 mU/L at the beginning of the year and 14.7 mU/L at the end of the year; those given T_4 had a fall in mean serum TSH from 10.8 to 2.6 mU/L. The T_4-treated patients had no change in weight, basal metabolic rate, water excretion, serum cholesterol or triglycerides, preejection period/left ventricular ejection time ratio (PEP:LVET), or QK_d (the interval from the Q wave on the electrocardiogram to the pulse arrival time at the brachial artery). A subgroup of patients with prolonged PEP:LVET ratios had normal values during therapy. The major finding of this study was that half the patients with subclinical hypothyroidism had fewer symptoms during treatment. The response of normal subjects to T_4 administration has not been assessed.

The second randomized trial was a 1-year double-blind crossover study.[21] Patients received either T_4 or placebo for each of two 6-month periods. Unlike the prior study, the dose of T_4 was not based on serum TSH measurements; all patients received 0.15 mg daily. Because this is an above-average replacement dose, some of the patients may have had subclinical thyrotoxicosis during treatment, and a reduction in systolic time intervals to subnormal values in this study may have reflected overzealous T_4 replacement (see chap 88). During the 6-month T_4 treatment period, there was a significant increase in serum procollagen II peptide concentrations, but no change

in heart rate, serum cholesterol, creatine kinase, or sex hormone-binding globulin concentrations, body mass, blood pressure, or hemoglobin. There was an improvement in psychometric test results and an improvement in hypothyroid symptoms during T_4 administration, and many patients correctly distinguished the treatment period from the placebo period. Thus, the major finding in this study confirmed that of the prior study; about half the patients felt better when they were receiving T_4.

Serum Lipid and Apoprotein Concentrations

The serum total cholesterol concentrations were no different from those in normal subjects in 10 cross-sectional studies of patients with subclinical hypothyroidism,[1,12,22–29] and they were not reduced by thyroid hormone therapy in 10 studies[19,21,24,28,30–35] (see Table 87-3). In one study serum cholesterol was reduced by T_4 treatment in a subgroup of seven women with subclinical hypothyroidism and type IIa hypercholesterolemia.[27] Serum TSH concentrations and cholesterol were positively correlated in one study; however, significant elevations in serum cholesterol concentrations occurred only when serum TSH concentrations exceeded 40 mU/L.[36]

There have been several reports of abnormalities in serum low-density lipoprotein (LDL) cholesterol and high-density lipoprotein (HDL) cholesterol or apoprotein concentrations in patients with subclinical hypothyroidism, as well as changes in these values with thyroid hormone therapy. In one study, patients with subclinical hypothyroidism and an average serum TSH concentration of 8.6 mU/L had a mean serum total cholesterol concentration that was no different from that of a control group matched for age, sex, and body mass index, but they did have a significant increase in serum LDL cholesterol and a decrease in serum HDL cholesterol concentrations.[22] In another study, patients with subclinical hypothyroidism had a low serum HDL cholesterol concentration.[28] In contrast, in three studies serum HDL or LDL cholesterol concentrations in patients with subclinical hypothyroidism were normal.[26,27,29]

Serum apoprotein A_1 (apoA_1) was increased in one study[29] and unchanged in two studies.[12,28] In three studies, serum apoprotein B (apoB) values were similar in patients with subclinical hypothyroidism and normal subjects.[12,28,29]

Thyroid hormone treatment of patients with subclinical hypothyroidism has resulted in inconsistent improvement in serum lipid subfraction and apoprotein concentrations (see Table 87-3). In one trial involving 13 patients, the mean serum TSH concentration decreased from 16.6 to 3.2 mU/L after T_4 treatment. Serum LDL cholesterol and apoB concentrations decreased, but there was no change in the serum concentrations of total cholesterol, HDL cholesterol, or or apoA_1.[34] Serum LDL concentrations were reduced by T_4 treatment in 7 women with subclinical hypothyroidism and type IIa hyperlipidemia.[27] In a study of 29 women, the mean serum TSH concentration decreased from 12 to 1.2 mU/L after T_4 treatment. Serum HDL cholesterol and apoA_1 concentrations increased, but there was no change in serum total cholesterol or apoB concentrations. In other studies, serum LDL[31,35] or HDL cholesterol[30,31,35] or apoA_1 and apoB[31] concentrations did not change in patients

TABLE 87-3.
Biologic Effects of Subclinical Hypothyroidism

	Cross-Sectional Studies			Effect of T₄ Therapy	
	INCREASED	DECREASED	NORMAL	IMPROVED	UNCHANGED
SERUM LIPID AND APOPROTEIN CONCENTRATIONS					
Total cholesterol			1,12,22–29	27*	19,21,24,28,30–35
Low-density lipoprotein cholesterol	22		26,27,29	27,* 34	31,35
High-density lipoprotein cholesterol		22,28	26,27,29	28	30,31,34,35
Apoprotein A₁	29		12,28	28	31,34
Apoprotein B			12,28,29	34	31,28
Apoprotein A₂			28		28
Lipoprotein lipase activity					31
CARDIAC EFFECTS					
Systolic time intervals			29,37,38	19,* 21,† 33,†‡ 38†	
Myocardial contractility				30,39	
Heart rate					21,30
Blood pressure					21
OTHER SYMPTOMS, SIGNS, AND BIOCHEMICAL VALUES					
Depression–psychiatric features	40–43				
Hypothyroid–somatic complaints	43			19,21,43	
Psychometric testing		43		21,43	
Achilles tendon reflex time	29,38			38†	
Serum procollagen II peptide				21	
Serum myoglobulin	29				
Serum α-subunit response to TRH	23,29§				
Serum prolactin response to TRH	29		44	19	
Basal metabolic rate					19
Body mass or weight					19,21,31,32
Nerve conduction velocity					30
Water excretion, day-to-night urinary sodium excretion					19,30
Serum insulin and glucagon					31
Serum sex hormone–binding globulin or hemoglobin					21
Serum creatine kinase			29		21

*Value improved in a subgroup of patients with abnormal baseline values.
†Some patients may have received excess doses of thyroid hormone.
‡Some patients may have had mild overt hypothyroidism.
§Values abnormal only in postmenopausal women.
TRH, thyrotropin-releasing hormone.

with subclinical hypothyroidism who received T₄ in a dose that normalized their serum TSH values.

Cardiac Function

Changes in systolic time intervals and cardiac contractility have been carefully studied in subclinical and overt hypothyroidism. In a study of patients with subclinical hypothyroidism and normal subjects there were no differences in the duration of electromechanical systole (Q-A₂), LVET, or PEP:LVET ratio.[37] In a second study, 20 patients with normal serum T₄ and elevated serum TSH concentrations given T₄ to normalize their serum TSH concentrations had a significant reduction in PEP:LVET ra-

tio and QK_d.[33] Five of the 20 patients initially had serum TSH concentrations over 40 mU/L, and 4 of the 20 had blunted or absent responses to TRH administration during treatment, suggesting that some patients had overt rather than subclinical hypothyroidism before therapy and subclinical thyrotoxicosis during therapy. In the randomized clinical trial discussed previously,[19] there was no change in PEP:LVET ratio or QK_d in patients with subclinical hypothyroidism who received T₄ therapy,[19] but a subgroup of patients initially had an increased PEP:LVET ratio that became normal during therapy. Two other trials are flawed due to possible overtreatment with thyroid hormone. Patients treated with 20 μg T₃ twice daily had a reduction in systolic time intervals, but so, too, did a group of normal subjects receiving the same regimen.[38] Finally, the other randomized trial discussed previously,[21] in which patients received a fixed daily dose of 0.15 mg T[4], the mean values for Q-A[2], PEP, and the PEP:LVET ratio all decreased, but some of the patients had subclinical thyrotoxicosis.[21]

Left ventricular ejection fraction (LVEF) also has been measured in patients with subclinical hypothyroidism before and during T[4] therapy.[30,39] There was no change in LVEF at rest or with moderate exercise, but LVEF at maximal exercise was improved by T[4] treatment. During therapy, there was also an increase in the slope of the ratio of systolic blood pressure/end-systolic volume at maximal exercise (but not at rest), indicating improved myocardial contractility.[39] Thus, at least some patients with subclinical hypothyroidism have subtle abnormalities in systolic time intervals and myocardial contractility that improve during T[4] treatment.

Neuropsychiatric Features

Reports of an increased prevalence of subclinical hypothyroidism in patients with depression or bipolar affective disorders need careful assessment due to frequently inadequate control groups, coincident lithium therapy, and the inclusion of patients with normal serum TSH values whose thyroid abnormality is limited to either an increased response of serum TSH to TRH administration or the presence of thyroid antibodies.[2] Nonetheless, several studies suggest an association of subclinical hypothyroidism with neuropsychiatric features. In one study the prevalence of hypothyroidism was 14.8% in patients with neurotic depression and 2.3% in those with senile and multi-infarct dementia, compared with 1.9% in nonpsychiatric inpatients.[40] Patients with depression and subclinical hypothyroidism may have a higher prevalence of associated panic disorder and a poorer response to antidepressant drug therapy than depressed euthyroid patients.[41] Randomly selected women with subclinical hypothyroidism, who had formal psychiatric assessment before assessment of thyroid function, were found to have a higher lifetime frequency of depression than euthyroid women.[42] Women found to have subclinical hypothyroidism after presenting to a clinic for assessment of goiter were found to have increased rates of free-flowing anxiety, somatic complaints, depressive features, and hysteria as compared with euthyroid patients with goiter, and these abnormalities improved following treatment with T[4].[43] Psychometric test results reported in this study were also abnormal and improved with therapy, confirming the results of one of the randomized trials of T[4] therapy discussed above.[21]

Other Measurements

Patients with subclinical hypothyroidism have a normal thyroidal response to TSH stimulation and no abnormality in sellar volume.[22] As expected, they do have a supranormal response of both serum TSHβ and α-subunit to TRH administration;[23] the serum prolactin response to TRH administration was increased in one study[29] and normal in another.[44] The Achilles reflex time is prolonged,[29,38] and treatment with T[3] restores it to normal.[38] Serum myoglobin concentrations are increased.[29] Abnormal day-to-night urinary sodium excretion and nerve conduction velocities failed to improve with treat-

ment.[30] Bone density was not reduced in patients with subclinical hypothyroidism after 14 months of T[4] treatment.[45] Subclinical hypothyroidism is not more prevalent among women with premenstrual syndrome.[44]

CONCLUSIONS

Subclinical hypothyroidism is common, especially among elderly women. Treatment may be indicated to prevent progression to overt hypothyroidism, especially in patients who have serum TSH values greater than 14 to 20 mU/L, and in patients who have anti-TPO antibody titers of 1:1600 or greater. Treatment is also indicated if a goiter is present. The major immediate benefit of treatment, based on two randomized studies, is an improvement in symptoms, and there may be improvements in cardiac contractility and lipid profiles in some patients.

Arguments against treatment include the costs of therapy and of monitoring therapy, as well as the lifelong commitment to daily medication in asymptomatic persons. In some patients, therapy may exacerbate angina pectoris or an underlying cardiac arrhythmia. If treatment is given, careful monitoring to avoid the adverse effects of subclinical hyperthyroidism is mandatory.

References

1. Evered DC, Ormston BJ, Smith PA, et al. Grades of hypothyroidism. BMJ 1973;1:657
2. Haggerty JJ Jr, Golden RN, Garbutt JC, et al. Subclinical hypothyroidism: a review of neuropsychiatric aspects. Int J Psychiat Med 1990;20:193
3. Bemben DA, Hamm RM, Morgan L, et al. Thyroid disease in the elderly. Part 2. Predictability of subclinical hypothyroidism. J Fam Pract 1994;38:583
4. Hamburger JI, Meier DA, Szpunar WE. Factitious elevation of thyrotropin in euthyroid patients. N Engl J Med 1985;313:267
5. Tunbridge WMG, Evered DC, Hall R, et al. The spectrum of thyroid disease in a community: the Whickham survey. Clin Endocrinol 1977;7:481
6. Tunbridge WMG, Harsoulis P, Goolden AWG. Thyroid function in patients treated with radioactive iodine for thyrotoxicosis. BMJ 1974;3:89
7. Toft AD, Irvine WJ, Hunter WM, Seth J. Plasma TSH and serum T[4] levels in long-term follow-up of patients treated with ¹³¹I for thyrotoxicosis. BMJ 1974;3:152
8. Evered D, Young ET, Tunbridge WMG, et al. Thyroid function after subtotal thyroidectomy for hyperthyroidism. BMJ 1975;1:25
9. Sawin CT, Geller A, Hershman JM, et al. The aging thyroid. The use of thyroid hormone in older persons. JAMA 1989;261:2653
10. Bagchi N, Brown TR, Parish RF. Thyroid dysfunction in adults over age 55 years. A study in an urban U.S. community. Arch Intern Med 1990;150:785
11. Sawin CT, Chopra D, Azizi F, et al. The aging thyroid. Increased prevalence of elevated serum thyrotropin levels in the elderly. JAMA 1979;242:247
12. Geul KW, van Sluisveld ILL, Grobbee DE, et al. The importance of thyroid microsomal antibodies in the development of elevated serum TSH in middle-aged women: associations with serum lipids. Clin Endocrinol 1993;39:275
13. Rosenthal MJ, Hunt WC, Garry PJ, Goodwin JS. Thyroid failure in the elderly. Microsomal antibodies as discriminant for therapy. JAMA 1987;258:209

14. Parle JV, Franklyn JA, Cross KW, et al. Prevalence and follow-up of abnormal thyrotrophin (TSH) concentrations in the elderly in the United Kingdom. Clin Endocrinol 1991;34:77

15. Gray RS, Borsey DQ, Seth J, et al. Prevalence of subclinical thyroid failure in insulin-dependent diabetes. J Clin Endocrinol Metab 1980;50:1034

16. Klein RZ, Haddow JE, Faix JD, et al. Prevalence of thyroid deficiency in pregnant women. Clin Endocrinol 1991;35:41

17. Tunbridge WMG, Brewis M, French JM, et al. Natural history of autoimmune thyroiditis. BMJ 1981;282:258

18. Kabadi UM. `Subclinical' hypothyroidism. Natural course of the syndrome during a prolonged follow-up study. Arch Intern Med 1993;153:957

19. Cooper DS, Halpern R, Wood LC, et al. L-Thyroxine therapy in subclinical hypothyroidism. A double-blind, placebo-controlled trial. Ann Intern Med 1984;101:18

20. Billewicz WZ, Chapman RS, Crooks J, et al. Statistical methods applied to the diagnosis of hypothyroidism. Q J Med 1969; 38:255

21. Nyström E, Caidahl K, Fager G, et al. A double-blind cross-over 12-month study of L-thyroxine treatment of women with `subclinical' hypothyroidism. Clin Endocrinol 1988;29:63

22. Althaus BU, Staub JJ, Ryff-de Léche A, et al. LDL/HDL-changes in subclinical hypothyroidism: possible risk factors for coronary artery disease. Clin Endocrinol 1988;28:157

23. Bigos ST, Ridgway EC, Kourides IA, Maloof F. Spectrum of pituitary alterations with mild and severe thyroid impairment. J Clin Endocrinol Metab 1978;46:317

24. Kutty KM, Bryant DG, Farid NR. Serum lipids in hypothyroidism—a re-evaluation. J Clin Endocrinol Metab 1978; 46:55

25. Tunbridge WMG, Evered DC, Hall R, et al. Lipid profiles and cardiovascular disease in the Whickham area with particular reference to thyroid failure. Clin Endocrinol 1977;7:495

26. Parle JV, Franklyn JA, Cross KW, et al. Circulating lipids and minor abnormalities of thyroid function. Clin Endocrinol 1992; 37:411

27. Bogner U, Arntz H-R, Peters H, Schleusener H. Subclinical hypothyroidism and hyperlipoproteinaemia: indiscriminate L-thyroxine treatment not justified. Acta Endocrinol 1993;128:202

28. Caron PH, Calazel C, Parra HJ, et al. Decreased HDL cholesterol in subclinical hypothyroidism: the effect of L-thyroxine therapy. Clin Endocrinol 1990;33:519

29. Staub J-J, Althaus BU, Engler H, et al. Spectrum of subclinical and overt hypothyroidism: effect on thyrotropin, prolactin, and thyroid reserve, and metabolic impact on peripheral target tissues. Am J Med 1992;92:631

30. Bell GM, Todd WTA, Forfar JC, et al. End-organ responses to thyroxine therapy in subclinical hypothyroidism. Clin Endocrinol 1985;22:83

31. Lithell H, Boberg J, Hellsing K, et al. Serum lipoprotein and apolipoprotein concentrations and tissue lipoprotein-lipase activity in overt and subclinical hypothyroidism: the effect of substitution therapy. Eur J Clin Invest 1981;11:3

32. Nilsson G, Norlander S, Levin K. Studies on subclinical hypothyroidism with special reference to the serum lipid pattern. Acta Med Scand 1976;200:63

33. Ridgway EC, Cooper DS, Walker H, et al. Peripheral responses to thyroid hormone before and after L-thyroxine therapy in patients with subclinical hypothyroidism. J Clin Endocrinol Metab 1981;53:1238

34. Arem R, Patsch W. Lipoprotein and apolipoprotein levels in subclinical hypothyroidism. Effect of levothyroxine therapy. Arch Intern Med 1990;150:2097

35. Franklyn JA, Daykin J, Betteridge J, et al. Thyroxine replacement therapy and circulating lipid concentrations. Clin Endocrinol 1993;38:453

36. Elder J, McLelland A, O'Reilly DS, et al. The relationship between serum cholesterol and serum thyrotropin, thyroxine and triiodothyronine concentrations in suspected hypothyroidism. Ann Clin Biochem 1990;27:110

37. Bough EW, Crowley WF, Ridgway EC, et al. Myocardial function in hypothyroidism. Relation to disease severity and response to treatment. Arch Intern Med 1978;138:1476

38. Ooi TC, Whitlock RM, Frengley PA, Ibbertson HK. Systolic time intervals and ankle reflex time in patients with minimal serum TSH elevation: response to triiodothyronine therapy. Clin Endocrinol 1980;13:621

39. Forfar JC, Wathen CG, Todd WTA, et al. Left ventricular performance in subclinical hypothyroidism. Q J Med 1985;57:857

40. Tappy L, Randin JP, Schwed P, et al. Prevalence of thyroid disorders in psychogeriatric inpatients. A possible relationship of hypothyroidism with neurotic depression but not with dementia. J Am Geriatr Soc 1987;35:526

41. Joffe RT, Levitt AJ. Major depression and subclinical (grade 2) hypothyroidism. Psychoneuroendocrinology 1992;17:215

42. Haggerty JJ, Stern RA, Mason GA, et al. Subclinical hypothyroidism: a modifiable risk factor for depression? Am J Psychiatry 1993;150:508

43. Monzani F, Del Guerra P, Caraccio N, Prunetti CA, Pucci E, Luisi M. Subclinical hypothyroidism: neurobehavioral features and beneficial effect of L-thyroxine treatment. Clin Invest 1993; 71:367

44. Casper RF, Patel-Christopher A, Powell AM. Thyrotropin and prolactin responses to thyrotropin-releasing hormone in premenstrual syndrome. J Clin Endocrinol Metab 1989;68:608

45. Ross DS. Bone density is not reduced during the short-term administration of levothyroxine to postmenopausal women with subclinical hypothyroidism: a randomized, prosepctive study. Am J Med 1993;95:385

Werner and Ingbar's The Thyroid, Seventh Edition,
edited by Lewis E. Braverman and Robert D. Utiger.
Lippincott–Raven Publishers, Philadelphia, © 1996

88

Subclinical Thyrotoxicosis

Douglas S. Ross

The introduction of serum thyrotropin (TSH) measurements into clinical practice during the early 1970s provided the necessary tool for defining subclinical hypothyroidism, although it took several years for our present understanding and an accepted definition of this entity to evolve (see chap 87). Similarly, the introduction within the past decade of sensitive immunometric TSH assays has allowed detection of subnormal TSH values. The term subclinical thyrotoxicosis refers to a usually asymptomatic state associated with normal serum free thyroxine (T_4) and triiodothyronine (T_3) and low serum TSH concentrations. Asymptomatic patients with slightly elevated serum free thyroid hormone concentrations have mild overt thyrotoxicosis. Before the introduction of sensitive TSH assays, subclinical thyrotoxicosis could be demonstrated by blunted responses of serum TSH to thyrotropin-releasing hormone (TRH) administration. TRH testing is currently unnecessary in these patients because the serum TSH response to TRH is generally proportional to the basal serum TSH concentration. The studies reviewed in this chapter document the biologic importance of subclinical thyrotoxicosis; however, there is not yet any consensus regarding the indications for therapeutic intervention.

ETIOLOGY

The major causes of subclinical thyrotoxicosis are listed in Table 88-1. Conceptually, there are two groups of patients: those who have subclinical thyrotoxicosis caused by exogenous thyroid hormone therapy and those in whom it is caused by slight endogenous overproduction of thyroid hormone.

Exogenous Subclinical Thyrotoxicosis

As many as 10 million people in the United States, and possibly as many as 200 million people worldwide, are taking thyroid hormone and are therefore at risk for subclinical thyrotoxicosis

either because of overzealous replacement therapy or intentional suppressive therapy. When sensitive methods for measuring serum TSH first became available, an estimated 40% to 50% of patients taking replacement T_4 therapy had subnormal serum TSH concentrations,[1] but their numbers have diminished as a result of the use of these assays to monitor therapy and recognition of the potential dangers of overzealous replacement. Patients with thyroid cancer, thyroid nodules, multinodular or diffuse goiter, or a history of neck irradiation who are treated with thyroid hormone to suppress TSH secretion to below normal have subclinical (if not overt) thyrotoxicosis. In these patients, the benefits of TSH suppression may exceed the potential risks of subclinical thyrotoxicosis.

Endogenous Subclinical Thyrotoxicosis

Endogenous subclinical thyrotoxicosis is most common in patients with an autonomously functioning thyroid adenoma or multinodular goiter. In one study, 6 of 15 patients had "patchy or irregular" uptake on thyroid radionuclide imaging, suggesting multinodular goiter and the possibility of autonomous thyroid secretion.[2] Subnormal serum TSH concentrations also have been found in apparently healthy people with no evidence of thyroid disease.

The prevalence of autonomously functioning thyroid adenomas and multinodular goiter and, thus, the prevalence of subclinical thyrotoxicosis varies considerably from one region of the world to another. This variation is presumably the result of differences in dietary iodine intake and possible genetic differences. For example, in a U.S. study, the ratio of patients with thyrotoxicosis caused by an autonomously functioning adenoma to those with thyrotoxicosis caused by Graves' disease was 1:50,[3] whereas in Switzerland it was 1:2.[4] In Europe, 22% of patients with nontoxic multinodular goiter had blunted serum TSH responses to TRH stimulation consistent with subclinical thyrotoxicosis and 28% had clear-cut autonomous area(s) on thyroid radionuclide imaging.[5]

TABLE 88-1.
Common Causes of Subclinical Thyrotoxicosis

EXOGENOUS SUBCLINICAL THYROTOXICOSIS

Overzealous thyroid hormone replacement therapy

Thyroid hormone suppressive therapy

ENDOGENOUS SUBCLINICAL THYROTOXICOSIS

Thyroid gland autonomy: autonomously functioning thyroid adenoma or multinodular goiter

Graves' disease

TSH SUPPRESSION NOT ASSOCIATED WITH SUBCLINICAL THYROTOXICOSIS

Secondary and central hypothyroidism

Severe nonthyroidal illness, glucocorticoid therapy, dopamine therapy

After treatment of thyrotoxicosis, before recovery of the pituitary–thyroid axis

Laboratory error

Subclinical thyrotoxicosis also occurs in patients with autoimmune thyroid disease. Sixty-three percent of patients with euthyroid Graves' disease (ophthalmic Graves' disease) in Japan had subnormal serum TSH responses to TRH,[6] and 4.1% of patients with Graves' disease in remission were also found to have subclinical thyrotoxicosis by TRH testing.[7] The thyrotropic activity of high serum chorionic gonadotropin concentrations during early pregnancy also may cause a transient rise in serum thyroid hormone concentrations and a reduction in serum TSH concentrations to subnormal values.[8]

Differential Diagnosis

Several causes of subnormal TSH concentrations do not reflect the presence of subclinical thyrotoxicosis (see Table 88-1). Patients with pituitary or hypothalamic disease who have hypothyroidism may have subnormal serum TSH concentrations. Serum TSH concentrations are frequently low in patients with severe nonthyroidal illness, especially those receiving glucocorticoid or dopamine therapy.[9] Low serum TSH values may be associated with low or normal serum thyroid hormone concentrations shortly after treatment or spontaneous resolution of overt thyrotoxicosis because of persistent suppression of pituitary TSH secretion.

EPIDEMIOLOGY AND NATURAL HISTORY

In a Swedish community-based study of 2000 consecutive adults, the prevalence of subnormal serum TSH concentrations without overt thyrotoxicosis was 3.3%.[10] Nine percent of the subjects with subclinical thyrotoxicosis had thyroid abnormalities (e.g., multinodular goiter, thyroiditis), and 40% had a normal serum TSH concentration on recall. In a U.S. study of 968 patients over age 55 years, 0.7% had endogenous subclinical thyrotoxicosis.[11] In another U.S. study, 46 of 2411 subjects (1.9%) over age 60 had subclinical thyrotoxicosis with serum

TSH values less than 0.1 mU/L[12]; during a 4-year follow-up period, only two of these subjects developed overt thyrotoxicosis and serum TSH concentrations became normal in the majority. In a similar study from England, 6.3% of women and 5.5% of men had low serum TSH concentrations (<0.5 mU/L); a year later the serum TSH values were normal in 60% of these subjects and only one patient (1.5%) developed overt thyrotoxicosis.[13] In Sweden, 1.8% of 886 subjects age 85 had subclinical thyrotoxicosis.[14] Thus, the prevalence of endogenous subclinical thyrotoxicosis in the community varies from 0.7% to 6.0%, depending on the criteria used and the age of the population. Over half these subjects, especially those with slightly subnormal serum TSH values, have normal serum TSH concentrations when retested during follow-up and few developed overt thyrotoxicosis (see also chap 26).

Although there are no long-term studies of the natural history of subclinical thyrotoxicosis, data are available regarding the natural history of autonomously functioning thyroid adenomas. In a U.S. study, 8.8% of initially euthyroid patients with these tumors developed overt thyrotoxicosis during follow-up for 6 years,[3] and in a European study, 18% of patients developed thyrotoxicosis during a 7-year follow-up period.[15]

BIOLOGIC IMPORTANCE

Physiology of Thyrotropin Suppression

Because the negative feedback relationship between serum TSH and thyroid hormone is log linear, even slightly excessive thyroid hormone therapy or endogenous thyroid hormone production will suppress serum TSH to subnormal concentrations.[16] Groups of patients with subnormal serum TSH values who receive slightly excessive doses of T_4 have serum T_4 and T_3 concentrations that are above the mean values for normal subjects but are within the normal ranges.

Presently, most clinicians accept serum TSH measurement as the most sensitive indicator of thyroid hormone status (in the absence of pituitary or hypothalamic disease). However, several experimental findings raise the question of whether this is always the case. In laboratory animals local deiodination of T_4 to T_3, a reaction that is catalyzed primarily by type II T_4-5'-deiodinase (see chap 8), contributes more of the T_3 bound to the T_3-nuclear receptors in the pituitary gland and serum T_3 contributes less than in most other organs.[17] Hence, the extent of T_3-induced inhibition, or lack thereof, of TSH secretion, may vary somewhat independently of the serum T_3 concentration. In addition, the concentrations of the different nuclear receptor isoforms differ in the pituitary and peripheral organs, and these concentrations are altered discordantly in states of thyroid hormone excess or deficiency.[18] Finally, some elderly patients with low serum T_4 and normal TSH concentrations appear to have a decreased set point for T_4- and T_3-mediated feedback inhibition of TSH secretion.[19]

Bone and Mineral Metabolism

Thyroid hormone has a direct resorptive effect on bone, and overt thyrotoxicosis is associated with increased bone resorption and to a lesser extent increased bone formation, and an increase in fracture rate[20] (Table 88-2). Cortical bone is affected more than trabecular bone. Patients with nodular goiter and subclinical thyrotoxicosis have reduced bone density compared with normal subjects,[21,22] although in one study significant reductions in bone density occurred only in sites rich in cortical bone in postmenopausal women.[22] The serum concentration of osteocalcin, a marker of bone turnover, is elevated in patients with nodular goiter and subclinical thyrotoxicosis and is inversely correlated with serum TSH concentrations.[23]

Controversy remains as to whether T_4 therapy in doses that result in subclinical thyrotoxicosis causes reduced bone density. Bone density may be reduced in premenopausal women receiving suppressive or overzealous replacement doses, but women receiving lower but still adequate or slightly excessive replacement doses have normal bone density.[20] As in endogenous subclinical thyrotoxicosis, bone density is more frequently reduced at sites rich in cortical bone (e.g., wrist and hip) than sites rich in trabecular bone (e.g., lumbar spine), and postmenopausal women are more likely to be affected than premenopausal women.[20] A meta-analysis concluded that reduced bone density occurs only in postmenopausal women.[24] The adverse effect of T_4 on bone density is associated with doses in excess of 1.6 μg/kg.[25] Estrogen

therapy appears to protect against T_4-induced bone loss among postmenopausal women.[25]

Other measures of bone mineral metabolism in addition to serum osteocalcin are abnormal in patients who have either exogenous or endogenous subclinical thyrotoxicosis. Urinary excretion of bone collagen-derived pyridinium cross-links and hydroxyproline is increased[26,27]; serum osteocalcin is inversely correlated with serum TSH in these patients.[28]

Data regarding the risk of fracture in patients with subclinical thyrotoxicosis are still preliminary. In one study of women over age 65 years, the overall fracture rate was 0.9% in those with normal serum TSH values, and it was 2.5% in those with subnormal serum TSH values; this difference was not statistically significant.[29] An interview-based study did not find an increased fracture risk in women taking T_4.[30] In a third study, the risk of hip fracture was increased twofold in women taking thyroid hormone; serum TSH values were not reported.[31]

Cardiac Function

The risk of atrial fibrillation is increased in patients with subclinical thyrotoxicosis (see Table 88-2). In a community-based study of 2007 subjects over 60 years of age who were followed for 10 years, the cumulative incidence of atrial fibrillation was

TABLE 88-2.
Biologic Effects of Subclinical Thyrotoxicosis

	CHANGE	REFERENCES
SKELETAL EFFECTS		
Bone density	↓	21,24,25
Biochemical markers of bone mineral metabolism		
Serum osteocalcin	↑	23,28
Urinary bone collagen-derived pyridinium cross-links	↑	26
Urinary hydroxyproline	↑	27
CARDIAC EFFECTS		
Heart rate	↑	36,37
Premature atrial contractions	↑	37
Atrial fibrillation	↑	32,33
Cardiac contractility	↑	37
Systolic intervals:		
Preejection period divided by left ventricular ejection time	↓	39,40
Isovolumetric contraction time	↓	38
Left ventricular mass index, intraventricular septal and posterior wall thickness	↑	37
OTHER EFFECTS		
Serum total and LDL cholesterol	↓	42
Erythrocyte oubain-binding capacity	↓	43
Serum liver enzymes: glutathionine S-transferase, alanine aminotransferase, γ-glutamyltransferase	↑	44
Serum creatine kinase	↓	44
Ratio of day-to-night urinary sodium excretion and urine flow	↓	36
Serum sex hormone–binding globulin	↑	23,24
Time asleep at night	↓	46
Mood (using multidimensional scale for state of well-being)	↑	46

28% for subjects with serum TSH concentrations of 0.1 mU/L or less, 16% for those with serum TSH concentrations of 0.1 to 0.4 mU/L, and 11% for those with normal serum TSH concentrations.[32] There was a threefold relative risk of atrial fibrillation in subjects with subnormal serum TSH concentrations, whether caused by endogenous and exogenous subclinical thyrotoxicosis. In a smaller study of 80 patients the prevalence of atrial fibrillation was twofold higher among patients with subclinical thyrotoxicosis as compared with matched control patients with normal serum TSH values.[33] During a 2-year follow-up period, 9% of the patients with subclinical thyrotoxicosis developed atrial fibrillation compared with none of the control group.

Patients presenting with atrial fibrillation may prove to have subclinical thyrotoxicosis. Of 126 consecutive patients presenting to a hospital with atrial fibrillation, 2 had overt thyrotoxicosis and 13 (10%) had subclinical thyrotoxicosis.[34] The arrhythmia may remit with antithyroid therapy.[35] Subclinical thyrotoxicosis also is associated with an increase in heart rate and an increase in atrial premature beats.[36,37]

Both increased cardiac contractility and left ventricular hypertrophy are found in patients with exogenous subclinical thyrotoxicosis. Echocardiography demonstrates higher values for the percentage of fractional shortening and the rate-adjusted mean velocity of shortening, and a reduction in the isovolumetric contraction time (the time between mitral value closure and aortic value opening).[37,38] Systolic time intervals, such as the preejection period/left ventricular ejection time (PEP:LVET) ratio, are also reduced in patients with subclinical thyrotoxicosis.[39,40] Left ventricular mass index, intraventricular septal thickness, and left ventricular posterior wall thickness are all increased in patients with subclinical thyrotoxicosis.[37] The increase in left ventricular mass index is proportional to the duration of subclinical thyrotoxicosis[37] and is prevented by β-adrenergic blocking drugs.[41] These results suggest that subclinical thyrotoxicosis could aggravate angina pectoris or congestive heart failure although there are no data that address these possibilities. Thyroid hormone therapy was associated with an increased risk of ischemic heart disease in patients under age 65 years, but this did not correlate with their serum TSH concentrations.[29] This observation may reflect undertreatment or poor compliance with thyroid hormone therapy because subclinical hypothyroidism is associated with abnormal serum lipid concentrations (see chap 87), whereas subclinical thyrotoxicosis is associated with reduced serum total and low-density lipoprotein cholesterol concentrations.[42]

Other Measurements

Erythrocyte sodium pump sites, estimated by measuring ouabain-binding capacity, were reduced by 15% in T_4-treated patients with subclinical thyrotoxicosis.[43] Serum glutathione S-transferase, alanine aminotransferase, and γ-glutamyltransferase values are increased.[44] Serum creatine kinase concentrations are reduced,[44] and there is a decrease in the ratio of day-to-night urinary sodium excretion and urine flow.[36] Serum sex hormone-binding concentrations are increased in patients with either endogenous or exogenous subclinical thyrotoxicosis.[23,45] Finally, patients with subclinical thyrotoxicosis sleep less than normal subjects and have a better mood.[46]

PREVENTION AND TREATMENT

Both reduced bone density and an increased risk of atrial fibrillation may result in substantial morbidity in older patients with subclinical thyrotoxicosis. Although the risk of these adverse effects may be small, exogenous subclinical thyrotoxicosis can and should be avoided or minimized by careful titration of thyroid hormone therapy using serum TSH measurements. Patients who are receiving T_4 replacement therapy should have the dose adjusted to maintain a normal serum TSH concentration. Subclinical thyrotoxicosis cannot be avoided in patients taking T_4 with the express goal of suppressing TSH secretion to decrease goiter size, prevent recurrent goiter, or prevent recurrence or minimize growth of thyroid carcinoma. The adverse effects of suppressive therapy can be minimized by using the smallest dose of T_4 necessary to meet the goal of therapy. The efficacy of suppressive therapy of goiter or thyroid nodules is controversial,[47] and no data are available to support specific goals for serum TSH concentrations. However, many thyroidologists suggest suppressing serum TSH to slightly subnormal values in patients with benign disease and to undetectable values (e.g., <0.05 mU/L) only in patients with extrathyroidal spread of cancer.

Few data are available to guide clinical decisions regarding the treatment of endogenous subclinical thyrotoxicosis. Because low serum TSH concentrations are often transient, a period of observation is appropriate. For patients with serum TSH concentrations that are very low or below the detection limit of the assay, or who have serum thyroid hormone concentrations near the upper limit of normal, antithyroid treatment (see chap 53) should be considered after careful assessment of cardiac status, skeletal integrity, and the coexistence of other risk factors for cardiac disease and osteoporosis.

References

1. Ross DS, Ardisson LJ, Meskell MJ. Measurement of thyrotropin in clinical and subclinical hyperthyroidism using a new chemiluminescent assay. J Clin Endocrinol Metab 1989;69:684
2. Stott DJ, McLellan AR, Finlayson J, et al. Elderly patients with suppressed serum TSH but normal free thyroid hormone levels usually have mild thyroid overactivity and are at increased risk of developing overt hyperthyroidism. Q J Med 1991;78:77
3. Hamburger JI. Evolution of toxicity in solitary nontoxic autonomously functioning thyroid nodules. J Clin Endocrinol Metab 1980;50:1089
4. Horst W, Rosler H, Schneider C, Labbart A. Three hundred six cases of toxic adenoma: clinical aspects, findings in radioiodine diagnostics, radiochromatography and histology; results of 131-I and surgical treatment. J Nucl Med 1967;8:515
5. Rieu M, Bekka S, Sambor B, et al. Prevalence of subclinical hyperthyroidism and relationship between thyroid hormonal status and thyroid ultrasonographic parameters in patients with nontoxic nodular goitre. Clin Endocrinol 1993;39:67
6. Kasagi K, Hatabu H, Tokuda Y, et al. Studies on thyrotropin receptor antibodies in patients with euthyroid Graves' disease. Clin Endocrinol 1988;29:357
7. Murakami M, Koizumi Y, Aizawa T, et al. Studies of thyroid function and immune parameters in patients with hyperthyroid Graves' disease in remission. J Clin Endocrinol Metab 1988;66:103
8. Glinoer D, De Nayer P, Bourdoux P, et al. Regulation of maternal thyroid during pregnancy. J Clin Endocrinol Metab 1990;71:276

9. Spencer C, Eigen A, Shen D, et al. Specificity of sensitive assays of thyrotropin (TSH) used to screen for thyroid disease in hospitalized patients. Clin Chem 1987;33:1391

10. Eggertsen R, Petersen K, Lundberg P-A, et al. Screening for thyroid disease in a primary care unit with a thyroid stimulating hormone assay with a low detection limit. BMJ 1988;297:1586

11. Bagchi N, Brown TR, Parish RF. Thyroid dysfunction in adults over age 55 years. A study in an urban U.S. community. Arch Intern Med 1990;150:785

12. Sawin CT, Geller A, Kaplan MM, et al. Low serum thyrotropin (thyroid stimulating hormone) in older patients without hyperthyroidism. Arch Intern Med 1991;151:165

13. Parle JV, Franklyn JA, Cross KW, et al. Prevalence and follow-up of abnormal thyrotropin (TSH) concentrations in the elderly in the United Kingdom. Clin Endocrinol 1991;34:77

14. Sundbeck G, Jagenburg R, Johansson P-M, et al. Clinical significance of low serum thyrotropin concentration by chemiluminometric assay in 85-year-old women and men. Arch Intern Med 1991;151:549

15. Sandrock D, Olbricht T, Emrich D, et al. Long-term follow-up in patients with autonomous thyroid adenoma. Acta Endocrinol 1993;128:51

16. Carr D, McLeod DT, Parry G, Thornes HM. Fine adjustment of thyroxine replacement dosage: comparison of the thyrotropin releasing hormone test using a sensitive thyrotrophin assay with measurement of free thyroid hormones and clinical assessment. Clin Endocrinol 1988;28:325

17. Silva JE, Larsen PR. Contributions of plasma triiodothyronine and local thyroxine monodeiodination to triiodothyronine to nuclear triiodothyronine receptor saturation in pituitary, liver, and kidney of hypothyroid rats. J Clin Invest 1978;61:1247

18. Hodin RA, Lazar MA, Chin WW. Differential and tissue-specific regulation of the multiple rat c-*erb*A messenger RNA species by thyroid hormone. J Clin Invest 1990;85:101

19. Lewis GF, Alessi CA, Imperial JG, Refetoff S. Low serum free thyroxine index in ambulatory elderly is due to a resetting of the threshold of thyrotropin feedback suppression. J Clin Endocrinol Metab 1991;73:843

20. Ross DS. Hyperthyroidism, thyroid hormone therapy, and bone. Thyroid 1994;4:319

21. Mudde AH, Reijnders FJL, Kruseman AC. Peripheral bone density in women with untreated multinodular goitre. Clin Endocrinol 1992;37:35

22. Földes J, Tarjan G, Szathmari M, et al. Bone mineral density in patients with endogenous subclinical hyperthyroidism: is this thyroid status a risk factor for osteoporosis? Clin Endocrinol 1993;39:521

23. Faber J, Perrild H, Johansen JS. Bone Gla protein and sex hormone-binding globulin in nontoxic goiter: parameters for metabolic status at the tissue level. J Clin Endocrinol Metab 1990;70:49

24. Faber J, Galloe AM. Changes in bone mass during prolonged subclinical hyperthyroidism due to L-thyroxine treatment: a meta-analysis. Eur J Endocrinol 1994;130:350

25. Schneider DL, Barrett-Connor EL, Morton DJ. Thyroid hormone use and bone mineral density in elderly women. Effects of estrogen. JAMA 1994;271:1245

26. Harvey RD, McHardy KC, Reid IW, et al. Measurement of bone collagen degradation in hyperthyroidism and during thyroxine replacement therapy using pyridinium cross-links as specific urinary markers. J Clin Endocrinol Metab 1991;72:1189

27. Krakauer JC, Kleerekoper M. Borderline-low serum thyrotropin level is correlated with increased fasting urinary hydroxyproline excretion. Arch Intern Med 1992;152:360

28. Ross DS, Ardisson LJ, Nussbaum SR, Meskell MJ. Serum osteocalcin in patients taking L-thyroxine who have subclinical hyperthyroidism. J Clin Endocrinol Metab 1991;72:507

29. Leese GP, Jung RT, Guthrie C, Waugh N, Browning MC. Morbidity in patients on L-thyroxine: a comparison of those with a normal TSH to those with a suppressed TSH. Clin Endocrinol 1992;37:500

30. Solomon BL, Wartofsky L, Burman KD. Prevalence of fractures in postmenopausal women with thyroid disease. Thyroid 1993;3:17

31. Bauer DC, Cummings SR, Tao JL, Browner WS. Study of Osteoporotic Fractures Research Group. Hyperthyroidism increases the risk of hip fractures. A prospective study. Am Soc Bone Miner Res 1992:Abstract 116

32. Sawin CT, Geller A, Wolf PA, et al. Low serum thyrotropin concentrations as a risk factor for atrial fibrillation in older persons. N Engl J Med 1994;331:1249

33. Tenerz A, Forberg R, Jansson R. Is a more active attitude warranted in patients with subclinical thyrotoxicosis? J Intern Med 1990;228:229

34. Monreal M, Lafoz E, Foz M, et al. Occult thyrotoxicosis in patients with atrial fibrillation and an acute arterial embolism. Angiology 1988;39:981

35. Forfar JC, Feek CM, Miller HC, Toft AD. Atrial fibrillation and isolated suppression of the pituitary-thyroid axis: response to specific antithyroid therapy. Int J Cardiol 1981;1:43

36. Bell GM, Sawers JSA, Forfar JC, et al. The effect of minor increments in plasma thyroxine on heart rate and urinary sodium excretion. Clin Endocrinol 1983;18:511

37. Biondi B, Fazio S, Carella C, et al. Cardiac effects of long term thyrotropin-suppressive therapy with levothyroxine. J Clin Endocrinol Metab 1993;77:334

38. Tseng KH, Walfish PG, Persaud JA, Gilbert BW. Concurrent aortic and mitral valve echocardiography permits measurement of systolic time intervals as an index of peripheral tissue thyroid functional status. J Clin Endocrinol Metab 1989;69:633

39. Jennings PE, O'Malley BP, Griffin KE, et al. Relevance of increased serum thyroxine concentrations associated with normal serum triiodothyronine values in hypothyroid patients receiving thyroxine: a case for "tissue thyrotoxicosis." BMJ 1984;289:1645

40. Banovac K, Papic M, Bilsker MS, et al. Evidence of hyperthyroidism in apparently euthyroid patients treated with levothyroxine. Arch Intern Med 1989;149:809

41. Biondi B, Fazio S, Cardella C, et al. Control of adrenergic overactivity by β-blockade improves the quality of life in patients receiving long term suppressive therapy with levothyroxine. J Clin Endocrinol Metab 1994;78:1028

42. Franklyn JA, Daykin J, Betteridge J, et al. Thyroxine replacement therapy and circulating lipid concentrations. Clin Endocrinol 1993;38:453

43. Wilcox AH, Levin GE. Erythrocyte ouabain binding in patients receiving thyroxine. Clin Endocrinol 1987;27:205

44. Gow SM, Caldwell G, Toft AD, et al. Relationship between pituitary and other target organ responsiveness in hypothyroid patients receiving thyroxine replacement. J Clin Endocrinol Metab 1987;64:364

45. Bartalena L, Martino E, Pacchiarotti A, et al. Factors affecting suppression of endogenous thyrotropin secretion by thyroxine treatment: retrospective analysis in athyreotic and goitrous patients. J Clin Endocrinol Metab 1987;64:849

46. Schlote B, Schaaf, L, Schmidt R, et al. Mental and physical state in subclinical hyperthyroidism: investigations in a normal working population. Biol Psychiatry 1992;32:48

47. Ross DS. Thyroid hormone suppressive therapy of sporadic nontoxic goiter. Thyroid 1992;2:263

Werner and Ingbar's The Thyroid, Seventh Edition,
edited by Lewis E. Braverman and Robert D. Utiger.
Lippincott–Raven Publishers, Philadelphia, © 1996

89

Thyroid Disease During and After Pregnancy

Charles H. Emerson

THYROID PHYSIOLOGY AND FUNCTION IN PREGNANCY

Maternal and Maternal-Fetal Thyroid Economy in Pregnancy

Pregnancy has sweeping effects on thyroid economy. There are alterations in iodine balance, thyroid gland activity, thyroid hormone transport in serum, and peripheral metabolism of thyroxine (T_4) and triiodothyronine (T_3). These perturbations have important consequences relating to the diagnosis and management of thyroid disease in pregnant women.

SERUM THYROXINE-BINDING PROTEINS

Serum T_4-binding globulin (TBG) concentrations increase about 2.5-fold during pregnancy, peak concentrations being reached at about the 21st week.[1,2] This increase is caused by the large amounts of estrogens that are secreted by the placenta. The affinity for T_4 of the TBG produced in response to increased estrogen secretion is normal, but it is rich in triantennary oligosaccharide chains of the N-acetylgalactosamine type, which cause it to be cleared from the circulation more slowly than the TBG of nonpregnant women. Serum transthyretin concentrations do not change or decline slightly during pregnancy. Hypoalbuminemia also occurs, but this has little effect on the overall binding or distribution of T_4 in serum.

CIRCULATING THYROID SIMULATORS

The serum of pregnant women contains thyroid-stimulating activity other than thyrotropin (TSH). This activity has been postulated to be due to human chorionic gonadotropin

(hCG), especially asialo-hCG, which has more thyrotropic activity than hCG.[3,4] Shortly after implantation of the ovum, serum hCG concentrations rise sharply, doubling every other day until peak concentrations are reached near the end of the first trimester. Thereafter, they decline, falling to 5% to 10% of the peak concentration at midgestation. At the same time that serum hCG concentrations are falling there is a shift to more negative isoforms, perhaps lowering thyrotropic potency.[5] There is a second increase as term approaches, but the values remain well below those in early gestation. Thus, insofar as serum hCG contributes to serum thyroid-stimulating activity, its effects are maximal in the first trimester.

IODINE METABOLISM

The thyroid radioactive iodine uptake is increased during pregnancy.[6] One reason for this is the increase in serum thyroid-stimulating activity, probably due to hCG. Another reason may be that renal iodide clearance increases, causing a decline in maternal serum inorganic iodide concentrations and secondarily, by autoregulation, an increase in thyroid inorganic iodide clearance. In iodine-sufficient regions, however, serum inorganic iodide concentrations are similar during pregnancy as compared with values several months after delivery.[7] It seems likely, therefore, that serum thyroid-stimulating activity is largely responsible for the increase in the thyroid radioiodine uptake during pregnancy.

Iodine is transferred from mother to fetus by diffusion across the placenta. Fetal demands probably have little impact on maternal iodine balance because the needs of the fetus could be met in less than 3 days if all the maternal intake were diverted to the fetus. Despite these relatively small requirements, the thyroid gland of the fetus is vulnerable to iodine deficiency because its ability to autoregulate iodine uptake is poorly developed.[8] Thus, neonatal and fetal thyroid iodine stores are decreased in direct proportion to the degree of maternal iodine deficiency.[9]

THE PLACENTA AND MATERNAL-FETAL THYROID ECONOMY

Administration of TSH to pregnant women does not stimulate fetal thyroid function, indicating that the placenta is impermeable to TSH.[8] It is permeable to thyrotropin-releasing hormone (TRH) because, with the exception of species with epitheliochorial placentation, exogenous administration of TRH to pregnant women stimulates fetal TSH secretion.[8] TRH is, however, also degraded by the placenta.

In humans and other species there are marked gradients for T_4 and T_3 between the maternal and fetal circulations.[2,8] In addition, administration of sufficient thyroid hormone to increase maternal serum T_3 or T_4 concentrations to supraphysiologic values does not prevent fetal hypothyroidism. These observations indicate that the transfer of T_4 and T_3 between the mother and fetus is limited. Nevertheless, maternal thyroid hormones may reach the fetus very early in pregnancy,[2] and infants with thyroid agenesis or total organification defects have cord serum T_4 concentrations that are about one-third of the normal concentration,[10] indicating that some maternal T_4 is transferred to the fetus late in pregnancy. This transfer is probably important in minimizing fetal brain damage in athyroid fetuses.

Thyroid Function Tests in Pregnancy

Table 89-1 summarizes the results of thyroid function tests in pregnant women. The results are listed as normal if they are usually within the reference ranges for nonpregnant women and men. This does not always mean, however, that the mean values are the same for pregnant and nonpregnant women.

SERUM THYROXINE, TRIIODOTHYRONINE, AND OTHER IODOTHYRONINES

Serum total T_4 concentrations increase early in gestation,[11] with peak values being reached just after midgestation (Fig 89-1). There may be a modest decline in serum T_4 late in

gestation, particularly if it is prolonged beyond 40 weeks. In some regions (e.g., the United States), more than 90% of women in the third trimester have serum T_4 concentrations that are greater than the upper limit of the normal range for nonpregnant women.[12] In regions of iodine deficiency, maternal serum T_4 concentrations are lower throughout pregnancy.[13] The pattern of changes in serum T_3 concentrations during pregnancy is similar.

Serum T_4 and T_3 concentrations increase during pregnancy primarily because of the increase in serum TBG (see above and chap 6). Therefore, thyroid function must be assessed by determining serum free hormone concentrations. Serum free T_4 and T_3 concentrations are usually within the normal range in most pregnant women throughout gestation, but the mean values are in the upper normal range (or just above it) early in pregnancy, when serum hCG concentrations are highest, and decrease to the lower normal range in the

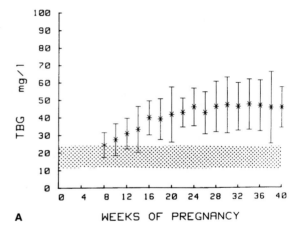

A

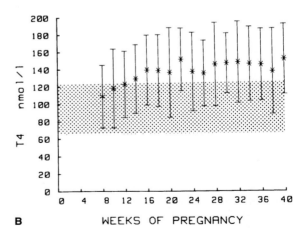

B

FIGURE 89-1. Mean (±2 SD) serum T_4 binding globulin (TBG) (*A*) and T_4 (*B*) concentrations during pregnancy in 290 normal women. The hatched area shows the normal range for nonpregnant women. To convert serum T_4 values to μg/dL divide by 12.9. (From Skjoldebrand L, Brundin J, Calstrom A, Pettersson T. Thyroid associated components in serum during normal pregnancy. Acta Endocrinol [Copenh] 1982;100:504)

TABLE 89-1.
Effect of Pregnancy on Thyroid-Function Tests

Test	Effect
Serum total T_4 concentration	Increased
Thyroid hormone–binding ratio (T_3-resin uptake)	Decreased
Serum free T_4 concentration	No change*
Serum total T_3 concentration	Increased
Serum TSH concentration	No change*
Serum thyroglobulin concentration	Increased

Serum free T_4 concentrations tend to decline and serum TSH concentrations tend to increase slightly during gestation, but most values are within the reference range for nonpregnant subjects.

third trimester. Mean serum reverse triiodothyronine (rT_3) concentrations are slightly higher in pregnant than in nonpregnant women.

SERUM THYROTROPIN AND THYROGLOBULIN CONCENTRATIONS

Serum TSH concentrations in most pregnant women are within the normal range for nonpregnant women and men.[1,2,13] Within this range, pregnancy has effects on serum TSH concentrations, suggesting that subtle alterations in thyroid secretion do occur. Specifically, serum TSH concentrations decline slightly during the first trimester,[13] probably because of the small increase in thyroid secretion engendered by hCG at this time (Fig 89-2), and then rise slightly. Serum thyroglobulin (Tg) concentrations also increase during the first trimester of pregnancy; about 50% of women have supranormal values at this time.[13,14]

Thyroid Status in Pregnancy

Thyroid hormone turnover is increased during pregnancy,[15] probably because of placental deiodination and transfer of maternal thyroid hormones.[2] In addition to the differences in thyroid status between pregnant and nonpregnant women, thyroid status changes during gestation.

FIRST TRIMESTER THYROID ACTIVATION

Serum free T_4 concentrations increase, albeit within the normal range, during the first trimester,[2,16] a change that is often accompanied by small decreases in serum TSH concentrations.[13] A few apparently normal women, as well as some women with hyperemesis gravidarum (see chap 33), have high serum free T_4 and low serum TSH concentrations, so-called gestational thyrotoxicosis. These women do not have symptoms of thyrotoxicosis, goiter, or any extrathyroidal manifestations of Graves' disease and their biochemical abnormal-

ities last no longer than a few weeks. Gestational thyrotoxicosis is probably caused by production of higher than normal amounts of asialo-hCG.[4,17]

THIRD TRIMESTER HYPOTHYROXINEMIA

Serum free T_4 and T_3 concentrations decline during the latter part of gestation,[13] due mostly to resolution of hCG-mediated thyroid activation. Serum total T_4:TBG ratios decline after the first trimester, both in iodine-sufficient regions[12] and in areas with marginal iodine deficiency.[13] Therefore, only near the end of the first trimester is the serum total T_4 concentration as high as would be expected on the basis of the increase in serum TBG. The physiologic importance of the marginal decline in serum free T_4 and T_3 concentrations in the latter part of gestation is not known. It becomes more pronounced if gestation extends beyond 40 weeks[12] and also occurs in laboratory animals.

THYROID DISEASES IN PREGNANCY

Goiter, Thyroid Nodules, and Thyroid Cancer

Goiter has been associated with pregnancy since antiquity. Thyroid volume increases by about 10% in iodine-sufficient regions, probably as a result of the increase in serum thyrotropic activity, and by approximately 30% in regions of mild iodine deficiency, where serum TSH concentrations tend to be higher as well. The ability of TSH and presumably other thyroid stimulators to promote thyroid growth is potentiated by iodine deficiency.

Palpable thyroid enlargement is abnormal in the pregnant woman whose iodine intake is adequate. If thyroid enlargement is detected and it is accompanied by clinical manifestations of hypothyroidism or thyrotoxicosis, prompt evaluation is indicated. If a discrete nodule is present a fine-needle aspi-

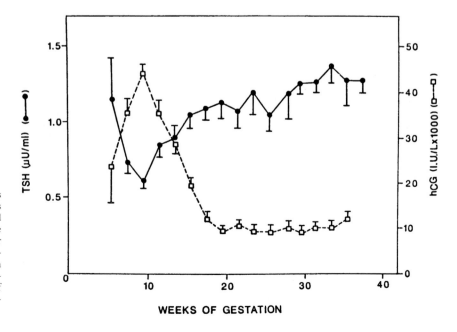

FIGURE 89-2. Serum TSH and hCG concentrations as a function of gestational age. Serum hCG was determined at the time of initial evaluation and serum TSH at the initial evaluation and during late gestation. Each symbol is the mean value (±SE) for samples pooled for 2 weeks of gestation and corresponds to the average of determinations for hCG in 33 women and for TSH in 49 women. (From Glinoer D, DeNayer P, Bourdoux P, et al. Regulation of maternal thyroid during pregnancy. J Clin Endocrinol Metab 1990;71:276)

ration biopsy should be performed, but thyroid imaging studies with radionuclides are contraindicated. Most thyroid nodules detected during pregnancy are not malignant; those that are malignant are usually papillary carcinomas. If the biopsy suggests thyroid carcinoma, the decision as to when to perform surgical resection should be individualized, based on the type of carcinoma, the stage of pregnancy, and tumor stage. Differentiated thyroid cancer is not thought to be adversely affected by pregnancy,[18] so that unless the tumor is growing rapidly or is highly malignant, it may be best for the fetus to delay surgery until after delivery.[19]

Hypothyroidism and Pregnancy

MATERNAL HYPOTHYROIDISM AND THE FETUS

Hypothyroidism is not a complete barrier to conception, but it decreases fertility in both humans and animals. In women who do become pregnant the first trimester miscarriage rate is increased. In the past there was a higher rate of preeclampsia, placental abruption, and perinatal morbidity. Now most hypothyroid women have a more favorable outcome, probably because their hypothyroidism is detected and they are treated earlier.[20] A poor outcome is correlated with the severity of maternal hypothyroidism.[21] Nevertheless, even subclinical hypothyroidism has been associated with increased rates of spontaneous miscarriage and premature delivery.[22] This may not be entirely due to hypothyroidism per se, however, but to the fact that thyroid autoimmunity, by far the most common cause of subclinical hypothyroidism, is associated with an increased risk of miscarriage.[23]

Maternal hypothyroidism also may have an adverse effect on fetal development. In one study, the incidence of motor and mental retardation in 8- to 12-month-old infants whose mothers had been severely hypothyroid during pregnancy was higher than in infants whose mothers were marginally hypothyroid or euthyroid.[24] In another study,[25] maternal hypothyroxinemia was associated with abnormal development of the progeny, and the frequency of these abnormalities was lower if the mother received thyroid hormone treatment during pregnancy. Some of the women in these studies, however, may not have been hypothyroid because the diagnosis of hypothyroidism was based on thyroid function tests that are now outdated and the incidence of hypothyroidism was much higher than would be expected from current studies that use more sensitive and specific thyroid function tests. A recent study revealed no evidence for impaired mental development in children whose mothers were hypothyroid for the first 13 to 28 weeks of gestation.[26]

DIAGNOSIS AND TREATMENT OF MATERNAL HYPOTHYROIDISM

The serum TSH concentration is the most sensitive test for primary hypothyroidism. If it is elevated, the serum free T_4 concentration should be determined, either by a direct method or by measuring the serum free T_4 index (see chaps 18 and 76). The combination of elevated serum TSH and low free T_4 values is virtually diagnostic of primary hypothyroidism. Borderline low serum free T_4 and slightly elevated serum TSH concentrations have been found in some pregnant women with preeclampsia and during the recovery phase of severe nonthyroidal illness. Central hypothyroidism should be diagnosed by the usual criteria (see chaps 59 and 76) but is very rare in pregnant women.

Women with symptoms or signs of hypothyroidism, a goiter, a history of thyroid disease, or who are taking a medication with antithyroid properties should have serum TSH concentrations determined at their first prenatal visit. Other findings that increase the possibility of hypothyroidism are a history of an autoimmune disorder or a family history of hypothyroidism, chronic autoimmune thyroiditis, or Graves' disease.

Pregnant women with newly diagnosed hypothyroidism, even subclinical hypothyroidism, should be treated with T_4 in a dose that is close to the anticipated requirement. This dose should be instituted immediately rather than, as is sometimes done in nonpregnant patients, beginning therapy with a relatively small dose and increasing the dose gradually. Serum TSH should be measured 4 to 6 weeks after the initiation of T_4 therapy and the dose of T_4 adjusted as necessary if the serum TSH is not normal.

Women with hypothyroidism receiving T_4 therapy should have measurements of serum TSH and free T_4 about 4 to 8 weeks after they become pregnant, even if the dosage had not been changed recently. The reason is that many hypothyroid women require a larger dose of T_4 to maintain the euthyroid state when they are pregnant.[2] The average increase is about 50%, but individual needs vary[15] (Fig 89-3). Serum TSH concentration should be measured approximately every 2 months

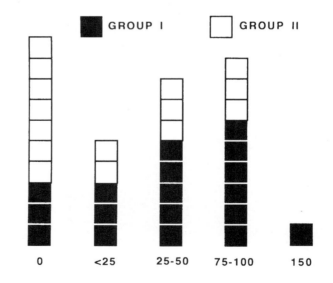

FIGURE 89-3. Increments in T_4 dose required to achieve a euthyroid state in pregnant women in whom the optimal dose was known both before and during pregnancy. Each square represents one women. The women in group 1 were hypothyroid because they had received ^{131}I therapy or had undergone thyroidectomy. The women in group 2 had hypothyroidism secondary to chronic autoimmune thyroiditis. (From Kaplan MM. Monitoring thyroxine treatment during pregnancy. Thyroid 1992;2:147)

during pregnancy to ensure that T_4 therapy is optimal.[27] After delivery the pre-pregnancy dose of T_4 can be resumed; serum TSH should be measured about 6 weeks later.

Severe iodine deficiency, an intake of less than 50μ of iodide per day, is the major cause of endemic goiter and is associated with varying degrees of maternal and fetal thyroid hormone insufficiency. Iodine supplementation is clearly needed for persons with this degree of iodine deficiency and should be instituted at the very beginning of pregnancy or preferably before conception to minimize fetal brain damage.[28] The optimal iodine intake for pregnant women has not been established but is probably about 150 to 200μ/d.[29,30] In a region of mild iodine deficiency where the iodine intake was 50 to 80μ/d, a daily supplement of 100μ during pregnancy normalized the marginally elevated serum TSH concentrations, minimized maternal thyroid growth during pregnancy, and was associated with lower thyroid weights in the neonates.[30]

DIAGNOSIS AND TREATMENT OF FETAL HYPOTHYROIDISM

The development of a goiter in the fetus can be associated with either fetal hypothyroidism or fetal hyperthyroidism. As noted below, fetal thyrotoxicosis is usually distinguished by fetal hyperactivity and tachycardia. There is currently no convenient and safe way to monitor fetal thyroid function during pregnancy although cordocentesis can be done to obtain fetal blood if absolutely necessary.[31] Amniotic fluid thyroid hormone or TSH measurements are not useful in the diagnosis of fetal hypothyroidism. Usually the diagnosis of congenital hypothyroidism is delayed until the time of neonatal screening but, even so, prompt institution of thyroid hormone treatment generally produces satisfactory results[2] (see section on congenital hypothyroidism in chap 85).

The possibility of fetal hypothyroidism (or hyperthyroidism) must be considered when treating pregnant women with a history of thyroid disease. This includes women who are euthyroid but have a past history of Graves' hyperthyroidism and those with chronic autoimmune thyroiditis. Fortunately, despite the high prevalence of the latter, very few women with this condition have hypothyroid infants, and those who do usually have high serum titers of TSH-blocking antibodies. Fetal hypothyroidism has, on rare occasions, been treated by intra-amniotic injection of T_4. This treatment may be beneficial in selected cases but, as noted recently, "whether treatment in utero of the occasional fetus with hypothyroidism is necessary or desirable remains to be demonstrated,"[2] and it is best instituted only after consultation with experts.

Thyrotoxicosis and Pregnancy

INCIDENCE AND DIFFERENTIAL DIAGNOSIS

Maternal thyrotoxicosis occurs in about 0.2% of all pregnancies.[1] Because thyrotoxicosis does not markedly impair fertility, all women in their childbearing years who are being treated for thyrotoxicosis should be counseled that their illness does not lessen their chances of becoming pregnant and that they should not become pregnant at a time when their thyroid function is abnormal. They should also be made aware

that pregnancy imposes additional complexities in the management of thyrotoxicosis and potential risks for the fetus. Certain treatments may reduce but not eliminate these risks, particularly if the cause of the thyrotoxicosis is Graves' disease. Except for hCG- mediated hyperthyroidism, the causes of thyrotoxicosis in pregnant women are the same as those in the general population. Among them, Graves' disease is by far the most common.

Maternal thyrotoxicosis predisposes to miscarriage. It is important, therefore, to treat these women with an antithyroid drug unless the thyrotoxicosis is mild or likely to be transient. For example, women with the hyperthyroidism of hyperemesis gravidarum rarely require antithyroid drug treatment, particularly because there is no evidence that such treatment alleviates hyperemesis.

CLINICAL FEATURES AND DIAGNOSIS

Healthy pregnant women have many of the physiologic changes and some clinical manifestations of thyrotoxicosis. These include increases in basal metabolic rate, respiratory rate, cardiac stroke volume, and heart rate; heat intolerance, excessive perspiration, emotional lability, palpitations, and tachycardia also occur. These symptoms and signs are more marked in pregnant women if they also have thyrotoxicosis. Features that are more specific for thyrotoxicosis in pregnant women are lid lag, muscle weakness, and goiter. Inadequate weight gain for gestational age or weight loss also occurs but appropriate weight gain does not exclude thyrotoxicosis.

The diagnosis of thyrotoxicosis can be established by the findings of low or undetectable serum TSH and high serum free T_4 values (see chap 52). Clinical features, serum tests, and, if need be, ultrasonography must be relied on to ascertain the cause of thyrotoxicosis because thyroid radionuclide scans and radioiodine (^{131}I or ^{123}I) uptake tests cannot be performed during pregnancy.

TREATMENT

Some methods for treating thyrotoxicosis cannot be used and others must be modified if the patient is pregnant. The antithyroid drugs methimazole (MMI), carbimazole (CBM), and propylthiouracil (PTU) all have the potential for causing fetal hypothyroidism. They have not, however, been implicated as a cause of impaired intellectual development in children whose mothers received them while pregnant.[32] The fetal bioavailability of MMI and CBM may be greater than that of PTU,[32,33] but there is little evidence that the incidence of neonatal hypothyroxinemia or goiter is greater in infants whose mothers received MMI or CBM as compared with PTU. Nevertheless, in part because of its decreased fetal bioavailability, PTU is used more frequently than MMI or CBM in North America.[1,32]

Another reason for this preference is the possible association between MMI and aplasia cutis in the fetus. Aplasia cutis is a focal circumscribed area of the neonatal scalp that lacks skin layers. Most lesions are less than 3 cm in diameter and heal with epithelialization of the skin but not necessarily hair growth. Approximately 17 cases of aplasia cutis were described between 1972 and 1994 in neonates of mothers who received MMI or CBM during pregnancy. A few of these women also received PTU. A confounding factor is that thyroid disease, in the absence of antithyroid drug treatment, has also been associated with aplasia cutis. Thus, the original report describing an association between aplasia cutis and MMI treatment included an additional woman whose only medication during pregnancy was thyroid extract.[34] In addition, the association of aplasia cutis with thyroid disease, and no antithyroid drug treatment, was noted in three successive generations.[35] No cases were found in a series of 117 infants whose mothers received MMI during their pregnancy,[36] and a significant association between maternal MMI or CBM therapy and aplasia cutis was not found in a survey of skin defects among 49,091 infants born at a large hospital during a 27-year period.[37] It is, therefore, uncertain whether there is a causal relationship between MMI and aplasia cutis.

Therapy with ^{131}I is absolutely contraindicated as a treatment for thyrotoxicosis in pregnancy because it is readily transferred across the placenta.[8] It is taken up by the fetal thyroid as early as the 12th week of gestation. It is not surprising, therefore, that inadvertent ^{131}I therapy during pregnancy has been associated with the development of congenital hypothyroidism. This therapy also is contraindicated because of the substantial radiation dose delivered to all fetal organs.

Stable iodine, in doses of 10 mg or greater, decreases thyroid hormone secretion and blood flow in patients with Graves' hyperthyroidism. Its therapeutic value is, however, limited. The administration of stable iodine to pregnant women with Graves' hyperthyroidism,[38] or the ingestion of pharmacologic doses of iodine in women with no thyroid disease,[8] may cause fetal goiter, probably due to immaturity of the system that mediates escape from the antithyroid actions of iodine (see section on effect of excess iodide in chap 14). In women with Graves' hyperthyroidism the development of fetal goiter may be potentiated by maternal TSH receptor-stimulating antibodies (TRAb).

Propranolol is not widely used in pregnant women with thyrotoxicosis. One reason is a retrospective study that suggested that it caused fetal growth retardation, although several prospective studies found no such effect.[39] Maternal propranolol administration at the time of delivery has been associated with delayed onset of spontaneous respiration, bradycardia, and hypoglycemia in the neonates. Prospective studies of pregnant women with cardiovascular disorders indicate that the incidence of these problems is low and may be unrelated to propranolol administration.[40] Even so, there seldom is any reason to use propranolol in pregnant women with thyrotoxicosis.

MANAGEMENT

Antithyroid drugs are the mainstay of treatment for pregnant women with thyrotoxicosis.[1,32] The primary goal is to control maternal thyrotoxicosis without adversely affecting fetal thyroid function. Occasionally an antithyroid drug is given to treat fetal hyperthyroidism caused by transplacental passage of maternal TRAb. Availability as well as preference influence the choice of MMI, CBM, or PTU in different parts of the world. If all three drugs are available and the patient has not yet received any of them, PTU is preferred. This recommendation is based on the impression that PTU is safer, because ma-

ternal-fetal transfer of MMI is greater, and the risk of aplasia cutis in the neonate is lower.[32] If a women is taking MMI or CBM when she becomes pregnant, changing to PTU might be considered.[32] The arguments in favor of PTU are noted above, but there are also reasons for continuing MMI or CBM. MMI, when given in low doses that are nonetheless effective, is probably less likely to cause agranulocytosis than PTU. In addition, control of thyrotoxicosis may be lost during the change in drug, for several reasons. The woman may be unable to tolerate PTU,[32] it may be difficult to find a bioequivalent dose of PTU, or compliance may be more difficult because PTU treatment often requires multiple daily doses, whereas MMI or CBM can usually be given once daily.

Therapy with PTU should be started in a dose of 150 to 200 mg every 12 hours. In severely symptomatic patients, it should be administered every 6 or 8 hours. Daily doses of more than 20 to 30 mg of MMI (or CBM) should not be used, not only because they increase the risk of fetal hypothyroidism, but also because higher doses increase the risk of agranulocytosis. Moreover, fairly rapid control of thyrotoxicosis can be achieved with low doses of MMI. Further guidelines and the indications for discontinuing or changing to a different antithyroid drug are described in chapter 53.

A response to PTU or MMI can be expected within 1 to 2 weeks after initiation of therapy. Lack of response is usually due to noncompliance rather than resistance to the antithyroid drug, and hospitalization may be needed to ensure compliance. As indexes of maternal thyroid function improve, the dose of antithyroid drug should be reduced to maintain the maternal serum free T_4 concentration or free T_4 index in the upper part of their respective normal range or the serum TSH concentration at the lower end of its normal range, or both. The only reason to supplement antithyroid drug therapy with T_4 in a pregnant woman is to treat maternal hypothyroidism if it develops in a mother who is receiving an antithyroid drug to treat fetal hyperthyroidism (see below). T_4 should not be added to the antithyroid drug regimen with the idea of preventing antithyroid drug-induced fetal hypothyroidism because doing so increases the dose of antithyroid drug required to control maternal thyrotoxicosis, thereby increasing the risk of fetal hypothyroidism.[41] A more recent rationale for combining T_4 with an antithyroid drug is that it may reduce the likelihood of postpartum relapse of Graves' disease.[42] Even if this is the case, however, the benefit to the mother is probably less than the risk of hypothyroidism in the fetus.

Subtotal thyroidectomy should be considered only if serious side effects are associated with antithyroid drug therapy. The optimal time for surgery is during the second trimester. Propranolol and iodide can be used to prepare the patient for surgery. Otherwise, these drugs should be reserved for severe or life-threatening thyrotoxicosis or for those patients who have a serious adverse reaction to antithyroid drugs and are poor surgical candidates. In this situation, relatively small doses of inorganic iodide, 5 to 40 mg daily, should be given to minimize the risk of fetal goiter.[43]

Regardless of whether or not the maternal response to antithyroid drug therapy is good, attention must also be directed toward fetal thyroid status, particularly during the last half of gestation. This is true even in euthyroid women with a history of treated Graves' hyperthyroidism. In them, TRAb production may persist or increase and cause fetal or neonatal thyrotoxicosis. Fetal tachycardia and hyperactivity are the hallmarks of fetal thyrotoxicosis.[44] Fetal thyrotoxicosis should be treated because it can cause intrauterine death and developmental abnormalities in survivors[44] (Fig 89-4). If fetal thyrotoxicosis is strongly suspected, a rational approach would be to give the mother an antithyroid drug (or increase the dose if she were already taking an antithyroid drug). If the clinical response in the fetus is satisfactory but hypothyroidism develops in a mother not already taking T_4, she should be given it. Fetal thyrotoxicosis requiring antithyroid drug therapy usually occurs in euthyroid or hypothyroid women who had received ablative treatment for Graves' hyperthyroidism before they became pregnant.

Thyroid receptor antibodies have been measured in an attempt to predict intrauterine or neonatal thyroid status, but the practical clinical value of the tests is less important than careful attention to the clinical manifestations of thyrotoxicosis in the fetus. Moreover, it is necessary to consider the clinical status of the mother and the method used for measurement of TRAb. In women with chronic autoimmune thyroiditis, high serum titers of TSH-blocking antibodies are associated with fetal hypothyroidism, not fetal thyrotoxicosis[45]; these antibodies cannot be distinguished from stimulating antibodies in TSH-binding inhibition assays (see chap 21). Measurements of TRAb are most useful in women who have a history of delivering infants with neonatal or fetal thyrotoxicosis. However, these assays are principally research tools and are generally not suitable for routine use. Less than 8% of pregnant women with Graves' disease have fetuses or neonates with thyrotoxicosis and in many its clinical and biochemical manifestations are not severe enough to require treatment.[46]

The clinical response to antithyroid drug treatment is satisfactory, in both mother and fetus, in most pregnant women with Graves' hyperthyroidism, and treatment often can be discontinued during pregnancy because the underlying activity of Graves' disease declines as gestation proceeds. It may be worthwhile, however, to continue a very low dose of antithyroid drug throughout gestation to reduce the risk for neonatal thyrotoxicosis and further reduce the very small risk of thyroid storm during labor and delivery if there is a relapse. It may be helpful to monitor fetal thyroid size by ultrasonography as an indication of overtreatment in women with a history of delivering goitrous infants,[47] or if there is fetal exposure to iodine or to an unusually large dose of antithyroid drug. At birth the infant should be examined carefully for signs of hypothyroidism or thyrotoxicosis and cord serum TSH concentration and free T_4 index measured (see chap 86).

After delivery, the dose of antithyroid drug may need to be increased because of the tendency for Graves' disease to worsen or relapse at this time. Studies of nursing infants whose mothers were taking an antithyroid drug are limited. No antithyroid effects were noted in one series in infants of women who took PTU while breast-feeding.[48] Even so, thyroid function should be evaluated periodically in any infant being nursed by a woman who is taking any antithyroid drug.

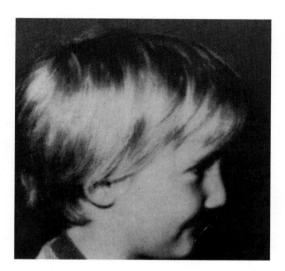

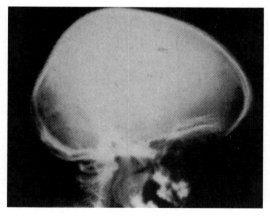

FIGURE 89-4. Skull abnormalities (frontal bossing and partial craniosynostosis) in a child who had fetal and neonatal thyrotoxicosis. The abnormality was attributed to the accelerating effect of thyroid hormone on skeletal maturation. (From Cove DH, Johnston P. Fetal hyperthyroidism: experience of treatment in four siblings. Lancet 1985;1:430)

POSTPARTUM THYROID DYSFUNCTION

Causes of Postpartum Thyroid Dysfunction

Postpartum thyroid dysfunction occurs in a relatively high percentage of recently pregnant women.[49] Postpartum pituitary infarction, a circulatory disorder, was the earliest cause of postpartum thyroid dysfunction to be identified. This syndrome is due to excessive vaginal bleeding and hypotension at the time of delivery. Hypothyroidism may develop insidiously and often is preceded by symptoms of prolactin and gonadotropin deficiency. Postpartum pituitary infarction is now rare in developed countries. Another unusual cause of postpartum thyroid dysfunction is lymphocytic hypophysitis. It is characterized by enlargement of the sella turcica, headache, and sometimes the development of secondary hypopituitarism. There may be signs of increased intracranial pressure or optic compression.

Postpartum thyroiditis and postpartum Graves' disease are far more common than either postpartum pituitary infarction or lymphocytic hypophysitis. Postpartum thyroiditis, postpartum Graves' disease, and lymphocytic hypophysitis are all immunologic disorders. The temporal aspect of their presentation is probably related to reequilibration of the immune system after pregnancy, either by natural delivery or by abortion.

Immune Function and Autoimmunity During and After Pregnancy

A fundamental question about pregnancy is why the fetus, which is endowed with paternal antigens, is not rejected by the mother. Pregnant women have fewer helper T cells (CD4) and more suppressor-cytotoxic T cells (CD8) during the latter part of pregnancy as compared with earlier in gestation.[50] As reflected by these changes in T cells, pregnancy may be considered a period of immune suppression. Blocking antibodies, disparity in HLA class II antigens between mother and father, differential endocrine and cytokine expression, and pregnancy-associated immunoregulatory proteins are all thought to contribute to the unique immune status of pregnancy.[51] In addition to its putative thyroid-stimulating properties, hCG may also have immunoregulatory properties.

Clinical observations, such as increased susceptibility to infection, enhancement of tumor growth, and prolongation of graft rejection, also suggest that generalized immunosuppression is characteristic for much of pregnancy.[51] Most autoimmune disorders, including Graves' disease and chronic autoimmune thyroiditis, tend to remit during gestation. Thus, in women with Graves' hyperthyroidism, the dose of antithyroid drug can usually be reduced or the drug discontinued in late pregnancy. In women with chronic autoimmune thyroiditis, antithyroid antibody titers decline and may become undetectable.[52]

The activity of autoimmune thyroid diseases as well as some nonendocrine autoimmune diseases[53] may be increased in the first trimester. Women with Graves' disease who are in remission tend to relapse soon after they become pregnant. This has been attributed to hCG, however, and not to a first trimester increase in TRAb.[54] On the other hand, natural killer cell activity is increased in the first trimester.[50] Whereas the incidence and titer of antithyroid antibodies are similar in nonpregnant women and in pregnant women in the third trimester,[55] both are clearly higher in the first trimester than in the third trimester.

Autoimmune diseases are prone to relapse after delivery. Women with low serum antithyroid antibody titers at the time of delivery have increases shortly thereafter, regardless of whether their underlying condition is Graves' disease or chronic autoimmune thyroiditis[50] (Fig 89-5). The antithyroid antibody titers are highest from 3 to 7 months after delivery and decline thereafter,[49] but they are still higher 1 year later than at term. The postpartum increase in antithyroid antibody titers is accompanied by a higher frequency of thyroid dysfunction than occurs in women without these antibodies,[56] and there is a good correlation between the timing of the changes in thyroid status and the increase in serum antithyroid antibody titers. CD45RA T cells also increase after delivery in normal women. The increase in these cells and antithyroid antibody titers is greater in women who subsequently develop postpartum thyroiditis.[50,52]

Postpartum Graves' Disease and Postpartum Thyroiditis

CLINICAL FEATURES AND DIFFERENTIAL ASPECTS

By definition, postpartum Graves' disease is Graves' disease presenting in the first year after delivery. Postpartum Graves' disease is a common cause of postpartum thyrotoxicosis. For example, more than half of Swedish women with Graves' disease who are in their active childbearing years are diagnosed within a year after they deliver.[57] An even more common cause of postpartum thyrotoxicosis is postpartum thyroiditis. The primary manifestations of either disorder are symptoms and signs of thyrotoxicosis. Thyroid enlargement may occur in both postpartum Graves' disease and postpartum thyroiditis, but is usually greater in the former. In postpartum thyroiditis, a rise in serum Tg concentration generally precedes the development of thyrotoxicosis by several weeks, whereas in postpartum Graves' disease this increase occurs at the time of the onset of thyrotoxicosis.[58] In Graves' disease the thyroid ^{131}I uptake is high, whereas in postpartum thyroiditis it is low. Postpartum thyroiditis may also occur at the same time as a relapse of Graves' hyperthyroidism, based on the finding of low thyroid ^{131}I uptake values in about 25%

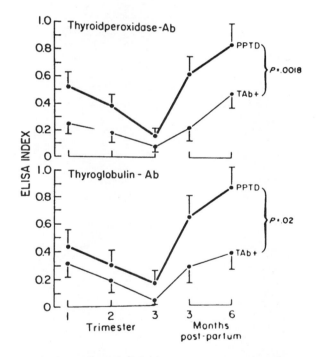

FIGURE 89-5. Antithyroid antibodies in serum during pregnancy and after delivery in thyroid antibody-positive women who did not develop postpartum thyroiditis (TAb+ group), and in thyroid antibody-positive women tho developed postpartum thyroiditis (PPTD group). In both groups there was a decline in antithyroid antibody titers during gestation and a rebound rise after delivery. The titers of thyroid autoantibodies were higher, however, in women who developed postpartum thyroiditis. (From Stagnaro-Green A, Roman SH, Cobin RH, El-Harazy E, Wallenstein S, Davies TF. A prospective study of lymphocyte-initiated immunosuppression in normal pregnancy: evidence of a T cell etiology for postpartum thyroid dysfunction. J Clin Endcrinol Metab 1992;74:645)

of women with a history of Graves' disease who developed postpartum thyrotoxicosis.[59]

Postpartum thyroiditis is more common than postpartum Graves' disease. The syndrome is in most respects similar to silent thyroiditis (see chap 34), except that the patients are women in their first year after delivery rather than other women or men. Early reports described the development of painless thyroid enlargement in women with goitrous autoimmune thyroiditis several months after childbirth. Many years later, the association of postpartum goiter, or enlargement of a preexisting goiter, transient hypothyroidism, and high titers of antithyroid antibodies was described. Shortly thereafter, similar women who had transient thyrotoxicosis before developing hypothyroidism were reported. Subsequent studies have shown that transient thyrotoxicosis alone, transient hypothyroidism alone, and thyrotoxicosis followed in several weeks by hypothyroidism occur with almost equal frequency in postpartum women.[49] The thyrotoxicosis usually occurs 2 to 4 months after delivery and lasts 2 to 6 weeks. The hypothyroidism, whether preceded by thyrotoxicosis or not, usually occurs 3 to 8 months after delivery and also lasts 2 to 6 weeks. The severity of the different phases of thyroid dysfunction varies. In most patients, the clinical manifestations of either thyrotoxicosis, hypothyroidism, or both, are mild, and thyroid function normalizes within 3 to 9 months after delivery. These women are prone to recurrence after subsequent pregnancies, however, as well as to the eventual development of permanent hypothyroidism.

There has been considerable interest in whether postpartum thyroiditis is an important cause of postpartum mental disturbances. No significant differences in thyroid function were found in hospitalized psychotic postpartum women and control postpartum women matched for age and time since delivery.[60] Although an association between antithyroid antibodies and postpartum depression has been reported,[61] no increase in the incidence of postpartum depression in women who had positive antithyroid antibodies during gestation was found in another study.[62] Despite these data it seems worthwhile to evaluate thyroid function in all women with postpartum mental disturbances.

EPIDEMIOLOGY AND PATHOGENESIS OF POSTPARTUM THYROIDITIS

Postpartum thyroiditis has been described in many regions of the world. Its incidence in postpartum women ranges from 3% to 16%, as determined by serial biochemical studies[49]; the frequency of clinical manifestations of thyroid dysfunction is lower. This diversity is probably related to the design of the screening programs, the diagnostic criteria used, and differences in susceptibility resulting from environmental and genetic factors. Patients with insulin-dependent diabetes mellitus have an even higher incidence of postpartum thyroiditis than the general population.[63] HLA status influences the incidence of postpartum thyroiditis. As is true for other organ-specific autoimmune diseases, it is associated with various HLA-B and HLA-D haplotypes in different populations.[64] As in other forms of autoimmune thyroiditis, a high iodine intake probably increases the incidence of postpartum thyroiditis.

Postpartum thyroiditis appears to be a specific, thyroid-directed process rather than a polyclonal activation of B cells.[65] The destructive nature of the process may be linked in part to the enhanced complement-fixing activity of antithyroid peroxidase antibodies.[66] Large-bore needle biopsies in the thyrotoxic phase of postpartum thyroiditis often show follicular disruption and focal or diffuse lymphocytic infiltration[67]; during recovery, focal infiltration with lymphocytes is characteristic. HLA-DR antigen expression is increased, especially on the cells of disrupted thyroid follicles.[67] These findings, the association of postpartum thyroiditis with positive tests for antithyroid antibodies, and the fact that women with a history of postpartum thyroiditis are at increased risk for developing permanent hypothyroidism are reasons why postpartum thyroiditis should be considered a form of chronic autoimmune thyroiditis. Unlike classic chronic autoimmune thyroiditis, however, oncocytic metaplasia is lacking and there is minimal to absent follicular atrophy and little or no fibrosis.[68]

DIAGNOSIS AND TREATMENT

It is worthwhile to warn pregnant women with a history of thyroid disease that their underlying disorder may worsen after delivery. Although postpartum thyroiditis is not responsible for most cases of postpartum psychosis, postpartum women with nervousness, depression, lethargy, or emotional lability should have thyroid function tests. There should be a high index of suspicion for testing women with a personal or family history of thyroid disease as well as those with insulin-dependent diabetes mellitus. Although testing for antithyroid antibodies during pregnancy has predictive value for the development of postpartum thyroiditis, the value of the test in clinical practice remains to be determined.

Thyroid function should be tested in the same way as it is in any patient suspected of having thyroid dysfunction. The serum TSH concentration should be measured; if abnormal, the serum free T_4 index or free T_4 concentration should be measured, preferably in the same sample used for the TSH measurement. Occasional patients with postpartum thyroiditis have serum antibodies that bind T_4 (or T_3), and therefore may have artefactually abnormal values in assays for serum total T_4 (or T_3)[69] (see chaps 18 and 21). In postpartum women with thyrotoxicosis in whom there is doubt about the cause—the thyroid gland is normal in size or minimally enlarged, there is no ophthalmopathy, and the woman is sufficiently symptomatic that some therapy is indicated (and she is not nursing)—thyroid ^{131}I uptake should be measured. A low value confirms a diagnosis of postpartum thyroiditis. A high value is usually indicative of Graves' hyperthyroidism, but the value also can be high transiently during the recovery phase in postpartum thyroiditis.

Most women with thyrotoxicosis caused by postpartum thyroiditis have relatively few symptoms, which usually do not last more than a few weeks, and therefore they do not require any treatment. Those who are more symptomatic can be treated with a β-adrenergic antagonist drug until their thyrotoxicosis subsides. Postpartum women with Graves' hyperthyroidism should be treated as they would be if their thyrotoxicosis had occurred at any other time (see chap 53).

Similarly, most women with postpartum hypothyroidism require no treatment, for the same reasons—the symptoms are mild and transient. More symptomatic women can be treated with small doses of T_4, for example 50 to 75 µg/d. If their serum TSH concentration remains high despite treatment with these doses of T_4 for several weeks, then the possibility that they have permanent hypothyroidism should be considered.

Close follow-up is important in all women with postpartum thyroiditis because, as is evident from this discussion, their thyroid function is unstable. Approximately one-fourth of them are found to be hypothyroid when tested 2 to 4 years later,[70] and others have a goiter. Therefore, they should be counseled about the need for long-term follow-up. Similar advice should be given to women with postpartum Graves' disease, even if their thyrotoxicosis remits.

Administration of T_4 during the latter part of pregnancy and the first year postpartum has been associated with a decreased incidence of postpartum relapse of Graves' hyperthyroidism.[42] The disadvantage of combining T_4 with an antithyroid drug during pregnancy has already been discussed. Whether T_4 supplementation would be equally effective in decreasing the incidence of postpartum relapse if it were started immediately after delivery, rather than during pregnancy, is not known.

References

1. Burrow GN. Thyroid function and hyperfunction during gestation. Endocr Rev 1993;14:194
2. Burrow GN, Fisher DA, Larsen PR. Maternal and fetal thyroid function. N Engl J Med 1994;331:1072
3. Hershman JM. Role of human chorionic gonadotropin as a thyroid stimulator. J Clin Endocrinol Metab 1992;74:258
4. Yamazaki K, Sato K, Shizume K, et al. Potent thyrotropic activity of human chorionic gonadotropin variants in terms of 125-I incorporation and de novo synthesized thyroid hormone release in human thyroid follicles. J Clin Endocrinol Metab 1995;80:473
5. Wide L, Lee JY, Rasmussen C. A change in the isoforms of human chorionic gonadotropin occurs around the 13th week of gestation. J Clin Endocrinol Metab 1994;78:1419
6. Aboul-Khair SA, Crooks J, Turnbull AC, Hytten FE. The physiological changes in thyroid function during pregnancy. Clin Sci 1964;27:195
7. Liberman C, Pino SC, Emerson CH. Pregnancy and serum non-protein bound iodine. Thyroid 1994;4:S-6
8. Roti E, Gnudi A, Braverman LE. The placental transport, synthesis and metabolism of hormones and drugs which affect thyroid function. Endocr Rev 1983;4:131
9. Delange F, Walfish P, Willgerodt H, et al. Reduction in the iodine stores of the thyroid in iodine deficient newborns. Horm Res 1989;31(suppl 1):75
10. Vulsma T, Gons MH, de Vijlder JJ. Maternal-fetal transfer of thyroxine in congenital hypothyroidism due to total organification defect or thyroid agenesis. N Engl J Med 1989;321:13
11. Skjoldebrand L, Brundin J, Carlstrom A, Pettersson T. Thyroid associated components in serum during normal pregnancy. Acta Endocrinol (Copenh) 1982;100:504
12. Guillaume J, Schussler GC, Goldman J, et al. Components of the total thyroid hormone concentrations during pregnancy: high free thyroxine and blunted thyrotropin (TSH) response to TSH-releasing hormone in the first trimester. J Clin Endocrinol Metab 1985;60:678
13. Glinoer D, De Nayer P, Bourdoux P, et al. Regulation of maternal thyroid during pregnancy. J Clin Endocrinol Metab 1990;71:276
14. Rasmussen NG, Hornnes PJ, Hegedus L, Feldt-Rasmussen U. Serum thyroglobulin during the menstrual cycle, during pregnancy, and postpartum. Acta Endocrinol (Copenh) 1989;121:168
15. Kaplan MM. Monitoring thyroxine treatment during pregnancy. Thyroid 1992;2:147
16. Kimura M, Amino N, Tamaki H, et al. Physiologic thyroid activation in normal early pregnancy is induced by circulating hCG. Obstet Gynecol 1990;75:775
17. Tsuruta E, Tada H, Tamaki H, et al. Pathogenic role of asialo human chorionic gonadotropin in gestational thyrotoxicosis. J Clin Endocrinol Metab 1995; 80:350
18. Choe W, McDougall IR. Thyroid cancer in pregnant women: diagnostic and therapeutic management. Thyroid 1994;4:433
19. Herzon FS, Morris DM, Segal MN, et al. Coexistent thyroid cancer and pregnancy. Arch Otolaryngol Head Neck Surg 1994;120:1191
20. Montoro M, Collea JV, Frasier SD, Mestman JH. Successful outcome of pregnancy in women with hypothyroidism. Ann Intern Med 1981;94:31
21. Davis LE, Leveno KJ, Cunningham FG. Hypothyroidism complicating pregnancy. Obstet Gynecol 1988;72:108
22. Glinoer D, Riahi M, Grun J, Kinthaert J. Risk of subclinical hypothyroidism in pregnant women with asymptomatic autoimmune thyroid disorders. J Clin Endocrinol Metab 1994;79:197
23. Stagnaro-Green A, Roman SH, Cobin RH, et al. Detection of at-risk pregnancy by means of highly sensitive assays for thyroid autoantibodies. JAMA 1990;264:1422
24. Greenman GW, Gabrielson MO, Howard-Flanders J, Wessel MA. Thyroid dysfunction in pregnancy. N Engl J Med 1962;267:426
25. Man EB, Serunian SA. Thyroid function in human pregnancy. IX. Development of retardation of 7-year-old progeny of hypothyroxinemic women. Am J Obstet Gynecol 1976;125:949
26. Liu H, Momotani N, Noh JY, et al. Maternal hypothyroidism during early pregnancy and intellectual development of the progeny. Arch Intern Med 1994;154:785
27. Mandel SJ, Brent G, Larsen PR. Levothyroxine therapy in patients with thyroid disease. Ann Intern Med 1193;119:492
28. Xue-Yi C, Xin-Min J, Zhi-Hong D, et al. Timing of vulnerability of the brain to iodine deficiency in endemic cretinism. N Engl J Med 1994;331:1739
29. Nohr SC, Laurberg P, Borlum KG, et al. Iodine status in neonates in Denmark: regional variations and dependency on maternal iodine supplementation. Acta Paediatr 1994; 83:578
30. Glinoer D, DeNayer P, DeLange F, et al. A randomized trial for the treatment of mild iodine deficiency during pregnancy: maternal and neonatal effects. J Clin Endocrinol Metab 1995;80:258
31. Thorpe-Beeston JG, Nicolaides KH, McGregor AM. Fetal thyroid function. Thyroid 1992;2:207
32. Mandel SJ, Brent GA, Larsen PR. Review of antithyroid drug use during pregnancy and report of a case of aplasia cutis. Thyroid 1994;4:129
33. Marchand B, Brownlie BEW, Hart DM, et al. The placental transfer of propylthiouracil, methimazole, and carbimazole. J Clin Endocrinol Metab 1977;45:1187
34. Milham S, Elledge W. Maternal methimazole and congenital defects in children. Teratology 1972;5:125
35. Fisher M, Schneider R. Aplasia cutis congenita in three successive generations. Arch Dermatol 1973;108:252
36. Momotani N, Ito K, Hamada N, et al. Maternal hyperthyroidism and congenital malformations in the offspring. Clin Endocrinol 1984;20:695
37. Van Dijke CP, Heydendael RJ, De Kleine MJ. Methimazole, carbimazole, and congenital skin defects. Ann Intern Med 1987;106:60
38. Senior B, Chernoff HL. Iodide goiter in the newborn. Pediatrics 1971;47:510

39. Rotmensch HH, Elkayam U, Frishman W. Antiarrhythmic drug therapy during pregnancy. Ann Intern Med 1983;98:487

40. Rubin PC. Beta-blockers in pregnancy. N Engl J Med 1981; 305:1323

41. Ramsay I, Kaur S, Krassas G. Thyrotoxicosis in pregnancy: results of treatment by antithyroid drugs combined with T_4. Clin Endocrinol 1983;18:73

42. Hashizume K, Ichikawa K, Nishi Y, et al. Effect of administration of thyroxine on the risk of postpartum recurrence of hyperthyroid Graves' disease. J Clin Endocrinol Metab 1992;75:6

43. Momotani N, Hisaoka T, Noh J, et al. Effects of iodine on thyroid status of fetus versus mother in treatment of Graves' disease complicated by pregnancy. J Clin Endocrinol Metab 1992;75:738

44. Cove DH, Johnston P. Fetal hyperthyroidism: experience of treatment in four siblings. Lancet 1985;1:430

45. Brown RS, Keating P, Mitchell E. Maternal thyroid-blocking immunoglobulins in congenital hypothyroidism. J Clin Endocrinol Metab 1990;70:1341

46. Tamaki H, Amino N, Aozasa M, et al. Universal predictive criteria for neonatal overt thyrotoxicosis requiring treatment. Am J Perinatol 1988;5:152

47. Perelman AH, Johnson RL, Clemons RD, et al. Intrauterine diagnosis and treatment of fetal goitrous hypothyroidism. J Clin Endocrinol Metab 1990;71:618

48. Momotani N, Yamashita R, Yoshimoto M, et al. Recovery from fetal hypothyroidism: evidence for the safety of breast-feeding while taking propylthiouracil. Clin Endocrinol 1989;31:591

49. Roti E, Emerson CH. Postpartum thyroiditis. J Clin Endocrinol Metab 1992;74:3

50. Stagnaro-Green A, Roman SH, Cobin RH, et al. A prospective study of lymphocyte-initiated immunosuppression in normal pregnancy: evidence of a T-cell etiology for postpartum thyroid dysfunction. J Clin Endocrinol Metab 1992;74:645

51. Abramsky O. Pregnancy and multiple sclerosis. Ann Neurol 1994;36(Suppl):S38

52. Amino N, Kuro R, Tanizawa O, et al. Changes of serum anti-thyroid antibodies during and after pregnancy in autoimmune thyroid diseases. Clin Exp Immunol 1978;31:30

53. Gleicher N. Pregnancy and autoimmunity. Acta Haematol 1986;76:68

54. Tamaki H, Itoh E, Kaneda T, et al. Crucial role of serum human chorionic gonadotropin for the aggravation of thyrotoxicosis in early pregnancy in Graves' disease. Thyroid 1993;3:189

55. Patton PE, Coulam CB, Bergstralh E. The prevalence of autoantibodies in pregnant and nonpregnant women. Am J Obstet Gynecol 1987;157:1345

56. Feldt-Rasmussen U, Hoier-Madsen M, Rasmussen NG, et al. Antithyroid peroxidase antibodies during pregnancy and postpartum. Relation to postpartum thyroiditis. Autoimmunity 1990; 6:211

57. Jansson R, Dahlberg PA, Winsa B, et al. The postpartum period constitutes an important risk for the development of clinical Graves' disease in young women. Acta Endocrinol (Copenh) 1987;116:321

58. Hidaka Y, Nishi I, Tamaki H, et al. Differentiation of postpartum thyrotoxicosis by serum thyroglobulin: usefulness of a new multisite immunoradiometic assay. Thyroid 1994;4:275

59. Momotani N, Noh J, Ishikawa N, Ito K. Relationship between silent thyroiditis and recurrent Graves' disease in the postpartum period. J Clin Endocrinol Metab 1994;79:285

60. Stewart DE, Addison AM, Robinson GE, et al. Thyroid function in psychosis following childbirth. Am J Psychiatry 1988; 145:1579

61. Hidaka Y, Amino N, Iwatani Y, et al. Changes in natural killer cell activity in normal pregnant and postpartum women: increases in the first trimester and postpartum period and decrease in late pregnancy. J Reprod Immunol 1991;20:73

62. Pop VJM, De Rooy H, Vader HL, et al. Microsomal antibodies during gestation in relation to postpartum thyroid dysfunction and depression. Acta Endocrinol (Copenh) 1993;129:26

63. Alvarez-Marfany M, Roman SH, Drexler AJ, et al. Long-term prospective study of postpartum thyroid dysfunction in women with insulin dependent diabetes mellitus. J Clin Endocrinol Metab 1994;79:10

64. Kologlu M, Fung H, Darke C, et al. Postpartum thyroid dysfunction and HLA status. Eur J Clin Invest 1990;20:56

65. Othman S, Amos N, Parkes AB, et al. Postpartum thyroiditis: an organ specific syndrome which is not associated with a postpartum polyclonal B-cell activation. Autoimmunity 1992; 13:333

66. Parkes AB, Othman S, Hall R, et al. The role of complement in the pathogenesis of postpartum thyroiditis. J Clin Endocrinol Metab 1994;79:395

67. Mizukami Y, Michigishi T, Nonomura A, et al. Postpartum thyroiditis. A clinical, histological, and immunopathologic study of 15 cases. Am J Clin Pathol 1993;100:200

68. LiVolsi VA. Postpartum thyroiditis. The pathology slowly unravels. Am J Clin Pathol 1993;100:193

69. John R, Othman S, Parkes AB, et al. Interference in thyroid-function tests in postpartum thyroiditis. Clin Chem 1991;37:1397

70. Othman S, Phillips DIW, Parkes AB, et al. A long-term follow-up of postpartum thyroiditis. Clin Endocrinol 1990;32:559

Werner and Ingbar's The Thyroid, Seventh Edition,
edited by Lewis E. Braverman and Robert D. Utiger.
Lippincott–Raven Publishers, Philadelphia, © 1996

90

Resistance to Thyroid Hormone

Samuel Refetoff

Resistance to thyroid hormone (RTH) is a syndrome of reduced responsiveness of target tissues to thyroid hormone. More than 500 cases that appear to fit this definition have been described.* In practice, patients are identified by their persistent elevation of serum free thyroxine (T_4) and free triiodothyronine (T_3) levels in association with normal thyrotropin (TSH) concentrations, in the absence of intercurrent illness, drugs, or alterations of thyroid hormone transport proteins in serum. More important, administration of supraphysiologic doses of thyroid hormone fail to produce the expected suppressive effect on the secretion of pituitary TSH and on the metabolic responses in peripheral tissues.

Although the apparent insensitivity to thyroid hormone may vary in severity, it is always partial. The variability in clinical manifestations may be due in part to the severity of the hormonal resistance, the effectiveness of compensatory mechanisms, the presence of modulating genetic factors, and the effects of prior therapy. Nevertheless, the syndrome appears to be invariably associated with mutations in the thyroid hormone receptor (TR)-β gene.[1]

Although the clinical presentation of RTH is variable, the common features characteristic of the syndrome are elevated serum levels of free T_4 and T_3, a normal or slightly increased TSH level that responds to thyrotropin-releasing hormone (TRH), absence of the usual symptoms and metabolic consequences of thyroid hormone excess, and goiter.

CLINICAL CLASSIFICATION

Until recently, the diagnosis was based solely on the clinical findings and results of standard laboratory tests. The proposed subclassification of RTH was thus based on symptoms, signs, and laboratory parameters of tissue responses to thyroid hormone. Not withstanding the assessment of TSH feedback regulation by thyroid hormone, the measurements of most other responses to the hormone are insensitive and relatively nonspecific. For this reason, all tissues other than the pituitary have been grouped together under the term *peripheral tissues*, on which the impact of thyroid hormone was roughly assessed by a combination of clinical observation and laboratory tests.

The majority of patients appeared to be eumetabolic and maintained a near-normal serum TSH concentration. They were classified as having *generalized resistance to thyroid hormone* (GRTH). In such individuals, the defect seemed to be compensated by the high levels of thyroid hormone. In contrast, patients with equally high levels of thyroid hormone and nonsuppressed TSH that appeared to be hypermetabolic or had sinus tachycardia were classified as having selective *pituitary resistance to thyroid hormone* (PRTH).[2] Finally, the occurrence of isolated *peripheral tissue resistance to thyroid hormone* (PTRTH) was reported in a single patient studied in detail.[3] In this individual with partial thyroid gland ablation, although serum TSH was suppressed with physiologic doses of L-T_3, supraphysiologic doses of this hormone failed to produce symptoms and signs of thyrotoxicosis or increased oxygen consumption and pulse rate.

Supported in part by U.S. Public Health Grants DK15070 and RR00055.

*A complete list of references and clinical and laboratory information on published cases can be obtained from the World-Wide Registry of RTH, which can be accessed by Internet connection. The Gopher address is "gopher.uchicago.edu" and the RTH Registry is located in the server "snakeoil.bsd.uchicago.edu". It is a "read only" file. Comments should be directed by e-mail to ".registry@medicine.bsd.uchicago.edu".

The earliest suggestion that PRTH may not constitute an entity distinct from GRTH can be found in a study by Beck-Peccoz and colleagues.[4] In a group of 15 patients with PRTH, these authors found that the serum level of a peripheral tissue marker of thyroid hormone action, sex hormone-binding globulin (SHBG), was not increased. In a recent comprehensive study involving 312 patients with GRTH and 72 patients with PRTH, it was conclusively shown that the response of this and other peripheral tissue markers of thyroid hormone action, were equally attenuated in both groups.[5] More importantly, identical mutations have been identified in individuals classified as having GRTH and PRTH. It appears that these two forms of RTH are the product of the subjective nature of symptoms and poor specificity of signs.

The existence of PTRTH is even less well founded. The original case has been found to have a normal TR-β gene sequence.[6] Because the putative defect in PTRTH spares the pituitary, the inability to upregulate thyroid hormone synthesis should produce sustained tissue hypothyroidism resulting in growth and mental retardation. This has not been observed. More common in clinical practice is the apparent tolerance of some individuals to the ingestion of supraphysiologic doses of thyroid hormone.

INCIDENCE AND INHERITANCE

The incidence of RTH is unknown. In the decade that followed its initial description in 1967,[7] 13 cases were reported. This contrasts with the publication of data on about 130 patients during the decade that followed. Of the 500 currently published cases, 349 have been reviewed in detail.[1] Thus, the syndrome appears to be more frequent than initially suspected. Because serum T_4 levels in affected subjects are elevated at birth,[8] this provides a unique opportunity to use the dried blood spots that are routinely obtained from neonates to screen for RTH. Such an approach would not only allow an early diagnosis but would also provide information on the prevalence of the syndrome.

Although most thyroid diseases occur more commonly in women, RTH has been found with equal frequency in both genders. The condition appears to have wide geographic distribution and has been reported in whites, blacks, and Asians. The prevalence may vary among different ethnic groups.

Familial occurrence of RTH has been documented in approximately 75% of cases; the incidence of true sporadic cases is 15%.[1] The reports of acquired RTH are seriously questioned. Two of the patients had antecedent thyrotoxicosis with low TSH levels and were treated with radioiodide. In these two patients[9,10] and in the two others with hypothyroidism,[11,12] the diagnosis was based on minimal elevation of serum T_4 and T_3 levels or on the requirement for hormone replacement slightly above the usual replacement doses to maintain a euthyroid state or to suppress the TSH response to TRH.

Inheritance is autosomal dominant. Transmission was clearly recessive in only one family.[7,13] Consanguinity in a family with dominant inheritance of RTH has produced a homozygous child with very severe resistance to the hormone.[14] The defect was present in two sets of identical twins,[15,16] whereas in another family, only one fraternal twin was affected.[17]

ETIOLOGY AND GENETICS

Early studies have shown that the excessive amounts of thyroid hormone secreted by patients with RTH[18-20] are normal stereochemically,[18] undergo degradation through normal pathways,[21,22] and adequately penetrate peripheral tissues.[18,23] Thus, soon after the description of the syndrome, it was postulated that the defect resides at the cellular level, probably at the receptor site.[18]

The opportunity to test this hypothesis arose with the demonstration of a putative TR.[24] Although the first study in a family with recessive inheritance suggested the presence of a receptor with reduced affinity for the hormone,[25] data derived from 48 patients belonging to 27 unrelated families and carried out in 14 laboratories have been disappointing. Abnormalities in affinity, capacity or both were detected in mononuclear cells and in fibroblasts of one-third and one-half of the cases studied, respectively.[1] Most disturbing was the report of discrepant results in several affected individuals belonging to the same family.[26] The inability to localize with consistency the defect at the level of the nuclear receptor, combined with the variable phenotype, suggested that the clinical syndrome of RTH represents the manifestations of a number of biochemical defects of thyroid hormone action, one of which may be at the level of the nuclear receptor.

Efforts to demonstrate receptor abnormalities resumed after the isolation of complementary DNAs that encode proteins with thyroid hormone-binding properties similar to those previously demonstrated in nuclear extracts.[27,28] These cellular homologues of the viral oncogene *erb*A mapped to the human chromosomes 17 and 3, and were named TR-α and TR-β, respectively. These two genes, of great structural similarity, generate several isoform products, of which the TR-β1 and TR-β2 (derived from the TR-β gene) and the TRα1 (derived from the TR-α gene) function as TRs.

Using the technique of restriction fragment length polymorphism, evidence for the implication of a TR in RTH was provided by the demonstration of linkage between the TR-β locus on chromosome 3 and the RTH phenotype in one family.[29] This was soon followed by the demonstration of point mutations, resulting in single amino acid substitutions in the hormone-binding domain of the TR-β.[30,31] In both families only one of the two alleles was involved, compatible with the apparent dominant mode of inheritance.

Mutations in the TR-β gene have been identified in subjects with RTH belonging to 98 families (Fig 90-1). All are located in functionally relevant areas of the T_3-binding domain (see Molecular Basis of RTH, below). Because only 58 of 98 mutations are unique, 40 occur in more than one family. Haplotyping by analysis of satellite DNA has established that in most instances identical mutations among families have occurred independently.[36,41] Furthermore, the frequency of de novo mutations (those that occurred within the last 50 years) is 15%. The majority of mutations involve a single nucleotide substitution resulting in the replacement of an amino acid and in two cases a truncated receptor protein due to a translation terminator codon. In three instances, a three-base deletion resulted in the loss of an amino acid and in three others a frame shift was caused by single nucleotide deletion or insertion and seven-base duplication, respectively. Deletion of all coding regions of

FAMILY ID	REFERENCES	NUCLEOTIDES	CODONS and AMINO ACIDS		CODON NUMBER and AMINO ACIDS	Ka Mutant / Ka Normal
[F1]	(13)	244-1704	**All deleted**			
T[F109]	(32)	985	(C) GCC → **Acc** Ala → **Thr**		**A234T**	0.34
no ID	(33)	1012	CGG → **Tgg** Arg → **Trp**		**R243W**	
no ID	(34)	1013	CGG → c**A**G Arg → **Gln**		**R243Q**	
*GP,8	(35,36)	1076	GTT → G**A**T Val → **Asp**		**V264D**	<0.01
(XV)[F99]	(37)	1214	ATG → A**C**G Met → **Thr**		**M310T**	
[F98]	(PO)	1223	ATG → A**C**G Met → **Thr**		**M313T**	
G-H deG(II); 9,10,11 *[F120]	(38) (35,36) (39,40)	1232	CGC → c**A**c Arg → **His**		**R316H**	0.019 <0.01 0.05
(XVIII) [F89] *[F52] *E-D[F100] Mlo AM *PC noID	(37,40,41) (40,41) (42) (PO) (36) (36) (43)	1234	(C) GCT → **ACT** Ala → **Thr**		**A317T**	0.16 0.16 0.22 0.16 0.13 0.13
W.R.[F54] [F88]	(44) (41)	1243	CGC → **Tgc** Arg → **Cys**		**R320C**	0.49
CL [F67] [F95] PM 7 4,5 no ID	(45) (40.41,46) (35,36) (35) (36)	1244	CGC → c**A**c Arg → **His**		**R320H**	0.46 0.42 0.38
SC GM	(36) (36)	1244	CGC → c**T**c Arg → **Leu**		**R320L**	0.10 0.10
ST	(36)	1247	TAT → T**G**T Tyr → **Cys**		**Y321C**	0.018
Mo	(47)	1249	GAC → **A**AC Asp → **Asn**		**D322N**	
I-R[F110]	(48)	1249	GAC → **C**AC Asp → **His**		**D322H**	0.39
Pt H	(49)	1275	TTG → TT**C** Leu → **Phe**		**L330F**	0.01
(VII) F-W) [F14]	(37,42)	1279	GGG → **A**GG Gly → **Arg**		**G332R**	
BB	(36)	1280	GGG → G**A**G Gly → **Glu**		**G332E**	0.02
So	(47)	1282	GAA → **C**AA Glu → **Gln**		**E333Q**	
no ID	(50)	1286	ATG → A**G**G Met → **Arg**		**M334R**	

FIGURE 90-1. Mutations in the TRβ gene associated with RTH, their location, and affinity for T_3.

the TR-β gene has been encountered in only one family (F1) representing the only example of recessive inheritance of RTH. Sixty-nine percent of mutations occur in CG-rich areas (four or more consecutive Cs or Gs) and in particular in CpG dinucleotide hot spots (47%),[36,41] which are frequent sites of poly-

morphism in man. It is, thus, not surprising that of the 13 mutations identified in more than one family, 9 occurred in CpG hot spots, which are also frequently the sites for de novo mutations. Most notable is the C-to-T transition in codon 338 replacing the normal Arg (CGG) with Trp (TGG), which has been detected in

FAMILY ID	REFERENCES	NUCLEOTIDES	CODONS and AMINO ACIDS		CODON NUMBER and AMINO ACIDS	Ka Mutant / Ka Normal
S[F66]	(51)	1295-1297	ACA CGG → AGG Thr Arg → Arg		T337Δ	0.001
[F29]	(40,41)	1297	CGG → TGG Arg → Trp		R338W	0.21
[106]	(40,41)					0.21
F.E.	(52)					0.019
*K-T [F111]	(48)					0.21
JM	(36)					0.10
*RM	(36)					0.10
LM	(36)					0.10
2 fam no ID	(36)					
L-F	(53)					0.23
A-O	(50)					
NM	(36)	1298	CGG → cTG Arg → Leu		R338L	0.26
D-C (D) [F56]	(54)	1305	CAG → caC Gln → His		Q340H	0.46
J-H	(55)	1210	AAA → ATA Lys → Ile		K342I	0.26
BK	(36)	1316	GGG → GAG Gly → Glu		G344E	<0.01
Mf [F44]	(30,56)	1318	GGT → CGT Gly → Arg		G345R	0.001
[F18]	(57)	1318	GGT → AGT Gly → Ser		G345S	<0.01
*G-S [F101]	(42)	1319	GGT → GTT Gly → Val		G345V	
(VIII) [F17]	(37)	1319	GGT → GAT Gly → Asp		G345D	
N-N [F102]	(42)	1325	GGG → GAG Gly → Glu		G347E	
SS	(36)	1330	GTG → ATG Val → Met		V349M	0.23
MS	(36)	1571	CGG → CAG Arg → Gln		R429Q	0.21
MA	(36)					0.21
no ID	(40,58)					0.9 (±0.2)
no ID,2	(35,36)	1573-1575 deletion	ATG Met		M430Δ	<0.01
[F51]	(PO)	1577	ATA → ACA Ile → Thr		I431T	0.05
*LO	(36)					0.01
no ID	(50	1579-1581 deletion	GGA Gly		G432Δ	<0.01
*Pt B [F34]	(59)	1589	CAT → cTT His → Leu		H435L	
Pt C	(59)	1590	CAT → CAA His → Gln		H435Q	
CMa	(36)	1597	CGC → TGC Arg → Cys		R438C	0.30
no ID	(36)					

FIGURE 90-1. Continued

10 families. Four different amino acid replacements have been identified in codons 345 and 453 (see Figure 90-1). Silent mutations (codons 319 and 417) were found in conjunction with missense mutations in two families, F100 and F45, respectively.

No mutations have been so far detected in the TR-α gene suggesting that either its products may play a minor role in TSH regulation or that TR-α defects are lethal.

MOLECULAR BASIS OF THE DEFECT

The α and β TR isoforms have in common a DNA-binding domain near their amino terminus and, with the exception of TR-

FAMILY ID	REFERENCES	NUCLEOTIDES	CODONS and AMINO ACIDS	CODON NUMBER and AMINO ACIDS	Ka Mutant / Ka Normal
(XII) Mt [F45]	(37,40,60)	1598	CGC → CAC / Arg → His	R438H	0.14 (0.25)
[F68]	(61)				
*[F114]	(62)				0.25
BW	(36)				0.23
CS	(36)				0.23
GS	(36)				0.23
JH	(36)				0.23
O-K [F103]	(42)	1609	ATG → GTG / Met → Val	M442V	0.17
K fam [F107]	(63)	1612	AAG → GAG / Lys → Glu	K443E	0.09 - 0.046
DiG [F117]	(47)	1614	AAG → AAC / Lys → Asn	K443N	
[F119]	(64)	1621	TGC → CGC / Cys → Arg	C446R	<0.03
[F108]	(65)	1623	TGC → TGA / Cys → Stop	C446X	
*P-V [F104]	(42)	1627 insertion	CCC ACA → CCC CAC AGA / Pro Thr → Pro His Arg	448fr shift463	<0.05
T-P [F112]	(48)	1634	CTC → CAC / Leu → His	L450H	0.39
*Pt A [F86]	(59)	1636	TTC → ATC / Phe → Ile	F451I	
*no ID	(66)	1637 1638	TTC → TAA / Phe → Stop	F451X	
BN	(36)	1638 7 base duplication	A CTC TTC ACT CTT Ccc ccc TTT / Leu Phe Thr Pro Pro Pro Phe	452fr shift463	<0.01
no ID	(67)	1639-1641 3 base deletion	TTC CCC CCT → TTC CCT / Phe Pro Pro → Phe Pro	P452Δ	
Q-W [F105]	(42)	1642	CCT → ACT / Pro → Thr	P453T	0.41
[F85]	(68)				0.46
*SH	(36)				0.20
PA	(36)				0.20
(X) [F27]	(37,69)	1642	CCT → TCT / Pro → Ser	P453S	
[F94]	(69)				
MC	(36)				0.36
noID	(36)				
TB	(36)	1642	CCT → GCT / Pro → Ala	P453A	0.17
A (Mh) [F22]	(31,37,70)	1643	CCT → CAT / Pro → His	P453H	0.16
no ID	(50)				
XI [F26]	(37)	1644 insertion	CCT TTG → CCC TTT GTT / Pro Leu → Pro Phe Val	454fr shift463	
R-L [F113]	(48	1661	TTC → TGC / Phe → Cys	F459C	0.33
MP	(36)	1663	(C) GAG → AAG / Glu → Lys	E460K	0.25

* De novo mutations; PO: personal observations.
Mutations in CpG dinucleotides are underlined
Numbers preceeded with F and in square brackets represent family members according Reffettoff et al[1]

FIGURE 90-1. (Continued)

α2, a thyroid hormone-binding domain at their carboxyl terminus. Evidence suggests that dimers of these TRs and heterodimers between a TR and a nuclear protein cofactor (e.g., the retinoid X receptor) associate with specific DNA sequences, termed thyroid hormone response elements (TREs), and function as activators or repressors of thyroid hormone-regulated genes. In the absence of hormone, TRs exert an opposite effect (inhibitory or stimulatory) compared with that observed in the presence of the hormone. The TR is activated by the hormone, probably through alteration of steric configuration, which results in changes in the rate of target gene transcription (see chap 9).

With the exception of the original family described in 1967 that had complete TR-β deletion,[13] all mutations are localized in the T_3-binding domain of the TR-β gene resulting in variable reduction of the affinity of the receptor for T_3 and interference with the function of the normal TRs. Most are clustered in two mutational "hot" areas spanning codons 310 to 349 and 429 to 460 (Fig 90-2). Not a single mutation has been so far identified in the "cold" area though it is not devoid of mutational CpG hot spots. Introduction of artificial mutations in this "cold" area according to the "hot spot" mutational rule yielded mutant TR-β with either normal T_3-binding affinity, or functional impairment of a lesser degree than that of natural mutations with the mildest functional and clinical defect.[40] Thus, natural mutations expected to occur in the "cold" region of the TR-β should fail to manifest as RTH and would escape detection.

The family with deletion of all coding sequences of the TR-β but intact TR-α exhibited an autosomal recessive inheritance of RTH. Thus, complete absence of the TR-β is compatible with life. Because some effects of thyroid hormone could be demonstrated in these subjects, it is logical to conclude that TR-α1, expressed in virtually all tissues, is capable of partially substituting for the function of TR-β. The deaf mutism and somatic abnormalities found in the affected homozygotes may be the consequence of the deletion of genetic material other than the TR-β. In all other families, RTH is inherited in a dominant fashion and affected individuals harbor mutations in only one of the two TR-β alleles. The finding that subjects with deletion of one of the two TR-β alleles have no clinical or laboratory abnormalities indicates not only that a single copy of the TR-β gene is sufficient for normal function but also that the dominant inheritance of RTH, caused by point mutations in the TR-β gene, is not simply due to a reduction in the amount of the normal TR-β. This finding supports the hypothesis that the mechanism of dominant inheritance of RTH requires the interference of a mutant TR with the function of the normal TR (*dominant negative effect*).

Early work has postulated three mechanisms to explain the dominant negative effect of a mutant TR (mTR) based on the cotransfection of mTR-β with normal TR.[71–73] They are a competition between a mTR and a normal TR at the level of TRE, heterodimer formation between a mTR and nuclear cofactors (TR auxiliary proteins, TRAPs) exhausting a limited amount of cofactors (squelching), and formation of inactive mTR/normal TR homodimers or mTR/TRAP heterodimers. It is likely that all three mechanism are operative though dimerization appears to play a central role because, when prevented by the introduction of a second mutation, the dominant negative effect of an mTR is abrogated.[74] It remains, however, unclear whether homodimerization of two mTRs[56,75] or heterodimers between a mTR with a cofactor[74,76] play a major role (Fig 90-3). The dominant negative effect of mTRs is undoubtedly more complex because preferential formation of the different dimeric forms appears to vary with the substituted amino acid in the mTR[77] and is influenced by other nuclear factors and the structure of the various TREs.

Of interest are the observations made in one subject with homozygous deletion of Thr-337 in the TR-β gene belonging to a family with dominantly inherited RTH (F66). This subject manifested the most severe form of RTH with signs of both hypothyroidism and thyrotoxicosis despite astronomical levels of thyroid hormone.[14,51] The severe hypothyroidism manifested in bone and brain of this subject is explained by the interference of the double dose mTR with the function of TR-α, a situation that does not occur in homozygous subjects with TR-β deletion. In contrast, manifestations of thyrotoxicosis in other tissues may be explained by the effect high thyroid levels have on tissues that normally express predominantly TR-α1.

The earlier expectation that differences in functional impairment resulting from a particular amino acid substitution in

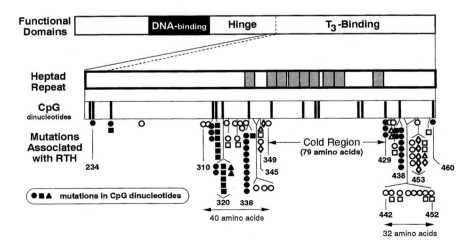

FIGURE 90-2. Location of natural mutations in the TR-β gene associated with RTH. Schematic representation of the TR-β and its functional domains for interaction with TREs (DNA-binding) and hormone (T_3-binding). The latter domain is expanded and the location of the 58 different mutations detected in each of 98 unrelated families are indicated by a symbol. Identical mutations in members of unrelated families are indicated by the same shading pattern of vertically placed symbols. Note the "cold region" of 79 amino acids, devoid of mutation associated with RTH. Amino acids are numbered consecutively starting at the amino terminus of the molecule.

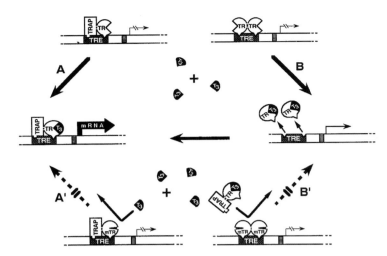

FIGURE 90-3. A model of thyroid hormone action and the dominant negative interaction of mutant TR (mTR) with a normal TR (TR). In the absence of T_3, TR heterodimers (TR-TRAP) and homodimers (TR-TR) bind to thyroid response element (TRE) on DNA and suppress target gene transactivation. T_3 activates transcription mediated by TR-TRAP heterodimers and favors the formation by dissociating TR-TR dimers occupying TREs. mTRs with reduced ability to bind T_3 produce an antagonistic (dominant negative) effect by persistent occupation of TREs as inactive dimers or heterodimers. (From Refetoff S, Weiss RE, Usala SJ. The syndromes of resistance to thyroid hormone. Endocr Rev 1993;14:348)

a mutant TR-β would explain the variable manifestations of RTH was not born out. In fact, the in vitro potency of dominant negative activity of mutant TRβs appear to correlate better with the RTH phenotype than the impairment of their T_3 binding.[75,78] Furthermore, the phenotype of RTH may vary among individuals harboring the same TR-β mutation, not only among families, but also in affected members of the same family.[38,41,46] The most striking example is the mutation R316H which, in family G.H., did not cosegregate with the RTH phenotype.[38] Indeed, only one of three members of this family harboring the TR-β mutation presented symptoms and serum thyroid hormone and TSH abnormalities typical of RTH. This variability in clinical and laboratory manifestations was not observed in affected members of two other families harboring the same mutation.[36,39] Although the precise mechanism of intrafamilial heterogeneity in RTH remains unknown, studies in a large family with the R320H TR-β mutation suggest that genetic variability of factors other than TR that contribute to the action of thyroid hormone may modulate the phenotype of RTH.[46]

Of interest is a recent study carried out with the TR-β mutant R429Q, which has normal affinity for T_3.[40,58] Although this mutant TR-β mediated a normal transactivation on positive TREs, it exhibited a reduced constitutive activation through a negative TRE and thus, a weaker T_3-mediated inhibition. This mutant TR-β possesses properties that could impair selectively the action of T_3 on thyrotrophs.

Over the past two decades, many attempts have been made to demonstrate tissue hyposensitivity in vitro. Measurements of the respiratory control of muscle mitochondria[18] and determination of the effect of thyroid hormone on low-density lipoprotein metabolism,[79] and glycosaminoglycan synthesis[80] in fibroblasts from patients with RTH showed poor reproducibility, no consistent abnormality, or studies were carried out on only a few patients with limited information on normal responses. Measurement of the normal inhibitory effect of T_3 on fibronectin synthesis,[81] or its messenger RNA[82] in fibroblasts of patients with RTH, showed more consistently attenuated or paradoxical responses. The latter results, which formerly were difficult to explain, are possibly the result of variable interaction of the mutant TR with the α and β isoforms of the normal TRs, variable expression of the α and β TR genes in different tissues, and differences in the regulation of expression of the

TR-α and TR-β genes by the hormone-activated TR, which in some tissues may be in opposite directions.[83–85]

Alternative causes giving rise to RTH have been considered. Defective plasma membrane transport of thyroid hormone has been suggested in one family.[86] This conclusion was based on the reduced ratio of cytosol to serum T_4 in red blood cells of an affected member of the family. Subsequently, fibroblasts from the same patients displayed a reduced response to T_3 manifested by decreased inhibition of glycosaminoglycan synthesis[80] and a mutation of the TR-β gene cosegregating with the RTH phenotype was identified.[37] Maxon and coworkers[87] reported the occurrence of familial elevations of serum T_4 and reverse T_3 (rT_3) concentrations in euthyroid subjects in whom the serum T_3 levels remained within the normal range. This finding is compatible with a primary abnormality in the extrathyroidal conversion of T_4 to T_3. Unfortunately, a direct proof is not available. Although this family does not have tissue insensitivity to thyroid hormone in the true sense, the findings indicate that inherited defects in the metabolism of thyroid hormone may exist. Ostensibly, the existence of such a defect was suggested in an early publication.[88]

PATHOGENESIS

There is no question that the thyroid gland hyperactivity and excessive thyroid hormone synthesis and secretion result from excess TSH secretion. Although the serum TSH concentration may not be above the upper limit of normal, it always is detectable and responds by a further increase to the administration of TRH. This persistence of TSH secretion in the face of high levels of free thyroid hormone contrasts with the low TSH levels in the more common forms of thyroid hormone hypersecretion that are TSH independent.

The evidence that TSH plays a central role in the maintenance of thyroid hormone hypersecretion and goiter in RTH is secure. The serum of these patients contains TSH that is identical immunologically to that secreted by the normal pituitary and to purified standard preparations.[89,90] It does not contain an excess of biologically inactive pituitary glycoprotein α-subunits (α-SU), typically found in the serum of patients with TSH-producing pituitary tumors.[90–93] It has normal[89,90] and even increased[35] biologic activity, as determined in heterologous bioassays and by its ability to stimulate thyroid hormone secretion and produce goiter in the patients. Indeed, administration of TRH to patients with RTH causes an increase in the serum T_4 and T_3 concentration[19,89–94] that is proportional to the TSH response.[94] Suppression of the endogenous TSH secretion has the opposite effect on the serum level of thyroid hormone and on the thyroidal radioiodide uptake. Administration of supraphysiologic doses of T_3 reduces the serum TSH and T_4 concentration in a dose-dependent manner.[89,90] TSH suppression results in goiter regression, which can be quite dramatic.[90,95]

In one patient who lacked TR-β, administration of 100 μg T_3 daily for 1 week caused an increase in the TRH-induced secretion of biologically active TSH.[94] An affected member of the same family also failed to respond to an antithyroid drug,[18] whereas in other cases studied, the expected reduction in serum thyroid hormone level and concomitant increase in TSH concentration have been observed.[15,23,89,95] Although dose and duration of drug administration have been implicated in the explanation of such discrepancies, it is more likely that they reflect the expression of this particular genetic defect. Indeed, the absence of TR-β may have uncovered minor effects of T_3 on the pituitary thyrotroph mediated through the TR-α, which resulted in the observed paradoxical effect.

When sought, TSH-binding antibodies could not be detected.[90,96] Thyroid-stimulating antibodies, responsible for the thyroid gland hyperactivity in Graves' disease, have been conspicuously absent in patients with RTH. Another potential thyroid stimulator, human chorionic gonadotropin, also is not involved.[89,91]

The selectivity of impaired responsiveness to thyroid hormone has been convincingly demonstrated. When tested at the pituitary level, both thyrotrophs and lactotrophs were less sensitive only to thyroid hormone. Thyrotrophs responded normally to the suppressive effects of the dopaminergic drugs L-dopa and bromocriptine,[90,92,97] as well as glucocorticoids.[23,90,92,94] Studies carried out in cultured fibroblasts confirm the in vivo findings of selective resistance to thyroid hormone. The responsiveness to dexamethasone, measured in terms of glycosaminoglycan[80] and fibronectin synthesis,[81] was preserved in the presence of T_3 insensitivity (Fig 90-4).

In patients with RTH, T_4 and T_3 are produced and degraded in excessive amounts.[18,19,22,91,92] Iodine kinetic studies indicate that their thyroid glands accumulate an excess of iodine in the presence of adequate dietary supply. It is stored in a large organic iodine pool, from which it is released at an increased rate, principally in the form of T_4.[7]

Several of the clinical features encountered in some patients with RTH may be the manifestation of selective tissue deprivation of thyroid hormone during early stages of development. These clinical features include retarded bone age, stunted growth, mental retardation or learning disability, emotional disturbances, attention deficit/hyperactivity disorder (ADHD), hearing defects, and nystagmus.[1] A variety of associated somatic abnormalities appear to be unrelated pathogenically and may be the result of involvement of other genes such as in major deletions of DNA sequences. However, no gross chromosomal abnormalities have been detected on karyotyping.[13,98]

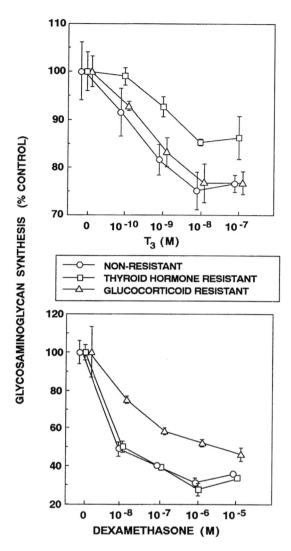

FIGURE 90-4. The inhibitory effect of T_3 and dexamethasone on glycosaminoglycan synthesis in fibroblasts from subjects with thyroid hormone and glucocorticoid resistance compared to that in fibroblasts from a normal (nonresistant) subject. Note that fibroblasts from the patient with RTH had an attenuated response to T_3 but not to dexamethasone, while those from the patient with glucocorticoid resistance showed an attenuated response to dexamethasone only. (From Refetoff S, Weiss RE, Usala SJ. The syndromes of resistance to thyroid hormone. Endocr Rev 1993;14:348)

PATHOLOGY

Little can be said about the pathologic findings in tissues other than the thyroid because of unavailability of autopsy data from patients with RTH. Electron microscopic examination of striated muscle obtained by biopsy from one patient revealed mitochondrial swelling also known to be encountered in thyrotoxicosis.[18] Light microscopy of skin fibroblasts stained with toluidine blue showed moderate to intense metachromasia.[18] Such deposition of extracellular metachromatic material in the upper layer of the dermis has been described in myxedema.[99] The presence of such material in the skin of patients with RTH is probably a manifestation of a decreased thyroid hormone action in this tissue. Furthermore, in contrast to patients with myxedema due to thyroid hormone deficiency, treatment with the hormone failed to induce a disappearance of the metachromasia in fibroblasts from patients with RTH.

Thyroid tissue, obtained by biopsy or at surgery, revealed various degrees of hyperplasia of the follicular epithelium.[90,92,93,96] The follicles may vary in size, from small to large. Some specimens have been described as "adenomatous goiters,"[92,96] others as "colloid goiters,"[91,100] and still others as normal thyroid tissue.[18] Lymphocytic infiltration has been reported in a single case, a finding not related to the syndrome but rather due to the fortuitous coexistence of thyroiditis in the patient and in other members of his family.[101]

CLINICAL FEATURES

Typical of the RTH syndrome is a paucity of specific clinical manifestations. When present, manifestations are variable from one patient to another. Investigation leading to the diagnosis has been undertaken because of the presence of goiter, hyperactive behavior or learning disabilities, developmental delay, and sinus tachycardia (Fig 90-5). With the exception of goiter, these features are common to a variety of unrelated congenital diseases. More recently, the fortuitous finding of elevated levels of thyroid hormone in serum in association with nonsuppressed TSH has been often responsible for the pursuit of further studies leading to the diagnosis.

The majority of untreated subjects maintain a normal metabolic state at the expense of high levels of thyroid hormone. The degree of this compensation of tissue hyposensitivity to the hormone is, however, variable among individuals as well as in different tissues. As a consequence, clinical and laboratory evidence of thyroid hormone deficiency and excess often coexist. For example, RTH can present with a mild to moderate growth retardation and delayed bone maturation suggestive of hypothyroidism along with hyperactivity and tachycardia, compatible with thyrotoxicosis. Frank symptoms of hypothyroidism are more common in individuals who, because of an erroneous diagnosis, have received treatment to normalize their circulating thyroid hormone levels. In such patients, symptoms of fatigue, somnolence, depression, weight gain, and bradycardia were

noted.[23,79,90] In children inappropriate treatment has aggravated the delay in growth and development.[1]

On physical examination, goiter is by far the most common abnormality, occurring in 85% of cases. In some patients, without clinically obvious thyroid gland enlargement, goiter could be either detected by ultrasonography, was absent due to prior surgery, or was present in other affected members of the family. Gland enlargement is usually diffuse; nodular changes and gross asymmetry are found in recurrent goiters after surgery.

Careful evaluation of subjects with RTH has shown that almost one-half have some degree of learning disability with or without ADHD.[1,1a,102] One-quarter have IQs less than 85, but frank mental retardation (IQ < 60) has been found only in 3% of cases. Impaired mental function was associated with impaired or delayed growth (<5th percentile) in 20% of subjects though growth retardation alone is rare (4%).[1] Despite the high prevalence of ADHD in patients with RTH, the occurrence of RTH in children with ADHD must be very rare, none having been detected in 330 such children studied.[103,104] Furthermore, current data do not support a genetic linkage of RTH with ADHD. Rather the association with low IQ scores may confer a higher likelihood for subjects with RTH to exhibit ADHD symptoms.[39]

A variety of physical defects that cannot be explained on the basis of thyroid hormone deprivation or excess have been recorded. These include major or minor somatic defects, such as winged scapulae, vertebral anomalies, pigeon breast, prominent pectoralis, birdlike facies, scaphocephaly, craniosynostosis, short fourth metacarpals, as well as Besnier's prurigo, congenital ichthyosis, and bull's eye type macular atrophy.[1] No particular defect appears to be prevalent in RTH. A distinct body habitus associated with the syndrome occurred in all three members of a single family with major gene deletion.[7] In all other instances, the associated defects were evident in one but not all affected subjects of the same family.

COURSE OF THE DISEASE

The course of the disease is as variable as its presentation. Some subjects have normal growth and development and lead a normal life at the expense of high thyroid hormone levels

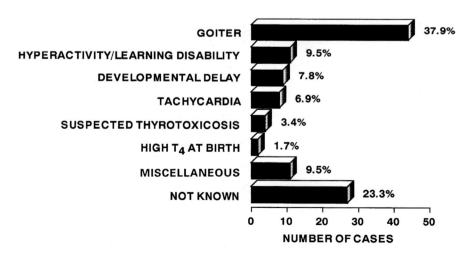

FIGURE 90-5. The reason prompting further investigation of the key member of each family with RTH.

and a small goiter. Others present variable degrees of mental and growth retardation. However, because of prior hormone reduction therapy, it is unknown to what extent this represents the natural course of the illness.

The thyroid gland of some patients with RTH appears to be resistant to thyroid therapy.[105] Goiter has recurred in every patient who underwent thyroid surgery. As a consequence, some subjects have been submitted to several consecutive thyroidectomies or treatments with radioiodide.[19,79,93,106]

In only one patient is RTH believed to have contributed to death. This child homozygous for a dominantly inherited TR-β mutation and a resting heart rate of 190 beats/min,[14,51] died from a cardiogenic shock complicating staphylococcal pneumonia (B. B. Bercu, personal communication). More recently, a 43-year-old woman with RTH died from severe, drug-resistant congestive failure without evidence of valvular or coronary artery heart disease (J. Lazarus et al., personal communication).

LABORATORY FINDINGS

Thyroid Hormone and Its Metabolites in Serum

In the untreated patient, elevation in the concentration of serum free T_4 is a sine qua non requirement for the diagnosis of RTH. It is accompanied by high serum concentrations of T_3. Serum thyroxine-binding globulin (TBG) and transthyretin concentrations are normal. The resin T_3 uptake is usually high because of saturation of TBG by the high concentration of T_4 and T_3.

Serum T_4 and T_3 values vary from just above to severalfold above the upper limit of normal. Although the levels may vary in the course of time in the same patient,[5] the degree of T_4 and T_3 elevation is usually congruent, resulting in a normal T_3:T_4 ratio.[1] This is in contrast to the disproportionate increase in serum T_3 concentration relative to that of T_4, characteristic of Graves' disease.[107] This observation has led some investigators to consider the possibility of reduced extrathyroidal conversion of T_4 to T_3 in patients with RTH.[93]

Reverse T_3 concentrations are also high in patients with RTH as are those of another product of T_4 degradation, 3,3'-T_2.[96] Serum thyroglobulin (Tg) concentration was 240 ng/mL (normal < 1–23) in a patient with RTH in whom the serum TSH level was very high due to prior thyroid surgery.[90] More modest increases were found in other patients who have not received prior treatment. In general, the degree of Tg elevation reflects the level of TSH-induced thyroid gland hyperactivity.

Thyrotropin and Other Thyroid Stimulators

A characteristic, if not pathognomonic, feature of the syndrome is the presence of TSH in serum and preservation of its response to TRH despite elevated thyroid hormone levels.[108] In most cases, the basal serum TSH concentration is normal and the circadian rhythm is unaltered.[15,109] TSH values above 10 mU/L have been reported in patients who, because of earlier diagnosis, have received treatment aimed at reducing their high level of thyroid hormone. The TSH response to TRH is either normal or exaggerated. TSH hyperresponsiveness to TRH is more common in patients receiving antithyroid drug therapy or in those with limited thyroidal reserve due to prior surgical or radioiodide therapy.

Thyrotropin circulating in the basal state and following TRH stimulation has normal[90] or increased[35] bioreactivity and the concentration of its free α-subunit is not disproportionately high.[1] Antibodies against TSH have not been detected[90,96] and the serum is free of thyroid-stimulating immunoglobulins. With the exception of a few cases with coincidental familial autoimmune thyroiditis,[110] serum of patients with RTH is devoid of antibodies against Tg and thyroid peroxidase.

Thyroid Gland Activity and Integrity of Hormone Synthesis

The fractional uptake of radioiodide by the thyroid gland is high. The absolute amount of iodide accumulated by the thyroid gland is also increased.[7] It appears to be normally organified because no discharge of trapped iodide has been observed after the administration of perchlorate.[7,19,95] Other inborn errors of thyroid hormone synthesis have been also ruled out by the failure to detect abnormal iodide-containing compounds in the circulation.[7,18]

Turnover of Thyroid Hormone

In vivo turnover kinetics of T_4 showed a normal or slightly increased volume of distribution and fractional disappearance rate of the hormone. However, because of the high concentration of T_4 in serum, the extrathyroidal pool and absolute daily production of T_4 have been clearly increased, up to twofold the upper limit of normal.[18—20,22,91] The production rate of T_3 was also increased by about twofold to fourfold.[18,22,91] The extrathyroidal conversion of T_4 to T_3 was, however, normal.[22]

In Vivo Effects of Thyroid Hormone

The impact of thyroid hormone on peripheral tissues has been assessed in vivo by a variety of tests. Results have been, by and large, normal, suggesting a reduced biologic response to the hormone.[1,5] The metabolic status has been evaluated by measurements of the basal metabolic rate (BMR), serum cholesterol, carotene, triglycerides, creatine kinase, alkaline phosphatase, angiotensin-converting enzyme, SHBG, ferritin, and osteocalcin, all of which usually have been within the normal range. Urinary excretion of magnesium, hydroxyproline, creatine, creatinine, carnitine, and cyclic adenosine monophosphate, all of which may be elevated in thyrotoxicosis, have been normal or low, suggesting normal or slightly reduced thyroid hormone effect. With the exception of increased resting pulse rate in more than one-half the patients with RTH, the cardiac contractility index has been normal. The Achilles tendon reflex relaxation time has been also normal or slightly prolonged. The prolactin response to TRH was not blunted as it is in patients with thyrotoxicosis. In fact, the prolactin hyperresponsiveness in some patients with RTH may be due to the functional thyroid hormone deprivation at the level of the lactotrophs.[108]

Other Endocrine Tests

Evaluation of endocrine function by a variety of tests has failed to reveal significant defects other than those related to the thyroid. The following laboratory analyses have been carried out in patients with RTH and were found to be within the normal range: serum levels of cortisol and its diurnal rhythm; testosterone, estrogens, and progesterone; gonadotropins and their response to gonadotropin-releasing hormone; adrenocorticotropic hormone; insulin; prolactin and its response to TRH, L-dopa, and glucocorticoids; growth hormone and its response to insulin hypoglycemia, arginine, and pyrogen; as well as the urinary excretion of 17-hydroxycorticoids, 17-ketosteroids, vanillylmandelic acid, adrenaline, and noradrenaline. Radiologic and magnetic resonance examinations of the pituitary gland and sella turcica have shown no anatomic abnormalities.

Bone Age

Radiologic evidence of delayed bone maturation has been observed in one-half the patients with RTH diagnosed during infancy or childhood.[1] However, the majority achieve normal adult stature. It is unclear whether the presence, in some cases, of stippled epiphyses is also the consequence of reduced thyroid hormone action in cartilage or the result of an associated genetic defect.

In Vitro Tests of Thyroid Hormone Action

The normal stimulatory effect of T_3 on the degradation rate of low-density lipoproteins was reduced in cultured fibroblasts obtained from three affected members of one family.[79] Similarly, T_3 and T_4, but not dexamethasone, failed to produce the normal inhibitory effect on the synthesis of glycosaminoglycans in fibroblasts from 4 of 6 patients with RTH.[80] In contrast, T_3 normally stimulated glucose consumption by cultured fibroblasts from a patient with RTH.[21,23] An in vitro study of striated muscle mitochondria from one patient was compatible with a normal response to thyroid hormone.[18] In vitro demonstration of RTH has been most consistent by measurement of the normal inhibitory effect of T_3 on the synthesis of fibronectin and its mRNA in skin fibroblasts maintained in culture. Of 12 patients with RTH who were studied, 11 showed either an attenuated or paradoxical response.[81,82]

RESPONSES TO THE ADMINISTRATION OF THYROID HORMONE

Because resistance to thyroid hormone plays a principal role in the pathogenesis of the syndrome, patients have been given exogenous thyroid hormone to observe their responses and thereby establish the presence of insensitivity to the hormone. Unfortunately, the data generated have been discrepant, not only because of differences in the relative degree of tissue hyposensitivity among patients but also because of lack of uniformity in the manner the hormone trials have been carried out. These include differences in hormonal preparations, dosages, duration of treatment, and the type of observa-

tions and measurements carried out, not to mention the conspicuous lack of adequate control studies. L-T_3 has been given in doses varying from 75 to 400 μ/d for durations of 7 days to 13 months. Administration of L-T_4 has also varied widely in dose (200–1000 μg/d), duration (10 days to several years), and age at initiation (1 month to 74 years).[1]

Administration of thyroid hormone ultimately suppresses TSH secretion, resulting in a decrease and eventually the abolition of the TSH response to TRH. The amount of thyroid hormone necessary to produce such an effect has been variable as has the relative effectiveness of L-T_3 as compared to L-T_4. Such observations have led to earlier speculations that some patients may have an abnormality in conversion of T_4 to T_3.[92,93] The decreased TSH secretion during the administration of supraphysiologic doses of thyroid hormone is accompanied by a reduction in the thyroidal radioiodide uptake,[19,79,89,93] and when exogenous T_3 is given, reduction in the pretreatment level of serum T_4.[89–91,93]

Various responses of peripheral tissues to the administration of thyroid hormone have been quantitated. Most notable are measurements of the BMR, pulse rate, reflex relaxation time, serum cholesterol, lipids, enzymes, and SHBG, and urinary excretion of hydroxyproline, creatine, and carnitine. Either no significant changes were observed, or they were much reduced relative to the amount of thyroid hormone given.[1]

Of great importance are observations on the catabolic effect of exogenous thyroid hormone. L-T_4 given in doses of up to 1000 μg/d and T_3 up to 400 μg/d failed to produce weight loss without a change in calorie intake nor did they induce a negative nitrogen balance.[18,89,90] In contrast, administration of these large doses of thyroid hormone over a prolonged period of time was apparently anabolic as evidenced by a dramatic increase in growth rate and accelerated bone maturation.[8,90]

Effects of Other Drugs

As expected, administration of the thyroid hormone analogue, 3,5,3'triiodo-L-thyroacetic acid (TRIAC) to patients with RTH produced attenuated responses.[18,109,111] Administration of glucocorticoids promptly reduced the TSH response to TRH and the serum T_4 concentration.[20,89,90,92,94]

Administration of L-dopa and bromocriptine produced a prompt, transient suppression of TSH secretion, as well as a diminution of the thyroidal radioiodide uptake and serum T_3 level.[90,92,97] Domperidone, a dopamine antagonist, caused a rise in the serum TSH concentration when given to patients with RTH.[109] These observations indicate that, in this syndrome, the normal inhibitory effect of dopamine on TSH is intact.

The response to antithyroid drugs has shown some variability. Methimazole and propylthiouracil, in doses usually effective in reducing the high serum thyroid hormone level of thyrotoxicosis, had no effect in two patients.[18] However, in other cases of RTH, antithyroid drugs induced some decrease in the circulating level of thyroid hormone, producing a reciprocal change in the TSH concentration.[17,30,95,98] Administration of 100 mg iodine daily had a similar effect in one patient,[91] but 4 mg potassium iodide per day produced no changes in another.[18]

Observations on the effect of other drugs such diazepam and chlorpromazine are limited. With one exception,[18] propranolol caused a reduction in heart rate.

DIFFERENTIAL DIAGNOSIS

Because the clinical presentation of RTH is variable, detection requires a high degree of suspicion. The differential diagnosis in essence includes all possible causes of hyperthyroxinemia. The sequence of diagnostic procedures listed in Table 90-1 is suggested.

The presence of elevated serum T_4 concentration with nonsuppressed TSH needs to be confirmed by repeating these tests. The possibility of an inherited or acquired increase in serum TBG must be excluded by direct measurement and by estimation of the circulating free T_4 level. The presence of a high serum T_3 level must also be documented for the following reasons. Reduced conversion of T_4 to T_3 by peripheral tissues may occasionally give rise to the elevation of total and free T_4 but not T_3 levels. This may occur transiently in a variety of nonthyroidal illnesses or during the administration of some drugs (see subchapters on effects of pharmacologic agents on thyroid hormones and nonthyroidal illness in chap 14). A familial form of hyperthyroxinemia presumably due to a defective T_4 monodeiodination has been also described.[87] The inherited abnormality of T_4 binding to an albumin-like serum protein typically presents with high serum T_4 but normal T_3 concentration (see chap 18). A rare cause of elevated serum T_4 and T_3 concentration is the endogenous production of antibodies directed against these hormones, which can be excluded by direct testing.

Most useful is the measurement of the serum TSH and response to the administration of TRH. Under most circumstances, patients with high concentrations of circulating free thyroid hormone have virtually undetectable serum TSH levels, which characteristically fail to increase in response to TRH. This is true even when the magnitude of thyroid hormone excess is minimal and therefore subclinical both on physical examination or by other laboratory tests (see chaps 12, 18 and 88). The combination of elevated serum levels of thyroid hormone, and not suppressed TSH, narrows the differential diagnosis to RTH and autonomous hypersecretion of TSH associated with pituitary tumors. The latter should be suspected when other members of the family, and particularly the parents of the patient, fail to exhibit thyroid test abnormalities.

TABLE 90-1.
Suggested Sequence of Diagnostic Procedures in Suspected Resistance to Thyroid Hormone

1. Usual presentation: high serum levels of free T_4 and T_3 with nonsuppressed TSH.
2. Confirm the elevated serum levels of free thyroid hormone (T_4 and T_3), and exclude thyroid hormone transport defects.
3. In the absence of similar thyroid hormone test abnormalities in other family members, exclude the presence of a pituitary adenoma by measurement of α-subunit in serum.
4. Demonstrate a blunted TSH suppression and metabolic response to the administration of supraphysiologic doses of thyroid hormone.
5. Perform linkage analysis and demonstrate a thyroid receptor gene defect.

In addition to symptoms and signs of thyrotoxicosis, some patients with TSH-producing (thyrotroph) pituitary adenomas may present with acromegaly due to the concomitant hypersecretion of growth hormone by the tumor. Galactorrhea and amenorrhea in association with hyperprolactinemia have also been reported (see chap 31). The tumor may be demonstrated by computerized tomography or by magnetic resonance imaging of the pituitary. A typical finding in patients with TSH-producing pituitary adenomas is a disproportionate abundance in serum of free α-subunit of TSH relative to whole TSH.[112] Moreover, with rare exceptions,[113] serum TSH fails to increase above the basal level in response to TRH or to decrease during the administration of thyroid hormone. Although tumors of trophoblastic origin produce thyroid-stimulating glycoproteins, ectopic production of TSH has not been unequivocally demonstrated (see chap 33). It is uncertain that endogenous TSH hypersecretion could maintain high thyroid hormone levels and induce hyperthyroidism.

Because the etiology of PRTH is not distinct from that of RTH, failure to demonstrate an anatomic defect in the pituitary gland by imaging does not exclude the presence of a small adenoma or thyrotroph hyperplasia. Furthermore, absence of conspicuous signs and symptoms of hypermetabolism are not sufficient to rule out thyrotoxicosis. The occurrence of an apparent selective hyposensitivity to thyroid hormone has been reported in one family.[114] It was probably due to a defect in type II 5'-deiodinase because administration of replacement doses of T_3 but not T_4 suppressed the inappropriate secretion of TSH. This enzyme is involved in the generation of T_3 from T_4 in the pituitary gland and central nervous tissue (see chap 8).

Proving the existence of peripheral tissue resistance to thyroid hormone, central to the diagnosis of RTH, is not simple. Lack of clinical symptoms and signs of hypermetabolism is not sufficient to establish the diagnosis, and no single test objectively proves the existence of eumetabolism. Because resistance to the hormone is variable in different tissues, no single test measuring a particular response to thyroid hormone is diagnostic. Furthermore, most tests that measure the effect of thyroid hormone on peripheral tissues give results with considerable overlap among thyrotoxic, euthyroid, and hypothyroid subjects. The value of these tests is enhanced if measurements are obtained before and after the administration of supraphysiologic doses of thyroid hormone.

A standardized diagnostic protocol, using short-term administration of incremental doses of L-T_3, is recommended (Fig 90-6). It is designed to assess several parameters of central and peripheral tissue effects of thyroid hormone in the basal state as compared to those elicited after the administration of L-T_3. The three doses given in sequence are a replacement dose of 50 μg/d and two supraphysiologic doses of 100 and 200 μg/d. The hormone is administered in a split dose every 12 hours and each incremental dose is given for the period of 3 days. Doses are adjusted in children and in adults of unusual size to achieve the same level of serum T_3. L-T_3, rather than L-T_4, is used because of its direct effect on tissues, bypassing potential defects of T_4 transport and metabolism that may also produce attenuated responses. In addition, the more rapid onset and shorter duration of T_3 action reduces the period required to complete the evaluation and shortens the du-

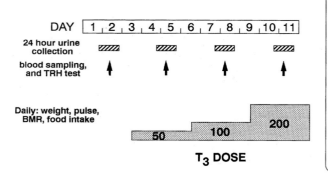

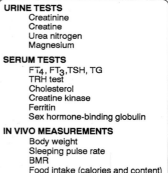

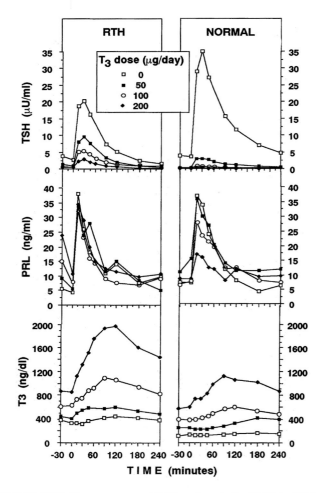

FIGURE 90-6. Schematic representation of a protocol for the assessment of the sensitivity to thyroid hormone using incremental doses of L-T$_3$. For details see text. (Adapted from Refetoff S, Weiss RE, Usala SJ. The syndromes of resistance to thyroid hormone. Endocr Rev 1993;14:348)

ration of symptoms that may arise in individuals with normal responses to the hormone.

Responses to each incremental dose of L-T$_3$ are expressed as increments and decrements or as a percent of the value measured at baseline. The results of such a study are shown in Figures 90-7 and 90-8.

Failure to differentiate RTH from ordinary thyrotoxicosis has resulted in the inappropriate treatment of nearly one-third of the patients. The diagnosis requires awareness of this entity usually suspected when high levels of circulating thyroid hormones are not accompanied by a suppressed TSH. Because of the development of sensitive and specific methods for the measurement of serum TSH, this test is being used with greater frequency in the diagnosis of thyrotoxicosis.

TREATMENT

Although no specific treatment is available to fully and specifically correct the defect, the ability to identify specific mutations in the TRs provides a means for prenatal diagnosis and appropriate family counseling. This is particularly important in families whose affected members show evidence of growth or mental retardation. Fortunately, in most cases of RTH, the partial tissue resistance to thyroid hormone appears to be adequately compensated for by an increase in the endogenous supply of thyroid hormone. Thus, treatment need not be given to such patients. This is not the case in patients with limited thyroidal reserve due to prior ablative therapy. In these patients, the serum TSH level can be used as a guideline for hormone dosage.

Not infrequently, some peripheral tissues in patients with RTH appear to be relatively more resistant than the pituitary. Thus, compensation for the defect at the level of peripheral tissues is incomplete. In such instances, judicious administration of supraphysiologic doses of the hormone is indicated. Because the dose varies greatly among cases, it should be individually determined by assessing tissue responses. In childhood, particular attention must be paid to growth, bone maturation, and mental development. It is suggested that thyroid hormone be given in incremental doses and that the BMR, nitrogen balance, and serum SHBG be monitored at each dose, and bone age and growth on a longer term. Development of a catabolic state is an indication of overtreatment.

FIGURE 90-7. The responses of TSH and prolactin (PRL) to TRH at baseline and at the completion of each dose of L-T$_3$. Measurements were begun before treatment and 15 minutes before the administration of the last incremental L-T$_3$ dose level. TRH was given 15 minutes after the administration of L-T$_3$ (time 0). Note the reduced suppressive effect of L-T$_3$ in the patient with RTH even though serum T$_3$ levels achieved were higher than in the normal subject. Data shown in Fig 90-7 are from the same study. (From Sakuri A, Takeda K, Ain K, et al. Generalizied resistance to thyroid hormone associated with a mutation in the ligand-binding domain of the human thyroid receptor b. Proc Natl Acad Sci USA 1989;86:8977)

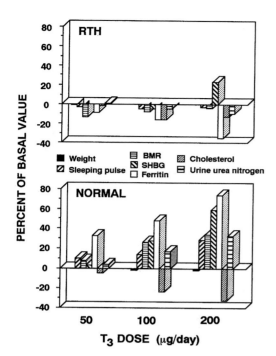

FIGURE 90-8. Responses of peripheral tissues to the administration of L-T₃. Each L-T₃ dose level was given for 3 consecutive days and was administered in 6 doses, every 12 hours. Average responses for each parameter and treatment period are expressed as percent increment (+) or decrement (−) from the corresponding mean basal value. Results of a patient with RTH are compared to those of a normal relative. Serum levels of T₃ achieved on each dose of L-T₃ were comparable to or higher than those of the normal subject. Yet, the responses in the patient with RTH are clearly attenuated. (From Sakuri A, Takeda K, Ain K, et al. Generalizied resistance to thyroid hormone associated with a mutation in the ligand-binding domain of the human thyroid receptor b. Proc Natl Acad Sci USA 1989;86:8977)

The exact criteria for treatment of RTH in infancy have not been established. This will become an issue in view of neonatal screening programs leading to early diagnosis. In infants with elevated serum TSH levels, subclinical hypothyroidism may be more harmful than treatment with thyroid hormone. Indications for treatment may include a TSH level above the upper limit of normal, retarded bone development, and failure to thrive. The outcome of affected older members of the family who did not receive treatment may serve as a guideline. Longer follow-up and psychological testing of infants who have been given treatment will determine the efficacy of early intervention.

Patients with more severe thyrotroph resistance and symptoms of thyrotoxicosis may require therapy. Usually symptomatic treatment with an β-adrenergic blocking agent, preferably atenolol, would suffice. Treatment with antithyroid drugs or thyroid gland ablation increase TSH secretion and may result in thyrotroph hyperplasia. Development of true pituitary tumors, even after long periods of thyrotroph overactivity, have not been reported.

Patients with presumed isolated peripheral tissue resistance to thyroid hormone present a most difficult therapeutic dilemma. The problem is, in reality, diagnostic rather than therapeutic. Many, if not most, patients falling into this category are habitual thyroid hormone users. Gradual reduction of the thyroid hormone dose and psychotherapy is recommended.

References

1. Refetoff S, Weiss RE, Usala SJ. The syndromes of resistance to thyroid hormone. Endocr Rev 1993;14:348
1a. Brucker-Davis I, Skarulis MC, Grace MB, et al. Genetic and clinical features of 42 kindreds with resistance to thyroid hormone: the National Institutes of Health prospective study. Ann Intern Med 1995;123:572
2. Weintraub BD, Gershengorn MC, Kourides IA, Fein H. Inappropriate secretion of thyroid stimulating hormone. Ann Intern Med 1981;95:339
3. Kaplan MM, Swartz SL, Larsen PR. Partial peripheral resistance to thyroid hormone. Am J Med 1981;70:1115
4. Beck-Peccoz P, Roncoroni R, Mariotti S, et al. Sex hormone-binding globulin measurement in patients with inappropriate secretion of thyrotropin (IST): evidence against selective pituitary thyroid hormone resistance in nonneoplastic IST. J Clin Endocrinol Metab 1990;71:19
5. Beck-Peccoz P, Chatterjee VKK. The variable clinical phenotype in thyroid hormone resistance syndrome. Thyroid 1994;4:225
6. Usala SJ. Molecular diagnosis and characterization of thyroid hormone resistance syndromes. Thyroid 1991;1:361
7. Refetoff S, DeWind LT, DeGroot LJ. Familial syndrome combining deaf-mutism, stippled epiphyses, goiter, and abnormally high PBI: possible target organ refractoriness to thyroid hormone. J Clin Endocrinol Metab 1967;27:279
8. Weiss RE, Balzano S, Scherberg NH, Refetoff S. Neonatal detection of generalized resistance to thyroid hormone. JAMA 1990; 264:2245
9. Salmerón de Diego J, Alonso Rodriguez C, Salazar Orlando A, et al. Syndrome of "inappropriate secretion of thyroid-stimulating hormone" by partial target organ resistance to thyroid hormones. Acta Endocrinol 1981;97:361
10. Sterling K, Aranow H. Acquired refractoriness to thyroid hormone action in treated toxic nodular goiter. JAMA 1981;245:1339
11. DeMeirleir K, Golstein J, Jonckheer MH, Vanhaelst L. Hypothyroidism with normal thyroid hormone levels as a consequence of autoimmune thyroiditis and peripheral resistance to thyroid hormone. Acta Clin Belg 1980;35:107
12. Connell JMC, McLaren EH. Partial end organ resistance to thyroid hormone in congenital hypothyroidism. Postgrad Med 1981;57:518
13. Takeda K, Sakurai A, DeGroot LJ, Refetoff S. Recessive inheritance of thyroid hormone resistance caused by complete deletion of the protein-coding region of the thyroid hormone receptor-β gene. J Clin Endocrinol Metab 1992;74:49
14. Ono S, Schwartz ID, Mueller OT, et al. Homozygosity for a "dominant negative" thyroid hormone receptor gene responsible for generalized resistance to thyroid hormone. J Clin Endocrinol Metab 1991;73:990
15. Kasai Y, Aritaki S, Utsunomiya M, Matsuno T. Twin sisters with Refetoff's syndrome. J Jap Pediatr Assoc 1983;87:1203
16. Sarne DH, Refetoff S, Rosenfield RL, Farriaux JP. Sex-hormone binding globulin in the diagnosis of peripheral tissue resistance to thyroid hormone: the value of changes following short-term triiodothyronine administration. J Clin Endocrinol Metab 1988; 66:740
17. Magner JA, Petrick P, Menezes-Ferreira MM, et al. Familial generalized resistance to thyroid hormones: report of three kindreds and correlation of patterns of affected tissues with the binding of (125I) triiodothyronine to fibroblast nuclei. J Endocrinol Invest 1986;9:459

18. Refetoff S, DeGroot LJ, Benard B, DeWind LT. Studies of a sibship with apparent hereditary resistance to the intracellular action of thyroid hormone. Metabolism 1972;21:723

19. Lamberg BA. Congenital euthyroid goitre and partial peripheral resistance to thyroid hormones. Lancet 1973;1:854

20. Gómez-Sáez JM, Fernández Castañer M, Navarro MA, et al. Resistencia parcial a las hormonas tiroideas con bocio y eutiroidismo. Med Clin 1981;76:412

21. Refetoff S, Matalon R, Bigazzi M. Metabolism of L-thyroxine (T₄) and L-triiodothyronine (T₃) by human fibroblasts in tissue culture: evidence for cellular binding proteins and conversion of T₄ to T₃. Endocrinology 1972;91:934

22. Gheri RG, Bianchi R, Mariani G, et al. A new case of familial partial generalized resistance to thyroid hormone: study of 3,5,3′-triiodothyronine (T₃) binding to lymphocyte and skin fibroblast nuclei and in vivo conversion of thyroxine to T₃. J Clin Endocrinol Metab 1984;58:563

23. Kaplowitz PB, D'Ercole AJ, Utiger RD. Peripheral resistance to thyroid hormone in an infant. J Clin Endocrinol Metab 1981;53:958

24. Oppenheimer JH, Koerner D, Schwartz HL, Surks MI. Specific-nuclear triiodothyronine binding sites in rat liver and kidney. J Clin Endocrinol Metab 1972;35:330

25. Bernal J, Refetoff S, DeGroot LJ. Abnormalities of triiodothyronine binding to lymphocyte and fibroblast nuclei from a patient with peripheral resistance to thyroid hormone action. J Clin Endocrinol Metab 1978;47:1266

26. Liewendahl K, Rosengård S, Lamberg BA. Nuclear binding of triiodothyronine and thyroxine in lymphocytes from subjects with hyperthyroidism, hypothyroidism and resistance to thyroid hormones. Clin Chem Acta 1978;83:41

27. Sap J, Muñoz A, Damm K, et al. The c-*erb*A protein is a high-affinity receptor for thyroid hormone. Nature 1986;324:635

28. Weinberger C, Thompson CC, Ong ES, et al. The c-*erb*A gene encodes a thyroid hormone receptor. Nature 1986;324:641

29. Usala SJ, Bale AE, Gesundheit N, et al. Tight linkage between the syndrome of generalized thyroid hormone resistance and the human c-*erb*Aβ gene. Mol Endocrinol 1988;2:1217

30. Sakurai A, Takeda K, Ain K, et al. Generalized resistance to thyroid hormone associated with a mutation in the ligand-binding domain of the human thyroid hormone receptor β. Proc Natl Acad Sci U S A 1989;86:8977

31. Usala SJ, Tennyson GE, Bale AE, et al. A base mutation of the c-*erb*Aβ thyroid hormone receptor in a kindred with generalized thyroid hormone resistance. Molecular heterogeneity in two other kindreds. J Clin Invest 1990;85:93

32. Behr M, Loos U. A point mutation (Ala²²⁹ to Thr) in the hinge domain of the c-*erb*Aβ thyroid hormone receptor in a family with generalized thyroid hormone resistance. Mol Endocrinol 1992;6:1119

33. Pohlenz J, Schönberger W, Wemme H, et al. A new point mutation (R243W) in the hormone-binding domain of the c-*erb*Aβ₁ gene in a family with generalized resistance to thyroid hormone. Hum Mutation 1996;7:79

34. Onigata K, Yagi H, Hagashima K, Kuroume T. Point mutation in exon of the c-*erb*Aβ thyroid hormone receptor gene in a family with generalized thyroid hormone resistance. 98th Meeting of the Japanese Pediatric Society. Yokohama, Japan, 1993

35. Persani L, Asteria C, Tonacchera M, et al. Evidence for secretion of thyrotropin with enhanced bioactivity in syndromes of thyroid hormone resistance. J Clin Endocrinol Metab 1994;78:1034

36. Adams M, Matthews C, Collingwood TN, et al. Genetic analysis of 29 kindreds with generalized and pituitary resistance to thyroid hormone: identification of thirteen novel mutations in the thyroid hormone receptor β gene. J Clin Invest 1994;94:506

37. Takeda K, Weiss RE, Refetoff S. Rapid localization of mutations in the thyroid hormone receptor-β gene by denaturing gradient gel electrophoresis in 18 families with thyroid hormone resistance. J Clin Endocrinol Metab 1992;74:712

38. Geffner ME, Su F, Ross NS, et al. An arginine to histidine mutation in codon 311 of the c-*erb*Aβ gene results in a mutant thyroid hormone receptor that does not mediate a dominant negative phenotype. J Clin Invest 1993;91:538

39. Weiss RE, Stein MA, Duck SC, et al. Low intelligence but not attention deficit hyperactivity disorder is associated with resistance to thyroid hormone caused by mutation R316H in the thyroid hormone receptor β gene. J Clin Endocrinol Metab 1994;78:1525

40. Hayashi Y, Sunthornthepvarakul T, Refetoff S. Mutations of CpG dinucleotides located in the triiodothyronine (T₃)-binding domain of the thyroid hormone receptor (TR) β gene that appears to be devoid of natural mutations may not be detected because they are unlikely to produce the clinical phenotype of resistance to thyroid hormone. J Clin Invest 1994;94:607

41. Weiss RE, Weinberg M, Refetoff S. Identical mutations in unrelated families with generalized resistance to thyroid hormone occur in cytosine-guanine-rich areas of the thyroid hormone receptor beta gene: analysis of 15 families. J Clin Invest 1993;91:2408

42. Parrilla R, Mixson AJ, McPherson JA, et al. Characterization of seven novel mutations of the c-*erb*Aβ gene in unrelated kindreds with generalized thyroid hormone resistance. Evidence for two "hot spot" regions of the ligand binding domain. J Clin Invest 1991;88:2123

43. Pohlenz J, Wirth S, Winterpacht A, et al. Phenotypic variability in patients with generalized resistance to thyroid hormone. J Med Genet 1995;32:393

44. Burman KD, Djuh YY, Nicholson D, et al. Generalized thyroid hormone resistance: identification of an arginine to cystine mutation in codon 315 of the c-*erb*A beta thyroid hormone receptor. J Endocrinol Invest 1992;15:573

45. Cugini CD Jr, Leidy JW Jr, Chertow BS, et al. An arginine to histidine mutation in codon 315 of the c-*erb*Aβ thyroid hormone receptor in a kindred with generalized resistance to thyroid hormones results in a receptor with significant 3,5,3′- triiodothyronine binding activity. J Clin Endocrinol Metab 1992;74:1164

46. Weiss RE, Marcocci C, Bruno-Bossio G, Refetoff S. Multiple genetic factors in the heterogeneity of thyroid hormone resistance. J Clin Endocrinol Metab 1993;76:257

47. Bartolone L, Regalbuto C, Benvenga S, et al. Three new mutations of thyroid hormone receptor-β associated with resistance to thyroid hormone. J Clin Endocrinol Metab 1994;78:323

48. Mixson AJ, Parrilla R, Ransom SC, et al. Correlations of language abnormalities with localization of mutations in the β-thyroid hormone receptor in 13 kindreds with generalized resistance to thyroid hormone: identification of four new mutations. J Clin Endocrinol Metab 1992;75:1039

49. Usala SJ, Menke JB, Hao EH, et al. Mutations in the c-*erb*A-beta gene in two different patients with selective pituitary resistance to thyroid hormones. 74th Annual Meeting of The Endocrine Society. San Antonio, Texas, 1992:135

50. Collingwood TN, Adams M, Tone Y, Chatterjee VKK. Spectrum of transcriptional, dimerization, and dominant negative properties of twenty different mutant thyroid hormone β-receptors in thyroid hormone resistance syndrome. Mol Endocrinol 1994;8:1262

51. Usala SJ, Menke JB, Watson TL, et al. A homozygous deletion in the c-*erb*Aβ thyroid hormone receptor gene in a patient with generalized thyroid hormone resistance: isolation and characterization of the mutant receptor. Mol Endocrinol 1991;5:327

52. Sasaki S, Nakamura H, Tagami T, et al. Pituitary resistance to thyroid hormone associated with a base mutation in the hormone-

binding domain of the human 3,5,3′-triiodothyronine receptor-β. J Clin Endocrinol Metab 1993;76:1254

53. Mixson AJ, Renault JC, Ransom S, et al. Identification of a novel mutation in the gene encoding the β-triiodothyronine receptor in a patient with apparent selective pituitary resistance to thyroid hormone. Clin Endocrinol 1993;38:227

54. Usala SJ, Menke JB, Watson TL, et al. A new point mutation in the 3,5,3′-triiodothyronine-binding domain of the c-*erb* Aβ thyroid hormone receptor is tightly linked to generalized thyroid hormone resistance. J Clin Endocrinol Metab 1991;72:32

55. Grace MB, Buzard GS. Mutant allele PCR and sequencing (MAPS): a novel method for identification of mutations of the human thyroid receptor-β (hTR-β) gene in patients with resistance to thyroid hormone. Thyroid 1994;4:S-83

56. Yen PM, Sugawara A, Refetoff S, Chin WW. New insights on the mechanism(s) of the dominant negative effect of mutant thyroid hormone receptor in generalized resistance to thyroid hormone. J Clin Invest 1992;90:1825

57. Adams M, Nagaya T, Tone Y, et al. Functional properties of a novel mutant thyroid hormone receptor in a family with generalized thyroid hormone resistance syndrome. Clin Endocrinol 1992;36:281

58. Flynn TR, Hollenberg AN, Cohen O, et al. A novel C-terminal domain in the thyroid hormone receptor selectively mediates thyroid hormone inhibition. J Biol Chem 1994;629:32713

59. Tsukaguchi H, Yoshimasa Y, Fujimoto K, et al. Three novel mutations of thyroid hormone receptor-β gene in unrelated patients with resistance to thyroid hormone: two mutations of the same codon (H435L and H453Q) produce separate subtypes of resistance. J Clin Endocrinol Metab 1995;80:3613

60. Sakurai A, Miyamoto T, Hughes IA, DeGroot LJ. Characterization of a novel mutant human thyroid hormone receptor β in a family with hereditary thyroid hormone resistance. Clin Endocrinol 1993;38:29

61. Boothroyd CV, Teh BT, Hayward NK, et al. Single base mutation in the hormone binding domain of the thyroid hormone receptor β gene in generalized thyroid hormone resistance demonstrated by single stranded conformation polymorphism analysis. Biochem Biophys Res Commun 1991;178:606

62. Gharib H, Nagaya T, Stelter A, et al. Characterization of the c-*erb*Aβ R438H mutant in generalized thyroid hormone resistance. Endocr J 1993;1:193

63. Sasaki S, Nakamura H, Tagami T, et al. A point mutation of the T₃ receptor beta 1 gene in a kindred of generalized resistance to thyroid hormone. Mol Cell Endocrinol 1992;84:159

64. Weiss RE, Chyna B, Duell PB, et al. A point mutation (C446R) in the thyroid hormone receptor-β gene of a family with resistance to thyroid hormone. J Clin Endocrinol Metab 1994;78:1253

65. Groenhout EG, Dorin RI. Generalized thyroid hormone resistance due to a deletion of the carboxy terminus of the c-*erb*Aβ receptor. Mol Cell Endocrinol 1994;99:81

66. Nakamura H, Sasaki S, Tagami T, et al. Identification and functions of abnormal T₃ receptors in patients with thyroid hormone resistance (abstract). Thyroid 1993;Suppl 3:T-3

67. Nakamura H, Sasaki S, Tagami T, et al. Analysis of the T₃ receptor genes in patients with generalized resistance to thyroid hormone and selective pituitary form. Thyroid 1992;2(Suppl 1):S-36

68. Shuto Y, Wakabayashi I, Amuro N, et al. A point mutation in the 3,5,3′-triiodothyronine-binding domain of thyroid hormone receptor β associated with a family with generalized resistance to thyroid hormone. J Clin Endocrinol Metab 1992;75:213

69. Refetoff S, Weiss RE, Wing JR, et al. Resistance to thyroid hormone in subjects from two unrelated families is associated with a point mutation in the thyroid hormone receptor β gene resulting in the replacement of the normal proline 453 with serine. Thyroid 1994;4:249

70. Usala SJ, Wondisford FE, Watson TL, et al. Thyroid hormone and DNA binding properties of a mutant c-*erb*Aβ receptor associated with generalized thyroid hormone resistance. Biochem Biophys Res Commun 1990;171:575

71. Sakurai A, Miyamoto T, Refetoff S, DeGroot LJ. Dominant negative transcriptional regulation by a mutant thyroid hormone receptor β in a family with generalized resistance to thyroid hormone. Mol Endocrinol 1990;4:1988

72. Chatterjee VKK, Nagaya T, Madison LD, et al. Thyroid hormone resistance syndrome. Inhibition of normal receptor function by mutant thyroid hormone receptors. J Clin Invest 1991;87:1977

73. Nagaya T, Madison LD, Jameson JL. Thyroid hormone receptor mutants that cause resistance to thyroid hormone. Evidence for receptor competition for DNA sequences in target genes. J Biol Chem 1992;267:13014

74. Nagaya T, Jameson JL. Thyroid hormone receptor dimerization is required for the dominant negative inhibition by mutations that cause thyroid hormone resistance. J Biol Chem 1993;268:15766

75. Hao E, Menke JB, Smith AM, et al. Divergent dimerization properties of mutant β1 thyroid hormone receptors are associated with different dominant negative activities. Mol Endocrinol 1994;8:841

76. Au-Fliegner M, Helmer E, Casanova J, et al. The conserved ninth C-terminal heptad in thyroid hormone and retinoic acid receptors mediates diverse responses by affecting heterodimer but not homodimer formation. Mol Cel Endocrinol 1993;13:5725

77. Zavacki AM, Harney JW, Brent GA, Larsen PR. Dominant negative inhibition by mutant thyroid hormone receptors is thyroid hormone response element and receptor isoform specific. Mol Endocrinol 1993;7:1319

78. Nagaya T, Eberhardt NL, Jameson JL. Thyroid hormone resistance syndrome: correlation of dominant negative activity and location of mutations. J Clin Endocrinol Metab 1993;77:982

79. Chait A, Kanter R, Green W, Kenny M. Defective thyroid hormone action in fibroblasts cultured from subjects with the syndrome of resistance to thyroid hormones. J Clin Endocrinol Metab 1982;54:767

80. Murata Y, Refetoff S, Horwitz AL, Smith TJ. Hormonal regulation of glycosaminoglycan accumulation in fibroblasts from patients with resistance to thyroid hormone. J Clin Endocrinol Metab 1983;57:1233

81. Ceccarelli P, Refetoff S, Murata Y. Resistance to thyroid hormone diagnosed by the reduced response of fibroblasts to the triiodothyronine induced suppression of fibronectin synthesis. J Clin Endocrinol Metab 1987;65:242

82. Sobieszczyk S, Refetoff S. Abnormal response of fibronectin messenger RNA to triiodothyronine in fibroblasts from patients with generalized resistance to thyroid hormone (abstract). 63rd Annual Meeting of the American Thyroid Association. Montreal, Quebec: 1987;121(Suppl):T-24

83. Hodin RA, Lazar MA, Chin WW. Differential and tissue-specific regulation of the multiple rat c-*erb*A messenger RNA species by thyroid hormone. J Clin Invest 1990;85:101

84. Sakurai A, Nakai A, DeGroot LJ. Expression of three forms of thyroid hormone receptor in human tissues. Mol Endocrinol 1989;3:392

85. Falcone M, Miyamoto T, Fierro-Renoy F, et al. Antipeptide polyclonal antibodies specifically recognize each human thyroid hormone receptor isoform. Endocrinology 1992;131:2419

86. Wortsman J, Premachandra BN, Williams K, et al. Familial resistance to thyroid hormone associated with decreased transport across the plasma membrane. Ann Intern Med 1983;98:904

87. Maxon HR, Burman KD, Premachandra BN, et al. Familial elevation of total and free thyroxine in healthy, euthyroid subjects without detectable binding protein abnormalities. Acta Endocrinol 1982;100:224

88. Hutchison JH, Arneil GC, McGerr EM. Deficiency of an extrathyroid enzyme in sporadic cretinism. Lancet 1957;2:314

89. Bode HH, Danon M, Weintraub BD, et al. Partial target organ resistance to thyroid hormone. J Clin Invest 1973;52:776

90. Refetoff S, Salazar A, Smith TJ, Scherberg NH. The consequences of inappropriate treatment due to failure to recognize the syndrome of pituitary and peripheral tissue resistance to thyroid hormone. Metabolism 1983;32:822

91. Tamagna EI, Carlson HE, Hershman JM, Reed AW. Pituitary and peripheral resistance to thyroid hormone. Clin Endocrinol 1979;10:431

92. Cooper DS, Ladenson PW, Nisula BC, et al. Familial thyroid hormone resistance. Metabolism 1982;31:504

93. Vandalem JL, Pirens G, Hennen G. Familial inappropriate TSH secretion: evidence suggesting a dissociated pituitary resistance to T_3 and T_4. J Endocrinol Invest 1981;4:413

94. Refetoff S, DeGroot LJ, Barsano CP. Defective thyroid hormone feedback regulation in the syndrome of peripheral resistance to thyroid hormone. J Clin Endocrinol Metab 1980;51:41

95. David L, Blanc JF, Chatelain P, et al. Goitre congéntal avec résistance péripherique partielle aux hormones thyroïdiennes. Ou syndrome de pseudo-hyperthyroïdie. Pédiatrie 1979;34:443

96. Lamberg B-A, Liewendahl K. Thyroid hormone resistance. Ann Clin Res 1980;12:243

97. Bajorunas DR, Rosner W, Kourides IA. Use of bromocriptine in a patient with generalized resistance to thyroid hormone. J Clin Endocrinol Metab 1984;58:731

98. Mäenpää J, Liewendahl K. Peripheral insensitivity to thyroid hormones in a euthyroid girl with goitre. Arch Dis Child 1980;55:207

99. Gabrilove JL, Ludwig AW. The histogenesis of myxedema. J Clin Endocrinol Metab 1957;17:925

100. Pagliara AS, Caplan RH, Gundersen CB, et al. Peripheral resistance to thyroid hormone in a family: heterogeneity of clinical presentation. J Pediatr 1983;103:228

101. Lamberg BA, Sandström R, Rosengård S, et al. Sporadic and familial partial peripheral resistance to thyroid hormone. In: Harland WA, Orr JS, eds. Thyroid hormone metabolism. London: Academic Press, 1975:139

102. Hauser P, Zametkin AJ, Martinez P, et al. Attention deficit-hyperactivity disorder in people with generalized resistance to thyroid hormone. N Engl J Med 1993;328:997

103. Weiss RE, Stein MA, Trommer B, Refetoff S. Attention-deficit hyperactivity disorder and thyroid function. J Pediatr 1993;123:539

104. Elia J, Gulotta C, Rose SR, et al. Thyroid function and attention-deficit hyperactivity disorder. J Am Acad Child Adolesc Psychiatry 1994;33:169

105. Ohzeki T, Egi S, Egawa M, Hachimori K. Thyroid hormone unresponsiveness in two siblings with intrauterine growth retardation and exophthalmos. Eur J Pediatr 1984;141:181

106. Bantle JP, Seeling S, Mariash CN, et al. Resistance to thyroid hormones: a disorder frequently confused with Graves' disease. Arch Intern Med 1982;142:1867

107. Schimmel M, Utiger R. Thyroidal and peripheral production of thyroid hormones: review of recent findings and their clinical implications. Ann Intern Med 1977;87:760

108. Sarne DH, Sobieszczyk S, Ain KB, Refetoff S. Serum thyrotropin and prolactin in the syndrome of generalized resistance to thyroid hormone: responses to thyrotropin-releasing hormone stimulation and triiodothyronine suppression. J Clin Endocrinol Metab 1990;70:1305

109. Hughes IA, Ichikawa K, DeGroot LJ, et al. Non-adenomatous inappropriate TSH hypersecretion and euthyroidism requires no treatment. Clin Endocrinol 1987;27:475

110. Lamberg BA, Rosengård S, Liwendahl K, et al. Familial partial peripheral resistance to thyroid hormones. Acta Endocrinol 1978;87:303

111. Kunitake JM, Hartman N, Henson LC, et al. 3,5,3'-triiodothyroacetic acid therapy for thyroid hormone resistance. J Clin Endocrinol Metab 1989;69:461

112. Beck-Peccoz P, Persani L, Faglia G. Glycoprotein hormone α-subunit in pituitary adenomas. Trends Endocrinol Metab 1992;3:41

113. Mornex R, Tommasi M, Cure M, et al. Hyperthyroidie associee a un hypopituitarisme au cours de l'evolution d'une tumeur hypophysaire secretant T.S.H. Ann d'Endocrinol (Paris) 1972;33:390

114. Rösler A, Litvin Y, Hage C, et al. Familial hyperthyroidism due to inappropriate thyrotropin secretion successfully treated with triiodothyronine. J Clin Endocrinol Metab 1982;54:76

Werner and Ingbar's The Thyroid, Seventh Edition,
edited by Lewis E. Braverman and Robert D. Utiger.
Lippincott–Raven Publishers, Philadelphia, © 1996

91

Infections of the Thyroid Gland

Nesli Basgoz

Morton N. Swartz

Infections of the thyroid gland are rare. The actual incidence is difficult to estimate because much of the early literature on acute or subacute thyroiditis assumed that it was infectious in etiology, and the lack of an identifiable infectious agent was attributed to early stages of infection or inability to identify or culture the microorganism.[1] Review of this early literature is further confounded by variability in the type of clinical information recorded, the availability of microbiologic techniques for diagnosis, and thyroid function testing. Advances in microbiology and pathology have made it possible to differentiate infectious from noninfectious cases of thyroiditis. Several excellent recent reviews have summarized the features of the proven infectious causes of thyroiditis.[2,3]

We present an overview of infections of the thyroid, including the pathogenesis of thyroid infection, the diagnosis and differential diagnosis of infectious thyroiditis, and the particular infectious agents associated with infectious thyroiditis.

PATHOGENESIS

Acute suppurative thyroiditis is rare. The low incidence of infection of the thyroid suggests that protective mechanisms must exist. They include a rich blood supply, an extensive system of lymph drainage,[1,4] high glandular concentrations of iodine, which may be bactericidal,[1,5] and separation of the gland from other structures in the head and neck by fascial planes.[1] In 1931, Womack and colleagues demonstrated this resistance to infection experimentally by injecting either staphylococci or streptococci into the carotid arteries (from which the arterial supply of the thyroid takes origin) of dogs, none of whom developed thyroid infections.[6]

The most common predisposing condition for thyroid infection appears to be preexisting thyroid disease.[1,2] It is noted in over two-thirds of women and one-half of men with infectious thyroiditis. Predisposing conditions include simple goiter, nodular goiter, adenoma, thyroiditis, and carcinoma. Infections of the thyroid gland with opportunisitic pathogens such as *Aspergillus* species or *Pneumocystis carinii* are associated with the same immunocompromising conditions that underlie other infections with these pathogens.[7–9]

Spread of infection from a contiguous focus may occur either in the setting of thyroid surgery or from communication with infections of other structures of the head and neck. Although wound infection may occur after thyroid surgery as after any other operation, it is exceedingly rare for this type of infection to involve the thyroid gland itself.[10] Infection may spread directly from embryologic cysts (primarily cysts at the terminations of internal fistulas originating in a pyriform sinus, and cysts of third or fourth branchial pouch origin) of the neck, as described below. In addition, infection may spread from the adjacent deep fascial spaces. Infections of the retropharyngeal spaces (from pharyngitis or tonsillitis) or of the lateral pharyngeal spaces (from pharyngitis, tonsillitis, odontogenic infection, parotitis, mastoiditis, or otitis) may rarely spread down posterior or lateral fascial planes into the neck and communicate with the anterior, pretracheal space that surrounds the esophagus, trachea, and thyroid. Infection may also arise directly in this pretracheal space, most commonly through perforations in the esophagus.[11]

Acute suppurative thyroiditis in children, particularly if recurrent, is associated in approximately 90% of cases with a left pyriform sinus fistula as the apparent route of infection[12,13] (Fig 91-1). The common involvement in pediatric acute suppurative

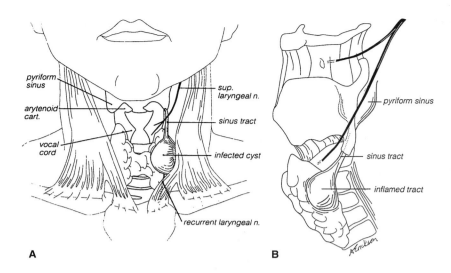

FIGURE 91-1. Fistulous tract extending from apex of the left pyriform sinus to infected cyst ending adjacent to or within left lobe of the thyroid. The tract passes deep to the superior laryngeal nerve and superficial to the recurrent laryngeal nerve. (*A*) Frontal view. (*B*) Lateral view. (Reproduced from Har-El G, Sasaki CT, Prager D, Krespi YP. Acute suppurative thyroiditis and the bronchial apparatus. Am J Otolaryngol 1991;12:6, with permission)

thyroiditis of aerobic and anaerobic bacteria indigenous to the upper respiratory tract is consistent with their passage via the fistula to the perithyroid space and the thyroid itself.

Hematogenous spread also occurs and is postulated to be the mechanism of infection in patients who had a preceding focus of infection in the skin, lower respiratory tract, or genitourinary or gastrointestinal tract. Positive cultures from the distant site, with or without positive blood cultures, suggest hematogenous dissemination of infection. A larger number of these cases occurs in adults than children, often in the presence of other underlying illnesses.[2]

DIAGNOSIS AND DIFFERENTIAL DIAGNOSIS

The differential diagnosis of infectious thyroiditis includes infections that involve other structures of the neck as well as other, noninfectious conditions of the thyroid gland itself.

Cervical adenitis is common and may present with a tender, warm, and enlarged mass in the neck. However, in most cases its anatomic location will easily distinguish it from infections of the thyroid.

A variety of cysts of the neck may become infected and be confused with infections of the thyroid.[3] Thyroglossal duct cysts are the most common congenital masses. They are almost always located in the midline. They result from embryologic anomalies in the descent of the thyroid into the neck and are located below the hyoid bone near the midline. They should move with swallowing and with protrusion of the tongue because they are attached both to the thyroid gland and to the tongue. They can cause respiratory obstruction or, if infected, formation of fistulous tracts in the neck. Suppurative thyroiditis has been reported to result from direct spread of infected material through a patent thyroglossal fistula.[1,14]

In addition to thyroglossal duct cysts, two other embryologic abnormalities, cystic hygromas and branchial cleft cysts, may present as infections of the neck. Cystic hygromas develop from the jugular lymph sac when it fails to communicate with the thoracic duct or internal jugular vein and become evident in the first 2 years of life, an uncommon time for

thyroid infections. Although cystic hygromas can appear anywhere in the neck, they typically involve the lower portion posterior to the sternocleidomastoid muscle and do not move on swallowing. Branchial cleft cysts can develop from the first, second, or third pharyngeal clefts, although the second is the most common origin. They usually present in childhood as masses or fistulous tracts posterior to the angle of the mandible. Dermoid cysts can occur anywhere in lines of fusion, including in the neck, most commonly above the hyoid. They also move with swallowing and protrusion of the tongue because they are related to the muscles at the base of the tongue.

Rarely, a bacterial infection in the anterior aspect of the neck (superficial fascial space or pretracheal space) may present as an erythematous warm, slightly swollen area over the thyroid. Such a swollen area does not move with swallowing, and thyroid radionuclide imaging does not reveal related hypofunctioning areas in the thyroid. Computed tomography (CT) and magnetic resonance imaging (MRI) can be valuable in distinguishing between thyroidal and adjacent fascial compartment infections.

It may be difficult to differentiate infections of the thyroid from more common conditions, especially subacute thyroiditis.[13] Subacute thyroiditis is characterized by pain and tenderness of the gland, which can be severe (see chap 34), although systemic manifestations are generally not as prominent as are those of bacterial thyroiditis. A sore throat is noted by most patients with acute suppurative thyroiditis; although it occurs also with subacute thyroiditis, it is less frequent. The active phase of subacute thyroiditis, unlike suppurative thyroiditis, is often accompanied by elevated serum thyroid hormone concentrations.[13] Other noninfectious conditions causing thyroid pain and tenderness include hemorrhage into a thyroid nodule, and occasionally chronic autoimmune thyroiditis and Graves' disease, if thyroid enlargement occurs rapidly. Conversely, slowly growing bacterial or nonbacterial causes of thyroid infection can mimic diffuse goiter, adenoma, or carcinoma clinically, with histologic examination and culture being required for differentiation.

Adjunctive studies may or not be helpful in diagnosis. Most patients with acute bacterial thyroiditis have a leukocytosis. There may be other culture evidence of bacterial infection. Serum thyroid hormone concentrations are usually normal, although there may be mild increases in serum triiodothyronine (T_3) and thyroxine (T_4) concentrations, due to excessive release of the hormones from the inflamed gland.[2] Thyroid radionuclide imaging may show a hypofunctioning area in the region of infection. Ultrasonography can help detect frank abscesses or cysts in the thyroid or in adjacent structures of the neck. Lateral soft tissue radiographs of the neck may show evidence of tissue edema or deviation of the tracheal air column. Anaerobic infection or esophageal perforation may be associated with air in the soft tissues of the neck.[2] CT and MRI of the thyroid define thyroid anatomy (see chap 22) and may delineate a localized infection or abscess.[15]

Bacterial infections are often diagnosed by needle aspiration of the thyroid, which may be facilitated if guided by ultrasonography. This technique has also been used successfully in the diagnosis of some mycobacterial and fungal abscesses.[2] However, many of the thyroid infections not associated with acute bacterial suppuration are diagnosed at surgery.[2]

BACTERIAL INFECTIONS OF THE THYROID GLAND

Acute Bacterial Infections of the Thyroid Gland

Recent reviews provide an excellent summary of the epidemiologic and clinical features of bacterial infections of the thyroid gland.[2,3] Most of these involve pyogenic bacteria, but a variety of other bacterial pathogens also have been described (Table 91-1). Although infection of the thyroid may occur at any age, an increased number of cases occur in certain age groups. One group consists of children under the age of 10 years; their infections are most often in the left lobe and associated with an embryologic remnant, a left pyriform sinus tract, but occasionally with other foci of infection in the head or neck. Among the children with acute suppurative thyroiditis associated with a pyriform sinus fistula who have been reported, the majority had had several episodes of thyroid infection before correct diagnosis and definitive surgical excision.[12,16]

Another group consists of young or middle-aged adults in whom the bacterial thyroiditis is often associated with other diseases of the gland. However, many adults also have a preceding or concurrent focus of infection, either contiguous, as in children, or distant, implying bacteremic spread. Distant infections include erysipelas, pleuropulmonary infections, postpartum sepsis, or infections of the genitourinary and gastrointestinal tracts. In most series over 50% of the adult patients were women, which may simply reflect the fact that most thyroid disorders are more common in women.

Most patients with acute bacterial thyroiditis have had symptoms for less than 1 to 2 weeks before diagnosis. The symptoms nearly always include pain and fever (Table 91-2) and the majority of patients have dysphagia and dysphonia, attributed to compression of local structures. The major signs of acute bacterial thyroiditis are tenderness to palpation, with associated erythema and warmth over the gland, and unilateral or bilateral thyroid lobar enlargement (Fig 91-2). The gland may be firm in one lobe, seemingly diffusely firm, or fluctuant, the latter indicating abscess formation. It is important to recognize that an initially firm thyroid may progress to fluctuance in several days, emphasizing the need for repeated examination. Pharyngitis or other upper or lower respiratory signs and symptoms may reflect associated sites of infection. Cervical lymphadenopathy may be present, particularly when associated with a predisposing pharyngitis, but is not a prominent feature.

Laboratory studies reveal leukocytosis in over two-thirds of patients and normal thyroid function studies in a similar majority. When thyrotoxicosis or hypothyroidism is present, it may be difficult to distinguish preceding thyroid disease from alterations due to the acute infection. Radionuclide imaging may reveal a hypofunctional area in the infected thyroid gland. Ultrasonography of a thyroid abscess shows an enlarged irregular mass of mixed echogenicity with sonolucent

---

TABLE 91-1.
Agents Associated With Bacterial Thyroiditis

ACUTE, SUPPURATIVE

Staphylococcus aureus
Other staphylococci
Streptococcus pyogenes
Streptococcus pneumoniae
Other streptococci
Enterobacteriaceae
Nonenteric gram-negative rods
Anaerobes
Other bacteria

MYCOBACTERIAL

Mycobacterium tuberculosis
Mycobacterium avium–intracellulare
Mycobacterium chelonei

SPIROCHETAL

Treponema pallidum

TABLE 91-2.
Signs and Symptoms of Acute Bacterial Thyroiditis

Pain
Tenderness
Fever
Dysphagia
Dysphonia
Erythema
Warmth
Unilateral thyroid mass or fluctuance (especially involving left lobe in children); deviation of trachea to the opposite side
Bilateral thyroid enlargement

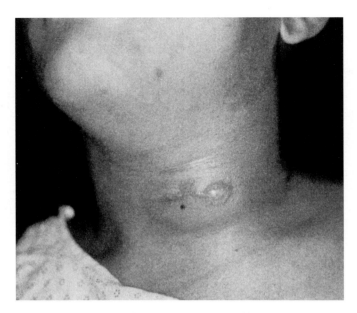

FIGURE 91-2. Neck swelling due to recurrent (three prior episodes) left thyroid abscess in a 43-year-old woman, found on exploration to have a fibrovascular mass extending from the left lobe of thyroid to the left pyriform sinus. The patient had further recurrences after removal of mass. (Reproduced from Har-El G, Sasaki CT, Prager D, Krespi YP. Acute suppurative thyroiditis and the bronchial apparatus. Am J Otolaryngeal 1991;12:6, with permission)

areas, and CT shows a cystic mass with an enhancing zone surrounding area(s) of low attenuation. Infection with anaerobic, gas-forming organisms can occasionally be detected by the presence of soft tissue gas on a radiograph of the neck.

Gram stains and cultures of material obtained by fine-needle aspiration (FNA) or surgical drainage reveal the causative agent in over 90% of cases in which they are performed. Blood cultures are positive in a substantial minority of patients, particularly adults, in whom hematogenous routes of infection appear clinically more likely. A small number of patients with acute bacterial thyroiditis have had sterile, sometimes foul-smelling pus drained from their lesions, presumably representing infection with anaerobic bacteria. The most common organisms isolated in cases of suppurative thyroiditis are listed in Table 91-1. *Staphylococcus aureus* is found in over one-third of cases in all series, usually in pure, but occasionally in mixed, culture. *Streptococcus pyogenes* is the next most commonly recovered organism and is more likely to be associated with a discernible focus of infection in the skin or respiratory tract. *Streptococcus pneumoniae* and other streptococci follow in frequency. In acute suppurative thyroiditis in children or recurrent suppurative thyroiditis in adults, associated with a pyriform sinus fistula, the bacteriology differs somewhat from the foregoing description.[13] In these patients, various streptococci (β-hemolytic, viridans, nonhemolytic, microaerophilic) are the most common isolates, followed in frequency by various anaerobic species (*Bacteroides* species, *Peptococcus* species); *S. aureus* and Enterobacteriaceae each comprise only 5% of isolates.

Enterobacteriaceae, particularly *Escherichia coli*, as well as nonenteric gram-negative bacilli such as *Pseudomonas*

aeruginosa, have been reported, particularly in older patients, but less frequently than gram-positive cocci. Although involvement of the thyroid occurred in less than 1% of patients with typhoid fever, *Salmonella typhi* was once a common enough infection that over 40 cases of salmonella thyroiditis were reported in the medical literature. *Salmonella enteritidis* thyroiditis has also been reported. Anaerobes of the oropharyngeal cavity such as *Bacteroides* and *Fusobacterium* species, usually in mixed culture, are uncommon pathogens in bacterial thyroiditis. Even rarer are infections with anaerobes thought to originate outside of the oral cavity, such as the one due to *Clostridium septicum* reported in a patient who also had colonic carcinoma. Similarly rare is infection with *Actinomyces* species, *Haemophilus* species, and *Actinobacillus actinomycetemcomitans*. Thyroiditis has also been reported in a patient diagnosed with cat-scratch disease, although the infection was not confirmed microbiologically.[18]

Treatment of acute suppurative thyroiditis involves antimicrobial therapy based on the findings of gram-stained smear and culture of a thin-needle aspirate of the enlarged portion of the thyroid or surgical drainage (or excision) of any area of fluctuance or abscess found on ultrasonography or other imaging procedures. Additional direction for antimicrobial selection may be provided by discovery of possible sources of infection elsewhere (e.g., urinary tract infection). If no organisms are seen on Gram stain of purulent aspirate from an adult, nafcillin (because of the high frequency of infection with *S. aureus* and other gram-positive cocci) along with gentamicin or a third-generation cephalosporin would be appropriate initial therapy while awaiting the results of culture. However, in children with acute suppurative thyroiditis or adults with recurrent episodes of the same process, initial antimicrobial therapy, pending Gram stain and culture results, should be directed against oropharyngeal flora because of the likelihood of infection arising via a pyriform sinus fistula. Antibacterial choices might include cefoxitin or clindamycin (active against streptococci and oral anaerobes). After recovery with antibiotic therapy and surgical drainage from an acute episode of suppurative thyroiditis in a child (or an adult with recurrent episodes), a barium swallow or CT scanning should be performed. If a pyriform sinus fistula is demonstrated, complete fistulectomy is warranted to prevent further episodes of thyroid infection.[16]

The residua from acute bacterial thyroiditis have been few but have included transient hypothyroidism and vocal cord paralysis.

Mycobacterial Infection of the Thyroid Gland

The first cases of tuberculous thyroiditis were documented pathologically in the 1860s, and by the turn of the century thyroiditis or thyroid abscess due to *Mycobacterium tuberculosis* had been recognized clinically. The true incidence of infection of the thyroid with *M. tuberculosis* is difficult to determine. Klassen reviewed the 130 cases reported in the world's literature before 1945.[19] He concluded that there were considerable differences in the criteria used to establish the diagnoses in these cases. The majority of the diagnoses were based on histologic changes such as lymphocytic infiltration or granulomata but without acid-fast bacilli having been seen either on smears, in the tissue, or on culture. Although these histologic changes are seen in tuberculosis, they are nonspecific and may be seen in sarcoidosis, syphilis, subacute thyroiditis, goitrous autoimmune thyroiditis, or other noninfectious conditions. It is likely, therefore, that some of these cases did not represent tuberculosis. Even with these nonspecific criteria, several series examining thyroid tissues reported the incidence of thyroidal tuberculosis to be between 0.0001% and 0.1%.[20,21,22] When Berger and colleagues applied strict diagnostic criteria for tuberculosis, requiring identifiable mycobacteria in thyroid tissue or classic histologic changes with mycobacteria at other sites, they were able to identify only 19 cases of thyroiditis due to *M. tuberculosis*.[2]

The pathogenesis of thyroid tuberculosis is not clear. However, many cases appear to be associated with disseminated or miliary infection.[20,23] In contrast to patients with bacterial thyroiditis, those with mycobacterial thyroiditis have symptoms for a much longer time—on average 3 to 4 months—and pain, tenderness, and fever are much less common in these patients than in those with acute bacterial thyroiditis. Resolution without residua usually follows appropriate antituberculous therapy, or, in the case of a fluctuant tuberculous abscess ready to drain spontaneously, the combination of surgical drainage (or resection) and antimycobacterial treatment.

Infections with atypical mycobacteria have also been reported in the thyroid gland.[2] Among them are reports of a 4-year-old girl with *Mycobacterium chelonei* thyroiditis presenting as a slowly enlarging mass[24] and a young girl with *Mycobacterium intracellulare* thyroiditis.[25] *Mycobacterium avium-intracellulare* has been found in the thyroid gland in patients with the acquired immunodeficiency syndrome (AIDS),[26] usually in the setting of widely disseminated infection. None of the patients described had specific symptoms or signs of infectious thyroiditis. Similarly, mycobacteria may be found in the thyroid gland in patients with lepromatous leprosy, in whom *Mycobacterium leprae* is widely disseminated throughout the body.[27] However, symptomatic thyroidal infection has not been described.

Syphilitic Infection of the Thyroid Gland

In the latter 1800s and early 1900s, many cases of thyroid disease were attributed to syphilis.[28] Secondary syphilis was thought to be commonly associated with pain and swelling of the thyroid. Both thyrotoxicosis and hypothyroidism were described in association with syphilitic infection of the gland. In addition, it was postulated that congenital syphilis might result in hypothyroidism in young children.[29] Goiter associated with a positive serologic test for syphilis was reported to respond favorably to therapy for syphilis; this therapy often included iodide.[30,31]

Microbiologic evidence for involvement of the thyroid gland with syphilis is lacking in most reports of congenital, secondary, or tertiary syphilis of the thyroid. Berger and coworkers found reports of seven gummata of the thyroid in the English language literature since 1900.[2] The symptoms and signs associated with acute bacterial thyroiditis were notably absent in these patients; the gummas presented as painless nodules resembling other slowly growing conditions of the gland. Symptoms of local compression were commonly noted, and hypothyroidism and ulceration of the overlying skin occurred in a few patients.

FUNGAL INFECTIONS OF THE THYROID GLAND

Infections of the thyroid with a limited number of fungal organisms have been reported (Table 91-3), but are rare.

Infection of the Gland with Aspergillus *Species*

Twenty-six cases of thyroiditis caused by *Aspergillus* species have been reported. Most were caused by *Aspergillus fumigatus*, with a smaller number of cases caused by *Aspergillus flavus*. These patients were all immunocompromised, with the most common underlying conditions being glucocorticoid therapy, leukemia, and lymphoma. The patients were very ill and had presented with evidence of disseminated aspergillosis. Involvement of the thyroid was detected postmortem, at which time focal abscesses, hemorrhagic lesions associated with invasion of blood vessels, or diffuse necrotizing thyroiditis were found. These pathologic findings are consistent with a hematogenous route of invasion of the gland. This view is supported by the vascular invasion, necrosis, and hemorrhage found in other tissues, such as the lung and brain, in immunocompromised patients with disseminated aspergillosis. Rare cases of aspergillosis of the thyroid have been associated with thyroid adenomas or goitrous autoimmune thyroiditis.[7,32]

Other Fungal Infections

Infections of the thyroid with the endemic fungi *Coccidioides immitis* and *Histoplasma capsulatum* have been described in a very small number of cases,[33,34] usually in association with disseminated disease. There is one case report each of infection of the thyroid with *Candida albicans* and *Allescheria boydii*.[2,35]

Pneumocystis carinii *Infection of the Thyroid Gland*

Although it was formerly classified as a protozoan parasite, this organism has now been reclassified as a fungus based on

TABLE 91-3.
Agents Associated With Fungal Thyroiditis

Yeasts and Molds
  Aspergillus sp
  Coccidioides immitis
  Histoplasma capsulatum
  Candida albicans
  Allescheria boydii
Pneumocystis carinii

ribosomal RNA sequencing.[36] *P. carinii* pneumonia is the most common opportunistic infection in patients with human immunodeficiency virus (HIV) infection, occurring in over 80% of patients not receiving prophylaxis. In the pre-AIDS era, pneumocystis infection was well described in patients with natural or iatrogenic defects in cellular immunity, particularly those with leukemia or lymphoma or those taking immunosuppressive drugs. In all these patients, pneumocystis infection most commonly presents as pneumonia. However, autopsy series reveal a 1% to 2% incidence of disseminated infection, with only a minority of the patients having evidence of pneumonia.[37–39] HIV infection itself does not seem to be associated with an increased incidence of extrapulmonary pneumocystosis. However, among patients with HIV infection, the use of aerosol pentamidine, which does not provide systemic protection, appears to be associated with occurrence of extrapulmonary pneumocystis disease.[8]

At autopsy, patients with extrapulmonary pneumocystis infection may have evidence of the organism in multiple organs or in only one or a few sites. The extrapulmonary sites, in order of involvement, include the liver and spleen, lymph nodes, bone marrow, adrenals, thyroid, eye, ear, and skin.[8,40] Infection of the thyroid is found in up to 20% of patients with disseminated pneumocystis infection at autopsy. However, symptomatic infection of the thyroid is rare.

Because pneumocystis infection is common, it may be useful to review in some detail the presentation of thyroidal infection with this organism. Gallant and colleagues reported an intravenous drug user with AIDS, receiving no prophylaxis, who presented with 2 weeks of left-sided neck swelling and dysphagia.[9] Physical examination revealed a diffusely enlarged (5 × 10 cm) and mildly tender left lobe of the thyroid, and a 3 × 5 cm right lobe that was more tender. On ultrasound examination of the neck, an enlarged left thyroid lobe with heterogenous echogenicity was seen. Calcification, reported in other cases of extrapulmonary pneumocystosis,[8,40] was not seen. Thyroid radionuclide imaging demonstrated nonvisualization of the left lobe of the thyroid; thyroid function was normal. FNA of the thyroid revealed the presence of *P. carinii* organisms. With trimethoprim-sulfamethoxazole therapy, the size of the thyroid decreased rapidly, and a repeat aspiration of the gland after 3 weeks of therapy revealed a smaller number of organisms. A third biopsy specimen after 7 weeks of therapy revealed no organisms. A subsequent series of patients with extrapulmonary pneumocystosis[40] included a brief report of a 49-year-old homosexual man with a prior episode of *P. carinii* pneumonia maintained on aerosol pentamidine secondary prophylaxis who developed a left-sided neck mass; a cold nodule was found on thyroid radionuclide imaging (Fig 91-3). FNA yielded pneumocystis organisms. In contrast to the prior patient, there was biochemical evidence of hypothyroidism.

PARASITIC INFECTIONS OF THE THYROID GLAND

Echinococcosis

Several parasitic agents have involved the thyroid on rare occasions (Table 91-4). Infection with the canine cestode (tape-worm) *Echinococcus granulosus* is common in most sheep- and cattle-farming regions of the world, including the Middle East, South America, Australia, New Zealand, Africa, and Eastern Europe. The liver and lungs are the most common sites for hydatid cyst formation in humans after ingestion of materials containing contaminated animal feces, but infection has been reported in virtually every organ of the body. Berger and colleagues[2] noted 31 cases of human thyroidal echinococcus infestation in the world literature before 1915 and described 9 recent patients. These patients had had symptoms for years before diagnosis and were often considered to have a goiter before surgical excision. Evidence suggesting echinococcal disease, such as abdominal calcifications or eosinophilia, was present in less than half the patients. The patients were treated with surgical resection and generally did well. Sequelae, when they occurred, were related to compression of vital structures by large masses or to postoperative complications.

If echinococcal infection is suspected, specific serologic testing should be obtained.[41] Diagnostic aspiration of intact cysts generally should not be performed because of the danger of rupture and spillage of cyst contents. Surgical removal is the preferred mode of therapy. Antiparasitic medications such as albendazole or praziquantel may have a role as an adjunct to surgery or for inoperable cases of echinococcal disease.[42]

Strongyloidiasis

Strongyloides stercoralis, a roundworm or nematode, is widely distributed in tropical climates, including the southeastern United States. Although most commonly associated with self-limited gastrointestinal symptoms, infection with this parasite is potentially lethal because of its unique "autoinfection" cycle.[43] Autoinfection results in an increasing worm burden, and immunocompromised patients may present with a hyperinfection syndrome, in which infection can be disseminated to the lung, liver, lymph nodes, central nervous system (CNS), and nearly every other organ in the body.[43] Involvement of the thyroid gland clinically or at autopsy has been reported, always in the setting of disseminated disease. The mortality of the hyperinfection syndrome is very high, and results from a combination of the patient's underlying disease, direct effects of the parasite, and secondary bacterial infections. Thiabendazole is an effective treatment. Prevention, however, remains the key, and all patients from endemic areas in whom increasing natural or iatrogenic immunosuppression is anticipated should have stool ova and parasite examinations for strongyloides.

Cysticercosis

Cysticercosis, an infection acquired by humans after ingestion of eggs of the pork (*Taenia solium*) tapeworm, occurs most commonly in Eastern Europe, Central and South America, Spain, Portugal and parts of Africa, China, and India. Although lesions can develop in almost any organ of the body, the most common clinical presentation is that of disease of the CNS.[44] A single patient with cysticercosis of the thyroid and the CNS has been reported.[45]

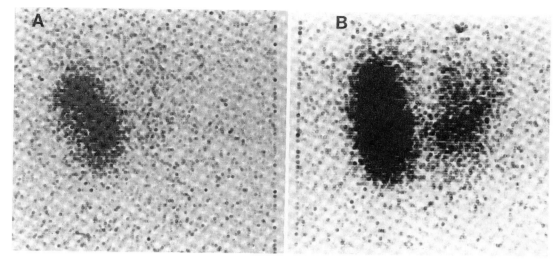

FIGURE 91-3. ^{123}I radionuclide scan of the thyroid showing (*A*) no uptake in the left lobe and homogeneous uptake in the right lobe of an HIV-infected patient receiving aerosolized pentamidine prophylaxis. *P. carinii* infection of an enlarged left lobe was demonstrated on fine-needle aspiration biopsy. (*B*) Repeat scan after 4 months of treatment with trimethoprim-sulfamethoxazole showing reappearance of radionuclide uptake in the left lobe. (Reproduced from Battan R, Mariuz P, Raviglone ML, et al. Pneumocystis Carini infection of the thyroid in a hypothyroid patient with AIDS: diagnosis by fine needle aspiration biopsy. J Clin Endocrinol Metab 1991;72:724, with permission)

VIRAL INFECTIONS OF THE THYROID GLAND

Thyroiditis on rare occasions has been temporally associated (often by serologic testing only) with infection by a variety of viral agents including the herpesviruses (Epstein-Barr virus and cytomegalovirus), measles, influenza, adenovirus, echovirus, mumps, and St. Louis encephalitis virus.[2] However, in most cases, because the presence of the viral agent in the thyroid gland was not demonstrated, a causal association is difficult to prove.

CONCLUSION

Infections of the thyroid are uncommon and may be difficult to differentiate from noninfectious thyroiditis. Although the epidemiologic setting, clinical features, adjunctive laboratory tests, and cultures from other sites and radiographic studies may be useful in suggesting the etiologic agent, FNA or surgical resection of involved thyroid tissue may be necessary in many cases, particularly in the more chronic forms of infection.

TABLE 91-4.
Agents Associated With Parasitic Thyroiditis

Echinococcus sp

Strongyloides sp

Taenia solium (cysticercosis)

References

1. Burhans EC. Acute thyroiditis. A study of sixty-seven cases. Surg Gynecol Obstet 1928;47:478
2. Berger SA, Zonszein J, Villamena P, Mittman N. Infectious diseases of the thyroid gland. Rev Infect Dis 1983;5:108
3. Brook I. The swollen neck. Cervical lymphadenitis, parotitis, thyroiditis, and infected cysts. Infect Dis Clin North Am 1988;2:221
4. Williamson GS. The applied anatomy and physiology of the thyroid apparatus. Br J Surg 1926;13:466
5. Thompson L. Syphilis of the thyroid. Am J Syphilis 1917;1:179
6. Womack NA, Cole WH. Normal and pathologic repair in the thyroid gland. Arch Surg 1931;23:466
7. Young RC, Bennett JE, Vogel CL, Carbone PP, DeVita VT. Aspergillosis. The spectrum of the disease in 98 patients. Medicine 1970;49:147
8. Northfelt DW, Clement MJ, Safrin S. Extrapulmonary pneumocystis: clinical features in human immunodeficiency virus infection. Medicine 1990;69:392
9. Gallant JE, Enriquez RE, Cohen KL, Hammers LW. *Pneumocystis carinii* thyroiditis. Am J Med 1988;85:250
10. Colcock BP, King ML. The mortality and morbidity of thyroid surgery. Surg Gynecol Obstet 1962;114:131
11. Jemerin EE, Aronoff JS. Foreign body in thyroid following perforation of esophagus. Surgery 1949;25:52
12. Har-El G, Sasaki CT, Prager D, Krespi YP. Acute suppurative thyroiditis and the branchial apparatus. Am J Otolaryngol 1991;12:6
13. Rich EJ, Mendelman PM. Acute suppurative thyroiditis in pediatric patients. Pediatr Infect Dis J 1987;6:936
14. Takai SI, Miyauchi A, Matsuzuka F, et al. Internal fistula as a route of infection in acute suppurative thyroiditis. Lancet 1979;1:751
15. Higgins CB, Auffermann W. MR imaging of thyroid and parathyroid glands: a review of current status. AJR Am J Roentgenol 1988;151:1095
16. Miyauchi A, Matsuzuka F, Kuma K, Takai S. Pyriform sinus fistula: an underlying abnormality common in patients with acute suppurative thyroiditis. World J Surg 1990;14:400

17. Joffe N, Schamroth L. Gas-forming infection of the thyroid gland. Clin Radiol 1966;17:95

18. Shumway M, Davis PL. Cat-scratch thyroiditis treated with thyrotropic hormone. J Clin Endocrinol 1954;14:742

19. Klassen KP, Curtis GM. Tuberculous abscess of the thyroid gland. Surgery 1945;17:552

20. Barnes P, Weatherstone R. Tuberculosis of the thyroid: two case reports. Br J Dis Chest 1979;73:187

21. Rankin FW, Graham AS. Tuberculosis of the thyroid gland. Ann Surg 1932;96:625

22. Levitt T. The status of lymphadenoid goitre, Hashimoto's and Riedel's diseases. Ann R Coll Surg Engl 1952;10:369

23. Johnson AG, Phillips ME, Thomas RJS. Acute tuberculous abscess of the thyroid gland. Br J Surg 1973;60:668

24. Gutman LT, Handwerger S, Zwadyk P, et al. Thyroiditis due to *Mycobacterium chelonei*. Am Rev Respir Dis 1974;110:807

25. Olin R, LeBien WE, Leigh JE. Acute suppurative thyroiditis. Report of two cases including one caused by *Mycobacterium intracellulare* (Battey Bacillus). Minn Med 1973;56:586

26. Horsburgh CR Jr. *Mycobacterium avium* complex infection in the acquired immunodeficiency syndrome. N Engl J Med 1991;324:1332

27. Hastings RC, Gillis TP, Krahenbuhl JL, Franzblau SG. Leprosy. Clin Microbiol Rev 1988;1:330

28. Netherton EN. Syphilis and thyroid disease with special reference to hyperthyroidism. American Journal of Syphilis 1932;16:479

29. Menninger WC. Congenital syphilis of the thyroid gland. Am J Syphilis 1929;13:164

30. Williams C, Steinberg B. Gumma of the thyroid. Surg Gynecol Obstet 1924;38:781

31. Storck JA. Syphilis of the thyroid. New Orleans Medical and Surgical Journal 1917;70:414

32. Winzelberg CG, Gore J, Yu D, et al. *Aspergillus flavus* as a cause of thyroiditis in an immunosuppressed host. Johns Hopkins Med J 1979;144:90

33. Loeb JM, Livermore BM, Wofsy D. Coccidioidomycosis of the thyroid. Ann Intern Med 1979;91:409

34. Goodwin RA Jr, Shapiro JL, Thurman GH, et al. Disseminated histoplasmosis: clinical and pathologic correlations. Medicine 1980;59:1

35. Rosen F, Deck JHN, Rewcastle NB. *Allescheria boydii*—unique systemic dissemination to thyroid and brain. Can Med Assoc J 1965;93:1125

36. Edman JC, Kovacs JA, Masur H, et al. Ribosomal RNA sequence shows *Pneumocystis carinii* to be a member of the fungi. Nature 1988;334:519

37. Awen CF, Baltzan MA. Systemic dissemination of *Pneumocystis carinii* pneumonia. Can Med Assoc J 1971;104:809

38. LeGolvan DP, Heidelberger KP. Disseminated, granulomatous *Pneumocystis carinii* pneumonia. Arch Pathol 1973;5:344

39. Burke BA, Good RA. *Pneumocystis carinii* infection. Medicine 1973;52:23

40. Raviglione MC. Extrapulmonary pneumocystosis: the first 50 cases. Rev Infect Dis 1990;12:1127

41. Williams JF. Cestode infections. In: Cohen S, Warren KS, eds. Immunology of parasitic infections. 2nd ed. London: Blackwell, 1982:676

42. Teggi A, Lastilla MG, DeRosa F. Therapy of human hydatid disease with mebendazole and albendazole. Antimicrob Agents Chemother 1993;37:1679

43. Scowden EB, Schaffner W, Stone WJ. Overwhelming strongyloidiasis. An unappreciated opportunistic infection. Medicine 1978;57:527

44. Loo L, Braude A. Cerebral cysticercosis in San Diego. A report of 23 cases and a review of the literature. Medicine 1982;61:341

45. Leelachaikul P, Chuahirun S. Cysticercosis of the thyroid gland in severe cerebral cysticercosis. Report of a case. J Med Assoc Thai 1977;60:405

Werner and Ingbar's The Thyroid, Seventh Edition,
edited by Lewis E. Braverman and Robert D. Utiger.
Lippincott–Raven Publishers, Philadelphia, © 1996

INDEX

NOTE: A *b* following a page number indicates boxed material; a *t* following a page number indicates tabular material; and an *f* following a page number indicates a figure.

variant forms, 586
viral antibody titers in, 584,
585f
syphilitic, 1053
thyroglobulin levels, 410
tuberculous, 1052-1053
Thyroid microsomal antigen. *See*
Thyroperoxidase
Thyroid peroxidase. *See*
Thyroperoxidase
Thyroid-stimulating activity, serum,
in pregnancy, 1021
Thyroid-stimulating antibody. *See*
Thyrotropin receptor antibody(ies)
Thyroid-stimulating hormone (TSH).
See Thyrotropin
Thyroid transcription factor(s)
thyroperoxidase gene
expression, 54
TTF-1, 12, 85, 911
in lungs, 617
ras oncogene and, 911
TTF-2, 85
Thyroperoxidase, 26-27, 30f, 52-54
abnormalities, hypothyroidism
and, 751-752
activity, iodide excess and, 245
amino acid sequence, 54f
antibodies to, 417-420
antithyroglobulin antibody
binding, 417
binding epitopes, 418-419
cDNA, 53
gene, 53, 752
mutations, 64, 752f
regulation of expression, 53-
54
immunodominant region, 419,
419f
iodination and. *See* Iodination
iodine organification,
thyrotropin and, 214
molecular biology, 53
porcine, 53, 54f, 55f
properties, 53
purification, 52-53
recombinant human, 53
resorcinol and, 269
specificity, 59-60
structure, 53, 54f
thioureylene inactivation of,
iodide concentration and, 67,
70f
Thyrotoxic crisis, 701-706

cardiac manifestations, 702
cardinal manifestations, 701
clinical features, 701-702
infection and, 701
laboratory findings, 702
liver in, 702
neurologic manifestations, 649
neuropsychiatric manifestations,
701
pathogenesis, 702-703
precipitating conditions, 701
treatment, 703t, 703-706, 727
antithyroid compounds,
703t, 703-704, 727
β-blockers, 727
for ongoing thyroid
hormone effects in
periphery, 704-705
potassium iodide, 727
for precipitating illness, 705-
706
propranolol, 666, 727
for systemic
decompensation, 703t,
704
Thyrotoxicosis. *See also*
Hyperthyroidism
adhesive capsulitis of shoulder in,
683
adrenocortical function in, 657-
659
age-specific hazard rate, 476f
amenorrhea in, 673
amiodarone-induced, 277, 323,
324t, 501
destructive, 323, 324t
iodine-induced, 323, 324t
androgens in, 658, 674
anemia in, 640t, 640-641, 695
anxiety in, 696
anxiety state vs., 697
apathetic, clinical presentation,
696-697
asthma and, 624
atrial fibrillation in, 611
stroke and, 649
autonomously functioning
thyroid nodule and, 566, 568
basal metabolic rate in, 687-688
behavioral and psychiatric
aspects. *See*
Neuropsychological disorders
behavioral syndromes
mimicking, 697-698

bone remodeling and, 680
carbohydrate metabolism in,
689
cardiovascular manifestations,
607-613
cardiac effects, 609
heart rate, 610-611
hemodynamic changes, 607-
608, 608t
left ventricular function, 612
mitral valve prolapse, 613
noninvasive cardiac
evaluation, 611-612
palpitations, 610
pathophysiology, 608f, 608-
610
peripheral circulatory
effects, 609-610
physical examination, 611
in pregnant patient, 613
pulmonary effects, 620-621
renal physiology and, 610
rhythm disturbances, 611
symptoms and signs, 610t,
610-611
thyroid hormone-
catecholamine interactions
and, 610, 664
treatment, 612-613
acute interventions, 612-
613, 613t
chronic therapy, 613
case finding, 710
catecholamine-thyroid hormone
interactions in, 664-665
cardiovascular responses,
664
mental state and, 699
metabolic responses, 664-
665
causes, 522, 523t, 524t, 708
diagnosis, 710-711, 711t
cerebral blood flow in, 650
chorea in, 649
clinical manifestations, 522, 523,
524t
coagulation proteins in, 640, 641
congestive heart failure in, 611
connective tissue in, 598-604
cortisol secretion and
metabolism in, 657f, 657-658,
659f
cutaneous alterations, 595-596,
596t